RADIATION ONCOLOGY
Rationale, Technique, Results

RADIATION ONCOLOGY
Rationale, Technique, Results

JAMES D. COX, M.D., F.A.C.R.
Professor and Head
Division of Radiation Oncology
The University of Texas M.D. Anderson Cancer Center
Houston, Texas

K. KIAN ANG, M.D., Ph.D.
Professor and Deputy Head
Division of Radiation Oncology
The University of Texas M.D. Anderson Cancer Center
Houston, Texas

EIGHTH EDITION

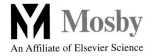 Mosby
An Affiliate of Elsevier Science

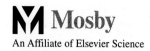

Mosby

An Affiliate of Elsevier Science

11830 Westline Industrial Drive
St. Louis, Missouri 63146

NOTICE

Medicine is an ever-changing field. Standard safety precautions must be followed, but as new
research and clinical experience broaden our knowledge, changes in treatment and drug therapy
may become necessary or appropriate. Readers are advised to check the most current product
information provided by the manufacturer of each drug to be administered to verify the
recommended dose, the method and duration of administration, and contraindications. It is the
responsibility of the licensed prescriber, relying on experience and knowledge of the patient, to
determine dosages and the best treatment for each individual patient. Neither the publisher nor the
author assumes any liability for any injury and/or damage to persons or property arising from this
publication.

The Publisher

Previous editions copyrighted 1959, 1965, 1969, 1973, 1979, 1989, 1994.

Library of Congress Cataloging-in-Publication Data

Radiation oncology: rationale, technique, results.—8th ed./[edited by] James D. Cox,
K. Kian Ang.
  p. ; cm.
  Includes bibliographical references and index.
  ISBN 0-323-01258-2 (alk. paper)
  1. Cancer—Radiotherapy. I. Cox, James D. (James Daniel), 1938-II. Ang,
K. K. (K. Kian)
  [DNLM: 1. Neoplasms—radiotherapy. QZ 269 R12803 2002]
RC271.R3 R3315 2002
616.99'40642—dc21

                                                                2002033756

Acquisitions Editor: Dolores Meloni
Publishing Services Manager: Patricia Tannian
Senior Project Manager: Suzanne C. Fannin
Design Manager: Gail Morey Hudson
Cover Design: Liz Rohne Rudder

Printed in the United States of America

Last digit is the print number: 9 8 7 6 5 4 3 2 1

Contributors

JAMES L. ABBRUZZESE, M.D.
Professor and Chairman
Department of Gastrointestinal Medical Oncology
The University of Texas M.D. Anderson Cancer Center
Houston, Texas

K. KIAN ANG, M.D., Ph.D.
Professor and Deputy Head
Division of Radiation Oncology
The University of Texas M.D. Anderson Cancer Center
Houston, Texas

JOHN A. ANTOLAK, Ph.D.
Assistant Professor, Department of Radiation Physics
The University of Texas M.D. Anderson Cancer Center
Houston, Texas

MATTHEW T. BALLO, M.D.
Assistant Professor, Department of Radiation Oncology
The University of Texas M.D. Anderson Cancer Center
Houston, Texas

JAMES D. BRIERLEY, M.B.B.S., M.R.C.P., F.R.C.R., F.R.C.P.(C)
Associate Professor, Department of Radiation Oncology
University of Toronto, Princess Margaret Hospital
Toronto, Ontario, Canada

THOMAS A. BUCHHOLZ, M.D.
Associate Professor, Department of Radiation Oncology
The University of Texas M.D. Anderson Cancer Center
Houston, Texas

ROGER W. BYHARDT, M.D.
Professor, Department of Radiation Oncology
Medical College of Wisconsin, Zablocki VA Hospital
Milwaukee, Wisconsin

JAY S. COOPER, M.D., F.A.C.R.
Department of Radiation Oncology
New York University Medical Center, Tisch Hospital
New York, New York

JAMES D. COX, M.D., F.A.C.R.
Professor and Head, Division of Radiation Oncology
The University of Texas M.D. Anderson Cancer Center
Houston, Texas

CHRISTOPHER H. CRANE, M.D.
Assistant Professor, Department of Radiation Oncology
The University of Texas M.D. Anderson Cancer Center
Houston, Texas

MARC E. DELCLOS, M.D.
Assistant Professor, Department of Radiation Oncology
The University of Texas M.D. Anderson Cancer Center
Houston, Texas

PATRICIA J. EIFEL, M.D.
Professor, Department of Radiation Oncology
The University of Texas M.D. Anderson Cancer Center
Houston, Texas

DOUGLAS B. EVANS, M.D.
Professor, Department of Surgical Oncology
The University of Texas M.D. Anderson Cancer Center
Houston, Texas

ADAM S. GARDEN, M.D.
Associate Professor, Department of Radiation Oncology
The University of Texas M.D. Anderson Cancer Center
Houston, Texas

MARY K. GOSPODAROWICZ, M.D., F.R.C.P.(C)
Professor, Department of Radiation Oncology
University of Toronto, Princess Margaret Hospital
Toronto, Ontario, Canada

CHUL S. HA, M.D.
Associate Professor, Department of Radiation Oncology
The University of Texas M.D. Anderson Cancer Center
Houston, Texas

ERIC J. HALL, D.Sc., F.A.C.R.
Director, Center for Radiological Research
Columbia University
New York, New York

WILLIAM F. HANSON, Ph.D.
Research Professor, Department of Radiation Physics
The University of Texas M.D. Anderson Cancer Center
Houston, Texas

KENNETH R. HOGSTROM, Ph.D.
Professor and Chair, Department of Radiation Physics
The University of Texas M.D. Anderson Cancer Center
Houston, Texas

JOHN L. HORTON, Ph.D.
Professor, Department of Radiation Physics
The University of Texas M.D. Anderson Cancer Center
Houston, Texas

DAVID H. HUSSEY, M.D., F.A.C.R.
Professor, Department of Radiology
The University of Texas Health Science Center at San Antonio
San Antonio, Texas

NORA A. JANJAN, M.D.
Professor, Department of Radiation Oncology
The University of Texas M.D. Anderson Cancer Center
Houston, Texas

ANUJA JHINGRAN, M.D.
Associate Professor, Department of Radiation Oncology
The University of Texas M.D. Anderson Cancer Center
Houston, Texas

RITSUKO KOMAKI, M.D.
Professor, Department of Radiation Oncology
The University of Texas M.D. Anderson Cancer Center
Houston, Texas

LARRY E. KUN, M.D.
Chairman, Department of Radiation Oncology
Co-Leader, Neurobiology and Brain Tumor Program
St. Jude Children's Research Hospital
Co-Chair, Children's Oncology Group Brain Tumor
    Consortium
Memphis, Tennessee

COLLEEN A. LAWTON, M.D., F.A.C.R.
Professor, Department of Radiation Oncology
Medical College of Wisconsin
Milwaukee, Wisconsin

VALERAE O. LEWIS, M.D.
Assistant Professor, Department of Radiation Oncology
The University of Texas M.D. Anderson Cancer Center
Houston, Texas

MARSHA D. McNEESE, M.D.
Associate Professor, Department of Radiation Oncology
The University of Texas M.D. Anderson Cancer Center
Houston, Texas

MARVIN L. MEISTRICH, Ph.D.
Ashbel Smith, Professor
Department of Experimental Radiation Oncology
The University of Texas M.D. Anderson Cancer Center
Houston, Texas

LUKA MILAS, M.D., Ph.D.
Professor and Chair
Department of Experimental Radiation Oncology
The University of Texas M.D. Anderson Cancer Center
Houston, Texas

MICHAEL F. MILOSEVIC, M.D., F.R.C.P.(C)
Assistant Professor, Department of Radiation Oncology
University of Toronto, Princess Margaret Hospital
Toronto, Ontario, Canada

WILLIAM H. MORRISON, M.D.
Associate Professor, Department of Radiation Oncology
The University of Texas M.D. Anderson Cancer Center
Houston, Texas

WILLIAM T. MOSS, M.D.
Professor Emeritus, Department of Radiation Oncology
The Oregon Health & Science University School of Medicine
Portland, Oregon

LINH N. NGUYEN, M.D.
Director, Radiation Oncology
Yakima Regional Cancer Center
Yakima, Washington

HARPER D. PEARSE, M.D.
Department of Radiation Oncology
The Oregon Health & Science University School of Medicine
Portland, Oregon

PETER W.T. PISTERS, M.D.
Associate Professor, Department of Surgical Oncology
The University of Texas M.D. Anderson Cancer Center
Houston, Texas

ALAN POLLACK, M.D., Ph.D.
Chair, Department of Radiation Oncology
Fox Chase Cancer Center
Philadelphia, Pennsylvania

ISAAC I. ROSEN, Ph.D.
Professor, Department of Radiation Physics
The University of Texas M.D. Anderson Cancer Center
Houston, Texas

NAOMI R. SCHECHTER, M.D.
Assistant Professor, Department of Radiation Oncology
The University of Texas M.D. Anderson Cancer Center
Houston, Texas

ALMON S. SHIU, Ph.D.
Associate Professor, Department of Radiation Physics
The University of Texas M.D. Anderson Cancer Center
Houston, Texas

LEWIS G. SMITH III, M.D.
Instructor, Department of Radiation Oncology
The University of Texas M.D. Anderson Cancer Center
Houston, Texas

GEORGE STARKSCHALL, Ph.D.
Professor, Department of Radiation Physics
The University of Texas M.D. Anderson Cancer Center
Houston, Texas

CRAIG W. STEVENS, M.D., Ph.D.
Associate Professor, Department of Radiation Oncology
The University of Texas M.D. Anderson Cancer Center
Houston, Texas

KENNETH R. STEVENS Jr., M.D., F.A.C.R.
Chairman, Department of Radiation Oncology
The Oregon Health & Science University
Portland, Oregon

ERIC A. STROM, M.D.
Associate Professor, Department of Radiation Oncology
The University of Texas M.D. Anderson Cancer Center
Houston, Texas

GILLIAN M. THOMAS, B.Sc., M.D., F.R.C.P.(C)
Professor of Radiation Oncology and Obstetrics and
    Gynecology
University of Toronto
Consultant Radiation Oncologist
Toronto Sunnybrook Regional Cancer Centre
Medical Director, GlaxoSmithKline
Toronto, Canada

ELIZABETH L. TRAVIS, Ph.D.
Professor, Department of Experimental Radiation Oncology
The University of Texas M.D. Anderson Cancer Center
Houston, Texas

RICHARD W. TSANG, M.D., F.R.C.P.(C)
Associate Professor, Department of Radiation Oncology
University of Toronto, Princess Margaret Hospital
Toronto, Ontario, Canada

B-CHEN WEN, M.D.
Professor, Division of Radiation Oncology
Department of Radiology
The University of Iowa Hospitals and Clinics
Iowa City, Iowa

RICHARD B. WILDER, M.D.
Professor, Department of Radiation Oncology
The University of Texas M.D. Anderson Cancer Center
Houston, Texas

ROBERT A. WOLFF, M.D.
Assistant Professor
Department of Gastrointestinal Medical Oncology
The University of Texas M.D. Anderson Cancer Center
Houston, Texas

GUNAR K. ZAGARS, M.D.
Professor, Department of Radiation Oncology
The University of Texas M.D. Anderson Cancer Center
Houston, Texas

To the residents
who ask the important questions—
our colleagues
who collaborate in providing the answers
for our patients, who deserve only the best

Preface

Radiation oncology has been extraordinarily exciting in the past few years. Developments in conforming the high-dose radiation region to the shape of the tumor have become quite advanced and widely available through the use of three-dimensional conformal radiation therapy and intensity-modulated radiation therapy. Adding to these advanced techniques for planning and delivering radiation therapy is a large body of evidence supporting the integration of cytotoxic chemotherapy and hormones with radiation therapy. The availability and potential use of molecular therapeutics are also on the horizon.

This eighth edition calls upon individuals to contribute who are highly specialized in the particular field about which they write. Several chapters are entirely new, and those that are revised have been profoundly altered. New chapters have been added that describe clinical radiation physics, palliative care, and emerging modalities.

We have strived for uniformity in the presentation of the chapters so as to serve better as a quick reference.

The importance of treatment effects on normal tissues is reflected in early presentation of this subject in each chapter. An emphasis has been placed on synthesis of large bodies of material in the interest of succinctness, conservation of space, and clarity.

Emphasis has been placed on the critical information needed by the radiation oncologist and clinicians from other specialties to care for patients.

The individuals who have contributed have toiled countless hours. We owe them a debt of gratitude. Our colleagues, our families, and our friends have borne the consequences of the commitment of time necessary to achieve the goal of a book in which we can take great pride. We are especially indebted to Christine Wogan of the Department of Scientific Publications at The University of Texas M.D. Anderson Cancer Center for a commitment to excellence and endurance that is barely imaginable.

James D. Cox
K. Kian Ang

Contents

RADIATION ONCOLOGY
Rationale, Technique, Results

PART I

Principles

CHAPTER 1

Physical and Biological Basis of Radiation Therapy

Eric J. Hall and James D. Cox

HISTORICAL BACKGROUND

Radiation has been an ever-present ingredient in the evolution of life on Earth. It is not something new, invented by human ingenuity in the technologic age; it has always been there. What *is* new, what is manmade, is the *extra* radiation to which we are subjected, largely for medical purposes, but also from journeys in high-flying jet aircraft and from the nuclear reactors that are used to generate electrical power.

X-rays were discovered in 1895 by the German physicist Wilhelm Conrad Roentgen. He found that "this new kind of ray" could blacken photographic film sealed in a container and stored in a drawer and could pass through materials opaque to light, including cardboard and wood. During a public demonstration of the production of x-rays, Roentgen asked his colleague, Herr Kölliker, to put his hand in front of the x-ray machine, and with a sheet of photographic film, he made the first radiograph displaying the bony structure of the hand. Roentgen was thus the father of diagnostic radiology as well as radiation physics. Some controversy exists as to who was the first to use x-rays therapeutically. In 1897, Professor Freund demonstrated before the Vienna Medical Society the disappearance of a hairy mole by the use of x-rays, and by the turn of the century x-rays had been used in Europe and America in primitive therapeutic applications.

Parallel to the discovery of x-rays, Becquerel discovered radioactivity in 1898. Three years later, he performed what is arguably the first radiobiological experiment when he inadvertently left a container with 200 mg of radium in his vest pocket for 6 hours. He subsequently described the erythema of the skin that became evident in 2 weeks and the ulceration that developed and required several weeks to heal.

During the early 1900s, radiobiological experiments were conducted with simple biological systems in parallel with the development of radiation therapy. One of the most well-known results, still cited today, was the so-called law of Bergonié and Tribondeau, which states that radiosensitivity is highest in tissues with the highest mitotic index and lowest in differentiated tissues. From 1912 to 1940, several investigators, first in Germany and later in the United Kingdom, demonstrated the dependence of radiation response on oxygen. The magnitude of the oxygen effect was determined by using seedlings of *Vicia faba*, and the possible implications for radiation therapy were discussed.

In Paris in the 1920s and 1930s, famous experiments were performed in which the testes of rams were irradiated with x-rays. It proved to be impossible to sterilize the animals in a single dose without causing a severe reaction in the skin of the scrotum; but if the dose was fractionated over some period, sterilization could be achieved with little apparent skin damage. It was argued that the testes were a model for a rapidly growing tumor, whereas the skin represented a normal tissue response. On this basis, fractionation was introduced into clinical radiation therapy.

Brachytherapy underwent a similar conceptual evolution after its first use in the early years of the twentieth century. As fractionation was recognized as being advantageous in external irradiation, protraction in brachytherapy (i.e., using low-activity sources for longer periods) was thought to improve the therapeutic ratio, although radiobiological studies of dose-rate effects were still decades away. This concept became the hallmark of the "Paris" approach to intrauterine and intravaginal radium therapy for cancer of the cervix. In Manchester, England, optimal arrangements of radium sources were sought to achieve a consistent dose rate and a more nearly homogeneous dose distribution through the tumor-bearing volume while sparing surrounding normal structures; this led to a more systematic application of the Paris concepts. In more recent times, afterloading systems have been developed in brachytherapy that use nonradioactive applicators so that the radioactive sources are introduced only after the desired relationships of sources are assured; the afterloading approach reduces radiation exposure to the administering personnel.

Large quantities of radium were gathered in some centers to produce a telecurietherapy unit (one that would permit the treatment of patients with gamma rays at a distance) in contrast to the placement of encapsulated radium in body cavities or directly into tumors (brachycurietherapy). Clinical experience with these units suggested advantages of high-energy radiation over the widely available 200 kilovolts-peak (kVp) x-ray generators. Between 1930 and 1950, technical advances permitted the development of much higher energy x-ray generators. In the 1950s, ^{60}Co teletherapy units became widely available, and the first generation of medical linear accelerators was developed.

In the wake of World War II and the use of atomic weapons on Hiroshima and Nagasaki, research in radiobiology developed rapidly. Significant milestones include the development of techniques to culture single mammalian cells in vitro in 1956 and to determine survival curves in vivo in 1959. These developments ushered in a greatly enhanced effort in radiation biology to understand conventional radiation therapy and suggested new horizons for improvements in treatment. In national laboratories on both sides of the Atlantic, radiation biology studies not related to radiation therapy were developing at the same time, involving basic studies of mutagenesis and carcinogenesis.

PHYSICAL BASIS
Types of Radiation

Types of radiation of concern in this book are those with the capacity to produce ionizations and excitations during the absorption of energy in biological material. The raising of an electron in an atom or molecule to a higher energy level, without the actual ejection of that electron from the atom or molecule, is called *excitation*. If the radiation has sufficient energy to eject one or more orbital electrons from the atom or molecule, this process is referred to as *ionization*, and the radiation is said to be *ionizing radiation*. The important characteristic of ionizing radiation is the localized release of large amounts of energy. The energy dissipated by an ionizing event is approximately 33 electron-volts (eV), which is more than enough to break a strong chemical bond; for example, the energy associated with a carbon-carbon bond is 4.9 eV. Ionizing radiation produces substantial biological effects for the relatively small total amounts of energy involved because the energy is released locally in "packets" large enough to break chemical bonds and initiate the chain of events that lead ultimately to a biological effect.

Electromagnetic Radiation

Electromagnetic radiation (x-rays and gamma rays) is *indirectly* ionizing. These types of radiation do not themselves produce chemical and biological damage, but when they are absorbed in the medium through which they pass, they give up their energy to produce fast-moving electrons by either the Compton, photoelectric, or pair-production processes (Fig. 1-1). X-rays and gamma rays are forms of electromagnetic radiation that

do not differ in nature or properties; the designation *x* or *gamma* reflects simply the way in which they are produced. X-rays are produced extranuclearly, which means that they are generated in an electric device that accelerates electrons to high energy and then stops them abruptly in a target, made usually of tungsten or gold. Part of the kinetic energy, or energy of motion of the electrons, is converted into photons of x-rays. Gamma rays, on the other hand, are produced intranuclearly (i.e., they are emitted by radioactive isotopes); they represent excess energy that is given off as the unstable nucleus breaks up and decays in its efforts to reach a stable form.

Particulate Radiation

Other forms of radiation that are used experimentally and used or contemplated for radiation therapy include electrons, protons, alpha particles, neutrons, negative pi-mesons, and high-energy heavy ions.

Electrons are light, negatively charged particles that can be accelerated to high energy and to a speed close to that of light by means of an electrical device such as a betatron or linear accelerator.

Protons are positively charged particles and are relatively massive, having a mass nearly 2000 times that of an electron. Protons require more complex and expensive equipment to accelerate them to useful energies. For example, 160-megaelectron volt (MeV) protons have a range of about 12 cm in tissue.

Alpha particles are nuclei of helium atoms, each consisting of two protons and two neutrons in close association. Because they have a net positive charge, they can be accelerated in large electrical devices similar to those used for protons. Alpha particles are also emitted during the decay of some radioactive isotopes.

Neutrons are particles having a mass similar to that of protons, but they carry no electrical charge. Because they are electrically neutral, they cannot be accelerated in an electrical device but rather are produced when a charged particle, such as a deuteron or proton, is accelerated to high energy and then made to impinge on a suitable target material. Neutrons are also emitted as a byproduct when heavy radioactive atoms undergo fission (i.e., split up to form two smaller atoms). Neutrons are indirectly ionizing because the first step in their absorption is for them to collide with nuclei of the atoms of the absorbing material and produce recoil protons, alpha particles, or heavier nuclear fragments. It is these charged particles that are responsible for the biological effects.

Negative pi-mesons are negatively charged particles with a mass 273 times that of the electron. They are produced by a complex process that necessitates a huge linear accelerator or synchrocyclotron capable of accelerating protons to energies of 400 to 800 MeV. When pi-mesons are absorbed in biological material,

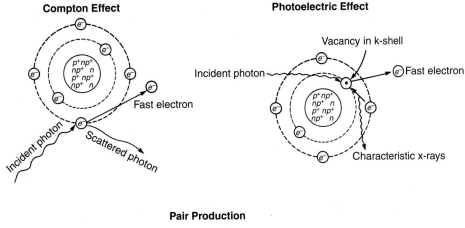

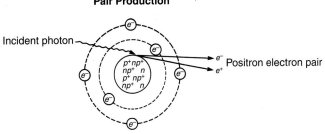

Fig. 1-1 The first step in the absorption of a photon of x-rays or gamma rays is the conversion of the energy of the photon into kinetic energy of an electron, or electron-positron pair. At higher energies, when the energy of the incident photon greatly exceeds the binding energy of the planetary electrons in the atoms of the absorber, the Compton process dominates. The photon interacts with the electron in a classic "billiard-ball" collision. Part of the photon energy is given to the electron as kinetic energy, whereas the photon is deflected and has reduced energy.

At lower energies, when the binding energy of the planetary electrons of the atoms of the absorber is not small compared with the photon energy, the photoelectric effect is most important. The photon disappears completely as it interacts with a bound electron. The electron is ejected with kinetic energy equal to the photon energy, less the energy required to overcome the electron bond. The vacancy caused by the removal of the electron must be filled by an electron dropping from an outer orbit, giving rise to a photon of characteristic radiation.

At sufficiently high photon energies, the photon may interact with the powerful nuclear forces to produce an electron-positron pair. The first 1.02 MeV of photon energy is used to create the rest mass of the pair, and the remainder is distributed equally between them as kinetic energy.

they behave like overweight electrons as long as they are relativistic (i.e., as long as their velocity is close to that of light). However, when they slow down, they spiral down the energy levels of an absorbing atom and are finally absorbed by the nucleus of that atom, which then explodes to produce fragments consisting of neutrons, alpha particles, and larger nuclear fragments.

Heavy ions are nuclei of elements such as nitrogen, carbon, neon, argon, or silicon that are positively charged because some or all of their planetary electrons have been stripped from them. To be useful, they must be accelerated to energies of thousands of millions of volts and can therefore be produced in only a very limited number of laboratories in the world.

Production of Radiation for Therapeutic Applications

When x-rays or gamma rays enter biological material, energy is converted into chemical damage and heat. At the energy levels of most x-ray and gamma-ray sources currently in use, the primary events are the interactions of photons with electrons in the outer shells, resulting in scattering of both the photons and the electrons (Compton scattering). With higher-energy photons, scatter of secondary electrons is more in the forward direction (i.e., in the direction of the primary beam). It takes some distance for the interactions to summate and reach a maximum, after which the energy of the beam dissipates by a constant fraction per unit depth. Figure 1-2 compares depth-dose characteristics of several radiation

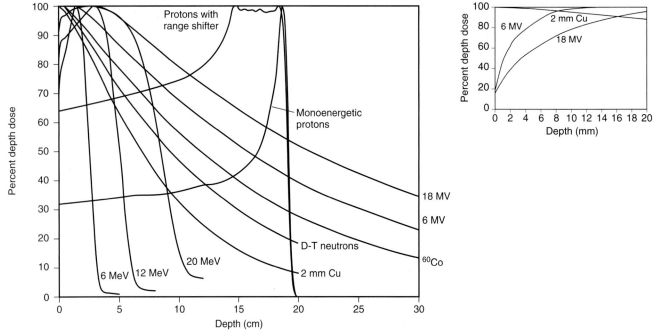

Fig. 1-2 Percentage depth-dose curves for a variety of radiation types used in radiation therapy. These include x-rays and γ-rays up to 18 MV, electrons of 6 to 20 MeV, and protons. The *inset* shows the pattern of absorption at shallow depths and provides a rationale for the skin-sparing effect.

beams commonly used in radiation therapy. The insert in this figure demonstrates the physical basis for skin sparing; the maximum dose occurs below the skin surface, unlike conventional x-rays.

The most commonly used sources for external irradiation are listed in Table 1-1. A great deal of overlap exists among the teletherapy sources. For example, there is relatively little difference in depth doses between the gamma rays from ^{60}Co and 2- to 6-megavolt (MV) x-rays. However, the edge of the beam produced by a linear accelerator is much sharper than that from cobalt units, which may be an important factor when radiation is delivered close to critical structures, such as the lens of the eye.

The sources most widely used for intracavitary or interstitial therapy are listed in Table 1-2. Again, the

various brachytherapy sources have overlapping capabilities, but some have specific advantages. For example, ^{192}Ir is the only isotope listed that has been widely and satisfactorily used with an afterloading

TABLE 1-2
Therapeutic Isotopes

Isotope	Half-life	Average Energy (keV)
PHOTON		
^{226}Ra	1620 yr	830
^{137}Cs	30 yr	662
^{198}Au	2.7 days	412
^{192}Ir	73.8 days	370
^{125}I	60 days	28
^{103}Pd	16.97 days	21

Isotope	Half-life	Maximum Energy (keV)
BETA		
^{32}P	14.3 days	1710
^{90}Sr/^{90}Y	28.5 yr/2.7 days	550/2280
^{188}W/^{188}Re	69.4 days/17 hr	350/2120
^{186}Re	3.8 days	1070
^{62}Zn/^{62}Cu	9.3 hr/9.7 min	660/2930
^{133}Xe	5.2 days	360
^{131}I	8.0 days	600
^{89}Sr	50.5 days	1495
^{166}Ho	26.8 hr	1850

keV, Kiloelectron volt.

TABLE 1-1
Teletherapy Sources

Unit	Mean Energy (MeV) Photons
150–440 kVp x-ray	0.06–0.14
^{137}Cs teletherapy	0.66
^{60}Co teletherapy	1.25
4 MV linear accelerator	1.3
6 MV linear accelerator	1.8
20–24 MV betatron and linear accelerator	6.2–7.0

MeV, Megaelectron volts; *kVp,* kilovolt peak; *MV,* megavolts.

technique for interstitial therapy. Radium and cesium can be used in afterloading intracavitary applicators. Gold and iodine can be used for permanent interstitial implants.

When used appropriately and meticulously, both teletherapy units and brachytherapy sources have had great success in the permanent control of a variety of malignant diseases. However, there is nothing inherent in any of these x-ray or gamma-ray generators that will ensure success independent of the expertise of the radiation oncologist.

Dose: Its Measurement and Meaning

Quantification of dose has been an important factor in the development of modern radiation therapy. The ability to prescribe and deliver specific amounts of radiation repeatedly with both precision and accuracy is essential if a given treatment is to be duplicated and if clinical data are to be accumulated and compared. Biological effects in laboratory research and in clinical practice correlate well with absorbed dose, expressed in energy per unit mass of tissue. This correlation holds true for all types of radiation used in conventional radiation therapy, such as x-rays, gamma rays, fast neutrons, and electrons, but is probably less satisfactory for very-high-energy heavy ions.

For many years, the unit of dose commonly used was the rad, defined to be an energy absorption corresponding to 100 ergs/g. This unit has been replaced by the gray (Gy), defined to be an energy absorption of 1 J/kg. One gray is equivalent to 100 rad.

Measurement of Dose

Dose can be measured directly, in terms of energy absorbed per unit mass, by measuring the temperature rise in the absorbing material. However, this can be done in only a few research centers because doses of several grays result in a temperature rise of only a few hundredths of a degree Celsius, which is exceedingly difficult to measure. Consequently, calorimeters designed to measure dose directly in absolute terms are not practical for everyday use, but rather are important in research. For practical day-to-day use, what is measured is the ability of the x-rays or gamma rays to ionize air because such measurements are sensitive and relatively easy to make. Absorbed dose is then calculated on the basis of the ionization measurements.

An ionization chamber consists of a cavity containing a gas that is surrounded by tissue-equivalent material. A central electrode within the cavity is maintained at a high voltage relative to the cavity walls. The gas is an insulator, so no charge will pass across the gas until x-rays or gamma rays pass through the cavity and produce ionizations. The collection of the charges produced leads to the current between the central electrode and cavity walls, which can be detected with a sensitive

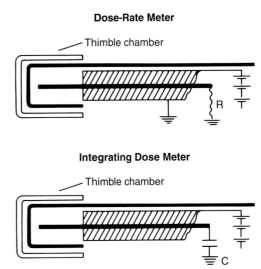

Fig. 1-3 An ionization chamber consists of a cavity fabricated from tissue-equivalent plastic and filled with an appropriate gas. A voltage is applied between the central electrode and the wall of the cavity. The gas is an insulator so that no current flows unless x-rays pass through the gas and ionize the gas into positive and negative ions that are collected by the voltage across the chamber. The charge generated is proportional to the x-ray intensity. If the charge is passed through a resistor *(R)*, the voltage generated across it is a measure of the instantaneous dose rate. It is then a *dose-rate meter*. If the charge is passed onto a condenser *(C)*, the change in voltage across the condenser is a measure of the total dose. It is then an *integrating dose meter*.

instrument. In practice, most of the ionizations occur in the cavity wall and result in electrons that pass through the cavity. If the ionization chamber is connected across a capacitor, then the dose meter will be an integrating dose meter (i.e., it will measure the total amount of radiation incident upon it) (Fig. 1-3). If the chamber is connected across a resistor and the current through that resistor is measured, then the dose meter will measure the instantaneous dose rate.

Patterns of Energy Deposition— Microdosimetry

Dose is an average quantity (i.e., the *average* energy deposited per unit mass of tissue). At a microscopic level, though, energy from ionizing radiation is not deposited uniformly but tends to be localized along the tracks of charged particles. What is critical, therefore, to the biological effect produced by a given amount of radiation is the *pattern* of energy deposition.

Figure 1-4 shows the tracks of secondary charged particles in cells irradiated with 1 centigray (cGy) of x-rays or 1 cGy of neutrons. In the case of x-rays, the charged particles set in motion are electrons, whereas in the case of neutrons, the secondary charged particles are protons. Obviously, a marked difference exists between the two. A dose of 1 cGy of x-rays results in essentially all cells

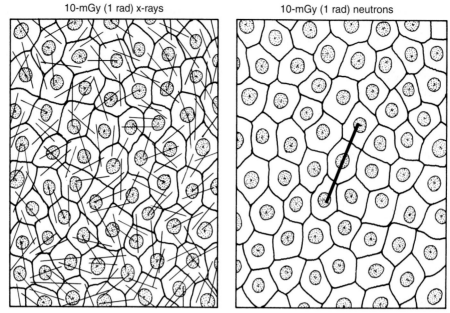

Fig. 1-4 When a population of cells is irradiated with 1 cGy of x-rays, a number of charged particle tracks traverse every cell. By contrast, in the case of neutrons, only a small proportion of the cells are traversed by a charged particle track. Consequently, when the x-ray dose is increased, the average energy deposited per cell is increased. When the neutron dose is increased, the number of cells in which energy is deposited is increased. This is a fundamental difference between x-rays and neutrons.

being traversed by several particles. For neutrons, only a few cells are traversed by a single particle. Consequently, when the dose of x-rays is doubled, the average energy per cell is increased; however, in the case of neutrons, the number of cells traversed is increased but the amount of energy per cell traversed does not change. This is a very vital and essential difference between the two types of radiation. Biological effects correlate with dose for a given type of radiation (i.e., a bigger dose leads to a bigger biological effect), but the same dose of a different type of radiation does *not* produce equal biological effects because of the considerations referred to above. In other words, the different relative biological effectiveness (RBE) of different types of radiation is largely a reflection of the different patterns of energy deposition.

Physical Basis for Choice of Treatment Techniques

The determinants for choosing particular techniques in clinical radiation therapy are (1) the limits of localization of the malignant tumor and especially its subclinical extensions and (2) the availability of particular sources of radiation. Except for the few institutions that have accelerators capable of producing beams of heavy charged particles, treatment choices are based on the external beams listed in Table 1-1 or the intracavitary sources listed in Table 1-2. The particular techniques that are suitable for individual malignant tumors are

found in chapters elsewhere in this book. A few generalizations are made here as follows.

The intent when administering ionizing radiation for the purpose of killing all cells in a malignant tumor is to deliver a dose that is sufficient to eradicate these cells but is limited with respect to the surrounding normal tissues. In light of the preceding discussion of dose and its meaning, it is worth noting the appropriate designations of dose in the clinical setting. The term *tumor dose* is inappropriate because dose distribution is rarely homogeneous throughout the tumor-containing volume. It is more appropriate to refer to *minimum tumor dose* because it is this dose that determines control of the tumor. Similarly, it is most meaningful to refer to *maximum doses* in specific normal tissues surrounding the tumor because these doses will determine the adverse effects of radiation therapy. In all cases, moreover, it is virtually meaningless to express a total dose without qualifying it by the fractionation regimen used (fractionation is discussed further later in this chapter).

A more detailed discussion of dose distributions, and the related subject of selection of single fields of specific radiation beams or the use of combinations of fields, is beyond the scope of this chapter. The reader is referred to standard texts for further discussion of these topics.

One principle of choosing treatment techniques can be noted. Given the contemporary availability of radiation beams, computers, and treatment-planning software, the temptation is to seek refinements of dose distribution that are conceptually satisfying but have little, if any, clinical importance. Such temptations are best resisted in the interest of daily reproducibility. To paraphrase a concept espoused by the fourteenth-century philosopher, William of Occam, "complexity is not to be assumed without necessity."

CANCER BIOLOGY

Cancer is thought to be a clonal disorder because most types of cancer seem to arise from a single cell that has suffered a disruption in its regulatory mechanisms for proliferation and self-elimination. Malignant cells differ from their normal tissue counterparts in several ways. First, they are often immortal, or at least have the ability to divide many more times than do cells from normal somatic tissues. Second, they often grow more rapidly than cells of the same tissue of origin. Third, they have abnormal cell-to-cell interactions, which result in their being able to invade, metastasize, and grow in foreign environments.

Mechanisms of Carcinogenesis

Carcinogenesis seems to be a multistep process, with multiple genetic alterations occurring over extended periods. Sometimes genetic alterations are carried in the germline and form cancer-predisposing syndromes, as described below; however, heritable mutations are the exception. Most of the alterations that lead to cancer are acquired in the form of somatic mutations.

Cell proliferation is controlled through a series of signals, both positive and negative, that affect cell division and differentiation. The acquisition of tumorigenicity results from changes that affect these signal-control points. The conversion of a cell to a malignant state can result from gain-of-function mutations that activate *oncogenes*, which are positive growth regulators; loss of function of a *tumor suppressor gene* product that normally acts as a negative growth regulator; or mutations that affect *death-regulating genes* that control apoptosis (programmed cell death).

Oncogenes are found in a mutated or abnormally expressed form in many human cancers.[1] Oncogenes can be activated by a point mutation, by a chromosomal rearrangement such as a translocation, or by gene amplification. Some human leukemias and lymphomas seem to be caused by specific chromosomal translocations that lead to oncogene activation in several different ways. Because oncogenes are gain-of-function mutations, only one of the two copies needs to be activated for their effects to be expressed, thus oncogenes act in a dominant (rather than a recessive) fashion.

The concept of tumor suppressor genes arose from the observation that the in vitro fusion of a normal human fibroblast with a HeLa cervical carcinoma cell suppressed the expression of the malignant phenotype of the HeLa cell. Of the many tumor suppressor genes whose location and function are now known, two of the most intensively studied are *p53* and *Rb*.[2,3] In contrast to oncogenes, tumor suppressor genes involve loss-of-function mutations, thus both copies of the gene must be lost for their effects to be expressed (i.e., they act in a recessive fashion). In practice, the loss of both copies of a gene occurs by somatic homozygosity, which is the process by which one chromosome of a pair is lost, a deletion occurs in the remaining chromosome, and the chromosome with the deletion replicates.

A third class of genes associated with some forms of cancer affects apoptosis. The most relevant example is the *bcl* family of genes, which includes *bcl-2*, *bcl-x*, and *bax*. *Bcl-2* is deregulated by the chromosomal translocation t(14;18), which blocks apoptosis and contributes to the development of follicular lymphoma.

The Multistep Nature of Cancer

The idea that carcinogenesis is a multistage process in which several distinct events occur, separated in time, is now almost 70 years old. Skin cancer experiments in mice led to the development of the concepts of initiation, promotion, and progression as being stages in tumor development. Genetic analysis of cells from solid tumors also suggests that multiple alterations, mutations, or deletions are needed in multiple signaling genes for the formation of cancer to occur. In the case of colorectal cancer, a model has been proposed that correlates a series of 6 to 12 chromosomal and molecular events producing changes in the histopathology of normal epithelium during the formation and metastasis of colorectal cancer.[4] These events are thought to involve a "mutator" phenotype in which multiple mutations are likely in cancer-associated genes (both oncogenes and tumor suppressor genes). This, in turn, leads to progression of the cancer and ultimately its invasive and metastatic properties.

Functions of Oncogenes and Tumor Suppressor Genes

The identification of genes associated with human cancer quickly led to studies of the function of these genes. Cells must repeatedly "decide" whether to divide, differentiate, or undergo apoptosis. All three outcomes affect cell number, and so it is not surprising that these decision pathways are the primary targets of oncogenes or tumor suppressor genes.

Most tumor suppressor genes can be classified as either *gatekeepers* or *caretakers*. Gatekeepers are genes that directly regulate the growth of tumors by inhibiting cell division or by promoting cell death. Thus the function of these genes is rate-limiting for tumor initiation and growth; both alleles (maternal and paternal) must be lost or inactivated for a tumor to develop. Predisposed individuals inherit one damaged copy of such a gene and so require only one additional mutation for tumor initiation. The identity of gatekeeper genes varies among tissues, such that inactivation of a given gene leads to predisposition to specific forms of cancer; for example, inherited mutations in the *APC* gene lead to colon cancer, and mutations in the *VHL* gene predispose an individual to develop kidney cancer. Because these gatekeeper genes are rate-limiting for tumor initiation, they often tend to be mutated in sporadic cancer through somatic mutations as well as in the germlines of predisposed individuals.

Inactivation of caretaker genes, in contrast, does not directly promote the growth of tumors but leads instead to genomic instability, thereby indirectly promoting growth by causing an increase in mutation rate. Such an increase in genetic instability can greatly accelerate the development of cancer, especially those types—such as colon cancer—that require numerous mutations for their full development. The targets of the accelerated mutation rate in cells with defective caretakers are the gatekeeper tumor suppressor genes, oncogenes, or both.

Signal Transduction

An elaborate system of biochemical communication networks exists in eukaryotic cells to provide information to the nucleus regarding the environment outside the cell. *Signal transduction* is the term used to describe the flow of information from the cell's outer membrane through the cytoplasm and into the nucleus. Multiple signal transduction cascades can operate simultaneously, with variable amounts of "cross-talk" between them. Even a weak signal can elicit a powerful response because it is amplified by biological processes in much the same way as a radio signal is amplified by an electronic device.

Signals, in the form of cytokines, low-molecular-weight hormones, growth factors, and other proteins that arrive at the outer plasma membrane, can affect the cell via two mechanisms. In the first, the signaling factor binds to a specific cell-surface receptor that spans the plasma membrane. Upon binding, these receptor molecules transduce a signal from the extracellular domain to the cytoplasmic domain on the inner surface of the plasma membrane; this transduction often leads to the activation of an enzyme such as a protein kinase. The second mechanism involves the migration of the signaling agent itself across the plasma membrane, followed by its binding to specific receptor molecules in the cytoplasm.

In either case, a biochemical cascade ultimately allows the signal to reach its destination—the nucleus—and alter cellular behavior. These signal transduction processes involve signaling molecules that are bound together by protein-protein interactions and by the production of second-messenger molecules. One important signaling pathway involves GTP-binding proteins such as those produced by the *ras* family; the *ras* gene is often mutated in human cancer. Another important pathway is that associated with protein kinase C (PKC). Ionizing radiation can activate both nuclear and membrane-cytoplasmic signal-transduction pathways; damage to deoxyribonucleic acid (DNA) modulates the transcriptional activity of *p53* through the activity of several kinases as well as by protein-protein interactions. These and other perturbations to signaling pathways can produce either cell cycle arrest or apoptosis.

The Cell Cycle

The ability of cells to produce exact, accurate copies of themselves is essential to the continuance of life; it is accomplished through highly organized processes, well conserved through evolution. Lack of fidelity in cellular reproduction, as manifested by alterations in DNA and chromosomes, is a hallmark of cancer. The division of the mammalian cell cycle into its constituent phases, M, G_1, S, and G_2, was accomplished by radiation biologists in the 1950s. As described in detail in the later section on "Tissue and Tumor Kinetics," it is now known that progression through the cell cycle is governed by protein kinases, which are activated by cyclins. Each cyclin protein is synthesized at a discrete phase of the cycle—cyclins D and E in G_1, cyclin A in S and G_2, and cyclin B in G_2 and M. Transitions in the cycle occur only when a given kinase activates the proteins required for progression.

The arrest of cells at various positions in the cycle by the action of "checkpoint genes" is an important response to DNA damage. The two principal checkpoints are the G_1/S and the G_2/M boundaries, but a checkpoint exists in S as well. G_2/M is the most well-known checkpoint after radiation damage; cells pause at G_2/M to repair damage before initiating the complex process of mitosis.

The hallmark of cancer is a lack of the ability to respond to signals that would normally cause the cell to stop progressing through the cycle and dividing. Of the tumor suppressor genes discovered so far in human cancers, only *pRb* and *p53* seem to be directly implicated in cell cycle control; clearly, much more remains to be learned on this topic.

Cancer Genetics

The link between cancer risk and genetic factors varies among tumor types. Up to 30% of rare childhood cancers occur in individuals who are predisposed to the condition, whereas only about 5% to 10% of common adult cancers are thought to be hereditary. Many instances of cancer predisposition are characterized by a distinctive pattern involving several different types of cancer in several different organs, sometimes accompanied by unusual physical features. In general, a family history of cancer, early age at onset, or multiple primary tumors strongly suggest the presence of a genetic disorder.

Germline mutations can result in a predisposition to cancer in any of four ways. Most cases of hereditary cancer predisposition can be traced to germline mutations in tumor suppressor genes. (Indeed, tumor suppressor genes were first discovered through a study of familial predisposition to retinoblastoma.) Germline mutations that activate oncogenes are another possible mechanism for hereditary predisposition to cancer, but the only disorders suspected of arising through this mechanism are multiple endocrine neoplasias. Medullary thyroid carcinoma and pheochromocytoma are a feature of these autosomal-dominant syndromes, and physical abnormalities often accompany the malignancy. Third, any syndrome that includes DNA-repair defects is likely to increase the probability of mutations in genes that lead to cancer. Xeroderma pigmentosum, ataxia telangiectasia, Bloom's syndrome, and Fanconi's anemia are all examples of relatively rare autosomal recessive syndromes that involve faulty DNA repair or replication. A particularly interesting member of this class is hereditary nonpolyposis colon cancer, which is caused by a mutation in one of five mismatch-repair genes; a mutation in one of these genes leads to a general instability known as the *mutator phenotype*. A fourth, less understood category of hereditary disorders predisposes to cancer through unusual sensitivity to common carcinogens. For example, lung cancer is usually considered to have only a small genetic component, but genetic variations in the metabolism of the carcinogens in tobacco smoke may be important in determining who develops a malignancy. Genetic variations also may influence susceptibility to hepatic cellular carcinoma caused by aflatoxins.

Several hereditary disorders are known to predispose to cancer, but understanding of those disorders at the molecular level is at various stages. Retinoblastoma displays the clearest pattern of a familial and sporadic form. Some researchers speculate that when all of the information is in, all common cancers will turn out to have familial and sporadic components, but that the genetics will be more complicated, and the pattern far less obvious, than those of retinoblastoma.

BIOLOGICAL BASIS OF RADIATION THERAPY
Radiation Chemistry

Some doubt still exists concerning exactly which critical targets in the mammalian cell must be damaged for a cell to lose its reproductive integrity. Strong circumstantial evidence indicates that DNA in the chromosomes is the critical target, although the nuclear membrane is also likely to be important. When x-rays or gamma rays are absorbed in biological material, the first step in the absorption process is the conversion of their energy to fast-moving recoil electrons. When neutrons are absorbed, the first step is the conversion of that energy into protons, alpha particles, or heavy nuclear fragments.

Radiochemical lesions in the DNA may result from the direct action of these charged particles or from indirect action mediated by highly reactive free radicals. Absorption of energy from direct action requires ionizations to occur within the DNA molecule itself. This is the dominant process for radiation of high linear energy transfer (LET), such as neutrons or alpha particles. (The concept of LET is discussed further later in this chapter under the heading "Radiation Quality.") Alternatively, the radiation may interact with other atoms or molecules in the cell, particularly water, to produce free radicals that can diffuse far enough to reach and damage the critical targets. A free radical is an atom or molecule carrying an unpaired electron in its outer shell. The most important of these is probably the hydroxyl radical OH•.

Free radicals have a lifetime of about 10^{-5} seconds, which is long relative to the time for the initial interaction of the radiation with the atoms and molecules of the absorber (10^{-15} seconds). Experiments in which free-radical scavengers are added to biological material during irradiation suggest that about two thirds of the damage produced by x-rays or gamma rays is mediated by free radicals. In the case of radiation of higher LET, the relative balance moves away from indirect action in favor of direct action.

The component of the radiation damage mediated by free radicals is readily amenable to modification by the presence or absence of oxygen or other chemical compounds. By contrast, direct action cannot be modified by chemical means.

DNA Breaks

DNA is a large molecule assembled as a double helix. Its two helical strands are held together by hydrogen bonds between the bases. The "backbone" of each strand consists of alternating sugar-phosphate groups. The sugar involved is deoxyribose. Attached to this backbone are four bases, the sequence of which specifies the genetic code. Two of the bases—thymine and cytosine—are single-ring groups (pyrimidines); the other bases—adenine and guanine—are double-ring groups (purines). The structure of a single strand of DNA is illustrated in Figure 1-5.

Bases on opposite strands must be complementary; adenine pairs with thymine, and guanine pairs with cytosine (Fig. 1-6, *A*). When cells are irradiated with x-rays, many breaks in single strands occur. These breaks

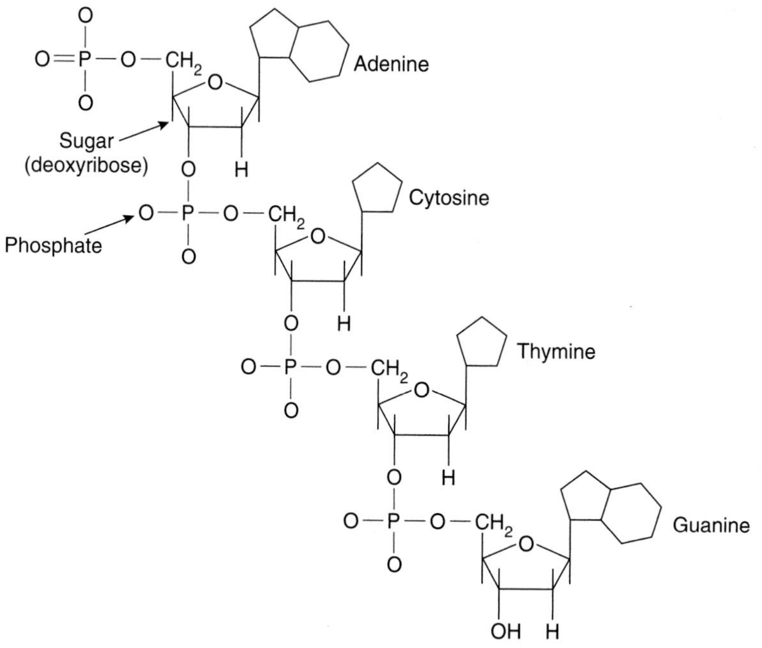

Fig. 1-5   Structure of a single strand of DNA.

can be observed and scored as a function of dose if the DNA is denatured and the supporting structure is stripped away. However, in intact DNA, single-strand breaks are of little biological consequence as far as cell death is concerned because single-strand breaks are readily repaired using the opposite strand as a template (see Fig. 1-6, *B*). If the repair is incorrect (misrepair), it may result in a mutation. If both strands of the DNA are broken but the breaks are well separated (see Fig. 1-6, *C*), repair again occurs readily because the two breaks are handled separately.

On the other hand, if the breaks in the two strands are opposite one another or are separated by only a few base pairs (see Fig. 1-6, *D*), this may lead to a double-strand break (DSB) (i.e., the piece of chromatin snaps into two pieces). When this occurs as the result of the passage of a charged particle, considerable damage can be produced in the region (a "locally multiple damaged site"[5]). A DSB is believed to be the most important lesion produced in chromosomes by radiation; as described in the next section, the interaction of two DSBs may result in cell death, mutation, or carcinogenesis.

Chromosome Aberrations

The most important of the chromosomal aberrations are exchange-type aberrations, which are formed when a DSB in each of two chromosomes, or chromosome arms, rejoins in an illegitimate way. A detailed discussion of cytogenetics is outside the scope of this chapter; a variety of complex aberrations can occur, but here attention focuses on *four* types of aberrations that are of special importance (Fig. 1-7).

The consequences of DSBs in two separate prereplication chromosomes are shown in Figure 1-7, *A* and *B*. In Figure 1-7, *A*, the rejoining occurs in such a way as to produce a symmetric *translocation*. This is compatible with cell viability but is occasionally associated with carcinogenesis by the activation of an oncogene. For example, if an oncogene is located on one of the chromosomes near the break point, the translocation may move it from a position where it is quiescent to a position where it is activated. A translocation between human chromosomes 2 and 8 is believed to be responsible for *myc* activation in Burkitt's lymphoma.

In Figure 1-7, *B*, the two broken chromosomes rejoin in such a way as to produce a dicentric fragment (i.e., a chromosome with two centromeres) and an acentric fragment. The acentric fragment will be lost at a subsequent mitosis because it has no centromere and thus cannot be segregated correctly to the daughter cells. The formation of a dicentric fragment is usually lethal to the cell. Another lethal aberration is the ring chromosome, the formation of which is illustrated in Figure 1-7, *C*. In this case, a DSB is produced in each arm of the *same* prereplication chromosome. The rejoining of the "sticky" ends may result in an acentric fragment and a ring. This aberration is usually not consistent with cell viability. Figure 1-7, *D*, illustrates the formation of an interstitial deletion in which two DSBs occur close together in the same arm of the same chromosome. This may lead to the loss of a section of genetic material, which may not affect cell viability. On the other hand, an interstitial deletion may be a mechanism of carcinogenesis if the deleted genetic material happens to be a tumor suppressor gene.

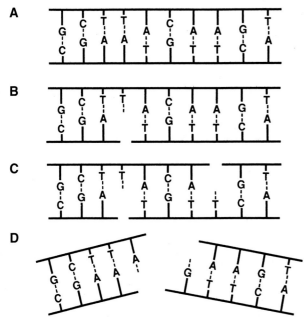

Fig. 1-6 Single- and double-strand breaks caused by radiation. **A,** Two-dimensional representation of the normal DNA double helix. The base pairs carrying the genetic code are complementary; adenine pairs with thymine, guanine pairs with cytosine, etc. **B,** A break in one strand is of little significance because it is readily repaired, using the opposite strand as a template. **C,** Breaks in both strands, if well separated, are repaired as independent breaks. **D,** If breaks occur in both strands and are directly opposite each other, or are separated by only a few base pairs, this may lead to a double-strand break where the chromatid snaps into two pieces.

Cell Survival Curves

A cell survival curve describes the relationship between the absorbed dose of radiation and the proportion of cells that "survive" in the sense that they are able to grow into a colony, thereby demonstrating retainment of their reproductive integrity.[6] With modern tissue culture techniques, it is possible to establish cell lines from many different tissues and tumors. If these cells are seeded as single cells and exposed to radiation or to some other cytotoxic agent, it is then possible to count the proportion of cells that are able to form macroscopic colonies after graded doses of the cytotoxic agent. Cell survival curves for mammalian cells have a characteristic shape. If surviving fraction is plotted on a logarithmic scale against dose on a linear scale, then the curve has an initial slope at low doses, where the surviving fraction seems to be an exponential function of dose (Fig. 1-8). As the dose is increased, the curve bends and becomes progressively steeper. At very high doses, the curve tends to become straight again (i.e., the surviving fraction returns to being an exponential function of dose). Over the first few decades of survival, survival curves for mammalian cells closely

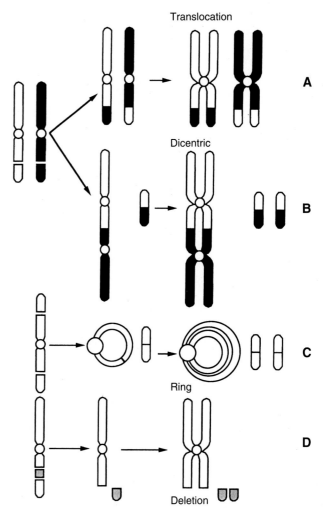

Fig. 1-7 Four types of chromosome aberrations. **A,** If breaks occur in two prereplication chromosomes, a symmetrical exchange may occur. This is consistent with cell viability; however, the process can lead to activation of an oncogene as described in the text. **B,** Breaks in two prereplication chromosomes may reconstitute to form a dicentric and an acentric fragment. This aberration is lethal to the cell at a subsequent division. **C,** Breaks in the two arms of a prereplication chromosome may rejoin to form a ring and an acentric fragment. This aberration is lethal to the cell. **D,** Two breaks in the *same* arm of a prereplication chromosome may result in a deletion. If the deletion is small, it may be consistent with cell viability. If the deleted piece of DNA includes a suppressor gene, it may result in carcinogenesis.

approximate that of a linear quadratic form expressed as follows:

$$S = e^{-\alpha D - \beta D^2}$$

where S is the fraction of cells surviving a dose (D), whereas α and β are constants.

Over a wider range of doses, a more complex relationship that contains at least three parameters usually proves to be a better fit. The parameters include an initial

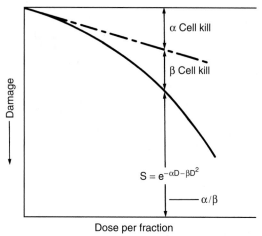

Fig. 1-8 Dose-response curves for mammalian cells are adequately fitted by the linear-quadratic relationship, at least over the range of doses of concern in radiation therapy. The form of the equation is

$$S = e^{-\alpha D - \beta D^2}$$

Where S is the fraction of cells surviving a dose D, and α and β are constants. Cell killing by the linear and quadratic term are equal when

$$\alpha D = \beta D^2.$$

This occurs when the dose D = α/β.

slope (D_1), a final slope (D_0), and some quantity that is a measure of the width of the shoulder. This quantity can be either the extrapolation number (n) or the quasi-threshold dose (Dq). For densely ionizing radiation, the shoulder of the survival curve tends to disappear, and the surviving fraction then approximates an exponential function of dose over the entire dose range. For a wide range of cells derived from normal tissue or from tumors investigated in vitro, the D_0 tends to be within the range of 1 to 2 Gy and the extrapolation number, n, varies from little more than 1 to about 20.

Effects on Normal Tissues
Clonogenic Survival Endpoints

As alluded to earlier in this chapter, normal tissue cells can be difficult to maintain in culture for long periods. In a limited number of instances, however, cell survival curves for normal tissues have been obtained through the use of ingenious techniques. The first example historically was for the survival of irradiated skin cells in the mouse. In this technique, devised by Withers,[7-9] a superficial x-ray machine is used to irradiate a circular annulus to the massive dose of 30 Gy to produce a moat of sterilized cells. In the center of this moat is an isolated island of intact skin, protected during the first exposure by means of a small metal sphere. This small area of intact

skin is then given a test dose, D, and subsequently observed for the regrowth of a nodule of skin. If one nodule regrows in half of the areas exposed, that indicates that a single cell survived. By varying the area of skin irradiated and dose of the radiation, it is possible to calculate the number of cells per square centimeter surviving various doses of radiation and thus to construct a cell survival curve. When this is done, the D_0 turns out to be about 1.35 Gy. Because the quantity scored is not the surviving fraction but rather the number of surviving cells per square centimeter of skin, no extrapolation number can be obtained. Instead, a second dose-response curve is constructed for split doses in which the radiation is administered in two equal fractions, 24 hours apart. The horizontal separation between the dose-response curve for single and split doses is then Dq. This value is about 3.5 Gy for mouse skin and is very similar for human skin.

Another normal tissue for which cell survival curves can be obtained is the "surviving crypts in the mouse jejunum system." The intestinal epithelium represents a classic self-renewing tissue. The crypts at the base of the villi contain dividing cells, which pass up the villi as they differentiate and become functional cells. A dose of radiation of several grays sterilizes a proportion of the dividing cells in the crypts but does not affect the mature, differentiated, functioning cells in the villi. After a dose of radiation, the villi shrink because no replacement cells from the crypts exist to take the place of those sloughed away from the tips of the villi. If the test animal is killed 3 or 4 days after the irradiation and sections are made of the jejunum, the number of regenerating crypts can be counted, giving a measure of surviving cells per circumference. This value can then be plotted as a function of dose. It turns out with this system that the D_0 is about 1.3 Gy, but the most interesting fact is that the Dq is very large, indicating the presence of a great deal of accumulation and repair of sublethal damage.

A third normal tissue system with which cell survival curves can be obtained was developed by McCullough and Till.[10] In this technique, a suspension of nucleated bone marrow cells is prepared from the bone marrow of a donor mouse and injected into a recipient mouse. Some of the circulating cells lodge in the spleen and produce nodules that can be counted after they have grown for 9 or 10 days; in effect, the investigator counts nodules in the spleen instead of colonies in a Petri dish. By comparing the number of spleen colonies resulting from cells taken from irradiated and unirradiated donor animals, the fraction of cells surviving a given dose can be calculated. The cell survival curve for these stem cells closely approximates an exponential function of dose (i.e., it has little or no shoulder and the D_0 is about 0.95 Gy). These cells represent the most radiosensitive mammalian cells that die a mitotic death. Dose-response curves for these three normal tissue systems are shown in Figure 1-9.

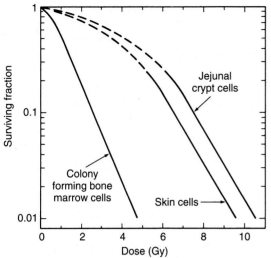

Fig. 1-9 Reconstructed x-ray survival curves for three mammalian cell types using in-vivo systems. Colony-forming units in the bone marrow are cultured according to the technique of JE Till and EA McCullough; skin colonies, by a technique devised by HR Withers; regenerating crypts in the intestinal epithelium, by a technique used by HR Withers and MM Elkind. The survival curves differ in slope, particularly in the width of the shoulder.

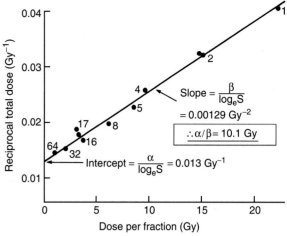

Fig. 1-10 Reciprocal of the total dose required to produce a given level of injury (acute skin reaction in mice) as a function of dose per fraction in multiple equal doses. The overall time of these experiments was sufficiently short that proliferation could be neglected; numbers of fractions are shown by each point. From the values of the "intercept" and "slope" of the best-fit line, the values of α and β, as well as the ratio α/β for the dose-response curve for organ function, can be determined. (Redrawn from Douglas BG, Fowler JF. *Radiat Res* 1976;66:401-426.)

Functional Endpoints

Although dose-response curves for clonogenic cell survival can be obtained in a limited number of circumstances, in many other situations it is practical to obtain a dose-response relationship for the loss of function of an organ or tissue. Organ function is obviously related more to the proportion of *functional* cells remaining in an irradiated organ at a particular time than to the proportion of clonogenic, or stem, cells. It is important to realize that it is the functional, and not the stem-cell, data that determine tolerance doses in multifraction radiation therapy. Functional dose-response curves can be constructed from multifraction experimental data by making several simple assumptions, namely that (1) the linear quadratic model is an adequate fit of the dose-response data, at least up to doses of a few grays; (2) the response of the tissue or organ is the same to each dose in a multifraction regimen; (3) the repair of sublethal damage is complete between multiple dose fractions; and (4) no cell division occurs during the fractionated regimen.

The basis of the method is to expose groups of animals to various numbers of fractions, with the dose per fraction titrated to produce a given functional impairment. The reciprocal of the total dose is then plotted against the dose per fraction, and the values of α and β corresponding to the linear quadratic form of the dose-response relationships can then be inferred from the intercept on the abscissa and from the slope of this plot. An example

is shown in Figure 1-10.[11] The extent to which the experimental data fit this straight-line plot, which is a transcription of the linear quadratic curve, is an indication of how well the linear quadratic relationship fits the basic dose-response data.

Acute functional effects for which multifraction techniques have been used to obtain the parameters of the dose-response relationship include the following:

    Acute desquamation in pig skin
    Acute desquamation in mouse skin
    Acute desquamation in rat skin
    Human skin "tolerance"
    Callus formation after bone breakage in mice
    Mouse tail necrosis
    Mouse $LD_{50/30}$ (the dose that is lethal to 50% of the animals within 30 days)
    Rat tail necrosis

For these acute effects, the ratio of $\alpha{:}\beta$ is usually close to 10 Gy, with the ratio being greater for the LD_{50} endpoints.

Late functional effects for which multifraction experiments have been performed to obtain the parameters of the dose-response curve include the following:

    Cervical and lumbar spinal cord function in rats
    Kidney function in the rabbit, pig, or mouse
    Lung LD_{50}
    Lung (number of breaths/min)
    Bladder (urination frequency)
    Skin of the pig (late contraction)

In these instances, the ratio of $\alpha{:}\beta$ usually falls in the range of 1.5 to 4 Gy.

Calculations of Tumor Cell Kill

Although the survival curve for cells exposed to graded single doses of radiation may be linear-quadratic, as described previously, the *effective* survival curve for a fractionated regimen delivered as daily 2-Gy fractions is an exponential function of dose. The D_0, the reciprocal of the slope of the curve and defined as the dose required to reduce the fraction of cells surviving to 37%, has a value of about 3 Gy for cells of human origin. This average value can differ significantly for different tumor types.

For calculation purposes, it is often useful to use the D_{10}, the dose required to kill 90% of the population:

$$D_{10} = 2.3 \times D_0$$

where 2.3 is the natural logarithm of 10.

Two sample calculations follow:

Example 1: A tumor consists of 10^9 clonogenic cells. The effective dose-response curve, given in daily dose fractions of 2 Gy, has no shoulder and a D_0 of 3 Gy. What total dose is required to give a 90% chance of tumor cure?

Answer: To give a 90% probability of tumor control in a tumor containing 10^9 cells requires a cellular depopulation of 10^{-10}. The dose to result in one decade of cell killing (D_{10}) is given by the following:

$$D_{10} = 2.3 \times D_0 = 2.3 \times 3 = 6.9 \text{ Gy}$$

Total dose for 10 decades of cell killing, therefore, is $10 \times 6.9 = 69$ Gy.

Example 2: Suppose that in the previous example the clonogenic cells underwent *three* cell doublings during treatment. Approximately what total dose would then be required to achieve the same probability of tumor control?

Answer: Three cell doublings would increase the cell number by $2 \times 2 \times 2 = 8$. Consequently, about one extra decade of cell killing would be required, corresponding to an additional dose of 6.9 Gy. Total dose is $69 + 6.9 = 75.9$ Gy.

Differential Effects on Normal Tissues

In both experimental animals and humans, normal tissues vary considerably in their sensitivity to ionizing radiation. Some of the least sensitive tissues (vagina, uterus, bile ducts) can tolerate a dose nearly 100 times that of very sensitive tissues (bone marrow, lens, gonads). The details of the effects that occur and the doses at which various effects can be seen are explored in the individual chapters of this text. However, some comparisons and generalizations of the biological effects of ionizing radiation can be made here.

Acute effects. Certain tissues manifest evidence of radiation effects in a matter of hours to days; they can be classified as acutely responding tissues. In approximate order of clinical significance, these tissues are as follows:

Bone marrow
Ovary
Testis
Lymph node
Salivary gland
Small bowel
Stomach
Colon
Oral mucosa
Larynx
Esophagus
Arterioles
Skin
Bladder
Capillaries
Vagina

Tissues that do not reveal acute effects of clinical significance but show evidence of damage of clinical significance in a matter of weeks to a few months after irradiation are often included with acutely responding tissues. Tissues such as these might be better categorized as "subacutely" responding tissues. Such tissues, in order of decreasing sensitivity, include the following:

Lung
Liver
Kidney
Heart
Spinal cord
Brain

Late effects. If given sufficient doses of radiation, all tissues can manifest late effects. However, several tissues are characterized as showing little, if any, evidence of acute effects but having well-recognized late effects. Such tissues include the following:

Lymph vessels
Thyroid
Pituitary
Breast
Bone
Cartilage
Pancreas (endocrine)
Uterus
Bile ducts

Effects on Tumors
Comparison of Normal and Malignant Cells

Malignant cells differ little from normal cells in their responses to ionizing radiation, tending to be most sensitive in the same phases of the cell cycle. Most cells seem to undergo repair of sublethal damage if sufficient time elapses between two doses of radiation. Depending again on the interval after irradiation, repopulation may result from the proliferation of clonogenic cells. Redistribution of cells as a function of their differing sensitivities in different phases of the cell cycle, with consequent radiation-induced synchrony, may occur in both benign and malignant cells. However, only malignant cells are thought to undergo reoxygenation after the administration of ionizing radiation. The radioprotective effect of hypoxia in tumors is an important reason for the failure to control tumors with irradiation. The concepts of reoxygenation and radioprotection are discussed further in the section on "Tissue and Tumor Kinetics."

Malignant tumors differ greatly in radiosensitivity. Although cell survival data suggest that different cell types have some inherent differences in radiosensitivity, the differences in sensitivities of tumors are the result of many factors, including inherent sensitivity, hypoxic fraction, vascularity, and changes in vascularity between repeated applications of radiation.

Both normal tissues and malignant tumors have sigmoid dose-response relationships (Fig. 1-11). A certain level of dose must be reached before any response is seen, after which the rate of response increases rapidly, followed by a diminishing rate of response at the highest dosage levels. As would be expected from the logarithmic reduction in the surviving fraction of cells after irradiation, higher doses are required to control larger tumors.

Unfortunately, the term *radiosensitivity* has often been used to describe the rapidity with which a tumor shrinks after irradiation. The rate of regression after irradiation is more appropriately termed *radioresponsiveness*; it has no relationship to radiosensitivity at the cellular level. Shrinkage is more related to the rate of cell removal (i.e., to the cell loss factor, as discussed later in this chapter).

Shrinkage, or "response" of a tumor, is an important element for determination of tumor control. *Complete response* is the only meaningful indicator of tumor control. Because of the heterogeneity of cells within a tumor,

there is no certainty of permanent tumor control after complete response. A *partial response* is a radiotherapeutic failure except in the infrequent cases of tumors that may reach a stable state after initial shrinkage, either because they have a large stromal component (e.g., desmoid) or because they have residual mature elements after the malignant component is eradicated (e.g., ganglioneuroblastomas or teratocarcinomas).

Assays for Transplantable Tumors in Laboratory Animals

Several assay systems have been developed for transplantable tumors in small laboratory rodents. These assay systems allow highly quantitative assessments to be made of the dose-response relationship for reproductive integrity of tumor cells exposed to radiation or to other cytotoxic agents. The first of these systems was based on lymphocytic leukemias, which can be propagated by inoculating a very few free cells. Subsequently, solid tumors of varying histologies have been developed in both rats and mice that can be propagated by the implantation of a small piece of tumor, or alternatively by the inoculation beneath the skin or into a muscle of a known number of cells, after disaggregation of the tumor by mechanical means and by the use of digestive enzymes such as trypsin. The advantage of these systems is that they are reproducible and highly quantitative. The disadvantage is that the tumors produced are highly anaplastic and undifferentiated, rapidly growing but remaining encapsulated, so that they show little resemblance to spontaneous tumors in humans.

The following paragraphs describe five basic assays that have been developed and used widely over the years. These assays vary in complexity and expense, and they have different advantages and disadvantages.

TCD$_{50}$ assay. The most direct experimental assay, which is parallel to the observation of patients treated with x-rays, is to determine the dose of radiation required to produce tumor control (tumor control dose [TCD]) in some proportion of irradiated animals.[12] In this assay, tumors are transplanted into a large number of animals and allowed to grow to a certain size, and then groups of animals are treated with graded doses of radiation. The animals are then observed for some period, and the dose is calculated that produces tumor control in half of the animals treated. This quantity is termed the *TCD$_{50}$*. The disadvantage of this system is that it is costly, inasmuch as perhaps 100 animals are required to produce this single-figure estimate of the TCD$_{50}$. The balancing advantage is that the tumor is treated in situ, with all of the complexities of the tumor-host response, and the tumor remains undisturbed after treatment.

Growth delay assay. In the growth delay assay, a large number of identical animals are used in which tumors of a given size are produced by transplantation.

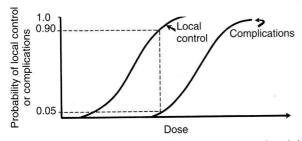

Fig. 1-11 Both the probability of local tumor control and the probability of complications are a sigmoid function of dose. If the two curves are well separated, it is possible to achieve a high rate of tumor control with a small complication rate. If the curves are closer together, as may be the case for large, resistant tumors, this favorable situation would not apply.

After irradiation, the tumors are measured daily so that the patterns of regression and regrowth can be established. The time in which a tumor grows back to its original size after irradiation is a measure of tumor response termed the *growth delay*. For tumors in which shrinkage does not occur, an alternative endpoint is to express the time for the tumor to grow from size A to size B (perhaps from 2 to 8 mm) in irradiated animals compared with the comparable time in unirradiated controls.

Dilution assay. The dilution assay technique devised by Hewitt and Wilson[13] was, in fact, the method by which the first in-vivo dose-response curve was obtained. In this technique, initially devised for lymphocytic leukemia and subsequently adapted for use with solid tumors, tumor-bearing animals are irradiated and then cells are withdrawn, diluted, and various numbers inoculated into recipient animals, which are then observed to see if they develop a tumor. The TD_{50} (i.e., the number of cells required to produce a tumor in half of the animals inoculated) is determined for control animals and irradiated animals. The ratio of TD_{50}s for control and irradiated animals is the surviving fraction of cells for that particular radiation dose. The strength of this system is that the tumor is irradiated in situ. An additional advantage of this assay over the two methods referred to above is that the reproductive integrity of individual cells is determined rather than the response of the tumor as a whole. The disadvantage of the dilution assay is that after the solid tumors are irradiated, the tumor must be broken up and disaggregated. Although this practice does not seem to produce any significant artifacts in the case of radiation, it may produce spurious results in evaluations of cytotoxic chemotherapy agents. This assay system is also time-consuming and expensive, inasmuch as many animals are required to produce a dose-response curve. For example, a control group of at least six animals and an irradiated group of six animals produces the same amount of information as that obtained from one control and one irradiated Petri dish in the in-vitro assay.

Lung colony assay. The lung colony assay system was developed and has been used largely in Canada.[14] In this system, solid tumors are irradiated in situ and then removed, disaggregated into a single-cell suspension, and inoculated into recipient animals that are killed some number of weeks later. The number of metastases in the animals' lungs is counted. This system, too, exploits the realism of in-vivo irradiation and assessment of the reproductive integrity of survivors, but it suffers the disadvantages of requiring large numbers of animals for a given amount of data and requiring that the tumor be disaggregated after treatment, before its assay.

In-vivo/in-vitro assay. In this assay, the tumor is irradiated in situ, removed, and disaggregated into a single-cell suspension. Various numbers of cells are then plated on Petri dishes, and their reproductive integrity is assessed by their ability to produce colonies in vitro. This technique combines the advantages and strengths of both the in-vivo and the in-vitro assays; the tumors are irradiated in situ with all of the complexities of the in-vivo milieu, and then they are assessed with the speed, accuracy, and economy of the in-vitro cell culture technique. Only a limited number of tumors have been developed that can be transferred back and forth between the animal and the Petri dish; unfortunately, these are all highly undifferentiated tumors. This technique also has the same limitation as the dilution assay and the lung colony assay systems in that it involves the disaggregation of the tumor after treatment.

These assay systems, developed initially for the assessment of response to x-rays, neutrons, and other types of radiation, have allowed a vast body of data to be accumulated for chemotherapy agents and hyperthermia as well. Use of these systems resulted in the development of the important concept that the presence of a proportion of hypoxic cells can limit the curability of a tumor with a single dose of x-rays, leading to the demonstration and explanation of the phenomenon of reoxygenation. Recently, models that involve the use of transplantable tumors in small rodents have fallen into disfavor to some extent because the dose-response curves obtained do not give much more information than an in-vitro survival curve that requires much less time and a fraction of the cost. Criticism levied against these models is that the tumors are highly undifferentiated and not at all like spontaneous human tumors. In addition, their response to hyperthermia and chemotherapy agents may give spurious results for various reasons that are described later in this chapter.

Tissue and Tumor Kinetics
The Cell Cycle

Mammalian cells propagate and increase in number by mitosis. The division cycle for mammalian cells is illustrated in Figure 1-12. The description of the principal phases of the cell cycle (M, G_1, S, G_2) dates from Howard and Pelc in 1953.[15] During a complete cell cycle, the cell must accurately replicate the DNA once during S phase and distribute an identical set of chromosomes equally to two progeny cells during M phase. Regulation of the cell cycle in eukaryotic cells occurs by the periodic activation of different members of the cyclin-dependent kinase (CDK) family. In its active form, each CDK is complexed with a particular cyclin. Different CDK-cyclin complexes are required to phosphorylate several protein substrates, and that phosphorylation drives cell-cycle events such as the initiation of DNA replication or the onset of mitosis. CDK-cyclin complexes are also vital in preventing the initiation of a cell-cycle event at the wrong time.

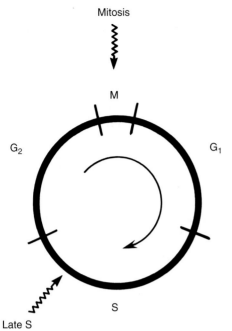

Fig. 1-12 The mammalian cell cycle. With a conventional microscope, the only phase of the cycle that can be identified is mitosis, in preparation for which the chromosomes condense and become visible. By the use of autoradiography, the DNA synthetic phase *(S)* can be identified to occupy a discrete length of time in the cycle.

Extensive regulation of CDK-cyclin activity by several transcriptional and posttranscriptional mechanisms ensures the perfect timing and coordination of cell-cycle events. The CDK catalytic subunit by itself is inactive, requiring association with a cyclin subunit and phosphorylation of a key threonine residue (usually T-160) to become fully active. The CDK-cyclin complex is reversibly inactivated either by phosphorylation on a tyrosine residue (usually Y-15) located in the ATP-binding domain, or by association with cyclin-dependent kinase inhibitor (CKI, also known as cell-directed inhibitor [CDI] proteins). After the completion of the cell-cycle transition, the complex is irreversibly inactivated by ubiquitin-mediated degradation of the cyclin subunit. The entry of cells into S phase is controlled by CDKs that are themselves sequentially regulated by cyclins D, E, and A. D-type cyclins act as growth-factor sensors, with their expression depending more on the extracellular cues than on the cell's position in the cycle. Mitogenic stimulation governs both their synthesis and formation of complexes with CDK4 and CDK6, and catalytic activity of the assembled complexes persists through the cycle as long as mitogenic stimulation continues. Cyclin E expression in proliferating cells is normally periodic and maximal at the G_1-S transition; throughout this interval, cyclin E enters into active complexes with its catalytic partner, CDK2. This view of the cell cycle and its regulation is illustrated in Figure 1-13.

The only phase of the cycle that can be observed with a light microscope is the process of division itself, in preparation for which the chromosomes condense and become visible. To visualize the DNA-synthesis (S) phase, the technique of autoradiography must be used. In this technique, cells are fed one of the precursors needed to build DNA that is labeled with a radioactive isotope such as tritium. Only those cells in the DNA-synthesis phase

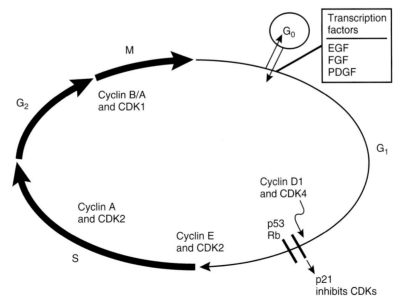

Fig. 1-13 Updated view of the phases of the cell cycle, showing how the phases are regulated by the periodic activation of different members of the cyclin-dependent kinase (CDK) family. Various CDK-cyclin complexes are required to phosphorylate several protein substrates that drive key events, including the initiation of DNA replication or the onset of mitosis. *EGF,* Epidermal growth factor; *FGF,* Fibroblast growth factor; *PDGF,* platelet-derived growth factor.

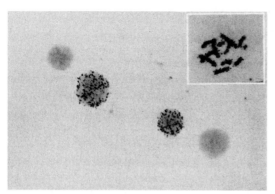

Fig. 1-14 Autoradiograph of a monolayer of mammalian cells flash-labeled with tritiated thymidine. Some cells are labeled, showing that they were synthesizing DNA at the time of the flash-labeling. The *inset* shows a labeled mitotic cell. The cell was in S phase at the time of flash-labeling but had moved to M phase before being fixed and stained. (Courtesy Dr. Charles Geard.)

take up the tritium. If those cells are later fixed, stained, and covered with a layer of nuclear emulsion, the beta particles from the tritium pass through the nuclear emulsion and produce an image that is visible when the emulsion is fixed and stained. Cells that have been labeled with tritiated thymidine are depicted in Figure 1-14; some cells are in interphase and some are in mitosis; some are labeled and some are not. To avoid using radioactivity, cells now are more often labeled by the incorporation of bromodeoxyuridine (BrdU), the presence of which can be detected by a fluorescent-labeled antibody. However, the principle remains the same.

The simplest experiment that can be done with a cell culture, a tissue, or a tumor is to flash-label it, that is, to expose the cells or tissues for 15 to 20 minutes with the labeled DNA precursor and then look at the samples after they have been autoradiographed. The labeling index (LI), the proportion of cells that are labeled,

reflects the ratio of the length of the DNA-synthesis phase (Ts) to that of the total cell cycle (Tc):

$$LI = \frac{Ts}{Tc}$$

From the same sample, it is also possible to observe the mitotic index (MI), defined as the proportion of cells in mitosis. This index represents the ratio of the length of the mitotic time (Tm) to that of the Tc:

$$MI = \frac{Tm}{Tc}$$

Thus it is possible, in a very simple experiment, to observe the ratio of the lengths of mitosis and the DNA-synthesis phase to that of the total cell cycle. However, these experiments involve the measurement of ratios and cannot be used to estimate the length of any phase of the cycle.

To determine the length of the various phases of the cell cycle, a much more complex procedure is necessary—the *percent-labeled mitoses technique*. The cell culture, tissue, or tumor is flash-labeled with tritiated thymidine, after which samples are taken, fixed, stained, and autoradiographed hourly for some period that is longer than the anticipated cell cycle. A typical percent-labeled mitoses curve is shown in Figure 1-15.[16] This technique follows the progress of the labeled cohort of cells through DNA synthesis, to the next mitosis, and through the cell cycle to another mitosis. The second wave of labeled mitoses is always smaller than the first because the cells in any population in vivo do not have a single cell-cycle time but rather are characterized by a range of cell-cycle times. In fact, a computer technique can be used to "unfold" the spectrum of cell-cycle times from the decrease in height of the second peak and thus to obtain an estimate of the range of cell cycles involved.

The width of the first wave of labeled mitoses at the 50% height gives an estimate of the Ts, and the time between the first and second peaks is an estimate of the average Tc. In many instances, particularly with normal

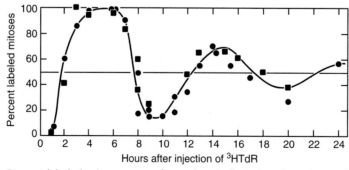

Fig. 1-15 Percent-labeled mitoses curve for a chemically induced carcinoma in the cheek pouch of a hamster. The *squares* and *circles* refer to two separate experiments. (From Brown JM. *Radiat Res* 1970;43:627–653.)

tissues, the second peak is too indistinct to be recognized; then the cell cycle cannot be estimated from the distance between consecutive peaks. In such cases, the Ts must be obtained from the width of the first peak and the cell cycle determined by the observation of the LI:

$$Tc = \frac{Ts}{LI}$$

Population Kinetics of Tumors

When animal tumors are studied with the percent-labeled mitoses technique, it becomes evident at once that the cell-cycle time is much shorter than the gross volume-doubling time. There are two reasons for this. First, not all cells in a growing tumor are actively cycling at any given time. By observing the uptake of tritium in mouse tumors, one can estimate that the *growth fraction (GF)*, defined as a proportion of cells that are actively cycling, ranges from 30% to 50%. From the cell cycle of individual cells and the growth fraction, it is possible to calculate the potential doubling time (T_{pot}). The potential doubling time is still much shorter than the actual gross volume-doubling time, and this difference is accounted for by the *cell loss fraction* (Φ), defined as the proportion of cells produced by mitosis that are lost from the tumor. These cells are lost largely into the necrotic "sinks" within the tumor, that is, areas where cells die because they are remote from a source of oxygen and nutrients.

The overall picture of tumor growth that emerges is that of a population of cells, some of which are dividing and others are quiescent, with the progeny of division largely being lost into necrotic areas of the tumor. For this reason, the gross volume-doubling time of the tumor, as a whole, is much longer than the cell-cycle time (Fig. 1-16).

In humans, a limited number of population kinetic studies have been performed because it is not possible in most countries to give large doses of tritiated thymidine to patients. In general, human tumors are observed to have gross volume-doubling times on the order of months, judging from repeated measurements of skeletal or pulmonary metastases. By contrast, 80% of human tumors have a cell cycle that lasts between 2 and 5 days. These numbers would be consistent with the estimate of Gordon Steel[17-19] that, on average, human tumors have a cell loss factor of 70% (i.e., almost three fourths of the cells produced by division are lost into necrotic areas within the tumor).

Clinical Applications

Although results from population kinetic studies performed in the past are illuminating and instructive, they cannot be applied to an individual patient because of the long periods required to perform cell cycle analyses. For example, an autoradiograph takes about 6 weeks to be produced, which includes the time necessary for sufficient beta particles to be emitted by tritium and incorporated within the cells and to produce a visible image in the nuclear emulsion above the cells. The breakthrough in this area has been the application of flow cytometry, as described in the following paragraphs.

Measurement of Potential Tumor Doubling Time

The growth rate of a tumor is slower than the growth rate of individual dividing cells for two reasons. First, as noted previously, most tumors contain a significant proportion of cells that are not cycling at any given time; the fraction of cells in cell cycle is the *growth fraction (GF)*. Second, many cells produced by division

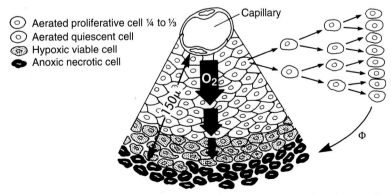

Fig. 1-16 Depiction of the overall pattern of growth of a tumor. Of the clonogenic cells, only a fraction, known as the *growth fraction* (GF), are actively proliferating at any given time. The remainder are quiescent but can be stimulated to return to a proliferating state. Of the cells produced by mitosis of the proliferating cells, some are lost from the tumor, largely into necrotic regions. The proportion lost is known as the *cell loss fraction* (Φ).

are lost, mainly in necrotic areas. The fraction of cells produced by mitosis that are lost from the tumor is known as the *cell loss fraction (Φ)*.

T_{pot} accounts for the proportion of dividing cells but not for cell loss. It is a measure of the rate of increase of cells capable of continued proliferation, and therefore it determines the outcome of a treatment delivered in fractions over an extended period.

Tumors with a short T_{pot} may repopulate if fractionation is extended over too long a period. T_{pot} can be calculated from the following relation:

$$T_{pot} = \frac{\lambda Ts}{LI}$$

where λ is a correction factor for the nonlinear distribution in time of the cells as they pass through the cycle (λ is between 1 and 0.67).

To measure T_{pot} precisely requires a knowledge of the Ts and the LI. The LI can be determined from a single sample, but measuring Ts requires labeling the cell population with tritiated thymidine or BrdU, taking samples hourly for some period approximately equal to the cell cycle, and counting the proportion of labeled mitoses as a function of time. From this percent-labeled mitoses curve, the Ts can be obtained. Although this sort of measurement can be done routinely for cells in culture or for tissues in animals, it is not practical for human tumors because it would entail a biopsy every hour or so for several days. An *estimate* of T_{pot} can be made from a single biopsy sample taken 4 to 8 hours after the injection of a trace amount of a thymidine analogue, usually BrdU or iododeoxyuridine (IdU). The biopsy specimen is treated with a fluorescent-labeled monoclonal antibody that detects the incorporation of the thymidine analogue into the DNA.[20,21]

The biopsy sample is also stained with propidium iodine to determine DNA content. A single-cell suspension of the biopsy specimen is then passed through a flow cytometer, which simultaneously measures DNA content (red fluorescence) and BrdU content (green fluorescence) (Fig. 1-17).[22]

The LI is simply the proportion of cells that show significant green fluorescence. The Ts can be calculated from the mean red fluorescence of S cells relative to G_1 and G_2 cells. The DNA content of cells in G_2 is double that in G_1. The method assumes that the red fluorescence of BrdU-labeled cells (i.e., the DNA content of cells in S) increases linearly with time (Fig. 1-18). If, for example, a biopsy sample was taken 6 hours after BrdU administration, and the relative DNA content of cells labeled with BrdU (i.e., in S) was 0.75, then midway between the DNA content characteristic of G_1 and that of G_2, the duration of Ts would be simply 12 hours. The method has been validated in several in vitro cell lines and also in animal tumor systems, where it can be checked with conventional cell kinetic studies. This technique gives an *average* value for T_{pot} of the cells in the biopsy specimen because the cells are disaggregated and made into a single-cell suspension. Evidence from animal experiments suggests that individual cells may

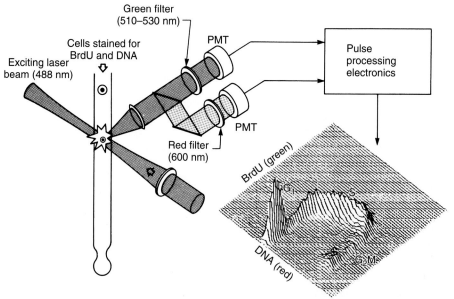

Fig. 1-17   Bromodeoxyuridine *(BrdU)*/deoxyribonucleic acid *(DNA)* analysis of Chinese hamster cells labeled with BrdU for 30 minutes and analyzed in a flow cytometer to investigate the distribution of cells in the various phases of the cycle. (From Gray SW, Dolbeare F, Pallavicini MG, et al. *Int J Radiat Biol* 1986;49:237-255.)

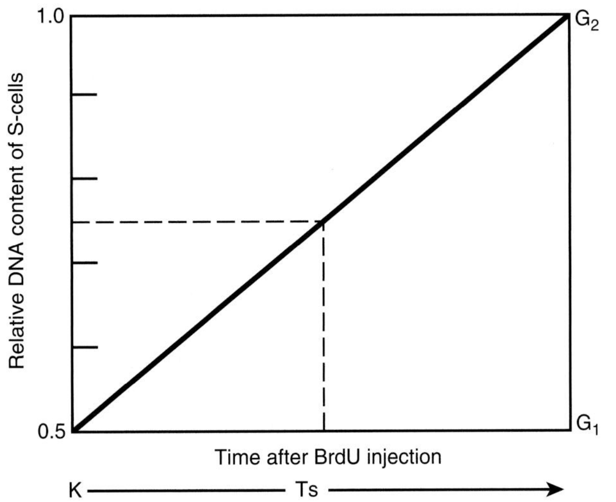

Fig. 1-18 The length of the deoxyribonucleic acid (DNA)-synthesis phase (Ts) can be estimated by flow cytometry of cells from a single tumor biopsy some hours after an injection of a thymidine analogue. Cells in S phase are identified by the green fluorescence from an antibody linked to the thymidine analogue. The relative DNA content is measured by the red fluorescence caused by the incorporated propidium iodide. The DNA content in G_2 cells is double that in G_1 cells. Ts can be estimated by the relative DNA content of the S-phase cells in relation to the time between the injection of the thymidine analogue and the biopsy. *BrdU*, Bromodeoxyuridine.

have much shorter T_{pot} values than those obtained from tissue specimens.

Systemic Effects

Systemic effects of ionizing radiation are determined by the proportion of the body irradiated, the specific organs included, and the dose received. At the extreme, lethal effects of total-body irradiation are well recognized. In addition to results from experiments with animals, especially experiments in which investigators are seeking the dose that results in the death of half the animals (lethal dose in 50%, or LD_{50}), limited data are available from accidental exposures to humans, such as that at Chernobyl. Three types of death from total-body exposures have been delineated. Doses on the order of 100 Gy or higher cause death in a matter of hours from effects on the central nervous system and cardiovascular collapse. Intermediate doses of 10 to 20 Gy result in death in several days caused by elimination of the intestinal epithelium with intractable diarrhea. Lower doses, from 1 to 5 Gy, result in depopulation of hematopoietic stem cells; death may occur several weeks after the exposure from infection or bleeding. The $LD_{50/60}$ for healthy young adults without medical intervention is between 3 and 4 Gy. Individuals can survive doses perhaps twice as large with supportive treatment, including antibiotics

and transfusions of blood products to help them over the nadir in peripheral blood counts.

In recent years, single-dose, total-body irradiation has been used either alone or with systemic cytotoxic drugs as ablative therapy to eradicate malignant cells from the bone marrow (especially in cases of leukemia) or from other parts of the body, followed by autologous, syngeneic, or allogeneic reconstitution of the bone marrow. In these clinical experiments, in which single, total-body doses of 5 to 10 Gy and fractionated doses of 12 to 16 Gy have preceded marrow transplants, it has become apparent that the limiting normal tissue is the lung; deaths have occurred weeks to months after irradiation from interstitial pneumonia.

The effects of irradiation on immune responses are complex. When total-body irradiation is given in doses that are potentially lethal, the immune mechanisms throughout the body, both humoral- and cell-mediated, are depressed. This is a direct result of the suppression of the progenitors of plasma cells and lymphocytes that produce immunoglobulins or participate in cell-mediated responses. The effects of local irradiation, particularly with regard to the volume irradiated and the amount of bone marrow within that volume, are only partially defined. Clearly, total lymphoid irradiation can have effects that are qualitatively similar to total-body irradiation but are quantitatively less similar. In the clinical setting, the malignant process itself may impair both humoral and cell-mediated immunity in humans, and hence the contributions of the primary disease and the therapy are difficult to separate. Irradiation of many of the common malignant conditions does not impair cellular immunity, as measured by the delayed hypersensitivity reaction. When very large volumes are irradiated, as in patients with Hodgkin's disease, cutaneous anergy may temporarily follow. Patients who have anergy, presumably related to the malignant process, often will recover their delayed hypersensitivity response after radiotherapeutic elimination of the tumor.

Depressions of the peripheral blood count from local irradiation are seen only when the volume irradiated is large and encompasses a significant portion of the active bone marrow. Irradiation of small areas does not significantly influence white blood cell count, platelet count, or hematocrit. The assumption that local irradiation is sufficient to cause profound pancytopenia can lead to serious delay in seeking the actual causes.

Nausea and vomiting have been considered by many, patients and physicians alike, to be a necessary accompaniment of any sort of radiation therapy. However, nausea and vomiting may also accompany irradiation as a function of the suggestibility of the patient. Undoubtedly, the range of individual sensitivities to these occasional side effects of irradiation is considerable, but nausea is most likely to occur when the stomach or significant portions of the intestine are included within the treatment volume. The irradiation of a very large volume of tissue, even when the gastrointestinal tract is excluded (e.g., treatment with the "mantle" field), also can result in nausea. Nausea that is truly related to irradiation for one of the above reasons occurs at the very start of a course of treatment. Serious delays in finding the causative factors can occur if it is assumed that nausea and vomiting that appear well into or near the end of a course of treatment are related to the irradiation when, in fact, they are not.

Fractionation

The earliest attempts at therapeutic uses of the newly discovered x-rays, especially in Germany, involved single, prolonged applications with profound effects on the tumor but severe injuries to normal tissues. More than 20 years passed before the advantages of repeated, brief applications of x-rays were appreciated. Indeed, the most important conceptual development in the history of clinical radiation oncology came from studies of spermatogenesis in the ram, reported by Regaud in the early 1900s.[23] Regaud demonstrated that a ram could not be sterilized by exposing its testes to a single dose of radiation without extensive damage to the skin of the scro-

tum, but if the radiation was given in a series of daily fractions, sterilization was possible without producing unacceptable skin damage. Reasoning that the testis was a model for a rapidly growing tumor, whereas the skin of the scrotum represented a dose-limiting normal tissue, the strategy of multifraction radiation therapy was born.

The efficacy of fractionation can now be understood in terms of radiobiological principles established with more relevant test systems. These principles have been described as the "four Rs" of radiobiology:

Repair
Reassortment of cells within the cell cycle
Repopulation
Reoxygenation

Repair

Sublethal damage repair and potentially lethal damage repair are both defined in operational terms. The molecular basis of either is not understood, nor is it known whether the two forms of repair involve the same or different molecular processes. *Sublethal damage repair* is defined as the increase in survival observed when a dose of radiation is split into two (or more) fractions with a time interval between. Figure 1-19, *A*, shows a dose-response curve for cells given single doses up to the

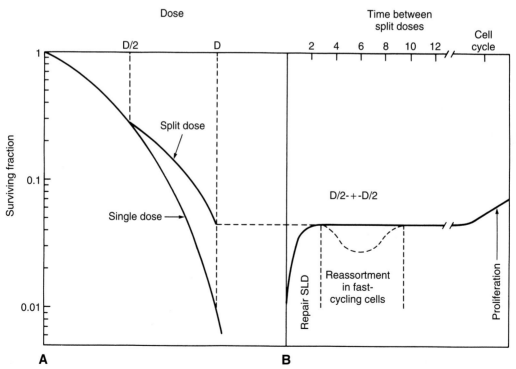

Fig. 1-19   A, Increase in cell survival observed when a dose of radiation is delivered in two fractions separated by a time interval adequate for repair of sublethal damage. When the dose is split into two fractions, the shoulder must be expressed each time. B, The fraction of cells surviving a split dose increases as the time interval between the two dose fractions increases. As the time interval increases from 0 to 2 hours, the increase in survival results from the repair of sublethal damage. In cells with a long cell cycle, or cells that are out of cycle, cell survival cannot be further increased by separating the dose by more than 2 or 3 hours.

dose value D (solid line). If a dose D/2 is given and a time interval of several hours is allowed to elapse before the remaining portion of the dose is delivered, then survival follows the dotted line as shown in Figure 1-19, *B* (i.e., the shoulder of the curve must be reexpressed). Figure 1-19, *B*, shows the result of an experiment in which two doses of D/2 were delivered, separated by various time intervals. It can be seen that repair takes place with a half-life of about an hour and is essentially complete by about 3 hours. Sublethal damage repair seems to be a ubiquitous phenomenon; it has been demonstrated in cells in culture, transplanted tumor systems, and normal tissue assay systems.

In the example quoted (i.e., rapidly dividing cells of rodent origin grown in vitro), the half-time of repair is about an hour. However, the rapidity of repair varies considerably. For cells of human origin cultured in vitro, it may vary from a few minutes to several hours.[24] Precise estimates for normal tissues in vivo are more difficult to make, but fractionation experiments suggest that the repair of sublethal damage may be very much slower in late-responding tissues.[25]

The extent of repair varies widely among different cells and tissues, tending to correlate with the size of the shoulder on the cell survival curve. One manifestation of sublethal damage repair is the effect of dose rate. Radiation delivered continuously at a low dose rate over some period approximates to an infinite number of infinitely small dose fractions. Sublethal damage repair occurs during the protracted exposure; as a consequence, the survival curve becomes shallower (the D_0 increases) and the shoulder has a tendency to disappear as the dose rate is progressively reduced (Fig. 1-20).

Potentially lethal damage repair is defined as the increase in cell survival that can be produced by manipulation of

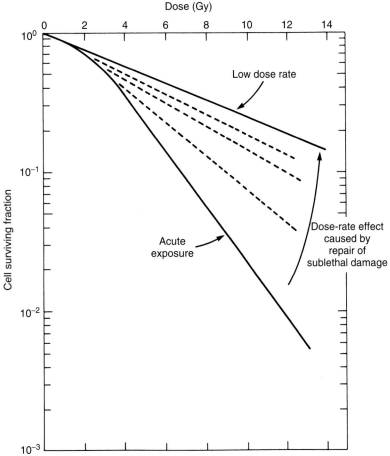

Fig. 1-20 The dose-rate effect. For sparsely ionizing types of radiation such as x-rays and gamma rays, the biological effectiveness of a given radiation dose decreases as the dose rate is lowered. This occurs when the exposure time becomes comparable to, or longer than, the halftime of repair of sublethal damage, so that sublethal damage is repaired during the protracted exposure. As the dose rate is progressively reduced, the slope of the survival curve gets shallower (the final slope [D_0] increases), and the shoulder of the survival curve disappears. The dose-response curve then approximates an exponential function of dose.

the postirradiation conditions. If, after irradiation, cells are kept in an environment that prevents cell division, more cells survive than if they are called on to divide soon after the exposure. This effect can be achieved with cells in culture by replacing the growth medium with saline or depleted medium, by lowering the temperature, or by maintaining the cells in plateau phase, that is, in culture conditions where they are confluent and have no room to proliferate. Potentially lethal damage repair occurs in cells of normal and malignant origin, and also has been demonstrated to occur in transplanted tumors in animals. If a tumor is left in situ for 6 to 24 hours after irradiation before being removed, subcultured, and transplanted, then more cells survive than if the tumor is transplanted immediately. The naive interpretation of these results is that some radiation damage that is potentially lethal can be repaired in a few hours, provided the cells are not called on to complete the complex task of mitosis during that time interval.

Presumably, potentially lethal damage repair also occurs in human tumors in vivo. It has been speculated that the ability to repair potentially lethal damage efficiently may be related to the resistance of some tumors, such as melanoma. Whether potentially lethal damage repair occurs in normal tissues in vivo is unknown because suitable assays are unavailable. However, it has been demonstrated in cells of normal tissue origin cultured in vitro.

Reassortment

The radiosensitivity of mammalian cells varies according to their position in the cell cycle. In fast-growing cells in culture, such as Chinese hamster cells, which have a cell cycle of only 9 or 10 hours, cells in mitosis (M) or late in G_2 are generally the most sensitive. They are characterized by a survival curve that is steep, with little or no initial shoulder. Cells late in the DNA-synthetic phase (late S) are most resistant and tend to have a survival curve with a broad shoulder. A similar pattern of radiosensitivity has been shown for the rapidly dividing crypt cells in the mouse intestinal epithelium, the only situation in vivo where good synchronization can be achieved by the use of a drug such as hydroxyurea. Cells cultured in vitro that have a longer cell cycle (e.g., 24 to 30 hours) and therefore a long G_1 phase seem to have a second period of resistance in G_1.

When an asynchronous population of cells is exposed to a single large dose of radiation, most of the survivors are in the resistant phases of the cell cycle (i.e., the surviving population is partially synchronized). A second dose of radiation would be less effective than the first because the population is resistant. If a time interval is allowed, however, cells tend to reassort themselves and become asynchronous again as cells move from resistant into sensitive phases of the cycle.

Repopulation

Repopulation refers to regrowth of cells after irradiation and was described earlier in the section on "Tissue and Tumor Kinetics."

Reoxygenation

Reoxygenation is the process whereby cells in a tumor that are hypoxic after a dose of radiation become oxygenated again as the tumor shrinks or as the demand for oxygen is reduced. This process has been demonstrated in many transplanted animal tumors. The extent and rapidity of reoxygenation vary considerably in animal tumors, but little is known about the process in humans. Reoxygenation is described in greater detail under the heading "Modifiers of Radiation Effects."

Fractionation and the Four Rs

Dividing a dose into fractions spares normal tissues because of the *repair* of sublethal damage between dose fractions and because of the *repopulation* of cells, if the overall time is sufficiently long. At the same time, dividing a dose into fractions increases damage to the tumor as a result of *reoxygenation.*

The effect of repopulation of normal tissue is rather complex. The extra dose that is required (because of fractionation) to produce a given level of damage does not increase until several weeks after the start of a multifraction regimen because proliferation does not occur until damage is expressed in the normal tissue. Once damage to normal tissue is apparent, compensatory proliferation is rapid. A further point to be made is that all normal tissues are not the same. In particular, a clear distinction exists between tissues that are rapidly responding, such as the skin, the intestinal epithelium, or the oral mucosa, and late-responding tissues, such as the spinal cord. It is important to realize, therefore, that prolonging overall treatment time within the normal radiation therapy range has little sparing effect on late reactions, but has a large sparing effect on early reactions. This axiom is of far-reaching importance in radiation therapy. Early reactions, including those in the skin and the mucosa, can be avoided by the simple expedient of prolonging the overall time. Although such a strategy avoids the problems of the early reactions, it has no effect whatsoever on the late reactions because compensatory proliferation in late-responding tissue does not occur during the time course of conventional radiation therapy.

Early- and Late-Responding Tissues

Differences in the repair and efficiency of reassortment of cells within the cell cycle lead to quite different shapes of the dose-response curves for early-responding and late-responding tissues. Dose-response relationships for late-responding tissues tend to be more curved

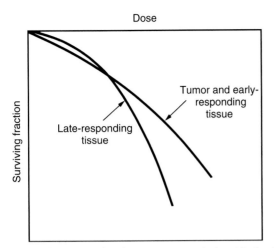

Dose

Surviving fraction

Tumor and early-responding tissue

Late-responding tissue

Fig. 1-21   Illustrating the dose-response relationship for late-responding tissue is "curvier" than for early-responding tissue. The dose at which cell killing is equal by the linear and quadratic components is α:β. This is about 2 Gy for late-responding and 8 to 10 Gy for early-responding tissue. (Based on ideas by HR Withers.)

TABLE 1-3	
Ratio of Linear to Quadratic Terms from Multifraction Experiments	
Reaction Sites	**α:β (Gy)**
EARLY REACTIONS	
Skin	9–12
Jejunum	6–10
Colon	10–11
Testis	12–13
Callus	9–10
LATE REACTIONS	
Spinal cord	1.7–4.9
Kidney	1.0–2.4
Lung	2.0–6.3
Bladder	3.1–7.0

From Fowler J. *Radiother Oncol* 1983;1:1-22.

than for early-responding tissues.[26] In terms of the linear-quadratic relationship between effect and dose, this translates into a larger ratio of α:β for early effects than for late effects. The difference in the shapes of the dose-response relationships is illustrated in Figure 1-21. Values of α:β for a range of tissues in experimental animals is shown in Table 1-3[27]; these data came from multifraction experiments with rats and mice. In general, the value of α:β is on the order of 2 Gy for late-responding tissues but is closer to 8 or 10 Gy for early-responding tissues.

Consideration of the shape of the dose-response relationship for early-responding and late-responding tissues leads to the important truism that fraction size is the dominant factor in determining late effects, whereas overall treatment time has little influence. By contrast, fraction size and overall treatment time both determine the response of acutely responding tissues.

The Strandqvist Plot

Early attempts to understand and account for fractionation in clinical radiation therapy gave rise to the well-known Strandqvist plot, in which the effective single dose was plotted as a function of the overall treatment time. Because all treatments were given as three or five fractions per week, overall time in these plots carried with it the implication of a certain number of fractions as well. These plots commonly showed that the slope of the isoeffect curve for skin was approximately 0.33.

The Nominal Standard Dose System

The most important contribution in the area of fractionation, made by Ellis and colleagues[28] with the

introduction of the nominal standard dose (NSD) system, was the recognition of the importance of separating overall treatment time from the number of fractions. According to this hypothesis, total dose for the tolerance of connective tissue is related to the number of fractions (N) and the overall time (T) as follows:

$$\text{Total dose} = \text{NSD} \times T^{0.11} \times N^{0.24}$$

The NSD system does allow some prediction to be made of equivalent dose regimens, provided the range of overall time and number of fractions is not too great and, further, that the dose regimen does not exceed the range over which the clinical data on which the system is based are available. An obvious weakness of the system is that time is represented in terms of a single power function with a nominal single dose proportional to $T^{0.11}$. On the other hand, biological experiments with small animals show quite clearly that proliferation does not affect the total dose required to produce a given biological effect until some time after irradiation begins, so that extra dose—because of proliferation—is a sigmoid function of time, not a power function of time. This represents a serious limitation of the NSD system. Perhaps the most significant limitation of the NSD system is that it is based on data for early reactions of skin and does not in any way predict late responses. Further, the NSD system does not provide any guidelines for dose-response in malignant tumors.

Tumor Control and Dose-Time Considerations

For many years, the basic determinant of total dose in the clinical setting was the tolerance of the surrounding normal tissues, especially the skin. With the advent of megavoltage treatment units and the attendant skin-sparing effect, greater attention has focused on the depth and distribution of dose correlated with permanent eradication of the disease. It is now apparent that tumor-control probability for epithelial tumors is profoundly affected by small changes in the time-dose relationships, and the size of the tumor greatly influences the dose necessary to achieve a high probability of control.

Although the time-dose relationships are of great importance for controlling epithelial tumors, the time factor seems to be of much less significance in the treatment of highly radiosensitive tumors (e.g., Hodgkin's disease, malignant lymphomas, seminoma, Wilms' tumor, neuroblastoma, and retinoblastoma). The total dose is a more important determinant in the control of Hodgkin's disease and nodular lymphomas, whereas the number of fractions and the time over which the dose is delivered are less important. Because deleterious effects on normal tissues are related not just to dose but also to fractionation and time, a greater margin of safety attends more fractionated irradiation delivered over a longer time.

Radiation in laboratory animals or humans is used, with rare exceptions, as a local-regional treatment. Although laboratory studies have consistently evaluated tumor control (TCD_{50}) as the endpoint, clinical results are often expressed in terms of survival or cancer-free survival. The only direct measure of the effectiveness of irradiation is control of the tumor within the irradiated volume (i.e., local control). Margin failure, the failure to appreciate the original extensions of the tumor, should be analyzed separately.

The only measure of failure of local control (i.e., true recurrence) is regrowth of the tumor within the irradiated volume. Identifying failure of local control requires careful evaluation of the patient over months and years, and attempts to predict failure of local control by other means have been unsuccessful. The rate at which the tumor regresses and, consequently, the extent of residual tumor at the completion of irradiation have been evaluated in animals and in humans and have not proven to correlate with ultimate control of disease. Suggestions that postirradiation biopsies might help were based on the expectation that "viability" could be assessed histologically. This has largely been proved incorrect in the immediate postirradiation period. However, if a high growth fraction is present and most cells are actively cycling, then eventual control might be predicted by repeat biopsies at the site of the original tumor.

Arriagada and colleagues[29] documented a high local failure rate of radiation to treat non–small cell carcinoma of the lung by using repeat bronchoscopy and biopsy 3 months after radiation therapy with and without induction chemotherapy. In that study, nearly every patient with positive biopsy results developed recurrent disease and eventually died, and all long-term survivors had negative bronchial biopsy results. By contrast, biopsies of the prostate 2 years or more after external beam radiation therapy are much less predictive of clinical local failure,[30] although they have been found to correlate with levels of prostate-specific antigen.[31]

Multiple Fractions Per Day

Most malignant tumors arising from the epithelium require total doses near, or even above, those tolerated by the surrounding normal tissues. Consideration of the different α:β ratios for early-responding tissues, including tumors, and late-responding tissues suggests an advantage to altered fractionation in the direction of increasing acute reactions while sparing late effects.

Prolongation of treatment has the advantage of avoiding acute reactions and allowing adequate reoxygenation in tumors. However, excessive prolongation can decrease acute reactions without necessarily sparing late injury, and it may allow surviving tumor cells to proliferate during treatment. Two separate strategies use multiple fractions per day, namely *hyperfractionation* and *accelerated fractionation*. The objectives of these two strategies are quite different, and they are discussed here in turn.

One thing that these two fractionation strategies have in common is that they both involve multiple fractions per day, and in this context it is important to ensure that the two fractions are separated by a sufficient time interval for the effects of the two doses to be independent, that is, for the repair of sublethal damage from the first dose to be complete before the second dose is delivered. With cells cultured in vitro, the half-time of repair is usually about an hour, but repair may be much slower in late-responding tissues. Clinical trials indicate that for a given total dose delivered in a given number of fractions, the incidence of late effect was *worse* for average interfraction intervals of less than 4.5 hours.[32] Current wisdom dictates an interfraction interval of 6 hours or more when multiple fractions per day are used.

Hyperfractionation. The basic aim of hyperfractionation is to further separate early and late effects. "Pure" hyperfractionation might be defined as keeping the same total dose as in a conventional regimen in the same overall time, but delivering it in twice as many fractions by the expedient of treating twice a day. However, this strategy would not be satisfactory because the total dose would have to be increased if the dose per fraction were decreased. In practice, then, "impure" hyperfractionation involves an increase in the total dose and sometimes a longer overall time, as well as many more fractions delivered twice a day. The intent of hyperfractionation is to reduce late effects while achieving the same or better tumor control and the same or slightly increased early effects.

A large controlled clinical trial of hyperfractionation for the treatment of head and neck cancer was conducted by the European Organization for Research and Treatment of Cancer (EORTC).[33] A hyperfractionated schedule of 80.5 Gy delivered in 70 fractions (1.15 Gy twice a day) over a period of 7 weeks was compared with a conventional regimen of 70 Gy delivered in 35 fractions of 2 Gy over 7 weeks. Local tumor control at 5 years after the hyperfractionated protocol increased from 40% to 59%, and this increase was reflected in improved survival. No increase in late effects or complications was reported. These results led to the conclusion that hyperfractionation confers an unequivocal advantage in the treatment of oropharyngeal cancer.

Two fractions per day may not be the limit of hyperfractionation; a further sparing of late effects by splitting the dose into more and more fractions of smaller and smaller size would occur as long as the dose fraction is still on the curved portion of the dose-response curve.

Accelerated treatment. The alternative strategy to hyperfractionation is *accelerated treatment*. "Pure" accelerated treatment might be defined as the same total dose delivered in half of the overall time by the expedient of giving two or more fractions each day. In practice, this can never be achieved because the acute effects become limiting. Either a rest period must be imposed in the middle of the treatment or the dose must be reduced slightly, with acute effects being the limiting factor. The intent of this accelerated treatment strategy is to reduce repopulation in rapidly proliferating tumors. Late effects should show little or no change because the number of fractions and the dose per fraction are unaltered.

In addition to the hyperfractionation trial noted above, the EORTC also conducted a large prospective randomized clinical trial of accelerated treatment for head and neck cancer (except that of the oropharynx).[34] The accelerated treatment consisted of 72 Gy given in 45 fractions (1.6 Gy in three fractions per day) over a 5-week span, with a 2-week rest in the middle. The conventional control condition involved 35 fractions of 2 Gy for a total dose of 70 Gy in 7 weeks. The results of this trial showed a 15% increase in local-regional control for accelerated fractionation, but this increase did not translate into a survival advantage. As expected, acute effects were significantly increased, but the observed increase in late effects was decidedly *not* expected; moreover, some of those effects involved complications that proved to be lethal.

This EORTC trial and several others testing accelerated treatment show that attempting to keep the total dose as high as 66 to 72 Gy while shortening the overall time by as much as 2 to 3 weeks from a conventional 6 or 7 weeks leads to serious problems with late complications. There are probably two reasons for this. First, the late effects observed are "consequential" late damage (i.e., late damage developing out of the very severe acute effects). Second, repair is probably incomplete between dose fractions, particularly for protocols involving three

fractions per day, because any unrepaired damage in the first interval would accumulate in the second interval in each day. Moreover, the interval between fractions in the early years of the EORTC trial was only 4 hours.

The continuous hyperfractionated accelerated radiation therapy protocol. The strategy underlying the Continuous Hyperfractionated Accelerated Radiation Therapy (CHART) trial was to use a low dose per fraction to minimize late effects and a very short overall time to minimize tumor proliferation.[35] In this unique study, conducted at the Mount Vernon Hospital in association with the Gray Laboratory, patients were given a total dose of 50.4 to 54 Gy in 36 fractions over 12 consecutive days, with three fractions delivered daily and an interfraction interval of 6 hours. The dose per fraction was 1.4 to 1.5 Gy. By conventional standards, the total dose was very low, but it was delivered in a very short time. This protocol produced good local tumor control; despite the severe acute reactions experienced, patients reportedly favored the protocol because treatment was concluded quickly. The incidence of late effects in general was not increased, and by some measures the incidence was actually decreased. The notable exception was damage to the spinal cord. Several myelopathies were recorded at total doses of 50 Gy, probably because an interfraction interval of 6 hours was not sufficient to allow full repair of sublethal damage in this tissue.

CHART is the only new fractionation schedule to date that resulted in a *lower* incidence of late complications. The severe but tolerable acute reactions associated with this protocol did not translate into late sequelae, probably because the total dose was relatively low. Effectiveness in tumor control was not lost, even at this low dose, because the overall treatment time was extremely short, minimizing tumor-cell proliferation. Compliance was also high because the acute reactions did not peak and become uncomfortable until after the end of treatment.

Radiation Therapy Oncology Group Trial 9003. In the largest fractionation trial yet conducted (1073 evaluable patients), trial 9003 by the Radiation Therapy Oncology Group (RTOG) compared a standard fractionation protocol (70 Gy delivered at 2.0 Gy per fraction) to three other fractionation protocols in patients with stage III to IV, M0 squamous carcinoma of the oral cavity, oropharynx, supraglottic larynx, or stage II to IV carcinoma of the base of the tongue or the hypopharynx.[36] Two of these protocols, one involving hyperfractionation of a total dose of 81.6 Gy given in 68 fractions twice daily over 7 weeks and the other involving accelerated fractionation via concomitant boost with 30 fractions of 1.8 Gy in 6 weeks plus a second fraction of 1.5 Gy during the last 12 treatment days (total dose of 72.0 Gy given in 42 fractions over 6 weeks), produced significantly higher local control rates than did standard fractionation. A third accelerated fractionation scheme with a total dose of 67.2 Gy given in 42 fractions over 6 weeks with an interruption after 38.4 Gy produced a local control rate similar to that of the standard fractionation protocol. The incidence of acute effects was higher among those treated with the nonstandard fractionation regimens than for those treated with the standard regimen, but the late effects were similar. These results provided immediate opportunities for mathematical modeling of radiation effects, especially the interplay of time and total dose in treatment outcome.[37,38]

Accelerated hyperfractionated radiation therapy with carbogen breathing and nicotinamide: the ARCON protocol. Also worthy of mention is a strategy involving accelerated hyperfractionated radiation therapy while the patient breathes carbogen (95% O_2 and 5% CO_2) with nicotinamide. The goals of this regimen, known by the acronym ARCON, were to accelerate treatment to avoid tumor proliferation, to hyperfractionate the doses (small doses per fraction) to minimize late effects, to add carbogen breathing to overcome chronic hypoxia, and to add nicotinamide to overcome acute hypoxia. Clinical trials of this complex but imaginative protocol are currently underway. Early results of a trial conducted in The Netherlands for patients with advanced laryngeal cancer were spectacular compared with historical controls. Results of a prospective randomized trial have yet to be published.

Lessons Learned from Fractionation Studies

Trials involving changes in fractionation patterns have produced several important results. The first of these "lessons learned" is that hyperfractionation seems to confer an unequivocal benefit in the treatment of head and neck cancer, in terms of both local control and survival, without producing any increase in late sequelae. On the other hand, accelerated treatment should be used cautiously given the findings from the EORTC trial of an unexpected increase in serious late complications. Particular caution is necessary if the spinal cord is in the treatment field for twice-a-day treatments because repair of sublethal damage is slow in this tissue. A second lesson is that late effects depend primarily on total dose and dose per fraction; the overall treatment time (within the usual therapeutic range) has little influence.

Another important lesson is that overall treatment time affects both acute effects and tumor control. Gaps in treatment should be avoided because they lead to an increase in overall treatment time and a concomitant decrease in tumor control.

The importance of overall treatment time was illustrated dramatically by Overgaard and colleagues[39] in their retrospective analysis of three consecutive trials of the Danish Head and Neck Cancer (DAHANCA) study (Fig. 1-22). All three trials involved a total dose of 66 to

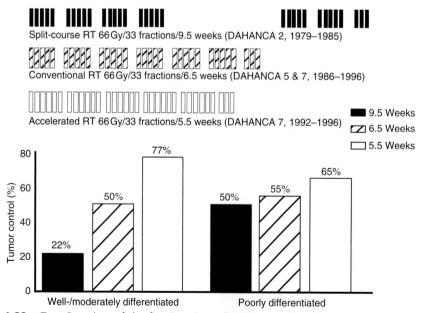

Split-course RT 66 Gy/33 fractions/9.5 weeks (DAHANCA 2, 1979–1985)

Conventional RT 66 Gy/33 fractions/6.5 weeks (DAHANCA 5 & 7, 1986–1996)

Accelerated RT 66 Gy/33 fractions/5.5 weeks (DAHANCA 7, 1992–1996)

■ 9.5 Weeks
▨ 6.5 Weeks
☐ 5.5 Weeks

Fig. 1-22 *Top,* Overview of the fractionation schedules used in the three Danish Head and Neck Cancer *(DAHANCA)* trials. *Bottom,* Relationship between histopathologic grade, overall treatment time, and local tumor control in the three trials. Only the well-differentiated or moderately differentiated tumors were significantly influenced by overall treatment time. *RT,* Radiation therapy. (Modified from Overgaard J, Sand Hansen H, Overgaard M, et al. *Proc ICRO/OGRO 6, 6th International Meeting on Progress in Radio-Oncology,* Salzburg, Austria; 13-17 May 1998. Bologna, Italy: Monduzzi Editore S.p.A.; 1998:743-752.)

68 Gy. The first trial, a split-course regimen that extended over a total of 9.5 weeks, produced a 3-year local control rate of 32%. The second trial, involving five fractions per week given over 6.5 weeks, had a 3-year local control rate of 52%. The most recent trial, in which six fractions were given per week and the overall treatment time was shortened to 5.5 weeks, produced a 3-year local control rate of 62%. No change in late effects was observed among the three treatment groups, but, as would be expected, the acute reactions became brisker as the overall treatment time became shorter. These intriguing findings must be viewed with some caution, however, because the three treatment groups came from different trials conducted over a period of several years; moreover, the initial purpose of the trials was to investigate the usefulness of hypoxic-cell radiosensitizers (discussed further in the section "Modifiers of Radiation Effects"). Nevertheless, in the case of relatively rapidly growing tumors such as head and neck cancer, overall treatment time can be a dominant factor in determining outcome.

Overall treatment time and local control. One of the most important lessons from fractionation studies is that local control is lost when overall treatment time is prolonged. For head and neck cancer in particular, local control is reduced by 0.4% to 2.5% for each day that the overall treatment time is prolonged.[37,38] In other words, after the first 4 weeks of a fractionated schedule, the first 0.61 Gy of each day's dose fraction is required to overcome proliferation from the previous day. Similar estimates can be made for carcinoma of the cervix, in which a mean of 0.5% local control (range, 0.3% to 1.1%) is lost for each day that the overall time is prolonged. On the other hand, the overall treatment time is not so critical for cancer of the breast or prostate in which tumor-cell proliferation is not so rapid. Although estimates of T_{pot} have not proven useful as predictors for individual patients, mean T_{pot} values for groups of patients are in accord with the importance—or lack thereof—of overall treatment time.

Accelerated Repopulation

Radiation or any other cytotoxic agent can trigger surviving clonogens in a tumor to divide faster than they did before treatment. This concept, accelerated repopulation, is illustrated for a rat rhabdomyosarcoma in Figure 1-23.[40] Figure 1-23, *A* (at left), shows the overall

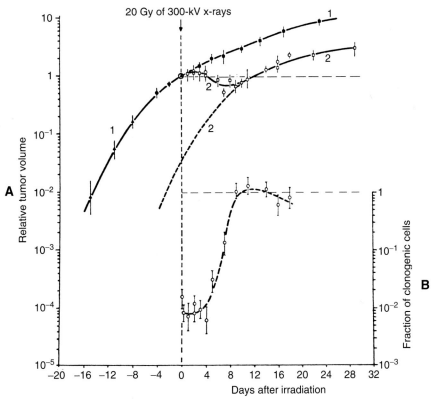

Fig. 1-23 Growth curves of a rat rhabdomyosarcoma showing shrinkage, growth delay, and subsequent recurrence after treatment with a single dose of 20 Gy of x-rays. **A,** *Curve 1* indicates growth curve of unirradiated control tumors; *curve 2*, growth curve of tumors irradiated at time t = 0, showing tumor shrinkage and recurrence. **B,** Variation in the fraction of clonogenic cells as a function of time after irradiation, obtained by removing cells from the tumor and assaying for colony formation in vitro. (From Hermens AF, Barendsen GW. *Eur J Cancer* 1969;5:173-189.)

growth curve for the tumor, as well as the shrinkage and regrowth that occurs after a single dose of 20 Gy. Figure 1-23, *B* (lower right), illustrates the repopulation of individual surviving cells, which, after treatment, are dividing with a cell cycle of only 12 hours—considerably faster than before irradiation. The rapid proliferation of surviving clonogens occurs while the tumor is overtly shrinking and regressing.

This same phenomenon also occurs in human tumors, although evidence to support this must be indirect. For example, from a survey of reports in the literature of radiation therapy of head and neck cancer, Withers and colleagues[41-43] concluded that the dose required to achieve local control in 50% of the cases (TCD$_{50}$) increased with overall treatment time beyond approximately 28 days. A dose increment of about 0.6 Gy/day is required to compensate for this accelerated repopulation of clonogens. Such a dose increment is consistent with a 4-day clonogen doubling time, compared with a median value of about 60 days for unperturbed growth.

The conclusion to be drawn from these findings is that radiation therapy, at least for head and neck cancer and probably in other instances, too, should be completed as soon as is practical after it has begun. It may be better to delay initiation of treatment than to introduce delays during treatment. If overall treatment time is too long, the effectiveness of later dose fractions will be prejudiced because the surviving clonogens in the tumor have been triggered into rapid repopulation.

The experimental data referred to above all relate to radiation therapy. However, similar considerations may well apply to chemotherapy or to a combination of radiation therapy and chemotherapy. As discussed in Chapter 4, some evidence exists to suggest that in some human malignancies, the results of radiation therapy are poorer if preceded by a course of chemotherapy. It may be that accelerated repopulation, triggered by the chemotherapy, is the explanation.

The Effect of Tumor Volume on Tumor Control by Irradiation

Presumably, larger tumors need larger irradiation doses to achieve tumor control. However, this topic cannot be dealt with rigorously by using radiobiological principles. Ultimately, the most pertinent information must be derived from clinical experience. Information from animal models cannot be extrapolated to the human situation because no information on scaling factors is available. Another problem is the absence of experimental data on volume-related variation in the tolerance of normal tissue to a given radiation dose because this tolerance ultimately limits the dose delivered and the strategy adopted.

The best that can be done to estimate the extra dose required to preserve a given level of tumor control as tumor volume increases is to perform a relatively naive calculation, results of which are shown in Figure 1-24. These calculations include several implicit assumptions, namely that (1) the number of clonogenic cells is proportional to volume; (2) the influence, if any, of hypoxic cells does not depend on tumor size; and (3) that the survival curve for multiple fractionated doses of 2 Gy can be represented by a simple exponential function of dose

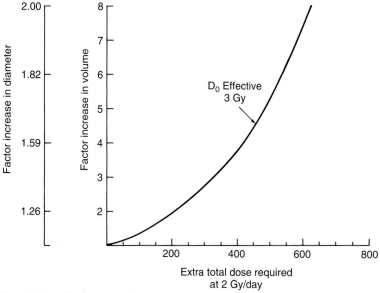

Fig. 1-24 Relationship between increased tumor size and the extra dose required in a fractionated regimen (2 Gy/day) to produce a given level of local tumor control. The final slope (*D$_0$*) of the effective dose-response curve for the fractionated regimen is assumed to be 3 Gy.

with a final slope (D_0) of about 3 Gy. This last assumption is itself based on the assumptions that each dose fraction kills the same proportion of cells and that 60 Gy, deiivered in 30 fractions, must result in a depopulation of about 10^{-9} because it controls some tumors.

Clinical experience with common epithelial tumors sheds some light on the issue of tumor control as a function of tumor volume. Because local control of very radiosensitive tumors (e.g., Hodgkin's disease, nodular lymphoma, seminoma) can be achieved readily regardless of tumor size, the most meaningful data come from irradiating less radiosensitive epithelial tumors such as squamous cell carcinomas and adenocarcinomas (Table 1-4). Although most larger tumors require higher doses for control, some exceptions exist such as squamous cell carcinoma of the glottis or the skin. In the glottis, the tumor volume is so small that sufficiently high doses have been used since the earliest years of radiation therapy. In the skin, the wide range of fractionation regimens used and the difficulty of comparing those regimens make these tumors poor models for other squamous cell carcinomas arising in the mucosal surfaces or viscera.

Assays for Predicting Tumor Sensitivity or Resistance to Radiation

Many laboratories around the world are actively seeking predictors of the success or failure of radiation therapy.[44] Investigators are attempting to determine which tumors have cells that are inherently less sensitive or are proliferating so rapidly as to overcome standard treatments. Predictive assays focus on one of three tumor characteristics—intrinsic radiosensitivity, oxygen status, and proliferative potential. Assays being studied include those at the subcellular level (DNA content,

percent of cells in S phase, nuclear antigens, micronuclei), the cellular level (T_{pot}, proliferation or clonogenicity after trial irradiation), and the tissue level (magnetic resonance spectroscopy, needle oximetry). Some of the techniques being evaluated for the ability to predict radiosensitivity are discussed briefly in the following paragraphs.

Intrinsic Radiosensitivity

Intrinsic cellular radiosensitivity can be assessed with clonogenic assays. In one pilot study, a correlation was found between the radiosensitivity of cultured normal tissue fibroblasts and the type of late reactions experienced after radiation therapy in the patients from whom the cells were taken; however, these results have yet to be duplicated. Cell lines from human tumors can be grown by conventional culture techniques; however, clonogenic assays take too long for them to realistically be used prospectively as a predictive assay. Nevertheless, two aspects of the initial region of cell-survival curves seem to correlate best with clinical radiosensitivity: SF_2, the fraction of cells surviving 2 Gy, and $\alpha:\beta$, the initial slope. West and colleagues[45-48] found that radiation therapy was associated with a lower probability of local tumor control in carcinoma of the cervix when the SF_2 (measured by the Courtenay assay) was greater than 0.55. To date, no other studies have shown such promising results.

Assays based on cell growth rather than clonogenicity also are being developed in which cells are cultured in microplates and exposed to radiation, after which their viability is assessed by staining for the ability to reduce compounds or by estimating total DNA or ribonucleic acid (RNA) content. These endpoints are surrogates for reproductive integrity. These assays are rapid, easy, and amenable to automation; they are suitable for screening drugs for their cytotoxic activity but are not suitable for predicting radiosensitivity. Another type of nonclonogenic assay assesses the ability of tumor cells to adhere and grow on a specially prepared matrix; the ability of this assay to predict tumor-cell radiosensitivity also has yet to be proven.

Oxygen Status

The oxygen status of a tumor can be assessed by the deposition of labeled nitroimidazoles in the tumor or with polarographic oxygen probes. Compounds labeled with the short-lived γ-emitting isotope ^{123}I also can be used in regions of low oxygen tension. The presence of hypoxia can be visualized by single photon emission computed tomography.[49] On the other hand, Eppendorf probes have a very fast response and can be moved quickly through a tumor under computer control to obtain an oxygen profile directly.

A clinical trial in Germany of patients with advanced carcinoma of the cervix treated with radiation therapy

TABLE 1-4

Interrelationship of Biological Dose, Tumor Size, and Control by Irradiation

Total Dose (Gy)*	Histology	Size	Control (%)
50	Squamous Adenocarcinoma	Subclinical (< 10^6 cells)	95+
60	Squamous	< 2 cm	85
		> 4 cm	50
65	Squamous	2-4 cm	70
70	Squamous	2-4 cm	90
	Adenocarcinoma	> 4 cm	60
75+	Squamous	> 4 cm	90

Data compiled from Fletcher and Shukovsky, Perez et al, Barker and Fletcher, Shukovsky and Fletcher.

*Approximation based on a minimum tumor dose of 2 Gy per fraction and five fractions per week.

has shown lower overall and recurrence-free survival in patients whose tumors exhibited median partial oxygen pressure (P_{O_2}) values less than or equal to 10 mm Hg as measured with the Eppendorf probe.[50] Although this evidence was initially interpreted to show that radioresistance caused by hypoxia was important, later studies indicated that hypoxia leads to more aggressive and malignant tumors.[51]

Proliferative Potential

The proliferative potential of a tumor can be expressed in terms of its T_{pot}, which, as noted earlier in this chapter, takes into account cell cycle time and growth fraction but not cell loss. As described in the section on tissue and tumor kinetics, T_{pot} can be measured by labeling tumor biopsy specimens with BrdU and then using flow cytometry to estimate doubling time. In a trial of head and neck cancer conducted by the EORTC, local control of fast-growing tumors (T_{pot} less than 4 days) was better after accelerated fractionation than after conventional therapy, but no difference was found in local control of slow-growing tumors from either type of therapy.[52] A later study found no correlation between T_{pot} and outcome after radiation therapy; although the LI and the length of the Ts phase correlated weakly with treatment outcome, that correlation was not strong enough for use as a predictor.[53]

In short, predictive assays are still in developmental stages. Although none of the markers explored thus far have been proven reliable for predicting the response of a tumor to radiation therapy, some may show promise for identifying groups of patients who may benefit from altered treatment protocols such as accelerated treatment, hyperfractionation, bioreductive drugs, or neutron therapy.

Modifiers of Radiation Effects
Oxygen

The sensitivity of biological material to sparsely ionizing radiation is critically dependent on the presence or absence of molecular oxygen. Survival curves for mammalian cells exposed to x-rays in the presence or absence of oxygen are shown in Figure 1-25. The ratio of doses needed under hypoxic and aerated conditions to achieve a given level of biological effect is said to be the *oxygen enhancement ratio* (OER). At high radiation doses, the OER has a value of between 2.5 and 3, and some evidence suggests that it may be reduced to about 2 for doses below 2 Gy. The magnitude of the oxygen effect seems to be the same for bacteria, plants, mammalian cells, and even some chemical systems, despite great differences in dose ranges.

For oxygen to act as a sensitizer, it must be present during the radiation exposure, or at least during the

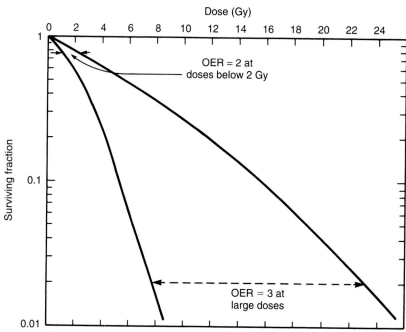

Fig. 1-25   Cells irradiated in the presence of molecular oxygen are more sensitive to killing by x-rays than cells that are hypoxic (deficient in oxygen). The ratio of doses that produce the same level of biological damage in the absence of oxygen and in the presence of oxygen is known as the *oxygen enhancement ratio (OER)*. At high doses, the OER has a value of about 3; its value seems to be smaller, close to 2, at doses below 2 Gy.

lifetime of the free radicals that are involved in the indirect action of radiation, which is about 10^{-5} seconds. According to the *oxygen fixation hypothesis*, in the absence of oxygen, the chemical changes produced in the target molecule may be repaired; if oxygen is present, the damage is "fixed" (i.e., made permanent and irreparable).

A question of obvious importance concerns the concentration of oxygen that is required to potentiate the effect of x-rays. The answer to this question is that only a very small amount of oxygen is necessary to produce a sensitizing effect. A P_{O_2} of about 3 mm Hg, corresponding to about 0.5%, is enough to take the radiation response halfway from fully hypoxic to fully oxygenated conditions. At concentrations characteristic of most normal tissues (i.e., about 30 mm Hg), the radiation response is essentially the same as that under fully aerated conditions, or, indeed, in the presence of 100% oxygen.

The importance of oxygen in tumor response. Oxygen was suspected of influencing the radiosensitivity of tumors in vivo as early as the mid 1930s. However, in 1955 a paper written by Thomlinson and Gray[54] led to overwhelming interest in the importance of oxygen in clinical radiation therapy. This paper, reporting results of a histologic study of bronchial carcinoma, concluded that tumor cords contained necrotic centers because of the limited distance that oxygen could diffuse in respiring tissue (100 to 180 μm). The authors proposed that, close to the end of the diffusion range of oxygen, there would be a region, possibly two cell layers thick, in which the oxygen tension would be low enough to be intransigent to killing by x-rays but high enough to be viable. (This concept would later be recognized as the mechanism underlying chronic hypoxia.) They went on to postulate that these cells might constitute a focus for tumor regrowth and so represent the limiting factor in the curability of some human tumors by x-rays. With the development of quantitative assay systems for transplanted tumors in experimental animals, by 1963 these tumors were shown to contain a proportion of viable hypoxic cells, and the resistance of these cells did indeed constitute a limit for the sterilization of these tumors by single large doses of x-rays.

Figure 1-26 shows a typical dose-response curve for the cells of an experimental animal tumor. Most of the cells have a dose response characteristic of fully aerated conditions, but some proportion of cells have a sensitivity characteristic of hypoxia. Many tumors of various histologic types have been evaluated in different animal species. The proportion of hypoxic cells in these tumors usually ranges from 10% to 15%. Although comparable data are not available for humans, experiments involving radiosensitizers indicate that the proportion of hypoxic cells in some skin nodules in humans may be similar.

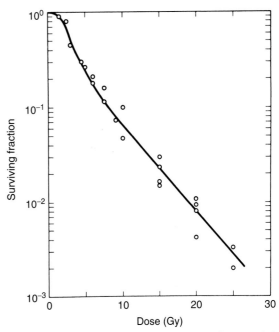

Fig. 1-26 A biphasic survival curve is characteristically obtained for tumors from air-breathing mice because aerated and hypoxic cells are both present in the tumors. (Courtesy Dr. Sarah Rockwell.)

Chronic and acute hypoxia. Hypoxia in tumors can result from two quite different mechanisms. As Thomlinson and Gray[54] surmised, *chronic hypoxia* results from the limited distance that oxygen can diffuse in respiring tissues. Regions of *acute hypoxia* within a tumor, by contrast, result from the temporary blockage of a blood vessel. If the blockage were permanent, the cells downstream would eventually die and be of no further consequence. However, good evidence exists to suggest that tumor blood vessels open and close randomly and thus that different regions of the tumor become hypoxic intermittently. Acute hypoxia is, in fact, the result of blood flow instability and is seldom a result of total stasis. Hence, at the moment when a radiation dose is delivered, some proportion of the tumor cells may be hypoxic; if the radiation were to be delayed, a different group of cells may be hypoxic. This concept of acute hypoxia was postulated in the late 1970s by Brown[55] and was later demonstrated unequivocally in rodent tumors.

Reoxygenation. When an animal tumor that consists of a mixture of aerated and hypoxic cells is irradiated, the aerated cells are killed preferentially because of their greater sensitivity, and the survivors will contain a preponderance of hypoxic cells. However, experimentation has shown that this situation is not static, but that over time after irradiation, the proportion of hypoxic cells tends to return to the preirradiation level. This shift of cells from the hypoxic to the aerated compartment is known as *reoxygenation*. Not surprisingly, the rapidity and extent of reoxygenation vary greatly among the different types of animal tumors that have been studied. In some tumors, such as mammary carcinomas, reoxygenation is rapid and complete. Predictably, such tumors can be readily eradicated, with acceptable normal tissue effects, by using a fractionated radiation schedule. Other animal tumors, such as the transplanted osteosarcoma, reoxygenate inefficiently and slowly; they cannot be eradicated with any fractionated schedule of x-rays without incurring substantial normal tissue damage. Reoxygenation simply cannot be studied in humans, and one is left to speculate on the patterns of reoxygenation in human tumors of different histologic types.

The effect of reoxygenation on a fractionated course of radiation is illustrated in Figure 1-27. Each dose of radiation reduces the aerated compartment but has comparatively little effect on hypoxic cells. If the interval between radiation doses is long enough to allow reoxygenation to take place, then hypoxic cells do not greatly affect the eventual outcome of the irradiation of the tumor. Few hypoxic cells are killed with each dose, but they are killed after they have become aerated as a result of the process of reoxygenation. To summarize, tumors that reoxygenate quickly and efficiently can be sterilized with a fractionated course of x-rays. They cannot be sterilized with a single dose, because the resistance of the hypoxic cells would dominate. However, if the radiation is split into fractions delivered over time, with the interval between the fractions being sufficient for reoxygenation to be complete, the presence of hypoxic cells has a minimal effect.

Hypoxia and tumor progression. Evidence that low-oxygen conditions play an important role in malignant progression comes from studies of the correlation between tumor oxygenation and treatment outcome in patients and in laboratory studies of cells and animals. Findings from these studies are summarized briefly here.

In a clinical study of radiation therapy for advanced cervical carcinoma performed in Germany, local control was found to be better for those tumors in which oxygen-probe measurements showed a Po_2 of 10 mm Hg than for tumors in which the Po_2 was less than 10 mm Hg. However, a similar improvement in outcome was also noted for better-oxygenated tumors that were treated *surgically* rather than radiologically.[51] This finding suggests that hypoxia may indicate tumor aggressiveness rather than conferring radioresistance to some cells.

In another clinical study, this one conducted in the United States, patients were given radiation therapy for soft tissue sarcoma; the extent of tumor oxygenation was found to be associated with the frequency of distant metastasis.[56] Among patients with tumors having a Po_2 of less than 10 mm Hg, 70% developed distant metastases as compared with 35% of those whose tumors had a Po_2 of more than 10 mm Hg. These findings were particularly compelling because the primary tumor was eradicated in all patients regardless of the level of oxygenation; only the incidence of metastasis varied between groups. The results from this study argue strongly that tumor oxygenation level influences tumor aggressiveness.

With regard to laboratory studies, at least three lines of evidence suggest a link between hypoxia and malignant progression.[57] First, hypoxia seems to destabilize the genome by inducing gene amplification and increasing gene mutation. Although the mechanisms by which this takes place are far from clear, genomic instability results in the production of transformed cells with

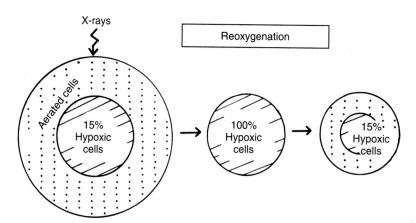

Fig. 1-27 Many animal tumors contain a mixture of aerated and hypoxic cells, with about 15% of the cells being deficient in oxygen. When a tumor is exposed to a dose of x-rays, a large proportion of the aerated cells is killed, and most of the surviving cells are hypoxic. If a time interval is allowed before a subsequent dose of radiation is administered, the initial pattern of aerated and hypoxic cells is restored. Consequently, if reoxygenation is rapid and complete between dose fractions, the presence of hypoxic cells does not affect the outcome of a multifraction regimen.

mutations that give them a survival advantage in adverse conditions. A second insight into how low-oxygen conditions may affect the aggressiveness of tumors is the observation that hypoxia initiates apoptosis in oncogenically transformed cells, thus functioning to enhance the selection of cells with reduced apoptotic sensitivity. Hence, cells with a defective apoptotic pathway, either from inactivation of the *p53* tumor suppressor gene or from overexpression of antiapoptotic genes such as *bcl-2*, have a survival advantage in a low-oxygen environment. The third consequence of hypoxia is the induction of proangiogenic stimulatory factors. Of the factors described to date, vascular endothelial growth factor is highly specific in stimulating endothelial cell proliferation and migration.

Radiosensitizers of Hypoxic Cells

Spurred largely by the efforts of radiation chemists (most notably Adams), a search was under way in the early 1960s for compounds that mimic oxygen in their ability to sensitize biological materials to the effects of x-rays.[58-60] Among the methods that have been proposed to eliminate foci of hypoxic cells within tumors, foci that are thought to lead to tumor regrowth after irradiation, are treatment in hyperbaric oxygen chambers; the use of chemical sensitizers; the use of hypoxic cytotoxins; and, conversely, the use of radioprotectant substances to protect normal tissue. These methods are reviewed briefly in the remainder of this section; another approach, the use of high-LET radiation such as neutrons or heavy ions, is discussed in further detail in the later section on "Radiation Quality."

Hyperbaric oxygen treatment. After hypoxia was identified as being a possible source of tumor resistance, the use of hyperbaric oxygen was explored for cancer treatment, first by Churchill Davidson at St. Thomas Hospital in London and later by others. Clinical trials were performed with patients sealed in a chamber filled with pure oxygen raised to a pressure of 3 atmospheres. Results from these trials were difficult to interpret given the small numbers of subjects and the use of unconventional fractionation schemes involving a few large fractions being given over short periods. The largest multicenter trials of hyperbaric oxygen, performed by the Medical Research Council in the United Kingdom, showed significant benefits in local control and survival for patients with carcinoma of the uterine cervix or advanced head and neck cancer but not for those with bladder cancer. Another overview of these trials revealed a 6.6% improvement in local control and perhaps an increase in late normal-tissue damage. Hyperbaric oxygen treatment fell into disuse, partly for its cumbersome nature and partly because drugs were thought to be able to achieve the same end by simpler means.

The notion of improving tumor oxygenation by breathing highly oxygenated air has been revived recently by experiments in which subjects breathe carbogen, a mixture of 95% O_2 and 5% CO_2 that does not produce the vasoconstriction associated with breathing 100% O_2. Breathing carbogen at atmospheric pressure is an attempt to overcome chronic (diffusion-limited) hypoxia through much simpler means than the use of hyperbaric chambers. Carbogen breathing also has been used in combination with nicotinamide, as described later in this section.

Chemical radiosensitizers. Instead of trying to "force" oxygen into tissues by the use of high-pressure chambers, the emphasis in the chemical-radiosensitizing approach focused on the use of oxygen substitutes that would diffuse into poorly vascularized areas of tumors and achieve the desired effect by chemical means. The vital difference between these drugs and oxygen, on which their success depends, is that the sensitizers are not rapidly metabolized by the cells in the tumor through which they diffuse. Thus they can penetrate further than oxygen and reach *all* of the hypoxic cells in the tumor, including those that are most remote from a blood supply.

The structures of three nitroimidazole-type radiosensitizers that have been tested in clinical trials are shown in Figure 1-28. The side chain determines position 1, and the position of the nitro group (NO_2) leads to the classification of the drug as a 2-nitroimidazole, 4-nitroimidazole, and so on. In general, 2-nitroimidazoles such as misonidazole and etanidazole have a higher electron affinity than 5-nitroimidazoles, the class that includes nimorazole.

Misonidazole produces appreciable sensitization of tumor cells, both in culture and in vivo. After encouraging results were found in laboratory studies, misonidazole was included in a large number of clinical trials involving many different types of human tumors in Europe and the United States. In general, the results have been disappointing. Of the 20 or so randomized prospective controlled clinical trials performed in the United States by the RTOG, none showed a statistically significant advantage for misonidazole, although several suggested a slight benefit. In a Danish DAHANCA study, the largest single trial of this sensitizer, the addition of

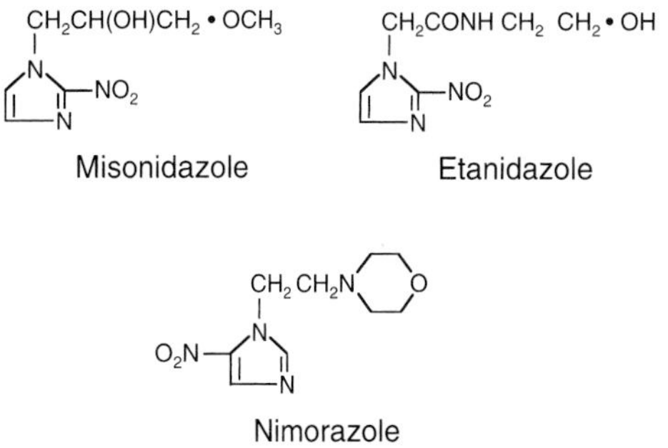

Fig. 1-28 The chemical structure of three compounds that have been tested as radiosensitizers in clinical trials.

misonidazole to radiation therapy conferred no significant advantage when all patients were analyzed as a group. Subgroup analysis, on the other hand, showed that male patients with high hemoglobin levels and cancer of the pharynx derived great benefit from the addition of misonidazole. The rate of tumor control at 3 years for this group was roughly twice that of patients given only radiation therapy.

In clinical use, the dose-limiting toxicity of misonidazole was found to be peripheral neuropathy, which progressed to central nervous system toxicity if use of the drug was continued. This effect precluded misonidazole being used at adequate levels throughout multifraction regimens.

Efforts to reproduce the laboratory success of misonidazole in the clinic led to the evaluation of etanidazole, another 2-nitroimidazole with equivalent sensitization but much less toxicity than misonidazole. The lower neurotoxicity of etanidazole is a function of its shorter half-life in vivo plus its lower partition coefficient, so it penetrates poorly into nerve tissue and does not cross the blood-brain barrier. Controlled clinical trials by the RTOG in the United States and by a multicenter consortium in Europe showed no benefit from adding etanidazole to conventional radiation therapy.

Nimorazole, a 5-nitroimidazole (see Fig. 1-28), is less effective as a radiosensitizer than either misonidazole or etanidazole, but it is much less toxic, allowing very large doses to be given. In a Danish DAHANCA trial, this compound produced significant improvement in both local-regional control rates and survival rates in patients with supraglottic or pharyngeal carcinoma relative to radiation therapy alone. Surprisingly, nimorazole has not been used elsewhere.

Nicotinamide and carbogen breathing. Hypoxic-cell radiosensitizers such as the nitroimidazoles were designed primarily to overcome *chronic* hypoxia, that is, diffusion-limited hypoxia resulting from the inability of oxygen to diffuse further than about 100 μm through respiring tissue. However, as noted earlier, hypoxia also arises through *acute* mechanisms (i.e., the intermittent blockage of blood vessels). Nicotinamide, a vitamin B_3 analogue, has been shown in mouse tumors to prevent the transient fluctuations in tumor blood flow that lead to the development of acute hypoxia.

The combination of nicotinamide to overcome acute hypoxia with carbogen breathing to overcome chronic hypoxia is the basis of the ARCON trials underway in several European centers. These trials also involve accelerated and hyperfractionated radiation therapy to avoid tumor proliferation and damage to late-responding normal tissues.

Compounds Cytotoxic to Hypoxic Cells

An alternative approach to designing drugs that preferentially radiosensitize hypoxic cells is to develop drugs that selectively kill hypoxic cells. It was pointed out at an early stage that the greater reductive environment of tumors might be exploited by developing drugs that are preferentially reduced to cytotoxic species in the hypoxic regions of tumors. Three classes of agents in this category are known: the quinone antibiotics, the nitroaromatic compounds, and the benzotriazine di-N-oxides. Mitomycin-C, a quinone antibiotic active against hypoxic cells, has been used as a chemotherapy agent for many years. However, the differential between aerated and hypoxic cells is relatively small for this and other quinone antibiotics. The nitroaromatics class has included dual-function agents developed by Adams and colleagues[60] at the British Medical Research Council. Thus far, toxicity to normal tissues has precluded clinical trials of these compounds. The lead compound of the third class, benzotriazine di-N-oxides, is tirapazamine (SR-4233), which shows highly selective toxicity towards hypoxic cells both in vitro and in vivo. Results from studies of this compound in laboratory and clinical trials are described in the following paragraphs.

Laboratory studies of tirapazamine. Survival curves for Chinese hamster cells treated with various doses of tirapazamine are illustrated in Figure 1-29. The ratio of cytotoxicity to hypoxic cells vs. aerated cells is about 100. In this system, tirapazamine is thought to be activated by the enzyme cytochrome P_{450}. The smaller cytotoxicity ratio for cell lines of human origin (about 20) presumably reflects a different spectrum, or different levels, of enzymes.[61]

Results of an experiment in which a transplanted mouse carcinoma was treated with x-rays, tirapazamine, or both are shown in Figure 1-30.[62] The drug was injected 30 minutes before each irradiation, which consisted of 2.5-Gy fractions given twice daily. The combination of tirapazamine and radiation was highly effective in reducing tumor volume; giving the drug before the radiation was slightly more effective than giving the treatments in the reverse order. The effect of the combination was greater than additive. In parallel experiments using the same x-ray and drug protocols, no evidence of radiosensitization or additive cytotoxicity (in terms of skin reactions) was produced by adding tirapazamine to the radiation treatments. This finding substantiates the tumor selectivity of the radiation enhancement.

Clinical trials of tirapazamine. Despite extensive laboratory findings in vitro and in vivo showing a greater-than-additive effect for the combination of x-rays and tirapazamine, only one phase II clinical trial has been conducted to test tirapazamine with radiation therapy in humans, perhaps because of nausea and severe muscle cramping associated with the tirapazamine. However, tirapazamine has shown some success in combination with chemotherapy. In a phase III trial comparing cisplatin or cisplatin combined with tirapazamine for advanced (stages IIIB and IV) non–small

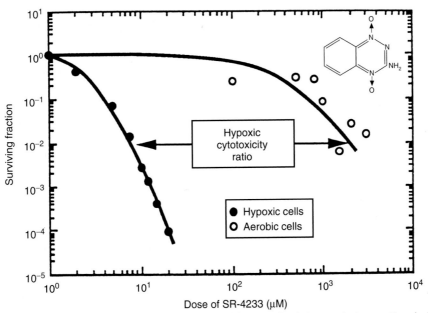

Fig. 1-29 Tirapazamine (SR-4233), synthesized by Stanford Research International, is a hypoxic cell cytotoxin. Its structure is shown in the *inset*. Dose-response curves in Chinese hamster cells are shown for cells exposed for 4 hours to graded concentrations of the drug under aerated and hypoxic conditions. Cells deficient in oxygen are preferentially killed. (Courtesy Dr. Martin Brown.)

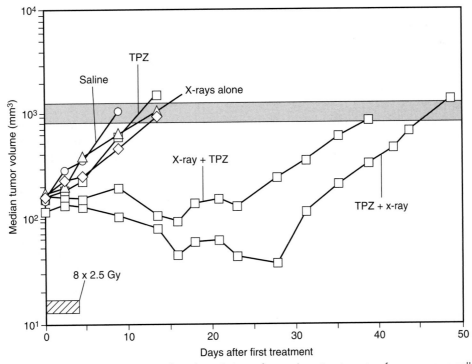

Fig. 1-30 Tumor volume as a function of time after various treatments of a squamous cell carcinoma (SCCVII) transplantable mouse carcinoma. Tirapazamine *(TPZ)* or radiation alone had little effect. The combination of TPZ and x-rays caused significant growth delay; giving radiation after the drug caused a slightly greater effect. (Redrawn from Brown JM, Lemmon MJ. *Int J Radiat Oncol Biol Phys* 1991;20:457-461.)

cell lung cancer,[63] patients given the combination had twice the response rate and significantly longer survival than patients given cisplatin alone. Although tirapazamine did not increase systemic cisplatin toxicity, some nausea and muscle cramping were reported.

Markers of Hypoxic Cells

A major development during the past two decades has been the synthesis of radiolabeled nitroimidazoles for use as markers of hypoxic cells. The technique is as follows. A dose of radiolabeled misonidazole or one of its analogues is administered. In tissues that are well aerated, the drug is quickly excreted without being metabolized, but under conditions of reduced oxygen tension, the drug *is* metabolized. In Edmonton, Chapman and colleagues[44] performed a study in which patients were given a nitroimidazole labeled with tritiated thymidine 22 hours before their tumors were surgically removed. In Figure 1-31, *A*, a section of a melanoma illustrates the density of grains, indicating the presence of hypoxic cells, over a region of the tumor. The interesting result of the study is that only four of nine patients had tumors with a significant proportion of hypoxic cells (see Fig. 1-31, *B*). In this small group of patients, biased by the fact that only accessible tumors could be studied, only melanoma and small cell lung cancer seemed to contain a proportion of hypoxic cells that would affect the outcome of radiation therapy.

Previously, only β-emitting isotopes could be used as labels, and those labels could be detected only by autoradiography after the tumor was removed and sectioned. More recently, Parliament and colleagues[49] successfully labeled a nitroimidazole by attaching a positron-emitting radionuclide (^{123}I) by means of a sugar molecule. The presence of hypoxia could then be detected noninvasively by single photon emission computed tomography. This exciting development opens the possibility of screening patients prospectively to select those in whom hypoxia is a problem for inclusion in protocols involving hypoxic cell sensitizers or bioreductive drugs.

Summary: meta-analysis of clinical trials. Of the dozens of clinical trials performed in attempts to overcome the perceived problem of hypoxic cells in tumors, most have shown inconclusive or borderline results. In 1996, Overgaard and Horsman[64] published the results of a meta-analysis of 10,602 patients treated in 82 randomized clinical trials involving hyperbaric oxygen, chemical sensitizers, carbogen breathing, or blood transfusions; the tumor sites studied included bladder, uterine cervix, central nervous system, head and neck, and lung. Overall, antihypoxic-cell treatments were found to improve local tumor control by 4.6% and survival rate by 2.8%. The complication rate increased by only 0.6%, which was not statistically significant. The largest number of trials involved head and neck tumors, which also showed the greatest benefit. Overgaard and Horsman also concluded

from the meta-analysis that the problem of hypoxia may be marginal in most adenocarcinomas and most important in squamous cell carcinomas.

Radiosensitization of Aerobic Cells

Much interest has been expressed over the years in the development of nonhypoxic-cell radiosensitizers. Indeed, a substantial list of chemical agents identified as sensitizers of aerobic cells has accumulated. Radiosensitization by these agents is mediated through a variety of mechanisms, including the inhibition of repair, modification of the DNA molecule, and perturbation of or redistribution in the cell cycle. Very few of these agents exhibit any tumor selectivity in vivo; perhaps the most successful example is the halogenated pyrimidines.

The halogenated pyrimidines. The van der Waals radius for the halogens is very similar to that of the methyl group, and consequently, the halogenated pyrimidines IdU and BrdU can replace thymidine in the DNA molecule. When this occurs, cells become more sensitive to both ultraviolet light and to x-rays, although the exact mechanism for this is not entirely clear. Because these agents require incorporation into cellular DNA before sensitization occurs, they also must be present for extended periods (comparable to several cycles) as the cells undergo DNA synthesis. As the percent replacement of thymidine bases with these halogenated bases increases, so does the extent of radiosensitization. Earlier studies were performed with BrdU, but more recently IdU has been used instead. The use of IdU produces approximately equal radiosensitization but significantly less photosensitization of the skin than does BrdU. The degree of sensitization produced in cultured mammalian cells by the incorporation of halogenated pyrimidines is shown in Figure 1-32.[65] The enhancement factor is approximately 2.

The potential usefulness of halogenated pyrimidines in clinical radiation therapy was realized in the early 1970s. Theoretically, because tumor cells may be cycling more rapidly than normal cells, more halogenated pyrimidines could be replaced in the tumor cell DNA, resulting in "selective" x-ray sensitization. It was perhaps unfortunate that head and neck tumors were selected for these early clinical trials, because these tumors tend to be surrounded by actively proliferating normal tissues. In these early clinical studies, good tumor responses were observed, but the damage to normal tissues was unacceptable. Tumors that might be more suitable for such studies would include those with a high growth fraction and rapid cell-cycling times. This idea was raised again in the early 1990s at the U.S. National Cancer Institute and elsewhere, and patients with high-grade gliomas and large, unresectable sarcomas were chosen for studies incorporating halogenated pyrimidines.[66,67] The results from these studies indicate that better information on LI and cell-cycling times in human tumors, compared with surrounding normal

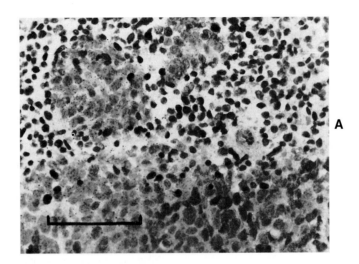

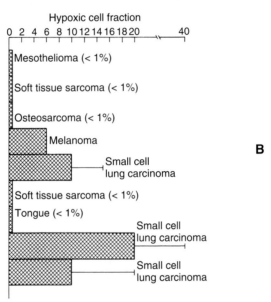

Fig. 1-31 **A,** Autoradiograph of a representative area from a histologic section of human small cell lung carcinoma. The patient was given misonidazole labeled with tritiated thymidine 22 hours before surgical resection. The intense labeling in some areas is consistent with a hypoxic cell fraction of 10% to 20%. **B,** Estimate of hypoxic cells in the first group of human tumors that were studied with radioactive-labeled misonidazole. Four of the first nine tumors show the presence of a significant proportion of hypoxic cells. (**A,** Courtesy Drs. J Donald Chapman, Raul Urtusan, Cameron Koch, Allan Franko, and James Raleigh, Cross Cancer Institute, Alberta, Canada. **B,** Drawn from data by Drs. J Donald Chapman and Raul Urtusan.)

tissues, is needed for such a choice to be made on a rational basis. A particularly promising idea is to incorporate halogenated pyrimidines with low-dose-rate interstitial implant therapy. The rationale for this is that the maintenance of a high level of halogenated pyrimidines throughout a 6-week course of beam therapy would be difficult, but high levels of the drug could be maintained readily for a few days during an implant.

Radioprotective Compounds

In 1948, Harvey Patt[68] and colleagues discovered that cysteine afforded mice considerable protection from death by whole-body irradiation. The dose required to produce lethality was almost doubled in animals that had been given the drug compared with those that had not. The structure of cysteine is illustrated as follows:

$$SH-CH_2-CH\diagup^{NH_2}_{\diagdown COOH}$$

Almost simultaneously in Europe, Bacq and colleagues[69] found that cysteamine was also a protector.

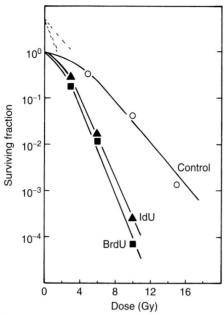

Fig. 1-32 Dose-response curves for Chinese hamster cells exposed to x-rays after incorporation of bromodeoxyuridine *(BrdU)* or iododeoxyuridine *(IdU)* compared with unlabeled control cells. (From Mitchell JB, Morstyn G, Russo A, et al. *Int J Radiat Oncol Biol Phys* 1984;10:1447-1451.)

The structure of this compound is illustrated as follows:

$$SH - CH_2 - CH_2 - NH_2$$

In the years that followed, many similar compounds were found to be effective protectors, and they all tended to have the same general structure: a free SH group (or potential SH group) at one end of the molecule and a strong basic function such as an amine or guanidine at the other end, separated by a straight chain of two or three carbon atoms. The problem with these simple compounds was their toxicity. In the years immediately after World War II, in the wake of the first use of atomic weapons, the possibility of a compound that would protect against whole-body irradiation was of great interest to the military. Over the years, the Walter Reed Army Hospital in Washington, DC, synthesized several thousand compounds that were similar in structure to cysteine and cysteamine, with the aim of finding something less toxic. The first breakthrough in this research was the discovery that covering the sulfhydryl group with a phosphate allowed the dose resulting in a given level of toxic effect to be doubled.

Amifostine and radiation therapy. Of the many compounds produced in the Walter Reed program, the one used most often in radiation therapy is WR-2721, recently dubbed *amifostine*. Amifostine is actually a prodrug; the presence of a terminal phosphorothioic acid group makes it relatively nonreactive, and it does not readily permeate cell membranes. Dephosphorylation by alkaline phosphatase, which is present in high concentrations in normal tissues and capillaries, converts amifostine to its active form, WR-1065. This metabolite readily enters normal cells by facilitated diffusion, where it scavenges free radicals generated by ionizing radiation or by some alkylating chemotherapeutic agents. It is taken up much more slowly by tumor tissues, perhaps because of the superior vascularization of normal tissues or by differences in the membrane structure of the tumor cells that impedes entry of this relatively hydrophilic compound. Whatever the underlying mechanism, the compound quickly floods normal tissues but penetrates tumors more slowly. Experiments with animal tumors have confirmed that concentrations of amifostine are high in several normal tissues shortly after drug administration but rise much more slowly in tumors.

The extent to which amifostine protects normal tissues from radiation effects varies considerably among tissue types (Table 1-5).[70] The hematopoietic system, the gut lining, and the salivary glands are generally well protected. However, because the drug does not cross the blood-brain barrier, it provides no protection to the brain and a disappointingly low level of protection to the lung.

Ideally, for the maximum radioprotective effect, radioprotectants such as amifostine should be administered at the maximum tolerable concentration immediately before the radiation dose is delivered, so that the drug can be present in and protect normal tissues—but not tumor cells—when the radiation is delivered.

TABLE 1-5

Summary of Normal Tissue Responsiveness to Protection by Amifostine (WR-2721)

Protected Tissues	Unprotected Tissues
Bone marrow (2.4-3.0)*	Brain
Immune system (1.8-3.4)	Spinal cord
Skin (2.0-2.4)	
Small intestine (1.8-2.0)	
Colon (1.8)	
Lung (1.2-1.8)	
Esophagus (1.4)	
Kidney (1.5)	
Liver (2.7)	
Salivary gland (2.0)	
Oral mucosa (>1)	
Testis (2.1)	

From Yuhas JM, Spellman JM, Culo F. The role of WR-2721 in radiotherapy and/or chemotherapy. In: Brady L, ed. *Radiation Sensitizers.* New York, NY: Masson; 1980.
*Numbers in parentheses are the dose-reduction factors or factor in resistance associated with amifostine injection.

Although radioprotectants such as amifostine have several potential applications in combination with radiation therapy, their clinical use has been slow in coming. Phase I toxicity trials of amifostine conducted in humans in the United States have shown that the dose-limiting toxicity is hypotension; this and other adverse effects such as sneezing and somnolence have tended to limit the amount of drug given to less than the dose needed to achieve maximum protection according to animal experiments. In a randomized clinical trial conducted in mainland China,[71] 100 patients with inoperable, unresectable, or recurrent adenocarcinoma of the rectum were stratified and randomly assigned to receive amifostine plus radiation therapy or radiation therapy only. The amifostine was administered 15 minutes before radiotherapy, 4 days a week, for 5 weeks. The amifostine group showed protection of the skin, mucous membranes, bladder, and pelvic structures against late, moderate, and severe reactions; none of the 34 evaluable patients in this group had such reactions, compared with 5 of 37 evaluable patients in the radiation-only group, a statistically significant difference. Moreover, amifostine afforded no apparent protection to the tumors.

One of the worrisome factors in the experimental use of radioprotectors in the clinic is that their use is not fail-safe. To exploit a benefit, radiation doses must be *increased*, with the confidence that the normal tissues are protected and that the extra dose will improve tumor response. If radioprotection does not occur, unacceptable normal tissue morbidity results.

A more modest but achievable goal is to use a radioprotectant to reduce the troublesome side effects of radiation therapy. The RTOG conducted a phase III randomized clinical trial in which amifostine was found to reduce xerostomia (dry mouth) without affecting early tumor control in patients with head and neck cancer given radiation therapy.[72] The drug was administered daily, 30 minutes before each dose fraction in a multifraction regimen. Three months after treatment, the incidence of xerostomia was significantly reduced in patients treated with amifostine; these patients also reported having less difficulty in eating or speaking and in the need for fluids and oral comfort aids. No difference was found in local-regional tumor control rates between patients given amifostine and those who were not.

Radioprotectors and chemotherapy. Although sulfhydryl compounds were initially developed as protectors against ionizing radiation, they also protect against the cytotoxic effects of several chemotherapeutic agents. Amifostine, for example, offers significant protection against the nephrotoxicity, ototoxicity, and neuropathy associated with cisplatin and against the hematologic toxicity associated with cyclophosphamide. The same studies indicated that amifostine had no obvious antitumor activity, again suggesting that its uptake by normal tissues may be different from that by malignant tissues.

Mechanism of action. The mechanisms most often implicated in sulfhydryl-mediated cytoprotection include free-radical scavenging, which would protect against oxygen-based free radicals generated by ionizing radiation or alkylating agents, and hydrogen-atom donation, which would facilitate direct chemical repair at sites of DNA damage. The protective effect of sulfhydryl compounds tends to parallel the oxygen effect, being maximal for sparsely ionizing, low-LET radiation such as x-rays or gamma rays and minimal for densely ionizing radiation such as low-energy alpha particles, which tend to damage DNA directly rather than generating free radicals. Presumably, if all free radicals are effectively scavenged, the highest possible dose-reduction factor would equal the OER, with a value of 2.5 to 3.0.

Radiation Quality

The energy deposited in biological materials by radiation is in the form of ionizations and excitations that are not distributed at random, but tend to be localized along the tracks of individually charged particles. The pattern of this energy deposition varies substantially with the type of ionizing radiation involved (Fig. 1-33). For example, photons give rise to fast electrons, particles carrying unit-negative electric charge and having a very small mass. Neutrons, on the other hand, give rise to recoil protons or alpha particles, that is, particles carrying 1 or 2 units of positive electric charge and having a mass approximately 2000 and 8000 times, respectively, that of the electron. The spatial distribution of the ionizing events they produce differ markedly. The tracks of energetic electrons, produced as a result of the absorption of x-ray photons, result in primary events that are well separated in space, and for this reason x-rays are described as sparsely ionizing. Alpha particles, on the other hand, give rise to individual ionizing events that occur close together, giving rise to tracks that consist of a column of ionizations; they are therefore said to be *densely ionizing*. Figure 1-33 is an attempt to illustrate the wide differences in ionization density associated with different types of radiation in common use. What is illustrated are computer simulations of ionizing events from several different types of radiation against the background of a strand of chromatin in a mammalian cell.

The Concept of Linear Energy Transfer

The quality of the radiation is described quantitatively in terms of LET, which is defined as the average energy imparted locally to the absorbing medium per unit length of track. The unit in which LET is commonly expressed is keV/μm (the kiloelectron volt being a unit

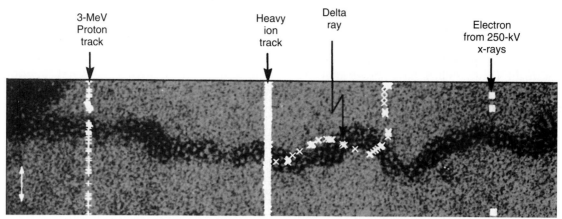

Fig. 1-33   Computer simulations of sections of charged-particle tracks produced by different types of radiation passing through a strand of chromatin. Each cross represents a single ionization of either the chromatin or the surrounding medium. *Right track,* Low-linear energy transfer (LET) 100-keV electron, typical of those produced by 250-kVp x-rays. *Center track,* High-LET, high-energy iron ion that produces a dense column of ionization; note the high-energy secondary delta ray coming out of the track. *Left track,* Medium-LET 3-MeV proton. The scale bar represents 50 nm. (Electron micrograph of the 30-nm chromatin fiber, courtesy Barbara Hamkalo, University of California; particle tracks were calculated and the diagram prepared by Dr. David Brenner, New York, NY.)

of energy and the micron a unit of length). It is evident from Figure 1-33 that LET is very much an average quantity. In some regions along the track, for a considerable distance on the microscopic scale, no energy at all is deposited. In other regions, a cluster of ionizations occurs, and thus a large amount of energy is deposited in a small distance. The LET of ^{60}Co gamma rays is about 0.2 keV/μm; that of 250-keV x-rays is about 2 keV/μm; that of 14-MeV neutrons is about 75 keV/μm; and that of heavy charged particles is anywhere from 100 to 2000 keV/μm. In general, for a given type of radiation, the LET goes down as the energy goes up. For example, 250-keV x-rays have a higher LET (and are more effective biologically) than are cobalt gamma rays. Likewise, for a given type of charged particle (e.g., an alpha particle), a high-energy particle has a lower LET and less biological effect per unit dose than a low-energy particle.

Linear Energy Transfer and Shape of Dose-Response Curve

Dose-response curves from mammalian cells exposed to low-energy (high-LET) neutrons and low-LET x-rays are shown in Figure 1-34. As the LET of the radiation increases, the slope of the survival curve gets progressively steeper, while the shoulder gets smaller. The relative biological effectiveness (RBE) of a given type of radiation is expressed in terms of a "standard radiation," usually taken to be low-LET photons having a LET value between 0.2 and 3 keV/μm. The RBE of neutrons is defined to be the ratio of doses of x-rays to neutrons required to produce a given biological effect. What biological effect? No particular biological effect is specified.

At a surviving fraction of 10^{-2}, the ratio of doses to produce the same effects is 2.7, whereas at a surviving fraction of 0.5, the RBE can be calculated to be 4.0. The important point to make, therefore, is that the value of the RBE for a given type of radiation (in this case, neutrons) varies with the level of biological damage involved or, what amounts to the same thing, the size of dose involved.

The effect of fractionation on RBE also is illustrated in Figure 1-34. When a dose of x-rays or of neutrons is split up into multiple fractions, separated by sufficient time to allow sublethal damage repair to be completed, the shoulder of the dose-response curve must be reexpressed with each fraction. For a given level of biological damage, it is at once obvious that the RBE is greater for a schedule that involves multiple fractions than for a single exposure. The reason for this is that the large shoulder of the dose-response curves for x-rays must be repeated with each exposure, whereas for neutrons only a small shoulder is repeated each time. It is not difficult to see that, for the fractionated regimen, the value of the RBE involved is that characteristic of the individual-dose fraction.

Relative Biological Effectiveness for Different Cells and Tissues

Even for a given dose per fraction, RBE values vary substantially according to the cell type or tissue. Dose-response curves for five different types of mammalian cells irradiated with x-rays or with neutrons are shown in Figure 1-35.[73] Two important points emerge. First, the overall variation of radiosensitivity is less for neutrons

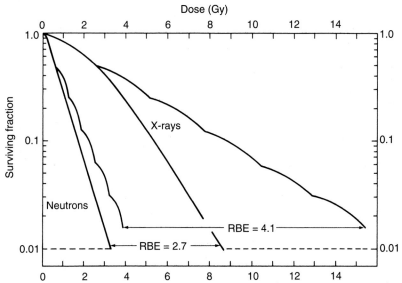

Fig. 1-34 The survival curve for x-rays is characterized by a broad initial shoulder, whereas for neutrons the survival curve has little or no shoulder. Consequently, the relative biological effectiveness *(RBE)* gets larger as the dose gets smaller. When a dose is fractionated, the RBE is larger for a given level of cell killing than if the dose is given in a single exposure because the large shoulder of the x-ray dose-response curve is repeated each time.

than for x-rays. The reason for this is not hard to see; variations of radiosensitivity for x-rays are a function more of the size of the shoulder than of the slope of the dose-response curve, and, because for neutrons the shoulder is less to start with, the overall variation is less. Second, the order of sensitivities is not the same for neutrons as it is for x-rays. Therefore, if the RBE is calculated using the data for the five different cell lines, the value of RBE would be different for each cell line. When an entire organism is irradiated with neutrons, each tissue will be characterized by a different RBE.

Relative Biological Effectiveness and Linear Energy Transfer

The variation of RBE as a function of LET has a characteristic shape (Fig. 1-36).[74] As LET increases from 1 to 10 keV/μm, RBE increases slowly but steadily, then increases more rapidly beyond 10 keV/μm to reach a peak at about 100 keV/μm, after which RBE tends to fall again for higher values of LET. The decrease of RBE at very high values of LET is generally attributed to the phenomenon of "overkill." At these very high LETs, the density of ionization is such that if a charged particle track passes through a cell, it deposits far more energy than is required to kill the cell. Consequently, much of this energy is "wasted" because the cell cannot be killed more than once. Because so much energy is deposited in each cell, the radiation is relatively inefficient and the killing effect per unit dose (which is what RBE amounts to) decreases.

Linear Energy Transfer and the Oxygen Enhancement Ratio

As LET increases, a corresponding decrease occurs in the dependence of cell killing on the presence of molecular oxygen, which is expressed in terms of the OER. This variation with LET also is illustrated in Figure 1-36.[74] As noted earlier in the section "Modifiers of Radiation Effects," low-LET forms of radiation, such as x-rays or gamma rays, are characterized by a large OER of between 2.5 and 3. Heavy charged particles with a LET of several hundred keV/μm have an OER of 1 (i.e., cell killing is independent of the presence or absence of oxygen). Between these two extremes, neutrons with an LET of about 70 keV/μm show an intermediate OER of about 1.6. As explained earlier in this chapter, the value of the OER reflects the relative importance of the direct-killing effect of the radiation vs. the indirect-killing effect, which is mediated by free radicals; this latter component of radiation damage depends on the presence or absence of oxygen.

Radiation Quality and Biological Effectiveness

In summary, RBE varies with radiation quality. In general, the more densely ionizing the radiation, the more biologically effective it is, at least up to a certain point. The biological effectiveness of a certain type of radiation depends on several factors, including radiation quality, dose per fraction, dose rate, the presence or absence of oxygen, and the biological system or cell type involved.

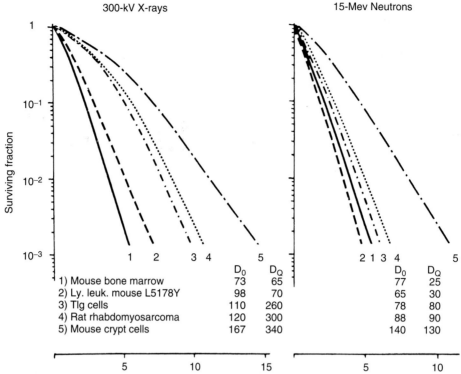

Fig. 1-35 Survival curves for various types of clonogenic mammalian cells irradiated with 300-kV x-rays or 15-MeV d⁺ → T neutrons. *Curve 1,* Mouse hematopoietic stem cells. *Curve 2,* Mouse lymphocytic leukemia *(Ly. leuk.)* L5178Y cells. *Curve 3,* Tlg cultured cells of human kidney origin. *Curve 4,* Rat rhabdomyosarcoma cells. *Curve 5,* Mouse intestinal crypt stem cells. The variation in radiosensitivity between different cell lines is markedly less for neutrons than for x-rays. (From Broerse JJ, Barendsen GW. *Curr Top Radiat Res Q* 1973;8:305-350.)

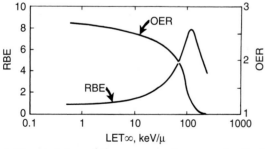

Fig. 1-36 Variation of the oxygen enhancement ratio *(OER)* and the relative biological effectiveness *(RBE)* as a function of the linear energy transfer *(LET)* of the radiation involved. The data were obtained by using T_1 kidney cells of human origin, irradiated with various naturally occurring alpha particles or with deuterons accelerated in the Hammersmith cyclotron. RBE increases rapidly and OER falls rapidly at about the same LET, namely, about 100 keV/μ. (Redrawn from Barendsen GW. In: *Proceedings of the Conference of Particle Accelerators in Radiation Therapy.* U.S. Atomic Energy Commission, Technical Information Center; 1972. LA-5180-C.)

In this context, radiation quality is measured in terms of the LET. The RBE depends on the dose level and the number of dose fractions—or, alternatively, the dose per fraction—because in general the shapes of the dose-response relationship are different for types of radiation that differ substantially in LET. The RBE can vary with dose rate, too, because the slope of the dose-response curve for sparsely ionizing radiations varies with changing dose rate. By contrast, the biological response to densely ionizing radiation depends little on the rate at which the radiation is delivered. The biological system, endpoint, or cell type chosen to determine RBE has a marked influence on the values obtained. In general, RBE values are high for tissues that accumulate and repair a great deal of sublethal damage and, consequently, have large shoulders to their x-ray dose-response relationships, and RBE values are low for those that do not.

Use of Neutrons in Radiation Therapy

Neutrons were first used in radiation therapy in the 1930s at the University of California at Berkeley. Their introduction was not based on any physical or radiobiological rationale, and they were abandoned because of severe late effects produced in many patients. After World War II, the use of neutrons was reintroduced at the Hammersmith Hospital in England because neutrons have a lower OER than x-rays and because of the premise that hypoxic cells limit the curability of tumors by x-rays.[75-77] After apparent early success, neutron machines also were used for therapy in the United States, continental Europe, and Japan. Controlled clinical trials for a wide range of tumors indicated little or no advantage for the new modality except perhaps in a few disease sites, specifically prostate cancer, salivary gland tumors, and possibly soft tissue sarcomas.[78,79]

The biological properties of neutrons differ from x-rays in several respects, apart from their lesser dependence on molecular oxygen for cell killing. Neutrons tend to be associated with less repair of both sublethal and potentially lethal damage, and they are associated with smaller variations in radiosensitivity according to the phase of the cell cycle. Perhaps because of these differences, neutron RBE values tend to be higher for slowly growing tumors. The rationale for the use of neutrons has evolved considerably over the years, but neutrons have not been widely adopted for radiation therapy.

Use of Protons in Radiation Therapy

The biological properties of high-energy protons do not differ significantly from x-rays. Protons produce ionizations and excitations in atoms along a track in much the same way as electrons are set in motion when x-rays are absorbed. The clinical use of protons is based on the superior dose distributions that can be obtained. Protons have an important place in the treatment of tumors for which dose localization is important, for example, tumors that are close to sensitive normal structures. In particular, protons have been widely used to treat choroidal melanoma of the eye, sarcoma of the base of the skull, and chordomas.

The increasingly impressive results of conformal radiation therapy, including intensity-modulated radiation therapy, both in decreasing effects on normal tissues and allowing much higher total doses than have been previously used, suggest wider applicability of proton therapy. This issue is discussed further in Chapter 2 of this book.

Adjuncts to Radiation
Hyperthermia

The use of hyperthermia to treat cancer has a history much longer than that of radiation. The first references are in an Egyptian papyrus roll dating from 5000 years ago. Just before the discovery of x-rays, it was noted that tumors regressed in patients with high fevers resulting from various bacterial infections.[80]

The interest in hyperthermia in modern times, however, results from experiments with cells in vitro and with animal tumors and normal tissues. The biological effects of heat that seem favorable for cancer therapy include the following:

- Heat kills; survival curves for heat are similar in shape to those for radiation, except that time at the elevated temperature replaces absorbed dose.
- The age-response function for heat complements that for x-rays. S-phase cells that are resistant to x-rays are sensitive to heat.
- Cells that are at low pH and nutritionally deprived (more likely to be in tumors) are more sensitive to heat, although cells can adapt to pH changes in 80 to 100 hours and can lose their sensitivity to heat.
- Hypoxia does not protect cells from heat as it does from x-rays.
- Heat preferentially damages tumor vasculature. After heating, blood flow goes down in tumors but increases in normal tissues. This may result in an enhanced temperature differential between tumors and normal tissues. Good evidence exists to support this contention in transplantable animal tumors, but it is less clear in spontaneous human tumors.
- Mild hyperthermia can promote tumor reoxygenation; this has been shown in animal experiments and in clinical studies.

Although the biological properties of heat seem favorable for its use in cancer therapy, physical devices to produce uniform heating at a particular depth are not well developed, and adequate thermometry is also difficult. The basic laws of physics make the desired end difficult or impossible to achieve. Microwaves provide good localization at shallow depths, but localization is poor at greater depths, where low frequencies are needed. With ultrasound, deep heating can be achieved with focused arrays, but bones or air cavities cause distortions. Because of these considerations, in practice, breast tumors, including recurrences and melanomas, can be heated adequately with microwaves, and deep-seated tumors below the diaphragm can be heated adequately with ultrasound. In any other site, however, the present methods of heating pose a major problem.

By contrast, the combination of interstitial implants of radioactive sources with hyperthermia generated by radiofrequency power applied to the implanted sources seems to be particularly promising because a good radiation dose distribution is combined with a good heat distribution.

Many thousands of patients have been treated with hyperthermia. The general consensus is that hyperthermia alone has no role in the curative treatment of cancer; its usefulness is limited to palliation or retreatment of recurrent tumors. On the other hand, several clinical studies have shown that the combination of hyperthermia plus radiation produces more complete and partial tumor responses than does radiation alone. Several phase III randomized trials have shown a clear and significant benefit for the addition of hyperthermia to standard radiation therapy.[81,82] The sites evaluated include superficial localized breast cancer, recurrent or metastatic melanoma, and nodal metastases from head and neck cancer. By contrast, trials involving advanced breast cancer and neck nodes with full-dose radiation therapy did not show any benefit from the addition of hyperthermia.

In summary, the clinical value of hyperthermia in the routine treatment of cancer is still not clear, despite its proven efficacy in a few specific instances. Notably, the situations in which hyperthermia seemed to be effective involved either its combination with external beam radiation therapy for the treatment of superficial tumors, where adequate heating is not so difficult, or its combination with brachytherapy, where heating is induced by implanted electrodes, inevitably involving all the complications and limitations of accessibility.

Cytotoxic Drugs

Drugs that are anticancer agents interact in complex and only partially understood ways with ionizing radiation. Although the combination is often used in clinical settings, such use is based on an empiric rationale with little regard for cellular interactions. Possible interactions of drugs with radiation are illustrated graphically in Figure 1-37.[83] The drugs under consideration in this section are those with known dose-response curves; thus, the interactions are considered at least potentially subadditive. However, they may be additive with regard to their effects on both tumors and normal tissues.

The object in combining anticancer drugs with ionizing radiation is to improve the therapeutic ratio relative to the use of either agent alone. It is beyond the scope of this chapter to consider cooperative interactions in which the effect of one agent is local, the other is systemic, and no interaction either on tumors or normal tissues is assumed. In general, little is known about the interactions of cytotoxic drugs and radiation at the subcellular or molecular levels. Although much is known about the mechanisms of action of the various classes of drugs, such as alkylating agents, antimetabolites, plant alkaloids, and antibiotics, little is known about specific drug-radiation interactions.

Several mechanisms by which cell death can be increased in vitro by the combined use of drugs and radiation can be identified: S-phase cytotoxicity, cell-cycle redistributions that increase either drug or radiation effects, and prevention of repair of potentially lethal damage. Cellular studies have suggested preferred sequencing and timing of drugs and radiation types, as well as interactions with other treatment modalities such as hyperthermia. However, no consistent correlation exists between interactions that are apparent at the cellular level and in-vivo effects. For example, hydroxyurea, a cell-cycle S-phase–specific agent, enhances radiation effects on cells in tissue culture. However, with few exceptions, the effects of this combination in vivo and in clinical settings have been disappointing.

Clinical data suggest that normal tissues are at least as likely as tumors, if not more so, to be affected by drug-radiation interactions. Notable examples of enhanced acute and late effects with radiation therapy include those seen with simultaneous administration of doxorubicin, dactinomycin, fluorouracil, methotrexate, bleomycin, nitrosoureas, and possibly etoposide.

In 1980, Tubiana[84] stated that 'the use of drugs during radiation therapy has never improved control of local lesions or reduced frequency of metastases from

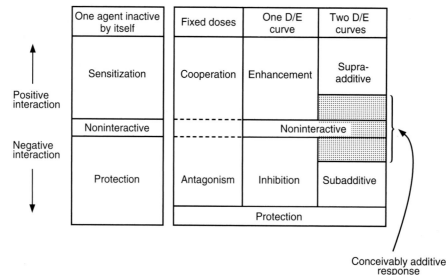

Fig. 1-37 Suggested terminology for drug-radiation interactions. Four experimental situations are envisaged: where the drug is inactive by itself, where fixed doses of drug and radiation are combined, where the dose-response (*D/E curve*) for one agent is studied with and without a fixed dose of another agent, and where dose-response curves for both agents are available. (From Steel GG. *Int J Radiat Oncol Biol Phys* 1979;5:1145-1150.)

any tumor.' Clinical data now convincingly show that local control can be enhanced with simultaneous chemotherapy and irradiation. Schaake-Koning and colleagues[85] reported statistically significant increases in local-regional control of non–small-cell carcinoma of the lung when cisplatin was given, either weekly or daily, simultaneously with thoracic irradiation. Concurrent 5-fluorouracil and pelvic irradiation has been shown to decrease local failure rates when given after resection of adenocarcinoma of the rectum.[86] Improved local control has resulted from the use of vincristine and cyclophosphamide (with or without dactinomycin and doxorubicin) for Ewing's sarcoma of bone and for embryonal rhabdomyosarcoma of the upper aerodigestive tract. Small-cell carcinoma of the lung has been controlled much more consistently with concurrent chemotherapy and radiation therapy than with either radiation therapy or chemotherapy alone. Finally, a French cooperative group[87] led by investigators from Tubiana's own institution showed a significant reduction in the frequency of distant metastasis and improved long-term survival with induction chemotherapy (vindesine, lomustine, cisplatin, and cyclophosphamide) followed by thoracic radiation therapy for non–small-cell carcinoma of the lung, despite local control not being improved. Herskovic and colleagues[88] reported significant decreases in rates of local failure and distant metastases and increases in survival when 5-fluorouracil and cisplatin were given concurrently with moderate-dose radiation therapy (50 Gy given in 25 fractions) compared with higher-dose radiation therapy alone (64.8 Gy in 36 fractions).

Biological Response Modifiers

Biological agents, once limited to derivatives of Calmette-Guérin bacillus, are being discovered at a rate unimaginable only a few years ago. They have been considered possibly restorative of cell-mediated immunity in patients with immune suppression, whether from cancer or the modalities with which cancer is treated. Very few laboratory studies are available describing possible interactions between local irradiation and biological agents. Clinical investigations are summarized in Chapter 39 of this book.

Gene Therapy

The term *gene therapy* covers several quite different approaches,[89] but all require some means of introducing a gene into tumor cells. At present, the most common of these means are viral vectors. Among the several types of vectors used, retroviruses are convenient to work with but can infect only dividing cells; adenoviruses can infect both dividing and quiescent cells, but they evoke an immune response that can make their repeated use difficult. Derivatives of the herpes simplex virus are attractive because of their large size, which

allows more material to be packaged in them, but they can be pathogenic and difficult to control.

In most cases, the virus is used as a simple vector to deliver a gene of interest to the cells. For safety's sake, the virus in these cases is usually engineered so that it cannot replicate. In a few cases, the virus itself is designed to be cytotoxic, and thus some means is needed to selectively limit its cytotoxicity to tumor cells. Several different forms of gene therapy currently being evaluated are described briefly below.

Tumor-suppressor gene therapy. In its purest form, gene therapy seeks to replace a gene in which a mutation initiates or otherwise enhances the malignant phenotype. The goal of such treatment may be to modify cell growth, invasiveness, or metastatic potential as much as it is to kill the cell. The *p53* gene has received a great deal of attention as a target for such therapy. The most commonly mutated gene in human cancer, *p53* can influence transcription, cell cycle checkpoints, DNA repair, apoptosis, and angiogenesis. In several tumor models, transducing cells with wild-type *p53* has inhibited growth and angiogenesis or initiated apoptosis.[90,91] In an early phase I clinical trial, patients with lung tumors that had not responded to conventional treatment were given a retrovirus carrying *p53* by direct injection; this treatment proved to be nontoxic and suppressed tumor growth in six of nine patients.[92]

The chief limitation to tumor-suppressor gene therapy is the paucity of target genes known to induce (or maintain) the malignant phenotype, or at least are necessary to maintain it; moreover, more than one genetic change is needed for carcinogenesis. Also, as is true for most forms of gene therapy, eradication of treated tumors is rare even in experimental systems because of the technical difficulty of transducing sufficiently large proportions of cells in the tumors.

Targeting a cytotoxic virus to mutated cells. Another strategy for treating tumors (both primary and metastatic) characterized by specific mutations involves the use of an adenovirus that replicates only within cells that have those mutations, killing them through cell lysis.[90,93] The basic biology involved in this strategy is as follows.

Two of the principal checks on normal cell growth are provided by *Rb* and *p53*. The product of the *Rb* gene, first discovered in retinoblastoma, prevents cells from entering the S (DNA-synthesizing) phase until the appropriate growth signal is received. The product of the *p53* gene, on the other hand, directs apoptosis of cells that contain damaged DNA. Cells are thought to become cancerous when one or both of these sentinel proteins are inactivated.

Adenovirus can be engineered to "home to" or target cells with deficiencies in *Rb* or *p53*. The wild-type adenovirus contains the *Ela* gene, which targets *Rb*, and the *Elb* gene, which targets and inactivates *p53*. Thus a virus in which the *Ela* gene is deleted or inactivated would grow only in *Rb*-deficient cells, whereas a virus in which the *Elb* gene is deleted or inactivated would grow only in *p53*-deficient cells. To date, only the latter idea has been exploited, that is, production of a virus that replicates only in cells deficient in *p53*. To the extent that mutant *p53* is a hallmark of cancer, this strategy preferentially targets the cytotoxic virus to cancer cells while sparing normal cells.

Designing a therapeutic modality that can distinguish between normal and malignant cells has been the "holy grail" of cancer research for decades. Although some debate still exists as to the extent to which these viruses proliferate and kill cells with normal *p53*, in early clinical trials the systemic inoculation of this vector significantly suppressed the growth of primary head and neck cancer.

Suicide gene therapy. The strategy in suicide gene therapy is to transduce cells with a gene that can convert an inert prodrug (administered separately) into a toxic agent. One such system that has been extensively investigated is the combination of the herpes simplex virus–thymidine-kinase gene (HSV-*tk*) with ganciclovir.[94] The virus containing the HSV-*tk* gene, which phosphorylates the ganciclovir, is injected into the tumor, and the ganciclovir is administered systematically. Phosphorylation of the ganciclovir converts it into a DNA-synthesis inhibitor, leading to cell death. Moreover, significant numbers of nontransduced cells are killed as well (the "bystander" effect) through various other transport and immune mechanisms. This therapy has been tested in more than 35 clinical trials for human malignancies as diverse as brain tumors, mesotheliomas, liver metastases, and peritoneal metastases. Suppression of tumor growth with this therapy has been impressive, but cure rates have been low. Moreover, although local treatments are well tolerated, systemic delivery of HSV-*tk* to target metastatic disease has been limited by liver damage caused by the hepatotropism of the virus. Because this form of gene therapy also seems to sensitize cancer cells to radiation, it may be useful as an adjuvant to radiation or chemotherapy.

Immunomodulatory gene therapy ("cancer vaccines"). The basis of the immunomodulatory gene therapy approach is to provoke or stimulate a cellular immune response to cancer cells that will be effective against metastatic lesions. Tumor vaccines are suspensions of irradiated tumor cells that have been genetically engineered to express cytokines or other molecules known to generate immune responses against tumor-specific antigens. Vaccination with tumor cells expressing cytokines such as interleukin-2, granulocyte-macrophage–colony-stimulating factor, or interferon-γ has been shown to induce an immunologic response in some animal model systems, resulting in growth arrest of local or metastatic tumors.[95] This approach has its problems, however. The molecular requirements for generating an immune response that would be capable of causing tumor rejection are not precisely known. Also, antitumor activity tends to be highest against small, subcutaneous tumor burdens.

Linking a radiation-inducible gene to a cytotoxic agent. In the linking of a radiation-inducible gene to a cytotoxic agent treatment strategy, the physics of radiation-targeting technology is combined with the molecular aspects of gene therapy.[96-98] A chimeric gene that can be activated by radiation is created and inserted into the genome of a nonreplicating adenovirus. The chimeric gene involves the human cDNA sequence that encodes the cytokine tumor necrosis factor-alpha and parts of the early growth response gene (*Egr-1*) promoter/enhancer, which is activated by a dose of radiation of about 0.5 Gy. The adenovirus is injected into the tumor, but the cytokine is activated only in the target volume delineated by the radiation field, thereby minimizing total-body toxicity. Released in the tumor, the tumor necrosis factor causes vascular destruction as well as apoptosis of tumor cells.

The key to the success of this strategy is the use of radiation-inducible promoters/enhancers, of which the early growth response (*Egr*) genes are an example. Elements within the promoters are activated by reactive oxygen intermediates, the triggering stimuli produced by radiation.

Radiogenetic therapy, as it is now called, has shown promise in a model system involving human laryngeal tumor-cell xenografts in the hind limbs of immunodeficient nude mice. This single demonstration of the technique may be just a preview of things to come.

The strategies described here have all had some measure of success in the treatment of localized and, occasionally, metastatic cancer in animal model systems. Although some progress has been made regarding treatment of cancer in humans, that progress is as yet less impressive. All of the strategies share a common problem, namely the difficulty of transducing therapeutic genes into sufficiently large proportions of tumor cells. A logical strategy would be to combine one or more of the gene-therapy approaches with standard radiation therapy or chemotherapy. The guiding principle must be to identify combinations that have additive or synergistic effect with regard to tumor cell kill but have tolerable, non-overlapping toxic effects on normal tissues.

Mutagenesis and Carcinogenesis

When radiation is absorbed in biological material, several biological consequences can result:

Cell death. This is the endpoint of principal concern in radiation therapy, in which the object of the treatment is to kill (in the sense of removing the reproductive integrity of) as many malignant cells as possible. It is also the endpoint of concern for some radiation effects on the developing embryo and fetus, which are cell-depletion phenomena.

Hereditary effects. Radiation may affect the germ cells in a way that does not kill the cells but allows them to survive and carry with them some legacy of the radiation exposure. Such effects will not be expressed until a later generation.

Carcinogenesis. The radiation may affect a somatic cell, leading to a point mutation or a chromosome rearrangement that results, for example, in the release or expression of an oncogene. This may result in leukemogenesis or carcinogenesis.

Hereditary effects and carcinogenesis, therefore, are potential hazards for people who are occupationally exposed to ionizing radiation and also for patients who are long-term survivors of radiation therapy. These effects are discussed in greater detail in the remainder of this chapter.

Hereditary Effects

Lymphocytes cultured from the peripheral blood of radiation workers characteristically show an incidence of gross chromosomal rearrangements, including dicentrics and rings. Because the gonads receive essentially the same dose of radiation as the bone marrow, the germ cells presumably carry similar chromosomal aberrations, although methods to score them are not available. Information concerning the hereditary effects of radiation comes principally from experimental studies in the mouse. Studies of the progeny of the Japanese survivors of Hiroshima and Nagasaki do not provide data that are statistically significant, but they do allow upper bounds to be set on the estimate of risk.

Mutations can be produced by radiation or they can occur spontaneously as a result of several different mechanisms. The first of these mechanisms is single-gene mutations, which may be dominant, recessive, or sex-linked. Second, chromosome rearrangements may result from incorrect rejoining of the "sticky ends" of chromosomes that have been broken. Third, an incorrect chromosome number, either too many or too few, may result in mutation.

Studies with *Drosophila*. Early estimates of genetic hazards came from the studies of *Drosophila*.[99] In this system, mutations that can be readily scored include a change of eye color, a change of body color, a shortening of the wing, or the production of recessive lethal genes. These studies, performed in the 1940s and 1950s, resulted in several important conclusions, namely that (1) the number of mutations was proportional to the radiation dose (i.e., if the dose was doubled, the number of mutations was doubled); (2) the number of mutations produced by a given dose was independent of the dose rate or fractionation pattern; and (3) the doubling dose, the dose of radiation required to produce a number of mutations equal to twice the spontaneous rate, was estimated to be in the range of 5 to 150 roentgens.

These experimental results led to the belief in the 1950s that the possibility of mutations was the most serious hazard for people occupationally exposed to radiation. This was based on two conclusions from the *Drosophila* data: (1) that genetic effects were cumulative because the number of mutations produced was independent of whether the dose was given in a single exposure or multiple exposures, and (2) that the lower end of the doubling dose (5 roentgens) was equal to the annual, maximum-permissible dose for occupational workers.

The megamouse project. Subsequent genetic experiments with mice have changed the perception of genetic hazards.[100,101] In the 1960s, relative mutation rates were assessed in the "megamouse project," in which about 7 million mice were used. A species was chosen that has seven easily identified specific locus mutations, six of which involved coat color changes and the seventh a shortened ear. Male and female animals were irradiated with graded doses, subsequently bred, and mutations scored in the offspring. Conclusions from this project are as follows:

1. The radiosensitivity of different mutations varies substantially, by a factor of about 20.

2. A dose-rate effect exists in the mouse, unlike *Drosophila*, such that spreading radiation over time greatly reduces the number of mutations observed.

3. The male mouse is much more sensitive than the female, and indeed, at low dose rate, essentially all of the genetic load is carried by the male. This may be an artifact of the species because, in the mouse, the oocytes are exquisitely sensitive to radiation, and of course, if they are killed by the radiation, mutations produced in them cannot be expressed.

4. The number of mutations produced by a given dose of radiation drops if a time interval is allowed to elapse between irradiation and mating. This finding is already used as a basis for human genetic counseling. If an individual is exposed to a large dose of radiation, either accidentally or as a consequence of medical procedures, then it is advisable that a planned conception be delayed so as to minimize the genetic consequences of the radiation.

5. The megamouse project indicates that the doubling dose is about 1 Gy.

These data from the mouse have, to some extent, reduced concerns about the genetic consequences of radiation for two reasons. In the first place, the lower end of the doubling dose is 10 times higher than was thought on the basis of the *Drosophila* data; second, given the clearly observed dose-rate effect, if radiation is spread over time (which in practice is the case for radiation workers occupationally exposed), then the genetic consequences are greatly reduced. Converting the estimates of mutation rates produced by the experimental mouse data into estimates of the probability of radiation-induced hereditary disorders in human populations requires using several assumptions and extrapolations. The animal data are expressed in terms of the doubling dose, that is, the amount of radiation necessary to produce twice as many mutations as those that occur naturally in a generation. This doubling dose is estimated to be about 1 Gy, based on mouse data and low-dose-rate exposure.

This is the estimate favored in the latest reports of both the Committee on the Biological Effects of Ionizing Radiation (BEIR V, 1990[102]) and the United Nations Scientific Committee on the Effects of Atomic Radiation (UNSCEAR, 1988[103]). This estimate includes hereditary disorders arising from autosomal and sex-linked mutations, as well as from changes in chromosome number or structure. It does not include any allowance for a genetic component to multifactorial disorders; both committees considered this an important effect of radiation, but were unable to make a realistic estimate.

The prevalence of naturally occurring genetic disorders in a typical Western population is about 10%. The severity of these different disorders varies over a wide range. About one third to one half of all the known naturally occurring hereditary disorders may be deemed severe and equivalent in severity to fatal cancer, either because they occur early in life or because they are as detrimental as lethal diseases in adult life.

For a working population, the International Commission on Radiological Protection[104] estimates the probability per caput for radiation-induced hereditary disorders to be about 0.006 per sievert (Sv). This is based on the doubling dose of 1 Gy plus a very approximate allowance for multifactorial diseases. This risk, of course, is additional to that for cancer.

Carcinogenesis

In sharp contradistinction to the situation for the genetic effects of radiation already discussed, an abundance of information exists concerning radiation carcinogenesis directly from humans. The human experience can be summarized as follows:

  Early workers, largely physicists and engineers working around accelerators, showed an increased incidence of skin cancer and other forms of tumors.

  Miners in Saxony at the turn of the century, and more recently uranium workers in the Central Colorado Plateau, showed an increased incidence of lung cancer as a result of inhaling radon in poorly ventilated mines.

  Workers who painted luminous dials on clocks and watches and who ingested radium by using their tongues to lick the tip of their brushes into a point, subsequently developed bone tumors.

  Patients in whom the contrast material Thorotrast (which contains radioactive thorium) was used subsequently developed liver tumors.

  The survivors of Hiroshima and Nagasaki have shown a whole spectrum of malignancies from leukemia to solid tumors.

  Children given therapeutic doses of radiation for infected tonsillar or nasopharyngeal lymphoid tissue or what was perceived to be an enlarged thymus subsequently developed benign and malignant thyroid tumors and leukemias.

  Children epilated by x-rays as part of the treatment for tinea capitis subsequently developed thyroid and skin tumors.

  Patients with ankylosing spondylitis who received x-rays for the relief of pain subsequently developed an increased incidence of leukemia.

  Women who underwent fluoroscopy many times during the management of tuberculosis showed an increased incidence of breast cancer.

The best quantitative data come from the Japanese atomic-bomb survivors. For solid tumors, risk seems to be a linear function of dose between about 0.2 and 2.5 Gy. For leukemia, a linear-quadratic relationship fits the data more closely. For protection purposes, it is assumed that these risks observed at high doses can be extrapolated linearly to low doses and that no dose threshold exists below which there is no risk.

The latent period. In leukemia, the latency period (i.e., the time between the radiation exposure and the appearance of the disease) is relatively short, with a peak excess incidence occurring by 7 to 10 years after radiation and with the radiation-induced incidence disappearing by about 15 years after radiation. In the case of solid tumors, the latent period may be considerably longer; for example, the excess incidence of solid tumors is still evident in the Japanese survivors nearly 50 years after the atomic bomb attacks. Part of the latency may have resulted from a form of induction period before the initially "transformed" cell or cells start to divide to form a tumor, or alternatively, to a period before the tumor assumes the malignant characteristics of growth and spread. For example, at short intervals after irradiation, the thyroid gland contains tumors that are of a benign histologic character, and malignant tumors become detectable only at later stages. It is widely believed from animal studies that tumorigenesis consists of three separate stages: initiation, promotion, and progression. Some chemicals can only initiate, whereas others can only promote. Radiation seems to be capable of both.

The perception of the latency period has changed in recent years. Radiation-induced tumors appear not at a fixed time after exposure, but rather at the age at which spontaneous tumors of the same type are most prevalent. For example, radiation-induced breast cancers in women appear in middle age, regardless of whether the radiation exposure occurred when the women were teenagers or in their thirties. This fact suggests that radiation may initiate the process at a young age but completion requires additional steps, some of which may depend on hormones.

Absolute vs. relative risk. The preceding information leads to the discussion of relative vs. absolute risk models in radiation carcinogenesis. Although they can seem unduly complex, use of one model over another can produce substantial differences in risk estimates of carcinogenesis, and thus some basic understanding of their principles is warranted. The absolute risk model assumes that radiation produces a discrete "crop" of malignancies that are unrelated to the natural or spontaneous incidence. This seems to be the case for leukemia; as noted in the previous paragraphs, radiation-induced leukemia in Japanese survivors of atomic-bomb blasts was observed for some period after the exposure, but the incidence subsequently returned to that characteristic of the control population. The relative risk model, by contrast, assumes that radiation increases the spontaneous incidence by some fixed factor. According to this model, the radiation-induced cancer incidence will increase with the age of the population as the spontaneous incidence increases. This seems to be the case for the Japanese atomic-bomb survivors as the population ages and the data mature; a relative risk model would predict a large number of tumors occurring late in the life of the irradiated population. The currently favored model is a relative risk model with allowance for age at exposure and time since exposure.

Another point of interest is that risk for three of the four common types of leukemia seems to be increased by radiation, but the risk of chronic lymphocytic leukemia has never been reported to increase from exposure to radiation.

Estimates of cancer risk for various organs, calculated by the Committee on BEIR and UNSCEAR, are summarized in Table 1-6.[102,103] These estimates are based on analyses of the Japanese atomic-bomb survivors and thus apply to high-dose-rate exposures to low-LET radiation. As the data from Japan have matured and more detailed information has become available, it has become evident that the risk of radiation-induced cancer varies considerably with age at the time of exposure. In most cases, individuals exposed at an early age are much more susceptible than are those exposed at older ages. This difference seems to be the most dramatic for female breast cancer; children exposed before 15 years of age are most susceptible, whereas women aged 50 or more at exposure show little or no excess risk. However, there

TABLE 1-6
Excess Cancer Mortality (Lifetime Risk/100,000, 0.1 Sv)

	BEIR V (U.S. POPULATION)		UNSCEAR 88 (JAPANESE POPULATION)	
	Males	Females		
Breast	–	70	Breast	60
Respiratory	190	150	Lung	151
Digestive system	170	290	Stomach	126
			Colon	79
Other solid	300	220	Other solid	194
Leukemia	110	80	Leukemia	100
TOTALS	770	810	TOTAL	710

are exceptions to this general rule. Susceptibility to radiation-induced leukemia is relatively constant throughout life, and susceptibility to respiratory cancers increases in middle age. However, the overall risk drops drastically with age; children and young adults are much more susceptible to radiation-induced cancer than are the middle-aged and old (Fig. 1-38).[102,104]

Use of these cancer risk estimates in a practical radiation protection situation requires the application of several correction factors, all of which involve uncertainties. First, the Japanese data reflect high doses, in an acute exposure, at high dose rates characteristic of an atomic bomb, whereas radiation workers are exposed to low doses, at low dose rates, over protracted periods. Second, the Japanese data refer only to gamma rays. The RBE values for neutrons and other forms of high-LET radiation must come from animal studies. Finally, risk estimates must be transferred from one population to another. For example, rates of stomach cancer are higher, and rates of breast cancer are lower, in the Japanese than in the U.S. populations. This transfer factor is important to consider in using the relative risk model.

Bearing all these uncertainties in mind, the International Commission on Radiological Protection recommends a figure of 0.5 per Sv as the probability of fatal cancer induction after low dose-rate irradiation of the total population.[104] A slightly lower value of 0.4 per Sv applies to a working population that excludes the young, who seem to be very sensitive to irradiation.

Second Malignancies in Patients Given Radiation Therapy

The risk of second malignancies after radiation therapy is a controversial topic for several reasons, among them that patients undergoing radiation therapy are often at high risk of a second cancer because of lifestyle factors, and these factors may be more dominant than the radiation risk. Although many single-institution studies involving radiation therapy for a variety of tumors have concluded that radiation is not associated

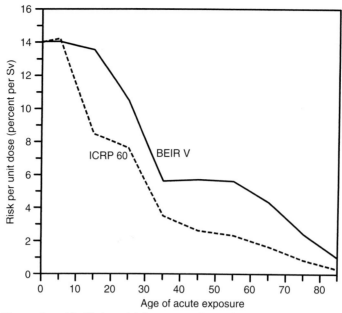

Fig. 1-38 The attributable lifetime risk from a single small dose of radiation to individuals at various ages at the time of exposure. Radiosensitivity decreases substantially with age. The higher risk for the younger age groups will not be expressed until late in life. These estimates are based on a multiplicative model and on a dose and dose-rate effectiveness factor (DDREF) of 2. *ICRP,* International Commission on Radiological Protection; BEIR, Biological Effects of Ionizing Radiation. (Modified from International Commission on Radiological Protection. *ICRP 60: 1990 Recommendations of the International Commission on Radiological Protection.* Oxford, England: Pergamon Press; 1990 and the Committee on the Biological Effects of Ionizing Radiation. *BEIR V: Health Effects of Exposure to Low Levels of Ionizing Radiation.* Washington, DC: National Academy of Sciences Press; 1990.)

with an increase in second malignancies, many such studies were much too small to detect any increased incidence of second malignancies induced by the treatment. Larger studies, however, have consistently indicated that radiation therapy is associated with a small but statistically significant enhancement in the risk of second malignancies, particularly among long-term survivors.

To credibly answer the question of whether radiation therapy is associated with a risk of second malignancies, a study must have (1) a sufficiently large number of patients, (2) a suitable control group, that is, patients with the same cancer treated by some means other than radiation, and (3) a sufficiently long follow-up period for radiation-induced solid tumors to become manifest. Studies that satisfy these criteria describing patients treated for prostate cancer, cervical cancer, and Hodgkin's disease are discussed briefly below.

Second malignancies after radiation therapy for prostate cancer. In the largest study of its kind published to date, Brenner and colleagues[105] used data from the National Cancer Institute's Surveillance Epidemiology and End Results (SEER) Program to evaluate outcome among 51,584 men with prostate cancer treated with radiation and 70,539 treated with surgery. No evidence was found of a difference in the risk of leukemia for radiation therapy vs. surgery patients, but the risk of a second solid tumor at any time after diagnosis was significantly greater after radiation therapy than after surgery by about 6%. This increased relative risk became greater with time, reaching 34% after 10 years or more. The greatest increases in relative risk were for tumors of the bladder (77%) and rectum (105%) 10 years or more after diagnosis. The increased risk of developing sarcoma in the heavily irradiated tissues within the field amounted to 145% at 5 years or more, compared with surgical patients.

Interestingly, the increase in relative risk for carcinoma of the lung, which was exposed to relatively low doses (about 0.5 Gy), was close to that for carcinoma of the bladder, rectum, or colon, all of which were subject to much higher doses (typically more than 5 Gy). This pattern may reflect the fact that carcinoma originating in actively dividing cells or cells under hormonal control can be efficiently induced by relatively low doses of radiation, as evidenced by the A-bomb survivors, but that the cancer risk at high doses decreases because of cell death. In contrast to this pattern for radiation-induced carcinomas, radiation-induced sarcomas generally appeared only in heavily irradiated sites (i.e., close to the treatment volume) where large radiation doses were needed to produce sufficient tissue damage to stimulate cellular renewal in otherwise dormant cells.

Second malignancies after radiation therapy for cervical cancer. In a landmark study, Boice and colleagues[106] studied the risk of second malignancies as a consequence of radiation treatment for carcinoma of the uterine cervix. This huge international study, involving 42 authors from 38 institutions, had not only a sample size of 150,000 patients but also an ideal control group for comparison because cervical cancer is equally well treated by radiation or surgery. Some of the pertinent findings from this large study are summarized below.

Very high doses (on the order of several hundred grays) were found to increase the risk of developing cancer of the bladder, vagina, possibly bone, uterine corpus, and cecum as well as non-Hodgkin's lymphoma. Risk ratios ranged from a high of 4.0 for bladder cancer to a low of 1.3 for bone cancer. A steep dose-response was observed for the risk of developing subsequent genital cancer, with a fivefold excess at doses of more than 150 Gy. Doses of several grays were found to increase the risk of stomach cancer and leukemia. Somewhat surprisingly, radiation therapy for cervical cancer did not increase the overall risk of subsequent cancer of the small intestine, colon, ovary, vulva, connective tissue, or breast, nor did it increase the risk of Hodgkin's disease, multiple myeloma, or chronic lymphocytic leukemia.

The overall conclusions of this study were that radiation therapy, unlike surgery, was certainly associated with a risk of excess cancer, and that the risks were highest among long-term survivors and concentrated among women who were irradiated at relatively young ages.

Second malignancies among long-term survivors of Hodgkin's disease treated with radiation therapy. In a 1996 report of the Late Effects Study Group, which followed 1380 children with Hodgkin's disease, 17 of 483 females in whom Hodgkin's disease was diagnosed before the age of 16 years subsequently developed breast cancer, with radiation therapy implicated in most cases.[107] The ratio of observed to expected cases in that study was 75.3. Another study involving 1641 patients treated for Hodgkin's disease as children in five Nordic countries reported 16 cases of breast cancer, for a relative risk 17 times that of the general population.[108] The largest study of this kind evaluated 3869 women in population-based registries participating in the SEER Program.[109] All of these women had been given radiation therapy as initial treatment for Hodgkin's disease. Breast cancer developed in a total of 55 patients, which represents a ratio of observed to expected cases of 2.24. However, the risk of subsequent breast cancer in women treated before the age of 16 years was 61%, with most tumors appearing 10 or more years after treatment. This finding agrees with those from previous studies showing the prepubertal and pubertal female breast to be very

radiosensitive. The risk of breast cancer decreased as the age at therapy increased and was only slightly elevated in women who were 30 years old or older when they were treated. In the most recent article on this subject,[110] 27 of 202 patients with Hodgkin's disease treated with radiation developed a second cancer. Most of the second tumors appeared within or near the treatment field, most commonly in the lung and breast; however, the spectrum was large and the risk was greatest among patients irradiated at young ages.

In summary, studies of large numbers of patients clearly indicate that radiation therapy induces an excess of second cancers. In the young, the breast is especially sensitive to the carcinogenic effects of radiation. The latency period for the development of excess cancers can range from 10 years to decades after the radiation treatment.

REFERENCES

1. Bishop JM. Cellular oncogene retroviruses. *Ann Rev Biochem* 1983;52:301-354.
2. Kundson AG. Mutation and cancer: statistical study of retinoblastoma. *Proc Natl Acad Sci U S A* 1971;68:820-823.
3. Knudson A. Anti-oncogenes and human cancer. *Proc Natl Acad Sci U S A* 1993;90:10914-10921.
4. Fearon ER, Vogelstein B. A genetic model for colorectal tumorigenesis. *Cell* 1990;61:759-767.
5. Ward JF. DNA lesions produced by ionizing radiation: locally multiplying damaged sites. In: Wallace SS, Painter RB, eds. *Ionizing Radiation Damage to DNA: Molecular Aspects.* New York, NY: Wiley-Liss; 1990.
6. Puck TT, Markus PI. Action of x-rays on mammalian cells. *J Exp Med* 1956;103:656-666.
7. Withers HR. The dose-survival relationship for irradiation of epithelial cells of mouse skin. *Br J Radiol* 1967;40:187-194.
8. Withers HR. Recovery and repopulation in vivo by mouse skin epithelium cells during fractionated irradiation. *Radiat Res* 1967;32:227-239.
9. Withers HR, Elkind MM. Microcolony survival assay for cells of mouse intestinal mucosa exposed to radiation. *Int J Radiat Biol* 1970;17:261-267.
10. McCullough EA, Till JE. The sensitivity of cells from normal mouse bone marrow to gamma radiation *in vitro* and *in vivo.* *Radiat Res* 1962;16:822-832.
11. Douglas BG, Fowler JF. The effect of multiple small doses of x-rays on skin reactions in the mouse and a basic interpretation. *Radiat Res* 1976;66:401-426.
12. Suit H, Wette R. Radiation dose fractionation and tumor control probability. *Radiat Res* 1966;29:267-281.
13. Hewitt HB, Wilson CW. A survival curve for mammalian leukaemia cells irradiated in vivo. *Br J Cancer* 1959;13:69-75.
14. Hill RP, Bush RS. A lung colony assay to determine the radiosensitivity of the cells of a solid tumor. *Int J Radiat Biol* 1969;15:435-444.
15. Howard A, Pelc SR. The synthesis of deoxyribose nucleic acid and its relationship to the chromosome damage induced by x-rays. *Heredity* 1953;6(suppl):261-273.
16. Brown JM. The effect of acute x-irradiation on the cell proliferation kinetics of induced carcinomas and their normal counterpart. *Radiat Res* 1970;43:627-653.
17. Steel GG. Cell loss as a factor in the growth rate of human tumors. *Eur J Cancer* 1967;3:381-387.
18. Steel GG. Cell loss from experimental tumors. *Cell Tissue Kinet* 1968;1:193-207.

19. Steel GG. The kinetics of cell proliferation in tumors. *Proceedings of the Carmel Conference on Time and Dose Relationships in Radiation Biology as Applied to Radiotherapy*. BNL 50203 (C-57). Upton, NY: Brookhaven National Laboratory; 1969.

20. Begg AC, McNally NJ, Shrieve D, et al. A method to measure the duration of DNA synthesis and the potential doubling time from a single sample. *Cytometry* 1985;6:620-625.

21. Begg AC, Moonen I, Hofland I, et al. Human tumor cell kinetics using a monoclonal antibody against iododeoxyuridine: intratumoral sampling variations. *Radiother Oncol* 1988;11:337-347.

22. Gray JW, Dolbeare F, Pallavicini MG, et al. Cell cycle analysis using flow cytometry. *Int J Radiat Biol* 1986;49:237-255.

23. Regaud C, Nogier T. Sterilization roentgenienne totale et definitive, sans radiodermite, des testicules du Belier adulte: conditions de sa realisation. *Compt Rend Soc Biol* 1911;70:202-203.

24. Brenner DJ, Hall E. Conditions for the equivalence of continuous to pulsed low dose rate brachytherapy. *Int J Radiat Oncol Biol Phys* 1991;20:181-190.

25. Thames HD, Ang KK, Stewart FA, et al. Does incomplete repair explain the apparent failure of the basic LQ model to predict spinal cord and kidney responses to low doses per fraction. *Int J Radiat Biol* 1988;554:13-19.

26. Withers HR, Peters LJ, Kogelnik HC. The pathobiology of late effects of irradiation. In: Meyn RE, Withers HR, eds. *Radiation Biology in Cancer Research*. New York, NY: Raven Press; 1980:439-448.

27. Fowler JF. The second Klaas Breur memorial lecture: La Ronde-radiation sciences and medical radiology. *Radiother Oncol* 1983;1:1-22.

28. Ellis F. Dose time and fractionation: a clinical hypothesis. *Clin Radiol* 1969;20:1-7.

29. Arriagada R, LeChevalier T, Quoix E, et al. Effect of chemotherapy on locally advanced non-small cell lung carcinoma: a randomized study of 3,553 patients. *Int J Radiat Oncol Biol Phys* 1991;20:1183-1190.

30. Cox JD, Stoffel TJ. The significance of needle biopsy after irradiation for stage C adenocarcinoma of the prostate. *Cancer* 1977;40:156-160.

31. Dugan TC, Shipley WU, Young RH, et al. Biopsy after external beam radiation therapy for adenocarcinoma of the prostate: correlation with original histological grade and current prostate specific antigen levels. *J Urol* 1991;146:1313-1316.

32. Cox JD, Pajak TF, Marcial VA, et al. Interfractional interval is a major determinant of late effects, with hyperfractionated radiation therapy of carcinomas of upper respiratory and digestive tracts: results from Radiation Therapy Oncology Group Protocol 8313. *Int J Radiat Oncol Biol Phys* 1991;20:1191-1195.

33. Horiot J-C, Le Fur R, N'Guyen T, et al. Hyperfractionation versus conventional fractionation in oropharyngeal carcinoma: final analysis of a randomized trial of the EORTC cooperative group of radiotherapy. *Radiother Oncol* 1992;25:231-241.

34. Horiot J-C, Bontemps P, van den Bogaert W, et al. Accelerated fractionation (AF) compared to conventional fractionation (CV) improves loco-regional control in the radiotherapy of advanced head and neck cancers: results of the EORTC 22851 randomised trial. *Radiother Oncol* 1997;44:111-121.

35. Dische S, Saunders M, Barrett A, et al. A randomized multicentre trial of CHART versus conventional radiotherapy in head and neck cancer. *Radiother Oncol* 1997;44:123-136.

36. Fu KK, Pajak TF, Trotti A, et al. A Radiation Therapy Oncology Group (RTOG) phase III randomized study to compare hyperfractionation and two variants of accelerated fractionation to standard fractionation radiotherapy for head and neck squamous cell carcinomas: first report of RTOG 9003. *Int J Radiat Oncol Biol Phys* 2000;48:7-16.

37. Fowler JF, Harari P. Confirmation of improved local-regional control with altered fractionation in head and neck cancer. *Int J Radiat Oncol Biol Phys* 2000;48:3-6.

38. Withers HR, Peters LJ. Transmutability of dose and time. Commentary on the first report of RTOG 9003. *Int J Radiat Oncol Biol Phys* 2000;48:1-2.

39. Overgaard J, Sand Hansen H, Overgaard M, et al. Importance of overall treatment time for the outcome of radiotherapy in head and neck carcinoma. Experience from the Danish Head and Neck Cancer Study. *Proc ICRO/ÖGRO 6, 6th International Meeting on Progress in Radio-Oncology*, Salzburg, Austria; 13-17 May 1998. Bologna, Italy: Monduzzi Editore S.P.A.; 1998: 743-752.

40. Hermens AF, Barendsen GW. Changes of cell proliferation characteristics in a rat rhabdomyosarcoma before and after irradiation. *Eur J Cancer* 1969;5:173-189.

41. Withers HR, Peters LJ, Thames HD, et al. Hyperfractionation. *Int J Radiat Oncol Biol Phys* 1982;8:1807-1809.

42. Withers HR, Mason K, Reid BO, et al. Response of mouse intestine to neutrons and gamma rays in relation to dose fractionation and division cycle. *Cancer* 1974;34:3947.

43. Withers HR, Taylor MMG, Maciejewski B, et al. The hazard of accelerated tumor clonogen repopulation during radiotherapy. *Acta Oncol* 1988;27:131-146.

44. Chapman JD, Peters LJ, Withers HR. *Prediction of Tumor Treatment Response*. New York, NY: Pergamon Press; 1989.

45. West CM. Intrinsic radiosensitivity as a predictor of patient response to radiotherapy. *Br J Radiol* 1995;68:827-837.

46. West CM, Davidson SE, Burt PA, et al. The intrinsic radiosensitivity of cervical carcinoma: correlations with clinical data. *Int J Radiat Oncol Biol Phys* 1995;31:841-846.

47. West CML, Davidson SE, Hendry JH, et al. Prediction of cervical carcinoma response to radiotherapy. *Lancet* 1991;338:818.

48. West CM, Davidson SE, Roberts SA, et al. Intrinsic radiosensitivity and prediction of patient response to radiotherapy for carcinoma of the cervix. *Br J Cancer* 1993;68:819-823.

49. Parliament MB, Chapman JD, Urtasun RC, et al. Noninvasive assessment of human tumour hypoxia with ^{123}I-iodoazomycin arabinoside: preliminary report of a clinical study. *Br J Cancer* 1992;65:90-95.

50. Höckel M, Knoop C, Schlenger K, et al. Intratumoral pO2 predicts survival in advanced cancer of the uterine cervix. *Radiother Oncol* 1993;26:45-50.

51. Höckel M, Schlenger K, Aral B, et al. Association between tumor hypoxia and malignant progression in advanced cancer of the uterine cervix. *Cancer Res* 1996;56:4509-4515.

52. Begg AC, Hofland I, Moonen L, et al. The predictive value of cell kinetic measurements in a European trial of accelerated fractionation in advanced head and neck tumors: an interim report. *Int J Radiat Oncol Biol Phys* 1990;19:1449-1453.

53. Begg AC, Haustermans K, Hart AAM, et al. The value of pretreatment cell kinetic parameters as predictors for radiotherapy outcome in head and neck cancer: a multicenter analysis. *Radiother Oncol* 1999;50:13-23.

54. Thomlinson RH, Gray LH. The histological structure of some human lung cancers and the possible implications for radiotherapy. *Br J Cancer* 1955;9:539-549.

55. Brown JM. Evidence for acutely hypoxic cells in mouse tumours, and a possible mechanism of reoxygenation. *Br J Radiol* 1979;52:650-656.

56. Brizel DM, Scully SP, Harrelson JM, et al. Tumor oxygenation predicts for the likelihood of distant metastases in human soft tissue sarcoma. *Cancer Res* 1996;56:941-943.

57. Giaccia AJ, Brown JM, Wouters B, et al. Cancer therapy and tumor physiology. *Science* 1998;279:12-13.

58. Adams GE. Chemical radiosensitization of hypoxic cells. *Br Med Bull* 1973;29:48-53.

59. Adams GE. Hypoxic cell sensitizers for radiotherapy. In: Becker FF, ed. *Cancer*. Vol 6. New York, NY: Plenum Press; 1977: 181-223.

60. Adams GE, Bremner J, Stratford IJ, et al. Nitroheterocyclic compounds as radiosensitizers and bioreductive drugs. *Radiother Oncol* 1991;20:85-91.
61. Brown JM, Siim BG. Hypoxia-specific cytotoxins in cancer therapy. *Semin Radiat Oncol* 1996;6:22-36.
62. Brown JM, Lemmon MJ. Tumor hypoxia can be exploited to preferentially sensitize tumors to fractionated irradiation. *Int J Radiat Oncol Biol Phys* 1991;20:457-461.
63. von Pawel J, von Roemeling R, Gatzemeier U, et al. Tirapazamine plus cisplatin in advanced non–small-cell lung cancer: a report of the international CATAPULT I study group. Cisplatin and Tirapazamine in Subjects with Advanced Previously Untreated Non–Small-Cell Lung Tumors. *J Clin Oncol* 2000;18:1351-1359.
64. Overgaard J, Horsman MR. Modification of hypoxia-induced radioresistance in tumours by the use of oxygen and sensitizers. *Semin Radiat Oncol* 1996;6:10-21.
65. Mitchell JB, Morstyn G, Russo A, et al. Differing sensitivity to fluorescent light in Chinese hamster cells containing equally incorporated quantities of BUdr versus IUdr. *Int J Radiat Oncol Biol Phys* 1984;10:1447-1451.
66. Cook JA, Glass J, Lebovics R, et al. Measurement of thymidine replacement in patients with high grade gliomas, head and neck tumors, and high grade sarcomas after continuous intravenous infusions of 5-iododeoxyuridine. *Cancer Res* 1992;52:719-725.
67. Sondak VK, Robertson JM, Sussman JJ, et al. Preoperative idoxuridine and radiation for large soft tissue sarcomas: clinical results with five-year follow-up. *Ann Surg Oncol* 1998;5:106-112.
68. Patt HM, Tyree EB, Straube RL, et al. Cysteine protection against x-irradiation. *Science* 1949;110:213.
69. Bacq ZM, Herve A, Lecompte J, et al. Protection contre le rayonnement x par la β-mercato-éthylamine. *Arch Intern Physiol* 1951;S9:442-447.
70. Yuhas JM, Spellman JM, Culo F. The role of WR2721 in radiotherapy and/or chemotherapy. In: Brady L, ed. *Radiation Sensitizers.* New York, NY: Masson Publishing; 1980.
71. Kligerman MM, Liu T, Liu Y, et al. Interim analysis of a randomized trial of radiation therapy of rectal cancer with/without WR-2721. *Int J Radiat Oncol Biol Phys* 1992;22:799-802.
72. Brizel D, Sander R, Wannenmacher M, et al. Randomized phase III trial of radiation ± amifostine in patients with head and neck cancer [abstract]. *Proc Am Soc Clin Oncol* 1998;17:1487.
73. Broerse JJ, Barendsen GW. Relative biological effectiveness of fast neutrons for effects on normal tissues. *Curr Top Radiat Res Q* 1973;8:305-350.
74. Barendsen GW. In: *Proceedings of the Conference of Particle Accelerators in Radiation Therapy.* U.S. Atomic Energy Commission, Technical Information Center; 1972. LA-5180-C.
75. Catterall M, Vonberg DD. Treatment of advanced tumors of head and neck with fast neutrons. *Br Med J* 1974;3:137-143.
76. Catterall M, Sutherland I, Bewley DK. First results of a clinical trial of fast neutrons compared with x or gamma rays in treatment of advanced tumors of the head and neck. *Br Med J* 1975;2:653-656.
77. Catterall M. Results of neutron therapy: differences, correlations, and improvements. *Int J Radiat Oncol Biol Phys* 1982;8:2141-2144.
78. Batterman JJ. Clinical Application of Fast Neutrons: the Amsterdam Experience. Amsterdam, The Netherlands: Rodipi; 1981.
79. Laramore GE, Krall JM, Thomas FJ, et al. Fast neutron radiotherapy for locally advanced prostate cancer: results of an RTOG randomized study. *Int J Radiat Oncol Biol Phys* 1985;11:1621-1627.
80. Coley WB. The treatment of malignant tumors by repeated inoculation of erysipelas: with a report of ten original cases. *Am J Med Sci* 1983;105:487.
81. Overgaard J, Gonzalez Gonzalez D, Hulschof MC, et al. Hyperthermia as an adjuvant to radiation therapy of recurrent or metastatic malignant melanoma. A multicentre randomized trial by the European Society of Hyperthermic Oncology. *Int J Hyperthermia* 1996;12:3-20.
82. Vernon CC, Hand JW, Field SB, et al. Radiotherapy with or without hyperthermia in the treatment of superficial localized breast cancer: results from five randomized controlled trials. International Collaborative Hyperthermia Group. *Int J Radiat Oncol Biol Phys* 1996;35:731-744.
83. Steel GG. Terminology in the description of drug-radiation interactions. *Int J Radiat Oncol Biol Phys* 1979;5:1145-1150.
84. Tubiana M. Les associations radiotherapie—chimeotherapie. *J Eur Radiother* 1980;1:107-114.
85. Schaake-Koning C, vanden Bogaert W, Dalesio O, et al. Effects of concomitant cisplatin and radiotherapy on inoperable nonsmall cell lung cancer. *N Engl J Med* 1992;326:524-530.
86. Krook JE, Moertel C, Gunderson L, et al. Effective surgical adjuvant therapy for high-risk rectal carcinoma. *N Engl J Med* 1991;324:709-715.
87. LeChevalier T, Arriagada R, Tarayre M, et al. Significant effect of adjuvant chemotherapy on survival in locally advanced nonsmall cell lung carcinoma. *J Natl Cancer Inst* 1992;84:58.
88. Herskovic A, Martz K, Al-Sarraf M, et al. Combined chemotherapy and radiotherapy compared with radiotherapy alone in patients with cancer of the esophagus. *N Engl J Med* 1992;326:1593-1598.
89. Hall SJ, Chen S-H, Woo SLC. Gene therapy 97: the promise and reality of cancer gene therapy. *Am J Hum Genet* 1997;61:785-789.
90. Fujiwara T, Cai DW, Georges RN, et al. Therapeutic effect of a retroviral wild-type of *p53* expression vector in an orthotopic lung cancer model. *J Natl Cancer Inst* 1994;86:1458-1462.
91. Nguyen DM, Spitz FR, Yen N, et al. Gene therapy for lung cancer: enhancement of tumor suppression by a combination of sequential systemic cisplatin and adenovirus-mediated *p53* gene transfer. *J Thorac Cardiovasc Surg* 1996;112:1372-1377.
92. Roth JA, Nguyen D, Lawrence DD, et al. Retrovirus-mediated wild-type *p53* gene transfer to tumors of patients with lung cancer. *Nat Med* 1996;2:985-991.
93. Gjerset RA, Turla ST, Sobol RE, et al. Use of wild-type *p53* to achieve complete treatment sensitization of tumor cells expressing endogenous mutant *p53*. *Mol Carcinog* 1995;14:275-285.
94. Tong X-W, Block A, Chen S-H, et al. In vivo gene therapy of ovarian cancer by adenovirus-mediated thymidine kinase gene transduction and ganciclovir administration. *Gynecol Oncol* 1996;61:175-179.
95. Porgador A, Gansbacher B, Bannerji R, et al. Anti-metastatic vaccination of tumor-bearing mice with IL-2-gene-inserted tumor cells. *Int J Cancer* 1993;53:471-477.
96. Hallahan DE, Mauceri HJ, Seung LP, et al. Spatial and temporal control of gene therapy using ionizing radiation. *Nat Med* 1995;1:786-791.
97. Datta R, Taneja N, Sukhatme VP, et al. Reactive oxygen intermediates target CC(A/T)6GG sequences to mediate activation of the early growth response 1 transcription factor gene by ionizing radiation. *Proc Natl Acad Sci U S A* 1993;90:2419-2422.
98. Weichselbaum RR, Hallahan DE, Sukhatme VP, et al. Gene therapy targeted by ionizing radiation. *Int J Radiat Oncology Biol Phys* 1992;24:565-567.
99. Muller HJ. Artificial transmutation of the gene. *Science* 1927;66:84-87.
100. Russell WL. The effect of radiation dose rate and fractionation on mutation in mice. In: Sobels FH, ed. *Repair of Genetic Radiation Damage.* New York, NY: Pergamon Press; 1963:205-217.
101. Russell WL. Effect of the interval between irradiation and conception on mutation frequency in female mice. *Proc Natl Acad Sci U S A* 1965;54:1552-1557.

102. Committee on the Biological Effects of Ionizing Radiation. *BEIR V. Health Effects of Exposure to Low Levels of Ionizing Radiation.* Washington, DC: National Academy Press; 1990.

103. United Nations Scientific Committee on the Effects of Atomic Radiation. *Sources and Effects of Ionizing Radiation.* New York, NY: United Nations; 1988.

104. International Commission on Radiological Protection. *ICRP 60: 1990 Recommendations of the International Commission on Radiological Protection.* Oxford, England: Pergamon Press; 1990.

105. Brenner DJ, Curtis RE, Hall EJ, et al. Second cancers after radiotherapy for prostate cancer. *Cancer* 2000;15:398-406.

106. Boice JD Jr, Engholm G, Kleinman RA, et al. Radiation dose and second cancer risk in patients treated for cancer of the cervix. *Radiat Res* 1988;116:3-55.

107. Bhatia S, Robison LL, Oberlin O, et al. Breast cancer and other second neoplasms after childhood Hodgkin's disease. *N Engl J Med* 1996;334:745-751.

108. Sankila R, Garwicz S, Olsen JH, et al. Risk of subsequent malignant neoplasms among 1,641 Hodgkin's disease patients diagnosed in childhood and adolescence: a population-based cohort study in the five Nordic countries. *J Clin Oncol* 1996;14:1442-1446.

109. Travis LB, Curtis RE, Boice JD Jr, et al. Late effects of treatment for childhood Hodgkin's disease. *N Engl J Med* 1996;335: 352-353.

110. Nyandoto P, Muhonen T, Joensuu H. Second cancers among long-term survivors from Hodgkin's disease. *Int J Radiat Oncol Biol Phys* 1998;42:373-378.

ADDITIONAL READINGS

Historical Background

del Regato JA. *Radiological Physicists.* New York, NY: American Institute of Physics; 1985.

Hall EJ. *Radiation and Life.* New York, NY: Pergamon Press; 1984.

Hall EJ. *Radiobiology for the Radiologist.* 4th ed. Philadelphia, Pa: JB Lippincott; 1994.

Types of Radiation

Goodwin PN, Quimby EH, Morgan RH. *Physical Foundations of Radiology.* New York, NY: Harper & Row; 1970.

Johns H, Cunningham J, eds. *The Physics of Radiology.* 4th ed. Springfield, Ill: Charles C Thomas; 1983.

Smith VP, ed. *Radiation Particle Therapy.* Philadelphia, Pa: American College of Radiology; 1976.

Production of Radiation for Therapeutic Applications

Hendee W, ed. *Radiation Therapy Physics.* St Louis, Mo: Mosby; 1981.

Johns H, Cunningham J, eds. *The Physics of Radiology.* 4th ed. Springfield, Ill: Charles C Thomas; 1983.

Dose: Its Measurement and Meaning

Rossi HH. Neutron and heavy particle dosimetry. In Reed GW, ed. *Radiation Dosimetry. Proceedings of the International School of Physics.* New York, NY: Academic Press; 1964.

Physical Basis for Choice of Treatment Techniques

Khan F, ed. *The Physics of Radiation Therapy.* Baltimore, Md: Williams & Wilkins; 1984.

Levitt SH, Khan FM, Potish RA. *Levitt and Tapley's Technological Basis of Radiation Therapy: Practical Clinical Applications.* 2nd ed. Philadelphia, Pa: Lea & Febiger; 1992.

Signal Transduction

Amundson SA, Myers TG, Fornace AJ. Roles of *p53* in growth arrest and apoptosis: putting on the brakes after genotoxic stress. *Oncogene* 1998;17:3287-3299.

The Cell Cycle

Hartwell LH, Weinert TA. Checkpoints: controls that ensure the order of cell cycle events. *Science* 1989;246:629-634.

Kastan MB, Zhan Q, El-Deiry WS, et al. A mammalian cell cycle checkpoint pathway utilizing p53 and GADD45 is defective in ataxia-telangiectasia. *Cell* 1992;71:587-597.

McKenna W, Iliakis G, Weiss MC, et al. Increased G_2 delay in radiation-resistant cells obtained by transformation of primary rat embryo cells with the oncogens H-*ras* and v-*myc*. *Radiat Res* 1991;125:283-287.

Oncogenes and Tumor Suppressor Genes

Bishop JM, Varmus HE. Functions and origins of retroviral transform- ing genes. In: Weiss R, Teich N, Varmus H, Coffinm J, eds. *RNA Tumor Viruses: Molecular Biology of Tumor Viruses.* 2nd ed. New York, NY: Cold Spring Harbor Laboratory; 1984:990-1108.

Cavanee WK. Tumor progression stage: specific losses of heterozygosity. *Int Symp Princess Takamatsu Cancer Res Found* 1989;20:33-42.

Cole M. The *myc* oncogene: its role in transformation and differentiation. *Annu Rev Genet* 1986;20:361-384.

Hartwell LH, Kastan MB. Cell cycle control and cancer. *Science* 1994;266:1821-1828.

Rous P. A sarcoma of fowl transmissible by an agent separable from the tumor cells. *J Exp Med* 1911;13:397.

Stanbridge EJ. Suppression of malignancy in human cells. *Nature* 1976;260:17-20.

Radiation Chemistry

Boag JW. The action of ionizing radiation on dilute aqueous solutions. *Phys Med Biol* 1965;10:457-476.

Ward JF. Biochemistry of DNA lesions. *Radiat Res* 1985;104:S103-S111.

Cell Survival Curves

Elkind MM, Sutton H. Radiation response of mammalian cells grown in culture. I. Repair of x-ray damage in surviving Chinese hamster cells. *Radiat Res* 1960;13:556-593.

Puck TT, Markus PI. Action of x-rays on mammalian cells. *J Exp Med* 1956;103:653-666.

Effects on Normal Tissues

Cox JD, Byhardt RW, Wilson JF, et al. Complications of radiation therapy and factors in their prevention. *World J Surg* 1986;10: 171-188.

Denekamp J. Cell kinetics and radiation biology. *Int J Radiat Biol* 1986;49:357-380.

Fowler JF, Kragt K, Ellis RE, et al. The effect of divided doses of 15 MeV electrons in the skin response of mice. *Int J Radiat Biol* 1965;9: 241-252.

Fowler JF, Morgan RL, Silvester JA, et al. Experiments with fractionated x-ray treatment of the skin of pigs. I. Fractionation up to 28 days. *Br J Radiol* 1963;36:188-196.

Hendry JH, Thames HD. The tissue-rescuing unit. *Br J Radiol* 1986;59:628-630.

Hopewell JW. Late radiation damage to the central nervous system: a radiobiological interpretation. *Neuropathol Appl Neurobiol* 1979;5:329-343.

Hopewell JW. Mechanisms of the action of radiation on skin and underlying tissues. *Br J Radiol* 1986;19(suppl):39-51.

Hopewell JW, Campling D, Calvo W, et al. Vascular irradiation damage: its cellular basis and likely consequences. *Br J Cancer* 1986;53:181-191.

Hopewell JW, Morris AD, Dixon-Brown A. The influence of field size on the late tolerance of the rat spinal cord to single doses of x-rays. *Br J Radiol* 1987;60:1099-1108.

Kerr JRF, Searle J. Apoptosis: its nature and kinetic role. In: Meyn RE, Withers HR, eds. *Radiation Biology in Cancer Research.* New York, NY: Raven Press; 1980:367-384.

Michalowsli A. A critical appraisal of clonogenic survival assays in the evaluation of radiation damage to normal tissues. *Radiother Oncol* 1984;1:241-246.

Phillips TL, Margolis L. Radiation pathology and the clinical response of lung and esophagus. *Front Radiat Ther Oncol* 1972;6:254-273.

Phillips TL, Ross G. A quantitative technique for measuring renal damage after irradiation. *Radiology* 1973;109:457-462.

Phillips TL, Ross G. Time-dose relationships in the mouse esophagus. *Radiology* 1974;113:435-440.

Rubin P. Late effects of chemotherapy and radiation therapy: a new hypothesis. *Int J Radiat Oncol Biol Phys* 1984;10:5-34.

Rubin P, Casarett GW. *Clinical Radiation Pathology.* Vol 1. Philadelphia, Pa: WB Saunders; 1968.

Stewart FA. Mechanism of bladder damage and repair after treatment with radiation and cytostatic drugs. *Br J Cancer* 1986;7(suppl): 280-291.

Travis EL, Liao Z-X, Tucker SL. Spatial heterogeneity of the volume effect for radiation pneumonitis in mouse lung. *Int J Radiat Oncol Biol Phys* 1997;38:1045-1054.

Travis EL, Tucker SL. Relationship between functional assays of radiation response in the lung and target cell depletion. *Br J Cancer Suppl* 1986;7:304-319.

van der Kogel AJ. Mechanisms of late radiation injury in the spinal cord. In: Meyn RE, Withers HR, eds. *Radiation Biology in Cancer Research,* New York, NY: Raven Press; 1980:461-470.

van der Kogel AJ. Central nervous system radiation injury in small animal models. In: Gutin PH, Leibel SA, Sheline GE, eds. *Radiation Injury to the Nervous System.* New York, NY: Raven Press; 1991: 91-112.

van der Schueren E, Landuyt W, Ang KK, et al. From 2 Gy to 1 Gy per fraction: sparing effect in rat spinal cord? *Int J Radiat Oncol Biol Phys* 1988;14:297-300.

Withers HR, Taylor JMG, Maciejewski B. Treatment volume and tissue tolerance. *Int J Radiat Oncol Biol Phys* 1988;14:751-759.

Withers HR, Thames HD, Peters LJ, et al. Keynote address: Normal tissue radioresistance in clinical radiotherapy. In: Fletcher GH, Nervi C, Withers HR, eds. *Biological Bases and Clinical Implications of Tumor Radioresistance.* New York, NY: Masson; 1983:139-152.

Effects on Tumors

Barendsen GW, Broerse JJ. Experimental radiotherapy of a rat rhabdomyosarcoma with 15 MeV neutrons and 300 kV x-rays. I. Effects of single exposures. *Eur J Cancer* 1969;5:373-391.

Hewitt HB. Studies in the quantitative transplantation of mouse sarcoma. *Br J Cancer* 1953;7:367-383.

Hewitt HB, Wilson CW. A survival curve for mammalian cells irradiated in vivo. *Nature* 1959;183:1060-1061.

Hewitt HB, Chan DPS, Blake ER. Survival curves for clonogenic cells of a murine keratinizing squamous carcinoma irradiated in vivo or under hypoxic conditions. *Int J Radiat Biol* 1967;12:535-549.

Hill EP, Bush RS. A lung colony assay to determine the radiosensitivity of the cells of a solid tumor. *Int J Radiat Biol* 1969;15: 435-444.

Powers WE, Tolmach LJ. A multicomponent x-ray survival curve for mouse lymphosarcoma cells irradiated in vivo. *Nature* 1963;197:710-711.

Tissue and Tumor Kinetics

Begg AC, McNally NJ, Schrieve DC, et al. A method to measure the duration of DNA synthesis and the potential doubling time from a single sample, *Cytometry* 1985;6:620-626.

Denekamp J. The cellular proliferation kinetics of animal tumors. *Cancer Res* 1970;30:393-400.

Dolbeare F, Beisker W, Pallavicini M, et al. Cytochemistry for BrdUrd/DNA analysis: stoichiometry and sensitivity. *Cytometry* 1985;6:521-530.

Dolbeare F, Gratzner H, Pallavicini M, et al. Flow cytometric measurement of total DNA content and incorporated bromodeoxyuridine. *Proc Natl Acad Sci U S A* 1983;80:5573-5577.

Frindel E, Malaise EP, Tubiana M. Cell proliferation kinetics in five human solid tumors. *Cancer* 1968;22:661-662.

Gray JW. Cell-cycle analysis of perturbed cell populations. Computer simulation of sequential DNA distributions. *Cell Tissue Kinet* 1976;9:499-516.

Mendelsohn ML. The growth fraction: a new concept applied to tumors. *Science* 1960;132:1496.

Mendelsohn ML. Principles, relative merits, and limitations of current cytokinetic methods. In: Drewinko B, Humphrey RM, eds. *Growth Kinetics and Biochemical Regulation of Normal and Malignant Cells.* Baltimore, Md: Williams & Wilkins; 1977.

Tubiana M, Malaise EP. Growth rate and cell kinetics in human tumors: some prognostic and therapeutic implications. In: Symington T, Carter RL, eds. *Scientific Foundations of Oncology.* St Louis, Mo: Mosby; 1976.

Systemic Effects

Bond VP, Fliedner TM, Archambeau JO. *Mammalian Radiation Lethality: A Disturbance in Cellular Kinetics.* New York, NY: Academic Press; 1965.

Hemplemann LH, Lisco H, Hoffman JG. The acute radiation syndrome: a study of nine cases and a review of the problem. *Ann Intern Med* 1952;36:279-510.

Lushbaugh CC. Reflections on some recent progress in human radiobiology. In: Augenstein LG, Mason R, Zelle M, eds. *Advances in Radiation Biology.* New York, NY: Academic Press; 1969.

Shipman TL, Lushbaugh CC, Peterson D, et al. Acute radiation death resulting from an accidental nuclear critical excursion. *J Occup Med* 1961;3:145-192.

Vriesendorp HM, van Bekkum DW. Role of total body irradiation in conditioning for bone marrow transplantation. In: Thierfelder S, Rodt H, Kolb HJ, eds. *Immunobiology of Bone Marrow Transplantation.* Berlin, Germany: Springer Verlag; 1980.

Vriesendorp HM, van Bekkum, DW. Total body irradiation. In: Broerse JJ, MacVittie T, eds. *Response to Total Body Irradiation in Different Species.* Amsterdam, The Netherlands: Martinus Nijhoff; 1984.

Wald N, Thoma GE. *Radiation Accidents: Medical Aspects of Neutron and Gamma-Ray Exposures.* Report ORNL-2748, Part B. Oak Ridge, Tenn: Oak Ridge National Laboratory; 1961.

Fractionation

Bedford JS, Hall EJ. Survival of HeLa cells cultured in vitro and exposed to protracted gamma irradiation. *Int J Radiat Biol* 1963;7: 377-383.

Bedford JS, Mitchell JB. Dose-rate effects in synchronous mammalian cells in culture. *Radiat Res* 1973;54:316-327.

Begg AC, Hofland I, Van Glabekke M, et al. Predictive value of potential doubling time for radiotherapy of head and neck tumor patients: results from the EORTC Cooperative Trial 22851. *Semin Radiat Oncol* 1992;2:22-25.

Belli JA, Shelton M. Potentially lethal radiation damage: repair by mammalian cells in culture. *Science* 1969;165:490-492.

Ben-Hur E, Elkind MM, Bronx BV. Thermally enhanced radiosensitivity of cultured Chinese hamster cells: inhibition of repair of sublethal damage and enhancement of lethal damage. *Radiat Res* 1974;55:38-51.

Dolbeare F, Beisker W, Pallavicini M, et al. Cytochemistry for BrdUrd/DNA analysis: stoichiometry and sensitivity. *Cytometry* 1985;6:521-530.

Dolbeare F, Gratzner H, Pallavicini M, et al. Flow cytometric measurements of total DNA content and incorporated bromodeoxyuridine. *Proc Natl Acad Sci U S A* 1983;80:5573-5577.

Elkind MM, Sutton H. Radiation response of mammalian cells grown in culture. I. Repair of x-ray damage in surviving Chinese hamster cells. *Radiat Res* 1960;13:556-593.

Fowler JF. Dose response curves for organ function or cell survival. *Br J Radiol* 1983;56:497-500.

Fowler JF. What next in fractionated radiotherapy? *Br J Cancer* 1984;49:285-300.

Fowler JF. Potential for increasing the differential response between tumors and normal tissues: can proliferation rate be used? *Int J Radiat Oncol Biol Phys* 12:641-645, 1986.

Fowler JF, Tepper JE, eds. Fractionation in radiation therapy. *Semin Radiat Oncol* 1992;2:1-72.

Hall EJ. Radiation dose-rate: a factor of importance in radiobiology and radiotherapy. *Br J Radiol* 1972;45:81-97.

Hall EJ. The biological basis of endocurietherapy. The Henschke Memorial Lecture, 1984, *Endocurie Hyperterm Oncol* 1985;1:141-151.

Hall EJ, Bedford JS. Dose rate: its effect on the survival of HeLa cells irradiated with gamma rays. *Radiat Res* 1964;22:305-315.

Hansen O, Overgaard J, Hansen HS, et al. Importance of overall treatment time for the outcome of radiotherapy of advanced head and neck carcinoma: dependency on tumor differentiation, *Radiother Oncol* 1997;43:47-51.

Hendry JH, Bentzen SM, Dale RG, et al. A modeled comparison of the effects of using different ways to compensate for missed treatment days in radiotherapy. *Clin Oncol* 1996;8:297-307.

Little JB, Hahn GM, Frindel E, et al. Repair of potentially lethal radiation damage in vitro and in vivo. *Radiology* 1973;106:689-694.

Mitchell JB, Bedford JS, Bailey SM. Dose-rate effects on the cell cycle and survival of S3 HeLa and V79 cells. *Radiat Res* 1979;79:520-536.

Nakatsugawa S, Kumar A, Ono K, et al. Increased tumor curability by radiotherapy combined with PLDR inhibitors in murine cancers. IAEA-SR, 62, prospective methods of radiation therapy in developing countries. *IAEA-TECDOC* 1982;266:77-86.

Nakatsugawa S, Sugahara T, Kumar A. Purine nucleoside analogues inhibit the repair of radiation induced potentially lethal damage in mammalian cells in culture. *Int J Radiat Biol* 1982;41:343-346.

Overgaard J, Hjelm-Hansen M, Johnsen LV, et al. Comparison of conventional and split-course radiotherapy as primary treatment in carcinoma of the larynx. *Acta Oncol* 1988;27:147-152.

Overgaard J, Sand Hansen H, Sapru W, et al. Conventional radiotherapy as the primary treatment of squamous cell carcinoma of the head and neck: a randomized multicenter study of 5 versus 6 fractions per week—preliminary report from the DAHANCA 6 and 7 trial. *Radiother Oncol* 1996;40:S31.

Peters LJ, Withers HR, Thames HD. Radiobiological bases for multiple daily fractionation. In: Kaercher KH, Kogelnik HD, Reinartz G, eds. *Progress in Radio-oncology*, Vol 2. New York, NY: Raven Press; 1982.

Phillips RA, Tolmach LJ. Repair of potentially lethal damage in x-irradiated HeLa cells. *Radiat Res* 1966;29:413-432.

Saunders MI, Dische S, Barrett A. et al. Randomised multicentre trials of CHART vs. conventional radiotherapy in head and neck cancer and non-small-cell lung cancer: an interim report. *Br J Cancer* 1996;73:1455-1462.

Saunders MI, Dische S, Hong A, et al. Continuous hyperfractionated accelerated radiotherapy in locally advanced carcinoma of the head and neck region. *Int J Radiat Oncol Biol Phys* 1989;17:1287-1293.

Sinclair WK. Cyclic x-ray responses in mammalian cells in vitro. *Radiat Res* 1968;33:620-643.

Sinclair WK. Radiation survival in synchronous and asynchronous Chinese hamster cells *in vitro*. In: *Biophysical Aspects of Radiation Quality*. Proceedings of the IInd IAEA Panel; Vienna; 1967. Vienna, Austria: IAEA; 1968.

Sinclair WK. Dependence of radiosensitivity upon cell age. In: *Proceedings of the Carmel Conference on Time and Dose Relationships in Radiation Biology as Applied to Radiotherapy*, BNL Report 50203 (C-57). Upton, NY: Brookhaven National Laboratory; 1969.

Sinclair WK, Morton RA. X-ray sensitivity during the cell generation cycle of cultured Chinese hamster cells. *Radiat Res* 1966;29:450-474.

Suit H, Urano M. Repair of sublethal radiation injury in hypoxic cells of a C3H mouse mammary carcinoma. *Radiat Res* 1969;37:423-434.

Terasima R, Tolmach LJ. X-ray sensitivity and DNA synthesis in synchronous populations of HeLa cells. *Science* 1963;140:490-492.

Tubiana N, Malaise E. Growth rate and cell kinetics in human tumors: some prognostic and therapeutic implications. In: Symington T, Carter RL, eds. *Scientific Foundations of Oncology*. St Louis, Mo; Mosby; 1976.

Weichselbaum RR, Little JB, Nove J. Response of human osteosarcoma in vitro to irradiation: evidence for unusual cellular repair activity. *Int J Radiat Biol* 1977;31:295-299.

Weichselbaum RR, Schmitt A, Little JB. Cellular repair factors influencing radiocurability of human malignant tumors. *Br J Cancer* 1982;45:10-16.

Withers HR. Isoeffect curves for various proliferative tissues in experimental animals. In: *Proceedings of Conference on Time-dose Relationships in Clinical Radiotherapy*. Madison, Wis: Madison Printing and Publishing; 1975.

Withers HR. Response of tissues to multiple small dose fractions. *Radiat Res* 1977;71:24-33.

Withers HR, Peters LJ, Taylor JMG, et al. Late normal tissue sequelae from radiation therapy for carcinoma of the tonsil: patterns of fractionation study of radiobiology. *Int J Radiat Oncol Biol Phys* 1995;33:563-568.

Modifiers of Radiation Effects

Adams GE. Chemical radiosensitization of hypoxic cells. *Br Med Bull* 1973;29:48-53.

Adams GE, Clarke ED, Gray P, et al. Structure-activity relationships in the development of hypoxic cell radiosensitizers. II. Cytotoxicity and therapeutic ratio. *Int J Radiat Biol* 1979;35:151-160.

Bagshaw MA, Doggett RL, Smith KC. Intra-arterial 5-bromodeoxyuridine and x-ray therapy. *AJR Am J Roentgenol* 1967;99:889-894.

Barendsen GW. Impairment of the proliferative capacity of human cells in culture by alpha particles with differing linear energy transfer. *Int J Radiat Biol* 1964;8:453-466.

Batterman JJ. *Clinical Application of Fast Neutrons: the Amsterdam Experience*. Amsterdam, The Netherlands: Rodipi; 1981.

Brown JM, Goffinet DR, Cleaver JE, et al. Preferential radiosensitization of mouse sarcoma relative to normal skin by chronic intra-arterial infusion of halogenated pyrimidine analogs. *J Natl Cancer Inst* 1971;47:75-89.

Brown JM, Lemmon MJ. Potentiation by the hypoxic cytotoxin SR4233 of cell killing produced by fractionated irradiation of mouse tumors. *Cancer Res* 1990;50:7745-7749.

Catterall M. The treatment of advanced cancer by fast neutrons from the Medical Research Council's cyclotron at Hammersmith Hospital, London. *Eur J Cancer* 1974;10:343.

Catterall M. Results of neutron therapy: differences, correlations, and improvements. *Int J Radiat Oncol Biol Phys* 1982;8:2141-2144.

Chapman JD, Whitmore GF. Chemical modifiers of cancer treatment. *Int J Radiat Oncol Biol Phys* 1984;10:1161-1813.

Coleman CN. Hypoxic cell radiosensitizers: expectations and progress in drug development. *Int J Radiat Oncol Biol Phys* 1985;11:323-329.

Deschner EE, Gray LH. Influence of oxygen tension on x-ray-induced chromosomal damage in Ehrlich ascites tumor cells irradiated in vitro and in vivo. *Radiat Res* 1959;11:115-146.

Elkind MM, Swain RW, Alescio T, et al. Oxygen, nitrogen, recovery and radiation therapy. In: Shalek R, ed. *Cellular Radiation Biology*. Baltimore, Md: Williams & Wilkins; 1965.

Field SB, Jones T, Thomlinson RH. The relative effect of fast neutrons and x-rays on tumor and normal tissue in the rat, II: fractionation recovery and reöxygenation. *Br J Radiol* 1968;41:597-607.

Fowler JF, Morgan RL. Pretherapeutic experiments with the fast neutron beam from the Medical Research Council cyclotron, VIII: general review. *Br J Radiol* 1963;36:115-121.

Fowler JF, Morgan RL, Wood CAP. Pretherapeutic experiments with fast neutron beam from the Medical Research Council cyclotron, I: the biological and physical advantages and problems of neutron therapy. *Br J Radiol* 1963;36:77-80.

Hall EJ. Radiobiology of heavy particle radiation therapy: cellular studies. *Radiology* 1973;108:119-129.

Hall EJ, Astor M, Geard C, et al. Cytotoxicity of Ro-07-0582; enhancement by hyperthermia and protection by cysteamine. *Br J Cancer* 1977;35:809-815.

Hall EJ, Graves RG, Phillips TL, et al. Particle accelerators in radiation therapy. *Int J Radiat Oncol Biol Phys* 1982;8:2041-2207.

Hall EJ, Roizin-Towle L. Hypoxic sensitizers: radiobiological studies at the cellular level. *Radiology* 1975;117:453.

Howes AE. An estimation of changes in the proportion and absolute numbers of hypoxic cells after irradiation of transplanted C3H mouse mammary tumors. *Br J Radiol* 1969;42:441-447.

Kallman RF, Jardine LJ, Johnson CW. Effects of different schedules of dose fractionation on the oxygenation status of a transplantable mouse sarcoma. *J Natl Cancer Inst* 1970;44:369-377.

Kinsella T, Mitchell J, Russo A, et al. Continuous intravenous infusions of bromodeoxyuridine as a clinical radiosensitizer. *J Clin Oncol* 1984;2:1144-1150.

Kinsella T, Mitchell J, Russo A, et al. The use of halogenated thymidine analogs as clinical radiosensitizers: rationale, current status, and future prospects: non-hypoxic cell sensitizers. *Int J Radiat Oncol Biol Phys* 1984;10:1399-1406.

Mitchell J, Kinsella T, Russo A, et al. Radiosensitization of hematopoietic precursor cells (CFUc) in glioblastoma patients receiving intermittent intravenous infusions of bromodeoxyuridine (BUdR). *Int J Radiat Oncol Biol Phys* 1983;9:457-463.

Mitchell J, Russo A, Kinsella T, et al. The use of non-hypoxic cell sensitizers in radiobiology and radiotherapy, *Int J Radiat Oncol Biol Phys* 1986;12:1513-1518.

Moulder JE, Rockwell S. Hypoxic fractions of solid tumors: experimental techniques, methods of analysis and a survey of existing data. *Int J Radiat Oncol Biol Phys* 1984;10:695-712.

Nordsmark M, Overgaard M, Overgaard J. Pretreatment oxygenation predicts radiation response in advanced squamous cell carcinoma of the head and neck. *Radiother Oncol* 1996;41:31-40.

Overgaard J, Horsman MR. Modification of hypoxia induced radioresistance in tumours by the use of oxygen and sensitizers. *Semin Radiat Oncol* 1996;6:10-21.

Overgaard J, Sand-Hansen H, Lindeløv B, et al. Nimorazole as a hypoxic radiosensitizer in the treatment of supraglottic larynx and pharynx carcinoma. First report from the Danish Head and Neck Cancer Study (DAHANCA) Protocol 5-85. *Radiother Oncol* 1991;20:143-150.

Overgaard J, Sand-Hansen H, Overgaard M, et al. The Danish Head and Neck Cancer Study Group (DAHANCA) randomized trials with radiosentizers in carcinoma of the larynx and pharynx. In: Dewey WC, Eddington M, Fry RJM, et al, eds. *Radiation Research. A Twentieth Century Perspective.* Vol II. New York, NY: Academic Press; 1992:573-577.

Powers WE, Tolmach LJ. A multicomponent x-ray survival curve for mouse lymphosarcoma cells irradiated in vivo. *Nature* 1963;197:710-711.

Report of the RBE Committee to the International Commissions on Radiological Protection and on Radiological Units and Measurements. *Health Phys* 1963;9:357.

Roizin-Towle LA, Hall EJ, Flynn M, et al. Enhanced cytotoxicity of melphalan by prolonged exposure to nitroimidazoles: the role of endogenous thiols. *Int J Radiat Oncol Biol Phys* 1982;8:757-760.

Rose CM, Millar JL, Peacock JH, et al. Differential enhancement of melphalan cytotoxicity in tumor and normal tissue by misonidazole. In: Brady LW, ed. *Radiation Sensitizers.* New York, NY: Masson Publishing; 1980.

Sutherland RM. Selective chemotherapy of non-cycling cells in an in vitro tumor model. *Cancer Res* 1974;34:3501.

Sutherland RM, ed. Conference on chemical modification: radiation and cytotoxic drugs; Key Biscayne, Florida; 17-20 September, 1981. *Int J Radiat Oncol Biol Phys* 1982;8:323-815.

Thomlinson RH. Changes of oxygenation in tumors in relation to irradiation, *Front Radiat Ther Oncol* 1968;3:109-121.

Thomlinson RH. Reoxygenation as a function of tumor size and histopathological type. In: *Proceedings of the Carmel Conference on Time and Dose Relationships in Radiation Biology as Applied to Radiotherapy.* BNL Report 50203 (C-57). Upton, NY: Brookhaven National Laboratory; 1969.

Thomlinson RH, Dische S, Gray AJ, et al. Clinical testing of the radiosensitizers Ro-07-0582, III: response of tumors. *Clin Radiol* 1976;27:167-174.

Utley JF, Marlowe C, Waddell WJ. Distribution of ^{35}S-labeled WR-2721 in normal and malignant tissues of the mouse. *Radiat Res* 1976;68:284-291.

van Putten LM. Tumor reoxygenation during fractionated radiotherapy: studies with a transplantable osteosarcoma. *Eur J Cancer* 1968;4:173-182.

Withers HR, Thames HD, Peters LJ. Biological bases for high RBE values for late effects of neutron irradiation. *Int J Radiat Oncol Biol Phys* 1982;8:2071-2076.

Wong TW, Whitmore GF, Gulyas S. Studies on the toxicity and radiosensitizing ability of misonidazole under conditions of prolonged incubation. *Radiat Res* 1978;75:541-555.

Yuhas J. Active versus passive absorption kinetics as the basis for selective protection of normal tissues by S-2-(3-aminopropylamino)-ethyl-phosphorothioic acid. *Cancer Res* 1980;40:1519-1524.

Adjuncts to Radiation

Cox JD, Byhardt RW, Komaki R, et al. Interaction of thoracic irradiation and chemotherapy on local control and survival in small cell carcinoma of the lung. *Cancer Treat Rep* 1979;63:1251-1255.

Dewey WC, Hopwood LE, Sapareto SA, et al. Cellular responses to combinations of hyperthermia and radiation. *Radiology* 1977;123:463-474.

Eddy HA. Alterations in tumor microvasculature during hyperthermia. *Radiology* 1980;137:515-521.

Elkind MM. Fundamental questions in the combined use of radiation and chemicals in the treatment of cancer. *Int J Radiat Oncol Biol Phys* 1979;5:1711-1720.

Gerner EW, Boone R, Conner WG, et al. A transient thermotolerant survival response produced by single thermal doses in HeLa cells. *Cancer Res* 1976;36:1035-1040.

Gerweck LE, Gillette EL, Dewey WC. Killing of Chinese hamster cells in vitro by heating under hypoxic or aerobic conditions. *Eur J Cancer* 1974;10:691-693.

Gerweck LE, Gillette EL, Dewey WC. Effect of heat and radiation on synchronous Chinese hamster cells: killing and repair. *Radiat Res* 1975;64:611-623.

Hahn GM, Braun J, Har-Kedar I. Thermochemotherapy: synergism between hyperthermia (42°-43°) and adriamycin (or bleomycin) in mammalian cell inactivation. *Proc Natl Acad Sci U S A* 1975;72:937-940.

Hall EJ, Roizin-Towle L. Biological effects of heat. *Cancer Res* 1984;44:4708-4713S.

Perez C, Brady L, Cox J, et al. Randomized study to evaluate efficacy of levamisole in patients with unresectable non-oat cell carcinoma of the lung treated with radiation therapy. *Int J Radiat Oncol Biol Phys* 1984;10:97-98.

Rubin P. The Franz Buschke Lecture. Late effects of chemotherapy and radiation therapy: a new hypothesis. *Int J Radiat Oncol Biol Phys* 1984;10:5-34.

Stewart JR. Past clinical studies and future directions. *Cancer Res* 1984;44:4902-4904S.

Tefft M, Chabora BMcC, Rosen G. Radiation in bone sarcomas. A re-evaluation in the era of intensive systemic chemotherapy. *Cancer* 1977;39:806-816.

Tubiana M. Les associations radiotherapiechemotherapie. *J Eur Radiotherapy* 1980;1:107-114.

Westra A, Dewey WC. Variation in sensitivity to heat shock during the cell cycle of Chinese hamster cells in vitro. *Int J Radiat Biol* 1971;19:467-477.

Mutagenesis and Carcinogenesis

Boice JD Jr, Land CE, Shore RE, et al. Risk of breast cancer following low-dose exposure. *Radiology* 1979;131:589-597.

Bond VP, Thiessens JW, eds. *Re-evaluation of Dosimetric Factors: Hiroshima and Nagasaki.* Proceedings Symposium. Springfield, Va: US Department of Energy, US Department of Commerce; 1982.

Cardis E, Gilbert ES, Carpenter L, et al. Effects of low doses and low dose rates of external ionizing radiation: cancer mortality among nuclear industry workers in three countries. *Radiat Res* 1995; 142:117-132.

Committee on the Biological Effects of Ionizing Radiation. *BEIR III Committee Report: Effects on Populations of Exposure to Low Levels of Ionizing Radiation.* Washington, DC: National Academy of Sciences, National Research Council; 1980.

Court-Brown WM, Doll R. Mortality from cancer and other causes after radiotherapy for ankylosing spondylitis. *Br Med J* 1965;2:1327-1332.

Court-Brown WM, Doll R, Hill AB. The incidence of leukemia following exposure to diagnostic radiation in utero. *Br Med J* 1960;2:1539.

Doll R, Smith PG. The long-term effects of x-irradiation in patients treated for metropathia haemorrhagic. *Br J Radiol* 1968;41: 362-368.

Doll R, Wakeford R. Risk of childhood cancer from fetal irradiation. *Br J Radiol* 1997;70:130-139.

Finkel AL, Miller CE, Hasterlik RJ: Radium-induced tumors in man. In: Mays CW, ed. *Delayed Effects of Bone-seeking Radionuclides.* Salt Lake City, Utah: University of Utah Press; 1969.

Jablon S, Belsky JL, Tachikawa K, et al. Cancer in Japanese exposed as children to atomic bombs. *Lancet* 1971;1:927-932.

Jablon S, Kato H. Childhood cancer in relation to prenatal exposure to atomic bomb radiation. *Lancet* 1970;2:1000-1003.

Hempelmann LH. Risk of thyroid neoplasms after irradiation in childhood. *Science* 1968;160:159-163.

Hempelmann LH, Pifer JW, Burke GJ, et al. Neoplasms in persons treated with x-rays in infancy for thymic enlargement: a report of third follow-up survey. *J Natl Cancer Inst* 1967;38:317-341.

IARC Study Group on Cancer Risk Among Nuclear Industry Workers. Direct estimates of cancer mortality due to low doses of ionizing radiation: an international study. *Lancet* 1994;344:1039-1043.

International Commission on Radiological Protection. *ICRP 60: 1990 Recommendations of the International Commission on Radiological Protection.* Oxford, England: Pergamon Press; 1990.

MacKenzie I. Breast cancer following multiple fluoroscopies. *Br J Cancer.* 1965;19:1-8.

MacMahon B. Prenatal x-ray exposure and childhood cancer. *J Natl Cancer Inst* 1962;28:1173-1191.

Modan B, Baidatz D, Mart H, et al. Radiation induced head and neck tumors. *Lancet* 1974;1:277.

Muller HJ. The nature of the genetic effects produced by radiation. In: Hollaender A, ed. *Radiation Biology.* New York, NY: McGraw-Hill; 1954.

Pierce DA, Shimizu Y, Preston DK, et al. Studies of the mortality of atomic bomb survivors, Report 12, Part I: Cancer: 1950-1990. *Radiat Res* 1996;146:1-27.

Rowland RE, Stehney AF, Lucas HF. Dose-response relationships for female radium dial workers. *Radiat Res* 1978;76:308.

Russell WL. X-ray-induced mutations in mice. Cold Spring Harbor Symp. *Quant Biol* 1951;16:327-336.

Russell WL. The nature of the dose-rate effect of radiation on mutation in mice. *Jpn J Genet* 1965;40:128-140.

Schull WL, Otake M, Neal JV. Genetic effects of the atomic bomb: a reappraisal. *Science* 1981;213:1220-1227.

Selby PB. Induced skeletal mutations, *Genetics* 92:127-133, 1979.

Selby PB. The doubling dose for radiation, or for any other mutagen, is actually several times larger than has been previously thought if it is based on specific-locus mutation frequencies in mice. *Environ Mol Mutagen* 1996;27:61.

Stewart A, Kneale GW. Changes in the cancer risk associated with obstetric radiography. *Lancet* 1968;1:104-107.

Stewart A, Webb J, Hewitt D. A survey of childhood malignancies. *Br Med J* 1958;1:1495-1508.

United Nations Scientific Committee on the Effects of Atomic Radiation. *Sources and Effects of Ionizing Radiation.* New York, NY: United Nations; 1977.

United Nations Scientific Committee on the Effects of Atomic Radiation. *Ionizing Radiation Sources and Biological Effects.* New York, NY: United Nations; 1988.

Upton AC. The dose response relation in radiation induced cancer. *Cancer Res* 1961;21:717-729.

Wolff S. Radiation genetics. *Annu Rev Genet* 1967;1:221-244.

CHAPTER 2

Clinical Radiation Physics

Kenneth R. Hogstrom, John A. Antolak, William F. Hanson, John L. Horton, Isaac I. Rosen, Almon S. Shiu, and George Starkschall

TECHNOLOGIC ADVANCES

The last decade of the twentieth century marked significant changes in the technical aspects of radiation oncology. These changes resulted largely from computer advances that have allowed the development of new technology related to diagnosis, planning, and treatment in radiation oncology. Most radiation oncologists have wanted to see this technology used in the clinic as rapidly as possible to improve patient care. This chapter presents for the radiation oncologist a view of this new technology from the perspective of the medical physicist.

Modern advances are best introduced by a vision of radiation oncology in the twenty-first century. The first step after diagnosis and decision to treat with radiation oncology is the physician's prescription of dose. The three-dimensional computed tomography (CT) data set will likely continue to be the patient data required for designing radiation treatments. Ancillary to the patient data set will be the dose prescription and outlines of normal tissue structures. With the use of multimodality imaging for functional and biological imaging[1,2] and with the knowledge of the extent of disease, the prescription of dose could become a complex three-dimensional distribution, significantly different than the present convention of a constant dose to a specified volume with perhaps one or two additional prescriptions to boost volumes. The second step will be to delineate volume outlines of normal tissue, a process that is now manual but will become automatic, as is already the case for lung and bone.[3,4] The third step will be to design a treatment that delivers the optimal arrangement of beams or radioactive sources for the available treatment modalities, which could be x-rays, electrons, protons, brachytherapy, or a combination of two or more of these. In some cases this is already becoming automated, as in the use of intensity-modulated radiation therapy (IMRT).[5] The ability of the treatment plan's computer-calculated dose distribution to meet the dose prescription is evaluated by the radiation oncologist and approved before treatment. The fourth step is for the patient to be positioned for treatment and, for fractionated treatment, to be repositioned automatically to account for daily errors in positioning or changes in anatomy.[6,7] The fifth step is for the treatment to be delivered under computer control, with its delivery synchronized to account for internal motion resulting from breathing, circulation, or other involuntary muscle movement.[8-11] The sixth step is to verify the proper delivery of treatment and patient positioning and then for that to be recorded by automated methods.

The radiation oncology community is in the early stages of refining this vision, and some institutions and vendors have progressed further than others. However, regardless of a particular institution's capability, a common set of questions and issues must be appreciated and addressed, including the value of the new technology to the patient and its cost and safety. Verifying the value of the new technology, which is the responsibility of the radiation oncologist, could take place over time through the use of randomized clinical trials and comparisons with historical data. This topic will not be discussed here; rather, the purpose of this chapter is to give the radiation oncologist an appreciation of the value of medical physics and dosimetry in the efficient, safe use of the new technology.

Adequate Support of Technology Endeavors

The presence of adequate, competent medical-physics support is necessary to support new technology in the radiation oncology clinic. For a medical physicist, competence is defined by certification in therapeutic radiation oncology by the American Board of Radiology, in radiation oncology physics by the American Board of Medical Physics or in an equivalent specialty by another board.[12] In some states (presently Texas, Florida, and Hawaii), licensure is required,[13] although other states may require board certification or other minimum qualifications. As the breadth and sophistication of the new technology increase, the need for residency training in radiation oncology physics will become more critical for a radiation therapy clinic to be able to deliver high-technology treatment safely and effectively.[14] When this chapter was written, at least six residency training

TABLE 2-1

Summary of Equipment and Physics and Dosimetry Costs for Special Procedures

	COSTS	
Procedures	Median	Mean ± S.D.
TOTAL-SKIN ELECTRON IRRADIATION		
Startup Costs and Effort		
Radiotherapy equipment ($)	2215	14,504 ± 6026
Physics equipment ($)	950	3885 ± 1083
Commissioning effort, medical physicist (h)	105	194 ± 45
Ongoing Effort		
Medical physicist (h/patient)	9	18 ± 4
Dosimetrist/technologist (h/patient)	5	11 ± 3
Total Costs, Equipment, and Effort		
Institutional distribution ($/patient)	2368	2796 ± 441
Patient-weighted mean ($/patient)	2079	
HIGH-DOSE-RATE REMOTE AFTERLOADING BRACHYTHERAPY		
Startup Costs and Effort		
Radiotherapy equipment ($)	480,980	446,832 ± 21,549
Physics equipment ($)	12,100	21,783 ± 3034
Commissioning effort, medical physicist (h)	170	331 ± 52
Ongoing Effort		
Medical physicist (h/patient)	8	11 ± 1
Dosimetrist/technologist (h/patient)	2	3 ± 0
Total Costs, Equipment, and Effort		
Institutional distribution ($/patient)	863	1069 ± 95
Patient-weighted mean ($/patient)	879	
TOTAL-BODY IRRADIATION		
Startup Costs and Effort		
Radiotherapy equipment ($)	2500	11,512 ± 5265
Physics equipment ($)	1250	9177 ± 2564
Commissioning effort, medical physicist (h)	85	161 ± 29
Ongoing Effort		
Medical physicist (h/patient)	9	18 ± 9
Dosimetrist/technologist (h/patient)	3	6 ± 1
Total Costs, Equipment, and Effort		
Institutional distribution ($/patient)	1062	2341 ± 1167
Patient-weighted mean ($/patient)	772	
LINEAR-ACCELERATOR-BASED STEREOTACTIC RADIOSURGERY		
Startup Costs and Effort		
Radiotherapy equipment ($)	285,170	281,170 ± 31,330
Physics equipment ($)	5000	19,047 ± 5488
Commissioning effort, medical physicist (h)	200	345 ± 51
Ongoing Effort		
Medical physicist (h/patient)	11	13 ± 1
Dosimetrist/technologist (h/patient)	3	5 ± 1
Total Costs, Equipment, and Effort		
Institutional distribution ($/patient)	1277	1646 ± 209
Patient-weighted mean ($/patient)	1168	

programs in radiation oncology physics were either accredited or seeking accreditation by the Commission on Accreditation of Medical Physics Education Programs. The rate of growth and acceptance of these programs will be significantly influenced by physician appreciation and support of professional training for medical physics that parallels physicians' professional training in radiation oncology.[15]

Two issues regarding medical-physics staffing are significant. The first is having an adequate number of

TABLE 2-1
Summary of Equipment and Physics and Dosimetry Costs for Special Procedures—cont'd

Procedures	COSTS	
	Median	Mean ± S.D.
INTRAOPERATIVE RADIATION THERAPY		
Startup Costs and Effort		
Radiotherapy equipment ($)	9400	290,707 ± 174,356
Physics equipment ($)	6000	7104 ± 2107
Commissioning effort, medical physicist (h)	225	399 ± 147
Ongoing Effort		
Medical physicist (h/patient)	6	15 ± 7
Dosimetrist/technologist (h/patient)	1	7 ± 7
Total Costs, Equipment, and Effort		
Institutional distribution ($/patient)	767	1830 ± 785
Patient-weighted mean ($/patient)	786	
ELECTRON-ARC IRRADIATION		
Startup Costs and Effort		
Radiotherapy equipment ($)	22,500	16,970 ± 5750
Physics equipment ($)	0	2689 ± 1585
Commissioning effort, medical physicist (h)	200	413 ± 158
Ongoing Effort		
Medical physicist (h/patient)	12	13 ± 3
Dosimetrist/technologist (h/patient)	9	14 ± 6
Total Costs, Equipment, and Effort		
Institutional distribution ($/patient)	3278	4144 ± 1078
Patient-weighted mean ($/patient)	2407	
STEREOTACTIC BRACHYTHERAPY		
Startup Costs and Effort		
Radiotherapy equipment ($)	27,500	34,958 ± 9285
Physics equipment ($)	0	1558 ± 907
Commissioning effort, medical physicist (h)	100	176 ± 52
Ongoing Effort		
Medical physicist (h/patient)	15	17 ± 2
Dosimetrist/technologist (h/patient)	3	3 ± 1
Total Costs, Equipment, and Effort		
Institutional distribution ($/patient)	1744	1981 ± 376
Patient-weighted mean ($/patient)	1300	
THREE-DIMENSIONAL TREATMENT PLANNING (EXTERNAL BEAM)		
Startup Costs and Effort		
Physics equipment ($)	380,625	483,770 ± 94,161
Commissioning effort, medical physicist (h)	425	1050 ± 379
Ongoing Effort		
Medical physicist (h/plan)	5.1	8.5 ± 2.0
Dosimetrist/technologist (h/plan)	7.1	8.9 ± 2.0
Plans per patient	1.37	1.57 ± 0.20
Total Costs, Equipment, and Effort		
Institutional distribution ($/plan)	1562	3271 ± 776
Patient-weighted mean ($/plan)	1035	

medical physicists to support the size and complexity of the radiation therapy clinic. Historically, the rule of thumb was that one medical physicist was required for every 400 new patients treated each year.[16] However, this number was based on data collected before the introduction of present-day technology and hence ignores the time required for the new high-technology procedures. The effort for medical physicists and dosimetrists that is required to support these new procedures should be determined differently because, at least for the time being, they require significantly greater resources. A task group from the American College of Medical Physics recently studied the amount of resources needed for selected high-technology procedures[17] (Table 2-1); a detailed discussion of the use of this report for planning three-dimensional treatment was provided by Hogstrom and Rosen.[18] One important finding from that analysis was the significant variation in manpower per patient attributable to the number of patients treated and the differences in technology.

The other significant issue regarding staffing for high technology is understanding the time and efforts not specifically related to patient care that are required to support new technology. Such efforts include specification and acquisition of equipment and space, commissioning of equipment and techniques, training of all members of the radiation oncology team, and ongoing provision of quality assurance for the equipment. The commissioning time is often long because manufacturers do not always provide adequate documentation of the new technology, the equipment often does not interface with other equipment in the clinic, temporary solutions must be devised to address deficiencies in equipment operation, and the medical physics staff may be inexperienced with the new technology. The last problem can be addressed through continuing education (e.g., by attending vendor-training classes, visiting institutions that have experience with the new technology, or attending scientific workshops). Some vendors also offer commissioning for a fee, which is often subcontracted to a medical physicist with expertise in this area. In such cases, the quality of commissioning is a concern. In the authors' experience, many medical physicists, including those that serve as subcontractors, might not use an adequate set of standards for the commissioning process. This can be problematic because fast commissioning times could result in inaccurate dose calculations outside normally acceptable ranges, inaccuracies of which both the medical physicist and radiation oncologist could be unaware.

Therefore before embarking on new high-technology endeavors, the radiation oncologist must specify his or her expectations; an adequate number of qualified medical physicists must be available to support these expectations; and adequate equipment, space, and time must be budgeted to commission the technique. These requirements put the onus on the radiation oncologist to be specific, the medical physicist to be able to justify staffing and operational plans, and the administrator to place safety and accuracy above clinical and economic pressures.

Medical physicists at The University of Texas M.D. Anderson Cancer Center work continually with radiation oncologists and administrative staff to bring new technology into the radiation oncology clinic, and such activity has been particularly fervent over the past several years. In the remainder of this chapter, the authors describe their insights and experiences with three-dimensional treatment planning and delivery, IMRT, stereotactic irradiation, electron conformal therapy, gated radiation therapy, high-dose-rate brachytherapy, and prostate implant therapy. Finally, the role of quality assurance in high-technology radiation oncology trials is discussed, particularly the use of a portal imaging and picture archival and communications systems (PACS) in the clinic and the support provided by the Radiological Physics Center for multi-institutional clinical trials.

THREE-DIMENSIONAL TREATMENT PLANNING AND DELIVERY

Three-dimensional treatment planning refers to the use of the patient's three-dimensional geometry to select beam directions, design beam apertures, compute doses, evaluate plans, and generate treatment verification images.[19] This term is an unfortunate misnomer that has sometimes been misinterpreted to mean the use of any beam arrangement that is not coplanar or not transaxial. Three-dimensional treatment planning also is not multislice two-dimensional planning.[20]

True three-dimensional treatment planning requires the direct involvement of the physician in the planning process; it requires complex software that is more difficult to commission for routine clinical use; it requires more training for physicians, physicists, and dosimetrists; and it often results in more complex plans that require careful implementation on therapy machines. Quality assurance for both the treatment planning and the daily treatment delivery also requires more effort and more knowledge than did previous techniques.[21]

The primary goal of three-dimensional treatment planning is to improve the therapeutic ratio, either by increasing the tumor dose without increasing morbidity or by reducing complications without sacrificing tumor control. To achieve either aim requires sparing normal tissue by confining the high-dose region to the target volume. Treatment techniques that accomplish this goal are generally called *conformal*.

Use of Volumetric Data

A key element in three-dimensional treatment planning is the use of a volumetric data set to delineate the patient's tumor and normal tissues. Parts of the three-dimensional surfaces of the prostate, rectum, and bladder, reconstructed from outlines drawn on the CT images, are shown in Figure 2-1 (see also Color Plate 1, after p. 80). Magnetic resonance (MR) images are often used in combination with the CT images for better tumor definition. Biological imaging using MR spectroscopy, positron

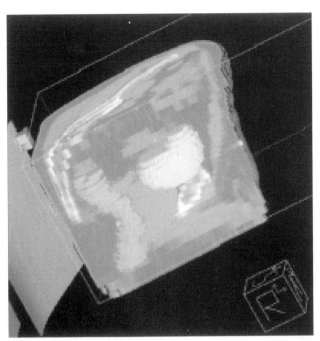

Fig. 2-1 Three-dimensional surfaces of the prostate *(green)*, rectum *(blue)*, and bladder *(yellow)* reconstructed from outlines drawn on the computed tomography images. (See Color Plate 1, after p. 80, for color reproduction.)

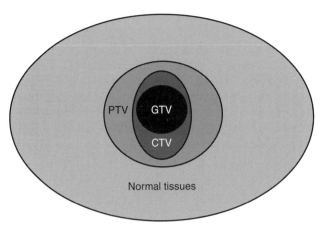

Fig. 2-2 The International Commission on Radiation Units and Measurements' Report 50 defined the gross target volume *(GTV)* as identified disease, the clinical target volume *(CTV)* as the GTV plus margin for microscopic disease, and the planning target volume *(PTV)* as the GTV plus margin for interfraction and intrafraction variations in tumor position.

emission tomography (PET), and single photon emission computed tomography (SPECT) are rapidly being incorporated into three-dimensional treatment planning.[1]

A standard method for defining target volumes was developed by the International Commission on Radiation Units and Measurement (ICRU) and published in its ICRU-50 report.[22,23] This standard was established with the goal of facilitating uniformity in prescribing, delivering, and reporting tumor doses so that clinical results from different institutions could be directly compared. The most important concepts introduced in the ICRU-50 are those of gross, clinical, and planning target volumes (Fig. 2-2). Use of these defined volumes, typically abbreviated as GTV, CTV, and PTV, requires the explicit delineation of subclinical microscopic disease and the quantitative incorporation of variation in patient set-up and organ or tumor motion. To escalate tumor doses without increasing the morbidity to normal tissue generally requires the use of more beams with smaller apertures. The margins defined in ICRU-50 attempt to distinguish those volumes that can be reduced without loss of local control through the use of better technology (e.g., repositioning and immobilization devices or motion-gated beam control) from those volumes that are biological and cannot be reduced without increased risk of recurrence. In 1999 the ICRU published its Report 62, in which some of the ICRU-50 concepts were refined and definitions added for internal margin, set-up margin, internal target volume, planning organ-at-risk volume, and conformity index.[24]

Numerous studies have been conducted worldwide on interfraction variations in patient set-up, interfraction mobility of tumor and normal tissues, and intrafraction organ motion.[25] The results, not surprisingly, depend on the type of immobilization used, the position of the patient, and the anatomic site of treatment. The authors studied set-up variation and organ mobility in prostate treatment by using online electronic portal imaging and multiple CT scans over the course of treatment.[26] Like others, the authors found that prostate mobility correlated significantly with rectal volume. These and other published results can be used in treatment planning when the same immobilization and set-up methods are used.

Knowledge of variations in set-up and mobility and motion of organs is used to determine the margin between the CTV and PTV. Typically, these variations are assumed to be normally distributed and independent so that they can be added in quadrature. They are usually reported in terms of the standard deviation of the mean. In theory, the treatment plan should deliver the prescribed tumor dose to the PTV so that the CTV receives the full dose regardless of where the CTV is within the PTV at any given time. In practice, the margin is set as some multiple of the measured uncertainty, which determines the probability of the CTV receiving the PTV dose. The margins suggested on the basis of a simple Gaussian distribution of motion often are too large relative to those suggested by clinical experience. A theoretical analysis was performed using more realistic assumptions, and it was found that using a margin of 1.65 times the standard deviation of the mean positional uncertainty in each direction of the CTV gives a PTV such that any point on the surface of the CTV is within the PTV 95% of the time.[27] For the prostate, this result matches well with the authors' clinical experience.

Beam Arrangement

The process of designing the best beam arrangement for a patient uses more information than does the conventional two-dimensional treatment planning process. In addition to selecting beam directions, treatment planners must create beam apertures from the projections of the target and normal tissues rather than from radiographs showing only bony anatomy. A beam's-eye view display used to draw the beam shape for treating the prostate from a lateral oblique direction is shown in Figure 2-3 (see also Color Plate 2, after p. 80). The margin around the PTV compensates for the finite penumbra of the beam. The treatment planning system is also used to generate digitally reconstructed radiographs for verifying the patient's position on the treatment machine. A digitally reconstructed radiograph for a conventional anterior prostate treatment beam is shown in Figure 2-4 (see also Color Plate 3, after p. 80). Such radiographs are produced by ray tracing through the CT images to compute a simulation of a radiograph taken from the beam direction and then superimposing a line drawing of the treatment beam shape. Portal images taken on the machine are compared with the reconstructed radiograph to assess the accuracy of the patient's position during treatment.

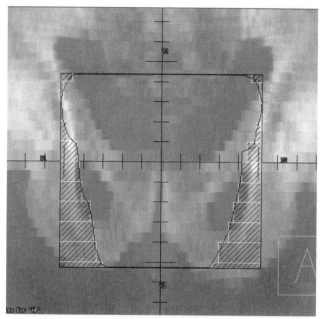

Fig. 2-4 Digitally reconstructed radiograph for a conventional anterior beam for prostate treatment. The beam aperture is superimposed on a gray-scale image reconstructed from the computed tomography data set and intended to approximate the image seen on a portal film. (See Color Plate 3, after p. 80, for color reproduction.)

After the beam arrangement (including directions, shapes, energies, and relative doses) is completed, doses within the patient are computed by using algorithms that include the effects of patient shape and tissue densities in all dimensions on the transport of both primary and secondary radiation. A variety of algorithms of varying accuracy and speed are commercially available (e.g., scatter-air ratio, pencil beam, convolution, or Monte Carlo).[28] In general, greater accuracy requires more computation time.

Evaluation of three-dimensional treatment plans uses not only multiple two-dimensional isodose displays but also three-dimensional dose surfaces and dose-volume histograms.[29] Isodose lines, color washes, and surface displays give detailed information about the physical locations of doses, but they give no information about irradiated volumes. Dose-volume histograms, on the other hand, clearly summarize the volumes irradiated to different dose levels but give no information about where doses occur within the organs. A dose-volume histogram for a patient receiving a conformal 10-field treatment to the prostate is shown in Figure 2-5. Dose-volume information has been found to correlate with clinical complications for many organs.[30-32] Isodose displays and dose-volume histograms provide complementary data that can be used by physicians to evaluate a treatment plan. Several biological models of tumor control and normal tissue complications have been developed with the goal of evaluating plans on the basis of

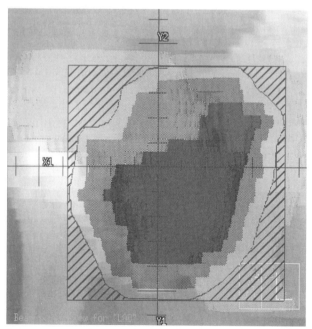

Fig. 2-3 Example of beam's-eye view display used to define the radiation beam aperture. The prostate *(magenta)*, bladder *(blue)*, and rectum *(green)* are shown from the perspective of the radiation beam. The beam aperture is drawn interactively on the computer to surround the target and avoid as much normal tissue as possible. (See Color Plate 2, after p. 80, for color reproduction.)

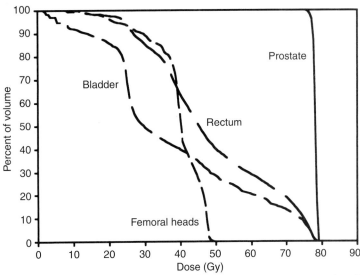

Fig. 2-5 Example of a dose-volume histogram for a prostate treatment using 10 coplanar beams. The histogram shows the percent volume of the target or organ receiving a given amount of radiation or more.

predicted clinical results. At present, these models are inadequate for treatment planning with patients.

Patient Positioning

Effective delivery of conformal treatments requires that the patient be immobilized and accurately repositioned for each fraction. Electronic portal imaging devices that allow patients to be imaged before each treatment have been applied to the problem of verifying conformal treatments.[33,34] There are two basic approaches to the routine clinical use of these devices. In interactive or online correction, the patient's position is adjusted before each treatment according to the results of a portal image. This approach removes both systematic and random variations in set-up. Studies have found that this approach can reduce set-up variations by up to a factor of two; however, treatment time is increased (by as much as 50% in some studies). An alternative method attempts to reduce only the systematic errors to a level below a clinically acceptable threshold. In this offline approach, the patient is imaged without correction for several fractions, and then the interfraction variation in set-up is computed and an adjustment is made to correct for the systematic component of the variation. This process is repeated throughout the course of treatment. Interfraction protocols achieve almost as good a result as the interactive approach and involve less effort. However, the use of automated or semiautomated algorithms for geometric registration of the portal image to the reference image in real time, coupled with the ability to adjust the patient position or beams remotely, improves the efficiency and appeal of the online method.

For some tumor sites, anatomic imaging methods other than x-ray are practical, more effective, or both. For treatments involving the head, for example, patient positions can be aligned by using video images of markers on the immobilization device[35] or images of the facial surface itself.[36] The rigidity of the anatomic structures and relative immobility of the target make surface-based positioning suitable for treatments to the head. As another example, x-ray portal images provide poor estimates of targeting accuracy of the prostate because the prostate is mobile relative to the skeleton. Sonography, however, can visualize the bladder, prostate, and rectum interfaces well. At the M.D. Anderson Cancer Center a specialized commercial sonography system is used to position patients being treated for prostate cancer before each treatment. The sonography system is interfaced to the treatment planning system so that the planned positions of the prostate, bladder, and rectum are superimposed on the sonograms. The therapist moves the patient until the prostate is in the proper position relative to the accelerator isocenter, as indicated by the combination of sonographic and treatment planning images.

Preparing a three-dimensional treatment planning system for clinical use is more difficult and time consuming than earlier, simpler treatment planning systems. Three-dimensional dose algorithms attempt to model the physical radiation transport and deposition processes and are therefore complex, with many parameters for which the values must be adjusted to give proper agreement between calculated and measured doses. Often parameter values cannot be directly determined by simple measurement. Therefore the modeling process can be a lengthy series of iterations in which parameter values are changed and then the effect on the computed doses is evaluated. The details of beam modeling, of course, depend on the details of the algorithm.[37,38]

Quality Assurance

Acceptance testing and quality assurance procedures for a three-dimensional treatment planning system focus on revealing significant software errors, determining the accuracy of geometric information, assessing the accuracy of dose calculation, and understanding the limitations of the system.[39,40] All sophisticated software systems have errors,[41] and three-dimensional treatment planning systems are no exception. Manufacturers go to considerable effort to avoid delivering systems that have errors that could potentially harm a patient. However, manufacturers can rarely predict all of the ways that a system will be used and cannot test all possible combinations of user operations. The medical physicist should test the treatment planning system with both extreme situations and with treatment techniques typical of the clinic in which the system is to be used to identify errors that could be encountered in routine use. Testing should be repeated after every software upgrade because major software revisions often contain errors in portions of the system that previously worked correctly.

The geometric accuracy of screen images and hard-copy graphics must be verified. Translations between the treatment planning coordinate system and the coordinate systems of the CT scanners and therapy machines must be clearly understood. Data output in digital form to other systems (e.g., those for recording and verification, multileaf collimators, block cutters, or milling machines) must be verified for geometric accuracy, correct orientation, and proper magnification.

The accuracy of the dose computation will depend on the inherent accuracy of the dose computation algorithm and the values of the beam model parameters. In particular, accuracy in the buildup and penumbra should be evaluated because these regions are the most difficult to model. The accuracy should be tested with measured data that were not part of the beam modeling data set.

Three-dimensional treatment planning and conformal radiation therapy produce dose distributions that are more focused, thereby sparing more normal tissues. For this advancement in technology to translate into improvement in clinical results, adequate resources must be dedicated to producing high-quality plans and to delivering them accurately and precisely. Analysis of a 1997 American College of Medical Physics survey[17] showed that experienced institutions (those that prepare more than 150 plans per year) were expending more than 7 hours of physics and dosimetry effort per three-dimensional plan, including maintenance of the planning system (Table 2-1). Moreover, efficiency in preparing plans was found to increase in tandem with the volume of plans prepared. Although the motivation for three-dimensional treatment planning and conformal treatments is the improved care of patients, such treatments can and must be financially self-supporting through appropriate billing and charge capture.

INTENSITY-MODULATED RADIATION THERAPY

For the purposes of this discussion, *IMRT* is defined as radiation therapy in which the intensity is modulated on a scale small enough to make forward planning impractical or impossible, thereby mandating inverse planning. Although use of a wedge or a field-in-field approach can be considered intensity modulation, the definition used here excludes the field-in-field approaches of Galvin and Chen[42] and Fraas and colleagues,[43,44] both of which can be used in the traditional forward-planning manner.

Inverse Treatment Planning

To define *inverse planning*, it is useful to first describe the traditional forward-planning approach. In forward planning, the planner proposes a possible arrangement of beams, including beam directions, shaping, modifiers, and weighting. The treatment planner calculates the results (using the treatment planning software), evaluates the results with or without the help of the radiation oncologist, and either accepts the plan or modifies the plan parameters. This process is repeated until a satisfactory plan is achieved. In inverse planning, the radiation oncologist specifies the desired dose constraints of the treatment plan, and the computer proposes a solution that is optimal in some sense. Notably, nothing in this definition implies that the solution has to be IMRT; for example, inverse planning could be used to find the best beam directions and weights for a set of open beams (this could also be done using a forward-planning approach). Because IMRT involves a large number of variables (beamlet weights), IMRT is impractical without some sort of inverse-planning approach. A general overview of treatment planning methods for IMRT has been written by Rosen.[45]

Beams for IMRT are divided into small independent elements usually referred to as *beamlets*. The size and shape of the beamlet depend on the nature of the IMRT delivery system but are usually rectangular in cross-section. The allowable intensities of the beamlets also depend on the delivery and treatment planning systems and can vary continuously or discretely.

Tomotherapy

Three major technologies are used for delivering IMRT: tomotherapy, dynamic multileaf collimation (DMLC), and beam attenuation. The tomotherapy concept originated with Mackie and colleagues[46] at the University of Wisconsin–Madison. The original concept involved a slice-by-slice treatment using arc delivery, similar to CT scanning. However, in the case of tomotherapy, the delivered fluence (analogous to the CT transmission profile) is the unknown variable, and the dose pattern (analogous to the CT attenuation map) is the known variable. The Nomos Corporation (Sewickley, Penn.) was the first company to commercialize tomotherapy with the Peacock system.[47-49] That system was first used to treat patients in 1994; at present, many sites throughout the world use the Nomos tomotherapy system (http://www.nomos.com).

The next major advance in tomotherapy will likely be the spiral tomotherapy system[50] being developed by Tomotherapy, Inc. (Madison, Wis.). One of the main technical challenges in the classical (or serial) tomotherapy approach is that couch movements must be extremely precise to avoid hot (or cold) junctions between the slices. In the authors' experience with the Nomos system, this requirement extends the treatment time because therapists must enter the room before each arc to position the treatment couch. A 1-mm error in couch positioning can cause a difference of up to 25% in the junction dose.[51] The spiral tomotherapy device uses a CT couch and gantry to provide a spiral delivery system that minimizes the dosimetric consequences of any couch translation imprecision, spreading any differences over a greater volume.

Dynamic Multileaf Collimation

Dynamic multileaf collimators are also used to deliver IMRT, but statistics on their use are difficult to gather. Although DMLC capability is included with most of the linear accelerators being sold today, it presumably is not being used by everyone who has it. The authors believe that as IMRT becomes more widely accepted, the use of DMLC will increase as well because it will be available from virtually all manufacturers as a relatively inexpensive option. Once a treatment center acquires the ability to generate an IMRT treatment plan and does the necessary commissioning and quality assurance of the DMLC device, then IMRT treatments can begin.

Treatment planning is again a key element in the use of DMLC for IMRT. Bortfeld and colleagues[52] first made the analogy between image reconstruction and IMRT dose delivery. Their approach for IMRT treatment planning uses an iterative back-projection of the desired dose distribution onto the beam intensity profiles. The number of beams and beam directions are chosen a priori, so some knowledge of desirable beam directions is required. Stein and colleagues[53] showed that for a small number of beams (five or fewer), the choice of beam directions is very important; as the number of

beams increases, the DMLC approach becomes similar to the tomotherapy approach, and satisfactory plans can be achieved with a standard set of beam angles. The authors' experience using the Corvus treatment planning system (Nomos Corporation) for DMLC treatment planning is similar to that described by Stein and colleagues.[53] Their current standard beam arrangement for prostate IMRT plans consists of 10 beams separated by approximately 30 degrees, covering from right posterior oblique to left posterior oblique. This beam arrangement has been sufficient for virtually all prostate treatment plans. Being able to control the accelerator gantry from outside the room means that the larger number of beams does not overly affect treatment time.

A variation on DMLC and tomotherapy is intensity-modulated arc therapy (IMAT).[54] In IMAT, the dynamic multileaf collimator is used in combination with arc rotation during the treatment so that the leaves of the collimator move while the gantry is in motion. If more than one arc is used, the total intensity pattern at each gantry angle can be modulated to produce dose distributions that are similar to those achieved in tomotherapy or DMLC.

Fixed Beam Attenuation

The third major technology for delivering IMRT is the use of fixed beam attenuators,[55,56] which are similar to but generally thicker than missing-tissue compensators. The process for treatment planning is similar to that used for DMLC. However, instead of translating the fluence pattern into a series of DMLC segments, the fluence pattern is converted into a physical attenuator profile in two dimensions. The biggest advantage of the attenuator system is that it is easy to understand and quality assurance is correspondingly simple.[57] For small fields, a single device (with multiple collimator angles) can be used to treat multiple fields without the therapist having to enter the treatment room,[56] overcoming one of the major shortcomings of DMLC.

Medical physicists at the M.D. Anderson Cancer Center have researched IMRT since the early 1990s. Thomas Bortfeld and Arthur Boyer showed that a DMLC device could deliver concave dose distributions, wrapping the high-dose region around the critical structure (Fig. 2-6).[58,59] Dr. Boyer's departure for Stanford slowed research into IMRT at the M.D. Anderson Cancer Center significantly, but in late 1997, implementing IMRT in the clinic at the M.D. Anderson Cancer Center became a high priority. After all of the commercial options were reviewed, the Nomos Peacock system was purchased, which was believed to offer the most straightforward path to implementing IMRT in the clinic. The system was delivered in June 1998, and the first patient was treated in December 1998. The dose distribution for one of the first patients treated with this device (Fig. 2-7; see

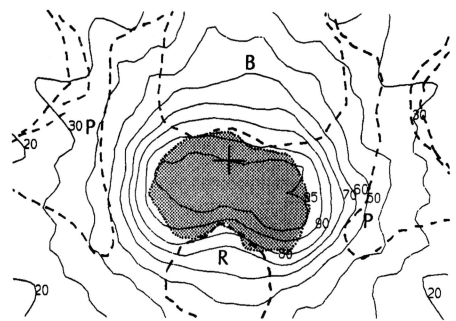

Fig. 2-6 Example of concave dose distribution using intensity-modulated radiation therapy. *B*, Bladder; *P*, pelvis; *R*, rectum. (From Bortfeld T, Boyer AL, Schlegel W, et al. *Int J Radiat Oncol Biol Phys* 1994;30:899-908.)

also Color Plate 4, after p. 80) illustrates how IMRT can be used to treat multiple targets simultaneously while avoiding multiple critical structures.

Increased Use of IMRT

To accommodate growth in the demand for IMRT, use of the Varian Clinac 2100C dynamic multileaf collimator was begun in May 2000. The number of patients treated with IMRT per quarter at the M.D. Anderson Cancer Center since December 1998 is shown in Figure 2-8; the doubling time has been approximately 6 months. As of September 2000, treatment for 20 to 25 patients per month had begun. By September 2001, the program plans to have the capacity to use IMRT for approximately 90 patients per month, or approximately 20% of all patients.

Approximately 70% of the patients undergoing IMRT to date are being treated for prostate carcinoma. Other institutions have also reported excellent results using IMRT for this purpose.[60,61] Because the position of the prostate and its target volume can vary greatly between fractions,[62-68] the Nomos BAT device is used, which uses transabdominal sonography to help position the prostate target volume relative to the radiation beams, before each fraction is delivered.[69,70] This practice allows the margin between the CTV and the PTV to be reduced, thereby increasing the dose to the prostate while maintaining the same minimum dose to the rectum.

The use of IMRT to treat tumors at other sites is increasing, especially in the time since DMLC was released for IMRT. As physicians become better able to define target volumes through the use of better imaging methods, the desire to conform the dose distribution to complex-shaped disease regions and to spare regions that are less likely to be involved will increase, and IMRT will be necessary to achieve the desired dose distributions.

Intensity-Modulated Radiation Therapy Treatment Process

The IMRT treatment process is similar to the three-dimensional treatment planning process. A means of immobilizing the patient is fabricated, and the patient undergoes CT scanning in the treatment position with a CT simulation system. The anatomy is outlined on the CT simulator, and the CT images and anatomy contours are transferred to the IMRT treatment planning computer. The radiation oncologist specifies dose goals for the targets, dose limits for other structures, and the treatment modality (e.g., tomotherapy or DMLC). A computer program then uses this information to compute an optimal solution. Dose goals and dose limits are adjusted by the radiation oncologist until the optimizer program achieves a satisfactory solution. Treatment settings are then transferred to the delivery and record-and-verify systems by using a floppy disk or local area network. The patient's control files are then loaded into the delivery system to deliver the treatment. For quality assurance, the same control files are used to deliver simulated treatments to phantoms. Such doses to the phantom are computed by the treatment planning system to verify the functionality of the dose delivery system. Sternick[71] provides additional details about

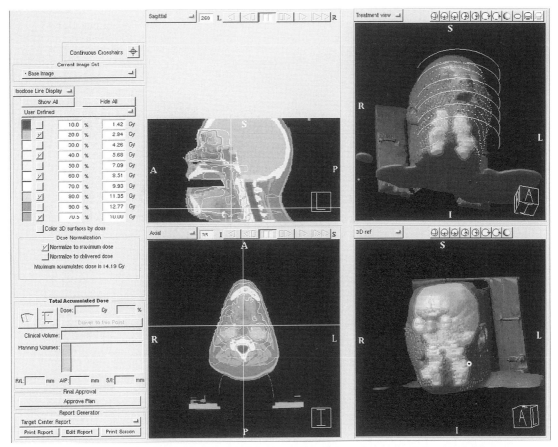

Fig. 2-7 Nasopharynx *(red)* and lymph node *(orange)* boost using tomotherapy intensity-modulated radiation therapy. The four panels show a sagittal slice through the nasopharynx target *(upper left)*, an axial slice through the lymph nodes *(lower left)*, the path of the tomotherapy arcs *(upper right, solid white lines)*, and a three-dimensional view of the targets relative to the critical structures *(lower right).* (See Color Plate 4, after p. 80, for color reproduction.)

IMRT delivery methods, treatment planning, quality assurance, and clinical use.

The biggest impediment to the efficient use of IMRT is the lack of tools with which to provide quality assurance for the many variables involved. For example, although electronic portal imaging devices have been around for many years, the reliability of these devices has not been very good. Adequate archival (PACS) capability for dealing with the large numbers of images generated for a typical treatment verification is also lacking.

At this time, quality assurance for IMRT is relatively labor intensive. Although learning about the reliability of the various components of IMRT will probably reduce the amount of quality assurance needed, automated tools will almost certainly be necessary as the number of patients treated with IMRT increases. The acceptability of IMRT in routine clinical practice also depends on the availability of efficient standard quality assurance methods.

Finally, the transition to IMRT depends on the radiation oncologist's current practice. For physicians who are familiar with routinely delineating target volumes and critical structures, the transition is quite straightforward, and the biggest change will be that from traditional forward treatment planning to inverse treatment planning. However, for physicians who do not routinely delineate structure volumes, the transition to IMRT may be more difficult because they must then decide exactly what portion of the anatomy is to be treated. Expecting too much from dose optimization and from IMRT can also be a problem. If the physician specifies an outcome that is impossible, then the computer algorithm must compute a trade-off between the dose goals for the target and critical structures. Thus the dose constraints should be prescribed as loosely as possible, giving the computer an achievable set of goals on which it can then try to improve.

The authors believe that IMRT and inverse treatment planning represent the next generation of tools for radiation oncology. With these tools, physicians will be able to free themselves from contemplating the mechanics so as to focus on the treatment objective—achieving the best outcome for patients. As imaging methods become

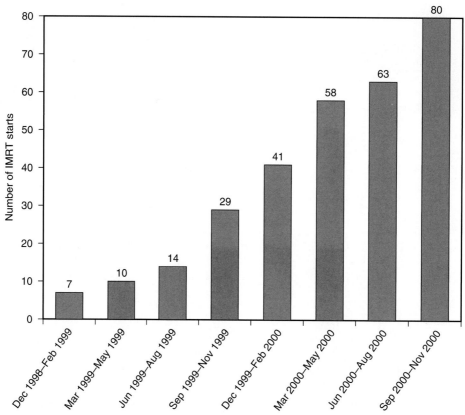

Fig. 2-8 Number of patients treated with intensity-modulated radiation therapy *(IMRT)* during the first 21 months of its use at the M.D. Anderson Cancer Center.

better able to localize and quantify disease and as biological models become better able to predict therapeutic results, radiation therapy can become more specific so that what needs to be treated can be treated as well as possible with fewer or less severe side effects.

STEREOTACTIC IRRADIATION

In 1951 Leksell[72] introduced the term *radiation surgery* to describe a technique in which narrow beams are stereotactically focused onto a target within the brain so as to achieve a high dose of localized irradiation. If the dose gradient is very steep at the edge of the volume chosen for irradiation, then a single dose that is sufficient to cause necrosis of the selected tissue volume can be administered. Hence, in radiation surgery, the most important factor is the physically determined concentration of the radiation on the target; this is in contrast to fractionated radiation therapy, which is based on differences in radiosensitivity between tumor cells and cells of the adjacent healthy tissue.

Three general approaches to radiosurgery are used today.[73-75] The first uses positively charged particles like protons or helium ions generated by large accelerators. Most of these accelerators were originally built for nuclear physics research, and only a few are in hospital-based

facilities. The second approach, popularly referred to as the *gamma knife*, makes use of the gamma radiation emitted from a fixed array of small ^{60}Co sources located within a large hemisphere that surrounds the patient's head. The third uses high-energy x-ray radiation produced by a medical linear accelerator (LINAC). The radiation oncology departments of most large hospitals now have LINAC units.

Stereotactic Radiosurgery

At the M.D. Anderson Cancer Center, LINAC-based stereotactic radiosurgery (SRS) has been under development since late 1989, and the first patient was treated with SRS in August 1991. The SRS system (Fig. 2-9) consists of variable collimation apertures that are inserted at the end of a circular collimator, a table-mounted docking device, a laser target-localization frame, and a couch top stabilizer. The head frame is attached to the docking device. The LINAC-based SRS system delivers a lethal, homogeneous dose to an approximately spherical treatment volume, which is surrounded by a region of rapid fall-off in dose. This form of treatment is best suited for small, spherical tumors.[76] Tumors that are more irregularly shaped are treated with larger circular collimators. Because these larger collimators expose a greater proportion of

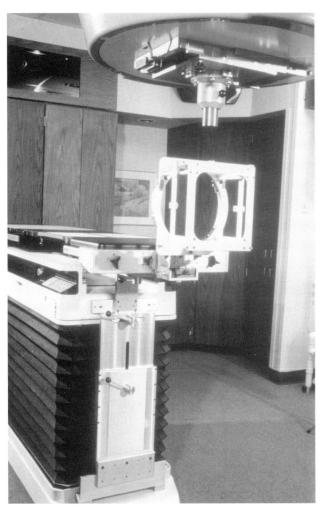

Fig. 2-9 The stereotactic radiosurgery system hardware at the M.D. Anderson Cancer Center.

healthy brain to high-dose irradiation, the doses that are to be delivered with large collimators are lower than those to be delivered with smaller collimators; for this reason, tumors larger than about 4 cm in diameter are inappropriate for SRS.

For irregularly shaped tumors, conformation of the radiation dose can be improved by delivering treatment with two or more overlapping isocenters. However, this practice can lead to the development of "hot" areas in the overlap region and increased complication rates.[77] Toxicity to normal tissues can be reduced by conforming the irradiated volume to the target volume and by ensuring that the dose distribution within the target is as uniform as possible. To achieve these goals, the authors developed a miniature multileaf collimator,[78,79] the technology for which was transferred in 1996 to Radionics, Inc. (Burlington, Mass.) and given 510(k) clearance by the U.S. Food and Drug Administration in 1998. That same year, development of a dedicated, integrated stereotactic radiosurgery and radiotherapy (SRS/SRT) delivery system[80] was begun jointly between Siemens Medical Systems, Radionics, and the M.D. Anderson Cancer Center, and in October 1999 the machine was released for clinical use (Fig. 2-10). Currently, the mini-multileaf and circular collimators are used for SRS, and the mini-multileaf collimator, along with a Gil-Thomas-Cosman frame or a noninvasive head-and-neck frame, is used for SRT.

An example of the use of the mini-multileaf collimator to treat a case of brain metastases with SRS is presented in the following section. A patient with metastases to the parietal occipital area of the brain was referred for SRS 3 months after having undergone a

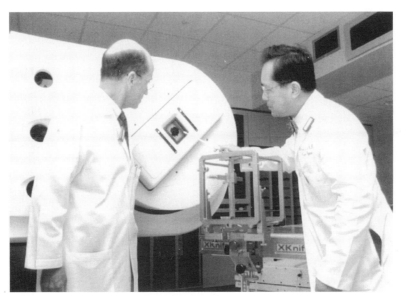

Fig. 2-10 The dedicated integrated stereotactic radiation surgery and radiation treatment delivery system.

craniotomy. Owing to the size (approximately 5 cm long) and irregular shape of the lesion, the mini-multileaf collimator was chosen to best conform the beam shape to the projected beam's-eye view of the target volume, thereby reducing the volume of normal tissue to be irradiated. A Radionics head ring was fixed securely to the patient's head with four adjustable head posts and fixation screws; this ring formed the base frame for determining the stereotactic coordinates and ensuring exact alignments during treatment. Next, a series of image scans was taken; in this case, CT scanning was used, but magnetic resonance imaging (MRI) or angiography can also be used as necessary. After a localizer frame was attached to the head ring, the images were transferred to the SRS/SRT treatment planning system. That system was used to identify the nine rods of the localizer frame, to transfer all images from CT coordinates to stereotactic frame coordinates, and to outline the critical structures of the head (e.g., brainstem, optic nerves, and optic chiasm) and tumor. A three-dimensional view through the LINAC beam collimator, with the shaped mini-multileaf collimator indicating the treatment portal, was then overlaid on the surrounding anatomy to allow the operator to select gantry angles and couch positions that would avoid critical structures. For this case, 15 multileaf collimation fields with four couch positions were chosen to deliver the treatment (Fig. 2-11; see also Color Plate 5, after p. 80, in which the green fields represent the entrance portals and the red fields represent the exit portals). These beam arrangements were selected to mimic four arc beams, usually used to simulate a 2π irradiation geometry.

The 14-Gy prescribed isodose surface distribution is illustrated in Figure 2-12 (see also Color Plate 6, after p. 80). The TVR (defined as *the total volume receiving the prescribed dose, including the lesion, divided by the lesion volume receiving the same dose*) was 1.6, indicating excellent conformity of dose distribution to lesion volume. The treatment delivery time for this case was approximately 30 minutes.

Quality Assurance

With regard to quality assurance, any stereotactic treatment requires verification that the isocenter has been placed at the correct target position and coincides with the center of the radiation field. Before each treatment, rigorous quality assurance procedures are followed, including a film test to ensure that the target center is aligned to the LINAC isocenter to within 0.5 mm.

In its first year of operation, the dedicated integrated auto-delivery system at the M.D. Anderson Cancer Center was used for 107 SRS cases and 17 SRT cases. The authors anticipate 180 SRS cases and 25 SRT cases per year thereafter and expect that 20% of the patients undergoing SRS will be treated with mini-multileaf collimators. Given the superiority of dose distribution and the brevity of treatment time of multileaf collimation over multi-isocenter treatments for irregularly shaped tumors, it is anticipated that the use of mini-multileaf collimators will surpass the use of circular collimators. Other plans for the future at the M.D. Anderson Cancer Center are to make the IMRT technique available for SRT and to "gate" the beam to synchronize stereotactic

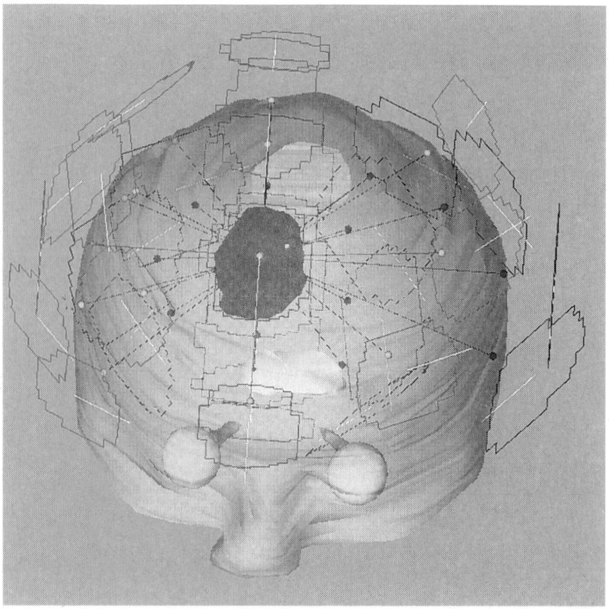

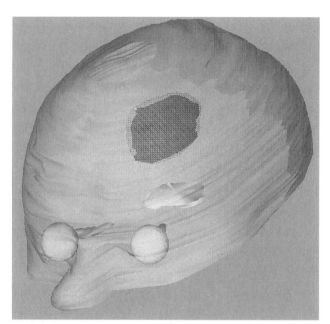

Fig. 2-11 Three-dimensional display of 15 mini-multileaf collimator fields. *Green,* Entrance fields; *red,* exit fields. (See Color Plate 5, after p. 80, for color reproduction.)

Fig. 2-12 Three-dimensional view of 14-Gy prescribed isodose surface distribution. (See Color Plate 6, after p. 80, for color reproduction.)

irradiation with the breath cycle for treating small lung or liver lesions (as discussed later in this chapter in the section on "Gated Radiation Therapy").

ELECTRON BEAM THERAPY

Radiation oncologists often underplay the significance of electron beam therapy, with many considering electrons to be simply a technique for delivering breast or off-cord boost doses, their most frequent applications. Although the number of patients that can benefit from electron techniques may be few, the use of electrons when needed is invaluable; consequently, electron beam therapy, as a whole, provides a formidable modality. Such has been the experience at the M.D. Anderson Cancer Center, a leader in electron beam therapy. Electrons have been beneficial for treatment of head, neck, and eye tumors[81]; total skin irradiation[68,82,83]; total limb irradiation[84]; intraoperative irradiation[85,86]; and chest wall irradiation using fixed beam[81] and arc therapy.[87] Electron fields, abutted to x-ray fields, have been invaluable in the treatment of the scalp[88] and spine in craniospinal irradiation.[89,90] Electrons have also been used in treating tumors of the nasal and parotid regions in an effort to spare the salivary glands and in treating the maxillary antrum to spare distal structures.[90,91] Many applications such as treatment of the nose or auditory canal have been improved through the use of bolus to improve dose homogeneity.[92,93]

Electron beam therapy differs from photon therapy in that a single beam can be used to irradiate a target volume that lies within approximately 6 cm of the body surface. This is possible because of the finite range of the electrons, which results in the dose falling off sharply with depth. However, this feature raises the need to consider the modification of range and dose distribution owing to heterogeneities of tissues. Also, the dose distribution within the 90% isodose surface area can be affected by surface and internal irregularities.[94] Therefore treatment planning must be done with dose algorithms that can account for the presence of heterogeneity.[94]

Since the early 1980s, pencil-beam algorithms have been the standard for commercial electron treatment planning systems. One of the most widely used of these algorithms was developed at the M.D. Anderson Cancer Center by Hogstrom and colleagues for fixed[95,96] and arced[97,98] electron beams. The fixed-beam algorithm has been implemented on three-dimensional planning systems by Starkschall and colleagues.[99] The accuracy of these algorithms for clinical situations has been well documented.[95,96,100] In some cases such as those involving sharp lateral air cavities like those in the nose and sinuses, the accuracy of the pencil-beam algorithm may be inadequate. However, newer, more accurate algorithms that include both analytical and Monte Carlo calculations are beginning to become available in commercial treatment planning systems.[100] One of these algorithms, the pencil-beam redefinition algorithm, is a significant improvement over the original pencil-beam algorithm.[101-103] Its ability to accurately predict the dose in the presence of tissue heterogeneity is illustrated in Figure 2-13 (see also Color Plate 7, after p. 80). However, both older and newer algorithms beg to be implemented by manufacturers so that they accurately simulate patient treatment methods (e.g., modeling skin collimators, bolus, and arc therapy).

Many electron treatments, with their ability to spare distal critical structures, are being rivaled by the increased availability of intensity-modulated x-ray therapy (IMXT). Although IMXT is highly valuable and in demand, x-ray beams still possess exit dose. Consequently, potential benefit remains from electron conformal therapy in which the exit dose (bremsstrahlung dose) is minimal. The remainder of this section describes the current state of electron conformal therapy at the M.D. Anderson Cancer Center and alludes to expected future technologic advances.

Electron Conformal Therapy

The objective of electron conformal therapy is to conform the 90% isodose surface to the distal surface of the target volume while keeping the dose inside the target volume as uniform as possible, or between 90% and 100%. In one method in which bolus is used for conforming the 90% isodose surface[104] the pencil-beam algorithm is used to calculate dose, and *bolus operators* are used to design a three-dimensional wax bolus, the bottom surface of which coincides with the patient's surface and the top surface of which produces the desired dose distribution. A bolus designed for a patient treated for sarcoma of the paraspinal muscle and a single plane image of the three-dimensional dose distribution are shown in Figure 2-14 (see also Color Plate 8, after p. 80).[105] The bolus is fabricated from a block of machineable wax by a computer-controlled milling machine[106] that receives the bolus design from the M.D. Anderson Cancer Center COPPER Plan three-dimensional treatment planning system.[107] One of the negative effects of the bolus is that its variable source-to-skin distance and sloping surfaces increase the dose spread within the 90% isodose contour, which typically contains the target volume.[105] However, dose homogeneity can be restored by using an x-ray multileaf collimator or some other device to modulate the intensity of the beam.[108]

Electron bolus has considerable potential in the clinic, with the most promising sites being the chest wall and head. As an example, in treating breast cancer that extends from a tumor in the right lower inner quadrant to the internal mammary chain into the chest wall, standard tangent fields with a fitted electron internal mammary

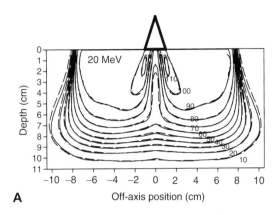

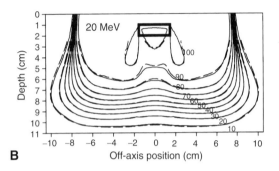

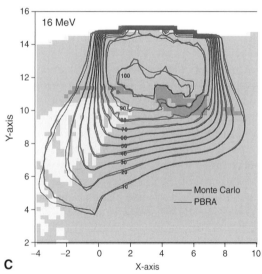

Fig. 2-13   Comparison of dose distributions calculated using the pencil-beam redefinition algorithm *(PBRA)* with those measured or calculated using the Monte Carlo method. PBRA calculations are shown as solid isodose contours; measured or Monte Carlo estimates of isodose contours are shown as dashed lines. **A,** Distribution of 20 MeV to be delivered to an irregular surface. **B,** Distribution of 20 MeV to account for bone heterogeneity. **C,** Distribution of 16 MeV to be delivered as internal mammary chain irradiation. (See Color Plate 7, after p. 80, for color reproduction.)

chain field can leave a cold abutment in the location of gross disease, and treatment with "deep" tangents can needlessly irradiate excess lung and the opposite breast. Bolus conformal therapy (Fig. 2-15; see also Color Plate 9,

after p. 80)[108a] can be quite helpful in this situation. Bawiec[109] also demonstrated the potential usefulness of electron conformal therapy in tumors of the head and neck, particularly for treating a target volume that extends to overlie the temporal lobe. The benefit of using a bolus to treat a squamous cell carcinoma in the right buccal mucosa region for a PTV that overlies the spinal cord and brain is illustrated in Figure 2-16.

Despite the availability of bolus technology, its commercial implementation has yet to become fashionable, in part because of the present focus on x-ray conformal therapy. As bolus technology becomes more acceptable, integrated tools for planning, fabrication, delivery, and quality assurance tools will be needed. At present, other alternatives to be considered are the use of multiple patched fields of different energies and beam weights[110,111] or the use of multiple intensity-modulated fields of differing electron energy.[112,113] Electron intensity modulation is possible through magnetic scanning[114] or through the use of an electron multileaf collimator.[115] As electron multileaf collimators become available, this technology and the use of bolus as described previously can be expected to meet most clinical needs for electron conformal therapy. Also, electron conformal therapy will most likely be used in conjunction with conventional radiation therapy or IMXT for many of the same reasons, such as skin sparing and increased depth of penetration, that were used to combine electron and x-ray fixed beam therapy.[116]

GATED RADIATION THERAPY

As described in the section on "Three-Dimensional Treatment Planning and Delivery," the ICRU's Report 50[22] defines the PTV as the CTV plus additional margins to account for variability in set-up and organ motion. Two kinds of organ motion enter into determinations of PTV: motion between treatments (intertreatment) and motion within treatments (intratreatment). Intertreatment motion can be resolved through the use of repeated imaging, typically with CT or sonography. Intratreatment organ motion results primarily from cardiac and respiratory motion. Radiographic and CT studies have been used to reveal the extent of tumor motion resulting from respiration (Fig. 2-17; see also Color Plate 10, after p. 80). MRI has also been considered for use in estimating treatment margins that account for respiratory motion and variation in set-up.[117] MRI has the advantages of being more reliable than CT or radiography for soft-tissue imaging and requiring less time for image acquisition, with the latter feature increasing the probability that a full image will be acquired during a breath-holding maneuver.

Once the extent of respiratory motion has been established, several options exist to account for this motion. A PTV that explicitly accounts for respiratory motion can

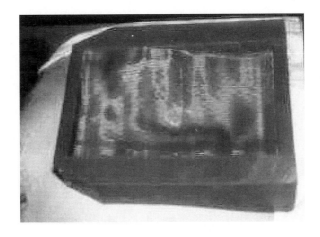

A

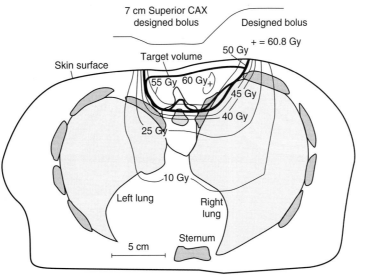

Fig. 2-14 Conformal electron therapy to the paraspinal muscles with the use of a custom-shaped wax bolus. The prescribed dose is 50 Gy. **A,** View of the patient with bolus in position. Isodose contours for a 20-MeV electron beam plotted in a superior transverse plane without bolus **(B)** or with bolus **(C).** (See Color Plate 8, after p. 80, for color reproduction.) (From Low DA, Starkschall G, Sherman NE, et al. *Int J Radiat Oncol Biol Phys* 1995;33:1127-1138.)

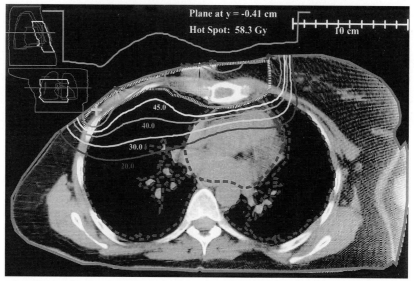

Fig. 2-15 View of isodose contours plotted on transverse computed tomography anatomy for conformal therapy using 16-MeV electron beam and custom-shaped wax bolus to irradiate the chest wall and internal mammary chain after mastectomy. The prescribed dose is 50 Gy. (See Color Plate 9, after p. 80, for color reproduction.) (From Perkins GH, McNeese MD, Antolak J, et al. *Int J Radiat Oncol Biol Phys* 2001;51:1142-1151.)

be defined, with the treatment portal design based on that volume. If the extent of respiratory motion can be quantified precisely rather than being merely estimated, the size of the PTV probably could be reduced, which would result, in turn, in smaller treatment portals and irradiation of less normal lung tissue. It may even be reasonable to design beam geometries so that the central axes of the radiation beams lie along the major extent of tumor motion, minimizing the extent of tumor motion in the plane perpendicular to the beam. This practice could also reduce the size of treatment portals and the amount of irradiation to uninvolved tissue.

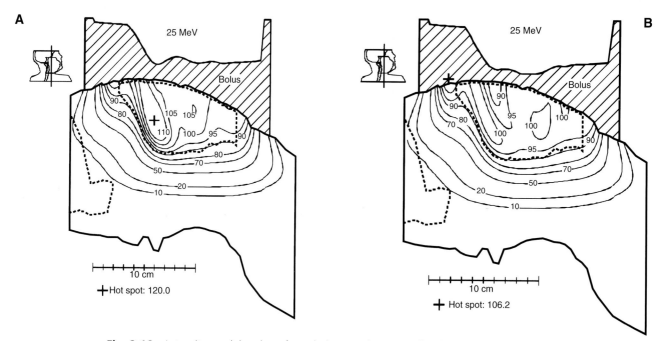

Fig. 2-16 Intensity-modulated conformal electron therapy with a bolus to irradiate a tumor of the right buccal mucosa with 25-MeV electrons. Plots of isodose contours in the sagittal plane (dose given is 100 Gy) show improved dose uniformity in the planning target volume (*dotted contour*) for the treatment plan that includes intensity modulation (**A**) relative to a treatment plan that does not include intensity modulation (**B**).

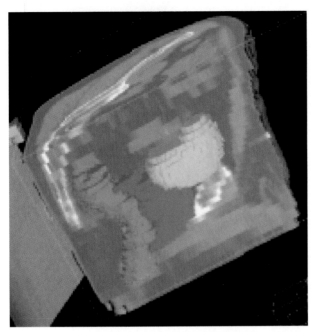

Color Plate 1 Three-dimensional surfaces of the prostate *(green)*, rectum *(blue)*, and bladder *(yellow)* reconstructed from outlines drawn on computed tomography images. (See also Figure 2-1.)

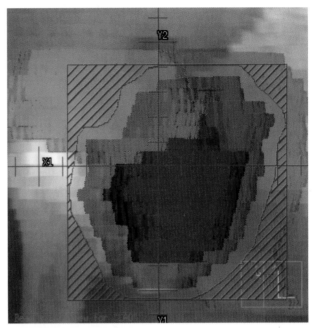

Color Plate 2 Example of beam's-eye view display used to define the radiation beam aperture. Prostate *(magenta)*, bladder *(blue)*, and rectum *(green)* are shown from the perspective of the radiation beam. Beam aperture is drawn interactively on the computer to surround the target and to avoid as much normal tissue as possible. (See also Figure 2-3.)

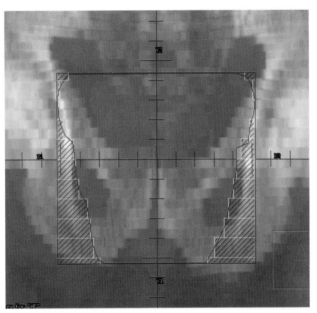

Color Plate 3 Digitally reconstructed radiograph for a conventional anterior beam for prostate treatment. Beam aperture is superimposed on a gray-scale image reconstructed from the computed tomography data set and is intended to approximate the image seen on a portal film. (See also Figure 2-4.)

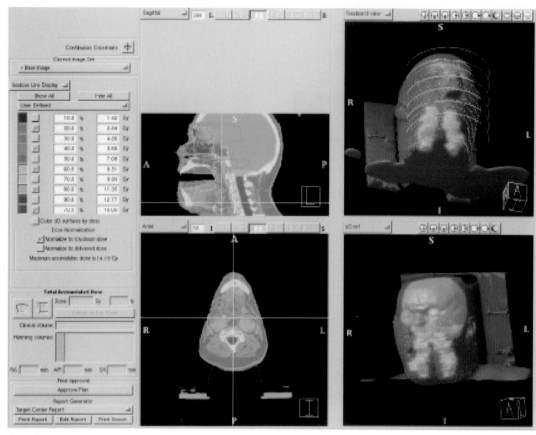

Color Plate 4 Nasopharynx *(red)* and lymph node *(orange)* boost using tomotherapy intensity-modulated radiation therapy. Four panels show a sagittal slice through the nasopharynx target *(upper left)*, an axial slice through the lymph nodes *(lower left)*, the path of the tomotherapy arcs *(upper right, solid white lines)*, and a three-dimensional view of targets relative to the critical structures *(lower right)*. (See also Figure 2-7.)

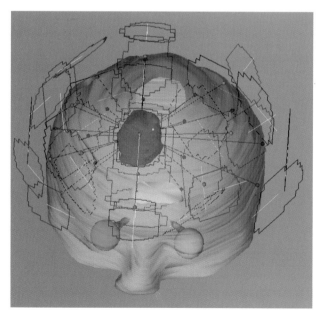

Color Plate 5 Three-dimensional display of 15 mini-multileaf collimator fields. *Green,* entrance fields; *red,* exit fields. (See also Figure 2-11.)

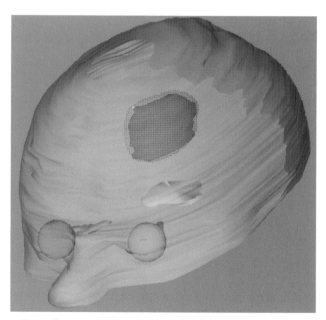

Color Plate 6 Three-dimensional view of 14-Gy pre-scribed iosodose surface distribution. (See also Figure 2-12.)

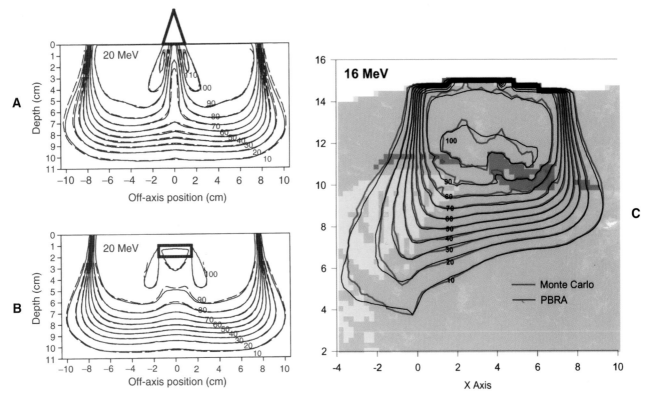

Color Plate 7 Comparison of dose distributions calculated using the pencil-beam redefinition algorithm *(PBRA)* with those measured or calculated using the Monte Carlo method. PBRA calculations are shown as solid isodose contours; measured or Monte Carlo estimates of isodose contours are shown as dashed lines. **A,** Distribution of 20 MeV to be delivered to an irregular surface. **B,** Distribution of 20 MeV to account for bone heterogeneity. **C,** Distribution of 16 MeV to be delivered as internal mammary chain irradiation. (See also Figure 2-13.)

Color Plate 8 Conformal electron therapy to the paraspinal muscles with the use of a custom-shaped wax bolus. Prescribed dose is 50 Gy. **A,** View of the patient with bolus in position. Isodose contours for a 20-MeV electron beam plotted in a superior transverse plane without bolus **(B)** or with bolus **(C).** (See also Figure 2-14.) (From Low DA, Starkschall G, Sherman NE, et al. *Int J Radiat Oncol Biol Phys* 1995;33:1127-1138.)

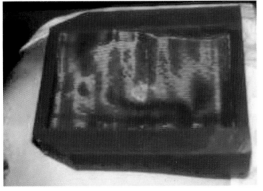

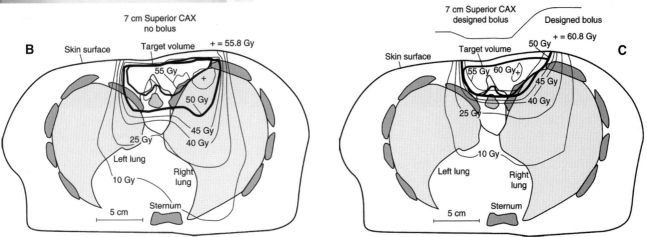

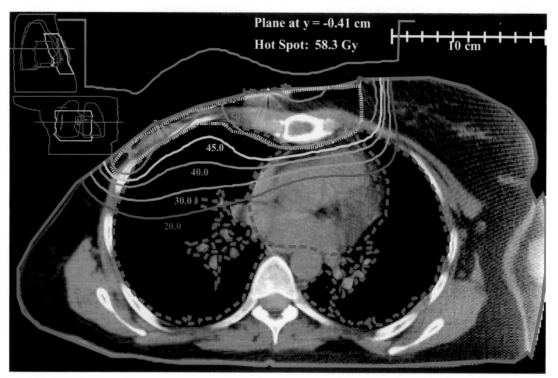

Color Plate 9 View of isodose contours plotted on transverse computed tomography scan of anatomy for conformal therapy using 16-MeV electron beam and custom-shaped wax bolus to irradiate the chest wall and internal mammary chain after mastectomy. Prescribed dose is 50 Gy. (See also Figure 2-15.) (From Perkins GH, McNeese MD, Antolak J, et al. *Int J Radiat Oncol Biol Phys* 2001;51:1142-1151.)

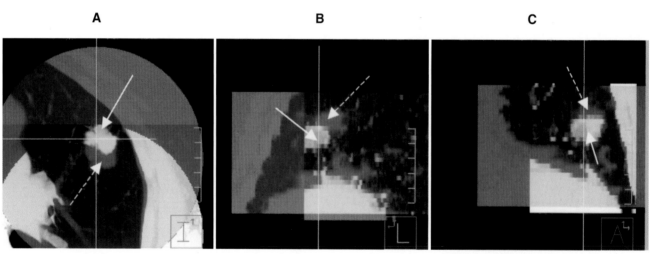

Color Plate 10 Merged computed tomography (CT) images at full inspiration and full expiration illustrating extent of tumor motion during respiratory motion. **A,** Transverse view; **B,** sagittal view; **C,** coronal view. *Solid arrows* point to the tumor on CT images obtained during full inspiration, and *dashed arrows* point to the tumor on CT images obtained during full expiration. The scale at the right of each image indicates 1-cm intervals. (See also Figure 2-17.)

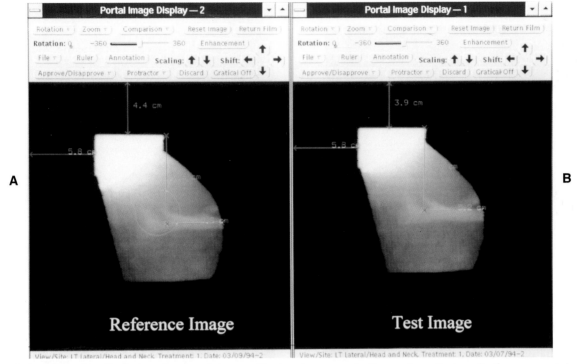

Color Plate 11 Radiation therapy picture archival and communication system display of reference portal image **(A)** and test portal image **(B)** of a head-and-neck treatment field used for image comparison. (See also Figure 2-20.)

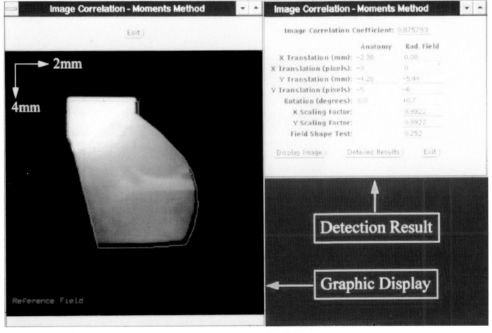

Color Plate 12 Display on a radiation therapy picture archival and communication system of the adjustments in patient positioning needed to bring the test image into alignment with the reference image. (See also Figure 2-21.)

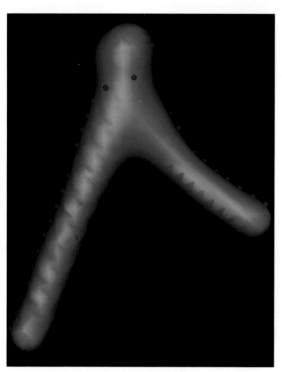

Color Plate 13 Plan for dual-catheter treatment of bronchogenic carcinoma. The *light blue* surface encloses the volume receiving at least 15 Gy. The *blue dots* on that surface are the points of dose specification. (See also Figure 2-22.)

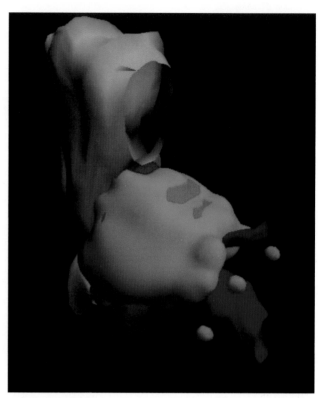

Color Plate 14 A ^{125}I computed tomography–based prostate treatment plan. The *light blue* surface demonstrates the 144-Gy surface; *yellow,* bladder; *dark blue,* rectum; *red,* prostate; *purple,* seminal vesicles; *green,* ureter. (See also Figure 2-23.)

Color Plate 15 Dose clouds surrounding a coronary stent implanted with 1 mCi of [103]Pd. **A,** 120 Gy. **B,** 90 Gy. **C,** 60 Gy. **D,** 40 Gy. (See also Figure 2-24.)

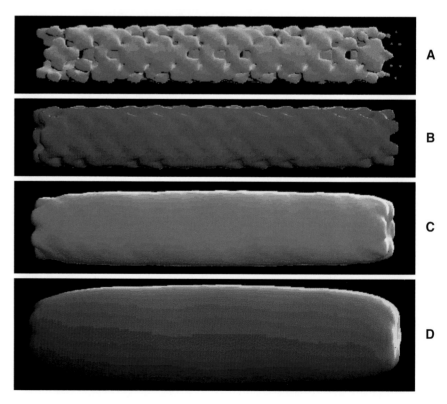
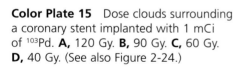

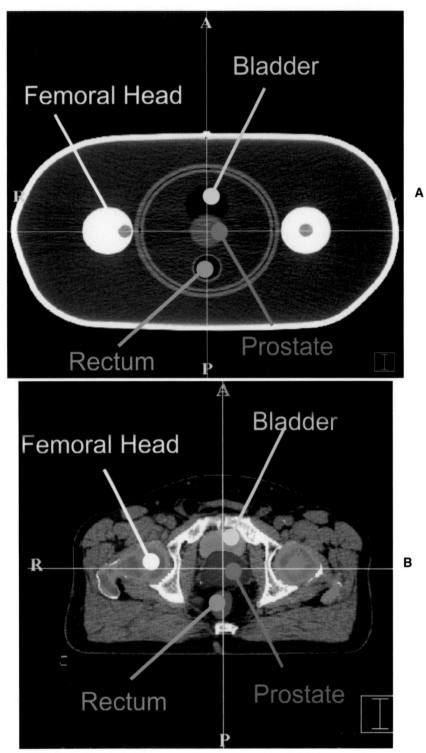

Color Plate 16 **A,** Cross-section of Radiological Physics Center's pelvic phantom for intensity-modulated radiation therapy showing the simulated organs. **B,** Transverse computed tomography scan of a male pelvis at same anatomic position as the phantom. (See also Figure 2-27.)

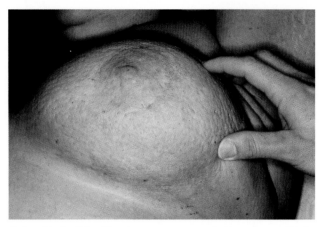

Color Plate 17 Classic appearance of skin edema: thickened skin with prominent hair follicles upon mild compression of the skin. This physical finding is called *peau d'orange* because appearance is similar to that of the skin of an orange. (See also Figure 15-4.)

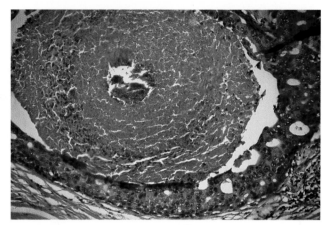

Color Plate 18 Histologic section of high-grade ductal carcinoma in situ with extensive comedo necrosis. (See also Figure 15-6.)

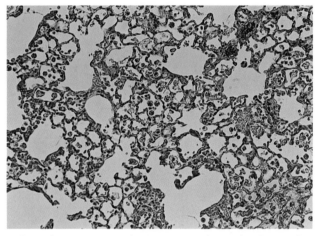

Color Plate 19 Histologic section from the lung of a C3Hf/Kam mouse irradiated to the whole thorax and killed 4 months later, showing classical radiation pneumonitis with inflammatory cell infiltrate and edema in the air spaces and interstitium. (See also Figure 17-1.)

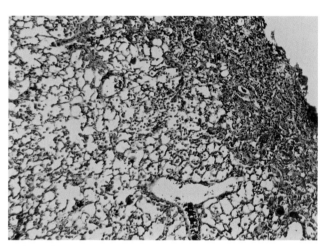

Color Plate 20 Histologic section from the lung of a C57Bl/6J mouse killed 5 months after administration of 16 Gy of radiation to the whole thorax, showing organizing alveolitis and collagen deposition. (See also Figure 17-2.)

Color Plate 21 Lymphatic drainage of the lobes of the lungs related to schema commonly used for classifying regional lymph nodes. Note crossover from the lingula of the left upper lobe and superior portion of the left lower lobe to right paratracheal nodes. Lymph node drainage does not parallel arteries or veins, nor does it remain distinct for each lobe. Node colors correspond to stations in the *AJCC Cancer Staging Manual.* (See also Figure 17-8.) (Modified from Nohl HC. *Thorax* 1956;11:172-185; Fleming I, Cooper JS, Henson DE, et al. *AJCC Cancer Staging Manual.* 5th ed. Philadelphia, Pa: Lippincott Williams & Wilkins; 1977:127-137.)

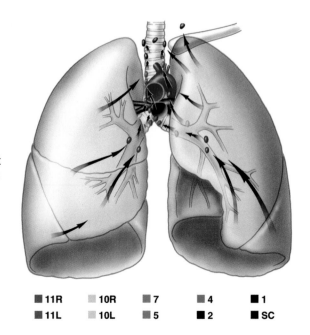

■ 11R	■ 10R	■ 7	■ 4	■ 1
■ 11L	■ 10L	■ 5	■ 2	■ SC

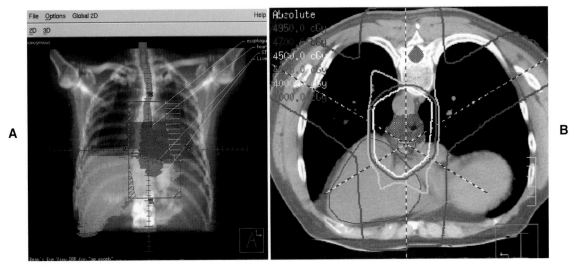

Color Plate 22 Treatment plans for adenocarcinoma of distal esophagus. **A,** Digitally reconstructed radiograph of esophageal tumor and surrounding normal structures. **B,** Dose distributions in the axial plane. (See also Chapter 18.)

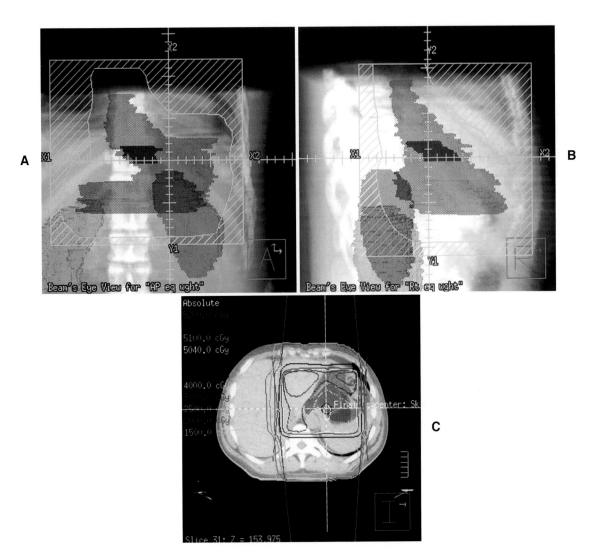

Color Plate 23 Typical anteroposterior **(A)** and lateral **(B)** fields for postoperative treatment of gastric cancer. Central axis dosimetry **(C)** is shown. The preoperative tumor volume is contoured as well as the entire nodal region at risk (clinical target volume). (See also Chapter 19.)

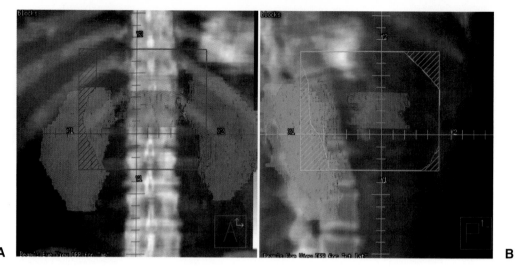

Color Plate 24 Typical anteroposterior **(A)** and lateral **(B)** simulation films for postoperative treatment of pancreatic cancer. Preoperative gross tumor volume and kidneys have been contoured and are shown. (See also Chapter 20.)

A

B

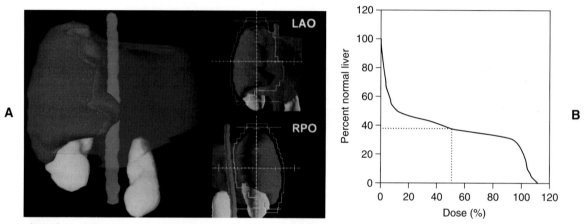

A

B

Color Plate 25 Treatment planning. **A,** Solid surface reconstruction of the target. Unresectable primary biliary cancer *(red),* liver *(purple),* kidneys *(orange),* and spinal cord *(green)* are shown at left, and beam arrangements are shown at right. *LAO,* Left anterior oblique; *RPO,* right posterior oblique. **B,** Dose-volume histogram of the normal liver treated in A. This patient would have received 48 Gy based on volume that received more than 50% of isocenter dose. Calculated V_{eff} for this plan was 38%, which led to a prescription dose of 69 Gy on current trial. (See also Chapter 21.) (From McGinn CJ, Ten Haken RK, Ensminger WD, et al. *J Clin Oncol* 1998;16:2246-2252.)

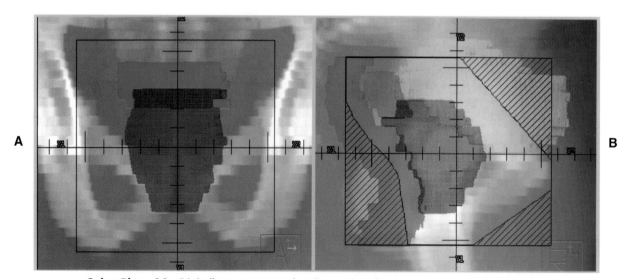

A

B

Color Plate 26 Digitally reconstructed radiographs of conventional anterior-posterior **(A)** and right lateral **(B)** fields (as part of the four-field technique) used at the M.D. Anderson Cancer Center. Prostate is shown in *red,* seminal vesicles in *blue,* rectum in *green,* and bladder in *yellow.* (See also Chapter 27.)

A   **B**

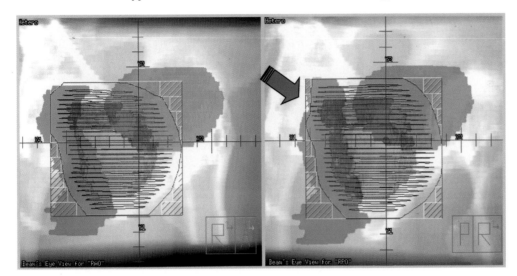

Color Plate 27
A, Digitally reconstructed right anterior oblique *(RAO)* and **B,** right posterior oblique *(RPO)* field radiographs used for conformal radiation therapy. Prostate is shown in *red,* seminal vesicles in *purple,* and planning target volumes as a *blue* wireframe. These fields were taken from a seven-field plan with one anterior, two lateral, and four oblique fields. Oblique fields were at 35 degrees above and below lateral positions. (See also Chapter 27.)

A

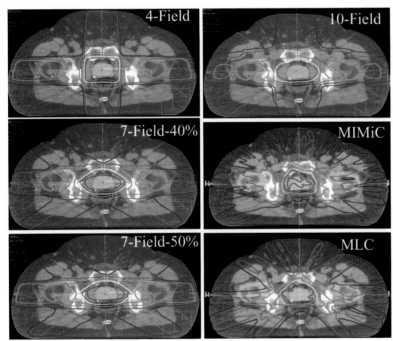

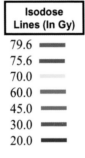

Isodose Lines (In Gy)	
79.6	▬
75.6	▬
70.0	▬
60.0	▬
45.0	▬
30.0	▬
20.0	▬

Color Plate 28   **A,** Dosimetry for a patient with favorable-risk prostate cancer generated by six contemporary conformal-based planning methods. Top row: *left,* 4-field plan with lateral field reduction posteriorly at 46 Gy; *right,* 10-field conformal boost plan (like that used in the M.D. Anderson Cancer Center dose-escalation trial). Middle row: *left,* 7-field conformal plan with 40% weighting of lateral fields; *right,* plan using the Peacock multileaf intensity-modulating collimator to deliver intensity-modulated radiation therapy. Bottom: *left,* a 7-field conformal plan with 50% weighting of lateral fields; *right,* plan using multileaf collimation *(MLC)* for intensity-modulated radiation therapy. Prescribed dose was 75.6 Gy to the planning target volume except in 10-field conformal boost plan, in which the dose was prescribed to isocenter (as was done in the M.D. Anderson Cancer Center protocol). **B,** Rectal dose-volume histogram analyses from six planning methods shown in **A.** Bars indicate standard error; asterisks indicate that percentage of rectum treated to more than 70 Gy was significantly less when intensity-modulated radiation therapy methods were used. (See also Chapter 27.)

B

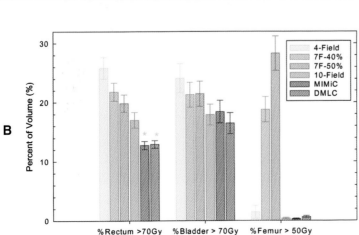

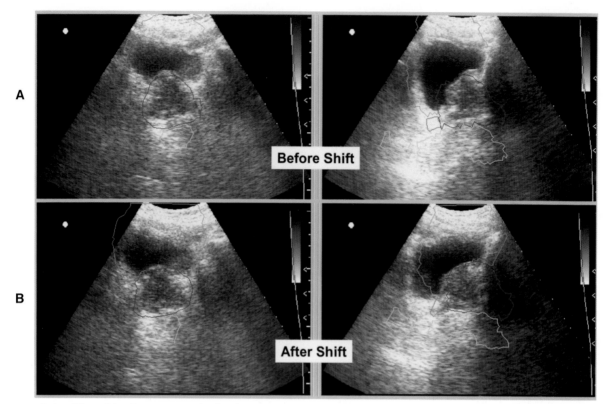

Color Plate 29 Sonograms obtained with Nomos Corporation's BAT system illustrating outlines of bladder, rectum, and prostate from planning computed tomography scan superimposed over sonogram taken before alignment **(A)** and after alignment **(B).** (See also Chapter 27.)

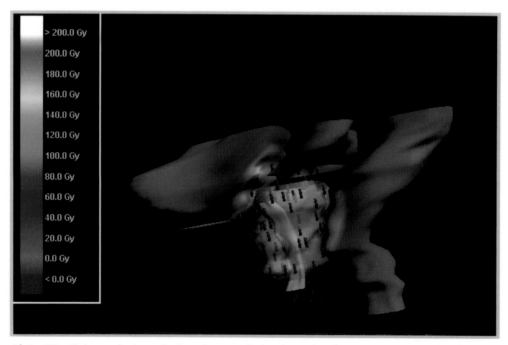

Color Plate 30 Colorwash dose display after needle implantation in prostate. Posterior apex of prostate receives less than the prescribed dose. (See also Chapter 27.)

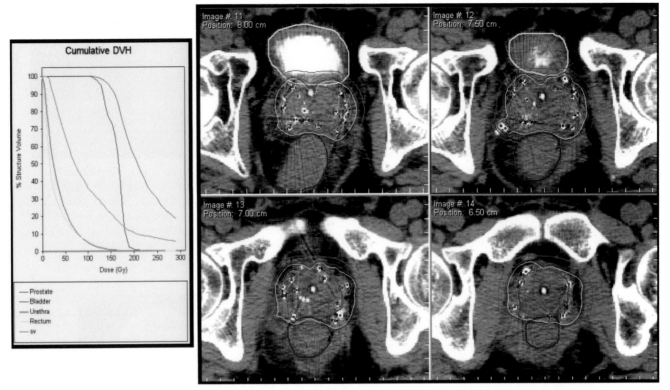

Color Plate 31 Transverse computed tomography scan images of pelvis with implant dosimetry superimposed. Yellow, red, and blue contours show bladder, prostate, and rectum, respectively; 144-Gy isodose line around prostate is shown in yellow. Dose-volume histogram analyses for prostate, bladder, urethra, and rectum are shown at left. (See also Chapter 27.)

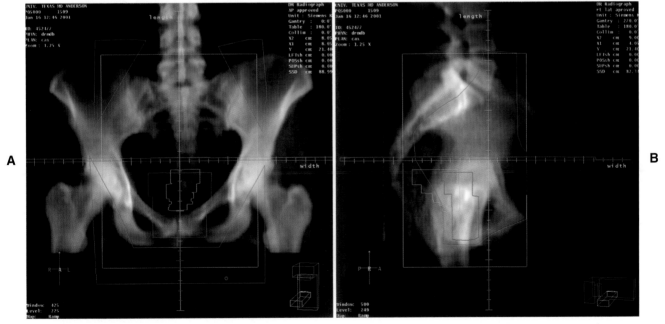

Color Plate 32 Typical anterior field **(A)** and lateral field **(B)** for treating carcinoma of endometrium. The rectum is outlined in *yellow,* and the vagina is outlined on an aquasimulation from computed tomography. (See also Figure 29-4.)

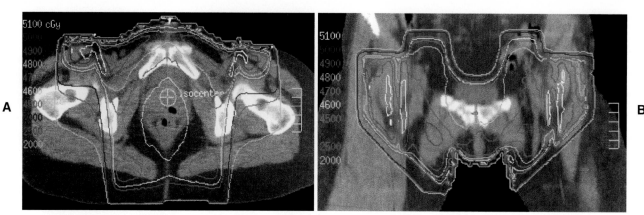

Color Plate 33 Transverse **(A)** and coronal **(B)** views of radiation dose distribution for vulvar carcinoma. A wide 6-MV anterior field encompassed the vulva and inguinal, external iliac, and internal iliac lymph nodes. A narrower 18-MV posterior field excluded femoral neck and part of femoral head. Dose to lateral inguinal lymph nodes was supplemented using electron fields matched to lateral borders of posterior field. Central block in superior portion of field reduced the amount of small bowel and rectum in treatment fields. A modified frog-leg position reduced skin dose in this patient, who had a posterior lesion. (See also Figure 30-2.)

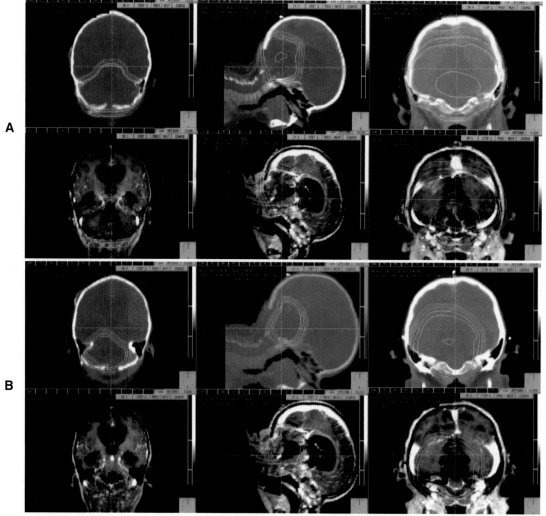

Color Plate 34 **A,** Treatment plans demonstrating ideal dose distribution for six-field, noncoplanar approach targeting entire posterior fossa. Anatomically, this approach includes the tentorium as it extends superiorly in posterior clinoid and then inferiorly to define anterior and superior margins of posterior fossa. Inferior and posterior margins are defined by calvarium and lower margin of foramen magnum. **B,** Conformal dose distribution covers operative bed after surgical resection of a medulloblastoma. Multifield, noncoplanar 6-MeV photons used for gross tumor volume outlining operative bed, expanded by 2 cm (modified by anatomic boundaries) to identify clinical target volume. A 5-mm planning target volume geometrically surrounds the clinical target volume. (See also Figure 32-4.)

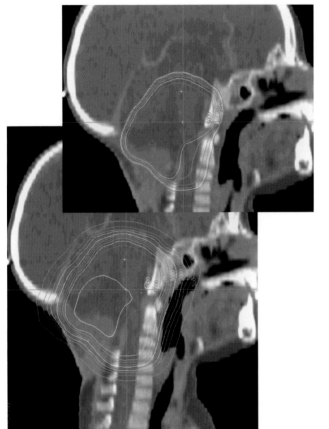

Color Plate 35 Treatment plan demonstrating isodose volumes for three-dimensional conformal approach, using multiple noncoplanar 6-MeV photon fields to encompass tumor within lower aspect of posterior fossa and uppermost spinal canal. Target volume in contemporary protocols more often addresses tumor bed or surgical bed than full posterior fossa. (See also Figure 32-10.)

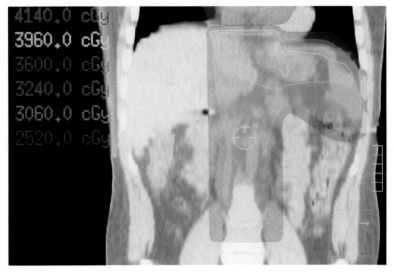

Color Plate 36 Dosimetry for paraaortic and spleen fields for patient in Figure 33-5, *A*.

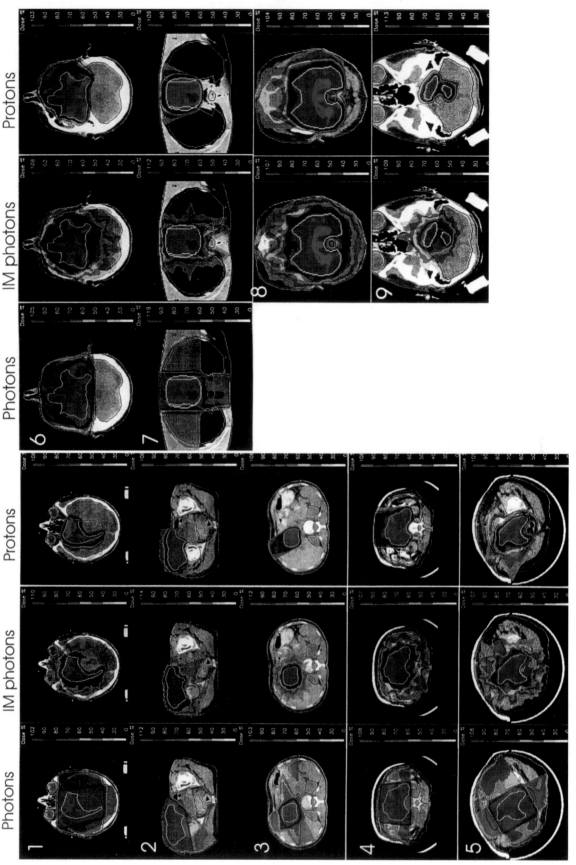

Color Plate 37 Comparison of therapy with standard photon therapy, intensity-modulated *(IM)* photon therapy, and protons. **A,** Central slices from each treatment plan for case 1 (meningioma), case 2 (malignant melanoma of right lumbar region), case 3 (hilar cholangiocarcinoma [Klatskin tumor]), case 4 (metastatic prostate carcinoma), and case 5 (cervical cancer). **B,** Central slices from each treatment plan for case 6 (chromophobic pituitary adenoma), case 7 (simulated thyroid carcinoma), case 8 (acinus cell carcinoma of right sublingual gland), and case 9 (relapsing medulloblastoma). Radiation dosages are indicated by colored bars at right of each panel. (See Chapter 39.) (From Lomax AJ, Bortfeld T, Goitein G, et al. *Radiother Oncol* 1999;51:257-271.)

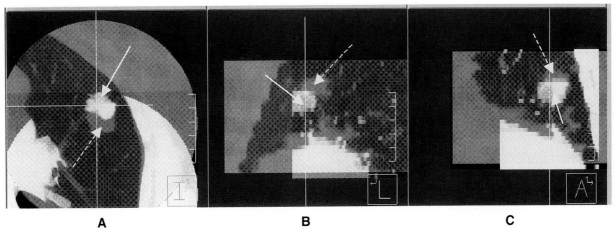

A   **B**   **C**

Fig. 2-17 Merged computed tomography (CT) images at full inspiration and full expiration illustrating the extent of tumor motion during respiratory motion. **A,** Transverse view; **B,** sagittal view; and **C,** coronal view. *Solid arrows* point to the tumor on the CT images obtained during full inspiration, and *dashed arrows* point to the tumor on the CT images obtained during full expiration. The scale at the right of each image indicates 1-cm intervals. (See Color Plate 10, after p. 80, for color reproduction.)

Forms of Gating

Another approach to account for the effects of respiratory motion is gating in which irradiation is delivered only at specified times in the patient's respiratory cycle. In one form of gating patients are instructed to hold their breath, thereby stopping respiratory motion, at a given point in the respiratory cycle, and irradiation is administered only at that point in the cycle. Figure 2-18 illustrates an example of a patient's respiratory cycle. In the deep-inspiration breath-hold technique,[118,119] patients are instructed to hold their breath at or slightly below deep inspiration. The output of the linear accelerator is increased, and the accelerator is turned on for 10 to 20 seconds during the period of breath-holding. Gating the radiation dose at the point of deep inspiration also maximizes lung volume, thereby minimizing the amount of lung tissue irradiated by a fixed-size treatment portal.

An alternative to the deep-inspiration technique is the active breathing control technique.[120] In this technique, the patient's respiratory cycle is monitored with a spirometer (Fig. 2-19). At a specified point in the respiratory cycle, a valve closes the air supply to the patient and the linear accelerator is turned on. After a predetermined period, the accelerator is turned off, the valve is opened, and the patient can resume breathing.

Both the deep-inspiration and active breathing control forms of gating require some training for the patients and the ability to comply with the breath-holding

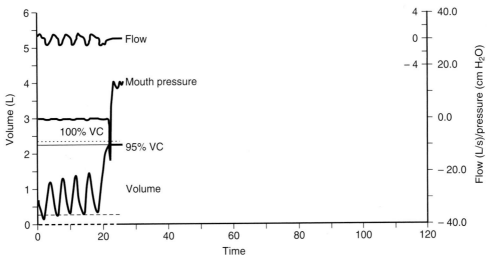

Fig. 2-18 Trace of respiratory cycle illustrating airflow, mouth pressure, and lung volume as a function of time. Note breath-hold at 95% ventilatory capacity *(VC)*.

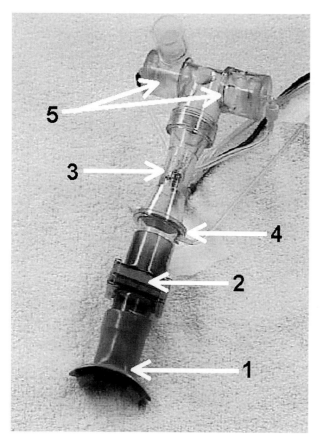

Fig. 2-19 A spirometer (SensorMedics; Yorba Linda, Calif.) used in respiratory gating. *1*, Mouthpiece; *2*, filter; *3*, flow sensor; *4*, pressure sensor; *5*, occlusion valves to control breath hold.

requirement. Ideally, a respiratory professional such as a respiratory therapist should be present to monitor the spirometry and train the patients in the breath-holding techniques.

Another approach is passive gating in which the patient's respiratory cycle is monitored and the accelerator is gated to turn on and off at specified points in the respiratory cycle. Typically, such techniques operate during the part of the respiratory cycle corresponding to full expiration.[121] Monitoring of external patient anatomy rather than respiratory cycle has also been considered as a gating cue, although the consistency of the correlation between external patient anatomy and respiratory cycle needs to be assessed.

Treatment planning for conformal radiation therapy of the lung in particular involves another dimension— that of the change in patient anatomy with regard to the respiratory cycle. In so-called four-dimensional treatment planning, the radiation dose distribution must be timed with regard to movement and changes in volume of the target.[122] Gateable multislice helical CT scanners are needed to accomplish this goal. New tools for analyzing radiation treatment plans may also be required. Moreover, because lung volumes change so dramatically

during respiration, the traditional dose-volume histogram may not be the most appropriate tool for evaluating treatment plans; rather, new analytical tools such as dose-mass histograms, which plot the mass of the lung that receives at least a certain dose, may be required.[118]

In summary, failure to account for intratreatment tumor motion may result in underirradiation of the target volume. Gating the treatment to the respiratory cycle can account for intratreatment tumor motion during lung irradiation and may result in a reduction in the volume of uninvolved tissue being irradiated. Such a reduction would allow higher doses to be delivered to the tumor volume while minimizing the risk of radiation-induced pulmonary complications.

PICTURE ARCHIVAL AND COMMUNICATION SYSTEMS IN RADIATION THERAPY

As its name implies, a radiation therapy picture archival and communication system (RT-PACS) is a system for acquiring, transmitting, storing, and using patient images and image-related information in radiation therapy.[123-125] An RT-PACS can provide a platform for the images and image functions used in both planning and delivering radiation treatment. For example, radiation treatment planning can be seen as an imaging application consisting of the following steps. A set of sequential CT images is consolidated to generate a three-dimensional representation of the patient's anatomy. Anatomic structures are delineated on the CT data set by manual or automatic segmentation. The data set is translated and rotated to determine optimal beam geometries for delivery of radiation. Treatment portals are determined on the basis of beam's-eye view projections of target volumes and anatomic structures. Dose distributions superimposed on the data set are reviewed, and the treatment plan is evaluated. The RT-PACS acquires the images from the CT scanner, displays them, and then stores them with the digitally reconstructed radiographs and dose distributions in a database. An RT-PACS can also be used to archive treatment plans and dose distributions for subsequent review.

An even more common image application in radiation oncology is the validation of treatment delivery, which involves comparing an image of the delivered radiation field with a reference image indicating the desired treatment portal. In these comparisons, portal images are taken during the course of treatment with simulation images (obtained as digitized simulator films or digitally reconstructed radiographs) or with an approved initial portal image. Although these image comparisons have traditionally been done manually with hard-copy films, the use of digital images on an RT-PACS allows computer-aided image comparisons.

Digital portal images acquired with electronic portal imaging devices are becoming more prevalent in the radiation oncology clinic. Two paradigms exist for the review of these digital portal images. The first is the traditional paradigm in which an initial portal image is reviewed against a simulation image to verify the initial patient treatment followed by regular review of on-treatment portal images as a continuing quality assurance check of treatment delivery. Portal images are typically reviewed at some time after image acquisition, often several hours to one day afterward. In the second paradigm, portal images are reviewed immediately on their acquisition and the patient set-up can be adjusted immediately on the basis of a comparison between the portal image and a reference image.[126] In both paradigms, the RT-PACS provides a necessary platform to support the review and storage of images. Moreover, in the first paradigm, the RT-PACS can provide a tasking queue in which images scheduled for review can be fetched and made available in a staging area to speed the image-review process.

Comparison Capabilities

At the very least, the capability of an RT-PACS to display images side by side allows physicians to compare images manually, much like comparing films in a conventional viewbox. As currently used at the M.D. Anderson Cancer Center, images are acquired by digitizing film with a computed radiography unit or from an electronic portal imaging device, and the images are displayed on an RT-PACS. Physicians review the portal image and the reference image, assess the alignment of the two images, and either approve the portal image or, if the image is unacceptable, transmit instructions to the radiation therapist by means of a messaging facility in the RT-PACS.

In the future, automatic image comparison tools will be incorporated into RT-PACSs. Comparison of portal images is a relatively straightforward task because the images are similar in quality, contrast, and noise, with the only significant differences being those of spatial orientation of anatomy with respect to field boundaries. Gradient search algorithms have been developed that efficiently align portal images and compute the magnitude and direction of translational and rotational misalignment.[127,128] In an example of such an alignment (Fig. 2-20; see also Color Plate 11, after p. 80), the test image on the right is aligned with a reference image on the left. After alignment, the translations and rotation required to align the image can be readily translated into specific instructions for the therapist to reposition the

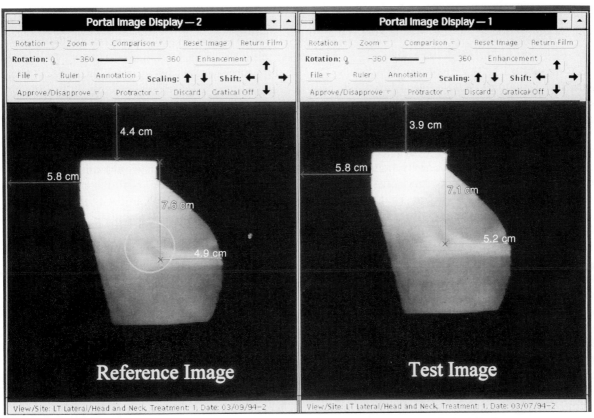

Fig. 2-20 Radiation therapy picture archival and communication system display of reference portal image *(left)* and test portal image *(right)* of a head-and-neck treatment field used for image comparison. (See Color Plate 11, after p. 80, for color reproduction.)

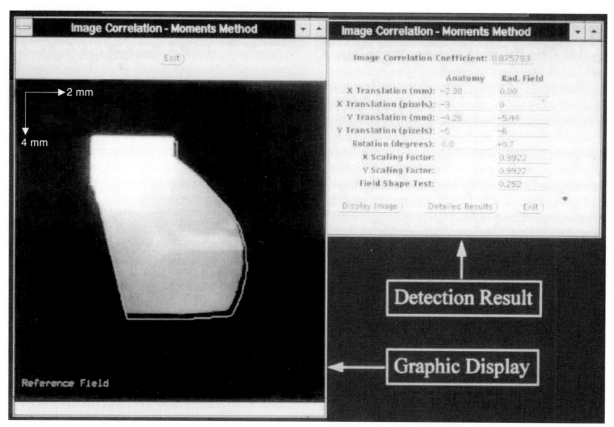

Fig. 2-21 Display on a radiation therapy picture archival and communication system of the adjustments in patient positioning needed to bring the test image into alignment with the reference image. (See Color Plate 12, after p. 80, for color reproduction.)

patient, if necessary (Fig. 2-21; see also Color Plate 12, after p. 80). Alternatively, edge-detection methods can be used to align portal images.[129]

A more difficult problem than assessing the alignment of portal images is the problem of assessing the alignment of simulator images with portal images. Because the mode of image acquisition is different, the two types of images differ significantly in contrast, detail, and noise. Methods that align the images, either through point matching[130] or line-segment matching,[131,132] seem promising. At present, points or line segments are manually identified on images, but research is currently under way to develop automated methods for identification and extraction of relevant points or line segments from the two types of images.

Incorporation of an RT-PACS in the radiation oncology clinic can greatly improve efficiency in clinical operations. Electronic images can be handled much more efficiently than can hard-copy images. Images can be retrieved much more quickly from an image database than from a film library; moreover, electronic images are never "checked out" from the database. Image processing tools such as gray-scale windows and leveling, histogram equalization, and image enhancement can aid

physicians in identifying details on a digital image that might not otherwise be visible on a film. Image alignment tools combined with decision criteria can be used to aid physicians in determining the quality of alignment of images used for treatment verification. Finally, the use of electronic images can save significant amounts of money that would otherwise be spent on the purchase and storage of film.

HIGH-TECHNOLOGY BRACHYTHERAPY

High-technology brachytherapy efforts being pursued at the M.D. Anderson Cancer Center include high-dose-rate, image-guided, and intravascular applications. Each of these efforts is described in further detail in the following paragraphs.

High-dose-rate Brachytherapy

At the M.D. Anderson Cancer Center, high-dose-rate brachytherapy is used mostly as an endobronchial treatment for lung cancer and airway tumors[133] and, with the use of vaginal dome cylinders, for uterine and vaginal tumors. The American Brachytherapy Society has drafted guidelines for high-dose-rate brachytherapy for lung carcinoma.[134] At the M.D. Anderson Cancer Center, either a single- or double-catheter technique is used, with the dose prescribed at the estimated position of the wall of the trachea or bronchus. Patients undergo bronchoscopy in a special procedures room and are then transported to a high-dose-rate treatment room. Treatment plans are created and optimized for each patient before delivery; a plan for dual-catheter treatment of bronchogenic disease is illustrated in Figure 2-22 (see also Color Plate 13, after p. 80). The prescribed dose is generally 15 Gy per fraction given in up to three fractions, usually at 2-week intervals.

High-dose-rate brachytherapy for gynecologic cancer is delivered by means of vaginal dome cylinders, with treatment prescribed at the surface of the dome. The dose and fractionation schedules vary depending on the disease and the intended treatment (monotherapy or a boost dose for external-beam therapy). Applicators for the domes are placed while the patient is in the radiation oncology department. Because the cylinders are of fixed geometry, most treatment plans are selected from an atlas and then modified as needed for each patient.

All high-dose-rate treatments that are not conducted during the course of surgery are performed with a

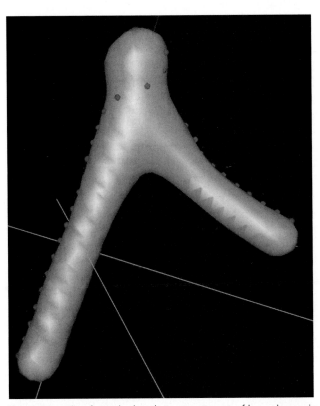

Fig. 2-22 Plan for a dual-catheter treatment of bronchogenic carcinoma. The *light blue* surface encloses the volume receiving at least 15 Gy. The *blue dots* on that surface are the points of dose specification. (See Color Plate 13, after p. 80, for color reproduction.)

high-dose-rate remote afterloader located in a simulator room within the radiation oncology department. This set-up allows the high-dose-rate applicators to be placed and treatment delivered without having to move patients between an x-ray localization site and a treatment site, thereby minimizing the time that the applicator remains in the patient.

Intraoperative high-dose-rate brachytherapy is an emerging treatment modality at the M.D. Anderson Cancer Center, where an operating suite houses both a LINAC and a high-dose-rate remote afterloader for delivering intraoperative radiation therapy. Having both machines in the same room allows radiation oncologists to choose the most appropriate modality for any intraoperative treatment. Initial use of this modality has focused on pelvic sidewall disease that cannot be accessed easily with an intraoperative electron applicator and, instead, is performed with the Harrison-Anderson-Mick applicator.[135] Treatment plans are selected from an atlas of plans based on the fixed geometry of the applicator device. The selected plan is then optimized for each patient. Experience gained with this new modality is expected to expand the ability to treat disease at other sites in the future.

Commissioning a high-dose-rate brachytherapy program requires a 2- to 4-month physicist effort for startup.[116,136] As an ongoing requirement after set-up, the American Association of Physicists in Medicine recommends one full-time equivalent physicist for a patient load averaging 10 fractions per week.[136]

Individuals administering high-dose-rate brachytherapy should be well trained in treatment planning, quality assurance, and emergency procedures, given the speed at which the treatment planning and delivery take place. At least one physicist and one dosimetrist (or two physicists) should participate in the treatment planning process, and these individuals should independently verify each other's work. Treatment time should be calculated using a method independent of the treatment planning computer before the treatment is administered.[137,138] The U.S. Nuclear Regulatory Commission regulations require that a radiation oncologist and physicist be present during each high-dose-rate brachytherapy treatment.

Image-Guided Brachytherapy

The M.D. Anderson Cancer Center has extensive experience with CT-guided [198]Au implants for the treatment of rectal carcinoma.[139] Another image-guided brachytherapy effort taking place is sonographically guided ^{125}I and [103]Pd implants for the treatment of prostate cancer. A typical CT-guided ^{125}I prostate treatment plan is displayed in Figure 2-23 (see also Color Plate 14, after p. 80). The authors recently initiated "real-time" treatment planning in the procedure room

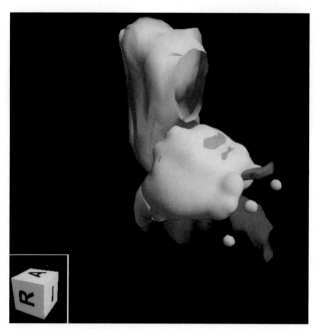

Fig. 2-23 A ^{125}I computed tomography–based prostate treatment plan. The *light blue* surface demonstrates the 144-Gy surface; *yellow*, bladder; *dark blue*, rectum; *red*, prostate; *purple*, seminal vesicles; and *green*, ureter. (See Color Plate 14, after p. 80, for color reproduction.)

using a laptop-based treatment planning computer. This procedure allows radiation oncologists to view the dose as the ^{103}Pd, ^{125}I, or ^{198}Au seeds are implanted and to adjust the planned location of each seed in light of this information. Future plans are to combine real-time treatment planning dosimetry with CT guidance and fluoroscopic verification of seed placement for permanent prostate implants. This procedure is currently limited by the size of the bore of current CT scanners.

Commissioning a permanent implant program for prostate treatment requires approximately 1 month of a full-time physicist's time. In addition, at least 10% of the seeds to be used in each seed implant should be assayed,[140] and the results of this assay should be within 5% of the manufacturer's specification.[141] Each implant requires approximately 2 hours of a physicist's or a dosimetrist's time in the operating room. As an ongoing requirement, the physicist's time required depends greatly on whether the treatment is preplanned and whether preloaded needles or a Mick applicator is used. Preplanned treatments require approximately 30 to 45 minutes per treatment; the use of preloaded needles requires 2 hours of a physicist's or dosimetrist's time for a typical case. Finally, the American Association of Physicists in Medicine recommends that physics personnel participating in a permanent-implant prostate treatment program perform at least five cases under the direct supervision of an experienced medical physicist before performing a case independently.[140]

Intravascular Brachytherapy

The M.D. Anderson Cancer Center, in collaboration with the Texas Heart Institute of St. Luke's Episcopal Hospital, is currently engaged in clinical trials to evaluate the role of intravascular brachytherapy radiation after percutaneous transluminal coronary angioplasty to inhibit restenosis in coronary arteries. Such angioplasty is used as an alternative to coronary artery bypass grafting to treat coronary artery disease. Angioplasty has lower initial costs and produces fewer complications than bypass surgery, but the effectiveness of the angioplasty is limited by restenosis appearing within 3 to 36 months in 30% to 50% of patients after treatment. Placement of coronary stents has been found to reduce the incidence of restenosis to 20% to 30%, but the total societal cost of even this reduced rate of restenosis has been estimated at up to $2 billion.[141,142] Recent studies indicate that the use of radiation may reduce the incidence of restenosis in such patients. The radiation dose can be delivered as either brachytherapy or external-beam therapy; however, external-beam therapy may be better suited for irradiation of peripheral vessels than coronary vessels because of cardiac motion.

Intravascular brachytherapy can be delivered by means of catheters or radioactive stents. The M.D. Anderson Cancer Center is currently using a ^{192}Ir catheter-based system consisting of a 3.3-mm linear array of ^{192}Ir seeds spaced on 4-mm centers, thus closely approximating a ^{192}Ir wire. Arrays in 6-, 10-, 14-, or 19-seed lengths are also available depending on the length of the area to be treated. The array is attached to a guide wire, inserted into a balloon catheter, and pushed into place in the stented area. A dose of 14 Gy is delivered 2 mm from the center of the source. Other catheter-based systems under development include several beta sources, with ^{32}P, ^{90}Y, and ^{90}Sr/^{90}Y sources being given the most consideration at this time.

Several radioactive stents are also under development, including stents incorporating ^{32}P, ^{103}Pd, ^{51}V, and other isotopes. Dose clouds surrounding a ^{103}Pd stent[143] are depicted in Figure 2-24 (see also Color Plate 15, after p. 80). These dose clouds were calculated with the Monte Carlo code EGS4. Conventional techniques for brachytherapy dosimetry are not applicable at the close treatment distances used for intravascular brachytherapy; rather, this modality requires that dosimetric calculations be performed with Monte Carlo techniques.

Intravascular radiation therapy is a rapidly emerging modality with potential applications for treating peripheral vessel angioplasty, bypass graft anastomoses, and arteriovenous dialysis grafts in addition to coronary vessels. Because dosimetric considerations differ for each of these treatment sites, no single delivery system is likely to be appropriate for all intravascular radiation therapy applications. Rather, use of any of these modalities

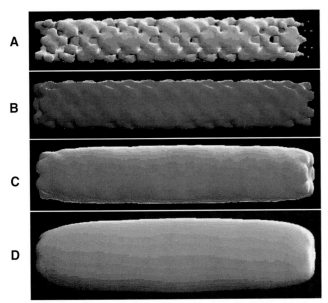

Fig. 2-24 Dose clouds surrounding a coronary stent implanted with 1 mCi of ^{103}Pd. **A,** 120 Gy. **B,** 90 Gy. **C,** 60 Gy. **D,** 40 Gy. (See Color Plate 15, after p. 80, for color reproduction.)

(external beam, catheter-based systems, and radioactive stents) will depend on the dosimetric and radiobiological considerations specific to each procedure site and each patient.

According to the American College of Medical Physics recommendations, intravascular brachytherapy after percutaneous transluminal coronary angioplasty requires a team consisting of an interventional cardiologist, a radiation oncologist, and a radiation physicist.[142] These individuals should spend at least 1 day of training with experienced personnel learning the basic techniques specific to any delivery system. An additional 2 to 4 weeks of physicist time will be required to develop and apply commissioning and quality assurance tools and techniques for the delivery system to be used. The amount of ongoing physicist time for quality assurance of sources or the afterloader depends greatly on the specific devices used. Physicist time required for each treatment is approximately 1 hour.

QUALITY ASSURANCE IN MULTI-INSTITUTIONAL TRIALS

Radiation oncology is an empirical science in which dose prescription and target volumes are based on previous experience gained either by the individual oncologist or from published studies. The importance of multi-institutional clinical trials in the advancement of this process has grown substantially over the past 30 years, and these trials are an essential component of the dramatic advances now being made with new high-technology

treatments. In 1969, at the urging of the Committee on Radiation Therapy Studies and the American Association of Physicists in Medicine, the U.S. National Cancer Institute funded the Radiological Physics Center (RPC) to standardize the technical components of radiation therapy. The following section begins with a brief history of the various players in quality assurance in Cooperative Oncology Groups, followed by brief reviews of past and future programs used by the RPC and programs to respond to the changing nature of radiation oncology.

A Brief History of Quality Assurance for Radiation Therapy Trials

The RPC at the M.D. Anderson Cancer Center has been continuously funded by the National Cancer Institute since 1969. From 1974 to 1986 the National Cancer Institute also funded six regional Centers for Radiological Physics to monitor and assist community hospitals that were becoming involved in cooperative clinical trials. The methods used by these centers were similar to those used by the RPC.

In the early days, the chairs of each protocol study were responsible for ensuring the quality of the clinical components of the protocols. In 1976 the National Cancer Institute funded the first in a series of clinical quality-assurance centers, which were charged with assisting the protocol study chairs and standardizing the clinical components of protocol treatment. Today, only three of these groups persist: the American College of Radiology program in Philadelphia, which serves the Radiation Therapy Oncology Group; the Quality Assurance Review Center in Providence, R.I., which serves the Children's Oncology Group, the Cancer and Acute Leukemia Group B, and the Eastern Cooperative Oncology Group; and the Southwest Oncology Group Quality Assurance Center at Wayne State University, which serves the Southwest Oncology Group.

In 1992 a Quality Assurance Center for three-dimensional conformal therapy was established at the Mallinckrodt Institute of Radiology in St. Louis to promote and provide quality assurance for the conformal radiation therapy protocols of the Radiation Therapy Oncology Group. This center developed procedures and tools for transferring volumetric target and dose data electronically between participating institutions and the center in St. Louis, and it has credentialed several institutions to participate in three conformal therapy protocols. The credentialing process involves an institution proving its ability by transferring "dry-run" data on a patient whose treatment was planned and delivered according to the conformal therapy protocol. The Mallinckrodt Quality Assurance Center also established a repository database for technical and clinical data on treated patients. In 1999 the National Cancer Institute funded an effort to extend the quality assurance program for high-technology radiation therapy to all cooperative groups, and at that time a consortium of the Mallinckrodt Quality Assurance Center, the American College of Radiology, the Quality Assurance Review Center in Providence, and the RPC in Houston was funded. The Resource Center for Emerging Technologies in Jacksonville, Fla., also received funding to establish a database system like that of the Mallinckrodt Quality Assurance Center. The Jacksonville program was intended to serve pediatric programs, and the Mallinckrodt Quality Assurance Center was intended to serve adult studies.

The Radiological Physics Center's Tools for Monitoring Conventional Therapy (1970 to 1995)

The primary responsibility of the RPC is to assure the National Cancer Institute and the cooperative groups that institutions participating in cooperative trials can be expected to deliver radiation treatments that are clinically comparable to those delivered at other participating institutions. According to RPC standards, institutions must demonstrate that they have the proper equipment, personnel, and quality-assurance procedures to deliver the prescribed dose to within ±5%. The RPC currently monitors nearly 1300 radiation therapy facilities that house more than 2500 megavoltage therapy units.

The RPC uses both on-site dosimetry reviews and various remote audit tools. During on-site reviews, key personnel are interviewed, physical measurements are made on therapy machines, dosimetry and quality assurance data are reviewed, treatment planning algorithms are tested, and patient dose calculations are evaluated. Remote audit tools include the use of thermoluminescent dosimeters (TLDs) for verifying output calibrations, standard data for verifying the dosimetry data, benchmark or actual patient calculations for verifying the treatment planning algorithms, and review of an institution's written quality assurance procedures and records.

Anthropomorphic phantoms are also used to verify tumor dose delivery for special treatment techniques. Any discrepancies found by the RPC are pursued to help the institution resolve them. Thus the RPC's overall quality assurance program affects not only patients in clinical trials but also the quality of dosimetry for all patients treated at the institution. Key aspects of on-site reviews and remote audit tools are reviewed briefly in the following paragraphs.

On-Site Reviews

On-site dosimetry reviews by the RPC have played a key role in achieving consistent dosimetry among institutions. By the mid-1990s, basic output calibration (i.e., the determination of dose rate delivered under reference conditions) was within the ±3% criterion for 98% of all photon beams and 93% of all electron beams measured by the RPC. (The comparable rates in the mid-1970s were around 75%.) Significant improvements in equipment and training of professional staff were instrumental in this improvement. In addition, the emphasis on quality assurance by the RPC, through the cooperative oncology groups, helped direct resources to improving quality. Although reference dose rate calibrations have become less of a concern, many concerns still exist regarding dosimetry. The RPC on-site review is comprehensive and includes the possibility that small errors in dosimetry could become compounded and could result in a major discrepancy. More than 90% of all participating institutions visited by the RPC receive at least one recommendation regarding improvements that could be made in dosimetry or quality assurance. Typical discrepancies encountered are listed in Table 2-2. In addition, at nearly half of all institutions visited during the past 3 years, the RPC identified at least one treatment combination for which the discrepancy in prescribed dose between the institution and the RPC exceeded 5%. The RPC works with the institution to resolve discrepancies such as these so that the quality of therapy improves at most institutions because of the visit by the RPC.

Asymmetric jaws on therapy machines were one of the first modern innovations or high-technology improvements in radiation oncology. The agreement between RPC measurements and institutional measurements of 97 asymmetric fields for photon beams are shown in Figure 2-25.[144] Most measurements fit into a tight Gaussian distribution, but approximately 5% of the measurements fall outside the ±5% criterion. Most of these values represent either measurement errors by the institution in regions of high dose gradient or a misunderstanding as to how the measured values should be used clinically.

Mailed Thermoluminescent Dosimeter Program

All institutions at which active clinical trials are taking place are subject to periodic monitoring with TLDs. This system, in which dosimeters are used and then mailed to the RPC, provides a mechanism for identifying potential problems at new institutions and allows remote surveillance of all participating institutions. The TLD program is designed to verify output and energy levels for electron beams and output levels for photons.[145,146] The results of the RPC assessment are reported to the institution. If the absorbed-dose measurements by the RPC and the institution disagree by more than 5%, the discrepancy is discussed by telephone with the participating physicist to identify the source of the discrepancy. A second set of dosimeters is then mailed immediately. If the discrepancy

TABLE 2-2	
Most Frequent Recommendations Resulting from On-Site Dosimetry Reviews at 80 Institutions between January 1996 and May 1998	
Recommendation Topic	**Number of Institutions Receiving Recommendation**
Wedge transmission	71 (89%)
Mechanical problems (lasers, optical distance indicator, collimator dial)	22 (28%)
Electron calibration	18 (23%)
Photon depth dose	16 (20%)
Review of quality assurance program	15 (19%)
Electron depth dose	15 (19%)
Photon calibration	10 (13%)
Off-axis factors	10 (13%)
Brachytherapy source calibration	9 (11%)
Patient dosimetry	8 (10%)
Beam asymmetry	7 (9%)
Using multiple sets of data	6 (8%)
Electron cone factors/ratio	6 (8%)
Temperature, pressure	6 (8%)

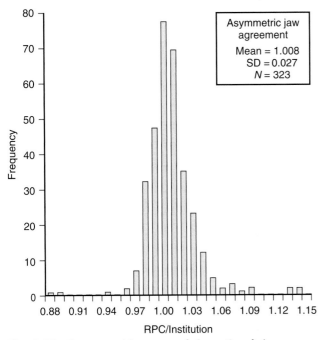

Fig. 2-25 Frequency histogram of the ratio of doses measured by the Radiological Physics Center *(RPC)* for asymmetric fields to the doses used at the institution being tested, for 6- to 20-MV photon beams.

persists, the RPC schedules an on-site dosimetry review. Approximately six institutions are visited annually to resolve apparent discrepancies that are identified by the dosimeters.

Evaluation of Patient Dosimetry

An institution's patient-dosimetry calculations are evaluated by reviewing data from benchmark cases or from treatment of patients on protocol. Benchmark cases are evaluated during an on-site review; such cases have included a parallel opposed-field brain treatment, a 90-degree wedged pair treatment, a three-field wedged rectal treatment, a lung or Hodgkin's mantle treatment including off-axis calculations, and a tangential-field breast treatment. These cases are intended to test the accuracy of the treatment planning algorithms used. The results over the past 10 years indicate that disagreement of more than 3% between the RPC and the institution measures occurs in about 1% of the brain, wedged-field, and lung-treatment benchmark cases, mostly for calculations on the central axis of the beam; 5% of the breast treatment cases; and 17% of the cases involving off-axis calculations. A major contributor to these discrepancies is a lack of understanding by the institution's medical physicist of the dose algorithms used in the treatment planning system. Most manufacturers of treatment planning systems consider their calculational algorithm to be proprietary, which adds to the problem. With the advent of convolution-based calculational models, an even greater lack of understanding of the algorithms and the data necessary to properly commission a treatment planning system for a therapy machine is anticipated.

The RPC also evaluates the treatment of individual patients entered in selected cooperative group studies. The object of this review is to verify that the patient was treated both as reported to the group and according to the specifications of the protocol. In a survey published in 1991, the RPC and institution could not agree with the dose at the prescription point to within ±5% among approximately 1% of the patient treatments reviewed; however, 6% of the patient treatments involved an error in dose reporting.[147] The RPC evaluation improved the dose data that had been reported to the cooperative group in 15% of the patient treatments reviewed.[147] Results over the ensuing 10 years have been comparable, except for a higher dosimetry-error rate for tangential breast treatments, as has continued to be the case for the benchmark cases.

Standard Data

The RPC has collected measurements of depth dose, output factors, wedge transmission, and other dosimetry parameters from several thousand radiation therapy machines, including photons and electron beams.[148–151] The RPC has five or more consistent data sets for 56 photon beams on 36 different models of accelerators built by multiple manufacturers. Review of these data suggests that machines of the same model have similar radiation characteristics (standard deviations of ±1%). The RPC has identified *standard data* (field size dependence, depth dose, and off-axis factors) for these 56 beams. Accumulated wedge transmission data for approximately 5300 wedges on more than 1000 accelerators since 1985 have been analyzed.[150] Like other dosimetry parameters for a particular model of accelerator, a standard wedge transmission factor can be assigned for each combination of wedge angle, nominal energy, and make and model of accelerator. The authors' data, with a few exceptions, can be used to predict the wedge transmission factor for most wedges in clinical use today to within ±2%. The data also showed that, over time, manufacturers have changed their wedge design and in some cases a particular wedge angle or energy and accelerator model may have up to three distinct standard wedge transmission factors. Moreover, identical or similar wedges are used on different models of accelerators by the same manufacturer, resulting in a single standard wedge transmission factor for several accelerators (Fig. 2-26). The RPC is trying to capitalize on standard data as a means of identifying institutions that would benefit from an on-site visit.[152]

Preapproval Processes

An increasing number of cooperative study groups (including the Radiation Therapy, Eastern Cooperative, Children's, and Gynecologic Oncology Groups) are developing protocols that involve advanced technology or specialized treatment techniques. Over the past 5 years the RPC has begun to play an increasing role in preapproving personnel and institutions to enter patients in these protocols. The process involves (1) completion of a knowledge assessment form regarding equipment and quality assurance procedures, knowledge of the protocol, and specification of dosimetry parameters; (2) completion of benchmark patient-treatment cases; and (3) verification of experience by having submitted at least one previous clinical case for review by the RPC. Although this preapproval program is a fairly new addition to the RPC program, compliance of the institutions that went through a required preapproval process to enter patients into a breast treatment study was good.[153] An additional impression is that the quality of cervical implants has

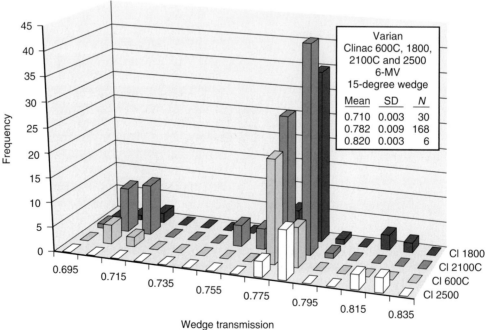

Fig. 2-26 Frequency histogram of the Varian Clinac models 600C, 1800, 2100C, and 2500 6-MV x-ray wedge transmission factors for the 15-degree wedge. The histograms indicate three possible mean wedge transmission factors.

improved since implementation of the preapproval program for high-dose-rate brachytherapy.

The Future

As radiation oncology begins to rely on image-based dynamic therapies and contemporary model-based dose-calculation algorithms, the effectiveness of monitoring tools developed for older conventional therapies is becoming unclear. The RPC has been developing a two-part approach to quality assurance for these newer concepts. The first part of this approach, to be implemented in collaboration with the Mallinckrodt Quality Assurance Center, involves the preapproval process; the RPC will address the dose-delivery issues, and the Mallinckrodt Quality Assurance Center will address the data transfer and analysis components. The second part of the approach involves using pseudo-anthropomorphic phantoms to test the entire treatment process from imaging to treatment planning to actual treatment delivery. Phantoms for four anatomic sites have been constructed or are under development.[154-157] All have the same basic design, including a water-filled outer plastic shell with inserts containing critical structures, imageable targets, and dosimeters (TLDs for measuring absolute dose and film to verify field placement and relative dose distributions).

The first of these phantoms was a stereotactic head phantom that was sent to institutions participating in Radiation Therapy Oncology Group SRS protocols. The head phantom has two inserts, the first of which contains a target that can be imaged with either CT or MRI; the second insert, which contains dosimeters, replaces the first without having to remove the phantom from the head frame. This phantom was designed to determine the dose with a precision of ±5% and to locate

the edge of the field in three dimensions to within ±1 mm. The results from the first 41 institutions monitored with the head phantom are as follows. First, all institutions met the ±5% criterion for delivery of dose to the middle of the target. The mean RPC:institution ratio for dose was 0.996 ±2.6%. Second, many institutions could not meet the ±1 mm criterion for field localization. The mean distance from the center of the target to the center of the radiation field was 1.3 ± 0.8 mm. Third, a measurably larger volume of tissue was being treated than is necessary. The mean ratio of the volume treated to the target volume was 1.6 ± 0.5. Fourth, the use of 3-mm slice spacing on the planning CT often resulted in larger geometric uncertainties along the superior–inferior axis. To date, three problems have been identified by use of the phantom and pursued to solution by the RPC. These problems included one malfunctioning MRI scanner, one institution using excessive slice spacing on the localization CT scan, and one software problem in transferring data from the CT scanner to the localization system.

Given the success of the head phantom, four other pseudo-anthropomorphic phantoms have been designed and are at various stages of construction: a modification of the head phantom to test IMRT treatments of the head and neck, a lung phantom, a pelvic phantom designed for Radiation Therapy Oncology Group conformal and IMRT treatments, and a breast phantom. A cross section of the pelvic phantom with a CT scan of a patient for comparison is shown in Figure 2-27 (see also Color Plate 16, after p. 80).

Summary

Quality assurance of both technical and clinical aspects of cooperative clinical trials has been effectively monitored by the RPC and various clinical quality assurance

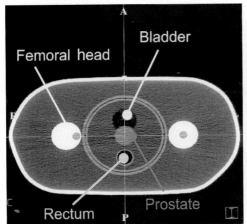 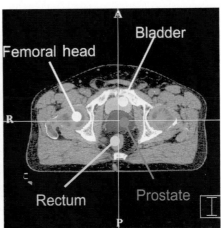

Fig. 2-27 Cross-section of the Radiological Physics Center's pelvic phantom for intensity-modulated radiation therapy showing the simulated organs *(left)*. A transverse computed tomography scan of a male pelvis at the same anatomic position as the phantom *(right)*. (See Color Plate 16, after p. 80, for color reproduction.)

centers for the past 30 years. The new challenges provided by high-technology radiation treatments are being addressed by the RPC, the Mallinckrodt Quality Assurance Center, the Resource Center for Emerging Technologies, the Quality Assurance Review Center, and the American College of Radiology. The tools being developed include anthropomorphic phantoms to audit the total planning/treatment process, Web-based tools for digital transmission of planning and treatment data, databases to collect and process patient treatment data, and treatment protocols to test new technologies and new dose-evaluation methods. As research enters the era of image-based radiation therapy, the challenge for all parties involved in quality assurance will be to apply well-established quality audit techniques wherever possible and to develop new quality audit techniques where none now exist.

REFERENCES

1. Ling CC, Humm J, Larson S, et al. Towards multidimensional radiotherapy (MD-CRT): biological imaging and biological conformality. *Int J Radiat Oncol Biol Phys* 2000;47:551-560.

2. Austin-Seymour M. Subjective target volume and normal structure segmentation. In: Hazle JD, Boyer AL, eds. *Imaging in Radiation Therapy*. Proceedings of the 1998 Summer School of the American Association of Physicists in Medicine, University of Wisconsin-Madison. Madison, Wis: Medical Physics; 1998:259-270. Medical Physics Monograph No. 24.

3. Kessler ML, Puff DT. Segmentation and visualization for treatment planning. In: Mackie TR, Palta JT, eds. *Teletherapy: Present and Future*. Proceedings of the 1996 Summer School of the American Association of Physicists in Medicine, University of British Columbia, Vancouver, Canada. Madison, Wis: Advanced Medical; 1996:63-83.

4. Chaney EL, Fritsch DS, Pizer SM. Objective GTV and normal structure segmentation. In: Hazle JD, Boyer AL, eds. *Imaging in Radiation Therapy*. Proceedings of the 1998 Summer School of the American Association of Physicists in Medicine, University of Wisconsin-Madison. Madison, Wis: Medical Physics; 1998:271-290. Medical Physics Monograph No. 24.

5. Mohan R. Intensity modulation in radiotherapy. In: Mackie TR, Palta JT, eds. *Teletherapy: Present and Future*. Proceedings of the 1996 Summer School of the American Association of Physicists in Medicine, University of British Columbia, Vancouver, Canada. Madison, Wis: Advanced Medical; 1996:761-803.

6. Dong L. Portal image correlation and analysis. In: Hazle JD, Boyer AL, eds. *Imaging in Radiation Therapy*. Proceedings of the 1998 Summer School of the American Association of Physicists in Medicine, University of Wisconsin-Madison. Madison, Wis: Medical Physics; 1998:415-444. Medical Physics Monograph No. 24.

7. Balter JM, McShan DL, Lam KL, et al. Incorporation of patient setup measurement and adjustment within a computer controlled radiotherapy system. In: Leavitt DD, Starkschall G, eds. Proceedings of the XIIth International Conference on the Use of Computers in Radiation Therapy, Salt Lake City, Utah, 27-30 May 1996. Madison, Wis: Medical Physics; 1997:182-184.

8. Wong JW, Yan D, Jaffray DA, et al. Interventional strategies to counter the effects of inter-fraction treatment variation. In: Schlegel W, Bortfeld T, eds. Proceedings of the XIIIth International Conference on the Use of Computers in Radiation Therapy, Heidelberg, Germany, 22-25 May 2000. New York, NY: Springer-Verlag; 2000:511-513.

9. Mageras GS. Interventional strategies for reducing respiratory-induced motion in external beam therapy. In: Schlegel W, Bortfeld T, eds. Proceedings of the XIIIth International Conference on The Use of Computers in Radiation Therapy, Heidelberg, Germany, 22-25 May 2000. New York, NY: Springer-Verlag; 2000:514-516.

10. Willoughby T, Kupelian P, Weinhous M. Ultrasound for patient positioning in radiation therapy. In: Schlegel W, Bortfeld T, eds. Proceedings of the XIIIth International Conference on The Use of Computers in Radiation Therapy, Heidelberg, Germany, 22-25 May 2000. New York, NY: Springer-Verlag; 2000:517.

11. Lu W, Mackie TR, Keller H, et al. A generalization of adaptive radiotherapy and the registration of deformable dose distributions. In: Schlegel W, Bortfeld T, eds. Proceedings of the XIIIth International Conference on The Use of Computers in Radiation Therapy, Heidelberg, Germany, 22-25 May 2000. New York, NY: Springer-Verlag; 2000:521-523.

12. Purdy JA. Medical physics certification: American Board of Radiology and American Board of Medical Physics. In: Hogstrom KR, Horton JL, eds. *Introduction to the Professional Aspects of Medical Physics*. Houston, Tex: The University of Texas M.D. Anderson Cancer Center; 1999:32-45.

13. Goff DL. Licensure and credentialing for medical physicists. In: Hogstrom KR, Horton JL, eds. *Introduction to the Professional Aspects of Medical Physics*. Houston: The University of Texas M.D. Anderson Cancer Center, 1999:48-55.

14. Hogstrom KR. Status of medical physics residency training programs. *Am Coll Radiol [ACR] Bull* 2000:56(3):40.

15. Hogstrom KR. Report from the Chairman of the Board. American Association of Physicists in Medicine Newsletter 2001:26(1):1a-1b.

16. Inter-Society Council for Radiation Oncology. *Radiation Oncology in Integrated Cancer Management (the "Blue Book")*. Philadelphia, Pa: American College of Radiology; 1991.

17. American College of Medical Physics. Survey of Physics Resources for Radiation Oncology Special Procedures. *ACMP Task Group Report*. Reston, VA: American College of Medical Physics; 22 April 1998.

18. Hogstrom KR, Rosen II. Resources needed to support 3-D radiation therapy treatment planning. In: Purdy JA, Starkschall G, eds. *A Practical Guide to 3-D Planning and Conformal Radiation Therapy*. Madison, Wis: Advanced Medical; 1999:341-358.

19. Starkschall G. What is 3-D radiation therapy treatment planning? In: Purdy JA, Starkschall G, eds. *A Practical Guide to 3-D Planning and Conformal Radiation Therapy*. Madison, Wis: Advanced Medical; 1999:1-6.

20. Starkschall G. 2D versus 3D radiotherapy treatment planning. In: Mackie TR, Palta JT, eds. *Teletherapy: Present and Future*. Proceedings of the 1996 Summer School of the American Association of Physicists in Medicine, University of British Columbia, Vancouver, Canada. Madison, Wis: Advanced Medical; 1996:17-36.

21. Rosen II. Quality assurance in conformal radiation therapy. In: Smith AR, ed. *Radiation Therapy Physics*. Berlin: Springer-Verlag; 1995.

22. International Commission on Radiation Units and Measurements. *Prescribing, Recording, and Reporting Photon Beam Therapy* (ICRU Report 50). Bethesda, Md: International Commission on Radiation Units and Measurements; 1993.

23. Purdy JA. A practical guide to ICRU 50 volume and dose specifications for 3-D conformal therapy. In: Purdy JA, Starkschall G, eds. *A Practical Guide to 3-D Planning and Conformal Radiation Therapy*. Madison, Wis: Advanced Medical; 1999.

24. International Commission on Radiation Units and Measurements. *Prescribing, Recording and Reporting Photon Beam Therapy* (Supplement to ICRU Report 50). Bethesda. Md: International Commission on Radiation Units and Measurement; 1999.

25. Verhey LJ. Patient immobilization for 3-D RTP and virtual simulation. In: Purdy JA, Starkschall G, eds. *A Practical Guide to 3-D*

Planning and Conformal Radiation Therapy. Madison, Wis: Advanced Medical; 1999:151-174.

26. Antolak JA, Rosen II, Childress CH, et al. Prostate target volume variations during a course of radiotherapy. *Int J Radiat Oncol Biol Phys* 1998;42:661-672.

27. Antolak JA. Planning target volumes for radiotherapy: how much margin is needed? *Int J Radiat Oncol Biol Phys* 1999;44: 1165-1170.

28. Starkschall G. Dose-calculation algorithms used in 3-D radiation therapy treatment planning. In: Purdy JA, Starkschall G, eds. *A Practical Guide to 3-D Planning and Conformal Radiation Therapy.* Madison, Wis: Advanced Medical; 1999:107-122.

29. Ten Haken RK. 3-D RTP plan evaluation. In: Purdy JA, Starkschall G, eds. *A Practical Guide to 3-D Planning and Conformal Radiation Therapy.* Madison, Wis: Advanced Medical; 1999:89-106.

30. Storey MR, Pollack A, Zagars G, et al. Complications from radiotherapy dose escalation in prostate cancer: preliminary results of a randomized trial. *Int J Radiat Oncol Biol Phys* 2000;48:635-642.

31. Graham MV, Purdy JA, Emami B, et al. Clinical dose-volume histogram analysis for pneumonitis after 3D treatment for non-small cell lung cancer (NSCLC). *Int J Radiat Oncol Biol Phys* 1999;45:323-329.

32. Armstrong JG, Zelefsky MJ, Leibel SA, et al. Strategy for dose escalation using 3-dimensional conformal radiation therapy for lung cancer. *Ann Oncol* 1995;67:693-697.

33. Herman MG. Clinical implementation of electronic portal imaging. In: Purdy JA, Starkschall G, eds. *A Practical Guide to 3-D Planning and Conformal Radiation Therapy.* Madison, Wis: Advanced Medical; 1999.

34. Mageras GS, Kutcher GJ. The role of EPIDs [electronic portal imaging devices] in conformal therapy. In: Hazle JD, Boyer AL, eds. *Imaging in Radiation Therapy.* Proceedings of the 1998 Summer School of the American Association of Physicists in Medicine, University of Wisconsin-Madison. Madison, Wis: Medical Physics; 1998:257-278. Medical Physics Monograph No. 24.

35. Menke M, Hirschfeld F, Mack T, et al. Photogrammetric accuracy measurements of head holder systems used for fractionated radiotherapy. *Int J Radiat Oncol Biol Phys* 1994;29:1147-1155.

36. Johnson LS, Milliken BD, Hadley SW, et al. Initial clinical experience with a video-based patient positioning system. *Int J Radiat Oncol Biol Phys* 1999;45:205-213.

37. Starkschall G, Steadham RE, Popple RA, et al. Beam-commissioning methodology for a three-dimensional convolution/superposition photon dose algorithm. *J Appl Clin Med Phys* 2000;1:8-27.

38. Starkschall G, Steadham RE, Wells NH, et al. On the need for monitor unit calculations as part of a beam commissioning methodology for a radiation treatment planning system. *J Appl Clin Med Phys* 2000;1:86-94.

39. Palta JR, Liu C, Li Z. Acceptance testing and commissioning a 3-D RTP system. In: Purdy JA, Starkschall G, eds. *A Practical Guide to 3-D Planning and Conformal Radiation Therapy.* Madison, Wis: Advanced Medical; 1999:133-150.

40. Ten Haken RK. Components of a 3-D CRT QA program. In: Purdy JA, Starkschall G, eds. *A Practical Guide to 3-D Planning and Conformal Radiation Therapy.* Madison, Wis: Advanced Medical; 1999:309-322.

41. Rosen II. Writing software for the clinic. *Med Phys* 1998;25:1-9.

42. Galvin JM, Chen XG. Combining multileaf fields to modulate fluence distributions. *Int J Radiat Oncol Biol Phys* 1993;27:697-705.

43. Fraass BA, McShan DL, Kessler ML, et al. A computer-controlled conformal radiotherapy system. I: Overview. *Int J Radiat Oncol Biol Phys* 1995;33:1139-1157.

44. Fraass BA, Kessler ML, McShan DL, et al. Optimization and clinical use of multisegment intensity-modulated radiation therapy for high-dose conformal therapy. *Semin Radiat Oncol* 1999;9: 60-77.

45. Rosen II. Treatment planning for IMRT. In: Sternick ES, ed. *The Theory and Practice of Intensity Modulated Radiation Therapy.* Madison, Wis: Advanced Medical; 1997:37-49.

46. Mackie TR, Holmes T, Swerdloff S, et al. Tomotherapy: a new concept for the delivery of dynamic conformal radiotherapy. *Med Phys* 1993;20:1709-1719.

47. Woo SY, Sanders M, Grant W, et al. Does the "peacock" have anything to do with radiotherapy? *Int J Radiat Oncol Biol Phys* 1994;29:213-214.

48. Woo SY, Grant WHI, Bellezza D, et al. A comparison of intensity modulated conformal therapy with a conventional external beam stereotactic radiosurgery system for the treatment of single and multiple intracranial lesions. *Int J Radiat Oncol Biol Phys* 1996;35:593-597.

49. Carol M, Grant WHI, Pavord D, et al. Initial clinical experience with the Peacock intensity modulation of a 3-D conformal radiation therapy system. *Stereotact Funct Neurosurg* 1996; 66:30-34.

50. Mackie TR, Balog J, Ruchala K, et al. Tomotherapy. *Semin Radiat Oncol* 1999;9:108-117.

51. Low DA, Mutic S, Dempsey JF, et al. Abutment region dosimetry for serial tomotherapy. *Int J Radiat Oncol Biol Phys* 1999;45: 193-203.

52. Bortfeld T, Burkelbach J, Boesecke R, et al. Methods of image reconstruction from projections applied to conformation radiotherapy. *Phys Med Biol* 1990;35:1423-1434.

53. Stein J, Mohan R, Wang XH, et al. Number and orientations of beams in intensity-modulated radiation treatments. *Med Phys* 1997;24:149-160.

54. Yu CX. Intensity-modulated arc therapy with dynamic multileaf collimation: an alternative to tomotherapy. *Phys Med Biol* 1995;40:1435-1449.

55. Frenzel T, Schmidt R, Scobel W. Application of modifiers for intensity modulated photon fields. In: Schlegel W, Bortfeld T, eds. Proceedings of the XIIIth International Conference on the Use of Computers in Radiation Therapy, Heidelberg, Germany, 22-25 May 2000. New York, NY: Springer-Verlag; 2000.

56. Popple R, Rosen II. Delivery of multiple IMRT fields using a single physical attenuator. In: Schlegel W, Bortfeld T, eds. Proceedings of the XIIIth International Conference on the Use of Computers in Radiation Therapy, Heidelberg, Germany, 22-25 May 2000. New York, NY: Springer-Verlag; 2000:191-193.

57. Low DA, Li Z, Klein EE. Verification of milled two-dimensional photon compensating filters using an electronic portal imaging device. *Med Phys* 1996;23:929-938.

58. Bortfeld TF, Kahler DL, Waldron TJ, et al. X-ray field compensation with multileaf collimators. *Int J Radiat Oncol Biol Phys* 1994;28:723-730.

59. Bortfeld T, Boyer AL, Schlegel W, et al. Realization and verification of three-dimensional conformal radiotherapy with modulated fields. *Int J Radiat Oncol Biol Phys* 1994;30: 899-908.

60. Zelefsky MJ, Leibel SA, Kutcher GJ, et al. Three-dimensional conformal radiotherapy and dose escalation: where do we stand? *Semin Radiat Oncol* 1998;8:107-114.

61. Zelefsky MJ, Cowen D, Fuks Z, et al. Long term tolerance of high dose three-dimensional conformal radiotherapy in patients with localized prostate carcinoma. *Cancer* 1999;85: 2460-2468.

62. Ten Haken RK, Forman JD, Heimburger DK, et al. Treatment planning issues related to prostate movement in response to differential filling of the rectum and bladder. *Int J Radiat Oncol Biol Phys* 1991;20:1317-1324.

63. Crook JM, Raymond Y, Salhani D, et al. Prostate motion during standard radiotherapy as assessed by fiducial markers. *Radiother Oncol* 1995;37:35-42.

64. van Herk M, Bruce AM, Kroes APG, et al. Quantification of organ motion during conformal radiotherapy of the prostate by

three-dimensional image registration. *Int J Radiat Oncol Biol Phys* 1995;33:1311-1320.

65. Rudat V, Schraube P, Oetzel D, et al. Combined error of patient positioning variability and prostate motion uncertainty in 3D conformal radiotherapy of localized prostate cancer. *Int J Radiat Oncol Biol Phys* 1996;35:1027-1034.

66. Melian E, Mageras GS, Fuks Z, et al. Variation in prostate position quantitation and implications for three-dimensional conformal treatment planning. *Int J Radiat Oncol Biol Phys* 1997; 38:73-81.

67. Roeske JC, Forman JD, Mesina CF, et al. Evaluation of changes in the size and location of the prostate, seminal vesicles, bladder, and rectum during a course of external beam radiation therapy. *Int J Radiat Oncol Biol Phys* 1995;33:1321-1329.

68. Antolak JA, Cundiff JH, Ha CS. Utilization of thermoluminescent dosimetry in total skin electron beam radiotherapy of mycosis fungoides. *Int J Radiat Oncol Biol Phys* 1998;42:661-672.

69. Lattanzi J, McNeeley S, Pinover W, et al. A comparison of daily CT localization to a daily ultrasound-based system in prostate cancer. *Int J Radiat Oncol Biol Phys* 1999;43:719-725.

70. Mohan DS, Kupelian PA, Willoughby TR. Short-course intensity-modulated radiotherapy for localized prostate cancer with daily transabdominal ultrasound localization of the prostate gland. *Int J Radiat Oncol Biol Phys* 2000;46:575-580.

71. Sternick ES, ed. *The Theory and Practice of Intensity Modulated Radiation Therapy*. Madison, Wis: Advanced Medical; 1997.

72. Leksell L. The stereotactic method and radiosurgery of the brain. *Acta Chirurgica Scandinavica* 1951;102:316-319.

73. Kjellberg RN, Preston WM. *The Use of the Bragg Peak of a Proton Beam for Intracerebral Lesions*. Proceedings of the IInd International Congress on Neurological Surgery, Washington, DC; 1961.

74. Leksell L. *Stereotactic and Radiosurgery: An Operative System*. Springfield, Ill: Charles C. Thomas; 1971.

75. Lutz W, Winston KR, Maleki N. A system for stereotactic radiosurgery with a linear accelerator. *Int J Radiat Oncol Biol Phys* 1988;14:373-381.

76. Kooy HM, Neszi LA, Loffer JS, et al. Treatment planning for stereotactic radiosurgery of intra-cranial lesions. *Int J Radiat Oncol Biol Phys* 1991;21:683-693.

77. Nedzi LA, Kooy HM, Alexander E, et al. Variables associated with the development of complications from radiosurgery of intracranial tumors. *Int J Radiat Oncol Biol Phys* 1991;21: 591-599.

78. Shiu AS, Kooy HM, Ewton JR, et al. Comparison of miniature multileaf collimation (MMLC) with circular collimation for stereotactic treatment. *Int J Radiat Oncol Biol Phys* 1997;37: 679-688.

79. Shiu AS, Wong J, Ewton JE, et al. Computer-controlled miniature multileaf colliator. In: Leavitt DD, Starkschall G, eds. Proceedings of the XIIth International Conference on the Use of Computers in Radiation Therapy, Salt Lake City, Utah, 27-30 May 1996. Madison, Wis: Medical Physics; 1997:83-85.

80. Shiu S, Parker B, Ye J, et al. An integrated treatment delivery system for SRS and SRT. In: Schlegel W, Bortfeld T, eds. Proceedings of the XIIIth International Conference on the Use of Computers in Radiation Therapy, Heidelberg, Germany, 22-25 May 2000. New York, NY: Springer-Verlag; 2000: 341-343.

81. Tapley N, ed. *Clinical Applications of the Electron Beam. Wiley Series in Diagnostic and Therapeutic Radiology*. New York, NY: John Wiley & Sons; 1976.

82. Almond P, Fraass B, Hogstrom KR, et al. Total skin electron therapy. In: American Association of Physicists in Medicine (AAPM), eds. *Technique and Dosimetry: Report of the AAPM Radiation Therapy Committee Task Group 23*. New York, NY: American Institute of Physics; 1988:1-55.

83. Antolak JA, Hogstrom KR. Multiple scattering theory for total skin electron beam design. *Med Phys* 1998;25:851-859.

84. Wooden KK, Hogstrom KR, Blum P, et al. Whole-limb irradiation of the lower calf using a six-field electron technique. *Med Dosim* 1996;21:211-218.

85. Hogstrom KR, Boyer AL, Shiu AS, et al. Design of metallic electron beam cones for an intraoperative therapy linear accelerator. *Int J Radiat Oncol Biol Phys* 1990;18:1223-1232.

86. Nyerick CE, Ochran TG, Boyer AL, et al. Dosimetry characteristics of metallic cones for intraoperative radiotherapy. *Int J Radiat Oncol Biol Phys* 1991;21:501-510.

87. Hogstrom KR, Leavitt D. Dosimetry of electron arc therapy. In: Elson H, Born C, eds. Proceedings of the 1985 Summer School of the American Association of Physicists in Medicine on Radiation Oncology Physics. New York, NY: American Institute of Physics; 1986:265-295.

88. Tung SS, Shiu AS, Starkschall G, et al. Dosimetric evaluation of total scalp irradiation using a lateral electron-photon technique. *Int J Radiat Oncol Biol Phys* 1993;27:153-160.

89. Maor MH, Fields RS, Hogstrom KR, et al. Improving the therapeutic ratio of craniospinal irradiation in medulloblastoma. *Int J Radiat Oncol Biol Phys* 1985;11:687-707.

90. Maor MH, Hogstrom KR, Fields RS, et al. New approaches to cerebrospinal irradiation in pediatric brain tumors. In: Brooks BF, ed. *Malignant Tumors of Childhood*. Austin: University of Texas Press; 1986:245-254.

91. Hogstrom KR, Fields RS. The use of CT in electron beam treatment planning, current and future development. In: Ling C, Rogers C, Morton R, eds. *Computerized Tomography in Radiation Therapy*. New York, NY: Raven Press; 1983:241-252.

92. McNeese MD, Chobe R, Weber RS, et al. Carcinoma of the nasal vestibule: treatment with radiotherapy. *Cancer Bull* 1989;41:84-87.

93. Morrison WH, Wong PF, Starkschall G, et al. Water bolus for electron irradiation of the ear canal. *Int J Radiat Oncol Biol Phys* 1995;33:479-483.

94. Hogstrom KR. Dosimetry of electron heterogeneities. In: Wright A, Boyer A, eds. *Advances in Radiation Therapy Treatment Planning*. New York, NY: American Institute of Physics; 1983:223-243. Medical Physics Monograph No. 9.

95. Hogstrom KR, Mills MD, Almond PR. Electron beam dose calculations. *Phys Med Biol* 1981;26:445-459.

96. Hogstrom KR. *Evaluation of Electron Pencil Beam Dose Calculations*. Proceedings of the 1985 Summer School of the American Association of Physicists in Medicine on Radiation Oncology Physics. New York, NY: American Institute of Physics; 1986:532-557.

97. Hogstrom KR, Kurup RG, Shiu AS, et al. A two-dimensional, pencil beam algorithm for calculation of arc electron dose distributions. *Phys Med Biol* 1989;34:315-341.

98. Kurup RG, Hogstrom KR, Otte VA, et al. Dosimetric evaluation of a two-dimensional, arc-electron, pencil-beam algorithm in water. *Phys Med Biol* 1992;37:127-144.

99. Starkschall G, Shiu AS, Bujnowski SW, et al. Effect of dimensionality of heterogeneity corrections on the implementation of a 3-dimensional electron pencil beam algorithm. *Phys Med Biol* 1991;36:207-227.

100. Hogstrom KR, Steadham RS. Electron beam dose computation. In: Mackie TR, Palta JT, eds. *Teletherapy: Present and Future*. Proceedings of the 1996 Summer School of the American Association of Physicists in Medicine, University of British Columbia, Vancouver, Canada. Madison, Wis: Advanced Medical; 1996:137-174.

101. Shiu AS, Hogstrom KR. A pencil-beam redefinition algorithm for electron dose distributions. *Med Phys* 1991;18:7-18.

102. Boyd RA, Hogstrom KR, Rosen II. Effects of using an initial polyenergetic spectrum with the pencil beam redefinition

algorithm for electron dose calculations in water. *Med Phys* 1998;25:2176-2185.

103. Boyd RA, Hogstrom KR. The effect of an initial monoenergetic versus a polyenergetic electron spectrum on the accuracy of dose calculated by the pencil-beam redefinition algorithm in heterogeneous media. In: Leavitt DD, Starkschall G, eds. Proceedings of the XIIth International Conference on the Use of Computers in Radiation Therapy, Salt Lake City, Utah, 27-30 May 1996. Madison, Wis: Medical Physics; 1997:197-200.

104. Low DA, Starkschall G, Bujnowski SW, et al. Electron bolus design for radiotherapy treatment planning: bolus design algorithms. *Med Phys* 1992;19:115-124.

105. Low DA, Starkschall G, Sherman NE, et al. Computer-aided design and fabrication of an electron bolus for treatment of the paraspinal muscles. *Int J Radiat Oncol Biol Phys* 1995;33:1127-1138.

106. Antolak JA, Starkschall G, Bawiec ER, et al. *Implementation of an Automated Electron Bolus Fabrication System for Conformal Electron Radiotherapy.* Proceedings of the XIth International Conference on the Use of Computers in Radiation Therapy. Manchester, UK: Handley Printers; 1994:162-163.

107. Starkschall G, Bujnowski SW, Antolak JA, et al. *Tools for 3-D Electron-beam Treatment Planning.* Proceedings of the XIth International Conference on the Use of Computers in Radiation Therapy. Manchester, UK: Handley Printers; 1994:126-127.

108. Kudchadker R, Hogstrom K, Boyd R. Multileaf collimation for electron intensity modulation. *Med Phys* 2000;27:1375.

108a. Perkins GH, McNeese MD, Antolak J, et al. A custom three-dimensional electron bolus technique for optimization of post-mastectomy irradiation. *Int J Radiat Oncol Biol Phys* 2001;51:1142-1151.

109. Bawiec ER. *The Effects of Accuracy of Milling of Electron Bolus on Dose Delivery.* Houston: The University of Texas Health Science Center at Houston Graduate School of Biomedical Sciences, Department of Radiation Physics; 1994.

110. Zachrisson B, Karlsson M. Matching of electron beams for conformal therapy of target volumes at moderate depths. *Radiother Oncol* 1996;39:261-270.

111. Klein E. Modulated electron beams using multi-segmented multileaf collimation. *Radiother Oncol* 1998;48:307-311.

112. Asell M, Hyodynmaa S, Gustafsson A, et al. Optimization of 3D conformal electron beam therapy in inhomogeneous media by concomitant fluence and energy modulation. *Phys Med Biol* 1997;42:2083-2100.

113. Ebert MA, Hoban PW. Possibilities for tailoring dose distributions through the manipulation of electron beam characteristics. *Phys Med Biol* 1997;42:2065-2081.

114. Karlsson MG, Karlsson MK, Zachrisson B. Intensity modulation with electrons: calculations, measurements and clinical applications. *Phys Med Biol* 1998;43:1159-1169.

115. Ma CM, Lee MS, Jiang SB, et al. Energy- and intensity-modulated electron beams for radiotherapy. *Phys Med Biol* 2000;45:2293-2311.

116. Fields RS, Hogstrom KR. A computer model for combining electron and photon beams. In: Paliwal B, ed. Proceedings of the Electron Dosimetry and Arc Therapy Symposium. New York, NY: American Institute of Physics; 1982:161-180.

117. Shimizu S, Shirato H, Aoyama H, et al. High-speed magnetic resonance imaging for four-dimensional treatment planning of conformal radiotherapy of moving body tumors. *Int J Radiat Oncol Biol Phys* 2000;48:471-474.

118. Hanley J, Debois MM, Mah D, et al. Deep inspiration breath-hold technique for lung tumors: the potential value of target immobilization and reduced lung density in dose escalation. *Int J Radiat Oncol Biol Phys* 1999;45:603-611.

119. Rosenzweig KE, Hanley J, Mah D, et al. The deep inspiration breath-hold technique in the treatment of inoperable non–small-cell lung cancer. *Int J Radiat Oncol Biol Phys* 2000;48:81-87.

120. Wong JW, Sharpe MB, Jaffray DA, et al. The use of active breathing control (ABC) to reduce margin for breathing motion. *Int J Radiat Oncol Biol Phys* 1999;44:911-919.

121. Kubo HD, Len PM, Minohara S, et al. Breathing-synchronized radiotherapy program at the University of California Davis Cancer Center. *Med Phys* 2000;27:346-353.

122. Shirato H, Shimizu S, Kitamura K, et al. Four-dimensional treatment planning and fluoroscopic real-time tumor tracking radiotherapy for moving tumor. *Int J Radiat Oncol Biol Phys* 2000;48:435-442.

123. Starkschall G. Design specifications for a radiation oncology picture archival and communication system. *Semin Radiat Oncol* 1997;7:21-30.

124. Starkschall G, Bujnowski SW, Li X-J, et al. A picture archival and communication system for radiotherapy. In: Purdy JA, Emami B, eds. Proceedings of an International Symposium on 3-D Radiation Treatment Planning and Conformal Therapy, Mallinckrodt Institute of Radiology, Washington University School of Medicine, St. Louis, Mo, 21-23 April 1993. Madison, Wis: Medical Physics; 1993.

125. Starkschall G, Bujnowski SW, Wong NW, et al. Implementation of image comparison methods in a radio-therapy PACS. In: Hounsell AR, Wilkinson JM, Williams PC, eds. Proceedings of the XIth International Conference on the Use of Computers in Radiation Therapy, Manchester, UK, 20-24 March 1994. North Western Medical Physics Department; 1994.

126. De Neve W, Van den Heuvel F, Coghe M, et al. Interactive use of on-line portal imaging in pelvic radiation. *Int J Radiat Oncol Biol Phys* 1993;25:517-524.

127. Dong L. *Development of Automated Image Analysis Tools for Verification of Radiotherapy Field Accuracy with an Electronic Portal Imaging Device.* Houston: The University of Texas at Houston Graduate School of Biomedical Sciences, Department of Radiation Physics; 1995.

128. Dong L, Boyer AL. A portal image alignment and patient setup verification procedure using moments and correlation techniques. *Phys Med Biol* 1996;41:697-723.

129. Petrascu O, Bel A, Linthout N, et al. Automatic on-line electronic portal image analysis with a wavelet-based edge detector. *Med Phys* 2000;27:321-329.

130. Bijhold J, van Herk M, Vijibrief R, et al. Fast evaluation of patient set-up during radiotherapy by aligning features in portal and simulator images. *Phys Med Biol* 1991;36:1665-1679.

131. Balter JM, Pelizzari CA, Chen GTY. Correlation of projection radiographs in radiation therapy using open curve segments and points. *Med Phys* 1992;19:329-334.

132. Gilhuijs KG, van Herk M. Automatic on-line inspection of patient setup in radiation therapy using digital portal images. *Med Phys* 1993;20:667-677.

133. Kelly JF, Delclos ME, Morice RC, et al. High-dose-rate endobronchial brachytherapy effectively palliates symptoms due to airway tumors: the 10-year M.D. Anderson Cancer Center experience. *Int J Radiat Oncol Biol Phys* 2000;48:697-702.

134. Nag S, Kelly JF, Horton JL, et al. Brachytherapy for carcinoma of the lung. *Oncology (Huntingt)* 2001;15:371-381.

135. Harrison LB, Enker WE, Anderson LL. High-dose-rate intraoperative radiation therapy for colorectal cancer. *Oncology* 1995;9:679-683.

136. Kubo HD, Glasgow GP, Pethel TD, et al. High dose rate brachytherapy treatment delivery: report of the American College of Medical Physics Radiation Therapy Committee Task Group No. 59. *Med Phys* 1998;25:375-403.

137. Miller AV, Davis MG, Horton JL. A method of verifying treatment times for simple high-dose-rate endobronchial brachytherapy procedures. *Med Phys* 1996;23:1903-1908.

138. Ezzell GA. A manual algorithm for computing dwell times for two-cathether endobronchial treatments using HDR brachytherapy. *Med Phys* 2000;27:1030-1033.

139. Janjan NA, Waugh KA, Skibber JM, et al. Control of unresectable recurrent anorectal cancer with Gold-198 seed implantation. *J Brachyther Int* 1999;15:115-129.

140. Yu Y, Anderson LL, Li Z, et al. Permanent prostate seed implant brachytherapy: report of the American Association of Physicists in Medicine Task Group No. 64. *Med Phys* 1999;26:2054-2076.

141. Pocock SJ, Henderson RA, Richards AF, et al. Meta-analysis of randomized trials comparing coronary angioplasty with bypass surgery. *Lancet* 1995;346:1184-1189.

142. Nath R, Amols H, Coffey C, et al. Intravascular brachytherapy physics: report of the American College of Medical Physics Radiation Therapy Committee Task Group No. 60. *Med Phys* 1999;26:119-152.

143. McLemore LB. *Dosimetric Characterization of a Palladium-103 Implanted Sent for Intravascular Brachytherapy.* Houston: The University of Texas Graduate School of Biomedical Sciences, Department of Radiation Physics; 2000.

144. Eglezopoulos L, Harris I, Aguirre JF, et al. Recent additions to the RPC routine dosimetry review measurements. *Med Phys* 1994;21:933.

145. Kirby TH, Hanson WF, Gastorf RJ, et al. Mailable TLD system for photon and electron therapy beams. *Int J Radiat Oncol Biol Phys* 1986;12:261-265.

146. Kirby TH, Hanson WF, Johnston DA. Uncertainty analysis of absorbed dose calculations from thermoluminescence dosimeters. *Med Phys* 1992;19:1427-1434.

147. Hanson WF. *Dosimetry Quality Assurance in the United States from the Experience of the Radiological Physics Center.* Proceedings of the American College of Medical Physics Symposium on Quality Assurance in Radiotherapy Physics, Galveston, TX, May 1991. Madison, Wis: Medical Physics; 1991:255-282.

148. Gastorf RJ, Hanson WF, Berkley LW, et al. A comparison of high-energy accelerator depth dose data. *Med Phys* 1983;10:881-885.

149. Kirby TH, Gastorf RJ, Hanson WF, et al. Electron beam central axis depth-dose measurements. *Med Phys* 1985;12:357-361.

150. Followill DS, Davis DS, Hanson WF. Standard wedge transmission for Varian, Siemens, Philips and AECL accelerators. *Med Phys* 1997;24:1076.

151. Davis DS, Followill DS, Hanson WF. Electron percent depth dose and cone ratio data for various machines. *Med Phys* 1995;22:1007.

152. BenComo JA, Followill DS, Cho SH, et al. *Comparison of On-site and Off-site Evaluations of Dosimetry Data.* Proceedings of the 2000 World Congress on Medical Physics and Biomedical Engineering, July 2000. College Park, Md: American Association of Physicists in Medicine; 2000.

153. Hanson WF, Martin B, Kuske RR, et al. Dose specification and quality assurance of RTOG protocol 95-17: a cooperative group study of Ir-192 breast implants as sole therapy. *Med Phys* 2001;28:1297.

154. Stovall M, Balter P, Hanson WF, et al. Quality audit of radiosurgery dosimetry using mailed phantoms. *Med Phys* 1995;22:1009.

155. Balter P, Stovall M, Hanson WF. An anthropomorphic head phantom for remote monitoring of stereotactic radiosurgery at multiple institutions. *Med Phys* 1999;26:1164.

156. Radford DA, Followill DS, Hanson W. *Design of an Anthropomorphic Intensity-Modulated Radiation Therapy Quality Assurance Phantom.* Proceedings of the 2000 World Congress on Medical Physics and Biomedical Engineering, July 2000. College Park, Md: American Association of Physicists in Medicine; 2000.

157. Cherry CPD, Followill DS, Hanson WF. *Design of a Heterogeneous Thorax Phantom for Remote Verification of Three-Dimensional Conformal Therapy.* Proceedings of the 2000 World Congress on Medical Physics and Biomedical Engineering, July 2000. College Park, Md: American Association of Physicists in Medicine; 2000.

CHAPTER 3

Principles of Combining Radiation Therapy and Surgery

Gunar K. Zagars

THE SIGNIFICANCE OF LOCAL–REGIONAL TUMOR CONTROL

Surgery and radiation therapy are local–regional treatment modalities. When they are successful, they permanently eradicate the primary tumor and regional nodal metastatic disease. Local–regional control of a tumor is an obvious prerequisite for cure. Conversely, failure to achieve local control not only signifies a failure to cure but also leaves the patient to face a variety of debilitating local–regional problems that ultimately become insoluble and may be fatal if death from distant metastases or intercurrent disease does not occur first. These virtues of local–regional control are self-evident; less conclusive is the potential salutary effect of effective regional treatment on the subsequent evolution of metastatic disease. Leaving aside the obvious systemic problems posed for the patient who already has gross hematogenous metastases, the potential presence of micrometastases complicates any evaluation of the effect of local treatment on the subsequent appearance of clinically evident metastases. The problem hinges on the time at which a primary tumor usually seeds its first metastasis—only in those tumors that initiate the metastatic cascade beyond the time of diagnosis and treatment can local–regional therapy have any effect on metastatic evolution by removing the source of potential metastatic dissemination. The time at which tumors first successfully shed metastases is unknown but clearly is highly variable, as reflected in the clinical recognition of a spectrum of metastatic potential from highly metastasizing cancers such as small cell lung cancer to infrequently metastasizing tumors such as dermatofibrosarcoma protuberans. Moreover, the time of first metastasis varies among patients with the same histopathologic tumor; although most women with a T1 breast cancer are free from clinically detectable metastases at diagnosis, some with ostensibly similar primary tumors already have overt metastatic disease. Despite these uncertainties, the high correlation between the size or extent of a primary tumor (T category) and the likelihood of subsequent metastatic relapse even after successful local treatment is prima facie evidence that the shedding of a first metastasis often occurs at a time corresponding to the growth of a T1 cancer to become a T4 cancer. Radiobiological evaluation of the response of hematogenous micrometastases to radiation also supports the idea that in a significant proportion of cancer in humans, the primary tumor seeds its first metastasis at or just before the time of its diagnosis.[1]

Indeed, the continuing drive for early diagnosis and prompt local treatment is based on the premise that early intervention not only eradicates the primary tumor but also removes the source for subsequent metastatic dissemination, thus achieving higher cure and survival rates than delayed treatment. This concept has been epidemiologically validated for breast,[2] cervix,[3] and colorectal[4] cancer. In keeping with these observations are many retrospective after-treatment studies in which a significant positive correlation between local recurrence and subsequent metastatic relapse has been found.[5-10] However, this finding has not been consistent, particularly among prospective randomized trials, where improvement in local control has often not translated into significant improvements in freedom from metastasis or survival.[11-15]

Prospective randomized trials are reliable arbiters for many controversies in therapeutics, but care must be taken in drawing inferences about endpoints for which such trials were not designed. Virtually all trials conducted to evaluate local–regional treatment alternatives are designed to detect differences in local–regional control. It is almost certain that such trials will fail to detect real differences in metastatic outcome between the evaluated treatment groups. A simple calculation demonstrates this concept. Suppose that, for the tumor in question, local control is associated with a true metastatic incidence of 30% (metastases seeded before treatment) and local relapse results in a true metastatic rate of 60% (including the excess metastases seeded from the locally persistent tumor). If one local treatment achieves an 80% local control rate and another achieves only 60%, this difference will be apparent in a randomized trial of approximately 200 patients (100 in each treatment group). Simple calculation reveals that the superior treatment will be associated with a 36% true incidence of metastatic relapse compared with a 42% incidence for the poorer treatment; this difference would require some 2000 patients (1000 in each group) to have an 80% chance of being detected as significant, despite the fact that the patient whose tumor recurs has a twofold excess risk of metastatic relapse. Because it would be unethical to continue accruing patients to a study where one treatment was demonstrably superior over another for local–regional control, randomized prospective trials provide no conclusive evidence on the relationship between local recurrence and metastatic dissemination.

Retrospective analyses that compare the correlation between local recurrence and metastasis are bedeviled by the possibility that those tumors that recur may well be those whose pathobiology also promotes early dissemination independently of any treatment effect. This is true to the extent that for many types of cancer, those pretreatment prognostic factors that correlate with local–regional relapse also correlate with metastatic dissemination. Nevertheless, given what is known about tumor biology and clinical outcomes, the onus of proof that local control has no effect on the likelihood of subsequent metastasis rests with those who uphold such a view. Common sense suggests that achievement of local–regional control not only avoids the problems of persistently growing local cancer but also abrogates the metastatic process, resulting in a lower likelihood of metastatic relapse in some proportion of patients.

THEORETICAL BASIS FOR COMBINING SURGERY AND RADIATION THERAPY

Surgery and radiation can be combined in two fundamentally different ways: (1) in a "salvage" fashion, where surgery is used after irradiation fails or irradiation is used after surgery fails, or (2) in a planned, combined bimodality fashion. The use of these modalities in a "salvage" fashion will not be discussed because this amounts to repeated single-modality treatment. The use of planned combinations of surgery and radiation evolved empirically as experience revealed the limitations of each modality when used alone in a variety of clinical circumstances and as the complementarity in their virtues became evident.[16-19] In parallel with clinical experience, experimental work in radiation and tumor biology has advanced the theoretical foundations for this combination and is increasingly influencing clinical practice.

SUBCLINICAL DISEASE

Locally invasive tumors, including all forms of cancer, infiltrate tissues around their primary site. Although

such local extension can occur in any direction, it typically follows the path of least resistance that is characteristic of different tumor types in different anatomic sites. Common pathways of local spread include those along fascial planes, muscle fibers, nerve sheaths, and periosteum. Important aspects of this spread are its microscopic character and potentially wide extent, creating a variable volume of grossly normal but tumor-bearing tissue around the primary tumor. This growth pattern is repeated at regional nodes harboring metastatic disease, if extracapsular extension occurs there, and at sites of hematogenous metastasis. The larger a primary tumor, the more extensive and dense the volume of microscopic infiltration because of the longer time that such a tumor is likely to have been present and because large tumors tend to be inherently more aggressive. Peripheral tumor infiltrates can contain any number of clonogenic cells from a few to as many as 10^9 or more before they become clinically evident. For example, if 10^6 cells, which occupy a volume of approximately 1 mm^3, were distributed in a tissue volume of 1 cm^3, then they may not be detected even under a microscope; if 10^9 cells, which occupy approximately 1 cm^3, were clustered, then they could be radiologically detected. However, in anatomic sites such as the abdomen, considerably larger deposits can be occult. Any tumor cell deposits or extensions that cannot be detected by clinical-radiographic means are called *subclinical disease*. Although the terms *subclinical* and *microscopic* are generally used interchangeably, it is important to understand that subclinical disease is not always microscopic (although advances in tumor imaging are bringing the two terms closer together). This distinction has implications for clinical practice because many of the basic concepts relating to subclinical disease and radiation were developed from experience with accessible and evaluable anatomic sites such as the head and neck, breast, and axilla and may not be directly applicable to less accessible areas such as the chest, abdomen, and pelvis, where subclinical disease can occupy a more substantial volume.[18,20-23]

The therapeutic problems posed by subclinical disease around a primary tumor are illustrated schematically in Figure 3-1. Surgery is a macroscopic, visual modality, and its selective therapeutic effect is for macroscopic tumor, with the surgeon guiding the scalpel around grossly evident tumor. Surgical removal of subclinical microscopic tumor entails resection of tissue, of which much is normal—a poor therapeutic ratio. Nevertheless, the importance of local–regional microscopic disease is reflected in the classical radical surgical techniques designed to deal with this problem. The Halsted radical mastectomy, the Wertheim radical hysterectomy, the classical radical neck dissection often combined with en bloc resection of the primary tumor (the so-called commando procedure), the abdominoperineal resection of Miles for low rectal cancer, and the radical

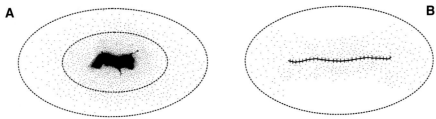

Fig. 3-1 Schematic illustration of subclinical disease around a primary tumor. **A,** A surgically undisturbed tumor surrounded by a zone of microscopic disease of decreasing density with increasing distance from the tumor. The dotted lines outline potential surgical resection planes. **B,** A resection of the tumor shown in **A** that passed through the inner ellipse with approximation of the excision margins. A significant amount of residual microscopic disease remains; complete surgical excision would require resection through the outer ellipse. The density of tumor cells in situations such as that on the right is usually so low that even careful microscopic examination will fail to reveal the residual cancer. As the microscopic disease grows, however, local recurrence will become clinically apparent. The illustrated situation is compounded for the worse in many epithelial cancers by metastatic regional nodal disease, when the problem is reiterated as tumor extends beyond the nodal capsule.

monobloc soft-part resection for soft tissue sarcoma were all developed in an attempt to deal with both the primary tumor and its local–regional extensions. The targeting of apparently normal tissues for therapy inherent in these radical surgical approaches leads to the concept of elective, adjuvant, or prophylactic treatment—treatment directed at disease that is assumed to be present. This assumption is based on prior knowledge that a significant fraction of patients with similar tumors had such disease. The application of radical surgical techniques significantly reduces but does not eliminate the likelihood of local–regional recurrence. However, these gains in local control are achieved at the expense of significant anatomic, functional, and cosmetic deficits. Furthermore, even radical surgical procedures often fail to achieve local control in large tumors (T3 and T4) at many anatomic sites.

Radiation Biology of Subclinical Disease

Radiation has a selective effect against cancer. Although the mechanisms for this selectivity are poorly understood, it is the cornerstone of radiation oncology. Radiation doses that have relatively little untoward effect on most normal tissues can eradicate significant deposits of most types of cancer cells. This ideal therapeutic ratio, however, depends on the amount of cancer present. Because of the random nature of cell killing by radiation, the local-control-vs.-dose curve (dose–response relationship) for any tumor is sigmoid,[24] and its location on the dose axis depends on many factors but principally on clonogen number (Fig. 3-2). The larger the clonogen number, the greater is the dose needed to achieve any level of local control and the closer is the dose-control relation to the dose–complication relation.

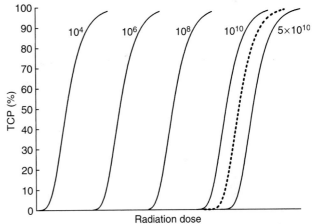

Fig. 3-2 Theoretical relationship between tumor control probability *(TCP)* and radiation dose for different numbers of clonogenic cells. Also shown is one possible relation between normal tissue complications and dose *(dashed line)*. As the number of clonogenic cells increases, the dose-control curve shifts to the right and higher doses are required to achieve control; a favorable therapeutic ratio becomes progressively less favorable as clonogen number increases. For the two largest clonogen numbers illustrated, no selectivity is present, and thus radiation becomes essentially equivalent to surgery (radiosurgery).

For large aggregates of tumor cells, radiation loses its therapeutic selectivity and tumor eradication requires destruction of normal tissue. Alternative ways of looking at the dependence between dose, tumor control, and clonogen number are illustrated in Figures 3-3 and 3-4. These theoretical conclusions have been extensively verified in clinical practice by Fletcher[25] and others (Table 3-1) and are the fundamental basis for the use of combined surgery and radiation therapy.

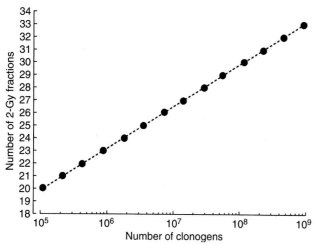

Fig. 3-3 A theoretical relationship between the number of 2-Gy fractions and the number of clonogens in which the goal is to achieve 90% local control. The relationship was modeled by assuming a surviving fraction of 0.5 after each fraction (SF$_2$). The TCP is equal to e^{-SN}, where S is the surviving fraction after F fractions (S = [SF$_2$]^F) and N is the clonogen number. The straight line is the relationship if dose were a continuous variable.

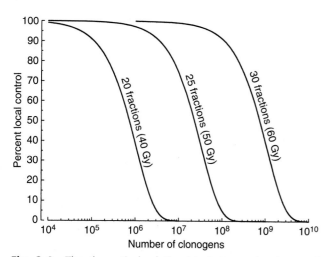

Fig. 3-4 The theoretical relationship between local control and clonogen number for different total doses delivered at 2 Gy per fraction. The parameters are the same as in Figure 3-3.

Surgery effectively removes large bulky tumors that even high doses of radiation often fail to control, whereas microscopic deposits around the primary tumor and in regional lymph nodes can be effectively eradicated by modest doses of radiation with minimal effects on normal tissue. This combined approach has the potential to achieve high local control rates with minimal disfiguration or disruption of anatomy or function.

When adjuvant radiation was first introduced, it seemed that a dose of 45 to 50 Gy given at 1.8 to 2.0 Gy per fraction would eradicate about 90% of microscopic

---

TABLE 3-1

Local Control Rates According to Tumor Size and Radiation Dose for Squamous Cell Carcinoma of the Head and Neck

Dose, Gy (Delivered at 10 Gy/wk)	Percent Control for Various Tumors
50	>90% for subclinical neck nodes
	About 50% for 2- to 3-cm neck nodes
60	80% to 90% for T1 pharynx and larynx
	About 50% for T3/T4 tonsil
70	About 90% for 1- to 3-cm neck nodes
	About 70% for 3- to 5-cm neck nodes

Modified from Fletcher GH, Shukovsky LJ. *J Radiol Electrol* 1975;56:383-400.

disease whether delivered before or after surgery.[16-18] However, it soon became evident that postoperative radiation delivered to surgically disturbed tissues had to be given in higher doses (approximately 60 Gy) to achieve equivalent control.[22,26-28] The reasons for this differential dose effect remain unclear. It is unlikely that the classical explanation invoking radioresistance as a result of hypoxia in surgically scarred tissue is valid because radiobiological hypoxia is extreme hypoxia that would be inconsistent with wound healing and tissue integrity. A more plausible explanation invokes accelerated clonogen repopulation after surgical resection.[29,30] Repopulation of clonogenic cells occurs during the irradiation of gross tumors, especially in head and neck cancer[31,32] but also in other types of cancer.[21,30] This accelerated repopulation typically begins after a lag period of approximately 3 to 4 weeks when gross tumors are treated and decreases the relative effectiveness of radiation delivered during the succeeding weeks (Fig. 3-5). Although relatively little is known about the repopulation kinetics of microscopic tumors after treatment, it is plausible to expect that they too may repopulate quickly after cytoreductive therapy, be it surgery, radiation, or chemotherapy. Some evidence exists to support acceleration of subclinical rectal adenocarcinoma after irradiation.[21,30] The adverse consequences of such early accelerated regrowth after surgery on the radiation response are illustrated in Figure 3-6.

Adjuvant radiation delivered preoperatively, or delivered to surgically undisturbed tissues postoperatively, is usually given to a dose of approximately 50 Gy over a period of 5 weeks; when surgically disturbed tissues are irradiated, the dose is typically increased to approximately 60 Gy given over 6 weeks. Because the density of clonogenic infestation decreases with distance from the

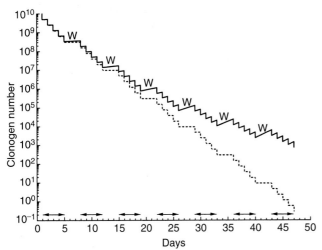

Fig. 3-5 The consequences of accelerated clonogen repopulation in a gross tumor (10^{10} cells) undergoing 7 weeks of radiation therapy (70 Gy given in 2-Gy fractions daily except on the weekends [W]). Each treatment reduces the surviving fraction by 50%. The dotted line shows the decline in clonogen number in the absence of repopulation; the approximately 0.3 cells left at the end of the treatment period corresponds to a control probability of approximately 75%. In the presence of repopulation (*solid line*), some 3000 clonogens remain at the end of treatment, precluding any chance for control.

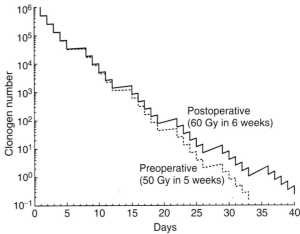

Fig. 3-6 Early accelerated repopulation from postoperative irradiation and lesser repopulation from preoperative irradiation. Postoperative conditions in the tumor bed and its surroundings are assumed to be particularly conducive to cell proliferation because of the local reparative tissue response and the release of microscopic tumor clonogens from restraining environmental conditions secondary to the preexisting gross tumor. In this example, 60 Gy given over a 6-week period after surgery produces effects that are approximately equivalent to 50 Gy given over a 5-week period before surgery. The surviving fraction after each dose is 0.5.

primary tumor (see Fig. 3-1), the last 10 Gy of the planned postoperative 60 Gy are delivered to a cone-down volume centered over the tumor bed itself—the shrinking field technique.

Although the optimal radiation dose for subclinical disease is often presented as an all-or-none quantity as in the previous discussion, it is important to understand that in some circumstances lesser or greater doses than 50 to 60 Gy may be optimal.[*] As already emphasized, the quantity of subclinical local–regional disease present in any patient can range anywhere from a few to as many as 10^9 or more cells. The optimal radiation dose therefore will vary accordingly between different patients. Unfortunately, no method has been found for quantifying clonogen density in individuals. Clinical judgment of factors such as the microscopic surgical margin and whether that margin is positive, negative, close, or wide is used to estimate likely clonogen density. Microscopically positive resection margins are a regularly documented predictor of increased recurrence rates in virtually all invasive tumors, and a dose of 65 Gy given by the shrinking field technique is widely used in this circumstance. Recent investigations of the response of subclinical disease to radiation have reaffirmed the great variation in clonogen density in different patients.[1,21,29,30] The numbers of patients with different

amounts of subclinical disease seem to be distributed across the spectrum of clonogen numbers from 1 to around 10^9, and the actual distribution is approximately log-normal (i.e., the fraction of patients with 10 to 10^2 cells is approximately the same as the fraction with 10^2 to 10^3 cells or 10^3 to 10^4 cells, and so on).[1] Although knowing the exact distribution of patients across this spectrum is not crucial, it is important to understand that such a wide distribution of clonogen number results in dose–response curves for the whole population that do not have a dose threshold, at least for doses greater than 10 Gy. However, some patients will have very few clonogens, and they will benefit even from relatively low radiation doses. This concept cannot in any way be taken as an endorsement of low-dose adjuvant radiation in general, but in some circumstances in which tissue tolerance is low, relatively low doses can be justified. In this regard, however, it is also good to emphasize that the effectiveness of conventional-dose adjuvant radiation is often not as impressive as initial inspection of clinical data might suggest.[1,29] For example, a not unusual outcome would be to find that combined surgery and radiation results in a very acceptable 90% local control rate; however, if the control rate with surgery alone is 70%, then only 20 of every 30 patients out of 100 would have had their subclinical disease eradicated by radiation—a less than great 60% local-control rate for radiation. In addition to noting overall local control rate, the radiation oncologist should pay

---

[*]References 1, 20, 25, 27, 29, 33.

close attention to the percentage reduction in recurrence rate, specifically, the following:

$$100 \times (\text{Failure rate without radiation} - \text{Failure rate with radiation}) \div \text{Failure rate without radiation}$$

This calculation provides the clearest index of the success of this treatment because not every patient judged to have subclinical disease actually has it.

Significantly, radiobiological evaluation of the dose–response relationship for subclinical disease reveals that the curves are quite steep.[21,29] This implies that relatively small increments in cytotoxicity should result in significant gains in control. Recent observations on the efficacy of combined chemotherapy and radiation (chemoradiation) as an adjuvant treatment may well reflect this observation.[12,34-39] Indeed, for many circumstances, chemoradiation is increasingly the preferred adjuvant treatment, as discussed in Chapter 4.

TOPOGRAPHIC RELATIONS BETWEEN SURGERY AND RADIATION

Surgery and radiation may be directed at the same area, or they can be used to treat different areas. When used to treat different areas, the plan usually is to use surgery for the primary tumor and adjuvant radiation for the clinically negative nodal drainage area instead of elective lymphadenectomy, thus sparing the patient some morbidity. This approach is often used for treating head and neck cancer and is standard practice for testicular seminoma. When both modalities are directed at more or less the same area, the rationale is either to improve control of large primary tumors (T3/T4) or to conserve organ anatomy and function and to minimize disfigurement for smaller tumors (T1/T2) by using conservative surgery for macroscopic tumor and radiation for occult local–regional disease. Lumpectomy and radiation for breast cancer is an example of this approach, as is the use of radiation and sphincter-sparing surgery for rectal cancer or the use of conservative resection and radiation for soft tissue sarcoma. Large primary tumors in many sites are treated with both modalities because local–regional control obtained with only one modality is often poor.

PREOPERATIVE VS. POSTOPERATIVE RADIATION

From general principles it is possible to provide a rationale for both preoperative and postoperative radiation; therefore it is not possible to definitively argue for one approach over the other. In practice, the decision to use one or the other of these sequences is dictated by clinical experience and tends to be site specific, as discussed in the appropriate sections in this book. However, it is instructive to review the virtues and limitations of each approach and to consider some aspects of intraoperative radiation therapy and brachytherapy.

Preoperative Radiation

Potential virtues of preoperative radiation are as follows:
1. An inoperable or borderline operable tumor may be rendered operable by destruction of peripheral tumor extensions that invade adjacent critical organs.
2. Destruction of peripheral tumor extensions decreases the likelihood of positive microscopic resection margins.
3. Inactivation of a large proportion of tumor clonogens decreases the likelihood of tumor cells being mechanically disseminated through vascular channels or being seeded throughout the surgical field.
4. Irradiation of a surgically undisturbed area allows the use of smaller radiation portals than would be possible postoperatively, when the whole surgical bed is potentially contaminated and requires irradiation.[40,41]
5. Irradiation of a surgically undisturbed tumor allows the use of a lower radiation dose (50 Gy) than that recommended postoperatively (60 Gy), thus potentially decreasing radiation complications.

Potential limitations of preoperative radiation are as follows:
1. Patients cannot be selected for adjuvant radiation on the basis of accurate surgical staging; depending on initial selection criteria, a significant fraction of patients treated preoperatively may not actually need both modalities.
2. The achievement of significant downstaging may preclude adequate selection of further treatment such as adjuvant chemotherapy; for example, preoperative radiation of the breast and axilla results in a high proportion of complete remission within the axilla.
3. Because surgery is delayed until about 4 weeks after the completion of radiation, a patient left with microscopically positive resection margins is faced with "split-course" radiation, which is known to be relatively ineffective.
4. Surgical complications are generally increased with preoperative radiation.[28,42-44]
5. The primary treatment (surgery) is delayed. (This common criticism is probably spurious—radiation is an effective modality, and tumors undergoing radiation cannot reasonably be deemed to remain untreated during this time.)

Postoperative Radiation

Potential virtues of postoperative radiation are as follows:
1. The extent of gross disease is accurately known and radiation can be specifically tailored to sites of special concern.

2. Microscopic margins are defined and positive margins, if present, are identified, thus allowing targeted boost radiation, ideally guided by surgical clips.
3. The likelihood of irradiating patients whose disease does not merit adjuvant treatment is reduced.
4. Increased surgical complications are avoided.

Potential limitations of postoperative radiation are as follows:

1. Delivery of radiation may be delayed by surgical complications, leading to significant clonogen repopulation and even occasionally gross recurrence.
2. Irradiation of a surgically disturbed tumor bed requires a higher dose than does preoperative irradiation.
3. The volume of tissue requiring irradiation is usually larger than for preoperative irradiation because the whole surgical bed and drain are potentially contaminated.
4. The surgical procedure may fix certain organs in or adjacent to the surgical bed, resulting in potentially significant radiation complications; fixation can be a particular problem for the small bowel after abdominopelvic surgery.

Very few clinical trials have addressed the issues posed by the previous summary, and the conclusions have been contradictory. A major problem in interpretation is posed by the often idiosyncratic preoperative radiation schedules, which emphasize the use of a few large fractions (e.g., 10 Gy given once or 3.7, 4, or 5 Gy given five times). Two prospective randomized trials that used conventional fractionation seem to have had a significant influence on the pattern of combined modality treatment for head and neck cancer. One of these trials compared 55 Gy given over 5.5 weeks either before or after surgery to patients with hypopharyngeal cancer and found a significant advantage for postoperative radiation with regard to overall survival.[45] Data on local–regional control were not clearly presented. The second trial comprised a much larger group of patients with advanced head and neck cancer and randomized them to undergo preoperative radiation (50 Gy at 1.8 to 2.0 Gy per fraction) or postoperative radiation (60 Gy at the same fraction size). Local–regional control was significantly better in the postoperative-radiation group.[46] Since then, postoperative radiation has become the standard for treating head and neck cancer. The only other disease for which preoperative radiation has been directly compared with postoperative radiation in randomized trials is rectal cancer, and, in that case, preoperative radiation emerged as the better sequence.[44] Thus neither considerations from first principles nor clinical results allows global conclusions to be reached regarding the superiority of preoperative or postoperative adjuvant radiation therapy.

Time Interval Between Treatment Modalities

Regardless of whether radiation is used before or after surgery, the time interval between the treatment modalities is of some significance in view of the possibility of tumor cell repopulation during that interval. Repopulation in the interval between preoperative radiation and surgery would seem to be of little consequence unless the operation was to be unreasonably delayed. If preoperative treatment eradicates all microscopic disease, then in situ repopulation is impossible, and reseeding of tissues by new clonogen outgrowth would be unlikely in the short term; if the treatment failed in this respect, then even prompt surgery would be of little avail. Thus the major determinant of the interval between modalities in this situation is the likelihood of surgical complications. When low-dose, high-dose-per-fraction radiation is used preoperatively, acute radiation reactions are insignificant and experience confirms that surgery can be safely accomplished within 1 to 2 weeks of the completion of radiation.

Several prospective trials involving hypofractionated preoperative radiation have showed no difference in postsurgical complications between patients treated with surgery alone and those treated with radiation followed by surgery within 2 weeks of the completion of radiation.[12,44,47-49] With intermediate radiation doses (about 40 Gy in 2.0-Gy fractions given over 4 weeks), modest acute reactions may occur, and surgery is usually delayed for 2 to 4 weeks until these reactions have more or less resolved. In this circumstance, surgical complications do not seem to be increased.[50-52] When 50 Gy is delivered over 5 weeks, acute radiation reactions are usual at the completion of therapy and surgery is delayed to the 4- to 6-week interval; with this practice, surgical complications such as delayed wound healing and wound breakdown are increased for some tumor sites[28,40,53,54] but not for others.[55]

Earlier studies had also noted an increase in surgical complications if surgery was performed less than 4 weeks after radiation,[19] and thus it is standard practice to delay surgery until 4 or 5 weeks after the completion of 50 Gy of preoperative radiation. One advantage of delaying surgery for this time is to allow the tumor time to regress (downstaging). In low rectal tumors, such downstaging increases the likelihood for sphincter-sparing surgery.[51]

It is a generally accepted principle that postoperative radiation must be delayed until the surgical wound has healed. Depending on the type of surgery performed, radiation is typically deferred for 3 to 6 weeks. Although accelerated clonogen repopulation may pose a problem even with these short time intervals, delays beyond 6 weeks raise the most concern. Some studies have reported poorer local–regional control in patients irradiated more than 6 weeks after surgery.[56-58] However, this finding has not been universal,[43] and it is possible that patients whose radiation is inordinately delayed by postsurgical wound problems are those with more advanced tumors that need more extensive surgery. This issue cannot be definitively resolved, but general principles suggest that radiation should commence as soon as feasible after surgery and that surgery should be optimized to avoid potential postoperative wound problems.

Intraoperative or Interstitial Radiation

Although preoperative or postoperative external beam radiation are the conventional forms of radiation integrated with surgery, the use of intraoperative or interstitial radiation has virtues as well. Intraoperative electron beam radiation has the advantage that patients can be selected on the basis of their tumor characteristics as defined at surgery and that the treatment can be directed to specific areas at high risk for harboring microscopic disease. However, its major disadvantage is that treatment is limited to one dose (typically 10 to 20 Gy), with all the attendant radiobiological disadvantages. Thus, intraoperative radiation is used as a boost to conventional external radiation. Few randomized clinical trials have evaluated the utility of this treatment. In one such trial for gastric carcinoma, the use of intraoperative irradiation (20 Gy) as sole adjuvant was associated with a significant reduction of local–regional recurrence compared with that achieved with surgery and conventional postoperative external irradiation.[59] For retroperitoneal sarcoma, the use of an intraoperative boost followed by external radiation was superior to the use of postoperative radiation with conventional boosting, but the gain in local control was small.[60] Adjuvant brachytherapy has the potential advantage of delivering a high dose to a limited volume and for delivering the radiation with minimal postsurgical delay. Adjuvant brachytherapy has been shown to significantly reduce the incidence of local recurrence for completely resected soft tissue sarcoma.[14] The use of brachytherapy as a boost form of radiation combined with more wide-field external radiation is an attractive strategy but has not been significantly explored as an adjuvant to surgery.

CLINICAL EXPERIENCES

Although this chapter was not intended to be a comprehensive review of clinical experience with combined radiation and surgery, it is useful to point out some clinical experiences that justify the theoretical arguments for combining these modalities. A large number of prospective trials have established that the use of radiation as a surgical adjuvant can significantly decrease local–regional recurrence rates for many types of cancer. For example, the current standard treatment for early

breast cancer is local excision (lumpectomy) and radiation; the addition of radiation to lumpectomy reduces the local recurrence rate from approximately 30% to approximately 10%.[11,13,61] For rectal cancer, the addition of radiation to surgery reduces local recurrence rates from approximately 30% to approximately 15%.[62-67] Most of the rectal carcinoma trials showing positive results have used preoperative hypofractionated radiation; in one trial of postoperative radiation, no benefit was found for radiation delivered in that sequence.[68] For soft tissue sarcomas managed with conservation surgery, postoperative radiation, whether external[15] or interstitial,[14] reduces local recurrence rates from approximately 30% to approximately 10%. Node-positive non–small-cell lung cancer with nodal disease has a local–regional recurrence rate of approximately 25% when managed surgically; the addition of postoperative radiation reduces this to 8%.[69] The risk of regional recurrence is reduced by a factor of 1.7 when preoperative radiation is added to surgery for esophageal cancer.[12] For gastric cancer, local–regional recurrences fall from 52% with surgery alone to 39% with adjuvant radiation.[50] Local–regional recurrence rates for patients with unfavorable cervical cancer fall from 19% with surgery alone to 13% when radiation is added postoperatively.[70] Survival duration of patients with malignant glioma increases from a median of 5 months with surgery alone to a median of 11 months with the addition of postoperative radiation.[71,72] Even metastatic disease can benefit from adjuvant radiation. The incidence of recurrence of resectable brain metastases falls from 70% with surgery alone to 18% when postoperative radiation is added.[73] However, for certain types of cancer, prospective trials have failed to find benefit from adjuvant radiation. For example, despite numerous studies, no conclusive evidence has been found that adjuvant preoperative radiation influences the outcome of bladder carcinoma.[48,49] Likewise, renal carcinoma does not seem to benefit from adjuvant radiation.[74,75] Indeed, one trial found that mortality among patients with right-sided primary tumors who received adjuvant treatment was increased because of radiation hepatitis.[74]

COMPLICATIONS

In general, the likelihood of complications increases when surgery and radiation are combined over that expected with either modality alone. As indicated previously, hypofractionated preoperative radiation does not seem to significantly increase surgical problems, but the incidence of immediate postsurgical wound complications is increased in many situations when 40 to 50 Gy is delivered preoperatively. Surgical procedures in irradiated areas should be modified to ensure healing, and appropriate surgical experience is important. In particular, suture lines should never be taut, and when hollow-organ reanastomosis is required unirradiated portions should be used if possible. In the head and neck region, trifurcate skin incisions for neck dissection should not be used because they often place the trifurcation point over the carotid artery, risking skin necrosis and carotid "blowout."[45] Handling tissues gently during the operation, maintaining meticulous hemostasis, avoiding closure under tension, and eliminating dead space through the use of drains and rotation flaps may decrease wound complication rates.[54] Similar attention should be paid to surgery for patients for whom postoperative radiation is planned. The incidence of long-term sequelae is often increased among patients given postoperative radiation. For example, long-term follow-up of women given adjuvant breast irradiation has revealed a significant incidence of cardiac morbidity that correlated directly with the proportion of the heart that was irradiated.[76] Even low-dose hypofractionated preoperative radiation has been found to have long-term effects on colon function.[67] Clearly, adjuvant radiation must be planned with all the attention to detail customarily used for definitive treatment because the lower doses used in the adjuvant setting do not preclude the development of significant long-term sequelae.

GENERAL GUIDELINES AND CONCLUSIONS

Not every patient with cancer needs combined modality treatment. Specific indications for the use of adjuvant radiation are presented elsewhere in this book. However, some general considerations are presented here. Combined radiation and surgery should be considered for the following circumstances:

1. Small tumors for which preservation of organs or functions are realistic treatment goals should be considered for conservative surgery and radiation. The sequence of modalities will often be dictated by patterns of current practice (e.g., breast cancer is usually managed with resection followed by radiation, whereas sarcoma is usually managed with radiation followed by resection).
2. Large tumors for which resection is expected to result in poor local control or the resectability of which is marginal should be considered for preoperative irradiation.
3. After resection, any one or more of the following adverse pathologic factors should at least lead to consideration of postoperative irradiation: microscopically positive resection margins; microscopically close margins (<5 mm); large primary tumors (T3/T4), regardless of margin status; tumors that invade beyond the capsule of their organ of origin; tumors with extensive lymph node involvement or extranodal extension; tumors with lymphatic permeation; tumors with perineural invasion, particularly of larger named nerves; and tumors with bone invasion.

Finally, it is worth reiterating that radiation, in modest doses (45 to 60 Gy), is a highly effective adjuvant to surgical resection of many types of cancer. Its efficacy in this respect rests not only on persuasive radiobiological grounds but has been confirmed for a variety of tumor types in many prospective randomized clinical trials.

REFERENCES

1. Withers HR, Peters LJ, Taylor JM. dose–response relationship for radiation therapy of subclinical disease. *Int J Radiat Oncol Biol Phys* 1995;31:353-359.
2. Fletcher S, Black W, Harris R, et al. Special article: report of the international workshop on screening for breast cancer. *J Natl Cancer Inst* 1993;85:1644-1656.
3. Hakama M. Potential contribution of screening to cancer mortality reduction. *Cancer Prev Det* 1993;17:513-520.
4. Selby JV, Friedman GD, Quesenberry CP, et al. A case-control study of screening sigmoidoscopy and mortality from colorectal cancer. *N Engl J Med* 1992;326:653-657.
5. Fuks Z, Leibel SA, Wallner KE, et al. The effect of local control in metastatic dissemination in carcinoma of the prostate: long-term results in patients treated with ^{125}I implantation. *Int J Radiat Oncol Biol Phys* 1991;21:537-548.
6. Zagars GK, von Eschenbach AC, Ayala AG, et al. The influence of local control on metastatic dissemination of prostate cancer treated by external beam megavoltage radiation therapy. *Cancer* 1992;6:2370-2377.
7. Vigliotti A, Rich TA, Romsdahl MM, et al. Postoperative adjuvant radiotherapy for adenocarcinoma of the rectum and rectosigmoid. *Int J Radiat Oncol Biol Phys* 1987;13:999-1006.
8. Trovik CS, Bauer HC. Local recurrence of soft tissue sarcoma a risk factor for late metastases: 379 patients followed for 0.5-20 years. *Acta Orthop Scand* 1994;65:553-558.
9. Chyle V, Zagars GK, Wheeler JT, et al. Definitive radiotherapy for carcinoma of the vagina: outcome and prognostic factors. *Int J Radiat Oncol Biol Phys* 1996;35:891-905.
10. Leibel SA, Scott CB, Mohiuddin M, et al. The effect of local–regional control on distant metastatic dissemination in carcinoma of the head and neck: results of an analysis from the RTOG head and neck database. *Int J Radiat Oncol Biol Phys* 1991;21:549-556.
11. Liljegren G, Holmberg L, Bergh J, et al. 10-year results after sector resection with or without postoperative radiotherapy for stage I breast cancer: a randomized trial. *J Clin Oncol* 1999; 17:2326-2333.
12. Bosset JF, Gignoux M, Triboulet JP, et al. Chemoradiotherapy followed by surgery compared with surgery alone in squamous-cell carcinoma of the esophagus. *N Engl J Med* 1997;337:161-167.
13. Fisher B, Anderson S, Redmond CK, et al. Reanalysis and results after 12 years of follow-up in a randomized clinical trial comparing total mastectomy with lumpectomy with or without irradiation in the treatment of breast cancer. *N Engl J Med* 1995;333:1456-1461.
14. Pisters PWT, Harrison LB, Leung DHY, et al. Long-term results of a prospective randomized trial of adjuvant brachytherapy in soft tissue sarcoma. *J Clin Oncol* 1996;14:859-868.
15. Yang JC, Chang AE, Baker AR, et al. Randomized prospective study of the benefit of adjuvant radiation therapy in the treatment of soft tissue sarcomas of the extremity. *J Clin Oncol* 1998;16:197-203.
16. MacComb WS, Fletcher GH. Planned combination of surgery and radiation in treatment of advanced primary head and neck cancers. *Ann Surg* 1957;77:397-414.

17. Bagshaw MA, Thompson RW. Elective irradiation of neck in patients with primary carcinoma of head and neck. *JAMA* 1971;217:456-458.

18. Fletcher GH. The evolution of the basic concepts underlying the practice of radiotherapy from 1949 to 1977. *Radiology* 1978;127:3-19.

19. White EC, Fletcher GH, Clark RL. Surgical experience with preoperative irradiation for carcinoma of the breast. *Ann Surg* 1962;155:948-956.

20. Fletcher GH. Implications of the density of clonogenic infestation in radiotherapy. *Int J Radiat Oncol Biol Phys* 1986;12:1675-1680.

21. Suwinski R, Taylor JM, Withers HR. Rapid growth of microscopic rectal cancer as a determinant of response to preoperative radiation therapy. *Int J Radiat Oncol Biol Phys* 1998;42:943-951.

22. Fletcher GH. Irradiation of subclinical disease in the draining lymphatics. *Int J Radiat Oncol Biol Phys* 1984;10:939-942.

23. Fletcher GH, Shukovsky LJ. The interplay of radiocurability and tolerance in the irradiation of human cancers. *J Radiol Electrol* 1975;56:383-400.

24. Zagars GK, Schultheiss TE, Peters LJ. Inter-tumor heterogeneity and radiation dose-control curves. *Radiother Oncol* 1987;8:353-362.

25. Fletcher GH. Irradiation of subclinical disease in the draining lymphatics. *Int J Rad Oncol Biol Phys* 1984;10:939-942.

26. Marcus RG, Million RR, Cassissi NJ, et al. Postoperative irradiation for squamous cell carcinomas of the head and neck: analysis of time-dose factors related to control above the clavicles. *Int J Radiat Oncol Biol Phys* 1979;5:1943-1949.

27. Amdur RJ, Parsons JT, Mendenhall WM. Postoperative irradiation for squamous cell carcinoma of the head and neck: an analysis of treatment results and complications. *Int J Radiat Oncol Biol Phys* 1989;16:25-36.

28. Pollack A, Zagars GK, Goswitz MS, et al. Preoperative radiotherapy in the treatment of soft tissue sarcomas: a matter of presentation. *Int J Radiat Oncol Biol Phys* 1998;42:563-572.

29. Peters LJ, Withers HR. Applying radiobiological principles to combined modality treatment of head and neck cancer—the time factor. *Int J Radiat Oncol Biol Phys* 1997;39:831-836.

30. Withers HR, Suwinski R. Radiation dose response for subclinical metastases. *Semin Radiat Oncol* 1998;8:224-228.

31. Withers HR, Taylor JMG, Maciejewski B. The hazard of accelerated tumor clonogen repopulation during radiotherapy. *Acta Oncol* 1988;27:131-146.

32. Awwad HK, Khafagy Y, Barsoum M, et al. Accelerated versus conventional fractionation in the postoperative irradiation of locally advanced head and neck cancer: influence of tumor proliferation. *Radiother Oncol* 1992;25:261-266.

33. Peters LJ, Ang KK, Byers RM, et al. Evaluation of the dose for postoperative radiation therapy of head and neck cancer: first report of a prospective randomized trial. *Int J Radiat Oncol Biol Phys* 1993;26:3-11.

34. El-Sayed S, Nelson N. Adjuvant and adjunctive chemotherapy in the management of squamous cell carcinoma of the head and neck region: a meta-analysis of prospective and randomized trials. *J Clin Oncol* 1996;14:838-847.

35. Munro AJ. An overview of randomized controlled trials of adjuvant chemotherapy in head and neck cancer. *Br J Cancer* 1995;71:83-91.

36. Heriot AG, Kumar D. Adjuvant therapy for resectable rectal and colonic cancer. *Br J Surg* 1998;85:300-309.

37. Klinkenbijl JH, Jeekel J, Sahmoud T, et al. Adjuvant radiotherapy and 5-fluorouracil after curative resection of cancer of the pancreas and periampullary region: phase III trial of the EORTC gastrointestinal tract cancer cooperative group. *Ann Surg* 1999;230:776-782.

38. Cox JD. Chemoradiation for malignant epithelial tumors. *Cancer Radiother* 1998;2:7-11.

39. Link KH, Staib L, Schatz M, et al. Adjuvant radiochemotherapy—what is the patient benefit? *Langenbecks Arch Surg* 1998;383:416-426.

40. O'Sullivan B, Davis A, Canadian Sarcoma Group, et al. Effect on radiotherapy field sizes in a recently completed Canadian Sarcoma Group and NCI Canada Clinical Trials Group randomized trial comparing pre-operative and post-operative radiotherapy in extremity soft tissue sarcoma [abstract 176]. *Int J Radiat Oncol Biol Phys* 1999;45(suppl):238-239.

41. Nielsen OS, Cummings B, O'Sullivan B, et al. Preoperative and postoperative irradiation of soft tissue sarcomas: effect on radiation field size. *Int J Radiat Oncol Biol Phys* 1991;21:1595-1599.

42. Suit HD, Makin HJ, Wood WC, et al. Preoperative, intraoperative, and postoperative radiation in the treatment of primary soft tissue sarcoma. *Cancer* 1985;55:2659-2667.

43. Taylor JMG, Mendenhall WM, Parson JT, et al. The influence of dose and time on wound complications following postradiation neck dissection. *Int J Radiat Oncol Biol Phys* 1992;23:41-46.

44. Frykholm GJ, Glimelius B, Pahlman L. Preoperative or postoperative irradiation in adenocarcinoma of the rectum: final treatment results of a randomised trial and an evaluation of secondary effects. *Dis Colon Rectum* 1993;36:564-572.

45. Vandenbrouck C, Sancho H, LeFur R, et al. Results of a randomized clinical trial of preoperative irradiation versus postoperative in treatment of tumors of the hypopharynx. *Cancer* 1977;39:1445-1449.

46. Tupchong L, Scott CB, Blitzer PH, et al. Randomized study of preoperative versus postoperative radiation therapy in advanced head and neck carcinoma: long-term follow-up of RTOG study 73-03. *Int J Radiat Oncol Biol Phys* 1991;20:21-28.

47. Hyams DH, Mamounas EP, Petrelli N, et al. A clinical trial to evaluate the worth of preoperative multimodality therapy in patients with operable carcinoma of the rectum: a progress report of National Adjuvant Breast and Bowel Protocol R-03. *Dis Colon Rectum* 1997;40:131-139.

48. Smith JA, Crawford ED, Paradelo JC, et al. Treatment of advanced bladder cancer with combined preoperative irradiation and radical cystectomy versus radical cystectomy alone: a phase III intergroup study. *J Urol* 1997;157:805-807.

49. Huncharek M, Muscat J, Geschwind JF. Planned preoperative radiation therapy in muscle invasive bladder cancer: results of a meta-analysis. *Anticancer Res* 1998;18:1931-1934.

50. Zhang ZX, Gu XZ, Yin WB, et al. Randomized clinical trial on the combination of preoperative irradiation and surgery in the treatment of adenocarcinoma of gastric cardia (AGC)—report on 370 patients. *Int J Radiat Oncol Biol Phys* 1998;42:929-934.

51. Francois Y, Nemoz CJ, Baulieux J, et al. Influence of the interval between preoperative radiation therapy and surgery on downstaging and on the rate of sphincter-sparing surgery for rectal cancer: the Lyon R90-01 trial. *J Clin Oncol* 1999;17:2396-2402.

52. Shipley WU, Cummings KB, Coombs LJ, et al. 4000 rad preoperative irradiation followed by prompt radical cystectomy for invasive bladder carcinoma: a prospective study of patient tolerance and pathologic downstaging. *J Urol* 1982;127:448-451.

53. Cheng EY, Dusenbery KE, Winters MR, et al. Soft tissue sarcomas: preoperative versus postoperative radiotherapy. *J Surg Oncol* 1996;61:90-99.

54. Bujko K, Suit HD, Springfield DS, et al. Wound healing after preoperative radiation for sarcoma of soft tissues. *Surg Gynecol Obstet* 1993;176:124-134.

55. Pollack A, Zagars GK, Dinney CP, et al. Preoperative radiotherapy for muscle-invasive bladder cancer: long term follow-up and prognostic factors for 338 patients. *Cancer* 1994;74:2819-2827.

56. Vikram B, Strong EW, Shah JP, et al. Failure in the neck following multimodality treatment for advanced head and neck cancer. *Head Neck Surg* 1984;6:724-729.

57. Vikram B. Importance of time interval between surgery and post-operative radiation therapy in the combined management of head and neck cancer. *Int J Radiat Oncol Biol Phys* 1979;5:1837-1840.

58. Byers RM, Clayman GL, Guillamondegui OM, et al. Resection of advanced cervical metastasis prior to definitive radiotherapy for primary squamous carcinomas of the upper aerodigestive tract. *Head Neck* 1992;14:133-138.

59. Sindelar WF, Kinsella TJ, Tepper JE, et al. Randomized trial of intraoperative radiotherapy in carcinoma of the stomach. *Am J Surg* 1993;165:178-186.

60. Sindelar WF, Kinsella TJ, Chen PW, et al. Intraoperative radiotherapy in retroperitoneal sarcomas: final results of a prospective, randomized, clinical trial. *Arch Surg* 1993;128: 402-410.

61. Recht A, Come SE, Gelman RS, et al. Integration of conservative surgery, radiotherapy and chemotherapy for the treatment of early stage node-positive breast cancer: sequencing, timing and outcome. *J Clin Oncol* 1991;9:1662.

62. Cohen AM. Has preoperative radiation therapy for resectable rectal cancer been proven effective. *J Surg Oncol* 1990;45:69-71.

63. Pahlman L, Glimelius B. Pre- or postoperative radiotherapy in rectal and rectosigmoid carcinoma: report from a randomized multicenter trial. *Ann Surg* 1990;211:187-192.

64. Glimelius B, Isacsson U, Jung G, et al. Radiotherapy in addition to radical surgery in rectal cancer: evidence for a dose–response effect favoring preoperative treatment. *Int J Radiat Oncol Biol Phys* 1997;37:281-287.

65. Dahlberg M, Glimelius B, Pahlman L. Improved survival and reduction in local rates after preoperative radiotherapy: evidence for the generalizability of the results of Swedish Rectal Cancer Trial. *Ann Surg* 1999;229:493-497.

66. Hoskins RB, Gunderson LL, Dosoretz DE, et al. Adjuvant postoperative radiotherapy in carcinoma of the rectum and rectosigmoid. *Cancer* 1985;55:61.

67. Dahlberg M, Glimelius B, Graf W, et al. Preoperative irradiation affects functional results after surgery for rectal cancer: results from a randomized study. *Dis Colon Rectum* 1998;41: 543-551.

68. Arnaud JP, Nordlinger B, Bosset JF, et al. Radical surgery and postoperative radiotherapy as combined treatment in rectal cancer: final results of a phase III study of the European Organization for Research and Treatment of Cancer. *Br J Surg* 1997;84:352-357.

69. Smolle-Juettner FM, Mayer R, Pinter H, et al. "Adjuvant" external radiation of the mediastinum in radically resected non-small cell lung cancer. *Eur J Cardiothorac Surg* 1996;10:947-950.

70. Sedlis A, Bundy BN, Rotman MZ, et al. A randomized trial of pelvic radiation therapy versus no further therapy in selected patients with stage IB carcinoma of the cervix after radical hysterectomy and pelvic lymphadenectomy. *Gynecol Oncol* 1999;73:177-183.

71. Walker MD, Alexander E, Hunt WE. Evaluation of BCNU and/or radiotherapy in the treatment of anaplastic glioma: a cooperative clinical trial. *J Neurosurg* 1978;49:333-343.

72. Kristiansen K, Hagen S, Kollevoid T, et al. Combined modality therapy of operated astrocytomas grade III and IV. Confirmation of the value of postoperative irradiation and lack of potentiation of bleomycin on survival time: a prospective multicenter trial of the Scandinavian Glioblastoma Study Group. *Cancer* 1981;47:649-652.

73. Patchell RA, Tibbs PA, Regine WF, et al. Postoperative radiotherapy in the treatment of single metastases to the brain: a randomized trial. *JAMA* 1998;280:1485-1489.

74. Finney R. An evaluation of postoperative radiotherapy in hypernephroma treatment—a clinical trial. *Cancer* 1973;32: 1332-1340.

75. Kjaer M, Frederiksen PL, Engelholm SA. Postoperative radiotherapy in stage II and III renal adenocarcinoma: a randomized trial by the Copenhagen Renal Cancer Study Group. *Int J Radiat Oncol Biol Phys* 1987;13:665-672.

76. Gyenes G, Rutqvist LE, Liedberg A, et al. Long-term cardiac morbidity and mortality in a randomized trial of pre- and postoperative radiation therapy versus surgery alone in primary breast cancer. *Radiother Oncol* 1998;48:185-190.

CHAPTER 4

Principles of Combining Radiation Therapy and Chemotherapy

Luka Milas and James D. Cox

In perhaps no other aspect of oncologic practice has a direction developed in the last decade of the twentieth century that is as clear and compelling as the use of chemotherapy in conjunction with radiation therapy or radiation therapy and surgery. The question of whether to use combined-modality treatment has changed to which sequence and which drugs are the best. Also, given the increasing availability of preclinical investigations that can be used to chart a course for combining radiation therapy with drugs, it is important to explore in some depth those preclinical findings that have pointed the way to the use of combined-modality therapy. Equally important is to clarify the essential steps by which clinical investigations establish the toxicity, the efficacy, and finally the proper place for chemotherapy in combined-modality therapies in standard practice. In this chapter, some basic concepts are introduced and defined, mechanisms of interaction between radiation and chemotherapy are outlined, theoretical principles underlying sequencing strategies are presented, and finally clinical applications of the combined-treatment strategies are reviewed.

THERAPEUTIC RATIO

Neither radiation nor chemotherapeutic drugs are particularly selective against tumors; both also damage normal tissues. This damage limits the dose of radiation, drugs, or a combination of both that can be given to patients. To be therapeutically beneficial, individual agents or their combination must be more effective against tumors than against normal tissues. In general, both antitumor efficacy and normal tissue injury are positively related to the dose of radiation or cytotoxic drugs, and this relationship is commonly described by a sigmoid curve (Fig. 4-1). The plots shown in Figure 4-1 provide information on the therapeutic ratio or index, which is defined as the ratio of the maximally tolerated drug (in this case, with regard to normal tissue damage, *curve C*) to the minimally curative or effective dose (in this case, the antitumor effect, *curve A* or *B*). Any level of probability can be used to calculate the therapeutic

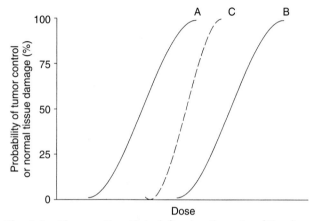

Fig. 4-1 *Therapeutic ratio* is defined as the ratio of the doses of an agent (or agents) that produce the same probability of normal tissue damage *(curve C)* and antitumor effect *(curves A and B)*. *Curve A* illustrates an agent with a positive (beneficial) therapeutic ratio, one that produces more damage to tumor than to normal tissue; *curve B* illustrates a negative (undesirable) therapeutic ratio in which the damage to normal tissue exceeds the damage to the tumor.

ratio; however, in experimental preclinical studies, 50% is the most commonly used.

The objective of any cancer treatment is to achieve a positive therapeutic ratio—that is, one in which the antitumor efficacy curve lies to the left of the curve representing normal tissue injury (see Fig. 4-1, *curve A*). Treatments for which the therapeutic ratio is negative (i.e., the antitumor response curve lies to the right of that for normal tissue damage [*curve B*], and hence normal tissue damage is more likely than tumor damage) are contraindicated, except perhaps for palliation in some circumstances.

In defining therapeutic ratio, the endpoints of tumor response and normal tissue injury must be appropriately categorized and quantified. The endpoints will vary depending on factors such as whether the treatment is intended to be curative or palliative and which tissues limit the doses that can be given. Damage to normal tissue must be within acceptable limits in terms of both the tissue type and the severity of the damage. The balance between complications arising from normal tissue damage and the probability of tumor control form the basis of the therapeutic ratio of a treatment.

IMPROVING THE THERAPEUTIC RATIO

The ultimate goal in combining chemotherapeutic drugs with radiation therapy is to improve the therapeutic ratio—that is, to enhance the antitumor effect while minimizing the toxicity of the treatment to critical normal tissues. Steel and Peckham[1] defined four principles by which therapeutic ratios of combined treatments can be improved: spatial cooperation, independence of toxicity, enhancement of tumor response, and protection of normal tissues. These principles are described briefly in the following paragraphs.

Spatial Cooperation

Treatments that act independently of each other at different anatomic sites are said to exhibit spatial coordination. For example, chemotherapy is commonly used to deal with tumor growth outside the radiation field, usually to eradicate metastases. Conversely, radiation can be used to treat neoplastic lesions in secluded sites that are poorly accessed by chemotherapeutic agents; an example of this strategy is the use of radiation to supplement chemotherapeutic treatment of leukemia that has spread to the brain.

Independence of Toxicity

Because toxicity to normal tissues is the principal dose-limiting factor both for chemotherapy and radiation therapy, the antitumor efficacy of a combined treatment theoretically would be improved more readily and tolerated more easily through the use of drugs with toxic effects that do not overlap or enhance those induced by radiation. Use of this principle requires thorough knowledge of the toxicity, pharmacology, and optimal administration of individual chemotherapeutic drugs to ensure that combining such drugs with radiation minimizes normal tissue damage while still retaining antitumor efficacy.

Enhancement of Tumor Response

Some drugs can enhance radiation-induced tumor damage, or radiation can make some cells more sensitive to chemotherapy, presumably through interactions between the agents at the molecular, cellular, or pathophysiologic (microenvironmental or metabolic) levels. Some of the more important mechanisms of drug-radiation interactions that increase tumor susceptibility are considered in more detail later in this chapter.

It should be noted that virtually all chemotherapeutic agents enhance radiation damage to normal tissues as well; consequently, therapeutic benefit will be achieved if the susceptibility of tumors rather than that of critical normal tissues were to be enhanced.

Protection of Normal Tissues

Some compounds are thought to increase the tolerance of normal tissues to radiation so that higher doses of radiation can be safely delivered to the tumor. Preclinical in vivo testing has shown that some chemicals can selectively or preferentially protect normal tissues.[2-4] Among the commonly tested protectors are thiol compounds such as WR-2721 that may be useful in clinical settings such as protecting salivary glands during radiation therapy delivered to the head and neck.[5] A major problem with concurrent chemoradiation therapy is the increase in the toxic effects on tissues that is conferred by radiation; however, radioprotectants and technical improvements in radiation therapy such as three-dimensional treatment planning, conformational radiotherapy, or the use of protons are likely to minimize tissue toxicity and consequently enhance the effectiveness of chemoradiation.

ADDITIVITY OF DRUG-RADIATION INTERACTIONS

Interactions between chemotherapeutic agents and radiation may result in additive, supra-additive, or subadditive effects, depending on whether the combination produces effects that are equal to, greater than, or less than, respectively, the sum of the activity produced by the individual agents. Evaluations of the additivity of a given combination must take into account the dose-response relationship of each individual agent. Such calculations are simple when both agents have effects that are exponentially related to the dose. However, the dose-effect relationship is rarely exponential. As described in Chapter 1, many radiation dose/cell survival curves have a "shoulder" of varying width at lower doses of irradiation and an exponential relationship at higher doses. The presence of a shoulder indicates that the cells can repair radiation damage. The dose-survival curves after chemotherapy tend to be more diverse; some have shoulders and some do not, and some show "tails" at higher drug doses. The presence of such tails implies the existence of cell subpopulations that are resistant to the chemotherapeutic agents. These nonlinear dose-related characteristics in cell killing imply that when two agents are combined, additive effects can be produced over a range of doses. Thus determinations of additivity on the basis of a combination of only one dose of each agent are inappropriate and can be misleading.

To overcome this problem, Steel and Peckham[1] introduced the concept of *isobologram analysis,* in which an isoeffect plot is generated for the dose-response to the combination of two agents (Fig. 4-2). Dose-response curves are generated for each agent, and those curves are used to generate isobolograms, which

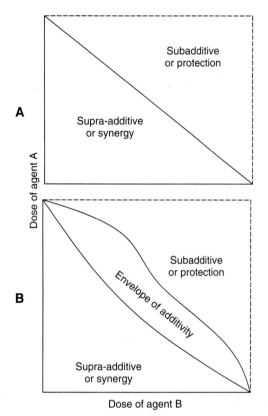

Fig. 4-2 Isobolograms for pairs of agents that either have linear dose response curves (**A**) or nonlinear dose response curves (**B**). Also shown are the envelope of additivity and regions of supra-additivity and subadditivity. (Modified from Steel GG, Peckham MJ. *Int J Radiat Oncol Biol Phys* 1979;5: 85-91.)

illustrate the expected additive response. In the simplest situation, that in which each agent produces a linear dose response, the isobologram is also linear (see Fig. 4-2, *A*). If the combination of the two agents has a supra-additive effect, then the response would appear to the left of the curve; if the combination has a subadditive effect, then the response would appear to the right of the curve. When the dose-response is nonlinear, an envelope of additivity appears in the isobologram (see Fig. 4-2, *B*), indicating a range of isoeffect curves that represent additive responses. In this situation, to obtain an additive effect, the doses of individual agents that produce the same biological effect lie within the envelope. If the doses lie to the left of the isobologram envelope, then the interaction is supra-additive or synergistic—that is, the effect is caused by lower doses of the two agents than the envelope of additivity would predict. In contrast, if the doses lie to the right side of the envelope, then the interaction is subadditive or antagonistic, meaning the effect requires higher doses of the two agents than predicted. The envelope of additivity becomes wider as the gap between the nonlinear dose-responses to individual agents becomes greater.

METHODS FOR ASSESSING DRUG-RADIATION EFFECTS

Many assays, both in vitro and in vivo, are used to assess the biological effects of drugs, radiation, and the combination of both.[6,7] In vitro assessments most commonly involve cell-survival or clonogenic assays, which involve measuring the ability of cells to survive and produce colonies of progeny of a defined minimum size (i.e., the ability to sustain reproductive integrity). Survival curves are usually presented by plotting the surviving fraction of cells on a logarithmic scale against the dose of radiation or drugs, which is plotted on a linear scale (Fig. 4-3). Established cell lines are usually used to assess clonogenic survival after treatment with

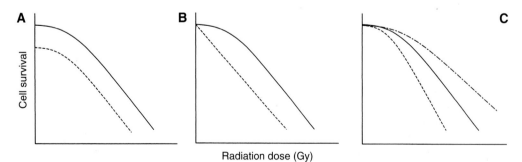

Fig. 4-3 The effects of chemotherapeutic drugs on cell survival after irradiation. Solid lines indicate radiation only; broken lines indicate drug plus radiation. **A,** Simple displacement of radiation survival curve, indicating additivity. **B,** Elimination of the shoulder, indicating inhibition of sublethal damage repair. **C,** Change in the slope of the radiation curve, indicating sensitization (displacement to the left) or protection (displacement to the right).

drugs or radiation in vitro, although a variation of the clonogenic cell-survival assay called the *excision assay* can also be used to study antitumor treatments given in vivo. In an excision assay, the tumor is excised at some specified time after treatment, and a single-cell suspension of tumor cells is prepared and plated for subsequent determination of cell survival.

The addition of drugs to radiation can influence survival curves in several ways (see Fig. 4-3). First, the drugs may simply shift the curve downward without changing its shape. The magnitude of this displacement corresponds to the amount of cells killed by the drugs (see Fig. 4-3, *A*). Second, the drugs may eliminate the shoulder of a radiation survival curve, which implies that the drugs are inhibiting the cellular radiation-repair process (see Fig. 4-3, *B*). Third, drugs may change the slope of the exponential portion of the survival curve (see Fig. 4-3, *C*); in this case, a steeper slope indicates sensitization and a more shallow slope indicates protection.

Many methods are also available for assessing the effects of chemotherapeutic drugs on tumors and normal tissues in vivo.[6,7] Two of the most common assays used to assess tumor response are the tumor growth delay assay[8] and the tumor-control dose (TCD_{50}) assay.[9] When the treatment endpoint is a delay in tumor growth, the size of untreated and treated tumors is measured as a function of time and plotted in growth curves. The *absolute growth delay* represents the difference in time (usually in days) needed for untreated and treated tumors to reach a defined size (Fig. 4-4, *A*). When a drug is given with radiation, the growth delay achieved by both modalities minus the delay caused by the drug alone is called the *normalized growth delay*. To determine if the addition of drugs enhances or reduces the antitumor efficacy of radiation requires determining normalized growth delay after at least three different doses of radiation. Then, both the normalized growth delays after the combined treatment and the absolute growth delays after radiation only are plotted as a function of radiation dose (see Fig. 4-4, *B*). The displacement of the normalized growth delay curve in relation to the absolute growth delay curve indicates the effect of drugs on tumor radioresponsiveness. No displacement indicates a simple additive effect, a shift to the left (to lower radiation doses) indicates enhancement of tumor radioresponse, and a shift to the right (to higher radiation doses) indicates a reduction in tumor radioresponse. The results shown in Figure 4-4, *B*, illustrate enhancement of radiation response of a mouse mammary carcinoma by the administration of docetaxel before irradiation.[10]

In the TCD_{50} assay, the endpoint is tumor control or cure in 50% of the treated subjects. In this assay, the proportion of tumors cured by radiation only or by a drug-radiation combination is plotted as a function of radiation

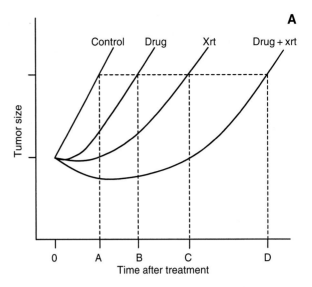

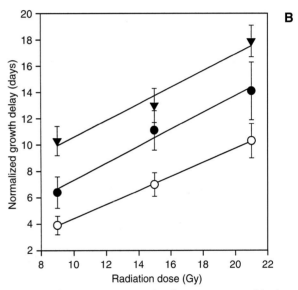

Fig. 4-4 Delay in tumor growth after treatment with drug, radiation, or a combination of both. In **A**, the points at *B*, *C*, and *D* are absolute growth delays after treatment with drug, radiation *(xrt)*, or drug plus radiation. Normalized growth delay is defined as *D* minus *B*. **B**, The interactions between the chemotherapeutic drug docetaxel and radiation in a murine mammary carcinoma. Addition of the drug displaced the radiation response curve to the left, indicating enhancement of tumor radioresponse. Open circles represent tumor response after radiation only; closed circles and triangles represent tumor radioresponse when docetaxel was given 9 or 48 hours before irradiation, respectively. (From Mason KA, Hunter NR, Milas M, et al. *Clin Cancer Res* 1997;3:2431-2438.)

dose. If the combination displaces the radiation-only curve to the left, then addition of the drug improves tumor curability; however, the displacement does not discriminate between improvement caused by independent cells killed by the drug and that caused by a supra-additive interaction between the drug and radiation.

TABLE 4-1

In Vivo Assays for Normal Tissue Damage in Drug-Radiation Combinations

	Clonogenic Endpoints	Functional Endpoints
Bone marrow	Exogenous and endogenous spleen colony assay	LD_{50}, depletion of different cell types
Skin	In situ skin colonies	Skin erythema and desquamation, hair loss, telangiectasia, skin contraction
Gastrointestinal tract	Jejunum and colon microcolonies	LD_{50}, weight loss, protein or electrolyte leakage
Lung		LD_{50}, breathing rate, CO uptake
Kidney	Kidney tubules	Urine output
Bladder		Urination frequency
Testis	Spermatogonial stem cell assay	Testis weight, sperm count, fertility
Central nervous system		LD_{50} (brain), paralysis (spinal cord)

LD_{50}, Lethal dose in 50%; *CO*, carbon monoxide.

Many assays can be used to quantify the radiation dose-response relationship for normal tissues and the influence of chemotherapeutic drugs on radiation response (Table 4-1). Some of these assays are clonogenic—that is, the endpoint depends directly on the reproductive integrity of individual cells. More frequently, however, dose-response relationships for normal tissues are based on functional endpoints. These endpoints tend to reflect the minimum number of functional cells remaining in tissues or organs rather than the proportion of cells that retain reproductive integrity.

MECHANISMS OF DRUG–RADIATION INTERACTIONS

As discussed in the remainder of this chapter, recent clinical experience has clearly shown that chemotherapy is most effective in improving local tumor control when it is given during the course of radiation therapy. This observation implies that chemotherapeutic drugs and radiation actively interact. The multiple mechanisms underlying that interaction, which undoubtedly occur at the cellular and tumor-microenvironment level, are complex; five major mechanisms are considered in the following paragraphs.

Initial Radiation Damage

As discussed in Chapter 1, the critical target for radiation injury is the deoxyribonucleic acid (DNA) molecule. Radiation induces several types of lesions, including single-strand breaks, double-strand breaks, base damage, and DNA-DNA or DNA-protein crosslinks. The most common type of lesion is the single-strand break, which is readily repaired. Double-strand breaks left unrepaired or misrepaired and associated chromosomal aberrations generally lead to cell death.[11] Certain drugs such as halogenated pyrimidines that become incorporated into DNA make the DNA more susceptible to radiation damage.[12] In addition to increasing the initial injury caused by radiation, halogenated pyrimidines can enhance cell radiosensitivity by interfering with cellular repair mechanisms,[12,13] as discussed in the next section.

Inhibition of Cellular Repair

Cells have the ability to repair both sublethal[14] and potentially lethal[15] radiation damage. Both types of repair are defined in operational terms. *Sublethal damage repair* is defined as the increase in survival observed when a dose of radiation is split into two (or more) fractions with some time interval between. Sublethal damage repair is manifested on cell-survival curves as restoration of a shoulder on the curve after the second dose. Repair takes place quickly, typically with a half-time of about 1 hour and a completion time of 4 to 6 hours after irradiation, and takes place in tumors, normal tissues, and cultured cells. Potentially lethal damage repair, in contrast, designates an increase in the proportion of cells that survived irradiation because of some modification of postirradiation conditions. In general, potentially lethal damage repair takes place under conditions that prevent cellular division for several hours, such as maintaining cultured cells in a plateau phase after irradiation or delaying removal of cells from tumors for clonogenic survival assay. Conceptually, repair of potentially lethal damage can be explained in terms of successful repair of DNA lesions that would have been lethal had the DNA undergone replication within several hours of irradiation. Repair can be achieved through several mechanisms such as restoration of damaged molecules by reducing species that donate electrons to oxidized substrates and through involvement of a variety of repair enzymes. Possible repair mechanisms for the various DNA lesions are summarized in Table 4-2.

TABLE 4-2

Radiation-Induced DNA Damage and Its Repair

Induced Lesions	Types of Repair
Single-strand breaks	Direct reversal
Double-strand breaks	Homologous and nonhomologous recombination
Base alterations	Base excision repair
DNA-protein crosslinks	Nucleotide excision repair

DNA, Deoxyribonucleic acid.

Many chemotherapeutic drugs can interact with cellular repair mechanisms, and in inhibiting those mechanisms the drugs may enhance the response of cells or tissues to radiation. As mentioned previously, halogenated pyrimidines can enhance cell radiosensitivity not only through increasing initial radiation damage but also by inhibiting cellular repair. Recently, significant research has focused on exploring the radioenhancing effects of nucleoside analogs such as fludarabine[16,17] and gemcitabine[16-18] that can inhibit the repair of radiation-induced DNA or chromosome damage. Fludarabine is a potent inhibitor of DNA primase, DNA polymerase-α, ε-DNA ligase, and ribonucleotide reductase, and it can cause DNA chain termination.[19] Fludarabine phosphate is rapidly dephosphorylated in vivo to form fludarabine, an adenine nucleoside analog that is transported by a carrier into cells, where it is converted to the active metabolite by the addition of adenosine triphosphate. Transport into cells and metabolic activation of fludarabine seem to differ among cell types, with malignant cells concentrating and metabolizing the drug more efficiently than do normal cells. Fludarabine is clinically active against leukemias and lymphomas but is not particularly effective against solid tumors.

Gemcitabine (2′-deoxy-2′,2′-difluorocytidine) is a fluorine-substituted cytarabine that also requires intracellular phosphorylation by deoxycytidine kinase to produce the active metabolites gemcitabine diphosphate (dFdCDP) and gemcitabine triphosphate (dFdCTP).[17,18,20] Compared with fludarabine, gemcitabine has greater membrane permeability and enzyme affinity, as well as longer intracellular retention.[17,20] dFdCDP interferes with DNA synthesis by inhibiting ribonucleotide reductase and hence reducing the deoxynucleotide pools. dFdCTP competes with deoxycytidine triphosphate for incorporation into elongated DNA strands; only one additional deoxynucleotide can be incorporated after the insertion of dFdCTP, thus halting DNA polymerization.[17,20] In contrast to fludarabine, gemcitabine is active against many common solid tumors in humans, including head and neck, lung, and pancreatic carcinoma.[16,17]

In general, nucleoside analogs like fludarabine and gemcitabine are potent radiosensitizers of mammalian cells in vitro[16-18,21] and enhancers of tumor radioresponse in vivo.[16,17,22-24] Investigations from our laboratory have demonstrated that both fludarabine and gemcitabine can significantly enhance the radioresponse of several mouse solid tumors, as assessed by tumor growth delay or local tumor cure, after single-dose or fractionated-dose irradiation.[16,17,22-24] Fludarabine in particular produced radioenhancement ranging from a factor of 1.2 to more than 2.0, depending on the timing of fludarabine administration relative to radiation, the dose of fludarabine, the type of tumor, and schedule of radiation. Although several mechanisms seem to have been responsible for the enhancement, inhibition of radiation damage repair seems to have been prominent. The effect of fludarabine on radiocurability of a murine sarcoma after single-dose or fractionated irradiation is illustrated in Figure 4-5. The enhancement was much greater when fludarabine was combined with fractionated irradiation, suggesting that the inhibition of sublethal (or potentially lethal) damage repair was a significant mechanism of enhancement of tumor radioresponse.

Cell Cycle Effects

The cytotoxicity of most chemotherapeutic agents and ionizing radiation is highly dependent on the proliferative state of the cells, with most agents being more effective against proliferating cells than nonproliferating cells. Sensitivity to such agents also varies depending on the phase of the cell cycle. The influence of cell cycle in response to radiation was first reported in 1963 by Terasima and Tolmach.[25] In general, cells in the G_2 and M phases are the most sensitive, and cells in the S phase are the most resistant. This variation in radiosensitivity over the cell cycle can be exploited for designing effective chemoradiation therapy strategies such as the use of drugs that either accumulate cells in a radiosensitive phase or eliminate radioresistant S-phase cells. Two recent examples illustrating these concepts are described in the following section.

Taxanes, of which paclitaxel and docetaxel are prototypes, are potent mitotic-spindle poisons. Taxanes inhibit tubulin depolymerization by binding to β-tubulin, increasing tubulin polymerization, and promoting microtubule assembly and stability, all of which leads to the cells becoming arrested in the radiosensitive G_2 and M phases of the cell cycle.[26] The ability of taxanes to block cells in G_2/M was the biological rationale that led to extensive testing of their radioenhancing properties. In the first report on the radioenhancing effect of taxanes,[27] the radiosensitivity of a human astrocytoma cell line was reportedly increased by a factor of 1.8 (Fig. 4-6). Radiosensitization was achieved only when the cells

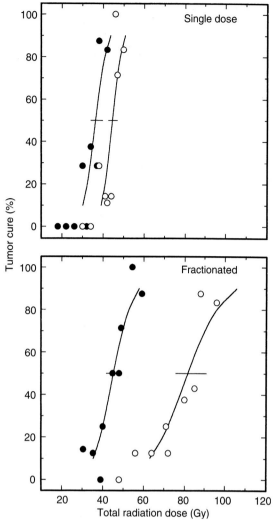

Fig. 4-5 Fludarabine-induced enhancement of response of the FSA mouse fibrosarcoma line to single-dose or fractionated-dose (16 fractions with a 6-hour interval between fractions) irradiation. Fludarabine (400 mg/kg) was given 3 hours before single-dose irradiation or daily during the 4-day fractionated treatment starting 3 hours before the first fractional dose of radiation. (From Gregoire V, Hunter NR, Brock WA, et al. *Radiat Res* 1996;146:548-553.)

were in phases G_2 and M at the time of irradiation, a result subsequently confirmed in many in vitro and in vivo studies.[28] Cells arrested in mitosis by taxanes often die by apoptosis (the underlying basis for the antitumor efficacy of these drugs), but they may overcome the mitotic block and continue with division. In that case, tumors are resistant to treatment with taxanes alone, but they can show an enhanced radioresponse if radiation is delivered at the time of mitotic arrest, usually between 6 and 12 hours after administration of the drug. (Tumor reoxygenation, another major mechanism of radioenhancement in tumors that respond to taxanes by both mitotic arrest and apoptosis, is discussed in more detail in the following section on "Hypoxia.") The histologic

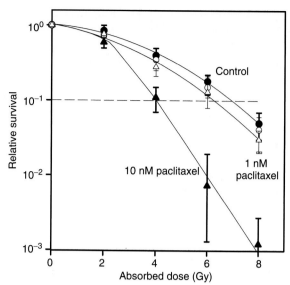

Fig. 4-6 Survival curves of astrocytoma cells treated with radiation and paclitaxel. Survival is presented at a particular radiation dose and expressed relative to that of nonirradiated controls given the same dose of paclitaxel. Points are means ± standard error. Symbols represent untreated control cells *(closed circles)* or cells treated with dimethylsulfoxide *(open circles)*, 1 nM paclitaxel *(open triangles)*, or 10 nM paclitaxel *(closed triangles)*. (From Tishler RB, Geard CR, Hall EJ, et al. *Cancer Res* 1992;52:3495-3497.)

appearance of mitotically arrested and apoptotic cells in murine MCa-4 tumors treated with docetaxel is shown in Figure 4-7.

Another approach for exploiting the cell-cycle effect in chemoradiation therapy is to use drugs that eliminate radioresistant S-phase cells. In addition to inhibiting radiation damage repair, nucleoside analogs such as fludarabine or gemcitabine become incorporated into

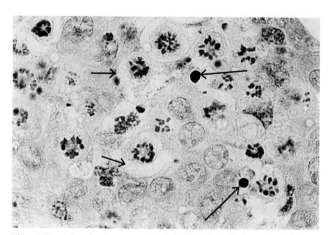

Fig. 4-7 Histologic appearance of mouse MCa-4 mammary tumors treated with 33 mg/kg docetaxel. *Short arrows,* Mitotically arrested cells; *long arrows,* apoptotic cells 12 hours after treatment with docetaxel. Mitotically arrested cells show characteristic coronal appearance. (×1000)

S-phase cells, many of which then die by apoptosis.[5,17,24,29] This preferential removal of the S-phase component from tumors leads to a parasynchronous movement of surviving cells through S phase and mitosis, resulting in accumulation of cells in G_2 and M phases of the cell cycle between 24 and 36 hours after administration of the drugs, when the highest radioenhancement values are observed. Thus both the elimination of radioresistant S-phase cells from the tumor cell population and the redistribution of surviving cells into more radiosensitive compartments of the cell cycle seem to be involved in the radioenhancement.

Hypoxia

The presence of oxygen has long been known to influence cell radiosensitivity; hypoxic cells are 2.5 to 3 times less sensitive to radiation than are well-oxygenated cells. Because tumors often include hypoxic areas but normal tissues usually do not, the radioresistant effect of hypoxia is generally restricted to tumors. Blood circulation within solid tumors tends to be poor because of abnormalities in the number, structure, and function of blood vessels within the tumor. Tumor blood vessels are commonly irregular and tortuous and have blind ends, arteriovenous shunts, incomplete endothelial linings, and basement membranes. All of these factors can limit intratumoral blood flow and hence the delivery of oxygen and nutrients, resulting in multiple tumor microregions becoming hypoxic, acidic, and eventually necrotic. Hypoxia develops in tissues when the distance from blood vessels exceeds some 100 to 150 μm; the proportion of hypoxic cells in tumors can often exceed 50%. Cells in hypoxic regions stop proliferating. In contrast, cells that are nearer to blood vessels are well oxygenated and actively proliferate.

Chemotherapeutic agents can improve the antitumor efficacy of radiation therapy by reducing or eliminating the negative (tumor-protective) effects of hypoxic cells. This improvement can be achieved by (1) eliminating tumor cells in oxygenated regions, (2) selectively eliminating hypoxic cells, or (3) sensitizing hypoxic cells to radiation. Elimination of cells in oxygenated regions leads to tumor reoxygenation (discussed in Chapter 1), and most chemotherapeutic drugs can achieve this effect because they preferentially kill well-oxygenated, proliferating cells. Eliminating oxygenated cells makes more oxygen available to the surviving cells through lowering the interstitial pressure on microvessels within the tumor, thereby reopening closed capillaries and increasing the intratumoral blood supply. Tumor shrinkage from cell loss and active migration of tumor cells also brings previously hypoxic microregions closer to blood vessels. Tumor reoxygenation was recently shown to be a major mechanism by which taxanes enhance tumor

radioresponsiveness[30] (Fig. 4-8). In that study, giving paclitaxel to mice bearing an adenocarcinoma within 3 days before local irradiation enhanced the radiosensitivity of the tumors. However, this enhancing effect was reduced when the tumors were rendered hypoxic by clamping the tumor-bearing legs at the time of irradiation. Paclitaxel's ability to increase tumor oxygenation was confirmed directly by measuring intratumoral partial pressure of oxygen (Po_2).[30]

Another chemotherapeutic approach that increases tumor radiosensitivity is to use drugs that selectively kill hypoxic cells. Several drugs with this property are available, including tirapazamine and mitomycin[31]; their cytotoxicity results from their reductive activation

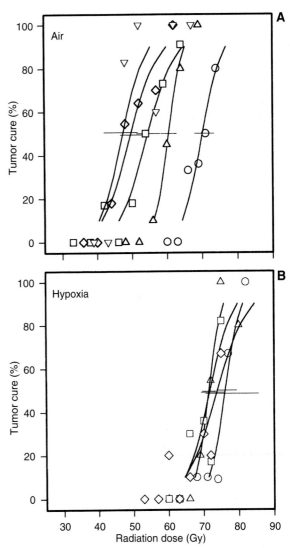

Fig. 4-8 Effect of paclitaxel on radiation dose-response curves for local control of murine MCa-4 tumors. Mice were irradiated under oxygenated (**A**) or hypoxic (**B**) conditions. Horizontal lines represent 95% confidence limits at the TCD$_{50}$ (radiation dose yielding local tumor control in 50% of the animals tested). (From Milas L, Hunter NR, Mason KA, et al. *Cancer Res* 1995;55:3564-3568.)

under hypoxic conditions. Some active metabolites can also diffuse into surrounding oxygenated regions and kill oxygenated cells. Hypoxia is associated with other metabolic alterations, including the development of low pH from the production of lactic acid through hypoxia-driven anaerobic metabolism.[32] Interestingly, the acidity is extracellular and does not seem to affect intracellular pH.[32] The acidic state of tumors can be therapeutically exploited by using drugs that selectively accumulate in acidic compartments or become activated at low pH values.[33]

Another approach to reducing the negative influence of hypoxic cells is to use drugs that selectively radiosensitize those cells.[34] Such drugs mimic the effect of oxygen in increasing radiation damage. Misonidazole and other hypoxic cell radiosensitizers are highly effective in enhancing the radioresponsiveness of tumors in rodents. Among the many clinical trials conducted to date, only a few have shown improved outcome from the combination of hypoxic-cell radiosensitizers with radiation therapy. The major limitation of these combinations in humans has been neurotoxicity, which precludes the use of effective doses of the hypoxic-cell radiosensitizers.

Cell Regeneration

In normal adult tissues, a balance is maintained between cell production and cell loss such that no net growth occurs. Radiation or chemotherapeutic drugs alter this balance by increasing cell loss; to restore the balance, the rate of cell production among the surviving cells increases. In clinical radiation therapy, which is typically given over several weeks, the cell loss that occurs after each fractional dose is counteracted by the compensatory cell regeneration (repopulation) that takes place between fractions. The extent of cell repopulation determines the tolerance of acutely responding tissues to radiation.

In malignant tumors, the balance between cell production and cell loss is shifted in favor of cell production, resulting in uncontrolled growth. In both tumors and normal tissues, radiation and other cytotoxic treatments produce massive cell loss, which in turn stimulates a compensatory regenerative response. Studies of cell regeneration in experimental tumors after single and fractionated radiation doses have shown that the rate of cell proliferation is generally higher in treated tumors than in untreated tumors, a phenomenon termed *accelerated cell proliferation*.[35-38] An example of accelerated proliferation after tumor irradiation is shown in Figure 4-9, where the rate of cell proliferation was measured by changes in TCD_{50} values. In this study, established 8-mm murine mammary carcinomas were irradiated with a single dose of 60 Gy, which allowed only a small number of tumor clonogens to survive. At different days thereafter, while

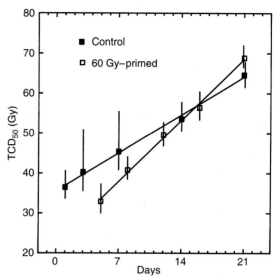

Fig. 4-9 TCD_{50} values for mouse MCa-4 tumors, with 95% confidence intervals, as a function of time after tumor cell inoculation *(open squares)* or after 8-mm established tumors had been exposed to 60 Gy *(closed squares)*. The linear increase in TCD_{50} is consistent with exponential growth, which was significantly faster in the preirradiated tumors. (From Milas L, Yamada S, Hunter N, et al. *Int J Radiat Oncol Biol Phys* 1991;21:1195-1202.)

the tumors regressed, transiently disappeared, or regrew, the tumors were irradiated again with graded doses to establish TCD_{50} values. The later doses were given under hypoxic conditions to exclude the influence of oxygen on tumor radioresponse. The TCD_{50} values of tumors, whether nonpalpable or of measurable size, that received no priming radiation dose served as controls. As shown in Figure 4-9, the slope of the TCD_{50} curve for the 60-Gy–primed tumors was significantly steeper than that for the control tumors, implying an increased rate of clonogen proliferation in the irradiated tumors. A similar accelerated repopulation was observed in murine tumors treated with cyclophosphamide.[39]

Accelerated proliferation of tumor clonogens also seems to occur during clinical radiation therapy. Withers and colleagues[40] reviewed the relationship between the probability of achieving local control of head and neck carcinoma and total radiation dose and treatment duration. In that study, the TCD_{50} increased progressively over time if the treatment period was prolonged beyond 30 days (Fig. 4-10). The increase in curative dose was greater than anticipated from estimates of pretreatment tumor volume and clonogen doubling rates. In that study, the dose increase needed to offset accelerated clonogen repopulation was about 0.6 Gy/day; however, that increase can exceed 1 Gy/day.[41]

In general, acutely responding normal tissues and tumors respond to radiation- or chemotherapy-induced

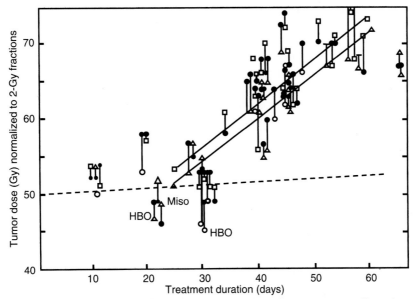

Fig. 4-10 TCD$_{50}$ as a function of overall treatment times for squamous cell carcinomas of the head and neck. Total doses were normalized to the dose equivalent of that of a regimen of 2-Gy fractions using an α/β value of 25 Gy. Doses and times are best estimates of median values. The dose and control rate reported in the literature from which the TCD$_{50}$ values were calculated are shown as closed circles to indicate the extent of the extrapolation. The rate of increase in TCD$_{50}$ was predicted from a 2-month clonogen-doubling rate *(dashed line)*. Estimated increases in TCD$_{50}$ *(solid lines)* over the radiation-treatment period are shown for T2 tumors *(open circles)*, T3 tumors *(open squares)*, and tumors of mixed T stage *(open triangles)*. *HBO,* Hyperbaric oxygen; *Miso,* misonidazole. (From Withers HR, Taylor JMG, Maciejewski B. *Acta Oncol* 1988;27:131-146.)

injury with increased clonogen production. Although accelerated cell proliferation can be beneficial in terms of sparing normal tissues, it also reduces the tumor-control efficacy of radiation. Thus any approach that reduces or eliminates accelerated clonogen proliferation in tumors would improve the efficacy of radiation therapy. This is likely one of the major mechanisms by which chemotherapeutic drugs improve local tumor control when given concurrently with radiation therapy. Even a small decrease in repopulation between radiation fractions can significantly improve tumor response to fractionated radiation. However, care must be taken to select drugs that preferentially affect rapidly proliferating cells and preferentially localize in malignant tumors. Another possibility is to supplement chemoradiation therapy with agents that have antiproliferative properties, such as those that block membrane receptors for growth factors or interfere with signaling pathways involved in cell proliferation.[42]

Increased repopulation of tumor cells may also play an important role in induction (neoadjuvant) chemotherapy. The rationale for this form of therapy is to reduce the number of clonogenic cells, improve tumor oxygenation, and eradicate tumor cells that are intrinsically resistant to radiation. According to radiobiological principles, all of these effects should improve tumor

response to radiation. Many clinical trials have been conducted in which induction chemotherapy has been combined with radiation therapy, but, in general, the results have not been greatly encouraging. Although large proportions of patients in these trials responded to chemotherapy by showing either complete or partial tumor regression, no significant improvement in treatment outcome has been achieved. Several possible explanations exist for the failure of induction chemotherapy to improve radiation therapy. One possibility is that response to chemotherapy simply predicts the response to radiation therapy. According to this reasoning, tumor cells that are sensitive or resistant to chemotherapeutic drugs are also sensitive or resistant to radiation, and therefore tumors that respond well to chemotherapy would be controlled with radiation therapy even if they had not been treated with chemotherapy. Another possibility is that chemotherapy induces or selects cell clones that are resistant to radiation; however, this explanation is not supported by the fact that most of the drugs that have been used for neoadjuvant chemotherapy do not produce cross-resistant effects with radiation. The most likely explanation seems to be that chemotherapy induces accelerated repopulation of tumor cell clonogens, an explanation for which some experimental evidence has been found.[39]

SEQUENCING OF CHEMOTHERAPY AND RADIATION THERAPY

Depending on the principal aim of chemoradiation therapy, drugs can be given before, during, or after the course of radiation therapy. According to this sequencing, chemotherapy is designated induction (neoadjuvant) chemotherapy when it is given before radiation, concurrent chemotherapy when it is given during radiation, and adjuvant chemotherapy when it is given after radiation. The goals of these three sequences are described further in the following paragraphs.

Induction Chemotherapy

Induction, or neoadjuvant, chemotherapy has two main objectives. One is to eradicate micrometastases while they contain small numbers of tumor cells. For this reason, induction chemotherapy is initiated soon after tumor diagnosis and can precede radiation therapy by weeks or months. The other objective of induction chemotherapy is to reduce the size of the primary tumor that is to be irradiated. Reducing the number of clonogenic cells in the tumor in this way increases the probability of tumor control by radiation. Also, chemotherapy-induced tumor shrinkage might allow a smaller tissue volume to be irradiated, thereby limiting normal tissue damage. The latter strategy is particularly important in treating lymphomas and tumors in children.

As discussed later in this chapter, induction chemotherapy generally has not provided the therapeutic benefits that might be expected from theoretical principles. Several reasons could account for this. One is that chemotherapy, like radiation, may accelerate the proliferation of tumor cell clonogens. Another possibility is that induction chemotherapy may select for or induce drug-resistant cells that might be cross-resistant to radiation. Development of drug resistance remains a significant problem in chemotherapy; nevertheless, evidence is still lacking to convincingly demonstrate that cells that acquire drug resistance are also resistant to radiation. Finally, chemotherapeutic drugs can, under certain conditions, increase the metastatic potential of tumor cells or damage normal tissues in such a way as to make them conducive to metastatic growth.

Concurrent Chemotherapy

In the concurrent mode of chemoradiation therapy, chemotherapeutic drugs are given during a course of radiation treatment so that the drug or drugs exert their effects during several radiation fractions. Even though drugs can act on both systemic and primary lesions, the main objective in concurrent chemotherapy is to use drug–radiation interactions to maximize tumor radioresponse. The optimal schedule for drug administration (e.g., once a week, daily, or at some other interval) depends on many factors, primarily the mechanisms of radioenhancement, the particular drug and conditions under which the enhancement is highest, and the toxicity of the treatment to normal tissue. In this type of chemoradiation therapy, therapeutic benefit occurs only when the enhancement of tumor response is greater than the toxic effects on critical normal tissues. As discussed in the following section, concurrent chemoradiotherapy has provided the best clinical results in terms of both local tumor control and patient survival.

In one mode of concurrent chemoradiation therapy, chemotherapy and radiation therapy are alternated rapidly (e.g., radiation is given one week and chemotherapy is given during the subsequent week, or vice versa), and this pattern is continued over the next few weeks. Alternating schedules such as these are given in an attempt to minimize excessive toxic effects on normal tissues (e.g., mucositis) and to enhance tumor response by exploiting some biological effect of an agent that renders tumor cells more responsive to the subsequent agent (e.g., through perturbing cell cycling or reoxygenation).

Adjuvant Chemotherapy

Adjuvant chemotherapy is given after a course of radiation therapy is completed. The primary objective of adjuvant chemotherapy is to eradicate disseminated disease, although drugs can eradicate surviving tumor cells in irradiated tumors as well.

CLINICAL APPLICATIONS OF COMBINED RADIATION THERAPY AND CHEMOTHERAPY

Laboratory investigations are providing important preclinical data regarding the interactions between combinations of cytotoxic drugs and radiation. However, sequential clinical investigations are required to establish the toxicity, effectiveness, and value of combined chemotherapy and radiation therapy for the care of human patients. The effects of drugs, given as single agents or in combination with other drugs, have usually been investigated without the addition of radiation therapy. On the other hand, for diseases in which radiation therapy is the standard of care, the addition of chemotherapy before irradiation is common, even when the value of such an addition is unknown. Separating the administration of the drug and the radiation by 2 weeks or more usually does not increase toxic reactions, and induction chemotherapy often produces some degree of response. However, the situation is quite different for concurrent chemotherapy and radiation therapy, where phase I clinical trials are needed to test either a standard dose of radiation with increasing doses of chemotherapy or a standard dose of chemotherapy with increasing doses of radiation. Once the maximum tolerated combination of chemotherapy and radiation therapy is established, then phase II trials can be used to test the efficacy of the combination in one or more diseases.

If phase II studies suggest that a particular combination is efficacious, then phase III comparative trials are required to compare the standard treatment against the new combination. Rarely, if ever, are phase II results sufficiently compelling to change practice throughout a nation or the world. Comparisons with historical control subjects are often undertaken, but known or unsuspected biases often influence the interpretation of such comparisons.

SEQUENTIAL CHEMOTHERAPY AND RADIATION THERAPY
Induction Chemotherapy

Induction chemotherapy relies heavily on the principle of spatial cooperation. For epithelial tumors, little evidence exists to suggest that the addition of chemotherapy before irradiation confers any benefit in controlling local–regional tumors; rather, the chemotherapy is directed at subclinical metastases. Only for malignant lymphomas does induction chemotherapy seem to be beneficial in terms of local tumor control. For example, for diffuse large-cell lymphomas that are less than 3.5 cm in their greatest dimension, induction chemotherapy that produces a complete response, coupled with subsequent irradiation, can lead to successful local control at a low total dose of radiation (e.g., 30 Gy). However, tumors 10 cm in diameter or larger that respond completely to induction chemotherapy nonetheless require substantially higher total doses (at least 45 Gy) than do smaller tumors.

In contrast to lymphomas, local–regional control of carcinomas is not improved by the addition of induction chemotherapy.[43,44] In fact, the response of local–regional tumors to induction chemotherapy can be misleading. Many investigators have been convinced that initial shrinkage of the tumor must eventually lead to improvements in local–regional control. However, this has not been borne out for carcinomas of the upper aerodigestive tract[44]; moreover, phase III comparative trials of induction chemotherapy for cancer of the cervix have shown survival to be better after radiation therapy alone than after induction chemotherapy followed by pelvic irradiation.[45,46]

Nonetheless, in some circumstances the use of induction chemotherapy before radiation can improve survival over that produced by radiation therapy alone. The best example of this is non–small-cell carcinoma of the lung, for which cisplatin-based induction chemotherapy has been shown to improve survival rates over those produced by radiation therapy alone in three independent studies.[47-49] Despite the fact that induction chemotherapy has not

been particularly effective in other diseases, many oncologists feel compelled to use chemotherapy before radiation. The rationales for this practice include the convenience of being able to start chemotherapy quickly rather than having to wait to plan radiation therapy, the ability to give the maximum doses of chemotherapy if no radiation therapy is to be given, and the longstanding belief that the subclinical burden is smallest at the time of diagnosis. However, induction chemotherapy does not affect local control of epithelial tumors, and in some circumstances such as carcinoma of the cervix, starting chemotherapy can delay effective local treatment and produce inferior results. Therefore induction chemotherapy should be used only when a phase III comparative trial has demonstrated a clear benefit.

The toxicity associated with combining chemotherapy and radiation therapy can be minimized by separating them in time, another feature that can make induction chemotherapy more attractive. Occasionally, induction chemotherapy can even increase the protection of normal tissues. This is true for patients with Hodgkin's disease who present with a large mediastinal mass; shrinking the mass with chemotherapy means that more lung can be protected in the course of subsequent radiation therapy.

Adjuvant Chemotherapy

With one exception, adjuvant chemotherapy (chemotherapy delivered after radiation therapy) is not particularly valuable. That exception is in the use of adjuvant hormonal therapy for prostate cancer. Disease-free and overall survival have been improved by following radiation therapy to the prostate with 2 to 3 years of androgen suppression therapy.[50,51]

Concurrent Chemotherapy and Radiation Therapy

As noted earlier in this chapter, the concurrent use of chemotherapy and radiation therapy tends to maximize the antitumor effect, even though it almost inevitably also increases the acute toxicity of the treatment. Nevertheless, concurrent chemoradiation therapy has been shown to improve survival in several types of carcinoma (see Table 4-3). In a study of carcinoma of the esophagus, cisplatin and 5-fluorouracil (5-FU) given concurrently with modest-dose irradiation (50 Gy) produced improved survival relative to high-dose radiation therapy (64 Gy) alone.[52] In another study, the use of cisplatin concurrent with radiation therapy followed by cisplatin and 5-FU improved survival over radiation therapy alone for patients with carcinoma of the nasopharynx.[53] Concurrent chemotherapy and radiation therapy also improved survival among patients with moderately advanced carcinoma of the cervix compared with radiation therapy alone.[54] Other supporting studies clearly confirmed the value of the combined treatment.[55]

Although the findings for carcinoma of the nasopharynx are compelling, the role of concurrent chemotherapy and radiation therapy for other sites in the upper aerodigestive tract is less clear. In one meta-analysis of head and neck squamous cell carcinoma,[44] an advantage was found for concurrent chemotherapy and radiation therapy but not for induction chemotherapy. In a trial comparing concurrent chemoradiation with hyperfractionated irradiation to a total dose of 75 Gy for patients with locally advanced head and neck cancer,[56] concurrent chemotherapy and radiation therapy proved superior to radiation alone in terms of local control and may have been beneficial for overall survival.

The improvement in survival produced by induction chemotherapy for unresectable non–small cell carcinoma of the lung is based entirely on control of distant metastasis. Two studies tested the hypothesis that concurrent chemoradiation would be superior to induction chemotherapy by virtue of improving control of both local disease and distant metastasis. In one such comparative study,[57] concurrent chemoradiation produced a statistically significant improvement in overall survival over that produced by induction chemotherapy. Preliminary results from the Radiation Therapy Oncology Group (RTOG) protocol 9410 also support the benefit of concurrent chemoradiation over induction chemotherapy followed by standard irradiation.[58]

The value of radiation therapy in combination with chemotherapy for small cell carcinoma of the lung is unclear; this type of cancer has been so responsive to combination chemotherapy that radiation therapy is considered by some to be unnecessary. Several trials comparing chemotherapy alone vs. chemotherapy with either concurrent or adjuvant radiation for small cell lung cancer have provided conflicting results. A meta-analysis suggested a small but statistically significant benefit to the use of radiation therapy over the use of chemotherapy alone. However, the optimal timing and sequencing of the treatments remain controversial. A study at the National Cancer Institute of Canada[59] indicated that early use of chemoradiation therapy was superior to delayed irradiation of the thorax. The best results found to date with regard to limited-stage small cell carcinoma of the lung have come from a national intergroup trial comparing accelerated fractionation to standard fractionation, both of which were given concurrently with chemotherapy; however, that study did not address the difference between induction vs. concurrent chemoradiation. To date, the only trial to have directly addressed that question indicated that the concurrent approach was superior.[60]

In contrast to the diseases described in the preceding paragraphs, carcinoma of the cervix has a relatively favorable prognosis after radiation therapy alone. The 5-year survival rate for patients with invasive cancer of the cervix (all stages combined) treated with radiation therapy is approximately 60%. As noted earlier in this chapter, induction chemotherapy not only does not improve this percentage but actually can have a deleterious effect on survival. However, a recent series of trials provided convincing evidence that concurrent chemoradiation therapy can improve on the results of radiation therapy. The RTOG protocol 9001 compared concurrent cisplatin and 5-FU with pelvic and intracavitary irradiation vs. radiation therapy alone for cervical cancer.[54] The concurrent chemoradiation strategy produced significantly better disease-free and overall survival rates and better local tumor control and freedom from distant metastasis. Other cooperative trials from the Gynecologic Oncology Group and the Southwest Oncology Group have also emphasized the importance of concurrent cisplatin in treating cervical cancer.[55]

Chemoradiation Plus Surgery

Chemotherapy and radiation have also been used in combination with surgery in attempts to produce better survival rates and organ conservation than can be obtained by surgical treatment alone. However, the results from trimodality treatments are difficult to compare and interpret by virtue of the complexities of treatment sequencing and timing, and the relative contributions of the modalities remain unclear. For example, the Gastrointestinal Tumor Study Group[61] reported that use of combined chemoradiation therapy after surgery prolonged disease-free survival time among patients with rectal carcinoma compared with those who had only surgery. In another study of rectal cancer,[62] postoperative chemotherapy delivered before, during, and after pelvic radiation therapy produced significantly better survival rates than did postoperative pelvic radiation therapy alone. The chemotherapy in that study included bolus-dose 5-FU; results from a later study indicated that protracted-infusion 5-FU produced better results than did bolus dosing.[63] However, another study by the National Surgical Adjuvant Breast and Bowel Project group found that, among patients with rectal cancer, survival after postoperative chemoradiation was no better than that after postoperative chemotherapy alone.[64] Controversies about the relative contributions of chemotherapy and radiation therapy for rectal cancer are not likely to be resolved any time soon, as new chemotherapeutic agents are tested in postoperative settings with or without pelvic irradiation and as more interest develops in preoperative administration of various combined treatments. Issues regarding the combination of radiation therapy with surgery are discussed in further detail in Chapter 3.

TABLE 4-3

Chemotherapy and Radiation Therapy for Carcinomas: Survival According to Therapy Sequence*

	Induction	Concurrent	Adjuvant
Head and neck[44]	±	+	
Nasopharynx[53]		+	
NSCLC[43,44,49,57,58]	+	+	
SCLC[44,59,68]	+	+	
Esophagus[52,66,67]	±S	+	
Stomach[69]		S+	
Rectum[62-64]		S+	
Prostate[50]			+(H)
Cervix[54,55]	−	+	
Breast[70,71]			S+

+, Increased survival compared with radiation therapy; −, decreased survival compared with radiation therapy; ±, conflicting results (increased, decreased, and no difference); *NSCLC*, non-small-cell lung cancer; *SCLC*, small-cell lung cancer; *S*, surgical adjuvant radiation and chemotherapy; *H*, hormone therapy.
*Based only on phase III comparative trials.

Combinations of surgery, chemotherapy, and radiation therapy have also been studied for potentially resectable carcinoma of the esophagus. To date, no prospective randomized trial has shown that postoperative radiation therapy produces better results than surgical resection alone for carcinoma of the esophagus. Nor has any evidence been found to suggest that preoperative irradiation or preoperative chemotherapy is beneficial in this disease.[65] However, considerable interest has been expressed with regard to induction chemotherapy given concurrently with radiation therapy followed by surgical resection. In one such study involving adenocarcinoma of the esophagus that included tumors of the gastric cardia, induction chemoradiation followed by surgery significantly improved survival rates relative to patients who underwent only surgery.[66] However, the survival rates for the surgery-only group in that trial were substantially lower than those reported in a later study.[65] A larger study of chemoradiation given before surgical resection for squamous cell carcinoma of the esophagus showed no evidence of benefit from this treatment.[67]

In summary, the sequence of combination treatment that has produced the best results seems to be concurrent chemoradiation therapy (Table 4-3),* but considerable variation is evident among disease sites and according to whether surgery was also used in the treatment.

Organ Conservation

Conservation of organ structure and function remains an important goal even when survival might not be improved by treatment. One of the earliest demonstrations of this principle was the use of radiation therapy to avoid the need for a permanent colostomy in patients with advanced anal carcinoma. Now, chemotherapy combined with radiation therapy is considered the treatment of choice for carcinoma of the anal canal.[72] A phase III comparative trial is underway to address whether mitomycin can improve outcome over the use of 5-FU and radiation for rectal cancer (RTOG protocol 8704).[73] Although some physicians prefer to use a combination of 5-FU and cisplatin with radiation therapy, the equivalence or superiority of these drugs to 5-FU and mitomycin has not yet been demonstrated.

Rectal Carcinoma

The success of chemoradiation therapy in preserving function in patients with anal carcinoma led to widespread interest in the use of preoperative chemoradiation for carcinoma of the distal rectum (lesions occurring less than 6 cm from the anal verge). Traditional treatment for such lesions involves abdominal peritoneal resection and permanent colostomy. However, for some patients preoperative chemoradiation (usually involving 5-FU, alone or in combination with other drugs) may reduce the tumor volume and peripheral extensions so that more limited surgical procedures that do not require a colostomy can be performed. No prospective studies have been done to compare chemoradiation followed by limited resection vs. limited resection alone vs. abdominoperineal resection.

Laryngeal Carcinoma

Total laryngectomy is accepted as being the single most effective treatment for laryngeal carcinoma. However, radiation therapy can be used to treat T1 and T2 lesions while allowing conservation of the larynx and hence laryngeal speech. Interest in laryngeal conservation for more advanced lesions was generated by results of a clinical trial within the U.S. Veterans Administration system.[74] In that trial, patients were randomized to receive standard laryngectomy followed by radiation therapy or to receive neoadjuvant therapy with cisplatin and 5-FU followed by radiation therapy for those who achieved a 50% or better tumor response to the chemotherapy. Survival among the first group (surgery plus radiation) was slightly (but not significantly) better than among those who had laryngectomy alone, but laryngeal function could be preserved in more than 60% of patients who underwent chemoradiation. These findings led to a large intergroup trial, coordinated by the RTOG, in which initial chemotherapy followed by radiation therapy was compared with radiation therapy alone and with a third arm in which radiation therapy was given concurrently with cisplatin. The results of this trial were not yet available when this chapter was written.

Bladder Carcinoma

Given sufficient motivation on the part of both patients and physicians, bladder conservation is possible in some cases of invasive bladder cancer through the use of chemotherapy, radiation therapy, and surgery. The most common sequence is to begin with transurethral resection of the bladder tumor, followed by two or more cycles of chemotherapy with methotrexate, cisplatin, and vinblastine, followed by pelvic irradiation with concomitant cisplatin. Careful follow-up using cystoscopy and biopsy is required, and cystectomy is reserved for persistent disease. In two studies of this approach, bladder conservation has been possible for 40% to 50% of patients with T2 to T4a carcinomas of the bladder.[75,76]

Toxicity Issues

All chemotherapeutic agents have clinically important toxic effects. An overview of the organ-specific toxicity of commonly used drugs or classes of drugs is provided in Table 4-4. Most chemotherapeutic agents are toxic to bone marrow; however, several are toxic to other organs as well, and that toxicity must be taken into account when combining chemotherapy with radiation therapy.

As noted earlier in this chapter, the sequential use of chemotherapeutic agents and radiation therapy usually does not increase toxicity. Although both modalities affect the bone marrow, the effects of radiation on bone tend to be localized unless the irradiated volume is very large. The sequential use of bleomycin and radiation therapy is an important exception, however, as the pulmonary toxicity of bleomycin can be greatly accentuated by subsequent radiation therapy. This effect is probably of greatest importance in the treatment of Hodgkin's disease.

Concurrent chemoradiation therapy is associated with much greater toxicity than is sequential use of either modality. Drugs such as doxorubicin and gemcitabine, when given at the doses usually used to treat systemic disease, profoundly increase the effects of radiation therapy. These combinations can lead to life-threatening toxic effects at total doses of radiation that are usually well tolerated. Similarly, the concurrent use of chemotherapy and irradiation can greatly increase esophageal reactions when cisplatin and etoposide are given concurrently with irradiation for carcinoma of the lung.

Two major strategies are available to enhance the effectiveness of concurrent treatment while avoiding its toxic effects. The first such strategy is to use conformal radiation therapy to specifically avoid irradiating normal tissues that have the most severe reactions. The second strategy is to use cytoprotective agents such as amifostine. These and other agents are being investigated for the degree of protection they produce during concurrent chemotherapy and radiation therapy. Newer cytoprotective drugs may become available within the next few years that may enhance the therapeutic ratio of concurrent chemotherapy and radiation therapy, which at present remains the most compelling chemoradiation strategy for achieving tumor control.

REFERENCES

1. Steel GG, Peckham MJ. Exploitable mechanisms in combined radiotherapy-chemotherapy: the concept of additivity. *Int J Radiat Oncol Biol Phys* 1979;5:85-91.
2. Yuhas JM, Storer JB. Differential chemo-protection of normal and malignant tissues. *J Natl Cancer Inst* 1969;42:331-335.
3. Milas L, Hanson WR. Eicosanoids and radiation. *Eur J Cancer* 1995;31A:1580-1585.
4. Hahn SM, Krishna MC, Samuni A, et al. Potential use of nitroxides in radiation oncology. *Cancer Res* 1994;54:2006S-2010S.

TABLE 4-4

Effects of Cytotoxic Drugs on Normal Tissues

Drugs of Classes	Bone Marrow	GI	Liver	Kidney	Lung	Heart	PNS/CNS	Gonads
Anthracycines	+++	+			+	+++		
Alkylators	+++	++		++	+	+		++
Antifolates	+++	++	+	++	+		+/+++	
Antipyrimidines	+++	+++	+	+		+	−/+	
Dacarbazine	+++							
Taxanes	+++	+				+	+++/+	
Podophyllotoxins	++	+				+		
Hydroxyurea	++	+						
Mitomycin	++			+++	++			+
Procarbazine	++							+
Vinca alkaloids	+	++					+++/+	
Cisplatin	+	+++		+++			++/+	
Bleomycin	+				+++			

GI, Gastrointestinal; *PNS*, peripheral nervous system; *CNS*, central nervous system.

+, Some reports of toxicity, usually not major; ++, major toxicity not unusual; +++, principal toxicity expected.

5. Buntzel J, Kuttner K, Frohlich D, et al. Selective cytoprotection with amifostine in concurrent radiochemotherapy for head and neck cancer. *Ann Oncol* 1998;9:505-509.

6. Hall EJ. *Radiobiology for the Radiologist.* 4th ed. Philadelphia, Pa.: J.B. Lippincott; 1993.

7. Kallman RF, ed. *Rodent Tumor Models in Experimental Cancer Therapy.* New York, NY: Pergamon Press; 1987.

8. Begg AC. Principles and practices of the tumor growth delay assay. In: Kallman RF, ed. *Rodent Tumor Models in Experimental Cancer Therapy.* New York, NY: Pergamon Press; 1987:114-121.

9. Suit HD, Sedlacek R, Thames HD Jr. Radiation dose-response assays of tumor control. In: Kallman RF, ed. *Rodent Tumor Models in Experimental Cancer Therapy.* New York, NY: Pergamon Press; 1987:138-148.

10. Mason KA, Hunter NR, Milas M, et al. Docetaxel enhances tumor radioresponse in vivo. *Clin Cancer Res* 1997;3:2431-2438.

11. Radford IR. Evidence for a general relationship between the induced level of DNA double-strand breakage and cell-killing after x-irradiation of mammalian cells. *Int J Radiat Biol* 1986;49:611-620.

12. Kinsella TJ, Dobson PP, Mitchell JB, et al. Enhancement of x-ray induced DNA damage by pretreatment with halogenated pyrimidine analogs. *Int J Radiat Oncol Biol Phys* 1987;13:733-739.

13. Wang Y, Pantelias GE, Iliakis G. Mechanism of radiosensitization by halogenated pyrimidines: the contribution of excess DNA and chromosome damage in BrdU radiosensitization may be minimal in plateau-phase cells. *Int J Radiat Biol* 1994;66:133-142.

14. Elkind MM, Sutton H. X-ray damage and recovery in mammalian cells in culture. *Nature* 1959;184:1293.

15. Little JB. Repair of potentially-lethal radiation damage in mammalian cells: enhancement by conditioned medium from stationary cultures. *Int J Radiat Biol* 1971;20:87.

16. Gregoire V, Hittelman WN. Nucleoside analogs as radiosensitizing agents. In: Cheson BD, Keating MJ, Plunkett W, eds. *Nucleoside Analogs in Cancer Therapy.* New York, NY: Marcel Dekker; 1997:315-358.

17. Gregoire V, Hittelman WN, Rosier JF, et al. Chemo-radiotherapy: radiosensitizing nucleoside analogues. *Oncology Reports* 1999; 6:949-957.

18. Lawrence TS, Chang EY, Hahn TM, et al. Radiosensitization of pancreatic cancer cells by 2′,2′difluoro-2′-deoxycytidine. *Int J Radiat Oncol Biol Phys* 1996;34:867-872.

19. Plunkett W, Huang P, Gandhi V. Metabolism and action of fludarabine phosphate. *Semin Oncol* 1990;17:3-17.

20. Plunkett W, Huang P, Xu YZ, et al. Gemcitabine: metabolism, mechanisms of actions, and self-potentiation. *Semin Oncol* 1995;22:3-10.

21. Lawrence TX, Eisbruch A, Shewach DS. Gemcitabine-mediated radiosensitization. *Semin Oncol* 1997;24:24-28.

22. Gregoire V, Hunter N, Milas L, et al. Potentiation of radiation-induced regrowth delay in murine tumore by fludarabine. *Cancer Res* 1994;54:468-474.

23. Gregoire V, Hunter NR, Brock WA, et al. Improvement in the therapeutic ratio of radiotherapy for a murine sarcoma by indomethacin plus fludarabine. *Radiat Res* 1996;146:548-553.

24. Milas L, Fujii T, Hunter N, et al. Enhancement of tumore radioresponse in vivo by gemcitabine. *Cancer Res* 1999;59:107-114.

25. Terasima T, Tolmach LJ. Variations in several responses of HeLa cells to x-irradiation during the cell cycle. *Biophys J* 1963;3:11-33.

26. Schiff PB, Fant J, Horwitz SB. Promotion of microtubule assembly in vitro by taxol. *Nature* 1979;277:665-667.

27. Tishler RB, Geard CR, Hall EJ, et al. Taxol sensitizes human astrocytoma cells to radiation. *Cancer Res* 1992;52:3495-3497.

28. Milas L, Milas MM, Mason KA. Combination of taxanes with radiation: preclinical studies. *Semin Radiat Oncol* 1999;9:12-26.

29. Gregoire V, Van NT, Brock WA, et al. The role of fludarabine-induced apoptosis and cell cycle synchronization in enhanced murine tumor radiation response in vivo. *Cancer Res* 1994;54:6201-6209.

30. Milas L, Hunter NR, Mason KA, et al. Role of reoxygenation in induction of enhancement of tumor radioresponse by paclitaxel. *Cancer Res* 1995;55:3564-3568.

31. Brown JM, Giaccia AJ. The unique physiology of solid tumors: opportunities (and problems) for cancer therapy. *Cancer Res* 1998;58:1408-1416.

32. Vaupel P, Kallinowski F, Okunieff P. Blood flow, oxygen and nutrient supply, and metabolic microenvironment of human tumors: a review. *Cancer Res* 1989;49:6449-6465.

33. Tannock IF, Rotin D. Acid pH in tumors and its potential for therapeutic exploitation. *Cancer Res* 1989;49:4373-4384.

34. Brown JM, Biaglow JE, Hall EJ, et al. Sensitizers and protectors to radiation and chemotherapeutic drugs. *Cancer Treatment Symposia* 1984;1:85-101.

35. Hermens AF, Barendsen GW. The proliferative status and clonogenic capacity of tumour cells in a transplantable rhabdomyosarcoma of the rat before and after irradiation with 800 rad of x-rays. *Cell Tissue Kinet* 1978;11:83-100.

36. Stephens TC, Steel GG. Regeneration of tumors after cytotoxic treatment. In: Meyn RE, Withers HR, eds. *Radiation Biology in Cancer Research.* New York, NY: Raven Press; 1980:385-395.

37. Trott KR. Cell repopulation and overall treatment time. *Int J Radiat Oncol Biol Phys* 1990;19:1071-1075.

38. Milas L, Yamada S, Hunter N, et al. Changes in TCD_{50} as a measure of clonogen doubling time in irradiated and unirradiated tumors. *Int J Radiat Oncol Biol Phys* 1991;21:1195-1202.

39. Milas L, Nakayama T, Hunter N, et al. Dynamics of tumor cell clonogen repopulation in a murine sarcoma treated with cyclophosphamide. *Radiother Oncol* 1994;30:247-253.

40. Withers HR, Taylor JMG, Maciejewski B. The hazard of accelerated tumor clonogen repopulation during radiotherapy. *Acta Oncol* 1988;27:131-146.

41. Taylor JMG, Withers HR, Mendenhall WM. Dose-time considerations of head and neck squamous cell carcinomas treated with irradiation. *Radiother Oncol* 1990;17:95-102.

42. Mendelsohn J, Fan Z. Epidermal growth factor receptor family and chemosensitization. *J Natl Cancer Inst* 1997;89:341-343.

43. Arriagada R, Le Chevalier T, Quiox E, et al. ASTRO Plenary: effect of chemotherapy on locally advanced non-small cell lung carcinoma: a randomized study of 353 patients. *Int J Radiat Oncol Biol Phys* 1991;20:1183-1190.

44. Pignon JP, Bourhis J, Domenge C, et al. Chemotherapy added to locoregional treatment for head and neck squamous-cell carcinoma: three meta-analyses of updated individual data. *Lancet* 2000;355:949-955.

45. Tattersall MH, Lorvidhaya V, Vootiprux V, et al. Randomized trial of epirubicin and cisplatin chemotherapy followed by pelvic radiation in locally advanced cervical cancer. *J Clin Oncol* 1995;13:444-451.

46. Souhami L, Gil RA, Allan SE, et al. A randomized trial of chemotherapy followed by pelvic radiation therapy in stage IIIB carcinoma of the cervix. *J Clin Oncol* 1991;9:970-977.

47. Dillman RO, Seagren SL, Propert KJ, et al. A randomized trial of induction chemotherapy plus high-dose radiation versus radiation alone in stage III non-small-cell lung cancer. *N Engl J Med* 1990;323:940-945.

48. Le Chevalier T, Arriagada R, Quoix E. Radiotherapy alone versus combined chemotherapy and radiotherapy in nonresectable non-small cell lung cancer: first analysis of a randomized trial in 353 patients. *J Natl Cancer Inst* 1991;83:417-423.

49. Sause WT, Scott C, Taylor S, et al. Radiation Therapy Oncology Group (RTOG) 88-08 and Eastern Cooperative Oncology Group (ECOG) 4588: preliminary results of a phase III trial in regionally advanced, unresectable non-small cell lung cancer. *J Natl Cancer Inst* 1995;87:198-205.

50. Pilepich MV, Caplan R, Byhardt RW, et al. Phase III trial of androgen suppression using goserelin in unfavorable-prognosis carcinoma of the prostate treated with definitive radiotherapy: report of Radiation Therapy Oncology Group Protocol 85-31. *J Clin Oncol* 1997;15:1013-1021.

51. Bolla M, Gonzalez D, Warde P, et al. Improved survival in patients with locally advanced prostate cancer treated with radiotherapy and goserelin. *N Engl J Med* 1997;337:295-300.

52. Herskovic A, Martz K, Al-Sarraf M, et al. Combined chemotherapy and radiotherapy compared with radiotherapy alone in patients with cancer of the esophagus. *N Engl J Med* 1992;326:1593-1598.

53. Al-Sarraf M, LeBlanc M, Giri PG, et al. Chemoradiotherapy versus radiotherapy in patients with advanced nasopharyngeal cancer: phase III randomized Intergroup study 0099. *J Clin Oncol* 1998;16:1310-1317.

54. Morris M, Eifel PJ, Lu J, et al. Pelvic radiation with concurrent chemotherapy compared with pelvic and para-aortic radiation for high-risk cervical cancer. *N Engl J Med* 1999;340:1137-1143.

55. Thomas GM. Improved treatment for cervical cancer: concurrent chemotherapy and radiotherapy. *N Engl J Med* 1999;340:1198-1200.

56. Brizel DM, Albers ME, Fisher SR, et al. Hyperfractionated irradiation with or without concurrent chemotherapy for locally advanced head and neck cancer. *N Engl J Med* 1998;338:1798-1804.

57. Furuse K, Fukuoka M, Kawahara M, et al. Phase III study of concurrent versus sequential thoracic radiotherapy in combination with mitomycin, vindesine, and cisplatin in unresectable stage III non-small-cell lung cancer. *J Clin Oncol* 1999;17:2692-2699.

58. Curran WJ, Scott C, Langer C, et al. Phase III comparison of sequential vs. concurrent chemoradiation for PTS with unresected stage III non-small cell lung cancer (NSCLC): initial report of Radiation Therapy Oncology Group (RTOG) 9410. *Proc Am Soc Clin Oncol* 2000;19:484a.

59. Murray N, Coy P, Pater JL, et al. Importance of timing for thoracic irradiation in the combined modality treatment of limited-stage small-cell lung cancer. *J Clin Oncol* 1993;11:336-344.

60. Goto K, Nishiwaki Y, Takada M, et al. Final results of a phase III study of concurrent versus sequential thoracic radiotherapy (TRT) in combination with cisplatin (P) and etoposide (E) for limited-stage small cell lung cancer (LD-SCLC): the Japan Clinical Oncology Group (JCOG) study [abstract]. *Proc Am Soc Clin Oncol* 1999;18:468a.

61. Gastrointestinal Tumor Study Group. Prolongation of the disease-free interval in surgically treated rectal carcinoma. *N Eng J Med* 1985;312:1465-1472.

62. Krook JE, Moertel CG, Gunderson LL, et al. Effective surgical adjuvant therapy for high-risk rectal carcinoma. *N Engl J Med* 1991;324:709-715.

63. O'Connell MJ, Martenson JA, Wieand HS, et al. Improving adjuvant therapy for rectal cancer by combining protracted-infusion fluorouracil with radiation therapy after curative surgery. *N Engl J Med* 1994;331:502-507.

64. Wolmark N, Wieand HS, Hyams DM, et al. Randomized trial of postoperative adjuvant chemotherapy with or without radiotherapy for carcinoma of the rectum: national surgical adjuvant breast and bowel project protocol R-02. *J Natl Cancer Inst* 2000;92:388-396.

65. Kelsen DP, Ginsberg R, Pajak TF, et al. Chemotherapy followed by surgery compared with surgery alone for localized esophageal cancer. *N Engl J Med* 1998;339:1979-1984.

66. Walsh TN, Noonan N, Hollywood D, et al. A comparison of multimodal therapy and surgery for esophageal adenocarcinoma. *N Engl J Med* 1996;335:462-467.

67. Bosset J-F, Gignou M, Triboulet J-P, et al. Chemoradiotherapy followed by surgery compared with surgery alone in squamous-cell cancer of the esophagus. *N Engl J Med* 1997;337:161-167.

68. Turrisi A, Kim K, Sause W, et al. Observations after 5 year follow-up of intergroup trial 0096: 4 cycles of cisplatin (P) etoposide (E) and concurrent 45 Gy thoracic radiotherapy (TRT) given in daily (QD) or twice-daily fractions followed by 25 Gy PCI. Survival differences and patterns of failure [abstract]. *Proc Am Soc Clin Oncol* 1998;17:457a.

69. Macdonald JS, Smalley S, Benedetti J, et al. Postoperative combined radiation and chemotherapy improves disease-free survival (DFS) and overall survival (OS) in resected adenocarcinoma of the stomach and GE junction. Results of intergroup study INT-0116 (SWOG 9008) [abstract]. *Proc Am Soc Clin Oncol* 2000;19:1a.

70. Overgaard M, Hansen PS, Overgaard J, et al. Postoperative radiotherapy in high-risk premenopausal women with breast cancer who receive adjuvant chemotherapy. *N Engl J Med* 1997;337:949-955.

71. Ragaz J, Jackson SM, Le N, et al. Adjuvant radiotherapy and chemotherapy in node positive premenopausal women with breast cancer. *N Engl J Med* 1997;337:956-962.

72. Bartelink H, Roelofsen F, Eschwege F, et al. Concomitant radiotherapy and chemotherapy is superior to radiotherapy alone in the treatment of locally advanced anal cancer: results of a phase III randomized trial of the European Organization for Research and Treatment of Cancer Radiotherapy Gastrointestinal Cooperative Groups. *J Clin Oncol* 1997;15:2040-2049.

73. Flam MS, Pajak TF, Haller D, et al. The role of mitomycin in combination with 5-fluorouracil and radiotherapy in the definitive nonsurgical treatment of epidermoid carcinoma of the anal canal: 5-year updated results of a phase III randomized study (RTOG 8704/ECOG 1289). Paper presented at: Japan/US Cancer Therapy Symposium; April, 1999; Hiroshima, Japan.

74. Spaulding MB, Fischer SG, Wolf GT. Tumor response, toxicity, and survival after neoadjuvant organ-preserving chemotherapy for advanced laryngeal carcinoma. The Department of Veterans Affairs Cooperative Laryngeal Cancer Study Group. *J Clin Oncol* 1994;12:1592-1599.

75. Kaufman DS, Shipley WU, Griffin PP, et al. Selective bladder preservation by combination treatment of invasive bladder cancer. *N Engl J Med* 1993;329:1377-1382.

76. Tester W, Caplan R, Heaney J, et al. Neoadjuvant combined modality program with selective organ preservation for invasive bladder cancer: results of Radiation Therapy Oncology Group phase II trial 8802. *J Clin Oncol* 1996;14:119-126.

PART II

Skin

CHAPTER 5

The Skin

K. Kian Ang and Richard B. Wilder

Basal and squamous cell carcinomas of the skin are the most common types of cancer in the United States, with an estimated annual incidence of about 1 million cases.[1] These carcinomas most often affect people with fair complexions, outdoor occupations, or both. Skin carcinomas may be disfiguring in certain locations but are rarely lethal. The American Cancer Society estimates that 1900 people in the United States die annually of cutaneous carcinoma.[1]

Cutaneous melanoma is largely a disease of individuals with fair complexions who have a tendency to sunburn even after relatively brief exposure to sunlight.[2,3] Approximately 53,600 cases of cutaneous melanoma will be diagnosed in the United States in 2002.[4] The incidence of malignant melanoma more than doubled between 1980 and 1990 and has continued to increase rapidly.[5] At present, 1 in 60 males and 1 in 80 females can be expected to develop malignant melanoma in their lifetime.[4] Increasing exposure to sunlight during recreational activities and additional ultraviolet (UV) radiation reaching Earth's surface are considered strong contributing factors to the epidemic. Fortunately, because of better public awareness of the disease, most new cases of melanoma are diagnosed early. Approximately 7400 people in the United States will die of cutaneous melanoma in 2002.[4]

Infrequent skin cancer includes Merkel cell carcinoma and adnexal carcinomas (sebaceous gland, eccrine, and apocrine carcinomas). Merkel cell carcinoma, also known as *primary cutaneous neuroendocrine carcinoma* or *trabecular carcinoma* of the skin, is a rare cancer originally described by Toker[6] in 1972. Sebaceous gland carcinoma accounts for fewer than 1% of all skin cancer.[7] Eccrine (sweat gland) carcinoma is rare, accounting for fewer than 0.01% of malignant epithelial neoplasms of the skin.[8] Apocrine carcinoma is equally rare. Data on the etiologic factors and epidemiology of Merkel cell and adnexal carcinomas are scarce. Likewise, information on prevention and early detection of these lesions is scanty.

ANATOMY OF THE SKIN

The skin is composed of three layers: epidermis, dermis, and subcutaneous tissue.[9] The epidermis is made up of stratified squamous epithelium that in most regions is only 0.05 to 0.15 mm thick. Cells in the basal layer of the epidermis regularly undergo mitotic division to replace epidermal cells lost from the surface. A thin basement membrane separates the epidermis from the dermis. The dermis, which is 1 to 2 mm thick, is composed of lymphatics, nerves, blood vessels, and sweat and sebaceous glands in a connective-tissue stroma. The portion of the dermis in contact with the epidermis is referred to as the *papillary layer*. The deeper portion of the dermis, which contains bundles of collagenous and elastic fibers, is called the *reticular layer*. Subcutaneous tissue lies underneath the dermis and supports the lymphatics, blood vessels, and nerves in loose connective tissue containing variable amounts of fat.

RESPONSE OF THE SKIN TO IRRADIATION

The extent of acute and chronic reactions of the skin to irradiation depends on several variables, including radiation dose and energy, number of days over which the dose is delivered, field size, and anatomic location.

Acute Reactions

Mitotic inhibition appears 30 minutes after a single dose of 4 to 5 Gy and is followed by a decrease in the proliferation of the germinal layer of the endothelium. The pathologic correlate of the erythema that begins to appear in the radiation therapy field within a few hours after irradiation is capillary dilatation and increased capillary permeability.[9] Higher-energy radiation requires a larger total dose than lower-energy radiation to produce a given degree of erythema.[10] If radiation is given in several fractions (as opposed to a single fraction), a higher total dose is required to cause erythema because of repair of injury between fractions. As the radiation therapy continues, swelling and proliferation of capillary endothelial cells appear. In the arterioles, the tunica intima and tunica media are disrupted after 2 to 3 weeks of radiation therapy. The basal cells enlarge and show nuclear pyknosis.[10] Maturing keratinocytes also show swelling, nuclear pyknosis, and cytoplasmic vacuolization. The moist desquamation phase of acute radiodermatitis begins 3 to 4 weeks after treatment begins and manifests as vascular dilatation and hyperemia, edema, and extravasation of erythrocytes and leukocytes. Approximately 4 weeks after treatment begins, small superficial blisters may form, coalesce, and rupture.

Similar acute changes are seen in the adnexal structures of the skin and are caused by death of the rapidly dividing germinal layer of the epithelium. In hair follicles, germinal epithelium dies after a single-fraction dose of 4 to 5 Gy, but hair loss does not occur until approximately 3 weeks after treatment because the hairs adhere to the follicles. The more active the hair growth, the more sensitive the hair follicles; thus hair follicles in the chin in men and the scalp in both genders are more sensitive to radiation than are hair follicles at other locations. The epithelial changes that develop in sebaceous and eccrine glands are similar to those in hair follicles, with sebaceous glands being about as sensitive as hair follicles and eccrine glands being slightly less so; these changes are responsible for the skin dryness that develops during treatment.

Epidermal necrosis and ulceration can occur as early as 2 months after the start of radiation therapy. Ulcers rarely develop when standard radiation therapy techniques are used; when soft tissue necrosis does occur, it is typically associated with trauma or infection. If irradiation produces mild necrosis of the subepidermis, the new epidermis that forms will be thinner than normal. If the necrosis is sufficient to cause disappearance of the basement membrane beneath the basal cells, the new epidermis will be highly susceptible to trauma, infection, and other stresses. With more extensive necrosis associated with greater damage to blood vessels and connective tissue, repair may be largely by secondary intention (i.e., by replacement fibrosis). When severe and deep necrosis of subepidermal supporting tissues and larger blood vessels occurs, an ulcer may take months or even years to heal.

Chronic Reactions

After radiation therapy, the decrease in the number of small blood vessels and the increase in the density and amount of fibrous tissue in irradiated regions gradually progress over time.[9] The damaged vasculature and connective tissue continue to deteriorate, partly because of the treatment and partly because of aging and other acquired insults. The irradiated epidermis remains chronically dry because of permanent damage to the sebaceous and eccrine glands. Microscopic atrophy of the epidermis occurs, with loss of epidermal rete (interpapillary) ridges and dermal papillae, a condition known as *poikiloderma*.[10] The basal layer shows few mitoses. Capillaries, venules, and lymphatic vessels are reduced in number and often show telangiectases. Telangiectases result from loss of microvascular endothelial cells and damage to the basement membrane, leading to contractions of multiple capillary

loops into a single distorted, sinusoidal channel. Total blood flow in the irradiated skin is reduced.

ETIOLOGY AND EPIDEMIOLOGY OF SKIN CANCER

The main cause of cutaneous carcinoma is exposure to sunlight.[8] Other contributory factors include exposure to chemical carcinogens (e.g., arsenic, tar, anthracene, and crude paraffin oil), chronic irritation or inflammation, and ionizing radiation. Several genetic syndromes are also associated with a higher incidence of cutaneous carcinoma. Individuals with xeroderma pigmentosum are prone to the development of basal cell and squamous cell carcinomas because of defective repair of UV light–induced deoxyribonucleic acid (DNA) damage.[11] The basal cell nevus syndrome is a genetic form of basal cell carcinoma inherited through an autosomal dominant gene.[12] People with epidermodysplasia verruciformis tend to develop squamous cell carcinomas within large verrucous plaques in the third and fourth decades of life.[13]

Like cutaneous carcinomas, cutaneous melanomas tend to develop in sun-exposed areas in fair-skinned people who burn rather than tan when outdoors.[2] Blistering sunburns during childhood increase the risk of melanoma later in life.[14] A patient with melanoma has a 3% to 5% lifetime risk of developing a second lesion, which is 900 times the risk of the general population.[15-17] A patient with multiple dysplastic nevi or the uncommon familial form of melanoma has an even higher lifetime risk (4% to 10%) of developing melanoma.[16] Individuals with occupational exposure to polyvinyl chlorides[18] or chemicals used in brewing and leather processing[19] are at increased risk for developing melanoma.

The incidence and aggressiveness of skin cancer are greatly increased in immunosuppressed individuals (e.g., organ transplant recipients and individuals with acquired immunodeficiency syndrome [AIDS]).

PREVENTION AND SCREENING

Skin cancer is an important target for preventive and screening measures because (1) most cancer is caused by exposure to UV light and (2) the impact of early detection and treatment on mortality and quality of life, particularly in melanoma, has been well documented.

A panel of the American College of Preventive Medicine recently performed a thorough review of the relevant medical literature and issued practice policy statements with regard to skin cancer prevention.[20] Recommended preventive measures include avoiding exposure to sunlight, particularly by limiting time spent outdoors between 10 AM and 3 PM, and wearing protective physical barriers such as hats and clothing. If exposure to sunlight cannot be limited because of occupational, cultural, or other factors, the use of sunscreen that either is opaque or blocks UVA and UVB is recommended. The College recommends discussing sun avoidance and sun protection measures with children and teenagers. For high-risk individuals (e.g., those with fair skin, multiple nevi, a family history of skin cancer, or a personal history of skin cancer), the College also recommends periodic screening, including 2- to 3-minute visual inspection of the entire integument, by an adequately trained physician.

CLINICAL MANIFESTATIONS, PATHOBIOLOGY, AND PATHWAYS OF SPREAD

Basal Cell Carcinoma

Clinical Presentation and Pathology

Basal cell carcinoma most commonly arises in the head and neck region, where it may present as an asymptomatic nodule, a pruritic plaque, or a bleeding sore that waxes and wanes.[21,22] Multiple synchronous lesions may be present. Approximately one third of patients treated for basal cell carcinoma develop at least one additional basal cell carcinoma.[23] Therefore careful evaluation of sun-exposed skin should be part of the follow-up examination. Each of the several subtypes of basal cell carcinoma has distinctive histologic and clinical features. The main subtypes are summarized in the following sections.

Nodulo-ulcerative subtype. Nodulo-ulcerative basal cell carcinoma, also referred to as a *rodent ulcer* because of its deeply infiltrating or burrowing nature, is the most commonly observed subtype. It begins as a papule. Central ulceration develops as the lesion grows. The margins of the lesion appear waxy and contain enlarged capillaries. Histologically, large islands of monomorphous basaloid cells, varying in size and shape, are embedded in a fibroblastic stroma in the dermis. The basaloid cells have large, oval, hyperchromatic nuclei, scant cytoplasm, and no intercellular bridges. The peripheral cell layer of the aggregate often demonstrates palisading, whereas the central cells are less organized. Depending on the number of melanocytes in the lesion, nodulo-ulcerative basal cell carcinomas may be blue, brown, or black. Consequently, they may be difficult to differentiate clinically from malignant melanomas.[24] Biopsy may be required to establish the correct diagnosis.

Superficial subtype. Superficial basal cell carcinomas present as red, scaly macules with an indistinct margin and are usually located on the trunk. They enlarge into a crusted, erythematous patch without induration and may be difficult to differentiate clinically from solar keratosis, psoriasis, squamous cell carcinoma in situ, or extramammary Paget's disease. Histologic examination shows multiple foci of neoplastic cells with peripheral palisading originating from the undersurface of the epidermis.[24]

Morphea-like subtype. Morphea-like basal cell carcinomas, also referred to as *sclerosing basal cell carcinomas*, appear as flat, indurated, ill-defined macules. The lesions generally have a smooth, shiny surface that becomes depressed as the lesions grow. Histologically, morphea-like basal cell carcinomas are characterized by the presence of small groups of narrow strands of basaloid cells embedded in a dense, fibrous connective tissue. Little peripheral palisading occurs.[24]

Infiltrative subtype. Infiltrative basal cell carcinomas have an opaque, yellowish appearance and blend subtly into the surrounding skin.[25] Histologically, the lesions are characterized by poorly circumscribed cell aggregates near the skin surface. Neoplastic cells infiltrate the reticular dermis and subcutis.

Basosquamous subtype. Basosquamous carcinomas, also known as *metatypical* or *keratotic basal cell carcinomas*, occur almost exclusively on the face and are uncommon. Histologically, they exhibit features of both basal and squamous cell carcinomas.

Terebrant subtype. Terebrant carcinomas present as small, ulcerated lesions and typically arise in the triangular region of the cheeks extending from the lower eyelids to the nasolabial folds.[26] Histologic examination usually reveals extensive infiltration of deeper structures by small nests of undifferentiated basal cells. This type of lesion may invade the orbit, nose, or maxilla, resulting in significant deformity. Therefore it should be treated at an early stage whenever possible.

Biology and Pattern of Spread

Between weeks 4 and 8 of embryologic development, anatomic regions grow together, and the covering epithelium subsequently migrates across junctional sites known as *embryologic fusion planes*. It has commonly been accepted that epithelial carcinomas spread along these embryologic fusion planes such as the nasolabial groove or the infranasal depression.[27,28] However, controversy has risen as to whether embryologic fusion planes persist in adults and influence the spread of skin tumors.[29]

The perineural space, the cleavage plane between a nerve and its sheath, provides a route of spread for skin cancer.[30] When perineural invasion is present at diagnosis,[31,32] basal cell carcinomas are often advanced and they tend to recur. Peripheral branches of the trigeminal and facial nerves are most commonly involved and provide a route for contiguous spread to the central nervous system.[33-35] In such cases, skip areas, areas where no carcinoma is identified in the pathologic specimen, may be present along the nerve between the primary tumor and the site of central nervous system involvement.[34] About two thirds of patients with cutaneous carcinoma with pathologic evidence of perineural invasion have no symptoms of this invasion.[34,36-38] Compression of a nerve may develop over a period of years, causing numbness, formication, burning, stinging, facial weakness, ptosis, or blurred or double vision.[34-37,39] Intraneural invasion is rare.[30,36,40]

The biological behavior of basal cell carcinomas varies with the histologic subtype. Nodulo-ulcerative basal cell carcinomas grow slowly over many years in people with normal immunity. They spread by peripheral and deep invasion, particularly along the perineural space, perichondrium, and periosteum. Superficial basal cell carcinomas may remain stable for a long period or enlarge gradually over a number of years. In contrast, morphealike, infiltrative, basosquamous, and terebrant carcinomas behave more aggressively.

Because the epidermis lacks lymphatics and blood vessels, basal cell carcinomas rarely spread to regional or distant sites. The overall incidence of metastasis is less than 0.01%.[41] Two thirds of metastases are detected in the regional lymphatics, and up to 20% of metastases involve the bones, lungs, or liver.[42] Metastases usually arise from large, ulcerated lesions in the head and neck region that have recurred after repeated surgeries and radiation therapy.[43]

Squamous Cell Carcinoma
Clinical Presentation and Pathology

Squamous cell carcinomas arise from malignant transformation of keratinocytes in the epidermis. This type of skin cancer most commonly develops as a result of damage from sunlight.[44] Much less frequently, it arises in an area of trauma or chronic irritation, such as a thermal burn scar (Marjolin's ulcer)[45] or a draining osteomyelitic sinus.[46]

The three main types of squamous cell carcinoma are squamous cell carcinoma in situ (Bowen's disease), superficial squamous cell carcinoma, and infiltrating squamous cell carcinoma. Pathologically, squamous cell carcinoma in situ exhibits a verrucous or papillated border. Atypical keratinocytes are confined to the epidermis. Clinically, squamous cell carcinoma in situ presents as a soft, erythematous, scaly, circumscribed patch. Superficial squamous cell carcinoma represents atypical keratinocyte proliferation confined to the upper reticular dermis, whereas infiltrating squamous cell carcinoma denotes extension into and beyond the lower reticular epidermis. Clinically, infiltrating squamous cell carcinoma presents as a firm, ulcerated mass with an elevated, nodular border.

Histologically, squamous cell carcinoma is described as well, moderately, or poorly differentiated on the basis of the magnitude of cellular polymorphism, keratinization, and mitosis. Diagnosis of the spindle cell subtype may require immunoperoxidase studies.

Biology and Pattern of Spread

Regional and distant metastases are uncommon in squamous cell carcinoma and are rare in basal cell carcinoma. At the time of diagnosis, metastatic spread is present in approximately 2% of patients with squamous cell carcinoma.[47] Factors determining the likelihood of metastasis include degree of differentiation, prior treatment, greatest dimension of the lesion, depth of invasion, and anatomic location.[48,49] Poorly differentiated or recurrent squamous cell carcinomas and those less than 3 cm in diameter, less than 4 mm thick, or arising on the lips are associated with lymph node metastases at diagnosis in approximately 10% of cases.[48,50-53] Reports conflict as to whether perineural spread by itself is associated with an increased risk of lymph node metastases.[37,54-56] Squamous cell carcinomas that arise in burn scars or osteomyelitic foci are associated with lymph node metastases at diagnosis in 10% to 30% of cases.[50]

Melanoma
Clinical Presentation and Pathology

Primary cutaneous melanoma may develop from preinvasive lesions such as lentigo maligna melanomas or dysplatic nevi, or it may arise de novo in normal skin. The four major subtypes are described in detail below.[57]

Superficial spreading melanoma. The most prevalent subtype is superficial spreading melanoma, which comprises about 70% of cases.[58,59] This subtype can occur in adults of any age and affects women more often than men. Superficial spreading melanoma often arises in a junctional nevus, where it first appears as a deeply pigmented lesion that progresses gradually to a flat, indurated macule over a period of years. Patches of amelanotic areas within the lesion are evident, apparently representing focal regression. As the lesion grows, the border may become irregular. Histologically, superficial spreading melanomas are characterized by a prominent intraepidermal proliferation of malignant melanocytes. The malignant cells resemble those of Paget's disease. Hence, this pattern is called *pagetoid melanoma*.[60] The malignant cells may be confined to the lower portion of the epidermis or may spread up into the granular cell layer of the epidermis, which is commonly hyperplastic. As the lesion enlarges, clusters of malignant cells invade the dermis and subcutaneous tissue.

Nodular melanoma. Nodular melanoma is the second most common subtype, comprising 15% to 25% of cases.[58,59] Nodular melanoma most often arises on the trunk or in the head and neck region and most often occurs in middle-aged individuals. In contrast to superficial spreading melanoma, nodular melanoma affects men more often than women. It presents as a raised or dome-shaped blue or black lesion. In general, nodular melanoma is darker than superficial spreading melanoma. About 5% of nodular melanomas have presenting symptoms of nonpigmented fleshy nodules and therefore are referred to as *amelanotic melanomas.*

Histologically, nodular melanoma appears as expanding lesions involving the papillary dermis with little or no epidermal component. Lesions are composed of epithelioid cells. Spindle cells and small epithelioid cells may also be present. Deeper invasion of the dermis and subcutaneous tissue occurs as lesions grow.

Lentigo maligna melanoma. The lentigo maligna subtype of melanoma comprises fewer than 10% of cases.[59,61] This subtype occurs mainly on the face or neck of fair-skinned women older than 50 years of age.[62] It typically presents as a relatively large (> 3 cm), flat, tan-colored (with different shades of brown) lesion that has been present for longer than 5 years. The border becomes irregular as the lesion enlarges. Histologically, lentigo maligna lesions are usually composed of spindlelike cells, which may be embedded in a connective tissue stroma with a desmoplastic pattern or may form fascicles displaying neural features and infiltrating the perineural space.[62,63]

Acral lentiginous melanoma. Acral lentiginous melanoma arises characteristically on the palms or soles or beneath the nail beds. However, some volar and plantar lesions are superficial spreading or nodular melanomas.[64-68] The relative frequency of acral lentiginous melanoma varies substantially with race. This subtype comprises only about 5% of melanomas in fair-skinned people but 35% to 60% in dark-skinned individuals.[69-71] Most acral lentiginous melanomas are brown and occur on the soles in individuals older than 60 years of age. Lesions generally evolve over a period of years and reach an average diameter of 3 cm before the diagnosis is established.[65,66] Histologically, early-stage acral lentiginous melanoma is composed of large, highly atypical, pigmented cells along the dermoepidermal junction in an area of hyperplasia. At the invasive stage, infiltrating cells may be epithelioid or spindle-shaped.[63] Infiltration may be present at diagnosis; if so, it occurs predominantly through the eccrine ducts.[60]

Biology and Pattern of Spread

Superficial spreading and lentigo maligna melanomas generally grow slowly over a period of many years (radial growth phase). Left untreated, these tumors gradually invade the dermis and subcutaneous tissue (vertical growth phase). In contrast, acral lentiginous and nodular melanomas progress more rapidly to a vertical growth phase.

As the depth of invasion increases, so does the risk of lymphatic and hematogenous spread. Therefore the maximum thickness and level of invasion of the primary lesion, as determined by histologic examination, are integral parts of staging for melanoma (see the section on "Patient Evaluation and Staging" later in this chapter). The risk of nodal spread is 25% for lesions 0.76 to 1.50 mm thick, 57% for lesions 1.51 to 4 mm thick, and 62% for lesions more than 4 mm thick. The corresponding risks for distant spread are 8%, 15%, and 72%, respectively.[72]

Merkel Cell Carcinoma
Clinical Presentation and Pathology

Merkel cell carcinoma, which is also known as *trabecular carcinoma* or *neuroendocrine carcinoma* of the skin, is a rare, aggressive neoplasm that was first described by Toker[6] in 1972. It typically presents as a firm, painless, red, pink, or blue cutaneous nodule involving the head and neck or extremities in people older than 60 years of age.[73,74] The median size of primary lesions at diagnosis is less than 2 cm, and the incidence of nodal involvement at presentation is approximately 20%.[75] The differential diagnosis includes poorly differentiated squamous cell carcinoma, melanoma, eccrine carcinoma, lymphoma, Langerhans' cell histiocytosis, and metastatic cancer, including islet cell carcinoma, medullary carcinoma of the thyroid, and small cell carcinoma of the lung.

The cell of origin is believed to be the dermal neurotactile Merkel cell, arising from the neural crest.[76] The lesion usually involves the reticular dermis and subcutaneous tissue, with minimal extension to the papillary dermis. The neoplastic cells possess cytoplasmic extensions and small, uniform, membrane-bound neurosecretory granules.[77] Several immunohistochemical markers have been identified in Merkel cell carcinoma. The neoplastic cells stain most consistently with polyclonal antisera to neuron-specific enolase and calcitonin; stains based on monoclonal antibodies bind to neurofilament and cytokeratin.[78-80]

Biology and Pattern of Spread

Merkel cell carcinoma has an aggressive course characterized by a propensity for contiguous spread and a high incidence of lymphatic and hematogenous dissemination.[74,75,81-83] The traditional treatment, wide local excision, results in local–regional recurrences in almost three quarters of patients[84]; in contrast, with surgery plus radiation therapy, the local–regional recurrence rate is only 15%.[73,75,80,85-87]

Assessment of patterns of failure in a series of 54 patients with Merkel cell carcinoma treated at The University of Texas M.D. Anderson Cancer Center revealed local and regional relapse rates of 35% and 67%, respectively.[75] Distant metastases occurred in 32 patients (59%). The median time to recurrence after surgical resection was 5 months, and 91% of relapses occurred within the first year. One patient died of uncontrolled primary disease, and 32 patients died of distant metastases. The 5-year disease-free survival rate was 11% for patients treated with surgery alone vs. 56% for patients treated with surgery and postoperative radiation therapy ($P = 0.002$).

Similarly, Meeuwissen and colleagues[87] reported that the 3-year disease-free survival rate was 0% for 38 patients treated with surgery alone vs. 68% for 34 patients treated with surgery and postoperative radiation therapy.

Adnexal Carcinomas: Sebaceous Carcinoma
Clinical Presentation and Pathology

Sebaceous carcinomas arise most commonly from the sebaceous glands of the ocular adnexa, the meibomian glands, and the glands of Zeis in the lid margin and the caruncle. Sites of origin, in decreasing frequency, are the head and neck, trunk and extremities, and external genitalia.[88-91]

Histologically, sebaceous carcinomas are composed of dermal-based lobules and cords of tumor cells with varying degrees of sebaceous differentiation and infiltration into the surrounding tissues. Differentiated cells contain foamy or vacuolated, slightly basophilic cytoplasm, whereas less differentiated cells contain more deeply basophilic cytoplasm. Clinical and pathologic features indicative of a poor prognosis include size greater than 1 cm (associated with a 5-year mortality rate of 50%), vascular and lymphatic invasion, poor sebaceous differentiation, highly infiltrative growth pattern, and carcinomatous changes in the overlying epithelium.[92]

Among the malignant neoplasms of the eyelids, sebaceous carcinomas are second only to basal cell carcinomas in frequency and second only to malignant melanomas in lethality.[92] The most common location of ocular sebaceous carcinomas is the upper eyelid; the second most common location is the lower eyelid and caruncle. Sebaceous carcinomas predominantly affect people older than 60 years of age, with a slight preponderance for women. Sebaceous carcinomas present as slowly growing, nontender, deep-seated, firm nodules. Often, they produce a chalazion or manifestations of inflammatory processes such as conjunctivitis, blepharitis, or tarsitis. Small primary tumors may be overlooked until orbital invasion or spread to preauricular or cervical nodes occurs. The differential diagnosis includes sebaceous adenoma and basal cell carcinoma with sebaceous differentiation (basosebaceous epithelioma).[93,94] Distinction between basosebaceous epithelioma and sebaceous carcinoma is important because of the difference between the two tumors in biological behavior.

Biology and Pattern of Spread

Sebaceous carcinoma behaves more aggressively than squamous cell carcinoma, with a propensity for nodal and hematogenous spread. Of 104 patients with sebaceous carcinoma registered by the Ophthalmic Pathology Branch of the Armed Forces Institute of Pathology,

23 patients (22%) experienced one local recurrence and 11 patients experienced two or more local recurrences. Twenty-three patients died of metastatic disease.[92]

Adnexal Carcinomas: Eccrine Carcinoma
Clinical Presentation and Pathology

Eccrine (sweat gland) carcinomas arise most often in the skin of the head and neck or the extremities and usually present as slow-growing, painless papules or nodules.[88] Eccrine carcinomas are usually diagnosed in people between 50 and 70 years of age.[94]

Histologically, eccrine carcinomas resemble carcinomas of the breast, bronchus, and kidney and thus may be difficult to differentiate from cutaneous metastases.[88,95] Histologic subtypes include ductal eccrine carcinoma, mucinous eccrine carcinoma, porocarcinoma, syringoid eccrine carcinoma, clear cell carcinoma, and microcystic adnexal carcinoma.[94,96-100]

Biology and Pattern of Spread

Eccrine carcinomas behave more aggressively than do basal cell and squamous cell carcinomas. In a series of 14 patients with eccrine carcinoma who underwent surgical excision with negative margins, 11 had at least one local recurrence, and five had recurrence in regional nodes or distant sites. One patient died of an uncontrolled local relapse, and four patients died of distant metastases 2 months to 10 years after diagnosis.[94]

Adnexal Carcinomas: Apocrine Carcinoma

Apocrine carcinoma arises most commonly from apocrine glands in the axilla. It can also originate from apocrine glands in the vulva or eyelids and from ceruminal glands in the external auditory canal.[101-103] Apocrine carcinoma usually presents as a reddish-purple nodule in elderly individuals. Because of the rarity of this lesion, its natural history is not well understood. Nodal and distant spread have been reported.[102a]

PATIENT EVALUATION AND STAGING

Clinical evaluation of skin cancer consists of inspection and palpation of the involved area and the regional lymph nodes. Imaging studies, such as chest radiographs, computed tomography scans, and magnetic resonance imaging scans, should be obtained when clinically indicated.

Carcinoma

The 1997 American Joint Committee on Cancer (AJCC) tumor-nodes-metastasis (TNM) staging system for carcinoma of the skin (Box 5-1) is based primarily on clinical findings.[102a]

BOX 5-1 American Joint Committee on Cancer Staging System for Carcinoma of the Skin (Excluding Eyelid, Vulva, and Penis)

PRIMARY TUMOR (T)

TX	Primary tumor cannot be assessed
T0	No evidence of primary tumor
Tis	Carcinoma in situ
T1	Tumor 2 cm or less in diameter
T2	Tumor more than 2 cm but not more than 5 cm in greatest dimension
T3	Tumor more than 5 cm in greatest dimension
T4	Tumor invades deep extradermal structures (e.g., cartilage, skeletal muscle, or bone)

REGIONAL LYMPH NODES (N)

NX	Regional lymph nodes cannot be assessed
N0	No regional lymph node metastasis
N1	Regional lymph node metastasis

DISTANT METASTASIS (M)

MX	Distant metastasis cannot be assessed
M0	No distant metastasis
M1	Distant metastasis

From Fleming I, Cooper JS, Henson DE, et al, eds. *AJCC Cancer Staging Manual*, 5th ed. Philadelphia, Pa: Lippincott Williams & Wilkins; 1997:157-161.

BOX 5-2 American Joint Committee on Cancer Staging System for Malignant Melanoma of the Skin

STAGE 0
Melanoma in situ (atypical melanocytic hyperplasia, severe melanocytic dysplasia), not an invasive malignant lesion (Clark's level I)

STAGE I
Localized ≤ 1.5 mm thick
≤ 0.75 mm thick or Clark's level II (pT1, N0, M0)
0.76-1.5 mm thick or Clark's level III (pT2, N0, M0)

STAGE II
Localized 1.5-4 mm thick or Clark's level IV (pT3, N0, M0)

STAGE III
Thick localized or nodal metastasis
> 4 mm thick, Clark's level V or satellite(s) within 2 cm of the primary tumor; no palpable nodes (pT4, N0, M0)
Nodal and/or in-transit metastasis (any pT, N1-2, M0)

STAGE IV
Distant metastasis (any pT, any N, M1)

Modified from Fleming I, Cooper JS, Henson DE, et al, eds. *AJCC Cancer Staging Manual*, 5th ed. Philadelphia, Pa: Lippincott Williams & Wilkins; 1997:163-170.
pT, Pathologic (rather than clinical) tumor stage.

Melanoma

Two surgical microstaging systems are used for melanoma: the Breslow system and the Clark method. Both of these systems are based on the recognition that, with melanomas, prognosis depends on the depth of invasion rather than the greatest dimension of the tumor.

The Breslow system classifies lesions by vertical thickness between the granular layer of the epidermis and the deepest part of the lesion as measured with an ocular micrometer. With ulcerated lesions, measurements are made from the surface of the skin to the deepest part of the primary tumor.[104]

The Clark method divides melanomas into five groups on the basis of the depth of invasion relative to normal tissue structures: level I is confined to the epidermis, level II invades the papillary dermis, level III invades the papillary-reticular dermal interface, level IV invades the reticular dermis, and level V invades the subcutaneous tissue.[58]

In 1988 the AJCC recommended a four-stage grouping based on the Breslow thickness and Clark's level of invasion, nodal involvement, and satellitosis or distant metastasis. A fifth group, stage 0, melanoma in situ, was added in 1997 (Box 5-2).[104a] When discordance is evident between thickness and level, thickness takes precedence because it is a better prognostic discriminator.[105] The AJCC stage grouping system has gained in popularity, which will facilitate comparison of treatment results.

PRIMARY THERAPY AND RESULTS
Carcinoma
Primary Tumor

The general strategy for treatment of the primary tumor is the same for basal cell and squamous cell carcinomas. A variety of treatment approaches are available, including curettage and electrodesiccation (not recommended for recurrent lesions[106]), Mohs' surgery, cryotherapy, surgical resection, and primary radiation therapy.[107,108]

A review of the literature indicates that nearly all treatment approaches result in 5-year recurrence rates of 1% to 10% for previously untreated cutaneous carcinomas.[106] The choice of treatment for individual patients is then determined on the basis of factors such as the location and size of the lesion; expected functional and cosmetic results; treatment time and cost; and patient age, occupation, and general physical condition.[109]

TABLE 5-1

Control Rates for Carcinomas of the Eyelid Treated with Radiation Therapy

| Histologic Subtype | NUMBER OF CASES TREATED | | | 5-Year Local Control Rate |
	Total	Previously Untreated	Recurrent	
Basal cell carcinoma	1062	686	376	1009 of 1062 (95%)
Squamous cell carcinoma	104	62	42	97 of 104 (92%)
TOTAL	1166	748	418	1106 of 1166 (95%)

From Fitzpatrick PJ, Thompson GA, Easterbrook WM, et al. *Int J Radiat Oncol Biol Phys* 1984;10:449-454.

Surgical modalities are preferred for most patients, particularly those with small lesions, for whom simple surgical procedures yield high cure rates. Primary radiation therapy is most often indicated for lesion s on or around the nose, lower eyelids, and ears, where radiation therapy yields better functional and cosmetic results than surgery. Similarly, primary radiation therapy is indicated for extensive lesions of the cheek, lip, or oral commissure that would require full-thickness resection.

In a series of more than 1000 patients with previously untreated and recurrent basal and squamous carcinomas of the eyelid who underwent primary radiation therapy, 5-year local control rates were more than 90% (Table 5-1).[110] The size of the primary lesion is the major determinant of local control after radiation therapy. In a series of 646 patients with carcinomas of the eyelid, pinna, nose, and lip treated with radiation, the 10-year local control rates were 98% for tumors measuring 2 cm or smaller, 79% for 2- to 5-cm lesions, and 53% (at 8 years) for carcinomas larger than 5 cm.[111] When results are adjusted for tumor size, local control rates seem to be slightly higher for basal cell carcinoma than for squamous cell carcinoma: 97% vs. 91% for lesions smaller than 1 cm and 87% vs. 76% for 1- to 5-cm lesions.[112] Recurrent basal and squamous cell carcinomas are more difficult to control than are previously untreated lesions.[85,107,113,114]

In general, radiation therapy is not recommended for patients younger than 50 years of age because the late effects after radiation therapy increase over time, as does the risk of a second cancer developing within the radiation portal.[115,116]

Postoperative radiation therapy may be beneficial in several clinical situations, including positive surgical margins, perineural spread, invasion of bone or cartilage, extensive skeletal muscle infiltration, a positive node measuring more than 3 cm in greatest dimension, extranodal spread, and multiple positive nodes.

Series published in the 1950s and 1960s reporting the use of orthovoltage x-rays and large daily doses of radiation[117-119] suggested that radiation therapy for carcinomas involving bone or cartilage resulted in an excessive risk of osteoradionecrosis or radiochondritis. However, data from more recent series using more fractionated, higher-energy radiation indicate that radiation therapy may in fact be the treatment of choice in selected patients with bone or cartilage involvement because the risk of complications is low with proper technique.[120,121]

Regional Nodes

Elective nodal treatment is not indicated for cutaneous basal cell carcinomas because of the low incidence of lymphatic spread. However, elective nodal treatment is indicated for large, infiltrative, ulcerative squamous cell carcinomas or recurrent squamous cell carcinomas.[122]

The choice of treatment for patients who present with nodal disease depends on the type of therapy selected for the primary lesion and the size of the involved lymph nodes. In general, single-modality therapy (surgery or radiation therapy) is sufficient for nodal disease up to 3 cm without evidence of extracapsular spread.[122]

Taylor and colleagues[123] reported on 37 patients treated with surgery and postoperative radiation therapy for lymph node metastases to the parotid region from cutaneous carcinomas. The overall regional control rate was 89%. All four recurrences occurred in patients with positive surgical margins and clinical evidence of facial nerve involvement. Epstein and colleagues[47] reported a 5-year survival rate of 25% in patients with preauricular metastases treated with surgery and postoperative radiation therapy.

Melanoma

For patients with localized cutaneous melanoma (stage I or II), wide local excision of the primary tumor is the standard treatment. For patients with known lymph node metastases at presentation (stage III), wide local excision plus therapeutic lymph node dissection is the accepted surgical approach.

Primary Tumor

The standard treatment for localized cutaneous melanoma (stages I and II) is wide local excision. Pathologic examination of the specimen is essential for establishment of a tissue diagnosis, assessment of the margins, and microstaging. The currently recommended skin margins are 1 cm for invasive lesions less than 1 mm thick and for lentigo maligna melanomas and 2 to 3 cm for melanomas at least 1 mm thick.

Melanoma thickness is the most powerful determinant of local control after wide local excision. In a large, multi-institutional trial, long-term local recurrence rates were 2.3% for melanomas 1 to 2 mm thick, 4.2% for melanomas 2 to 3 mm thick, and 11.7% for melanomas 3 to 4 mm thick.[124] Local recurrence is a poor prognostic sign; most patients with local recurrence ultimately die of their disease.

Several prognostic factors are independent of tumor thickness and level of invasion.[105] These are, in decreasing order of importance, the presence of ulceration (associated with a lower survival rate), location of the primary tumor (patients with extremity melanomas fare better than those with trunk and head and neck primary tumors), sex (women have a higher survival rate than men), and age (younger patients fare better than older patients). A complex interrelationship exists between primary tumor thickness, ulceration, and primary tumor location. Men have a higher proportion of thick, ulcerated lesions that are located on the trunk or in the head and neck region. Independent prognostic variables in patients with stage III disease are the number of involved nodes (the fewer the better), primary tumor location, and ulceration.

Radiation therapy is rarely indicated as the definitive treatment for primary malignant melanomas, except in the case of large facial lentigo maligna melanomas, wide local excision of which might necessitate extensive reconstruction. In a series of patients with lentigo maligna melanomas treated with primary radiation therapy at the Princess Margaret Hospital and followed for a period of 6 months to 8 years (median, 2 years), local control was achieved in 23 (92%) of 25 patients.[125] The median time to complete regression of lesions was 8 months, although some lesions took 2 years to disappear. Radiation therapy was delivered with orthovoltage x-rays (100 to 250 keV) and consisted of 35 Gy in 5 fractions over 1 week for lesions smaller than 3 cm, 45 Gy in 10 fractions over 2 weeks for lesions measuring 3 to 4.9 cm, and 50 Gy in 15 to 20 fractions over 3 to 4 weeks for lesions measuring 5.0 cm or more.

Regional Nodes

Elective lymph node dissection. The role of elective lymph node dissection (ELND) in malignant melanoma has long been disputed. Results of a prospective, nonrandomized study at the Sydney Melanoma Unit involving 1319 patients suggested that ELND improves the survival of patients with intermediate-thickness (0.76 to 4 mm) melanomas.[126] However, a prospective phase III trial conducted by the World Health Organization (WHO) Melanoma Program in which 553 patients with stage I disease were randomly assigned to receive wide local excision and ELND or wide local excision and delayed therapeutic lymphadenectomy (i.e., lymph node dissection only if regional nodes became clinically detectable) showed no difference in the survival rate between the two groups.[127] It should be noted that these two studies did not enroll entirely similar patient populations. The Sydney Melanoma Unit trial included melanomas at all anatomic sites, whereas the WHO study was only open to patients with melanomas of the distal two thirds of the extremities.

Two multicenter trials, one sponsored by the National Cancer Institute of the United States (Intergroup Melanoma Surgical Program)[128] and the other sponsored by the WHO Melanoma Program,[129] were launched in an effort to resolve the controversy. The Intergroup Melanoma Surgical Trial, results of which were published in 1996, included 740 patients with clinically localized melanomas 1 to 4 mm thick. No significant difference in 5-year overall survival was evident between patients assigned to ELND and those assigned to observation (86% vs. 82%, $P = 0.25$). However, significant differences in 5-year survival rates were observed among patients 60 years of age or younger (88% vs. 81%, $P = 0.04$), particularly when they had nonulcerative melanomas (95% vs. 84%, $P = 0.01$) or had melanomas 1 to 2 mm thick (97% vs. 87%, $P = 0.005$). The WHO Melanoma Program trial, results of which were published in 1998, included 240 eligible patients with truncal melanomas at least 1.5 mm thick who had no clinical evidence of regional or distant metastases. Multivariate analysis revealed that routine use of immediate ELND had no effect on 5-year overall survival (hazard ratio, 0.72; 95% confidence interval, 0.5–1.02). The sample size did not allow for subgroup analysis.

Morton and colleagues[130] have developed a minimally invasive intraoperative lymphatic mapping technique that allows for identification of the "sentinel" node, defined as the first node in the regional nodal basin into which the primary tumor drains. With this procedure, patients with clinically occult nodal disease can be identified who may benefit from lymph node dissection.[131] Until the results of the ongoing international randomized study assessing the efficacy of selective lymphadenectomy are available,[132] ELND will remain controversial.

Therapeutic lymph node dissection. Therapeutic nodal dissection along with wide local excision is the accepted surgical approach for patients with known nodal metastases.[133] However, surgery alone does not control local–regional disease in many cases. Data from the M.D. Anderson Cancer Center and the Sydney Melanoma Unit indicate that 34% to 50% of patients presenting with palpable lymphadenopathy (stage III disease) have a regional relapse after therapeutic nodal dissection.[86,134] Although most of these patients die as a consequence of distant spread, which usually manifests less than 2 years after treatment,[135] local–regional relapses are significant because they are often refractory to therapy and can cause substantial morbidity because of pain, infection, and disfigurement. Local–regional relapse from cutaneous melanoma of the head and neck can be particularly distressing because of compression of vital organs. Therefore prevention of local–regional failure is desirable from a quality-of-life standpoint even though overall survival may not be significantly improved.

Radiation Therapy

Investigators at the M.D. Anderson Cancer Center have studied the role of elective, postoperative radiation therapy in the treatment of various subgroups of melanoma patients at high risk for local–regional recurrence. Between 1983 and 1992, 174 patients (132 men and 42 women) with head and neck melanomas were enrolled in a phase II study.[136] Three groups of patients were eligible: (1) patients with primary tumors of at least 1.5 mm thick or classified as Clark's level IV disease without palpable lymphadenopathy (i.e., AJCC stage II and IIIA) who underwent wide local excision; (2) patients with primary tumors of any size and palpable regional lymphadenopathy (stage IIIB) who underwent wide local excision and limited neck dissection; and (3) patients who had primary lesions excised and underwent a neck dissection for nodal relapse without evidence of distant metastases. Each of these three subgroups of patients had a projected local–regional recurrence rate of 35% to 50%. Patients received postoperative radiation therapy consisting of 6 Gy per fraction twice a week to a total dose of 30 Gy.

Tolerance of adjuvant radiation therapy was excellent. The most commonly observed acute reaction was transient parotid swelling, which usually lasted for about a day, mainly after the first radiation fraction was delivered. Moist skin desquamation and confluent mucositis of short duration were observed in fewer than 5% of patients. Late radiation complications were observed in only three patients. The complications were neck fibrosis, mild ipsilateral hearing impairment, and transient cartilage exposure.

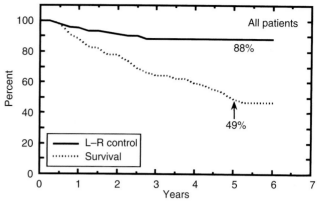

Fig. 5-1 Actuarial local–regional (L–R) control and survival rates for patients with high-risk melanoma treated with adjuvant radiation therapy. (Modified from Ang KK, Peters LJ, Weber RS, et al. Int J Radiat Oncol Biol Phys 1994;30:795-798.)

At a median follow-up time of 35 months (range 3 to 112 months), 111 of 174 patients were alive. Patterns of failure for the whole population and the patient subgroups are shown in Table 5-2. Figure 5-1 shows the corresponding actuarial local–regional control and survival rates. This study established the safety of the hypofractionated radiation regimen as adjuvant therapy for melanoma. The local–regional control rate obtained in selected high-risk patients treated with postoperative radiation therapy is encouraging. The Eastern Cooperative Oncology Group activated a randomized trial testing the efficacy of such adjuvant radiation therapy in combination with interferon (see the following section on "Systemic Adjuvant Therapy") for patients with nodal metastases and extracapsular spread.

Systemic Adjuvant Therapy

Because distant metastasis is the main pattern of relapse in melanoma, numerous attempts have been made to develop effective systemic therapy for this disease. However, none of the regimens tested has been found to improve overall survival in a phase III setting with the exception of interferon-alpha (IFN-α). An

---

TABLE 5-2

Patterns of Recurrence by Patient Group

Group	No. of Patients	NED	Dermal	Nodal	Dermal and Nodal	Dermal and DM	Nodal and DM	Dermal, Nodal, and DM	DM Only
					TYPE OF RECURRENCE				
Group 1	79	51	2	2	1	—	2	—	21
Group 2	32	17	—	—	—	2	—	—	13
Group 3	63	33	1	—	—	2	1	2	24
TOTAL	174	101	3	2	1	4	3	2	58

NED, No evidence of disease; *DM*, distant metastasis.

Eastern Cooperative Oncology Group trial enrolled 280 patients with the following disease characteristics: primary melanoma more than 4 mm thick without palpable nodes, metastasis detected at ELND, primary melanoma of any stage with clinically palpable regional lymph nodes, or nodal recurrence at any interval after surgery for primary melanoma of any depth.[137] Patients received IFN-α2b intravenously five times a week for 4 weeks and then subcutaneously three times a week for 48 weeks. This treatment significantly increased 5-year actuarial relapse-free survival rates (37% vs. 26%, $P = 0.0023$) and 5-year actuarial overall survival rates (46% vs. 37%, $P = 0.024$). The overall benefit of treatment in this trial correlated with tumor burden and the presence of palpable regional lymph node metastases. The benefit of therapy with IFN-α2b was greatest among patients with either palpable nodal metastases at presentation or nodal recurrence.

A French multi-institutional trial accrued 489 eligible patients with no palpable lymph nodes and no evidence of distant metastasis who underwent wide local excision of melanomas more than 1.5 mm thick.[138] This phase III trial showed that patients treated with subcutaneous IFN-α2a three times per week for 18 months had a significantly longer relapse-free interval than that of patients in the control group ($P = 0.035$). The hazard ratio of relapse in treated patients was 0.75 (0.57 to 0.98), and the 5-year relapse rate was 43% in the IFN-α group vs. 51% in the group that did not receive IFN. There was a trend toward improved overall survival in IFN-α2a–treated patients compared with the control group ($P = 0.059$). IFN-α2a remains the only Food and Drug Administration–approved systemic therapy for patients with high-risk disease.[139]

Cisplatin-based chemotherapy has resulted in 12% to 30% response rates in randomized trials with no improvement in the overall survival of patients with metastatic melanoma.[140] Numerous phase II trials have combined tamoxifen with different chemotherapeutic agents. Because results have been conflicting, the benefit of tamoxifen remains unclear.[140]

A large number of melanoma vaccines are in development or clinical testing.[141] Autologous and allogeneic tumor cell vaccines yielded interesting results in initial studies. However, subsequent randomized trials (e.g., trials of vaccinia melanoma oncolysate vaccine) did not show improved survival. Progress in immunology and molecular biology has led to a newer generation of vaccines that are currently undergoing clinical testing (e.g., GM_2 ganglioside keyhole limpet hemocyanin (KLH) conjugate vaccine).

Merkel Cell Carcinoma

The initial treatment for Merkel cell carcinoma is usually surgery to establish a tissue diagnosis. The role of radiation therapy in the management of Merkel cell carcinoma has been evaluated since the early 1980s because of the poor local–regional control rates obtained with surgery alone. Several studies have demonstrated the radiosensitivity of Merkel cell carcinoma.[73,75,80,86,142] Pacella and colleagues[80] reported that local control was achieved in 35 of 36 fields irradiated in 19 patients (gross disease was present in 23 of the fields). Similarly, in-field control was obtained in 30 of 31 patients treated in a series at the M.D. Anderson Cancer Center.[75] However, marginal recurrences developed in three patients.[75] This finding indicates that the target volume should include a wide margin around gross disease.

Between 1982 and 1987, as the natural history of Merkel cell carcinoma became more apparent, elective postoperative local–regional radiation therapy was given to five of six patients referred to the M.D. Anderson Cancer Center after local excision.[75] The primary tumor bed and draining lymphatics were irradiated with an electron beam to cumulative doses of 50 to 55 Gy and 45 to 55 Gy, respectively, using daily 2- to 2.5-Gy fractions. At a minimum follow-up time of 3 years, none of these patients had experienced a local or regional recurrence. Although patient numbers in this study were small because of the rarity of Merkel cell carcinoma, many retrospective series support the use of surgery and postoperative radiation therapy for previously untreated or recurrent primary tumors.* The available data are insufficient to permit detailed dose-response analysis. However, it appears that in-field recurrence is rare after a total dose of 50 Gy to microscopic disease using daily 2- to 2.5-Gy fractions.[75]

Data on the responsiveness of Merkel cell carcinoma to cytotoxic agents are emerging.[144-146] So far, the most active drugs are doxorubicin, cyclophosphamide, and vincristine. Responses of metastatic deposits to multiagent chemotherapy can be dramatic, but, unfortunately, such responses are often of short duration.[146,147]

The treatment policy for localized Merkel cell carcinoma at the M.D. Anderson Cancer Center can be summarized as follows. For patients presenting with no evidence of regional or distant metastases, surgical excision of the primary tumor followed by elective irradiation of the surgical bed with generous margins and the draining lymphatics is recommended.[107] The excision margin need not be wide, and ELND is not done because of the routine administration of postoperative radiation therapy. Given the radiosensitivity of Merkel cell carcinoma,[75,80,85] patients who, for medical reasons, cannot undergo surgery are treated with primary radiation therapy to higher doses. For gross, unresected disease, 56 to 66 Gy is recommended.[75] For patients presenting with regional lymph node metastases, the

---

*References 55, 73, 75, 80, 85, 86, 143.

current practice is local excision of the primary tumor, therapeutic nodal dissection, and postoperative irradiation of the surgical bed, including the draining lymphatics. Patients with large primary tumors or adenopathy are also considered for investigational chemotherapy.

Adnexal Carcinomas

The standard treatment for sebaceous carcinoma is wide local excision and therapeutic nodal dissection if lymphadenopathy is present. The role of adjuvant therapeutic modalities has not been explored systematically. As is the case for other types of skin cancer, indications for postoperative irradiation include positive surgical margins, perineural spread, invasion of bone or cartilage, extensive skeletal muscle infiltration, a positive node measuring more than 3 cm in greatest dimension, extranodal spread, and multiple positive nodes.

For eccrine and apocrine carcinomas, wide excision of the primary lesion is accepted as the standard treatment in patients with no lymphadenopathy at diagnosis. Postoperative radiation therapy to the surgical bed with 2- to 3-cm margins is indicated, particularly for eccrine carcinoma, because of the high incidence of local recurrence after surgery alone. The role of elective treatment of regional lymphatics is controversial. Treatment for patients with palpable lymphadenopathy consists of wide local excision, lymph node dissection, and postoperative irradiation of the surgical bed.

TREATMENT OF ADVANCED DISEASE AND PALLIATIVE THERAPY

Radiation therapy administered to total doses of 60 to 70 Gy (depending on tumor size, location, and anticipated toxicity) can result in local control in some patients with advanced skin carcinomas. Lee and colleagues[148] reported a 5-year local control rate of 67% in 33 patients with previously untreated T4 skin carcinomas who underwent radiation therapy to doses of 60 to 75 Gy over 6 to 8 weeks. Bone invasion or perineural spread reduced the likelihood of local control in this small series of patients.

Radiation can reduce symptoms for most patients with locally advanced inoperable or metastatic skin cancer. The recommended dose-fractionation schedules depend on the tumor location and the patient's life expectancy. The most commonly used regimens are 30 Gy in 10 fractions over 2 weeks, 45 to 50 Gy in 18 to 25 fractions over 4 to 5 weeks, and 36 Gy in 6 fractions over 3 weeks. The last regimen is used for the treatment of melanoma. In patients with one or two brain metastases, particularly from melanoma, and good performance status with stable extracranial disease, stereotactic radiosurgery (15 to 20 Gy in a single fraction) is delivered to treat the brain metastases.[149]

RADIATION THERAPY

The general principles of radiation therapy for skin cancer are discussed in this section. The technical details of radiation treatment for skin cancer are described elsewhere.[150]

Carcinoma

In radiation therapy for skin carcinoma, the target volume is determined mainly by the size of the lesion and the type of growth. Infiltrative lesions and those with ill-defined borders (e.g., morphea-like carcinomas) require more generous margins. Orthovoltage x-rays or an electron beam is generally used. With the electron beam, the field size at the skin surface is 0.5 cm larger because of constriction of the isodose lines in the depth.[107] Typically, the portal is designed to encompass the visible or palpable tumor, along with 0.5 to 1 cm of surrounding normal-appearing skin in the case of carcinomas smaller than 1 cm and up to 2 cm of normal-appearing skin for larger or ill-defined carcinomas.[122] The field size may be reduced after the delivery of a dose sufficient to sterilize microscopic disease. Margins may be smaller when areas close to the eye are treated.

In occasional patients (almost exclusively those with squamous cell carcinoma who present with either small [≤3 cm] involved lymph nodes or advanced primary tumors) the initial field is designed to encompass the primary tumor and regional lymphatics. The target volume is subsequently reduced to cover the areas of gross disease with adequate margins.

Perineural invasion typically extends 1 to 2 cm along the nerve sheath[151] but may rarely extend up to 14 cm.[36] Consequently, in the presence of major nerve invasion, the target volume should encompass the involved nerve to the skull base.[55,56,152,153] In patients undergoing postoperative irradiation for pathologically proven perineural invasion or lymph node involvement, the initial target volume includes the primary tumor bed plus the potential route of perineural spread or the regional lymphatics. The target volume is then reduced to include the primary tumor and nodal beds.

Several fractionation schedules have been used to treat skin carcinomas. In general, the more protracted schedules produce the best cosmetic results.[154,155] The recommended radiation regimen for individual patients depends on the size and location of the carcinoma. For most skin cancer, 40 Gy in 10 fractions, 45 Gy in 15 fractions, or 50 Gy in 20 fractions are appropriate and effective regimens.[155] If the patient is elderly and in generally poor health, 32 Gy in four fractions or a single dose of 20 Gy may be used. For large lesions close to the eye, however, 60 to 70 Gy in 30 to 35 fractions is recommended.[155] Patients with positive nodes usually receive 2-Gy fractions because of the large irradiated volume. Similarly, postoperative radiation therapy is delivered using 2-Gy fractions.

The dose for orthovoltage x-rays is prescribed to D_{max}, whereas the dose for electrons is prescribed to the 90% isodose line to take into account the difference in relative biological effectiveness between the beams.[156,157]

Melanoma

The target volume for patients with stage I to III melanoma includes the tumor or surgical bed with margins of at least 2 cm and the ipsilateral neck nodes down to the clavicle. The target volume for patients with nodal recurrence includes the ipsilateral neck nodes. The primary tumor bed is also irradiated if regional relapse occurs less than 1 year after excision of the primary tumor.

Elective adjuvant radiation therapy is administered in 6-Gy fractions prescribed to D_{max} twice a week to a total dose of 30 Gy. If microscopic residual disease is present, an additional fraction may be given through a smaller portal, for a cumulative dose of 36 Gy. Care is taken to ensure that the dose to the spinal cord does not exceed 24 Gy in four fractions over 2 weeks.

Merkel Cell and Adnexal Carcinoma

In radiation therapy for Merkel cell carcinoma, the target volume consists of the primary tumor bed with 4- to 5-cm margins except when the lesion is situated at or close to critical structures (e.g., the optic apparatus). In the case of Merkel cell carcinoma of the head and neck region, the whole ipsilateral neck is irradiated. In radiation therapy for adnexal carcinomas, the target volume consists of the primary tumor bed with 2- to 3-cm margins and the draining lymphatics.

Radiation is administered, preferably with electrons, in 2-Gy daily fractions. For Merkel cell carcinoma, a dose of 46 to 50 Gy is delivered to the region of elective radiation, followed by a boost consisting of 10 Gy in five fractions to the gross disease. At the M.D. Anderson Cancer Center, a cumulative dose of 66 Gy is given in the case of bulky primary tumors. For adnexal carcinomas, a dose of 60 Gy is generally administered in the postoperative setting.

Patient Care During and After Radiation Therapy

A tumoricidal dose of radiation generally produces moist desquamation. The skin reaction usually reaches a peak 3 to 6 weeks after the start of radiation therapy and resolves spontaneously within 6 weeks. Irradiated skin should be protected from heat, cold, sunlight, friction, and other sources of irritation to avoid additional tissue injury. Patients are instructed to use sun blocks with a sun protection factor of at least 15 over the irradiated area and, in the case of facial lesions, to wear a hat when outdoors after the completion of treatment. Once moist desquamation occurs, the area should be cleaned with aluminum subacetate (Domeboro) soaks or 1% hydrogen peroxide to prevent secondary infection.

Patients should also be informed about the specific acute and late side effects of treatment such as mucositis of the nasal passages and lips, nasal dryness, synechiae (when nostril lesions are treated), conjunctivitis, and loss of eyelashes (when eyelid cancer is treated). When the lacrimal canaliculi are treated, irrigation of the ducts during the healing phase after treatment helps prevent synechiae.

Late side effects include hypopigmentation, hyperpigmentation, telangiectasia, and skin atrophy, which may develop gradually over a period of years. Hair loss and loss of sweat gland function are usually permanent. Irradiated skin is more sensitive to trauma. Blood flow in the irradiated tissues may decrease. As a result, healing may be delayed after surgery on an irradiated region. Skin retraction at the lower eyelid may result in ectropion. Fibrosis of the lacrimal duct may result in epiphora. These side effects are rarely serious after properly administered radiation therapy. Cataracts can occur after irradiation of lower-eyelid lesions, but when appropriate shielding is used, this side effect is uncommon.

The long-term cosmetic results after radiation therapy depend on the fraction size, total dose, and volume of tissue irradiated. When the previously described techniques are used, the risk of soft tissue necrosis is less than 3% and the risk of osteoradionecrosis is approximately 1%. Radiochondritis is rare and is usually a sign of recurrent disease.[158]

Regular follow-up examinations include evaluation of the treated area for late complications, and because one third of treated patients will develop metachronous skin cancer, inspection for new lesions is also included.

REFERENCES

1. American Cancer Society. *Cancer Facts & Figures-2001*. Atlanta, Ga: American Cancer Society; 2001.
2. Beral V, Evans S, Shaw H, et al. Cutaneous factors related to the risk of malignant melanoma. *Br J Dermatol* 1983;109:165-172.
3. Gellin GA, Kopf AW, Garfinkel L. Malignant melanoma. A controlled study of possibly associated factors. *Arch Dermatol* 1969;99:43-48.
4. Jemal A, Thomas A, Murray T, et al. Cancer statistics, 2002. *CA Cancer J Clin* 2002;52:23-47.
5. Rigel DS, Kopf AW, Friedman RJ. The rate of malignant melanoma in the United States: are we making an impact? *J Am Acad Dermatol* 1987;17:1050-1053.
6. Toker C. Trabecular carcinoma of the skin. *Arch Dermatol* 1972;105:107-110.
7. Urban FH, Winkelmann RK. Sebaceous malignancy. *Arch Dermatol* 1961;84:63-72.
8. Tulenko JF, Conway H. An analysis of sweat gland tumors. *Surg Gynecol Obstet* 1965;121:343-348.

9. Rubin P, Casarett G. *Clinical Radiation Pathology*. Philadelphia, Pa: WB Saunders; 1968.

10. Fajardo LG, Berthrong M, Anderson RE. Skin. In: *Radiation Pathology*. New York, NY: Oxford University Press; 2001: 411-420.

11. Cleaver JE. Defective repair replication of DNA in xeroderma pigmentosum. *Nature* 1968;218:652-656.

12. Anderson DE, Taylor WB, Falls HF, et al. The nevoid basal cell carcinoma syndrome. *Am J Hum Genet* 1967;19:12-22.

13. Lutzner MA. Epidermodysplasia verruciformis: an autosomal recessive disease characterized by viral warts and skin cancer. A model for viral oncogenesis. *Bull Cancer* 1978;65:169-182.

14. Lew RA, Sober AJ, Cook N, et al. Sun exposure habits in patients with cutaneous melanoma: a case control study. *J Dermatol Surg Oncol* 1983;9:981-986.

15. Scheibner A, Milton GW, McCarthy WH, et al. Multiple primary melanoma—a review of 90 cases. *Australas J Dermatol* 1982;23:1-8.

16. Bellet RE, Vaisman I, Mastrangelo MJ, et al. Multiple primary malignancies in patients with cutaneous melanoma. *Cancer* 1977;40:1974-1981.

17. Veronesi U, Cascinelli N, Bufalino R. Evaluation of the risk of multiple primaries in malignant cutaneous melanoma. *Tumori* 1976;62:127-130.

18. Lundberg I, Gustavasson A, Holmberg B, et al. Mortality and cancer incidence among PVC-processing workers in Sweden. *Am J Ind Med* 1993;23:313-319.

19. Linat MS, Malker HS, Chow WH, et al. Occupational risks for cutaneous melanoma among men in Sweden. *J Occup Environ Med* 1995;37:1127-1135.

20. Hill L, Ferrini RL. Skin cancer prevention and screening: summary of the American College of Preventive Medicine's practice policy statements. *CA Cancer J Clin* 1998;48:232-235.

21. Kopf AW. Computer analysis of 3531 basal cell carcinomas of the skin. *J Dermatol* 1979;6:267-281.

22. Rahbari H, Mehregan AH. Basal cell epitheliomas in usual and unusual sites. *J Cutan Pathol* 1979;6:425-431.

23. Robinson JK. Risk of developing another basal cell carcinoma: a 5-year prospective study. *Cancer* 1987;60:118-120.

24. Patterson JAK, Geronemus RG. Cancers of the skin. In: DeVita VT, Hellman S, Rosenberg SA, eds. *Cancer: Principles and Practice of Oncology*, 3rd ed. Philadelphia, Pa: JB Lippincott; 1989: 1469-1498.

25. Siegle RJ, MacMillan J, Pollack S. Infiltrative basal cell carcinoma: a nonsclerosing subtype. *J Dermatol Surg Oncol* 1986;12:830-836.

26. Battle RJV, Patterson TJS. The surgical treatment of basal-celled carcinoma. *Br J Plast Surg* 1960;13:118-135.

27. Mohs FE, Lathrop TG. Modes of spread of cancer of the skin. *Arch Dermatol Syphilol* 1952;66:427-439.

28. Panje WR, Ceilley RI. The influence of embryology of the midface on the spread of epithelial malignancies. *Laryngoscope* 1979;89:1914-1920.

29. Wentzell JM, Robinson JK. Embryologic fusion planes and the spread of cutaneous carcinoma: a review and reassessment. *J Dermatol Surg Oncol* 1990;16:1000-1006.

30. Dodd GD, Dolan PA, Ballantyne AJ, et al. The dissemination of tumors of the head and neck via the cranial nerves. *Radiol Clin North Am* 1970;8:445-461.

31. von Domarus H, Stevens PJ. Metastatic basal cell carcinoma: report of five cases and review of 170 cases in the literature. *J Am Acad Dermatol* 1984;10:1043-1060.

32. Binkley GW, Rauschkolb RR. Basal-cell epithelioma metastasizing to lymph nodes. *Arch Dermatol* 1962;86:332-342.

33. Carlson KC, Roenigk RK. Know your anatomy: perineural involvement of basal and squamous cell carcinoma on the face. *J Dermatol Surg Oncol* 1990;16:827-833.

34. Hanke CW, Wolf RL, Hochman SA, et al. Chemosurgical reports: perineural spread of basal-cell carcinoma. *J Dermatol Surg Oncol* 1983;9:742-747.

35. Smith JB, Bishop VL, Francis IC, et al. Ophthalmic manifestations of perineural spread of facial skin malignancy. *Aust N Z J Ophthalmol* 1990;18:197-205.

36. Ballantyne AJ, McCarten AB, Ibanez M. The extension of cancer of the head and neck through peripheral nerves. *Am J Surg* 1963;106:651-657.

37. Goepfert H, Dichtel WJ, Medina JE, et al. Perineural invasion in squamous cell skin carcinoma of the head and neck. *Am J Surg* 1984;148:542-547.

38. Mendenhall WM, Parsons JT, Mendenhall NP, et al. Carcinoma of the skin of the head and neck with perineural invasion. *Head Neck* 1989;11:301-308.

39. Clouston PD, Sharpe DM, Corbett AJ, et al. Perineural spread of cutaneous head and neck cancer. Its orbital and central neurologic complications. *Arch Neurol* 1990;47:73-77.

40. Mark GJ. Basal cell carcinoma with intraneural invasion. *Cancer* 1977;40:2181-2187.

41. Paver K, Poyzer K, Burry N, et al. The incidence of basal cell carcinomas and their metastases in Australia and New Zealand. *Australas J Dermatol* 1973;14:53.

42. Cannon JR, Schneidman DW. Recent developments in adnexal pathology. In: Moschella SL, ed. *Dermatology Update: Reviews for Physicians*. New York, NY: Elsevier; 1982:217-252.

43. Soffer D, Kaplan H, Weshler Z. Meningeal carcinomatosis due to basal cell carcinoma. *Hum Pathol* 1985;16:530-532.

44. Epstein JH. Photocarcinogenesis, skin cancer, and aging. *J Am Acad Dermatol* 1983;9:487-502.

45. Akguner M, Barutcu A, Yilmaz M, et al. Marjolin's ulcer and chronic burn scarring. *J Wound Care* 1998;7:121-122.

46. Hejna WF. Squamous-cell carcinoma developing in the chronic draining sinuses of osteomyelitis. *Cancer* 1965;18:128-132.

47. Epstein E, Epstein NN, Bragg K, et al. Metastases from squamous cell carcinomas of the skin. *Arch Dermatol* 1968;97:245-251.

48. Friedman HI, Cooper PH, Wanebo HJ. Prognostic and therapeutic use of microstaging of cutaneous squamous cell carcinoma of the trunk and extremities. *Cancer* 1985;56:1099-1105.

49. Immerman SC, Scanlon EF, Christ M, et al. Recurrent squamous cell carcinoma of the skin. *Cancer* 1983;51:1537-1540.

50. Møller R, Reymann F, Hou-Jensen K. Metastases in dermatological patients with squamous cell carcinoma. *Arch Dermatol* 1979;115:703-705.

51. Modlin JJ. Cancer of the skin: surgical treatment. *Mo Med* 1954;51:364-367.

52. Dinehart SM, Pollack SV. Metastases from squamous cell carcinoma of the skin and lip. An analysis of twenty-seven cases. *J Am Acad Dermatol* 1989;21:241-248.

53. Binder SC, Cady B, Catlin D. Epidermoid carcinoma of the skin of the nose. *Am J Surg* 1968;116:506-512.

54. Mohs FE. *Chemosurgery: Microscopically Controlled Surgery for Skin Cancer*. Springfield, Ill: Charles C. Thomas; 1978.

55. Bourne RG. The Costello Memorial Lecture. The spread of squamous cell carcinoma of the skin via the cranial nerves. *Australas Radiol* 1980;24:106-114.

56. Loeffler JS, Larson DA, Clark JR, et al. Treatment of perineural metastasis from squamous carcinoma of the skin with aggressive combination chemotherapy and irradiation. *J Surg Oncol* 1985;29:181-183.

57. Gruber SB, Barnhill RL, Stenn KS, et al. Nevomelanocytic proliferations in association with cutaneous melanoma: a multivariate analysis. *J Am Acad Dermatol* 1989;21:773-780.

58. Clark WH, Ainsworth AM, Bernardino EA. The developmental biology of primary human malignant melanomas. *Semin Oncol* 1975;2:83-103.

59. McGovern VJ, Murad TM. Pathology of melanoma: an overview. In: Balch CM, Milton GW, eds. *Cutaneous Melanoma: Clinical Management and Treatment Results Worldwide*. Philadelphia, Pa: JB Lippincott; 1985:29-53.

60. Barnhill RL, Mihm MC. Histopathology of malignant melanoma and its precursor lesions. In: Balch CM, Houghton AN, Milton GW, et al, eds. *Cutaneous Melanoma*. Philadelphia, Pa: JB Lippincott; 1992:234-263.

61. Urist MM, Balch CM, Soong SJ. Head and neck melanoma in 534 clinical stage I patients: a prognostic factor analysis and results of surgical treatment. *Ann Surg* 1984;200:769-775.

62. Clark WH, Mihm MC. Lentigo maligna and lentigo-maligna melanoma. *Am J Pathol* 1969;55:39-67.

63. Reed RJ. The pathology of human cutaneous melanoma. In: Costanzi JJ, ed. *Malignant Melanoma*. The Hague, The Netherlands: Martinus Nijhoff; 1983:85-116.

64. Arrington JH, Reed RJ, Ichinose H, et al. Plantar lentiginous melanoma: a distinctive variant of human cutaneous malignant melanoma. *Am J Surg Pathol* 1977;1:131-143.

65. Coleman WP, Loria PR, Reed RJ, et al. Acral lentiginous melanoma. *Arch Dermatol* 1980;116:773-776.

66. Krementz ET, Feed RJ, Coleman WP, et al. Acral lentiginous melanoma. A clinicopathologic entity. *Ann Surg* 1982;195:632-645.

67. Feibleman CE, Stoll H, Maize JC. Melanomas of the palm, sole and nailbed: a clinicopathologic study. *Cancer* 1980;46:2492-2504.

68. Patterson RH, Helwig EB. Subungual malignant melanoma: a clinical-pathologic study. *Cancer* 1980;46:2074-2087.

69. Seiji M, Takahashi M. Acral melanoma in Japan. *Hum Pathol* 1982;13:607-609.

70. Balch CM, Urist MM, Maddox WA, et al. Melanoma in the southern United States: experience at the University of Alabama in Birmingham. In: Balch CM, Milton GW, eds. *Cutaneous Melanoma: Clinical Management and Treatment Results Worldwide*. Philadelphia, Pa: JB Lippincott; 1985:397-418.

71. Reintgen DS, McCarty KM, Cox E, et al. Malignant melanoma in black American and white American populations: a comparative review. *J Am Med Assoc* 1982;248:1856-1859.

72. Balch CM. Surgical management of regional lymph nodes in cutaneous melanoma. *J Am Acad Dermatol* 1980;3:511-524.

73. Cotlar AM, Gates JO, Gibbs FA. Merkel cell carcinoma: combined surgery and radiation therapy. *Am Surg* 1986;52:159-164.

74. Sibley RK, Dehner LP, Rosai J. Primary neuroendocrine (Merkel cell?) carcinoma of the skin. I. A clinicopathologic and ultrastructural study of 43 cases. *Am J Surg Pathol* 1985;9:95-108.

75. Morrison WH, Peters LJ, Silva EG, et al. The essential role of radiation therapy in securing locoregional control of Merkel cell carcinoma. *Int J Radiat Oncol Biol Phys* 1990;19:583-591.

76. Merkel F. Tastzellen und tastkoerperchen bei den haushieren und beim menschen. *Arch Mikr Anat* 1875;11:636-652.

77. Silva EG, Mackay B, Goepfert H, et al. Endocrine carcinoma of the skin (Merkel cell carcinoma). *Pathol Annu* 1984;19:1-30.

78. Bonfiglio TA. Neuroendocrine carcinoma of the skin: diagnostic and management considerations. *Int J Radiat Oncol Biol Phys* 1988;14:1321-1322.

79. Drijkoningen M, De Wolf-Peeters C, van Limbergen E, et al. Merkel cell tumor of the skin: an immunohistochemical study. *Hum Pathol* 1986;17:301-307.

80. Pacella J, Ashby M, Ainslie J, et al. The role of radiotherapy in the management of primary cutaneous neuroendocrine tumors (Merkel cell or trabecular carcinoma): experience at the Peter MacCallum Cancer Institute (Melbourne, Australia). *Int J Radiat Oncol Biol Phys* 1988;14:1077-1084.

81. Bourne RG, O'Rourke MG. Management of Merkel cell tumour. *Aust N Z J Surg* 1988;58:971-974.

82. Hitchcock CL, Bland KI, Laney RG, et al. Neuroendocrine (Merkel cell) carcinoma of the skin. Its natural history, diagnosis and treatment. *Ann Surg* 1988;207:201-207.

83. Meland NB, Jackson IT. Merkel cell tumor: diagnosis, prognosis, and management. *Plast Reconstr Surg* 1986;77:632-638.

84. Rice RD Jr, Chonkich GD, Thompson KS, et al. Merkel cell tumor of the head and neck. Five new cases with literature review. *Arch Otolaryngol Head Neck Surg* 1993;119:782-786.

85. Wilder RB, Shimm DS, Kittelson JM, et al. Recurrent basal cell carcinoma treated with radiation therapy. *Arch Dermatol* 1991;127:1668-1672.

86. O'Brien PC, Denham JW, Leong AS. Merkel cell carcinoma: a review of behaviour patterns and management strategies. *Aust N Z J Surg* 1987;57:847-850.

87. Meeuwissen JA, Bourne RG, Kearsley JH. The importance of postoperative radiation therapy in the treatment of Merkel cell carcinoma. *Int J Radiat Oncol Biol Phys* 1995;31:325-331.

88. Civatte J, Tsoitis G. Adnexal skin carcinomas. In: Andrade R, Gumport SL, Popkin GL, et al, eds. *Cancer of the Skin*. Vol 2. Philadelphia, Pa: WB Saunders; 1976:1045-1068.

89. Rulon DB, Helwig EB. Cutaneous sebaceous neoplasms. *Cancer* 1974;33:82-102.

90. Oppenheim AR. Sebaceous carcinoma of the penis. *Arch Dermatol* 1981;117:306-307.

91. Batsakis JG, Littler ER, Leahy MS. Sebaceous cell lesions of the head and neck. *Arch Otolaryngol* 1972;95:151-157.

92. Rao NA, Hidayat AA, McLean IW, et al. Sebaceous carcinomas of the ocular adnexa: a clinicopathologic study of 104 cases, with five-year follow-up data. *Hum Pathol* 1982;13:113-122.

93. Boniuk M, Zimmerman LE. Sebaceous carcinoma of the eyelid, eyebrow, caruncle and orbit. *Trans Am Acad Ophthalmol Otolaryngol* 1968;72:619-642.

94. Wick MR, Goellner JR, Wolfe JT, et al. Adnexal carcinomas of the skin. II. Extraocular sebaceous carcinomas. *Cancer* 1985;56:1163-1172.

95. Berg JW, McDivitt RW. Pathology of sweat gland carcinomas. *Pathol Annu* 1968;3:123-144.

96. Mishima Y, Morioka S. Oncogenic differentiation of the intraepidermal eccrine sweat duct: eccrine poroma, poroepithelioma and porocarcinoma. *Dermatologica* 1969;138:238-250.

97. Lipper S, Peiper SC. Sweat gland carcinoma with syringomatous features: a light microscopic and ultrastructural study. *Cancer* 1979;44:157-163.

98. Mendoza S, Helwig EB. Mucinous (adenocystic) carcinoma of the skin. *Arch Dermatol* 1971;103:68-78.

99. Liu Y. The histogenesis of clear cell papillary carcinoma of the skin. *Am J Pathol* 1949;25:93-99.

100. Nickoloff BJ, Fleischmann HE, Carmel J, et al. Microcystic adnexal carcinoma: immunohistologic observations suggesting dual (pilar and eccrine) differentiation. *Arch Dermatol* 1986;122:290-294.

101. Pawlowski A, Haberman HF, Menon IA. Junctional and compound pigmented nevi induced by 9, 10-demethyl, benzanthracene in skin of albino guinea pigs. *Cancer Res* 1976;36:2813-2821.

102. Kripke ML, Fisher MS. Immunologic parameters of ultraviolet carcinogenesis. *J Natl Cancer Inst* 1976;57:211-215.

102a. Fleming I, Cooper JS, Henson DE, et al, eds. *AJCC Cancer Staging Manual*, 5th ed. Philadelphia, Pa: Lippincott Williams & Wilkins; 1997:157-161.

103. Crombie IK. Variation of melanoma incidence with latitude in North America and Europe. *Br J Cancer* 1979;40:774-781.

104. Breslow A. Thickness, cross-sectional areas and depth of invasion in the prognosis of cutaneous melanoma. *Ann Surg* 1970;172:902-908.

104a. Fleming I, Cooper JS, Henson DE, et al, eds. *AJCC Cancer Staging Manual*, 5th ed. Philadelphia, Pa: Lippincott Williams & Wilkins; 1997:163-170.

105. Balch CM, Soong SJ, Shaw HM, et al. An analysis of prognostic factors in 8500 patients with cutaneous melanoma. In: Balch CM, Houghton AN, Milton GW, et al, eds. *Cutaneous Melanoma*. Philadelphia, Pa: JB Lippincott; 1992:165-187.

106. Rowe DE, Carroll RJ, Day CL Jr. Mohs surgery is the treatment of choice for recurrent (previously treated) basal cell carcinoma. *J Dermatol Surg Oncol* 1989;15:424-431.

107. Wilder RB, Margolis LW. Skin cancer. In: Leibel SA, Phillips TL, eds. *Textbook of Radiation Oncology*. Philadelphia, Pa: WB Saunders; 1998:1165-1182.

108. Morrison WH, Garden AS, Ang KK. Radiation therapy for nonmelanoma skin carcinomas. *Clin Plast Surg* 1997;24:719-729.

109. von Essen CF. Indicators for radiation therapy of skin cancer. In: Cumley RW, ed. *Tumors of the Skin*. Chicago, Ill: Year Book Medical; 1964:285-298.

110. Fitzpatrick PJ, Thompson GA, Easterbrook WM, et al. Basal and squamous cell carcinoma of the eyelids and their treatment by radiotherapy. *Int J Radiat Oncol Biol Phys* 1984;10:449-454.

111. Petrovich Z, Parker RG, Luxton G, et al. Carcinoma of the lip and selected sites of head and neck skin. A clinical study of 896 patients. *Radiother Oncol* 1987;8:11-17.

112. Lovett RD, Perez CA, Shapiro SJ, et al. External irradiation of epithelial skin cancer. *Int J Radiat Oncol Biol Phys* 1990;19:235-242.

113. Wilder RB, Kittelson JM, Shimm DS. Basal cell carcinoma treated with radiation therapy. *Cancer* 1991;68:2134-2137.

114. Shimm DS, Wilder RB. Radiation therapy for squamous cell carcinoma of the skin. *Am J Clin Oncol* 191;14:383-386.

115. Preston DS, Stern RS. Nonmelanoma cancers of the skin. *N Engl J Med* 1992;327:1649-1662.

116. Janse GT, Westbrook KC. Cancer of the skin. In: Suen JY, Myers EN, eds. *Cancer of the Head and Neck*. New York, NY: Churchill Livingstone; 1981:212-241.

117. Metcalf PB Jr. Carcinoma of the pinna. *N Engl J Med* 1954;251:91-95.

118. Fredricks S. External ear malignancy. *Br J Plast Surg* 1956;9:136-160.

119. Schewe EJ Jr, Pappalardo C. Cancer of the external ear. *Am J Surg* 1962;104:753-755.

120. Petrovich Z, Kuisk H, Langholz B, et al. Treatment of carcinoma of the skin with bone and/or cartilage involvement. *Am J Clin Oncol* 1988;11:110-113.

121. Avila J, Bosch A, Aristizabal S, et al. Carcinoma of the pinna. *Cancer* 1977;40:2891-2895.

122. Ang KK. Altered fractionation trials in head and neck cancer. *Semin Radiat Oncol* 1998;8:1-15.

123. Taylor JBW, Brant TA, Mendenhall NP, et al. Carcinoma of the skin metastatic to parotid area lymph nodes. *Head Neck* 1991;13:427-433.

124. Karakousis CP, Balch CM, Urist MM, et al. Local recurrence in malignant melanoma: long-term results of the multi-institutional randomized surgical trial. *Ann Surg Oncol* 1996;3:446-452.

125. Harwood AR. Conventional fractionated radiotherapy for 51 patients with lentigo maligna and lentigo maligna melanoma. *Int J Radiat Oncol Biol Phys* 1983;9:1019-1021.

126. Milton GW, Shaw HM, McCarthy WH, et al. Prophylactic lymph node dissection in clinical stage I cutaneous malignant melanoma: results of surgical treatment in 1319 patients. *Br J Surg* 1982;69:108-111.

127. Veronesi U, Adamus J, Bandiera DC, et al. Stage I melanoma of the limbs: immediate versus delayed node dissection. *Tumori* 1980;66:373-396.

128. Balch CM, Soong SJ, Bartolucci AA, et al. Efficacy of an elective regional lymph node dissection of 1 to 4 mm thick melanomas for patients 60 years of age and younger. *Ann Surg* 1996;224:255-266.

129. Cascinelli N, Morabito A, Santinami M, et al. Immediate or delayed dissection of regional nodes in patients with melanoma of the trunk: a randomised trial. *Lancet* 1998;351:793-796.

130. Morton DL, Wen DR, Wong JH, et al. Technical details of intraoperative lymphatic mapping for early stage melanoma. *Arch Surg* 1992;127:392-399.

131. Lang PG Jr. Malignant melanoma. *Med Clin North Am* 1998;82:1325-1358.

132. Ross MI. Surgical management of stage I and II melanoma patients: approach to the regional lymph node basin. *Semin Surg Oncol* 1996;12:394-401.

133. Singletary SE, Balch CM, Urist MM, et al. Surgical treatment of primary melanoma. In: Balch CM, Houghton AN, Milton GW, et al, eds. *Cutaneous Melanoma*. Philadelphia, Pa: JB Lippincott; 1992:269-274.

134. Byers RM. The role of modified neck dissection in the treatment of cutaneous melanoma of the head and neck. *Arch Surg* 1986;12:1338-1341.

135. Balch CM, Soong SJ, Murad TM, et al. A multifactorial analysis of melanoma. IV. Prognostic factors in 200 melanoma patients with distant metastases (stage III). *J Clin Oncol* 1983;1:126-134.

136. Ang KK, Peters LJ, Weber RS, et al. Postoperative radiotherapy for cutaneous melanoma of the head and neck region. *Int J Radiat Oncol Biol Phys* 1994;30:795-798.

137. Kirkwood JM, Strawderman MH, Ernstoff MS, et al. Interferon alfa-2b adjuvant therapy of high-risk resected cutaneous melanoma: the Eastern Cooperative Oncology Group trial EST 1684. *J Clin Oncol* 1996;14:7-17.

138. Grob JJ, Dreno B, de la Solmoniere P, et al. Randomised trial of interferon alpha-2a as adjuvant therapy in resected primary melanoma thicker than 1-5 mm without clinically detectable node metastases. *Lancet* 1998;351:1905-1910.

139. Mays SR, Nelson BR. Current therapy of cutaneous melanoma. *Cutis* 1999;63:293-298.

140. Rusthoven JJ. The evidence for tamoxifen and chemotherapy as treatment for metastatic melanoma. *Eur J Cancer* 1998;34:S31-S36.

141. Livingston P, Sznol M. Vaccine therapy. In: Balch CM, Houghton AN, Sober AJ, et al, eds. *Cutaneous Melanoma*, 3rd ed. St. Louis, Mo: Quality Medical; 1998:437-450.

142. Pilotti S, Rikle F, Bartoli C, et al. Clinicopathologic correlations of cutaneous neuroendocrine Merkel cell carcinoma. *J Clin Oncol* 1988;6:1863-1873.

143. Kokoska GR, Kokoska MS, Collins BT, et al. Early aggressive treatment for Merkel cell carcinoma improves outcome. *Am J Clin Oncol* 1997;174:688-693.

144. Feun LG, Savaraj N, Legha SS, et al. Chemotherapy for metastatic Merkel cell carcinoma. Review of the M.D. Anderson Hospital's experience. *Cancer* 1988;62:683-685.

145. Wynne CJ, Kearsley JH. Merkel cell tumor: a chemosensitive skin cancer. *Cancer* 1988;62:28-31.

146. Grosh WW, Giannone L, Hande KR, et al. Disseminated Merkel cell tumor. Treatment with systemic chemotherapy. *Am J Clin Oncol* 1987;10:227-230.

147. Fenig E, Lurie H, Klein B, et al. The treatment of advanced Merkel cell carcinoma. A multimodality chemotherapy and radiation therapy treatment approach. *J Dermatol Surg Oncol* 1993;19:860-864.

148. Lee WR, Mendenhall WM, Parsons JT, et al. Radical radiotherapy for T4 carcinoma of the skin of the head and neck: a multivariate analysis. *Head Neck* 1993;15:320-324.

149. Joseph J, Adler JR, Cox RS, et al. Linear accelerator-based stereotactic radiosurgery for brain metastases: the influence of number of lesions on survival. *J Clin Oncol* 1996;14:1085-1092.

150. Ang KK, Kaanders JHAM, Peters LJ. *Radiotherapy for Head and Neck Cancers: Indications and Techniques*. Philadelphia, Pa: Lea & Febiger; 1994.

151. Carter RL, Foster CS, Dinsdale EA, et al. Perineural spread by squamous carcinomas of the head and neck: a morphological study using antiaxonal and antimyelin monoclonal antibodies. *J Clin Pathol* 1983;36:269-275.

152. Barrett TL, Greenway HT Jr, Massullo V, et al. Treatment of basal cell carcinoma and squamous cell carcinoma with perineural invasion. In: Callen JP, Dahl MV, Golitz LE, et al, eds. *Advances in Dermatology.* St. Louis, Mo: Mosby; 1993;277-306.

153. Cottel WI. Perineural invasion by squamous-cell carcinoma. *J Dermatol Surg Oncol* 1982;8:589-600.

154. Traenkle HL, Mulay D. Further observations on late radiation necrosis following therapy of skin cancer. *Arch Dermatol* 1960;81:908-913.

155. Petrovich Z, Kuisk H, Langholz B, et al. Treatment results and patterns of failure in 646 patients with carcinoma of the eyelids, pinna, and nose. *Am J Surg* 1987;154:447-450.

156. Williams PC, Hendry JH. The RBE of megavoltage photon and electron beams. *Br J Radiol* 1978;51:220.

157. Boland J. Human skin reaction. *Br J Radiol* 1957;30:351-352.

158. Wang CC. Cancer of the skin. In: Wang CC, ed. *Radiation Therapy for Head and Neck Neoplasms: Indications, Techniques, and Results.* Chicago, Ill: Year Book Medical;1990:85.

PART III

Head and Neck

CHAPTER 6

The Salivary Glands

Adam S. Garden

The salivary glands consist of major and minor glands. The major glands consist of paired parotid, submandibular, and sublingual glands. The hundreds of minor salivary glands are evident, and they reside in the oral cavity, pharynx, and paranasal sinuses. The primary purpose of the major salivary glands is to secrete, store, and excrete saliva. Flow rates of saliva vary among individuals, but the average person excretes approximately 1 L of saliva per day. The salivary glands are highly radiosensitive, and many patients undergoing radiation treatment for head and neck tumors can develop xerostomia, a side effect that can lead to secondary oral complications and can significantly affect quality of life.

Neoplasms of the salivary glands are uncommon, and most tumors are benign. Primary tumors of the parotid contribute the largest proportion of salivary gland tumors, representing approximately two thirds of all salivary gland neoplasms. The submandibular glands are the next most common site; together with the parotid glands, they account for 90% of salivary gland neoplasms. Sublingual primary malignancies are rare and can be difficult to distinguish from minor primary salivary gland tumors of the anterior floor of the mouth.

In this chapter, the anatomy of the salivary glands and the effect of radiation on the normal glands are described first, followed by brief descriptions of the epidemiology, clinical presentation, staging, and pathology of salivary gland tumors. Finally, treatment options, including radiation, are reviewed.

ANATOMY

Embryologically, the major salivary glands are derived from the ectoderm. Epithelial buds originate from the oral cavity and eventually differentiate into the glands, which consist of ducts and secretory end pieces. On histologic examination, the salivary glands appear as lobules separated by connective tissue. The lobules consist primarily of acini, intercalated ducts, and small striated ducts. The ductal system continues in the connective tissue as larger striated ducts, interlobular ducts, and a main excretory duct (Fig. 6-1).

The acini consist of serous cells, mucinous cells, or both types of cells. The parotid glands are predominantly composed of serous cells, whereas the submandibular glands are mostly mucinous cells. The excretory ducts are lined with epithelial cells.

The precise cell of origin of salivary gland neoplasms is not universally agreed upon. A widely believed hypothesis is that neoplasms arise from stem cells originating in the intercalated ducts or excretory ducts. Salivary gland carcinomas can be either poorly differentiated or better differentiated depending on whether they develop early or late in the differentiation pathway. Acinic cell carcinoma, adenoid cystic carcinoma, and mixed tumors (benign and malignant) mainly arise from stem cells of intercalated ducts, whereas mucoepidermoid carcinomas mainly arise from excretory ducts.

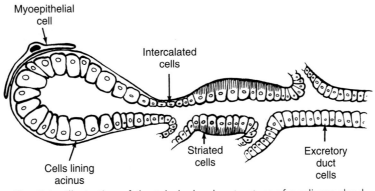

Fig. 6-1 Illustration of the tubuloalveolar structure of a salivary gland.

Parotid Glands

The parotid glands are pyramidal. Each gland lies below the zygomatic arch, in front of and below the external acoustic meatus, and in front of the mastoid process. The inferior border of the gland rests between the angle of the mandible and the anterior border of the sternocleidomastoid muscle. The anterior edge is somewhat C-shaped because of the gland's relationship with the ascending ramus of the mandible. The gland abuts the ramus, extending anterolaterally around the edge of the bone and then onto the lateral edge of the masseter muscle to lie between this muscle and the skin. The parotid duct, which is 5 cm long, emerges from the parotid gland through the masseter muscle to open opposite the upper second molar. Anteromedially, the parotid gland extends between the medial edge of the ascending ramus and the medial pterygoid muscle. The posterior medial edge of the parotid gland abuts the styloid process. The medial edge of the gland lies close to the retropharyngeal space and may even come in contact with the lateral pharyngeal wall (Figs. 6-2 and 6-3).

The parotid glands are divided into superficial and deep lobes by the facial nerve and its branches.

Submandibular and Sublingual Glands

The submandibular glands lie mainly under the cover of the horizontal ramus of the mandible. Medially they are related to the mylohyoid, hyoglossus, and digastric

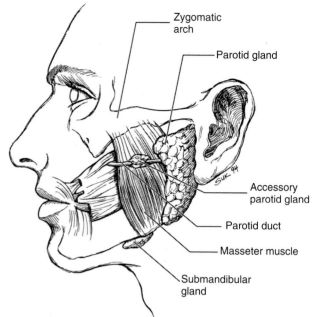

Fig. 6-2 Anatomic illustration of the parotid gland and its relationship to adjacent structures.

muscles. The deep portion of each gland lies inferior to the lingual nerve and superior to the hypoglossal nerve (Figs. 6-4 and 6-5).

The sublingual glands lie in the floor of the mouth, below the mucous membrane and above the muscular floor, anterior to the submandibular glands.

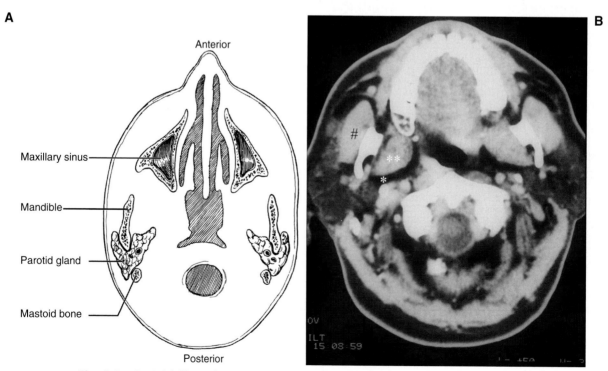

Fig. 6-3 **A,** Axial illustration and **B,** computed tomographic image of the parotid gland curving around the posterior ascending ramus of the mandible. Note the relationship between the gland and the masseter (#) and pterygoid (**) muscles and the parapharyngeal space (*).

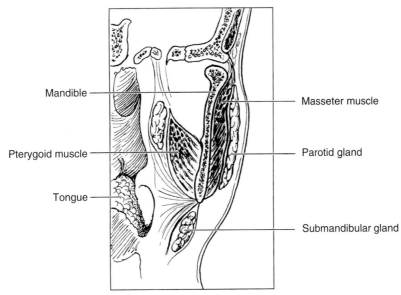

Fig. 6-4 Anatomic coronal illustration of the submandibular gland and its relationship to adjacent structures.

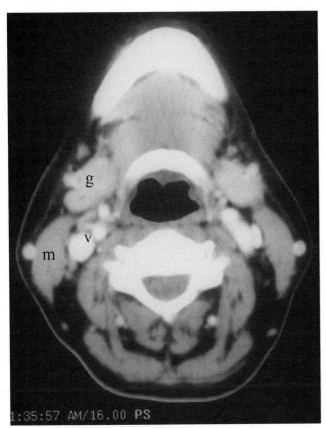

Fig. 6-5 Axial computed tomographic image of the submandibular gland *(g)* and its relationship in the neck to the sternocleidomastoid muscle *(m)* and vessels *(v)*.

RADIATION EFFECTS ON NORMAL SALIVARY GLANDS

The two main cells of the major salivary glands, serous and mucinous, differ in their sensitivity to radiation injury.

Despite their slow turnover rate, the serous cells are highly radiosensitive. Stephens and colleagues[1] studied the effects of radiation on the acinar serous cells of rhesus monkeys, which are quite similar to the salivary gland cells of humans. Injury to irradiated serous cells was expressed within 24 hours of irradiation, with cells exhibiting destruction secondary to apoptosis and an acute inflammatory response. In submandibular glands, the selective destruction of serous acini was particularly apparent within the normal mix of cells. Although acinar cells can recover and repopulate, the typical therapeutic radiation doses eventually damage the ducts, ductal stem cells, and the mucinous and supporting stromal and vascular cells. This damage often results in xerostomia and fibrosis.

Swelling occurs and pain occasionally is experienced during the first week of irradiation, particularly when doses per fraction are relatively high, but these symptoms are almost always self-limiting. The primary effect of radiation on the salivary glands is xerostomia. Because xerostomia not only affects quality of life but also can increase the risk of dental caries and oral infections, early involvement of a dental oncologist is essential when patients are to undergo radiation to the head and neck that includes the major salivary glands.

Defining a threshold dose (TD) in clinical situations is complicated because most tumoricidal doses exceed the radiation threshold of the salivary glands. Estimates of $TD_{5/5}$ and $TD_{50/5}$ (the threshold doses at which 5% and 50% of the population, respectively, experience sequelae 5 years after treatment) vary widely in the literature and often have been based on anecdotal observations rather than large prospective trials. This variability also results from inconsistent or unclear definitions of xerostomia or different ways of measuring salivary flow rates. Estimates of $TD_{5/5}$ range from 30 to 50 Gy; for

$TD_{50/5}$ the range is greater—from 30 to 70 Gy.[2-6] Evidence from recent literature suggests that threshold doses are at the lower end of this range. Several investigators have found the $TD_{100/5}$ to be 50 Gy, with all or nearly all patients who receive this or a higher dose to all major salivary glands experiencing xerostomia.[2]

Xerostomia develops relatively quickly and consistently. After treatment with 10 Gy (given in 5 fractions over a period of 1 week), dryness of the mouth is evident subjectively, and objective flow measurements demonstrate reductions in flow rate of about 50%. Additional irradiation continues to diminish flow rate; at the completion of a full course of radiation, flow rates are only 10% of their original baseline values. Dreizen and colleagues,[7] documenting changes in salivary flow rates over time, suggested that salivary flow levels show little or no recovery after having reached this nadir.

The late recovery process is controversial. Leslie and Dische[8] argued that sparing either part of the gland or maintaining the dose below threshold levels conferred a reasonable expectation of recovery. In their studies, flow rates declined to less than 20% of their baseline values when more than 80% of the gland was in the radiation field; in contrast, flow rates could be maintained at 80% or more of baseline levels if less than 30% of the gland was in the radiation field.[8] This observation has led to exploratory use of conformal and intensity-modulated radiation therapy to partially spare the parotid glands and thereby reduce the risk of xerostomia. Eisbruch and colleagues[9] used intensity-modulated radiation therapy to define a mean dose of 24 Gy or less to one gland as being sufficient to maintain salivary flow rates after treatment near the pretreatment baseline levels. Using a more complex model, Chao and colleagues[10] determined that stimulated saliva secretion is reduced exponentially at a rate of 4%/Gy of mean dose to the parotid, with a threshold of 32 Gy.

The use of amifostine, a radioprotectant preferentially taken up by the salivary glands, may also decrease the incidence of radiation-induced xerostomia. In one randomized trial, the incidence of grade 2 or higher xerostomia was reduced from 57% in controls to 35% in patients given amifostine.[11] Amifostine is currently approved for postoperative treatment of squamous cell carcinoma of the head and neck.

Xerostomia can be difficult to manage. Once the symptom develops, effective therapies are limited. Saliva substitutes can be helpful for some patients; others respond well to induction or overstimulation of residual functioning glands by cholinergic agonists such as pilocarpine.[12]

EPIDEMIOLOGY OF SALIVARY GLAND CANCER

Salivary gland neoplasms account for approximately 3% to 7% of head and neck tumors. Because most salivary gland neoplasms are benign, they most likely account for 1% to 2% of head and neck malignancies. Unlike most cases of head and neck cancer, salivary gland carcinomas are not associated with tobacco exposure. A strong association is evident between parotid carcinomas and prior radiation exposure. Alcohol use and exposure to hair dye are also linked to these carcinomas.[13] No predilection is evident for a particular sex or age group, but the median age of patients with salivary gland neoplasms is younger than that of patients with more common malignancies of the head and neck. Interestingly, younger patients (those less than 40 years old) tend to be female, whereas older patients are more often male.

A controversial association is the finding in some studies of a higher incidence of salivary gland tumors among women with breast cancer. This finding, considered together with the fact that both salivary gland tumors and breast tumors arise in organs consisting of lobules and ducts, has led some investigators to use breast cancer therapies, mainly hormonal therapies, for patients with salivary gland malignancies.

A general rule of thumb for salivary gland neoplasms is that the size of the gland is directly proportional to the likelihood that a neoplasm will develop but is inversely proportional to the likelihood that a neoplasm will be malignant. Hence, at most one third of parotid gland tumors are malignant, but approximately two thirds of minor salivary gland tumors are malignant. The rate of malignancy for submandibular gland tumors is between the rates for the other two sites.

CLINICAL PRESENTATION
Parotid Gland Tumors

More than 80% of parotid tumors develop in the superficial lobe (Fig. 6-6). The most typical presentation is a painless mass located over or behind the ascending ramus of the mandible. It is unusual for patients with parotid tumors to present with pain, and pain is a poor prognostic sign. Deep lobe tumors (Fig. 6-7) can be indolent and can be present for a long time before symptoms appear. As they grow, they invade the retropharyngeal space. Deep lobe tumors are usually detected when the mass fills the pharyngeal space enough to interfere with swallowing or speech.

Facial nerve paralysis is an uncommon finding that usually indicates a malignant tumor and is believed to correlate with a poorer prognosis. Other cranial nerve palsies are extremely rare. Although deep lobe tumors can invade the retropharyngeal space, involvement of the cranial nerves that traverse this space is unusual.

Lymph node metastases develop in 10% to 15% of patients with parotid malignancies (Fig. 6-8). Metastases are most common in patients with higher-grade tumors, particularly high-grade mucoepidermoid carcinomas or adenocarcinomas. The parotid glands drain first to

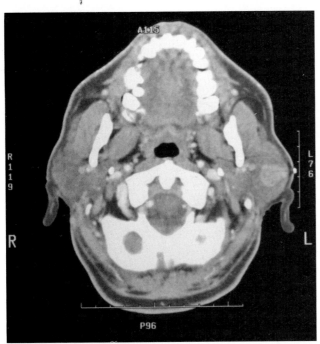

Fig. 6-6 Axial computed tomographic image showing adenoid cystic carcinoma of the superficial lobe of the left parotid gland.

lymph nodes within the superficial gland and overlying superficial fascia and then to the jugulodigastric lymph nodes in the neck.

Submandibular Gland Tumors

Submandibular gland tumors present as painless masses in the submandibular triangle. Malignant submandibular gland tumors, particularly neurotropic adenoid cystic carcinoma, may present with nerve palsy, with either sensory or motor changes in the tongue depending on the nerve involved. Lymph node metastases develop in 10% to 15% of cases. The submandibular glands drain first to the submandibular nodes and then to nodes in the jugular chain.

Minor Salivary Gland Tumors

Minor salivary gland tumors usually present as painless masses that may become symptomatic on further growth. Paranasal sinus tumors may present with obstructive breathing symptoms, and base-of-tongue and palatal tumors may interfere with swallowing. Because about two thirds of minor salivary gland tumors are malignant and because a very high proportion of those tumors are adenoid cystic carcinomas, symptoms related to cranial nerve deficits are not uncommon. Whether lymph node metastases occur depends greatly on the site of origin of the tumor and the richness of lymphatics at that site. Thus paranasal sinus tumors rarely metastasize to

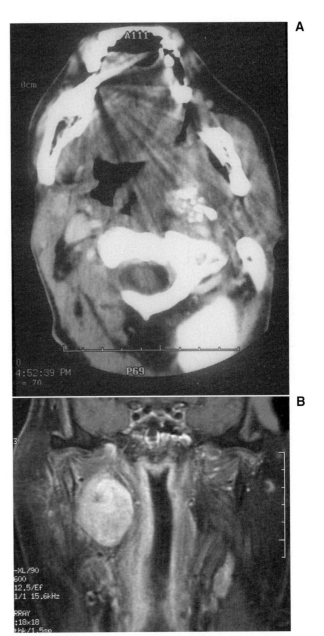

Fig. 6-7 **A,** Axial computed tomographic image of a benign pleomorphic adenoma of the deep lobe of the left parotid gland. **B,** Coronal magnetic resonance image of a poorly differentiated carcinoma of the deep lobe of the right parotid gland.

lymph nodes in less than 5% of cases, whereas tongue and floor-of-mouth tumors metastasize in more than 35% of cases.[14] Overall, neck metastases develop in 10% to 15% of patients with minor salivary gland tumors.

STAGING

Major salivary gland tumors are staged using the American Joint Committee on Cancer (AJCC) tumor-nodes-metastasis (TNM) staging system in which the primary tumor is

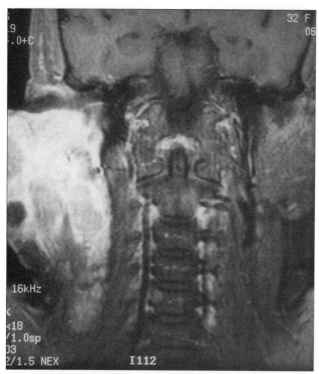

Fig. 6-8 High-grade mucoepidermoid carcinoma of the right parotid gland with lymph node metastases.

staged on the basis of size and local extension (Box 6-1).[3,15] Both larger size of the primary tumor and invasion into local tissues, particularly major nerves (facial, hypoglossal, or lingual), correlate with a poorer prognosis.[16] Minor salivary gland tumors are staged using the systems for squamous cell cancer of the respective sites. The nodal staging system is the same as that used for other head and neck mucosal sites (other than nasopharynx).[15]

PATHOLOGY AND NATURAL HISTORY
Benign Tumors

The most common benign tumor of the parotid gland is the benign mixed (or pleomorphic) adenoma, which accounts for 75% of benign parotid tumors and more than 50% of all parotid neoplasms. Most commonly, benign mixed adenomas develop in the superficial lobe of the parotid gland and consist of a mixture of ductal, myoepithelial, and mesenchymal cells. These tumors have a very low recurrence rate after surgery, but when they do recur, they can give rise to carcinomas and must be examined very carefully microscopically.

The second most common benign parotid tumor is the Warthin's tumor (papillary cystadenoma lymphomatosum), which represents 2% to 6% of all parotid tumors.

BOX 6-1   American Joint Committee on Cancer Staging System for Salivary Gland Tumors

PRIMARY TUMOR (T)

TX	Primary tumor cannot be assessed
T0	No evidence of primary tumor
T1	Tumor 2 cm or less in greatest dimension without extraparenchymal extension
T2	Tumor more than 2 cm but not more than 4 cm in greatest dimension without extraparenchymal extension
T3	Tumor having extraparenchymal extension without seventh nerve involvement and/or more than 4 cm but not more than 6 cm in greatest dimension
T4	Tumor invades base of skull seventh nerve, and/or exceed 6 cm in greatest dimension

REGIONAL LYMPH NODES (N)

NX	Regional lymph nodes cannot be assessed
N0	No regional lymph node metastasis
N1	Metastasis in a single ipsilateral lymph node, 3 cm or less in greatest dimension
N2	Metastasis in a single ipsilateral lymph node, more than 3 cm but not more than 6 cm in greatest dimension; or in multiple ipsilateral lymph nodes, none more than 6 cm in greatest dimension; or in bilateral or contralateral lymph nodes, none more than 6 cm in greatest dimension
N2a	Metastasis in single ipsilateral lymph node more than 3 cm but not more than 6 cm in greatest dimension
N2b	Metastasis in multiple ipsilateral lymph nodes, none more than 6 cm in greatest dimension
N2c	Metastasis in bilateral or contralateral lymph nodes, none more than 6 cm in greatest dimension
N3	Metastasis in a lymph node more than 6 cm in greatest dimension

DISTANT METASTASIS (M)

MX	Distant metastasis cannot be assessed
M0	No distant metastasis
M1	Distant metastasis

STAGE GROUPING

Stage I	T1–T2	N0	M0
Stage II	T3	N0	M0
Stage III	T1–T2	N1	M0
Stage IV	T4	N0	M0
	T3–T4	N1	M0
	Any T	N2	M0
	Any T	N3	M0
	Any T	Any N	M1

From Fleming I, Cooper JS, Henson DE, et al, eds. *AJCC Cancer Staging Manual*, 5th ed. Philadelphia, Pa: Lippincott Williams & Wilkins; 1997:51-58.

It is extremely rare for a Warthin's tumor to undergo malignant transformation. Less common benign tumors include lymphoepithelial lesions and monomorphic adenomas, including basal cell adenomas, myoepitheliomas, oncocytomas, and salivary duct adenomas.

Malignant Tumors

Malignant salivary gland tumors are a diverse group with regard to their histologic type, but their prognosis and behavior can generally be predicted by their grade. Higher-grade tumors tend to be more invasive locally, are more prone to lymphatic and hematogenous metastases, and, even in the case of appropriate surgical treatment, have high local recurrence rates.

Mucoepidermoid carcinoma is the most common malignancy of the parotid glands but develops less often in other salivary glands. These tumors exhibit a wide variation in their differentiation and behavior, although lower-grade lesions are most common. Mucoepidermoid carcinomas consist of a combination of mucin-producing and epidermoid cells. Mucin-producing cells are more prevalent in well-differentiated lesions. Mucin-producing cells are much less common in higher-grade lesions, and thus these tumors rarely may be classified as squamous cell carcinomas. The incidence of nodal and distant metastases and perineural invasion increases with increasing grade of mucoepidermoid carcinoma.

Acinic cell carcinomas are the second most common malignant tumors of the parotid gland. These tumors rarely develop in other salivary glands. Acinic cell carcinomas are nearly always well-differentiated tumors. When treated appropriately, they are associated with an excellent prognosis.

Adenoid cystic carcinoma is the most common malignancy of the major and minor salivary glands with the exception of the parotid gland, where it ranks in frequency behind mucoepidermoid and acinic cell carcinomas[16,17] (Table 6-1). Adenoid cystic carcinomas represent 10% of parotid malignancies and 30% to 50% of malignancies of the other glands. Although histologically these tumors often have a low-grade appearance, they can behave similarly to high-grade lesions. They tend to grow slowly but are notorious for infiltrating adjacent tissue. They often spread along perineural spaces. Some classify adenoid cystic carcinomas as having tubular, cribriform, or solid patterns. These patterns have some correlation with prognosis, with the tubular pattern associated with a favorable outcome and the solid pattern often associated with an aggressive course. Another important pathologic prognostic factor is tumor ploidy: aneuploid tumors often metastasize, whereas diploid tumors rarely do.[18]

Adenocarcinomas, although not rare, represent a minority of malignant salivary gland tumors. They are a heterogeneous group in terms of both type and grade.

TABLE 6-1

Histologic Findings in Primary Malignant Tumors of the Parotid and Submandibular Glands

	NUMBER OF PATIENTS (%)	
Histologic Characteristics	**Parotid Gland Tumors**	**Submandibular Gland Tumors**
Mucoepidermoid	55 (36)	15 (18)
Acinic	17 (11)	1 (1)
Adenoid cystic	17 (11)	37 (44)
Adenocarcinoma	15 (10)	9 (10)
Unclassified/ undifferentiated	13 (8)	6 (7)
Salivary duct	13 (8)	0
Myoepithelial	9 (6)	0
Malignant mixed	8 (5)	9 (10)
Squamous/ adenosquamous	6 (4)	9 (10)
Oncocytic/basaloid	2 (1)	0
TOTAL	155 (100)	86 (100)

Modified from Frankenthaler RA, Luna MA, Lee SS, et al. *Arch Otolaryngol Head Neck Surg* 1991;117:1251-1256; Weber RS, Byers RM, Petit B, et al. *Arch Otolaryngol Head Neck Surg* 1990;116:1055-1060.

They fall into two well-defined clinicopathologic groups. Terminal duct adenocarcinomas are low-grade malignancies arising from intercalated ducts. They most commonly are found in the palate. Salivary duct adenocarcinomas account for 5% to 10% of malignancies and typically metastasize early. They most commonly arise from major glands.

Malignant mixed tumors also tend to behave aggressively and must be diligently sought in cases of recurrent benign tumors. The most common malignant mixed tumor is carcinoma ex pleomorphic adenoma, which arises from its benign counterpart and is a high-grade tumor. Less common are true mixed malignant tumors, which are a mix of carcinoma and sarcomatous elements. These too are aggressive malignancies.

Finally, squamous cell carcinomas represent 1% to 2% of primary parotid malignancies. Histologically, squamous cell tumors of the parotid gland may be difficult to distinguish from metastatic squamous cell carcinoma within an intraparotid lymph node, a situation seen most often in the case of primary skin cancer. In the absence of a known skin tumor, squamous cell carcinoma in the parotid gland should be managed as a primary malignancy of the parotid gland.

OUTCOME

Ten-year survival rates for patients with major salivary gland tumors range from 50% to 70%. Most series[16,17,19-22] have found that primary tumor stage (or size) and tumor grade are strong predictors of outcome, with low-grade and small tumors associated with low recurrence rates. Lymph node involvement and involvement of large or eponymous nerves are predictors of disease recurrence and poorer survival.

Rates of distant metastasis vary from series to series. Metastases develop in approximately 25% to 30% of cases.[16,23,24] Lung metastases are most common, accounting for more than half of distant recurrences. The bones are the second most common site of distant metastases. Although most recurrences happen within 5 years of treatment, late recurrences can occur. In several long-term analyses, the disease-free survival curves flatten but do not reach a plateau past 10 years.[23]

TREATMENT OPTIONS
Surgery

Surgery is the treatment of choice for salivary gland tumors. For parotid tumors, surgery at a minimum consists of gross tumor removal through superficial or total parotidectomy depending on the tumor location and size. Surgery alone is often sufficient for low-grade malignancies. Higher-grade tumors necessitate removal of the lymph nodes in continuity with the gland.

In the case of positive lymph nodes, a more complete neck dissection is required. Radiation therapy is effective in controlling microscopic disease (as described in the following sections). Thus the entire facial nerve or its main trunk can often be spared, provided that the nerve is not invaded and that all gross tumor can be removed without removal of the nerve. In the case of very extensive lesions, sacrifice of the facial or auriculotemporal nerve or removal of skin or bone may be required to achieve a gross total removal.

Surgical management of submandibular tumors consists of a regional dissection of the submandibular triangle, including the gland and the adjacent submandibular, submental, and facial lymph nodes. Extensive disease may require removal of additional structures such as muscle, mandible, or a portion of the floor of the mouth. In the case of clinically apparent adenopathy, more extensive lymph node dissection, the details of which are dictated by the extent of nodal disease, is necessary.

For minor salivary gland tumors, the location of the primary tumor and the extent of tumor involvement determine the extent of resection.

Postoperative Radiation Therapy

The role of radiation in the treatment of salivary gland tumors is most often adjunctive. Before 1965, postoperative radiation therapy was rarely used because salivary gland tumors were thought to be radioresistant; unless inoperable, tumors were treated with surgery only.

However, patients with high-grade malignancies were noted to have high local recurrence rates. On the basis of these observations, Fletcher started to use radiation therapy as an adjunctive treatment and found that the addition of postoperative radiation therapy improved local control relative to surgery alone. Moreover, control of subclinical disease was no different for epithelial salivary gland malignancies and squamous cell carcinomas.[25] In 1975 Guillamondegui and colleagues[26] reported the results of surgery alone for patients with parotid cancer and compared those results with outcomes in a later cohort treated with surgery followed by radiation. The authors concluded that the addition of postoperative radiation therapy dramatically improved local control for high-grade malignancies. This favorable experience with postoperative radiation therapy for parotid tumors was extrapolated to the treatment of all salivary gland cancer.

In 1976 Tapley and Fletcher[27] outlined the indications for postoperative radiation therapy. These have not significantly changed over the years and include gross residual disease, positive or close (less than 5 mm) margins, high tumor grade, squamous cell subtype, extraglandular involvement, perineural invasion, recurrent disease, and lymph node involvement.

Outcomes with Surgery and Postoperative Radiation Therapy

Over the past three decades, numerous series have demonstrated improved local control rates in patients with salivary gland tumors treated with postoperative irradiation compared with patients treated with surgery alone (Table 6-2).[14,28-32] Fu and colleagues[28] described a series of patients with major and minor salivary gland tumors treated with either surgery alone or surgery and postoperative irradiation. In patients with inadequate surgical margins, the addition of postoperative radiation therapy significantly improved local control rates. Simpson and colleagues[33] reported improved local–regional control rates in patients with adenoid cystic carcinomas, from less than 15% without radiation therapy to more than 80% with radiation therapy and surgery. At The University of Texas M.D. Anderson Cancer Center, in a series of 198 patients with adenoid cystic carcinoma, 70% of whom had either inadequate surgical margins or perineural spread, postoperative irradiation resulted in a 10-year local control rate of 86%.[34]

Local–regional control rates in patients with parotid malignancies treated with surgery and radiation are high—more than 80% in most series. Selected series are summarized in Table 6-3.[35-45]

Bissett and Fitzpatrick[41] reported an improvement in local–regional control with the addition of postoperative radiation therapy to surgical resection of submandibular gland malignancies. The local–regional control rate was 30% with surgery alone, compared with 69% when radiation was added. Weber and colleagues[17]

TABLE 6-2

Local–Regional Control Rates in Series of Patients with Major and Minor Salivary Gland Tumors Treated with Surgery and Postoperative Radiation Therapy

Study and Reference	Glands	Number of Patients	Local–Regional Control Rate*	Follow-up Period
Fu et al, 1977[28]	Major	29	86%	Minimum 3 yr
Tran et al, 1986[29]	Major	57	75%	30 mo-10 yr
Harrison et al, 1990[30]	Major	46	73% (actuarial)	Median 5.8 yr
North et al, 1990[31]	Major	64	92%	NS
Garden et al, 1994[14]	Minor	160	82%	Median 110 mo
Parsons et al, 1996[32]	Minor	40	88%	Minimum 2 yr

NS, Not stated.
*All rates shown are crude except as indicated.

TABLE 6-3

Local–Regional Control Rates in Series of Patients with Parotid Gland Tumors Treated with Surgery and Postoperative Radiation Therapy

Study and Reference	Number of Patients	Local–Regional Control Rate*	Median Follow-up Period
Theriault et al, 1986[35]	167	75%	10 yr
Spiro et al, 1992[36]	57	87% (actuarial)	66 mo
Sykes et al, 1995[37]	104	68% (actuarial)	51 mo
Garden et al, 1997[38]	166	87%	155 mo
Leverstein et al, 1998[39]	51	80%	90 mo
Renehan et al, 1999[40]	66	85%	12 yr

*All rates shown are crude except as indicated.

similarly described an improvement in local–regional control with the addition of radiation therapy to surgery in patients whose tumors invaded the extraglandular soft tissues. Storey and colleagues[42] recently updated an experience with 83 patients with submandibular tumors treated with combined surgery and radiation therapy at the M.D. Anderson Cancer Center; the 10-year local–regional control rate was 88%.

The author's group at the M.D. Anderson Cancer Center reported a crude local recurrence rate of 12% in patients treated with surgery and radiation for minor salivary gland cancer.[14] Two thirds of these recurrences were diagnosed more than 5 years after treatment. Parsons and colleagues[32] reported a 74% actuarial 15-year local control rate, which was similar to the rate in the author's series.

Postoperative Radiation Therapy for Benign Pleomorphic Adenomas

Benign pleomorphic adenomas are the most common neoplasms of the parotid gland. Like their malignant counterparts, they are treated by surgical resection. The more thorough the surgical procedure, the lower the recurrence rate. A review of several series found that the recurrence rate was more than 20% in patients who underwent simple enucleation, compared with less than 0.5% in patients who underwent total parotidectomy.[43]

The role of postoperative radiation therapy in the treatment of benign pleomorphic adenomas is controversial, and some authors believe that radiation therapy should be avoided even in patients with incomplete resections and residual microscopic disease. This management algorithm involves waiting for recurrence and managing any recurrence with repeated and more aggressive surgical resections. Samson and colleagues[44] have advocated radiation therapy for microscopic disease in patients with benign tumors adherent to but resectable from the facial nerve. Indications for postoperative irradiation in 55 patients with benign pleomorphic adenomas treated at the Princess Margaret Hospital[45] included multifocality, nerve involvement, tumor "spill," residual disease (gross or microscopic), and recurrent disease (disease that recurred after a first surgery and was treated with a second operation). The risk of a third recurrence is high in most series reporting the management of recurrent pleomorphic adenoma.[46] In the Princess Margaret Hospital series, control rates in patients with recurrent disease were 81% in patients

---

TABLE 6-4

Local–Regional Control Rates in Series of Patients with Benign Pleomorphic Adenomas of the Parotid Gland Treated with Surgery and Postoperative Radiation Therapy

Study and Reference	Number of Patients	Crude Local–Regional Control Rate*	Follow-up Period
Dawson, 1989[47]	20	90%	1-26 yr
Samson et al, 1991[44]	21	90%	Mean 5.9 yr
Barton et al, 1992[48]	187	95%	Median 14 yr
Liu et al, 1995[45]	55	95%	Median 21.5 yr
Renehan et al, 1996[49]	51	92%	Median 14 yr

---

treated with postoperative irradiation vs. 6% in patients treated with surgery alone.

Overall control rates for patients with benign pleomorphic adenomas treated with surgery and postoperative irradiation range from 90% to 95%.[44,45,47-49] Results of several series are summarized in Table 6-4. One reason for the reluctance to use radiation is the fear of inducing a second malignant tumor either in the remaining gland or in other organs in the head and neck. However, series reviewing the outcome of patients undergoing irradiation for benign pleomorphic adenoma have found that the incidence of second primary tumors is negligible.

Primary Radiation Therapy

Occasionally, patients with salivary gland tumors present with unresectable disease or are medically inoperable. These patients can be treated with radiation therapy alone. Several small retrospective series[28,50] describe control rates of approximately 30% with this approach. Although this control rate seems low when compared with outcomes of surgical series, it must be remembered that patients treated with primary radiation therapy by selection have an unfavorable prognosis. Wang and Goodman[51] have reported control rates of more than 80% for unresectable parotid and minor salivary gland tumors treated with radiation alone, but findings from this small retrospective series have yet to be reproduced. Parsons and colleagues[32] reported a control rate of 50% for minor salivary gland tumors treated with radiation alone. This was a worse control rate than that achieved in patients treated with surgery and postoperative irradiation. However, the authors argue that for selected patients in whom the morbidity of surgery may be unacceptable, radiation is certainly a reasonable and sometimes preferable treatment option.

RADIATION TECHNIQUES

Techniques of irradiation for salivary gland tumors vary depending on the location of the primary tumor.

Parotid gland and submandibular gland tumors, with their lateral locations, often lend themselves to ipsilateral treatment. This allows normal tissue, particularly the contralateral salivary glands, to be spared and reduces the incidence of radiation-induced xerostomia. Treatment of minor salivary gland tumors is more individualized and depends greatly on the site of origin. Techniques tend to be similar to those used for squamous cell cancer arising from these sites, although issues regarding coverage of the base of the skull and the neck need to be addressed on a case-by-case basis.

Parotid Gland Tumors

The two most common techniques used for treating parotid tumors are a wedged-pair technique (two photon beams) and a single ipsilateral field using a mixed beam of electrons and photons. At the M.D. Anderson Cancer Center, the single ipsilateral field technique is favored because it treats less normal tissue and because this technique is thought to be easier to reproduce on a daily basis (Fig. 6-9).

Both techniques can exceed spinal cord tolerance if care is not taken. The posterior field in the wedged pair must be off the spinal cord. The mixed beam technique, despite the shallow range of electrons, can also exceed cord tolerance if the spinal cord is within a high-depth dose curve. This is particularly true today with the availability of very high electron energies (18 to 25 MeV) that have 90% dose curves at depths of 4 to 7 cm. A second concern with the wedged pair technique is that the beam can exit through the contralateral eye if the proper precautions are not taken.

For patients treated with superficial parotidectomy, a combination of high-energy electrons and photons is used and a dose of 50 Gy at the ipsilateral edge of the pharyngeal wall is planned to ensure coverage of the entire parotid bed. Weightings that heavily favor the high-energy electrons are used. The photons in the mix allow some skin sparing (high-energy electrons have high skin doses) and add some depth to the distribution.

When a patient has a parotid tumor involving the deep lobe, especially one invading deep into the parapharyngeal space, the wedged-pair technique may be preferred. This technique may give a better dose distribution when deep tissues are at risk.

Depending on the degree of risk, doses of 55 to 65 Gy are recommended. In patients with recurrent low-grade tumors (e.g., low-grade mucoepidermoid or acinic cell carcinomas), the lower end of this dose range may be recommended. In contrast, higher doses are preferable for patients with high-grade lesions with close or positive margins. When a mixed beam technique is used, the prescribed dose is typically to the 90% isodose line with the appropriate energy selected to keep the target within the distal aspect of the 90% volume. In this way, the target gets the prescribed dose, but within this volume the tissues at risk will be getting up to a 10% higher dose. Elective irradiation with matched ipsilateral fields designed to cover the mid to low neck is used for patients with high-grade lesions or neck disease found at surgery (Fig. 6-10).

Several devices and techniques are used to help with dosimetry and help reduce acute reactions. An acrylic stent (Fig. 6-11) with cerrobend shielding is used intraorally to protect the tongue.[52] When fields must be superior to the zygomatic arch, bolus material is sometimes used to reduce the depth of electron beam penetration and thus minimize the risk of temporal lobe necrosis. One area of particular dose inhomogeneity, particularly with electrons, is the ear. To reduce these inhomogeneities, the ear is taped against the skull. Occasionally, the ear canal is filled with a mild acetic acid solution to avoid the inhomogeneities in this structure.[53]

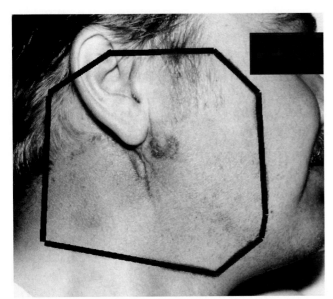

Fig. 6-9 This 39-year-old man underwent a superficial parotidectomy in 1982. He had an acinic cell carcinoma that was dissected off the branches of the facial nerve. From October through November 1982 he received 60 Gy delivered to the parotid bed using a mixed-beam technique. He was alive without evidence of disease 15 years after treatment.

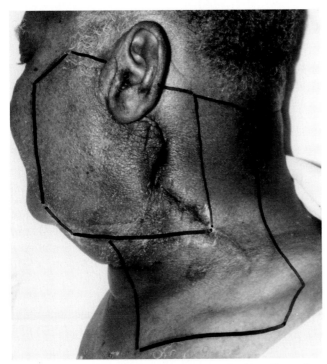

Fig. 6-10 This 76-year-old man presented with salivary duct carcinoma of the parotid gland. He underwent parotidectomy and neck dissection, which revealed perineural invasion of the cancer into the buccal branch of the facial nerve and 2 lymph nodes containing tumor. A 65-Gy dose was delivered to the parotid bed with a mix of 20-MeV electrons and 18-MV photons weighted 3:1. A separate neck field received 50 Gy with 9-MeV electrons. The patient died 5 years later from a second malignancy without recurrence of his parotid cancer. (From Garden AS, El-Naggar A, Morrison W, et al. *Int J Radiat Oncol Biol Phys* 1997;37:79-85.)

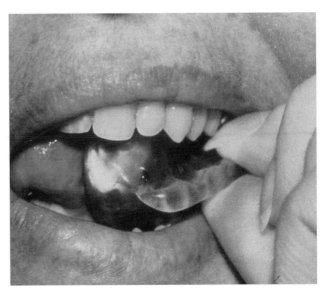

Fig. 6-11 Placement of an intraoral acrylic stent demonstrating medial displacement of the tongue away from the range of an appositional electron beam.

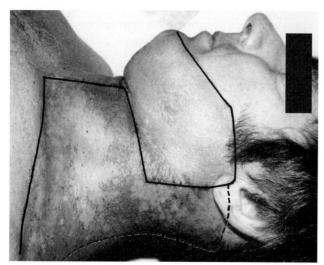

Fig. 6-12 This 46-year-old man presented with a submandibular mass. Excision in January 1985 revealed an adenoid cystic carcinoma with perineural and lymphatic space invasion. Findings at reexcision and selective neck dissection in February 1985 were negative for disease. From March through April 1985, radiation therapy was given as a 13-MeV electron-beam appositional field covering the submandibular gland bed and a 9-MeV electron-beam field covering the lower neck (operative bed). The glandular bed received 60 Gy dosed to the 90% isodose line, and the lower neck received 50 Gy dosed to the 100% line. The patient was alive without evidence of disease 14 years after treatment.

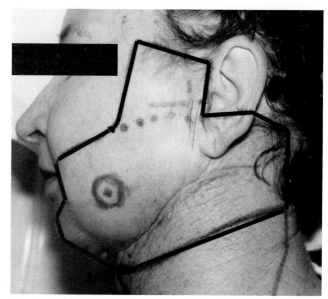

Fig. 6-13 This 60-year-old woman with adenoid cystic carcinoma of the left submandibular gland underwent resection of her tumor with neck dissection in 1986. Section margins were microscopically positive, and tumor had invaded into the strap muscles and lingual nerve. The initial postoperative portal arrangement was through parallel-opposed fields with a final dose to the base of the skull of 55 Gy. The submandibular bed received 60 Gy. The patient was alive without evidence of disease 13 years after treatment.

Submandibular Gland Tumors

Submandibular gland tumors, like parotid gland tumors, can be treated with a unilateral technique. As is done with parotid tumors, we treat submandibular tumors (Fig. 6-12) by using a single appositional field with electrons only or a mixture of photons and electrons. It is important to remember that the submandibular gland extends medially and sits behind bone. Therefore higher energies of electrons may be needed to provide adequate coverage of the glandular bed. Occasionally, even higher-energy electrons may not be sufficient, and then parallel-opposed fields may be desirable (Fig. 6-13). This is particularly true if coverage of the base of the skull is a concern (see the section on "Coverage in Cases of Spread along Nerves" later in this chapter). As is the case for parotid tumors, a matching low-neck field is used for high-grade lesions or known nodal disease.

Minor Salivary Gland Tumors

Techniques for irradiation of minor salivary gland tumors are highly dependent on the primary site of origin. Techniques tend to be similar to those used for squamous cell tumors arising from the same sites: parallel opposed fields for tongue (Fig. 6-14) and palate lesions, two or three wedged fields for sinus tumors, and ipsilateral fields for buccal tumors.

Unlike squamous cell carcinoma, perineural spread of minor salivary gland tumors to the base of the skull is of greater concern than is lymphatic spread to the neck. In a review of 160 patients treated with postoperative irradiation for minor salivary gland malignancies,[14] the incidence of recurrence in the neck was extremely low (< 5%), even in patients who did not undergo elective irradiation of the neck. The incidence of nodal disease at presentation was also low (8%), and nodal disease was detected predominantly in patients with primary lesions in the tongue and floor of mouth. Thus adjunctive or elective treatment of the neck is recommended only if (1) nodal involvement is present, (2) the primary lesion arises from the tongue or floor of mouth, or (3) removal of the primary tumor required surgery on the neck. Coverage of the base of the skull is discussed in the next section.

Coverage in Cases of Spread along Nerves

Salivary gland tumors, particularly adenoid cystic carcinomas, can spread along nerves. When such spread is discovered on pathologic examination, it raises the question of how far to follow the nerve pathways with the radiation fields. Parotid tumors do not present much controversy; the fields need to be large enough to cover

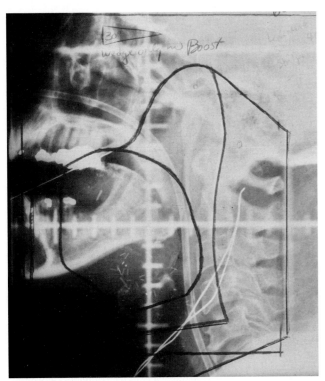

Fig. 6-14 This 51-year-old man presented in September 1994 with an adenoid cystic carcinoma that occupied the entire right base of the tongue and crossed the midline. He underwent a resection of the primary tumor with an ipsilateral modified neck dissection. The tongue was reconstructed by using a soft-tissue free-flap transfer. Findings at pathologic examination included involvement of the lingual and hypoglossal nerves and positive margins. He was treated with lateral fields to 44 Gy. Fields were reduced off the spinal cord to 50 Gy, and then the tongue dose was boosted to 66 Gy. The initial portals were designed to include the base of the skull. The patient was alive without evidence of disease 6 years after treatment.

the facial nerve from the stylomastoid foramen, but this does not involve a significant change in field size. A wedged pair technique may be more effective than the mixed-beam technique for covering the facial canal or the temporal bone.

The question is more difficult when the nerve involved or at risk is relatively distant from the gland, as in the common case of a submandibular gland tumor with lingual nerve involvement. Covering the perineural pathways to the base of skull in this case would result in a substantial increase in field size. As a general policy at the M.D. Anderson Cancer Center, the nerve pathways to their origin are covered from the skull base if major nerve involvement is present, as documented by clinical examination, findings at surgery, or findings on pathologic examination. Following these guidelines has resulted in a recurrence rate at the base of the skull of less than 2%.[34]

Locally Advanced and Inoperable Tumors

Several trials[54,55] have investigated the use of fast neutrons for the treatment of locally advanced and inoperable salivary gland tumors. Battermann and colleagues[56] demonstrated that the relative biological effectiveness of irradiation with neutrons was higher in metastatic adenoid cystic carcinomas than in other metastatic tumors. It is believed that cells with long cell cycles are more sensitive to neutrons than photons, and salivary gland tumors with many cells remaining in the G_0 phase of the cell cycle are selectively sensitive to neutrons.

The role of neutrons has been studied in a prospective randomized cooperative trial[57] conducted by the Radiation Therapy Oncology Group in the United States and the Medical Research Council in Great Britain. This study evaluated whether neutrons were more advantageous than photons for inoperable salivary gland tumors. Neutrons proved to be superior with respect to control of primary disease: 2-year local–regional control rates were 67% for patients treated with neutrons compared with 17% for patients treated with photons. However, the high rate of distant metastases in the overall group canceled out any potential survival advantage. Ultimately, the study evaluated only 25 patients.

The University of Washington has one of the largest experiences in using neutrons to treat salivary gland tumors. Investigators there report relatively high control rates for their patients with parotid gland and minor salivary gland tumors. Douglas and colleagues[58] reported on the use of neutrons for gross tumors of major salivary glands and described a 5-year actuarial local–regional control rate of 59%. A separate study by Douglas and colleagues[59] evaluating the use of neutrons for adenoid cystic carcinomas reported an overall 5-year actuarial local control rate of 47%. In the case of lesions close to the brain, the dose may be limited because neutrons are more neurotoxic than photons; Douglas and colleagues found that the control rate was only 15% when the tumor involved the nasopharynx, cavernous sinus, or base of the skull. However, the development of improved conformal techniques may allow better dosing in these areas. These studies suggest that in the uncommon situation of a patient with an inoperable salivary gland tumor, referral to a center with neutron capabilities may be appropriate.

REFERENCES

1. Stephens L, Schultheiss T, Price R, et al. Radiation apoptosis of serous acinar cells of salivary and lacrimal glands. *Cancer* 1991;67:1539-1543.
2. Emami B, Lyman J, Brown A, et al. Tolerance of normal tissue to therapeutic radiation. *Int J Radiat Oncol Biol Phys* 1991;21:109-122.
3. Fajardo LF, Berthrong M, Anderson RE. Salivary glands. In: *Radiation Pathology.* New York, NY: Oxford University Press; 2001:265-270.

4. Marks J, Davis C, Gottsman V, et al. The effects of radiation on parotid salivary function. *Int J Radiat Oncol Biol Phys* 1981;7: 1013-1019.

5. Mira J, Wescott W, Starcke E, et al. Some factors influencing salivary function when treating with radiotherapy. *Int J Radiat Oncol Biol Phys* 1981;7:535-541.

6. Rubin P, Casarett G. *Clinical Radiation Pathology*, Philadelphia, Pa: WB Saunders; 1968:242-262.

7. Dreizen S, Brown L, Handler S, et al. Radiation-induced xerostomia in cancer patients. *Cancer* 1976;38:273-278.

8. Leslie MD, Dische S. The early changes in salivary gland function during and after radiotherapy given for head and neck cancer. *Radiother Oncol* 1994;30:26-32.

9. Eisbruch A, Ten Haken R, Kim H, et al. Dose, volume, and function relationships in parotid salivary glands following conformal and intensity-modulated irradiation of head and neck cancer. *Int J Radiat Oncol Biol Phys* 1999;45:577-587.

10. Chao K, Deasy J, Markman J, et al. A prospective study of salivary function sparing in patients with head-and-neck cancers receiving intensity-modulated or three-dimensional radiation therapy: initial results. *Int J Radiat Oncol Biol Phys* 2001;49: 907-916.

11. Brizel D, Wasserman T, Henke M, et al. Phase III randomized trial of amifostine as a radioprotector in head and neck cancer. *J Clin Oncol* 2000;18:3339-3345.

12. LeVeque FG, Montgomery M, Potter D, et al. A multicenter, randomized, double-blind, placebo-controlled, dose-titration study of oral pilocarpine for treatment of radiation-induced xerostomia in head and neck cancer patients. *J Clin Oncol* 1993;11:1124-1131.

13. Spitz M, Fueger J, Goepfert H, et al. Salivary gland cancer. A case-control investigation of risk factors. *Arch Otolaryngol Head Neck Surg* 1990;116:1163-1166.

14. Garden AS, Weber RS, Ang KK, et al. Postoperative radiation therapy for malignant tumors of minor salivary glands. *Cancer* 1994;73:2563-2569.

15. Fleming I, Cooper JS, Henson DE, et al, eds. *AJCC Cancer Staging Manual*, 5th ed. Philadelphia, Pa: Lippincott Williams & Wilkins; 1997:51-58.

16. Frankenthaler RA, Luna MA, Lee SS, et al. Prognostic variables in parotid gland cancer. *Arch Otolaryngol Head Neck Surg* 1991;117:1251-1256.

17. Weber RS, Byers RM, Petit B, et al. Submandibular gland tumors. Adverse histologic factors and therapeutic implications. *Arch Otolaryngol Head Neck Surg* 1990;116:1055-1060.

18. Luna M, El-Naggar A, Batsakis J, et al. Flow cytometric DNA content of adenoid cystic carcinoma of submandibular gland. Correlation of histologic features and prognosis. *Arch Otolaryngol Head Neck Surg* 1990;116:1291-1296.

19. Hicks MJ, El-Naggar AK, Flaitz CM, et al. Histocytologic grading of mucoepidermoid carcinoma of major salivary glands in prognosis and survival: a clinicopathologic and flow cytometric evaluation. *Head Neck* 1995;17:89-95.

20. Spiro RH, Thaler HT, Hicks WF, et al. The importance of clinical staging of minor salivary gland carcinoma. *Am J Surg* 1991;162:330-336.

21. Spiro RH, Huvos AG. Stage means more than grade in adenoid cystic carcinoma. *Am J Surg* 1992;164:623-628.

22. Vander Poorten VL, Balm AJ, Hilgers FJ, et al. Prognostic factors for long-term results of the treatment of patients with malignant submandibular gland tumors. *Cancer* 1999;85:2255-2264.

23. Fordice J, Kershaw C, El-Naggar A, et al. Adenoid cystic carcinoma of the head and neck: predictors of morbidity and mortality. *Arch Otolaryngol Head Neck Surg* 1999;125:149-152.

24. Spiro R. Salivary neoplasms: overview of a 35-year experience with 2,807 patients. *Head Neck Surg* 1986;8:177-184.

25. King J, Fletcher G. Malignant tumors of the major salivary glands. *Radiology* 1971;100:381-384.

26. Guillamondegui OM, Byers RM, Luna MA, et al. Aggressive surgery in treatment for parotid cancer: the role of adjunctive postoperative radiotherapy. *Am J Roentgenol* 1975;123:49-54.

27. Tapley N, Fletcher G. Malignant tumors of the salivary gland. In: Tapley N, ed. *Clinical Applications of the Electron Beam*. New York, NY: John Wiley & Sons; 1976:141-171.

28. Fu KK, Leibel SA, Levine ML, et al. Carcinoma of the major and minor salivary glands. *Cancer* 1977;40:2882-2890.

29. Tran L, Sadeghi A, Hanson D, et al. Major salivary gland tumors: treatment results and prognostic factors. *Laryngoscope* 1986; 96:1139-1144.

30. Harrison LB, Armstrong JG, Spiro RH, et al. Postoperative radiation therapy for major salivary gland malignancies. *J Surg Oncol* 1990;45:52-55.

31. North C, Lee D, Piantadosi S, et al. Carcinoma of the major salivary glands treated by surgery or surgery plus postoperative radiotherapy. *Int J Radiat Oncol Biol Phys* 1990;18:1319-1326.

32. Parsons J, Mendenhall W, Stringer S, et al. Management of minor salivary gland carcinomas. *Int J Radiat Oncol Biol Phys* 1996;35:443-454.

33. Simpson J, Thawley S, Matsuba H. Adenoid cystic salivary gland carcinoma: treatment with irradiation and surgery. *Radiology* 1984;151:509-512.

34. Garden A, Weber R, Morrison W, et al. The influence of positive margins and nerve invasion in adenoid cystic carcinoma of the head and neck treated with surgery and radiation. *Int J Radiat Oncol Biol Phys* 1995;32:619-626.

35. Theriault C, Fitzpatrick PJ. Malignant parotid tumors. Prognostic factors and optimum treatment. *Am J Clin Oncol* 1986;9:510-516.

36. Spiro I, Wang C, Montgomery W. Carcinoma of the parotid gland. *Cancer* 1992;1:2699-2705.

37. Sykes A, Logue J, Slevin N, et al. An analysis of radiotherapy in the management of 104 patients with parotid carcinoma. *Clin Oncol* 1995;7:16-20.

38. Garden AS, El-Naggar A, Morrison W, et al. Postoperative radiotherapy for malignant tumors of the parotid gland. *Int J Radiat Oncol Biol Phys* 1997;37:79-85.

39. Leverstein H, van der Waal J, Tiwari R, et al. Malignant epithelial parotid gland tumours: analysis and results in 65 previously untreated patients. *Br J Surg* 1998;85:1267-1272.

40. Renehan A, Gleave E, Slevin N, et al. Clinico-pathological and treatment-related factors influencing survival in parotid cancer. *Br J Cancer* 1999;80:1296-1300.

41. Bissett RJ, Fitzpatrick PJ. Malignant submandibular gland tumors. A review of 91 patients. *Am J Clin Oncol* 1988;11:46-51.

42. Storey M, Garden A, Morrison W, et al. Postoperative radiotherapy for malignant tumors of the submandibular gland. *Int J Radiat Biol Oncol Phys* 2001;51:952-958.

43. Henriksson G, Westrin K, Carlsoo B, et al. Recurrent primary pleomorphic adenomas of salivary gland origin. Intrasurgical rupture, histopathologic features and pseudopodia. *Cancer* 1998; 82:617-620.

44. Samson MJ, Metson R, Wang CC, et al. Preservation of the facial nerve in the management of recurrent pleomorphic adenoma. *Laryngoscope* 1991;101:1060-1062.

45. Liu F, Rotstein L, Davison A, et al. Benign pleomorphic adenomas: a review of the Princess Margaret Hospital experience. *Head Neck* 1995;17:177-183.

46. Piorkowski R, Guillamondegui O. Is aggressive surgical treatment indicated for recurrent benign mixed tumors of the parotid gland? *Am J Surg* 1981;142:434-436.

47. Dawson A. Radiation therapy in recurrent pleomorphic adenoma of the parotid. *Int J Radiat Oncol Biol Phys* 1989;16: 819-821.

48. Barton J, Slevin N, Gleave E. Radiotherapy for pleomorphic adenoma of the parotid gland. *Int J Radiat Oncol Biol Phys* 1992; 22:925-928.

49. Renehan A, Gleave N, McGurk M. An analysis of the treatment of 114 patients with recurrent pleomorphic adenomas of the parotid gland. *Am J Surg* 1996;172:710-714.

50. Fitzpatrick P, Theriault C. Malignant salivary gland tumors. *Int J Radiat Oncol Biol Phys* 1986;12:1743-1747.

51. Wang C, Goodman M. Photon irradiation of unresectable carcinomas of salivary glands. *Int J Radiat Oncol Biol Phys* 1991;21:569-576.

52. Fleming T, Rambach S. A tongue-shielding radiation stent. *J Prosthet Dent* 1983;49:389-392.

53. Morrison WH, Wong PF, Starkschall G, et al. Water bolus for electron irradiation of the ear canal. *Int J Radiat Oncol Biol Phys* 1995;33:479-483.

54. Catterall M, Errington R. The implications of improved treatment of malignant salivary gland tumors by fast neutron radiotherapy. *Int J Radiat Oncol Biol Phys* 1987;13:1313-1318.

55. Griffin T, Pajak T, Laramore G, et al. Neutron vs photon irradiation of inoperable salivary gland tumors: results of an RTOG-MRC cooperative randomized study. *Int J Radiat Oncol Biol Phys* 1988;15:1085-1090.

56. Battermann JJ, Breur K, Hart GA, et al. Observations on pulmonary metastases in patients after single doses and multiple fractions of fast neutrons and cobalt-60 gamma rays. *Eur J Cancer* 1981;17:539-548.

57. Laramore GE, Krall J, Griffin T, et al. Neutron versus photon irradiation for unresectable salivary gland tumors: final report of an RTOG-MRC randomized clinical trial. *Int J Radiat Oncol Biol Phys* 1993;27:235-240.

58. Douglas JG, Lee S, Laramore GE, et al. Neutron radiotherapy of the treatment of locally advanced major salivary gland tumors. *Head Neck* 1999;21:255-263.

59. Douglas JG, Laramore GE, Austin-Seymour M, et al. Treatment of locally advanced adenoid cystic carcinoma of the head and neck with neutron radiotherapy. *Int J Radiat Oncol Biol Phys* 2000;46:551-557.

CHAPTER 7

The Nasal Fossa and Paranasal Sinuses

K. Kian Ang and Linh N. Nguyen

Neoplasms arising in the nasal cavity and paranasal sinuses (sinonasal cancer) are relatively uncommon, accounting for fewer than 1% of all cases of cancer. Fewer than 4100 people in the United States are diagnosed with these neoplasms each year.[1] The incidence of sinonasal cancer in the United States is about 0.75 cases per 100,000 individuals per year.[2] The incidence is higher in some regions outside the United States, including Japan and South Africa.[3] Tumors of the maxillary sinus are twice as common as those of the nasal cavity, and tumors of the ethmoid, sphenoid, and frontal sinuses are extremely rare. Sinonasal neoplasms are twice as common in men as in women.

In general, sinonasal neoplasms present a difficult therapeutic challenge. Such tumors have a distinctive pattern of spread, and most have an indolent clinical course. However, as a consequence of their rarity, clinical experience with sinonasal tumors is limited and many are diagnosed at an advanced stage. The problem of advanced stage is compounded by the proximity of primary tumors to critical structures (e.g., the eye, brain, and cranial nerves) and by esthetic considerations that complicate radical surgical resection and delivery of radiation treatment.

The clinical presentation of epithelial neoplasms originating in the nasal cavity or paranasal sinuses, the natural history of these lesions, treatment options, and patient outcomes are summarized in this chapter. Other types of tumors that may arise in the nasal cavity or paranasal sinuses, for example, soft tissue sarcomas, osteogenic sarcomas, lymphomas, and plasmacytomas, are discussed in chapters devoted to those types of tumors.

ANATOMY
Nasal Cavity

The nasal cavity is divided into three regions: the nasal vestibule, the nasal cavity, and the olfactory region.[4]

The nasal vestibule is a triangular space situated anterior to the limen nasi and defined laterally by the alae nasi, medially by the membranous septum—the distal end of the cartilaginous septum—and columella nasi, and inferiorly by the adjacent floor of the nasal cavity. The nasal vestibule is covered by skin, and therefore lesions at this location are essentially squamous cell skin cancer.[5]

The nasal cavity (nasal fossa) begins at the limen nasi anteriorly, ends at the choana posteriorly, and extends from the hard palate inferiorly to the base of the skull superiorly. The lateral walls consist of thin bony structures with three shell-shaped projections (superior, middle, and inferior conchae or turbinates) into the nasal cavity. The septum divides the nasal cavity into right and left halves. The nasal cavity is connected with a number of structures.

The olfactory nerves penetrate the roof of the nasal cavity and the cribriform plate and innervate the superior nasal concha and the upper third of the septum. The superior nasal concha and the upper third of the septum are referred to as the olfactory region. The remainder of the cavity, the respiratory region, contains orifices connecting the nasal cavity with the paranasal sinuses. The superior meatus connects the nasal cavity with the posterior ethmoid air cells, the middle meatus connects the nasal cavity with the anterior and middle ethmoid air cells and the frontal sinus, and the inferior meatus connects the nasal cavity with the nasolacrimal duct. The sphenoid sinus drains into the nasal cavity through an opening in the anterior wall. Knowledge of nasal cavity anatomy facilitates comprehension of the pattern of spread of tumors of this region.

Paranasal Sinuses

The paranasal sinuses are air-filled outgrowths of the nasal cavity into a number of cranial bones. They are named according to the bones in which they are located (i.e., maxillary, ethmoid, frontal, and sphenoid sinuses). Mucosal secretions from these sinuses drain to the nasal cavity through orifices situated at the lateral wall of the nasal cavity (Fig. 7-1). The maxillary sinuses, the largest of the paranasal sinuses, are pyramid-shaped cavities located in the maxillae.[6] The base of each maxillary sinus forms the inferior part of the lateral wall of the nasal cavity. The roof of each maxillary sinus is formed by the floor of the orbit, which contains the infraorbital canal, and the floor of each maxillary sinus is composed of the

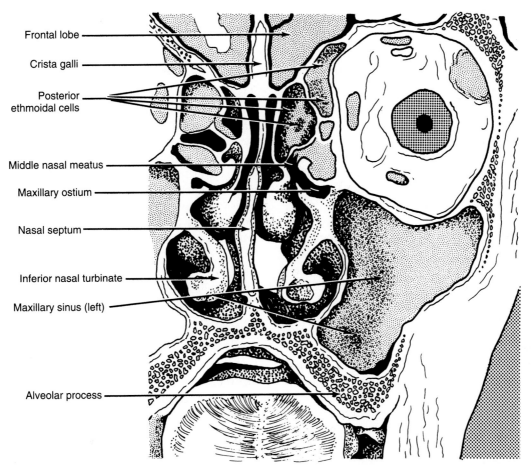

Frontal lobe

Crista galli

Posterior
ethmoidal cells

Middle nasal meatus

Maxillary ostium

Nasal septum

Inferior nasal turbinate

Maxillary sinus (left)

Alveolar process

Fig. 7-1 Diagram of a frontal section through the head illustrating the relationships of the nasal fossa to the paranasal sinuses, orbit, and hard palate.

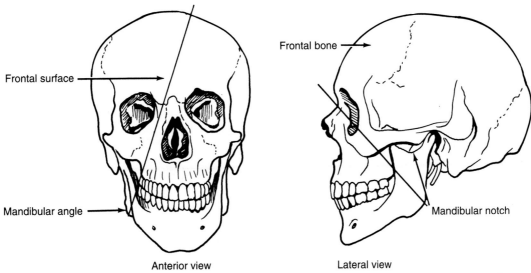

Frontal bone

Frontal surface

Mandibular angle

Mandibular notch

Anterior view

Lateral view

Fig. 7-2 Diagram of Ohngren's line, which divides the maxillary sinus into a superolateral suprastructure and an inferomedial infrastructure. The line passes through the medial canthus of the eye and the angle of the mandible.

alveolar process. The apex extends toward and commonly into the zygomatic bone. Maxillary sinus secretions drain into the middle meatus through the hiatus semilunaris. Ohngren's line divides the maxillary sinuses into the suprastructure and infrastructure (Fig. 7-2).

The ethmoid sinuses consist of several small cavities called *ethmoid air cells* within the ethmoidal labyrinth located below the anterior cranial fossa and between the nasal cavity and the orbit.[6] The ethmoid air cells are separated from the orbital cavity by a thin, porous bone called the *lamina papyracea* and from the anterior cranial fossa by a portion of the frontal bone, the fovea ethmoidalis. The ethmoid sinuses are divided into anterior, middle, and posterior groups of air cells. The middle cells open directly into the middle meatus. The anterior cells may drain indirectly into the middle meatus through the infundibulum. The posterior cells open directly into the superior meatus.

ETIOLOGY AND EPIDEMIOLOGY OF SINONASAL CANCER

In most patients diagnosed with sinonasal carcinoma, the cause is unclear. Several types of nasal cavity and paranasal sinus cancer are relatively more common in individuals engaged in certain occupations or exposed to certain chemical compounds. Adenocarcinoma of the nasal cavity and ethmoid sinus, for instance, occurs more often in carpenters and sawmill workers who are exposed to wood dust, and squamous cell carcinoma of the nasal cavity develops more often in nickel workers. Maxillary sinus carcinoma was associated with receipt of thorium oxide (Thorotrast), a radioactive thorium-containing contrast material used for radiographic study of the maxillary sinuses.[3,7,8] Occupational exposure in the production of chromium, mustard gas, isopropyl alcohol, or radium also increases the risk of sinonasal carcinoma.[2]

PREVENTION AND EARLY DETECTION

No specific recommendations regarding prevention and early detection of sinonasal tumors can be issued to the general population at present because the etiologic factors for these rare neoplasms are not well known. In general, carpenters, sawmill workers, and workers involved in the production of nickel, chromium, mustard gas, isopropyl alcohol, or radium should use appropriate face masks to reduce occupational exposure to potential carcinogens. Individuals in these professions who develop persistent nasal or sinus symptoms should see otolaryngologists to rule out sinonasal cancer.

NATURAL HISTORY

The clinical course of sinonasal cancer and the prognosis of affected patients depend on the anatomic site,

histologic type, and tumor stage. This section describes the natural history of sinonasal cancer by disease site.

Nasal Vestibule Tumors

Nasal vestibule carcinoma can spread by invasion of the upper lip, gingivolabial sulcus, premaxilla, or nasal cavity. Vertical invasion may result in septal (membranous or cartilaginous) perforation or destruction of alar cartilage. Lymphatic spread from nasal vestibule carcinoma is usually to the ipsilateral facial (buccinator and mandibular) and submandibular lymph nodes. Large lesions extending across the midline may spread to the contralateral facial or submandibular lymph nodes. In published series, the average incidence of nodal metastasis at diagnosis is about 5%.[9-11] Without elective treatment of the lymphatics, about 15% of patients have nodal relapse.[9-12] Hematogenous metastasis is rare.[11]

Nasal Cavity and Ethmoid Air Cell Tumors
Respiratory Region and Ethmoid Air Cells

Neoplasms originating in the respiratory region of the nasal cavity and the ethmoid air cells are squamous cell carcinoma, adenocarcinoma, and adenoid cystic carcinoma. Carcinoma may arise from inverted papilloma. The pattern of contiguous spread of carcinoma varies with the location of the primary lesion. Tumors arising in the upper nasal cavity and ethmoid air cells extend to the orbit through the lamina papyracea and to the anterior cranial fossa through the cribriform plate or grow through the nasal bone to the subcutaneous tissue and skin. Lateral-wall primary tumors invade the maxillary antrum, ethmoid air cells, orbit, pterygopalatine fossa, and nasopharynx. Primary tumors of the floor of the nasal cavity and lower septum may invade the palate and maxillary antrum. Spreading also may occur through perineural spaces; this phenomenon is most often seen in adenoid cystic carcinoma.

Lymphatic spread is rare in the case of primary tumors of the respiratory region. In a series at The University of Texas M.D. Anderson Cancer Center of 51 patients with such primary tumors, only one patient had palpable subdigastric lymphadenopathy at diagnosis.[13] Of the 36 patients who did not undergo elective lymphatic irradiation, only two (6%) experienced subdigastric nodal relapse. Hematogenous dissemination is also rare. In the M.D. Anderson Cancer Center series, for example, distant metastasis to bone, brain, or liver occurred in 4 of 51 patients.[13]

Olfactory Region

The olfactory region is the site of origin of esthesioneuroblastoma and, occasionally, adenocarcinoma. Esthesioneuroblastoma is a tumor of neural-crest origin first reported by Berger and Luc[14] in 1924 as "esthesioneuroepithelioma olfactif." Since that time, the tumor has been given a variety of names, including *olfactory neuroblastoma, esthesioneurocytoma,* and, most commonly, *esthesioneuroblastoma.* This very rare tumor constitutes approximately 3% of all intranasal neoplasms. About 250 cases were reported in the literature between 1924 and 1990.[15] Esthesioneuroblastoma typically consists of round, oval, or fusiform cells containing neurofibrils with pseudorosette formation and diffusely increased microvascularity.[16] Perivascular palisading of cells can be observed in the absence of pseudorosette formation. The route of contiguous spread of esthesioneuroblastoma is similar to that of ethmoidal carcinoma. In a 1979 review of 97 cases by Elkon and colleagues,[17] the incidence of lymph node involvement at diagnosis was 11%, and the incidence of distant metastasis at diagnosis was 1%.

Maxillary Sinus Tumors

The most common maxillary sinus cancer is squamous cell carcinoma, and the second most common is adenoid cystic carcinoma. Other histologic types arising in the maxillary sinus are adenocarcinoma, mucoepidermoid carcinoma, undifferentiated cancer, and occasionally, malignant melanoma.

The pattern of spread of maxillary sinus cancer varies somewhat according to the site of origin within the antrum. Neoplasms of the suprastructure tend to spread into the nasal cavity, ethmoid air cells, orbit, pterygopalatine fossa, infratemporal fossa, and base of skull. It is sometimes difficult to differentiate tumors originating from the infrastructure from those of the upper gum and hard palate. Neoplasms of the infrastructure tend to spread into the palate, alveolar process, gingivobuccal sulcus, soft tissue of the cheek, nasal cavity, masseter muscle, pterygopalatine space, and pterygoid fossa.

Overall, clinical lymphadenopathy is relatively uncommon at diagnosis in patients with tumors of the maxillary sinus. In an M.D. Anderson Cancer Center series, only 6 (8%) of 73 patients had palpable lymphadenopathy at diagnosis.[18] The incidence of nodal spread, however, varied with the histologic type: 17% (5 of 29) for patients with squamous cell or poorly differentiated carcinoma vs. 4% (1 of 27) for patients with adenocarcinoma, adenoid cystic carcinoma, or mucoepidermoid carcinoma. The incidence of subclinical spread, reflected in the rate of nodal relapse without elective neck treatment, also varied with histologic type: 38% (9 of 24) for patients with squamous cell or poorly differentiated carcinoma vs. 8% (2 of 26) for patients with adenocarcinoma, adenoid cystic carcinoma, or mucoepidermoid carcinoma. The cumulative incidence of nodal involvement (gross and microscopic) for patients with squamous cell and poorly differentiated

carcinoma was thus about 30%.[18] Ipsilateral subdigastric and submandibular nodes are the most frequently involved. Hematogenous spread is rather uncommon.

CLINICAL MANIFESTATIONS, EVALUATION, AND STAGING
Nasal Vestibule Tumors

Small carcinomas of the nasal vestibule usually present as asymptomatic plaques or nodules, often with crusting and scabbing. Advanced lesions may fill the vestibule or extend beyond it and may cause pain, bleeding, or ulceration. Large ulcerated lesions may become infected, leading to severe tenderness that hinders complete clinical assessment.

Contiguous spread is best detected by bimanual palpation and examination through a nasal speculum or fiberoptic telescope. Local anesthesia and decongestion of nasal mucosa facilitate assessment of contiguous extension. Early buccinator and submandibular nodal involvement are also best discovered by bimanual palpation. Nasal vestibule carcinoma is staged according to the American Joint Committee on Cancer (AJCC) tumor-nodes-metastasis classification system for the skin (described in Chapter 5).

Nasal Cavity and Ethmoid Air Cell Tumors
Carcinoma

Clinical manifestations. The presenting symptoms and signs of nasal cavity tumors usually consist of chronic unilateral nasal discharge, nasal ulcer, nasal obstruction, anterior headache, and intermittent epistaxis. The similarity between these symptoms and signs and those of nasal polyps often leads to a delay in diagnosis because many patients have a history of treatment for nasal polyps. In 45 patients with nasal cavity tumors referred to the M.D. Anderson Cancer Center between 1969 and 1985, the first symptom or sign was nasal obstruction in 23 patients (51%) and epistaxis in 7 (16%); the remaining 15 patients had a variety of symptoms, including nasal ulcer, discharge, tenderness, facial swelling, and pain.[13]

Additional symptoms and signs develop as the lesion enlarges, and their nature depends on the pattern of spread. Invasion of the orbital cavity, for instance, may produce a palpable medial orbital mass, proptosis, and diplopia. Obstruction of the nasolacrimal duct causes epiphora. Involvement of the olfactory region may produce anosmia (loss of the sense of smell) and expansion of the bridge of the nose. Extension through the cribriform plate results in frontal headache.

The presenting symptoms and signs of ethmoid air cell tumors are sinus ache and referred pain to the nasal or retrobulbar region, subcutaneous nodule at the inner canthus, nasal obstruction, nasal discharge, diplopia, and proptosis.

Evaluation and staging. Physical assessment to determine the extent of nasal cavity and ethmoid air cell tumors should include fiberoptic examination of the nasal cavity and nasopharynx after mucosal decongestion and application of topical anesthesia; evaluation of cranial nerves (particularly cranial nerves III, IV, V, and VI); and palpation of the nose bridge, cheek, and medial orbital cavity. Computed tomography (CT) or, preferably, magnetic resonance imaging (MRI) is essential to determine the disease extent and invasion of adjacent structures (e.g., orbital cavity and anterior cranial fossa).

The AJCC has not issued a staging system for nasal cavity tumors. The classification system proposed by the University of Florida[19] is simple and, therefore, can be use in the interim. In this system, stage I represents lesions limited to the nasal fossa, stage II represents lesions extending to adjacent sites (i.e., paranasal sinuses, skin, orbit, pterygomaxillary fossa, and nasopharynx), and stage III represents lesions extending beyond these structures.[19]

Tumors of the lateral wall and floor of the nasal cavity tend to be diagnosed at more advanced stages. Among patients with nasal cavity tumors referred to the M.D. Anderson Cancer Center between 1969 and 1985, 3 (21%) of 14 patients with septal lesions and 20 (65%) of 31 patients with lateral wall or floor lesions had disease extension beyond the nasal cavity (stages II and III).[13]

The T-stage description in the 1997 AJCC staging system for ethmoid sinus neoplasms,[20] which is based on clinical and radiologic evidence of involvement of various adjoining anatomic structures, is the following:

T1   Tumor confined to the ethmoid with or without bone erosion

T2   Tumor extends into the nasal cavity

T3   Tumor extends to the anterior orbit and/or maxillary sinus

T4   Tumor with intracranial extension, orbital extension including apex, involving sphenoid, and/or frontal sinus and/or skin of external nose

Esthesioneuroblastoma

Because of the rarity of esthesioneuroblastoma, the natural history of this disease was not well known until Elkon and colleagues[17] conducted a thorough literature review of the characteristics of 97 patients reported between 1969 and 1977. These authors found the age distribution to be bimodal, with a first peak incidence occurring between 11 and 20 years and a second, higher peak incidence occurring between 51 and 60 years. There is a slight preponderance for women.

The most common presenting symptoms are nasal obstruction and epistaxis. Spaulding and colleagues[21] found that anosmia can precede diagnosis by many years. Other symptoms include symptoms related to contiguous disease extension into the orbit (proptosis, visual field defects, orbital pain, and epiphora), paranasal

sinuses (medial canthus mass and facial swelling) and anterior cranial fossa (headache) and manifestations of inappropriate antidiuretic hormone secretion.

The recommended physical evaluation and staging work-up for esthesioneuroblastoma are similar to those for nasal cavity tumors. The commonly used staging system, proposed by Kadish and colleagues,[16] is as follows:

Stage A   Disease confined to the nasal cavity

Stage B   Disease confined to the nasal cavity and one or more paranasal sinuses

Stage C   Disease extending beyond the nasal cavity and paranasal sinuses, which includes involvement of the orbit, base of skull or intracranial cavity, or cervical lymph nodes or distant metastasis

The stage distribution at diagnosis for the 97 patients reviewed by Elkon and colleagues[17] was as follows: stage A, 30%; stage B, 42%; and stage C, 28%. Of the 22 patients with stage C disease, 9 had orbital involvement, 6 had invasion of the cribriform plate or cranial fossa, 11 had palpable neck nodes, and only 1 patient had distant metastasis.

Maxillary Sinus Tumors

Maxillary sinus tumors tend to have an indolent course and therefore are usually diagnosed at advanced stages. Of the 73 patients referred to the M.D. Anderson Cancer Center for treatment between 1969 and 1985, for example, 26 (36%) sought medical attention because of symptoms and signs induced by disease extension to the premaxillary region such as facial swelling, pain, or paresthesia of the cheek. Twenty patients (27%) had symptoms related to tumor spread to the nasal cavity (e.g., epistaxis, nasal discharge, or nasal obstruction), and 19 patients (26%) had symptoms related to tumor spread to the oral cavity (e.g., ill-fitting denture, alveolar or palatal mass, or unhealed tooth socket after extraction). Five patients (7%) presented with symptoms and signs of orbital invasion, such as proptosis, diplopia, impaired vision, or orbital pain.[18]

Physical examination should include assessment of the oral and nasal cavities, palpation of the cheek, evaluation of eye movement and function, and assessment of the trigeminal nerve, particularly the branches of V_2 (infraorbital nerve, anterior superior alveolar nerve, posterior superior alveolar nerve, and greater palatine nerve). Biopsy with a Caldwell-Luc operation should be avoided because this can result in numbness of the incisor teeth and upper lip. CT or, preferably, MRI is essential to determine the disease extent and invasion of adjacent structures (e.g., orbital cavity and infratemporal, pterygopalatine, and anterior cranial fossae).

The T-stage description in the 1997 AJCC staging system,[20] which is based on clinical and radiologic evidence of involvement of various adjoining anatomic structures, is the following:

TX Primary tumor cannot be assessed

T0 No evidence of primary tumor

Tis Carcinoma in situ

T1 Tumor limited to the antral mucosa with no erosion or destruction of bone

T2 Tumor causing bone erosion or destruction, except for the posterior antral wall, including extension into the hard palate and/or the middle nasal meatus

T3 Tumor invades any of the following: bone of the posterior wall of maxillary sinus, subcutaneous tissues, skin of cheek, floor or medial wall of orbit, infratemporal fossa, pterygoid plates, ethmoid sinuses

T4 Tumor invades orbital contents beyond the floor or medial wall including any of the following: the orbital apex, cribriform plate, base of skull, nasopharynx, sphenoid, frontal sinuses

Of the 73 patients with maxillary sinus tumors referred to the M.D. Anderson Cancer Center between 1969 and 1985, 3 had T1 tumors, 16 had T2 tumors, 32 had T3 tumors, and 22 had T4 tumors.

PRIMARY THERAPY
Nasal Vestibule Tumors

Radiation therapy is generally preferred over surgery for carcinoma of the nasal vestibule because radiation produces a better cosmetic outcome. Depending on the location and size of the primary lesion, radiation therapy can be accomplished by using external-beam irradiation, brachytherapy, or a combination of the two techniques. Cartilage invasion per se is not a contraindication for radiation therapy because the risk of necrosis is low with fractionated irradiation.[22]

Surgery can yield a high control rate with excellent cosmetic results in selected small superficial lesions. The rare cases of large primary tumors with extensive tissue destruction and distortion are best managed by resection in combination with preoperative or postoperative radiation therapy. Experienced prosthodontists can design custom-made nasal prostheses.

Of the 32 patients with newly diagnosed nasal vestibule carcinoma who received primary radiation therapy at the M.D. Anderson Cancer Center between 1967 and 1984, 11 patients with small tumors were given interstitial brachytherapy, and the remaining 21 patients were given external-beam radiation therapy to the primary tumor.[12] In 14 of these 21 patients, the draining lymphatics were also irradiated.[12] Local control was achieved in 11 of 11 patients treated with brachytherapy and 20 of 21 patients treated with external-beam therapy, resulting in an overall local primary-tumor control rate of 97%. None of the 11 patients with well-delineated small lesions treated with brachytherapy

had a nodal recurrence. Four of nine patients who underwent external-beam radiation therapy to the primary lesion (including two patients who also had undergone radiation therapy to the facial lymphatics) experienced a neck node recurrence. In contrast, none of 12 patients who received local treatment with elective neck node irradiation had nodal failure.

Table 7-1 summarizes the results of relatively large series of patients with nasal vestibule tumors treated with radiation therapy. Selected patients in the M.D. Anderson Cancer Center and University of Florida series received brachytherapy,[12,23] whereas all patients in the Princess Margaret Hospital series underwent external-beam irradiation.[11] Several conclusions can be reached from these findings. First, brachytherapy or external-beam irradiation cures, on average, about 90% of patients with nasal vestibule lesions smaller than 2 cm. Second, given in adequate doses, external-beam irradiation can control 70% to 80% of tumors 2 cm or larger. Third, the rate of occult nodal spread is extremely low in lesions smaller than 2 cm but can be as high as about 40% in the case of larger primary tumors. Finally, the incidence of severe late complications is low with proper radiation technique and fractionation schedules.

Nasal Cavity and Ethmoid Air Cell Tumors
Carcinoma

Radiation therapy and surgery are equally effective in curing stage I lesions of the respiratory region. Therefore, the choice of therapy depends on the size and location of the tumor and the expected cosmetic outcome. For example, posterior nasal septum lesions are easily treated with surgery without cosmetic impairment. In contrast, small (≤ 1.5 cm) anterior-inferior septal lesions are best treated with interstitial brachytherapy ^{192}Ir wire implant to avoid deformity from surgical removal of the anterior nasal septum. Also for cosmetic reasons, external-beam irradiation is the preferred treatment for lateral wall lesions extending to the ala nasi. Stage II and operable stage III neoplasms of the nasal cavity are best treated with surgery and, in most cases, postoperative irradiation.

Nasal cavity tumors—the M.D. Anderson Cancer Center experience. Between 1969 and 1985, 51 patients with carcinoma of the nasal cavity proper were referred to the M.D. Anderson Cancer Center, of whom 45 received curative treatment and were followed for 2.8 to 16.8 years (median, 11 years).[13] Eighteen patients received radiation therapy only (interstitial brachytherapy in 5 and external-beam therapy in 13), and 27 underwent surgery and postoperative radiation therapy. The site of origin of the primary lesion was the nasal septum in 14 patients and the lateral wall or floor of the cavity in 31 patients. All 14 lesions of the nasal septum were squamous cell carcinoma. Of the 31 nonseptal

---

TABLE 7-1

Reported Local and Regional Control Rates for Nasal Vestibule Carcinomas Treated with Definitive Radiation Therapy

Institution and Reference	Local Control	Regional Control	Late Complications
M.D. Anderson Cancer Center[12]	Brachytherapy: 11/11 External-beam radiation therapy: 20/21 (95%) TOTAL: 31/32 (97%)	Small lesions: 11/11 Large lesions: ELI: 12/12 (100%) No ELI: 5/9 (56%) TOTAL: 28/32 (88%)	Osteonecrosis at area of hot spot: 1 Nosebleeds: 1
University of Florida[23]	Brachytherapy: 9/9 External-beam radiation therapy: 8/11 (73%) Combination: 12/16 (75%) TOTAL: 29/36 (81%)	ELI: 3/3 No ELI: 23/27 (85%); 4 relapses were salvaged TOTAL: 26/30* (87%)	Transient soft tissue necrosis after implants: 4 Nasal stenosis: 1
Princess Margaret Hospital[11]	< 2 cm (n = 34): 97%[†] ≥ 2 cm (n = 16) and size not recorded (n = 6): 57%[†] • < 55 Gy/5 wk: 30%[‡] • ≥ 55 Gy/5 wk: 82%[‡]	No ELI: 51/54 (94%) (2 patients presented with positive nodes)	Osteonecrosis: 2 (1 resulting in fistula) Nasal stenosis: 2 Massive epistaxis: 1

ELI, Elective lymphatic irradiation.
*Eligible for 2-year follow-up.
[†]5-Year actuarial rates.
[‡]2.5 to 3 Gy per fraction.

---

nasal cavity tumors, 16 were squamous cell carcinoma, 9 were adenocarcinoma, 5 were adenoid cystic carcinoma, and 1 was undifferentiated cancer.

Table 7-2 shows the pattern of failure in this series of patients. All 14 patients with carcinoma of the nasal septum had the disease controlled (10 after initial therapy and 4 after salvage therapy). Nine of 31 patients with lesions of the lateral wall or floor died of disease—five of uncontrolled local disease, two of distant metastases, and two of both. The disease-specific survival rates at 5 and 10 years were 83% and 80%, respectively. The corresponding overall survival rates were 69% and 58%, respectively.

Two patients underwent required orbital exenteration, and two others had radiation injury to the cornea

and optic pathway. Other infrequent side effects were bone necrosis, dental decay, nasal stenosis, and septal perforation. However, these complications occurred predominantly in patients treated before implementation of individual portal shaping.

This study indicated that the prognosis of patients with nasal cavity carcinoma was better than that of patients with maxillary sinus cancer treated during the same era (see the section on "Maxillary Sinus Tumors"). In addition, the study showed that carcinoma of the nasal septum was diagnosed at an earlier stage than carcinoma of the lateral wall and nasal floor so excellent control could be achieved by primary radiation therapy. When accessible, interstitial brachytherapy might be the

---

TABLE 7-2

Patterns of Failure of Nasal Cavity Carcinomas

Timing of Relapse and Location of Primary Tumor	TYPE OF RELAPSE				
	Number of Patients	Local	Nodal	Local and Distant	Distant Only
After primary therapy					
Septum	14	2	2	0	0
Lateral wall or floor	31	9	0	1	2
After salvage therapy					
Septum	4	0	0	0	0
Lateral wall or floor	5	1	0	1	0

Modified from Ang KK, Jiang GL, Frankenthaler RA, et al. *Radiother Oncol* 1992;24:163-168.

treatment of choice in patients with early-stage carcinoma of the nasal septum.

Nasal cavity tumors—outcomes in large series. Comparing findings in the literature on nasal cavity lesions is difficult because the patient populations vary among the reported series. Table 7-3[13,24-26] summarizes the results of relatively large series focusing on nasal cavity tumors. Local–regional control rates obtained with definitive irradiation in patients with tumors confined to the nasal cavity and with combined surgery and radiation therapy in patients with more advanced disease range from 60% to 80%. The control rate is thus higher for nasal cavity lesions than for maxillary sinus tumors (as discussed later in this chapter). The incidence of isolated regional recurrence in patients who had no palpable lymphadenopathy at diagnosis and did not receive elective nodal treatment was about 5% in the M.D. Anderson Cancer Center series. Treatment morbidity was proportional to extent of disease, which dictated the magnitude of surgical resection and the target volume for radiation therapy. The most frequent complications were soft tissue necrosis, nasal stenosis, and visual impairment (see Table 7-3).

Ethmoid air cell tumors—the M.D. Anderson Cancer Center experience. Between 1969 and 1985, 17 patients with carcinoma of the ethmoid air cells were referred to the M.D. Anderson Cancer Center for therapy. Nine patients received primary radiation therapy, and eight underwent surgical resection preceded (two patients) or followed (six patients) by radiation therapy. None of the patients received elective nodal treatment.

Results were evaluated with regard to disease control, survival, and tolerance. At the last follow-up, 11 patients had no evidence of disease, 4 patients had developed local recurrence, and 2 patients had distant metastasis (one of whom experienced regional relapse that was subsequently controlled by nodal dissection and postoperative radiation therapy). The 5-year actuarial local control, overall survival, and relapse-free survival rates for this group of patients were 70%, 55%, and 61%, respectively. Treatment complications were vision impairment (three patients), frontal lobe necrosis (two patients), bone necrosis (one patient), and nasal stenosis (one patient).

Esthesioneuroblastoma

Literature overview. Because of the low incidence of esthesioneuroblastoma, it is not possible to define the optimal therapy on the basis of prospective studies. Elkon and colleagues[17] reviewed case reports of patients treated before 1977 (see the following paragraph). They found that single-modality therapy with either radiation therapy or surgery yielded ultimate local–regional control rates of more than 90% for stage A lesions, although several patients had to undergo salvage therapy for local or regional relapse. The optimal therapy for stage B disease is unclear, partly because this stage represents a heterogeneous group of tumors. Combinations of surgery and radiation therapy seem to have a slight advantage for this patient subset. For patients with stage C lesions, the evidence suggests better results from the combination of surgery and radiation therapy. The available data do not justify routine

---

TABLE 7-3

Outcomes in Patients with Nasal Cavity Tumors Treated with Radiation, Surgery, or Both

Institution and Reference	Treatment: Number of Patients	Survival	Late Complications: Number of Patients
M.D. Anderson Cancer Center[13]	Radiation therapy only: 18 Radiation therapy followed by surgery: 2 Surgery followed by radiation therapy: 25	5-year actuarial: 75% All 14 nasal septum lesions and 22/31 tumors of lateral wall or floor were controlled	Radiation-induced blindness: 2 Surgical blindness: 2 Maxilla necrosis: 2 Stenosis/perforation: 3
Roswell Park Memorial Institute[24]*	Radiation therapy only: 30 Surgery only: 13 Surgery and radiation therapy: 14	5-year actuarial: 67% Patients with well-differentiated squamous cell carcinoma had the best outcome	Not presented
University of Puerto Rico[25]*	Radiation therapy only: 34 Surgery only: 6	5-year overall: 56%	Not presented
Mallinckrodt Institute of Radiology[26]*	Radiation therapy only: 28 Radiation therapy followed by surgery: 18 Surgery followed by radiation therapy: 10	5-year actuarial: 52% Survival not significantly affected by histology Neck relapse occurred in 10/52 with N0 disease	Complications (soft tissue necrosis, cataract, synechiae, otitis media) requiring surgery: 5

*Included patients with nasal vestibule carcinomas.

TABLE 7-4

Outcomes in Patients with Esthesioneuroblastoma by Stage and Treatment Modality

		PATIENT OUTCOME (NUMBER OF PATIENTS)				
Kadish Stage	Therapy	Local Recurrence	Nodal Relapse	Salvage with Subsequent RT or S	Distant Metastasis	Died of Disease
A	RT	2/5	1/5	3/3	0/5	0/5
(N= 24)	S	4/9	1*/9	4/4	0/9	0/9
	S + RT	1/10	2/10	2/2	1†/10	1/10
TOTALS	All	7/24 (29%)	4/24 (17%)	9/9	1/24 (4%)	1/24 (4%)
B	RT	1/7	2/7	0/1	0/7	3/7
(N= 33)	S	3/6	0/6	1/2	0/6	2/6
	S + RT	5/20	1/20	3/4	3/20	5/20
TOTALS	All	9/33 (27%)	3/33 (9%)	4/7	3/33 (9%)	10/33 (30%)
C	RT	3/5	0/5	0/0	1/5	4/5
(N= 21)	S	0/1	0/1	0/0	0/1	0/1
	S+RT‡	6/15	1/15	1/1	1/15	8/15
TOTALS	All	9/21 (43%)	1/21 (5%)	1/1	2/21 (10%)	12/21 (57%)

Modified from Elkon D, Hightower SI, Lim ML, et al. *Cancer* 1979;44:1087-1094.
RT, Radiation therapy; *S*, surgery.
*Along with local recurrence.
†Along with nodal relapse.
‡Site of relapse not specified in two patients.

elective nodal treatment because the incidence of isolated nodal relapse is less than 15%.

Table 7-4 summarizes the literature on patients with esthesioneuroblastoma treated by various modalities between 1969 and 1977, as compiled by Elkon and colleagues.[17] The treatment outcome of patients with stage A lesions was excellent. Although 42% of these patients developed local or regional recurrence after initial treatment, salvage therapy was successful in all nine patients in whom it was attempted. Consequently, only one of 24 patients with stage A tumors died of the disease (as a result of neck node recurrence and lung metastasis).

The prognosis of patients with stage B disease was also relatively good. The local–regional recurrence rate in patients with stage B tumors after initial therapy was not higher than that of patients with stage A lesions, but salvage therapy was less successful. Overall, 30% of patients with stage B tumors died of the disease.

About 60% of patients with stage C tumors died of the disease. It is important to note that most of these patients succumbed to local tumor progression. Distant metastasis is a rare failure pattern (≤ 10%) even in local–regionally advanced esthesioneuroblastoma.

Results of individual series. Several large series of patients with esthesioneuroblastoma have been reported in the past few years. Between 1957 and 1988, 21 patients were treated for esthesioneuroblastoma at the M.D. Anderson Cancer Center. Two patients had stage A disease, 13 had stage B disease, and 6 had stage C disease. Four patients underwent surgery, 5 received radiation therapy, and 12 received combined surgery

and irradiation. Five patients had local recurrence, three had regional failure, and one had distant metastasis. Salvage treatment was successful in two of five patients with local recurrence and in all three patients with regional relapse. At last follow-up, 17 (81%) of 21 patients had no evidence of disease. The median survival time for the group overall was 6.3 years. The 5-year actuarial overall survival and disease-specific survival rates were 78% and 84%, respectively.

Spaulding and colleagues[21] reported one of the largest single-institution series of patients with esthesioneuroblastoma. These authors retrospectively reviewed the records of 25 patients treated at the University of Virginia Medical Center between 1959 and 1986. Twenty-four patients had stage B or C tumors and were followed for 2 or more years after treatment. Treatment policy and technique had gradually evolved over the study period, with progressive introduction of craniofacial resections, complex field megavoltage radiation, and—for stage C disease—the addition of chemotherapy to radiation therapy and surgery. Therefore, patients were divided into two groups on the basis of treatment era for comparative analysis.

Group I consisted of 10 patients (six stage B and four stage C) treated between 1959 and 1975. Seven patients were treated with a combination of radiation therapy (40 to 60 Gy) and wide local excision, two received radiation therapy only (50 Gy and 55 Gy, respectively), and one received radiation therapy (23 Gy) with vincristine.

Group II consisted of 15 patients (one stage A, six stage B, and eight stage C) treated between 1976 and

1985. Five patients with stage B disease underwent preoperative radiation therapy (50 Gy) and craniofacial resection, and the other patient with stage B disease, who had a synchronous lung cancer, received cyclophosphamide, doxorubicin, and vincristine followed by radiation therapy (63.3 Gy). The treatment of patients with stage C disease was more varied: two underwent preoperative radiation therapy with 50 Gy or 55 Gy and craniofacial resection, one had subtotal excision followed by radiation therapy (56 Gy), and five underwent two to four cycles of chemotherapy (vincristine and cyclophosphamide) plus radiation therapy (50 Gy) and craniofacial resection.

Among patients with stage B disease, those in groups I and II had identical local control (83%) and 2-year disease-specific survival (83%) rates. Among patients with stage C disease, however, group II patients had a higher local control rate (57% vs. 25%). Because salvage therapy for local recurrence was successful in several group II patients, the 5-year disease-specific survival rate was also higher in group II (~70% vs. 0%).

Although the series was relatively small, two important conclusions can be drawn from this retrospective analysis. First, extensive craniofacial resection does not seem to confer a major advantage over wide local excision for patients with stage B lesions. Second, the addition of chemotherapy to craniofacial resection and radiation therapy for patients with stage C tumors may yield a higher disease-specific survival rate than that achievable with wide local excision and radiation therapy.

Maxillary Sinus Tumors

In patients presenting with T1 or T2 tumors of the infrastructure, surgery alone is often sufficient for local control. Depending on the location and size of the lesion, surgery can in most cases be limited to a partial maxillectomy. For patients with more advanced but resectable disease who are fit to undergo resection, the combination of surgery and radiation therapy, usually postoperative radiation therapy, is the treatment of choice. Radical maxillectomy with or without orbital exenteration is necessary in most of these patients. Primary

radiation therapy should be reserved for patients who are medically inoperable or who refuse radical surgery.

Postoperative Radiation Therapy

According to published series, the combination of surgery and irradiation in patients with maxillary sinus tumors yields 5-year local control rates of 53% to 78% and 5-year survival rates of 39% to 64%.[27-36] These rates are better than those achieved with surgery or radiation therapy alone.

In a 1989 report, outcomes of the 73 patients with maxillary sinus carcinoma who underwent postoperative radiation therapy at the M.D. Anderson Cancer Center between 1969 and October 1985 were analyzed. The AJCC T-stage distribution was as follows: T1, 3 patients; T2, 16 patients; T3, 32 patients; and T4, 22 patients. Only six patients had palpable nodal disease at diagnosis. All patients underwent partial or radical maxillectomy followed by radiation therapy delivered using a wedged-pair or three-field technique. The radiation doses ranged from 50 to 60 Gy except in three patients who received lower doses. Elective nodal irradiation was given to 17 patients. The results of this retrospective study are presented in Tables 7-5 through 7-8.

Several conclusions can be drawn from this retrospective analysis. First, local recurrence and distant metastasis were the major causes of death. Second, the local recurrence rate was significantly higher in the presence of perineural invasion by the primary tumor (36% vs. 10%). Third, the nodal relapse rate in patients with squamous cell and undifferentiated carcinoma who did not undergo elective lymphatic irradiation was more than 30%. (This observation was confirmed by data from two more recently reported series.[37,38]) Finally, major complications occurred predominantly in patients treated during the earlier part of the study period, when large wedged-pair portals were used, radiation was administered in fractions of greater than 2 Gy, and significant dose heterogeneity existed within the target volume. Survival rates from combined treatment with surgery and postoperative radiation therapy are shown in Figure 7-3.

Several modifications to treatment policy were introduced in August 1989 on the basis of these findings.

TABLE 7-5

Patterns of Failure in 73 Patients with Maxillary Sinus Carcinoma

	SITE OF RELAPSE					
Timing of Relapse	Local	Nodal	Local and Nodal	Distant Metastasis	Local and Distant Metastasis	Nodal and Distant Metastasis
After initial therapy	10	10	1	8	3	1
After salvage therapy	11	0	1	11	4	1

Modified from Jiang GL, Ang KK, Peters LJ, et al. *Radiother Oncol* 1991;21:193-200.

TABLE 7-6

Incidence of Nodal Metastasis by Histologic Type in 73 Patients with Maxillary Sinus Carcinoma*

Histologic Type	Number of Patients Who Presented with Positive Neck Nodes	Number of Patients Who Developed Nodal Recurrence
Squamous cell carcinoma	5/23	6/18
Undifferentiated tumor	0/6	3/6
Adenocarcinoma	1/6	1/5
Adenoid cystic carcinoma	0/19	1/19
Mucoepidermoid carcinoma	0/2	0/2

Modified from Jiang GL, Ang KK, Peters LJ, et al. *Radiother Oncol* 1991;21:193-200.
*Excludes 17 patients who received elective neck irradiation.

TABLE 7-7

Influence of Disease and Treatment Variables on Treatment Outcome in 73 Patients with Maxillary Sinus Carcinoma

Variable	Number of Patients	5-Year Local Control (%)	5-Year Nodal Control (%)*	5-Year Distant Metastasis (%)	5-Year Relapse-Free Survival (%)	5-Year Disease-Specific Survival (%)
PATHOLOGIC T STAGE[†]						
T1+2	12	91	71	17	64	75
T3	28	77	80	25	57	69
T4	29	65	93	37	44	59
N STAGE						
N0	67	74	84	27[‡]	53	66[‡]
N1-2	6	67	82	48[§]	33	33
HISTOLOGIC TYPE						
Squamous cell carcinoma	36	62	86	17[‡]	49	53
Undifferentiated	9	89	67	50	53	42
Adenocarcinoma	6	80	67	39	42	60
Adenoid cystic carcinoma	20	82	94	31	60	84
Mucoepidermoid	2	(2/2)	(2/2)	(0/2)	(2/2)	(2/2)
NERVE INVASION[†]						
No	29	90[‡]	86	20	74[‡]	78
Yes	42	64	80	36	37	57
MARGIN OF RESECTION[†]						
Negative	54	74	86	17	58	66
Positive	17	77	76	32	38	66
ELECTIVE NODAL RADIATION						
No	50	77	80	31[‡]	51	58
Yes	17	61	100	0	61	68

Modified from Jiang GL, Ang KK, Peters LJ, et al. *Radiother Oncol* 1991;21:193-200.
*Including salvage treatment.
[†]Excluding patients for whom pathology reports were not complete.
[‡]Significant at 0.05 level.
[§]Including 11 patients who did not receive elective neck treatment and developed nodal recurrence.

TABLE 7-8

Type and Incidence of Treatment Complications Occurring in 73 Patients with Maxillary Sinus Carcinoma

Complication	Number of Patients (%)	Latent Period: Range in Months After Radiation Therapy
Ipsilateral blindness*	13 (30)	1-36
Bilateral blindness	4 (5)	13-36
Brain necrosis	5 (7)	5-73
Bone necrosis requiring debridement	4 (5)	1-17
Soft tissue necrosis/fistula	2 (3)	17-74
Trismus	9 (12)	0-4
Pituitary insufficiency	3 (4)	60-72
Hearing loss	3 (4)	3-48

Modified from Jiang GL, Ang KK, Peters LJ, et al. *Radiother Oncol* 1991;21:193-200.
*Assessed in 44 patients who did not undergo ipsilateral enucleation.

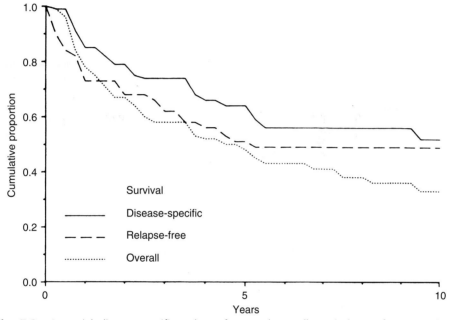

Fig. 7-3 Actuarial disease-specific, relapse-free, and overall survival rate for 73 patients treated by surgery and postoperative irradiation for cancer of the maxillary sinus. (From Jiang GL, Ang KK, Peters LJ, et al. *Radiother Oncol* 1991;21:193-200.)

First, radiation portals were designed to more generously encompass the base of the skull, including the trigeminal ganglion, in patients with evidence of perineural invasion and patients with adenoid cystic carcinoma. Second, elective irradiation was delivered to the ipsilateral upper neck nodes in patients with T2 to T4 squamous cell or undifferentiated carcinoma. Third, measures were taken to improve dose distribution within the target volume; these included the use of a water-filled balloon to reduce the size of the air cavity.

In 1996 the first interim analysis was undertaken to assess how the change in the treatment policy affected patient outcome. Patients who were treated between 1969 and 1993 were studied. Of a total of 115 patients, 90 received treatment before and 25 received treatment after implementation of the revised treatment policy. The two groups were balanced with regard to age, T and N stage, histologic subtype, surgical margins (proportion of patients with microscopic residual disease: 23% vs. 20%), and median nominal radiation dose. However, the group treated under the revised treatment policy had a lower proportion of women and, obviously, a shorter follow-up time (medians, 18 months vs. 47 months). The two groups had identical 4-year actuarial local control rates (76%). Among patients with squamous cell or undifferentiated carcinoma, the regional control rate was slightly higher among patients who received elective nodal irradiation (revised treatment policy) than among those who did not (4-year actuarial regional control rates, 90% vs. 80%). Patients treated under the revised policy had a slightly higher 4-year actuarial relapse-free survival rate (68% vs. 55%) and a slightly lower 4-year actuarial incidence of distant metastasis (10% vs. 24%). The most striking difference between the two groups was in the incidence of severe complications. None of the 25 patients treated under the revised policy developed severe complications, whereas the actuarial cumulative incidence of severe complications among patients treated under the earlier policy (see Table 7-8) was 15% at 1 year, 30% at 2 years, 38% at 3 years, and 40% at 4 years.

Primary Radiation Therapy

Compilation of data from the published literature reveals that in patients with maxillary sinus tumors, definitive radiation therapy yields 5-year local control rates of 22% to 39% and 5-year survival rates of 22% to 40%.[27,28,33,35,39-41]

Locally Advanced Disease

At the M.D. Anderson Cancer Center, a pilot study was designed to address the role of chemotherapy combined with radiation therapy in the treatment of patients with mostly advanced maxillary sinus cancer. Between 1969 and 1985, 23 patients (12 men and 11 women) who refused surgery or were medically unfit for surgical resection were enrolled in the study. The patients ranged in age from 23 to 75 years, with a median of 57 years. In 18 patients, chemotherapy consisted of intraarterial fluorouracil infusion delivered concurrently with radiation therapy at a dose of 4 to 6 mg/kg, 5 days a week for 2 to 4 weeks depending on the severity of acute reactions. The remaining five patients received induction chemotherapy consisting of bleomycin, fluorouracil, and cyclophosphamide administered intravenously (four patients) or bleomycin and cisplatin administered intraarterially (one patient). Although the acute reactions were severe, 14 of 18 patients were able to tolerate radiation doses of 60 to 61 Gy. The remaining four patients received 50 to 55 Gy delivered in 2-Gy fractions.

The 5-year overall survival and relapse-free survival rates were 18% and 35%, respectively. The 5-year rate of disease control above the clavicle was 39%. The incidences of local recurrence, nodal relapse, and distant metastasis as a function of T stage and histologic type are shown in Table 7-9. Of the 15 patients whose entire ipsilateral orbital content was encompassed in the radiation portals, two had corneal injury leading to vision impairment and eight had blindness as a result of retinal or optic nerve injury. One patient developed bilateral blindness as a consequence of optic chiasm injury. Bone necrosis occurred in three patients, trismus occurred in two patients, and pituitary insufficiency occurred in one patient.

The results of this trial are within the range of those achieved with radiation therapy alone. It can thus be

TABLE 7-9

Treatment Outcome by T Stage and Histologic Type in 17 Patients with Advanced Maxillary Sinus Carcinoma

Variable	Local Control	Nodal Control*	Distant Metastasis
T STAGE			
T2	0/1	0/1	0/1
T3	5/8	8/8	2/8
T4	3/8	7/8	0/8
HISTOLOGIC TYPE			
Squamous cell carcinoma	7/14	12/14	2/14
Undifferentiated cancer	0/1	1/1	0/1
Adenocarcinoma	1/1	1/1	0/1
Adenoid cystic carcinoma	0/1	1/1	0/1

*All 17 patients had no palpable nodes at presentation and did not receive elective neck irradiation.

concluded that administration of intraarterial fluorouracil during radiation therapy as used in this pilot study does not improve the rate of control above the clavicle.

Future Directions

Studies are ongoing that address the role of induction chemotherapy (e.g., intraarterial administration of cisplatin and fluorouracil or combinations of newer agents) given before or during radiation therapy in improving local–regional control or reducing the extent of surgery and thus leading to better functional and cosmetic outcomes in patients with maxillary sinus tumors. The roles of conformal and intensity-modulated radiation therapy in improving local control and preserving organ structure and function also are being investigated.

TECHNIQUES OF IRRADIATION

The general radiation therapy policies and techniques currently used at the M.D. Anderson Cancer Center are presented in this section. All radiation therapy is administered in 2-Gy fractions at five fractions per week unless otherwise specified. More detailed information has been presented elsewhere.[42]

Nasal Vestibule Tumors
Radiation Target Volume and Dose

Small (≤1.5 cm), circumscribed, well-differentiated nasal vestibule tumors are treated with a therapeutic dose of 60 to 66 Gy to the primary tumor with a 1- to

2-cm margin. A small portal reduction is sometimes made after 50 Gy. Alternatively, accessible lesions can be treated with brachytherapy with an ^{192}Ir wire implant to 60 to 65 Gy delivered over 5 to 7 days.

Larger (>1.5 cm) and all poorly differentiated nasal vestibule tumors without palpable lymphadenopathy are treated with irradiation of the primary tumor with margins of at least 2 to 3 cm (wider margins for infiltrative tumor) and irradiation of the bilateral facial nodes (the "mustache" area), submandibular nodes, and subdigastric nodes. When upper neck lymph node involvement is present at diagnosis, the lower neck nodes are also treated with elective irradiation. After an elective radiation dose of 50 Gy is reached, the radiation volume is reduced to cover the original gross disease with 1- to 2-cm margins to deliver a boost dose of 16 to 20 Gy by external beam. Alternatively, when the tumor is accessible, it is reasonable to deliver a boost dose of 20 to 25 Gy over about 2 days by low-dose-rate brachytherapy.

External-Beam Radiation Therapy Set-up

For external-beam irradiation, the patient is immobilized while lying supine with the head positioned slightly flexed so that the anterior surface of the maxilla is parallel to the top of the couch. This set-up facilitates irradiation of the primary lesion through a vertical appositional field matching with appositional portals to cover the facial lymphatics and with opposed lateral photon fields to cover the upper neck lymph nodes. Lower neck nodes are irradiated, when necessary, with an anterior field matched to the lateral upper neck field.

Radiation is usually administered using a combination of electrons and photons in a ratio of 4:1. Skin collimation is used to minimize scatter irradiation to the eye. For electron treatments, bolus material (beeswax) is applied to smooth the surface contour of the nose and fill the nares, thus improving dose homogeneity. The bolus is removed for photon treatments to achieve skin sparing.

Nasal Cavity and Ethmoid Air Cell Tumors
Radiation Target Volume and Dose

For primary radiation therapy for tumors of the nasal cavity or ethmoid air cells, the initial portals encompass the primary tumor with 2- to 3-cm margins. Once a dose of 50 Gy is reached, the margins are reduced to 1 to 2 cm, and an additional 16 to 20 Gy is delivered depending on the size of the tumor.

For postoperative radiation therapy, the initial target volume consists of the surgical bed with 1- to 2-cm margins, depending on the surgical pathology findings and the proximity of critical structures, to a dose of 54 Gy. A boost of 6 to 12 Gy is then given. The boost volume consists of areas at higher risk for recurrence, such as the regions of close or positive section margins or extensive

perineural invasion. Elective nodal irradiation is not routinely given.

For very selected nasal cavity carcinomas, for example, those of the anterior-inferior nasal septum, low-dose-rate brachytherapy may be appropriate. The dose schedule is 60 to 65 Gy given over 5 to 7 days.

The optimal radiation therapy dose-fractionation schedule for the treatment of esthesioneuroblastoma has not been well established. It seems reasonable to prescribe 60 Gy in 30 fractions for primary radiation therapy and 50 to 56 Gy in 25 to 28 fractions for postoperative radiation therapy.

External-Beam Radiation Therapy Set-up

For external-beam radiation therapy, patients are generally immobilized in a supine position with the head positioned such that the hard palate is perpendicular to the couch. An intraoral stent is used to open the mouth and depress the tongue out of the radiation fields. The tumor location and extent determine the appropriate portal arrangement. In general, for tumors located in the anterior lower half of the nasal cavity, anterior oblique wedged-pair photon fields are appropriate. For tumors of the posterior nasal fossa without extension to ethmoid air cells, opposed lateral fields may be more appropriate because these can avoid the optic pathway. For irradiation of the upper nasal cavity and ethmoidal neoplasms, a three-field technique[42] is best (Fig. 7-4). This set-up allows coverage of ethmoid air cells without delivery of high doses to the optic apparatus. CT-based treatment planning is necessary to determine the appropriate intersection angle between the two beams, the appropriate wedge angle, and the relative loading of the fields.

Maxillary Sinus Tumors
Radiation Target Volume and Dose

For postoperative radiation therapy for maxillary sinus carcinoma, the initial portals encompass the surgical bed with margins of 1 to 2 cm depending on the surgical pathology findings and the proximity of critical structures, generally to a dose of 54 Gy. The normal tissues of particular concern are the eye and the optic pathways. The cornea usually can be shielded in patients with limited involvement of the medial or inferior orbital wall to avoid vision impairment resulting from iatrogenic keratitis. If the tumor invades the orbital cavity but does not necessitate orbital exenteration, the lacrimal gland is shielded whenever possible to prevent the occurrence of painful dry eye. Cataract is no longer a major concern because it is relatively easy to correct this side effect.

The boost portals cover areas where the risk of recurrence is higher, such as regions of close or positive margins or extensive perineural invasion. The boost dose is generally an additional 6 to 12 Gy. Prudence dictates that

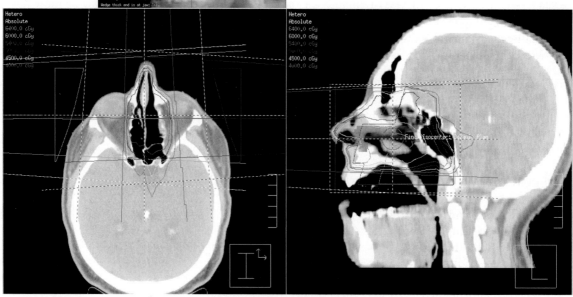

Fig. 7-4 A patient with a nasal cavity tumor who underwent endoscopic sinus surgery, including exploration of the left maxillary and ethmoid sinuses, before referral to our institution. A three-field technique was used to encompass the nasal cavity, left maxillary, and ethmoid sinus regions. *Top:* The typical three-field technique. Anteroposterior, right lateral, and left lateral are weighted 1:0.07:0.07, respectively. *Bottom:* Isodose lines are shown for the axial plane in the region of the optic chiasm and the midsagittal plane. A total of 60 Gy was delivered to the tumor bed after surgery. A reduction off the optic apparatus is made after 50 to 54 Gy to limit the dose to the optic nerves and chiasm to 54 Gy or less.

the contralateral optic nerve and optic chiasm be excluded from the volume receiving more than 54 Gy to minimize the risk of bilateral blindness. For tumors extending through the posterior ethmoid air cells to abut the optic chiasm, the risks and benefits of delivering a dose of up to 60 Gy, which is associated with a 5% to 10% risk of optic nerve injury, should be discussed with the patient.

The guidelines for primary radiation therapy for maxillary sinus carcinoma are, in general, similar to those for postoperative radiation therapy, and the total dose ranges from 66 to 70 Gy depending on the stage. Normal tissue doses to the eye and optic pathway as mentioned previously are generally applied to minimize complications.

Patients with squamous cell or poorly differentiated carcinoma presenting with no clinical evidence of lymphadenopathy receive elective irradiation of the ipsilateral submandibular and subdigastric nodes to a dose of 50 Gy. Patients in whom nodal dissection reveals multiple positive nodes or the presence of extracapsular extension receive adjunctive postoperative radiation therapy to 60 Gy.

External-Beam Radiation Therapy Set-up

For external-beam radiation therapy, patients are immobilized in a supine position, usually with the head slightly hyperextended to bring the floor of the orbit perpendicular to the couch. This position allows irradiation of the entire orbital floor while sparing the cornea and most of the globe. An intraoral stent helps open the mouth and depress the tongue out of the radiation fields. Marking the lateral canthi, the medial and inferior parts of the limbus while the patient gazes straight ahead, and the oral commissures, external auditory canals, and external scar before simulation films are taken is helpful in designing radiation portals.

When surgical resection includes the palate, the stent can be designed to hold a water-filled balloon, which occludes the surgical defect and minimizes the dose heterogeneity produced by a large air cavity. In the case of orbital exenteration, the defect is filled directly with the water-filled balloon to decrease the dose delivered to the temporal lobe.

A three-field technique with an anterior portal and two lateral fields (usually with 60-degree wedges) is preferable for most patients, particularly for those with tumors involving the suprastructure or extending to the roof of the nasal cavity and ethmoid air cells (see Fig. 7-4). The relative loading of the anteroposterior, right lateral, and left lateral fields is usually 1:0.07:0.07 but may vary slightly depending on the tumor location. Anterior and ipsilateral wedged-pair (usually with 45-degree wedges) photon fields may be adequate for tumors of the infrastructure with no extension into the orbit or ethmoid air cells. If necessary, the lateral portal can be designed with a 5-degree inferior tilt to avoid beam divergence into the contralateral eye. Lateral-opposed fields may be preferred for tumors of the infrastructure spreading across the midline through the hard palate. If necessary, the fields can be slightly oblique (5-degree inferior tilt from ipsilateral side and 5-degree superior tilt from contralateral side) to avoid irradiation of the contralateral eye. In addition, the use of half-beam technique with the isocenter at the level of the orbital floor also minimizes exposure of the eyes caused by beam divergence.

Ipsilateral upper neck irradiation is accomplished through a lateral appositional electron field (usually 12 MeV) matched to the inferior border of the primary portal posteriorly. A small triangle over the cheek is not irradiated except when there is involvement of the soft tissues of the cheek, in which case a triangular abutting electron field is added.

Bilateral neck treatment is indicated in patients presenting with extensive nodal involvement. A proper field matching technique is essential to minimize dose inhomogeneity and to prevent overdose to the spinal cord and mandible as a result of beam divergence. This can be accomplished by treating both the primary tumor bed and the upper neck with asymmetric jaw matching. The central axes of the primary fields and the opposed-lateral upper-neck fields are all placed in the plane of the inferior border of the maxillary fields (usually 1 cm below the floor of the maxillary sinus). It is prudent to move the junction line between the primary and neck fields during the course of treatment to minimize overdosing or underdosing. The mid neck and lower neck are irradiated with an anterior appositional photon field matched to the opposed upper-neck fields.

Patient Care During and After Radiation Therapy

It is common practice to give patients specific information about acute and late side effects of radiation therapy—such as skin desquamation, mucositis, nasal dryness, and, when applicable, the risk of visual impairment—before treatment is begun. It is also prudent to monitor the skin and mucosal reactions during treatment, particularly when radiation therapy is administered with a combination of electrons and photons with surface bolus. When moist skin desquamation or confluent mucositis occurs, proper care (e.g., pain medication, measures to prevent infection) is prescribed. Saline nasal rinses are begun during the period of confluent mucositis to prevent crusting and secondary infection. A topical antibiotic (neomycin and polymyxin B [Neosporin ointment]) is prescribed when infection develops. Patients are instructed to use sun block over the irradiated area after completion of treatment. Regular follow-up examinations include evaluation of the treated area for late complications.

NEW THERAPY DIRECTIONS AND CLINICAL STUDIES
Surgical Techniques

Craniofacial surgical techniques have been refined and applied in the treatment of sinonasal tumors at an increasing number of centers. These techniques provide better access for complete tumor resection, particularly resection of neoplasms extending to the skull base, while preserving some functionally important structures.

Conformal Radiation Therapy

Technical innovations in radiation therapy in the form of three-dimensional conformal treatment planning and delivery enable dose escalation to the tumor or surgical bed without overdosing the critical adjacent normal tissues. Several centers are applying conformal techniques in the treatment of patients with sinonasal carcinoma.[43,44] The objective is to reduce normal tissue radiation exposure to minimize complications and to escalate the dose of radiation to more than 75 to 78 Gy over 7 to 8 weeks to increase the local control rate. No long-term results were available at the time of this review.

Chemoradiation Therapy

The efficacy of new cytotoxic drugs in the treatment of sinonasal cancer is being assessed. As mentioned earlier, these agents are being used in the induction setting. Some are administered intraarterially instead of intravenously to enhance tumor regression. Ongoing clinical studies are addressing questions such as whether the extent of surgery can be reduced when good tumor response is achieved with chemotherapy and whether surgery can be avoided altogether in those who achieve a complete response. Several investigators are also assessing the role of concurrent chemoradiation therapy in the management of sinonasal carcinoma. The role of chemotherapy in the management of esthesioneuroblastoma is also being addressed.

Unfortunately, because of the rarity of sinonasal cancer, it will take many years to assess the relative value of these new developments in improving the overall outcome of patients with this disease.

REFERENCES

1. Greenlee RT, Hill-Harmon MB, Murray T, et al. Cancer statistics, 2001. *CA Cancer J Clin* 2001;51:15-36.
2. Roush GC. Epidemiology of cancer of the nose and paranasal sinuses. *Head Neck Surg* 1979;2:3-11.
3. Torjussen W, Solberg LA, Hgetviet AC. Histopathological changes of nasal mucosa in nickel workers: a pilot study. *Cancer* 1979;44:963-974.
4. Fletcher GH. Nasal and paranasal sinus carcinoma. In: Fletcher GH, ed. *Textbook of Radiotherapy*. Philadelphia, Pa: Lea & Febiger; 1980:408-425.
5. Goepfert H, Guillamondegui OM, Jesse RH, et al. Squamous cell carcinoma of nasal vestibule. *Arch Otolaryngol Head Neck Surg* 1974;100:8-10.
6. Moore KL, Dalley AF. *Clinically Oriented Anatomy*. 4th ed. Baltimore, Md: Lippincott Williams & Wilkins; 1999.
7. Acheson ED, Hadfield EH, Macbeth RG. Carcinoma of the nasal cavity and accessory sinuses in woodworkers. *Lancet* 1967;1:311-312.
8. Acheson ED, Cowdell RH, Hadfield E, et al. Nasal cancer in woodworkers in the furniture industry. *Br Med J* 1968;2:587-596.
9. Bars G, Visser AG, van Andel JG. The treatment of squamous cell carcinoma of the nasal vestibule with interstitial iridium implantation. *Radiother Oncol* 1985;4:121-125.
10. McNeese MD, Chobe R, Weber RS, et al. Carcinoma of the nasal vestibule: treatment with radiotherapy. *Cancer Bull* 1989;41:84-87.
11. Wong CS, Cummings BJ, Elhakim T, et al. External irradiation for squamous cell carcinoma of the nasal vestibule. *Int J Radiat Oncol Biol Phys* 1986;12:1943-1946.
12. Chobe R, McNeese MD, Weber R, et al. Radiation therapy for carcinoma of the nasal vestibule. *Otolaryngol Head Neck Surg* 1988;98:67-71.
13. Ang KK, Jiang GL, Frankenthaler RA, et al. Carcinomas of the nasal cavity. *Radiother Oncol* 1992;24:163-168.
14. Beitler JJ, Fass DE, Brenner HA, et al. Esthesioneuroblastoma: is there a role for elective neck treatment? *Head Neck* 1991;13:321-326.
15. Goldsweig HG, Sundaresan N. Chemotherapy of recurrent esthesioneuroblastoma: case report and review of the literature. *Am J Clin Oncol* 1990;13:139-143.
16. Kadish S, Goodman M, Wine CC. Olfactory neuroblastoma: a clinical analysis of 17 cases. *Cancer* 1976;37:1571-1576.
17. Elkon D, Hightower SI, Lim ML, et al. Esthesioneuroblastoma. *Cancer* 1979;44:1087-1094.
18. Jiang GL, Ang KK, Peters LJ, et al. Maxillary sinus carcinomas: natural history and results of postoperative radiotherapy. *Radiother Oncol* 1991;21:193-200.
19. Parsons JT, Mendenhall WM, Mancuso AA, et al. Malignant tumors of the nasal cavity and ethmoid and sphenoid sinuses. *Int J Radiat Oncol Biol Phys* 1988;14:11-22.
20. Fleming I, Cooper JS, Henson DE, et al, eds. *AJCC Cancer Staging Manual*. 5th ed. Philadelphia, Pa: Lippincott-Raven; 1997:47-52.
21. Spaulding CA, Kranyak MS, Constable WC, et al. Esthesioneuroblastoma: a comparison of two treatment eras. *Int J Radiat Oncol Biol Phys* 1988;15:581-590.
22. Million RR. The myth regarding bone or cartilage involvement by cancer and the likelihood of cure by radiotherapy. *Head Neck Surg* 1989;11:30-40.
23. McCollough WM, Mendenhall NP, Parsons JT, et al. Radiotherapy alone for squamous cell carcinoma of the nasal vestibule: management of the primary site and regional lymphatics. *Int J Radiat Oncol Biol Phys* 1993;26:73-79.
24. Badib AO, Kurohara SS, Webster JH, et al. Treatment of cancer of the nasal cavity. *Am J Roentgenol* 1969;106:824-830.
25. Bosch A, Vallecillo L, Frias Z. Cancer of the nasal cavity. *Cancer* 1976;37:1458-1463.
26. Hawkins RB, Wynstra JH, Pilepich MV, et al. Carcinoma of the nasal cavity—results of primary and adjuvant radiotherapy. *Int J Radiat Oncol Biol Phys* 1988;15:1129-1133.
27. Beale FA, Garrett PG. Cancer of paranasal sinus with particular reference to maxillary sinus cancer. *J Otolaryngol* 1983;12:377-382.
28. Bush SE, Bagshaw MA. Carcinoma of the paranasal sinuses. *Cancer* 1982;50:154-158.
29. Gadeberg CC, Hjelm HM, Sgaard H, et al. Malignant tumors of the paranasal sinuses and nasal cavity. *Acta Radiol Oncol* 1984;23:181-187
30. Hordiji GJ, Brons EN. Carcinoma of maxillary sinus: a retrospective study. *Clin Otolaryngol* 1985;10:285-288.
31. Hu Y, Tu G, Qi Y, et al. Comparison of pre- and postoperative irradiation in the combined treatment of carcinoma of maxillary sinus. *Int J Radiat Oncol Biol Phys* 1982;8:1045-1049.
32. Lindeman P, Eklund U, Petruson B. Survival after surgical treatment in maxillary neoplasm of epithelial origin. *J Laryngol Otol* 1987;101:564-568.
33. Sakai S, Hohki A, Fuchihata H, et al. Multidisciplinary treatment of maxillary sinus carcinoma. *Cancer* 1983;52:1360-1364.

34. Schlappack OK, Dobrowsky W, Schratter M, et al. Radiotherapy for carcinoma of the paranasal sinuses. *Strahlenther Onkol* 1986; 162:291-299.

35. St-Pierre S, Baker S. Squamous cell carcinoma of the maxillary sinus. *Head Neck Surg* 1983;5:508-513.

36. Tsujii H, Kamada T, Arimoto T, et al. The role of radiotherapy in the management of maxillary sinus carcinoma. *Cancer* 1986; 57:2261-2266.

37. Le Q-T, Fu KK, Kaplan MJ, et al. Lymph node metastasis in maxillary sinus carcinoma. *Int J Radiat Oncol Biol Phys* 2000;46: 541-549.

38. Paulino AC, Fiosher SG, Marks JE. Is prophylactic neck irradiation indicated in patients with squamous cell carcinoma of the maxillary sinus? *Int J Radiat Oncol Biol Phys* 1997;39: 283-289.

39. Amendola BE, Eisert D, Hazra TA, et al. Carcinoma of the maxillary antrum: surgery or radiation therapy? *Int J Radiat Oncol Biol Phys* 1981;7:743-746.

40. Frich JC. Treatment of advanced squamous carcinoma of the maxillary sinus by irradiation. *Int J Radiat Oncol Biol Phys* 1982;8:1453-1459.

41. Olmi P, Cellai E, Chiavacci A, et al. Paranasal sinuses and nasal cavity cancer: different radiotherapeutic options, results and late damages. *Tumori* 1986;72:589-595.

42. Ang KK, Kaanders JHAM, Peters LJ, eds. *Radiotherapy for Head and Neck Cancers: Indications and Techniques*. Philadelphia, Pa: Lea & Febiger; 1994.

43. Krasin MJ, King S, Sethi A, et al. Significant reduction in critical structure doses in paranasal sinus and nasopharynx patients planned with intensity modulated radiotherapy compared with 3-D conformal radiotherapy [abstract 1036]. *Int J Radiat Oncol Biol Phys* 1999;45(suppl):275.

44. Pommier P, Ginestet C, Sunyach M-P, et al. Conformal radiotherapy for paranasal sinus and nasal cavity tumors: three-dimensional treatment planning and preliminary results in 40 patients. *Int J Radiat Oncol Biol Phys* 2000;48:485-492.

CHAPTER 8

The Nasopharynx

Adam S. Garden

In the nasopharynx, as in other head and neck sites, carcinomas are the most common type of malignancy. However, malignancies in the nasopharynx differ from malignancies at other head and neck sites with respect to epidemiology, histopathologic features, patterns of disease spread, and management. These differences are what prompted the American Joint Committee on Cancer (AJCC) to create a separate staging system for nasopharyngeal carcinoma (NPC) (see the section on "Staging" later in this chapter).[1]

NPC is uncommon in the United States compared with parts of Asia. In Hong Kong, NPC was the third most common cancer diagnosis among men.[2] The cause of NPC remains unclear, although it is strongly associated with the Epstein-Barr virus. NPC is often undifferentiated, and it has the highest rates of both regional and distant metastasis of all of the types of cancer that originate from head and neck sites.

The management of NPC has been of great interest to radiation oncologists. Surgery has had a limited role, and radiation is necessary for almost all patients. The local control rates achieved by radiation suggest that NPC may be more radiosensitive than carcinomas arising from other head and neck sites. Nevertheless, management remains a challenge because high doses are needed for cure and the tumors are often adjacent to critical neural structures, irradiation of which could lead to devastating side effects. Recent advancements in the management of NPC are the use of conformal radiation therapy and the integration of systemic therapies with radiation.

ANATOMY

The nasopharynx is the superior of the three subdivisions of the pharynx. It is a cuboidal cavity formed by muscle and fascia with an epithelial mucosal covering.

The roof of the soft palate forms the inferior border of the nasopharynx and creates the junction between the nasopharynx and the oropharynx. Defining this junction clinically can be difficult because the palate slopes; thus both clinical and radiographic definition of disease extent into the oropharynx is challenging. The nasopharynx is bound anteriorly by the posterior end of the nasal septum and the choanae; posteriorly by the vertebral bodies, the

atlas, and the axis; and superiorly by the sphenoid sinus and the basisphenoid (Fig. 8-1).

The muscular component of the nasopharynx is the superior constrictor muscle of the pharynx, which emanates from the pharyngeal tubercle. Lateral to the nasopharynx are the parapharyngeal space and the masticator space (Fig. 8-2). These spaces are separated from the nasopharynx by the pharyngobasilar fascia. The fascia arises from the base of the skull and fans laterally just anterior to the carotid canal. The fascia then continues anteriorly and medially and inserts into the posterior aspect of the medial pterygoid plate.

The eustachian tubes descend medially to enter the lateral nasopharynx. The posterior aspect of each tube's orifice creates a protrusion called the *torus tubarius* (Fig. 8-3). Posterior to the torus is the lateral recess known as the *pharyngeal recess,* or *Rosenmüller's fossa.*

ROUTES OF DISEASE SPREAD

NPC most commonly arises in Rosenmüller's fossa (Fig. 8-4, *A*). Anterior tumor extension along the lateral wall of the nasopharynx can partially or completely occlude the pharyngeal orifice of the eustachian tube, causing hearing loss, otitis media, or both. In the United States, where NPC is uncommon, these presenting symptoms often go undiagnosed for months because of a low index of suspicion. Further anterior tumor extension or growth causes nasal obstruction or epistaxis (see Fig. 8-4, *B*).

Superior extension of NPC can result in bone erosion. Destruction of the clivus (see Fig. 8-4, *C*) often results in headache. Further extension can involve either the second or third division of the trigeminal nerve by infiltration into the superior maxillary foramen or the oval foramen of the sphenoid bone. Another mechanism of perineural involvement is invasion into the cavernous sinus (see Fig. 8-4, *D*). In this scenario, the abducent nerve is usually damaged, resulting in diplopia. Extension of disease into the orbital apex (see Fig. 8-4, *E*) can have further effects on vision. Direct intracranial extension (see Fig. 8-4, *F*) is seen in fewer than 10% of cases.

Despite the lack of a barrier against spread, inferior extension into the oropharynx is not common. Occasionally, an examiner will note a submucosal asymmetry or bulging of the posterior pharyngeal wall that may

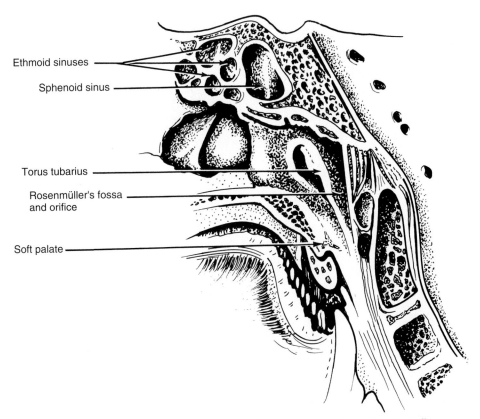

Ethmoid sinuses

Sphenoid sinus

Torus tubarius

Rosenmüller's fossa
and orifice

Soft palate

Fig. 8-1 Diagram of a sagittal view of the nasopharynx illustrating its walls.

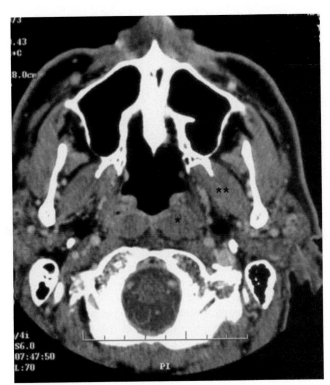

Fig. 8-2 Axial image of a normal nasopharynx and its relationships to the masticator muscles. *, Nasopharynx; **, pterygoid muscle.

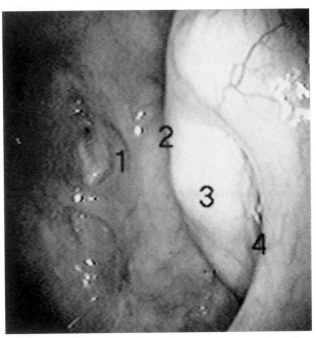

Fig. 8-3 Photograph of the nasopharynx as seen through a fiberoptic scope. *1*, posterior wall; *2*, fossa of Rosenmüller; *3*, torus tubarius; *4*, eustachian tube orifice.

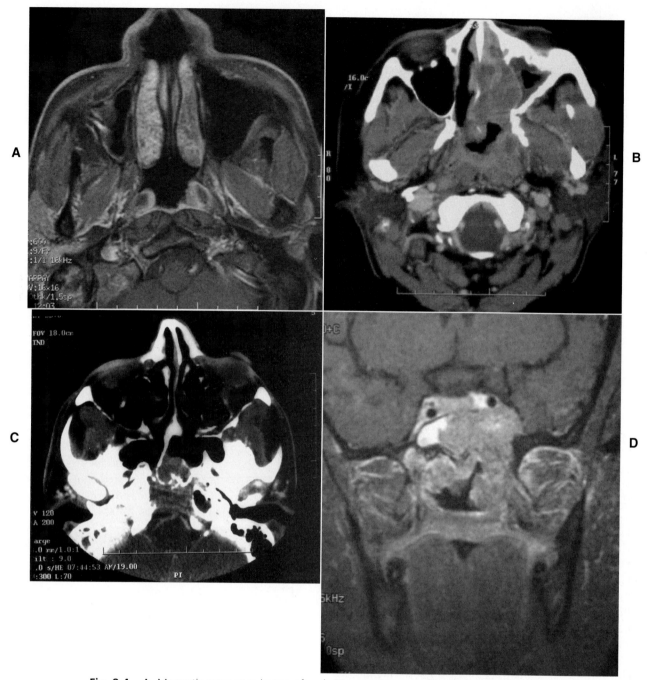

Fig. 8-4 **A,** Magnetic resonance image of early T1 nasopharyngeal carcinoma. **B,** Extension of tumor originating in the left fossa of Rosenmüller into the nasal cavity. **C,** Clival destruction by tumor. **D,** Invasion of the cavernous sinus by tumor.

be a result of submucosal spread of tumor (Fig. 8-5, *A*) or a clinical manifestation of extensive retropharyngeal adenopathy.

Posterior and lateral infiltration beyond the pharyngobasilar fascia can result in involvement of cranial nerves IX to XII as they exit the jugular foramen and hypoglossal canal (see Fig. 8-5, *B*), leading to cranial neuropathies. Direct lateral extension can result in invasion of the masticator space (see Fig. 8-5, *C*), with trismus as a presenting symptom.

STAGING

The current staging system for NPC is the tumor-node-metastasis classification outlined in the fifth edition of the *AJCC Cancer Staging Manual* (Box 8-1).[1] The current staging system, published in 1997, is substantially different from the previous staging system, which was published in 1992. Because of reports suggesting that subsite within the nasopharynx was not prognostically relevant, the 1997 staging system does not recognize subsite

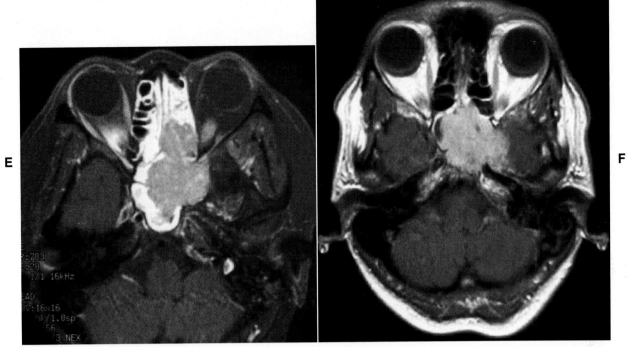

Fig. 8-4, cont'd **E,** Orbital invasion by tumor. **F,** Intracranial extension of tumor.

divisions. In addition, on the basis of natural history, several presentations were downgraded in the 1997 staging system. Tumors with oropharynx and nasal cavity involvement are now considered T2 rather than T3. Bony erosion of the base of the skull without cranial nerve involvement is now believed to be a more favorable presentation than perineural or intracranial involvement and was therefore downgraded from T4 to T3.

The nasopharynx has a rich submucosal network of lymphatics, and clinical lymphadenopathy is common in NPC. It is present in 70% of patients at presentation, and some suggest that if subclinical nodal metastases are included, as many as 90% of patients with NPC have nodal involvement at presentation. Involvement of retropharyngeal lymph nodes (Fig. 8-6, *A*), posterior cervical nodes (see Fig. 8-6, *B*), and jugular-chain nodes is common. Clinical lymphadenopathy without other signs or symptoms is a common presentation for patients with NPC.

Because patterns of nodal spread in NPC are different from patterns of nodal spread in other head and neck cancer and because the implications of nodal involvement are different in NPC than in other head and neck cancer, NPC has a unique nodal staging scheme. Notable differences between N staging for NPC and other head and neck cancer include the following: (1) the nasopharynx is considered a midline structure, so in staging for NPC there is no reference to contralateral nodes; (2) size differences are not as critical in NPC, so only a 6-cm cutoff is used; and (3) nodal levels are significant in NPC, and staging based on involvement of the supraclavicular fossa is included.

Because the 1997 staging system for NPC is greatly different not only from the previous edition but also from staging systems for other head and neck cancer, it may initially cause confusion at centers where NPC represents a small proportion of treated cancer. However, several studies have already demonstrated that the new system accomplishes the goals of staging. Cooper and colleagues[3] showed that, in their experience, the 1997 staging system separated patients into cohorts of more equal size than those in the 1992 system, which classified 90% of tumors as stage IV. Also, in the new system, the correlation between stage and likelihood of survival was as good as, if not better than, the correlation in the previous staging system.

HISTOPATHOLOGIC TYPES

Carcinomas are the most common malignancies of the nasopharynx, accounting for about 90% of all cases. Because the nasopharynx is part of Waldeyer's tonsillar ring and is rich in lymph tissue, lymphomas occasionally arise in the nasopharynx, and many carcinomas in the nasopharynx have a lymphoid stroma. A separate entity, lymphoepithelioma, has also been described in the nasopharynx; lymphoepithelioma is essentially a squamous carcinoma with a benign lymphoid component. Historically, compared with carcinoma, lymphoepithelioma was thought to be associated with higher local–regional control rates because of its more pronounced radiosensitivity but with equivalent survival rates because of its higher rate of distant recurrence.

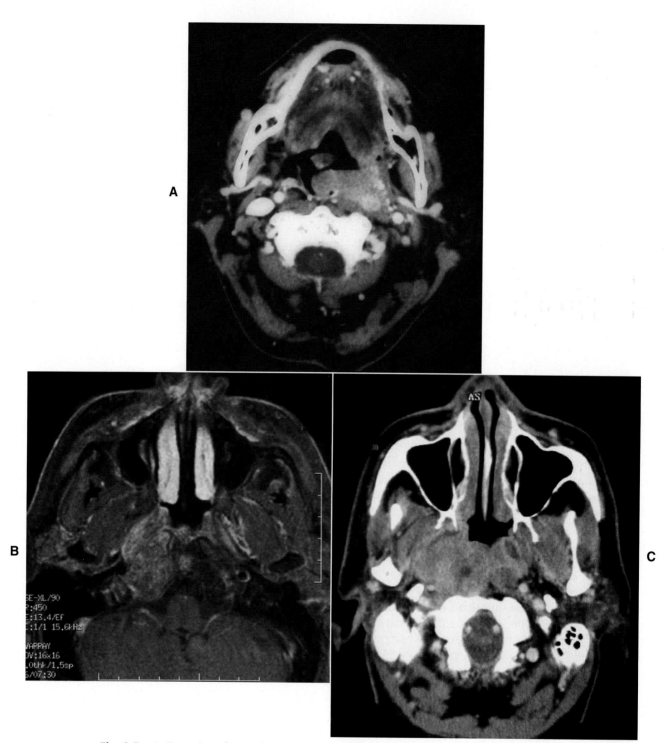

Fig. 8-5 **A,** Extension of nasopharyngeal carcinoma into the oropharynx. **B,** Posterior extension beyond the pharyngobasilar fascia to invade cranial nerves ix to xii. **C,** Invasion into the masticator space.

However, the significance of lymphoepithelioma is now thought to be less than previously described.

The World Health Organization (WHO) histopathologic classification is the recommended histopathologic classification for NPC. The WHO classification describes three types of NPC: (1) squamous cell carcinoma, (2) nonkeratinizing squamous cell carcinoma, and

(3) undifferentiated carcinoma.[1] As acceptance of the WHO classification becomes more widespread, the description of lymphoepithelioma is becoming less common. Lesions that previously would have been classified as lymphoepitheliomas are classified in the WHO system as either type 2 or type 3 disease. Type 3 is the most common subtype. Among populations where NPC

BOX 8-1   American Joint Committee on Cancer Staging System for Nasopharyngeal Carcinoma

PRIMARY TUMOR (T)

TX	Primary tumor cannot be assessed
T0	No evidence of primary tumor
Tis	Carcinoma in situ
T1	Tumor confined to the nasopharynx
T2	Tumor extends to soft tissues of oropharynx and/or nasal fossa
	T2a Without parapharyngeal extension
	T2b With parapharyngeal extension
T3	Tumor invades bony structures and/or paranasal sinuses
T4	Tumor with intracranial extension and/or involvement of cranial nerves, infratemporal fossa, hypopharynx, or orbit

REGIONAL LYMPH NODES (N)

NX	Regional lymph nodes cannot be assessed
N0	No regional lymph node metastasis
N1	Unilateral metastasis in lymph node(s), 6 cm or less in greatest dimension, above the supraclavicular fossa
N2	Bilateral metastasis in lymph node(s), 6 cm or less in greatest dimension, above the supraclavicular fossa
N3	Metastasis in a lymph node(s)
	N3a greater than 6 cm in dimension
	N3b extension to the supraclavicular fossa

DISTANT METASTASIS (M)

MX	Distant metastasis cannot be assessed
M0	No distant metastasis
M1	Distant metastasis

STAGE GROUPING: NASOPHARYNX

Stage 0	Tis	N0	M0
Stage I	T1	N0	M0
Stage IIA	T2a	N0	M0
Stage IIB	T1	N1	M0
	T2	N1	M0
	T2a	N1	M0
	T2b	N0	M0
	T2b	N1	M0
Stage III	T1	N2	M0
	T2a	N2	M0
	T2b	N2	M0
	T3	N0	M0
	T3	N1	M0
	T3	N2	M0
Stage IVA	T4	N0	M0
	T4	N1	M0
	T4	N2	M0
Stage IVB	Any T	N3	M0
Stage IVC	Any T	Any N	M1

From Fleming I, Cooper JS, Henson DE, et al, eds. *AJCC Cancer Staging Manual*, 5th ed. Philadelphia, Pa: Lippincott Williams & Wilkins; 1997:31-39.

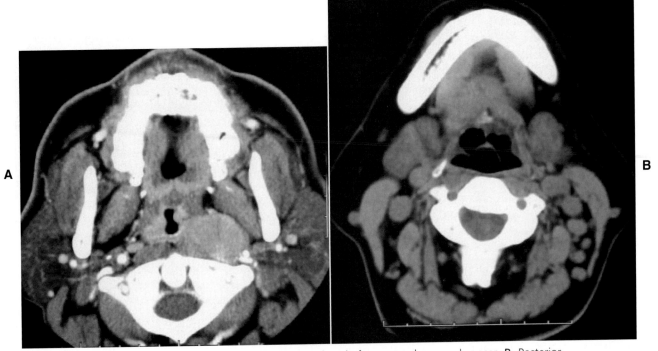

Fig. 8-6   A, Metastasis to a retropharyngeal node from nasopharyngeal cancer. B, Posterior cervical node involvement from nasopharyngeal cancer.

is endemic, type 3 accounts for almost 99% of cases of NPC. WHO type 1 is more common in the United States, where it accounts for approximately 20% of cases.

EPIDEMIOLOGY

NPC is endemic in China, where the incidence approaches 80 cases per 100,000 people per year. In contrast, in the United States, the incidence of NPC is fewer than two cases per 100,000 people per year. Other areas across Southeast Asia, North Africa, and Saudi Arabia have an intermediate incidence.[4]

NPC has a male predominance, although the male:female incidence ratio is lower for NPC than for other types of head and neck cancer. The disease also affects a younger population than other types of head and neck cancer; the median age at diagnosis is 50 to 60 years.[2]

A strong association exists between Epstein-Barr virus and endemic NPC.[5] In a study performed at the National Taiwan University Hospital, immunoglobulin A (IgA) antiviral capsid antigen was detected in more than 80% of patients with NPC compared with only 2% of control subjects.[6] However, the therapeutic and prognostic significance of Epstein-Barr virus in NPC is unclear; studies of the relationship between antibody titer levels and prognosis have produced mixed results.

The high rates of NPC seen in China may be the result of a genetic predisposition. Several cytogenetic abnormalities have been described in NPC, including changes on the human leukocyte antigen major histocompatibility complex alleles.[7] Alterations in the tumor suppressor gene *p16* have also been described in 35% of patients with primary undifferentiated NPC.[8] However, the *p53* mutations seen in other types of head and neck cancer are less common in endemic NPC.[9]

Finally, environmental factors may play a role in NPC. Various dietary components have been studied in populations at risk[10] and have been implicated as direct carcinogens or Epstein-Barr virus activators. Further evidence of an environmental influence is that the incidence of NPC in United States–born descendants of Chinese is much lower than the incidence of the disease in immigrants from China.[11]

In the United States approximately 20% of cases of NPC are WHO type 1. It is believed that these keratinizing squamous cell carcinomas may be caused in part by alcohol and tobacco use[12] and may behave similarly to the tobacco-related squamous cell carcinomas seen in other head and neck sites.

THERAPEUTIC APPROACHES

Primary therapy for NPC is radiation. Over the past several decades, the role of systemic therapy in improving treatment outcome in NPC has been investigated, and concurrent chemotherapy and radiation therapy is now considered by most investigators to be the approach of choice for treatment of NPC.

Radiation Therapy

The basic goal of radiation therapy in patients with NPC is to treat both clinically apparent disease and sites of subclinical lymphatic spread. Defining these sites of subclinical spread is a challenge.

Treatment Planning

In 1980 Fletcher and Million,[13] who did not have access to the high-tech tools available today, used knowledge of patterns of metastasis in NPC to define targets to ensure adequate coverage of the sites of potential tumor spread. These targets are still used today, more than 20 years later. For early-stage tumors, the radiation portals encompass the nasopharynx proper; the posterior 2 cm of the nasal cavity; the posterior ethmoid sinuses; the entire sphenoid sinus and basiocciput; the cavernous sinus; the base of the skull, including the oval foramen, spinous foramen, and carotid canal; the pterygoid fossae; the posterior third of the orbit; the posterior third of the maxillary sinus; the lateral and the posterior oropharyngeal wall to the mid-tonsillar level; and the retropharyngeal nodes. In patients with base-of-skull or intracranial nerve involvement, the superior border is raised to include all of the pituitary fossa, the base of the brain in the suprasellar area, the adjacent middle cranial fossa, and the posterior portion of the anterior cranial fossa.[13]

The basic radiation therapy technique for NPC consists of a three-field technique: lateral opposed fields for the primary tumor and upper neck and a matching anterior low-neck portal (Fig. 8-7). The use of computed tomography (CT) and magnetic resonance imaging (MRI) has allowed better definition of the extent of disease. Fields are designed so that 2 cm of tissue beyond the gross disease outlined on imaging receives a subclinical dose of 50 Gy. A reduction is made to approximately 42 Gy off the posterior border to shield the spinal cord. These posterior tissues are then treated with electron beams that target the superficial node-bearing posterior tissues while limiting the dose to the deeper spinal cord. Boost fields are designed to deliver 66 to 70 Gy to gross disease with a 1- to 1.5-cm margin. These boost fields can continue through lateral fields, but the challenge is to adequately cover the tumor while limiting the dose to adjacent normal structures, particularly the normal neural structures, including the spinal cord, brainstem, and, in advanced cases with significant superior extension, the optic chiasm.

In the current (1997) staging system for NPC, a separate category, *T2b*, was defined as tumor extension into

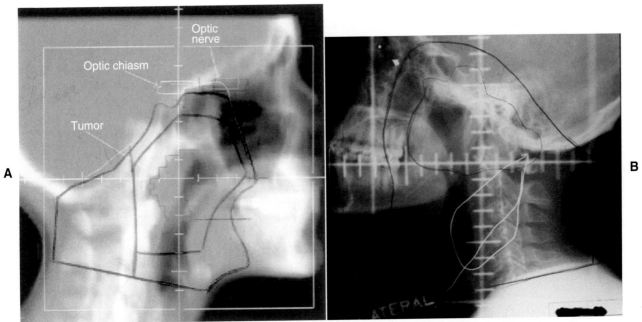

Fig. 8-7 Lateral simulation films for a T2 N0 nasopharyngeal cancer (**A**) and a T4 node-positive nasopharyngeal cancer (**B**).

the parapharyngeal space (i.e., posterolateral infiltration beyond the pharyngobasilar fascia). The prognostic significance of parapharyngeal extension is controversial; some authors contend that parapharyngeal extension is associated with an increased risk of local recurrence.[14] The question is whether this increased risk reflects more advanced disease or increased likelihood of a geographic miss.

For NPC that extends posteriorly to the same coronal level as critical neural tissue, more creative field arrangements are required. Simple methods such as the use of parallel fields that are delivered at oblique angles off the spinal cord and brainstem may be effective when the disease is well lateralized. However, this approach is often difficult in the case of a horseshoe-shaped tumor with bilateral retropharyngeal or parapharyngeal extension. Historically, this problem was addressed using antral fields—anterior oblique fields that entered through the maxillary sinuses and treated the nasopharynx through an oblique approach. This technique was a crude forerunner to the conformal approaches that are being used today (discussed later in this section).

In certain circumstances, cold spots (regions in which the dose is lower than desired) can be treated supplementally with higher-energy electrons; however, this approach requires extremely careful planning. This technique may be necessary in patients with significant anterior disease extension into the ethmoid sinuses, where the nearness to the optic chiasm limits the ability to deliver high doses with photons. This technique may also be necessary in patients with posterior high nodal disease that can be reached with electrons while limiting the dose to the spinal cord.

More recently, various conformal radiation therapy systems of various degrees of sophistication have become available to solve the problem of achieving a complex dose distribution that will cover disease while limiting the radiation dose to normal tissues. Most conformal systems use a general conceptual approach in which the dose to the tumor is distributed by using multiple beams entering the patient at different angles. The number of beams can range from 7 to as many as 20 (Fig. 8-8, *A*), and the beams can be coplanar or non-coplanar. The use of newer three-dimensional planning systems allows improved visualization of the tumor and optimization of the angles of entry and the shape of individual beams. A single axial slice of an isodose distribution obtained with a seven-field coplanar plan is shown in Figure 8-8, *B*.

The latest approach to radiation therapy for NPC is intensity-modulated radiation therapy. This approach improves on conformal radiation systems by dynamically changing the shape and output of the beam as it is delivered. Intensity-modulated radiation therapy builds on the conformal approach by using either multiple beams with a dynamic multileaf delivery system or a MiMic system—that is, an arc rotational system. A potential further advantage of these systems is their advanced software treatment algorithms that allow inverse planning, planning that allows the radiation dose distributions to be optimized on the basis of dose priorities specified by the treating physician.

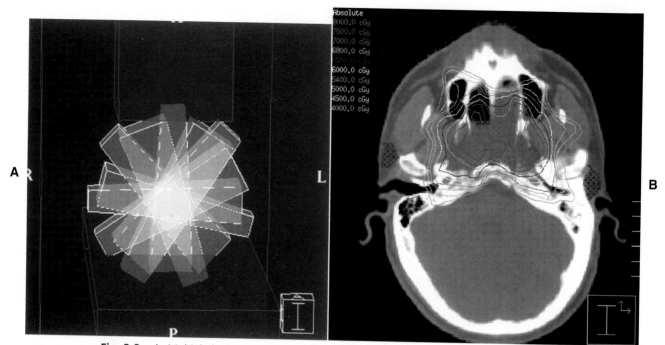

Fig. 8-8   **A,** Multiple beam arrangement for conformal treatment of nasopharyngeal cancer. **B,** Isodose distribution from a seven-beam conformal radiation therapy plan used to treat nasopharyngeal cancer.

Regardless of the techniques used, the anterior low-neck field is matched to the inferior border of the fields used to treat the upper neck and nasopharyngeal disease. A block is placed centrally to shield the larynx and to help avoid accidental overlap on the spinal cord. If the treatment is directed at subclinical metastases only, then 50 Gy is sufficient. If gross disease is present, then that disease needs to receive a boost to 66 to 70 Gy. Because nodal disease is often present in the spinal accessory chain, a posterior field is often required.

Dose and Fractionation

NPC is generally treated with conventional fractionation at 2 Gy/day once daily. The recommended total radiation dose for the primary tumor is 66 to 70 Gy, with the higher dose advised for most patients except those with T1 disease. Dose recommendations for nodal disease are as follows: 50 Gy for subclinical nodal metastases, 66 Gy for nodes smaller than 3 cm, and 70 Gy for nodes 3 cm or larger.

In NPC, as in other types of cancer of the head and neck, prolonging or interrupting radiation therapy can compromise outcome. Kwong and colleagues[15] reported a 3.3% decrease in the local–regional control rate for each day of treatment interruption in their patients treated with radiation. So far, however, unlike the case in other head and neck cancer, no firm evidence is available to support the use of altered fractionation for patients with NPC outside of the setting of clinical trials.[16,17] Teo and colleagues[18] are conducting a randomized trial comparing hyperfractionated

radiation (70 Gy in 40 fractions over 30 days) with conventional fractionation (60 Gy in 26 fractions over 30 days) in patients with NPC. Preliminary reports demonstrate the feasibility of hyperfractionation, but no obvious advantage of this approach has been seen to date. A recent report on hyperfractionation cautions that late effects, specifically temporal lobe necrosis, may be more common with this approach because of incomplete repair of brain tissue, even with a 6-hour interfraction interval.[19]

At The University of Texas M.D. Anderson Cancer Center, most patients with NPC are treated with conventional fractionation. This approach is based on the finding that results in a small cohort of patients treated with a concomitant boost fractionation schedule were equivalent to results in patients treated with conventional schedules.[20] Several explanations were proposed for the lack of benefit of accelerated fractionation in this series. The simplest was that the series was too small to demonstrate a benefit. It was also postulated that the tumor biology of NPCs is different from that of other head and neck squamous cell carcinomas and that, as a result, an accelerated schedule is not as critical for NPC. Finally, because of the proximity of NPC to critical tissues, the boost fields have extremely small margins, resulting in poorer coverage of the macroscopic tumor. The lack of benefit with the concomitant boost schedule was mainly seen in patients with T4 disease (1992 AJCC staging system). Local control for patients with T2 and T3 disease treated with concomitant boost fractionation approached 90%.[20]

Over the years, the total radiation dose used to treat NPC has gradually been escalated. In the 1950s and 1960s, patients treated at the M.D. Anderson Cancer Center received an average dose of 61 Gy. Fletcher, recognizing that the location of the nasopharynx within typical portal arrangement created cold spots,[13] recommended a makeup dose of 5 to 7.5 Gy. This resulted in an average dose to the primary tumor of 67 Gy during the 1970s and an average dose of 70 Gy more recently.

The literature is mixed regarding the existence of a dose-effect relationship for treatment of NPC. Analysis of dose in 378 patients treated with radiation alone at the M.D. Anderson Cancer Center revealed no clear trend for higher control rates with higher doses; the best control rates were seen in patients who received either 60 to 65 Gy or more than 70 Gy. Kaasa and colleagues[21] reported no correlation between radiation dose and survival time in 122 patients treated at the Norwegian Radium Hospital. In contrast, Perez and colleagues[22] at the Mallinckrodt Institute of Radiology in St. Louis, Mo., reported a clear benefit in local control when doses of greater than 66 Gy were used for T1 to T3 disease. However, no advantage was seen for higher doses in T4 disease (1988 AJCC staging system).[22] A recent study by Willner and colleagues[23] found that correcting the dose-response curve for tumor volume created a steep dose-response relationship and found that tumors larger than 64 mm^3 were unlikely to be controlled with 72 Gy. However, this study did not correct for the influence of histologic type on outcome.

Results of Radiation Therapy

Outcomes for patients with NPCs have improved over the past four decades, in part because of improvements in treatment techniques but also because of progress in diagnostic imaging, which has enabled better disease staging.

Survival rates differ from series to series[22,24-35] (Table 8-1) and are dependent on the stage distribution in the treated population and the type of treatment delivered. Series from China and Hong Kong are composed almost exclusively of patients with undifferentiated NPC. In areas where NPC is endemic, a greater proportion of patients have earlier-stage disease because the symptoms and signs of NPC are more likely to be recognized in a timely manner. One of the largest series reported to date is from Queen Elizabeth Hospital in Hong Kong. This retrospective analysis of more than 5000 patients found a 10-year overall survival rate of 43%.[24] At the M.D. Anderson Cancer Center, the 10-year actuarial survival rate in 378 patients treated between 1954 and 1992 was 34%.[28]

Local recurrence is the dominant relapse pattern in patients with NPC treated with radiation therapy alone. The 10-year local control rates in the Queen Elizabeth Hospital and the M.D. Anderson Cancer Center series were similar at 61% and 66%, respectively.[24,28] Numerous series have demonstrated the association between advanced tumor stage and poorer local control. Perez and colleagues[22] reported 10-year primary tumor control rates of 85% for T1 disease and 40% for T4 disease (disease staged according to the 1988 AJCC staging system). At the M.D. Anderson Cancer Center, 10-year primary tumor control rates were 87% for T1 disease and 45% for T4 disease.[28]

Among patients with T4 disease, those with cranial nerve involvement have a lower probability of local control. Parapharyngeal space infiltration is also correlated with a poorer prognosis, although this relationship is not universally accepted. In series from areas where NPC

TABLE 8-1

Results of Selected Series of Radiation Therapy Only for Treatment of Nasopharyngeal Cancer

Study and Reference	Year(s) of Study	Number of Patients	Survival Rate (%)	Local Control Rate (%)
Lee et al, 1992[24]	1976–1985	5037	43 (10 yr)	61 (10 yr)
Huang, 1980[25]	1958–1973	1605	32 (5 yr)	84 (5 yr)
Qin et al, 1988[26]	1958–1978	1379	41 (5 yr)	NS
Zhang et al, 1989[27]	1974	604	33 (10 yr)	NS
Sanguinetti et al, 1997[28]	1954–1992	378	48 (5 yr)	71 (5 yr)
Wang, 1997[29]	1970–1994	259	59 (5-yr DSS)	65 (5 yr)
Johansen et al, 1992[30]	1975–1984	167	37 (10 yr)	54 (10 yr)
Laramore et al, 1988[31]	1975–1985	166	23–39 (4 yr)	64 (crude rate)
Olmi et al, 1992[32]	1978–1991	165	53 (5-yr DSS)	72 (5 yr)
Perez et al, 1992[22]	1956–1986	143	10–40 (10 yr)	40–85 (10 yr)
Dickson and Flores, 1985[33]	1971–1980	134	38 (5 yr)	NS
Vikram et al, 1985[34]	1970–1980	107	NS	69 (crude rate)
Bailet et al, 1992[35]	1955–1990	103	58 (5 yr) 30 (5 yr DFS)	68 (crude rate)

yr, Year; *NS,* not stated; *DSS,* disease-specific survival; *DFS,* disease-free survival.

is not endemic, the WHO type 1 subtype (keratinizing squamous cell carcinoma) is often regarded as unfavorable. In the M.D. Anderson Cancer Center series, the 10-year actuarial control rate for squamous cell carcinoma was only 54% compared with 79% for lymphoepithelioma and 71% for unclassified carcinoma.[28]

With comprehensive nodal irradiation, the regional control rate for NPC is relatively high. The 10-year regional control rate of 64% reported from Queen Elizabeth Hospital[24] was, in part, the result of a policy of not electively treating the neck in the absence of palpable lymph nodes. The regional failure rate in the subset of 906 patients who did not undergo irradiation of the neck was 40%.[24] In the M.D. Anderson Cancer Center experience, systematic irradiation of the neck produced a 10-year regional control rate of 83%.[28] Chow and colleagues[36] at the Princess Margaret Hospital in Toronto compared regional control rates in patients with NPC and known lymph node metastases and patients with lymph node metastases from other head and neck mucosal sites. The study was a matched case study, and the authors reported that, stage for stage, regional control was better for patients with NPC than for those with other types of cancer.

Distant metastases are more common in squamous cell carcinomas of the nasopharynx than in this type of tumor at other head and neck sites. The bones and lungs are the most common sites. Nodal status is the strongest predictor of distant failure. The highest rate of metastases reported by Lee and colleagues,[24] 57%, was in patients with Ho's stage N3 disease (nodes involving the supraclavicular region or the skin). In the M.D. Anderson Cancer Center series, the actuarial 10-year rate of distant disease was 32%, and the risk increased greatly in the presence of advanced neck disease and low-neck disease.[37]

Complications of Radiation Therapy

The large portals used in radiation therapy for NPC can induce acute reactions, dermatitis, mucositis, and late complications. Treating the masticator spaces can result in trismus. Radiation therapy for NPC often causes xerostomia, and in younger patients, who are less likely to have lost all of their natural teeth, this can lead to late osteoradionecrosis of the mandible and maxilla. Chronic skin and soft tissue ulceration occur infrequently.

Endocrine sequelae should not be underestimated. Neck irradiation can result in hypothyroidism. Large fields encompassing the sphenoid sinus, base of skull, and cavernous sinus can result in hypopituitarism.

The most severe sequelae of radiation therapy for NPC are neurologic sequelae. The presence of large tumors (T3 or T4) often necessitates coverage of the orbits and optic chiasm. If the dose to these structures is not kept within the limits of tolerance, blindness can result. Hearing loss not only is a common presenting symptom but also can be a complication of radiation therapy. Hearing loss is more common in patients treated with the combination of cisplatin, which is ototoxic, and radiation.[38] Cranial nerve damage, particularly to nerves IX to XII, can occur, and bilateral damage can be devastating. The brainstem and spinal cord are potentially at risk, particularly in cases of bilateral parapharyngeal disease extension. Treating patients to 70 Gy or greater can lead to memory loss and temporal lobe necrosis, resulting in seizure or strokelike presentations. Better tumor definition with more tailored fields, the use of conformal techniques, and the use of a brachytherapy boost may all help reduce the incidence of these potentially severe complications.

Brachytherapy

The nasopharynx is essentially a cavity lined by mucosa and is therefore a site amenable to brachytherapy. The appeal of brachytherapy for delivering the boost dose in the nasopharynx is the ability to lessen external-beam doses to normal adjacent structures, particularly the brainstem and temporal lobes. Brachytherapy can be delivered by either interstitial or intracavitary implant techniques. Interstitial approaches use ^{198}Au grain implants or permanent ^{125}I or ^{192}Ir wires. A group at Memorial Sloan-Kettering Cancer Center in New York developed a transpalatal flap technique that permits better access to the nasopharynx for implantation of radioactive sources.[39] Intracavitary techniques place radioactive sources in the nasopharynx within ingeniously modified endotracheal tubes or Foley catheters, providing low-dose-rate or, more recently, high-dose-rate irradiation.

Intracavitary approaches are preferred because of their practicality. Wang[29] has described using a cesium boost technique as a portion of therapy for patients with T1 to T3 (1988 staging) disease. In general, these patients received 60 to 64 Gy external-beam irradiation followed by a 10- to 15-Gy boost to the mucosal surface. Wang reported a significant improvement in local control with intracavitary boosts compared with external-beam radiation therapy alone (to doses of 65 to 70 Gy), although the control rates of patients treated with external-beam therapy alone were low (54% to 64%).

The intracavitary boost technique has been used less often at the M.D. Anderson Cancer Center because the emphasis has been to improve control rates with accelerated fractionation or multimodality therapy. Brachytherapy boosts have been used in patients with T1 to T2 tumors with residual primary tumor masses at the completion of external-beam therapy. In these cases brachytherapy was delivered with an "afterloadable" nasopharyngeal applicator. Designed by Delclos, Moore, and Sampiere,[40] the applicator consists of a spherical Teflon ball anchored in the nasopharynx by two pediatric endotracheal tubes placed into each of the nares (Fig. 8-9, *A*). A ^{137}Cs point source is afterloaded through one of the endotracheal tubes. A 10- to 15-Gy surface dose is delivered with the intracavitary applicator (see Fig. 8-9, *B*).

In recent years, great interest has come about for using high-dose-rate brachytherapy to treat NPC. The combination of easily insertable, commercially available applicators and rapid treatment minimizes the discomfort associated with this therapy. A lateral radiograph illustrating dummy sources inserted into a brachytherapy nasopharyngeal applicator to deliver a boost with high-dose-rate ^{192}Ir to the roof of the nasopharynx is shown in Figure 8-9, *C*.

Levendag and colleagues[41] in Rotterdam, Netherlands, have reported using a protocol involving high-dose-rate brachytherapy after external-beam radiation therapy. Patients with T1 to T3 tumors received 60 Gy followed by six fractions of 3 Gy, whereas patients with T4 disease received 70 Gy followed by four fractions of 3 Gy. Using this approach, the authors reported a 3-year local relapse-free survival rate of 86%. This was significantly better than the rate in their historical controls treated with external-beam therapy alone. Severe complications were uncommon and consisted of nasal synechiae in three patients.

Chang and colleagues[42] described their experience treating 133 patients with T1 to T2 NPC with 64.8- to 68.4-Gy external-beam radiation therapy followed by 1 to 3 fractions of 5- to 5.5-Gy high-dose-rate brachytherapy. These authors also reported improvement in local control with brachytherapy but found a moderate incidence of tissue perforation and necrosis, which correlated with the total dose, brachytherapy fraction number, and size of tumor. They concluded that total doses should range from 72.5 to 75 Gy with high-dose-rate brachytherapy given in 2.5-Gy sessions. Notably, these authors prescribed their boost doses at 2 cm from the central axis, which results in a high mucosal surface dose and most likely contributed to the high incidence of complications.

The advantage of brachytherapy—the ability to limit the dose to the mucosa with rapid fall-off—is actually a limitation in patients with disease that extends posteriorly into the parapharyngeal space or superiorly into the clivus or brain. In such patients, one potential means of delivering additional therapy is by a stereotactic radiosurgical boost. This method can deliver a boost to sites of disease remote from the nasopharynx while limiting the dose to normal nearby tissue. At Stanford University in Palo Alto, Calif., patients have been treated with external-beam radiation combined with chemotherapy followed by a stereotactic radiosurgical boost within 4 weeks of their external-beam treatment. After a median dose of 66 Gy, a single fraction of 12 Gy using one to four isocenters is delivered as a boost. Tate and colleagues[43] reported a local control rate of 100% and no complications in 23 patients treated with this approach.

Chemotherapy

Chemotherapy has been used in patients with NPC with hematogenous spread since the 1970s. Chemotherapy in these patients yields fairly high overall response rates—almost 80% in some series—and complete response rates ranging from 14% to 27%.[44-47] Better responses are seen in patients treated with platinum-based regimens. The chemosensitivity of NPCs has led to numerous trials attempting to improve outcome by combining chemotherapy with radiation in the neoadjuvant (preoperative) or adjuvant (postoperative) settings or concurrently with radiation.

Neoadjuvant Chemotherapy

Theoretically, neoadjuvant chemotherapy has two potential benefits: eradication of subclinical distant metastases and reduction of local tumor volume, which could potentially improve the efficacy of radiation therapy. Because NPCs are associated with high recurrence rates and because these tumors are chemosensitive, neoadjuvant therapy is an attractive option for treatment of this disease. This strategy has been investigated in numerous phase II trials, the results of which have been encouraging.

A phase II study at the M.D. Anderson Cancer Center involving patients with NPC that had been staged by CT showed that neoadjuvant chemotherapy with cisplatin and fluorouracil followed by radiation therapy resulted in a 5-year survival rate of 68% compared with 56% with radiation alone (*P* = 0.02).[20] This improvement in survival seemed to result from improvements in local control and a reduction in distant metastases, primarily in a subgroup of patients with undifferentiated NPC. These results were subsequently substantiated in a matched cohort study.[48]

Unfortunately, phase III trials have not confirmed the promising results from phase II trials[49-53] (Table 8-2). The first reported phase III trial of neoadjuvant chemotherapy in NPC was a single-institution trial performed at Prince of Wales Hospital in Hong Kong.[50] The experimental treatment consisted of two cycles of fluorouracil and cisplatin before radiation therapy plus four cycles of systemic therapy with the same drugs after the completion of radiation therapy. No difference in the 2-year survival rate was detected between the chemotherapy-plus-radiation and radiation-alone treatment groups (about 80% for both groups). The authors pointed out two weaknesses of their study: small sample size (*N* = 77) and inadequate intensity of neoadjuvant chemotherapy (only two cycles and 3 days of fluorouracil). Subsequently, the authors performed a retrospective analysis of more than 200 patients treated with induction chemotherapy and concluded that contrary to the results of their randomized trial, a benefit was evident in terms of local control in patients who received chemotherapy,

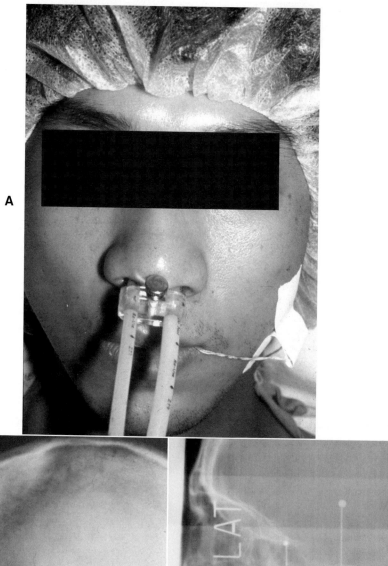

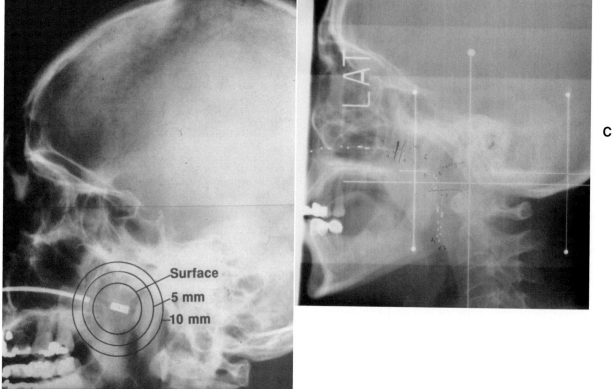

Fig. 8-9 **A,** Patient with an intracavitary brachytherapy system for treating nasopharyngeal cancer. **B,** Radiograph showing ^{137}Cs point source in place. **C,** Lateral radiograph with high-dose-rate iridium sources in the nasopharynx to deliver a boost dose.

TABLE 8-2
Results of Randomized Trials of Chemotherapy and Radiation Therapy for Nasopharyngeal Cancer

Study and Reference	Number of Patients	Approach	Drugs	Survival Rate (Experimental vs. Control)*	Relapse-Free Survival Rate (Experimental vs. Control)*
CNR, 1988[49]	229	Adjuvant (6 cycles)	Vincristine, cyclophosphamide, and doxorubicin	59% vs. 67% $(P = 0.13)$	58% vs. 56% $(P = 0.045)$
Prince of Wales Hospital, 1995[50]	82	Neoadjuvant (2 cycles) plus adjuvant (4 cycles)	Cisplatin and fluorouracil Cyclophosphamide	80% vs. 81% $(P = NS)$	68% vs. 72% $(P = NS)$
INCS, 1996[51]	339	Neoadjuvant (3 cycles)	Bleomycin, epirubicin, and cisplatin	63% vs. 60% $(P = NS)$	54% vs. 40% $(P < 0.01)$
Intergroup 0099, 1998[52]	147	Concurrent (3 cycles) plus adjuvant (3 cycles)	Cisplatin Cisplatin and fluorouracil	78% vs. 47% $(P = 0.05)$	69% vs. 24% $(P < 0.001)$
AOCOA, 1998[53]	334	Neoadjuvant (2-3 cycles)	Epirubicin and cisplatin	78% vs. 71% $(P = 0.57)$	48% vs. 42% $(P = 0.45)$

CNR, National Research Council of Italy; *NS*, not significant; *INCS*, International Nasopharynx Cancer Study; *AOCOA*, Asian-Oceanic Clinical Oncology Association.
*Control groups were patients treated with radiation only.

particularly among patients with node-positive Ho's stage T3 disease, which is roughly equivalent to AJCC stage T3 or T4 disease.[54] The authors believe that the discrepancy between the results of their randomized study and retrospective analysis was, in part, the result of the separation in the curves between years 3 and 5 after treatment. In patients treated with chemotherapy, the local recurrence rate appeared to plateau after 2 years, whereas in patients treated with radiation alone, local recurrences continued to occur more than 2 years after treatment.

The Asian-Oceanic Clinical Oncology Association randomly assigned 334 patients with NPC to receive either induction cisplatin and epirubicin followed by radiation or radiation alone.[53] Overall, relapse-free and overall survival did not differ between the groups. However, a subgroup analysis demonstrated an improvement in relapse-free and overall survival in favor of chemotherapy in patients with bulky nodal disease.

The International Nasopharynx Cancer Study Group conducted the third randomized study of neoadjuvant chemotherapy for NPC.[51] In this study, 339 patients with undifferentiated NPC were randomly assigned to neoadjuvant bleomycin, epirubicin, and cisplatin plus radiation or radiation alone. An excess of deaths was seen in the chemotherapy group (8%). The relapse-free survival rate was higher in the chemotherapy group, but overall survival was no different in the two groups.

Adjuvant Chemotherapy

Adjuvant chemotherapy has been included in trials of neoadjuvant chemotherapy for NPC and in trials of concurrent chemotherapy and radiation therapy for NPC,

but adjuvant chemotherapy has rarely been tested by itself in the treatment of NPCs. Rossi and colleagues[49] treated patients with radiation therapy alone or radiation therapy plus adjuvant vincristine, cyclophosphamide, and doxorubicin and found that adjuvant treatment produced no benefit in survival. The study, however, did not test drugs more commonly used for NPC, particularly cisplatin.

Concurrent Chemotherapy and Radiation Therapy

For head and neck carcinomas in general, several randomized trials have shown an improvement in outcome when chemotherapy is delivered concurrently with radiation. More recent trials have demonstrated that the improvement in outcome is the result of improved local–regional control.[55-57]

The data on concurrent therapy in NPC are quite controversial. No pure randomized study has been conducted comparing concurrent radiation therapy and chemotherapy with radiation alone. The main body of evidence comes from the Intergroup trial 0099.[51] In that study, patients were randomly assigned to concurrent chemotherapy and radiation therapy followed by adjuvant chemotherapy or to radiation therapy alone. The experimental treatment called for delivery of 100 mg/m^2 of cisplatin on days 1, 21, and 42 of radiation therapy, followed by three courses of adjuvant cisplatin (100 mg/m^2 on day 1) and fluorouracil (1000 mg/m^2/day on days 1 through 5). In both treatment groups, radiation therapy consisted of 70 Gy delivered over a period of 7 weeks.

The trial was stopped early because of a highly significant survival benefit in the experimental-therapy group. The 3-year disease-free survival rate was 69% in the chemotherapy group compared with 24% in the radiation-only group. Because of the overwhelming evidence of the benefits of concurrent chemotherapy and radiation therapy in other head and neck sites and because most trials of adjuvant and neoadjuvant chemotherapy in NPC showed no survival benefit, the benefit of the experimental therapy in the Intergroup trial has been attributed to the concurrent therapy component. However, several criticisms have been raised regarding this trial. Only 150 of the 193 entered patients were eligible. The authors performed a separate analysis to address this problem and concluded that it did not influence the results. The second criticism regards the poor results seen in the control group. Many argue that the control rates seen were 20% to 25% lower than expected for radiation therapy alone. Because of these questions, a second, confirmatory trial of concurrent chemotherapy and radiation therapy for NPC is being conducted outside the United States. However, most authors currently consider this approach to be the standard for managing NPC.

Reports corroborating the Intergroup experience have recently been published. Cooper and colleagues[58] at New York University reported a 3-year survival rate of 93% for patients with stage III and IV NPC treated with a regimen similar to that used by the Intergroup. The 3-year survival rate for the historical control patients treated with radiation alone was only 61%. Cheng and colleagues[59] from Taipei reported a 3-year primary tumor control rate of 97% and an overall survival rate of 80% in 74 patients treated with concurrent and adjuvant cisplatin and fluorouracil. Clival invasion and an elevated lactate dehydrogenase level predicted poorer outcome.

Salvage Therapy for Local Recurrence

Despite aggressive radiation therapy, local recurrence happens in 10% to 30% of patients with NPC. In patients with extensive local relapse, particularly in the skull base, treatment options may be limited to palliative therapy with chemotherapy or radiation. However, in a subset of patients with small, superficial recurrences, disease can potentially still be cured with aggressive local therapy.

Although rarely used in the initial treatment of NPC, surgery can yield good results in selected patients with local recurrence. Tumors have been resected through transpalatal, transcervical, and transmaxillary approaches. Recently, King and colleagues[60] from the Prince of Wales Hospital in Hong Kong reported a 5-year survival rate of 42% in 31 patients with recurrent T1 to T3 tumors treated with nasopharyngectomy. Postoperative irradiation was used in some patients and seemed to be beneficial. The authors reported few complications. Wei and colleagues[61] reported a similar outcome: local control was obtained in 19 of 45 patients after resection of recurrent NPCs. Brachytherapy was used in 22% of the patients in this series who had inadequate margins. Despite the relatively high control rates, these authors also reported a 6% mortality rate. Fee and colleagues[62] also advocated surgery in selected cases of recurrent NPC but described a high rate of skull base osteomyelitis secondary to this procedure.

Reirradiation is often recommended for treatment of relatively small recurrent nasopharyngeal tumors. No conclusive data exist regarding the value of chemotherapy in this clinical setting. Reported local–regional control rates with reirradiation range from 15% to 40%. Table 8-3 compares different series reporting results of retreatment of NPC.[29,60,62-71] The wide range of results is the result

---

TABLE 8-3

Results of Retreatment of Recurrent Nasopharyngeal Cancer

Study and Reference	Approach	Number of Patients	5-Year Actuarial Survival Rate (%)	5-Year Actuarial Local Control Rate (%)
Lee et al, 1993[63]	EBRT ± IRT	706	14	32
Chang et al, 2000[64]	EBRT ± SRT	186	12	NS
Teo et al, 1998[65]	EBRT ± IRT	103	8	15
Hwang et al, 1998[66]	XRT	74	37	40 (LRPF)
Pryzant et al, 1992[67]	EBRT ± IRT	53	21	35
Wang, 1997[29]	EBRT ± IRT	38	59 (DSS)	40
Syed et al, 2000[68]	EBRT + IRT*	34	30	93
McLean et al, 1998[69]	EBRT + IRT	17	65 (crude rate)	65
Orecchia et al, 1999[70]	SRT	13	31 (3 yr)	NS
King et al, 2000[60]	Surgery	31	47	43
Hsu et al, 1997[71]	Surgery	24	NS	46 (crude rate)
Fee et al, 1991[62]	Surgery	15	80 (crude rate)	46 (crude rate)

EBRT, External-beam radiation therapy; *IRT,* interstitial or intracavitary brachytherapy; *SRT,* stereotactic radiation; *NS,* not stated; *XRT,* external-beam radiation therapy, brachytherapy, heavy-charged-particle-beam therapy, and/or gamma knife therapy; *LRPF,* local–regional progression-free; *DSS,* disease-specific survival.
*Chemotherapy and/or hyperthermia.

reflects a combination of patient selection and radiation techniques. The use of external-beam radiation therapy alone to doses of 60 Gy or more produced a control rate of 15% in a series reported from the Prince of Wales Hospital.[64] Reirradiation to these doses also resulted in a more than 20% rate of temporal lobe encephalopathy.

The 5-year actuarial local control rate in the M.D. Anderson Cancer Center reirradiation series was 35%.[66] The control rate in patients treated with brachytherapy, most of whom had smaller recurrent tumors, was 67%. The author believes that patients with disease confined to the nasopharynx are best treated with a combination of external-beam irradiation and intracavitary brachytherapy. A total dose of 70 to 80 Gy to the nasopharynx is recommended, which generally consists of 20 to 30 Gy delivered with external-beam techniques and 40 to 50 Gy with low-dose-rate brachytherapy to the mucosal surface. Similar to the findings in the Hong Kong experience, it was found that delivery of cumulative doses of more than 100 Gy to the temporal lobe resulted in a 39% incidence of severe neurotoxicity, compared with 4% with doses of 100 Gy or less.

The stage of the recurrent tumor was found in many series to be a predictor of outcome. Wang[29] reported a control rate of only 15% for recurrent T3 to T4 tumors compared with 38% for recurrent T1 to T2 tumors. Stereotactic radiosurgery and radiation therapy may help improve control in patients with more advanced recurrences. Cmelak and colleagues[72] at Stanford University reported local control in seven of 12 patients treated with single-fraction (median, 18 Gy) stereotactic radiosurgery for skull base recurrences of NPC. Using stereotactic radiation therapy, Mitsuhashi and colleagues[73] controlled four of five cases of small recurrent NPC (median tumor size, 3.2 cm^3).

NASOPHARYNGEAL CARCINOMAS IN CHILDREN

Epidermoid carcinoma, particularly of the head and neck, is rare in children and adolescents. The annual incidence in North America is estimated to be approximately one case per 100,000 people per year. NPC accounts for most of these head and neck neoplasms. Carcinomas account for 85% to 90% of NPCs in adults but only 20% to 50% of NPCs in children. Most childhood nasopharyngeal tumors are sarcomas and lymphomas.

NPC in the young is closely associated with Epstein-Barr virus. Most cases present as WHO type 3 disease (advanced disease), with most series reporting nodal involvement in more than 90% of cases. In a combined report from the M.D. Anderson Cancer Center and Stanford University, only four of 57 patients with NPC, ages 4 to 21 years, did not have clinically evident nodal involvement.[74]

In children, as in adults, radiation therapy is the primary treatment modality for NPC. However, because the disease is much less common in children, the appropriate radiation dose for the treatment of childhood NPC is unclear. Several authors reported good control rates with doses in the range of 45 to 50 Gy with or without chemotherapy.[75] At the M.D. Anderson Cancer Center it is recommended that children older than 10 years be treated with doses similar to those used in adults, with 66 Gy delivered for stage T3 to T4 undifferentiated carcinoma. Also, a 10% dose reduction is recommended for children less than 10 years old.

Local–regional control rates are high in children with NPC. In the M.D. Anderson Cancer Center and Stanford University series, only six patients (14%) had local–regional recurrences during a median follow-up period of 93 months (range, 6 to 178 months). In another series, Ayan and Altun[76] reported a local–regional control rate of 79% in 50 patients with NPC, ages 5 to 16 years (follow-up period, 6 to 195 months). Many of the recurrences in this series occurred during an early era of treatment, and the authors suggested that these recurrences were in part the result of poor tumor definition. At the Princess Margaret Hospital, only one of 32 patients treated between 1975 and 1990 had an isolated local–regional recurrence.[77]

The primary failure pattern for children with NPC is distant metastasis. Five-year survival rates are similar to those for adults, ranging from 30% to 60%. Interest has been expressed in combining chemotherapy with radiation therapy in the treatment of NPC in children, but extrapolation from adult series is difficult, primarily because of the different patterns of recurrence. Concurrent chemotherapy and radiation is more difficult to rationalize in children than adults, but the question of whether a concurrent approach can lower the effective radiation dose needs to be addressed. Pao and colleagues[75] achieved high local control rates in children with NPC with the use of 50 Gy plus adjuvant chemotherapy.

Results of trials testing induction and adjuvant chemotherapy are mixed, and, unfortunately, no randomized trials and few prospective trials have been reported to date. Most authors advocate chemotherapy because many trials have suggested improvement in disease control with chemotherapy and because NPC in children is primarily systemic.

Chronic side effects from radiation therapy are a problem in children with NPC. Late sequelae include hypopituitarism, hypothyroidism, trismus, advanced dental decay, arrested development (particularly of clavicular growth), skin and soft tissue fibrosis, and second malignancies.

REFERENCES

1. Fleming I, Cooper JS, Henson DE, et al, eds. *AJCC Cancer Staging Manual*, 5th ed. Philadelphia, PA: Lippincott Williams & Wilkins; 1997:31-39.

2. Huang DP, Low KW. Aetiological factors and pathogenesis. In: Van Hasselt CA, Gibb AG, eds. *Nasopharyngeal Carcinoma.* 2nd ed. Hong Kong: Chinese University Press, Sha Tin NT; 1999:31-60.

3. Cooper J, Cohen R, Stevens R. A comparison of staging systems for nasopharyngeal carcinoma. *Cancer* 1998;83:213-219.

4. Yu MC. Nasopharyngeal carcinoma: epidemiology and dietary factors. *IARC Sci Publ* 1991;105:39-47.

5. Pathmanathan R, Prasad U, Sadler R, et al. Clonal proliferations of cells infected with Epstein-Barr virus in preinvasive lesions related to NPC. *N Engl J Med* 1995;333:693-698.

6. Lynn TC, Tu SM, Kawamura A Jr. Long-term follow-up of IgG and IgA antibodies against viral capsid antigens of Epstein-Barr virus in nasopharyngeal carcinoma. *J Laryngol Otol* 1985;99: 567-572.

7. Burt R, Vaughan T, Nisperos B, et al. A prospective association between the HLA-A2 antigen and nasopharyngeal carcinoma in US caucasians. *Int J Cancer* 1994;56:465-467.

8. Lo K, Huang D, Lau K. *p16* gene alterations in nasopharyngeal carcinoma. *Cancer Res* 1995;15:2039-2043.

9. Effert P, McCoy R, Abdelmalid M. Alteration of the p53 gene in NPC. *J Virol* 1992;37:63-75.

10. Lee H, Gourley L, Duffy S, et al. Preserved foods and nasopharyngeal carcinoma: a case-control study among Singapore Chinese. *Int J Cancer* 1994;59:585-590.

11. Buell P. The effect of migration on the risk of nasopharyngeal cancer among Chinese. *Cancer Res* 1974;34:1189-1191.

12. Chow W, Mclaughlin J, Hrubec Z, et al. Tobacco use and nasopharyngeal carcinoma in a cohort of US veterans. *Int J Cancer* 1993;55:538-540.

13. Fletcher GH, Million RR. Nasopharynx. In: Fletcher GH, ed. *Textbook of Radiotherapy.* 3rd ed. Philadelphia, PA: Lea & Febiger; 1980:364-383.

14. Teo P, Shiu W, Leung S, et al. Prognostic factors in nasopharyngeal carcinoma investigated by computer tomography—an analysis of 659 patients. *Radiother Oncol* 1992;23:79-93.

15. Kwong D, Sham J, Chua D, et al. The effect of interruptions and prolonged treatment time in radiotherapy for nasopharyngeal carcinoma. *Int J Radiat Oncol Biol Phys* 1997;39:703-710.

16. Fu K, Pajak T, Trotti A, et al. A Radiation Therapy Oncology Group (RTOG) phase III randomized study to compare hyperfractionation and two variants of accelerated fractionation to standard fractionation radiotherapy for head and neck squamous cell carcinomas: first report of RTOG 9003. *Int J Radiat Oncol Biol Phys* 2000;48:7-16.

17. Horiot J, Le Fur R, N'Guyen T, et al. Hyperfractionation versus conventional fractionation in oropharyngeal carcinoma: final analysis of a randomized trial of the EORTC cooperative group of radiotherapy. *Radiother Oncol* 1992;25:231-241.

18. Teo P, Kwan W, Leung S, et al. Early tumour response and treatment toxicity after hyperfractionated radiotherapy in nasopharyngeal carcinoma. *Br J Radiol* 1996;69:241-248.

19. Lee A, Sze W, Fowler J, et al. Caution on the use of altered fractionation for nasopharyngeal carcinoma. *Radiother Oncol* 1999; 52:207-211.

20. Garden A, Lippman S, Morrison W, et al. Does induction chemotherapy have a role in the management of nasopharyngeal carcinoma? Results of treatment in the era of computerized tomography. *Int J Radiat Oncol Biol Phys* 1996;36: 1005-1112.

21. Kaasa S, Kragh-Jensen E, Bjordal K, et al. Prognostic factors in patients with nasopharyngeal carcinoma. *Acta Oncol* 1993;32: 531-536.

22. Perez C, Devineni V, Marcial-Vega V, et al. Carcinoma of the nasopharynx: factors affecting prognosis. *Int J Radiat Oncol Biol Phys* 1992;23:271-280.

23. Willner J, Baier K, Pfreundner L, et al. Tumor volume and local control in primary radiotherapy of nasopharyngeal carcinoma. *Acta Oncol* 1999;38:1031-1035.

24. Lee A, Poon Y, Foo W, et al. Retrospective analysis of 5037 patients with nasopharyngeal carcinoma treated during 1976-1985: overall survival and patterns of failure. *Int J Radiat Oncol Biol Phys* 1992;23:261-270.

25. Huang S. Nasopharyngeal cancer: a review of 1605 patients treated radically with cobalt 60. *Int J Radiat Oncol Biol Phys* 1980;6:401-407.

26. Qin D, Hu Y, Yan J, et al. Analysis of 1379 patients with nasopharyngeal carcinoma treated by radiation. *Cancer* 1988;61: 1117-1124.

27. Zhang E-P, Lian P-G, Cai K-L, et al. Radiation therapy of nasopharyngeal carcinoma: prognostic factors based on a 10-year follow-up of 1302 patients. *Int J Radiat Oncol Biol Phys* 1989;16:301-305.

28. Sanguinetti G, Geara F, Garden A, et al. Carcinoma of the nasopharynx treated by radiotherapy alone: determinants of local and regional control. *Int J Radiat Oncol Biol Phys* 1997;37: 985-996.

29. Wang CC. *Radiation Therapy for Head and Neck Neoplasms.* New York, NY: Wiley-Liss; 1997:257-280.

30. Johansen L, Mesre M, Overgaard J. Carcinoma of the nasopharynx: analysis of treatment results in 167 consecutively admitted patients. *Head Neck* 1992;14:200-207.

31. Laramore G, Clubb B, Quick C, et al. Nasopharyngeal carcinoma in Saudi Arabia: a retrospective study of 166 cases treated with curative intent. *Int J Radiat Oncol Biol Phys* 1988;15:1119-1127.

32. Olmi P, Cellai E, Fallai C. Nasopharyngeal carcinoma: an analysis of 308 patients treated with curative radiotherapy. Presented at the IVth International IST Symposium on Interaction of Chemotherapy and Radiotherapy in Solid Tumours, Geneva, 1992.

33. Dickson R, Flores A. Nasopharyngeal carcinoma: an evaluation of 134 patients treated between 1971-1980. *Laryngoscope* 1985; 95:276-283.

34. Vikram B, Mishra UB, Strong E, et al. Patterns of failure in carcinoma of the nasopharynx: I. Failure at the primary site. *Int J Radiat Oncol Biol Phys* 1985;11:1455-1459.

35. Bailet J, Mark R, Abemayor E, et al. Nasopharyngeal carcinoma: treatment results with primary radiation therapy. *Laryngoscope* 1992;102:965-972.

36. Chow E, Payne D, Keane T, et al. Enhanced control by radiotherapy of cervical lymph node metastases arising from nasopharyngeal carcinoma compared with nodal metastases from other head and neck squamous cell carcinomas. *Int J Radiat Oncol Biol Phys* 1997;39:149-154.

37. Geara F, Sanguineti G, Tucker S, et al. Carcinoma of the nasopharynx treated by radiotherapy alone: determinants of distant metastasis and survival. *Radiother Oncol* 1997;43:53-61.

38. Kwong D, Wei W, Sham J, et al. Sensorineural hearing loss in patients treated for nasopharyngeal carcinoma: a prospective study of the effect of radiation and cisplatin treatment. *Int J Radiat Oncol Biol Phys* 1996;36:281-289.

39. Harrison L, Nori D, Hilaris B, et al. Nasopharynx: brachytherapy experience. In: Anderson LL, Nath R, Weaver, KA, et al, eds. *Interstitial Brachytherapy: Physical, Biological, and Clinical Considerations.* New York, NY: Raven Press; 1990:95-109.

40. Delclos L, Moore B, Sampiere V. A disposable "afterloadable" nasopharyngeal applicator for radioactive point sources. *Endocuriether/Hyperther Oncol* 1994;10:43-47.

41. Levendag P, Schmitz P, Jansen P, et al. Fractionated high-dose-rate brachytherapy in primary carcinoma of the nasopharynx. *J Clin Oncol* 1998;16:2213-2220.

42. Chang J, See L-C, Tang S, et al. The role of brachytherapy in early stage nasopharyngeal carcinoma. *Int J Radiat Oncol Biol Phys* 1996;36:1019-1024.

43. Tate D, Adler J, Chang S, et al. Stereotactic radiosurgical boost following radiotherapy in primary nasopharyngeal carcinoma: impact on local control. *Int J Radiat Oncol Biol Phys* 1999;45: 915-921.

44. Cvitkovic E. Neoadjuvant chemotherapy (NACT) with epirubicin (EPI), cisplatin (CDDP), bleomycin (BLEO) (BEC) in undifferentiated nasopharyngeal cancer (UCNT): preliminary results of an international (Int) phase (PH) III trial [abstract]. *Proc Am Soc Clin Oncol* 1994;13:283a.

45. Decker D, Drelichman A, Al-Sarraf M, et al. Chemotherapy for nasopharyngeal carcinoma. a ten-year experience. *Cancer* 1983;52:602-605.

46. Choo R, Tannock I. Chemotherapy for recurrent or metastatic carcinoma of the nasopharynx. a review of the Princess Margaret Hospital experience. *Cancer* 1991;68:2120-2124.

47. Boussen H, Cvitkovic E, Wendling J, et al. Chemotherapy of metastatic and/or recurrent undifferentiated nasopharyngeal carcinoma with cisplatin, bleomycin, and fluorouracil. *J Clin Oncol* 1991;9:1675-1681.

48. Geara F, Glisson B, Sanguineti G, et al. Induction chemotherapy followed by radiotherapy versus radiotherapy alone in patients with advanced nasopharyngeal carcinoma. *Cancer* 1997;79: 1279-1286.

49. Rossi A, Molinari R, Boracchi P, et al. Adjuvant chemotherapy with vincristine, cyclophosphamide, and doxorubicin after radiotherapy in local-regional nasopharyngeal cancer: results of a 4-year multicenter randomized trial. *J Clin Oncol* 1988;6:1401-1410.

50. Chan A, Teo P, Leung T, et al. A prospective randomized study of chemotherapy adjunctive to definitive radiotherapy in advanced nasopharyngeal carcinoma. *Int J Radiat Oncol Biol Phys* 1995;33:569-577.

51. International Nasopharynx Cancer Study Group. Preliminary results of a randomized trial comparing neoadjuvant chemotherapy (cisplatin, epirubicin, bleomycin) plus radiotherapy vs. radiotherapy alone in stage IV (≥N2, M0) undifferentiated nasopharyngeal carcinoma: a positive effect on progression-free survival. VUMCA I trial. *Int J Radiat Oncol Biol Phys* 1996;35: 463-469.

52. Al-Sarraf M, LeBlanc M, Giri S, et al. Chemoradiotherapy versus radiotherapy in patients with advanced nasopharyngeal cancer: phase III randomized intergroup study 0099. *J Clin Oncol* 1998;16:1310-1317.

53. Chua D, Sham J, Choy D, et al. Preliminary report of the Asian-Oceanian Clinical Oncology Association randomized trial comparing cisplatin and epirubicin followed by radiotherapy versus radiotherapy alone in the treatment of patients with locoregionally advanced nasopharyngeal carcinoma. *Cancer* 1998;83:2270-2283.

54. Teo P, Chan A, Lee W, et al. Enhancement of local control in locally advanced node-positive nasopharyngeal carcinoma by adjunctive chemotherapy. *Int J Radiat Oncol Biol Phys* 1999;43:261-271.

55. Calais G, Alfonsi M, Bardet E, et al. Randomized trial of radiation therapy versus concomitant chemotherapy and radiation therapy for advanced-stage oropharynx carcinoma. *J Natl Cancer Inst* 1999;91:2081-2086.

56. Brizel DM, Albers ME, Fisher SR, et al. Hyperfractionated irradiation with or without concurrent chemotherapy for locally advanced head and neck cancer. *N Engl J Med* 1998;338:1798-1804.

57. Adelstein D, Lavertu P, Saxton J, et al. Mature results of a phase III randomized trial comparing concurrent chemoradiotherapy with radiation therapy alone in patients with stage III and IV squamous cell carcinoma of the head and neck. *Cancer* 2000;88:876-883.

58. Cooper J, Lee H, Torrey M, et al. Improved outcome secondary to concurrent chemoradiotherapy for advanced carcinoma of the nasopharynx: preliminary corroboration of the intergroup experience. *Int J Radiat Oncol Biol Phys* 2000;47:861-866.

59. Cheng S, Jian J-M, Tsai S, et al. Prognostic features and treatment outcome in locoregionally advanced nasopharyngeal carcinoma following concurrent chemotherapy and radiotherapy. *Int J Radiat Oncol Biol Phys* 1998;41:755-762.

60. King W, Ku P, Mok C, et al. Nasopharyngectomy in the treatment of recurrent nasopharyngeal carcinoma: a 12-year experience. *Head Neck* 2000;22:215-222.

61. Wei W. Salvage surgery for recurrent primary nasopharyngeal carcinoma. *Crit Rev Oncol Hematol* 2000;33:91-98.

62. Fee W Jr, Roberson J, Goffinet D. Long-term survival after surgical resection for recurrent nasopharyngeal cancer after radiotherapy failure. *Arch Otolaryngol Head Neck Surg* 1991;117: 1233-1236.

63. Lee A, Law S, Foo W, et al. Retrospective analysis of patients with nasopharyngeal carcinoma treated during 1976-1985: survival after local recurrence. *Int J Radiat Oncol Biol Phys* 1993; 26:773-782.

64. Chang J, See L, Liao C, et al. Locally recurrent nasopharyngeal carcinoma. *Radiother Oncol* 2000;54:135-142.

65. Teo P, Kwan W, Chan A, et al. How successful is high-dose (≥60 Gy) reirradiation using mainly external beams in salvaging local failures of nasopharyngeal carcinoma? *Int J Radiat Oncol Biol Phys* 1998;40:897-913.

66. Hwang J-M, Fu K, Phillips T. Results and prognostic factors in the retreatment of locally recurrent nasopharyngeal carcinoma. *Int J Radiat Oncol Biol Phys* 1998;41:1099-1111.

67. Pryzant R, Wendt C, Delcos L, et al. Re-treatment of nasopharyngeal carcinoma in 53 patients. *Int J Radiat Oncol Biol Phys* 1992;22:941-947.

68. Syed A, Puthawala A, Damore S, et al. Brachytherapy for primary and recurrent nasopharyngeal carcinoma: 20 years' experience at Long Beach Memorial. *Int J Radiat Oncol Biol Phys* 2000;47:1311-1321.

69. McLean M, Chow E, O'Sullivan B, et al. Re-irradiation for locally recurrent nasopharyngeal carcinoma. *Radiother Oncol* 1998;48:209-211.

70. Orecchia R, Redda M, Ragona R, et al. Results of hypofractionated stereotactic re-irradiation on 13 locally recurrent nasopharyngeal carcinomas. *Radiother Oncol* 1999;53:23-28.

71. Hsu MM, Ko JY, Sheen TS, et al. Salvage surgery for recurrent nasopharyngeal carcinoma. *Arch Otolaryngol Head Neck Surg* 1997;123:305-309.

72. Cmelak A, Cox R, Adler J, et al. Radiosurgery for skull base malignancies and nasopharyngeal carcinoma. *Int J Radiat Oncol Biol Phys* 1997;37:997-1003.

73. Mitsuhashi N, Sakurai H, Katano S, et al. Stereotactic radiotherapy for locally recurrent nasopharyngeal carcinoma. *Laryngoscope* 1999;109:805-809.

74. Ingersoll L, Woo S, Donaldson S, et al. Nasopharyngeal carcinoma in the young: a combined M.D. Anderson and Stanford experience. *Int J Radiat Oncol Biol Phys* 1990;19:881-887.

75. Pao W, Hutsu O, Douglass E, et al. Pediatric nasopharyngeal carcinoma: long-term follow-up of 29 patients. *Int J Radiat Oncol Biol Phys* 1989;17:299-305.

76. Ayan I, Altun M. Nasopharyngeal carcinoma in children: retrospective review of 50 patients. *Int J Radiat Oncol Biol Phys* 1996;35:485-492.

77. Ahern V, Jenkin D, Banerjee D, et al. Nasopharyngeal carcinoma in the young. *Clin Oncol (R Coll Radiol)* 1994;6:24-30.

CHAPTER 9

The Oropharynx

William H. Morrison

The oropharynx consists of the tongue base, tonsillar fossa, soft palate, and lateral and posterior oropharyngeal walls (Fig. 9-1). These structures play an essential role in swallowing and speech. Extensive neoplasms arising in the oropharynx can impede swallowing and speech by infiltrating muscles or nerves or obstructing the oropharyngeal air space. Treatments administered to cure oropharyngeal tumors also can cause structural deformity and functional impairment. Radiation therapy is generally preferred over surgery for the management of early-stage to moderately advanced oropharyngeal tumors because tumoricidal doses can be given with a relatively high likelihood of preserving swallowing and speech.

Carcinoma of the oropharynx constitutes a good model in which to investigate the radiobiology of human tumors. Because oropharyngeal carcinomas are readily accessible to examination, staging and evaluations of response to therapy can be performed accurately. A large body of time-dose fractionation data has been obtained from studying the response of oropharyngeal tumors to irradiation.[1-3]

PATHOLOGY

Approximately 95% of oropharyngeal tumors are squamous cell carcinomas. Less common epithelial neoplasms originating in the oropharynx are minor salivary gland tumors[4] and squamous carcinoma with lymphoid stroma (lymphoepithelioma).[5] Malignant lymphomas occasionally occur in the lymphoid tissue of the oropharynx (part of Waldeyer's ring).[6]

ANATOMY AND PATHWAYS OF SPREAD

The route of spread of oropharyngeal cancer varies somewhat with the subsite. Knowledge of the anatomy of the subsites facilitates insight into the pathways of spread.

Tongue Base

The tongue base is the posterior, vertical component of the tongue and includes the valleculae. It starts behind the terminal sulcus of the tongue, borders the glossopharyngeal sulcus laterally, and ends at the junction between the valleculae and the base of the epiglottis inferiorly. The tongue base contains numerous submucosal lymphoid follicles, which give its surface an irregular appearance. This lymphoid tissue can enhance on contrast-enhanced computed tomography (CT), producing a radiologic appearance that can be confused with tumor.

The tongue base has a different embryologic origin than the oral tongue. The main sensory innervation of the tongue base is from the lingual branch of the glossopharyngeal nerve. The hypoglossal nerve provides the motor innervation of the entire tongue, including the base. The main lymphatic drainage pathway of the tongue base is to the jugular chain of lymph nodes.

Early tongue base tumors tend to grow either in an exophytic manner or, more often, with a prominent submucosal infiltrative component that invades the intrinsic tongue muscles. At a later stage, tongue base tumors can extend anteroinferiorly through the intrinsic tongue muscles to involve the extrinsic muscles, causing tongue deviation or impaired tongue mobility; spread laterally through the glossopharyngeal sulcus to the tonsillar fossa and pharyngeal wall; or grow inferiorly into the pre-epiglottic space, hypopharynx, and larynx. Very advanced tongue base tumors can extend into the soft tissues of the neck. Invasion through the mandibular cortex is unusual.

The incidence of nodal involvement at diagnosis in patients with tongue base tumors referred to The University of Texas M.D. Anderson Cancer Center between 1948 and 1965 was 78%.[7] Figure 9-2 shows the distribution of nodal disease at presentation in 185 patients with tongue base carcinoma. Bilateral nodal disease was present in 29% of patients, which is as expected for a tumor arising in a midline structure. In a series of patients with no palpable lymphadenopathy who underwent neck dissection at Mayo Clinic, the incidence of subclinical nodal involvement was 44%.[8]

Tonsillar Fossa

The tonsillar fossa is located between the anterior and posterior palatoglossal arches (faucial pillars). The palatine tonsil has a surface mucosa of stratified squamous

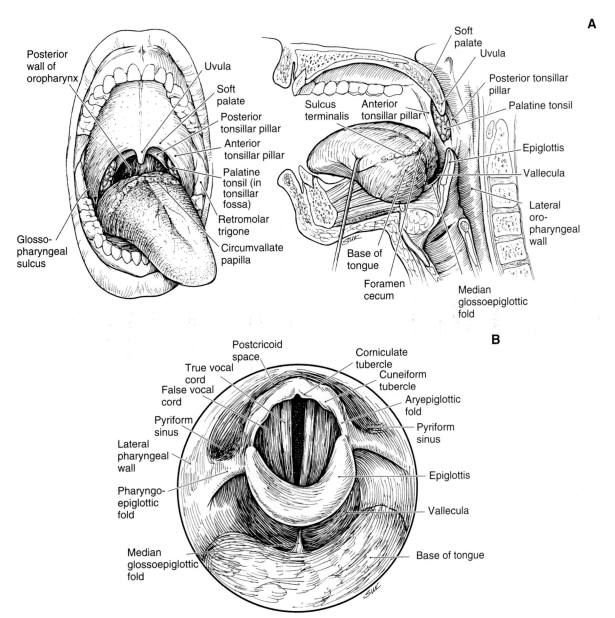

Fig. 9-1 Normal anatomy of the oropharynx. **A,** Anterior view and lateral view of the oropharynx with left lateral structures removed. **B,** Oropharynx as viewed through a fiberoptic endoscope.

epithelium overlying lymphatic nodules. A fibrous capsule forms the lateral surface of the tonsil, and underneath this capsule are the superior pharyngeal constrictor muscle, the pterygoid muscles, and the mandible. The internal carotid artery is located approximately 2 cm lateral and posterior to the tonsil in the parapharyngeal space. The sensory innervation of the tonsil is from the middle and posterior palatine branches of the maxillary nerve.

Tumors originating in the tonsillar fossa often grow as an exophytic mass into the oropharyngeal air space. Other tonsillar tumors spread anteriorly in the anterior palatoglossal arch, medially along the soft palate, across the glossopalatine sulcus into the tongue base, and posteriorly to the posterior palatoglossal arch and lateral pharyngeal wall. More advanced tumors can extend laterally into the pterygoid muscles, superiorly into the nasopharynx, and inferiorly into the pyriform sinus. Invasion of the extrinsic muscles of the root of the tongue can impair tongue mobility, and significant infiltration of the pterygoid muscles will cause trismus. Very advanced tonsillar fossa tumors can extend into the neck, encase the carotid artery, or erode the cortex of the mandible.

The pattern of local extension for 160 patients with carcinoma of the tonsil referred to the M.D. Anderson Cancer Center between 1968 and 1979 is shown in Table 9-1.[9] In this series, nodal disease was present at diagnosis in 69% of patients. Figure 9-3 shows the sites

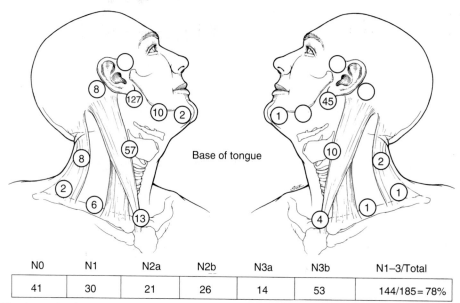

Base of tongue

N0	N1	N2a	N2b	N3a	N3b	N1–3/Total
41	30	21	26	14	53	144/185 = 78%

Fig. 9-2 Distribution of nodal metastases at presentation in patients with squamous carcinoma of the tongue base seen at the M.D. Anderson Cancer Center between 1948 and 1965. (From Lindberg R. *Cancer* 1972;29:1446-1449.)

TABLE 9-1

Sites of Local Extension of Carcinoma of the Tonsil in 160 Patients Seen at M.D. Anderson Cancer Center Between 1968 and 1979

Site	Percent of Patients
Tonsil and pillars only	23
Tongue base	38
Lateral pharyngeal wall	31
Soft palate	23
Retromolar triangle	10
Oral tongue	4
Posterior pharyngeal wall	3
Buccal mucosa	3
Lateral floor of mouth	2
Pterygoid muscles	2
Mandibular or maxillary bone	1

From Remmler D, Medina JE, Byers RM, et al. *Head Neck Surg* 1985;7:206-211.

of nodal involvement in these patients. In a series of patients with tonsillar fossa tumors and no palpable lymphadenopathy who underwent neck dissections at Mayo Clinic between 1970 and 1988, the incidence of subclinical nodal involvement was 32%.[10]

Soft Palate

The soft palate consists of five muscles (levator veli palatini, tensor veli palatini, uvulae, palatoglossus, and palatopharyngeus) covered with stratified squamous epithelium on the oral surface and most of the nasal surface. The soft palate has an important role in speech and swallowing. It closes off the nasopharynx during swallowing to prevent nasal reflux and during phonation to produce certain sounds. The lesser palatine nerve, a branch of the maxillary nerve, provides sensory innervation to the soft palate. The tensor veli palatini muscle is innervated by the mandibular nerve through the branch to the medial pterygoid muscle. The other soft palate muscles are innervated by the contribution of the vagus nerve to the pharyngeal plexus.

Almost all soft palate tumors arise on the oral surface. Early tumors tend to grow superficially along mucosal surfaces and often appear as regions of erythroplasia with indistinct borders. The erythroplasia may be multifocal. Common routes of spread are down the anterior palatoglossal arches, into the tonsillar fossa and pharyngeal wall, and anteriorly onto the hard palate. Locally advanced tumors are not as common as in other oropharyngeal sites.

The frequency of nodal involvement at diagnosis in patients with soft palate carcinoma who presented to the M.D. Anderson Cancer Center between 1948 and 1965 was 40%,[7] which was lower than the incidences for tongue base and tonsillar region tumors. Because of the midline nature of soft palate tumors, bilateral nodal disease at presentation is common.

Oropharyngeal Walls

The lateral and posterior oropharyngeal walls consist of squamous epithelium overlying the superior and middle pharyngeal constrictor muscles. Located behind the epithelium of the posterior pharyngeal wall are the retropharyngeal space, longus capitis and longus colli muscles, prevertebral fascia, and vertebral bodies.

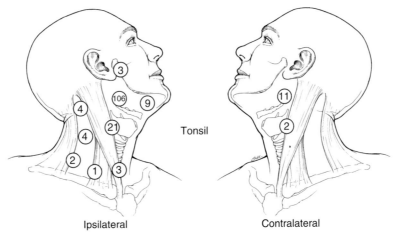

Fig. 9-3 Distribution of nodal metastases at presentation in patients with squamous carcinoma of the tonsil seen at the M.D. Anderson Cancer Center between 1968 through 1979. (From Remmler D, Medina JE, Byers RM, et al. *Head Neck Surg* 1985;7:206-211.)

Tumors of the posterior oropharyngeal wall usually grow anteriorly into the pharyngeal cavity and posteriorly into the prevertebral muscles. However, invasion through the prevertebral fascia and into the vertebral bodies rarely occurs. Tumors of the lateral pharyngeal wall extend anteriorly and posteriorly along the mucosa and parapharyngeal space, can grow as exophytic masses into the pharyngeal cavity, and in advanced stages can directly invade the neck. The incidence of nodal involvement at presentation among 164 patients with oropharyngeal wall squamous carcinomas treated at the M.D. Anderson Cancer Center between 1954 and 1974 was 57%.[11]

CLINICAL MANIFESTATIONS, EVALUATION, AND STAGING

Early-stage oropharyngeal tumors cause few symptoms. Pain, which can be local or radiate to the ear, is a common first symptom. The initial sign of disease is often an asymptomatic neck mass located in the jugulodigastric region. Masses in the tonsil and soft palate can be seen easily on direct examination. Patients with advanced-stage disease can present with trismus, odynophagia, dysphagia, dysarthria, and necrotic odor.

Physical examination includes assessment of the local extent of the primary tumor and the presence and location of lymphadenopathy. The size of the primary tumor and nodal disease should be measured because these measurements form the basis of the American Joint Committee on Cancer (AJCC) staging system for oropharyngeal cancer.[12] Impairment of tongue protrusion is a sign of root-of-tongue involvement. Trismus, a consequence of infiltration of the pterygoid muscles, is documented by measuring the distance between the upper and lower incisors or alveolar ridges. Tumor extension into the pyriform sinus should be noted because this finding has an important impact on the radiation portal. Documentation of the anterior tumor border in relation

to the position of radio-opaque anatomic structures, such as the retromolar triangle, hard palate, and various teeth, also is useful for radiation portal design.

In addition to a complete history and physical examination, the staging work-up for oropharyngeal tumors includes chest radiography, a complete blood count, and routine serum chemistry studies. CT and magnetic resonance imaging (MRI) are useful in defining the anatomic extensions of the primary tumor and nodal disease; low-volume nodal disease that is not evident on physical examination often can be detected with these imaging techniques. Other tests are performed as indicated by the clinical findings.

The current AJCC staging system for oropharyngeal carcinomas is shown in Box 9-1. All available information obtained before treatment, including CT and MRI findings, can be used to designate the T stage. The distinction between T1, T2, and T3 is based simply on tumor size. Tumors are classified as T4 on the basis of invasion into adjacent structures, such as pterygoid muscle(s), mandible, hard palate, deep muscle of tongue, and larynx. At the M.D. Anderson Cancer Center, tumors are staged T4 only if there is extensive infiltration of one of these adjacent structures. Minor clinical extensions to the listed structures (e.g., extension of soft palate tumors onto the hard palate or superficial extension of tongue base tumors onto the lingual surface of the epiglottis) should not result in classification of disease as T4. For a tumor to be staged T4, invasion of the pterygoid muscles should be extensive enough to cause some trismus. Invasion into the deep muscles of the tongue is a difficult clinical call because the boundary of the deep muscles cannot be seen or palpated. Tumors that cause tongue fixation or significant tongue deviation on protrusion can be assumed to be invading the deep tongue muscles. Tongue base tumors that involve the deep tongue muscles usually can be palpated through the posterolateral floor of the mouth. Staging of

---

Box 9-1   American Joint Committee on Cancer Staging System for Tumors of the Oropharynx

PRIMARY TUMOR (T)

TX   Primary tumor cannot be assessed
T0   No evidence of primary tumor
Tis Carcinoma in situ
T1   Tumor 2 cm or less in greatest dimension
T2   Tumor more than 2 cm but not more than 4 cm in greatest dimension
T3   Tumor more than 4 cm in greatest dimension
T4   Tumor invades adjacent structures (e.g., pterygoid muscle[s], mandible, hard palate, deep muscle of tongue, larynx)

REGIONAL LYMPH NODES (N)

NX   Regional lymph nodes cannot be assessed
N0   No regional lymph node metastasis
N1   Metastasis in a single ipsilateral lymph node, 3 cm or less in greatest dimension
N2   Metastasis in a single ipsilateral lymph node, more than 3 cm but not more than 6 cm in great dimension, or in multiple ipsilateral lymph nodes, none more than 6 cm in greatest dimension, or in bilateral or contralateral lymph nodes, none more than 6 cm in greatest dimension
N2a Metastasis in a single ipsilateral lymph node more than 3 cm but not more than 6 cm in greatest dimension

N2b Metastasis in multiple ipsilateral lymph nodes, none more than 6 cm in greatest dimension
N2c Metastasis in bilateral or contralateral lymph nodes, none more than 6 cm in greatest dimension
N3   Metastasis in a lymph node more than 6 cm in greatest dimension

DISTANT METASTASIS (M)

MX   Distant metastasis cannot be assessed
M0   No distant metastasis
M1   Distant metastasis

STAGE GROUPING: OROPHARYNX

Stage 0	Tis	N0	M0
Stage I	T1	N0	M0
Stage II	T2	N0	M0
Stage III	T3	N0	M0
	T1	N1	M0
	T2	N1	M0
	T3	N1	M0
Stage IVA	T4	N0	M0
	T4	N1	M0
	Any T	N2	M0
Stage IVB	Any T	N3	M0
Stage IVC	Any T	Any N	M1

From Fleming I, Cooper JS, Henson DE, et al, eds. *AJCC Cancer Staging Manual*, 5th ed. Philadelphia, Pa: Lippincott Williams & Wilkins; 1997:35.

---

nodal disease using the AJCC system is relatively straightforward; the N classification is based on the size, number, and location of involved nodes.

PRIMARY THERAPY
General Principles of Treatment

The goal of treatment of oropharyngeal tumors is to maximize the tumor control rate while minimizing functional impairment and cosmetic deformity. The choice of treatment depends on the stage and site of the disease.

Early Carcinomas

For early oropharyngeal carcinomas (T1, N0-1 disease and small T2, N0-1 disease), primary radiation therapy and primary surgery (often with the judicious use of postoperative radiation therapy as indicated by the pathologic findings) produce similar local and regional control rates. Consequently, treatment selection is based on the anticipated cosmetic and functional outcome and the need for and extent of nodal therapy. For example, surgery is an option for the treatment of small and superficial tumors of the anterior palatoglossal

arches, particularly when resection can be done through a transoral approach and the likelihood of obtaining tumor-free resection margins is high. In contrast, radiation therapy is more suitable for the treatment of most T1 and early T2 N0-1 carcinomas of the tonsillar fossa with minimal extension onto the soft palate because unilateral irradiation in this situation results in local–regional control without causing permanent xerostomia. Radiation therapy (bilateral irradiation) also is indicated for the treatment of small tonsil tumors that extend onto the soft palate because resection of the soft palate would impair swallowing function. Patients with early-stage oropharyngeal carcinoma who require bilateral irradiation are candidates for parotid-sparing techniques using intensity-modulated radiation therapy.

Intermediate-Stage Carcinomas

Intermediate-stage carcinomas (larger T2, nonextensive T3, or any T stage with N2-3 disease) are best treated with primary radiation therapy because most patients with intermediate-stage carcinomas treated with primary surgery end up requiring postoperative radiation therapy because of multiple positive nodes, extranodal extension, or close resection margins. Patients with tongue base or soft palate carcinomas will have significantly worsened functional outcomes if a major component of the affected organ is resected. Approaches to the treatment of nodal disease are presented in the section on "Integration of Treatment of Primary Tumor and Nodal Disease."

Advanced Infiltrative Primary Tumors

Advanced infiltrative primary tumors (advanced infiltrative T3, T4) have traditionally been treated with the combination of composite primary resection, nodal dissection, and postoperative irradiation. Because of the morbidity of surgery in this setting, many patients are being enrolled in protocols investigating the role of chemotherapy in combination with radiation therapy, surgery, or both modalities.

Integration of Treatment of Primary Tumor and Nodal Disease

Three general strategies are commonly used in patients with resectable nodal disease whose primary tumor is being treated with definitive radiation therapy: radiation therapy as the initial treatment, with subsequent neck dissection only in patients with persistent nodal disease after radiation therapy; neck dissection followed by radiation therapy; and radiation therapy as the initial treatment, with neck dissection planned for all patients regardless of the response to radiation. The last strategy is used most often in patients with N2-3 neck disease. At the M.D. Anderson Cancer Center, the strategy used depends in part on whether extensive dental extractions are necessary before radiation therapy. If extensive dental procedures are planned and the patient is deemed likely to require neck dissection after irradiation, then neck dissection and dental surgery are performed during the same period of general anesthesia. At the M.D. Anderson Cancer Center, most patients treated with preradiation-therapy neck dissections have nodes 4 cm or larger.[13]

Treatment Policies by Subsite
Tongue Base Carcinomas

Many centers regard primary radiation therapy as the treatment of choice for T1, T2, and favorable T3 tongue base carcinomas. In such cases, nonpalpable lymph nodes on both sides of the neck need to be electively irradiated because tongue base tumors are situated at or close to the midline and thus have a high propensity for bilateral nodal spread. In selected cases the boost dose to the primary tumor or a supplemental dose to a slowly regressing tumor is delivered by interstitial therapy. Using new technologies, many clinicians are investigating whether the bilateral nodes at risk can be irradiated while the dose to the parotid glands is limited to a moderate dose that does not cause xerostomia.

The standard therapy for more advanced tongue base tumors is surgery and postoperative radiation therapy. Surgery for advanced tumors commonly requires a laryngectomy to prevent aspiration. Patients who have had a glossectomy may have difficulty swallowing solid food. These patients, with rehabilitated speech and varying degrees of dysphagia, generally have a poor quality of life. This unsatisfactory outcome has led to trials of tissue-conserving approaches using systemic therapies combined with radiation.

Tonsillar Fossa Carcinomas

Tumors of the tonsillar fossa are known to be radiosensitive, and high local control rates can be achieved with radiation therapy alone. At many centers, radiation therapy is the preferred treatment for T1, T2, and moderately advanced T3 tonsillar fossa carcinomas. To avoid radiation-induced permanent xerostomia, unilateral irradiation has been increasingly used in the treatment of T1 and early T2, N0-1 carcinomas of the tonsillar fossa with minimal extension onto the soft palate. More advanced tumors (larger T2 and exophytic T3 carcinomas) are treated with bilateral irradiation. In selected cases in which primary tumor extension into the tongue base persists after external-beam radiation therapy, a boost dose designed to eradicate the remaining tumor is administered by brachytherapy. An additional dose of 10 to 15 Gy can be given in this manner.[14]

The standard therapy for more advanced tumors (infiltrative T3 and T4 carcinomas) is surgery and comprehensive postoperative radiation therapy. Infiltrative tumors tend to invade deeply into the pterygoid muscles, neck, and tongue base, causing tongue deviation on protrusion. These tumors are less likely to grow prominently into the air cavities or superficially along mucosal surfaces and are more likely to cause pain. Because tonsillar tumors are radiosensitive, many centers are investigating the role of altered fractionation and chemoirradiation as an alterative to surgery for these patients.

Soft Palate Carcinomas

The overall treatment strategy for soft palate carcinomas is similar to that for tongue base carcinomas. Soft palate tumors often have indistinct margins and are associated with other areas of erythroplasia. Consequently, surgeons can have difficulty achieving negative surgical margins if they attempt to perform a limited excision. In addition, surgical excision of all but the smallest soft palate carcinomas will cause velopharyngeal incompetence and speech dysfunction that cannot be adequately corrected with prosthetic devices. Therefore, radiation therapy is generally considered to be the treatment of choice.

In a small fraction of patients with accessible, well-delineated T1 and T2 tumors, the boost dose can be delivered through an intraoral cylindrical applicator to

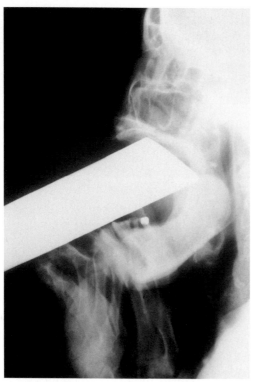

Fig. 9-4 A 71-year-old woman presented in January 1994 with a recurrent squamous carcinoma at the junction of the hard and soft palates. The patient was treated initially through a 3.5-cm intraoral applicator with 250-KeV x-rays to a dose of 10 Gy in four fractions. The radiograph shows the positioning of the intraoral applicator. After the intraoral therapy was completed, the patient was treated with 6-MV photons to 60 Gy to the primary tumor site and 50 Gy to the neck using 2-Gy fractions and shrinking field technique. The patient remained free of head and neck disease but died of a primary lung carcinoma.

spare the mandible and mastication muscles from receiving more than 50 to 55 Gy. This approach is most applicable for edentulous patients, in whom there is more room for the applicator. The boost dose, usually in the range of 15 to 18 Gy in five to six fractions, is generally administered before external-beam irradiation, when the tumor borders can be clearly visualized. Another reason for delivering the boost dose before external-beam therapy is that patient tolerance of the applicator is better if it is used before mucositis develops. A soft palate tumor that was treated with an intraoral applicator is shown in Figure 9-4.

Oropharyngeal Wall Carcinomas

Radiation therapy is generally the preferred treatment for oropharyngeal wall tumors. Because the posterior pharyngeal wall is immediately adjacent to the prevertebral fascia and prevertebral muscles, surgeons have difficulty resecting tumors of the posterior oropharyngeal wall with wide margins, with the possible exception of very small, superficial tumors. Surgical treatment of the

retropharyngeal nodes also is difficult because these nodes extend up to the skull base. With radiation therapy, the primary tumor and nodal beds can be treated with a wide margin until spinal cord tolerance is reached. After this, the posterior field border is placed near the posterior aspect of the vertebral body, and the treatment is continued with this narrower but adequate margin until the final tumor dose is achieved. Multiple portal films must be taken in these patients to verify that the field has been set up accurately and the spinal cord is excluded from irradiation.

Treatment Results by Subsite

This section summarizes data from relatively large series of radiation therapy for treatment of oropharyngeal carcinoma. The information is organized by disease site and radiation therapy strategy. The available data on prognostic factors and the results of phase III trials of altered fractionation are also briefly summarized.

Tongue Base Carcinomas

External-beam radiation therapy. Reported local control rates after radiation therapy for treatment of tongue base carcinomas are shown in Table 9-2.[15-20] According to data published by Spanos and colleagues (M.D. Anderson Cancer Center),[15] Foote and colleagues (University of Florida),[16] and Wang (Massachusetts General Hospital),[17] radiation delivered in standard daily 2-Gy fractions yields a control rate of approximately 90% for T1 tongue base tumors. The dose per fraction and total dose used varied somewhat among series, but the results were similar. For T2 tumors, the local control rates ranged from 70% to 90%. A wide range of local control rates have been reported for T3 tumors; this may be due in part to heterogeneity of patient selection because there is no upper size limit for the T3 classification.

With once-daily fractionation, Foote and colleagues[16] reported a 4% incidence of moderate to severe bone exposure and a 7% incidence of moderate soft tissue necrosis. The main complication in the large series reported from the M.D. Anderson Cancer Center in 1976 was mandibular exposure and necrosis.[15] Of patients in this series, 5% had mandibular exposure that healed with conservative management, and an additional 3% of patients required resection of the mandible because of necrosis. The risk of mandibular necrosis was highest when the tumor extended to the mucosa overlying the mandible. The risk of significant mandibular complications also increased as larger field sizes were used. Mendenhall and colleagues,[18] reporting on a series in which patients were treated predominantly with hyperfractionation, noted that 4% of patients experienced severe late complications, including severe dysphagia requiring a permanent gastrostomy (2%) and osteonecrosis (1%).

TABLE 9-2

Reported Local Control Rates for Squamous Carcinoma of the Tongue Base

Study	Institution	T1	T2	T3	T4	Comments
Spanos et al[15]	M.D. Anderson Cancer Center	91%	71%	78%	52%	1954–1971, varied once-daily fractionation
Foote et al[16]	University of Florida	89%	90%	81%	36%	Once-daily fractionation
Wang[17]	Massachusetts General Hospital	87%	74%	28%	17%	Once-daily fractionation
Weber et al[19]	M.D. Anderson Cancer Center	100%	86%	59%	44%	Interstitial boosts in 14 patients (8%); once-daily fractionation
Wang[17]	Massachusetts General Hospital	90%	84%	64%	28%	Accelerated split course fractionation
Mak et al[20]*	M.D. Anderson Cancer Center	100%†	98%	76%	0%‡	Concomitant boost fractionation
Mendenhall et al[18]	University of Florida	96%	91%	81%	38%	Once-daily fractionation: 31% Hyperfractionation: 69%
Harrison et al[21]*	Memorial Sloan-Kettering Cancer Center	87%	93%	82%	100%§	External-beam radiation therapy plus interstitial radiation therapy

*5-Year actuarial control rates.
†Three of three patients.
‡None of one patient.
§Two of two patients.

External-beam radiation therapy plus brachytherapy. High rates of local and regional control of tongue base carcinomas also can be achieved using a combination of external-beam radiation therapy and brachytherapy. Harrison and colleagues[21] reported on 68 patients treated with this approach at Memorial Sloan-Kettering Cancer Center. Forty-eight patients (71%) had tumors classified as T1 or T2. Patients were considered unsuitable candidates for brachytherapy if their disease extended below the hyoid bone, eroded the mandible, or involved the epiglottis. Patients were treated with 50 to 54 Gy of external-beam radiation to the primary tumor site and upper neck followed by a 20- to 30-Gy boost to the primary tumor using a ^{192}Ir implant. All patients underwent surgery to create a temporary tracheostomy. The 5-year actuarial local control rates were 87%, 93%, and 82%, respectively, for T1, T2, and T3 tumors. The 5-year actuarial regional control rate was 96%. Complications, including soft tissue ulceration, mandibular osteonecrosis, and bleeding at the time of catheter removal, occurred in 19% of the patients.

Puthawala and colleagues[22] reported a series of 70 patients treated with a combination of external-beam radiation therapy and brachytherapy. The median follow-up was 5 years (range for living patients, 2 to 10 years). Crude local control rates in this experience were 88%, 75%, and 67% for T2, T3, and T4 tumors, respectively. Late complications, including soft tissue necrosis and osteonecrosis, occurred in 11% of the patients.

Surgery alone for early-stage tumors. Foote and colleagues[10] reported on a series of 55 patients with tongue base carcinomas who were treated with surgery alone at Mayo Clinic between 1971 and 1986. All 55 patients underwent partial glossectomy, and 11 of the patients also underwent partial or complete laryngectomy. The median follow-up for living patients was 9.4 years (range, 5 to 21 years). The crude rates of local control were as follows: T1, 77%; T2, 81%; and T3, 75%. The crude rate of regional control was 56%, and the rate of disease control above the clavicles was 49%. Sixteen patients required further surgery to manage complications: fistula and abscess formation (eight patients), osteomyelitis with bone necrosis (six patients), pectoralis myocutaneous flap failure (two patients), and hemorrhage (two patients). Five patients required permanent gastrostomy tubes. The surgical mortality rate was 4%. In summary, the local–regional control rate in this experience using surgery alone seems to be worse than local–regional control rates achieved with radiation therapy, and the complication rate was substantial.

Surgery and radiation therapy in combination. Extensive (> 6 cm), infiltrative T3 and T4 tumors of the tongue base have a tendency for local recurrence when treated with radiation therapy alone. Therefore these tumors are usually treated with a combination of surgery and postoperative radiation therapy. De Los Santos and colleagues[23] reported a series of 51 patients with advanced tongue base carcinoma who were treated with surgery and postoperative radiation therapy at the M.D. Anderson Cancer Center between 1980 and 1997. Of the patients, 86% had T3 (21 patients) or T4 (23 patients) tumors. All patients underwent glossectomy, and this was accompanied by laryngectomy in 51% of patients and mandibulectomy in 35%. The median radiation therapy dose was 63 Gy. The 5-year actuarial local–regional control rate was 74%, and the 5-year rate of distant metastases was 35%. Although swallowing function was not formally assessed, chronic swallowing deficits of various degrees were noted in 21 patients. Because of the significant functional problems seen after treatment with surgery plus radiation therapy, patients with advanced tongue base carcinomas are currently being treated on clinical trials of radiation therapy and chemotherapy.

Quality of life. Harrison and colleagues[24] at Memorial Sloan-Kettering Cancer Center have performed detailed quality-of-life studies on patients with tongue base carcinoma treated with radiation therapy. The authors found that after radiation therapy, most patients were able to return to work and maintain approximately the same income level as they had before treatment. In addition, validated tests of speech, swallowing, and diet showed that the patients had good functional outcomes after radiation therapy.

Tonsillar Fossa Carcinoma

External-beam radiation therapy: M.D. Anderson Cancer Center series. Wong and colleagues[25] reported on 150 patients with tonsillar fossa carcinoma treated with external-beam radiation therapy with 2-Gy fractionation at the M.D. Anderson Cancer Center between 1968 and 1983. The mean tumor doses were as follows: T1, 64 Gy; T2, 68 Gy; and T3, 70 Gy. Boosts were usually given through ipsilateral reduced fields, most often with a combination of high-energy electrons and photons. In 26 patients, a neck dissection was performed approximately 6 weeks after the completion of radiation therapy. The local control rates after radiation therapy were 94%, 79%, and 58%, respectively, for T1, T2, and T3 tumors (Table 9-3). The ultimate local control rates after surgical salvage therapy were 100%, 85%, and 60% for T1, T2, and T3 tumors, respectively. The regional control rate, calculated after exclusion of patients who had a local recurrence, was 96%. Seventeen severe complications developed in 14 patients, including bone necrosis requiring mandibular resection (seven patients), soft tissue necrosis (four patients), trismus (five patients), and cranial nerve palsies (one patient). All 14 patients received doses of greater than 67.5 Gy.

At this writing, 98 patients with intermediate-stage tonsillar fossa carcinoma (41 with T2 tumors and 57 with T3 tumors) have been treated at the M.D. Anderson Cancer Center with a concomitant boost fractionation schedule. This schedule involves giving 54 Gy in 1.8-Gy fractions over a period of 6 weeks to lateral fields that include the primary tumor and the draining lymphatics. Subclinical disease can usually be eradicated with this dose. The fields are generally reduced off the spinal cord after 41.4 Gy, with the goal of limiting the spinal cord dose from the entire treatment to 45 Gy. At the beginning

---

TABLE 9-3

Local Control Rates for Patients with Squamous Carcinoma of the Tonsil Treated with Standard 2-Gy Fractionation at M.D. Anderson Cancer Center Between 1968 and 1983*

Tumor Stage	ALL PATIENTS Local Control After XRT (%)	EVALUABLE PATIENTS† Local Control After XRT (%)	Salvage Surgery	Local Control After Surgery	Ultimate Local Control (%)
T1	16/17 (94)	15/16 (94)	1	1/1	16/16 (100)
T2	48/59 (81)	41/52 (79)	6	3/6	44/52 (85)
T3	44/66 (67)	30/52 (58)	10	1/10	31/52 (60)
T4	5/8 (63)	3/6 (50)	1	0/1	3/6 (50)
TOTAL	113/150 (75)	89/126 (71)	18	5/18	94/126 (75)

Modified from Wong CS, Ang KK, Fletcher GH, et al. *Int J Radiat Oncol Biol Phys* 1989;16:657-662.
*Note: Patients treated between July 1968 and December 1983. Analysis performed December 1986.
†Twenty-four patients who died within 2 years after irradiation without local failure were excluded from the analysis of local control. Length of follow-up after salvage therapy ranged from 26 to 162 months.

of the fourth week of treatment, a boost of 15 to 18 Gy (given in 1.5-Gy fractions twice a day, with an interfraction interval of 6 hours) is then delivered to the primary tumor and clinical nodal disease. The final dose is 69 to 72 Gy, given over 6 weeks, and the maximum dose point on the isodose plan is limited to 75 Gy. The 5-year actuarial local control rates for T2 and T3 tumors treated with this schedule are 86% and 83%, respectively (Morrison WH, unpublished data).

External-beam radiation therapy: non–M.D. Anderson Cancer Center series. Over a 33-year interval, 400 patients with squamous carcinoma of the tonsillar region were treated at the University of Florida with either once-daily fractionation schedules (40% of patients) or twice-daily fractionation schedules (60% of patients).[26] Hyperfractionation to a median dose of 76.8 Gy was used in 60% of the patients; the other 40% were treated with standard fractionation. In addition to the external-beam radiation therapy, 27% of the patients received a brachytherapy boost of 10 to 15 Gy, usually to the tongue base component of the tumor. Planned neck dissections were performed in 125 patients after completion of radiation therapy. The minimum follow-up for living patients was 2 years. The local control rates were as follows: T1, 83%; T2, 81%; T3, 74%; and T4, 60%. When tumors of the anterior palatoglossal arches were excluded, the local control rates for the tonsillar fossa and posterior palatoglossal arch tumors that remained were as follows: T1, 90%; T2, 88%; T3, 66%; and T4, 58%. Nineteen patients experienced severe late complications. The most common of these were osteonecrosis necessitating a segmental mandibulectomy (eight patients) and swallowing difficulty necessitating a permanent gastrostomy (six patients); other complications were bone exposure requiring debridement and hyperbaric oxygen (three patients), orocutaneous fistula (one patient), and fatal aspiration (one patient).

Bataini and colleagues[27] reported on a series of 465 patients with squamous carcinoma of the tonsillar region who were treated almost exclusively with external-beam radiation therapy at the Institut Curie. Mean radiation doses were 65 Gy for T1 and T2 tumors, 67 Gy for T3 tumors, and 68 Gy for T4 tumors. The minimum follow-up interval for living patients was 5 years. The local control rates for T1, T2, T3, and T4 tumors were 89%, 84%, 63%, and 43%, respectively. These authors reported that tumors of the tonsillar fossa had higher local control rates than tumors originating in other sites of the tonsillar region (P < 0.01).

Moderate-dose external-beam irradiation with brachytherapy boost. Several investigators have reported good results treating tonsillar fossa tumors with external-beam radiation therapy to doses in the range of 45 to 50 Gy followed by an interstitial brachytherapy boost. Pernot and colleagues[28] reported a series of 343 patients with velotonsillar carcinomas who were treated with external-beam irradiation to 50 Gy in 5 weeks followed by a brachytherapy boost of 20 to 30 Gy. The median follow-up period was 4 years (range, 3 to 13 years). Local control rates for T1, T2, and T3 tumors were 89%, 85%, and 67%, respectively. A multivariate analysis showed that the overall duration of the combined therapy significantly correlated with tumor control. Patients whose treatment was completed within 55 days had a local control rate of 89%, whereas patients whose treatment lasted longer had a local control rate of 78% (P = 0.008). The complication rates were higher in patients who were treated at a dose rate exceeding 0.6 Gy/hr (P = 0.001). Mazeron and colleagues[29] treated 33 patients with selected T1 and T2 tonsil tumors with external-beam radiation therapy to 45 Gy followed by a 30-Gy interstitial boost. At a minimum follow-up time of 2 years (median > 5 years), only 2 of the 69 patients had local–regional recurrence.

Soft Palate Carcinoma

External-beam radiation therapy. Outcomes of various radiation therapy approaches to the treatment of soft palate carcinoma are shown in Table 9-4.[17,30-33] At the Netherlands Cancer Institute,[30] 146 patients with soft palate carcinoma were treated with either external-beam radiation therapy alone (71%) or an intraoral applicator followed by external-beam radiation therapy (29%). The mean total dose was 68 Gy, and the mean treatment duration was 45 days. As would be predicted, patients who received boost doses with the intraoral cylinder had fewer normal tissue complications. For T3 and T4 tumors, control rates did not increase when doses were escalated from 60 to 75 Gy; however, doses were sometimes increased when persistent tumor was present at the completion of the initially planned dose. The authors recommended limiting the external-beam radiation dose to 70 Gy to minimize complications.

Lindberg and Fletcher[31] reported on a series of patients with soft palate tumors who were treated at the M.D. Anderson Cancer Center between 1964 and 1973. The local control rates after radiation therapy were 100%, 88%, 77%, and 83% for T1, T2, T3, and T4 tumors, respectively. Some of the patients with T2 and T3 tumors who had a recurrence subsequently had their disease controlled with surgery; the ultimate control rates for T2 and T3 tumors were 100% and 82%, respectively.

Brachytherapy. Several groups, mostly from France, have achieved good results treating soft palate tumors with interstitial irradiation, usually in combination with external-beam radiation therapy. Mazeron and colleagues[32] reported delivering a mean external-beam dose of 47 Gy and a mean brachytherapy dose of 31 Gy. The crude local control rates with this approach were 93% and 87% for T1 and T2 tumors, respectively. The incidence of soft tissue necrosis was low, and in most

TABLE 9-4

Local Control of Soft Palate Tumors Treated with Radiation Therapy

Author and Institution	TUMOR STAGE			
	T1	T2	T3	T4
Keus et al,[30] Netherlands Cancer Institute	92%	67%	58%	37%
Lindberg and Fletcher,[31] M.D. Anderson Cancer Center (once-daily fractionation)	100%	88%	77%	83%
Wang,[17] Massachusetts General Hospital (1970–1994)	96%	81%	55%	24%
Fein et al,[33] University of Florida (once-daily fractionation)	9/11 (81%)	13/20 (65%)	5/10 (50%)	1/4
Mazeron et al,[32] Henry Mondor Hospital	13/14	20/23	—	—
Fein et al,[33] University of Florida (twice-daily fractionation)	1/1	10/10 (100%)	6/10 (60%)	0/3
Wang,[17] Massachusetts General Hospital (accelerated split course)	91%	79%	68% (T3 + T4)	
Morrison, M.D. Anderson Cancer Center, unpublished data	2/2	21/22 (95%)	13/20 (65%)	—

cases complications could be managed conservatively. An additional six patients with small tumors were treated with interstitial therapy alone, all of whom had their disease locally controlled. At the Institut Gustave-Roussy,[34] 43 patients with early-stage soft palate carcinoma were treated with interstitial irradiation with or without external-beam irradiation. All 34 patients with T1 tumors had their disease locally controlled, and the actuarial local control rate for all patients was 92%.

Oropharyngeal Wall Carcinoma

Standard fractionated and concomitant boost radiation therapy. Meoz-Mendez and colleagues[11] reported a series of patients with pharyngeal wall tumors treated at the M.D. Anderson Cancer Center between 1954 and 1974 with standard fractionation to 70 to 75 Gy in 7 to 7.5 weeks. Local control rates after radiation therapy were 91%, 73%, 61%, and 37%, respectively, for TI, T2, T3, and T4 tumors. No improvement in local control was seen at doses higher than 70 Gy, but patients selected to receive 75 Gy had more massive tumors. The ultimate local control rates after surgical salvage therapy were 100%, 78%, 71%, and 41%, respectively, for T1, T2, T3, and T4 tumors.

Also at the M.D. Anderson Cancer Center, 26 patients with intermediate-stage oropharyngeal wall carcinoma (15 with T2 disease and 11 with T3 disease) have been treated with a concomitant boost schedule.[35] The 5-year actuarial local control rates for the T2 and T3 tumors are 93% and 82%, respectively (Morrison WH, unpublished data).

Concurrent chemotherapy. A phase III trial conducted by the Groupe d'Oncologie Radiothérapie Tête et Cou (GORTEC)[36,37] compared the role of radiation

therapy with or without concurrent chemotherapy in patients with advanced-stage carcinoma of the oropharynx. A total of 226 patients were randomly assigned to radiation therapy alone (70 Gy in 2-Gy fractions) or the same radiation therapy schedule plus concurrent chemotherapy (three cycles of carboplatin and fluorouracil). The median follow-up time was 35 months (range, 12 to 56 months). Acute side effects, particularly mucositis, were worse in the combined-modality arm. The crude local recurrence rates were 51% in patients who received radiation therapy alone and 33% in patients who received combined-modality therapy. Distant metastases occurred in 11% of the patients of both arms. The 3-year actuarial overall survival rates were 51% in the combined-modality arm and 31% in the radiation-therapy-only arm ($P = 0.02$). Disease-free survival also was better in the concurrent chemotherapy arm (42% vs. 20%; $P = 0.04$). The trial was updated in 2001,[37] when the median follow-up was 63 months. At that time, the local–regional control rates were 53% in the combined-modality group and 27% in the radiation-only group.[37] The incidence of grade 3 to 4 late toxic reactions was higher in the combined-modality group (8%) than in the radiation-only group (4%) because of a higher incidence of cervical fibrosis among those given the combined-modality therapy. The investigators concluded that the results of this study support the use of concurrent chemotherapy and radiation therapy for patients with carcinoma of the oropharynx.

Brizel and colleagues[38] at Duke University performed a phase III trial testing concurrent and adjuvant chemotherapy in 116 patients with head and neck carcinoma, 45% of whom had carcinoma of the oropharynx. Eligible patients had T3 or T4 primary tumors of the tonsillar fossa or oropharyngeal wall or T2 N0 tongue base carcinomas. Of the primary tumors, 53% were believed to be unresectable, and 44% of the primary tumors were classified as T4. Patients were randomly assigned to hyperfractionated radiation therapy alone (75 Gy in 1.25-Gy twice-daily fractions) or hyperfractionated radiation therapy at a lower dose (70 Gy in 1.25-Gy twice-daily fractions with a 1-week treatment break) plus two cycles of concurrent cisplatin and fluorouracil. Most patients assigned to receive concurrent chemotherapy also received two cycles of adjuvant chemotherapy after the completion of radiation therapy. The local–regional control rates at 3 years were 70% in the combined-modality arm and 44% in the radiation-therapy-only arm ($P = 0.01$). The 3-year survival rates were 55% in the combined-therapy group and 34% in the radiation-therapy-only group ($P = 0.07$). The authors concluded that concurrent chemoradiation and adjuvant chemotherapy is more efficacious than radiation therapy alone for advanced head and neck carcinoma.

Other phase III studies investigating the role of concurrent chemoradiation in treating carcinoma of the oropharyngeal wall have completed accrual, and the initial published reports should be available soon. The Eastern and Southwest Oncology Groups have completed a phase III study in which patients were randomly assigned to standard fractionated radiation therapy, the same radiation schedule with concurrent cisplatin, or a split-course chemoirradiation schedule.[39] A phase III multicenter German trial compared hyperfractionated accelerated radiation therapy with the same radiation therapy regimen plus concurrent fluorouracil and carboplatin.[40] This trial contained a second randomization for granulocyte colony-stimulating factor.

In summary, two completed randomized trials have shown a benefit for concurrent chemoradiation with cisplatin- and carboplatin-based regimens, and results of other trials are to be published soon. Evidence is increasing that adding concurrent chemotherapy to radiation therapy can improve local–regional control rates in patients with advanced-stage carcinoma of the oropharyngeal wall. The current practice at the M.D. Anderson Cancer Center is to treat patients with advanced-stage (infiltrative T3 and T4) disease with concurrent chemoradiation.

Clinical trials are being performed by many groups to investigate how best to optimize the addition of chemotherapy to radiation therapy in the treatment of carcinoma of the oropharyngeal wall. For example, the Radiation Therapy Oncology Group (RTOG) has recently completed a phase II trial exploring the combination of concurrent cisplatin (100 mg/m^2 on days 1 and 22) and a concomitant boost fractionation schedule.[35]

Control of Nodal Disease

The treatment policy for regional disease from oropharyngeal cancer varies among institutions. At Memorial Sloan-Kettering Cancer Center, patients with tongue base carcinoma and palpable nodes have routinely been treated with neck dissection after irradiation.[41] In these patients the primary tumor and neck lymphatics are initially treated with external-beam radiation therapy to 54 Gy given in 1.8-Gy fractions. Nodal disease is then further irradiated with an electron beam to 60 Gy. The primary tumor is treated with a boost dose using an interstitial implant, and patients undergo a modified radical neck dissection during the same operation to place the implant. In a series of 50 patients treated with this approach, 70% of the patients had pathologically negative neck dissection specimens. Rates of complete pathologic response were similar in patients who presented with advanced nodal stage and patients with more limited nodal disease. The 5-year actuarial rate of regional control was 96%.[24] Morbidity from neck dissection was minimal. The authors noted that their treatment policy might lead to overtreatment of some patients. However, the strategy of giving 60 Gy followed by neck dissection is particularly beneficial when significant nodal disease is present in the low neck because high radiation doses given to the region of the brachial plexus could cause brachial plexopathy.

At the M.D. Anderson Cancer Center, regional disease is treated according to one of two pathways. Patients who will require general anesthesia for extensive dental extractions and who may require a neck dissection after radiation therapy (usually patients with nodal disease ≥4 cm at presentation) are sometimes treated with a preradiation-therapy neck dissection. All other patients are treated initially with definitive radiation therapy. In these patients, disease is reassessed with clinical examination and CT approximately 6 weeks after completion of radiation therapy. Patients who have persistent nodal masses undergo a limited modified neck dissection consisting of removal of the residual mass and immediate surrounding nodes; patients who have a complete clinical and radiologic response are observed.

An analysis of an M.D. Anderson Cancer Center series of patients treated with one concomitant boost schedule[13,35] revealed that 17 patients who underwent preradiation-therapy neck dissection had slightly larger nodes at presentation than did 75 patients who were treated initially with radiation therapy (median nodal size, 4 cm vs. 3 cm). Four (23%) of the 17 patients who were initially treated with neck dissection had a regional recurrence. Of the 75 patients who were initially treated with radiation therapy, 13 underwent a planned neck dissection for persistent nodal masses. Nodal size at presentation was larger than 3 cm in 12 of these 13 patients. None of these 13 patients had a regional recurrence. The remaining 62 patients had a complete response in the neck and therefore did not undergo neck dissection after radiation therapy. Subsequent nodal recurrence occurred in seven (11%) of these 62 patients, of whom three had an isolated regional relapse.

No difference in nodal control was found between the different oropharyngeal subsites, and no relationship was found between initial nodal size and the risk of subsequent recurrence in the neck. The actuarial 2-year probability of control of neck disease was 87% for patients who had initial nodal size less than 3 cm and 85% for patients who had initial nodal size greater than 3 cm. However, the probability of complete response to radiation therapy was less in those patients who presented with larger initial node size. It was concluded that neck dissection could be omitted in patients whose nodes are included in the high-dose volume and who respond completely to treatment.

The current strategy at the M.D. Anderson Cancer Center is to treat nodes 2 cm or larger with radiation to a dose of 69 to 72 Gy over 6 weeks using the concomitant boost fractionation schedule.[13,35] Smaller palpable nodes are treated to doses between 66 and 69 Gy depending on their size. Nodal disease located in the upper jugular region can often be encompassed in the field used to treat the primary tumor, especially when oblique boost fields are used. When a boost dose is delivered to nodes located outside the primary tumor fields, attempts are made to exclude as much of the mucosal surfaces as possible by using electron-beam or glancing photon fields. In addition, when midneck photon fields are used, the volume of the midneck treated to a high dose is limited by giving at least 4.5 Gy with an appositional electron field that encompasses the nodal disease with an appropriate margin.

Distant Metastasis

In analyzing the outcome of a series of 751 patients with oropharyngeal carcinoma treated with radiation therapy at the M.D. Anderson Cancer Center between 1960 and 1974, Lindberg[42] found that distant metastasis was the first site of relapse in 7.7% of the patients. The crude incidence of distant metastases was 2% for patients with stage I to III disease and 13% for those with stage IV disease. In 200 patients treated at the M.D. Anderson Cancer Center with the concomitant boost schedule,[43] the 5-year actuarial incidence of distant metastases was 12% for all patients and 16% for patients who presented with nodal disease.[44] The 5-year actuarial rate of distant metastases was 9% for the 156 patients with local–regional disease control, as opposed to 25% for the 44 patients who experienced a local–regional recurrence ($P = 0.007$). For all 200 patients, the 5-year actuarial incidences of distant metastases were 5%, 17%, 15%, and 18%, respectively, for patients with N0, N1, N2, and N3 neck disease. In the RTOG 9003 study in which 62% of the 1073 patients had oropharyngeal cancer and 31% had T4 primary tumors, the actuarial incidence of distant metastases at 2 years was 17%.[45]

Prognostic Factors

Bataini and colleagues[27] performed a multivariate analysis of the data on 465 patients with carcinoma of the tonsillar region who were treated at the Institut Curie between 1958 and 1976. The authors found that T stage and radiation therapy duration, as a continuous variable, were highly significantly correlated with local control ($P < 0.0001$ for both factors). When stratified by T stage, treatment duration was inversely correlated with local control of T3 tumors ($P = 0.002$) and T4 tumors ($P = 0.04$).

Withers and colleagues[3,46] investigated the effectiveness of various fractionation schemes at nine institutions in North America and England in the treatment of 676 patients with tonsil carcinoma irradiated with external-beam photons alone between 1976 and 1985. Fractionation schedules used varied from 51 Gy in 16 fractions to 75 Gy in 37 fractions. The mean treatment duration was 37 days, and treatment duration was between 20 and 56 days in 90% of the patients. Treatment parameters that significantly correlated with local control were total dose and treatment duration. For a constant treatment duration, the probability of local control increased by nearly 2% for every 1-Gy increase in total dose, and for a constant dose, the probability of local control decreased by 1%/day of treatment prolongation. The estimated extra dose required to compensate for each day of treatment prolongation was in the range of 0.5 to 0.7 Gy/day. Fraction size by itself did not emerge as an independent prognostic factor for tumor control.

An inverse relationship was found between treatment duration and mucosal complications. Higher total dose correlated with a higher incidence of bone, muscle, and mucosal complications, and for a given total dose, larger fraction size was associated with an increased risk of bone and muscle (but not mucosal) complications. Field size correlated significantly with the rate of mandibular complications. Withers and colleagues[46] concluded that the radiobiological characteristics of bone and muscle were similar to the characteristics of other late-responding tissues, whereas the radiobiological characteristics of mucosa were similar to those of acute-responding tissues.

Altered Fractionation

For approximately 3 decades, the standard fractionation schedule for irradiation of head and neck cancer was 2 Gy/fraction given once daily, to a total dose of 66 to 70 Gy. In the late 1970s and early 1980s investigators began to devise different fractionation schedules based on radiobiological principles that were emerging at that time. Early enthusiasm with the results led to the initiation of several randomized trials designed to compare the results from the new fractionation schedules with those from the standard schedule. The best-designed and most carefully conducted of these trials are described in the following paragraphs. The results of these studies do support the superiority of altered fractionation schedules over the previous "standard" schedule.

The European Organization for Research and Treatment of Cancer undertook a prospective randomized trial to address the value of hyperfractionation in the treatment of oropharyngeal carcinoma.[47] This phase III trial compared a hyperfractionated regimen (two 1.15-Gy fractions per day to a total dose of 80.5 Gy in 7 weeks) with a conventional schedule (daily 2-Gy fractions to a total dose of 70 Gy in 7 weeks). The authors showed that hyperfractionation significantly improved the local control rate for T3 tumors ($P = 0.001$; 5-year actuarial control rate, ~52% vs. ~18%) but not for T2 tumors ($P = 0.67$; 5-year actuarial control rate, ~62% vs. ~60%) without appreciably increasing the incidence of grade 2 or worse side effects. Noteworthy, however, was that the control rate in the conventional-fractionation arm of the study for T3 tumors was extremely low.

The RTOG has recently reported the results of a phase III trial (9003) comparing various altered fractionation schedules.[45] The regimens tested were the concomitant boost, hyperfractionation, and accelerated split-course fractionation regimens.[17] The standard treatment was 70 Gy in 2-Gy fractions over 7 weeks. The hyperfractionation regimen was 81.6 Gy in 1.2-Gy fractions twice daily. The concomitant boost regimen consisted of 1.8-Gy fractions to 54 Gy to the large fields plus 18 Gy delivered to the boost field in 12 fractions as a second daily treatment during the last 2.5 weeks of treatment.

The study accrued 1073 analyzable patients, of whom 60% had tumors of the oropharynx. At 2 years, both the hyperfractionation and concomitant boost arms had significantly increased local–regional control rates compared to rates in the standard fractionation arm ($P < 0.05$). The accelerated split-course regimen and standard fractionation had similar local–regional control rates. No significant difference was found in overall survival between the various arms. Compared to standard fractionation, all three altered fractionation schedules were associated with a significantly increased incidence of grade 3 or worse acute side effects. However, when side effects were scored at 6 to 24 months after treatment, no significant difference in the frequency of grade 3 or worse late effects was found between the arms.

As a result of this study, the RTOG has changed their standard radiation schedule for head and neck cancer. Both the concomitant boost fractionation schedule and hyperfractionation produced essentially equivalent results with regard to tumor control and side effects and produced higher tumor control rates than the old standard (70 Gy in 7 weeks). Because the concomitant boost schedule can be completed in 26 fewer treatments than hyperfractionation, it has been adopted by the RTOG as their new standard regimen.

At the M.D. Anderson Cancer Center, 66 Gy in 2-Gy daily fractions is believed to be adequate to treat T1 oropharyngeal tumors because this regimen produces control rates greater than 90% and is associated with lower rates of acute side effects than accelerated fractionation. For the remaining tumors, the concomitant boost schedule is preferred.

The concomitant boost accelerated-fractionation schedule, conceived at the M.D. Anderson Cancer Center by Peters,[35] delivers the reduced field boost in 10 to 12 fractions (depending on tumor volume) of 1.5 Gy as second daily treatments. The interfraction interval is a minimum of 6 hours. This results in shortening the overall time required to administer 69 to 72 Gy from 7 to 8 weeks to 6 weeks without increasing the fraction size.

By October 1997, 276 patients with oropharyngeal carcinoma had been treated at the M.D. Anderson Cancer Center with the concomitant boost schedule with the boost given during the final phase of treatment.[44] The data were updated and analyzed in 1999, when the minimum follow-up for living patients was 2 years. Of the 276 patients, 120 had T2 tumors and 117 patients had T3 tumors. The primary tumor sites were as follows: tonsil, 120 patients; base of tongue, 87 patients; soft palate, 41 patients; and pharyngeal wall, 28 patients. Although mucositis was severe, only 3% of patients required a treatment interruption of more than one scheduled treatment day. The 5-year actuarial disease-specific and overall survival rates for the whole group were 76% and 64%, respectively. The 5-year actuarial local control rates after radiation therapy were 95%, 93%, and 76%, respectively, for T1, T2, and T3 tumors. After surgery for recurrence, the local control rate for T3 tumors was 79%. The local–regional control rate for all patients was 79%. No significant difference was found in the local control rates between the various oropharyngeal subsites.[44]

The long-term rate of persistent late complications, while remaining low, has increased over time. In the M.D. Anderson Cancer Center series in 1999, five patients were dependent on gastrostomy tubes. Three of the tubes were inserted between 5 and 8 years after the completion of treatment. Six patients were unable to swallow solid foods and were on a liquid diet. The rate of chronic dysphagia was higher when the cricopharyngeal muscles were treated in the lateral fields and not excluded from treatment by the larynx block. Other late complications included osteonecrosis requiring partial mandibulectomy (four patients), esophageal stricture (three patients), severe trismus (two patients), and cranial neuropathy (two patients).

Locally Advanced Disease and Palliation

Patients with locally advanced, resectable squamous carcinomas of the oropharynx can be treated with surgery and postoperative radiation therapy. The morbidity of surgery for advanced oropharyngeal carcinomas varies by the site in the oropharynx. Resection of advanced tongue base tumors often requires a concomitant laryngectomy because of the high risk of aspiration after this procedure. Patients with chronic lung disease are more likely to require a concomitant laryngectomy because they tolerate aspiration poorly. If the entire soft palate is resected, a prosthetic replacement device must be fabricated in an attempt to at least partially duplicate the function of the soft palate. In contrast, resection of advanced tonsil tumors that do not extend onto the soft palate or tongue base, usually with a concomitant partial mandibulectomy, leaves patients with adequate retention of speech and swallowing function.

The patient must weigh the potential morbidity of surgery against the option of entering a trial of tissue conservation therapies. The favored alternate treatment strategy for patients who prefer nonsurgical therapy is concomitant chemotherapy and irradiation. For patients with unresectable tumors, chemoradiation can sometimes make surgery possible. Advances in reconstruction have made resection of large tumors more feasible.

Patients who have obviously incurable tumors may benefit from receiving a short course of palliative radiation therapy. The favored regimens at the M.D. Anderson Cancer Center include 30 Gy in 10 fractions and 14 Gy in 4 fractions given over 2 days for three cycles, with an off–spinal-cord reduction after the second cycle. The cycles are separated by 3 to 4 weeks. The 14-Gy regimen has the advantage of being below the dose threshold for acute mucositis.

Postoperative Radiation Therapy

Zelefsky and colleagues[48] reported a series of 51 patients with oropharyngeal carcinoma who were treated at Memorial Sloan-Kettering Cancer Center with postoperative radiation therapy. Indications for radiation therapy were advanced stage (66% of patients had T3 or T4 tumors), close or positive margins (64% of patients), and multiple positive neck nodes (84% of patients). Of the patients with tongue base tumors, 25% required total laryngectomy and 9% required supraglottic laryngectomy.

The 7-year actuarial local and regional control rates were 82% and 81%, respectively, and the 7-year actuarial distant metastasis rate was 28%. The local control rate for patients with close or positive margins who received 60 Gy was 93%. A treatment interruption of at least 1 week because of severe mucositis was allowed in 41% of the patients; in those patients, the treatment was prolonged for a median time of 11 days. Patients who had an interruption in treatment had a 7-year actuarial local control rate of 63%, compared to 93% for those who had no break ($P = 0.05$). Thus good local and regional control rates can be achieved using

surgery and postoperative radiation therapy. However, the authors recommend radiation therapy as the primary therapeutic modality for patients with tongue base tumors because primary radiation therapy in these patients produces tumor control rates similar to those achieved with primary surgery and postoperative radiation therapy and results in superior functional outcomes.

Treatment of Recurrence After Radiation Therapy

Treatment of locally recurrent oropharyngeal carcinomas after radiation therapy is a vexing problem. The standard therapy for postirradiation recurrence is surgical resection, but the salvage rate is usually low.[14] In addition, many patients will not be candidates for surgery or will refuse surgery.

Some encouraging results have been reported from France with the use of salvage irradiation with brachytherapy. Peiffert and colleagues[49] reported on 73 patients with recurrent velotonsillar carcinomas treated with this approach. The stage of the recurrent tumors corresponded to T1 N0 or T2 N0 in 89% of the patients. The mean interstitial dose was 60 Gy, and the mean dose rate was 10.7 Gy/day. After reirradiation, 10 patients had a local recurrence, and 5 patients had a regional recurrence. The disease-specific survival rate was 64% at 5 years. However, a third or fourth primary tumor occurred in half of these patients. The reirradiation was well tolerated, with the main complication being soft tissue necrosis. All cases of necrosis were successfully managed with conservative therapy.

Mazeron and colleagues[50] used brachytherapy to treat 70 patients with new or recurrent oropharyngeal carcinomas in previously irradiated fields. The actuarial 5-year local and regional control rates were 69% and 90%, respectively. However, the 5-year actuarial survival rate was only 14% because of deaths from multiple causes.

Haraf and colleagues[51] have reported the outcomes in 45 patients with recurrent head and neck tumors who underwent external-beam reirradiation with concurrent fluorouracil, hydroxyurea, and cisplatin given on an alternate-week schedule. The patients were treated in four consecutive phase I dose escalation studies; both the chemotherapy dose and the radiation dose were increased with each subsequent study. The median dose of radiation was 50 Gy (range, 9 to 75 Gy) given in 1.8- to 2.0-Gy fractions. The local control rate was 38% for the 20 patients who received more than 58 Gy, compared to 0% for those who received lower doses. Five patients had fatal complications. In a recent update, Haraf and colleagues[52] reported that treatment had been intensified by increasing the reirradiation dose to 75 Gy in 1.5-Gy twice-daily fractions (after a median first-course dose of 68 Gy) and substituting paclitaxel for cisplatin. The full results of this aggressive reirradiation program have not been reported yet.

RADIATION TECHNIQUES
Primary Radiation Therapy: Treatment Set-up and Portal Arrangement
T1-2 N0-1 Tonsillar Fossa Carcinoma

In many centers, early cancer of the tonsillar region is treated with unilateral irradiation encompassing the primary tumor and ipsilateral nodes. A series of 228 patients treated with unilateral irradiation at the Princess Margaret Hospital was reported in 2001[53]; 191 (84%) of the patients had T1 and T2 tumors. The patients were treated predominantly with unilateral wedge-pair technique. Only eight patients (3.5%) experienced a contralateral nodal relapse. Jackson and colleagues[54] reported on 155 patients with N0-1 tonsillar fossa carcinoma who were treated in Vancouver with ipsilateral radiation therapy. The incidence of contralateral nodal recurrence was 2.6%. In a smaller series[10] of 56 patients (45 of whom had T1-2 tumors) treated with surgical procedures not including contralateral neck dissection, 6 patients (11%) had a contralateral nodal recurrence. Given the data from these three series, ipsilateral treatment for patients with tonsillar fossa carcinoma with limited nodal disease seems reasonable. The goals are to minimize morbidity, particularly xerostomia, for patients with tonsillar fossa carcinoma confined to the tonsil or extending to the anterior tonsillar pillar or lateral pharyngeal wall.

Unilateral irradiation of the primary tumor and upper neck can be done with appositional combined electron-photon beams (weighted 4:1 for electron: photon) (Fig. 9-5), wedge-pair photon beam technique, or intensity-modulated radiation therapy. The initial portals should encompass the primary tumor with at least 2.5-cm margins, most of the ipsilateral pterygoid muscles, and the ipsilateral upper jugular nodes. After delivery of the dose required for eradication of subclinical disease (e.g., 50 to 54 Gy in 25 to 30 fractions), the fields are reduced in size to include the primary tumor with 2-cm margins and the involved upper neck nodes. An appositional electron or anterior photon portal is used for elective irradiation of the midneck and lower neck nodes.

A CT-based dosimetric treatment plan is essential. Heterogeneity correction is of particular importance in the case of electron beam therapy. Because the mandible absorbs more of the electron beam than does the soft tissue, the range of the electron beam will decrease by approximately 1 cm distal to the mandible. Electron beam constriction occurring at depth must be taken into account when the portals are designed. If

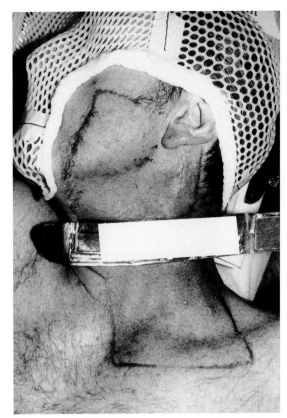

Fig. 9-5 This 53-year-old man presented to the M.D. Anderson Cancer Center in May 1995 with a diagnosis of unknown primary carcinoma after a left neck dissection showed squamous carcinoma in one node located in the subdigastric region. A diagnostic tonsillectomy performed at the M.D. Anderson Cancer Center showed squamous carcinoma. The patient was treated with unilateral 20-MeV electron and 6-MV photon beams, weighted 4:1 in favor of the electron beam. Lead skin collimation was used to block out the electron beam penumbra at the interior field border. The upper and lower neck fields are shown in the photograph. The tonsil bed was treated with 66 Gy in 33 fractions (specified as a minimum tumor dose to the tonsil using full heterogeneity corrections on the dosimetric plan). In December 2000 the patient was free of disease and had experienced no complications of treatment.

intensity-modulated radiation therapy is used, the dose distribution can be configured so that the primary tumor receives a higher dose than the surrounding normal tissues, especially the contralateral parotid glands.

Other Oropharyngeal and More Advanced Tonsillar Fossa Carcinomas

For all tongue base, soft palate (Fig. 9-6), and oropharyngeal wall carcinomas and for more advanced stage tonsillar fossa carcinomas, comprehensive irradiation encompassing the primary tumor and bilateral neck nodes is recommended. The primary tumor is generally treated with parallel-opposed fields with 3-cm margins (Fig. 9-7). Photon beam energies should be in the range

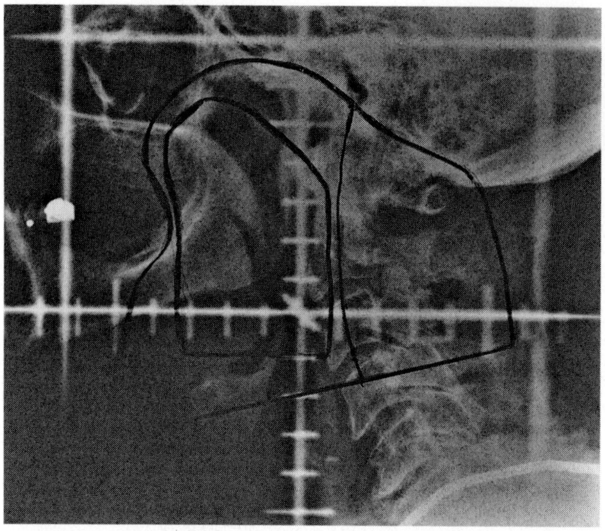

Fig. 9-6 Fields used to treat a T2 N0 squamous carcinoma of the soft palate.

of 1 to 6 MV because higher beam energies may result in an insufficient dose to superficial nodal disease. The superior border of the initial portals should be high enough to cover the retropharyngeal nodes and high jugular nodes approaching the jugular fossa, especially in patients with advanced nodal disease. In patients with tonsillar fossa carcinoma, the ipsilateral pterygoid muscles should be treated. The anterior border of the initial portals is determined by the extent of the primary tumor, and for tonsil tumors this border should always be anterior to the retromolar triangle. The posterior border should be just behind the spinous processes or, in the presence of large posterior cervical nodal masses, more posterior. The inferior border, which matches the anterior lower neck field, should be placed above the arytenoid cartilages unless a more inferior border is necessary to encompass extension of the primary tumor into the laryngeal or hypopharyngeal region.

In patients who have cervical adenopathy extending inferior to the arytenoid level, an asymmetric jaw match is generally done through the nodal disease to avoid unnecessary irradiation of the larynx and cricopharyngeal muscles. The isocenter is placed just above the arytenoid cartilages, and the lateral primary fields and low neck field are matched using an asymmetric jaw technique. When massive neck disease is present, particularly when the disease is displacing the larynx, the junctions are moved inferiorly, and the arytenoid cartilages and cricopharyngeal muscles are included in the lateral fields for the first 44 Gy. Irradiating the larynx below the arytenoid cartilage and cricopharyngeal muscles–upper esophagus during the first 44 Gy increases the risk that gastrostomy tube feeding will be needed in the acute period and increases the risk of chronic dysphagia.

Large upper jugular nodal disease often will be located in the junction between the photon field and the posterior cervical electron portals if horizontal off-cord fields are used. The coverage of upper jugular nodal disease may be improved by using oblique off-cord and boost fields angled so as not to transect the nodal disease. An oblique angle is selected that will provide a 1- to 1.5-cm margin behind the nodal mass (Fig. 9-8). Parallel opposed oblique beam angles of 20 to 35 degrees above and below the horizontal are often necessary to achieve this.

If large nodes are present on one side of the neck and smaller nodes are on the contralateral side, then an oblique beam angle is chosen through which the larger nodes are fully encompassed in the photon field. If the contralateral smaller nodes are located posterior to the oblique photon field or are transected by it, then these nodes can be treated with a boost dose using an electron beam field located posterior to the oblique photon fields.

Tumors of the Posterior Pharyngeal Wall

Because of their proximity to the spinal cord, tumors of the posterior pharyngeal wall are particularly challenging to treat. It is critical to assess anatomic relationships between the tumor, the vertebral body, and the spinal cord using CT or MRI. In many cases the posterior border of the off-cord field needs to be only millimeters in front of the posterior aspect of the vertebral body (Fig. 9-9). When the tumor extends in a posterolateral direction along the lateral aspect of the vertebral body, coverage of the tumor may be improved by using shallow oblique fields or intensity-modulated radiation therapy. Multiple portal films need to be taken to assure that the set-up is accurate.

Anterior field: midneck and lower neck nodes. An anterior appositional photon field is used for treatment of the midneck and lower neck nodes bilaterally. A boost dose to nodal disease located in the midneck or lower neck can be given through an appositional electron portal or glancing anterior-posterior fields or both depending on the size and location of the node(s).

Boost fields: primary or nodal. Boost doses to the primary tumor and involved upper neck node(s) are usually administered using external-beam irradiation with photons, electrons of appropriate energy, or a combination of both. In selected patients with residual tongue base disease after completion of the planned external-beam therapy, a supplemental boost dose of 10 to 15 Gy can be administered by interstitial implant. Patients are selected to receive an interstitial boost if their clinical rate of tumor regression is deemed to be inadequate. The decision to deliver a boost dose by brachytherapy must be made early enough that the overall duration of treatment is not overly prolonged. Only 4 of the first 200 patients treated with the

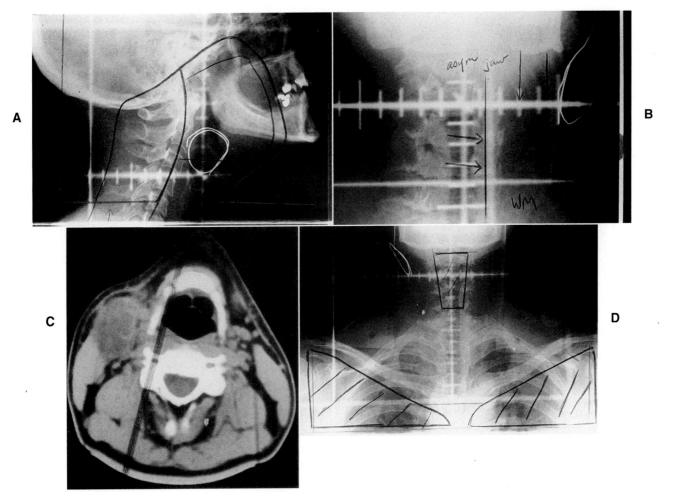

Fig. 9-7 Fields used to treat a T3 N1 squamous carcinoma of the tonsil. The primary tumor extended 0.5 cm anterior to the retromolar triangle and along the soft palate to the uvula. Wire was placed on the skin over the palpable neck node. **A,** The initial lateral field portals. The fields are matched to the lower neck portal at the isocenter, using an asymmetric jaw technique. To reduce the volume of epiglottis and mucosal surfaces treated to high dose, the isocenter of the primary tumor boost field is located 1 cm superior to the initial isocenter. (In other patients it is feasible to move the isocenter more superiorly, depending on the disease anatomy, and spare more of the epiglottis from the boost photon field.) The inferior border of the lateral boost field is located within the nodal disease. **B,** A typical midneck oblique boost field that is matched to the primary boost field using an asymmetric jaw technique. An oblique angle is chosen to position the beam lateral to the spinal cord but medial to the thyroid cartilage, which is visible on the film. Wider coverage of jugular chain disease can be achieved by angling the oblique field. **C,** A sketch on a computed tomography scan of a typical medial beam edge used in the oblique midneck field to deliver a boost dose to an involved node. **D,** The supraclavicular field. A 3-cm-long larynx block is tapered to shield the structures within the thyroid cartilages. The patient was treated with the concomitant boost fractionation schedule to a dose of 72 Gy to the primary tumor and neck node. The patient had a complete response to irradiation and remained without disease 2 years after treatment.

concomitant boost schedule at the M.D. Anderson Cancer Center were given an interstitial boost.

In patients with tongue base carcinoma, treatment set-up may be improved if a tongue-depressing stent is used. Figure 9-10 demonstrates exclusion of the soft palate during the boost in a patient who had a tumor in the inferior component of the tongue base. During the boost phase of treatment in patients with tongue base tumors, the use of a stent often can make it possible to exclude varying amounts of the superior oropharynx and oral cavity.

Dose-fractionation schedules for external-beam radiation therapy. For patients with T1 oropharyngeal carcinoma, a conventionally fractionated regimen

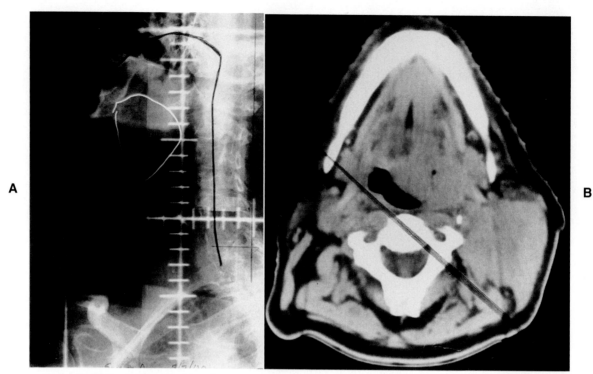

Fig. 9-8   A 60-year-old patient presented with a T2 N3 squamous carcinoma of the tongue base and left neck in July 2000. He was treated with the concomitant boost fractionation schedule and concurrent cisplatin and docetaxel. **A,** The oblique primary boost field. An angle of 33 degrees above and below the horizontal was chosen for the photon beams so the opposed fields would encompass the node with a minimum margin of 1 cm. **B,** The anterior and posterior field margins of the photon field are sketched on a transverse cut of the patient's planning computed tomography (CT) scan. The primary tumor and involved nodes are fully encompassed in the photon fields. Only fibrosis was evident on the CT scans obtained 6 weeks and 4 months after treatment. No neck dissection was performed. He was without disease and well on last follow-up in December 2001.

of 2-Gy fractions, five fractions per week over 6.5 weeks to a total dose of 66 Gy yields a control rate of 90% or greater; thus this regimen is still considered the standard radiation therapy regimen. With this fractionation schedule, the recommended dose for elective nodal irradiation is 50 Gy in 25 fractions, and the recommended dose for therapeutic irradiation of palpable involved nodes ranges from 64 to 70 Gy in 32 to 35 fractions depending on the nodal size.

For patients with T2 and T3 oropharyngeal carcinomas who are treated outside a protocol setting, the concomitant boost fractionation schedule is used. The recommended dose to the primary tumor is 69 to 72 Gy in 40 to 42 fractions over 6 weeks, with smaller tumors receiving the lower dose. With proper supportive care, no more than 2% of patients will require prolongation of treatment beyond 6 weeks because of acute mucosal reactions. It is now considered unethical to interrupt planned treatment to reduce acute toxicity if such interruption will result in an overall treatment time of more than 6 weeks. Protocols are ongoing that are designed to study the optimal way to add concurrent chemotherapy to the concomitant boost schedule.

Treatment of intermediate-stage oropharyngeal carcinoma with static parallel-opposed fields has been standard therapy for the past half-century. All patients treated with these fields develop xerostomia. Many centers are investigating the role of intensity-modulated radiation therapy for patients with intermediate-stage oropharyngeal carcinoma. It is often possible to treat oropharyngeal primary tumors and the nodal beds at risk while limiting the dose to the superficial lobe of the parotid gland to doses below the dose that causes xerostomia (approximately 30 Gy) (Fig. 9-11). When intensity-modulated radiation therapy is delivered with machines equipped with a dynamic multileaf collimator, it is feasible to use an asymmetric jaw technique to match a static supraclavicular field to an intensity-modulated upper neck and primary tumor field. The static supraclavicular field is preferred for the lower neck because the arytenoid cartilages and cricopharyngeal muscles can be completely excluded from the treatment fields. Irradiation techniques for oropharyngeal carcinoma are expected to evolve significantly in the next few years as radiation delivery technology advances.

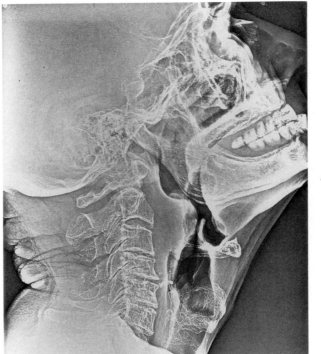

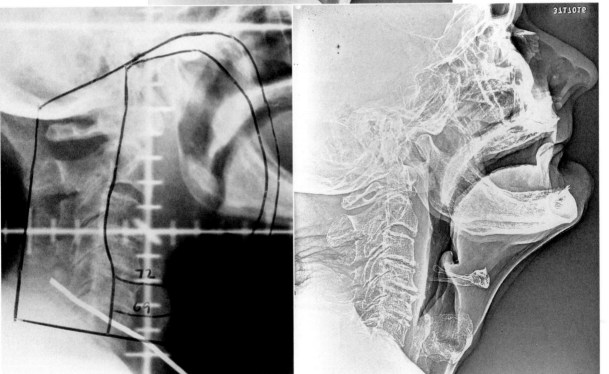

Fig. 9-9 This 77-year-old man presented with a posterior pharyngeal wall squamous carcinoma in March 1993. **A,** Soft tissue xerogram showing the tumor. **B,** The patient was treated with the concomitant boost fractionation schedule with the fields as shown to 72 Gy. The posterior borders of the off-cord and boost fields were located close to the posterior aspect of the vertebral bodies. **C,** Repeat xerogram taken 1 month after the completion of treatment shows an excellent tumor response. The patient had no recurrences but died of complications of Alzheimer's disease in March 1996.

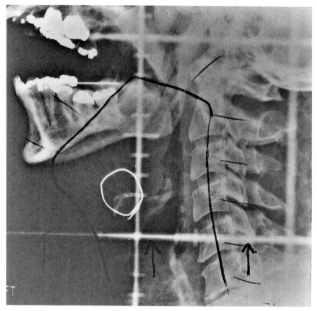

Fig. 9-10 Boost field of a patient with a T2 N2b squamous carcinoma of the inferior aspect of the tongue base. A tongue-depressing stent (see wire) is used to depress the tongue away from the soft palate. Using this technique, the soft palate was excluded from the boost field.

Postoperative Radiation Therapy
Treatment Set-up and Portal Arrangement

The general technique for postoperative radiation therapy is similar to that for primary external-beam radiation therapy. The initial target volume covers the entire surgical bed and all nodal areas of the neck at risk, and the boost volume encompasses areas that harbored known disease. The disease spread and extent of surgery (scar/flap) determine the portal borders.

Lateral-opposed photon fields are used for treating the primary tumor and upper neck nodes, and a matching anterior photon field is used to cover the midneck and lower neck. The location of the lower border of the lateral fields is determined predominantly by the extent of the nodal disease. It is desirable to place this border above the arytenoids whenever possible to avoid irradiating the larynx; a midline shielding block can be placed in the anterior low neck field to exclude the larynx from the beam. The skin and subcutaneous tissue over the larynx, if in the surgical bed, are irradiated with low-energy electrons.

Dose Fractionation Schedules

When postoperative radiation therapy is given in 2-Gy fractions, a dose of 56 Gy is administered to the operative bed, and 60 Gy is administered to regions of clonogenic density, such as regions of positive margins, multiple positive nodes, or extracapsular extension.[55] Higher doses may be needed in selected patients, such as

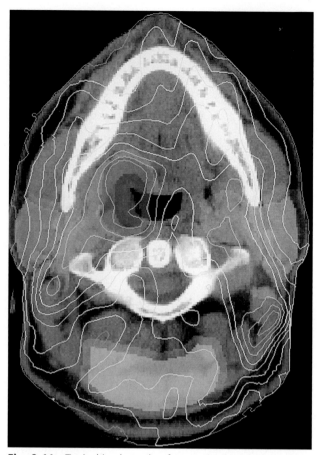

Fig. 9-11 Typical isodose plan for treating a right lateral pharyngeal wall tumor with intensity-modulated radiation therapy techniques. The primary tumor in this case would be treated to 66 Gy in 30 fractions, and the dose to the parotid gland would be 28 to 30 Gy.

those who have tumor dissected off of the carotid artery or those with gross residual disease after surgery.

FUTURE POSSIBILITIES

Early-stage squamous carcinomas of the oropharynx have a high cure rate when they are treated with radiation therapy. Efforts to decrease the morbidity of therapy for patients with such tumors are warranted. With modern technology, the volume of the high-dose region can be limited with techniques such as intensity modulation, three-dimensional treatment planning, and proton beams. For patients with early-stage oropharyngeal carcinoma, use of intensity-modulated radiation therapy allows the contralateral parotid dose to be limited to less than 25 Gy and preserves the ability to treat the contralateral nodes at risk.

The optimal way to sequence chemotherapy with irradiation, surgery, or both and the optimal doses of chemotherapy drugs in these settings remain subjects of intense investigation. Research conducted over the next decade will establish more effective approaches for integrating available drugs into current regimens. The role of biological agents also is expected to increase, given the intensive research currently being done on these agents. Currently a phase III trial is being conducted to investigate the efficacy of the antiepidermal growth factor C225 administered in combination with radiation therapy.

REFERENCES

1. Coutard H. Roentgen therapy of epitheliomas of the tonsillar region, hypopharynx, and larynx from 1920 to 1926. *Am J Roentgenol* 1932;28:313-331.
2. Fletcher GW, MacComb WS, Chau PM, et al. Comparison of medium voltage and supervoltage roentgen therapy in the treatment of oropharynx cancers. *Am J Roentgenol* 1959;81:375-401.
3. Withers HR, Peters LJ, Taylor JM, et al. Local control of carcinoma of the tonsil by radiation therapy: an analysis of patterns of fractionation in nine institutions. *Int J Radiat Oncol Biol Phys* 1995;33:549-562.
4. Garden AS, Weber RS, Ang KK, et al. Postoperative radiation therapy for malignant tumors of minor salivary glands. *Cancer* 1994;73:2563-2569.
5. Dubey P, Ha CS, Ang KK, et al. Nonnasopharyngeal lymphoepitheliomas of the head and neck. *Cancer* 1998;82:1556-1562.
6. Kong JS, Fuller LM, Butler JJ, et al. Stages I and II non-Hodgkin's lymphomas of Waldeyer's ring and the neck. *Am J Clin Oncol* 1984;7:629-639.
7. Lindberg R. Distribution of cervical lymph node metastases from squamous cell carcinoma of the upper respiratory and digestive tracts. *Cancer* 1972;29:1446-1449.
8. Foote RL, Olsen KD, Davis DL, et al. Base of tongue carcinoma: patterns of failure and predictors of recurrence after surgery alone. *Head Neck* 1993;15:300-307.
9. Remmler D, Medina JE, Byers RM, et al. Treatment of choice for squamous carcinoma of the tonsillar fossa. *Head Neck Surg* 1985;7:206-211.
10. Foote RL, Schild SE, Thompson WM, et al. Tonsil cancer. *Cancer* 1994;73:2638-2647.
11. Meoz-Mendez RT, Fletcher GH, Guillamondegui OM, et al. Analysis of the results of irradiation in the treatment of squamous cell carcinomas of the pharyngeal walls. *Int J Radiat Oncol Biol Phys* 1978;4:579-584.
12. Fleming I, Cooper JS, Henson DE, et al, eds. *AJCC Cancer Staging Manual*, 5th ed. Philadelphia, Pa: Lippincott Williams & Wilkins; 1997:35.
13. Peters LJ, Weber RS, Morrison WH, et al. Neck surgery in patients with primary oropharyngeal cancer treated by radiotherapy. *Head Neck* 1996;18:552-559.
14. Gwozdz JT, Morrison WH, Garden AS, et al. Concomitant boost radiotherapy for squamous carcinoma of the tonsillar fossa. *Int J Radiat Oncol Biol Phys* 1997;39:127-135.
15. Spanos WJ, Shukovsky LJ, Fletcher GH. Time, dose, and tumor volume relationships in irradiation of squamous cell carcinomas of the base of the tongue. *Cancer* 1976;37:2591-2599.
16. Foote RL, Parsons JT, Mendenhall WM, et al. Is interstitial implantation essential for the successful radiotherapeutic treatment of base of tongue carcinoma? *Int J Radiat Oncol Biol Phys* 1990;18:1293-1298.
17. Wang CC. *Radiation Therapy for Head and Neck Neoplasms*. 3rd ed. New York, NY: Wiley-Liss; 1997:187-203.
18. Mendenhall WM, Stringer SP, Amdur RJ, et al. Is radiation therapy a preferred alternative to surgery for squamous cell carcinoma of the base of tongue? *J Clin Oncol* 2000;18:35-42.
19. Weber RS, Gidley P, Morrison WH, et al. Treatment selection for carcinoma of the base of the tongue. *Am J Surg* 1990;160:415-419.
20. Mak AC, Morrison WM, Garden AS, et al. Base-of-tongue carcinoma: treatment results using concomitant boost radiotherapy. *Int J Radiat Oncol Biol Phys* 1995;33:289-296.
21. Harrison LB, Zelefsky MJ, Pfister DG, et al. Detailed quality of life assessment in patients treated with primary radiotherapy for squamous cell cancer of the base of the tongue. *Head Neck* 1997;19:169-175.
22. Puthawala A, Syed AMN, Eads DL, et al. Limited external beam and interstitial 192 iridium irradiation in the treatment of carcinoma of the base of the tongue: a ten year experience. *Int J Radiat Oncol Biol Phys* 1988;14:839-848.
23. De Los Santos JF, Morrison WH, Garden AS, et al. Surgery and postoperative radiation therapy for advanced squamous cell carcinoma of the base of tongue [abstract]. *Cancer J* 2000;6:411. Abstract 53.
24. Harrison LB, Lee HJ, Pfister DG, et al. Long-term results of primary radiotherapy with/without neck dissection for squamous cell cancer of the base of tongue. *Head Neck* 1998;20:668-673.
25. Wong CS, Ang KK, Fletcher GH, et al. Definitive radiotherapy for squamous cell carcinoma of the tonsillar fossa. *Int J Radiat Oncol Biol Phys* 1989;16:657-662.
26. Mendenhall WM, Amdur RJ, Stringer SP, et al. Radiation therapy for squamous cell carcinoma of the tonsillar region: a preferred alternative to surgery? *J Clin Oncol* 2000;18:2219-2225.
27. Bataini JP, Asselain B, Jaulerry C, et al. A multivariate primary tumour control analysis in 465 patients treated by radical radiotherapy for cancer of the tonsillar region: clinical and treatment parameters as prognostic factors. *Radiother Oncol* 1989;14:265-277.
28. Pernot M, Malissard L, Taghian A, et al. Velotonsillar squamous cell carcinoma: 277 cases treated by combined external irradiation and brachytherapy—results according to extension, localization, and dose rate. *Int J Radiat Oncol Biol Phys* 1992;23:715-723.
29. Mazeron JJ, Lusinchi A, Marinello G, et al. Interstitial radiation therapy for squamous cell carcinoma of the tonsillar region: the Creteil experience (1971–1981). *Int J Radiat Oncol Biol Phys* 1986;12:895-900.
30. Keus RB, Pontvert D, Brunin F, et al. Results of irradiation in squamous cell carcinoma of the soft palate and uvula. *Radiother Oncol* 1988;11:311-317.
31. Lindberg RD, Fletcher GH. The role of irradiation in the management of head and neck cancer: analysis of results and causes of failure. *Tumori* 1978;64:313-325.
32. Mazeron JJ, Belkacemi Y, Simon JM, et al. Place of iridium 192 implantation in definitive irradiation of faucial arch squamous cell carcinomas. *Int J Radiat Oncol Biol Phys* 1993;27:251-257.
33. Fein DA, Lee WR, Amos WR, et al. Orpharyngeal carcinoma treated with radiotherapy: a 30-year experience. *Int J Radiat Oncol Biol Phys* 1996;34:289-296.
34. Esche BA, Haie CM, Gerbaulet AP, et al. Interstitial and external radiotherapy in carcinoma of the soft palate and uvula. *Int J Radiat Oncol Biol Phys* 1988;15:619-625.
35. Peters LJ. Accelerated fractionation using the concomitant boost: a contribution of radiobiology to radiotherapy. *Br J Radiol* 1992;24:200-203.
36. Calais G, Alfonsi M, Bardet E, et al. Randomized trial of radiation therapy versus concomitant chemotherapy and radiation therapy for advanced-stage oropharynx carcinoma. *J Natl Cancer Inst* 1999;91:2081-2086.
37. Calais G, Alfonsi M, Bardet E, et al. Radiation alone (RT) versus RT with concomitant chemotherapy (CT) in stages III and IV oropharynx carcinoma. Final results of the 94-01 GORTEC randomized study [abstract]. Presented at the 43rd annual meeting of the American Society for Therapeutic Radiology and Oncology; November 4-8, 2001; San Francisco, Calif.
38. Brizel DM, Albers ME, Fisher SR, et al. Hyperfractionated irradiation with or without concurrent chemotherapy for locally advanced head and neck cancer. *N Engl J Med* 1998;338:1798-1804.

39. Adelstein DJ, Adams GL, Li Y, et al. A phase III comparison of standard radiation therapy (RT) versus RT plus concurrent cisplatin versus split-course RT plus concurrent cisplatin and 5-fluorouracil in patients with unresectable squamous cell head and neck cancer: an intergroup study. In: *Program and Abstracts of the 36th Annual Meeting of the American Society of Clinical Oncology;* May 20-23, 2000; New Orleans, La. Abstract 1624.

40. Staar S, Rudat V, Dietz A, et al. Hyperfractionated (HF) acceler-ated (ACC) radiochemotherapy versus HF/ACC radiotherapy in advanced head and neck cancer—a multicentric randomized German trial. In: *Program and Abstracts of the 36th Annual Meeting of the American Society of Clinical Oncology;* May 20-23, 2000; New Orleans, La. Abstract 1628.

41. Lee HJ, Zelefsky MJ, Kraus DH, et al. Long-term regional control after radiation therapy and neck dissection for base of tongue car-cinoma. *Int J Radiat Oncol Biol Phys* 1997;38:995-1000.

42. Lindberg RD. Sites of first failure in head and neck cancer. *Cancer Treat Symp* 1983;2:21-31.

43. Gwozdz JT, Morrison WH, Garden AS. Concomitant boost radio-therapy for squamous cell carcinoma of the oropharynx. In: *Program and Abstracts of the 4th International Conference on Head and Neck Cancer;* July 1996; London, England. Abstract 54.

44. Morrison WH, Garden AS, Ang KK, et al. Long-term results of the concomitant boost fractionation schedule for treatment of oropharyngeal carcinoma. *Int J Radiat Oncol Biol Phys* 1999; 45(suppl 3):98.

45. Fu KK, Pajak TF, Trotti A, et al. A Radiation Therapy Oncology Group (RTOG) phase III randomized study to compare hyper-fractionation and two variants of accelerated fractionation to standard fractionation radiotherapy for head and neck squamous cell carcinomas: first report of RTOG 9003. *Int J Radiat Oncol Biol Phys* 2000;48:7-16.

46. Withers HR, Peters LJ, Taylor JM, et al. Late normal tissue seque-lae from radiation therapy for carcinoma of the tonsil: patterns of fractionation study of radiobiology. *Int J Radiat Oncol Biol Phys* 1995;33:563-568.

47. Horiot JC, Le Fur R, N'Guyen T. Hyperfractionation vs. conven-tional fractionation in oropharyngeal carcinoma: final analysis of a randomized trial of the EORTC cooperative group of radiotherapy. *Radiother Oncol* 1992;25:231-241.

48. Zelefsky MJ, Gaynor J, Kraus D, et al. Long-term subjective func-tional outcome of surgery plus postoperative radiotherapy for advanced stage oral cavity and oropharyngeal carcinoma. *Am J Surg* 1996;171:258-262.

49. Peiffert D, Pernot M, Malissard L, et al. Salvage irradiation by brachytherapy of velotonsillar squamous cell carcinoma in a pre-viously irradiated field: results of 73 cases. *Int J Radiat Oncol Biol Phys* 1994;29:681-686.

50. Mazeron JJ, Langlois D, Glaubiger D, et al. Salvage irradiation of oropharyngeal cancer using iridium 192 wire implants: 5-year results of 70 cases. *Int J Radiat Oncol Biol Phys* 1987;13: 957-962.

51. Haraf DJ, Weichselbaum RR, Vokes EE. Re-irradiation with con-comitant chemotherapy of unresectable recurrent head and neck cancer: a potentially curable disease. *Ann Oncol* 1996;7: 913-918.

52. Haraf DJ, Chung T, Stenson K, et al. High dose reirradiation with concomitant chemotherapy for local/regionally recurrent head and neck cancer: results in 48 patients. In: *Program and Abstracts of the 36th Annual Meeting of the American Society of Clinical Oncology;* May 20-23, 2000; New Orleans, La. Abstract 1630.

53. O'Sullivan B, Warde P, Grice B, et al. The benefits and pitfalls of ipsilateral radiotherapy in carcinoma of the tonsillar region. *Int J Radiat Oncol Biol Phys* 2001;51:332-343.

54. Jackson SM, Hay JH, Flores AD, et al. Cancer of the tonsil: the results of ipsilateral radiation treatment. *Radiother Oncol* 1999;51:123-128.

55. Peters LJ, Goepfert H, Ang KK, et al. Evaluation of the dose for postoperative radiation therapy of head and neck cancer: first report of a prospective randomized trial. *Int J Radiat Oncol Biol Phys* 1993;26:3-11.

CHAPTER 10

The Oral Cavity

Jay S. Cooper

Carcinomas of the oral cavity will be detected in approximately 21,700 United States residents in 2001 (Table 10-1).[1] These tumors account for approximately 2% of all neoplasms (excluding basal and squamous cell carcinomas of the skin) in the United States.[1] Only about 50% of patients with carcinoma of the oral cavity survive for more than 5 years after diagnosis. Despite improvements in imaging and therapy, the survival rate for patients with these tumors has not changed substantially for many years. Furthermore, the residual effects of smoking and alcohol consumption are likely to keep the incidences of these tumors at their current levels for the foreseeable future.

ACUTE EFFECTS OF IRRADIATION ON NORMAL TISSUES

Changes in the salivary glands are usually the first sign of radiation-related damage in the region of the oral cavity. Salivary flow decreases markedly after administration of a few grays, and many patients complain of dryness of the mouth after receiving a single fraction of radiation. As radiation therapy continues, salivary flow continues to decrease, and the saliva takes on a stickier quality. Food and debris adhere tenaciously to the teeth and gums. A minority of patients experience self-limited swelling of the submandibular or parotid glands for the first few days of treatment. Most patients experience a temporary increase in serum amylase levels as a result of the effects of radiation on the salivary glands.[2]

Irradiation of the oral cavity also affects the taste buds and produces a decrease in the ability to distinguish the taste of foods. As a result, patients often choose sweeter foods, which stick to the teeth and foster decay.

Because cellular turnover is more rapid in mucosa than in skin, the mucosa tends to show changes before reactions are apparent in the skin. After 15 to 20 Gy, delivered in conventional fractions of 2 Gy/day, the mucosa becomes erythematous. After an additional 10 Gy, small white areas of mucositis begin to appear. In their early stages, these patches tend to be scattered throughout the treatment field, leading to the term *patchy mucositis*. As treatment continues, the patches begin to coalesce, potentially leading to *confluent mucositis*, wherein few areas of normal intact mucosa remain.

While the mucosa progresses through the erythema-patchy mucositis-confluent mucositis continuum, the skin begins to demonstrate the effects of radiation. Initially, erythema appears, and in some patients the skin becomes hyperpigmented. Both erythema and hyperpigmentation may be difficult to detect in dark-skinned patients. Many patients subsequently experience desquamation of the skin in which coarse flakes of skin are shed but the skin beneath remains intact, known as *dry desquamation*. Some patients have a more severe reaction in which the shedding of the overlying skin leaves a weeping, eroded site, known as *moist desquamation*. In some patients, moist desquamation is promoted by friction such as that from a shirt collar against the skin of the neck.

To facilitate comparisons among studies of the degree and type of side effects during treatment, the Radiation Therapy Oncology Group (RTOG) created a scale to describe acute toxic effects (e.g., those experienced within 90 days of treatment) (Table 10-2).[2a]

TABLE 10-1

Estimated Incidence of and Deaths from Oral Cavity Cancer in the United States in 2001

Tumor Site	ESTIMATED INCIDENCE			ESTIMATED DEATHS		
	Total	Male	Female	Total	Male	Female
Tongue	7100	4800	2300	1700	1100	600
Mouth	10,500	6000	4500	2300	1300	1000
Other	4100	3100	1000	1700	1200	500

Data from Greenlee RT, Hill-Harmon MB, Murray T, et al. *CA Cancer J Clin* 2001;51:15-36.

TABLE 10-2

Radiation Therapy Oncology Group (RTOG) Criteria for Acute Toxic Effects

Site	TOXIC EFFECTS				
	Grade 0	Grade 1	Grade 2	Grade 3	Grade 4
Skin	No change from baseline	Follicular, faint, or dull erythema Epilation Dry desquamation Decreased sweating	Tender or bright erythema, patchy moist desquamation Moderate edema	Confluent, moist desquamation other than skin folds, pitting edema	Ulceration, hemorrhage, necrosis
Mucous membranes	No change from baseline	Redness May experience mild pain not requiring analgesics	Patchy mucositis that may produce an inflammatory serosanguinous discharge May experience moderate pain requiring analgesia	Confluent fibrinous mucositis May include severe pain requiring narcotic	Ulceration, hemorrhage, or necrosis
Salivary gland	No change from baseline	Mild mouth dryness; slightly thickened saliva May have slightly altered taste such as metallic taste Changes not reflected in alteration in baseline feeding behavior, such as increased use of liquids with meals	Moderate to complete dryness Thick, sticky saliva Markedly altered taste	[RTOG classification does not describe grade 3 salivary-gland effects]	Acute salivary gland necrosis

Modified from Cox JD, Stetz J, Pajak TF. *Int J Radiat Oncol Biol Phys* 1995;31:1341-1346.

ETIOLOGY

The vast majority of tumors in the oral cavity are epithelially derived squamous cell carcinomas. The entire oral cavity can be visually inspected and palpated, and screening for tumors is simple and inexpensive because many invasive tumors are preceded by dysplastic or in situ lesions that are white (leukoplakia) or red (erythroplakia). However, comprehensive screening programs for oral cancer have not garnered the level of attention afforded screening programs for other types of cancer (e.g., prostate-specific antigen measurement for prostate cancer and mammography for breast cancer). Consequently, at present, many cases of oral cancer are not detected until they are fairly far advanced.

The risk of developing an oral cancer is higher in men than women, although the male:female incidence ratio has decreased from approximately 10:1 several decades ago to about 2:1 now. The typical patient is a man in his 50s or 60s who smokes tobacco heavily or consumes large amounts of alcohol. The amount smoked is directly correlated with the likelihood of dying of oral cancer, and cigarette, cigar, and pipe smoking appear to be equally dangerous.[3] Smoking more than 20 cigarettes daily correlates with a sixfold increase in the risk of developing intraoral cancer compared with the risk in nonsmokers.[4] Drinking more than 6 ounces of hard liquor daily increases the risk of intraoral cancer tenfold.[5] Other kinds of smoking and alcohol consumption also seem to predispose to oral cancer; habitual use of marijuana[6] and habitual use of alcohol-containing mouthwashes[7,8] have been implicated as risk factors for oral-cavity tumors. Moreover, the deleterious effects of smoking and alcohol consumption may be more than additive.[9]

Several risk factors have been identified that are associated with tumors in specific oral-cavity subsites. Chewing a mixture of betelnut, tobacco, and slaked lime,[10] the use of smokeless "chewing" tobacco,[11] and "snuff dipping"[11,12] are associated with carcinomas of the buccal mucosa, gingiva, lip, and floor of the mouth. Smoking cigars in a reversed position (lit end inside the mouth) is associated with tumors of the hard palate.[13,14] Poor dental hygiene may contribute to the induction of intraoral tumors[4]; carcinomas of the oral tongue often arise directly adjacent to decayed or broken teeth. Carcinomas of the lip are caused in large part by sunlight exposure.[15]

Host factors also seem to be important. Schantz and colleagues[16] have demonstrated that lymphocytes from young adults with squamous cell carcinoma have greater chromosomal fragility on exposure to bleomycin than do lymphocytes from age- and sex-matched controls. However, once an oral squamous cell carcinoma develops, the virulence of the disease is not related to the patient's smoking or drinking history.[17]

ANATOMY

The oral cavity (Figs. 10-1 and 10-2) is composed of the mucosal portion of the lips, the buccal mucosa, the upper and lower gingivae, the floor of the mouth, the retromolar trigones, the hard palate, and the anterior two thirds of the tongue, up to the vallate papillae.

Beneath the mucosa, the relationships among the muscles, nerves, and mandible are complex. At the insertion of the genioglossus and geniohyoid muscles on the mandible, bony projections (the genial tubercles) encroach on the floor of the mouth. The degree of encroachment varies from patient to patient, and in some patients the tubercles are sufficiently prominent to impede brachytherapy. The submandibular ducts (Wharton's ducts) course from the submandibular glands both anteriorly and superiorly for approximately

5 cm to enter the floor of the mouth anteriorly near the midline. The lumen of these ducts can be obstructed by tumor, resulting in enlargement of the submandibular glands that clinically simulates tumor infiltration. The lingual nerve (cranial nerve V), which provides sensory fibers to the oral tongue, traverses the foramen ovale to meet the auriculotemporal nerve in the gasserian ganglion. Because the auriculotemporal nerve supplies sensory fibers to the helix and tragus of the ear and the anterior wall of the external auditory canal, lesions of the oral cavity not infrequently produce referred pain that is attributed to the ear (Fig. 10-3).

Anatomic barriers induce tumors to grow locally in relatively predictable patterns. Tumors presumably take the paths of least resistance, both on the mucosal surfaces from which they arise and in the submucosal tissues that they invade. Spread of disease through the loose fibrofatty tissue planes that envelop muscles from their origin to insertion can often be detected with computed tomography (CT) or magnetic resonance imaging (MRI) even when such spread is not evident on physical examination. Tumors also tend to extend along neurovascular bundles, along periosteal surfaces, and rarely, if tumors penetrate the cortex of the mandible, through the marrow space.

WORK-UP AND DIAGNOSIS

Table 10-3 summarizes the typical work-up for oral cancer and the rationale for each element of the work-up.

Clinical Presentation

Because tumors in the oral cavity nearly always arise from the mucosal surfaces, they generally are first

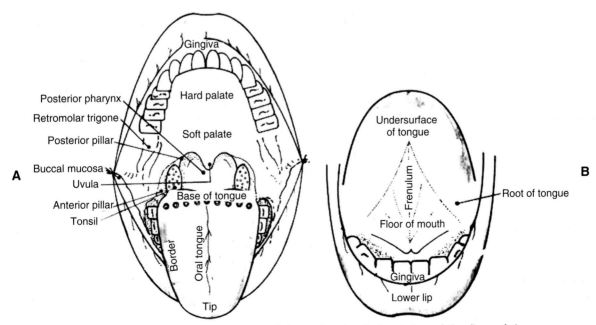

Fig. 10-1 **A,** Front (open-mouth) view of the oral cavity. **B,** Front view of the floor of the mouth with the tongue raised.

Fig. 10-2 Lateral view of the oral cavity.

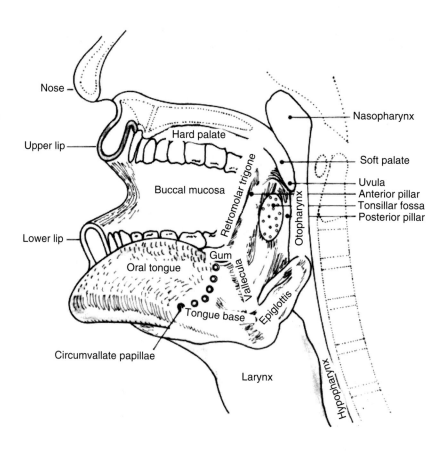

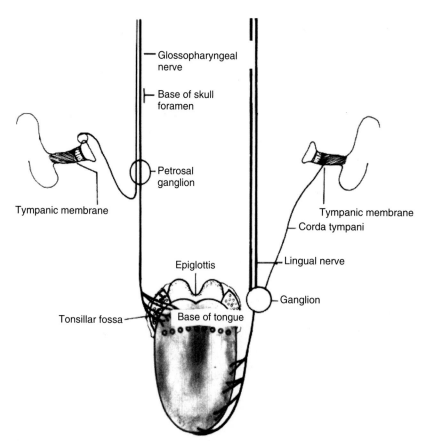

Fig. 10-3 Diagram of the nerve pathways that account for referred pain in the region of the ear from primary neoplasms of the oral cavity.

TABLE 10-3

Typical Work-up for Oral Cancer

Procedure	Purpose
Inspection	Evaluate extent of disease
Palpation	Evaluate extent of disease
Direct or indirect examination of entire head and neck mucosa	Evaluate extent of disease; rule out second primary tumor
Biopsy	Confirm diagnosis and histologic type
MRI or CT of oral cavity (multiplanar)	Evaluate extent of disease; rule out mandibular involvement
Dental evaluation with or without dental therapy	Reduce toxicity of treatment
CT of chest	Rule out metastases and second primary tumor
Esophagography or esophagoscopy	Rule out second primary tumor

MRI, Magnetic resonance imaging; *CT*, computed tomography.

detectable as mucosal irregularities. Common signs and symptoms of oral cavity tumors are listed in Table 10-4.

Typically, tumors in the oral cavity initially appear as slightly discolored regions (white or red). As lesions progress, they acquire a distinct thickness and induration. Eventually the mucosa can become eroded or ulcerated, the growing edges of the visible lesion become more apparent, and the lesion may take on a whiter or a redder color. Some lesions develop deep central ulceration, whereas others take on a multilobulated, cauliflower-like appearance. Bleeding may occur. Tumors of the floor of the mouth often appear as slitlike crevasses and are best appreciated by palpation of the involved area. When an oral tumor is suspected but is not obvious or when the borders of an oral tumor are indistinct, vital staining with tolonium chloride (toluidine blue) may help demarcate the lesion.[18]

Physical Examination

All subregions of the oral cavity are accessible for digital examination in patients who are able to cooperate with

TABLE 10-4

Common Signs and Symptoms of Oral Cancer

Early Disease	Advanced Disease
Leukoplakia	Pain
Erythroplakia	Level I, II, or III adenopathy
Asymptomatic mass	Slurred speech
Persistent sore or ulceration	Difficulty chewing or swallowing
Bleeding mass	

the examiner. As tumors grow, the difference in their texture compared to the texture of adjacent normal tissues becomes more apparent on palpation. For lesions of the lip, floor of the mouth, or buccal mucosa, bimanual examination should be routine; a gloved finger is inserted in the mouth, and the tumor is gently pressed against the examiner's other hand, which is held outside the mouth. In the case of tumors that have invaded into deeper tissues, infiltration into nerves can cause local pain, dysesthesias, paresthesias, and referred pain in the ipsilateral ear. More advanced lesions can cause loosening of the teeth, dysarthria, dysphagia, and trismus.

Imaging Studies

For all oral cavity tumors except clearly superficial, small lesions, CT and MRI have become standard elements of the diagnostic work-up. Images of the primary tumor site, likely routes of spread, and regional nodal drainage pathways are capable of demonstrating extensions of disease that are otherwise clinically imperceptible.

In the current era of cost-conscious medicine, physicians often must carefully consider whether to order CT, MRI, or both. Although CT and MRI can be viewed as alternative or even competitive technologies, they are in fact complementary and supplement the physical examination for mapping and staging tumors. (*Mapping* refers to the spatial localization of all aspects of a tumor, whereas *staging* refers to the application of rules that group lesions of similar prognosis.) Both techniques have advantages (Table 10-5). Within the oral cavity,

TABLE 10-5

Relative Advantages of CT and MRI for Mapping Tumors of the Oral Cavity

Advantages of CT	Advantages of MRI
Metastatic nodal disease is more readily assessed	Direct sagittal, coronal, and axial images are obtained, facilitating mapping
Integrity of cortical bone (mandible) is more accurately assessed	Intravenous contrast agents (e.g., gadolinium-DTPA) are safer than the iodinated agents used for CT
Examination time is shorter	Images of the oral cavity are less likely to be degraded by artifacts
Cost is often substantially less	Perineural spread of tumors is more accurately assessed
Suitable for patients who have pacemakers or aneurysm clips	Integrity of medullary bone (mandible) is more accurately assessed

CT, Computed tomography; *MRI*, magnetic resonance imaging; *DTPA*, diethylenetriaminepentaacetic acid.

MRI is generally better than CT in delineating the size of primary tumors.[19]

Evaluation of Tumor Extent

CT or MRI cannot be used to confirm a strictly mucosal abnormality that is obvious on visual examination. However, when tumors are sufficiently thick and invade below the mucosa, CT and MRI are useful because they provide the clinician with a detailed picture of the submucosal tissues. This improved view of tumor extent can be a critical factor in determining the most appropriate treatment for a particular patient. For example, mandibular invasion (Fig. 10-4) from lesions of the floor of the mouth generally implies the need to resect the affected bone. In contrast, posterior lesions that cross the midline lingual septum (Fig. 10-5) generally cannot be resected with partial glossectomy, and CT or MRI evidence of such spread argues in favor of radiation therapy.

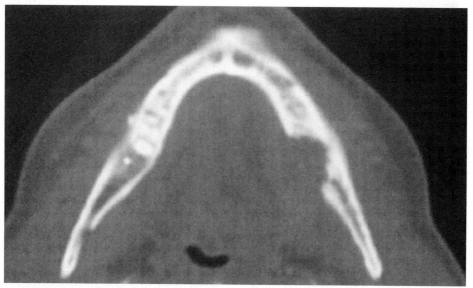

Fig. 10-4 Axial computed tomography image at the level of the mandible demonstrating a destructive lesion predominantly involving the lingual cortex.

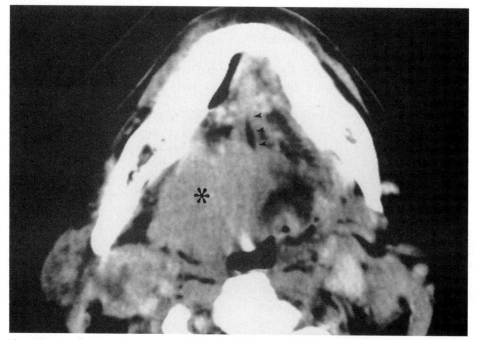

Fig. 10-5 Axial contrast-enhanced computed tomography scan demonstrating pathologic-appearing enhancing mass involving the oral and oropharyngeal portions of the right side of the tongue (*). Note the obliteration of the normal fatty lingual septum *(arrowheads)*, indicating extension across the midline.

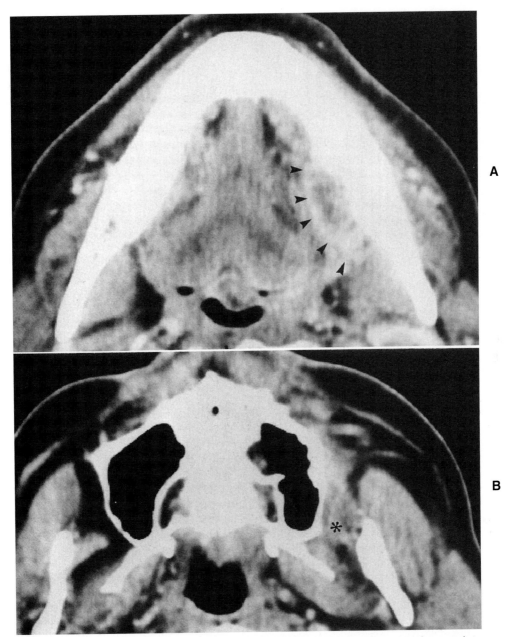

Fig. 10-6 A, Contrast-enhanced computed tomography (CT) scan (same patient as in Fig. 10-4) demonstrating an enhancing mass in the posterior left side of the floor of the mouth extending to the retromolar trigone *(arrows)*. B, Contrast-enhanced CT scan (same patient as in Fig. 10-6, *A*) at the level of the maxilla demonstrating submucosal infiltration along the pterygomandibular raphe to the posterior aspect of the normally fat-filled buccinator space (*). This was clinically occult disease identified only by imaging.

Sometimes the information obtained by imaging studies is unexpected and cannot be discerned by other means. For example, some lesions of the retromolar triangle invade the pterygomandibular raphe, a path of little resistance that courses from the mandible, just deep to the retromolar trigone and up to the pterygoids at the base of the skull. These lesions can extend to the base of the skull via the raphe in a manner that is radiographically obvious but undetectable by other means (Fig. 10-6). Knowledge of such spread can prevent ill-advised surgery and influence the size and placement of radiation therapy portals.

Evaluation of Regional Adenopathy

Imaging can also reveal regional adenopathy that cannot be detected by physical examination. Sectional imaging can supplement the physical examination by revealing the location of nonpalpable involved lymph nodes. One commonly used system divides the relevant cervical lymph nodes into five levels. Level I includes the submandibular and submental lymph nodes. Levels II, III, and IV correspond to the upper (jugulodigastric), middle (jugulo-omohyoid), and lower (jugulocarotid) nodes, respectively, of the anterior deep jugular cervical chain. Level V designates nodes in the posterior triangle of the neck.

Level I nodes are inferior and lateral to the myelohyoid muscle in close proximity to the submandibular glands (Fig. 10-7). Nodes in levels II, III, and IV are located near the internal jugular vein, typically anterior or deep to the anterior aspect of the sternocleidomastoid muscle. Technically, levels II, III, and IV are demarcated by the level of the bifurcation of the carotid artery and the level of the intersection of the internal jugular vein and the omohyoid muscle. Because the carotid bifurcation and omohyoid muscle can be difficult to find on axial images, the hyoid bone and cricoid cartilage, which lie at approximately the same levels as the carotid

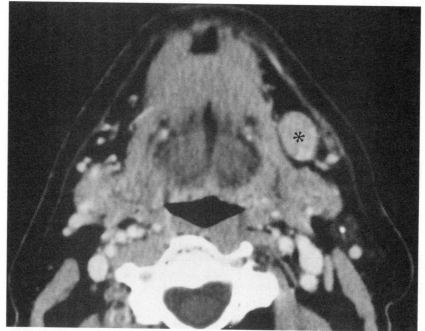

Fig. 10-7 Axial contrast-enhanced computed tomography scan demonstrating a single enlarged level I lymph node (*) anterior to the left submandibular gland.

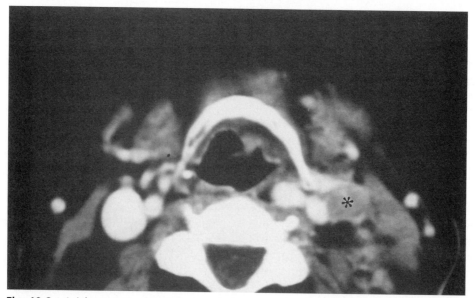

Fig. 10-8 Axial contrast-enhanced computed tomography scan at the level of the hyoid bone demonstrating a single pathologic-appearing lymph node (*) lateral to the left common carotid artery. This lymph node is at the boundary between levels II and III.

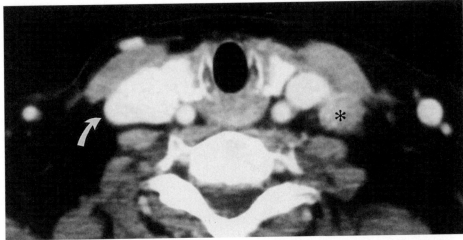

Fig. 10-9 Axial contrast-enhanced computed tomography scan at the level of the cricoid cartilage demonstrating a single pathologic-appearing lymph node (*) immediately posterior to the right internal jugular vein. This lymph node is at the boundary between levels III and IV. The left internal jugular vein *(curved white arrow)* is markedly larger than the right. This is a normal anatomic variant.

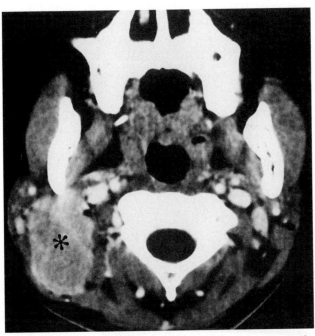

Fig. 10-10 Axial contrast-enhanced computed tomography scan demonstrating an abnormal mass deep to the sternocleidomastoid muscle. This is an example of a level V (spinal accessory chain, posterior triangle) lymph node.

bifurcation and the omohyoid muscle, respectively, can be used as boundaries between levels II and III and levels III and IV (Figs. 10-8 and 10-9). Level V nodes are located predominantly posterior to the sternocleidomastoid muscle (Fig. 10-10).

In general, uninvolved lymph nodes are 1 cm or less in diameter. Thus it is prudent to consider any node longer than 1.5 cm along its long axis or 1.0 cm along its short axis to be abnormal.[20,21] (Nodes smaller than 1.5 cm may well be invaded by tumor, but these nodes cannot be distinguished on the basis of size.) However, some nodes larger than 1.5 cm are enlarged secondary to hyperplasia rather than tumor. A better indicator of tumor is therefore a hypodense nodal center, commonly called a *necrotic center*, even though histopathologic examination of such nodes often does not disclose necrosis of the cells. The appearance of central necrosis is sufficiently diagnostic of neoplastic invasion that nodes of any size with central lucency must be considered neoplastic (Fig. 10-11).

Imaging can also assess the integrity of the nodal capsule. When lymph nodes are invaded by tumor, the fascial planes surrounding the node remain intact unless tumor ruptures the capsule. A node with central lucency and an indistinct periphery should therefore be interpreted as a tumor-bearing node with extracapsular extension of disease (see Fig. 10-11).

The presence of central necrosis and evidence of extracapsular extension of disease are readily detected on contrast-enhanced CT. Recent studies suggest that contrast-enhanced MRI is a reasonable alternative to CT for the evaluation of metastasis to level I and II nodes if appropriate pulse sequences are used.[19]

Ruling Out Second Malignancies

The diagnostic work-up in patients with oral-cavity tumors must include a search for coincident second malignancies of the upper aerodigestive tract. Bronchoscopy, esophagoscopy or esophagography, and chest radiography are used for this purpose. In approximately 10% of cases, depending on the thoroughness of the search, a synchronous second malignancy is detected.[22]

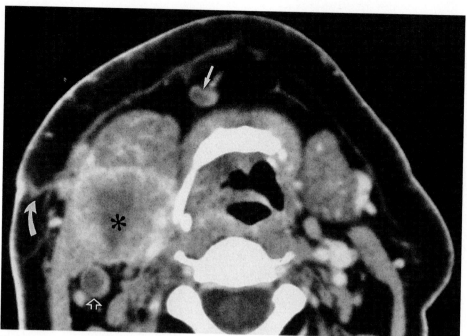

Fig. 10-11 Axial contrast-enhanced computed tomography scan at the level of the hyoid bone demonstrating a 5-cm necrotic internal jugular chain lymph node (*) with extracapsular extension and a fistulous tract *(curved white arrow)* extending to the skin. Note the additional 1-cm necrotic lymph nodes posterior to the largest nodal mass *(open white arrow)* and in the submental triangle *(short white arrow)*.

PATTERNS OF SPREAD
Lymphatic Metastases

Spread of disease by way of regional lymphatics occurs relatively often with carcinomas of the oral cavity. To a considerable degree, the likelihood of lymphatic metastases can be predicted on the basis of the primary tumor's size, histologic grade, and location and the presence or absence of perineural and vascular invasion.[23] The lymph drainage of the oral cavity filters predominantly through the submandibular and upper anterior cervical (jugulodigastric) nodes. However, some anatomic subsites have unique drainage patterns. The lymphatics of the upper lip drain into the submandibular and preauricular nodal beds (Fig. 10-12), and the lymphatics of the midlip and lower lip and the anterior floor of the mouth drain into the submental nodal group (Fig. 10-13). The lymphatics of the oral tongue drain into the anterior cervical chain; lesions located more anteriorly drain lower in the neck than lesions located more posteriorly (Fig. 10-14). Crossing lymphatics can lead to contralateral nodal metastases (Fig. 10-15). The consistency of nodal drainage from oral cavity carcinomas means that previously hidden primary tumors are sometimes discovered because of unusual patterns of nodal disease.

The incidence and the location of lymph node metastases vary only slightly among the different tumor subsites in the oral cavity.[24] Overall, the risk of lymph node

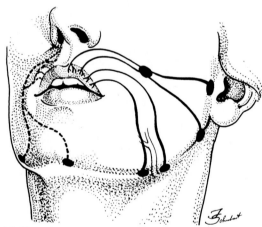

Fig. 10-12 The lymphatics of the upper lip drain into the buccal, parotid, upper cervical, and submandibular nodes. The lymphatics of the skin of the upper lip *(dotted line)* may cross the midline to terminate in submental and submandibular nodes on the contralateral side.

involvement over the course of the disease is approximately 35%. The ipsilateral upper jugular nodes (level II), submandibular nodes (level I), and midjugular nodes (level III) account for the vast majority of sites of spread (Fig. 10-16). Contralateral spread is much less likely, but when it occurs, it involves the same nodal levels.

The relative predictability of drainage pathways permits physicians to design treatment plans that

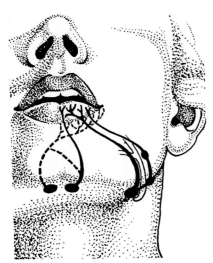

Fig. 10-13 The lymphatics of the lower lip drain to the submental and submandibular nodes. Sometimes disease involves facial nodes. The lymphatics of the skin of the lower lip *(dotted line)* may cross the midline to end in submental or submandibular nodes on the contralateral side.

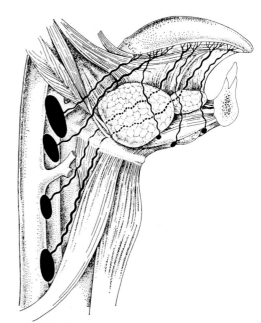

Fig. 10-14 Lymphatics of the tongue. The more anteriorly these lymphatics originate in the tongue, the lower in the neck their draining nodes may lie.

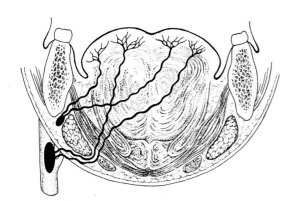

Fig. 10-15 The lymphatics of the tongue in frontal section illustrating both ipsilateral and contralateral drainage in submandibular and cervical lymph nodes.

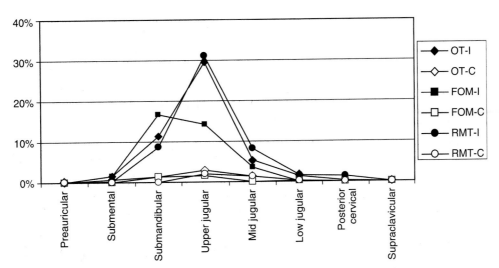

Fig. 10-16 Incidence of ipsilateral and contralateral adenopathy at presentation by site of primary disease and nodal level. *I,* Ispilateral adenopathy; *C,* contralateral adenopathy; *OT,* oral tongue; *FOM,* floor of mouth; *RMT,* retromolar trigone. (From Lindberg RD. *Cancer* 1972; 29:1446-1450.)

rationally target both clinically apparent and clinically undetectable (subclinical) disease. When regional lymph nodes are enlarged by tumor, they may be the deciding factor in determining the manner of treatment. The risk of subclinical nodal disease also must be taken into account in decisions about treatment. As a general rule, elective nodal irradiation is justified when the risk of involvement by subclinical disease exceeds 10% (i.e., when the likelihood that treatment will benefit the patient exceeds the risk that the treatment will cause serious permanent damage to the patient). In most series, the risk of subclinical disease in the regional lymph nodes is approximately 30% overall.[25]

August and Gianetti[26] found a benefit of elective nodal irradiation in patients with oral cancer: in a series of 73 patients with surgically treated oral cancer, the recurrence rate was 3% in patients who were given elective nodal irradiation after surgery vs. 31% in patients who underwent only observation after surgery. The 5-year survival rates were 90% in the group that received elective nodal irradiation vs. 40% in the group that was observed. In a series of patients treated with radical neck dissection, Shah[27] found that levels I and II were the most likely to be involved but that all nodal levels had some degree of risk (Table 10-6). However, these data should be interpreted as approximate only. They certainly reflect some selection bias (e.g., why were elective dissections done?). The data also may be somewhat out of date because newer imaging techniques may detect previously undetectable disease, thus rendering therapeutic a surgical procedure that would previously have been considered elective. Friedman and colleagues[28] suggest that the rate of occult disease varies substantially by the method of evaluation. On the basis of physical examination only, the likelihood of occult disease in their patients was 31%, but when CT or MRI was added, the rate dropped to 12%. Finally, because the size of the primary tumor strongly correlates with the incidence of clinically detectable nodal disease at presentation, it is reasonable to assume that a similar relationship exists between the size of the primary tumor and the likelihood of subclinical nodal disease at presentation. Thus clinical judgment must be exercised in decisions regarding elective irradiation of clinically unremarkable nodal drainage sites.

Hematogenous Metastases

Distant metastasis occurs relatively late in the development of carcinomas of the oral cavity. The risk of distant disease is best predicted by the degree of lymph node involvement. Patients who have no clinically appreciable adenopathy virtually never develop distant metastases as their first site of treatment failure. In contrast, many current series show that in patients who present with N2 or N3 disease, the incidence of distant metastasis approaches the incidence of local–regional recurrence. In one such series, Merino and colleagues[29] reviewed the records of 5019 patients with head and neck tumors who had no clinical evidence of hematogenous metastasis at presentation. Distant metastases subsequently occurred in 10% of these patients. The lungs and bones were the most commonly affected sites. The risk of distant metastasis seems to be substantially greater when the local–regional manifestations of tumor are not controlled,[30] implying that distant spread often occurs after tumors have been brought to medical attention. As local–regional therapies become more effective and patients live longer, the rate of distant metastasis is likely to rise to 15% to 20%.

STAGING

Staging of head and neck cancer is based on information obtained by clinical examination and imaging studies (by CT, MRI, or both). The American Joint Committee on Cancer (AJCC) staging system[31] is the standard classification for carcinomas of the oral cavity. In the AJCC system, disease stage is determined on the basis of the size of the primary tumor and whether or not it invades adjacent structures; the number, size, and location (unilateral or bilateral) of involved lymph nodes; and the presence or absence of distant metastases. The staging system, published in 1997, is shown in Box 10-1.

PATHOLOGY

Within the oral cavity, a spectrum of progression from seemingly normal cells to dysplastic regions, carcinoma in situ, and, finally, frankly invasive cancer can be observed, suggesting that oral cavity tumors are the result of a multistep process that occurs over many years. Preexistent or coincident leukoplakia (a clinical descriptor implying only that the tissues are white and cannot easily be scraped off the mucosa; histologically, leukoplakia is

TABLE 10-6	○
Likelihood of Subclinical Nodal Metastases from Oral Cavity Tumors by Nodal Group	
Nodal Group	**Rate of Involvement (%)**
Level I nodes	20
Level II nodes	17
Level III nodes	9
Level IV nodes	3
Level V nodes	1
Any regional nodes	34

Modified from Shah JP. *Am J Surg* 1990;160:405-409.

BOX 10-1 American Joint Commitee on Cancer Staging System for Tumors of the Lip and Oral Cavity

PRIMARY TUMOR (T)

TX	Primary tumor cannot be assessed
T0	No evidence of primary tumor
Tis	Carcinoma in situ
T1	Tumor 2 cm or less in greatest dimension
T2	Tumor more than 2 cm but not more than 4 cm in greatest dimension
T3	Tumor more than 4 cm in greatest dimension
T4 (lip)	Tumor invades adjacent structures (e.g., through cortical bone, inferior alveolar nerve, floor of mouth, skin of face)
T4 (oral cavity)	Tumor invades adjacent structures (e.g., through cortical bone, into deep [extrinsic] muscle of tongue, maxillary sinus, skin. Superficial erosion alone of bone/tooth socket by gingival primary is not sufficient to classify as T4)

REGIONAL LYMPH NODES (N)

NX	Regional lymph nodes cannot be assessed
N0	No regional lymph node metastasis
N1	Metastasis in a single ipsilateral lymph node, 3 cm or less in greatest dimension
N2	Metastasis in a single ipsilateral lymph node, more than 3 cm but not more than 6 cm in greatest dimension; or in multiple ipsilateral lymph nodes, none more than 6 cm in greatest dimension; or in bilateral or contralateral lymph nodes, none more than 6 cm in greatest dimension
N2a	Metastasis in single ipsilateral lymph node more than 3 cm but not more than 6 cm in greatest dimension
N2b	Metastasis in multiple ipsilateral lymph nodes, none more than 6 cm in greatest dimension
N2c	Metastasis in bilateral or contralateral lymph nodes, none more than 6 cm in greatest dimension
N3	Metastasis in a lymph node more than 6 cm in greatest dimension

DISTANT METASTASIS (M)

MX	Distant metastasis cannot be assessed
M0	No distant metastasis
M1	Distant metastasis

STAGE GROUPING

Stage 0	Tis	N0	M0
Stage I	T1	N0	M0
Stage II	T2	N0	M0
Stage III	T3	N0	M0
	T1–T3	N1	M0
Stage IVA	T4	N0–N1	M0
	Any T	N2	M0
Stage IVB	Any T	N3	M0
Stage IVC	Any T	Any N	M1

From Fleming I, Cooper JS, Henson DE, et al, eds. *AJCC Cancer Staging Manual*, 5th ed. Philadelphia: Lippincott Williams & Wilkins; 1997:24-30.

---

characterized by hyperplasia of keratinocytes that are associated with normal or neoplastic adjacent cells) can be seen adjacent to frank oral cavity tumors in approximately 20% of cases.[32] The presence of erythroplakia even more strongly suggests invasive tumor.[33]

Dysplasia is primarily defined by cytologic atypia such as cellular pleomorphism, increased nuclear size, hyperchromatism, dyskeratosis, and abnormal-appearing mitotic figures. When such changes are confined to the basal or parabasal epithelium, dysplasia is considered mild; involvement of the midspinous layer of the epithelium renders the dysplasia moderate. If such changes are evident in the surface epithelium, the dysplasia is termed *severe*, and if the full thickness of the epithelium is involved, the lesion is classified as *carcinoma in situ*. Whether such changes precede the development of all cases of oral cancer is unknown. However, certainly some forms of invasive oral cancer can arise without a clinically detectable premalignant precursor.

The molecular events that correlate with premalignant and malignant changes in the oral cavity are now becoming known. These molecular changes may provide targets for antitumor therapy.

Alteration of the tumor suppressor gene *p53* and mutations of chromosome 9 (*9p21-22*) have often been associated with oral cancer.[34-36] Nuclear expression of *p53* and cyclin D1 increases along the spectrum from normal epithelium to low-grade oral leukoplakia (mild to moderate dysplasia) to high-grade leukoplakia (severe dysplasia).[37] As cells then progress to frank carcinoma, a further increase in *p53* expression is apparent, often associated with a decrease in expression of the cyclin-dependent kinase inhibitors *p21* (*CIP1/WAF1*) and *p27* (*Kip1*).[38-40] Overexpression, or alteration, of *p53* is detectable not only in approximately 40% to 50% of oral squamous cell carcinomas but also in a substantial percentage of histologically normal-appearing cells adjacent to these tumors.[41]

The S-phase protein cyclin A and the M-phase protein cyclin B1 both have increased expression in squamous cell carcinomas of the floor of the mouth as compared with normal epithelium from the same site.[42] The percentage of cells with detectable cyclin D1 is smaller in samples taken from the basal and suprabasal epithelium of oral cancer than in samples of nontumorous basal and suprabasal epithelium.[43] Expression of integrin subunits (α2 and β1) and nuclear retinoid receptors (RAR-β) also seems to be lower in oral squamous cell carcinomas than in normal oral epithelium.[44,45] Epidermal growth factor receptor has been reported to be amplified in oral cancer,[46] elevated in poorly differentiated tumors,[47] associated with larger primary tumors,[48] and related to tumor progression[49]; in addition, downregulation of its membrane-associated form has been reported to correlate with tumor recurrence.[50]

In one study, human papillomavirus (HPV) was detected in approximately half of a series of 102 oral lesions (21 cases of oral hyperplasia and 81 cases of oral squamous cell carcinoma), raising the possibility that HPV is a cocarcinogen.[51] HPV-16 and HPV-18 are the most common subtypes associated with oral cancer.[51,52]

The vast majority (more than 90%) of invasive tumors arising from structures within the oral cavity are squamous cell carcinomas (Figs. 10-17 and 10-18). Grossly, lesions range from exophytic masses (at any site) to deeply ulcerated, slitlike crevasses (most typically in the floor of the mouth). Generally, tumors of the oral cavity are moderately to well differentiated. However, the degree of differentiation tends not to be a major independent determinant of a tumor's biological behavior. Vascular invasion, on the other hand, portends a poorer outcome.[53]

Salivary gland tumors (typically mucoepidermoid carcinomas), arising from minor salivary glands located in the hard palate, tongue, or retromolar region, account for a small percentage of oral cavity tumors.[54] The significance of salivary gland tumors lies in their penchant for perineural spread (particularly adenoid cystic carcinomas), often to relatively great distances from their site of origin. The hard palate, it should be remembered, is unique among the sites in the oral cavity because it is the only site in which the predominant histopathologic tumor type is of salivary origin. In fact, squamous cell carcinomas of the hard palate are sufficiently rare that when this diagnosis is being considered, special care should be taken to rule out the more common situation

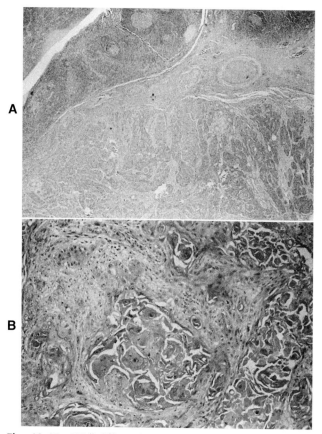

Fig. 10-17 Well-differentiated squamous cell carcinoma. **A,** Low power. **B,** High power. (Photographs courtesy Dr. J. Jagadar.)

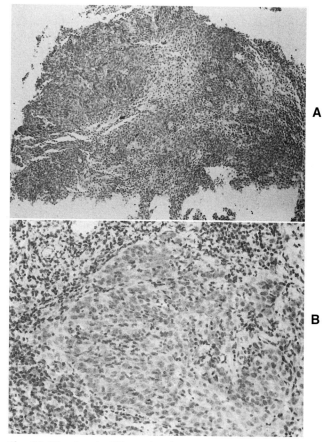

Fig. 10-18 Poorly differentiated squamous cell carcinoma. **A,** Low power. **B,** High power. (Photographs courtesy Dr. J. Jagadar.)

of a gingival tumor that has extended or a maxillary sinus tumor that has penetrated the floor of the antrum to present on the palate.

Other malignancies rarely encountered in the oral cavity include those arising from soft tissue, bone, cartilage, melanocytes, and odontogenic structures.

TREATMENT: GENERAL CONCEPTS

Carcinomas of the oral cavity can be treated with surgery, radiation therapy, or a combination of surgery and radiation therapy. For early-stage lesions, either modality produces a high likelihood of cure, whereas for advanced-stage lesions, neither modality by itself is sufficient. Recent data suggest that chemotherapy may have a role in the treatment of advanced disease.

More than one optimal treatment plan may be available for an individual patient, and no absolute guidelines exist regarding the best treatment for a given presentation of disease. Lesions treated effectively with surgery at one institution may be treated effectively with radiation therapy at another and vice versa. To some degree, this choice of treatment reflects physicians' preferences or biases, the degree of expertise available at a particular institution, and the nature of the patient population receiving care at an institution. Treatment choice therefore depends on the complications, cosmetic changes, and functional consequences that the treatment is expected to cause.

Treatment options for each stage of disease at each anatomic site are summarized in Table 10-7. Table 10-8 provides representative local control and survival rates for the spectrum of available therapies for oral cancer. The greater likelihood of lesions arising from the lips to be localized at presentation (Fig. 10-19) translates into a commensurate benefit in overall survival (Fig. 10-20).

Surgery permits the patient's tumor to be treated most quickly, allows the pathologist to assess the likelihood

that the entire tumor was extirpated (i.e., whether the margins of the specimen contain tumor), and causes few dental or salivary flow problems. Conceptually, surgery must encompass not only the gross disease but the presumed microscopic (subclinical) extensions of tumor as well. As tumors become larger, the applicability of surgery becomes limited by functional and cosmetic factors despite the availability of reconstructive techniques and prostheses. In addition, in the case of relatively medial lesions in which the regional lymphatics in both sides of the neck are at risk of invasion and may therefore need to be treated, surgery tends to be associated with more morbidity than is radiation therapy.

TABLE 10-7
Overview of Treatment Options by Tumor Site

Tumor Site	TREATMENT OPTIONS			
	Stage I	Stage II	Stage III	Stage IV
Lip	S, R	S, R	SR, R, C	SR, R, C
Tongue	S, SR, R	R, SR	R, SR, C	SR, R, C
Buccal mucosa	S, R	R, S, SR	S, R, SR, C	S, R, SR, C
Floor of mouth	S, R	S, R, SR	S, R, C	S, R, C
Lower gingiva	S, R	S, R	RS, SR, C	S, R, SR, C
Retromolar trigone	S, R, RS	S, R, RS	SR, C, R	SR, C, R
Upper gingiva	S, SR, R	SR	R, SR, C	SR, C, R

Modified from the National Cancer Institute PDQ Database. Available at: http://cancernet.nci.nih.gov/pdq.html. Accessed February 2000.
S, Surgery; R, radiation therapy; SR, surgery followed by radiation therapy; C, chemotherapy with or without surgery, with or without radiation therapy as part of clinical trial; RS, radiation therapy followed by surgery.

TABLE 10-8
Local Control and 5-Year Survival Rates by Tumor Site and Disease Stage

Tumor Site	LOCAL CONTROL RATE (%)/5-YEAR SURVIVAL RATE (%)			
	Stage I	Stage II	Stage III	Stage IV
Lip	90/90	90/90	NS/NR	NS/NR
Anterior tongue	96-100/100	85-93/70	50-65/35	40-45/NS
Buccal mucosa	90+/NS	90/NS	NR	NR/NS
Floor of mouth	88-100/NS	70-90/NS	70/NS	30-50/NS
Retromolar trigone	90-100/NS	90/NS	90/NS	60-89/NS
Upper gingiva	NR	NR	NR	NR
Lower gingiva	90+/NS	90+/NS	< 90/NS	30-55/NS

Modified from the National Cancer Institute PDQ Database, May 1992. Available at: http://cancernet.nci.nih.gov/pdq.html.
NS, Not stated; NR, not reported.

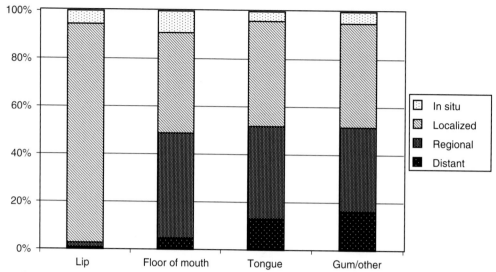

Fig. 10-19 Extent of tumor at presentation by anatomic site. (Data from SEER*Stat 2.0, National Cancer Institute, Bethesda, Md; April 1999.)

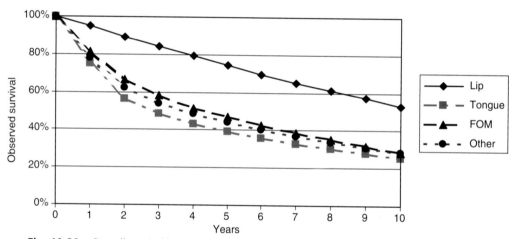

Fig. 10-20 Overall survival by anatomic site of primary disease. Note the similarities between all sites except the lip. (Data from SEER*Stat 2.0, National Cancer Institute, Bethesda, Md; April 1999.)

Radiation therapy takes somewhat longer (brachytherapy) or considerably longer (teletherapy) than surgery to complete. Although radiation therapy preserves both the anatomy and the function of most irradiated tissues, teletherapy often imposes some degree of xerostomia and, at least temporarily, alters taste. Also, some patients treated with radiation therapy will develop necrosis of soft tissue or bone, particularly after brachytherapy, just as some patients treated with surgery will develop fistulous tracts.

The selection of therapy must therefore be based not only on advice from a head and neck surgical oncologist and a radiation oncologist but also, optimally, on input from a diagnostic radiologist, a surgical pathologist, a medical oncologist, a dentist, and the patient. A variety of

tumor and host factors need to be considered. The anatomic location and size of the lesion, potential involvement of adjacent tissues, clinical evidence of regional lymph node spread, the histologic type and grade of the tumor, the nature of the tumor margins ("pushing" vs. infiltrating), the patient's Karnofsky performance status and estimated physical reserve, psychosocial factors that might influence care or outcome (alcohol abusers and smokers who cannot or will not change are relatively worse candidates for radiation therapy), any personal preferences that a patient may hold, and any prior therapy (either surgery or radiation therapy) in the volume of interest may individually or in combination tip the decision toward a particular form of treatment. Such factors notwithstanding, some general concepts apply.

T1 and T2 Lesions

Limited-size lesions (T1 and T2) generally can be controlled with single-modality therapy, and surgery and radiation therapy generally produce equivalent results. For such small tumors, brachytherapy will control 85% to 90% of tumors initially, and with salvage surgery for treatment of recurrences, an ultimate local control rate of 95% is feasible.[55]

Small T3 Lesions

Some small T3 lesions that just cross the T2 to T3 border and are not associated with adenopathy (i.e., small T3 N0 M0 lesions) may also be suitable for single-modality treatment.

Larger T3 and T4 Lesions

Relatively large lesions (most T3 and T4) usually are not well controlled either with surgery or with radiation therapy (local control rates ≤ 50%). Combined-modality therapy generally represents the treatment of choice if surgery can extirpate all gross evidence of tumor and is reasonable given the patient's overall status. If tumor has invaded bone, surgical resection of the affected bone in conjunction with the primary tumor and regional lymph nodes is indicated. Despite prior debate about the relative merits of preoperative vs. postoperative radiation therapy, in most situations, postoperative irradiation is the preferred choice. The RTOG conducted a prospective randomized trial of preoperative (50 Gy) vs. postoperative (60 Gy) radiation therapy for advanced operable tumors of the oral cavity, oropharynx, supraglottic larynx, or hypopharynx.[56] After a median follow-up of 10 years, local control rates were superior in the group that received postoperative radiation therapy.

Lesions of the Lips

Lesions of the lips are often amenable to either surgery or radiation therapy. Small lesions, particularly of the lower lip, can often be simply excised. In the case of larger lesions and those close to a commissure, more complex plastic surgery is generally required to permit patients to open their mouths relatively widely, either to eat or to insert their dentures; radiation therapy is the simpler alternative. The choice between surgery and radiation therapy generally should be made on the basis of the anticipated cosmetic and functional result. Younger patients who are destined to receive considerable additional sun exposure should preferentially be treated with surgery.

Radiation therapy for tumors of the lip can be delivered by any of several different techniques. Superficial lesions can be treated with superficial x-ray therapy and

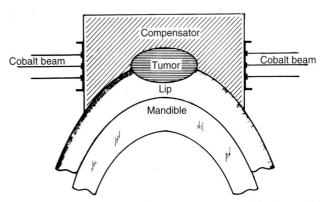

Fig. 10-21 Use of a tissue compensator to provide dose uniformity from tangential megavoltage irradiation of a large tumor of the lip.

somewhat larger or thicker lesions can be treated with en face electron beams. Custom-made, coated lead shields are placed behind the lip to absorb transmitted radiation. Alternatively, brachytherapy (interstitial implants or surface moulds) can be used for small lesions. When lesions are very thick or wrap sufficiently far around the lip that their shape makes treatment by en face techniques or brachytherapy less desirable, tangential megavoltage external-beam techniques can be used. A compensator is built to fit over the lip to eliminate skin sparing and provide homogeneity of dose (Fig. 10-21).

Lesions of the Buccal Mucosa

Tumors of the buccal mucosa can be treated with surgical excision, radiation therapy, or a combination of both modalities. Very small lesions can be excised and closed primarily, whereas larger tumors typically require a split-thickness skin graft for closure. For larger lesions of the buccal mucosa, combined surgery and radiation therapy is the best treatment; however, local–regional recurrence remains the predominant mode of treatment failure despite combined therapy.[57] Tumors that involve the commissure of the lips generally are not treated surgically because of the risk of subsequent microstomia unless reconstruction is done. These tumors and moderate-sized (i.e., small T2) lesions tend to be well suited for brachytherapy.[58] Somewhat larger lesions generally require external-beam radiation therapy, preferably with a technique that limits the dose to the opposite side of the mouth (e.g., mixed electron/photon beam or wedged-pair photon techniques). Large lesions (i.e., T3 and T4) usually are best treated with surgery and postoperative irradiation.

Lesions of the Oral Tongue

Small lesions of the oral tongue, particularly those of the anterior tip, are readily managed with transoral surgical excision and generally should be treated with surgery.

However, as lesions increase in size, the increasing functional deficits that are imposed by surgical management limit the usefulness of surgery and argue for radiation therapy. Brachytherapy should be considered for relatively small lesions that cannot be excised without a substantial functional deficit.[59] Some authors[60,61] advocate peroral cone therapy for small lesions. Still others advocate surgery followed by external-beam irradiation.[62] Large lesions generally are best treated with resection followed by postoperative irradiation. When this approach is not feasible, definitive external-beam irradiation and an interstitial boost can sometimes be effective.[63] Remote high-dose-rate brachytherapy is emerging as yet another alternative. High-dose-rate brachytherapy, either alone or as a supplement to surgery or conventional radiation therapy, seems to have some efficacy in the treatment of oral-tongue and floor-of-mouth cancer (see the next paragraph).[64,65]

Lesions of the Floor of the Mouth

Treatment options for lesions of the floor of the mouth are the same as those for lesions of the oral tongue (see the preceding paragraph), although results of radiation therapy are better in the floor of the mouth. Surgery is favored for lesions that are adherent to the mandible, whereas radiation therapy should be considered for lesions that invade the tongue. Proponents of elective neck dissection point to data suggesting improved cure rates (as compared with rates in patients who are only observed)[66]; however, elective radiation therapy most likely produces a similar benefit.

Lesions of the Upper or Lower Gingiva

Small lesions of the upper or lower gingiva should generally be excised. The relative scarcity of tissue in these areas forces the surgeon to excise adjacent bone as lesions advance in size; however, this usually does not have functional or cosmetic sequelae. Radiation therapy provides an alternative for small lesions when surgery is not possible, but proximity to bone essentially limits radiation therapy options to external-beam techniques or moulds. Advanced lesions generally are best treated with surgery and postoperative irradiation.

Lesions of the Retromolar Triangle

Small tumors of the retromolar trigone can be treated with either radiation therapy or surgery, but large lesions require combined management. Hard palate lesions are usually of salivary gland origin and should be treated surgically. Postoperative irradiation of the tumor bed and the most likely route of spread of salivary gland tumors, particularly those displaying perineural spread, is generally advisable.

Regional Lymph Nodes

Not infrequently, the mode of treatment selected for the primary oral cavity tumor influences the treatment applied to the draining lymph nodes. However, the following principles of management for regional nodes apply to the extent that they do not conflict with the required management of the primary tumor.

Nodal groups that have a high likelihood of containing only occult disease should be treated with radiation therapy when the primary tumor is treated with radiation therapy. Elective neck dissection is warranted only when the position of the primary tumor necessitates surgical manipulation of the regional nodes anyway or a limited dissection is sought for its prognostic value (e.g., a supraomohyoid neck dissection for carcinomas of the floor of the mouth). The reader should be aware of overly enthusiastic advocates of "elective" neck dissections; when such procedures reveal no evidence of disease, they represent unnecessary surgery, and when they reveal metastatic disease, this is often considered an indication for subsequent radiation therapy (in which case the cancer is effectively treated twice).

Relatively small involved nodes (e.g., 0.5 to 2.5 cm) can usually be effectively treated with either surgery or radiation therapy. Often the modality most appropriate for the primary tumor is used.

Larger involved nodes tend to require combined-modality treatment. Once tumor cells have expanded a node to beyond 3 cm in diameter, the nodal capsule is often transgressed, and tumor in adjacent soft tissues generally cannot be removed with surgery. Conversely, nodes larger than 3 cm typically contain too much viable disease to be controlled reliably with radiation therapy alone. Multiple enlarged nodes also represent an indication for combined therapy. Chemotherapy is currently being tested as an adjuvant to postoperative radiation therapy for high-risk tumors (see Chapters 3 and 4).

Recurrent Disease

The influence and effects of primary treatment preclude simple strategies for treatment of recurrent disease. In general, treatment of recurrence is most successful when it relies on a different modality from the primary modality (i.e., surgery for recurrence after radiation therapy and vice versa). However, attempts at surgical salvage of recurrences after radiation therapy are more likely to succeed than are attempts at radiotherapeutic salvage of recurrences after surgery. In the select subgroups wherein postsurgical recurrent disease can be encompassed by using brachytherapy techniques, Vikram and colleagues[67] have documented a reasonable prospect of radiotherapeutic salvage. Aggressive combinations of surgery and radiation therapy or chemotherapy and radiation therapy offer the best prospects for control of advanced tumors.[68]

CHEMOPREVENTION

With increasing progress in the treatment of oral cavity carcinomas, more patients will live long enough to develop second independent malignancies. At present, chemoprevention remains a greater hope than reality, but chemoprevention may improve the survival of patients with oral cavity tumors in the next decade.

The progression from normal to dysplastic to malignant tissue that is often seen for oral cavity tumors offers a target for early intervention. Administration of 13-cis-retinoic acid (13-CRA, Isotretinoin), a synthetic analogue of vitamin A, has been shown to cause regression of oral leukoplakia. Hong and colleagues[69] reported that 13-CRA, given orally in daily doses of 1 to 2 mg/kg for 3 months, reduced the size of leukoplakic patches in 67% of patients. Unfortunately, about two thirds of the patients experienced side effects (mostly dryness of the skin and mucous membranes and elevation of serum triglyceride levels), and the beneficial effects were only temporary (patch regrowth occurred in 50% of patients within 3 months of cessation of 13-CRA). Hong and colleagues[70] have also used 13-CRA to try to prevent the appearance of second independent malignancies in patients already treated for a head and neck cancer. In that study, daily 50 to 100 mg/m^2 doses of 13-CRA given for 1 year were associated with a significantly decreased rate of second malignancies at a median follow-up time of 32 months. However, only two thirds of the patients completed a full year of treatment, and second malignancies seemed to be only suppressed and delayed, not eliminated, by treatment. A successor trial (RTOG 91-15) of a smaller dose of 13-CRA for a longer period (30 mg daily for 3 years) has completed accrual of more than 1300 patients, and follow-up is currently maturing.

Other agents may also be effective. The combination of the antioxidants β-carotene, α-tocopherol, and vitamin C has been reported to induce redifferentiation of dysplastic oral mucosa, possibly mediated by decreases in the S-phase fraction and decreases in the number of micronuclei.[71] Similar effects can possibly be produced by common foods. Green tea may be able to produce a temporary G$_1$ block that retards cell cycle progression in dysplastic tissues.[72] In one prospective double-blind intervention trial, a specially blended tea was more effective than placebo in reducing the size of oral leukoplakic lesions and in decreasing toward normal the number of cells having micronuclei.[73]

RADIATION THERAPY TECHNIQUES

Discussion of radiation therapy techniques for tumors arising in the oral cavity must include both brachytherapy (implants and moulds) and teletherapy (conventional external-beam treatment, intraoral cones, and, increasingly, 3-dimensionally planned, intensity-modulated, conformal techniques). For small lesions, brachytherapy, delivered by means of radioactive implants, or less often by means of a surface mould, is preferable. Intraoral cone irradiation, a unique form of teletherapy for small lesions, has its advocates as well. External-beam radiation therapy provides the most versatility and becomes mandatory for large tumors for which it is usually given postoperatively. Selection among these modalities depends on the anatomic tumor site; the extent of tumor involvement; and the treating physician's experience, expertise, and preferences.

Brachytherapy

Ideally, as long as the tumor volume is relatively small (< 2.5 cm), brachytherapy can deliver lethal doses of radiation to a target tumor volume relatively quickly (brachytherapy is a form of accelerated radiation therapy) while at the same time limiting the radiation dose to adjacent normal tissues. Local control rates of 85% to 90% are typical; however, they are accompanied by self-limited soft-tissue ulceration during the first 18 months after treatment in approximately 30% of patients.[74]

The technical limitations of source implantation are such that for practical purposes, if a tumor has a maximum diameter of more than 2.5 cm, it is difficult to place radioactive sources without creating cold spots that are underdosed. Because of the rapid fall-off in dose from each radioactive source, the need for supplemental external-beam radiation therapy to "cobble" the dose homogeneity increases in proportion to the implant volume. (External-beam radiation therapy supplements the dose at each cold spot and thereby increases dose homogeneity.) In addition, as the implant volume increases, so too does the risk of mandibular osteonecrosis.[74] Simon and colleagues[75] have shown the spacing between sources (9 to 14 mm vs. 15 to 20 mm) to be related to rates of local control at 5 years (86% vs. 76%, $P = 0.13$) and necrosis at 5 years (33% vs. 46%, $P = 0.04$).

When brachytherapy is used as the exclusive method of treatment, doses of 65 to 75 Gy (delivered at approximately 0.5 Gy/hr, resulting in 10 to 15 Gy/day) are commonly used. When lesions exceed 2.5 cm, a typical combined treatment plan delivers 50 Gy over 5 weeks by teletherapy and 30 Gy over 5 weeks by brachytherapy.

Although the rules of source placement for brachytherapy established years ago for preloaded radium or cesium needles still apply, temporary ^{192}Ir afterloading techniques have become today's standard. [192]Ir sources in the United States consist of rice-sized iridium seeds that are manufactured at precisely spaced increments from each other within flexible nylon tubes. (In Europe, solid iridium wires serve the same purpose.) Rarely, the lack of tissue to hold an iridium implant will favor use of a permanent radioactive iodine seed implant (gold grains were previously used for this purpose) or a temporary surface mould.

Many different ways are available for implanting sources through either submental or intraoral routes. Pierquin and colleagues[76] describe nearly a dozen afterloading techniques that can be used to place radioactive materials in desired geometric patterns. The techniques have in common the introduction of nonradioactive rigid or nonrigid guides into tissues in such a way that the subsequently placed iridium sources must conform to the same pattern as the guides. Because these guides can be slowly and accurately positioned, the subsequently placed radioactive sources are more likely to yield a homogeneous dose pattern. In addition, the relative speed of placement of the afterloaded radioactive sources decreases the exposure of medical personnel.

Different philosophies of source arrangement are also evident. Initially, idealized plans were required because of the difficulty of manually calculating isodose distributions from multiple sources of radiation. The Manchester system[77] provided the practitioner with a set of rules for both source position and source strength that permitted prediction of the distribution of isodose curves generated. An alternative approach, the Paris system,[78,79] used sources of uniform linear activity placed in equidistant parallel lines and planes. This approach was well suited for ^{192}Ir ribbons. In reality, any of these historically derived systems can be viewed as a starting point; computerized dosimetry systems can calculate dose distributions from virtually any arrangement of sources to permit individualization of implants for individual patient's needs.

Most brachytherapy source arrangements can be viewed as a series of parallel lines, often connected by looping from one line to the other the flexible iridium sources that make up each line (previously, separate radioactive needles, known as *crossing sources,* provided the same function as the top of the loop). Figure 10-22 illustrates several arrangements of radioactive sources that are suitable for treatment of oral-tongue lesions of various sizes and in various locations. Although the sources are drawn as rigid needles, the concepts are equally applicable for flexible sources. A blind-end iridium ribbon implant is essentially equivalent to a noncrossed rigid needle implant; a looped iridium implant is functionally equivalent to a needle implant with one crossed end. It should be noted that most of the sources in Figure 10-22, *A* and *F,* are oriented so that they are being viewed on end (i.e., they run from the dorsum of the tongue down through the substance of the tongue into the floor of the mouth). This orientation is illustrated in Figure 10-23 using cesium needles and in Figure 10-24 using iridium ribbons. Note the use of a protector (Figs. 10-22, *D,* and 10-25) that is placed over the mandible to shield it from radiation and thus decrease the risk of subsequent osteonecrosis.

Tumors of the floor of the mouth, as long as they are not too close to the mandible, can be treated in a similar

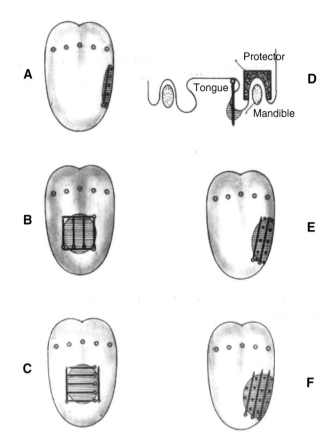

Fig. 10-22   **A,** Diagram of a single-plane implant suitable for a carcinoma of the border of the tongue of 1-cm thickness and 4 cm in the anteroposterior dimension. Five needles are implanted vertically with 1-cm separation between needles; a single needle is used to cross the superior end of the vertical needles, implanting it 0.5 cm below the mucosa, in an anteroposterior direction. **B,** Diagram of a single-plane implant suitable for a carcinoma of the dorsum of the tongue. The needles are placed 0.5 cm deep to the mucosa, and both ends are crossed. **C,** Diagram of a single plane implant for a carcinoma of the dorsum of the tongue with both ends crossed. The needles are placed 0.5 cm deep to the mucosa. **D,** Diagram of a dental plastic protector to reduce the dose to the gingiva and mandible, as used in a single-plane implant for a carcinoma of the floor of the mouth. Note that the needles are inserted through the tongue and the ends are not crossed. **E,** Diagram of a two-plane implant suitable for an advanced (2.5-cm–thick) carcinoma of the tongue. **F,** Diagram of a volume implant suitable for very advanced (more than 2.5-cm–thick) carcinoma of the tongue.

fashion. However, placement of radioactive implants too close to the mandible leads to an unacceptable rate of osteonecrosis. Patients who have protruding genial tubercles may not have sufficient space in their mouths to permit successful brachytherapy. Lesions of the lip or buccal mucosa generally are thin enough to be treated with single plane implants. In all cases, the parallel sources are spaced approximately 1 cm apart, and the sources physically encompass the entire gross extent of the tumor

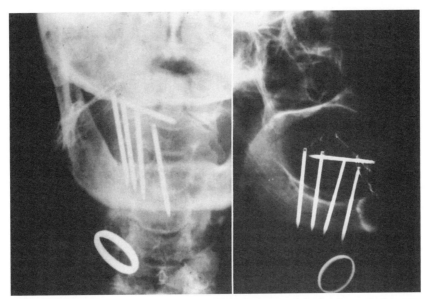

Fig. 10-23 Radiographs of rigid cesium needles placed in a single-plane configuration for treatment of a tongue lesion.

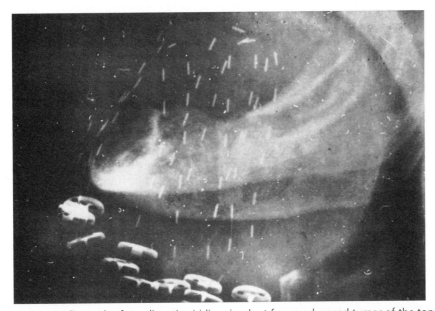

Fig. 10-24 Radiograph of a radioactive iridium implant for an advanced tumor of the tongue and floor of the mouth. The iridium seeds are contained in flexible nylon threads that are inserted through hollow metal guides placed in a submental and submaxillary approach. Once the iridium-containing threads are inserted (afterloading technique), the guides are removed. Hairpin-shaped iridium wire can be used as a substitute for needles or for flexible iridium-containing threads.

plus 1 cm to provide a margin that will encompass subclinical disease.

Intraoral Cone Therapy

An intraoral cone permits treatment of small volumes with external-beam irradiation that is more concentrated, or more like brachytherapy, than with typical teletherapy techniques. Although current cones have a periscope to permit visualization of the tumor in the treatment position, the cone requires a cooperative patient who will keep his or her mouth open widely and work to keep the lesion immobile despite any inherent soreness. This technique is not available universally, but, in experienced hands, it can yield results for selected lesions (e.g., T1 and T2 oral tongue) that rival and perhaps exceed results achieved with interstitial implant techniques.[60,61]

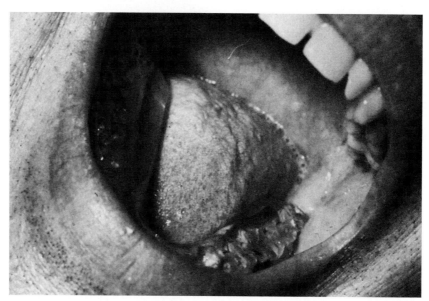

Fig. 10-25 Plastic gum protector (separator) prepared in anticipation of a needle implant for a carcinoma of the floor of the mouth. The needles will be implanted through the substance of the tongue. The protector will increase the separation of needles from gum and decrease the risk of excessive irradiation of the adjoining gum and mandible.

Conventional External-Beam Radiation Therapy

Definitive primary irradiation of oral cavity tumors with external-beam techniques is a difficult task because these tumors are less likely to respond to treatment than are their counterparts in most other head and neck sites. Although the concept of a dose-response relationship holds true in the oral cavity, the range of doses that can actually be used in this region is constrained. Even small lesions that for some reason cannot be excised or treated with brachytherapy typically require 66 Gy, establishing the lower end of the range. Large lesions, which in theory would benefit from doses in excess of 70 Gy delivered by conventional fractionation, cannot be treated to substantially larger doses because of the limitations imposed by surrounding normal tissues. Thus doses in the range of 66 to 70 Gy delivered over 6.5 to 7 weeks, conventionally fractionated at 2 Gy per daily treatment session, have traditionally been used for unresected disease. However, recent findings suggest that better control of advanced tumors can be achieved with altered-fractionation regimens.

Altered-Fractionation Regimens

The optimum altered-fractionation approach at present is either a concomitant boost approach in which 72 Gy is delivered in 42 fractions over 6 weeks (1.8 Gy per fraction per day to a large field plus 1.5 Gy per fraction per day to a boost field during the final 12 treatment days) or a hyperfractionated regimen in which 81.6 Gy is delivered in 68 fractions over 7 weeks (1.2 Gy per fraction, twice daily, 6 hours apart).[80] At the 2-year mark, both of these altered-fractionation regimens seem to improve local–regional control and disease-free survival at the cost of greater acute toxicity (approximately 50% more grade 3+ toxicity) but no increase in late toxicity.

The addition of concurrent chemotherapy may further improve outcome. For example, Brizel and colleagues[81] compared hyerfractionated radiation therapy alone to hyperfractionated radiation therapy plus concurrent and adjuvant cisplatin and fluorouracil and observed that, at 3 years of follow-up, the combined treatment was associated with improved local–regional control, improved disease-free survival, and improved overall survival. Equally important, with the regimen used (70 Gy in 1.25-Gy fractions twice daily plus 12 mg/m^2/day of cisplatin and 600 mg/m^2/day of fluorouracil for 5 days during weeks 1 and 6 of irradiation), the rate of severe complications was not significantly different between the groups. Further improvements in the integration of altered-fractionation radiation therapy with chemotherapy will most likely provide the next major advance in the treatment of oral cavity tumors.[82,83] Identification of precisely which tumors will respond optimally to combinations of radiation therapy and chemotherapy will most likely be one of the major advances in cancer care over the next decade.

Postoperative Regimens

In the postoperative setting, where all grossly detectable disease has been removed, smaller radiation doses are adequate. Although 90% of undisturbed microscopic epithelial tumors in a variety of anatomic sites are controlled when treated with 45 to 50 Gy,[84] subclinical disease in a bed that has been surgically altered is somewhat more difficult to control. Peters and colleagues[85] conducted a prospective randomized dose-seeking trial of postoperative external-beam radiation therapy for head and neck cancer. They demonstrated that 52 to 54 Gy delivered in 1.8-Gy increments was insufficient even for tumors that were excised with uninvolved margins. In common practice, undissected tissues with a low risk of tumor involvement receive 50 Gy, dissected tissues with clean margins receive 60 Gy, and dissected tissues with involved margins receive 66 Gy. The necessity of adequate dose is particularly important for tumors with features that place the patient at high risk for local recurrence—that is, two or more involved lymph nodes, extracapsular extension of disease, or microscopically involved mucosal margins.[86] In fact, the relatively high risk of recurrence of such tumors prompted the design of a prospective national trial (RTOG 95-01) that is currently testing the value of concurrent cisplatin chemotherapy with radiation therapy.

Treatment Set-up and Portal Arrangement

Lesions of the oral cavity often are treated with a three-field technique consisting of lateral parallel opposed photon fields and an anterior low neck field. (However, far lateral tumors [e.g., tumors confined to the buccal mucosa] are better treated with wedged-pair or mixed electron-photon techniques that spare contralateral normal tissues mated to an ipsilateral or bilateral low neck field.) The arrangement generally should encompass the primary tumor and the first echelon of draining nodes in a single portal. For most oral cavity subsites, these first echelon nodes are located in levels I and II. If other lymph nodes are clinically involved, they generally should also be included in the primary treatment portals.

In general, for tumors of the oral tongue or floor of the mouth, the lateral fields encompass the primary tumor, the submandibular nodes, and the upper jugular nodes. Irradiation of the posterior chain is not required unless clinically positive cervical nodes are present.

For tumors of the retromolar trigone, the ipsilateral posterior cervical nodes are usually irradiated only if the primary tumor is T3 or T4. The posterior cervical nodes generally should be irradiated (for any primary tumor site) if clinically involved nodes are in the anterior chain. Figures 10-26 and 10-27 depict typical treatment portals.

Tissue compensators may be needed to produce relative homogeneity of dose throughout the treatment volume. For lesions of the floor of the mouth, inferior gingiva, or oral tongue, a bite-block spacer, also known as a *stent* or *lollypop*, should be placed inside the patient's mouth so that the tongue is depressed and the maxilla is

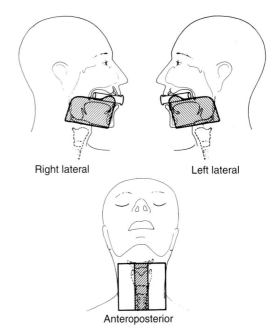

Fig. 10-26 Schematic representation of anatomic sites included in radiation fields used for extensive tumors in the lower aspect of the oral cavity. For small, well-differentiated tumors, the field treating the low anterior neck should be omitted in the absence of palpable disease.

moved up and out of the fields. For all tumors except very small tumors that have no demonstrable associated adenopathy, the primary tumor portals generally are mated to an anterior low neck field that irradiates the nodal stations that lie between the inferior edge of the primary treatment portals and the inferior edge of the clavicles. The philosophic intent is to encompass all nodal stations that have a probability of subclinical involvement (based on the characteristics of the primary tumor) while minimizing the risk of treatment complications. For lesions of the oral cavity that do not have bulky associated adenopathy, a midline block is generally used in the anterior neck field to shield the underlying larynx and spinal cord. To maximize the patient's comfort, the primary portals should be as small as possible, and the anterior portal should be commensurately as large as possible without excluding gross disease from the lateral portals.

As they traverse tissue, the inferior edges of the lateral treatment portals diverge downward, and the superior edge of the anterior portal diverges upward. Therefore if the lateral and anterior fields are abutted on the skin, a small area of overlap occurs. Because the midline block in the anterior field protects the spinal cord from irradiation, the area of overlap generally is not clinically important. However, the match can be improved either by using a half-beam block (treating the lateral fields with the upper, unblocked half of the portal and treating the anterior neck with the lower, unblocked half of a portal, using a common central axis) or by angling the anterior

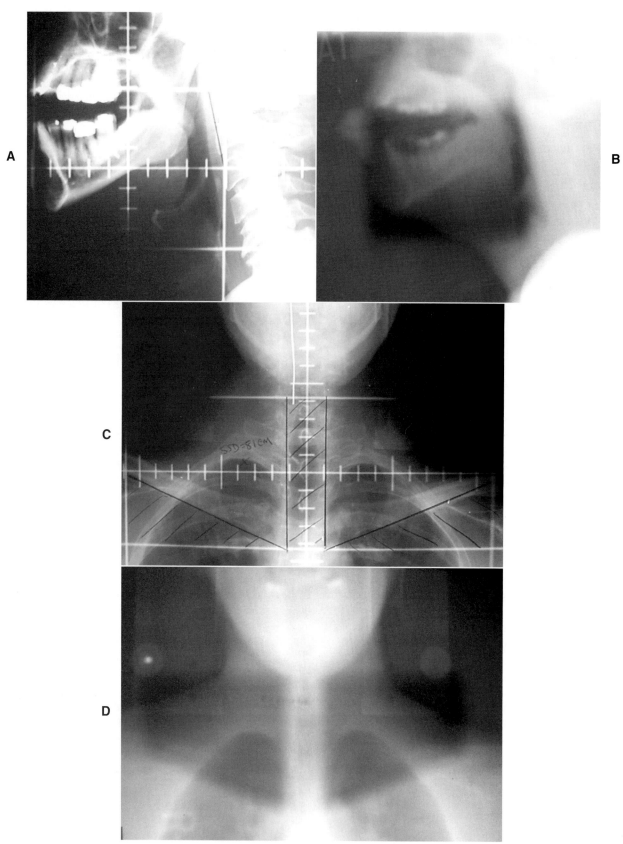

Fig. 10-27 **A,** Representative volume included in the lateral treatment portals for postoperative irradiation of a tumor of the floor of the mouth (corresponding to schematic Fig. 10-26). **B,** Anterior neck field for the same patient. **C,** Portal film of the lateral field. **D,** Portal film of the anterior neck field.

TABLE 10-9

Simplified Schema for Radiation Therapy of the Lip

Disease Stage	Modality	Dose	Boost Dose	Neck Treatment
T1–T2 N0	Choice of XRT or brachytherapy	50 Gy, 25 fractions	6-10 Gy in 3-5 fractions	No RT
		60-65 Gy, 5-7 days	None	No RT
T3 N0	XRT	50 Gy, 25 fractions	10-20 Gy in 5-10 fractions	Levels I and II
T1–T3, positive nodes	XRT	50 Gy, 25 fractions	16-20 Gy in 8-10 fractions	Levels I-IV

XRT, External-beam radiation therapy; *RT,* radiation therapy.

field toward the patient's feet (easily done by turning the couch 90 degrees and angling the gantry approximately 3 degrees, depending on field sizes and source-to-skin distance, to eliminate cephalad divergence). If bulky adenopathy is present in the low neck field, a half-beam blocked combination of lateral opposed fields superiorly mated to anteroposterior-posteroanterior opposed fields inferiorly often produces an appropriate plan.

At simulation, a radio-opaque paste or marker may be used to demarcate grossly evident tumor for fluoroscopic visualization. The patient's head should be immobilized sufficiently to prevent movement during treatment (e.g., with tape or Aquaplast). Contours should be taken at the central axis close to the cephalad and the caudad edges of the lateral portals to check for homogeneity of dose throughout the treated volume. Before treatment, critical structures must be identified on the treatment plan, and steps must be taken to ensure that the doses to be received are within the tolerance of the normal tissues. Simulation films and portal (beam) films should be taken of all new fields to ensure accurate placement. Verification films taken periodically through treatment help ensure that the portals have remained accurate.

Tables 10-9 and 10-10 present simplified radiation therapy schema for common sites and categories of oral cavity tumors.

Three-Dimensional Conformal Radiation Therapy

The development of computers that can calculate dose distributions from noncoplanar fields in three dimensions within a time frame congruent with appropriate patient care has given birth to conformal radiation therapy. As suggested by the name, the goal of conformal treatment is to shape the dose to the tumor as tightly as possible, sparing the normal tissues as much as possible. Consequently, for such plans, the traditional concept of describing boundaries of treatment portals is replaced by definitions of three-dimensional tumor volumes that need to receive specified dose minimums and three-dimensional normal tissue volumes that ideally should receive less than specified dose maximums. The concept of three-dimensional conformal therapy is discussed in further detail in Chapter 2 of this text. Within the oral cavity, conformal therapy is the approach most likely to permit protection of normal tissues (most

TABLE 10-10

Simplified Schema for Radiation Therapy of the Oral Tongue and Floor of the Mouth

Disease Stage	Modality	Dose	Boost Dose	Neck Treatment
T1 N0	Brachytherapy	65-75 Gy, 6-7 days	None	No XRT
T2 N0	XRT	50 Gy, 25 fractions	6-10 Gy, 3-5 fractions	Levels I and II
T3–T4 N0 or N+	Surgery + XRT or altered-fractionation XRT or chemotherapy + XRT	60-66 Gy, 30-33 fractions	None	All levels
		72 Gy, 42 fractions, 6 weeks	Included in 72 Gy	
		70 Gy, 35 fractions	None	

XRT, External-beam radiation therapy.

importantly the salivary glands; see the section on "Xerostomia" later in this chapter) and may also result in better tumor control through escalation of the dose to small volumes.

RESULTS OF RADIATION THERAPY

The success rate of radiation therapy for carcinomas of the oral cavity is best measured by local control of disease. The lifestyles often associated with oral cancer can also lead to other neoplastic and nonneoplastic causes of death that obscure the efficacy of treatment.[87] In addition to the cardiovascular consequences of smoking and drinking, second independent malignancies are now commonly appreciated as important causes of morbidity and mortality in these patients. However, local–regional recurrence of tumor remains the principal cause of morbidity and mortality for these patients.[88] Local recurrence after radiation therapy is more common for oral cavity tumors than for tumors in most other head and neck sites.[89-91]

Failure to control primary tumors becomes apparent relatively quickly; 80% to 90% of local recurrences are detected within 2 years after completion of treatment, and virtually all other recurrences become apparent over the next year. Beyond 3 years, local recurrences are rare and second independent malignancies begin to pose an increasingly greater problem. In each successive year, approximately 3% of patients who are cured of their first tumor develop a second independent tumor, most often arising in the upper aerodigestive tract.[87]

Three years of follow-up is also adequate to detect the vast majority of distant metastases. Thus patients who are disease-free 3 years after treatment can be considered "cured" of their disease.

Factors Influencing the Likelihood of Local Control of Disease

The probability of tumor control is influenced by various tumor and host factors. The best correlates of outcome are the anatomic measures of primary tumor, nodal, and distant metastatic involvement that form the basis of the AJCC staging system. The likelihood of control is also influenced, but to a lesser degree, by the anatomic subsite of disease (see Table 10-8). Vascular invasion seems to predict increased risk of local recurrence and diminished likelihood of survival.[53] Suggestions have also been made in some analyses that tumor control correlates with the primary tumor's thickness[92]; the tumor's histologic grade (with control less likely for well-differentiated tumors than for moderately or poorly differentiated lesions); the patient's hemoglobin level; and the patient's sex, with control more likely in women than in men.[93] In general, lesions that originate more anteriorly have a better prognosis than lesions

that arise more posteriorly (i.e., as one goes from the lips toward the base of tongue). In addition, local control is directly related to the total dose of radiation delivered and inversely related to the duration of treatment.[93]

Patterns of Disease Regression

Primary tumors generally regress more rapidly than do involved regional lymph nodes. However, the rate of tumor response is only a weak predictor of eventual local control. Tumors that have not regressed completely by the completion of radiation therapy may yet resolve over the next few weeks. Sobel and colleagues[94] suggest that the most accurate time to assess the degree of tumor clearance is 30 to 90 days after the completion of radiation therapy.

Overall, complete regression of disease can be expected in 65% to 75% of all patients who present with tumors of the oral cavity. From 1977 to 1980, the RTOG prospectively registered all patients who had tumors of the head and neck region who had been seen in member institutions.[95] A total of 217 patients who had cancer of the oral cavity (excluding tumors of the lips, which are known to have a better prognosis) were followed, and, in these patients, a complete response rate of 67% was

TABLE 10-11

Percentage of Patients in whom Oral Cavity Tumors and Involved Lymph Nodes Were Cleared by Radiation Therapy, by Disease Stage

Patients with Clearance of Tumor (%)

All T categories	76
T1	97
T2	87
T3	61
T4	38

Patients with Clearance of Lymph Node Involvement (%)

All N categories	68
N1	83
N2	58
N3	55

Patients with Clearance of Primary Tumor and Lymph Node Involvement (%)

Stage I	97
Stage II	87 (6)*
Stage III	51 (14)*
Stage IV	39 (5)*

Modified from Marcial V, Amato D, Pajak T. *Cancer Treatment Symposia* 1983;2:33-40.
*In parentheses, clearance achieved with radiation therapy and surgical salvage therapy.

TABLE 10-12

Rates of Complete Response to Radiation Therapy and Local–Regional Control at 3 Years and 5 Years among Patients with Oral Cavity Tumors in the Radiation Therapy Oncology Group Head and Neck Cancer Registry

Disease Stage	Number of Patients	Complete Response Rate (%)	LOCAL CONTROL RATE (%)	
			3 Years	5 Years
I	36	97	74	65
II	71	87	49	49
III	51	51	11	*
IV	59	39	*	*

*Too few patients for reliable estimate.

observed. In addition, salvage surgery eliminated residual disease in an additional 6% of patients, for a total complete response rate of 73%.

It is instructive to examine disease clearance rates in the primary tumor and regional lymph nodes separately (Table 10-11). In the RTOG study, complete clearance of the primary tumor was observed in 97% of T1 lesions of the oral cavity, 87% of T2 lesions, 61% of T3 lesions, and 38% of T4 lesions.[95] In similar fashion, rates of clearance of metastatic disease in regional lymph nodes decreased as nodal size increased. Disease was completely cleared in approximately 83% of patients with N1 disease, 58% with N2 disease, and 55% with N3 disease.[95] Little, if any, difference was noted in the response of nodes based on the exact site of origin of the primary tumor.

Data from the RTOG's registry for patients with head and neck cancer treated with radiation therapy clearly demonstrate decreases in local control and survival rates with increases in disease stage (Tables 10-12 and 10-13). Also notable is the greater difference between 3-year and 5-year survival rates than between 3-year and 5-year local–regional control rates, a pattern reflecting the relatively high rate of death from nonneoplastic causes and second independent malignancies in this patient population.

TABLE 10-13

Estimated Absolute Survival at 3 Years and 5 Years among Patients with Oral Cavity Cancer in the Radiation Therapy Oncology Group Head and Neck Cancer Registry

Disease Stage	Number of Patients	ABSOLUTE SURVIVAL RATE (%)	
		3 Years	5 Years
I	36	68	53
II	71	52	39
III	51	33	*
IV	59	*	*

*Too few patients for reliable estimate.

Because of the diversity of tumors that are grouped within each stage category, even for single anatomic subsites, the expected outcome of treatment (ultimate local control or survival) can only be approximated. In addition, recent RTOG trials have shown a clear trend toward improving control and survival for advanced tumors.[88] With this understanding, rates of local control of early-stage tumors of the oral cavity can be expected to be in the range of 80% to 90%.[96] Moderately advanced lesions typically have a 60% to 70% likelihood of local control, whereas far-advanced lesions are controlled 35% to 45% of the time. It is perhaps surprising, but also instructive, to review the variations in reported outcome by stage and anatomic site and to note how many categories do not have reliable (nonanecdotal) data available (see Table 10-8).

Site-Specific Results
Lesions of the Lip

Carcinomas of the lip have the most favorable outcome of all the oral cavity tumors. Most lesions are detected when they are relatively small, and cure rates exceeding 90% are possible with either radiation therapy or surgery.

Beauvois and colleagues[97] treated 237 patients with squamous cell carcinoma of the lower lip (158 T1, 61 T2, 17 T3, and 1 T4) with low-dose-rate ^{192}Ir brachytherapy alone. With 5 years of follow-up, the local control rate was 95%, the overall survival rate was 74%, and the cause-specific survival was 91%. Fongione and colleagues[98] treated 69 patients with lip tumors (36 T1, 12 T2, 2 T3, and 19 recurrent tumors) with interstitial brachytherapy alone and reported only 1 persistent tumor and no local recurrences. At 5 years, the overall survival rate was 77%, and the disease-specific survival rate was 91%. Orecchia and colleagues[99] treated 47 patients with lip tumors (21 T1 and 26 T2) and obtained local control in 94%.

Lesions of the Buccal Mucosa

Relatively small carcinomas of the buccal mucosa generally are considered suitable for either surgery or irradiation. However, Strome and others[100] observed a startling 100% local recurrence rate after wide local excision alone for stage I and II tumors. Sakai and colleagues[101] reported the outcome of a variety of treatments for 55 buccal carcinomas. As assessed by multivariate analysis, the local control rate was 85% in patients treated with preoperative radiation therapy followed by surgery; interstitial implant; or electron beam therapy. In contrast, the local control rate was approximately 30% in patients treated with external photon beam therapy or external photon beam therapy followed by mould therapy. The authors concluded that the success of interstitial brachytherapy rivals that of surgery for T1 to early T3 buccal carcinomas that do not invade the bucco-alveolar sulci or retromolar trigone regions. Lapeyre and colleagues[58] obtained local control in 91% of 22 buccal carcinomas treated with a looping (encircling) technique. Fang and colleagues[57] reported a 3-year actuarial local–regional control rate of 64% and an overall survival rate of 55% after surgery and postoperative radiation therapy for 6 stage II, 21 stage III, and 30 stage IV buccal cancer cases. Mishra and colleagues[92] found that tumor thickness predicted the risk of local–regional recurrence of buccal carcinomas.

Lesions of the Gingiva, Hard Palate, and Retromolar Triangle

Relatively little current information is available about radiation therapy for carcinomas of the gingiva, hard palate, or retromolar trigones. It seems fortunate that relatively few squamous cell carcinomas arise on the upper gingiva or hard palate, as bone often tends to be involved and the outcome after any type of therapy tends to be poor.[102] However, Cengiz and colleagues[103] reported two early-stage carcinomas of the upper gingiva that were locally controlled with high-dose-rate brachytherapy delivered by a surface mould. Fuchihata and colleagues[104] treated 162 squamous cell carcinomas of the lower gingiva with external-beam radiation therapy and simultaneous bleomycin or peplomycin chemotherapy. Sixty-seven percent of T1 and T2 tumors responded completely as opposed to only 35.5% of T3 and T4 tumors. Local control rates at 5 years (including salvage therapy) were 91% for T1 tumors, 89% for T2 tumors, 76% for T3 tumors, and 61% for T4 tumors. Five-year cause-specific survival rates were 75% for stage I, 87% for stage II, 71% for stage III, and 51% for stage IV tumors.

Carcinomas of the retromolar trigones are often grouped with carcinomas of the anterior faucial pillar, and relatively few series clearly separate these two entities. However, Lo and colleagues[105] reported that local control was achieved in 66% of a variety (T1 through T4) of retromolar trigone lesions treated essentially with 60 to 75 Gy external-beam radiation therapy.

Lesions of the Floor of the Mouth

Small, centrally located carcinomas of the floor of the mouth respond well to brachytherapy. Pernot and colleagues[106] treated 102 carcinomas of the floor of the mouth with brachytherapy only and treated 105 lesions with external-beam radiation therapy plus brachytherapy. At 5 years, local control rates were 97% for T1 lesions, 72% for T2 lesions, and 51% for T3 lesions. This translated into 5-year overall survival rates of 71%, 42%, and 35% and 5-year cause-specific survival rates of 88%, 47%, and 36%, respectively. Grade 2 or more severe complications occurred in 19% of patients. The authors concluded that brachytherapy alone is the preferable treatment for T1 N0 and T2 N0 tumors. Mazeron and colleagues[107] reported primary tumor control rates of 93.5% and 74.5% for T1 N0 and T2 N0 tumors, respectively, after ^{192}Ir brachytherapy, which resulted in 5-year cause-specific survival rates of 94% and 62%. In contrast, once lesions extended to the gingiva or exceeded 3 cm, control rates were only 50% and 58%, respectively. Consequently, larger tumors and those located close to the mandible should be considered for surgery or external-beam radiation therapy (either alone or with a limited brachytherapy boost) or both modalities depending on their size and location.

Inoue and colleagues[108] compared the outcomes in 41 patients with floor-of-mouth tumors treated with low-dose-rate [198]Au grain implants and 16 patients with similar tumors treated with high-dose-rate interstitial therapy and found no significant differences in local control rates (75% for low-dose-rate therapy and 94% for high-dose-rate therapy at 2 years) or rates of late-occurring bone exposure or ulceration. (32% for low-dose-rate therapy and 38% for high-dose-rate therapy).

Lesions of the Oral Tongue

For oral-tongue tumors, surgery is often the preferred form of treatment.[109] However, when small carcinomas of the oral tongue can be encompassed within the high-dose envelope produced by brachytherapy and the envelope avoids irradiation of the mandible, results comparable to surgery can be obtained.[110] Pernot and colleagues[111] treated 125 T1 and 186 T2 tumors with brachytherapy with or without external-beam radiation therapy and obtained 5-year local control rates of 93% and 65%, respectively. Five-year disease-specific survival rates were 78% and 43%, respectively, and overall survival rates were 69% and 41%, respectively, for T1 and T2 tumors. Mazeron and colleagues[112] obtained a local control rate of 87% for 70 T1 N0 and 83 T2 N0 tumors treated with [192]Ir. This corresponded to 5-year actuarial survival rates of 52% for the T1 N0 tumors and 44% for the T2 N0 tumors. Yoshida and colleagues[113] reported a 5-year local control rate of 78% for 498 T1 and T2 oral-tongue tumors treated with brachytherapy alone or brachytherapy and external-beam radiation therapy. Similarly, in a series of 207 squamous carcinomas of the oral tongue treated with brachytherapy alone (127 tumors) or combined brachytherapy and external-beam radiation therapy (80 tumors), Fujita and colleagues[114] reported 5-year local control rates of 93% for T1 tumors, 82% for T2a tumors, and 72% for T2b tumors.

When implants are combined with external-beam radiation therapy, several series[111,114,115] report better control when a greater percentage of the dose is delivered by brachytherapy. However, the retrospective nature of these series raises the possibility that larger lesions were more often treated with combined therapy and that the outcome thus reflects selection as much as it does modality. Nevertheless, this observation has been sufficiently common that it seems prudent to heed its implicit warning. Similarly, Pernot and colleagues[111] compared outcomes in 152 T2 N0 tumors treated in a nonrandomized fashion with either brachytherapy alone or brachytherapy and external-beam radiation therapy. Both local control (90% vs. 50%, $P = 0.0000$) and cause-specific survival (60% vs. 31%, $P = 0.01$) were better after brachytherapy alone, although these data must be interpreted with caution because of the hazards inherent in comparing nonrandomized groups.

Definitive irradiation of oral-tongue tumors is associated with both soft-tissue and bone complications. Pernot and colleagues[111] reported grade 1 complications in 19% of patients (15% soft tissue and 3% bone), grade 2 complications in 6% of patients (2% soft tissue and 4% bone), and grade 3 complications in 3% of patients (1% soft tissue and 2% bone). Fein and colleagues[109] reported some degree of soft-tissue necrosis or bone exposure in approximately one third of patients and severe complications in 11% of patients with oral-tongue tumors treated mostly with brachytherapy and external-beam radiation therapy.

The combination of surgery and postoperative external-beam radiation therapy is not a panacea either. Despite gross total resection and microscopically clean margins, Zelefsky and colleagues[116] reported a 38% local recurrence rate and a corresponding overall survival rate of 55% at 5 years.

LATE EFFECTS AND COMPLICATIONS OF RADIATION THERAPY

Although many squamous cell carcinomas of the head and neck can be eradicated without inducing serious long-term complications in surrounding normal tissues, the relative sensitivities of tumors and the surrounding normal tissues are such that complications (Box 10-2) are inevitable in a small percentage of patients. As valid instruments have been developed for measuring quality of life, a more precise estimate of the toxicity of conventional treatment has been

---

BOX 10-2 Side Effects and Complications of Treatment of Oral Cavity Tumors

Xerostomia
Mucositis
Diminished taste acuity
Sensitivity to spicy foods
Enhanced dental decay
Susceptibility to infection
Impaired nutrition
Surgically induced difficulty eating, speaking, and swallowing
Relative stiffness of tissues
Osteonecrosis

---

obtained. To facilitate comparison of the degree and type of side effects after treatment, the RTOG has created a late (beyond 90 days after treatment) toxicity scale (Table 10-14).

Xerostomia

With conventional radiation therapy, virtually all patients experience some degree of persistent xerostomia if a substantial part of the parotid glands is included within the radiation portal. Scintigraphic evaluation of parotid gland function suggests that a dose of less than 33 Gy will result in subacute xerostomia (xerostomia occurring within the first 6 months) in 50% of patients and that a dose of less than 52 Gy will result in chronic xerostomia (after 12 months) in 50% of patients.[117] In one study, most glands irradiated with doses of 40 to 50 Gy had recovered approximately 70% of their pretreatment salivary flow rate by 18 months after the completion of treatment.[118] Epstein and colleagues[119] documented complaints of dry mouth in 92% of patients, changes in taste in 75%, dysphagia in 63%, altered speech in 51%, difficulty using dentures in 49%, and increased dental decay in 31% of dentate patients.

The advent of conformal, intensity-modulated radiation therapy techniques offers the prospect of avoiding acute and subacute xerostomia if the mean dose delivered to one parotid gland can be kept below 26 Gy.[120] Alternatively, pharmacologic agents may be able to protect patients to some degree from radiation-induced damage. Pilocarpine, a parasympathomimetic drug, may be able to degranulate secretory cells and possibly decrease their radiosensitivity.[121] However, at the conventional radiation doses required for control of human tumors, the predominant mechanism of action by which pilocarpine restores saliva is stimulation of the parts of the salivary glands that are not encompassed within the treatment portals.[122] In glands totally

TABLE 10-14

Radiation Therapy Oncology Group Criteria for Late Toxic Effects

Site	Grade 0	Grade 1	Grade 2	Grade 3	Grade 4
			TOXIC EFFECTS		
Skin	None	Slight atrophy Pigmentation change Some hair loss	Patch atrophy Moderate telangiectasia Total hair loss	Marked atrophy Gross telangiectasia	Ulceration
Subcutaneous tissue	None	Slight induration (fibrosis) and loss of subcutaneous fat	Moderate fibrosis but without symptoms Slight field contracture (< 10% reduction in linear measurement)	Severe induration and loss of subcutaneous tissue Moderate field contracture (> 10% reduction in linear measurement)	Necrosis
Mucous membranes	None	Slight atrophy and dryness	Moderate atrophy and telangiectasia Little mucus	Marked atrophy with complete dryness Severe telangiectasia	Ulceration
Salivary gland	None	Slight dryness of mouth Good response on stimulation	Moderate dryness of mouth Poor response on stimulation	Complete dryness of mouth No response on stimulation	Fibrosis

Modified from Cox JD, Stetz J, Pajak TF. *Int J Radiat Oncol Biol Phys* 1995;31:1341-1346.

irradiated to tumoricidal doses, the administration of 5 mg of pilocarpine four times a day during and after radiation therapy for a total of 3 months had no beneficial effect.[122] Amifostine, a free-radical scavenger, has been shown in a small prospective randomized phase II trial of carboplatin plus radiation therapy (with or without amifostine) to decrease the severity of induced xerostomia and mucositis.[123] As the ability to overcome the toxic effects of progressively more aggressive therapy improves, strategies for amelioration of toxic effects will play an increasingly prominent role in the decision-making processes involved in day-to-day patient care.

In addition to causing discomfort associated with the sensation of dryness, xerostomia makes it more difficult for patients to chew and swallow their food. Artificial saliva improves the comfort level of some patients. Others simply carry a small bottle of water with them and rinse their mouths at frequent intervals. Other patients find that chewing gums specially formulated for dry mouths (e.g., Biotene) or sucking on sugar-free candy is soothing. Rinsing with a solution of baking soda in water (1 teaspoon baking soda dissolved in half a glass of room-temperature water) is relatively bland and soothing and helps dissolve sticky saliva. Baking soda can also be used with a soft toothbrush to clean the teeth and tongue. Commercial mouthwashes (e.g., Biotene) have also been developed for patients who have undergone irradiation of the oral cavity.

Fungal, Viral, and Bacterial Infections

Because the dry mouth is prone to opportunistic attack, patients may require specific therapy for fungal, viral, or bacterial infections. *Candida albicans* is the most common opportunistic organism. It classically appears as a fluffy off-white growth that can be partially scraped off the involved tissues by using a tongue blade. Sometimes this organism is less obvious, appearing only as fissuring of the angles of the lips. Patients who demonstrate marked erythema or mucositis earlier in treatment than anticipated should be examined particularly closely for such infection.

In most instances, candidal infections can be managed with topical suspensions (e.g., nystatin) or, if necessary, with systemic therapy (e.g., fluconazole). When nystatin is chosen, patients must be instructed to swish the medication in the mouth vigorously for at least 5 minutes four times per day. Some patients are unwilling to do this, some patients are unable to do this because of soreness, and some patients simply cannot get the medication far enough back in their mouth to come in contact with the fungus. Therefore, theoretically, systemic therapy provides advantages over topical therapy. However, patients should be informed of the potential side effects of systemic therapy, including potentially severe hepatic toxicity, and should be allowed to participate in choosing their medication.

Herpes simplex is the most common viral infection. Classically appearing as small vesicles, the infection typically lasts approximately 1 week and is self-limited. In patients who are more immunocompromised, the lesions may ulcerate and may be extremely painful. Treatment typically involves an antiviral medication such as acyclovir.

Overt bacterial infections are relatively uncommon. Despite the existence of gingivitis or periodontitis in many adults, clinically significant bacterial infections are uncommon. When they do occur, mild infections can be treated with a topical rinse such as chlorhexidine. However, chlorhexidine tends to stain dental plaque, and, in some patients who are already experiencing severe soreness from treatment or tumor, an unacceptable burning sensation prevents the use of this drug. In cases of more severe infection, systemic antibiotics are required.

Mucositis and Pain

Mucositis currently represents the most common dose-limiting side effect of modern aggressive altered-fractionation and chemoradiation therapy regimens, and mucositis persists longer after treatment with these regimens than with traditional regimens.[80,82,83] Mucositis primarily reflects direct injury of the irradiated mucosa; however, to some degree, mucositis may be mediated by irradiation of the parotid glands. Christensen and colleagues[124] reported a significant decrease in the salivary content of epidermal growth factor after radiation therapy and speculated that the drop in this mitogenic peptide, implicated in mucosal regeneration, may contribute to the development of mucositis.

Pain, generally secondary to mucositis, is common by the midpoint of conventionally fractionated radiation therapy regimens and can last for many weeks after treatment. For mild pain, simple analgesics like aspirin crushed and dissolved in water or Aspergum provide relief. Some patients find that coating the mouth with olive oil or swallowing 1 teaspoon of olive oil before they eat and as necessary during meals makes them more comfortable. For more severe pain, stronger measures are required. Viscous lidocaine (Xylocaine) often provides effective pain relief, but patients tend to experience a burning sensation until the medication "takes." To ameliorate this sensation, the drug can be dispensed in a mixture with soothing agents (e.g., a mixture of Xylocaine, Mylanta, and Benadryl). Systemic medications such as acetaminophen with codeine (Tylenol No. 3) or Percocet may be necessary.

Nutritional Problems

Nutrition tends to suffer as treatment progresses. Patients require nutritional counseling and encouragement. Most patients can tolerate six half-size meals per day better than three full meals. Nutritional supplements (e.g., Ensure) should be considered between meals. Capable patients can be instructed in the preparation of homemade nutritional supplements that they can vary to suit their taste. Patients who have advanced mucositis essentially have to rely on a soft, bland diet that is served at room temperature without added spices. Beverages should be similarly bland. Some patients fail to realize that oranges and tomatoes are relatively acidic and usually are best avoided during and for some time after treatment.

When changing the diet and blending food are insufficient to permit the patient to consume an adequate diet, placement of a percutaneous gastrostomy tube provides an alternative means of supporting the patient's nutritional requirements during and after radiation therapy. As treatment regimens have become more aggressive, the nutritional demands on patients have become more difficult to satisfy orally, and a general trend toward more frequent insertion of percutaneous gastrostomy tubes can be seen. Many chemoradiation therapy regimens are sufficiently aggressive that percutaneous gastrostomy tubes should be placed prophylactically.

Osteonecrosis

Osteonecrosis (also known as *osteoradionecrosis*) typically involves the mandible and represents a late-appearing manifestation of injury beyond the reparative capacity of the normal cells. Radiation most likely produces hypocellular, hypovascular, hypoxic tissue, which leads to tissue breakdown and a chronic nonhealing wound.[125] The role of infection in fostering osteonecrosis is subject to debate. Although the necrosis by itself is nonspecific, the development of periosteal thickening, mottled areas of resorption, osteoporosis, sclerosis, lysis, or fracture of bone occurring 6 months to several years after treatment is generally diagnostic.

Osteonecrosis typically is thought of as a consequence of brachytherapy applied close to the mandible. Mazeron and colleagues[107] treated 95 evaluable patients who had T1 or T2 cancer of the floor of the mouth with iridium brachytherapy alone. Grade 1 complications (spontaneously healing exposure that did not interfere with the patients' sense of well-being) occurred in soft tissues 15 times and in bone seven times. Grade 2 complications (requiring hospitalization and usually antibiotics and steroids) occurred in soft tissues eight times and in bone three times. Grade 3 complications (requiring surgery or leading to substantial disability or death) occurred in soft tissues eight times and in bone seven times. However, osteonecrosis can also occur after external-beam radiation therapy. Niewald and colleagues[126] reported an 8.6% rate of osteonecrosis after conventionally fractionated external-beam radiation therapy (60 to 70 Gy delivered at 2 Gy in one fraction per day) and a

22.9% rate of osteonecrosis after aggressive hyperfractionated therapy (82.8 Gy delivered at 1.2 Gy in each of two daily fractions at least 4 hours apart).

Although patients who are edentulous may have a more difficult time chewing their food during treatment, they are at a relative advantage in having a lesser risk of osteonecrosis. To a large degree, having all patients undergo dental evaluation before radiation therapy is begun can eliminate this difference. Healthy teeth should not be extracted even if they will be within the radiation portals; teeth that are irradiated do not experience worse damage than adjacent nonirradiated teeth. Broken, badly decayed teeth or preexistent gingival disease needs to be corrected before radiation therapy begins. When teeth are so badly decayed that caries cannot be repaired quickly, extraction is appropriate. The socket should be rongeured smooth, and the mucosa overlying the socket should be sutured closed. Approximately 2 weeks should be allowed for healing before radiation therapy is begun. Ideally, the incidence of osteonecrosis could be decreased by waiting 3 weeks after extraction,[127] but the need to start treatment as quickly as possible renders 2 weeks a suitable compromise for most patients.

Dental Decay

Failure to protect teeth from the changes produced by radiation therapy over time leads to dental decay, which characteristically occurs along the gumline (Fig. 10-28, *A*). Even when decay is relatively far advanced, appropriate intervention and restoration is worthwhile and can salvage the situation (see Fig. 10-28, *B*). Aside from its salutary effect on the patient's appearance, restoration

removes one portal of entry for infection. On the other hand, dental manipulation by itself may be sufficiently traumatic to produce osteonecrosis in previously marginally viable mandibular bone. Prevention of decay is therefore preferable. A prospective randomized trial has shown that if teeth must be extracted from a previously irradiated mandible, hyperbaric oxygen is more successful than penicillin in preventing subsequent osteonecrosis (5% vs. 30%).[128]

If, despite all efforts, osteonecrosis does occur, antibiotic therapy and patience should be the first line of management. Hyperbaric oxygen can help in some cases by stimulating angiogenesis, increasing neovascularization, and optimizing cellular oxygen levels to enhance osteoblast and fibroblast proliferation.[129] Only when it becomes apparent that osteonecrosis will be progressive or persistent should surgical management be undertaken.

FOLLOW-UP CARE

Head and neck tumors that are not controlled with initial treatment tend to recur within 2 years after radiation therapy. Follow-up care, therefore, needs to be offered to patients on an intensive basis for the first few years after treatment. For the typical patient who has no complicating factors that require earlier medical intervention, it is prudent to schedule the first follow-up appointment approximately 2 weeks after the completion of treatment. At that time, the acute reaction from radiation therapy should have peaked, and the patient should verify and examination should demonstrate the onset of recovery. As soon as the radiation-induced soreness subsides, daily fluoride therapy should be initiated to protect

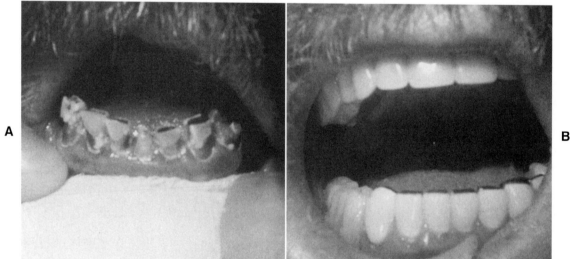

Fig. 10-28   **A,** Characteristic radiation-induced dental decay, predominantly along the gum line. The patient was placing fluoride gel in dental trays, but instead of placing the trays over his teeth, the patient was dipping his toothbrush into the trays and then brushing. **B,** Same patient following dental restoration.

against future dental decay. The use of custom-shaped plastic trays that are fitted over the upper and lower teeth is preferable. A solution of approximately 1% fluoride is prescribed. Patients place three or four drops of fluoride in each tray and then place the trays over their teeth for 10 min/day every day for the rest of their lives.

During the first year of follow-up, patients tend to have concerns because of xerostomia, and many become frightened when a benign submental collection of lymphatic fluid in sagging skin (i.e., a dewlap) becomes evident 1 to 4 months after treatment. Patients should be offered palliative agents for xerostomia and should be reassured both that the dewlap does not represent recurrent tumor and that its appearance will improve over time without intervention. Patients generally are seen every 2 to 3 months for the first year.

During the second year, patients tend to feel relatively well, and follow-up appointments can be spaced to once every 3 months. However, the period around 18 months after completion of treatment constitutes the time of greatest risk of recurrence, and patients should be dissuaded from thinking that extending the interval between follow-up examinations suggests that they should become lax in their care.

By the third year, most recurrences have already become evident, and follow-up can be extended to once every 3 to 4 months. After 3 years, the chance of recurrence is very small, and patients can be seen only twice per year. At that point, follow-up care is justified by the need to detect second independent malignancies as early as possible.

SUMMARY

Radiation oncologists play a major role in the treatment of carcinomas of the oral cavity. The wide range in the size and behavior of lesions challenges physicians to use virtually all of their armamentarium to achieve optimum management of lesions. Fortunately, treatment of oral cavity lesions is often successful. The importance of multimodal care in the management of oral cavity carcinomas demands that radiation oncologists have a close working rapport with diagnostic radiologists, surgical pathologists, head and neck surgeons, medical oncologists, and dentists. The possibility of applying recently described principles of tumor biology and recently pioneered strategies of fractionation and sensitization raises the hope that radiation care now stands on the threshold of better tumor control and decreased cosmetic and functional consequences for these lesions.

REFERENCES

1. Greenlee RT, Hill-Harmon MB, Murray T, et al. Cancer statistics, 2001. *CA Cancer J Clin* 2001;51:15-36.
2. Borok TL, Cooper JS. Time course and significance of acute hyperamylasemia in patients receiving fractionated therapeutic radiation to the parotid gland region. *Int J Radiat Oncol Biol Phys* 1982; 8:1449-1451.
2a. Cox JD, Stetz J, Pajak TF. Toxicity criteria of the Radiation Therapy Oncology Group (RTOG) and the European Organization for Research and Treatment of Cancer (EORTC). *Int J Radiat Oncol Biol Phys* 1995;31:1341-1346.
3. US Department of Health and Human Services. *The Health Consequences of Smoking: Cancer. A Report of the Surgeon General.* Rockville, Md: US Department of Health and Human Services, Public Health Service; 1982, DHHS Publication No. PHS 82-50179.
4. Graham S, Dayal H, Roher T, et al. Dentition, diet, tobacco and alcohol in the epidemiology of oral cancer. *J Natl Cancer Inst* 1977;59:1611-1618.
5. Wynder EL, Bross IJ, Feldman RM. A study of the etiological factors in cancer of the mouth. *Cancer* 1957;10:1300-1323.
6. Zhang Z-F, Morgenstern H, Spitz MR, et al. Marijuana use and increased risk of squamous cell carcinoma of the head and neck. *Cancer Epidemiol Biomarkers Prev* 1999;8:1071-1078.
7. Weaver A, Fleming SM, Smith DB, et al. Mouthwash and oral cancer. Carcinogen or coincidence? *J Oral Surg* 1979;37:250-253.
8. Winn DM, Blot WJ, McLaughlin JK, et al. Mouthwash use and oral conditions in the risks of oral and pharyngeal cancer. *Cancer Res* 1991;5:3044-3047.
9. Morse DE, Katz RV, Pendrys DG, et al. Smoking and drinking in relation to oral epithelial dysplasia. *Cancer Epidemiol Biomarkers Prev* 1996;5:769-777.
10. Hirayama T. An epidemiological study of oral and pharyngeal cancer in central and southeast Asia. *Bull World Health Organ* 1966;34:41-69.
11. Vogler WR, Lloyd WJ, Milmore BK. A retrospective study of aetiological factors in cancer of the mouth, pharynx and larynx. *Cancer* 1962;15:246-258.
12. Rosenfeld L, Callaway J. Snuff dippers' cancer. *Am J Surg* 1963; 106:840-844.
13. Pindborg JJ, Mehta FS, Gupta PC, et al. Reverse smoking in Andhra Pradesh, India: a study of palatal lesions among 10,169 villagers. *Br J Cancer* 1971;25:10-20.
14. Reddy DG, Rao VK. Cancer of the palate in coastal Andhra due to smoking cigars with the burning end inside the mouth. *Indian J Med Sci* 1957;11:791-798.
15. Dorn HF, Cutler SJ. Morbidity from cancer in the United States. Public Health Monographs, No. 56, Washington, D.C.; 1959, Public Health Service publication No. PHS 590.
16. Schantz SP, Hsu TC, Ainslie N, et al. Young adults with head and neck cancer express increased susceptibility to mutagen-induced chromosome damage. *JAMA* 1989;262:3313-3315.
17. Bundgaard T, Wildt J, Elbrond O. Oral squamous cell cancer in nonusers of tobacco and alcohol. *Clin Otolaryngol* 1994;19:320-326.
18. Silverman S Jr, Miglioratti C, Barbosa J. Toluidine blue staining in the detection of oral precancerous and malignant lesions. *Oral Surg Oral Med Oral Pathol* 1984;57:379-382.
19. Daura Saez A, Rodriguez San Pedro F, Asenjo Garcia B, et al. Magnetic resonance imaging in the diagnosis of oral carcinoma [in Spanish]. *Acta Otorrinolaringol Esp* 1999;50:283-290.
20. van den Brekel MWM, Castelijns JA. Radiologic evaluation of neck metastases: the otolaryngologist's perspective. *Semin Ultrasound CT MR* 1999;20:162-174.
21. Som PM, Curtin HD, Mancuso AA. Imaging-based classification for the cervical lymph nodes designed as an adjunct to clinically based nodal classifications. *Arch Otolaryngol Head Neck Surg* 1999;125:388-396.
22. Black RJ, Gluckman JL, Shumrick DA. Multiple primary tumours of the upper aerodigestive tract. *Clin Otolaryngol* 1983;8:277-281.
23. Woolgar JA, Scott J. Prediction of cervical lymph node metastasis in squamous cell carcinoma of the tongue/floor of mouth. *Head Neck* 1995;17:463-472.

24. Lindberg RD. Distribution of cervical lymph node metastases from squamous cell carcinoma of the upper respiratory and digestive tracts. *Cancer* 1972;29:1446-1450.

25. Mendenhall WM, Million RR, Cassisi NJ. Elective neck irradiation in squamous-cell carcinoma of the head and neck. *Head Neck Surg* 1980;3:15-20.

26. August M, Gianetti K. Elective neck irradiation versus observation of the clinically negative neck of patients with oral cancer. *J Oral Maxillofac Surg* 1996;54:1050-1055.

27. Shah JP. Patterns of cervical lymph node metastasis from squamous carcinomas of the upper aerodigestive tract. *Am J Surg* 1990;160:405-409.

28. Friedman M, Mafee MF, Pacella BL, et al. Rationale for elective neck dissection in 1990. *Laryngoscope* 1990;100:54-59.

29. Merino OR, Lindberg RD, Fletcher GH. An analysis of distant metastases from squamous cell carcinoma of the upper respiratory and digestive tracts. *Cancer* 1977;40:145-151.

30. Leibel SA, Scott CB, Mohiuddin M, et al. The effect of local-regional control on distant metastatic dissemination in carcinoma of the head and neck: results of an analysis from the RTOG head and neck database. *Int J Radiat Oncol Biol Phys* 1991;21:549-556.

31. Fleming I, Cooper JS, Henson DE, et al, eds. *AJCC Cancer Staging Manual*, 5th ed. Philadelphia, Pa: Lippincott Williams & Wilkins; 1997:24-30.

32. Langdon JD, Harvey PW, Rapidis AD, et al. Oral cancer: the behaviour and response to treatment of 194 cases. *J Maxillofac Surg* 1977;5:221-237.

33. Shafer WG, Waldron CA. Erythroplakia of the oral cavity. *Cancer* 1975;36:1021-1028.

34. Shin DM, Kim J, Ro JY, et al. Activation of p53 gene expression in premalignant lesions during head and neck tumorigenesis. *Cancer Res* 1994;54:321-326.

35. Nawroz H, van der Riet P, Hruban RH, et al. Allelotype of head and neck squamous cell carcinoma. *Cancer Res* 1994;54:1152-1155.

36. van der Riet P, Nawroz H, Hruban RH, et al. Frequent loss of chromosome *9p21-22* early in head and neck cancer progression. *Cancer Res* 1994;54:1156-1158.

37. Liu SC, Hu Y, Sauter ER, et al. Image analysis of *p53* and cyclin D1 expression in premalignant lesions of the oral mucosa. *Anal Quant Cytol Histol* 1999;21:166-173.

38. Kerdpon D, Rich AM, Reade PC. Expression of *p53* in oral mucosal hyperplasia, dysplasia and squamous cell carcinoma. *Oral Dis* 1997;3:86-92.

39. Kudo Y, Takata T, Ogawa I, et al. Expression of *p53* and *p21CIP1/ WAF1* proteins in oral epithelial dysplasias and squamous cell carcinomas. *Oncol Rep* 1999;6:539-545.

40. Jordan RC, Bradley G, Slingerland J. Reduced levels of the cell-cycle inhibitor *p27Kip1* in epithelial dysplasia and carcinoma of the oral cavity. *Am J Pathol* 1998;152:585-590.

41. Shintani S, Yoshihama Y, Emilio AR, et al. Overexpression of *p53* is an early event in the tumorigenesis of oral squamous cell carcinomas. *Anticancer Res* 1995;15:305-308.

42. Kushner J, Bradley G, Young B, et al. Aberrant expression of cyclin A and cyclin B1 proteins in oral carcinoma. *J Oral Pathol Med* 1999;28:77-81.

43. Kotelnikov VM, Coon JS IV, Mundle S, et al. Cyclin D1 expression in squamous cell carcinomas of the head and neck and in oral mucosa in relation to proliferation and apoptosis. *Clin Cancer Res* 1997;3:95-101.

44. Maragou P, Bazopoulou-Kyrkanidou E, Panotopoulou E, et al. Alteration of integrin expression in oral squamous cell carcinomas. *Oral Dis* 1999;5:20-26.

45. Xu XC, Ro JY, Lee JS, et al. Differential expression of nuclear retinoid receptors in normal, premalignant, and malignant head and neck tissues. *Cancer Res* 1994;54:3580-3587.

46. Yamamoto T, Kamata N, Kawano H, et al. High incidence of amplification of the epidermal growth factor receptor gene in human squamous carcinoma cell lines. *Cancer Res* 1986;46:414-416.

47. Scambia G, Panici PB, Battaglia F, et al. Receptors for epidermal growth factor and steroid hormones in primary laryngeal tumors. *Cancer* 1991;67:1347-1351.

48. Santini J, Formento JL, Francoual M, et al. Characterization, quantification, and potential clinical value of the epidermal growth factor receptor in head and neck squamous cell carcinomas. *Head Neck* 1991;13:132-139.

49. Kannan S, Balaram P, Chandran GJ, et al. Co-expression of ras p21 and epidermal growth factor receptor during various stages of tumour progression in oral mucosa. *Tumour Biol* 1994;15:73-81.

50. Maiorano E, Favia G, Maisonneuve P, et al. Prognostic implications of epidermal growth factor receptor immunoreactivity in squamous cell carcinoma of the oral mucosa. *J Pathol* 1998;185:167-174.

51. Aggelopoulou EP, Skarlos D, Papadimitriou C, et al. Human papilloma virus DNA detection in oral lesions in the Greek population. *Anticancer Res* 199;19:1391-1395.

52. Sugerman PB, Shillitoe EJ. The high risk human papillomaviruses and oral cancer: evidence for and against a causal relationship. *Oral Dis* 1997;3:130-147.

53. Close LG, Brown PM, Vuitch MF, et al. Microvascular invasion and survival in cancer of the oral cavity and oropharynx. *Arch Otolaryngol Head Neck Surg* 1989;115:1304-1309.

54. Lopes MA, Kowalski LP, da Cunha Santos G, et al. A clinicopathologic study of 196 intraoral minor salivary gland tumours. *J Oral Pathol Med* 1999;28:264-267.

55. Henk JM. Treatment of oral cancer by interstitial irradiation using iridium-192. *Br J Oral Maxillofac Surg* 1992;30:355-359.

56. Tupchong L, Scott CB, Blitzer PH, et al. Randomized study of preoperative versus postoperative radiation therapy in advanced head and neck carcinoma: long-term follow-up of RTOG study 73-03. *Int J Radiat Oncol Biol Phys* 1991;20:21-28.

57. Fang FM, Leung SW, Huang CC, et al. Combined-modality therapy for squamous carcinoma of the buccal mucosa: treatment results and prognostic factors. *Head Neck* 1997;19:506-512.

58. Lapeyre M, Peiffert D, Malissard LH. An original technique of brachytherapy in the treatment of epidermoid carcinomas of the buccal mucosa. *Int J Radiat Oncol Biol Phys* 1995;33:447-454.

59. Lambin P, Haie-Meder C, Gerbaulet A, et al. Curietherapy versus external irradiation combined with curietherapy in stage II squamous cell carcinoma of the mobile tongue. *Radiother Oncol* 1992;23:55-56.

60. Wang CC. Radiotherapeutic management and results of T1N0, T2N0 carcinoma of the oral tongue: evaluation of boost techniques. *Int J Radiat Oncol Biol Phys* 1989;17:287-291.

61. Wang CC. Intraoral cone for carcinoma of the oral cavity. *Front Radiat Ther Oncol* 1991;25:128-131.

62. Wendt CD, Peters LJ, Delclos L, et al. Primary radiotherapy in the treatment of stage I and II oral tongue cancers: importance of the proportion of therapy delivered with interstitial therapy. *Int J Radiat Oncol Biol Phys* 1990;18:1287-1292.

63. Mazeron JJ, Grimard L, Benk V. Curietherapy versus external irradiation combined with curietherapy in stage II squamous cell carcinomas of mobile tongue and floor of mouth. *Recent Results Cancer Res* 1994;134:101-110.

64. Leung TW, Wong VY, Wong CM, et al. Technical hints for high dose rate interstitial tongue brachytherapy. *Clin Oncol (R Coll Radiol)* 1998;10:231-236.

65. Klein M, Menneking H, Langford A, et al. Treatment of squamous cell carcinomas of the floor of the mouth and tongue by interstitial high-dose-rate irradiation using iridium-192. *Int J Oral Maxillofac Surg* 1998;27:45-48.

66. McGuirt WF Jr, Johnson JT, Myers EN, et al. Floor of mouth carcinoma. The management of the clinically negative neck. *Arch Otolaryngol Head Neck Surg* 1995;121:278-282.

67. Vikram B, Strong EW, Shah JP, et al. Intraoperative radiotherapy in patients with recurrent head and neck cancer. *Am J Surg* 1985;150:485-487.

68. Spencer SA, Wheeler RH, Peters GE, et al. Concomitant chemotherapy and reirradiation as management for recurrent cancer of the head and neck. *Am J Clin Oncol* 1999;22:1-5.

69. Hong WK, Endicott J, Itri LM, et al. 13-cis-retinoic acid in the treatment of oral leukoplakia. *N Engl J Med* 1986;315:1501-1505.

70. Hong WK, Lippman SM, Itri LM, et al. Prevention of second primary tumors with isotretinoin in squamous-cell carcinoma of the head and neck. *N Engl J Med* 1990;323:795-801.

71. Barth TJ, Zoller J, Kubler A, et al. Redifferentiation of oral dysplastic mucosa by the application of the antioxidants beta-carotene, alpha-tocopherol and vitamin C. *Int J Vitam Nutr Res* 1997;67:368-376.

72. Khafif A, Schantz SP, al-Rawi M, et al. Green tea regulates cell cycle progression in oral leukoplakia. *Head Neck* 1998;20:528-534.

73. Li N, Sun Z, Han C, et al. The chemopreventive effects of tea on human oral precancerous mucosa lesions. *Proc Soc Exp Biol Med* 1999;220:218-224.

74. Lozza L, Cerrotta A, Gardani G, et al. Analysis of risk factors for mandibular bone radionecrosis after exclusive low dose-rate brachytherapy for oral cancer. *Radiother Oncol* 1997; 44:143-147.

75. Simon JM, Mazeron JJ, Pohar S, et al. Effect of intersource spacing on local control and complications in brachytherapy of mobile tongue and floor of mouth. *Radiother Oncol* 1993;26:19-25.

76. Pierquin B, Wilson JF, Chassagne D. Basic techniques of endocurietherapy. In: *Modern Brachytherapy*. New York, NY: Masson; 1987.

77. Paterson R, Parker HM. A dosage system for gamma-ray therapy. *Br J Radiol* 1934;7:592-633.

78. Pierquin B, Dutreix A. Pour une nouvelle methodologie en curietherapie: le Systeme de Paris (endo et plesio-radiotherapie avec preparation non radio-active). *Ann Radiol* 1966;9:757-760.

79. Pierquin B, Dutreix A, Paine CH, et al. The Paris system in interstitial radiation therapy. *Acta Radiol Oncol* 1978;17:33-48.

80. Fu KK, Pajak TF, Trotti A, et al. A Radiation Therapy Oncology Group (RTOG) phase III randomized study to compare hyperfractionation and two variants of accelerated fractionation to standard fractionation radiotherapy for head and neck squamous cell carcinomas: preliminary results of RTOG 9003. *Int J Radiat Oncol Biol Phys* 2000;48:7-16.

81. Brizel DM, Albers ME, Fisher SR, et al. Hyperfractionated irradiation with or without concurrent chemotherapy for locally advanced head and neck cancer. *N Engl J Med* 1998;338: 1798-1804.

82. Vokes EE. Combined-modality therapy of head and neck cancer. *Oncology* 1997;11:27-30.

83. Brizel DM. Radiotherapy and concurrent chemotherapy for the treatment of locally advanced head and neck squamous cell carcinoma. *Semin Radiat Oncol* 1998;8:237-246.

84. Fletcher GH. Clinical dose-response curves of human malignant epithelial tumours. *Br J Radiol* 1973;46:1-12.

85. Peters LJ, Goepfert H, Ang KK, et al. Evaluation of the dose for postoperative radiation therapy of head and neck cancer: first report of a prospective randomized trial. *Int J Radiat Oncol Biol Phys* 1993;26:3-11.

86. Cooper JS, Pajak TF, Forastierre A, et al. Precisely defining high-risk operable head and neck tumors based on RTOG #85-03 and #88-24: targets for post-operative radiochemotherapy. *Head Neck* 1998;21:588-594.

87. Cooper JS, Pajak TF, Rubin P, et al. Second malignancies in patients who have head and neck cancers: incidence, effect on survival and implications for preventive medicine based on the RTOG experience. *Int J Radiat Oncol Biol Phys* 1989; 17:449-456.

88. Lee DJ, Cosmatos D, Marcial VA, et al. Results of an RTOG phase III trial (RTOG 85-27) comparing radiotherapy plus etanidazole with radiotherapy alone for locally advanced head and neck carcinomas. *Int J Radiat Oncol Biol Phys* 1995;32:567-576.

89. Kramer S, Gelber RD, Snow JB, et al. Combined radiation therapy and surgery in the management of advanced head and neck cancer: final report of study 73-03 of the Radiation Therapy Oncology Group. *Head Neck Surg* 1987;10:19-30.

90. Griffin TW, Pajak TF, Gillespie BW, et al. Predicting the response of head and neck cancers to radiation therapy with a multivariate modeling system: an analysis of the RTOG head and neck registry. *Int J Radiat Oncol Biol Phys* 1984;10:481-487.

91. Zelefsky MJ, Harrison LB, Armstrong JG. Long-term treatment results of postoperative radiation therapy for advanced stage oropharyngeal carcinoma. *Cancer* 1992;70:2388-2395.

92. Mishra RC, Parida G, Mishra TK, et al. Tumour thickness and relationship to locoregional failure in cancer of the buccal mucosa. *Eur J Surg Oncol* 1999;25:186-189.

93. Bentzen SM, Johansen LV, Overgaard J, et al. Clinical radiobiology of squamous cell carcinoma of the oropharynx. *Int J Radiat Oncol Biol Phys* 1991;20:1197-1206.

94. Sobel S, Rubin P, Keller B, et al. Tumor persistence as a predictor of outcome after radiation therapy of head and neck cancers. *Int J Radiat Oncol Biol Phys* 1976;1:873-880.

95. Marcial V, Amato D, Pajak T. Patterns of failure after treatment for cancer of the upper respiratory and digestive tracts: a Radiation Therapy Oncology Group report. *Cancer Treat Symp* 1983;2:33-40.

96. Wallner PE, Hanks GE, Kramer S. Patterns of care study: analysis of outcome survey data—anterior two-thirds of tongue and floor of mouth. *Am J Clin Oncol* 1986;9:50-57.

97. Beauvois S, Hoffstetter S, Peiffert D, et al. Brachytherapy for lower lip epidermoid cancer: tumoral and treatment factors influencing recurrences and complications. *Radiother Oncol* 1994;33:195-203.

98. Fongione S, Signor M, Beorchia A. Interstitial brachytherapy in carcinoma of the lip. Case histories and results [in Italian]. *Radiol Med (Torino)* 1994;88:657-660.

99. Orecchia R, Rampino M, Gribaudo S, et al. Interstitial brachytherapy for carcinomas of the lower lip. Results of treatment. *Tumori* 1991;77:336-338.

100. Strome SE, To W, Strawderman M, et al. Squamous cell carcinoma of the buccal mucosa. *Otolaryngol Head Neck Surg* 1999;120:375-379.

101. Sakai M, Hatano K, Sekiya Y, et al. Radiotherapy for carcinoma of the buccal mucosa: analysis of prognostic factors [in Japanese]. *Nippon Igaku Hoshasen Gakkai Zasshi* 1998;58:705-711.

102. Kryst L, Piekarczyk J, Miosek K, et al. Results of treatment of upper gingiva and palate carcinomas [in Polish]. *Czas Stomatol* 1990;43:62-67.

103. Cengiz M, Ozyar E, Ersu B, et al. High-dose-rate mold brachytherapy of early gingival carcinoma: a clinical report. *J Prosthet Dent* 1999;82:512-514.

104. Fuchihata H, Furukawa S, Murakami S, et al. Results of combined external irradiation and chemotherapy of bleomycin or peplomycin for squamous cell carcinomas of the lower gingiva. *Int J Radiat Oncol Biol Phys* 1994;29:705-709.

105. Lo K, Fletcher GH, Byers RM, et al. Results of irradiation in the squamous cell carcinomas of the anterior faucial pillar-retromolar trigone. *Int J Radiat Oncol Biol Phys* 1987;13:969-974.

106. Pernot M, Hoffstetter S, Peiffert D, et al. Epidermoid carcinomas of the floor of mouth treated by exclusive irradiation: statistical study of a series of 207 cases. *Radiother Oncol* 1995; 35:177-185.

107. Mazeron JJ, Grimard L, Raynal M, et al. Iridium-192 curietherapy for T1 and T2 epidermoid carcinomas of the floor of mouth. *Int J Radiat Oncol Biol Phys* 1990;18:1299-1306.

108. Inoue T, Inoue T, Yamazaki H, et al. High dose rate versus low dose rate interstitial radiotherapy for carcinoma of the floor of mouth. *Int J Radiat Oncol Biol Phys* 1998;41:53-58.

109. Fein DA, Mendenhall WM, Parsons JT, et al. Carcinoma of the oral tongue: a comparison of results and complications of treatment with radiotherapy and/or surgery. *Head Neck* 1994; 16:358-365.

110. Shibuya H, Hoshina M, Takeda M, et al. Brachytherapy for stage I & II oral tongue cancer: an analysis of past cases focusing on control and complications. *Int J Radiat Oncol Biol Phys* 1993; 26:51-58.

111. Pernot M, Malissard L, Hoffstetter S, et al. The study of tumoral, radiobiological, and general health factors that influence results and complications in a series of 448 oral tongue carcinomas treated exclusively by irradiation. *Int J Radiat Oncol Biol Phys* 1994;29:673-679.

112. Mazeron JJ, Crook JM, Benck V, et al. Iridium 192 implantation of T1 and T2 carcinomas of the mobile tongue. *Int J Radiat Oncol Biol Phys* 1990;19:1369-1376.

113. Yoshida K, Koizumi M, Inoue T, et al. Radiotherapy of early tongue cancer in patients less than 40 years old. *Int J Radiat Oncol Biol Phys* 1999;45:367-371.

114. Fujita M, Hirokawa Y, Kashiwado K, et al. Interstitial brachytherapy for stage I and II squamous cell carcinoma of the oral tongue: factors influencing local control and soft tissue complications. *Int J Radiat Oncol Biol Phys* 1999;44:767-775.

115. Mendenhall WM, Van Cise WS, Bova FJ, et al. Analysis of time-dose factors in squamous cell carcinoma of the oral tongue and floor of mouth treated with radiation therapy alone. *Int J Radiat Oncol Biol Phys* 1981;7:1005-1011.

116. Zelefsky MJ, Harrison LB, Fass DE, et al. Postoperative radiotherapy for oral cavity cancers: impact of anatomic subsite on treatment outcome. *Head Neck* 1990;12:470-475.

117. Kaneko M, Shirato H, Nishioka T, et al. Scintigraphic evaluation of long-term salivary function after bilateral whole parotid gland irradiation in radiotherapy for head and neck tumour. *Oral Oncol* 1998;34:140-146.

118. Funegard U, Franzen L, Ericson T, et al. Parotid saliva composition during and after irradiation of head and neck cancer. *Eur J Cancer B Oral Oncol* 1994;30:230-233.

119. Epstein JB, Emerton S, Kolbinson DA, et al. Quality of life and oral function following radiotherapy for head and neck cancer. *Head Neck* 1999;21:1-11.

120. Eisbruch A, Ten Haken RK, Kim HM, et al. Dose, volume, and function relationships in parotid salivary glands following conformal and intensity-modulated irradiation of head and neck cancer. *Int J Radiat Oncol Biol Phys* 1999; 45:577-587.

121. Beer KT. Campaign against radio-xerostomia [in German]. *Ther Umsch* 1998;55:453-455.

122. Valdez IH, Wolff A, Atkinson JC, et al. Use of pilocarpine during head and neck radiation therapy to reduce xerostomia and salivary dysfunction. *Cancer* 1993;71:1848-1851.

123. Buntzel J, Kuttner K, Frohlich D, et al. Selective cytoprotection with amifostine in concurrent radiochemotherapy for head and neck cancer. *Ann Oncol* 1998;9:505-509.

124. Christensen ME, Hansen HS, Poulsen SS, et al. Immunohistochemical and quantitative changes in salivary EGF, amylase and haptocorrin following radiotherapy for oral cancer. *Acta Otolaryngol* 1996;116:137-143.

125. Marx RE. Osteoradionecrosis: a new concept of its pathophysiology. *J Oral Maxillofac Surg* 1983;41:283-288.

126. Niewald M, Barbie O, Schnabel K, et al. Risk factors and dose-effect relationship for osteoradionecrosis after hyperfractionated and conventionally fractionated radiotherapy for oral cancer. *Br J Radiol* 1996;69:847-851.

127. Marx RE, Johnson RP. Studies in the radiobiology of osteoradionecrosis and their clinical significance. *Oral Surg Oral Med Oral Pathol* 1987;64:379-390.

128. Marx RE, Johnson RP, Kline SN. Prevention of osteoradionecrosis: a randomized prospective clinical trial of hyperbaric oxygen versus penicillin. *J Am Dent Assoc* 1985;111:49-54.

129. Myers RA, Marx RE. Use of hyperbaric oxygen in postradiation head and neck surgery. *NCI Monogr* 1990;9:151-157.

CHAPTER 11

The Larynx and Hypopharynx

Adam S. Garden

ANATOMY
Larynx

The larynx is the organ responsible for speech and airway protection. It consists of cartilage, joints, ligaments, muscles, and mucosa, all of which interact to permit its important functions. Although the larynx is not critical for survival, its functions are important for good quality of life. Thus the larynx is often the benchmark in oncologic studies examining the role of organ preservation.

Most of the larynx is within and connected to the hypopharynx (Fig. 11-1). Inferiorly, the larynx is connected to the trachea at the same level at which the hypopharynx is connected to the esophagus. Posteriorly, the larynx lies anterior to the posterior pharyngeal wall, prevertebral fascia and muscles, and cervical vertebral bodies. Lateral to the larynx are the lateral walls of the pharynx. Anteriorly, the larynx is relatively superficial, and the anterior commissure can lie within 1 cm of the skin surface (Fig. 11-2). Inferolaterally, the larynx is very close to the thyroid gland. This can be of concern in patients undergoing treatment for thyroid disease because the recurrent laryngeal nerve, which innervates most of the laryngeal

muscles, lies adjacent to the medial portion of each lobe of the gland.

The larynx is divided into three regions: the supraglottis, the glottis, and the subglottis. The natural history and optimal management of laryngeal tumors differ depending on the region in which the tumor arises. The supraglottis lies above the level where the mucosa of the upper surface of the true vocal cords turns upward to form the lateral wall of the ventricle. The supraglottis consists of the epiglottis, aryepiglottic folds, arytenoids, and false vocal cords; essentially the lateral walls of the aryepiglottic folds are the medial walls of the pyriform sinuses (Fig. 11-3). The epiglottis is leaf-shaped. Superiorly, it sits in air within the pharynx and coordinates with the base of the tongue to permit proper swallowing. The midepiglottis is connected to the tongue by two membranes, the valleculae, one on either side. The inferior epiglottis becomes a stalk, the petiolus epiglottidis, which inserts into the anterior aspect of the thyroid cartilage. Just inferior to this is the anterior commissure, which is formed by the joining of the two vocal ligaments. For staging

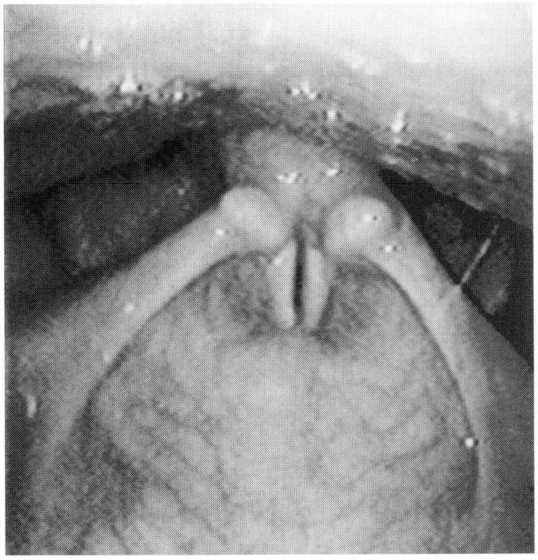

Fig. 11-1 Photograph of the larynx and hypopharynx.

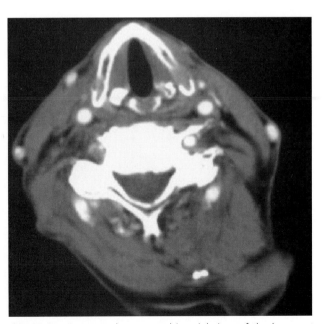

Fig. 11-2 Computed tomographic axial view of the larynx at the true vocal cords.

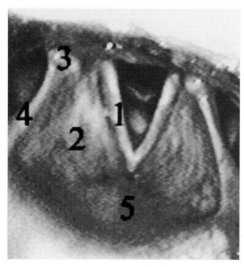

Fig. 11-3 Photograph of the structures of the supraglottic larynx: *1*, true vocal cord; *2*, false vocal cord; *3*, arytenoid; *4*, aryepiglottic fold; *5*, infrahyoid epiglottis.

purposes, the epiglottis is often further divided into a suprahyoid and an infrahyoid epiglottis, although this is not a true anatomic division. The glottis consists of the true vocal cords and the region extending 0.5 cm below the true vocal cords. The subglottis extends from the lower boundary of the glottis to the superior aspect of the trachea.

The laryngeal framework consists of nine cartilages. The largest are the epiglottic, thyroid, and cricoid cartilages. Three pairs of smaller cartilages—the arytenoid, cuneiform, and corniculate cartilages—complete the

cartilaginous composition of the larynx. The arytenoid, thyroid, and cricoid cartilages are composed of hyaline cartilage, which in most people undergoes calcification or ossification beginning around 20 years of age. This often aids in the radiographic localization of these structures. The pattern of ossification in the anterior aspect of the thyroid cartilage is often referred to as *"figure 8" ossification* because of its unique appearance on lateral radiographs. The thyrohyoid membrane connects the hyoid bone and thyroid cartilage. Schematically, on a sagittal view, the hyoid bone, infrahyoid epiglottis, and thyrohyoid membrane form a triangular space filled with fat and referred to as the pre-epiglottic space. Because the pre-epiglottic space is filled only with fat, it offers little resistance to laryngeal tumors.

The thyroid cartilage is a V-shaped structure formed by the fusion of two laminae. The anterior borders of these laminae diverge superiorly to form the thyroid notch. The inferior constrictors of the pharynx attach to the laminae. Posteriorly, the cartilage is prolonged upward and downward to form the superior and inferior horns of the thyroid cartilage. Inferior to the thyroid cartilage lies the cricoid cartilage, a complete ring. The inferior border of the cricoid cartilage marks the inferior extent of the larynx and hypopharynx and the beginning of the trachea and esophagus.

Hypopharynx

The hypopharynx extends from the hyoid bone to the cricoid cartilage. It is the most inferior of the anatomic subdivisions of the pharynx, beginning at the inferior

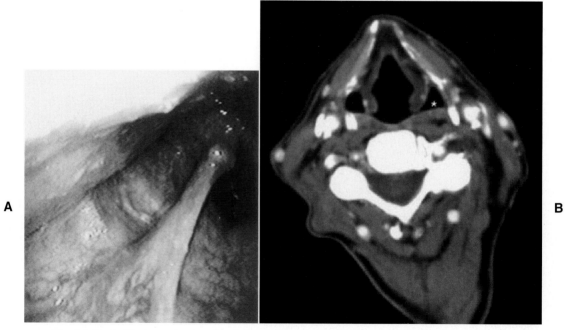

Fig. 11-4 **A,** Photograph of a direct view of the pyriform sinus. **B,** Computed tomographic axial view of the pyriform sinus (***).

border of the oropharynx and eventually connecting with the cervical esophagus at the cricopharyngeal muscle.

The hypopharynx has three anatomic subsites: the pyriform sinuses, the pharyngeal walls, and the postcricoid region. The pyriform sinuses are formed by the invagination of the larynx into the hypopharynx. Each sinus consists of three walls: a lateral wall, a medial wall, which superiorly becomes the aryepiglottic fold, and an anterior wall (Fig. 11-4). Posteriorly, each pyriform sinus is open. Superior to each pyriform sinus is the vestibule formed by the rim of the three walls. Inferiorly, the three walls taper to form the apex.

The pharyngeal walls of the hypopharynx are indistinguishable from the walls of the oropharynx (they are simply a continuation) and are defined by their relationship with neighboring anatomic structures. The separation between the oropharyngeal and hypopharyngeal walls is at the valleculae, pharyngoepiglottic folds, and lateral projections of the aryepiglottic folds.

The postcricoid region, as its name implies, is the region of the hypopharynx posterior to the larynx, beginning at the level of the arytenoids and continuing until the transition into the esophagus. The anterior border of the postcricoid region is formed by the posterior larynx, and the posterior border of the postcricoid region is formed by the posterior pharyngeal wall.

PATTERNS OF TUMOR SPREAD
Tumors of the Supraglottis

Tumors of the supraglottis account for 25% to 33% of all laryngeal neoplasms. Suprahyoid epiglottic tumors can either grow in an exophytic pattern off the tip of the epiglottis or spread inferiorly to infiltrate and ulcerate the epiglottic cartilage (Fig. 11-5). Because of their destructive nature, suprahyoid epiglottic tumors can, even with effective tumoricidal therapy, render the epiglottis ineffective with respect to its function of airway protection, resulting in aspiration.

Infrahyoid epiglottic tumors can invade directly through the base of the epiglottis into the pre-epiglottic space and onto the lingual epiglottis. If they remain undetected, infrahyoid epiglottic tumors can invade the valleculae, pharyngoepiglottic folds, and tongue base. Sometimes these tumors spread onto one or both of the aryepiglottic folds, at times creating a semicircular formation. They then spread either inferiorly onto the false vocal cords or anteriorly onto the anterior commissure and glottis. Advanced tumors can invade the tongue or extend directly into the neck.

Lesions originating on the aryepiglottic folds can spread onto the other components of the supraglottis, including the epiglottis, arytenoids, and false vocal cords. These tumors also can spread laterally into the pyriform sinuses, and in such cases it is sometimes difficult to distinguish the true origin of the tumor (aryepiglottic fold vs. medial pyriform sinus). Lesions originating on the aryepiglottic folds are often infiltrative, and they have easy access to the paraglottic space, which lies between the external frame of the larynx and its internal components. This space is filled with adipose tissue and offers little resistance to growing tumors. From this space, infiltrative tumors can break through ligaments above or below the thyroid cartilage into the neck or invade the cartilage directly. Once invasion into the paraglottic space takes place, the mobility of the larynx often becomes impaired.

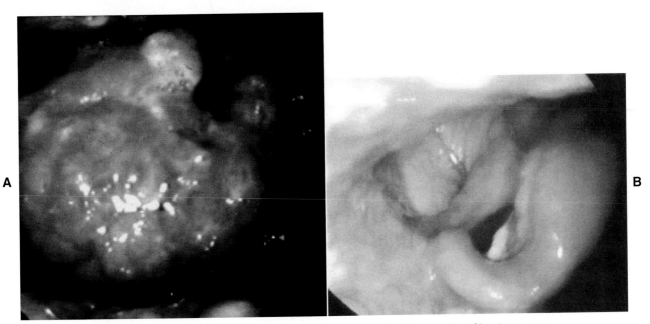

Fig. 11-5   Photographs of tumors of the epiglottis. **A,** Exophytic tumor. **B,** Infiltrative tumor.

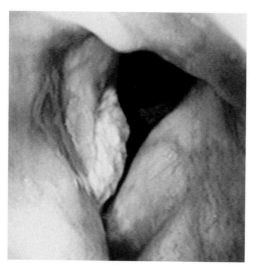

Fig. 11-6 Photograph of tumor of the true vocal cord.

Like lesions of the aryepiglottic folds, lesions of the false vocal cords face few barriers to their spreading. These tumors can extend inferiorly to invade the glottic larynx, and they can easily invade the paraglottic space, laryngeal musculature, and nerves to cause either impaired mobility or fixation of the hemilarynx.

Tumors of the Glottis

Although the glottis is the smallest component of the larynx, most laryngeal cancer originates in this region,

on the true vocal cords. Most tumors of the true vocal cords arise on the free margin and the upper surface of the anterior two thirds of the vocal cords (Fig. 11-6). Lesions often remain confined to the mucosa of the true cords but, if untreated, can eventually spread into the supraglottis or subglottis. Even small lesions can cause hoarseness by limiting either the vibratory ability of the cord or the ability of the cord to completely adduct and oppose the contralateral cord.

If lesions of the true vocal cords are left unattended, they can invade into the intrinsic musculature and joints of the larynx, resulting in decreased vocal cord mobility and, ultimately, vocal cord fixation. Anterior lesions can extend from the commissure directly into the thyroid cartilage and eventually the neck (Fig. 11-7).

Tumors of the Subglottis

Subglottic tumors are very uncommon, accounting for fewer than 1% of all cases of laryngeal cancer. These tumors can spread inferiorly to the trachea, extend through the cricothyroid membrane into the neck, or directly invade the cricoid cartilage. Differentiating between a tumor originating from the subglottis and a tumor originating from the true vocal cords can be difficult because subglottic tumors often involve the under-surface of the glottis. Typically, laryngeal tumors are judged to originate from the subglottis if the bulk of the disease is below the true vocal cords and the upper surfaces of the true vocal cords are free of tumor. Identifying

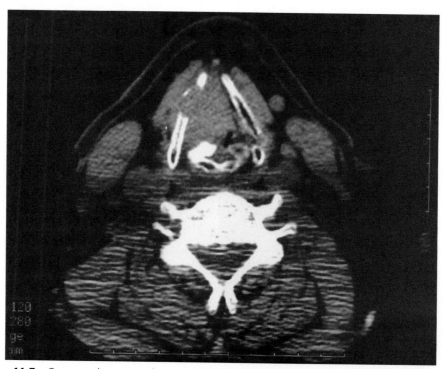

Fig. 11-7 Computed tomography scan of an advanced carcinoma of the glottis obstructing the airway and invading the neck.

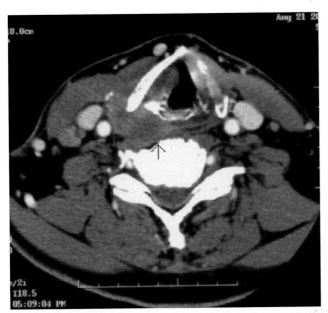

Fig. 11-8 Computed tomography scan of carcinoma of the pyriform sinus with invasion of the larynx and neck.

the subsite of origin is really of academic interest only and should not affect management decisions.

Tumors of the Hypopharynx

Pyriform sinus tumors account for 70% of cancer that originates in the hypopharynx. In contradistinction to glottic tumors, pyriform sinus tumors often present in advanced stages (Fig. 11-8).

Medial wall tumors have few barriers to tumor extension posteriorly along the sinus walls and into the postcricoid space. These tumors easily infiltrate the larynx, often resulting in fixation. Lateral wall tumors also have few barriers to growth. They can extend along the mucosa to involve the posterior hypopharyngeal wall. These tumors often fill the apex and extend deep to the sinus submucosally to involve other adjacent structures, including the laryngeal framework and the thyroid gland. Lateral wall tumors can eventually invade directly into the neck. Submucosal extension can continue inferiorly into the cervical esophagus, and it is sometimes difficult to identify precisely the extent of disease even with direct visualization and radiographic imaging. The patterns of spread can be similar to those of esophageal tumors, with extensive spread along lymphatic spaces and with skip lesions.

Postcricoid tumors are rare and almost always present in advanced stages. They can extend laterally into the pyriform sinuses or anteriorly, directly invading laryngeal structures.

Lymphatic Metastasis

The lymphatic drainage patterns differ significantly among the subsites of the larynx and the hypopharynx.

The true vocal cords have a sparse lymphatic supply and therefore have a low propensity for lymphatic spread. The incidence of lymphadenopathy at diagnosis in patients with glottic carcinomas is low and most likely only increases with increasing stage as a manifestation of the tumor gaining access to lymphatics beyond the true cords. Fewer than 2% of patients with T1 disease have involved lymph nodes. The incidence of nodal involvement is still relatively low in advanced glottic disease; only about 20% of patients who present with T3 or T4 disease are node-positive. The frequency of occult nodal involvement is also low; Byers and colleagues[1] found microscopic nodal involvement in fewer than 20% of patients with T3 N0 or T4 N0 disease who underwent elective nodal dissection at the same time as laryngectomy.

The subglottic lymphatic supply is also poor. The lymphatic capillaries drain through the cricothyroid membrane to either the Delphian node or the prelaryngeal node as well as to the midjugular and lower jugular nodes and the paratracheal and supraclavicular nodes.

In contrast to the lack of lymphatic capillaries in the glottis, the supraglottis has a moderately rich supply of lymphatic drainage. Lymphatic vessels in the supraglottis collect in channels that pass through the pyriform sinuses to drain to nodes along the jugular chain, particularly the upper jugular and midjugular lymph nodes. The incidence of clinically involved lymph nodes in patients with primary supraglottic cancer is 55%.[2] In a study of patients undergoing neck dissection in addition to supraglottic laryngectomy at The University of Texas M.D. Anderson Cancer Center for treatment of T2 or T3 disease, nearly two thirds of patients had lymph node involvement.[3] One third of patients had palpable nodes at presentation, and nearly an additional one third of patients had pathologic nodal involvement.[3]

Hypopharyngeal cancer also commonly presents with nodal metastases because the pharynx has an extensive lymphatic network. Lindberg[2] reported an overall 75% incidence of nodal metastases in patients presenting to the M.D. Anderson Cancer Center with hypopharyngeal tumors. The incidence of positive lymph nodes in a series of patients with early (T1-T2) hypopharyngeal cancer treated with radiation at the M.D. Anderson Cancer Center was 52%.[4] The jugular chain, particularly the subdigastric and midjugular nodes, is the area most often found to have metastases. Bilateral lymphadenopathy is seen in 15% of patients.[2] Hypopharyngeal tumors also have access to deep jugular, posterior cervical, and retropharyngeal lymph nodes.

Distant Metastasis

Distant metastases from glottic cancer are extremely rare. The hypopharynx represents the other end of the spectrum: of all the types of head and neck mucosal cancer, it is the cancer most likely to metastasize to distant sites.

A study of more than 5000 patients at the M.D. Anderson Cancer Center found that the incidence of distant failure was 1%, 13%, and 23% for patients with carcinomas of the true vocal cords, supraglottis, and hypopharynx, respectively.[5] This pattern is most likely the result of the extent of local and regional disease at presentation rather than the site of origin. The incidence of clinically evident metastases is approximately 20% in patients with stage IV disease.[5]

The lungs are the most common site for the development of distant metastases from both laryngeal and hypopharyngeal cancer, and the lungs are the first site of presentation of hematogenous metastases in nearly 60% of patients. Bones are the next most common sites, with bone metastases developing in 20% of patients with distant disease. Liver metastases occur in 10% of patients with hematogenous spread of disease from the larynx and hypopharynx. Spread to mediastinal lymph nodes, the brain, or other organs is rare.

PATHOLOGY

Most cases of laryngeal and hypopharyngeal cancer are squamous cell carcinomas. Laryngeal carcinomas, particularly those originating on the true vocal cords, are usually well differentiated. Hypopharyngeal cancer tends to be less well differentiated.

Pathologic tissue changes seen in the larynx range from premalignant atypia or dysplasia to carcinoma in situ to microinvasion. Carcinoma in situ is a pathologic entity in which the carcinomatous changes are confined to the thickened epithelium and do not penetrate the lamina propria. Clinically, carcinoma in situ appears as a whitish, thickened, irregular area on the mucosa. Pathologically, penetration through the basement membrane is necessary to make the diagnosis of invasive carcinoma. Invasion can be missed if biopsy samples are too small or too superficial for proper histologic evaluation.

Variants of squamous cell carcinoma represent approximately 3% of all laryngeal malignancies. The most common variant is verrucous carcinoma, a slow-growing tumor with an exophytic warty appearance. This tumor is often low grade and has a low metastatic potential. Another variant is squamous cell carcinoma with spindle cell features, also known as *pseudosarcoma*. On microscopic examination, squamous carcinoma cells are seen along with spindle cells. The nature of these spindle cells is controversial: they are believed to be either benign or highly malignant. On clinical examination, squamous cell carcinomas with spindle cell features often present as large polypoid lesions that sometimes act as ball valves in the larynx. Basaloid squamous cell carcinoma and lymphoepithelioma also can be seen in the larynx and hypopharynx.

Malignancies more commonly found in other locations are occasionally seen in the larynx and hypopharynx. These malignancies include types of minor salivary gland cancer such as adenocarcinoma and adenoid cystic carcinoma; neuroendocrine carcinomas, including true small cell and oat cell carcinoma; sarcomas; and lymphomas.

CLINICAL MANIFESTATIONS
Lesions of the Glottis

In patients with carcinoma of the glottis, hoarseness is the most common presenting system. Pain, dysphagia, and ultimately airway obstruction can occur but not until the disease is advanced. Involvement of the recurrent laryngeal nerve can lead to referred otalgia.

Lesions of the Supraglottis

In patients with supraglottic cancer, as in patients with glottic cancer, voice changes are often the presenting symptom. The quality of the changes depends on the location of the tumor within the supraglottis. Patients with false vocal cord lesions often present with hoarseness, whereas patients with epiglottic tumors often have voice changes often referred to as *supraglottic ("hot potato") voice*. Odynophagia and dysphagia are other common presenting symptoms of supraglottic carcinoma. Referred otalgia also can be a presenting symptom. Rarely, patients may present with an asymptomatic neck metastasis. As tumors become more advanced, they can cause airway obstruction or aspiration as a result of dysfunction of the epiglottis.

Lesions of the Subglottis

Early disease of the subglottis can present as hoarseness. However, because the subglottis is a "silent" region, often no symptoms are evident until tumors reach advanced stages. Symptoms of advanced subglottis tumors include dyspnea and stridor because of respiratory obstruction and, occasionally, hemoptysis.

Lesions of the Hypopharynx

The most common presenting symptom of hypopharyngeal cancer is throat pain with or without referred otalgia. Dysphagia and weight loss often develop in patients with carcinoma of the hypopharynx, who often have malnutrition and poor performance status. Hoarseness can occur when invasion of the larynx results in impairment of vocal cord motion. Because of the very high incidence of nodal involvement, patients with hypopharyngeal cancer can occasionally present with asymptomatic neck masses.

PATIENT EVALUATION

Clinical evaluation of patients with laryngeal or hypopharyngeal cancer includes a complete medical history and thorough physical examination. The examination must include good visualization of the larynx and hypopharynx, which can be accomplished with indirect laryngoscopy with a mirror and fiberoptic endoscopy. The examination includes an assessment of the size of the lesion, its morphology, extension into adjacent structures, and vocal cord motion. The examination also should include assessment for indirect signs of pre-epiglottic space invasion, such as fullness of the valleculae or ulceration of the infrahyoid epiglottis.

It is important to examine the neck so that any lymphadenopathy can be detected and its extent can be assessed in terms of mobility or fixation of nodal disease, the size of nodal disease, and the number of nodal groups involved. Palpation of the neck also can reveal direct tumor extension, indicated by tenderness of the thyroid cartilage or the presence of a subcutaneous mass. Absence of the thyroid click may indicate a large posterior lesion displacing the larynx anteriorly.

As indicated in the section on "Distant Metastasis" earlier in this chapter, the lungs are the most likely site of distant metastases. Therefore examination of the chest is a crucial part of the clinical examination in patients with laryngeal and hypopharyngeal cancer. At a minimum, a chest radiograph is required not only to rule out hematogenous spread but also to assess for a synchronous second primary cancer involving the lungs.

A complete blood count and liver function tests also should be obtained to assess for anemia and liver dysfunction. Although these tests will have a low yield in identifying distant disease, they nevertheless are simple screening tests that should be part of the initial work-up. Many believe that anemia may be an indicator of poor outcome with radiation therapy,[6] but it is unclear whether correcting this abnormality improves outcome or whether anemia should influence the choice of treatment modality.

Radiologic studies supplement the clinical evaluation of the primary tumor site and the neck. Computed tomography (CT) and magnetic resonance imaging (MRI) scans are both used, and the modality of choice is controversial. Often the choice of scan type is based on the experience of the evaluating team, particularly the diagnostic radiologist. Scans are useful for identifying involved lymph nodes that were not detected by palpation. Scans also are useful for assessing the pre-epiglottic space, tongue base, paraglottic region, and subglottis, areas sometimes difficult to visualize on direct examination. Thyroid cartilage invasion, particularly if not through the full thickness of the cartilage, may be detected only on CT or MRI scans. The inferior extent of hypopharyngeal cancer is also difficult to detect on clinical examination, and radiographic scans are critical in determining disease extent. Evaluation of this area can be supplemented by a barium swallow study. Finally, for hypopharyngeal cancer, it is impera-

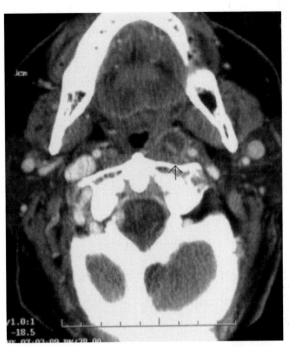

Fig. 11-9 Computed tomography scan of retropharyngeal node metastasis from carcinoma of the pyriform sinus.

tive that the scan include the retropharyngeal region to rule out the possibility of metastatic disease in this region (Fig. 11-9).

A tissue diagnosis is ultimately required, and this is obtained at direct laryngoscopy. This evaluation also permits an opportunity to directly visualize the disease and determine its extent. Some physicians still perform triple endoscopy (laryngoscopy, bronchoscopy, and esophagoscopy) as a component of the initial work-up, but the yield in terms of finding a synchronous primary lesion in patients without symptoms suggestive of such a lesion is low.

STAGING

The staging system for cancer of the larynx and hypopharynx is the American Joint Committee on Cancer (AJCC) tumor-node-metastasis (TNM) system,[7] which includes separate tumor classification systems for each of the three subsites of the larynx. The nodal classification system is the same for all three laryngeal subsites and the hypopharynx and is, in fact, the same system used for head and neck cancer in general (except for the nasopharynx). The nodal classification system is based on the size, number, and laterality of nodes. The 1997 TNM system is shown in Box 11-1.

Larynx

In the case of laryngeal cancer, primary tumor stage is determined on the basis of sites of extension and vocal

BOX 11-1   American Joint Committee on Cancer Staging System for Cancer of the Larynx and Hypopharynx

PRIMARY TUMOR (T)

TX   Primary tumor cannot be assessed
T0   No evidence of primary tumor
Tis   Carcinoma in situ

SUPRAGLOTTIS

T1   Tumor limited to one subsite of supraglottis with normal vocal cord mobility
T2   Tumor invades mucosa of more than one adjacent subsite of supraglottis or glottis or region outside the supraglottis (e.g., mucosa of base of tongue, vallecula, medial wall of pyriform sinus) without fixation of the larynx
T3   Tumor limited to larynx with vocal cord fixation and/or invades any of the following: postcricoid area, pre-epiglottic tissues
T4   Tumor invades through the thyroid cartilage, and/or extends into soft tissues of the neck, thyroid, and/or esophagus

GLOTTIS

T1   Tumor limited to the vocal cord(s) (may involve anterior or posterior commissure) with normal mobility
   T1a   Tumor limited to one vocal cord
   T1b   Tumor involves both vocal cords
T2   Tumor extends to supraglottis and/or subglottis, and/or with impaired vocal cord mobility
T3   Tumor limited to the larynx with vocal cord fixation
T4   Tumor invades through the thyroid cartilage and/or to other tissues beyond the larynx (e.g., trachea, soft tissues of neck, including thyroid, pharynx)

SUBGLOTTIS

T1   Tumor limited to the subglottis
T2   Tumor extends to vocal cord(s) with normal or impaired mobility
T3   Tumor limited to larynx with vocal cord fixation
T4   Tumor invades through cricoid or thyroid cartilage and/or extends to other tissues beyond the larynx (e.g., trachea, soft tissues of neck, including thyroid, esophagus)

HYPOPHARYNX

T1   Tumor limited to one subsite of hypopharynx and 2 cm or less in greatest dimension
T2   Tumor involves more than one subsite of hypopharynx or an adjacent site, or measures more than 2 cm but not more than 4 cm in greatest diameter without fixation of hemilarynx
T3   Tumor measures more than 4 cm in greatest dimension or with fixation of hemilarynx
T4   Tumor invades adjacent structures (e.g., thyroid/cricoid cartilage, carotid artery, soft tissues of neck, prevertebral fascia/muscles, thyroid and/or esophagus)

REGIONAL LYMPH NODES (N)

NX   Regional lymph nodes cannot be assessed
N0   No regional lymph node metastasis
N1   Metastasis in a single ipsilateral lymph node, 3 cm or less in greatest dimension
N2   Metastasis in a single ipsilateral lymph node, more than 3 cm but not more than 6 cm in greatest dimension, or in multiple ipsilateral lymph nodes, none more than 6 cm in greatest dimension, or in bilateral or contralateral lymph nodes, none more than 6 cm in greatest dimension
   N2a   Metastasis in single ipsilateral lymph node more than 3 cm but not more than 6 cm in greatest dimension
   N2b   Metastasis in multiple ipsilateral lymph nodes, none more than 6 cm in greatest dimension
   N2c   Metastasis in bilateral or contralateral lymph nodes, none more than 6 cm in greatest dimension
N3   Metastasis in a lymph node more than 6 cm in greatest dimension

DISTANT METASTASIS (M)

MX   Distant metastasis cannot be assessed
M0   No distant metastasis
M1   Distant metastasis

STAGE GROUPING

Stage 0	Tis	N0	M0
Stage I	T1	N0	M0
Stage II	T2	N0	M0
Stage III	T3	N0	M0
	T1–T3	N1	M0
Stage IVA	T4	N0–N1	M0
	Any T	N2	M0
Stage IVB	Any T	N3	M0
Stage IVC	Any T	Any N	M1

Modified from Fleming I, Cooper JS, Henson DE, et al, eds. *AJCC Cancer Staging Manual.* 5th ed. Philadelphia, Pa: Lippincott Williams & Wilkins; 1997:31-46.

cord mobility (a surrogate of disease extension) but not tumor size. Few modifications have been made to the staging system over the years. The latest system considers patients with supraglottic tumors with mucosal involvement of the base of the tongue or involvement of the medial wall of the pyriform sinus to have more favorable disease, and such tumors are currently classified as T2 disease.

Hypopharynx

The primary tumor stage for hypopharyngeal tumors is based on sites of involvement and larynx motion as well as the size of the tumor, although in this region an accurate clinical assessment of tumor size can be difficult. However, the 1997 AJCC system, in which size was added as a component of staging, helps address the problem of large tumors originating in the pharyngeal walls, which were previously classified as T1 disease because of the lack of involvement of additional subsites or invasion into the larynx.

SELECTION OF TREATMENT

The primary goal in the treatment of cancer of the larynx and hypopharynx is to maximize the cure rate. However, preservation of speech and swallowing is also desirable. Establishing algorithms that accomplish these two goals is a challenge. Different strategies have been pursued, including a greater reliance on radiation therapy instead of surgery for treatment of local disease, improvements in partial laryngeal surgery to lessen the amount of laryngeal tissue removed and to improve the natural voice, and exploration of the use of systemic therapies to either enhance radiation therapy or identify patients for whom more limited or no surgical resection is required. Although beyond the scope of this chapter, improvements in rehabilitative techniques also have been significant in improving the functional outcome of these patients.

Early-Stage Disease

Both radiation therapy and surgery have been used in the management of laryngeal and hypopharyngeal cancer. Early-stage disease often can be cured with either modality, and single-modality therapy is preferred. The choice of modality is often based on the perception of the quality of function that can be achieved and is determined by the experience of the managing physicians.

Limited surgery, including laser excision, stripping, laryngofissure, and cordectomy, can potentially be successful for early-stage laryngeal cancer. Larger laryngeal lesions still considered early-stage disease (T2 disease) can be managed with partial laryngeal surgery. A small hypopharyngeal tumor can sometimes be managed with a limited pharyngectomy.

Radiation therapy is also an effective treatment for early laryngeal and hypopharyngeal cancer. In particular, high success rates are achieved with radiation therapy for early glottic tumors. Because the volume of tissue irradiated for these tumors is small, chronic side effects are minimal. For patients with early hypopharyngeal tumors located such that surgery would leave the patient with poor function, radiation therapy may be

the best choice. Another advantage of radiation therapy in patients with early laryngeal or hypopharyngeal tumors is that it addresses subclinical disease, including potential retropharyngeal nodal disease.

One important factor in the choice between surgery and radiation therapy is the quality of voice expected after therapy. Laser excision of a mid–vocal-cord lesion often leaves patients with excellent voice quality, comparable to voice quality after radiation therapy.[8] However, laser excision, particularly of lesions in the region of the anterior commissure, can result in hoarseness as a permanent side effect.[9] Harrison and colleagues[10] studied voice quality in irradiated patients and concluded that the resultant voice quality was excellent.

An additional factor in treatment decision-making is cost, particularly when other factors such as curability and resultant function are believed to be equivalent. Foote and colleagues[11] evaluated the cost of radiation therapy for early laryngeal cancer and concluded that the cost was similar to that of limited surgery when salvage therapy was factored in. Other studies also have suggested that radiation is cost-effective in comparison to surgery.[12]

Advanced Disease

Advanced laryngeal and hypopharyngeal cancer often requires the use of combination therapies. Locally advanced disease can be treated with a single modality, but often clinical or pathologic features are present that are predictive of a high rate of recurrence if the disease is not treated with radiation and surgery in combination. This is particularly true for patients with advanced hypopharyngeal cancer, in whom the rate of regional metastasis is high.

In the United States total laryngectomy is still considered the standard for managing advanced laryngeal cancer and is often the control condition for studies evaluating other therapies. Disease control rates with total laryngectomy are moderately high (70% to 80%),[13-15] and with tracheoesophageal punctures for voice restoration, patients can regain their verbal communication skills. This treatment is still ideal for patients in whom surveillance will be difficult or those who may not be fit for or have the social support needed to undergo more aggressive or protracted treatments.

In addition to local therapies (surgery and radiation), systemic therapies, primarily cytotoxic chemotherapy, are becoming an important component of the management of advanced laryngeal and hypopharyngeal cancer. Three randomized studies[16-18] have investigated induction chemotherapy as an initial treatment vs. immediate surgery consisting of total laryngectomy, and two of the studies have concluded that induction chemotherapy does not compromise survival rates and allows larynx

TABLE 11-1

Randomized Trials of Induction Chemotherapy Followed by Surgery vs. Immediate Surgery for Advanced Laryngeal and Hypopharyngeal Carcinomas

Study and Reference	Primary Tumor Site	Number of Patients	T Stage Distribution	% Node Positive	5-Year Survival Rates
VA[18]	Larynx	332	T1-2, 11% T3, 65% T4, 24%	48	Surgery first, 45% Induction chemotherapy, 42% (P = 0.35)
EORTC[17]	Hypopharynx	194	T1-2, 21% T3, 76% T4, 3%	65	Surgery first, 35% Induction chemotherapy, 30% (Relative risk = 0.86)
GETTEC[16]	Larynx	68	T3, 100%	23	Surgery first, 62% Induction chemotherapy, 30% (P = 0.02)

VA, U.S. Department of Veterans Affairs; *EORTC*, European Organization for Research and Treatment of Cancer; *GETTEC*, Groupe d'Etudes des Tumeurs de la Tete et du Cou.

preservation in some percentage of patients (Table 11-1). Systemic therapy has particularly strong appeal in the management of hypopharyngeal cancer, which is associated with a high rate of distant metastasis. More recently, other investigators have studied concurrent chemotherapy and radiation therapy and compared this strategy with radiation therapy alone.[19,20] Although these studies have focused on head and neck cancer in general as opposed to laryngeal and hypopharyngeal cancer, concurrent chemoradiation for advanced resectable and unresectable laryngeal and hypopharyngeal cancer is becoming an accepted treatment of choice.

Ultimately, it must be remembered that patients must make the decisions regarding their treatment. In a survey of patient preferences with regard to treatment of laryngeal cancer, McNeil and colleagues[21] found that 20% of respondents chose radiation therapy over surgery, even with a compromise in survival, to maintain their voices. Involving patients in treatment decisions and ensuring that patients understand possible function and rehabilitation after laryngectomy is critical. van der Donk and colleagues[22] found that, although 83% of clinicians preferred radiation therapy over laryngectomy for managing T3 laryngeal cancer, only 50% of former laryngeal cancer patients shared this preference.[2] It is important to realize that larynx preservation is feasible and in most cases does not affect survival, but when laryngeal preservation is not prudent or desired, voice restoration is still achievable, and the change in voice does not have as great an effect on patients' quality of life as people might believe.

Carcinoma of the Glottis

Controversies regarding optimal management exist for all presentations of carcinoma of the glottis, including carcinoma in situ of the true vocal cords. Management practices for carcinoma in situ range from after-biopsy observation to vocal cord stripping, cordectomy, or open partial laryngectomy to primary radiation therapy.[23] Results of conservative surgical approaches such as microexcision, laser ablation,[24,25] and vocal cord stripping[26] are often excellent. In the management of carcinoma in situ, we favor a limited surgical procedure as the initial treatment of choice. However, in the event of recurrence, further surgery, even if limited to strippings or laser excisions, can cause a significant degradation in voice quality, and radiation therapy is therefore an ideal treatment. Radiation therapy is also an effective initial treatment for carcinoma in situ and is recommended by some authors.

T1 and T2 Tumors

T1 tumors of the glottis respond well to radiation therapy, and in most centers radiation therapy is the treatment of choice for these lesions. Other options include laser excision,[27] laryngofissure,[28] and partial laryngectomy,[29,30] but these often result in poorer voice quality.

Many groups consider radiation therapy to be the treatment of choice for T2 lesions as well, although partial laryngeal surgery is also an option for these lesions. Results with partial vertical laryngectomy are similar to those achieved with radiation therapy, although again voice quality is an issue. At the University of Florida, a review of patients with T2 disease revealed that more than 50% of the patients who underwent radiation therapy would have required total laryngectomy if a surgical approach had been chosen (voice-preserving surgery would not have been feasible).[31] Recently surgical groups have reported using a horizontal partial laryngectomy with cricohyoidopexy to maintain voice and achieve high control rates.[32] Some groups have used induction chemotherapy followed by limited surgery for patients with T2 tumors, with promising results.[33]

T3 Tumors

The management of T3 carcinoma of the glottis is highly controversial. The traditional standard therapy consists of total laryngectomy followed by postoperative irradiation therapy if high-risk pathologic features (poor differentiation, extensive subglottic extension, or cartilage invasion) are identified.[34] Postoperative irradiation is also advised in patients who require tracheostomy as a separate surgical procedure before laryngectomy and in patients with the uncommon finding of multiple nodes in the neck or extracapsular invasion. For some patients and for some practitioners, this traditional standard approach is still the treatment of choice.

The findings of a study by the Department of Veterans Affairs (VA) of patients with advanced laryngeal cancer who were given induction chemotherapy followed by radiation therapy (for those who responded) or surgery (for those who did not) led many groups to consider induction chemotherapy to be the standard of care for patients with advanced glottic cancer.[18] The VA study included a large group of patients with supraglottic disease, as well as a relatively large group of patients who had node-positive disease. A multi-institutional European trial of similar design involving mostly patients with negative nodes and advanced glottic disease found a negative effect of induction chemotherapy on survival and disease-free survival.[16] However, these findings should be interpreted cautiously because of the small patient numbers in this study, which was closed early because of poor accrual.[16]

Because the impact of induction chemotherapy on cure is uncertain, some oncologists find it difficult to endorse this treatment strategy, believing that the chemotherapy is just an expensive and potentially toxic assay used to select an appropriate local therapy. Another factor making it difficult to advocate induction chemotherapy is that randomized studies in head and neck cancer have not shown improvements in survival from the addition of induction chemotherapy to radiation therapy or surgery.

The appeal of the VA trial for some physicians, however, is in part based on the unproven bias that radiation therapy (with surgery to be used as salvage in the case of treatment failure) is inferior to total laryngectomy with respect to survival. Some nonrandomized analyses, primarily from non-American sites where definitive radiation therapy is used more commonly for advanced glottic disease, suggest that the bias against radiation therapy is unfounded and that up-front radiation therapy, particularly for T3 glottic cancer, can offer voice preservation without compromising survival. Unfortunately, a randomized trial of surgery vs. radiation

therapy has not been done, and in light of the survival equivalency demonstrated by the VA trial, induction therapy is appealing to some groups. However, the appropriateness of induction chemotherapy may be called into question by a recent meta-analysis suggesting that the use of induction chemotherapy for laryngeal cancer has a negative effect on patient outcome.[35]

Radiation therapy alone can produce moderately high local control rates in patients with T3 disease and is the treatment of choice at some centers, although it is uncommon practice in the United States. The Radiation Therapy Oncology Group (RTOG) recently completed accrual for a trial to compare induction chemotherapy with immediate laryngectomy or radiation (depending on response) to either radiation alone or concurrent chemotherapy and radiation. The goal of this trial was organ preservation. Preliminary analyses suggest that concurrent chemoradiation prolonged the time to laryngectomy and improved the laryngectomy-free survival rate relative to induction chemotherapy.[36] The addition of chemotherapy did not improve overall survival rates. The authors concluded that concurrent chemoradiation therapy should be considered the standard of care. Moreover, they agree with conclusions from other studies[20] that the concurrent delivery of chemotherapy and radiation can improve organ preservation rates. However, quality of life, a critical component in considering the choice of treatment, has yet to be analyzed in the RTOG study.

T4 Tumors

For patients with T4 glottic cancer, total laryngectomy remains the treatment of choice. Postoperative irradiation is almost always required. Definitive radiation therapy is still an option for patients who are medically inoperable or decline to undergo total laryngectomy. The outcome of patients with T4 disease treated with induction chemotherapy and surgery seems poorer than expected for patients treated with surgery alone, thus induction chemotherapy is not recommended.[37] Concurrent chemotherapy and radiation therapy may be beneficial in patients with T4 tumors, but at present this approach should be considered experimental and should be offered only in the context of a clinical trial.

Carcinoma of the Supraglottis
Early-Stage Disease

Both radiation therapy and surgery can offer cure and voice preservation for patients with early supraglottic cancer. Endoscopic removal of early lesions is becoming a recommended procedure in some centers, particularly in Germany, where the procedure has been used for many years.[38] Patients with larger lesions can undergo supraglottic laryngectomy. The success rate of supraglottic laryngectomy is high, but patient selection is critical. Patients must be motivated for the rehabilitation that is required, and they also must have sufficient pulmonary reserve to tolerate the procedure. Aspiration is a problem because the protection from the epiglottis is removed, and patients must be fit enough to combat this. The need for a permanent tracheostomy is uncommon, although in some patients it takes months before decannulation is possible.

Radiation therapy is often the treatment of choice for patients with early supraglottic carcinomas. Results of many series are comparable to results of series of patients treated with supraglottic laryngectomies. Most radiation therapy series include patients who were medically unable to undergo a voice-preserving treatment or whose tumors were not amenable to partial laryngectomy.

In the treatment of supraglottic cancer, management of the neck is a significant issue that must be considered in addition to management of the primary tumor. In patients who are clinically node-negative, the neck must be managed with the same modality that is chosen for management of the primary tumor. A neck dissection should accompany laryngectomy. One third of patients without clinical adenopathy have subclinical nodal disease revealed by the neck dissection. If multiple nodes or extracapsular nodal disease is found on pathologic review, postoperative irradiation to lessen the risk of recurrence is recommended. Findings from surgical series[1,39] suggest that patients who are clinically node-negative and will undergo irradiation as definitive therapy must have their necks included in the treatment fields. The nodal basins at risk are levels II and III.

Patients with clinically evident adenopathy may require radiation therapy and surgery. If a patient requires dental extractions, the neck dissection can be done at that time, and then radiation therapy can be delivered to the neck (as postoperative therapy) and to the primary tumor (as primary therapy with curative intent). Radiation therapy is often required for patients undergoing laryngectomy and neck dissection because nearly two thirds have pathologic nodal disease.

Patients with N1 supraglottic disease often can be treated with radiation alone to the primary tumor and neck. A postirradiation neck dissection may be required if the nodal disease persists after therapy. For patients with more extensive nodal disease, many groups argue that a neck dissection after irradiation should be mandatory, whereas others advocate observation in the event of complete disappearance of nodal disease after irradiation.

T3 Disease

T3 supraglottic carcinoma encompasses an extremely heterogeneous mix of tumors. The current staging system has shifted tumors with involvement of the medial wall of the pyriform sinus into the T2 category, but the current T3 category still includes a subgroup of disease (particularly exophytic tumors) for which radiation therapy is the treatment of choice. Recently, the use of CT-based tumor volume measurements has been advocated as a useful tool for determining suitability for radiation. Freeman and colleagues[40] from the University of Florida found 6 cm^3 to be a valid volume cutoff—tumors smaller than this size were highly radiocurable, but larger tumors would more likely benefit from surgery. In our practice, if tumors are amenable to voice-preserving surgery, then this should be the treatment of choice. However, if total laryngectomy is required, then radiation remains an option.

For patients with bulky T3 disease, supraglottic laryngectomy may be the treatment of choice, especially for disease with significant involvement of the pre-epiglottic space.[41] This procedure is theoretically feasible if no significant subglottic involvement is present and one arytenoid cartilage is uninvolved and can be spared. Again, the caveats regarding the patient being willing to undergo rehabilitation and having sufficient pulmonary reserve apply.

Currently, the optimal management of T3b disease (fixation of the hemilarynx) remains unclear, and the questions that remain to be answered are similar to those regarding management of T3 glottic cancer. Total laryngectomy is still the standard for most patients with T3b disease. They often will require postoperative irradiation because of inadequate margins, perineural or vascular spread, cartilage involvement, or subglottic involvement of more than 1 cm. The finding of multiple nodes or extracapsular nodal spread also will dictate the need for postoperative irradiation.

The VA study of induction chemotherapy[18] included a large subgroup of patients with supraglottic disease who were node-positive. These patients may benefit the most from induction chemotherapy because they are slightly more prone to distant failure and chemotherapy has been shown to result in modest reductions of hematogenous metastases in numerous trials of adjuvant and induction therapy. Concurrent chemotherapy is speculated to be more beneficial than adjuvant or induction chemotherapy, but its role is still evolving.

T4 Disease

T4 supraglottic disease is usually best managed with total laryngectomy. Postoperative irradiation is used in most cases because of cartilage invasion, subglottic spread, or inadequate margins. Some patients have disease classified as T4 disease because of involvement of the base of the tongue. Many of these patients may do well with primary radiation therapy or, for very bulky disease, chemotherapy combined with radiation therapy. These tumors tend to behave more like oropharyngeal carcinomas, which some groups speculate have better outcomes than laryngeal or hypopharyngeal cancer in terms of stage-for-stage local control.

Carcinoma of the Subglottis

Carcinomas of the subglottis are very uncommon and are often best managed with surgery. A partial laryngectomy is rarely possible, so these patients are usually treated with total laryngectomy. The finding of nodal disease, which necessitates adjuvant radiation therapy, is uncommon. Postoperative irradiation is needed in cases of inadequate margins and cartilaginous extension. Small tumors may be treated with radiation therapy alone, but these are very rare and most often are actually glottic tumors that originate from the undersurface of the true vocal cord.

Carcinoma of the Hypopharynx

Early tumors of the hypopharynx are uncommon and can be treated with definitive radiation therapy. Infrequently, a partial pharyngectomy with or without a partial laryngectomy can be done, but radiation therapy often will result in better function as well as addressing the lymphatics in the clinically node-negative patient. Posterior wall lesions in particular are better suited for radiation therapy because it is often difficult to obtain negative surgical margins in the region of the prevertebral fascia and muscles.

Because most patients with hypopharyngeal tumors have node-positive disease, the neck usually requires both surgery and radiation therapy. One option is to irradiate the primary hypopharyngeal tumor and the neck nodes and to follow the radiation therapy with a neck dissection. The second option, especially for small primary tumors, is to do the neck dissection first. In this case radiation therapy would be the definitive treatment for the primary tumor and postoperative adjuvant treatment for the neck. This second option is often preferred for patients who require dental extractions, a procedure that necessitates a delay in irradiation of the primary tumor. When the primary tumor is small, this second option also may allow a reduction in the high-dose volume because the neck does not require a dose of 70 Gy or greater.

Advanced tumors of the hypopharynx are often best managed with total laryngectomy and partial or total pharyngectomy. The feasibility of this extensive surgical procedure has been enhanced by the use of free tissue transfer using either stomach or intestine (jejunum) to fill the defect and allow return of swallowing. Postoperative radiation therapy is almost always required to improve local and regional control. In the case of large hypopharyngeal tumors, it is often difficult to get generous margins, and these patients, particularly those with advanced primary disease, usually have significant nodal disease as well.

In a study similar to the VA study of induction chemotherapy in patients with laryngeal cancer in the United States,[18] the European Organization for Research and Treatment of Cancer (EORTC) studied initial surgery and postoperative irradiation vs. induction chemotherapy for hypopharyngeal cancer.[17] One difference between the two studies is that in the VA trial, patients with either a complete or partial response to chemotherapy went on to undergo irradiation, whereas in the EORTC trial, a complete response was required to avoid surgery and be treated with radiation alone. Interestingly, in the EORTC trial, the complete response rate was high, greater than 50%. However, survival rates between the two study groups were believed to be equivalent, and laryngeal preservation was achieved in more than one third of the patients treated with induction chemotherapy. Most patients had T2 or T3 disease. Induction chemotherapy is accepted as a method of care for patients with advanced hypopharyngeal disease. It should be noted that few patients with T4 disease were treated in this study, and surgery and postoperative irradiation should be considered the appropriate treatment for those patients unless they are either medically inoperable or have unresectable disease.

For patients with unresectable disease, concurrent chemotherapy and radiation therapy seems to produce better outcomes than radiation therapy alone, although the treatment is more toxic and patients must be more highly selected for this approach. Few data exist regarding radiation alone for unresectable T4 hypopharyngeal cancer, although the impression is that control with this approach is poor.

RADIATION THERAPY TECHNIQUES
Beam Energies

^{60}Co is often the ideal mode of radiation for treating patients with laryngeal cancer. For primary treatment of laryngeal cancer, ^{60}Co allows adequate dosing of the superficial tissues. Historically, great concern has been expressed that 6-MV photons have too large a build-up region and can potentially underdose superficial tissues. Most radiation oncology centers today have only linear accelerators. If a ^{60}Co unit is not available, 4-MV photon beams are adequate. However, many centers have units whose lowest energy is 6-MV photons. Recent series have reviewed experiences with 6-MV photons and have concluded that control rates for early lesions remain high and use of this "higher" energy does not compromise treatment.[42]

At the University of Florida, a dosimetric comparison between ^{60}Co and 6-MV beams was performed.[43] The authors concluded that the dose distribution for the two beams was similar except for the most anterior tissues

(3 mm below the surface), where underdosing occurred with the 6-MV beam. On the basis of their results, the authors cautioned against using 6-MV beams for lesions in the anterior commissure. However, when there is concern about the anterior extent of disease, tissue-equivalent bolus material for build-up or a beam spoiler can be used.

In patients with more posterior lesions, such as supraglottic tumors epicentered on the posterior aryepiglottic folds or arytenoids, hypopharyngeal lesions involving the posterior pharyngeal wall, or postcricoid lesions, energies of 4 to 6 MV are used. Bolus material may be required for very thin patients and for patients whose lesions extend anteriorly (e.g., to the pre-epiglottic tissues), such that there would be a potential danger of disease being present in the build-up region. Bolus material also may be required for clinically apparent nodal disease that lies in the superficial tissues. If disease in the build-up region is a concern, then ^{60}Co remains a good alternative.

Although many of our patients begin treatment on a ^{60}Co unit, when it is time to treat off–spinal-cord fields, we typically use a linear accelerator. This practice allows the patient to be treated on one unit because electrons of 6 to 12 MeV often are used in addition to photons. The electrons treat tissues in the posterior cervical chains that are missed in the off–spinal-cord fields. Also, the sharper edge of the photon beams is preferred at the posterior edge, particularly for posterior pharyngeal wall tumors, where it is sometimes necessary to have a tight posterior edge adjacent to the spinal cord.

For patients with node-negative disease, occasionally a boost can be done with higher-energy photons (15 to 22 MV) to minimize the dose to the lateral tissues. Often, however, the gain from this approach is minimal because it is uncommon to have patients who are so wide as to get a large benefit from this approach. More often 6 MV will give the best distribution for these tumors.

Most of our patients who present for postoperative radiation therapy are treated with ^{60}Co. This energy is ideal for the superficial tissues that may have been seeded by the surgical procedure. Again, in the absence of a ^{60}Co unit, the lowest energy available, 4 to 6 MV, should be used. It is necessary to deliver a bolus dose to the tissues violated by surgery to avoid dermal or subcutaneous underdosing, which could result in a recurrence. In some cases, the choice of beams is subordinate to the technique chosen. For example, if an asymmetric jaw technique (described in the following section) is needed to adequately cover disease, photons will be used because this matching technique is not available on most ^{60}Co units. Energies higher than 6 MV are rarely needed for postoperative therapy.

Simulation and Field Arrangements

Simulation is required before treatment is begun so as to allow establishment of a reproducible treatment set-up. Simulation also allows delineation of fields before therapy and determination of the parameters necessary for treatment planning.

Patients are treated in the supine position with the head extended, which often elevates the larynx slightly away from the shoulders and thoracic inlet. Straps are commonly used so that the patients' shoulders are pulled to a more inferior position, thereby avoiding penetration of the shoulders by lateral beams (Fig. 11-10, *A*).

The head is immobilized with the use of individualized thermoplastic masks. For patients who are being treated with small laryngeal fields, the authors prefer to cup the mask around the chin and demarcate the field borders and set-up points on the skin (see Fig.

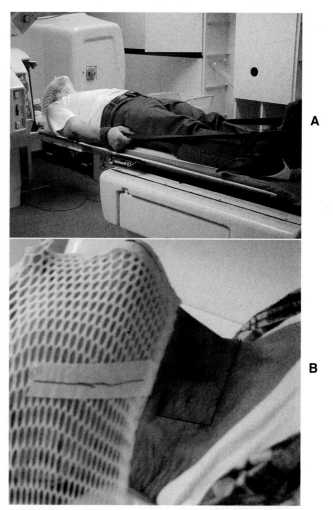

A

B

Fig. 11-10 Photographs of a patient with laryngeal cancer being treated with radiation therapy. **A,** Use of straps to optimize shoulder placement. **B,** Immobilization of the head with a thermoplastic mask.

11-10, *B*). This allows clinical verification of the field borders in addition to radiographic portal imaging. In patients who are treated postoperatively or have supraglottic or hypopharyngeal tumors, the mask encompasses the head and neck, and most set-up points and points delineating the fields are marked on the mask. Historically, immobilization was accomplished with bite blocks, and this technique is still used in a few centers. As the technology continues to evolve, newer noninvasive immobilization techniques are being developed that use combinations of older techniques, including bite blocks, face masks, and immobilization cradles.

Although CT treatment planning often will identify involved lymph nodes, it is still found to be useful while developing a treatment plan to delineate the clinically apparent nodal disease with solder wire before simulation films are obtained. Use of wire to delineate the anterior skin is also useful to ensure fall-off or, if fall-off is not required, to block a strip of skin. Wire is also used to delineate scars and the stoma in the postoperative setting. A thick wire placed at the region where the neck widens to become the shoulder is also useful. This wire helps determine whether the central structures that need to be treated will be missed because the beam is going through the trapezius muscles or the shoulder. This wire is also useful for determining a good location for matching the lateral fields and the anterior

field. More recently, the external auditory canals have been located on the lateral radiographs to facilitate the design of fields that avoid the ears if possible.

Set-up Techniques

Parallel opposed fields may suffice in certain situations. However, when the intended targets include the primary tumor and draining lymphatics, a three-field set-up is used. In this set-up, lateral opposed fields to treat the primary tumor and nodes of the upper and middle neck are matched to an anterior portal to cover the lower neck and supraclavicular nodes.

The set-up technique for the three-field match relies on angling the inferior border of the lateral fields (Fig. 11-11). The anterior field is then clinically matched to the light field on the skin. This allows treatment of the superficial tissues at risk at the junction while creating a gap that is deep and central at the level of the spinal cord. We tend to avoid placing safety blocks on the inferior-posterior aspect of the lateral fields over the spinal cord. In postoperative treatment, safety blocks can block the operative bed, and in the case of hypopharyngeal cancer, the posterior cervical chain is a significant lymphatic drainage site that should not be blocked.

The asymmetric jaw-matching technique, also known as a *mono-isocentric technique*, is used to avoid overlap created by the divergence of the lateral and

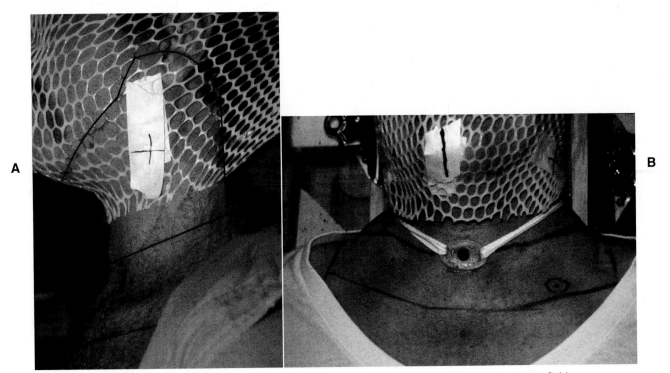

Fig. 11-11 Photographs of a three-field set-up: two lateral fields **(A)** and an anterior field **(B)** matched on the skin.

anterior fields commonly used in three-field set-ups for treating head and neck cancer. The asymmetric jaw-matching technique is very useful for treating cancer of the oropharynx and nasopharynx, where the anterior field will have a central larynx block that also serves as a safety block for avoiding overlap between the fields at the spinal cord. The technique also can be used to treat laryngeal or hypopharyngeal cancer, but it is not as facile in these settings. The lateral fields can be quite long, creating fields that have great divergence superiorly and thus treat a greater extent of tissue. Thus with this technique, application of wire to delineate structures that need to be encompassed or avoided is useful. In the postoperative setting, it is desirable to treat the stoma, and so localizing a central block can be complicated. Similarly, in patients with a larynx, the central block may lie over the Delphian nodes.

Three-dimensional planning and conformal techniques allow more creative solutions for difficult problems. One such problem is the localization of safety blocks in a three-field set-up. Sometimes a safe block over the spinal cord cannot be identified because of concern that disease might be blocked. In such a case, more sophisticated planning is required. A simple solution is to use fields that are caudally oriented so that junctions can be avoided (Fig. 11-12). The ability to

visualize these beams in a treatment planning system allows the beam weightings and distribution to be optimized. Most important, the ability to plan these treatments allows appropriate wedging or tissue compensation to be selected in areas that are anatomically heterogeneous. Caudally oriented beams are also an ideal solution when the larynx sits between the shoulders in a short-necked individual.

Treatment Volumes and Radiation Fields
Carcinoma of the Glottis

T1 and T2 carcinomas of the true vocal cords can be treated with a pair of small, lateral, opposed photon fields that encompass only the larynx (Fig. 11-13). Typical field sizes range from 25 cm^2 (5 cm × 5 cm) to 36 cm^2 (6 cm × 6 cm). The fields are defined by anatomic landmarks. The isocenter is located at the middle of the true cord. Anteriorly, the fields should fall off the skin surface. The posterior border is the anterior edge of the vertebral bodies. The superior border is above the thyroid notch, and the inferior border is inferior to the cricoid cartilage. In patients with T2 lesions, the borders are increased to appropriately encompass the disease. Involvement of the supraglottis necessitates increasing the superior border, and conversely, subglottic disease extension requires increasing the inferior border, often to encompass the upper trachea. For T2 disease, unless extensive supraglottic involvement is present, we use small fields that do not encompass the draining lymphatics.

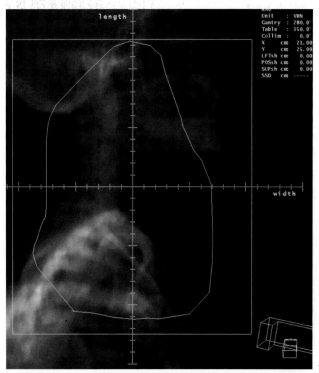

Fig. 11-12 Digitally reconstructed radiograph of a caudally tilted (angled down) field used to avoid a match when use of a safety block over the spinal cord with a three-field technique would potentially block disease.

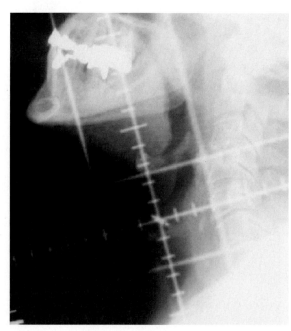

Fig. 11-13 Simulation film of opposed fields used to treat a patient with early glottic cancer.

Occasionally other techniques are required for T1 or T2 glottic cancer. This may involve caudally orienting the beams. Sometimes using a pair of left and right anterior oblique fields (wedged pair) with or without a straight anterior field may provide a better arrangement for encompassing the larynx and providing an improved distribution. Wang has described a four-field technique.[44]

A dosimetric plan is obtained to evaluate the dose distribution. This can be done either with a contour or with a CT plan. Given the triangular shape of the larynx and surrounding tissues, tissue compensation, usually in the form of wedges, is required to optimize the dose distribution. Treating without wedges results in a less homogeneous distribution, but this may be advantageous for anterior lesions where the built-in dose differential (5% to 10%) is desirable. Occasionally, lateralized lesions can be treated with a single appositional field, but treating these lesions with opposed beams and unequally weighting the fields (e.g., 3:2) to favor the side of the lesion is preferred.

Because of the moderate incidence of subclinical lymphadenopathy in patients with T3-T4 N0 glottic carcinomas, both the primary lesion and the draining lymphatics are treated. This is accomplished with parallel opposed lateral portals covering the primary tumor and upper jugular and midjugular lymph node chains (Fig. 11-14). The superior border is located approximately 2 cm superior to the angle of the mandible. Posteriorly, the fields are more generous to encompass the jugular nodes, and the posterior border is placed behind the spinous processes. The inferior border is determined by the inferior extent of disease and is adjusted to encompass any subglottic extension. A matching anterior portal encompassing the lower jugular and supraclavicular lymph nodes is also used with techniques described previously.

Because the initial fields include the spinal cord, a field reduction from the posterior border must be done before 45 Gy is delivered. Tissues excluded from the reduced fields may contain nodes at risk for subclinical metastases and can be supplemented with narrow electron-beam fields to bring the dose to those regions to 50 Gy. After 50 Gy is delivered to the primary tumor with margin and the electively treated draining lymphatics, a boost dose is delivered to the primary site. The dose is delivered by using parallel opposed fields with a 1- to 1.5-cm margin surrounding the gross disease.

The field design for postoperative treatment of T3 and T4 glottic carcinoma is similar to that used for definitive treatment of such lesions (Fig. 11-15). A three-field technique is preferred, with the stoma included in the low neck field. The operative bed and neopharynx are

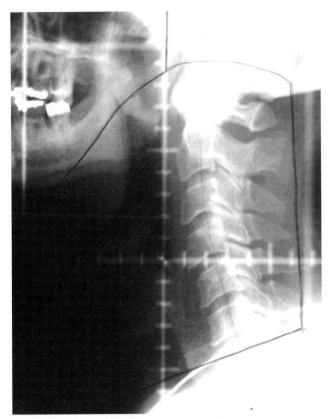

Fig. 11-14 Simulation film of opposed fields used to treat a patient with advanced laryngeal cancer without regional metastases.

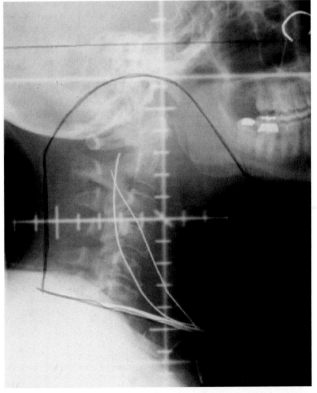

Fig. 11-15 Simulation film of opposed fields used for postoperative irradiation of a patient who had undergone laryngectomy for advanced glottic cancer.

included in the opposing lateral fields, with fields adjusted to appropriately cover any clinical or pathologic adenopathy. The inferior border is set to ensure that all preclinical extensions of disease are encompassed in the lateral fields with a 1.5- to 2-cm margin. If this is not possible because of the patient's anatomy, then caudally oriented fields can be used. Areas of high risk are boosted through parallel opposed fields. If any area in the neck requires a higher dose than the neopharynx, that dose can be delivered by using an appositional electron field.

Carcinoma of the Supraglottis

Supraglottic carcinoma requires treatment of the draining lymphatics. In patients with T1 N0 lesions, the low jugular and supraclavicular nodes need not be treated. Two parallel fields are used (Fig. 11-16). The superior border encompasses the subdigastric nodes. The posterior border is located at the posterior spinous processes to ensure coverage of the nodes along the jugular vein. The inferior border is set below the larynx. Fall-off may be required for anterior lesions. For posterior lesions, pulling the anterior neck skin out of the field by using clothespins may spare skin and thus avoid chronic problems with lymphatic drainage, resulting in less dewlap and perhaps less chronic laryngeal edema. A reduction off the spinal cord is necessary before 45 Gy is delivered. The posterior cervical strips are supplemented with electrons to 50 Gy. After a subclinical dose of 50 Gy is delivered, fields are reduced to treat the primary lesion with a 1- to 1.5-cm margin.

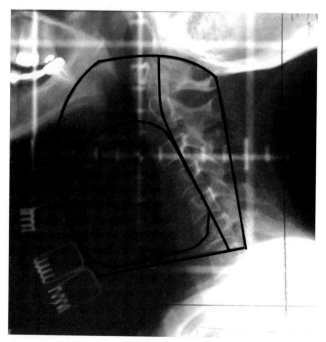

Fig. 11-16 Simulation film of opposed fields used to treat a patient with early supraglottic cancer.

Boost fields for these early lesions can be small, but from a dosimetric standpoint, these fields should not be less than 4 cm in any dimension.

The field design for T2-T3 lesions is similar to the field design for T1 disease. The low neck is treated with a matching anterior neck field. The superior border is adjusted in patients with clinical adenopathy. The superior border must cover the entire jugular chain and follow the inner table of the skull posteriorly. The mastoid tip is included, and then the superior border sweeps forward to encompass the anterior superior jugular nodes that are close to the angle of the mandible.

Nodes may lie at a level parallel to and posterior to the spinal cord such that if true lateral fields were used for the off–spinal-cord fields and boost fields, then only a portion of each node would be treated. Although the posterior aspect of the nodes can potentially be encompassed in electron fields, we prefer, when possible, to use parallel oblique fields that fully encompass the nodes in the photon fields. Care must be taken with this field arrangement, however, to ensure that treatment of the primary tumor is not compromised. When the patient has bilateral positive nodes, the decision becomes more difficult. If one side has deep adenopathy that would be difficult to encompass with electrons, using oblique fields to fully encompass the deep nodes and primary tumor in the photon fields while encompassing the smaller nodes in an appositional electron field is one alternative to best encompass all disease. These field designs are only guidelines; treatment in the complicated scenarios described here must be individualized.

Radiation techniques following a supraglottic laryngectomy are similar to those used in patients with an intact larynx. Parallel opposed fields are used to encompass the larynx and operative bed. In the setting of positive pathologic nodal involvement, the entire jugular chain is included. Anteriorly, the fields should fall off the skin surface. The stoma is included in the anterior low neck field. Fields are reduced off the spinal cord before 45 Gy is delivered. A boost is delivered to the neck if the indication for radiation therapy was based on adverse pathologic features involving the lymph nodes. If the risk is on one side, an appositional electron field is used. If both sides of the neck require a boost dose, anterior or anteroposterior parallel opposed fields with midline blocking can be used.

The techniques for postoperative radiation therapy for supraglottic carcinomas are similar to those for postoperative radiation therapy for glottic carcinoma, with the following exceptions. In the case of supraglottic carcinomas, the draining lymphatics may need to be covered more comprehensively because they are more likely to have pathologic involvement. If nodes are involved, the superior aspect of the field must cover to the jugular foramen. Boost fields also may need to be more generous superiorly if there was base-of-tongue involvement.

Carcinoma of the Hypopharynx

Fields used to treat hypopharyngeal carcinomas are designed to encompass the primary tumor and draining lymphatics regardless of the primary tumor stage (Fig. 11-17). The nodal levels at risk include levels II through V and the retropharyngeal nodes. Large lateral portals cover the primary disease, the upper jugular nodes, and the midjugular nodes. High junctional nodes, posterior cervical nodes, and retropharyngeal nodes are all included. The classic retropharyngeal nodes lie anterior to C1 and C2. To treat all these nodes, the superior border should extend to the base of the sphenoid sinus. For pyriform sinus tumors, the inferior border of the lateral fields must cover the entire pyriform sinus, including the apex. Thus the entire cricoid cartilage must be encompassed with a 1-cm margin in the lateral fields. For post-cricoid tumors and posterior pharyngeal wall tumors, even more generous coverage is required, often including the upper cervical esophagus. This may require a different field arrangement if the lateral fields cannot be extended inferiorly to encompass this target without the shoulders' interfering. The posterior border is drawn to cover the posterior cervical nodes. Anteriorly, a strip of skin can often be spared by pulling it forward out of the field with clothespins or another device. The anterior border must adequately cover the anterior jugular nodes and the larynx, including the pre-epiglottic space, but can exclude the oral cavity.

A matching anterior portal encompassing the lower jugular and supraclavicular lymph nodes is also used. We usually use a technique that matches the fields on the skin. The inferior borders of the lateral fields are angled such that the posterior border is more superior than the anterior border. The field design is such that despite divergence, a central gap exists at the spinal cord. If creating a cold region in the lower neck near nodal disease is a concern, matching using a mono-isocentric technique may be a better approach, although the field length may limit the capability of using wedging or tissue compensators on some treatment units. Using a true horizontal isoplane also may be disadvantageous because it may make it more difficult to get adequate coverage of the inferior aspect of the primary tumor without treating through the shoulder. One solution is to rotate the collimation on the lateral fields such that the posterior border is more superior than the anterior border, possibly allowing for avoidance of the shoulders. The exact match is maintained by using a cephalad tilt on the anterior field with the exact angle as the collimation on the lateral fields. The challenge remains that of where best to put a safety block over the spinal cord because even though the fields are "exactly" matched and theoretically there is no divergence, the individual units' collimation may create hot regions at the match at the spinal cord. If there are concerns that the safety block may shield disease, then the technique may not be appropriate, and a pair of caudally oriented beams may be a better technique for ensuring disease coverage without overlap over the spinal cord.

Field design for postoperative radiation in general follows the same concepts with the same targets—the primary tumor bed and all the lymphatics, including the retropharyngeal nodes (Fig. 11-18). The stoma is included as well, either in the lateral fields, if it can be encompassed in the generous inferior border of these fields, or in the anterior field.

Dose and Fractionation
Carcinoma of the Glottis

T1 tumors of true vocal cords are treated to doses of 60 to 66 Gy. The lower dose is used for patients whose diagnostic procedure has removed all visible tumor, whereas higher doses are used when visible gross disease is still present. Occasionally doses as high as 70 Gy may be appropriate for a very bulky lesion. Similar doses are used for carcinoma in situ. The precise dose per fraction is controversial, and the literature abounds with studies evaluating different dose schedules. It is

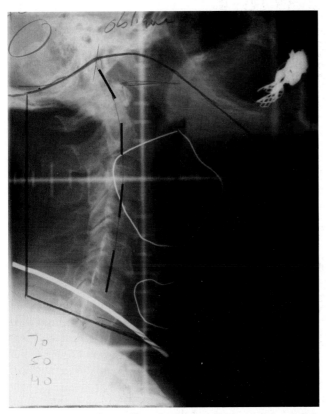

Fig. 11-17 Simulation film of opposed fields used for definitive irradiation of a patient with carcinoma of the pyriform sinus.

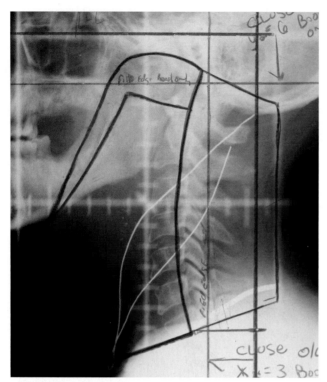

Fig. 11-18 Simulation film of opposed fields used for post-operative irradiation of a patient who had undergone laryn-gopharyngectomy for advanced pyriform sinus cancer.

clear from the literature that doses lower than 2 Gy/fraction result in lower control rates, thus the fraction size should not be less than 2 Gy. The greater efficacy of higher doses per fraction is less clear, although some series recommend between 2.1 and 2.5 Gy/fraction, with total doses of 60 to 63 Gy.[45-47]

The standard dose schedule for T2 glottic carcinoma is 70 Gy in 35 fractions. The role of larger fraction sizes for that stage of disease is unclear. Several centers, including the M.D. Anderson Cancer Center, have advocated hyperfractionation for that stage of disease. Treatment consists of 76.6 Gy at 1.2 Gy/fraction with twice-daily treatments and a 6-hour interval between treatments. Although hyperfractionation has generally been shown to improve local control for advanced cancer of the head and neck, outcome data for hyperfractionation for T2 disease are less compelling. The RTOG is currently studying the value of hyperfractionation in this setting in a randomized trial comparing 70 Gy in 35 fractions to 79.2 Gy in 68 fractions.

T3 and T4 glottic cancer treated with curative intent are usually treated to 70 Gy in 35 fractions. This was the dose schedule used in the RTOG larynx preservation trial.[36] At the same time as the larynx preservation trial, the RTOG conducted a separate trial investigating the effect of different fractionation schedules. Although patients with glottic cancer were excluded, the results for the remaining head and neck sites are compelling

enough to suggest that either hyperfractionation or accelerated fractionation with a concomitant boost schedule may enhance local control in patients with glottic cancer. Primarily because it involves fewer fractions and completes the treatment sooner, we have begun to use accelerated fractionation with a concomitant boost for our patients with advanced laryngeal cancer who are to be treated with radiation alone.

The appropriate dose and fractionation to use when chemotherapy is involved is less clear. In the RTOG larynx preservation trial, all patients received 70 Gy in 35 fractions. No data exist to support lowering the dose after induction therapy, even in the case of an excellent response. The role of altered schedules after induction therapy is less clear because the tumor kinetics after chemotherapy are different from those in patients whose treatment starts with radiation. Although efficacy is expected to increase with concurrent chemotherapy and radiation therapy, the ability to lower the total dose in this setting is unproven. Therefore, if concurrent chemoradiation is used, we favor standard fractionation, 70 Gy in 35 fractions. At present, studies are evaluating more efficacious schedules, such as concomitant boost with chemotherapy, recognizing that tolerance is a key endpoint of potentially toxic therapies.

On the basis of findings from a dose-seeking trial, we recommend that 63 Gy in 7 weeks be given as the optimal dose for patients with head and neck cancer treated with postoperative radiation therapy.[48] Doses of 57.6 Gy were considered sufficient if the risk of recurrence as judged by pathologic findings was not considered high, but postoperative irradiation was indicated nevertheless. Complex formulas for determining risk were designed; these formulas can be summarized as follows: high-risk patients were those with multiple nodes, extracapsular spread of nodal disease, soft tissue extension of the primary tumor, or inadequate margins. Because of our belief that time is critical and influential on outcome, we studied shortening the schedule to 5 weeks by using twice-daily fractionation for 2 weeks. We also decided that the difference in the rate of acute complications between patients treated at 1.8 Gy and 2 Gy/fraction was minimal, and our standard postoperative dose has been 60 Gy in 30 fractions. One secondary finding of our study of accelerating the radiation was the importance of the overall treatment time. Patients whose therapy from surgery to completion of radiation therapy lasted 13 weeks or longer had a poorer outcome. Many groups advocate higher doses for patients with positive margins or extracapsular spread of disease, but few data are available to support this practice.

We treat the operative bed to 56 Gy, reducing off the spinal cord at 42 or 44 Gy to ensure that the dose is less than 45 Gy. Additional boosts to the high-risk areas are given to the final desired dose.

Carcinoma of the Supraglottis

Definitive radiation therapy for T1 supraglottic carcinoma consists of 66 Gy in 33 fractions. This stage presentation is actually fairly uncommon, so dose fractionation data are limited.

Definitive radiation therapy for T2 and T3 lesions consists of 70 Gy in 35 fractions. The RTOG fractionation study did include a cohort of patients with supraglottic tumors. The hyperfractionation and concomitant boost schedules were equivalent in their efficacy and superior to standard fractionation. A retrospective review of our experience with hyperfractionation suggested that it was superior to conventional once-daily schedules, and some groups also advocate hyperfractionation for T2 and T3 lesions. We continue to use hyperfractionation for patients with T2 disease. For patients with T3 disease, we use concomitant boost fractionation, although most patients with T3 disease are not treated with radiation alone, but rather with radiation in combination with chemotherapy.

Shrinking-field techniques are used. An off–spinal-cord reduction is made between 41 and 43 Gy. The posterior cervical strips are supplemented to 50 to 55 Gy depending on the fractionation. To reduce set-up time, we rarely treat the electron strips twice per day if they are being treated for subclinical disease. Boost fields to gross disease are treated after 50 Gy (for conventional fractionation) or after 55 Gy (for hyperfractionation) to the final dose. The uninvolved low neck is treated to 50 Gy at 2 Gy/fraction with the dose prescribed as a maximal dose.

Patients who undergo postoperative irradiation after supraglottic laryngectomy receive 55 Gy in 6 weeks to the larynx. If significant nodal disease is present, the neck is boosted to 63 Gy. Higher doses to the larynx after supraglottic laryngectomy are of great concern, even though few data are available to support this concern. Some groups believe that the risk of significant complications, particularly laryngeal necrosis, is increased after partial laryngectomy. For the rare cases in which positive margins are encountered, we recommend treating the larynx to 60 Gy.

The dose and fractionation issues for postoperative radiation therapy after total laryngectomy for supraglottic carcinoma are similar to those described for glottic carcinomas. In a maximum of 6 weeks, 60 Gy are delivered with off–spinal-cord reductions made at 42 Gy and boosts delivered after the surgical bed has received 56 Gy. If the low neck is uninvolved, it is treated to 50 Gy, although if portions of the operative bed are within the low-neck field, these areas are supplemented to 56 Gy.

Carcinoma of the Hypopharynx

Dose and fractionation issues for cancer of the hypopharynx are similar to those for carcinoma of the supraglottis. T1 disease is treated to 66 Gy in 33 fractions. We have favored hyperfractionation for T2 disease and have found a significantly improved control rate with twice-daily treatment compared to conventional fractionation.[4] Most patients with T3 disease are either treated on study with chemotherapy or are treated postoperatively. Patients treated with radiation alone can be treated with either hyperfractionation or concomitant boost.

Shrinking-field techniques are used. An off–spinal-cord reduction is made between 41 and 43 Gy. The posterior cervical strips are supplemented to 50 to 55 Gy depending on the fractionation. To reduce set-up time, we rarely treat the electron strips twice per day if they are being treated for subclinical disease. Boost fields to gross disease areas are treated after 50 to 55 Gy (the former dose is used with conventional fractionation and the latter dose is used with hyperfractionation) to the final dose. The uninvolved low neck is treated to 50 Gy at 2 Gy/fraction with the dose prescribed as a maximal dose.

After total laryngectomy, partial pharyngectomy, and neck dissection, 60 Gy is delivered over a maximum of 6 weeks. When jejunal grafts are used for restoration of the pharynx, the doses are not altered, and we have found that if the graft has not been rejected before radiation therapy begins, then the graft is not at a significantly high risk of rejection despite higher doses being used for these restorations, which are used in the treatment of abdominal malignancies. Off–spinal-cord reductions are made at 42 Gy, and boosts are delivered after the surgical bed has received 56 Gy. If the low neck is uninvolved, it is treated to 50 Gy, although if portions of the operative bed are within the low-neck field, these areas are supplemented to 56 Gy. Unless specific concerns are noted regarding disease in the peristomal tissues or the stoma is incorporated in the boost because of its proximity to the primary bed, we limit the stoma to 50 Gy.

RESULTS OF RADIATION THERAPY
Carcinoma of the Glottis

Reported local control rates for patients with carcinoma in situ of the glottis treated with primary radiation therapy are high. Most series report control rates of 90% or more.[44,49-52] Pene and Fletcher[53] reported a local control rate of 86%, but it was suspected that several of the treated patients had invasive carcinoma because, although invasion was not seen on their biopsy specimens, the clinical appearance of their tumors suggested T2 disease.

T1 Disease

The control rates with irradiation for T1 disease are similar to those achieved with irradiation for carcinoma in situ. Most series describing radiation therapy in patients with T1 disease report control rates of 85% to 95% (Table 11-2).[31,44,47,49,54-62] Although local control rates are equivalent for carcinoma in situ and T1 disease, the time to local failure is generally longer for carcinoma in situ; most series report recurrences developing between 2 and 5 years after radiation therapy for in situ disease, whereas recurrence of T1 disease tends to develop within 3 years.[49,53,63-66] Successful salvage therapy is the norm after local failure, and ultimate control rates are greater than 95%. In addition, for some patients, voice preservation is still possible with partial laryngectomy. However, many patients who require salvage therapy require a total laryngectomy to treat their recurrent tumor. Wang and McIntyre[67] reported a small series of reirradiation for recurrence of glottic tumors after radiation therapy. They reported a moderately high success rate, with a lower than anticipated rate of complications.

T2 Disease

Local control rates for T2 glottic cancer treated with radiation range from 65% to 80%, and the ultimate local control rate is about 90% (Table 11-3).* The wide range in local control rates is, in part, a result of the

*References 37, 44, 54, 55, 57, 58, 61, 68-70, 72, 73.

TABLE 11-2
Results of Radiation Therapy for T1 Glottic Carcinomas

Study and Reference	Number of Patients	Local Control Rate, %*	Local Control Rate After Salvage, %*
Wang, 1997[44]	665	93 (5-year actuarial)	98 (5-year disease-specific)
Hendrickson, 1985[54]	364	90	ND
Lustig et al, 1984[55]	342	90 (3-year actuarial)	ND
Harwood et al, 1979[49]	333	86 (5-year actuarial)	ND
Fletcher and Goepfert, 1980[56]	332	89	84
Le et al, 1997[57]	315	84	83
Schwaab et al, 1994[58]	194	86	89
Mendenhall et al, 1988[31]	171	93	58
Akine et al, 1991[59]	154	89	94
Olszewski et al, 1985[60]	137	80	82
Klintenberg et al, 1996[61]	129	90	75
Yu et al, 1997[47]	126	79	88
Pellitteri et al, 1991[62]	113	93	75

ND, No data.
*Rates are crude unless otherwise specified.

TABLE 11-3
Results of Radiation Therapy for T2 N0 Glottic Carcinomas

Study and Reference	Number of Patients	Local Control Rate, %*	Local Control Rate After Salvage, %*
Barton et al, 1992[68]	327	69 (5-year actuarial)	ND
Wang, 1997[44*,†]	237	71-77 (5-year actuarial)	84-92 (5-year disease-specific)
Karim et al, 1987[69]	156	68 (5-year actuarial)	92[‡]
Howell-Burke et al, 1990[70]	114	68	76
Lustig et al, 1984[55]	109	78 (3-year actuarial)	ND
Mendenhall et al, 1988[32]	108	75	74
Klintenberg et al, 1996[61]	94	74	38
Van den Bogaert et al, 1983[73]	83	76	65
Le et al, 1997[57]	83	67	74
Hendrickson, 1985[54]	76	73	50
Wiggenraad et al, 1990[72]	71	76	65
Schwaab et al, 1994[58]	65	66	55

ND, No data.
*Rates are crude unless otherwise specified.
†Data given for T2a and T2b separately.
‡Ultimate local control probability after salvage surgery for failures after radiation therapy.

subtleties of the relatively imprecise staging system, which lead to a moderate amount of subjective variation with respect to identifying clinical impairment, but not fixation, of vocal cord motion. The staging system also does not account for tumor volume, which has greater variability with increasing stage.

The need for a separate substage based on vocal cord mobility within the classification of T2 disease is controversial. Numerous series demonstrate a decrease in control ranging from 20% to 30% for T2 lesions with impaired vocal cord mobility compared to lesions associated with mobile vocal cords.[57,61,73,74] However, equally numerous series have not demonstrated a difference in outcome based on impairment of vocal cord motion.[44,69,70,72]

Hyperfractionated radiation therapy has been used as an attempt to improve control rates for T2 glottic carcinoma. Although this strategy has been shown to improve local control in oropharyngeal cancer and in advanced nonglottic head and neck cancer, data supporting the use of hyperfractionated radiation therapy in the treatment of T2 glottis carcinoma are sparse. Both the University of Florida and the M.D. Anderson Cancer Center have reported nonsignificant trends of improved local control for patients with T2 disease treated with hyperfractionation.[75,76] The RTOG is conducting a separate fractionation trial specifically addressing the role of twice-daily radiation for this disease site and stage.

T3 Disease

Not surprisingly, in patients treated with radiation alone, local control rates decrease with increasing stage. Thus reported local control rates for patients with T3 glottic carcinoma treated with radiation alone range from 45% to 70% (Table 11-4).[44,54,55,77-81] The feasibility of successful surgical salvage therapy also decreases with increasing initial stage; only half to two thirds of patients with T3 glottic carcinoma who are not cured with radiation therapy are ultimately cured with surgery.

Several studies have argued that when the endpoint for comparison is survival, expected results for patients treated with radiation therapy and surgical salvage therapy are similar to those that could be obtained with total laryngectomy and postoperative radiation therapy.[79,82] However, a randomized study to answer this question has not been done, and it is unlikely that such a trial will ever be performed. The VA randomized study for advanced laryngeal cancer concluded that the strategy of induction chemotherapy followed by radiation therapy for responders did not compromise survival and resulted in a substantial gain in voice preservation.[18] A European trial studying the same question reported that induction therapy did seem to compromise survival outcome, but its closure before completion makes its results more questionable.[16] Because no trial has demonstrated an improvement in survival with induction chemotherapy added to radiation therapy, the role of induction chemotherapy in this cohort of patients with a low likelihood of distant failure is questioned by many groups. To try to resolve this issue, the RTOG has begun a study comparing radiation alone vs. radiation plus chemotherapy, either induction or concurrent.

Another approach is not to use stage as the only factor for treatment selection but rather, within a stage, to attempt to determine which patients would most likely do well with a larynx-preserving approach and which patients would be better off with surgery. At the University of Florida, CT volume measurements have been studied as a predictor of outcome with radiation therapy. Using 3.5 cm^3 as a categorical cutoff point, the investigators found that patients with T3 disease with a volume of less than 3.5 cm^3 had very high local control rates with radiation therapy compared to rates in patients with larger tumors, for whom total laryngectomy may be

---

TABLE 11-4
Results of Radiation Therapy Alone for T3 Glottic Carcinomas

Study and Reference	Number of Patients	Local Control Rate, %*	Local Control Rate After Salvage, %*
Lundgren et al, 1988[77]	141	44	59
Terhaard et al, 1991[78]	104[†]	53 (3-year actuarial)	53
Wang, 1997[44]	65	57 (5-year actuarial)	75
Bryant et al, 1995[79]	55	55	ND
Lustig et al, 1984[55]	47	65 (3-year actuarial)	ND
Pameijer et al, 1997[80]	42	62	ND
Hendrickson, 1985[54]	39	56	47
Croll et al, 1989[81]	30	70	66

ND, No data.

*Rates are crude unless otherwise specified.

†Includes patients with cancer in any region of larynx.

best.[80] An indirect measure of tumor volume is respiratory distress and the need for emergent tracheotomy. The control rates of patients treated with radiation alone who had an emergent tracheotomy are significantly worse, sometimes less than 20%, and similarly, total laryngectomy may be the treatment of choice for these patients.[79]

T4 Disease

Surgery is the treatment of choice for patients with T4 glottic disease. Although the VA study[18] suggested that induction chemotherapy may be appropriate for advanced laryngeal cancer in general, the experience at the M.D. Anderson Cancer Center[37] suggests that patients with T4 disease do not benefit from this approach, and we recommend total laryngectomy as the standard of care. Few radiation series describe results for patients with T4 disease. Karim and colleagues[83] reported crude local control in 63% of 38 patients treated; similarly, Harwood and colleagues[84] reported disease control in 56% of 39 patients with T4 disease treated with radiation therapy alone.

Control rates for patients with T3 N0 and T4 N0 glottic cancer treated with total laryngectomy are high. At the M.D. Anderson Cancer Center, patients treated with surgery and postoperative irradiation had local control rates of greater than 90%. Similar control rates were achieved with surgery alone in the absence of the following adverse features: poor differentiation, subglottic extension of greater than 1 cm, or tracheotomy done emergently before the laryngectomy.[34] When these features were present, the control rate was less than 75%; thus the addition of postoperative irradiation is recommended in such situations.

Carcinoma of the Supraglottis

T1 tumors of the supraglottis are uncommon. Reported control rates for patients with T1 tumors treated with radiation alone range from 84% to 100%.[44,56,75] In 1974, Bataini and colleagues[85] reported an overall local–regional control rate of 76% for a relatively large series of patients with T1-T2 N0-N2 supraglottic carcinomas treated with radiation therapy alone.

Control rates for patients with T2 disease range from 61% to 90%.[44,75,86] The worst control rates are from series describing experiences with conventional fractionation. In 1980, Fletcher and Goepfert[56] demonstrated the importance of dose escalation to 70 Gy for T2 supraglottic tumors. Studies done at the M.D. Anderson Cancer Center, the University of Florida, and Massachusetts General Hospital have all suggested that twice-daily fractionation improves the control rate in this subgroup of patients.[44,75,86]

T3 disease comprises an extremely heterogeneous group of tumors. Control rates with radiation therapy alone range from 40% to 75%.[44,75,86] The improvement in control with twice-daily fractionation seen in T2 disease also has been demonstrated for T3 disease.

Several authors have suggested that not only primary tumor stage but also the presence of nodal disease is an important determinant of outcome. Both Wall and colleagues[87] at the M.D. Anderson Cancer Center and Wang and colleagues[88] have reported a lower incidence of local control in the presence of regional disease. However, these experiences were not replicated at the University of Florida.[89]

Radiographic volumetric measurements also have been found to be predictive of control with radiation therapy for supraglottic cancer. At the University of Florida, tumors less than 6 cm^3 had excellent control rates, but results were poorer when larger tumors were treated with radiation alone.[40]

Most patients with large or infiltrative T3 supraglottic primary tumors, particularly T3b tumors (vocal cord fixation), are treated with surgery. Some patients have lesions amenable to supraglottic laryngectomy, whereas others require total laryngectomy. Control rates for patients undergoing supraglottic laryngectomy are 80% to 90%.[3,39,90] Many of these patients receive postoperative radiation therapy because of either inadequate margins or the presence of nodal disease. However, results are rarely reported separately for this subgroup, and thus it is difficult to determine the value of radiation therapy for these patients. In patients with stage IV supraglottic cancer treated with total laryngectomy, Goepfert and colleagues[91] reported a 2-year control rate of 37% for surgery alone as opposed to 63% for combined surgery and postoperative radiation therapy. However, salvage was possible in 50% of the unirradiated patients but was rare in patients treated with initial combined therapy.

The VA study included many patients with supraglottic cancer, although a subsite analysis was not reported. A moderate incidence of patients with positive regional disease was noted, however, and these patients most likely had supraglottic rather than glottic tumors. The patients with supraglottic tumors may have accounted for most of the reduction in distant failure in the chemotherapy arm of the study, but this interpretation is only speculative.

Carcinoma of the Hypopharynx

Few series have reported outcome data for early hypopharyngeal carcinoma. Control rates range from 74% to 90% for T1 disease and 59% to 79% for T2 disease.[4,92,93] More recent results have suggested an improvement in control rates with the use of hyperfractionated radiation. At the M.D. Anderson Cancer Center, the local control rate for patients with early hypopharyngeal carcinoma treated with hyperfractionated radiation was 86%.[4] At the University of Florida, Mendenhall and colleagues[93] reported local control in

94% of patients with T2 pyriform sinus cancer treated with twice-a-day radiation therapy. Wang[92] reported a 5-year actuarial local control rate of 76% for patients with T2 pyriform sinus cancer treated with split-course accelerated radiation therapy.

The treatment of choice for patients with T3-T4 hypopharyngeal cancer is surgery. Most patients are advised to receive radiation postoperatively. Vandenbrouck and colleagues[94] performed a randomized trial comparing preoperative and postoperative radiation therapy in the treatment of hypopharyngeal tumors and demonstrated a significant improvement in survival when the radiation was delivered after surgery. Local–regional control rates in the multiple reported series range from 51% to 89%.[94-96] Despite this relatively wide range, 5-year survival rates seem relatively consistent across series, ranging from 22% to 43%. Analyzing patients treated at the M.D. Anderson Cancer Center between 1949 and 1976, El Badawi and colleagues[95] found that patients who received surgery and radiation therapy had significantly higher local control and 5-year survival rates than did patients who underwent surgery alone. A more recent study by Frank and colleagues[96] found that patients with hypopharyngeal cancer who received postoperative irradiation had only a 14% local–regional failure rate, compared to 57% in those treated with surgery only, despite the fact that patients treated with combined therapy had more advanced disease.

The EORTC conducted a voice preservation study for patients with hypopharyngeal cancer that was similar to the larynx preservation trial conducted by the VA.[17,18] Induction chemotherapy followed by radiation therapy for complete responders or surgery for noncomplete responders was compared to immediate pharyngolaryngectomy and postoperative irradiation. Survival rates were equivalent in the two treatment groups, but patients in the chemotherapy group had a 5-year voice preservation rate of 35%. Interestingly, the complete response rate to cisplatin and fluorouracil was more than 50%. Also, even though the trial was for patients with stage III or IV cancer, only a minority had T4 disease.

COMPLICATIONS

Complications of radiation therapy depend on both dose and volume. Patients with T1 laryngeal disease treated with fields ranging from 25 cm^2 to 36 cm^2 and doses of 66 Gy have few late complications. Fletcher and Goepfert[56] described a 1% crude incidence of late edema in patients with T1 disease treated between 1962 and 1979. Howell-Burke and colleagues[70] at the M.D. Anderson Cancer Center analyzed 114 patients with T2 glottic tumors and described a 5-year actuarial incidence of late complications of 4.6%. (The complications were four cases of moderate to severe late edema

and one case of laryngeal webbing, one of laryngeal stenosis, and one of soft tissue or cartilage necrosis.)

Complication rates are higher after radiation therapy for supraglottic and hypopharyngeal tumors than after radiation therapy for early-stage glottic carcinomas, probably because of the difference in the volumes of tissue being irradiated. Investigators at the University of Florida reported a 6% incidence of severe acute and late complications in patients receiving primary radiation therapy for supraglottic carcinomas.[75] In a series of 236 patients with head and neck cancer treated with hyperfractionation at the M.D. Anderson Cancer Center, the crude severe late complication rate was 9%. Two deaths were attributed to complications, and two patients who had been rendered free of disease required total laryngectomy for management of their complications.[76] Many of these severe complications occurred during the early days of using hyperfractionation. These early experiences led to recognition of the importance of increasing the interfraction interval to at least 6 hours. Since this adjustment was made, complication rates have decreased.

REFERENCES

1. Byers RM, Wolf PF, Ballantyne AJ. Rationale for elective modified neck dissection. *Head Neck Surg* 1988;10:160-167.
2. Lindberg RD. Distribution of cervical lymph node metastases from squamous cell carcinoma of the upper respiratory and digestive tracts. *Cancer* 1972;29:1446-1449.
3. Lee NK, Goepfert H, Wendt CD. Supraglottic laryngectomy for intermediate stage cancer: M.D. Anderson Cancer Center experience with combined therapy. *Laryngoscope* 1990;100:831-836.
4. Garden AS, Morrison WH, Clayman GL, et al. Early squamous cell carcinoma of the hypopharynx: outcomes of treatment with radiation alone to the primary disease. *Head Neck* 1996;18:317-322.
5. Merino OR, Lindberg RL, Fletcher GH. An analysis of distant metastases from squamous cell carcinoma of the upper respiratory and digestive tracts. *Cancer* 1977;40:145-151.
6. Warde P, O'Sullivan B, Bristow R, et al. T1/T2 glottic cancer managed by external beam radiotherapy: the influence of pretreatment hemoglobin on local control. *Int J Radiat Oncol Biol Phys* 1988;41:347-353.
7. American Joint Committee on Cancer. The pharynx and the larynx. In: Fleming I, Cooper JS, Henson DE, et al, eds. *AJCC Cancer Staging Manual*. 5th ed. Philadelphia, Pa: Lippincott Williams & Wilkins; 1997:31-46.
8. McGuirt WF, Blalock D, Koufman JA, et al. Comparative voice results after laser resection or irradiation of T1 vocal cord carcinoma. *Arch Otolaryngol Head Neck Surg* 1994;120:951-955.
9. Hirano M, Hirade Y, Kawasaki H. Vocal function following carbon dioxide surgery for glottic carcinoma. *Ann Otol Rhinol Laryngol* 1985;94:232-235.
10. Harrison LB, Solomon B, Miller S, et al. Prospective computer-assisted voice analysis for patients with early stage glottic cancer: a preliminary report of the functional result of laryngeal irradiation. *Int J Radiat Oncol Biol Phys* 1990;19:123-127.
11. Foote R, Buskirk S, Grado G, et al. Has radiotherapy become too expensive to be considered a treatment option for early glottic cancer? *Head Neck Surg* 1997;19:692-700.
12. Mittal B, Rao DV, Marks JE, et al. Comparative cost analysis of hemilaryngectomy and irradiation for early glottic carcinoma. *Int J Radiat Oncol Biol Phys* 1983;9:407-408.

13. DeSanto LW. T3 glottic cancer: options and consequences of the options. *Laryngoscope* 1984;94:1311-1315.

14. Hao SP, Myers EN, Johnson JT. T3 glottic carcinoma revisited. Transglottic vs pure glottic carcinoma. *Arch Otolaryngol Head Neck Surg* 1995;121:166-170.

15. Kowalski LP, Batista MB, Santos CR, et al. Prognostic factors in T3,N0-1 glottic and transglottic carcinoma. A multifactorial study of 221 cases treated by surgery or radiotherapy. *Arch Otolaryngol Head Neck Surg* 1996;122:77-82.

16. Richard J, Sancho-Garnier H, Pessey J, et al. Randomized trial of induction chemotherapy in larynx carcinoma. *Oral Oncol* 1998;34:224-228.

17. Lefebvre JL, Chevalier D, Luboinski B, et al. Larynx preservation in pyriform sinus cancer: preliminary results of a European Organization for Research and Treatment of Cancer phase III trial. EORTC Head and Neck Cancer Cooperative Group. *J Natl Cancer Inst* 1996;88:890-899.

18. Department of Veterans Affairs Laryngeal Cancer Study Group. Induction chemotherapy plus radiation compared with surgery plus radiation in patients with advanced laryngeal cancer. *N Engl J Med* 1992;324:1685-1690.

19. Brizel D, Albers M, Fisher S, et al. Hyperfractionated irradiation with or without concurrent chemotherapy for locally advanced head and neck cancer. *N Engl J Med* 1998;338:1798-1804.

20. Adelstein D, Lavertu P, Saxton J, et al. Mature results of a phase III randomized trial comparing concurrent chemoradiotherapy with radiation therapy alone in patients with stage III and IV squamous cell carcinoma of the head and neck. *Cancer* 2000;88:876-883.

21. McNeil B, Weichselbaum R, Pauker S. Speech and survival: trade-offs between quality and quantity of life in laryngeal cancer. *N Engl J Med* 1981;305:982-987.

22. van der Donk J, Levendag P, Kuijpers A, et al. Patient participation in clinical decision-making for treatment of T3 laryngeal cancer: a comparison of state and process utilities. *J Clin Oncol* 1995;13:2369-2378.

23. Ferlito A, Polidoro F, Rossi M. Pathological basis and clinical aspects of treatment policy in carcinoma in situ of the larynx. *J Laryngol Otol* 1981;95:141-154.

24. McGuirt WF, Browne JD. Management decisions in laryngeal carcinoma in situ. *Laryngoscope* 1991;101:125-129.

25. Wolfensberger M, Dort JC. Endoscopic laser surgery for early glottic carcinoma: a clinical and experimental study. *Laryngoscope* 1990;100:1100-1105.

26. Maran AG, Mackenzie IJ, Stanley RE. Carcinoma in situ of the larynx. *Head Neck Surg* 1984;7:28-31.

27. Strong MS. Laser excision of carcinoma of the larynx. *Laryngoscope* 1975;85:1286-1289.

28. Neel HB III, Devine KD, DeSanto LW. Laryngofissure and cordectomy for early cordal carcinoma: outcome in 182 patients. *Otolaryngol Head Neck Surg* 1980;88:79-84.

29. Soo KC, Shah JP, Gopinath KS, et al. Analysis of prognostic variables and results after supraglottic partial laryngectomy. *Am J Surg* 1988;156:301-305.

30. Laccourreye O, Weinstein G, Brasnu D, et al. Vertical partial laryngectomy: a critical analysis of local recurrence. *Ann Otol Rhinol Laryngol* 1991;100:68-71.

31. Mendenhall WM, Parsons JT, Stringer SP, et al. T1-T2 vocal cord carcinoma: a basis for comparing the results of radiotherapy and surgery. *Head Neck Surg* 1988;10:373-377.

32. Laccourreye H, Laccourreye O, Weinstein G, et al. Supracricoid laryngectomy with cricohyoidopexy: a partial laryngeal procedure for selected supraglottic and transglottic carcinomas. *Laryngoscope* 1990;100:735-741.

33. Laccourreye O, Brasnu D, Bassot V, et al. Cisplatin-fluorouracil exclusive chemotherapy for T1-T3N0 glottic squamous cell carcinoma complete clinical responders: five-year results. *J Clin Oncol* 1996;14:2331-2336.

34. Yuen A, Medina J, Goepfert H, et al. Management of stage T3 and T4 glottic carcinomas. *Am J Surg* 1984;148:467-472.

35. Pignon J, Bourhis J, Domenge C, et al. Chemotherapy added to locoregional treatment for head and neck squamous-cell carcinoma: three meta-analyses of updated individual data. *Lancet* 2000;355;949-955.

36. Forastiere AA, Berkey B, Maor M, et al. Phase III trial to preserve the larynx: induction chemotherapy and radiotherapy versus concomitant chemoradiotherapy versus radiotherapy alone. Intergroup trial R91-11 [abstract]. *Proceedings of the American Society of Clinical Oncology* 2001;20:4a.

37. Shirinian MH, Weber RS, Lippman SM, et al. Laryngeal preservation by induction chemotherapy plus radiotherapy in locally advanced head and neck cancer: the M.D. Anderson Cancer Center experience. *Head Neck* 1994;16:39-44.

38. Steiner W. Results of curative laser microsurgery of laryngeal carcinomas. *Am J Otolaryngol* 1993;14:116-121.

39. Bocca E, Pignataro O, Oldini C. Supraglottic laryngectomy: 30 years of experience. *Ann Otol Rhinol Laryngol* 1983;92:14-18.

40. Freeman DE, Mancuso AA, Parsons JT, et al. Irradiation alone for supraglottic larynx carcinoma: can CT findings predict treatment results? *Int J Radiat Oncol Biol Phys* 1990;19:485-490.

41. Robbins KT, Davidson W, Peters LJ, et al. Conservation surgery for T2 and T3 carcinomas of the supraglottic larynx. *Arch Otolaryngol Head Neck Surg* 1988;114:421-426.

42. Foote RL, Grado GL, Buskirk SJ, et al. Radiation therapy for glottic cancer using 6-MV photons. *Cancer* 1996;77:381-386.

43. Sombeck MD, Kalbaugh KJ, Mendenhall WM, et al. Radiotherapy for early vocal cord cancer: a dosimetric analysis of 60-Co versus 6 MV photons. *Head Neck* 1996;18:167-173.

44. Wang CC. *Radiation Therapy for Head and Neck Neoplasms*. New York, NY: Wiley-Liss; 1997:221-255.

45. Burke LS, Greven KM, McGuirt WT, et al. Definitive radiotherapy for early glottic carcinoma: prognostic factors and implications for treatment. *Int J Radiat Oncol Biol Phys* 1997;38:37-42.

46. Rudoltz MS, Benammar A, Mohiuddin M. Prognostic factors for local control and survival in T1 squamous cell carcinoma of the glottis. *Int J Radiat Oncol Biol Phys* 1993;26:767-772.

47. Yu E, Shenouda G, Beaudet MP, et al. Impact of radiation therapy fraction size on local control of early glottic carcinoma. *Int J Radiat Oncol Biol Phys* 1997;37:587-591.

48. Peters LJ, Goepfert H, Ang KK, et al. Evaluation of the dose for postoperative radiation therapy of head and neck cancer: first report of a prospective randomized trial. *Int J Radiat Oncol Biol Phys* 1993;26:3-12.

49. Harwood AR, Hawkins NV, Rider WD, et al. Radiotherapy of early glottic cancer. I. *Int J Radiat Oncol Biol Phys* 1979;5:473-476.

50. Kalter PO, Lubsen H, Delemarre JFM, et al. Squamous hyperplasia of the larynx (a clinical follow-up study). *J Laryngol Otol* 1987;101:579-588.

51. Fernberg JO, Ringborg U, Silfversward C, et al. Radiation therapy in early glottic cancer: analysis of 177 consecutive cases. *Acta Otolaryngol* 1989;108:478-481.

52. Smitt MC, Goffinet DR. Radiotherapy for carcinoma-in-situ of the glottic larynx. *Int J Radiat Oncol Biol Phys* 1994;28:251-255.

53. Pene F, Fletcher GH. Results in irradiation of the in situ carcinoma of the vocal cord. *Cancer* 1976;37:2586-2590.

54. Hendrickson FR. Radiation therapy treatment of larynx cancers. *Cancer* 1985;55:2058-2061.

55. Lustig RA, MacLean CJ, Hanks GE, et al. The patterns of care outcome studies: results of the national practice in carcinoma of the larynx. *Int J Radiat Oncol Biol Phys* 1984;10:2357-2362.

56. Fletcher GH, Goepfert H. Larynx and pyrifom sinus. In: Fletcher G, ed. *Textbook of Radiotherapy*. 3rd ed. Philadelphia, Pa: Lea & Febiger; 1980:330-363.

57. Le QX, Fu KK, Kroll S, et al. Influence of fraction size, total dose, and overall time on local control of T1-T2 glottic carcinoma. *Int J Radiat Oncol Biol Phys* 1997;39:115-126.

58. Schwaab G, Mamelle G, Lartigau E, et al. Surgical salvage treatment of T1/T2 glottic carcinoma after failure of radiotherapy. *Am J Surg* 1994;168:474-475.

59. Akine Y, Tokit N, Ogino T, et al. Radiotherapy of T1 glottic cancer with 6 MeV x-rays. *Int J Radiat Oncol Biol Phys* 1991;20:1215-1218.

60. Olszewski SJ, Vaeth JM, Green JP, et al. The influence of field size, treatment modality, commissure involvement and histology in the treatment of early vocal cord cancer with irradiation. *Int J Radiat Oncol Biol Phys* 1985;11:1333-1337.

61. Klintenberg C, Lundgren J, Adell G, et al. Primary radiotherapy of T1 and T2 glottic carcinoma—analysis of treatment results and prognostic factors in 223 patients. *Acta Oncol* 1996;35(suppl 8):81-86.

62. Pellitteri PK, Kennedy TL, Vrabec DP, et al. Radiotherapy—the mainstay in the treatment of early glottic carcinoma. *Arch Otolaryngol Head Neck Surg* 1991;117:297-301.

63. Hintz BL, Kagan AR, Nussbaum H, et al. A watchful waiting policy for in situ carcinoma of the vocal cords. *Arch Otolaryngol* 1981;107:746-751.

64. MacLeod PM, Daniel F. The role of radiotherapy in in-situ carcinoma of the larynx. *Int J Radiat Oncol Biol Phys* 1990;18:113-117.

65. Sung DI, Chang CH, Harisiadis L, et al. Primary radiotherapy for carcinoma in situ and early invasive carcinoma of the glottic larynx. *Int J Radiat Oncol Biol Phys* 1979;15:467-472.

66. Elman AJ, Goodman M, Wang CC, et al. In situ carcinoma of the vocal cords. *Cancer* 1979;43:2422-2428.

67. Wang C, McIntyre J. Re-irradiation of laryngeal carcinoma—techniques and results. *Int J Radiat Oncol Biol Phys* 1993;26:783-785.

68. Barton MB, Keane TJ, Gadalla T, et al. The effect of treatment time and treatment interruption on tumor control following radical radiotherapy of laryngeal cancer. *Radiother Oncol* 1992;23:137-143.

69. Karim ABMF, Kralendonk JH, Yap LY, et al. Heterogeneity of stage II glottic carcinoma and its therapeutic implications. *Int J Radiat Oncol Biol Phys* 1987;13:313-317.

70. Howell-Burke D, Peters LJ, Goepfert H, et al. T2 glottic cancer. *Arch Otolaryngol Head Neck Surg* 1990;116:830-835.

71. Van den Bogaert W, Ostyn F, van der Schueren E. The significance of extension and impaired mobility in cancer of the vocal cord. *Int J Radiat Oncol Biol Phys* 1983;9:181-184.

72. Wiggenraad RG, Terhaard CH, Horidjik GJ, et al. The importance of vocal cord mobility in T2 laryngeal cancer. *Radiother Oncol* 1990;18:321-327.

73. Harwood AR, Beale FA, Cummings BJ, et al. T2 glottic cancer: an analysis of dose-time-volume factors. *Int J Radiat Oncol Biol Phys* 1981;7:1501-1505.

74. Kelly MD, Hahn SS, Spaulding CA, et al. Definitive radiotherapy in the management of stage I and II carcinomas of the glottis. *Ann Otol Rhinol Laryngol* 1989;98:235-239.

75. Mendenhall WM, Parsons JT, Mancuso AA, et al. Radiotherapy for squamous cell carcinoma of the supraglottic larynx: an alternative to surgery. *Head Neck* 1996;18:24-35.

76. Garden AS, Morrison WH, Ang KK, et al. Hyperfractionated radiation in the treatment of squamous cell carcinomas of the head and neck: a comparison of two fractionation schedules. *Int J Radiat Oncol Biol Phys* 1995;31:493-502.

77. Lundgren JAV, Gilbert RW, Van Nostrand AWP, et al. T3N0M0 glottic carcinoma—a failure analysis. *Clin Otolaryngol* 1988;13:455-465.

78. Terhaard CHF, Karim AB, Hoogenraad WJ, et al. Local control in T3 laryngeal cancer treated with radical radiotherapy, time dose relationship: the concept of nominal standard dose and linear quadratic model. *Int J Radiat Oncol Biol Phys* 1991;20:1207-1214.

79. Bryant GP, Poulsen MG, Tripcony L, et al. Treatment decision in T3N0M0 glottic carcinoma. *Int J Radiat Oncol Biol Phys* 1995;31:285-293.

80. Pameijer FA, Mancuso AA, Mendenhall WM, et al. Can pretreatment computed tomography predict local control in T3 squamous cell carcinoma of the glottic larynx treated with definitive radiotherapy? *Int J Radiat Oncol Biol Phys* 1997;37:1011-1021.

81. Croll GA, Gerritsen GJ, Tiwari RM, et al. Primary radiotherapy with surgery in reserve for advanced laryngeal carcinoma: results and complications. *Eur J Surg Oncol* 1989;15:350-356.

82. Mendenhall W, Parsons J, Mancuso A, et al. Definitive radiotherapy for T3 squamous cell carcinoma of the glottic larynx. *J Clin Oncol* 1997;15:2394-2402.

83. Karim A, Kralendonk J, Njo K, et al. Radiation therapy for advanced (T3-T4N0-N3M0) laryngeal carcinoma: the need for a change of strategy. A radiotherapeutic viewpoint. *Int J Radiat Oncol Biol Phys* 1987;13:1625-1633.

84. Harwood A, Beale F, Cummings B, et al. T4N0M0 glottic cancer: an analysis of dose-time volume factors. *Int J Radiat Oncol Biol Phys* 1981;7:1507-1512.

85. Bataini JP, Ennuyer A, Poncet P, et al. Treatment of supraglottic cancer by radical high dose radiotherapy. *Cancer* 1974;33:1253-1262.

86. Wendt CW, Peters LJ, Ang KK, et al. Hyperfractionated radiotherapy in the treatment of squamous cell carcinomas of the supraglottic larynx. *Int J Radiat Oncol Biol Phys* 1989;17:1057-1062.

87. Wall TJ, Peters LJ, Brown BW, et al. Relationship between lymph nodal status and primary tumor control probability in tumors of the supraglottic larynx. *Int J Radiat Oncol Biol Phys* 1985;11:1895-1902.

88. Wang CC, Nakfoor BM, Spiro IJ, et al. Role of accelerated fractionated irradiation for supraglottic carcinoma: assessment of results. *Cancer J Sci Am* 1997;3:88-91.

89. Freeman DE, Mendenhall WM, Parsons JT, et al. Does neck stage influence local control in squamous cell carcinomas of the head and neck? *Int J Radiat Oncol Biol Phys* 1992;23:733-736.

90. Ogura JH, Marks JE, Freeman RB. Results of conservation surgery for cancers of the supraglottis and pyriform sinus. *Laryngoscope* 1980;90:591-600.

91. Goepfert H, Jesse RH, Fletcher GH, et al. Optimal treatment for the technically resectable squamous cell carcinoma of the supraglottic larynx. *Laryngoscope* 1975;85:14-32.

92. Wang CC. *Radiation Therapy for Head and Neck Neoplasms*. New York, NY: Wiley-Liss; 1997:205-220.

93. Mendenhall WM, Parsons JT, Stringer SP, et al. Radiotherapy alone or combined with neck dissection for T1-T2 carcinoma of the pyriform sinus: an alternative to conservation surgery. *Int J Radiat Oncol Biol Phys* 1993;27:1017-1027.

94. Vandenbrouck C, Sancho H, Le Fur R, et al. Results of a randomized clinical trial of preoperative irradiation versus postoperative in treatment of tumors of the hypopharynx. *Cancer* 1977;39:1445-1449.

95. El Badawi SA, Goepfert H, Fletcher GH, et al. Squamous cell carcinoma of the pyriform sinus. *Laryngoscope* 1982;92:357-364.

96. Frank JL, Garb JL, Kay S, et al. Postoperative radiotherapy improves survival in squamous cell carcinoma of the hypopharynx. *Am J Surg* 1994;168:476-480.

CHAPTER 12

The Orbit

Linh N. Nguyen and K. Kian Ang

A variety of benign and malignant diseases either primarily or secondarily involve the orbit. Radiation therapy can be used to treat many of these diseases. Late effects of radiation therapy, although rare with modern techniques and careful treatment planning, can have drastic effects on visual function. Consequently, for benign orbital diseases, radiation therapy is typically used as an adjunct to surgery or is reserved for cases in which other treatments have failed. For malignant orbital diseases, however, radiation therapy has emerged as the initial treatment of choice because the alternative typically includes surgery that ranges from local excision to enucleation, leaving the patient with significant morbidity. In all cases, treatment decisions should be individualized, and desirable results can be achieved through careful patient selection.

ANATOMY

The outer covering of the eyeball is composed of three main tissue layers (Fig. 12-1).[1] The external fibrous coat consists of the sclera, cornea, and corneal limbus. The middle vascular coat (the uvea) consists of the choroid, ciliary body, and iris. The inner neural coat, the retina, is the sensory region. Within the outer covering of the eyeball lie the crystalline lens, vitreous humor, and aqueous humor. The six extraocular muscles controlling eye movement insert into the sclera. The orbital contents that hold the eyeball in place consist of the extraocular muscles, the nerves and vessels that serve the globe, and in-filling fatty tissues. The orbital contents reside in a protective cone consisting of seven bones of the skull that together compose the bony orbit (Figs. 12-2 and 12-3).[2]

In the treatment of orbital diseases, detailed knowledge of the spatial relationships between anatomic structures allows radiation oncologists to spare as much normal tissue as possible without compromising coverage of the target volume. From topographic measurements using computed tomography (CT) scans with eyelid markers on 66 patients, Karlsson and colleagues[3] determined that the mean distance from the anterior surface of the superior eyelid to the posterior surface of the

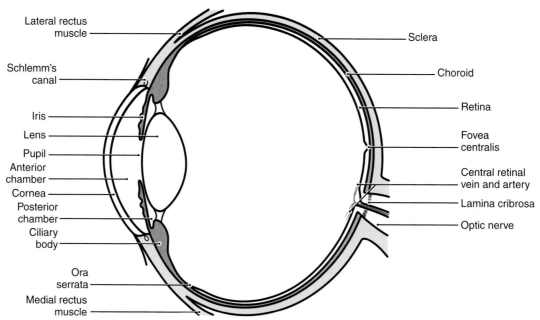

Fig. 12-1 Horizontal section of the right eye. (From Saude T. The outer coats of the eye. In: Saude T, ed. *Ocular Anatomy and Physiology.* Oxford, England: Blackwell Science; 1993:11-25.)

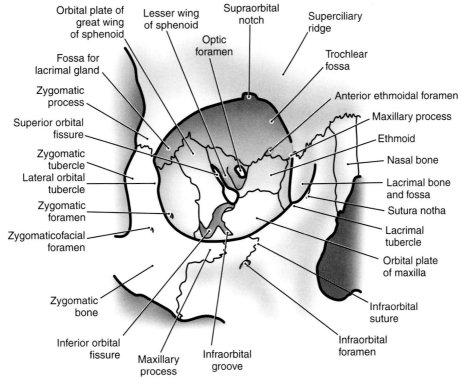

Fig. 12-2 The right orbit viewed along its axis. (From Bron AJ, Tripathi RC, Tripathi BJ. *Wolff's Anatomy of the Eye and Orbit.* 8th ed. London, England: Arnold; 1997.)

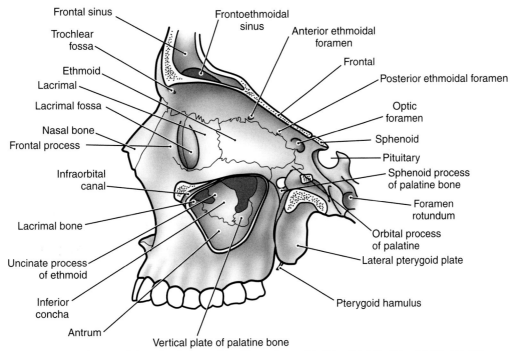

Fig. 12-3 The medial wall of the orbit. (From Bron AJ, Tripathi RC, Tripathi BJ. *Wolff's Anatomy of the Eye and Orbit.* 8th ed. London, England: Arnold; 1997.)

lens was 10.1 mm ± 1 mm and that the mean distance from the posterior surface of the lens to the intercanthal line was 8.5 mm ± 2.6 mm. The median sagittal globe diameter was 24.6 mm.

RESPONSE OF NORMAL ORBITAL STRUCTURES TO IRRADIATION

The various orbital tissues each respond differently to irradiation. In general, a gradient of decreasing radiosensitivity is found going from the anterior structures to the posterior structures. Rohrschneider,[4] one of the first to address the topic, reported that the most radiosensitive structures, in order of decreasing sensitivity, were the lens, conjunctiva, cornea, uvea, and retina and that the least radiosensitive structure was the optic nerve. More recent findings regarding the radiosensitivity of orbital structures[5] (discussed below) confirm Rohrschneider's early findings.

Eyelashes and Eyelid

The eyelashes are end organs of touch and, upon contact, initiate a blink reflex to protect the eye. Doses of 20 to 30 Gy or more given in 2- to 3-Gy fractions cause alopecia of the eyelashes and thus abolish this protective mechanism, resulting in irritation of the conjunctiva and corneal surfaces.[6] Occasionally, regrowth of the lashes may produce trichiasis and entropion requiring intervention.[7]

Irradiation of the eyelid produces observable effects similar to those produced by irradiation of other skin and mucosa in the body, and, with commonly prescribed radiation doses, healing is typically complete. However, the skin and mucosa of the eyelid are among the more delicate tissues in the body, and side effects occurring in this region are more uncomfortable for the patient than those arising in other regions.

Lacrimal Gland

Radiation treatment fields that include the lacrimal gland can cause atrophy and loss of glandular function, leading to dry eye syndrome. Nowadays, dry eye symptoms can usually be sufficiently treated with artificial tears or lubricants. Chronic irritation of the cornea by the eyelid, however, may lead to a painful eye with vision loss resulting from corneal laceration and subsequent ulceration with infection, opacification, or vascularization. Parsons and colleagues[8] examined the dose-response relationship for dry-eye complications using data from the University of Florida and from the literature. No complications occurred with doses up to 30 Gy. The incidence of injury was 5% to 25% in the range of 30 to 40 Gy and increased steeply for doses above 40 Gy, reaching 100% for doses of 57 Gy or greater.

With doses of radiation in the curative range, stenosis or even obstruction of the nasolacrimal duct may occur. The main symptom is epiphora, which may be remedied with recanalization of the duct.

Cornea

It is difficult to distinguish direct radiation injury to the cornea from indirect injury resulting from dry eye syndrome because in most reported series, the entire eye is included in the treatment volume.[9-11] Radiation-induced keratitis with varying amounts of tearing may develop during treatment but also may manifest a few weeks or months after treatment.[9] Radiation-induced corneal injury manifests as multiple tiny ulcers in the corneal epithelium seen under fluorescein staining. This type of injury typically occurs after doses of 30 to 50 Gy given over 4 to 5 weeks[12,13] and gradually resolves over 4 to 6 weeks with conservative treatment without sequelae. Corneal ulceration may occur with doses greater than 50 Gy in 4 to 5 weeks.

Merriam and colleagues[9] reported three severe corneal ulcerations in 25 patients treated for rhabdomyosarcoma of the orbit with 60 Gy (22.5 MeV) in 5 to 6 weeks. The cornea received the full dose, and in two patients perforation occurred, necessitating enucleation. Chan and Shukovsky[10] reported that with a follow-up time of 2 years, corneal lesions occurred in 15% of patients treated with 60 Gy over 6 weeks to the entire eye for nasal cavity and paranasal sinus tumors. When intra-arterial fluorouracil was given along with radiation, all patients developed corneal lesions. Bessell and colleagues[11] reported corneal ulceration in 2 of 13 patients treated with 40 to 49 Gy over 3 or 4 weeks for orbital lymphoma. However, both patients also had tear film instability, which most likely contributed to the ulcerative process. In both cases, the corneal ulcer eventually healed.

Corneal stromal edema may be seen with doses of 40 to 50 Gy in 2 to 3 weeks.[9] The edema is typically self-limiting, resolving over 2 to 4 weeks, and may be adequately treated with topical antibiotics and steroids. Prolonged edema of the stroma is uncommon but is more likely with doses greater than 50 Gy—usually on the order of 70 to 80 Gy.

Reporting on a series of patients treated at The University of Texas M.D. Anderson Cancer Center, Jiang and colleagues[14] suggested that visual impairment from corneal injury most likely resulted from a combination of lacrimal gland injury and direct effects of radiation on the cornea. In that series, no patients who had both lacrimal and corneal shielding during irradiation developed visual impairment. In contrast, 2 of 8 patients treated with lacrimal shielding only and 2 of 12 patients treated with cornea-lens shielding only developed corneal injury. The incidence of visual impairment at

2 years was 81% to 88% with doses of 56 to 74.5 Gy to the lacrimal gland (corneal dose, 31 to 41 Gy) with or without chemotherapy as opposed to 17% for doses of 42 to 45 Gy (corneal dose, 23 to 30 Gy) without chemotherapy. Overall treatment time ranged from 29 to 52 days. The median time to manifestation of visual impairment was 9 months (range, 1 to 31 months).

If the cornea and conjunctiva are not at risk for harboring subclinical disease, a practical, useful strategy for decreasing the incidence of corneal complications is to irradiate patients with their eyelids open for the anterior field such that the cornea and conjunctiva are located in the build-up region of the megavoltage beams.

Lens

The lens is the most radiosensitive organ in the body. The lens itself consists largely of fiber cells covered anteriorly by an epithelium and is enclosed in a capsule.[15] Cell division in the lens continues throughout a person's lifetime. With radiation injury to the dividing cells, the resulting abnormal fibers migrate toward the posterior pole, where they constitute the beginning of a cataract.

Definitive studies from Merriam and colleagues[9] shed light on the dose-response relationship for cataracts. These authors analyzed the available dose estimates to the lens for a total of 233 patients who received radiation therapy to the eye. Radiation cataracts developed in 128 patients. The minimum cataractogenic doses were 2 Gy for single-dose radiation, 4 Gy for multiple doses given over a period ranging from 3 weeks to 3 months, and 5.5 Gy for multiple doses given over a period longer than 3 months. Higher doses decreased the latent period and increased the severity of the cataracts. In patients who received 2.5 to 6.5 Gy, the latent period was 8 years and 7 months, and one third of the patients developed progressive cataracts. In patients who received 6.51 to 11.5 Gy, the latent period was 4 years and 4 months, and two thirds of the patients developed progressive cataracts.

Sclera

The sclera is extremely radioresistant, as illustrated by its tolerance of the high doses of radiation used for the treatment of ocular melanomas. However, doses in the range of 200 to 300 Gy may cause atrophy after a latency of several years.[9]

Retina

Radiation damage to the retina is primarily seen in the endothelium of the retinal capillaries.[16] Ophthalmoscopic findings include retinal hemorrhages, microaneurysms, hard exudates, cotton-wool spots, and telangiectases.[17] In the M.D. Anderson Cancer Center series from Jiang and colleagues,[14] the onset of visual impairment caused by retinopathy occurred 5 to 30 months (median, 11 months) after radiation treatment. With doses of 50 to 60 Gy given over 29 to 62 days, the overall actuarial incidence of retinopathy was 20%.[14] However, this was most likely an underestimation because not all patients underwent systematic ophthalmologic evaluation.

Limited data are available in the literature on the dose-response relationship for radiation retinopathy. Parsons and colleagues[18] reported no retinopathy in 33 eyes treated with doses less than 45 Gy. For higher doses, the incidences of retinopathy were as follows: 50% (6 of 12) for doses of 45 to 55 Gy; 83% (10 of 12) for doses of 55 to 65 Gy, and 100% (11 of 11) for doses above 65 Gy. Several anecdotal reports have suggested that patients with diabetes mellitus are at increased risk of developing radiation retinopathy.[19-21] In our practice, we prefer to limit the retinal dose to 50 Gy when possible to minimize complications.

Optic Nerve and Chiasm

In an M.D. Anderson Cancer Center series, Jiang and colleagues[14] reported that visual impairment resulting from damage to the optic nerve and chiasm occurred 7 to 50 months (median, 27 months) after radiation therapy. Optic neuropathy was not observed after doses of less than 56 Gy, and the incidence of this complication remained low (< 5% at 10 years) with doses up to 60 Gy in fractions not exceeding 2.5 Gy. However, with doses higher than 60 Gy, the incidence of optic neuropathy increased considerably, to 34% at 10 years. In a University of Florida series from Parsons and colleagues,[22] optic neuropathy was not observed in 106 optic nerves that received a total dose of less than 60 Gy. With doses of 60 Gy or more, the incidence of optic neuropathy increased, and a suggestion was made that the incidence depended on dose per fraction. With doses of 60 Gy or more, the 15-year actuarial risk of optic neuropathy was 11% with fractions of less than 1.9 Gy vs. 47% with fractions of 1.9 Gy or greater.

Optic chiasm injury resulting in bilateral blindness is one of the most devastating complications of radiation therapy. In the series of Jiang and colleagues,[14] none of 32 patients who received total doses of less than 50 Gy and only 4 of 110 patients (8% actuarial rate at 10 years) who received doses of 50 to 60 Gy in fractions of 2.6 Gy or less developed optic chiasm injury. Total doses of 61 to 76 Gy were associated with a higher complication rate (24% at 10 years). For treatment planning, we prefer to limit the dose to the optic nerve and chiasm to 54 Gy. In the presence of gross tumor in close proximity that requires higher doses, we limit the dose to the optic nerve and chiasm to 60 Gy, and we ensure that the patient understands that the risk of blindness with this treatment approaches approximately 10%.

BENIGN ORBITAL DISEASES
Graves' Ophthalmopathy

Graves' disease is an autoimmune disorder with three major manifestations: hyperthyroidism, ophthalmopathy, and dermopathy. Graves' ophthalmopathy occurs in 20% to 40% of patients with Graves' disease and manifests as exophthalmos with ophthalmoplegia and congestive oculopathy characterized by chemosis, conjunctivitis, periorbital swelling, and the potential complications of corneal ulceration, optic neuritis, and optic atrophy.[23]

Pathologic examination reveals an inflammatory infiltrate of the orbital contents and enlargement of the extraocular muscles. Although the pathogenesis of Graves' ophthalmopathy is still not fully understood, one proposed mechanism is the development of antibodies against specific antigens in the extraocular muscles. The disease has a benign course in most patients and, interestingly, is independent of the course of the hyperthyroidism. More severe cases of Graves' ophthalmopathy require medical intervention. The first line of treatment is high-dose steroids (e.g., prednisone 100 to 120 mg/day). Surgical decompression of the orbit is sometimes performed to relieve compression of the optic nerve and orbital blood vessels and to reduce pain. Surgical correction of the eye muscles can diminish diplopia, and surgical correction of the eyelids can improve the function of the distorted edematous lids to lessen corneal damage.

Although the indications for orbital irradiation in the treatment of Graves' ophthalmopathy are still controversial, this treatment is generally reserved for ophthalmopathy refractory to steroids. Bilateral irradiation is preferred because of the high incidence of bilateral involvement detectable by diagnostic imaging, even in patients with minimal symptoms and signs in the contralateral eye.[24] Moreover, when a one-sided lateral photon portal is used, subsequent treatment of the contralateral eye is problematic because of the relatively high exit dose received (approximately 60%).[25] Therefore opposed lateral fields with half-beam technique have been used.[24,25] With this technique the dose to the lens can be drastically reduced, to reportedly 4% of the prescribed dose, by placing the anterior border at the lateral fleshy canthus. For more severe cases, however, the anterior border should be adjusted according to the degree of exophthalmos.

Evidence of the efficacy of radiation therapy for Graves' ophthalmopathy is derived mostly from retrospective analyses of patients to whom radiation was given as second-line treatment.[24,26-29] The recommended dose is 20 Gy in 10 fractions.[24,26-29] Between 76% and 90% of patients are able to discontinue steroid therapy after irradiation.[24,26]

Petersen and colleagues[27] attempted to improve outcome by giving a higher dose—30 Gy in 15 fractions—but observed no improvement relative to outcomes with the lower dose of 20 Gy in their retrospective series of 311 patients. Improvements were noted in soft tissue involvement (e.g., redness, chemosis, or periorbital edema) (experienced by 80% of patients), corneal involvement (77%), sight loss (61%), eye muscle function (61%, but only 32% of patients had a complete response), and exophthalmos (51%). Importantly, the lens-shielding technique did not lead to an increase in cataract formation.

Prummel and colleagues[29] performed a randomized double-blind study comparing the efficacy of prednisone plus sham irradiation against placebo plus 20 Gy irradiation in 56 patients. The overall treatment efficacy was similar in the two groups, with response rates of approximately 50% and 75% for patients undergoing subsequent rehabilitative surgery. Patients who received radiation therapy had greater improvement in extraocular muscle involvement, whereas patients treated with prednisone responded more rapidly but at a cost of more frequent and more severe side effects from the medication.

An Italian group conducted two randomized studies comparing the combination of radiation therapy and systemic steroids with either systemic steroids or radiation therapy alone in the treatment of Graves' ophthalmopathy.[28,30] Both studies found a benefit for combined treatment, although patient numbers were small in both studies (24 patients and 26 patients). These authors recommended that combined therapy be considered for the initial treatment of severe ophthalmopathy.

No reports of radiation-induced orbital tumors in patients with Graves' ophthalmopathy have been noted, although some authors have estimated a theoretical risk of tumor induction of 0.3% to 1.2%.[31,32]

Orbital Pseudotumor

Orbital pseudotumor (idiopathic orbital inflammatory disease) is a nongranulomatous acute or subacute inflammatory disease usually occurring in the anterior orbit or midorbit, often involving the lacrimal gland.[33] This condition is idiopathic by definition, and thus neoplastic, infectious, and systemic inflammatory or immunologic causes are excluded.[34] Generally the disease is unilateral, although occasionally it may be bilateral.

Clinical symptoms consist of abrupt pain, conjunctival redness, chemosis, lid edema, exophthalmos, and restriction of eye movement. Pathologic examination reveals a gray rubbery mass composed of a polymorphic infiltrate of lymphocytes, eosinophils, plasma cells, and polymorphonuclear leukocytes.[35] The clinical course is variable, and spontaneous regression may occur in a minority of patients.

First-line treatment consists of steroids and typically produces a dramatic response in 30% to 60% of patients.[34,36] In refractory cases, radiation therapy is highly effective, yielding control rates of 65% to 75% after doses of 10 to 30 Gy given in one of several fractionation schedules.[34,36-39] For anterior lesions, Donaldson and Findley[40] described an electron beam technique with lens shielding that uses a centrally placed lead eye shield suspended 1 cm above the lens. The field size should be at least 4 × 4 cm to reduce dose inhomogeneity. The authors recommend 9- to 16-MeV beams for superficial lesions. At our institution, we prefer to mount the block on a contact lens to place the shield directly over the lens and cornea as described later in this chapter in the section on "Orbital Lymphomas." The treatment planning should be individualized with the aid of CT scans.

Pterygium

A pterygium is a conjunctival growth over the sclera and onto the cornea; it occurs more often on the nasal side in the palpebral fissure area.[41] Exposure to ultraviolet light and exposure to dust have been reported as causative factors.[41] Treatment is warranted when pterygia cause visual or cosmetic impairment. First-line therapy is surgical excision of the pterygium. However, because the incidence of recurrence after excision alone is relatively high (20% to 39%,[42,43] with most recurrences happening in the first year after excision[44]), surgery is usually accompanied by adjuvant treatment in an attempt to prevent recurrence. Nonradiation treatment modalities include mitomycin C application and conjunctival autotransplantation.

Experience with treatment of pterygia with strontium 90/yttrium 90 beta-ray surface applicators is extensive.[43,45-47] The maximum surface dose and rapid dose fall-off make beta-rays ideally suited for adjuvant treatment of pterygia. The first application is typically given within 12 to 24 hours after surgery. A variety of radiation schedules have been used, ranging from 20 Gy in one fraction to 24 to 60 Gy given in weekly fractions of 8 to 10 Gy.[43,45-47] With the addition of adjuvant radiation therapy to surgery, the control rate is excellent: the recurrence rate is less than 5%.[43,45-47] The main concern with radiation therapy is the risk of late scleral necrosis and the attendant risks of corneoscleral ulceration and infection. However, with fractionated radiation therapy, the late complication rate is usually less than 1%.[45,47,48] The higher reported complication rates have generally been associated with the use of large single fractions.[43,49,50] To minimize late complications, it is also imperative to carefully calibrate plaques to ensure an accurate dose rate because calibrated rates may be 30% to 57% higher than dose rates provided by the manufacturer.[51,52]

A reasonable schedule comes from Paryani and colleagues[47] of the North Florida Pterygium Study Group, who reported on the largest series of patients in North America. Adjuvant beta-ray therapy was given within 24 hours after complete surgical excision of primary or recurrent pterygia in 690 patients. The source was calibrated by the National Bureau of Standards, and the regimen was 60 Gy in 6 weekly fractions of 10 Gy. At a median follow-up time of greater than 8 years, the recurrence rate was 1.7%, with most of the recurrences occurring in patients who received fewer than five of the prescribed fractions. No major late complications were reported with this regimen.

MALIGNANT ORBITAL DISEASES

Basal and squamous cell carcinoma and melanoma of the eyelids have a natural history similar to that of their counterparts in other skin locations. Therefore these neoplasms are discussed in the chapter on the skin (Chapter 5).

Ocular Melanoma

The most common primary malignant tumor of the eye is melanoma. Like its cutaneous counterpart, ocular melanoma originates from melanocytes derived from neural crest tissue. However, ocular melanomas are not related to sun exposure.[53] Melanomas of the uveal tract (iris, ciliary body, and choroid) are 20 to 40 times more common than those of the conjunctiva.

Uveal Melanoma

Although melanoma is the most common primary malignant tumor of the eye, the overall incidence of uveal melanoma is only five to seven cases per million people per year.[53] The average age at diagnosis is 55 years.[54] Tumors of the posterior uvea account for more than 90% of cases, with the majority being choroidal melanomas. In the past the misdiagnosis rate was high because of the difficulties in obtaining biopsy material. With the emergence of ancillary investigations such as fluorescein angiography, sonography, color Doppler imaging, phosphorus-32 uptake testing, CT, and magnetic resonance imaging (MRI), the error rate has been reduced to less than 1%, as reported by the multicenter Collaborative Ocular Melanoma Study (COMS).[55] Prognostic factors include age, cell type, tumor size, tumor location, integrity of Bruch's membrane (the lamina between the choriocapillaris and the pigmented layer of the retina), scleral invasion, and pigmentation.[56] As reflected by the American Joint Committee on Cancer staging system (Box 12-1),[57] tumor size seems to be the most important prognostic factor, with tumor dimension greater than 10 mm conferring a poor prognosis.

BOX 12-1   American Joint Committee on Cancer Tumor (T) Staging System for Choroidal Melanomas

TX	Primary tumor cannot be assessed
T0	No evidence of primary tumor
T1*	Tumor 10 mm or less in greatest dimension with an elevation 3 mm or less

    T1a Tumor 7 mm or less in greatest dimension with an elevation of 2 mm or less

    T1b Tumor more than 7 mm but not more than 10 mm in greatest dimension with an elevation of more than 2 mm but not more than 3 mm

T2*	Tumor more than 10 mm but not more than 15 mm in greatest dimension with an elevation of more than 3 mm but not more than 5 mm
T3*	Tumor more than 15 mm in greatest dimension or with an elevation of more than 5 mm
T4	Tumor with extraocular extension

When dimension and elevation show a difference in classification, the highest category should be used for classification.

From Fleming I, Cooper JS, Henson DE, et al, eds. *AJCC Cancer Staging Manual.* 5th ed. Philadelphia, Pa: Lippincott Williams & Wilkins; 1997:267.

*In clinical practice the tumor base may be estimated in optic disc diameters (dd) (average: 1 dd = 1.5 mm). The elevation may be estimated in diopters (average: 3 diopters = 1 mm). Other techniques used, such as ultrasonography and computerized stereometry, may provide a more accurate measurement.

For many years, all patients with uveal melanoma underwent enucleation; thus little is known about the natural history of this disease. Most tumors arise from the pigmented cells in the choroid. Tumor spread is mainly local. With inward growth, the tumor may displace the retina or rupture Bruch's membrane and spread over the retinal surface. Outward growth of the tumor may lead to extrascleral infiltration of tumor into orbital soft tissues. Anterior choroidal and ciliary-body tumors may involve the lens and seed the posterior chamber.[6,58,59]

Because the uvea has no lymphatic drainage, metastasis occurs by hematogenous routes. The overall metastasis rate is approximately 50%, and metastases have a particular predilection for the liver. Doubling times range from a few months to several years. Sato and colleagues[60] reported that the median time from treatment to systemic metastasis was 20 months for the group with the most unfavorable prognosis (age >60, male, tumor diameter >10 mm), in contrast with 76 months for the group with the most favorable prognosis (age ≤60, female, diameter ≤10 mm).

The traditional practice of enucleation of the involved eye was questioned in the 1970s by Zimmerman and colleagues,[61,62] who suggested that enucleation may worsen prognosis by promoting metastasis caused by dissemination of tumor cells during the surgical procedure. Although this theory has been questioned by others[63-65] and the best treatment remains elusive, the trend at many centers has shifted toward more conservative treatment and preserving visual acuity when possible. Shields and Shields[66] reserved enucleation for large melanomas (>10 mm in thickness and >15 mm in diameter), treatment of which with radiation therapy would be expected to cause considerable visual morbidity. However, if the melanoma is located in the patient's only useful eye, it is reasonable to attempt control with radiation therapy despite the expected poor visual outcome.

A variety of radiation therapy techniques are used for conservative management of uveal melanoma, including plaque therapy with ^{222}Rn, ^{198}Au, ^{60}Co, ^{192}Ir, ^{182}Ta, ^{125}I, and ^{106}Ru. In the United States, ^{125}I has become widely used because its lower energy allows less shielding of normal tissues and medical personnel without compromising the dose distribution in the target volume.[67]

Because of the continued controversies regarding the relative indications for enucleation and radiation therapy, the multicenter COMS[68] in the United States and Canada was launched in 1986. Patients with medium-sized tumors (2.5 to 10 mm in apical height and ≤ 16 mm in basal diameter) were randomly assigned to treatment with ^{125}I brachytherapy or enucleation. The COMS trial uses ^{125}I plaques, the size of which is chosen to cover the tumor base (defined to include all pigmented areas) plus a margin of 2 to 3 mm. Tumors contiguous with the optic disc are excluded because vision would be compromised because of radiation damage to the optic nerve. A dose of 100 Gy is delivered at a rate of 0.5 to 1.25 Gy/hr. Accrual ended in July 1998, and follow-up is expected to continue for up to 10 more years.[69]

In the absence of prospective data, Augsburger and colleagues[70] in Philadelphia have published their results extensively. In a recent matched-pair analysis of 448 patients (from an original group of 734 patients), the 15-year survival rates were 57% in the enucleation group and 62% in the plaque-radiation-therapy group.[70] The 15-year local relapse rate was 18.9% with plaque radiation therapy. Although the study did not have sufficient power to show a small difference in survival, a large difference in survival between the treatment groups would be unlikely.

A second COMS randomized trial compared enucleation with and without preoperative external-beam radiation therapy (20 Gy in five daily fractions) for patients with large tumors (>10 mm in apical height or >16 mm in basal diameter). Mortality findings were published in 1998.[71] With 5-year results known for 80% of enrolled patients, pre-enucleation radiation therapy did not yield a statistically significant improvement in survival. The estimated 5-year survival rates were 57% for enucleation alone and 62% for pre-enucleation radiation therapy. Serious complications were infrequent and were not increased with pre-enucleation radiation.[72] So far, routine preoperative irradiation does not seem to have a role in the treatment of large uveal melanomas.

Particle beam therapy has emerged as an alternative to brachytherapy. By taking advantage of the Bragg peak effect (see Chapter 1), particle beam therapy has been refined so as to deposit radiation in the target while limiting the dose to noninvolved structures. Results achieved with proton beam therapy are promising; a group at the Massachusetts General Hospital reported local control rates of more than 95% and eye retention rates of 97% for small tumors and 78% for large tumors.[73] Retrospective comparison with enucleation has not shown a compromise in survival with proton beam therapy.[74,75] Fractionated stereotactic radiation therapy also has been used, and preliminary results are encouraging.[76,77]

Conjunctival Melanoma

Conjunctival melanomas are rare, accounting for 2% of ocular melanomas. These tumors are treated with local excision or cryotherapy. The role of radiation therapy in this disease is unclear.[78]

Orbital Lymphomas

Primary non-Hodgkin's lymphoma of the orbit is a rare disease, accounting for 1% of cases of non-Hodgkin's lymphoma[79] and 10% of all orbital tumors.[80] Primary non-Hodgkin's lymphomas of the orbit are distinct from intraocular lymphomas involving the vitreous humor, retina, or choroid, which have a high rate of central nervous system involvement.[81] Usually arising from the conjunctiva, non-Hodgkin's lymphomas of the orbit present as a smooth, shiny, salmon-colored swelling, which often is asymptomatic.[79] Retrobulbar lesions restrict extraocular movement and cause exophthalmos, diplopia, edema, chemosis, and pain. Vision is usually preserved. In addition to using CT or MRI to evaluate the local disease extent, diagnostic evaluation should include the ancillary evaluations typically done in patients with lymphoma (e.g., bone marrow biopsies and CT scanning of the chest, abdomen, and pelvis) to evaluate the systemic extent of disease.

Treatment selection depends on the pathologic subtype and disease stage. Radiation therapy alone is an accepted treatment for low-grade lymphomas confined to the orbit. Because high-grade lymphomas are associated with high distant relapse rates (60%),[82,83] treatment usually consists of initial chemotherapy followed by consolidative irradiation. Several reports have shown that local control rates with radiation doses of 25 to 40 Gy given in the 1.5- to 2.0-Gy fractions typical for lymphoma are excellent (90% to 100%).[82-85] In the M.D. Anderson Cancer Center series, none of the patients with low-grade lymphomas treated with 30 Gy in 20 fractions had a local relapse.[85] For high-grade lesions, we recommend initial chemotherapy followed by 30 Gy in 20 fractions if there is a complete response to chemotherapy or 36.0 to 39.6 Gy in 20 to 22 fractions if there is a partial response.

Electron beam therapy, typically 6 to 9 MeV with a 0.5- to 1.0-cm bolus, is adequate for anterior lesions involving the eyelid or conjunctiva. A lens or eye shield can be used if its use does not compromise tumor coverage. For eyelid tumors, commercial lead eye shields, 1.7 mm thick, provide inadequate protection for electron beam energies of 6 MeV or greater, with 50% dose transmission on the surface (cornea) and 27% dose transmission at a depth of 6 mm (lens).[86] In place of lead, we use a tungsten eye shield, 3 mm thick, which reduces the transmission dose to the cornea and lens to less than 5% for 6- to 9-MeV electrons (Fig. 12-4).[87] Conjunctival tumors require irradiation of both the palpebral and bulbar conjunctiva. In these cases the lens may be protected by using a suspended lead eye bar as outlined earlier in the chapter in the section on "Orbital Pseudotumor." With this technique, it is essential that the patient fix his or her gaze on the block while the treatment beam is on. However, we prefer to mount the block on a contact lens so that the shielding is placed directly over the lens and cornea (Fig. 12-5). The dose to the cornea with this technique has been calculated to be approximately 5% of the total dose. Posterior lesions usually require treatment with photon beams to achieve sufficiently deep dose distribution.

METASTASIS TO THE ORBIT

Although metastasis to the orbit is uncommon, metastatic tumors are the most common intraocular malignancy. Metastases to the orbit most often originate from primary breast carcinoma or lung cancer.[86,88-90] Given the increasing survival times of cancer patients, the incidence of orbital metastasis can be expected to increase as well. Metastases to the eye can involve any orbital structure. Intraocular metastases are typically located in the choroid. Presenting symptoms include decreased vision, exophthalmos, pain, heaviness, and double vision. Ophthalmoscopic examination often reveals retinal detachment.[90] CT or MRI delineates the extent of the metastatic deposit.

9-MeV Electron beam

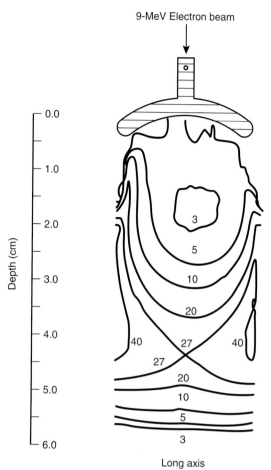

Fig. 12-4 Isodose distribution beneath a tungsten eye shield for a 9-MeV electron beam from a linear accelerator. (Redrawn from Block R, Gartner S. *Arch Ophthalmol* 1971;85:673-675.)

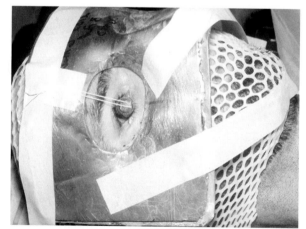

Fig. 12-5 Field set-up for an anteriorly located orbital lymphoma treated with an electron beam with shielding of the lens and cornea through use of a brass shield mounted on a contact lens.

In most cases, a history of prior malignancy, multiple lesions in one eye, or bilateral tumors establishes the diagnosis. In other cases, metastatic choroid tumors can be differentiated from other tumors—mainly choroidal

melanomas, benign lesions such as hemangiomas, and inflammatory granulomas[91]—by using ancillary studies as described earlier in the chapter in the section on "Uveal Melanoma." Bilateral involvement is found in 20% to 25% of cases.[89,90] The initial evaluation should include MRI of the brain because synchronous brain metastases are infrequently found.

Unilateral radiation therapy with a lateral electron portal of sufficient energy is adequate. The anterior border should be placed just behind the anterior chamber of the eye, and a posterior tilt should be placed to avoid the lens. For bilateral metastases, posteriorly tilted opposing photon fields can be used.

Radiation therapy is very effective in relieving symptoms and controlling tumor growth. With doses of at least 30 Gy in daily fractions of 2 to 3 Gy, symptomatic improvement and tumor control are seen in approximately 90% of patients.[90,92] Doses less than 30 Gy may be less effective. In a report by Maor and colleagues,[92] none of the nine patients who received 30 Gy in 10 fractions had tumor regrowth after therapy. In contrast, 2 of 10 patients treated with 25 Gy in 10 fractions had tumor regrowth. In a series reported by Reddy and colleagues,[89] 30% of patients treated with doses of 21 to 30 Gy had no response. The median survival time after detection of choroidal metastases is 8.5 to 12 months, and, in most patients, the benefit in vision produced by radiation therapy lasts for the remainder of their lives.

REFERENCES

1. Saude T. The outer coats of the eye. In: Saude T, ed. *Ocular Anatomy and Physiology.* Oxford, England: Blackwell Science; 1993:11-25.
2. Bron AJ, Tripathi RC, Tripathi BJ. *Wolff's Anatomy of the Eye and Orbit.* 8th ed. London, England: Arnold; 1997.
3. Karlsson U, Kirby T, Orrison W, et al. Ocular globe topography in radiotherapy. *Int J Radiat Oncol Biol Phys* 1995;33:705-712.
4. Rohrschneider W. Experimentelle Untersuchungen uber die Veranderungen normaler Augengewebe nach Rontgenbestrahlung. III. Mitteilung. Beranderungen der Linse der Netzhaut und des Sehnerven nach Rontgenbestrahlung. *Graefes Arch Ophthal* 1929;122:282.
5. Fajardo LF, Berthrong M, Anderson RE. Eye and its adnexa. In: *Radiation Pathology.* New York, NY: Oxford University Press; 2001:399-408.
6. Hungerford J. Current management of choroidal malignant melanoma. *Br J Hosp Med* 1985;34:287-293.
7. Brady L, Shields J, Augusburger J, et al. Complications from radiation therapy to the eye. *Front Radiat Ther Oncol* 1989;23:238-250.
8. Parsons J, Bova FJ, Fitzgerald CR, et al. Severe dry-eye syndrome following external beam irradiation. *Int J Radiat Oncol Biol Phys* 1994;30:775-780.
9. Merriam G, Szechter A, Focht E. The effects of ionizing radiations on the eye. In: Vaeth JM, ed. *Radiation Effect and Tolerance, Normal Tissue.* Baltimore, Md: University Park Press; 1972:346-385.
10. Chan R, Shukovsky L. Effects of irradiation on the eye. *Radiology* 1976;120:673-675.
11. Bessell E, Henk JM, Whitelocke RA, et al. Ocular morbidity after radiotherapy of orbital and conjunctival lymphoma. *Eye* 1987;1:90-96.

12. Merriam G. Late effects of beta radiation on the eye. *Arch Ophthalmol* 1955;53:708.

13. Merriam G. The effects of β-radiation on the eye. *Radiology* 1956; 66:240.

14. Jiang G, Tucker SL, Guttenberger R, et al. Radiation-induced injury to the visual pathway. *Radiother Oncol* 1994;30:17-25.

15. Hall EJ. Radiation cataractogenesis. In: Hall EJ, ed. *Radiobiology for the Radiologist.* Philadelphia, Pa: Lippincott; 1994:379-384.

16. Archer D. Doyne lecture: responses of retinal and choroidal vessels to ionizing radiation. *Eye* 1993;7:1-13.

17. Brown G, Shields JA, Sanborn G, et al. Radiation retinopathy. *Ophthalmology* 1982;89:1494-1501.

18. Parsons J, Bova FJ, Fitzgerald CR, et al. Radiation retinopathy after external-beam irradiation: analysis of time-dose factors. *Int J Radiat Oncol Biol Phys* 1994;30:765-773.

19. Dhir S, Joshi A, Banerjee A. Radiation retinopathy in diabetes mellitus. *Acta Radiol Oncol* 1982;21:111-113.

20. Mewis L, Tang R, Salmonsen P. Radiation retinopathy after "safe" levels of irradiation. *Invest Ophthalmol Vis Sci* 1982;22:222.

21. Viebahn M, Barricks M, Osterloh M. Synergism between diabetic and radiation retinopathy: case report and review. *Br J Ophthalmol* 1991;75:629-632.

22. Parsons J, Bova FJ, Fitzgerald CR, et al. Radiation optic neuropathy after megavoltage external-beam irradiation: analysis of time-dose factors. *Int J Radiat Oncol Biol Phys* 1994;30:755-763.

23. Wartofsky L. Diseases of the thyroid. In: Isselbacher KJ, Braunwald E, Wilson JD, et al., eds. *Harrison's Principles of Internal Medicine.* 13th ed. New York, NY: McGraw-Hill; 1994:1930-1953.

24. Olivotto I, Ludgate CM, Allen LH, et al. Supervoltage radiotherapy for Graves' ophthalmopathy: CCABC technique and results. *Int J Radiat Oncol Biol Phys* 1985;11:2085-2090.

25. Donaldson S, McDougall I, Kriss J. Grave's disease. In: Alberti WE, Sagerman RH, eds. *Medical Radiology: Radiotherapy of Intraocular and Orbital Tumors.* Berlin, Germany: Springer-Verlag; 1993:192-197.

26. Palmer D, Greenberg P, Cornell P, et al. Radiation therapy for Graves' ophthalmopathy: a retrospective analysis. *Int J Radiat Oncol Biol Phys* 1987;13:1815-1820.

27. Petersen I, Kriss JP, McDougall IR, et al. Prognostic factors in the radiotherapy of Graves' ophthalmopathy. *Int J Radiat Oncol Biol Phys* 1990;19:259-264.

28. Marcocci C, Bartalena L, Bogazzi F, et al. Orbital radiotherapy combined with high dose systemic glucocorticoids for Graves' ophthalmopathy is more effective than radiotherapy alone: results of a prospective randomized study. *J Endocrinol Invest* 1991;14:853-860.

29. Prummel M, Mourits MP, Blank L, et al. Randomised double-blind trial of prednisone versus radiotherapy in Graves' ophthalmopathy. *Lancet* 1993;342:949-954.

30. Bartalena L, Marcocci C, Chiovato L, et al. Orbital cobalt irradiation combined with systemic corticosteroids for Graves' ophthalmopathy: comparison with systemic corticosteroids alone. *J Clin Endocrinol Metab* 1983;56:1139-1144.

31. Snijders-Keilholz A, De Keizer RJ, Goslings BM, et al. Probable risk of tumour induction after retro-orbital irradiation for Graves' ophthalmopathy. *Radiother Oncol* 1996;38:67-71.

32. Blank L, Barendsen GW, Prummel MF, et al. Probable risk of tumour induction after retro-orbital irradiation for Graves' ophthalmopathy [letter]. *Radiother Oncol* 1996;40:187-188.

33. Dutton J. Orbital diseases. In: Yanoff M, Duker JS, eds. *Ophthalmology.* London, England: Mosby; 1999:7.14.1-7.14.18.

34. Char D, Miller T. Orbital pseudotumor. Fine needle aspiration biopsy and response to therapy. *Ophthalmology* 1993;100: 1702-1710.

35. Kennerdell J, Dresner S. The nonspecific orbital inflammatory syndromes. *Surv Ophthalmol* 1984;29:93-103.

36. Leone C, Lloyd W. Treatment protocol for orbital inflammatory disease. *Ophthalmology* 1985;92:1325-1331.

37. Sergott R, Glaser J, Charyulu K. Radiotherapy for idiopathic inflammatory orbital pseudotumor. *Arch Ophthalmol* 1981;99: 853-856.

38. Orcutt J, Garner A, Henk JM, et al. Treatment of idiopathic inflammatory orbital pseudotumours by radiotherapy. *Br J Ophthalmol* 1983;67:570-574.

39. Gunalp I, Gunduz K, Yazar Z. Idiopathic orbital inflammatory disease. *Acta Ophthalmol Scand* 1996;74:191-193.

40. Donaldson S, Findley D. Treatment of orbital lymphoid tumors with electron beams. *Front Radiat Ther Oncol* 1991;25:187-200.

41. Sugar A. Conjunctival and corneal degenerations. In: Yanoff M, Duker JS, eds. *Ophthalmology.* London: Mosby; 1999:5.6.1-5.6.8.

42. Cameron M. *Pterygium Throughout the World.* Springfield, Ill: Charles C. Thomas; 1965.

43. Bahrassa F, Datta R. Postoperative beta radiation treatment of pterygium. *Int J Radiat Oncol Biol Phys* 1983;9:679-684.

44. Hirst L, Sebban A, Chant D. Pterygium recurrence time. *Ophthalmology* 1994;101:755-758.

45. Van Den Brenk H. Results of prophylactic postoperative irradiation in 1,300 cases of pterygium. *Am J Roentgenol* 1968;103:723-733.

46. Wilder R, Buatti JM, Kittelson JM, et al. Pterygium treated with excision and postoperative beta irradiation. *Int J Radiat Oncol Biol Phys* 1992;23:533-537.

47. Paryani S, Scott WP, Wells JW, et al. Management of pterygium with surgery and radiation therapy. *Int J Radiat Oncol Biol Phys* 1994;28:101-103.

48. Alaniz-Camino F. The use of postoperative beta radiation in the treatment of pterygium. *Ophthalmic Surg* 1982;13:1022-1025.

49. MacKenzie F, Hirst LW, Kynaston B, et al. Recurrence rate and complications after beta irradiation for pterygia. *Ophthalmology* 1991;8:1776-1781.

50. Moriarty A, Crawford GJ, McAllister IL, et al. Severe corneoscleral infection: a complication of beta irradiation scleral necrosis following pterygium necrosis. *Arch Ophthalmol* 1993;111: 947-951.

51. Dusenbery K, Alul IH, Holland EJ, et al. β-irradiation of recurrent pterygia: results and complications. *Int J Radiat Oncol Biol Phys* 1992;24:315-320.

52. Goetsch S. Strontium-90 ophthalmic applicators: use with caution [letter]. *Ophthalmic Surg* 1988;19:827-828.

53. Scotto J, Fraumeni JJ, Lee J. Melanomas of the eye and non-cutaneous sites: epidemiologic aspects. *J Natl Cancer Inst* 1976;56: 489-491.

54. Egan K, Seddon JM, Glynn RJ, et al. Epidemiological aspects of uveal melanoma. *Surv Ophthalmol* 1988;32:239-251.

55. Collaborative Ocular Melanoma Study Group. Accuracy of diagnosis of choroidal melanoma in the Collaborative Ocular Melanoma Study: COMS report no. 1. *Arch Ophthalmol* 1990;108:1268-1273.

56. Shammas H, Blodi F. Prognostic factors in choroidal and ciliary body melanomas. *Arch Ophthalmol* 1977;95:63-69.

57. Fleming I, Cooper JS, Henson DE, et al, eds. *AJCC Cancer Staging Manual.* 5th ed. Philadelphia, Pa: Lippincott Williams & Wilkins; 1997:267.

58. Moss W. The orbit. In: Cox JD, ed. *Moss' Radiation Oncology: Rationale, Technique, Results.* 7th ed. St. Louis, Mo: Mosby; 1994:246-259.

59. Sahel J, Earle J, Albert D. Intraocular melanomas. In: DeVita VT Jr, Hellman S, Rosenberg SA, eds. *Cancer: Principles and Practice of Oncology.* 4th ed. Philadelphia, Pa: JB Lippincott; 1993:1662.

60. Sato T, Babazono A, Shields JA, et al. Time to systemic metastases in patients with posterior uveal melanoma. *Cancer Invest* 1997;15:98-105.

61. Zimmerman L, McLean I. Changing concepts concerning the malignancy of ocular tumors. *Arch Ophthalmol* 1975;78:487-494.

62. Zimmerman L, McLean I, Foster W. Does enucleation of the eye containing a malignant melanoma prevent or accelerate the

dissemination of tumour cells? *Br J Ophthalmol* 1978;62: 420-425.

63. Seigel D, Myers M, Ferris F, et al. Survival rates after enucleation of eyes with malignant melanoma. *Am J Ophthalmol* 1979;87: 761-765.

64. Manschot W, van Peperzeel H. Choroidal melanoma: enucleation or observation? A new approach. *Arch Ophthalmol* 1980;98:71-77.

65. Manschot W, Van Strik R. Is irradiation a justifiable treatment of choroidal melanoma? Analysis of published results. *Br J Ophthalmol* 1987;71:348-352.

66. Shields J, Shields C. Management of posterior uveal melanoma. In: Shields JA, Shields CL, eds. *Intraocular Tumors: A Textbook and Atlas.* Philadelphia, Pa: WB Saunders; 1992:171-205.

67. Earle J, Kline R, Robertson D. Selection of iodine 125 for the Collaborative Ocular Melanoma Study. *Arch Ophthalmol* 1987;105:763-764.

68. Collaborative Ocular Melanoma Study Group. *COMS Manual of Procedures.* Springfield, Va: National Technical Information Service; 1995.

69. Earle JFTC. Results from the Collaborative Ocular Melanoma Study (COMS) of enucleation versus preoperative radiation therapy in the management of large ocular melanomas. *Int J Radiat Oncol Biol Phys* 1999;43:1168-1169.

70. Augsburger J, Schneider S, Freire J, et al. Survival following enucleation versus plaque radiotherapy in statistically matched subgroups of patients with choroidal melanomas: results in patients treated between 1980 and 1987. *Graefes Arch Clin Exp Ophthalmol* 1999;237:558-567.

71. Collaborative Ocular Melanoma Study Group. The Collaborative Ocular Melanoma Study (COMS) randomized trial of pre-enucleation radiation of large choroidal melanoma II: initial mortality findings. COMS report no. 10. *Am J Ophthalmol* 1998;125:779-796.

72. Collaborative Ocular Melanoma Study Group. The Collaborative Ocular Melanoma Study (COMS) randomized trial of pre-enucleation radiation of large choroidal melanoma III: local complications and observations following enucleation. COMS report no. 11. *Am J Ophthalmol* 1998;126:362-372.

73. Munzenrider J. Proton therapy for uveal melanomas and other eye lesions. *Strahlenther Onkol* 1999;175(suppl 2):68-73.

74. Seddon J, Gragoudas ES, Albert DM, et al. Comparison of survival rates for patients with uveal melanoma after treatment with proton beam irradiation or enucleation. *Am J Ophthalmol* 1985;99:282-290.

75. Seddon J, Gragoudas ES, Egan KM, et al. Relative survival rates after alternative therapies for uveal melanoma. *Ophthalmology* 1990;97:769-777.

76. Tokuuye K, Akine Y, Sumi M, et al. Fractionated stereotactic radiotherapy for choroidal melanoma. *Radiother Oncol* 1997;43: 87-91.

77. Zehetmayer M, Dieckmann K, Kren G, et al. Fractionated stereotactic radiotherapy with linear accelerator for uveal melanoma—preliminary Vienna results. *Strahlenther Onkol* 1999;175(suppl 2): 74-75.

78. Rennie I. Diagnosis and treatment of ocular melanomas. *Br J Hosp Med* 1991;46:144-156.

79. Fitzpatrick P, Macko S. Lymphoreticular tumors of the orbit. *Int J Radiat Oncol Biol Phys* 1984;10:333-340.

80. Reese A. Orbital neoplasms and lesions simulating them. In: Hoeber PB, ed. *Tumours of the Eye.* New York, NY: Harper & Row; 1976:434-440.

81. Char D, Ljung BM, Miller T, et al. Primary intraocular lymphoma (ocular reticulum cell sarcoma) diagnosis and management. *Ophthalmology* 1988;95:625-630.

82. Bessell E, Henk JM, Wright JE, et al. Orbital and conjunctival lymphoma treatment and prognosis. *Radiother Oncol* 1988;13: 237-244.

83. Bolek T, Moyses HM, Marcus RB, et al. Radiotherapy in the management of orbital lymphoma. *Int J Radiat Oncol Biol Phys* 1999; 44:31-36.

84. Smitt M, Donaldson S. Radiotherapy is successful treatment for orbital lymphoma. *Int J Radiat Oncol Biol Phys* 1993;26:59-66.

85. Pelloski CE, Wilder RB, Ha CS, et al. Clinical stage IEA-IIEA orbital lymphomas: outcomes in the era of modern staging and treatment. *Radiother Oncol* 2001;59:145-151.

86. Shiu A, Tung SS, Gastorf RJ, et al. Dosimetric evaluation of lead and tungsten eye shields in electron beam treatment. *Int J Radiat Oncol Biol Phys* 1996;35:599-604.

87. Block R, Gartner S. The incidence of ocular metastatic carcinoma. *Arch Ophthalmol* 1971;85:673-675.

88. Ferry A, Font R. Carcinoma metastatic to the eye and orbit I. A clinicopathologic study of 227 cases. *Arch Ophthalmol* 1974;92: 276-286.

89. Reddy S, Saxena VS, Hendrickson F, et al. Malignant metastatic disease of the eye: management of an uncommon complication. *Cancer* 1981;47:810-812.

90. Glassburn J, Klionsky M, Brady L. Radiation therapy for metastatic disease involving the orbit. *Am J Clin Oncol* 1984;7:145-148.

91. Gragoudas E. Current treatment of metastatic choroidal tumors. *Oncology* 1989;3:103-110.

92. Maor M, Chan R, Yound S. Radiotherapy of choroidal metastases. *Cancer* 1977;40:2081-2086.

CHAPTER 13

The Temporal Bone, Ear, and Paraganglia

David H. Hussey and B-Chen Wen

Primary tumors of the ear are rare, and consequently they are seen only infrequently in most radiation oncology practices. Nevertheless, these tumors deserve special consideration because they involve an important sensory organ and lie close to critical structures, such as the dura mater, brain, cranial nerves, carotid artery, temporomandibular joint, and parotid gland. Any of these structures may be invaded by tumors of the ear. Furthermore, the functions of the ear—hearing and balance—can be disturbed by either cancer or treatment of cancer.

ANATOMY

Anatomists divide the ear into three parts—the outer ear, the middle ear, and the inner ear. The outer ear comprises the auricle and the external auditory canal (EAC) (Fig. 13-1). The EAC extends from the auricle laterally to the tympanic membrane medially and is approximately 2.5 cm long. The EAC has a cartilaginous lateral portion and a bony medial portion. The cartilaginous portion is pierced by fissures through which tumors can spread anteriorly into the temporomandibular joint or the parotid gland. The EAC is lined with skin that is closely adherent to the perichondrium and periosteum. The lymphatic drainage of the auricle and the EAC is to the preauricular, postauricular, and subdigastric lymph nodes.

The middle ear is composed of the tympanic cavity, the eustachian tube, and the mastoid process of the temporal bone. The tympanic cavity is an air-containing chamber lined with predominantly squamous epithelium and bounded by the tympanic membrane laterally and the osseous labyrinth medially. The tympanic cavity contains the auditory ossicles (the malleus, incus, and stapes), the tensor muscle of the tympanum, the stapedius muscle, and the chorda tympani nerve. The tympanic cavity communicates posteriorly with the tympanic antrum and mastoid air cells. It is continuous anteromedially with the eustachian tube, which opens into the nasopharynx. The eustachian tube is approximately 3.5 cm long. It is lined with pseudostratified ciliated columnar epithelium. Nodal metastasis is uncommon for tumors of the middle ear, suggesting that this region has few lymphatics.

The inner ear comprises the osseous labyrinth, which is a series of cavities in the dense petrous part of the temporal bone, and the membranous labyrinth, which is an intricate series of membranous ducts suspended within the osseous labyrinth. The labyrinthine system has three parts—the cochlea, the vestibule (which contains the utricle and saccule), and the semicircular canals. Each of these structures has a specific function. The cochlea is responsible for sound detection, the utricle is responsible for static equilibrium, and the three semicircular canals are responsible for dynamic equilibrium.

The cochlea is a spiral chamber surrounding a central hollow post, called the *modiolus*, through which passes the cochlear nerve (see Fig. 13-1, *B*). This chamber is divided into three parts by the thin bony spiral lamina, the basilar membrane, and the vestibular membrane. Upon the basilar membrane lies the organ of Corti (spiral organ). The organ of Corti contains hair cells that make synaptic contact with the auditory nerve fibers. It is the structure that is responsible for converting fluid waves to nerve impulses.

The tympanic membrane vibrates when it receives sound waves, and this vibration is transmitted through the chain of ossicles to the oval window. Vibration of the footplate of the stapes covering the oval window produces traveling waves within the perilymph. These traveling waves cause the basilar membrane to oscillate, leading to deformity of the hair cells of the organ of Corti. When the hair cells are deformed, the nerve endings are stimulated, producing nerve impulses that are transmitted to the brain by the eighth cranial nerve.

RESPONSE OF THE NORMAL EAR TO IRRADIATION
Outer Ear

The skin of the outer ear responds to irradiation in a fashion similar to that of the skin in other parts of the body. However, skin reactions in the auricle tend to be more severe than skin reactions elsewhere in the body

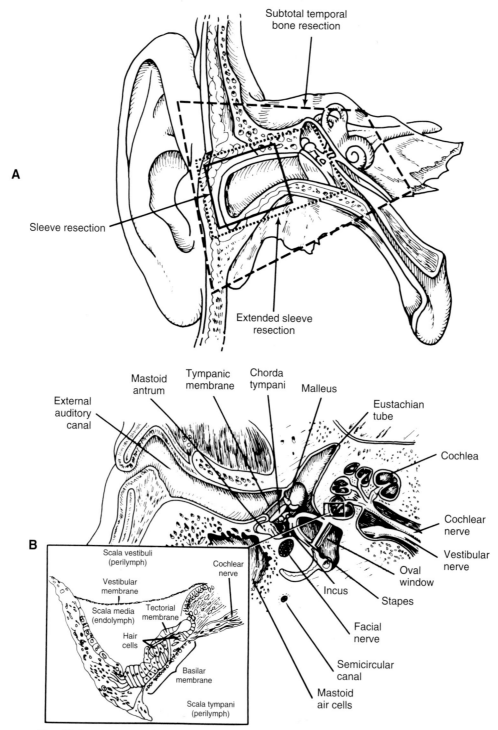

Fig. 13-1   Anatomy of the ear and related structures. **A,** Oblique coronal view. **B,** Axial view. The organ of Corti is shown in detail.

because the auricle has an irregular surface, which interferes with skin sparing, and has been sensitized by years of exposure to the sun. The most severe skin reactions are usually seen on the dorsum of the helix and in the sulci, where skin sparing is most impaired.

The EAC commonly develops a moist desquamation during radiation therapy, and this can lead to considerable drainage or bleeding. Depression of ceruminous gland function usually occurs, and late reactions such as stenosis and even necrosis have been reported. However, these changes are uncommon and are usually associated with extensive tumors or prior surgery.[1]

Chondronecrosis is rare after fractionated megavoltage irradiation. When this side effect does occur, it usually appears within the first year after treatment.[2] However, it may develop years later if the tissues are challenged by subsequent trauma. As with bone necrosis in the oral cavity, chondronecrosis usually occurs as a result of an overlying soft tissue necrosis.

Middle Ear

Serous otitis media may develop after radiation therapy for cancer in the vicinity of the ear. This side effect is thought to be caused by swelling of the mucosa that leads to obstruction of the eustachian tube and transudation of a sterile serous fluid.[3] Serous otitis media is characterized clinically by ear discomfort, a sensation of fullness in the ear, a conductive hearing loss, and occasional tinnitus. This complication usually resolves with the administration of nasal decongestants but sometimes necessitates a myringotomy.

The incidence of serous otitis media caused solely by irradiation is not clearly established, but this side effect has been reported in 15% to 50% of cases in some series.[4,5] Many of these cases are the result of obstruction of the eustachian tube resulting from tumor or prior surgery.[6]

In general, the ossicles tolerate radiation therapy well, and necrosis of the ossicular chain after conventionally fractionated radiation therapy is very rare. However, at least one case of osteoradionecrosis of the ossicles has been reported.[7]

Inner Ear

In the past, sensorineural hearing loss resulting from radiation therapy for head and neck cancer was believed to be very uncommon. However, this side effect is probably more common than previously thought, particularly when high doses have been delivered. Leach[8] reported a 36% incidence of sensorineural hearing loss after fractionated doses of 30 to 80 Gy, and Grau and colleagues[9] found a 29% incidence of this side effect after doses of 29 to 68 Gy. Moretti[10] reported a higher incidence of sensorineural hearing loss (7 of 13 patients) in a small series of patients treated to doses of 60 to 240 Gy for nasopharyngeal cancer. However, these doses are much higher than those usually employed clinically.

A dose-response relationship for radiation-induced sensorineural hearing loss seems to be evident. The threshold for this injury occurs at a dose of approximately 50 to 60 Gy in 5 to 6 weeks. Thibadoux and colleagues[11] found no hearing loss in children with acute leukemia who received prophylactic cranial irradiation to a dose of 24 Gy in 12 fractions. Similarly, Evans and colleagues[12] found no hearing impairment in the irradiated ear compared with the nonirradiated ear in patients with cancer of the parotid gland who received unilateral irradiation to doses of 55 to 60 Gy in 5 to 6 weeks.

However, neither of those studies required baseline studies of auditory function before irradiation. Grau and colleagues[9] tested patients' hearing both before and after irradiation. They found an 8% (1 in 13) incidence of sensorineural hearing loss with fractionated doses up to 50 Gy and a 44% (8 in 18) incidence after doses of 59 Gy or more (Fig. 13-2). These results correlate well with results of animal studies, which showed significant degeneration of the sensory and supporting cells of the organ of Corti and loss of fibers of the eighth nerve after fractionated doses in excess of 60 Gy.[13]

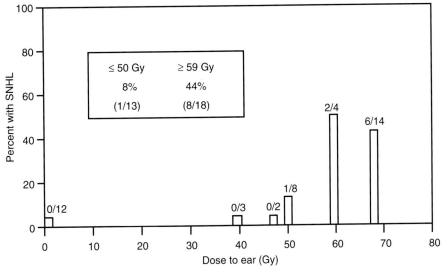

Fig. 13-2 The incidence of sensorineural hearing loss *(SNHL)* as a function of radiation dose delivered to the ear. Only 8% of patients who received a dose of 50 Gy or less developed SNHL, compared with 44% of those who received a dose of 59 Gy or more. (Modified from Grau C, Moller K, Overgaard M, et al. *Int J Radiat Oncol Biol Phys* 1991;21:723-728.)

Drugs such as cisplatin also have ototoxic effects, and the injury is greater in the setting of prior or concurrent irradiation.[14] However, radiation therapy delivered after chemotherapy does not worsen the side effects of chemotherapy. This suggests that the synergistic effect of irradiation may be caused by hyperemia or chemosensitization.[15]

Little is known about the effects of irradiation on vestibular function, but vestibular damage appears to be very rare after conventionally fractionated doses.[16] Moskovskaya[17] reported increased excitability of the labyrinth during irradiation, and Gamble and colleagues[18] found that the endolymphatic spaces of the semicircular canals became distended after large single doses of radiation. However, vestibular damage has not been reported with commonly used fractionated doses.[3,8]

Temporal Bone Necrosis

Necrosis of the temporal bone occurs occasionally after high-dose radiation therapy for cancer of the ear. However, this side effect is rarely seen when the temporal bone is incidentally irradiated during the course of treatment for cancer of other head and neck sites.

Osteoradionecrosis may be confined to the EAC, or it may involve the entire temporal bone diffusely. Focal osteoradionecrosis usually presents as an area of exposed bone that ultimately forms a sequestrum. When necrosis is limited, the healing process may be slow, but the necrosis almost always heals eventually. Diffuse osteoradionecrosis is more difficult to manage. Symptoms of necrosis of the temporal bone include severe boring pain, nausea, vertigo, and otorrhea. An area of exposed or dead bone is usually present, and there may be a fistula extending intracranially or to the skin.

The risk of temporal bone radionecrosis is greater with orthovoltage irradiation than it is with megavoltage irradiation because of differences in the way kilovoltage and megavoltage beams are absorbed by bone. This complication is also more likely to develop if high total doses have been delivered, if the treatment has not been well fractionated, or if there have been focal areas of overdosage such as can occur with poorly designed wedged portal field arrangements. Wang and Doppke[19] reported a 60% incidence of osteoradionecrosis in patients with tumors of the ear who received doses greater than 2000 rets (rad equivalent therapeutics) (70 Gy). This would be approximately 74 Gy at 2 Gy/fraction if the treatment were given in a standard fashion. Other factors that increase the likelihood of temporal bone necrosis include prior surgery and a long history of ear infections.

MALIGNANT TUMORS OF THE EAR

Malignant tumors of the EAC and middle ear are very rare. Only approximately two cases per million people in the United States occur each year.[1] However, the incidence of skin cancer involving the auricle is much greater. In one series,[20] approximately 60% of tumors of the ear originated from the auricle, 28% originated in the EAC, and fewer than 12% were primary tumors of the middle ear.

Tumors of the ear are much more common in the elderly than in the young and are slightly more common in women than in men. In most series, the ratio of EAC and middle-ear neoplasms to benign ear disease is in the range of 1:5000 to 1:20,000; thus most otolaryngologists will see only one or two cases of carcinoma of the ear during their entire career.[21]

Because carcinomas of the ear are uncommon, they are usually diagnosed late in the course of the disease. Many patients are treated for chronic otitis for long periods before cancer is suspected. The location of these tumors—deep within the EAC or in the middle ear—also makes early diagnosis difficult. Consequently, many of these carcinomas are extensive when first diagnosed, and, therefore, the results of treatment in most series are understandably poor.

Pathology

Malignant tumors of the ear are predominantly squamous or basal cell carcinomas. However, the relative incidence of these two histopathologic types differs for various subsites. Approximately 55% of tumors involving the auricle are squamous cell carcinomas, and 45% are basal cell carcinomas,[22] whereas 90% of the tumors involving the EAC and almost all of those involving the middle ear are squamous cell carcinomas. Other tumors that can originate in the ear include melanomas, adenoid cystic carcinomas, adenocarcinomas of the sebaceous and ceruminous glands, Ewing's sarcomas, osteosarcomas, and rhabdomyosarcomas.

Routes of Spread
External Auditory Canal

Basal cell carcinomas of the EAC tend to originate at the entrance of the cartilaginous portion of the canal, whereas squamous cell carcinomas of the EAC may develop anywhere along the canal. Both types of tumors tend to fill the canal before invading the perichondrium or periosteum. Once the cartilage is invaded, however, the tumor can spread anteriorly to the parotid gland or posteriorly into the posterior auricular area. Carcinomas of the bony portion of the canal usually spread longitudinally before infiltrating the middle ear.

Squamous cell carcinomas of the EAC metastasize to regional lymph nodes in 10% to 20% of cases.[23,24] The most common sites of regional metastasis are the preauricular, subdigastric, and postauricular lymph nodes. There are no reports of metastasis from basal cell carcinomas of the EAC.

Middle Ear

Tumors of the middle ear may grow medially along the eustachian tube to the nasopharynx or erode through the wall of the eustachian tube to involve the petrous apex and carotid canal. They may extend posteriorly through the mastoid antrum to the mastoid air cells, ultimately reaching the sigmoid sinus and posterior cranial fossa. The petrous part of the temporal bone resists invasion because it is very dense. However, the roof of the tympanic cavity (tegmen tympani) is thin, and thus access to the middle cranial fossa through this route is relatively easy. Middle-ear tumors also can erode through the floor of the hypotympanum into the tail of the parotid gland or the soft tissues of the upper neck.

Middle-ear tumors often spread to nearby structures by growing along the nerves and blood vessels that course through the temporal bone. Middle-ear tumors may grow along the chorda tympani and the facial nerve to reach the posterior cranial fossa. They also may reach the posterior cranial fossa by eroding through the medial wall of the tympanic cavity and growing along the acoustic nerve. Middle-ear tumors may spread to the middle cranial fossa by growing along the tympanic nerve (Jacobson's nerve) or the lesser superficial petrosal nerve, both of which are branches of cranial nerve IX.

Regional metastasis from middle ear tumors is uncommon in most series, occurring only late in the course of the disease.[1] Boland and Paterson,[25] for example, reported only a 12% (10 of 86) incidence of regional lymph node metastasis from middle-ear tumors.

Presenting Symptoms

Patients with carcinomas of the EAC and the middle ear usually present with granulation tissue and a chronic draining ear or a polypoid mass visible in the EAC. The tympanic membrane is often perforated, and considerable purulent drainage usually occurs. As the disease progresses, the patient may develop facial nerve paralysis, vertigo, tinnitus, or deep boring pain. If the tumor invades the parotid gland or the soft tissues of the neck, it may be palpable as preauricular induration or an upper neck mass.

Clinical Evaluation

Clinical evaluation of patients with tumors of the ear should include careful examination of the auricle, the EAC, and the tympanic membrane. A neurologic examination should be performed to detect facial nerve paralysis or other cranial nerve palsies. The facial nerve may be affected even if the tumor is confined within the temporal bone. However, involvement of cranial nerves IX to XI usually means that the tumor has spread beyond the temporal bone. The patient should be evaluated for trismus, which, if present, indicates the possibility of invasion of the pterygoid muscles or the temporomandibular joint. The neck should be examined for lymphadenopathy, especially in the subdigastric, preauricular, and postauricular areas. Hearing should be tested with a tuning fork, and baseline audiometry should be performed before treatment.

In the past, most tumors of the ear were studied with plain roentgenograms and laminar tomograms of the skull and temporal bone. These studies have been replaced for the most part with high-resolution computed tomography (CT) and magnetic resonance imaging (MRI), which are better able to delineate local tumor extension. Often both studies are necessary. CT is superior for detecting bone erosion, and MRI is better for assessing intracranial extension. Directly acquired coronal CT images (as opposed to reconstructed images) should be obtained for this evaluation, along with standard axial sections.

CT and MRI are usually adequate for assessing the status of the carotid canal and the sigmoid and transverse sinuses. However, carotid angiography with balloon occlusion may be necessary if sacrifice of a carotid artery is being considered.

Staging

The American Joint Committee on Cancer (AJCC) staging system has no specific classification for carcinoma of the ear. However, several staging systems for carcinoma of the ear have been proposed that are based on a variety of prognostic factors.[26,27] The staging system outlined in Table 13-1 is a modification of a classification proposed by Goodwin and Jesse.[26]

In general, carcinomas that are limited to the EAC have a better prognosis than those that involve the middle ear (Table 13-2).[26,28-33] For example, Crabtree and colleagues[28] reported a 91% (20 of 22) survival rate 1 to 5 years after treatment for patients with tumors confined to the EAC. This is much better than the 30% to 40% 5-year survival rates usually reported for patients with tumors involving the middle ear.[30,34,35]

Survival correlates well with the extent of the disease. Goodwin and Jesse,[26] for example, reported absolute 5-year survival rates of 57% for patients with cancer involving the cartilaginous portion of the EAC or the adjacent concha, 45% for patients with tumors involving the bony portion of the EAC or the mastoid cortex, and 29% for patients with tumors involving the deep structures of the temporal bone.

Resectability is one of the most important prognostic indicators. In Goodwin and Jesse's series,[26] 11 (58%) of 19 patients who had complete resection of their middle-ear tumors (T3) had local tumor control, compared with none of 13 patients who had incomplete resection with or without radiation therapy (T4) (Table 13-3).[26]

TABLE 13-1

General Policies for Treatment of Carcinomas of the External, Middle, or Inner Ear

Tumor Extent*	Treatment
T1 Carcinoma of the external auditory canal ± invasion of the cartilaginous portion of the canal or pinna (no involvement of the bony canal or tympanic membrane)	Sleeve resection[†] or local radiation therapy alone
T2 Tumor of the external auditory canal with minimal invasion of the bony canal or extension to tympanic membrane	Extended sleeve resection[†] with or without postoperative radiation therapy, depending on margins
T3 Technically resectable cancer that extends beyond the external auditory canal, including tumors of the middle ear and mastoid	Subtotal temporal bone resection[†] and postoperative radiation therapy
T4 Technically unresectable tumor (extension to apex of petrous bone, cavernous sinus, internal auditory canal, internal carotid artery, middle or posterior cranial fossa, Cl or C2, or base of occiput)	Radiation therapy or no treatment

*Text modified from Goodwin WJ, Jesse RH: *Arch Otolaryngol* 1980;106:675-679.
[†]See Figure 13-3.

TABLE 13-2

Local Control Rates in the Treatment of Carcinoma of the External Auditory Canal and Middle Ear

| Study | LIMITED DISEASE (T1-T2) | | EXTENSIVE DISEASE (T3-T4) | |
	S	S + RT	S	S + RT
Arriaga et al[29]	3 of 4	4 of 9	1 of 2	10 of 20
Hahn et al[30]	3 of 4	2 of 2	1 of 8	4 of 10
Goodwin and Jesse[26]	T1 37 of 56*	—	6 of 13	5 of 19
	T2 5 of 11	5 of 5	—	—
Lesser et al[31]	5 of 7[†]	—	3 of 17[†]	—
Crabtree et al[28]	20 of 22	3 of 3	0 of 5	3 of 9
Wang[32]	—	4 of 4	—	7 of 19
Gacek and Goodman[33]	3 of 3	7 of 8	—	8 of 18
SUBTOTAL	71 of 100 (71%)	30 of 38 (79%)	8 of 28 (29%)	40 of 112 (36%)
TOTAL	101 of 138 (73%)		48 of 140 (34%)	

S, Surgery; *RT*, radiation therapy.
*Includes five patients treated with radiation therapy alone.
[†]Includes nine patients treated with radiation therapy alone.

TABLE 13-3

Comparison of Local Control Rates Achieved with Surgery Alone or Surgery Followed by Irradiation

Stage	Surgery (%)	Surgery + Radiation Therapy (%)	Total (%)
Group I (confined to cartilaginous canal concha—T1)	—	—	37 of 56 (66)*[†]
Group II (involving bony canal or mastoid cortex—T2)	5 of 11 (45)	5 of 5 (100)	10 of 16 (62.5)[†]
Group III (involving middle ear, facial canal, or base of skull—T3 and some T4)			
Complete resection	6 of 13 (46)	5 of 6 (83)	11 of 19 (58)
Incomplete resection	—	0 of 13 (0)	0 of 13 (0)

From Goodwin WJ, Jesse RH. *Arch Otolaryngol* 1980;106:675-679.
*Mainly treated with surgery.
[†]Surgery patients (groups I and II) classified as having persistent local tumor received salvage treatment.

Treatment

Treatment options by stage for carcinomas of the ear are shown in Table 13-1. Patients with small tumors confined to the EAC usually can be treated satisfactorily with a single modality—either surgery or radiation therapy. Patients with larger EAC tumors or tumors originating in the middle ear are usually best treated with combined surgery and radiation therapy. Massive tumors are usually best managed palliatively with radiation therapy, although some patients with massive tumors will not benefit from any form of treatment.

Patients with tumors of the ear should be evaluated for signs of technical inoperability. These include evidence of disease extension to the internal auditory canal, the middle or posterior cranial fossa, the body of the atlas or axis, or the base of the occiput. Tumors of the ear are usually not technically resectable if cranial nerves IX to XI are involved, and, although resection of the carotid artery is technically feasible in some cases, it usually results in undesirable long-term sequelae.[24] Tumor extension to the parotid gland, the ascending ramus of the mandible, or the soft tissues of the upper neck is not a sign of technical unresectability, nor is limited involvement of the dura.[24]

The technical details of radiation therapy for carcinomas of the ear are described in the section on "Radiation Therapy Technique" later in this chapter.

T1 Disease

Tumors confined to the cartilaginous portion of the EAC and adjacent concha without extension to the bony portion of the EAC or tympanic membrane can be treated with either surgery or radiation therapy alone. Surgery for these lesions usually consists of a sleeve resection of the auditory canal, which means removal of a core of skin, cartilage, and possibly some bone (Fig. 13-3). The defect is covered with a split-thickness skin graft. T1 tumors also can be treated with radiation therapy alone. The appropriate radiation dose is determined by the size of the tumor and ranges from 60 Gy in 6½ weeks to 70 Gy in 7 to 7½ weeks.

T2 Disease

Cancer that involves the bony portion of the EAC can be treated with an extended sleeve resection, which consists of removal of a core of skin, cartilage, and bone; the tympanic membrane; and the malleus or incus or both structures. The adjacent mastoid also may be removed (see Fig. 13-3). Postoperative radiation therapy is added if the resection margins are close or positive. The postoperative dose is 60 Gy in 6 to 6½ weeks if the margins are negative and 65 to 70 Gy in 6½ to 7 weeks if residual disease is present.

T3 Disease

If the middle ear is involved, subtotal temporal bone resection (see Fig. 13-3) and postoperative radiation therapy is required. This treatment involves removal of the entire temporal bone en bloc except for the petrous apex. The tumor may have to be dissected off the dura of the middle and posterior cranial fossa, and the ipsilateral sigmoid sinus may have to be sacrificed. This can be accomplished if the contralateral sinus is patent. Tumor extension to the parotid gland, the mandible, or the neck may necessitate a parotidectomy, partial mandibulectomy, or radical neck dissection.

Postoperative radiation therapy is almost always recommended for patients with T3 disease regardless of the resection margins because the local failure rate after treatment with surgery alone is high (see Table 13-3).[26] The radiation therapy doses are determined by the margins of resection, the volume of residual disease, and the tolerance of adjacent normal tissues and usually range from 60 Gy in 6 to 6½ weeks to 70 Gy in 7 to 7½ weeks.

T4 Disease

Patients with technically unresectable tumors of the ear are usually treated with high doses of radiation, although the goal of treatment is often only palliation. The doses are usually in the range of 60 to 70 Gy or greater in 6½ to 7½ weeks.

Radiation Therapy Technique

For temporal bone malignancies, a shrinking field technique is used most often. The initial treatment portals should include all clinically detectable tumor and areas at risk for subclinical disease. If the treatment is being given after surgery, the entire surgical bed must be encompassed in the treatment portals. After 45 to 50 Gy, the fields are reduced to include only the areas of gross tumor involvement with a small margin. Care is taken to limit the dose to critical normal structures, such as the optic chiasm, brainstem, temporal lobe, and spinal cord.

If the tumor is confined to the cartilaginous portion of the EAC, the treatment fields should encompass the EAC with a 2- to 3-cm margin. A variety of field arrangements may be used depending on the clinical situation, including ipsilateral electron beams, mixed electron and photon beams, and wedged photon beams. The electron beam energy should be determined on the basis of the depth of the disease.

Tumors involving the middle ear are usually more advanced, with a larger target volume. Patients with middle-ear tumors may be treated with combined photon and electron beam portals if no bone invasion is present. However, if temporal bone involvement has occurred, wedged photon beams should be used rather

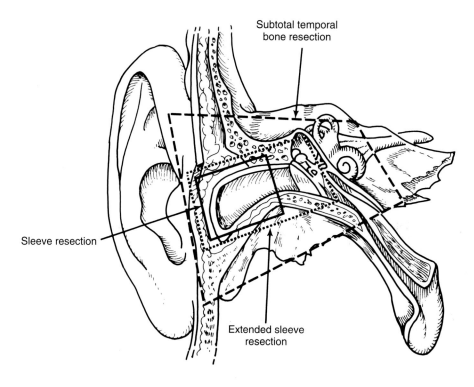

Subtotal temporal bone resection

Sleeve resection

Extended sleeve resection

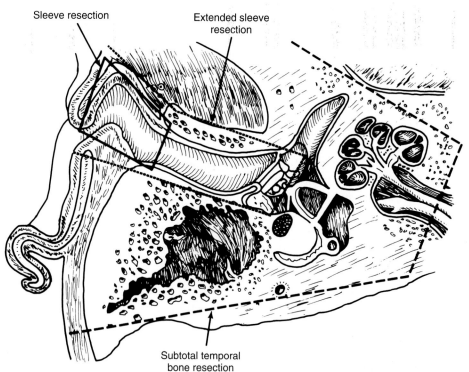

Sleeve resection

Extended sleeve resection

Subtotal temporal bone resection

Fig. 13-3 Surgical procedures for carcinomas of the ear.

than an electron-photon combination because the distribution of the electron beam dose in the dense temporal bone is uncertain.

Both anteroposterior and superoinferior wedged portal arrangements have been used for tumors of the temporal bone (Fig. 13-4). An anteroposterior orientation is usually preferred because the isotope distribution conforms to the general shape of the temporal bone and makes it easier to exclude the brainstem (Figs. 13-5 and 13-6). However, the posterior oblique field must be angled inferiorly to avoid exit through the contralateral eye. The brainstem is usually included in the anterior oblique portal but excluded from

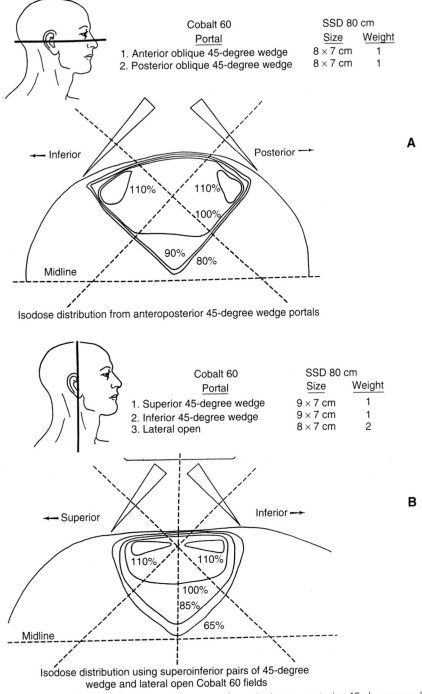

Fig. 13-4 Isodose distribution for two treatment plans. **A,** Anteroposterior 45-degree wedge filtered portals. **B,** A three-field technique using superior-inferior wedge filtered portals and a lateral open field.

the posterior oblique portal. This results in a triangular isodose distribution with the apex of the distribution situated anterior to the spinal cord.

Results

Survival rates for tumors of the ear correlate well with the location and the extent of the disease. Five-year survival rates are usually in the range of 70% to 75% for patients with early cancer of the EAC (T1 and T2), compared with 40% to 45% for patients with technically resectable cancer involving the middle ear (T3). The results for patients with technically unresectable cancer (T4) are very poor, with only 0% to 20% of patients surviving 5 years.

The results achieved with surgery alone, radiation therapy alone, and combined surgery and radiation therapy

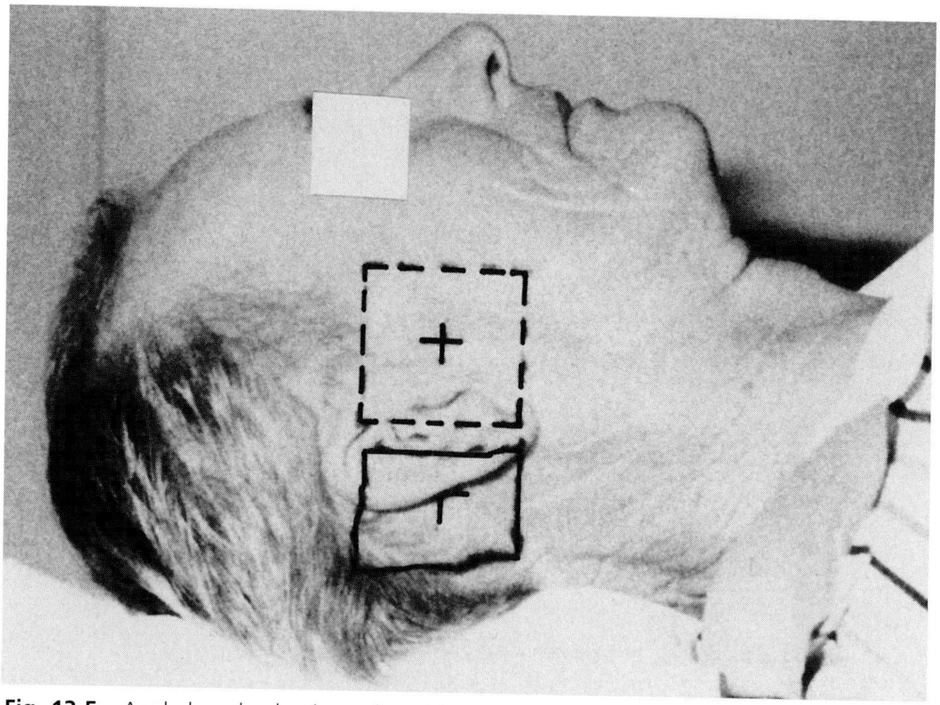

Fig. 13-5 Angled wedged pair used to deliver high dose to the right temporal bone while sparing the underlying brain.

are difficult to compare because treatment methods are selected on the basis of the extent of the tumor. Surgery is not chosen unless the tumor is thought to be technically resectable and the patient is medically operable. On the other hand, radiation therapy is often used to treat patients palliatively, and postoperative radiation therapy is usually added when there is a significant risk of residual disease after surgery (see Table 13-2). In general, patients who have been treated with surgery alone have had less extensive disease than those treated with either radiation therapy or combined surgery and radiation therapy.

In the M.D. Anderson Cancer Center series,[26] 66% of patients with Tl tumors had local tumor control after treatment with a single modality (see Table 13-3). The overall local control rate for patients with T2 disease was similar (62%). However, the patients who received postoperative radiation therapy had a much higher local control rate than those who were treated with surgery alone (5 of 5 vs. 5 of 11). Similarly, the local control rate was better when postoperative radiation therapy was added for patients with T3 cancer of the middle ear (5 of 6 vs. 6 of 13). None of those who had incompletely resected middle ear tumors (T4) had local tumor control (0 of 13), even with the addition of postoperative irradiation (see Table 13-3).

CHEMODECTOMAS

Chemodectomas are a group of rare tumors that arise from the chemoreceptor system. They are also called *nonchromaffin paragangliomas* and *glomus tumors*. Chemodectomas are 3 to 4 times more common in women than in men. The peak incidence is in the fifth decade of life, but tumors have been reported in patients as young as 22 months and as old as 85 years.[36]

Chemodectomas cause symptoms by progressive enlargement and compression or by infiltration of adjacent bone, nerves, and blood vessels. Although histologically benign, these tumors have been reported to metastasize in 2% to 6% of cases.[37] They are the second most common benign neoplasm of the base of the skull, with acoustic neuromas being the most common.

Anatomy

The normal glomus bodies, or paraganglia, are derived from neural crest cells. They are found in all parts of the body, but they are much more common in the head and neck and mediastinum than elsewhere. The glomus bodies of the head and neck and mediastinum are termed the *branchiomeric paraganglia* because they are located near the great vessels and cranial nerves of the primitive branchial arches. The branchiomeric paraganglia include the jugulotympanic, intercarotid, subclavian, laryngeal, coronary, aortopulmonary, and pulmonary glomus bodies.

Normal glomus bodies are very small, ranging from 0.1 to 1.5 mm in diameter.[38] They are composed of two primary cell types: granule-storing chief cells and Schwann-like satellite cells. These cells are intermixed

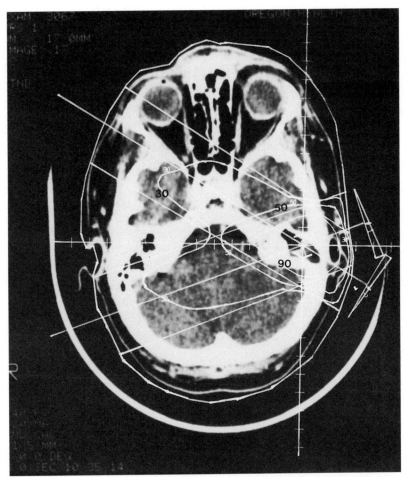

Fig. 13-6 Isodose curves of a patient treated with a portal arrangement similar to that shown in Figure 13-5.

with a rich capillary network. The chief cells are thought to be the functional cells. They contain dense granules and numerous organelles that contain acetylcholine, catecholamines, and serotonin.

The glomus bodies are an important part of the chemoregulatory system. They respond to a variety of chemical changes within the body and thus help keep the body in physiologic balance. The carotid bodies, for example, appear to serve as initiators of increased ventilation when oxygen tension is low and as suppressors of ventilation when oxygen tension is high.[39,40] In addition to being hypoxic receptors, the paraganglia are thought to be receptors for monitoring changes in pH, carbon dioxide concentration, blood flow, and possibly temperature.[38]

Pathology

The distribution of chemodectomas throughout the body corresponds to the anatomic distribution of the normal paraganglia. In the head and neck, chemodectomas are seen most commonly near the carotid bifurcation (carotid body tumors), the jugular bulb (glomus jugular tumors), the tympanic and auricular nerves (glomus tympanicum tumors), and the vagus nerve at the base of the skull (vagal body tumors). Glomus body tumors also may be found in the nasal cavity, orbit, pharynx, and larynx.

Grossly, chemodectomas may appear as small, well-localized, reddish-purple masses or as deeply infiltrating tumors destroying bone and adjacent vital structures. Histopathologically, chemodectomas are benign—similar in appearance to the normal paraganglia. They tend to form nests of 15 to 20 chief cells arranged haphazardly within a rich vascular stroma. On electron microscopy, the chief cells are seen to contain neurosecretory-like granules.

Approximately 10% of chemodectomas are multicentric, and there is a high association with other neoplasms, especially other neural crest tumors.[41,42] Chemodectomas can be familial, and the incidence of multicentric tumors is greater in patients with a familial history of the disease than in sporadic cases.[43] In one series, 33% of 209 patients with familial glomus tumors had multicentric tumors.[38]

Presenting Symptoms

The most common presenting symptoms of a temporal bone chemodectoma are mild hearing loss, pulsatile tinnitus, and facial nerve paralysis. These symptoms are usually gradual in onset but become more severe as the disease progresses. Other common symptoms include bloody or purulent otorrhea, vertigo, and palsy of cranial nerves IX to XII. The differential diagnosis for a glomus tumor includes chronic otitis media, cholesterol granuloma, carcinoma of the middle ear, vascular anomalies, and primary brain tumors.[36]

Clinical Evaluation

Clinical evaluation of a patient with a suspected chemodectoma should include an otoscopic examination of the EAC and tympanic membrane. In most cases a reddish-purple discoloration of the tympanic membrane is seen. However, an aural polyp or tumor may obscure the tympanic membrane. The mass commonly pulsates, and it may blanch when external pressure is applied with a pneumatic otoscope (Brown's sign).[44]

A complete neurologic examination should be performed to evaluate for cranial nerve deficits. The facial nerve is the cranial nerve most commonly involved because of its location within the temporal bone. The incidence of paralysis of the facial nerve with glomus tumors ranges from 10% to 40%.[38] Cranial nerves IX to

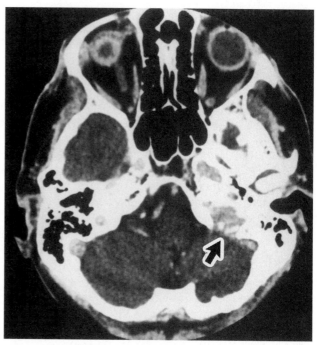

Fig. 13-7 Computed tomography scan of a 70-year-old woman with an enhancing destructive lesion in the region of the left jugular foramen with marked expansion and bony destruction.

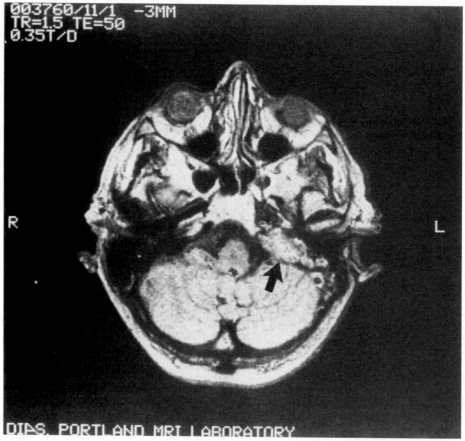

Fig. 13-8 Magnetic resonance imaging scan of the same patient shown in Figure 13-7.

XII also are commonly involved, and cranial nerves V and VI may be impaired if the tumor extends to the middle cranial fossa. This usually is seen only when the disease is advanced.

Radiographic studies should include a high-resolution CT scan to evaluate for bone destruction and to delineate the soft tissue mass and an MRI scan to determine whether intracranial extension is present (Figs. 13-7 and 13-8). Angiography should be performed to evaluate the arterial supply if the patient is being considered for surgery or embolization. Arteriography can be used to differentiate a glomus tumor from other vascular and nonvascular lesions of the temporal bone and may eliminate the need for a biopsy (Fig. 13-9).[36]

Clinical Staging

The prognosis for a patient with a glomus tumor is closely related to the size of the tumor and its anatomic location. The following classification was proposed by McCabe and Fletcher[45]:

Group I Tympanic tumors, characterized by absence of bone destruction on radiographs of the mastoid bone and jugular fossa, absence of facial nerve weakness, an intact eighth nerve with conductive deafness only, and intact jugular foramen nerves (cranial nerves IX, X, and XI)

Group II Tympanomastoid tumors, characterized by radiographic evidence of bone destruction confined to the mastoid bone and not involving the petrous bone, a normal or paretic seventh nerve, intact jugular foramen nerves, and no evidence of involvement of the superior bulb of the jugular vein on retrograde venogram

Group III Petrosal and extrapetrosal tumors, characterized by evidence of destruction of the petrous bone, jugular fossa, and/or occipital bone on radiograph, positive findings on retrograde jugulography, evidence of destruction of the petrous occipital bone on arteriography, jugular foramen syndrome (paresis of cranial nerve IX, X, or XI), or presence of metastasis

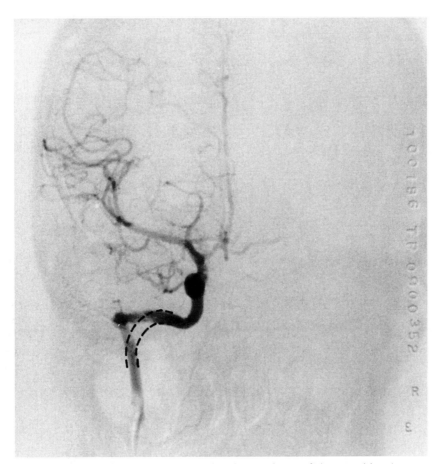

Fig. 13-9 A 17-year-old woman presented with complaints of decreased hearing, a sensation of aural fullness, and pulsatile tinnitus. On otoscopic examination she was found to have a blue mass bulging behind the tympanic membrane. Plain films were suggestive of a glomus jugulare tumor. Angiography revealed an aberrant carotid artery. Dashed lines indicate the normal course of the vessel. Biopsy of similar lesions has occasionally been fatal.

TABLE 13-4

Local Control with Surgery for Chemodectoma of the Temporal Bone: Literature Review

Institution	Local Control Rate
Royal Marsden Hospital[46]	0 of 4
University of Virginia[47]	17 of 20
University of Iowa[48]	6 of 13
University of Florida[49]	4 of 6
Mount Sinai Hospital[50]	16 of 17
University of Kansas Medical Center[51]	3 of 13
Washington University, St. Louis[52]	10 of 11*
	35 of 45†
Geisinger Medical Center[53]	4 of 8
Arthus Municipal Hospital, Denmark[54]	4 of 6
University of California, San Francisco[55]	3 of 14
Massachusetts General Hospital[56]	8 of 16
Mount Sinai Hospital (New York)[57]	14 of 23‡
TOTAL	124 of 196 (63%)

*Glomus tympanicum.
†Glomus jugulare.
‡One patient lost to follow-up was excluded.

Treatment

The treatment for chemodectomas of the temporal bone is controversial. For limited chemodectomas, otolaryngologists often prefer surgery, and radiation oncologists usually prefer radiation therapy. Most agree that surgery is effective treatment for early tumors that can be completely excised. For example, surgery is usually adequate for small glomus tympanicum tumors of the middle ear (group I). These tumors usually can be excised through the ear canal or the mastoid with reasonable assurance of complete removal. However, surgery is less likely to be successful for more extensive glomus tympanicum tumors or for glomus jugulare tumors (groups II and III). These tumors often are resected in a piecemeal fashion, and, therefore, residual disease is a significant risk. Hemorrhage is a significant risk as well. The difficulties associated with surgery for glomus jugulare tumors are reflected in a poor initial local control rate with surgery alone (Table 13-4)[46-57] and a high complication rate (up to 60% in the surgical literature).[50] Complications of surgery include hemorrhage, cranial nerve deficits, dysphagia, wound infections, cerebrospinal fluid leaks, and meningitis.

TABLE 13-5

Local Control with Radiation Therapy* for Chemodectomas of the Temporal Bone: Review of Literature

Institution	Local Control Rate	Nominal Dosage Schedule
Royal Marsden Hospital[46]	52 of 59	35-66 Gy in 4-6 wk
University of Virginia[47]	25 of 29	30-60 Gy in 3-6 wk
University of Iowa[48]	14 of 14†	29-67.5 Gy in 2½-7 wk
University of Florida[49]	19 of 19	40-50 Gy in 4-5 wk
University of Kansas[51]	4 of 4	22-56 Gy in 3-6 wk
Geisinger Medical Center[53]	20 of 22	40-50 Gy‖
Arthus Municipal Hospital, Denmark[54]	13 of 15	50-60 Gy in 5-6 wk
University of California, San Francisco[55]	6 of 6	46-55 Gy in 4½-5½ wk
Massachusetts General Hospital[56]	13 of 16	15-45 Gy in 2-5 wk
Washington University, St. Louis[58]	12 of 15	30-55 Gy in 3-5½ wk
Princess Margaret Hospital, Toronto[59]	42 of 45‡	35 Gy in 3 wk
Rotterdamsch Radio-Therapeutisch Institute, The Netherlands[60]	19 of 19	40-60 Gy in 4-6 wk
University of Washington[61]	10 of 13	28-65 Gy in 4-7 wk
University Hospital of Wales, Cardiff[62]	2 of 14	42.5-55 Gy in 15 fractions
Queen Elizabeth Hospital, UK[63]	22 of 23§	45-50 Gy in 4-5 wk
M.D. Anderson Cancer Center[64]	16 of 17	45-50 Gy in 4½-5 wk
Mount Sinai Hospital (New York)[65]	6 of 6	40-50 Gy in 4-5 wk
University of Minnesota[66]	13 of 14	30-60 Gy in 4-6 wk
TOTAL	308 of 350 (88%)	

*Includes patients treated with radiation therapy alone or a combination of surgery and radiation therapy.
†Previously untreated patients. If patients treated for recurrent disease are included, the local control rate is 16 of 19 (84%).
‡Includes two patients in whom the initial treatment failed but salvage therapy was successful.
§One patient in whom the initial treatment failed had successful salvage radiation therapy.
‖Fraction schedule not specified.

Groups II and III chemodectomas of the temporal bone are usually better treated with radiation therapy because it is very effective in ameliorating symptoms and in halting the progression of the disease. However, a persistent mass often is present clinically and angiographically after radiation therapy, and some surgeons have interpreted this as evidence of a lack of effectiveness of radiation therapy for chemodectomas.

In most radiation therapy series, patients have been considered to have local tumor control if no evidence of disease progression is found clinically or radiographically at the time of the analysis or until death from intercurrent disease. Using these criteria, the overall local control rate with radiation therapy is in the range of 90% (Table 13-5).[46-49,51,53-56,58-66] The incidence of complications after radiation therapy is low because the radiation dose required for local tumor control is only 45 to 50 Gy in $4\frac{1}{2}$ to 5 weeks.

Wang and colleagues[48] compared the results achieved with radiation therapy with those attained with surgery alone. In their series, 13 patients were treated with surgery alone, 15 with radiation therapy alone, and 4 with combined surgery and radiation therapy. In general, the patients treated with radiation therapy or combined surgery and radiation therapy had more advanced disease than those treated with surgery alone. The initial local control rate with surgery was 46% (85% after salvage with additional treatment); 31% of patients developed complications, and 78% survived 10 years. The initial local control rate with radiation therapy was 84%; 11% of patients developed complications, and 76% survived 10 years. These results show that radiation therapy is an effective treatment for chemodectomas of the temporal bone.

Radiation Therapy Technique

The treatment portals for chemodectomas of the temporal bone are similar to those outlined earlier in this chapter for carcinomas of the ear. Most often small portals can be used for relatively localized glomus tympanicum tumors (group I). However, larger portals must be used for the more advanced tympanomastoid, petrosal, and extrapetrosal tumors (groups II and III). Most patients are treated with photons using a wedged field portal arrangement (see Fig. 13-4). Either superoinferior or anteroposterior wedge portal arrangements may be employed. Sometimes a three-field portal arrangement including two wedge fields and a lateral open field (weighted 1:1:33) is useful (see Fig. 13-4). The treatment is usually delivered with daily fraction sizes of 1.8 to 2 Gy to a total tumor dose of 45 Gy in 5 to $5\frac{1}{2}$ weeks.

REFERENCES

1. Stell PM. Carcinoma of the external auditory meatus and middle ear. *Clin Otolaryngol* 1984;9:281-299.

2. Parsons JT. The effect of radiation on normal tissues of the head and neck. In: Million RR, Cassisi NJ, eds. *Management of Head and Neck Cancer.* Philadelphia, Pa: Lippincott; 1984:173-207.

3. Borsanyi SJ, Blanchard CL. Ionizing radiation and the ear. *JAMA* 1962;181:958-961.

4. O'Neill JV, Katz AH, Skolnik EM. Otologic complications of radiation therapy. *Otolaryngol Head Neck Surg* 1979;87:359-363.

5. Brill AH, Martin MM, Fitz-Hugh GS, et al. Postoperative and postradiotherapeutic serous otitis media. *Arch Otolaryngol* 1974;99:406-408.

6. Myers EN, Beery QC, Bluestone CD, et al. Effect of certain head and neck tumors and their management on the ventilatory function of the eustachian tube. *Ann Otol Rhinol Laryngol* 1984; 114(suppl):3-16.

7. Kveton JF, Sotelo-Avila C. Osteoradionecrosis of the ossicular chain. *Am J Otol* 1986;7:446-448.

8. Leach W. Irradiation of the ear. *J Laryngol Otol* 1965;79:870-880.

9. Grau C, Moller K, Overgaard M, et al. Sensorineural hearing loss in patients treated with irradiation for nasopharyngeal carcinoma. *Int J Radiat Oncol Biol Phys* 1991;21:723-728.

10. Moretti JA. Sensorineural hearing loss following radiotherapy to the nasopharynx. *Laryngoscope* 1976;85:598-602.

11. Thibadoux GM, Pereira XW, Hodges JM, et al. Effects of cranial radiation on hearing in children with acute lymphocytic leukemia. *J Pediatr* 1980;96:403-406.

12. Evans RA, Liu KC, Azhar T, et al. Assessment of permanent hearing impairment following radical megavoltage radiotherapy. *J Laryngol Otol* 1988;102:588-589.

13. Bohne BA, Marks JE, Glasgow GP. Delayed effects of ionizing radiation on the ear. *Laryngoscope* 1985;195:818-828.

14. Kretschmar CS, Warren MP, Lavally BL, et al. Ototoxicity of preradiation cisplatin for children with central nervous system tumors. *J Clin Oncol* 1990;8:1191-1198.

15. Walker DA, Pillow J, Waters KD, et al. Enhanced cisplatinum ototoxicity in children with brain tumors who have received simultaneous or prior cranial irradiation. *Med Pediatr Oncol* 1989;17: 48-52.

16. Berg NO, Lindgren M. Dose factors and morphology of delayed radiation lesions of the internal and middle ear in rabbits. *Acta Radiol* 1961;56:305-319.

17. Moskovskaya NV. Effect of ionizing radiation on function of vestibular analyzer. *Otorinolaringologie* 1960;22:43-49.

18. Gamble JE, Peterson EA, Chandler JR. Radiation effects on the inner ear. *Arch Otolaryngol* 1968;88:156-161.

19. Wang CC, Doppke K. Osteoradionecrosis of the temporal bone: consideration of nominal standard dose. *Int J Radiat Oncol Biol Phys* 1976;1:881-883.

20. Lewis JS. Cancer of the ear: a report of 150 cases. *Laryngoscope* 1960;50:551-579.

21. Kinney SE. Squamous cell carcinoma of the external auditory canal. *Am J Otol* 1989;10:111-116.

22. Hyams VJ. Pathology of tumors of the ear. In: Thawley SE, Panje WR, eds. *Comprehensive Management of Head and Neck Tumors.* Philadelphia, Pa: WB Saunders; 1987:168-180.

23. Lewis JS. Cancer of the ear. *CA Cancer J Clin* 1987;37:78-87.

24. Jesse RH. External auditory canal, middle ear, and mastoid. In: MacComb WS, Fletcher GS, eds. *Cancer of the Head and Neck.* Baltimore, Md: Williams & Wilkins; 1967:412-427.

25. Boland J, Paterson R. Cancer of the middle ear and external auditory meatus. *J Laryngol* 1955;69:468-478.

26. Goodwin WJ, Jesse RH. Malignant neoplasms of the external auditory canal and temporal bone. *Arch Otolaryngol* 1980;106:675-679.

27. Stell PM, McCormick MS. Carcinoma of the external auditory meatus and middle ear. *J Laryngol Otol* 1985;99:847-850.

28. Crabtree JA, Britton BH, Pierce MK. Carcinoma of the external auditory canal. *Laryngoscope* 1976;86:405-415.

29. Arriaga M, Hirsch BE, Kamerer DB, et al. Squamous cell carcinoma of the external auditory meatus (canal). *Otolaryngol Head Neck Surg* 1989;101:330-337.

30. Hahn SS, Kim JA, Goodchild N, et al. Carcinoma of the middle ear and external auditory canal. *Int J Radiat Oncol Biol Phys* 1983;9:1003-1007.

31. Lesser RW, Spector GJ, Deviveni VR. Malignant tumors of the middle ear and external auditory canal: a 20-year review. *Otolaryngol Head Neck Surg* 1987;96:43-47.

32. Wang CC. Radiation therapy in the management of carcinoma of the external auditory canal, middle ear, or mastoid. *Radiology* 1975;116:713-715.

33. Gacek RR, Goodman M. Management of malignancy of the temporal bone. *Laryngoscope* 1977;87:1622-1634.

34. Sinha PP, Aziz HI. Treatment of carcinoma of the middle ear. *Radiology* 1978;126:485-487.

35. Lederman M. Malignant tumors of the ear. *J Laryngol Otol* 1965;79:185-199.

36. Zak FG, Lawson W. *The Paraganglionic Chemoreceptor System: Physiology, Pathology, and Clinical Medicine.* New York, NY: Springer-Verlag; 1982.

37. Irons GB, Weiland LH, Brown WL. Paragangliomas of the neck: clinical and pathologic analysis of 116 cases. *Surg Clin North Am* 1977;57:575-583.

38. Smith PG, Schwaber MK, Goebel JA. Clinical evaluation of glomus tumors of the ear and the base of the skull. In: Panje WR, Thawley SE, eds. *Comprehensive Management of Head and Neck Tumors.* Philadelphia, Pa: WB Saunders; 1987:207-218.

39. Arias-Stella J, Valcarcel J. Chief cell hyperplasia in the human carotid body at high altitudes: physiologic and pathologic significance. *Hum Pathol* 1976;7:361-373.

40. Lack EE. Carotid body hypertrophy in patients with cystic fibrosis and cyanotic congenital heart disease. *Hum Pathol* 1977;8:39-51.

41. Hayes HM Jr, Fraumeni JF Jr. Chemodectomas in dogs: epidemiologic comparison with man. *J Natl Cancer Inst* 1974;52:1455-1458.

42. Spector GJ, Ciralsky R, Maisel RH, et al. Multiple glomus tumors in the head and neck. *Laryngoscope* 1975;85:1066-1075.

43. Cook PL. Bilateral chemodectomas in the neck. *J Laryngol Otol* 1977;91:611-618.

44. Brown LA. Glomus jugulare tumor of the middle ear: clinical aspects. *Laryngoscope* 1953;53:281-292.

45. McCabe BF, Fletcher M. Selection of therapy of glomus jugulare tumors. *Arch Otolaryngol* 1969;89:156-159.

46. Powell S, Peters N, Harmer C. Chemodectoma of the head and neck: results of treatment in 84 patients. *Int J Radiat Oncol Biol Phys* 1992;22:919-924.

47. Larner JM, Hahn SS, Spaulding CA, et al. Glomus jugulare tumors. *Cancer* 1992;69:1813-1817.

48. Wang ML, Hussey DH, Doornbos JF, et al. Chemodectoma of the temporal bone: a comparison of surgical and radiotherapeutic results. *Int J Radiat Oncol Biol Phys* 1988;14:643-648.

49. Friedland JL, Mendenhall WM, Parsons JT, et al. Chemodectomas arising in temporal bone structures. *Head Neck Surg* 1988;10:552-555.

50. Cece JA, Lawson W, Biller HF, et al. Complications in the management of large glomus jugulare tumors. *Laryngoscope* 1987;97:152-157.

51. Reddy EK, Mansfield CM, Hartman GV. Chemodectomas of glomus jugulare. *Cancer* 1983;52:337-340.

52. Spector GJ, Fierstein J, Ogura JH. A comparison of therapeutic modalities of glomus tumors in the temporal bone. *Laryngoscope* 1976;86:690-696.

53. Cole JM. Glomus jugulare tumor. *Laryngoscope* 1977;87:1244-1258.

54. Thomsen K, Elbrond O, Andersen AP. Glomus jugulare tumors (a series of 21 cases). *J Laryngol Otol* 1975;89:1113-1121.

55. Newman H, Rowe JF Jr, Phillips TL. Radiation therapy of the glomus jugulare tumor. *AJR Am J Roentgenol* 1973;118:663-669.

56. Hatfield PM, James AE, Schultz MD. Chemodectomas of the glomus jugulare. *Cancer* 1972;30:1164-1168.

57. Rosenwasser H. Glomus jugulare tumors: long-term tumors jugulare. *Arch Otolaryngol* 1969;89:186-192.

58. Konefal JB, Pilepich MV, Spector GJ, et al. Radiation therapy in the treatment of chemodectomas. *Laryngoscope* 1987;97:1331-1335.

59. Cummings BJ, Beale FA, Garrett PG, et al. The treatment of glomus tumors in the temporal bone by megavoltage radiation. *Cancer* 1984;53:2635-2640.

60. Lybeert MLM, Van Andel JG, Eijkenboom WMH, et al. Radiotherapy of paragangliomas. *Clin Otolaryngol* 1984;9:105-109.

61. Simko TG, Griffin TW, Gerdes AJ, et al. The role of radiation therapy in the treatment of glomus jugulare tumors. *Cancer* 1978;42:104-106.

62. Gibbin KP, Henk JM. Glomus jugulare tumors in South Wales: a 20-year review. *Clin Radiol* 1978;29:607-609.

63. Arthur K. Radiotherapy in chemodectoma of the glomus jugulare. *Clin Radiol* 1977;28:415-417.

64. Tidwell TJ, Montague ED. Chemodectomas involving the temporal bone. *Radiology* 1975;116:147-149.

65. Silverstone SM. Radiation therapy of glomus jugulare tumors. *Arch Otolaryngol* 1973;97:43-48.

66. Maruyama Y. Radiotherapy of tympanojugular chemodectomas. *Radiology* 1972;105:659-663.

ADDITIONAL READINGS

Antoniades J. *Uncommon Malignant Tumors.* New York, NY: Masson; 1982.

Brown JS. Glomus jugulare tumors revisited: a 10-year statistical follow-up of 231 cases. *Laryngoscope* 1985;95:284-287.

Burres SA, Wilner HL. Nonsurgical management of a large recurrent glomus jugulare tumor. *Otolaryngol Head Neck Surg* 1983;91:312-314.

Cannon CR, McLean WC. Adenoid cystic carcinoma of the middle ear and temporal bone. *Otolaryngol Head Neck Surg* 1983;91:96-98.

Kabnick EM, Serchuk L. Metastatic chemodectoma. *J Natl Med Assoc* 1985;77:750-756.

Lo WWM, Solti-Bohman LG. High-resolution CT in the evaluation of glomus tumors of the temporal bone. *Radiology* 1984;150:737-742.

Lybeert MLM, Van Andel JG. Radiotherapy of paragangliomas. *Clin Otolaryngol* 1984;9:105-109.

Mikhael MA, Wolff AP. Current concepts in neuroradiological diagnosis of acoustic neuromas. *Laryngoscope* 1987;97:471-476.

Moss WT. *Radiation Oncology: Rationale, Technique, Results.* 6th ed. St Louis, Mo: Mosby; 1989.

Olson LE, Cox JD. Chemodectomas. In: Laramore GE, ed. *Radiation Therapy of Head and Neck Cancer.* New York, NY: Springer-Verlag; 1989:171-179.

Pallach JF, McDonald TJ. Adenocarcinoma and adenoma of the middle ear. *Laryngoscope* 1982;92:47-53.

Pansky B. *Review of Gross Anatomy.* 5th ed. New York, NY: Macmillan; 1984.

Patel M, Cronin J: Primary adenocarcinoma of the middle ear. *Ear Nose Throat J* 1981;60:527-529.

Perez CA, Brady LW, eds: *Principles and Practice of Radiation Oncology.* Philadelphia, Pa: JB Lippincott; 1987.

Phelps PD, Lloyd GA. Vascular masses in the middle ear. *Clin Radiol* 1986;37:359-364.

Pritchett JW. Familial concurrence of carotid body tumor and pheochromocytoma. *Cancer* 1982;49:2578-2579.

Reddy EK, Mansfield CM. Chemodectoma of glomus jugulare. *Cancer* 1983;52:337-340.

Sataloff RT, Kemink JL. Total en bloc resection of the temporal bone and carotid artery for malignant tumors of the ear and temporal bone. *Laryngoscope* 1984;94:528-533.

Schuller DE, Conley JJ. Primary adenocarcinoma of the middle ear. *Otolaryngol Head Neck Surg* 1983;91:280-283.

Sinha PP, Aziz HI. Treatment of carcinoma of the middle ear. *Radiology* 1978;126:485-487.

Strauss M, Nichols GG. Malignant catecholamine-secreting carotid body paraganglioma. *Otolaryngol Head Neck Surg* 1983;91:315-321.

Thabet JH, Ali F. Unusual presentations of carotid body tumors. *Ear Nose Throat J* 1983;62:316-320.

Tidwell TJ, Montague ED. Chemodectomas involving the temporal bone. *Radiology* 1975;116:147-149.

Wang CC. *Radiation Therapy for Head and Neck Neoplasms: Indications, Techniques and Results*. Boston, Mass: John Wright; 1983.

Wang CC, Doppke K. Osteoradionecrosis of the temporal bone: consideration of nominal standard dose. *Int J Radiat Oncol Biol Phys* 1976;1:881-883.

CHAPTER 14

The Thyroid

Richard W. Tsang and James D. Brierley

EFFECTS OF IRRADIATION ON THE NORMAL THYROID

The thyroid is incidentally irradiated during mantle radiation therapy and many head and neck treatment plans, which can result in thyroid dysfunction and neoplasia, both benign (goiter, nodular disease) and malignant (thyroid carcinoma). Sonographic examination of 47 patients treated in childhood for Hodgkin's disease revealed that all had thyroid abnormalities; 95% had diffuse thyroid atrophy, 5% had a goiter, 42% had focal or multifocal abnormalities, and 5% had a carcinoma.[1] The incidence of hypothyroidism after irradiation varies from 10% to 45% depending on radiation dose, age at the time of irradiation, and length of follow-up.[2,3] Similarly, the risk of developing a second malignancy depends on age at the time of radiation exposure and the length of time since the irradiation. The relative risk of developing thyroid cancer after irradiation for Hodgkin's disease has been reported to be 15.6% (95% confidence interval, 6.3 to 32.5).[3] Such tumors are usually well differentiated (the papillary type is more common than the follicular type, and anaplastic tumors are rare) and behave similarly to spontaneous thyroid cancer. Secondary thyroid cancer is often multifocal. Given the prolonged latency period from the time of radiation to the development of thyroid dysfunction or malignancy, it is prudent to provide periodic clinical examination and biochemical testing for patients who have undergone thyroid irradiation. Suspicious lesions can be investigated by cytologic examination of fine-needle aspiration (FNA) samples.

THYROID CANCER

Thyroid diseases, including various inflammatory, autoimmune, and benign neoplasms, are common in the general population, yet cancer arising from the thyroid gland is rare, accounting for only 1% of all malignancies and 0.2% of cancer deaths in the United States. Thyroid cancer is important, however, because of its unique clinical features, the wide range in prognosis depending on its histology, the role of oncogenes in its pathogenesis, and the therapeutic effectiveness of radioactive iodine. Exposure to radiation is a significant etiologic factor in the development of differentiated thyroid carcinoma, the most common type of thyroid cancer. Differentiated thyroid cancer has a high cure rate; in contrast, anaplastic cancer commonly presents as extensive localized disease and therefore poses a challenge of special interest to radiation oncologists. Anaplastic thyroid cancer has such a poor prognosis that all cases are classified as stage IV by the American Joint Committee on Cancer (AJCC) and the International Union Against Cancer (UICC).[4,5]

The management of thyroid cancer is primarily influenced by the histology of the tumor, the age of the patient, and the extent of the disease. Because low-risk disease is characterized by a long natural history and a high survival rate, an important goal of therapy for low-risk disease is to minimize the toxicity of that therapy. Surgery, with or without radiolabeled iodine, remains the standard treatment for low-risk disease; the involvement of experienced thyroid surgeons is essential for achieving the best results. High-risk disease often requires a coordinated multidisciplinary approach, with the participation of surgeons, endocrinologists, nuclear medicine physicians, and radiation oncologists, to optimally control the disease.

Two caveats should be considered in discussions of the management of thyroid cancer. First, few randomized phase III studies have been done in thyroid oncology, and therefore treatment decisions are based on reports of historically treated, uncontrolled patient populations. Second, because the prognosis for differentiated thyroid cancer is generally excellent, most retrospective reviews that include prolonged clinical follow-up are based on pathologic diagnoses made many years before. Changes in pathology classifications, as discussed below, make comparisons between previous and current classifications difficult. This chapter reviews the various types of thyroid cancer and their management, emphasizing the role of radiolabeled iodine and external radiation therapy. Technical aspects of the delivery of radiolabeled iodine and external beam radiation and results of those treatments will be discussed. Lymphomas of the thyroid gland will not be covered here, because the principles of their management are different, being more in keeping with other non-Hodgkin's lymphomas.

INCIDENCE AND EPIDEMIOLOGY

The incidence of thyroid cancer in the United States has been increasing. Data collected in the Surveillance, Epidemiology, and End Results program indicated a rise in the incidence of thyroid cancer from 3.6 per 100,000 in 1973 to 5.8 per 100,000 in 1997, an increase of 61% in 24 years.[6] The increase may reflect earlier diagnosis of the disease, as sophisticated diagnostic tools such as sonography and cytologic analysis of fine-needle aspirates become available, or perhaps radiation exposure during childhood (as discussed in the next section). Thyroid cancer is more common in females, with a female-to-male ratio of 3:1, especially between the ages of 15 and 40 years, when the incidence among women peaks. Geographic variations are evident, with the highest incidence rate being in Hawaii (7.2 per 100,000 during the period 1993 to 1997). Racial differences are also apparent, with lower incidence rates among blacks and native Americans (2.9 per 100,000 and 2.2 per 100,000, respectively, in 1990 to 1997).[6,7] Despite a slow, steady rise in the overall incidence of thyroid cancer during the past 3 decades, the mortality rate has remained fairly stable over that period at roughly 0.4 per 100,000. Thus the proportion of diagnosed patients dying of thyroid cancer has decreased over time, with 5-year relative survival rates of 95% for 1986 to 1996 and 92% for 1974 to 1979.[6]

ETIOLOGY AND CAUSATIVE FACTORS

Despite an increasing understanding of the genetic and phenotypic events underlying the development and progression of thyroid cancer, in most cases the causative agent has not been identified. About 20% to 30% of cases of medullary thyroid cancer (MTC) are familial.[8-11] Mutation in the germline proto-oncogene *RET* has been shown to be associated with familial MTC and multiple endocrine neoplasia (MEN) types 2A and 2B. The *RET* gene, located on chromosome 10q11.2, encodes for a tyrosine kinase receptor. Mutations of codons 609, 611, 618, 620 in exon 10, and most commonly, codon 634 in exon 11 of the *RET* gene, usually by a single substitution of cysteine by another amino acid, is the causative event leading to constitutive activation of the tyrosine kinase receptor, giving rise to familial MTC and MEN2A.[12,13] The classic MEN2A syndrome is associated with pheochromocytoma in 30% to 50% of cases and parathyroid diseases in 10% to 15%. Mutations of codon 918 are associated with MEN2B, a rare syndrome involving a marfanoid habitus in combination with ganglioneuromas of the mucosa and gastrointestinal tract. Somatic mutations of the *RET* proto-oncogene have also been reported in 30% to 40% of cases of sporadic MTC.[14-16] The importance of identifying the mutated gene in patients with MTC relates to the high penetrance of the gene and the need for genetic screening of family members; the lifetime risk of carriers developing MTC is approximately 90%. Treating identified carriers promptly with total thyroidectomy before the disease becomes clinically manifest produces a cure rate of more than 90%.[17,18]

Although the papillary and follicular forms of thyroid cancer are generally not considered to be hereditary, several families have been documented to have a high incidence of the disease.[19-21] Candidate genes under study in these families include the *RET* proto-oncogene. Inherited syndromes associated with papillary thyroid carcinoma include Gardner's syndrome (familial adenomatosis polyposis)[22] and Cowden's syndrome, which is characterized by multiple harmartomas and other benign or malignant lesions of the breast, ovary, and uterus.[23] Less well characterized are genetic factors related to the racial differences in disease incidence mentioned in the previous section on Incidence and Epidemiology.

The main environmental factor linked to thyroid carcinogenesis is radiation exposure.[24] At the Princess Margaret Hospital in Toronto, the proportion of patients with differentiated thyroid cancer in whom a history of excessive radiation exposure was elicited was 14%.[25] These exposures included treatments for other types of cancer (e.g., Hodgkin's disease) or for benign disease (e.g., ringworm, acne, or tuberculosis) and the use of radioiodine for the treatment of thyrotoxicosis. The nuclear accident at Chernobyl, Ukraine, in 1986 has attested to the powerful carcinogenic effects of radiation, particularly for young children.[26,27] Radiation fallout after nuclear weapons testing on the Bikini atoll resulted in an increased relative risk of 4.5.[28] Most radiation-induced thyroid cancer is of the papillary type and the latency period exceeds 10 years; however, the latency period in children, especially those exposed in the Chernobyl incident, can be much shorter.[26]

The association between low iodine intake and follicular carcinoma has suggested that iodine insufficiency results in chronic overproliferation of follicular cells. This overproliferation results in follicular adenomas, from which follicular carcinoma can develop. A multistep clonal evolution involving somatic mutations may explain the development of this type of cancer. Mutations of the *p53* tumor-suppressor gene are also common features of anaplastic thyroid cancer and may be a critical event that transforms a differentiated thyroid cancer into an undifferentiated one.[29] Unlike follicular carcinoma, papillary thyroid cancer has no histologic precursor; however, the *RET/PTC* oncogene has been found to be associated with papillary thyroid cancer.[30] *RET* rearrangements are common in children with papillary thyroid carcinoma, although such rearrangements have been found in less than half of adult cases. *RET/PTC3* in particular has been associated with the solid follicular subtype of papillary carcinoma in children exposed in the Chernobyl accident.[27] Findings such as these have led to the suggestion that radiation, in combination with deoxyribonucleic acid (DNA) strand breaks, activates *RET*. *RET* rearrangement on its own is probably not sufficient to cause papillary thyroid cancer and secondary genetic changes are needed.

PATHOLOGY CLASSIFICATION

The thyroid contains two main types of cells, follicular epithelial cells and C cells. Most cases of thyroid cancer develop from cells of follicular origin and are usually classified as differentiated (papillary and follicular carcinomas) or undifferentiated (anaplastic carcinoma). Insular carcinoma is intermediate between the differentiated and undifferentiated types and probably represents a point on a continuum.[31] MTC originates from C cells and thus is clinically, pathologically, and etiologically distinct from differentiated and anaplastic cancer.

Papillary Carcinoma

Papillary carcinoma manifests histologically as follicular differentiation with papillary or follicular architecture and characteristic nuclear features (Fig. 14-1) including enlargement, crowding, overlapping, and either a hyperchromatic with finely dispersed chromatin (ground glass) or a clear (Orphan Annie) appearance (Fig. 14-2). Extrafollicular psammoma bodies, caused by calcification arising from damaged papillae, are observed in about 50% of papillary tumors. Multicentricity, which may reflect multiple primary sites or lymphatic spread within the thyroid, is common. Immunohistochemical staining for thyroglobulin and cytokeratins is positive. Most papillary carcinomas have both papillary and follicular architecture, but even if the predominant architecture is follicular they behave and are characterized as papillary tumors. The follicular variant of papillary carcinoma has a follicular architecture but the nuclear

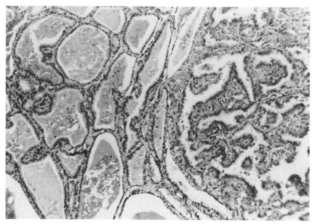

Fig. 14-1 Papillary thyroid carcinoma containing both papillary *(right)* and follicular *(left)* elements. (×100)

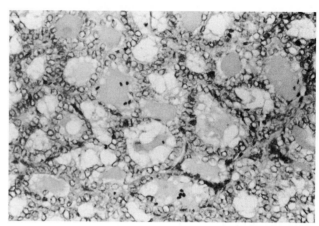

Fig. 14-2 Ground glass or Orphan Annie nuclei characteristic of papillary thyroid carcinoma in an area of follicular architecture. (×250)

features of papillary carcinoma, and it behaves similarly to pure papillary carcinoma. In the past, tumors with mostly follicular architecture have often been classified as follicular tumors; thus the change in classification has resulted in an apparent increase in the relative ratio of papillary to follicular carcinomas.[32]

In the so-called tall-cell variant of papillary carcinoma, between 30% and 50% of cells are twice as high as they are wide. Tall-cell variants are said to be more aggressive because they can present at a higher stage, typically with more extensive local disease, but stage for stage the prognosis associated with tall-cell disease seems to be similar to that for pure papillary carcinoma.[33] A rare columnar cell variant has the distinctive feature of nuclear stratification, like tumors of the colon; columnar cell cases are more common in males than females and tend to present at advanced stages.[34,35] The diffuse sclerosing variant is characterized by diffuse involvement of one or both thyroid lobes with dense sclerosis and by scattered foci of papillary carcinoma. This variant occurs in young patients, and although it usually presents as advanced disease at diagnosis, it has a relatively low mortality rate.[36]

Follicular Neoplasms

Follicular adenomas are common benign neoplasms of the thyroid. The adenoma cells resemble normal follicular cells; they stain positively for thyroglobulin and cytokeratins and are invariably encapsulated. Minimally invasive follicular carcinomas tend to have thicker capsules and are characterized by their invasion through the tumor capsule or into blood vessels. No cytologic features distinguish benign adenomas from minimally invasive carcinomas. In the past, many minimally invasive follicular carcinomas may have been misdiagnosed as benign neoplasms.[32] In contrast, widely invasive

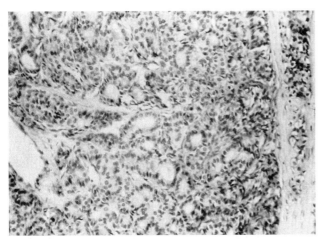

Fig. 14-3 Follicular thyroid carcinoma showing invasion of the tumor capsule. (×100)

follicular carcinomas are characterized by gross extension into the surrounding thyroid parenchyma, a poorly identified tumor capsule, necrosis, high mitotic rate, and nuclear atypia (Fig. 14-3).

Hürthle Cell Tumors

Hürthle probably described C cells; however, the name Hürthle (or Askanazy) is used to refer to *oncocytic neoplasms*, characterized by abundant granular cells rendered eosinophilic from numerous mitochondria. Hürthle cell carcinomas, unlike Hürthle cell adenomas, show capsular or vascular invasion.[37] Those rare cases that exhibit papillary architecture throughout are classified as papillary Hürthle cell carcinomas.

Insular Carcinomas

Poorly differentiated or insular carcinomas are intermediate between well-differentiated and anaplastic carcinomas, and probably represent part of a continuum from differentiated to anaplastic thyroid cancer.[31,38] Insular carcinomas are composed of a population of homogenous small cells with round nuclei and areas of necrosis, and they stain positively for thyroglobulin and cytokeratins.

Anaplastic Carcinomas

Anaplastic (undifferentiated) thyroid carcinomas (ATC) are partially or completely composed of undifferentiated cells (Fig.14-4, *A*). The cells can have a sarcomatoid or spindle-cell pattern, or a giant-cell or squamoid pattern.[39] All have high mitotic rates and often have areas of necrosis (see Fig. 14-4, *B*), lack of follicular formation, and intravascular tumor invasion. Positive staining for cytokeratins is typical, but positive staining for thyroglobulin is variable. Areas of relatively well-differentiated tumor

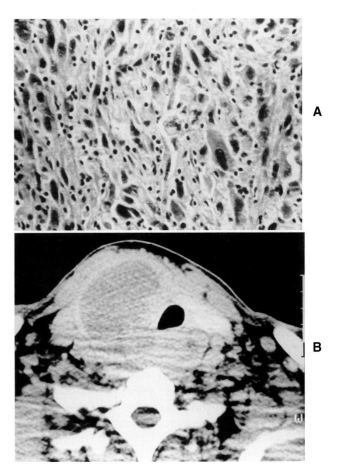

Fig. 14-4 **A,** Anaplastic thyroid cancer with spindle cells, bizarre giant cells, and mitoses. (×250) **B,** Axial computed tomography slice of anaplastic thyroid carcinoma demonstrating extensive extrathyroidal infiltration of neck tissues by tumor, with displacement of the trachea and areas of necrosis.

are occasionally present. The differential diagnosis includes thyroid lymphoma or MTC; in the era before routine immunohistochemical staining, making an accurate diagnosis could be difficult.

Medullary Thyroid Carcinoma

The malignant cells in MTC are derived from C cells, the parafollicular cells of the thyroid gland. MTCs can exhibit a wide range of growth patterns, the most common being uniform nests of cells separated by fibrovascular stroma (Fig. 14-5). The appearance of the cells also varies widely, the most common being round or oval, but spindle cells are not uncommon. Amyloid, detected by Congo red staining, is present in at least 80% of cases (see Fig. 14-5). The characteristic immunohistochemical findings are positive staining for calcitonin and carcinoembryonic antigen (CEA), but staining for cytokeratins and neuroendocrine markers (e.g., neuron-specific enolase) can be positive as well.

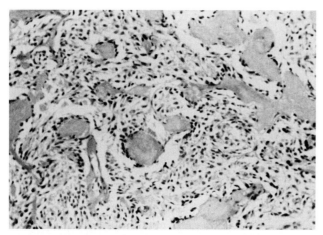

Fig. 14-5 Medullary thyroid carcinoma with uniform cells and large amounts of amyloid that stains with Congo red. (×100)

DIFFERENTIATED THYROID CANCER
Clinical Manifestations and Evaluation

Thyroid nodules are common, found at 50% of autopsies, but the prevalence of palpable thyroid nodules in the United States ranges from 4% to 7%. Of these nodules, only about 4% are malignant. Most thyroid nodules are asymptomatic. Local tumor growth can cause pain, and the presence of local compressive symptoms would suggest extrathyroidal extension of disease. Hoarseness caused by recurrent laryngeal nerve paralysis is an important finding in more advanced cases. Rarely, carcinoma can present in a thyroglossal duct or cyst higher in the neck,[40,41] usually close to the midline. Some cases present with cervical lymph node metastasis. The most commonly involved nodes are those in the central compartment (level 6) and the jugular chain (levels 2, 3, and 4). Occasionally, low inferior cervical lymph nodes (level 5) are affected, but rarely are level 1 nodes. Infrequently, the nodes are cystic.

The most important diagnostic tool for a palpable thyroid nodule is cytologic analysis of FNA samples by experienced physicians and cytologists. In a review of the accuracy of FNA cytology from two different institutions, 84.3% of 16,574 specimens were diagnostic, 3.5% of which were malignant; the sensitivity was 98%, the specificity 99%, and the accuracy 98%.[42] Cytologic findings can be classified as benign, suspicious, malignant, or unsatisfactory. Because follicular carcinoma cannot be diagnosed cytologically, a suspicious or indeterminate finding in an FNA sample does not exclude a follicular carcinoma, and malignancy may be present in up to 30% of such cases.[43] Although radioisotope scanning is highly sensitive, its specificity is low, and hence it is most useful as an adjunct rather than a primary diagnostic test. Sonographic examination of the thyroid can reveal nodules as small as 2 to 3 mm; although it cannot distinguish benign from malignant tumors, sonography is useful in aiding FNA biopsy of small lesions and in following up lesions being treated conservatively.

Staging

The UICC/AJCC staging classification for thyroid cancer[4,5] (Box 14-1) is unique in that the classification varies depending on the age of the patient as well as the histology of the tumor. Because the prognosis for differentiated thyroid cancer in young patients is excellent, patients younger than 45 years are classified as having stage I disease unless distant metastasis is present, in which case the classification is stage II. Unfortunately, a plethora of alternative staging and prognostic indices exist for thyroid cancer. The most common in North America are AMES,[44] the AGES,[45] which subsequently evolved into the MACIS,[46] and clinical class.[47] The AMES score depends on age (A), the presence or absence of metastasis (M) or extrathyroidal extension (E), and size of the tumor (S). The MACIS scale depends on metastasis (M), age (A), completeness of excision (C), invasion beyond the thyroid (I), and size (S). These and other prognostic-factor indices represent attempts to distinguish low-risk from high-risk disease. Our analysis of 10 classification systems demonstrated that the AJCC/UICC tumor-node-metastasis (TNM) classification was as effective in predicting outcome as was the AGES and MACIS systems and was better than the others.[48] Thus because the TNM classification is universally available and widely accepted for other disease sites, the authors recommend that it be used for all reports of treatment and outcome in thyroid cancer.[48]

Prognostic Factors

Although the cancer-specific survival rate for differentiated thyroid cancer is high (94% at 20 years in one series of 1353 patients[48]), several adverse prognostic factors have been identified. Age is the most important prognostic factor in determining survival[25,44-46,48-50]; older patients tend to present with other high-risk factors.[51] Other independent factors for cause-specific survival include tumor size, histologic grade, postoperative presence of macroscopic residual disease, and presence of distant metastases.[25] For local–regional recurrence, the most significant factor is age, with additional factors being tumor size, multifocality within the thyroid gland, lymph node involvement, surgical treatment consisting of a less-than-total thyroidectomy, and lack of use of radioiodine.[25] Although recurrence rates are highest at extremes of age, survival with treatment is excellent in the young.[49,52]

Principles of Management

Many aspects of managing differentiated thyroid carcinoma are controversial. The minimum surgical treatment

---

BOX 14-1   American Joint Committee on Cancer and the International Union Against Cancer Tumor-Node-Metastasis Classification for Carcinoma of the Thyroid Gland

PRIMARY TUMOR (T)

All categories may be subdivided: (a) solitary tumor; (b) multifocal tumor (the largest determines the classification)

TX	Primary tumor cannot be assessed
T0	No evidence of primary tumor
T1	Tumor 1 cm or less in greatest dimension limited to the thyroid
T2	Tumor more than 1 cm but not more than 4 cm in greatest dimension limited to the thyroid
T3	Tumor more than 4 cm in greatest dimension limited to the thyroid
T4	Tumor of any size extending beyond the thyroid capsule

REGIONAL LYMPH NODES (N)

NX	Regional lymph nodes cannot be assessed
N0	No regional lymph node metastasis
N1	Regional lymph node metastasis
	N1a Metastasis in ipsilateral cervical lymph node(s)
	N1b Metastasis in bilateral, midline, or contralateral cervical or mediastinal node(s)

DISTANT METASTASIS (M)

MX	Distant metastasis cannot be assessed
M0	No distant metastasis
M1	Distant metastasis

UICC STAGE GROUPINGS FOR DIFFERENTIATED THYROID CARCINOMA*

	Age < 45 years			Age 45 years and older		
Stage I	Any T	Any N	M0	T1	N0	M0
Stage II	Any T	Any N	M1	T2	N0	M0
				T3	N0	M0
Stage III				T4	N0	M0
				Any T	N1	M0
Stage IV				Any T	Any N	M1

From Fleming I, Cooper JS, Henson DE, et al, eds. *AJCC Cancer Staging Manual*, 5th ed. Philadelphia, Pa: Lippincott Williams & Wilkins; 1997:59-64.

*For medullary thyroid carcinoma, refer to the UICC staging manual. For anaplastic (undifferentiated) thyroid carcinomas, all cases are classified as stage IV.

---

is thyroid lobectomy and isthmusectomy,[53] and some centers routinely perform total thyroidectomy for all patients.[54] The prognosis for patients younger than 45 years whose tumors are smaller than 4 cm is excellent, with virtually 100% cause-specific survival at 10 years after limited surgery without the use of radioactive iodine.[25,45,46,55,56] However, a risk of local–regional recurrence remains, most commonly in cervical lymph nodes, in up to 10% of patients whose disease is managed conservatively.[56,57] This risk can be minimized by using, as initial treatment, total thyroid ablation—surgical total thyroidectomy, followed by routine postoperative thyroid-remnant ablation with radioiodine.[25,49,58] These two approaches—limited surgery without radioiodine vs. total thyroid ablation—have never been compared in a randomized trial. The concerns regarding the use of thyroidectomy for low-risk patients are the small but nonnegligible risk of recurrent laryngeal nerve paralysis (1% to 4%, depending on surgical expertise) and the 5% to 10% risk of permanent hypoparathyroidism requiring lifelong calcium therapy. The risk associated with giving postoperative radioiodine once is minimal; ^{131}I is typically given in doses of 1100 MBq (30 mCi) to 7400 MBq (200 mCi). In general, if surgical expertise is available and the philosophy of management is to minimize the long-term recurrence rate, total thyroid

ablation is used. Successful management also requires appropriate preparation, including thyroxine withdrawal (to achieve a high thyrotropin or thyroid-stimulating hormone [TSH] level), a low-iodine diet, and a gamma camera scan (either before or after therapy) to document the location of abnormal areas of uptake and to screen for metastases (Fig. 14-6, *A*). The availability of recombinant TSH (rTSH) allows scanning without thyroxine withdrawal, and several studies have confirmed the validity of diagnostic scans after 2 or 3 days of rTSH stimulation.[59-61] However, uncertainty remains as to whether the uptake or the therapeutic activity of the radioiodine is as effective after rTSH stimulation as after thyroid hormone withdrawal. Until such data are available, patients who undergo scanning with subsequent plans for radioiodine treatment should undergo thyroxine withdrawal.

After radioiodine therapy, patients require lifelong thyroid replacement therapy, not only to prevent hypothyroidism but also to suppress thyrotropin, which might stimulate tumor growth. Although suppressing thyrotropin may improve survival,[49,62,63] overaggressive suppression can lead to cardiac arrhythmias and osteopenia. In the authors' practice, for low-risk patients, suppressing thyrotropin to below-normal levels in a sensitive assay is the aim, but for high-risk

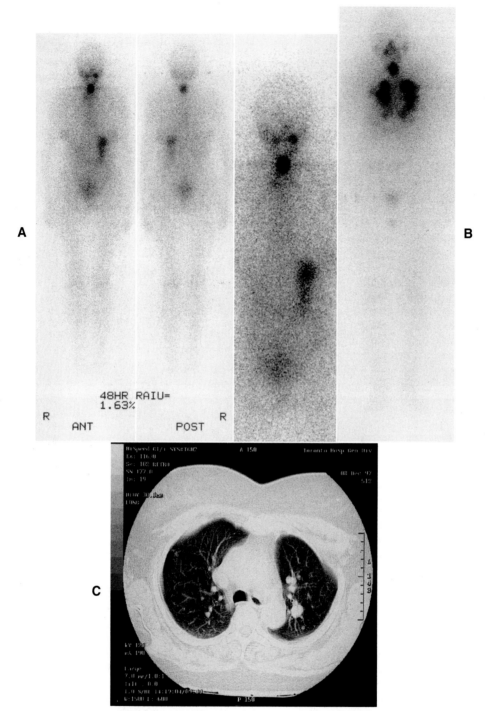

Fig. 14-6 **A,** Diagnostic scans after total thyroidectomy, with the patient under hypothyroid conditions, performed 48 hours after a tracer dose of ^{131}I (3 mCi). The panel at far right is an enlarged view of the anterior scan *(at left)*; the middle panel is the posterior view. The extent of the radioiodine uptake in the neck and its location are compatible with a small thyroid remnant. Physiologic uptake is seen in the submandibular salivary glands *(anterior views on the left and right panels)*, gastrointestinal tract, and urinary bladder. **B,** Iodine scan *(anterior view)* showing concentration of the radionuclide by residual disease in the thyroid bed. The most superior areas of mild uptake are most compatible with iodine being concentrated in the salivary glands. **C,** Computed tomography scan of patient in **B** showing radionuclide uptake by lung metastases.

patients, the aim is for an undetectable level. The level of suppression can be relaxed after 10 years of disease-free survival. Patients are followed with regular physical examinations; measurements of thyrotropin, free tri-iodothyronine (T_3), and thyroglobulin; and sonography of the neck. After radioiodine therapy, it recommended that patients be scanned every 6 to 12 months until documentation of one negative scan. Others recommend scanning until two scans are negative[64] or even scanning at regular intervals regardless of the number of negative scans obtained. The disadvantage of performing iodine scans as part of routine follow-up is the clinical hypothyroidism associated with thyroxine withdrawal, but this condition can be mitigated by using rTSH and not stopping the thyroxine.

The thyroglobulin level in the blood should be undetectable after complete thyroid ablation; a detectable or raised level, even in the absence of symptoms, indicates persistent or recurrent disease.[65-67] Care is required in interpreting thyroglobulin levels, as the presence of thyroid antibodies interferes with some thyroglobulin assays, often producing a false-positive result.[68] In addition, some patients can have undetectable thyroglobulin levels despite the presence of disease,[69] a finding that suggests that the tumor has dedifferentiated into a higher histologic grade or an anaplastic cancer.

External Beam Radiation Therapy
Adjuvant Radiation to the Neck

Most cases of differentiated thyroid cancer can be adequately treated with thyroidectomy and radioiodine. However, some locally invasive tumors do not concentrate radioiodine when they recur.[70] This finding raises the opportunity to adopt another approach, one involving external radiation therapy, to control local disease in patients judged to be at high risk of local recurrence, such as those with extrathyroidal extension of disease.

Many investigators have reported the significance of extrathyroidal extension (designated T4 in the UICC/AJCC TNM classification) as a poor prognostic factor,[25,44,45,48] especially among patients older than 45 years.[71] Mazzaferri and Jhiang[49] found that local tumor invasion into the neck structures (present at diagnosis in 8% of 1077 patients with papillary carcinoma and 12% of 278 patients with follicular carcinoma) was associated with higher 20-year recurrence rates (38% for those with tumor invasion vs. 25% for those without, $P < 0.001$) and higher 20-year cancer mortality rates (20% for those with invasion vs. 5% for those without, $P = 0.001$). Extrathyroidal extension at diagnosis or recurrence can be asymptomatic or can present as a neck mass, hoarseness, cough, dysphagia, hemoptysis, or dyspnea. A review of 262 patients with invasive papillary cancer found the site of invasion to be the muscle in 53% of cases, the laryngeal nerve in 47%, the trachea in 37%, the esophagus in 21%, and the larynx in 12%.[72]

Because radiation therapy for thyroid cancer has not been studied in randomized trials, its potential benefit can be assessed only from interpreting series of patients at adverse risk, comparing outcome in patients who were treated with radiation therapy vs. those who were not. In one such trial at the Princess Margaret Hospital, patients who underwent external radiation therapy for microscopic residual disease had a better 10-year actuarial local control rate than those who did not (93% vs. 78%, $P = 0.01$).[25] The prescribed doses used were 40 Gy given in 15 or 16 daily fractions or 50 Gy given in 20 fractions.[25,62,73] Many investigators have reached similar conclusions in retrospective reviews[74-78] (Table 14-1).

Patients with postoperative gross residual disease, or patients older than 45 years with extensive T4 lesions and grossly complete resection, are at high risk of local recurrence and may benefit from adjuvant external radiation therapy after surgery and radioiodine treatment. Extensive T4 disease implies that the disease has infiltrated one

TABLE 14-1

Ten-Year Local Recurrence Rates after Adjuvant External Radiation Therapy for High-Risk Disease: Retrospective Studies

	TREATMENT	
Study and Reference	Surgery with Radioactive Iodine (%)	Radioactive Iodine with Radiation Therapy (%)
Tubiana et al, 1985[77]	21	14
Simpson et al, 1988[62]*	18	14
Esik et al, 1994[78]	60[†]	20[†]
Phlips et al, 1993[76]	21	3
Farahati et al, 1996[75]	50[‡]	10[‡]
Tsang et al, 1998[25] (papillary only)	22	7

*Local recurrence rate after surgery alone was 74%.
[†]No radioactive iodine, compares low-dose vs. higher-dose radiation therapy.
[‡]Includes distant failures.

or more of the critical structures of the neck, such as the carotid sheath, nerve, larynx, trachea, or esophagus. In general, lymph node involvement by itself is not an indication for external radiation therapy because regional control is usually achieved with initial neck dissection in combination with postoperative radioiodine. Radiation therapy, when recommended at all, should be given after the radioiodine to avoid the possibility of stunting (impairing the ability of the thyroid to take up radioiodine in subsequent therapy). However, the effect of stunting when external radiation is given before radioiodine has not been adequately studied.

Gross Residual Disease

Grossly palpable disease occasionally remains in the thyroid bed after surgery. In general, radioiodine is unlikely to eradicate gross local disease, and thus patients with this condition could benefit from planned combination radioiodine and external radiation therapy. In a series at Princess Margaret Hospital in of 46 patients with gross disease after surgery, this combined approach produced 5-year cause-specific survival and local control rates of 65% and 62%.[25] Other authors have reported disease control rates of 30% to 60%.[77,79-82] The planned radiation therapy volume should cover the gross disease generously, to a dose of at least 60 Gy. The time to response can be as long as 8 to 12 months after completion of the radiation therapy.

Local or Regional Recurrence of Thyroid Cancer

Most differentiated thyroid cancer that recurs in the neck appears in the cervical lymph nodes (regional recurrence) rather than in the thyroid bed (local recurrence).[25,83] Lymph node recurrence should be treated with neck dissection followed by additional radioiodine; such a combination has been highly successful in tumor control.[83] Occasionally, nodal disease recurs in the superior mediastinum, requiring a superior mediastinal dissection. In that case, radioiodine alone, without surgery, may be adequate if the tumor burden is low (e.g., the nodes are smaller than 2 cm). External radiation therapy is recommended only if the nodal disease persists or recurs despite a full modified neck dissection and radioiodine therapy. In this situation, the planned target volume should cover the bilateral cervical lymph nodes and the superior mediastinal lymph nodes to a total dose of 50 Gy, with consideration of a boost to the main areas of involvement to a further 10 to 16 Gy.

Locally recurrent disease in the thyroid bed usually has a more ominous prognosis than does lymph node recurrence, largely because the disease is less likely to concentrate radioiodine.[70] This condition generally occurs in older patients with T4 lesions at initial diagnosis that had not been adequately treated with radioiodine or adjuvant external radiation therapy. Recurrence under these

conditions is managed by a combination of surgical resection (if the disease is resectable), followed by routine postoperative iodine and external radiation therapy. The prescribed radiation volume and dose would be as described above for the treatment of gross residual disease. Because survival can be prolonged even in the presence of metastatic disease,[83] surgery may still be appropriate to prevent life-threatening complications from local disease, such as airway obstruction or hemorrhage.[84]

Metastatic Disease

In a large French study of 2200 patients treated for differentiated thyroid cancer, 17.9% developed metastases to lung or bone at some stage of the disease; an additional eight patients had metastases to the brain, four to the skin, and three to the liver.[85] Survival of patients with metastatic disease depends on age, site of involvement, and tumor burden. Patients younger than 20 years have a 100% survival rate at 10 years, but survival among those older than 40 years falls to 20%. Metastases in older patients are less likely to concentrate iodine and therefore respond poorly to radioiodine therapy.[85] Survival times are longest among patients with diffuse lung metastases that concentrate radioiodine (and thus can be seen on ^{131}I imaging) but are too small to be seen on chest x-ray.[45,51,85,86] The mainstay of therapy is radioiodine, but this treatment is effective only if a total or near-total thyroidectomy has been performed (see Fig. 14-6, B).

Failure to achieve complete remission in metastatic differentiated thyroid cancer can be predicted by failure to concentrate radioiodine, age older than 40, and the presence of bone metastases.[85,86] In the large French study mentioned above, patients with lung metastases had a complete response rate of 50% and a 10-year survival rate of 60%; however, the corresponding values for patients with bone metastases were only 10% and 20%.[85] In view of this poor response to radioiodine and radiation therapy among patients with bone metastases, surgical resection of a solitary bone lesion may be appropriate.[87] For patients expected to survive for long periods, the addition of high-dose radiation therapy (e.g., 40 to 50 Gy in 1.8- to 2-Gy fractions) to radioiodine therapy can prolong local control.

Even patients who present with distant metastatic disease can survive for prolonged periods. In one series of 44 such patients, the 20-year survival rate was 43%.[88] Ideally, treatment should consist of total thyroidectomy, both to resect the primary lesion and to facilitate the use of radioiodine.

Thyroglobulin-Positive, Scan-Negative Disease

When high thyroglobulin levels are present without evidence of disease on a radioisotope scan, other diagnostic tools can be used to locate the disease, including sonography; computed tomography (CT); magnetic resonance imaging; or thallium, tetrofosmin, sestamibi, or positron emission tomography scanning.[89,90] Measurable recurrence in the neck should be treated surgically. Because whole-body scanning after a therapeutic dose of radioactive iodine is more sensitive than diagnostic scanning, it has been argued that all patients with scan-negative, thyroglobulin-positive disease should be given a therapeutic dose of iodine. Others argue that if the diagnostic scan is negative, then the uptake of a therapeutic dose will be too low to be of value.[91] The authors' practice is usually to give such patients a therapeutic trial of 7400 MBq (200 mCi).

When the Thyroid Does Not Take Up Iodine

Little effective therapy is available for disease that has not responded to the combination of surgery, radioiodine, and external radiation therapy.[92] The most effective chemotherapeutic regimen is single-agent doxorubicin, which produces response rates of only 25% to 40%.[93,94] Combination chemotherapy does not seem to be any more effective; in a small, randomized study that included advanced thyroid cancer of all histologic types, no difference in overall response rate was found when doxorubicin alone was compared with doxorubicin and cisplatin,[94] although the complete remission rate was higher in the group given both drugs. In another study, retinoid therapy given with chemotherapy for disease that did not respond to radioiodine resulted in increased uptake of radioiodine and tumor redifferentiation[95]; these interesting observations need to be confirmed in larger studies.

MEDULLARY THYROID CANCER
Clinical Manifestations and Evaluation

Sporadic MTC generally presents as a thyroid nodule. If cytologic analysis of an FNA sample yields a definitive diagnosis of MTC, a careful history and physical examination should be done, with particular attention to family history and any symptoms related to hypercalcitoninemia (e.g., watery diarrhea) or pheochromocytoma (e.g., episodic hypertension). Laboratory studies should include measurements of serum calcitonin and calcium, and catecholamines and their metabolites should be assayed in urine and serum to screen for pheochromocytoma. Blood lymphocytes should be tested for germline mutations of the *RET* oncogene. If biochemical tests are suggestive of pheochromocytoma, then abdominal imaging should be done and endocrinologists and anesthesiologists consulted to prepare the patient for surgical treatment of the pheochromocytoma first. Often, however, MTC is diagnosed only after definitive

thyroid surgery from analysis of the histologic sections. In that case, the postoperative evaluation should include the same investigations as those noted above. If the basal calcitonin level is normal, a challenge test involving injection of pentagastrin (a gastric secretion stimulant) is a sensitive means of detecting residual disease.[96,97] If calcitonin levels remain normal despite the challenge, the prognosis is good and the disease is probably cured. However, significant numbers of patients have residual disease after surgical resection, as evidenced by high serum calcitonin and CEA levels or metastasis.[98,99] Abnormal calcitonin or CEA levels should prompt further investigations to look for regional or metastatic disease. Nodal involvement of the neck and superior mediastinum is relatively common, occurring in approximately 50% of cases, and is often subclinical, with the only detected abnormality being elevated serum calcitonin.[9,11] CT scanning of the neck, chest, and abdomen should be performed. A bone scan will help rule out skeletal metastases. Scans with octreotide, a somatostatin analogue, are highly specific for MTC and may help locate the disease even if CT scans are negative. It is important to distinguish local–regional disease from distant metastasis because the prognoses and management strategies for the two conditions differ. Gross disease in the neck can cause local compressive symptoms, as discussed in the previous section on differentiated thyroid cancer.

Patients who show a germline mutation in the *RET* oncogene should be offered genetic counseling, with appropriate screening of first-degree relatives (siblings, parents, and children). The clinical probability that a *RET*-mutation–positive person will develop MTC is very high (lifetime risk of more than 90%); prophylactic thyroidectomy is recommended and has a high cure rate.[17,18]

Prognostic Factors

Survival among patients with familial MTC and MEN2A is better than that among patients with sporadic MTC,[9,11,100] although this difference disappears when patients are matched for age, extent of tumor, and lymph node involvement.[9,11] MEN2B presents at earlier ages and more advanced stages than MEN2A and is associated with poorer survival.[101] A multivariate analysis of 73 patients treated at the Princess Margaret Hospital revealed that extrathyroidal invasion and postoperative gross residual disease were predictive of poor outcome.[8] In another series of 53 patients, clinical stage (UICC/AJCC) was the only prognostic factor.[102]

Principles of Management

The main treatment for MTC is surgery, with total thyroidectomy and cervical lymph node dissection as necessary. Radioactive iodine has no role in the management of MTC. Residual hypercalcitoninemia after thyroidectomy can be cured in some proportion of patients by meticulous nodal microdissection.[98,99]

Patients with gross or microscopic residual disease after surgery or extensive regional lymph node involvement are at high risk for recurrence; without further treatment, about 50% will experience recurrence. Postoperative adjuvant external radiation therapy to the thyroid bed and regional nodal tissue can be considered for patients with high-risk disease. A radiation dose of 40 Gy, given in 2-Gy fractions, to lymph nodes in the neck and upper mediastinum followed by a boost to the thyroid bed to a total dose of 50 Gy, produced a local–regional control rate of 86% at 10 years.[8] Although radiation treatment does not affect overall survival rates, local–regional control is important because relapse in the cervical nodes can negatively affect the patient's quality of life.[103-105] No role has been established for adjuvant chemotherapy. For patients with gross residual disease after surgery, the local control rate after radiation therapy is as low as 20%.[8] Therefore every attempt should be made to completely extirpate disease surgically; when this is not possible, external radiation may result in long-term local control in a few patients.

Hypercalcitoninemia Without Clinically Detectable Metastasis

Even after adequate surgical therapy, high levels of calcitonin can persist with no clinical evidence of metastasis. Imaging with radionuclides such as metaiodobenzylguanidine (MIBG) or octreotide may reveal abnormalities and can help direct therapy,[106,107] perhaps by facilitating the decision to offer local–regional radiation to the neck. Selective venous catheterization has been used to detect calcitonin gradients and thus locate occult tumor foci as being the source of the calcitonin.[108] Calcitonin and CEA levels correlate with tumor bulk; it is not unusual to see elevated but stable calcitonin or CEA levels for long periods (e.g., 5 to 10 years) without obvious progression of disease.[109] Thus cytotoxic treatment for an asymptomatic patient should be considered carefully. Diarrhea resulting from hypercalcitoninemia can be palliated with nonspecific drugs (e.g., diphenoxylate, loperamide) or a somatostatin analogue[110] with or without interferon.[111] A drop in the serum calcitonin level can indicate dedifferentiation and herald a more aggressive clinical course.[100]

Metastatic Disease

The most common sites of metastatic MTC are liver, lung, and bone. Treatment is palliative and includes supportive measures; analgesic drugs; and consideration of chemotherapy, hormonal therapy, and local radiation.

Chemotherapy involving doxorubicin, given alone or with cisplatin,[94] or drug combinations including 5-fluorouracil[112-115] or other drugs[93,116] can produce response rates of 15% to 30%. Hormonal therapy with octreotide has been reported to lessen symptoms and reduce calcitonin levels but generally does not induce tumor shrinkage.[110,117-120] A combination of octreotide and interferon-α was shown to improve response rates.[110,111] Local radiation is best suited for symptomatic osseous metastases. Experimental therapies to target tumor cells by linking monoclonal antibodies (e.g., anti-CEA) to radionuclides (e.g., ^{111}In-octreotide) are under active study.[121-124]

ANAPLASTIC THYROID CARCINOMA
Clinical Manifestations and Evaluation

ATC accounts for less than 2% of thyroid cancer cases.[125,126] The cardinal clinical features include a rapidly enlarging thyroid mass (typically over a few weeks) in an elderly person (see Fig. 14-4, *B*). Some patients may have a history of goiter or thyroid mass consistent with prior undiagnosed differentiated thyroid cancer. Compressive symptoms of the upper aerodigestive tract are common in ATC. Some tumors invade and ulcerate through the skin of the neck. Metastases are found at diagnosis in 30% to 50% of cases, typically in the lung.[127-131] It is important to evaluate the integrity of the upper airway and the need for tracheostomy. Chest radiography or CT and bone scanning can be useful in detecting metastatic disease.

Prognostic Factors

All ATCs are classified as stage IV by the AJCC/UICC.[4,5] Many ATCs coexist with areas of differentiated thyroid carcinoma in the gland, suggesting that the anaplastic component arises from preexisting differentiated disease (dedifferentiation).[126,131,132] An analysis by the thyroid cancer study group of the European Organization for Research and Treatment of Cancer (EORTC) showed that the prognosis for patients with any element of anaplasia within a differentiated thyroid cancer was no different than that for patients with anaplastic tumor throughout, with a 1-year survival rate of only 10%. Nevertheless, the prognosis for patients with small tumors (less than 5 cm), no extrathyroidal extension, and no lymph node involvement has been described as relatively good.[129] Occasional long-term survival has been described for patients with completely resected tumors and extrathyroidal disease that extends only into the adjacent soft tissues.[133]

Principles of Management

Complete surgical resection gives the best chance of cure, but this is possible for only a few patients.[127,133,134]

Most amenable to this approach are those tumors that consist predominantly of differentiated thyroid carcinoma with only a small focus of ATC.[134,135] Radical surgery is not warranted for patients with more extensive invasion of adjacent structures, as such surgery has a significant negative effect on quality of life and does not seem to prolong survival.[133] Surgery should be considered only when the extent of local disease allows thyroidectomy without undue morbidity.[133] ATC in most patients is unresectable at diagnosis; the main role for surgery is biopsy to confirm the diagnosis and tracheostomy as needed to alleviate airway obstruction.

Because ATC does not concentrate radioiodine, radiation is usually given in the form of external beam radiation, with the goal of improving local control. Because the expected 5-year survival is only about 5% with any currently available treatment approach,[127,128,130,133-136] the main goals of treatment are to achieve local control in the neck and to palliate any symptomatic metastatic disease so as to maintain quality of life.

Local control remains a major problem even after external beam radiation; however, even those patients in whom local control is achieved still die from distant metastatic disease.* The ineffectiveness of radiation alone for ATC prompted the development of novel fractionation schedules and concurrent chemotherapy regimens. Because ATC grows quickly, hyperfractionated and accelerated radiation schedules have been used, sometimes in combination with chemotherapy and surgical resection. Phase II studies of hyperfractionated radiation therapy combined with doxorubicin reported local control rates of 68%,[139,140] but a similar approach in patients with unresectable disease gave a local control rate of only 25%.[137]

The most successful regimen for obtaining local control, described by a Swedish group,[128,136] involves combined preoperative hyperfractionated radiation, chemotherapy, and subsequent surgical resection. However, despite a local control rate of 48%, only four patients from that study lived for 2 years or more.[128] Other approaches to intensify radiation therapy have had limited success because of increased damage to normal tissues.[137,141] In a study of hyperfractionated radiation therapy in 17 patients (60.8 Gy given in 32 twice-daily fractions over 20 to 24 days), complete response was reported in 3 patients (17.6%) and partial response in 7 (41.2%).[141] Nevertheless, the median survival time was only 10 weeks and the toxic effects were unacceptable, with most patients developing grade 3 or 4 toxicity and five dying before the toxicity resolved.

Even when local control is achieved, the metastatic rate for ATC remains high. Theoretically, giving chemotherapy beyond the course of radiation could improve survival if it eliminates micrometastases. Unfortunately, no known chemotherapy is effective against this type of cancer. Schlumberger and colleagues gave doxorubicin every 4 weeks for up to nine courses, in addition to radiation, and achieved only 15% survival at 20 months.[142]

At the Princess Margaret Hospital, patients with good performance status are prescribed a course of accelerated hyperfractionated radiation: 60 Gy given in 40 fractions, 1.5 Gy per fraction, twice a day over 4 weeks—without chemotherapy. To avoid the significant toxicity that others have encountered in using hyperfractionated radiation, no attempt is made to include all of the regional lymph nodes. For patients with poor performance status or known metastases, radiation is given with palliative intent at 20 Gy in five fractions, with the option of a second course 4 weeks later for those who respond to this treatment. Because the prognosis of ATC is extremely poor and because current therapies are ineffective, innovative approaches are needed for the treatment of this disease.

RARE TYPES OF THYROID CANCER

Rare primary tumors arising from the thyroid gland include squamous cell carcinomas, sarcomas, and even germ cell tumors. Lymphomas are occasionally seen, typically in elderly women who have a history of Hashimoto's thyroiditis. In general, the discovery of a rare tumor type involving the thyroid gland requires expert pathology review to rule out tumors of nonthyroid origin that may have infiltrated the thyroid gland (e.g., primary squamous cell carcinoma of the trachea or esophagus). Parathyroid carcinomas are occasionally seen, although they account for less than 1% of parathyroid neoplasms. Invasion into neck tissues or the thyroid gland, together with hypercalcemia from elevated parathyroid hormone production, should raise suspicion of a parathyroid carcinoma. For extensive local disease, a combination of surgery and postoperative local radiation therapy[143] generally produces a favorable outcome for parathyroid carcinoma. In contrast, primary squamous cell carcinoma of the thyroid is equally rare but highly malignant, with extensive local–regional invasion and a moderately high rate of metastatic spread. Treatment for this disease should consist of thyroidectomy with surgical extirpation of all gross disease, followed by postoperative radiation therapy.[144,145] Patients with unresectable disease can be treated with palliative radiation. Despite aggressive management, most patients (70% to 80%) will succumb to the disease. Lymphomas and sarcomas are treated according to the principles established for each histologic type, as discussed in Chapters 33 and 34 of this book.

---

*References 127, 128, 130, 131, 133-135, 137, 138.

RADIATION THERAPY TECHNIQUES
Radioiodine

Radioactive iodine can be given either as adjuvant treatment to ablate thyroid remnants after surgery or to treat residual, recurrent, or metastatic differentiated thyroid cancer. The rationale for giving ablative radioactive iodine postoperatively can be summarized as follows: (1) to ablate residual thyroid tissue that may contain microfoci of carcinoma (i.e., to treat multifocal disease); (2) to ablate residual thyroid tissue to remove the source of thyroglobulin so that the serum thyroglobulin assay can be used as a marker of thyroid cancer in follow-up (any rise in thyroglobulin can be assumed to be of malignant origin); and (3) to enable the detection of micrometastasis with iodine scanning that would otherwise be masked by absorption of radioiodine by the thyroid remnant. Many retrospective studies have indicated that postoperative iodine is beneficial in reducing the recurrence rate and improving the survival rate.

As discussed earlier, identifying patients who would benefit from radioactive iodine ablation remains controversial. It has been argued that the prognosis for patients younger than 45 years with tumors smaller than 4 cm is excellent and that these patients can be effectively treated by surgery alone. However, the authors believe that all adults probably benefit from radioactive iodine for the reasons listed above, unless they have unifocal tumors less than 1.5 cm or minimally invasive follicular carcinomas.

No consensus exists as to the best way of preparing patients for radioiodine therapy or the optimal activity level to be given in such therapy. The current approach at the Princess Margaret Hospital is as follows. Although thyroid remnants can be ablated after a less-than-total or near-total thyroidectomy, the success rate for this procedure is low (approximately 60%)[146] and can be associated with acute toxicity. The authors therefore recommend a completion thyroidectomy in the event of a previous thyroid lobectomy. The serum thyrotropin level should be above 30 μU/ml to maximize the uptake of radioiodine by the remnant thyroid tissue. To achieve this level, thyroxine is stopped for 6 weeks and L-T_3 is given for the first 3 weeks and then discontinued. The thyrotropin level peaks at 2 to 3 weeks after cessation of the T_3. The resulting clinical hypothyroidism can be significant, and about 50% of patients may have to stop work for this reason.[147] Reducing the length of time of thyroxine and T_3 withdrawal, especially in elderly patients with cardiac disease, can lessen the effect. An alternative is the use of rTSH, which allows patients to continue taking their normal dose of thyroxine.[59-61] Because consuming a low-iodine diet can increase 24-hour iodine uptake, a simplified low-iodine diet for 1 week before radioiodine therapy is recommended. (However, many patients find the diet unpleasant, and some physicians do not routinely recommend a low-iodine diet.) The use of iodinated contrast media in diagnostic imaging should be avoided for at least 3 months before radioiodine therapy. Medications containing high amounts of iodine such as amiodarone can also prevent successful iodine therapy.

When the patient is under hypothyroid conditions, we perform a 74- or 110-MBq (2 or 3 mCi of ^{131}I) diagnostic scan and quantify the radioiodine uptake in the neck before iodine therapy to assess the extent of thyroid remnants and the presence of any metastatic disease (see Fig. 14-6). If the 48-hour scan shows thyroid remnants and less than 2% uptake in the neck, then less than 1100 MBq (29.9 mCi) is prescribed, to be taken on an outpatient basis, for patients who have no adverse prognostic factors. For those with a neck uptake greater than 2%, 100 mCi is prescribed. This policy results in an effective rate of ablation of 80%.[146,148] If the scan indicates the presence of uptake in cervical lymph nodes superior to the thyroid bed or if extrathyroidal extension of disease is present (UICC T4 lesion), 5550 to 7400 MBq (150 to 200 mCi) is prescribed, as is also done in the rare case in which distant metastatic disease exists at the diagnostic scan. The therapeutic dose should be given as soon as possible, typically within 5 days of the diagnostic scan. Some physicians do not recommend a scan before therapy, either because of concern about stunting (as has been shown in a small proportion of patients exposed to 185 to 1100 MBq [5 to 30 mCi] of radioiodine[149,150]) or because some physicians empirically prescribe some fixed dose of radioiodine (e.g., 1100 MBq [100 mCi]) and therefore find it unnecessary to perform a scan before therapy. After radioiodine therapy, the usual practice is to scan 7 to 10 days later to locate the abnormal areas of radioiodine uptake. It is not unusual to find additional foci of uptake not previously visible on the pretherapy scan,[151] such as in the neck, indicating disease in the cervical lymph nodes, or occasionally diffuse uptake in the lungs, indicating iodine-avid micrometastasis.

To radiation oncologists, it is more attractive to prescribe an absorbed dose to the target than to prescribe an empirical dose of radioiodine, but this practice requires estimating both the mass of remnant thyroid tissue *and* the effective half-life of the retained radioactivity. The maximum tolerated activity is limited by the total blood dose, which should not exceed 2 Gy. Detailed dosimetric studies have demonstrated that 300 Gy resulted in ablation of 80% of remnants, and 100 ± 20 Gy resulted in 80% complete response of nodal or soft tissue metastases.[152,153] However no comparative studies have been done to verify the superiority of this approach in terms of improving recurrence rate or survival.

The need to admit patients to a hospital facility depends on the recommendations of the local regulatory body. Although many centers require that patients given 1100 MBq (30 mCi) or more be admitted until the retained activity drops below 1100 MBq, recent changes in the U.S. Nuclear Regulatory Commission Guidelines[154] allow much larger activity levels to be administered on an outpatient basis. This practice requires careful measurement and documentation of neck and whole-body retention, effective half-life, patients' living conditions, and time spent with other people.

External Beam Radiation Therapy

The main consideration regarding external radiation therapy techniques for thyroid cancer is deciding whether to treat the thyroid bed alone or the thyroid bed plus the lymph nodes (bilateral, cervical, and superior mediastinum). The thyroid bed volume curves around the vertebral body and includes the air column in the trachea. This U-shaped volume presents a challenge for adequately treating the thyroid bed while sparing the spinal cord. If the lymph nodes are considered to be at risk, then at least two phases of treatment are required to stay within spinal-cord tolerance limits. Several techniques have been described to overcome these difficulties,[155] but some degree of compromise is invariably necessary. Additional details regarding treatment techniques are provided in the following paragraphs.

Thyroid Bed Alone

If only the thyroid bed is to be treated, then the target volume extends from the hyoid superiorly to just below the suprasternal notch, and that volume is adjusted according to the surgical and pathology findings. (This is the most common volume when radiation therapy is to be given after thyroidectomy and radioiodine for differentiated thyroid carcinoma with extensive extrathyroidal extension of disease [UICC/AJCC T4 lesion]). The characteristic rapid fall-off of a direct electron beam and the effect of the neck contour can produce an acceptable high-dose volume if only the thyroid bed is to be treated (Fig. 14-7). Planning CT scanning should be performed to aid the choice of electron energy and obtain an isodose distribution. The Princess Margaret Hospital technique commonly uses 12- to 20-MeV beams or a mixed beam of two energies (see Fig. 14-7, B and C). In the absence of gross disease, 40 Gy, given in 15 or 16 fractions over 3 weeks, is prescribed. If gross disease is present, a higher dose of 50 Gy is given in 20 fractions over 4 weeks.[25,73] The dose is prescribed at 100% and the maximum spinal cord dose is limited to 60% of the prescribed dose (see Fig. 14-7, B and C). The authors use this conservative limit because of the uncertainty in the actual dose received, given the complex three-dimensional nature of the tissue inhomogeneities, the presence of air in the trachea, the bone density of the vertebra, and the changing contour. This

technique produces a brisk skin reaction because of the lack of skin sparing. An immobilization shell is usually not necessary, but if one is used, it should be limited to the face and mandible to maintain a reproducible neck position and should not cover the irradiated area so as to minimize the skin dose. An alternative technique is to use two anterolateral oblique wedged fields such as those used for laryngeal cancer.[155] The posterior border is placed so as to exclude the spinal cord. The advantage of this technique over a single anterior electron beam is additional skin sparing, but it comes at the cost of underdosing the posterior lateral part of the volume. It is important to plan this technique with CT scanning before treatment and to examine the axial dose distributions that are off the central slice so as to ensure the spinal cord position. Shielding of the spinal cord may be required because its anteroposterior position will vary throughout the treatment volume.

For most patients with ATC and significant tumor bulk, the anterior electron beam or the anterolateral wedged-pair techniques are inadequate for tumor coverage. The therapy should then take place in two phases as described below, with the upper and lower borders adjusted depending on the necessity to cover the extent of disease.

Thyroid Bed with the Cervical and Superior Mediastinal Lymph Nodes

Large-volume treatment involving the cervical and superior lymph nodes and the thyroid bed is typical for MTC and for differentiated thyroid cancer that either persists after neck dissection and radioiodine therapy or has extensive nodal extracapsular extension (Fig. 14-8). Such treatment also applies to ATC if regional nodes are involved in addition to the local thyroid disease. This technique consists of a minimum of two phases. The initial volume (phase 1) includes the regional lymph nodes from the mastoid tip to the carina, including the thyroid bed (see Fig. 14-8, A), and consists of parallel opposing anteroposterior-posteroanterior fields to 40 to 46 Gy. The patient is treated while supine with the neck extended to avoid the parotid glands and the oral cavity. Because of variation in the thickness of the volume, obtaining a sagittal isodose distribution is important for ensuring an accurate spinal cord dose. The mandible and lung tissue should be routinely shielded. In ATC, the target volume is usually smaller, planned to cover the gross disease with a 2- to 3-cm margin. The aim of phase 1 is to deliver a dose of 45 to 46 Gy before starting the off-cord treatment. Depending on the phase 2 technique and the spinal cord dose in that phase, the phase 1 treatment dose may need to be adjusted to less than 46 Gy. This can be done by terminating the phase 1 arrangement at a lower dose (e.g., 40 Gy). Alternatively, phase 1 can be continued to 46 Gy with the insertion of a full-length, posterior-only spinal cord shield

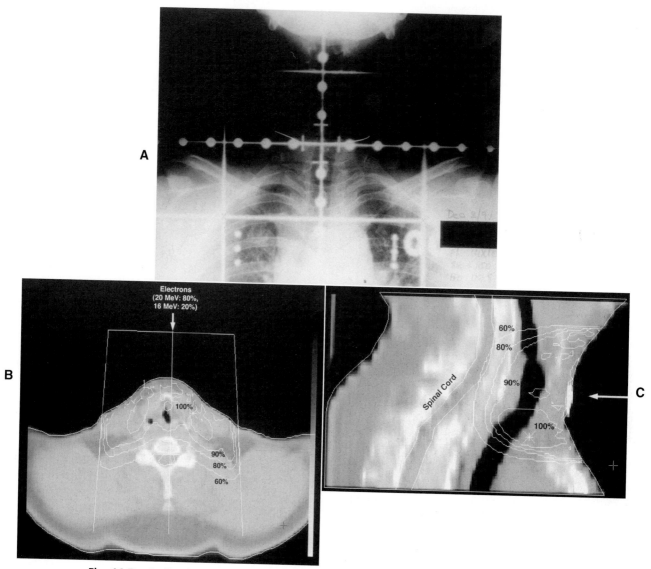

Fig. 14-7   **A,** Simulator film for a typical field of direct electrons to the thyroid bed. Isodose distributions in an axial computed tomography image **(B)** and a sagittally reconstructed image **(C)** show the maximum spinal cord dose to be 60% of the prescribed dose.

for the final few treatments to reduce the spinal cord dose to 40 to 45 Gy, but this practice compromises the midline dose.

The phase 2 volume should include those tissues considered to be at the highest risk of relapse—that is, any gross residual disease and any areas of extrathyroidal extension documented during surgery or imaging. The principal aim is to boost the high-risk tissue to a total dose of 14 Gy (cumulative total dose of 60 Gy) while keeping the maximum cumulative spinal cord dose to 50 Gy, with the dose per fraction not exceeding 2 Gy. A phase 1 dose of 46 Gy would allow an additional maximum of 4 Gy to be delivered to the spinal cord from the

phase 2 boost. The phase 2 planning process should be completed as early as possible, preferably before initiation of phase 1, so that the overall plan can be scrutinized for the safety of all critical normal tissues such as spinal cord, esophagus, and salivary gland tissues. Any dose adjustments and placement of shielding can then be effected early in the course of therapy, so that subsequent phase 2 therapy need not be compromised because of excessive phase 1 treatment for a particular critical organ.

For a phase 2 boost to the thyroid bed alone, the technique can be a direct anterior electron beam, as described above, or anterolateral oblique wedged fields. Another alternative is a lateral pair of angled-down

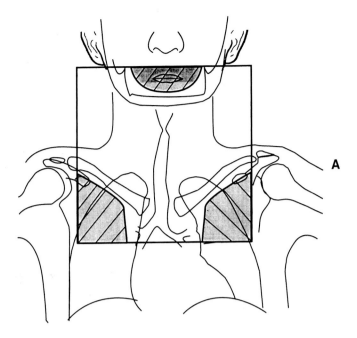

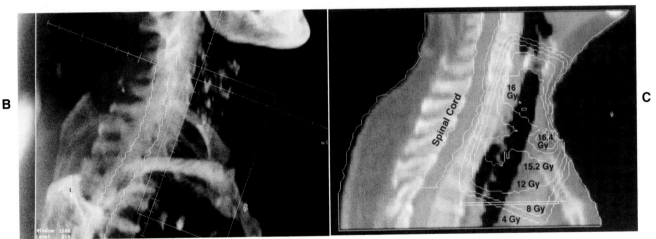

Fig. 14-8 **A,** Typical phase 1 large field (to maximum dose of 46 Gy). **B,** Digital subtraction radiograph of the field borders and shielding. **C,** Isodose distribution of phase 2 boost with lateral angled-down wedged-pair fields (couch rotation 20 degrees).

oblique fields, achieved with a couch rotation of 10 to 20 degrees aiming inferiorly to avoid the shoulders, off the spinal cord (see Fig. 14-8, *B* and *C*). Planning CT is indispensable. Beam's eye views are helpful in ensuring exclusion of the spinal cord. The degree of couch rotation depends on the position of the shoulders and the inferior extent of the mediastinal volume. With a couch rotation of 20 degrees, all of the superior mediastinal lymph nodes can be included to the level of the carina. The main disadvantage of this technique is possible exposure of the parotid glands because of the higher entrance point of the lateral beams.

Because the thyroid bed target volume is U-shaped and because regional lymph nodes often must be included, conformal radiotherapy, or intensity-modulated radiation therapy if it is available, is ideal for treatment planning for this difficult volume.

Palliative Radiation Therapy for Metastatic Disease

The principal sites of metastatic disease are bone and lung, with occasional involvement of soft tissues and lymph nodes. Liver metastasis is common in MTC.

In general, for differentiated thyroid cancer, radioiodine should be considered first, and radiation should be used only for disease in which iodine cannot be concentrated or is ineffective. The main role of external radiation therapy is to palliate painful bone metastases. It is important to establish the goal of palliative therapy, particularly with regard to distinguishing whether it is offered for local control or purely to alleviate symptoms. Because the natural history of thyroid cancer is long, patients can live for many years despite the presence of metastatic disease. Therefore patients for whom maximal control of metastatic disease site is desirable should be offered a radical course of therapy to doses of 40 to 50 Gy. It is also important to consider the contributing dose from cumulative radioiodine therapy, particularly for vertebral lesions in direct contact with the spinal cord. Additional management considerations include the possibility of surgical resection of solitary metastases or resection and internal fixation of bones at risk of pathologic fracture. Pure symptom relief for patients whose life expectancy is short can be achieved with 8 Gy given as a single dose, 20 Gy given in 5 fractions, or 30 Gy given in 10 fractions, as is commonly used for other types of metastatic disease.

COMPLICATIONS OF RADIATION THERAPY
Radioiodine

Nausea, headache, and vomiting resulting from radiation sickness occurs in 60% to 70% of patients given 7400 MBq (200 mCi) of radioactive iodine. Parotid swelling, altered sense of taste, and dry mouth can occur but are rare after doses of 3700 MBq (100 mCi) or less. Reversible bone marrow depression is most severe at 6 weeks. At cumulative activity levels of 18,500 to 37,000 MBq (500 to 1000 mCi), the incidence of chronic bone marrow depression is less than 1.5%; at cumulative activity levels exceeding 1000 mCi, the incidence rises to 25% or more.[156] Leukemia has been associated with cumulative doses of more than 29,400 MBq (800 mCi), and an increased risk of breast and bladder cancer has been reported after average cumulative doses of about 37,000 MBq (1000 mCi).[157] Men can experience reversible or irreversible gonadal failure, especially after higher cumulative doses. In a study of 2113 pregnancies among women previously given radioiodine, the rates of miscarriages or preterm births, stillbirths, or congenital defects were no higher than those among women given thyroid surgery without iodine therapy.[158] Radiation pneumonitis or fibrosis is rare, having been reported in less than 2% of patients treated for lung metastases.

External Beam Radiation Therapy

Well-planned external beam radiation therapy produces acceptable levels of acute toxicity, rarely produces serious complications, and does not preclude future surgical intervention. During the course of radiation therapy, moderate skin erythema develops, with higher doses causing dry or, rarely, moist desquamation. Mucositis of the esophagus, trachea, and larynx can occur toward the end of the irradiation and may require consumption of a soft diet and use of analgesics. Depending on the superior extent of the fields, changes in taste sensation and xerostomia are possible. Late toxicity is infrequent, consisting mostly of skin telangiectasias, skin pigmentation, soft tissue fibrosis, and mild lymphedema, usually appearing just below the chin. Esophageal or tracheal stenosis is extremely rare. Tsang and colleagues[25] reported no grade IV toxic effects (using the Radiation Therapy Oncology Group scale) among patients given doses of 40 to 50 Gy in 2- to 2.5-Gy fractions to the neck and superior mediastinum. Farahati and colleagues[75] observed no irreversible late toxic effects among 99 patients given doses of 50 to 60 Gy in 1.8- to 2.0-Gy fractions to a large volume.

REFERENCES

1. Shafford E, Kingston J, Healy J, et al. Thyroid nodular disease after radiotherapy to the neck for childhood Hodgkin's disease. *Br J Cancer* 1999;80:808.
2. Grande C. Hypothyroidism following radiotherapy for head and neck cancer: multivariate analysis of risk factors. *Radiother Oncol* 1992;25:31.
3. Hancock S, McDougal I, Constine L. Thyroid abnormalities after therapeutic radiation. *Int J Radiat Oncol Biol Phys* 1995;31:1165.
4. Fleming I, Cooper JS, Henson DE, et al, eds. *AJCC Cancer Staging Manual*, 5th ed. Philadelphia, Pa: Lippincott Williams & Wilkins; 1997:59-64.
5. Sobin LH, Wittekind C, eds. *TNM Classification of Malignant Tumours*, 5th ed. New York, NY: Wiley-Liss; 1997.
6. Ries LAG, Eisner MP, Kosary CL, et al. *SEER Statistics Review, 1973-1997.* Bethesda, Md: National Cancer Institute; 2000.
7. Franceschi S, Boyle P, Maisonneuve P, et al. The epidemiology of thyroid carcinoma. *Crit Rev Oncog* 1993;4:25.
8. Brierley JD, Tsang RW, Gospodarowicz MK, et al. Medullary thyroid cancer—analyses of survival and prognostic factors and the role of radiation therapy in local control. *Thyroid* 1996;6:305.
9. Raue F. German medullary thyroid carcinoma/multiple endocrine neoplasia registry. German MTC/MEN Study Group. Medullary Thyroid Carcinoma/Multiple Endocrine Neoplasia Type 2. *Langenbecks Arch Surg* 1998;383:334-336.
10. Bergholm U, Bergstrom R, Ekbom A. Long-term follow-up of patients with medullary carcinoma of the thyroid. *Cancer* 1997;79:132.
11. Samaan NA, Schultz PN, Hickey RC. Medullary thyroid carcinoma: prognosis of familial versus sporadic disease and the role of radiotherapy. *J Clin Endocrinol Metab* 1988;67:801.
12. Eng C. RET proto-oncogene in the development of human cancer. *J Clin Oncol* 1999;17:380.
13. Eng C. Seminars in medicine of the Beth Israel Hospital, Boston. The RET proto-oncogene in multiple endocrine neoplasia type 2 and Hirschsprung's disease. *N Engl J Med* 1996;335:943.
14. Mulligan LM, Kwok JB, Healey CS, et al. Germ-line mutations of the RET proto-oncogene in multiple endocrine neoplasia type 2A. *Nature* 1993;363:458.

15. Mulligan LM, Eng C, Healey CS, et al. Specific mutations of the RET proto-oncogene are related to disease phenotype in MEN 2A and FMTC. *Nat Genet* 1994;6:70.

16. Eng C, Clayton D, Schuffenecker I, et al. The relationship between specific RET proto-oncogene mutations and disease phenotype in multiple endocrine neoplasia type 2. International RET mutation consortium analysis. *JAMA* 1996;276:1575.

17. Wells SA, Chi DD, Toshima K, et al. Predictive DNA testing and prophylactic thyroidectomy in patients at risk for multiple endocrine neoplasia type 2A. *Ann Surg* 1994;220:237.

18. Modigliani E, Cohen R, Campos JM, et al. Prognostic factors for survival and for biochemical cure in medullary thyroid carcinoma: results in 899 patients. The GETC Study Group. Groupe d'Etude des Tumeurs a Calcitonine. *Clin Endocrinol (Oxf)* 1998;48:265.

19. Hemminki K, Dong C. Familial relationships in thyroid cancer by histo-pathological type. *Int J Cancer* 2000;85:201.

20. Malchoff CD, Malchoff DM. Familial nonmedullary thyroid carcinoma. *Semin Surg Oncol* 1999;16:16.

21. Lupoli G, Vitale G, Caraglia M, et al. Familial papillary thyroid microcarcinoma: a new clinical entity. *Lancet* 1999;353:637.

22. Cetta F, Toti P, Petracci M, et al. Thyroid carcinoma associated with familial adenomatous polyposis. *Histopathology* 1997;31:231.

23. Lynch ED, Ostermeyer EA, Lee MK, et al. Inherited mutations in PTEN that are associated with breast cancer, cowden disease, and juvenile polyposis. *Am J Hum Genet* 1997;61:1254.

24. Shore RE. Issues and epidemiological evidence regarding radiation-induced thyroid cancer. *Radiat Res* 1992;131:98.

25. Tsang RW, Brierley JD, Simpson WJ, et al. The effects of surgery, radioiodine and external radiation therapy on the clinical outcome of patients with differentiated thyroid cancer. *Cancer* 1998;82:375.

26. Astakhova LN, Anspaugh LR, Beebe GW, et al. Chernobyl-related thyroid cancer in children of Belarus: a case-control study. *Radiat Res* 1998;150:349-356.

27. Thomas GA, Bunnell H, Cook HA, et al. High prevalence of RET/PTC rearrangements in Ukrainian and Belarussian post-Chernobyl thyroid papillary carcinomas: a strong correlation between RET/PTC3 and the solid-follicular variant. *J Clin Endocrinol Metab* 1999;84:4232.

28. Hamilton H, van Belle G, LoGerfo J. Thyroid neoplasia in Marshall Islanders exposed to nuclear fallout. *JAMA* 1987;258:629.

29. Fagin J, Matsuo K, Karmakar A, et al. High prevalence of mutations of the *p53* gene in poorly differentiated human thyroid carcinomas. *J Clin Invest* 1993;91:179.

30. Sugg SL, Ezzat S, Rosen IB, et al. Distinct multiple *RET/PTC* gene rearrangements in multifocal papillary thyroid neoplasia. *J Clin Endocrinol Metab* 1998;83:4116.

31. van den Brekel MW, Hekkenberg RJ, Asa SL, et al. Prognostic features in tall cell papillary carcinoma and insular thyroid carcinoma. *Laryngoscope* 1997;107:254.

32. LiVolsi V, Asa S. The demise of follicular carcinoma of the thyroid. *Thyroid* 1994;4:233.

33. Johnson TL, Lloyd RV, Thompson NW, et al. Prognostic implications of the tall cell variant of papillary thyroid carcinoma. *Am J Surg Pathol* 1988;12:22.

34. Evans H. Columnar-cell carcinoma of the thyroid. A report of two cases of an aggressive variant of thyroid carcinoma. *Am J Clin Pathol* 1986;85:77.

35. Sobrinho-Simoes M, Nesland JM, Johannessen JV. Columnar-cell carcinoma. Another variant of poorly differentiated carcinoma of the thyroid. *Am J Clin Pathol* 1988;89:264.

36. Carcangiu ML, Bianchi S. Diffuse sclerosing variant of papillary thyroid carcinoma. Clinicopathologic study of 15 cases. *Am J Surg Pathol* 1989;13:1041.

37. Carcangiu ML, Bianchi S, Savino D, et al. Follicular Hurthle cell tumors of the thyroid gland. *Cancer* 1991;68:1944.

38. Rodriguez JM, Parrilla P, Moreno A, et al. Insular carcinoma: an infrequent subtype of thyroid cancer. *J Am Coll Surg* 1998;187:503.

39. Carcangiu ML, Steeper T, Zampi G, et al. Anaplastic thyroid carcinoma. A study of 70 cases. *Am J Clin Pathol* 1985;83:135.

40. Fernandez JF, Ordonez NG, Schultz PN, et al. Thyroglossal duct carcinoma. *Surgery* 1991;110:928.

41. O'Connell M, Grixti M, Harmer C. Thyroglossal duct carcinoma: presentation and management, including eight case reports [published erratum appears in Clin Oncol (R Coll Radiol) 1998; 10(4):following table of contents]. *Clin Oncol (R Coll Radiol)* 1998;10:186.

42. Giuffrida D, Gharib H. Controversies in the management of cold, hot, and occult thyroid nodules. *Am J Med* 1995;99:642.

43. Tyler DS, Winchester DJ, Caraway NP, et al. Indeterminate fine-needle aspiration biopsy of the thyroid: identification of subgroups at high risk for invasive carcinoma. *Surgery* 1994;116: 1054.

44. Cady B, Rossi R. An expanded view of risk-group definition in differentiated thyroid carcinoma. *Surgery* 1988;104:947.

45. Hay ID. Papillary thyroid carcinoma. *Endocrinol Metab Clin North Am* 1990;19:545.

46. Hay ID, Bergstralh EJ, Goellner JR, et al. Predicting outcome in papillary thyroid carcinoma: development of a reliable prognostic scoring system in a cohort of 1779 patients surgically treated at one institution during 1940 through 1989. *Surgery* 1993; 114:1050.

47. DeGroot LJ, Kaplan EL, Straus FH, et al. Does the method of management of papillary thyroid carcinoma make a difference in outcome? *World J Surg* 1994;18:123.

48. Brierley JD, Panzarella T, Tsang RW, et al. A comparison of different staging systems predictability of patient outcome. Thyroid carcinoma as an example. *Cancer* 1997;79:2414.

49. Mazzaferri EL, Jhiang SM. Long-term impact of initial surgical and medical therapy on papillary and follicular thyroid cancer. *Am J Med* 1994;97:418.

50. Simpson WJ, McKinney SE, Carruthers JS, et al. Papillary and follicular thyroid cancer. *Am J Med* 1987;83:479.

51. Coburn MC, Wanebo HJ. Age correlates with increased frequency of high risk factors in elderly patients with thyroid cancer. *Am J Surg* 1995;170:471.

52. Vassilopoulou-Sellin R, Goepfert H, Raney B, et al. Differentiated thyroid cancer in children and adolescents: clinical outcome and mortality after long-term follow-up. *Head Neck* 1998;20:549.

53. Pasieka JL, Rotstein LE. Consensus conference on well-differentiated thyroid cancer: a summary. *Can J Surg* 1993;36:298.

54. Kebebew E, Clark OH. Differentiated thyroid cancer: "complete" rational approach. *World J Surg* 2000;24:942-951.

55. Shaha AR, Shah JP, Loree TR. Low-risk differentiated thyroid cancer: the need for selective treatment. *Ann Surg Oncol* 1997; 4:328.

56. Sanders LE, Cady B. Differentiated thyroid cancer: reexamination of risk groups and outcome of treatment. *Arch Surg* 1998; 133:419.

57. Shaha AR, Shah JP, Loree TR. Patterns of failure in differentiated carcinoma of the thyroid based on risk groups. *Head Neck* 1998; 20:26.

58. Mazzaferri EL. An overview of the management of papillary and follicular thyroid carcinoma. *Thyroid* 1999;9:421.

59. Ladenson PW, Braverman LE, Mazzaferri EL, et al. Comparison of administration of recombinant human thyrotropin with withdrawal of thyroid hormone for radioactive iodine scanning in patients with thyroid carcinoma. *N Engl J Med* 1997;337:888.

60. Ladenson PW. Recombinant thyrotropin versus thyroid hormone withdrawal in evaluating patients with thyroid carcinoma. *Semin Nucl Med* 2000;30:98.

61. Haugen BR, Pacini F, Reiners C, et al. A comparison of recombinant human thyrotropin and thyroid hormone withdrawal for the detection of thyroid remnant or cancer. *J Clin Endocrinol Metab* 1999;84:3877.

62. Simpson WJ, Panzarella T, Carruthers JS, et al. Papillary and follicular thyroid cancer: impact of treatment in 1578 patients. *Int J Radiat Oncol Biol Phys* 1988;14:1063.

63. Cooper DS, Specker B, Ho M, et al. Thyrotropin suppression and disease progression in patients with differentiated thyroid cancer: results from the National Thyroid Cancer Treatment Cooperative Registry. *Thyroid* 1998;8:737.

64. Sherman S. Adjuvant therapy and long-term management of differentiated thyroid carcinoma. *Semin Surg Oncol* 1999;16:30.

65. Ozata M, Suzuki S, Miyamoto T, et al. Serum thyroglobulin in the follow-up of patients with treated differentiated thyroid cancer. *J Clin Endocrinol Metab* 1994;79:98.

66. Pineda JD, Lee T, Ain K, et al. Iodine-131 therapy for thyroid cancer patients with elevated thyroglobulin and negative diagnostic scan. *J Clin Endocrinol Metab* 1995;80:1488.

67. Schlumberger M, Baudin E. Serum thyroglobulin determination in the follow-up of patients with differentiated thyroid carcinoma. *Eur J Endocrinol* 1998;138:249.

68. Hjiyiannakis P, Mundy J, Harmer C. Thyroglobulin antibodies in differentiated thyroid cancer. *Clin Oncol (R Coll Radiol)* 1999;11:240.

69. Westbury C, Vini L, Fisher C, et al. Recurrent differentiated thyroid cancer without elevation of serum thyroglobulin. *Thyroid* 2000;10:171.

70. Vassilopoulou-Sellin R, Schultz PN, Haynie TP. Clinical outcome of patients with papillary thyroid carcinoma who have recurrence after initial radioactive iodine therapy. *Cancer* 1996;78:493.

71. Anderson P, Kinsella J, Loree TR, et al. Differentiated carcinoma of the thyroid with extrathyroid extension. *Am J Surg* 1995;170:467.

72. McCaffrey TV, Bergstralh EJ, Hay ID. Locally invasive papillary thyroid carcinoma: 1940-1990. *Head Neck* 1994;16:165.

73. Brierley JD, Tsang RW. External radiation therapy in the treatment of thyroid cancer. In: Burman KD, ed. *Thyroid Cancer II, Endocrinol Metab Clin North Am*, Vol. 25. Philadelphia, Pa: WB Saunders;1996:141.

74. Benker G, Olbricht T, Reinwein D, et al. Survival rates in patients with differentiated thyroid carcinoma. Influence of postoperative external radiotherapy. *Cancer* 1990;65:1517.

75. Farahati J, Reiners C, Stuschke M, et al. Differentiated thyroid cancer. Impact of adjuvant external radiotherapy in patients with perithyroidal tumor infiltration (stage pT4). *Cancer* 1996;77:172.

76. Phlips P, Hanzen C, Andry G, et al. Postoperative irradiation for thyroid cancer. *Eur J Surg Oncol* 1993;19:399.

77. Tubiana M, Haddad E, Schlumberger M, et al. External radiotherapy in thyroid cancers. *Cancer* 1985;55:2062.

78. Esik O, Nemeth G, Eller J. Prophylactic external irradiation in differentiated thyroid cancer: a retrospective study over a 30-year observation period. *Oncology* 1994;51:372.

79. Sheline GE, Galante M, Lindsay S. Radiation therapy in the control of persistent thyroid cancer. *Am J Roentgenol Radium Ther Nucl Med* 1966;97:923.

80. Harmer CL. External beam radiotherapy for thyroid cancer. *Ann Radiol (Paris)* 1977;20:791.

81. O'Connell M, Hern R, Harmer CL. Results of external beam radiotherapy in differentiated thyroid carcinoma: a retrospective study from the Royal Marsden Hospital. *Eur J Cancer* 1994;30A:733.

82. Glanzmann C, Lutolf UM. Long-term follow-up of 92 patients with locally advanced follicular or papillary thyroid cancer after combined treatment. *Strahlenther Onkol* 1992;168: 260.

83. Coburn M, Teates D, Wanebo HJ. Recurrent thyroid cancer. Role of surgery versus radioactive iodine (I-131). *Ann Surg* 1994;219:587.

84. Gillenwater AM, Goepfert H. Surgical management of laryngotracheal and esophageal involvement by locally advanced thyroid cancer. *Semin Surg Oncol* 1999;16:19.

85. Schlumberger M, Challeton C, De Vathaire F, et al. Radioactive iodine treatment and external radiotherapy for lung and bone metastases from thyroid carcinoma. *J Nucl Med* 1996;37:598.

86. Casara D, Rubello D, Saladini G, et al. Distant metastases in diffentiated thyroid cancer: long term results of radioiodine treatment. *Tumori* 1991;77:432.

87. Proye CA, Dromer DH, Carnaille BM, et al. Is it still worthwhile to treat bone metastases from differentiated thyroid carcinoma with radioactive iodine? *World J Surg* 1992;16:640.

88. Shaha AR, Shah JP, Loree TR. Differentiated thyroid cancer presenting initially with distant metastasis. *Am J Surg* 1997;174:474.

89. Lind P. 131I whole body scintigraphy in thyroid cancer patients. *Q J Nucl Med* 1999;43:188.

90. Grunwald F, Briele B, Biersack H-J. Non-131I-scintigraphy in the treatment and follow-up of thyroid cancer. Single-photon-emitters or FDG-PET? *Q J Nucl Med* 1999;43:195.

91. Robbins J. Management of thyroglobulin-positive, body scan-negative thyroid cancer patients: evidence for the utility of I-131 therapy. *J Endocrinol Invest* 1999;22:808.

92. Dinneen SF, Valimaki MJ, Bergstralh EJ, et al. Distant metastases in papillary thyroid carcinoma: 100 cases observed at one institution during 5 decades. *J Clin Endocrinol Metab* 1995;80:2041.

93. Ekman ET, Lundell G, Tennvall J, et al. Chemotherapy and multimodality treatment in thyroid carcinoma. *Otolaryngol Clin North Am* 1990;23:523.

94. Shimaoka K, Schoenfeld DA, DeWys WD, et al. A randomized trial of doxorubicin versus doxorubicin plus cisplatin in patients with advanced thyroid carcinoma. *Cancer* 1985;56:2155.

95. Haugen BR. Management of the patient with progressive radioiodine non-responsive disease. *Semin Surg Oncol* 1999;16:34.

96. Wells SA, Baylin SB, Linehan WM, et al. Provocative agents and the diagnosis of medullary thyroid carcinoma. *Ann Surg* 1978;188:139.

97. Simpson WJ, Carruthers JS, Malkin D. Results of a screening program for C-cell disease (medullary thyroid cancer and C-cell hyperplasia). *Cancer* 1990;65:1570.

98. Moley JF, Wells SA, Dilley WG, et al. Reoperation for recurrent or persistent medullary thyroid cancer. *Surgery* 1993;114:1090.

99. Tisell LE, Hansson G, Jansson S, et al. Reoperation in the treatment of asymptomatic metastasizing medullary thyroid carcinoma. *Surgery* 1986;99:60.

100. Saad M, Orddonez N, Rashid R, et al. Medullary carcinoma: Prognostic factors and treatment. *Int J Radiat Oncol Biol Phys* 1984;9:161.

101. O'Riordain D, O'Brien T, Crotty TB, et al. Multiple endocrine neoplasia type 2B: more than an endocrine disorder. *Surgery* 1995;118:936.

102. Dottorini ME, Assi A, Sironi M, et al. Multivariate analysis of patients with medullary thyroid carcinoma. Prognostic significance and impact on treatment of clinical and pathologic variables. *Cancer* 1996;77:1556.

103. Fife KM, Bower M, Harmer CL. Medullary thyroid cancer: the role of radiotherapy in local control. *Eur J Surg Oncol* 1996;22:588.

104. Mak A, Morrison W, Garden A, et al. The value of postoperative radiotherapy for regional medullary carcinoma of the thyroid. *Int J Radiat Oncol Biol Phys* 1994;30:234.

105. Nguyen TD, Chassard JL, Lagarde P, et al. Results of postoperative radiation therapy in medullary carcinoma of the thyroid: a

retrospective study by the French Federation of Cancer Institutes—the Radiotherapy Cooperative Group. *Radiother Oncol* 1992;23:1.

106. Baudin E, Lumbroso J, Schlumberger M, et al. Comparison of octreotide scintigraphy and conventional imaging in medullary thyroid carcinoma. *J Nucl Med* 1996;37:912.

107. Tisell LE, Ahlman H, Wangberg B, et al. Somatostatin receptor scintigraphy in medullary thyroid carcinoma. *Br J Surg* 1997; 84:543.

108. Abdelmoumene N, Schlumberger M, Gardet P, et al. Selective venous sampling catheterisation for localisation of persisting medullary thyroid carcinoma. *Br J Cancer* 1994;69:1141.

109. Girelli ME, Nacamulli D, Pelizzo MR, et al. Medullary thyroid carcinoma: clinical features and long-term follow-up of seventy-eight patients treated between 1969 and 1986. *Thyroid* 1998;8:517.

110. di Bartolomeo M, Bajetta E, Buzzoni R, et al. Clinical efficacy of octreotide in the treatment of metastatic neuroendocrine tumors. A study by the Italian Trials in Medical Oncology Group. *Cancer* 1996;77:402.

111. Lupoli G, Cascone E, Arlotta F, et al. Treatment of advanced medullary thyroid carcinoma with a combination of recombinant interferon alpha-2b and octreotide. *Cancer* 1996;78:1114.

112. Schlumberger M, Abdelmoumene N, Delisle MJ, et al. Treatment of advanced medullary thyroid cancer with an alternating combination of 5 FU-streptozocin and 5 FU-dacarbazine. The Groupe d'Etude des Tumeurs a Calcitonine (GETC). *Br J Cancer* 1995;71:363.

113. Orlandi F, Caraci P, Berruti A, et al. Chemotherapy with dacarbazine and 5-fluorouracil in advanced medullary thyroid cancer. *Ann Oncol* 1994;5:763.

114. Bajetta E, Rimassa L, Carnaghi C, et al. 5-Fluorouracil, dacarbazine, and epirubicin in the treatment of patients with neuroendocrine tumors. *Cancer* 1998;83:372.

115. Di Bartolomeo M, Bajetta E, Bochicchio AM, et al. A phase II trial of dacarbazine, fluorouracil and epirubicin in patients with neuroendocrine tumours. A study by the Italian Trials in Medical Oncology (ITMO) Group. *Ann Oncol* 1995;6:77.

116. Wu LT, Averbuch SD, Ball DW, et al. Treatment of advanced medullary thyroid carcinoma with a combination of cyclophosphamide, vincristine, and dacarbazine. *Cancer* 1994;73:432.

117. Frank-Raue K, Ziegler R, Raue F. The use of octreotide in the treatment of medullary thyroid carcinoma. *Horm Metab Res Suppl* 1993;27:44.

118. Mahler C, Verhelst J, de Longueville M, et al. Long-term treatment of metastatic medullary thyroid carcinoma with the somatostatin analogue octreotide. *Clin Endocrinol (Oxf)* 1990;33:261.

119. Modigliani E, Cohen R, Joannidis S, et al. Results of long-term continuous subcutaneous octreotide administration in 14 patients with medullary thyroid carcinoma. *Clin Endocrinol (Oxf)* 1992;36:183.

120. Vitale G, Tagliaferri P, Caraglia M, et al. Slow release lanreotide in combination with interferon-alpha2b in the treatment of symptomatic advanced medullary thyroid carcinoma. *J Clin Endocrinol Metab* 2000;85:983.

121. Behr TM, Sharkey RM, Juweid ME, et al. Phase I/II clinical radioimmunotherapy with an iodine-131–labeled anti-carcinoembryonic antigen murine monoclonal antibody IgG. *J Nucl Med* 1997;38:858.

122. Juweid M, Sharkey RM, Behr T, et al. Radioimmunotherapy of medullary thyroid cancer with iodine-131–labeled anti-CEA antibodies. *J Nucl Med* 1996;37:905.

123. Stein R, Juweid M, Zhang CH, et al. Assessment of combined radioimmunotherapy and chemotherapy for treatment of medullary thyroid cancer. *Clin Cancer Res* 1999;5:3199s.

124. Juweid ME, Hajjar G, Stein R, et al. Initial experience with high-dose radioimmunotherapy of metastatic medullary thyroid cancer using 131I-MN-14 F(ab)2 anti-carcinoembryonic antigen MAb and AHSCR. *J Nucl Med* 2000;41:93.

125. Hundahl SA, Fleming ID, Fremgen AM, et al. A National Cancer Data Base report on 53,856 cases of thyroid carcinoma treated in the U.S., 1985-1995. *Cancer* 1998;83:2638.

126. Ain KB. Anaplastic thyroid carcinoma: a therapeutic challenge. *Semin Surg Oncol* 1999;16:64.

127. Junor E, Paul J, Reed N. Anaplastic thyroid carcinoma: 91 patients treated by surgery and radiotherapy. *Eur J Surg* 1992; 18:83.

128. Nilsson O, Lindeberg J, Zedenius J, et al. Anaplastic giant cell carcinoma of the thyroid gland: treatment and survival over a 25-year period. *World J Surg* 1998;22:725.

129. Nel CJ, van Heerden JA, Goellner JR, et al. Anaplastic carcinoma of the thyroid: a clinicopathologic study of 82 cases. *Mayo Clin Proc* 1985;60:51.

130. Lo CY, Lam KY, Wan KY. Anaplastic carcinoma of the thyroid. *Am J Surg* 1999;177:337.

131. Ain KB. Anaplastic thyroid carcinoma: behavior, biology, and therapeutic approaches. *Thyroid* 1998;8:715.

132. van der Laan BFAM, Freeman JL, Tsang RW, et al. The association of well-differentiated thyroid carcinoma with insular or anaplastic thyroid carcinoma: evidence for dedifferentiation in tumor progression. *Endocr Pathol* 1993;4:215.

133. Passler C, Scheuba C, Prager G, et al. Anaplastic (undifferentiated) thyroid carcinoma (ATC). A retrospective analysis. *Langenbecks Arch Surg* 1999;384:284.

134. Voutilainen PE, Multanen M, Haapiainen RK, et al. Anaplastic thyroid carcinoma survival. *World J Surg* 1999;23:975.

135. Demeter JG, De Jong SA, Lawrence AM, et al. Anaplastic thyroid carcinoma: risk factors and outcome. *Surgery* 1991;110:956.

136. Tennvall J, Lundell G, Hallquist A, et al. Combined doxorubicin, hyperfractionated radiotherapy, and surgery in anaplastic thyroid carcinoma. Report on two protocols. The Swedish Anaplastic Thyroid Cancer Group. *Cancer* 1994;74:1348.

137. Wong CS, Van Dyk J, Simpson WJ. Myelopathy following hyperfractionated accelerated radiotherapy for anaplastic thyroid carcinoma. *Radiother Oncol* 1991;20:3.

138. Tan RK, Finley RK III, Driscoll D, et al. Anaplastic carcinoma of the thyroid: a 24-year experience. *Head Neck* 1995;17:41.

139. Kim JH, Leeper RD: Treatment of anaplastic giant and spindle cell carcinoma of the thyroid gland with combination Adriamycin and radiation therapy. A new approach. *Cancer* 1983;52:954.

140. Kim JH, Leeper RD. Treatment of locally advanced thyroid carcinoma with combination doxorubicin and radiation therapy. *Cancer* 1987;60:2372.

141. Mitchell G, Huddart R, Harmer C. Phase II evaluation of high dose accelerated radiotherapy for anaplastic thyroid carcinoma. *Radiother Oncol* 1999;50:33.

142. Schlumberger M, Parmentier C, Delisle MJ, et al. Combination therapy for anaplastic giant cell thyroid carcinoma. *Cancer* 1991;67:564.

143. Chow E, Tsang RW, Brierley JD, et al. Parathyroid carcinoma: the Princess Margaret Hospital experience. *Int J Radiat Oncol Biol Phys* 1998;41:569.

144. Cook AM, Vini L, Harmer C. Squamous cell carcinoma of the thyroid: outcome of treatment in 16 patients. *Eur J Surg Oncol* 1999;25:606.

145. Simpson WJ, Carruthers J. Squamous cell carcinoma of the thyroid gland. *Am J Surg* 1988;156:44.

146. Logue JP, Tsang RW, Brierley JD, et al. Radioiodine ablation of residual thyroid tissue in thyroid cancer: relationship between administered activity, neck uptake, and outcome. *Br J Radiol* 1994;67:1127.

147. Maxon HR. Detection of residual and recurrent thyroid cancer by radionuclide imaging. *Thyroid* 1999;9:443.

148. Hodgson DC, Brierley JD, Tsang RW, et al. Prescribing 131Iodine based on neck uptake produces effective thyroid ablation and reduced hospital stay. *Radiother Oncol* 1998;47:325.

149. Park HM, Perkins OW, Edmondson JW, et al. Influence of diagnostic radioiodines on the uptake of ablative dose of iodine-131. *Thyroid* 1994;4:49.

150. Park HM. Stunned thyroid after high-dose I-131 imaging. *Clin Nucl Med* 1992;17:501.

151. Fatourechi V, Hay ID, Mullan BP, et al. Are posttherapy radioiodine scans informative and do they influence subsequent therapy of patients with differentiated thyroid cancer? *Thyroid* 2000;10:573.

152. Maxon HR. Quantitative radioiodine therapy in the treatment of differentiated thyroid cancer. *Q J Nucl Med* 1999;43:313.

153. Maxon HR, Thomas SR, Hertzberg VS, et al. Relation between effective radiation dose and outcome of radioiodine therapy for thyroid cancer. *N Engl J Med* 1983;309:937.

154. Regulatory Guide 8.39: *Release of Patients Administered Radioactive Material.* US Nuclear Regulatory Commission, Washington, DC, April 1997.

155. Harmer C, Bidmead M, Shepherd S, et al. Radiotherapy planning techniques for thyroid cancer. *Br J Radiol* 1998; 71:1069.

156. Grunwald F, Schomburg A, Menzel C, et al. Changes in the blood picture after radioiodine therapy of thyroid cancer. *Med Klin* 1994;10:522.

157. Maxon H. The role of radioiodine in the treatment of thyroid cancer. *Thyroid Today* 1993;16.

158. Dottorini ME, Lomuscio G, Mazzucchelli L, et al. Assessment of female fertility and carcinogenesis after iodine-131 therapy for differentiated thyroid cancer. *J Nucl Med* 1995;36: 21-27.

PART IV

Breast

CHAPTER 15

The Breast

Thomas A. Buchholz, Eric A. Strom, and Marsha D. McNeese

ANATOMY OF THE BREAST AND DRAINING LYMPHATICS

Depending on clinical and pathologic findings and the type of surgery performed, radiation oncologists may need to treat any or all of the following areas in patients with nonmetastatic breast cancer: the breast or chest wall, the axilla, and the ipsilateral supraclavicular and internal mammary lymph nodes. Designing radiation therapy fields so that they not only cover the areas at risk for disease but also spare as much normal tissue as possible by avoiding areas with a low risk of microscopic involvement requires an understanding of the breast's lymphatic drainage pathways and the risk of disease spread to the surrounding nodal basins. The design of radiation fields depends not only on the prior surgical procedure, the stage of the disease, and the equipment available but also on the anatomy of the individual being treated. A brief review of the anatomy of the breast and surrounding nodal areas is necessary so that explanations of radiation techniques and field design can be more easily understood.

Breast

A thin layer of mammary tissue extends from the midline laterally to the latissimus dorsi muscle and superiorly to the clavicle. However, the majority of protuberant breast tissue extends medially to the lateral edge of the sternum and laterally to near the midaxillary line. The caudal and cranial borders of the breast are typically the sixth anterior rib and the second anterior rib, respectively, although the breast may extend higher in the anterolateral region as it nears the axilla. This axillary extension of the breast is commonly known as the *tail of Spence*. The glandular tissue is supported by fibrous septa (Cooper's suspensory ligaments) and contains blood vessels, nerves, lymphatics, and adipose tissue intermingled so that no surgical planes are within the gland itself.[1] The ligamentous structures attach to the pectoralis major muscle, the overlying fascia of which serves as the deep boundary of the breast.

Primary breast tumors occur most often in areas with the largest volume of breast tissue. The most common location is the upper outer quadrant. In carefully documented series reported by Haagensen[1] and Donegan,[2] 40% to 48% of primary breast tumors were located in the upper outer quadrant, 17% to 27% were located in the central region, 16% were located in the upper inner quadrant, 10% to 11% were located in the lower outer quadrant, and 6% to 7% were located in the lower inner quadrant.[1,2]

The breast parenchyma is composed of a series of ductal and lobular units. The ductal system of the breast is divided into segments. Each segment has a series of branching ducts that converge into major lactiferous ducts near the nipple-areola complex. The opposite end of the ductal system is at an interface with lobular breast parenchyma. This interface is known as the terminal ductal-lobular unit and is the most common location for the development of breast cancer. The lobular units of the breast are responsible for the production of breast milk.

The breast has a rich lymphatic plexus with primary drainage to the lymph nodes of the axilla, internal mammary chain, and supraclavicular fossa (Fig. 15-1).[3] Lymph nodes draining the breast can also be identified within the substance of the breast (intramammary nodes) and below the pectoralis major muscle (subpectoral or interpectoral [Rotter's] nodes).

Axillary Lymph Nodes

The axilla is bordered medially by the serratus anterior muscle, anteriorly by the pectoralis major and minor muscles, and posteriorly by the converging muscles and fascia of the subscapular region. The apex of the axilla lies below the midclavicle. Within this space, lymph nodes lie in proximity to the vascular structures. Axillary lymph nodes are customarily divided into three levels according to the following anatomic guidelines: level I (low axillary) nodes are those below the inferolateral border of the pectoralis minor muscle, level II (midaxillary) nodes are those directly beneath the pectoralis minor muscle, and level III (apical or subclavicular) nodes are those superior to the pectoralis minor muscle.

The axillary nodes provide the major drainage for the breast tissue, and the disease status of these nodes is the most important prognostic factor in patients with breast cancer. Generally, a level I to II axillary dissection is adequate for accurate staging. Skip metastases (metastases

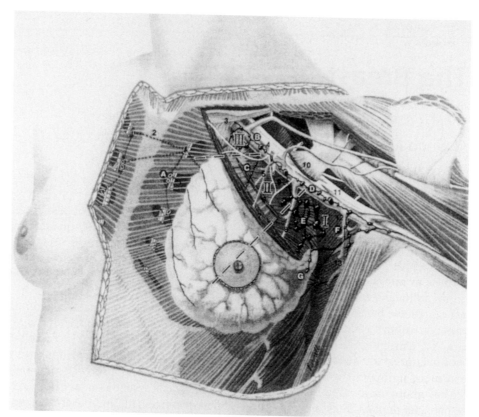

Fig. 15-1 Anatomy of the breast and lymphatics. *1*, Internal mammary artery and vein. *2*, Substernal cross drainage to contralateral internal mammary lymphatic chain. *3*, Subclavius muscle and Halsted ligament. *4*, Lateral pectoral nerve (from the lateral cord). *5*, Pectoral branch from thoracoacromial vein. *6*, Pectoralis minor muscle. *7*, Pectoralis major muscle. *8*, Lateral thoracic vein. *9*, Medial pectoral nerve (from the medial cord). *10*, Pectoralis minor muscle. *11*, Median nerve. *12*, Subscapular vein. *13*, Thoracodorsal vein. *A*, Internal mammary lymph nodes; *B*, apical lymph nodes; *C*, interpectoral (Rotter's) lymph nodes; *D*, axillary vein lymph nodes; *E*, central lymph nodes; *F*, Scapular lymph nodes; *G*, external mammary lymph nodes. *Level I lymph nodes:* lateral to lateral border of pectoralis minor muscle. *Level II lymph nodes:* behind pectoralis minor muscle. *Level III lymph nodes:* medial to medial border of pectoralis minor muscle. (From Osborne MP, Kinne DW. Breast development and anatomy. In: Harris JR, Hellman S, Henderson KC, eds. *Breast Disease.* Philadelphia, Pa: JB Lippincott; 1987:1-14.)

in higher-level nodes in the absence of metastases in lower-level nodes) are rare; in an analysis of 539 patients who underwent complete axillary dissection, Veronesi reported that skip metastases occurred in only 3.8% of patients.[4] In this same series, when level I nodes were positive, higher-level nodes were also involved in 40% of cases.[4] In a series of 1228 patients who underwent complete axillary dissection at Memorial Sloan-Kettering Cancer Center in New York, Rosen and colleagues[5] found skip metastases in 1.6% of patients overall and in 3% of those with lymph node metastases.

Full axillary dissection, including stripping of the axillary vein, has been shown to increase the incidence of arm edema. Larson and colleagues[6] reviewed the records of 475 women with early breast cancer treated between 1968 and 1980, 91% of whom received axillary irradiation to 50 Gy. Edema of the arm was scored on clinical grounds and ranged from mild hand swelling to an 8-cm

increase in arm circumference. At 6 years, the actuarial risk of developing arm edema was 8% for the entire study population. This risk was 13% for the 240 patients who had axillary surgery and 4% for the 235 patients who did not undergo axillary surgery ($P = 0.006$). For patients who underwent axillary surgery, the risk of arm edema was 37% with full dissection and 8% with less extensive dissection ($P = 0.03$). The risk of arm edema at 6 years was 28% if more than 10 nodes were removed and 9% if 1 to 10 nodes were removed ($P = 0.03$). However, the extent of axillary dissection was a stronger predictor of subsequent edema than was the number of nodes removed.[6] Clarke and colleagues[7] reported that the degree of postsurgical edema in the intact breast also correlated with the extent of axillary nodal dissection.

At The University of Texas M.D. Anderson Cancer Center, to decrease the risk of arm and breast edema, only the level I and II axillary nodes are dissected. Level III nodes are not routinely removed unless gross involvement is present. For patients with nodal involvement at levels I and II, postoperative radiation therapy to the axillary apex has been shown to be highly effective in controlling microscopic nodal involvement and is associated with only minimal risk of arm edema.

Supraclavicular Lymph Nodes

The major route by which cancer spreads to the supraclavicular nodes is through the axillary chain. In rare cases, patients can present with supraclavicular adenopathy without axillary involvement; however, supraclavicular node involvement is generally thought to indicate advanced regional disease and as such is associated with a grave prognosis. Large lymphatic trunks pass from the subclavicular nodes at the axillary apex medially through the small anatomic triangle formed by the subclavian vein, the subclavian muscle tendon, and the chest wall to terminate into the jugular-subclavian venous confluence, either directly or by lymphatic ducts. As lymph nodes in this region become obstructed with tumor, retrograde spread may occur into other supraclavicular nodes located more laterally. The supraclavicular lymph nodes at greatest risk of involvement are often difficult to palpate because of their location behind the sternocleidomastoid muscle, whereas the secondary, more lateral nodes are easier to examine.

Internal Mammary Lymph Nodes

The internal mammary lymphatic trunks are located along the intercostal spaces and contain small nodes, usually 2 to 5 mm in diameter, and loose aggregates of lymphoid tissue that do not form clearly defined nodes. In most patients these nodes and lymphatics lie within 3 cm of the sternal edge on the parietal pleura, separated from the pleura by a thin fascia. Nodes can usually be identified in the first three intercostal spaces, and in a study by Urban and Marjani,[8] nodes were also identified in the fourth and fifth interspaces in 47% and 12%, respectively, of patients undergoing extended radical mastectomy. The internal mammary lymphatic trunks empty into the great veins by way of the right lymphatic duct or, on the left, the thoracic duct or directly through the jugular vein–subclavian vein confluence. Nodes behind the manubrium connect the right and left lymphatic trunks at the first interspace in approximately 50% of patients.[1] Despite this anatomic finding, clinical manifestations of contralateral internal mammary node involvement are rare.

Lymphatic Drainage to the Contralateral Breast and Axilla

The lymphatics of the breast and surrounding nodal areas generally tend to follow the course of associated blood vessels. However, when normal paths become obstructed, retrograde lymphatic flow can occur, resulting in tumor involvement of the opposite breast, chest wall, or axilla. Therefore examination of the contralateral breast and nodal basins is extremely important in the staging, treatment, and follow-up care of patients with breast cancer.

RESPONSE OF THE NORMAL BREAST TO IRRADIATION

In adult women, the breast is very tolerant of high-dose irradiation, and, provided that standard techniques and dosages are used, radiation therapy for treatment of breast cancer is unlikely to cause serious normal tissue injury. The most common complications after irradiation of the breast are excessive subcutaneous fibrosis and atrophy of breast tissue. However, complications such as these are unusual, with several series reporting that 80% to 95% of patients have good to excellent aesthetic outcomes after breast irradiation to total doses of 45 to 50.4 Gy in daily fractions of 1.8 to 2.0 Gy.[9-11]

A steep dose-response gradient for complications seems to be evident in the normal breast between whole-breast doses of 50 and 60 Gy. In a series of 458 patients treated with breast-conserving surgery and breast irradiation, Taylor and Meltzer[9] reported that the percentage of women with good to excellent aesthetic outcomes decreased with increasing radiation dose. A good to excellent result was seen in 85% of women who received 50 Gy to the breast, 73% of women who received 50 to 52 Gy, and 20% of women who received 52 to 62 Gy.[9] Other authors have reported that the use of a tumor bed boost, which typically escalates the dose to a particular region of breast tissue to 60 Gy or greater, also can have an adverse effect on aesthetic outcome.[10,12]

The daily dose per fraction seems to be as important as total dose in determining the response of the normal breast to irradiation. Van Limbergen and colleagues[13] noted that increasing the dose per fraction beyond 2 Gy negatively influenced the final cosmetic outcome. From their results, they estimated the alpha/beta ratio (defined in Chapter 1) for breast tissue to be 2.5 Gy. These findings suggest that the breast is a late-responding normal tissue and that increases in the dose per fraction beyond 2 Gy will decrease the therapeutic ratio.

Cosmetic complications of breast irradiation likely result from damage to the supportive connective tissue elements of the breast rather than to the breast parenchyma. Information on how therapeutic doses of radiation affect the breast parenchyma is largely derived from studies of mastectomy specimens from patients who received preoperative breast irradiation. Schnitt and colleagues[14] compared 36 irradiated breast specimens with 35 nonirradiated control breast specimens and found that the most common postirradiation change was atypical epithelial cells in the terminal ductal-lobular unit associated with lobular sclerosis and atrophy.

Lactation and breast-feeding are possible after radiation therapy for breast cancer. In a survey of 53 patients who became pregnant after a course of breast irradiation for breast cancer, Tralins[15] reported that 34% were able to lactate and 25% were able to successfully breast-feed from the treated breast.

Perhaps the most important potential negative effect of breast irradiation is an increase in the risk of subsequent breast cancer development. Some of the first evidence of the carcinogenic effect of radiation came from longitudinal studies of Japanese atomic bomb survivors. Among women exposed to 1 Sv of radiation from the atomic bomb in Hiroshima, Tokunaga and colleagues[16] reported increases in the relative risks of breast cancer of thirteenfold for women younger than 35 years and twofold for women older than 35 years at the time of exposure. The importance of radiation as a breast carcinogen was further confirmed by the findings of increased breast cancer rates in women treated with radiation for nonmalignant conditions such as tuberculosis and enlargement of the thymus.[16-18] The use of radiation as a cancer treatment has also been shown to carry carcinogenic risks. In a large study of girls treated with mantle irradiation (treatment of the neck, axilla, and mediastinal lymph nodes) for Hodgkin's disease, the risk of developing breast cancer was increased seventy-fivefold compared with the risk in the general population, and the 30-year actuarial risk of developing breast cancer approached 35%.[19] The lifetime risk was projected to be much higher than the risk in nonirradiated women and close to that of women with a germline mutation in the *BRCA1* gene.[19] The age of the patient at the time of radiation therapy and the total radiation dose were important contributors to breast cancer risk, with adolescent age (10 to 16 years) at exposure and radiation doses of 20 to 40 Gy conferring the highest relative risk.

Whether radiation therapy for treatment of breast cancer increases the risk of new breast tumors is much less clear. This uncertainty is due in part to the difficulty of distinguishing ipsilateral new primary breast tumors from local recurrence of the disease and the difficulty of showing a relationship between new primary breast tumors and previous irradiation. Evidence exists to suggest that breast irradiation may increase the incidence of contralateral breast cancer in women 45 years of age or younger: in an analysis based on the Connecticut cancer registry database of 41,109 breast cancer patients, Boice and colleagues[20] reported that women who survived for at least 10 years after diagnosis and who were treated with radiation had a relative risk of a second breast tumor of 1.33 compared with the risk in 10-year

survivors not treated with radiation. However, this finding has not been reproduced in the clinical studies that have evaluated outcomes after breast conservation therapy (BCT).[21,22]

Finally, irradiation of the breast bud before adolescence can prevent subsequent breast growth. Treatment of lung metastases from Wilms' tumor and other pediatric malignancies with dosages as low as 12 Gy delivered over 2 weeks has resulted in impairment of breast development during adolescence.[23] Radiation has been used therapeutically in the past for prevention of breast engorgement and discomfort in men with prostate cancer treated with estrogens.

EPIDEMIOLOGY OF BREAST CANCER

Breast cancer is the most common nondermatologic cancer among women in the United States. The American Cancer Society[24] estimated that 193,700 women would be diagnosed with an invasive breast cancer in 2001. According to current statistics, approximately one in eight women (12.83% of all women) will develop breast cancer at some point during her lifetime.[24]

The incidence of invasive breast cancer steadily increased during the 5 decades up until 1988 (Fig. 15-2).[25] Since 1988, the annual incidence of invasive breast cancer has been relatively constant. However, over this same period, the incidence of noninvasive breast cancer has significantly increased. The American Cancer Society estimates that between 1982 and 1988, the incidence of ductal carcinoma in situ (DCIS) increased 28% per year, in part reflecting the increasing use of screening mammography. Since 1988, the incidence of DCIS has continued to increase, at a rate of approximately 6% per year (Fig. 15-3).[25]

The combined incidence of invasive and noninvasive breast cancer is expected to continue to increase over the next two decades. One reason for the expected increase is the dramatic change in breast cancer risk factors that occurred during the middle of the twentieth century. Specific changes included a decrease in age at menarche, an increase in age at first pregnancy, and an increase in the percentage of nulliparous women. Another factor expected to contribute to an increase in breast cancer incidence is expansion in the population at risk owing to an increase in the percentage of women in their 50s and 60s. A final factor sure to increase breast cancer incidence is the effect of advances in other aspects of medical care in decreasing the competing risks of death from cardiovascular disease and other illnesses.

Mortality Rates

Even though the percentage of women with noninvasive breast cancer and early-stage invasive disease has

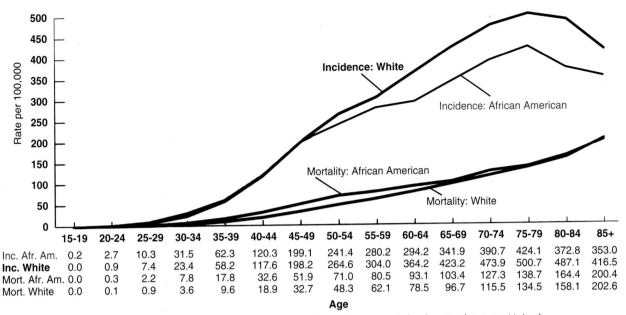

Age	15-19	20-24	25-29	30-34	35-39	40-44	45-49	50-54	55-59	60-64	65-69	70-74	75-79	80-84	85+
Inc. Afr. Am.	0.2	2.7	10.3	31.5	62.3	120.3	199.1	241.4	280.2	294.2	341.9	390.7	424.1	372.8	353.0
Inc. White	0.0	0.9	7.4	23.4	58.2	117.6	198.2	264.6	304.0	364.2	423.2	473.9	500.7	487.1	416.5
Mort. Afr. Am.	0.0	0.3	2.2	7.8	17.8	32.6	51.9	71.0	80.5	93.1	103.4	127.3	138.7	164.4	200.4
Mort. White	0.0	0.1	0.9	3.6	9.6	18.9	32.7	48.3	62.1	78.5	96.7	115.5	134.5	158.1	202.6

Fig. 15-2 Breast cancer in women: age-specific incidence and death rates by race, United States, 1992-1996. (From American Cancer Society. *Breast Cancer Facts and Figures 1999-2000.* Atlanta, Ga: American Cancer Society; 2000.)

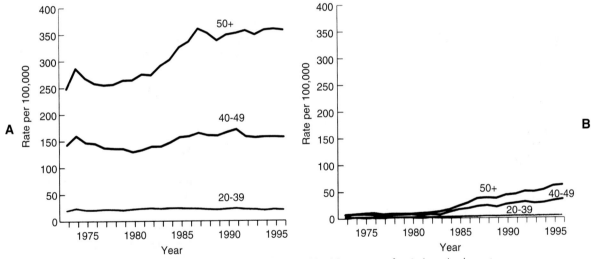

Fig. 15-3 Breast cancer in women: age-adjusted incidence rates for **A,** invasive breast cancer and **B,** ductal carcinoma in situ by age, United States, 1973-1996. Rates are age-adjusted to the 1970 U.S. standard population. (From American Cancer Society. *Breast Cancer Facts and Figures 1999-2000.* Atlanta, Ga: American Cancer Society; 2000.)

increased relative to the percentage of women with advanced disease, breast cancer remains the second leading cause of cancer deaths in women. In 2001 approximately 40,600 deaths were estimated to result from breast cancer.[24] Breast cancer is estimated to be the most common cause of cancer deaths among women age 20 to 59 years. In the past decade, however, a consistent, 1.8% annual decline in breast cancer death rates has occurred—the first decline in breast cancer death rates seen in United States history.

This decrease in mortality is most pronounced in younger women.[24]

Death rates from breast cancer vary significantly around the world. In general, western industrialized nations have much higher breast cancer incidence and mortality rates than do nations of the Far East. For example, between 1994 and 1997 the age-adjusted death rate from breast cancer in China and Japan was approximately 25% that of the death rates in the United States, western Europe, and the Scandinavian countries.[24]

Risk Factors

Table 15-1 lists risk factors for developing breast cancer.

Female Sex

The strongest risk factor for breast cancer is being female. Breast cancer in men accounts for fewer than 1% of all new breast cancer cases (approximately 1400 cases annually).[24]

Older Age

The second most important risk factor for breast cancer development is an individual's age. The annual risk increases exponentially up to the age of menopause, at which time the rate of increase in the annual risk slows significantly. After the age of 80, the annual incidence of breast cancer begins to show a slight decline.[25] Table 15-2 shows the risk of developing either invasive or noninvasive breast cancer as a function of age. For women in their late 30s, the annual risk of developing breast cancer is approximately 0.07% per year. This increases to 0.44% per year for women in their late 70s. Although these percentages may seem low, they represent only the risk for a given year. The lifetime risk is a summation of the annual breast cancer risks. Because younger women have a longer life expectancy than older women, younger women have a greater lifetime risk. Only 0.43% of women develop breast cancer before the age of 40, whereas 4% of women develop breast cancer between the ages of 40 and 59 and 6.88% of women develop breast cancer between the ages of 60 and 79.[24]

Reproductive and Hormonal Factors

The risk of breast cancer development is also determined by age at menarche, age at first pregnancy, and age at menopause. In a recent large study of Swedish women, the risk of breast cancer increased approximately 13% for every 5-year increase in age at first birth.[26] Originally, it was thought that pregnancy early in life afforded protection against breast cancer by causing differentiation of the terminal ductal-lobular units of the breast. More recently, however, this mechanism has been questioned. It is clear that the short-term high levels of circulating estrogen associated with pregnancy are protective against breast cancer later in life, but the mechanism of this protective effect is still unknown. Paradoxically, chronic exposure to low-dose estrogen increases breast cancer risk. The length of exposure of

---

TABLE 15-1

Breast Cancer Risk Factors

Significant Risk Factors	Moderate Risk Factors	Unlikely Risk Factors
Female sex Older age Family history of breast cancer Nulliparity Older age at menarche Personal history of breast cancer Personal history of lobular carcinoma in situ Personal history of atypical ductal hyperplasia Germline mutation in *BRCA1* or *BRCA2*	Higher alcohol consumption Low amounts of exercise Use of hormone replacement therapy Lack of breast-feeding	Higher fat intake Fibrocystic breast disease Fibroadenoma Simple breast cysts Use of oral contraceptives Use of tobacco

---

TABLE 15-2

Estimated New Breast Cancer Cases and Deaths in Women by Age in the United States in 1999

Age	Cases of In Situ Disease	Percent	Cases of Invasive Disease	Percent	Deaths	Percent
<30	100	0.3	800	0.5	100	0.2
30-39	1400	3.5	7400	4.2	1200	2.8
40-49	9000	22.6	32,100	18.3	5600	12.9
50-59	10,000	25.1	37,400	21.4	7000	16.2
60-69	8500	21.3	32,600	18.6	7100	16.4
70-79	8200	20.6	40,700	23.2	11,000	25.4
80+	2700	6.8	24,000	13.7	11,300	26.1
TOTAL*	39,900	99.9	175,000	99.9	43,300	100.0

Data from American Cancer Society. *Breast Cancer Facts and Figures 1999-2000.* Atlanta, Ga: American Cancer Society; 2000.
*Because of rounding, percentages in some cases do not equal 100%.

the breast to these lower estrogen levels is determined by a woman's lifetime menstruation history. A woman with natural menopause at age 44 years has half the breast cancer risk of the general United States population, in which the median age at menopause is 52 years.

Postmenopausal estrogen replacement therapy also modestly increases the risk of breast cancer. The Collaborative Group on Hormonal Factors in Breast Cancer performed a meta-analysis of 51 epidemiologic studies that included 52,705 women with breast cancer and 108,411 women without breast cancer.[27] The authors reported that postmenopausal hormone replacement therapy increased the annual relative risk of developing breast cancer by 2.3% for each year of hormonal therapy. A more recent study of 46,000 women reported that the combined use of estrogen and progesterone increased the relative risk of breast cancer 8% compared with the risk in nonusers, whereas the use of estrogen alone increased the relative risk only 1%.[28] Hormone replacement therapy after menopause has a number of benefits, such as prevention of osteoporosis and possible protection against cardiovascular death, that may outweigh the drawback of increased risk of breast cancer development. For women who have undergone hysterectomy, it seems that hormone replacement therapy with estrogen alone rather than estrogen and progesterone has a minimal effect on breast cancer risk.[29] For women who have not undergone hysterectomy, combined estrogen and progesterone remains the standard for hormone replacement therapy to avoid the risk of endometrial cancer that is associated with unopposed estrogen replacement. The use of oral contraceptives has not been associated with breast cancer development.[30]

An understanding of the effects of estrogen and progesterone on breast cancer risk permits the development of strategies to minimize breast cancer risk. In an innovative research program, Guzman and colleagues[31] explored chemoprevention of breast cancer through estrogen modulation. Using a rat model, they showed that induction of a false pregnancy with estradiol and progesterone early in life has high efficacy in protecting against carcinogen-induced mammary cancer.[31] The implication of their work is that a similar strategy used in young adolescent girls might markedly reduce the risk of breast cancer in later life, although it is unlikely that modulation of hormonal levels in healthy adolescent females will be studied any time soon.

Family History of Breast Cancer

Family history is another important determinant of an individual's breast cancer risk. Women with a first-degree relative (mother or sister) with a history of breast cancer have an increased risk of developing the disease.[32] This increased risk can be explained in part by inheritance of a genetic condition that predisposes an individual to breast cancer development (e.g., mutations in *BRCA1* or *BRCA2*); shared lifestyle; and inheritance of genes that affect risk factors, such as body habitus and age at menarche. Between 20% and 25% of women diagnosed with breast cancer have a positive family history of the disease, and approximately 10% of women with breast cancer are from families that display an autosomal dominant pattern of breast cancer inheritance.

The actual risk that family history conveys depends on the number of relatives affected and their age at diagnosis (having a first-degree relative with premenopausal breast cancer conveys a greater risk than does having a first-degree relative with postmenopausal cancer). Women with one first-degree relative affected by the disease have an increased relative risk of developing breast cancer two to three times that of women with no family history.[32] Women with two or more first-degree relatives with a diagnosis of breast cancer have a still greater risk, four to six times that of women with no family history (or two to three times that of the average-risk population).

Environmental Factors

Few environmental agents consistently demonstrate an association with breast cancer development. The clearest example of a breast cancer carcinogen is ionizing radiation. The carcinogenic effects of radiation on the normal breast were discussed earlier in this chapter in the section on "Response of the Normal Breast to Irradiation."

Dietary Factors

It was once believed that increases in dietary fat intake could help explain why rates of breast cancer are dramatically higher among women of Asian heritage who live in the United States than among Asian women living in Asia. However, carefully conducted studies, including a large study of 30,000 nurses that carefully evaluated diet,[33] indicate that dietary fat does not affect breast cancer risk.

An association between alcohol use and breast cancer has consistently been demonstrated in large studies correlating dietary habits with breast cancer risk. Alcohol increases the relative risk of developing breast cancer in a dose-dependent fashion, with three to four alcoholic drinks per day increasing the relative risk fourfold.[34]

Exercise and Body Weight

Like dietary factors, exercise and body weight have a moderate impact on breast cancer risk and are risk factors that can be controlled by individuals. Recently, large studies have demonstrated that daily exercise, particularly early in life, can decrease the risk of breast cancer for both premenopausal and postmenopausal women.[35,36] Exercise is believed to reduce the risk of breast cancer by decreasing circulating estrogen levels, although this association has yet to be definitively established. Obesity can increase circulating levels of estrogen, and associations have been found between abdominal body fat and adult weight gain and breast cancer risk.[37]

Lactation

Another risk factor that may make a moderate contribution to the risk of breast cancer development is lactation. In a study of more than 3600 breast cancer patients who were age-matched with controls, a suggestion was evident that women who breast-fed for at least 2 weeks had a modest decrease in breast cancer risk compared with women who never lactated.[38]

Pathologic Factors

In addition to patient and environmental factors, several pathologic factors increase breast cancer risk. Personal history of breast cancer and personal history of DCIS are strong risk factors for the development of new breast cancer. Atypical ductal hyperplasia and lobular carcinoma in situ (LCIS) are also associated with increased risk of breast cancer development. In contrast, a history of simple cysts or fibrocystic breast parenchyma does not seem to increase breast cancer risk.

Determining an Individual's Risk

It is important to consider the combination of risk factors when a generalized risk profile is determined. For example, combining age and family history indicates that a 40 year old with two or more first-degree relatives with breast cancer has approximately the same annual risk of developing breast cancer as a 60 year old with no risk factors.[39,40] As mentioned earlier, despite this equivalence in annual risk, the 40 year old used in this example has a much higher overall lifetime risk. Gail and colleagues[39,40] have used these epidemiologic risk factors to derive a model for predicting an individual's annual and lifetime risks of breast cancer. In this model, an individual's annual risk of breast cancer is based on her present age, number of first-degree relatives with breast cancer, age at first birth, age at menarche, number of breast biopsies, and history of atypical ductal hyperplasia. The use of exogenous hormones is not considered in this model.

BREAST CANCER PATHOGENESIS AND PREVENTION
Breast Cancer Development

All forms of breast cancer are believed to develop as a consequence of unregulated cell growth and the development of phenotypic changes such as the ability to invade, recruit a new blood supply, and metastasize. These changes in phenotypes are secondary to the development

of aberrations in genetic pathways. Some of these aberrations are inherited (germline mutations), whereas others develop during the life of a breast cell (somatic mutations). It is currently believed that most breast cancer is a consequence of a series of somatic mutations. As previously noted, only 20% to 25% of breast cancer patients have a history of breast cancer in a first-degree relative. However, it is possible that some women without a first-degree relative with breast cancer still inherit a genetic background that predisposes to breast cancer. These mutations may be insufficient to cause breast cancer unless accompanied by other mutations and therefore would be predicted to have a low penetrance. Historically, it has been much more difficult to discover low-penetrance mutations than to discover germline mutations that result in an autosomal dominant pattern of breast cancer development. However, with newer molecular techniques, such as deoxyribonucleic acid (DNA)–array assays, the identification of low-penetrance predisposing mutations may be more feasible.

Approximately 10% of breast cancer patients have familial breast cancer, typically defined as breast cancer showing an *autosomal dominant inheritance pattern*. During the 1990s, germline mutations in three important tumor suppressor genes—*p53*, *BRCA1*, and *BRCA2*— were discovered in family members of individuals with familial breast cancer. All three genes have been shown unequivocally to predispose to breast cancer.

Mutations in p53

Germline mutations in the *p53* gene are very rare and result in *Li-Fraumeni syndrome*, named after two investigators who made significant contributions to the understanding of this condition.[41] *p53* is one of the most important tumor suppressor genes and has been called the "guardian of the genome" because of its critical role in cellular pathways that recognize and direct a response to DNA injury. *p53* is a transcription regulator of a number of important genes. Through regulation of *p21*, *GAD45*, and other genes, *p53* can promote cell cycle arrest after DNA injury, allowing cells sufficient time for DNA repair before S phase, G_2, and mitosis.[42] Alternatively, through regulation of the *bcl-2* family of genes, *p53* can direct a cell toward apoptosis to prevent propagation of damage to progeny cells.[43] One consequence of a germline mutation in *p53* is cancer development. Individuals with Li-Fraumeni syndrome are at increased risk for a variety of cancer, including childhood sarcomas, gynecologic tumors, and breast cancer. Breast cancer is the most common malignancy in patients with Li-Fraumeni syndrome; the lifetime risk is estimated to be 90%.[44]

Mutations in BRCA1 and BRCA2

Studies of patients with familial breast cancer led to the discovery of *BRCA1* in 1995 and *BRCA2* in

1996.[45,46] Similar to *p53*, both *BRCA1* and *BRCA2* are tumor suppressor genes that contribute to the stability of the genome by mediating the effects of the cellular response to DNA injury. The *BRCA1* and *BRCA2* proteins have been found to play important roles in the processing of double-strand DNA damage. The proteins encoded by these genes colocalize with *Rad51* to form a complex important in the repair of double-strand breaks.[47,48] In addition, *BRCA1* has been found to play a role in transcription-coupled repair, homologous repair, and end rejoining.[49,50] One consequence of loss of function of either *BRCA1* or *BRCA2* is increased radiosensitivity.[47-50] This radiosensitivity is directly related to dysregulation of the double-strand DNA damage pathway.

Individuals with a germline mutation in *BRCA1* have a lifetime risk of breast cancer of 65% to 85%.[51,52] In addition, these individuals have a lifetime risk of ovarian cancer approaching 50%.[51,52] Other types of cancer that develop more frequently in *BRCA1* carriers include colon cancer and prostate cancer.[51]

The lifetime risk of breast cancer for women with germline *BRCA2* mutations mirrors that for women with *BRCA1* mutations.[46] *BRCA2* mutation carriers are also at increased risk for ovarian cancer compared with the general population, but their risk is much less than the risk in women with *BRCA1* mutations. *BRCA2* is also associated with male breast cancer.[53,54]

Genetic screening for germline mutations in *BRCA1* and *BRCA2* is now possible. Testing should be performed only in centers equipped with genetic counseling programs designed to properly inform individuals of the social, economic, and legal consequences associated with genetic testing. Germline mutations in *BRCA1* and *BRCA2* are rare, occurring in fewer than 7% of patients with breast cancer.[46,51] Thus, only a minority of breast cancer patients with a family history of the disease would be predicted to carry a mutation in one of these genes. Table 15-3 contains data concerning the probability of carrying a *BRCA1* mutation based on an individual's age at cancer diagnosis, personal cancer history, and family cancer history and whether the individual is of Ashkenazi Jewish descent.[55] Both treating physicians and patients have consistently been found to overestimate the probability of having a germline mutation in a *BRCA* gene.[56]

No definitive data exist on which to base screening recommendations for individuals with a proven germline mutation in a gene predisposing to the development of breast cancer. The American Society of Clinical Oncology has published a consensus statement recommending that these individuals undergo annual mammography and clinical and self-breast examination beginning at the age of 25 to 35 years. In addition, annual pelvic examinations with transvaginal sonography, color Doppler examinations of the ovaries, and

TABLE 15-3

Probability of *BRCA1* Germline Mutations in Various Clinical Scenarios

Scenario	Probability
Mother or father proven carrier	50%
40-year-old with breast cancer and a first-degree relative with breast cancer	
Ashkenazi	5%
Non-Ashkenazi	20%
60-year-old with bilateral breast cancer and a first-degree relative with breast cancer	
Ashkenazi	5%
Non-Ashkenazi	20%
30-year-old with breast cancer and a first-degree relative with ovarian cancer	
Ashkenazi	20%
Non-Ashkenazi	50%

Data from Shattuck-Eidens D, Oliphant A, McClure M, et al. *JAMA* 1997;278:1242-1250.

measurement of serum CA-125 levels are recommended beginning at age 25 to 35 years.[57]

Breast Cancer Prevention Strategies
Tamoxifen

One of the most exciting areas of breast cancer research is breast cancer prevention. Understanding of the role of estrogens and progesterones in breast cancer development has led to the development of pharmacologic strategies that could significantly decrease the incidence of breast cancer over the next two decades.

Several pharmaceuticals that affect the estrogenic pathways have been studied as chemopreventive agents, but the only agent for which mature data from clinical trials are available is tamoxifen. Interest in tamoxifen as a chemopreventive agent arose after a number of randomized trials designed to test the efficacy of hormonal therapy for invasive breast cancer reported that tamoxifen reduced the incidence of contralateral breast cancer.[58-60] On the basis of these data, in 1992 the National Surgical Adjuvant Breast and Bowel Project (NSABP) began a randomized, placebo-controlled study (the P-1 trial) to test the efficacy of 5 years of tamoxifen in the prevention of breast cancer.[61] Between 1992 and 1997, 13,388 women with a 1.67% or greater predicted risk of developing breast cancer within 5 years were enrolled in this trial. Risk was assessed using a modification of the Gail model, which permitted enrollment of any woman older than 60 years of age and selected women younger than 60 years with additional risk factors that increased their annual risk to at least that of a 60-year-old. In addition, women with a history of LCIS were included because their risk was believed to exceed the cutoff risk of 1.67%. Women were not allowed to use estrogen replacement therapy during their participation in the trial.

The results of the P-1 trial indicated that tamoxifen reduced the rates of invasive and noninvasive breast cancer by 49% and 50%, respectively.[61] The benefit of tamoxifen was seen in all age groups (≤ 49 years, 50 to 59 years, ≥ 60 years). In addition, women with a history of atypical ductal hyperplasia had an 86% risk reduction, and women with a history of LCIS had a 56% risk reduction. Finally, the benefit was seen across all subgroups specified according to family history of breast cancer. Tamoxifen selectively reduced the incidence of estrogen receptor–positive tumors; estrogen receptor–negative tumors developed at an equal rate in the tamoxifen and placebo groups. No evidence of a cardioprotective effect of tamoxifen was found in this trial, but the number of osteoporosis-related fractures was reduced in the tamoxifen-treated cohort. Tamoxifen increased the risk of developing stage I endometrial cancer (risk ratio of 2.53).

Although this study indicated that 5 years of tamoxifen use decreased the 5-year risk of developing breast cancer by about 50%, whether this result warrants the widespread use of tamoxifen for breast cancer prevention is controversial. In the NSABP report, 5 years of tamoxifen therapy in 6576 women reduced the number of invasive or noninvasive breast cancer by 120 compared with the expected number.[61] With the relatively short follow-up period of this important study, however, it was not possible to determine whether tamoxifen actually prevented this number of cases of breast cancer or rather simply delayed the onset of the disease.

Prophylactic Surgery

An alternative strategy used to prevent breast cancer development is prophylactic surgical intervention. Hartmann and colleagues[62] analyzed outcomes in women with a family history of breast cancer who underwent bilateral prophylactic mastectomy at Mayo Clinic between 1960 and 1993. With a median follow-up time of 14 years, only 4 of the 639 treated patients developed breast cancer. According to the Gail model, 37.4 cases of breast cancer would have been expected to develop in this population, so the prophylactic surgery resulted in an 89.5% risk reduction ($P < 0.001$).[62]

Future Directions

Breast cancer prevention strategies will continue to be a dynamic area of preclinical and clinical research in the near future. New selective estrogen receptor modulators, such as raloxifene, are being discovered that should prove to have a greater impact than tamoxifen in preventing breast cancer with a lower risk of endometrial cancer. The current NSABP prevention trial for women at risk for breast cancer is the Study of Tamoxifen and

Raloxifene (STAR trial), which is designed to compare the efficacy and side effects of these two drugs.

DIAGNOSIS AND STAGING
Diagnosis

Breast cancer most commonly presents as an asymptomatic mammographic finding or an asymptomatic palpable breast mass. All women who present with either of these conditions require pathologic confirmation of the absence or presence of breast cancer.

For women presenting with a new palpable breast mass, the initial step in evaluation should be a careful history and physical examination. The breast should be inspected while the woman lies in the supine position and in the prone position, both with the pectoralis major muscle contracted and with this muscle relaxed. The presence of breast asymmetry, skin retraction, erythema, or edema should be noted. Skin edema is a sign of advanced disease and typically appears as thickened skin with prominent follicles (peau d'orange), particularly when the skin is compressed between two fingers (Fig. 15-4; see also Color Plate 17, after p. 80). If a palpable mass is present, it should be measured, and its consistency should be described. The axilla and supraclavicular regions should be carefully examined for suspicious adenopathy. If the clinical findings are suggestive of breast cancer, bilateral diagnostic mammograms should be obtained. Sonographic examination is also helpful in confirming or ruling out the presence of a simple fluid-filled cyst. Even when radiographic findings are normal, diagnostic biopsies are required to rule out malignancy in the case of a palpable mass. Either fine-needle aspiration or core needle biopsy can be used. Fine-needle aspiration is useful for ruling out simple cysts and establishing a diagnosis of

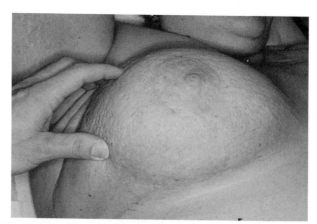

Fig. 15-4 Classic appearance of skin edema: thickened skin with prominent hair follicles upon mild compression of the skin. This physical finding is called peau d'orange because the appearance is similar to that of the skin of an orange.

malignancy, but because this method yields disaggregated cells rather than intact tissue, this method does not permit pathologists to distinguish invasive disease from noninvasive breast cancer.

For women presenting with mammographic abnormalities without a palpable mass, tissue can be obtained with stereotactic core biopsy or needle localization excisional biopsy. A stereotactic core biopsy is typically done in a radiology department under mammographic guidance. A needle localization biopsy also uses mammograms to localize the suspicious region but requires an operative procedure. The advantages of stereotactic core biopsy over needle localization excisional biopsy are the avoidance of a breast scar and the avoidance of an additional operative procedure. In addition, in most cases in which cancer is diagnosed, excisional biopsy must be followed by re-excision to obtain adequate margins because surgeons are reluctant to perform wide excisions before the establishment of a cancer diagnosis.

Staging

Once a diagnosis of invasive cancer is established, a series of tests are helpful to determine the extent of disease. These include chest radiography, liver function tests, biochemical profile, and a complete blood count. In addition, bone scans and liver imaging with sonography or computed tomography (CT) are standard for women with lymph node–positive disease or large primary tumors.

Previous staging systems for breast cancer were based on clinical and radiographic findings because many women presented with advanced, inoperable disease. The Columbia Clinical Classification (Table 15-4)[63] was one of the first widely used staging classifications for breast cancer. In this system, tumor size was not taken into consideration, and stage C or D disease (locally advanced) was considered inoperable.[63]

In 1960 the International Union Against Cancer published the first tumor-nodes-metastasis (TNM) staging system for breast cancer, which was adopted, with modifications, by the American Joint Committee for Cancer (AJCC) Staging and End Results Reporting in 1962. The 1983 version of this staging system achieved worldwide acceptance; revisions in 1988 and the early and mid-1990s led to the 1997 staging system (Box 15-1).[64] One of the most important benefits of this staging system is that it includes both clinical and pathologic staging. N1 disease is subcategorized pathologically according to disease extent, the number of involved lymph nodes, and extracapsular extension. This is an important advantage because clinical examination of the axilla is inaccurate in at least 30% of cases and also because prognosis varies according to the extent of nodal involvement.[65] The clinical and pathologic tumor stages may differ at the primary site as well as the axilla because surgical staging includes only the invasive portion of the tumor

TABLE 15-4

The Columbia Clinical Classification for Breast Cancer

Stage	Defining Features
Stage A	No skin edema, ulceration, or solid fixation of tumor to chest wall Axillary nodes not clinically involved
Stage B	No skin edema, ulceration, or solid fixation of tumor to chest wall Clinically involved nodes but less than 2.5 cm in transverse diameter and not fixed to overlying skin or deeper structures of axilla
Stage C	Any two of the following five *grave signs* of advanced breast carcinoma: 1. Edema of skin of limited extent (involving less than one third of the skin over the breast) 2. Skin ulceration 3. Solid fixation of tumor to chest wall 4. Massive involvement of axillary lymph nodes (measuring ≥ 2.5 cm in transverse diameter) 5. Fixation of the axillary nodes to overlying skin or deeper structures of axilla
Stage D	All other more advanced breast carcinoma, including the following: 1. A combination of any two or more of the five *grave signs* listed under Stage C 2. Extensive edema of skin (involving more than one third of the skin over the breast) 3. Satellite skin nodules 4. Inflammatory type of carcinoma 5. Clinically involved supraclavicular lymph nodes 6. Internal mammary metastases as evidenced by a parasternal tumor 7. Edema of the arm 8. Distant metastases

Modified from Haagensen CD, Stout AP. *Ann Surg* 1943;118: 859-870, 1032-1051.

whereas clinical examination does not distinguish invasive from in situ disease.

RADIATION THERAPY FOR DUCTAL CARCINOMA IN SITU

Noninvasive carcinoma of the breast is defined by the presence of malignant cells that are contained within the breast lobules or ducts and have not invaded through the basement membrane. The most common type of noninvasive breast cancer, DCIS, is a premalignant condition. It is difficult to accurately estimate the risk of progression of DCIS to invasive breast cancer because few data are available on patients with DCIS who received no treatment after biopsy. The studies that address this issue have been hampered by small patient

---

BOX 15-1   American Joint Commitee on Cancer Staging System for Breast Cancer

PRIMARY TUMOR (T)

TX	Primary tumor cannot be assessed
T0	No evidence of primary tumor
Tis	Carcinoma in situ: intraductal carcinoma, lobular carcinoma in situ, or Paget's disease of the nipple with no tumor
T1	Tumor 2 cm or less in greatest dimension

	T1mic	Microinvasion 0.1 cm or less in greatest dimension
	T1a	Tumor more than 0.1 but not more than 0.5 cm in greatest dimension
	T1b	Tumor more than 0.5 cm but not more than 1 cm in greatest dimension
	T1c	Tumor more than 1 cm but not more than 2 cm in greatest dimension

T2	Tumor more than 2 cm but not more than 5 cm in greatest dimension
T3	Tumor more than 5 cm in greatest dimension
T4	Tumor of any size with direct extension to (a) chest wall or (b) skin, only as described below

	T4a	Extension to the chest wall
	T4b	Edema (including peau d'orange) or ulceration of the skin of the breast or satellite skin modules confined to the same breast
	T4c	Both (T4a and T4b)
	T4d	Inflammatory carcinoma

REGIONAL LYMPH NODES (N)

NX	Regional lymph node(s) cannot be assessed (e.g., previously removed)
N0	No regional lymph node metastasis
N1	Metastasis to movable ipsilateral axillary lymph nodes
N2	Metastasis to ipsilateral axillary lymph node(s) fixed to one another or to other structures
N3	Metastasis to ipsilateral internal mammary lymph node(s)

DISTANT METASTASIS (M)

MX	Distant metastasis cannot be assessed
M0	No distant metastasis
M1	Distant metastasis (includes metastasis to ipsilateral supraclavicular lymph node[s])

STAGE GROUPING

Stage 0	Tis	N0	M0
Stage I	T1*	N0	M0
Stage IIA	T0	N1	M0
	T2	N0	M0
Stage IIB	T2	N1	M0
	T3	N0	M0
Stage IIIA	T0	N2	M0
	T1*	N2	M0
	T2	N2	M0
	T3	N1	M0
	T3	N2	M0
Stage IIIB	T4	Any N	M0
	Any T	N3	M0
Stage IV	Any T	Any N	M1

From Fleming I, Cooper JS, Henson DE, et al, eds. *AJCC Cancer Staging Manual*, 5th ed. Philadelphia, Pa: Lippincott Williams & Wilkins; 1997:171-180.
*T1 includes T1mic.
†The prognosis of patients with pN1a is similar to that of patients with pN0.

---

numbers and selection bias. It is likely that 30% to 50% of women with untreated DCIS will develop invasive disease within 10 years after diagnosis.

DCIS is distinct from LCIS, the other type of noninvasive breast cancer, because DCIS is a true premalignant condition that can progress to invasive disease, but LCIS is considered a marker of increased risk of breast cancer rather than a true premalignant condition and is more appropriately called *lobular neoplasia*. Whereas DCIS increases the risk of invasive cancer in the ipsilateral breast, LCIS increases the risk of invasive cancer equally in both breasts.

The distinction between DCIS and LCIS has important therapeutic relevance. Because LCIS is not a premalignant condition, specific therapy to eradicate the LCIS is not routinely recommended. Rather, careful screening for breast cancer or discussion of prevention strategies

(chemoprevention or bilateral prophylactic mastectomy) is appropriate. In contrast, in patients with DCIS, local therapies are generally recommended to eradicate the region of DCIS and thus minimize the risk of evolution to an invasive breast cancer.

Common Presentations and Pathologic Subtypes

The diagnosis of DCIS has become much more common over the past decade because of the increase in mammographic screening of asymptomatic women. Before screening mammography, DCIS was uncommon. This is because by the time DCIS has grown large enough to be palpable, it has usually developed a component of invasive disease. Previously, the most common presentation of DCIS was a palpable mass, but today the vast majority of cases of DCIS

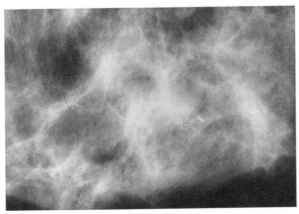

Fig. 15-5 Typical mammographic appearance of untreated ductal carcinoma in situ of the breast. The microcalcifications can be described as clustered, pleomorphic, and branching.

are nonpalpable lesions detected during mammographic screening. The most common mammographic findings are branching microcalcifications localized to a small region of the breast. The classic mammographic appearance of DCIS is shown in Figure 15-5.

DCIS includes a spectrum of pathologic entities. Well-differentiated DCIS closely resembles atypical ductal hyperplasia of the breast, whereas high-grade DCIS is cytologically indistinguishable from invasive breast cancer. A pathology consensus conference in 1997 recommended that all cases of DCIS be categorized to reflect the biological potential of the disease.[66] Accordingly, information on nuclear grade, the presence or absence of necrosis, tissue architecture, and polarization or radial orientation should be provided. Tissue architecture can range from the more indolent papillary, micropapillary, and cribriform patterns to the more biologically aggressive solid and comedo subtypes. Comedo necrosis represents necrotic debris centrally located in the duct. An example of high-grade DCIS with comedo necrosis is shown in Figure 15-6; see also Color Plate 18, after p. 80.

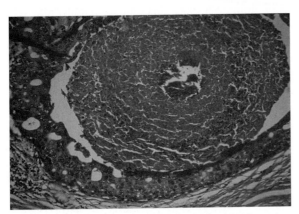

Fig. 15-6 Histologic section of high-grade ductal carcinoma in situ with extensive comedo necrosis.

Treatment

BCT has become the standard treatment for women with DCIS. Mastectomy is now reserved for the less common cases that present with diffuse microcalcifications throughout the entire breast or large volumes of palpable disease, or cases in which surgical margins free of carcinoma cannot be obtained with breast-conserving surgery.

A randomized clinical trial has never been designed to directly compare mastectomy and BCT for patients with DCIS. In the NSABP B-06 trial, which compared mastectomy and BCT for women with invasive breast cancer, a small percentage of women enrolled were later recognized to have DCIS. Within this relatively small subset of patients, an overall survival rate of 96% was the same in the conservatively treated patients and the patients treated with mastectomy.[67] This very low probability of breast cancer death after BCT for DCIS has been confirmed in several subsequent publications, and thus a randomized trial comparing this treatment against mastectomy is unnecessary.

Role of Radiation Therapy

With the historical change from mastectomy to BCT as the preferred therapeutic approach for DCIS, controversy has arisen over the need for radiation therapy and tamoxifen as standard components of treatment. Although randomized data are available that address both of these questions, these data have not led to resolution of the current controversies. In part, the continuing controversy is attributable to the fact that the follow-up periods of these studies, particularly those involving the question of tamoxifen use, are relatively short.

NSABP B-06 trial. The first data defining the role of radiation therapy in the management of DCIS came from the NSABP B-06 trial. The B-06 trial was designed for patients with invasive disease, but 76 patients were subsequently found to have pure DCIS with no evidence of invasion. With a median follow-up time of 83 months, the local recurrence rates were 7% for patients treated with lumpectomy and radiation vs. 43% for patients treated with lumpectomy alone ($P = 0.01$).[67]

NSABP B-17 trial. Although data from the B-06 trial provided the first suggestion that radiation plays a critically important role in BCT for DCIS, that trial was specifically designed to study invasive disease. Therefore the NSABP began a new trial in 1985, designed specifically to define the role of radiation therapy in the treatment of DCIS. The B-17 trial was a dual-arm prospective trial that enrolled 818 women who were randomly assigned to the use or omission of radiation therapy after breast-conserving surgery.[68] To be eligible for this trial, women had to have negative surgical margins. Postoperative mammograms or specimen radiographs were not required. The overall survival rates at 8 years were equivalent in the two treatment arms (radiation, 94%; no radiation, 95%). Radiation reduced the 8-year overall rate of recurrence in the ipsilateral breast (12.1% vs. 26.8%; $P < 0.000005$). Radiation proved to reduce both the rates of noninvasive disease recurrence and the rates of invasive disease recurrence. Among the patients who developed recurrent disease, 51% of the lumpectomy-alone patients and 36% of the lumpectomy-plus-radiation patients developed an invasive recurrence.[68]

The NSABP B-17 study included a wide spectrum of pathologic subtypes of DCIS. It has been argued that the results of this trial are most relevant to patients with disease at the more biologically aggressive end of the spectrum. To address this criticism, the NSABP carefully analyzed the patient and pathologic characteristics of the trial to determine whether the trial was representative of the types of cases currently being diagnosed.[68,69] With respect to patient and presenting characteristics, 83% of the patients presented with nonpalpable disease, and fewer than 5% of patients had disease larger than 2 cm, detected either by gross assessment of the pathology specimen or by mammography. Approximately 50% of the study participants had DCIS diagnosed from a 1-cm or smaller cluster of microcalcifications found on routine mammography. Furthermore, the benefit of radiation therapy was significant for both tumors measuring 1.0 cm or smaller and tumors larger than 1.0 cm.[68] In the 623 cases in which central pathology review was possible, the presence and degree of comedo necrosis was the strongest predictor of recurrence in both treatment groups. Most important, radiation produced a reduction in recurrences in the breast in both the patients with high-risk pathologic features and the patients with low-risk pathologic features.[69] The B-17 trial has been criticized for the fact that although negative margins were required, margins were considered clear even if a single normal cell separated the disease from the margin.

EORTC 10853 trial. The European Organization for Research and Treatment of Cancer (EORTC) has also completed an important randomized prospective clinical trial that compared breast-conserving surgery with or without radiation therapy for patients with DCIS (trial 10853).[70] More than 1000 patients with DCIS of less than 5 cm that was treated with breast-conserving surgery were randomly assigned to radiation therapy vs. no further therapy. In this trial, re-excision was required in the 34% of patients with initially positive margins. The final margin status was positive in only seven cases, although the degree of margin negativity was not provided. Approximately 20% of the patients presented with palpable disease, with a mean tumor diameter of 2.1 cm. The results from this study confirmed those of the B-17 trial. Patients treated with radiation had a lower 4-year rate of overall recurrence (i.e., recurrence of invasive or noninvasive disease) in the breast (9% vs. 16%,

TABLE 15-5

Rates of Recurrence in the Ipsilateral Breast in the NSABP B-17 and EORTC 10853 Trials of Treatment for Ductal Carcinoma In Situ of the Breast

Trial	RECURRENCE RATE (%)		
	No Radiation	Radiation	P Value
NSABP B-17[69] (8-YEAR RESULTS)			
Overall	26.8	12.1	<0.000005
Invasive	13.4	3.9	<0.0001
Noninvasive	13.4	8.2	0.007
EORTC 10853[70] (4-YEAR RESULTS)			
Overall	16	9	0.005
Invasive	8	4	0.04
Noninvasive	8	5	

NSABP, National Surgical Adjuvant Breast and Bowel Project; *EORTC*, European Organization for Research and Treatment of Cancer.

$P = 0.005$) and a lower rate of invasive recurrence in the breast. Table 15-5[69,70] summarizes the results of the NSABP B-17 and EORTC 10853 trials. The median follow-up period at the time of publication of the EORTC trial was 4.25 years, so the long-term data from this study were less reliable. However, the local recurrence rates continued to increase at an annual rate of 2% (irradiation) and 3.5% (no irradiation) through the 10 years of available data. Only 11 deaths occurred as a result of recurrence in the ipsilateral breast in the 1002 enrolled patients, and no difference in overall survival was evident between the two randomized groups.[70]

Van Nuys data. Although the benefit of radiation therapy was clearly demonstrated for all subsets of patients analyzed in the NSABP B-17 trial, the routine use of radiation therapy for DCIS has not become standard in the United States. In 1998 it was estimated that 55% of DCIS patients treated with BCT were treated with surgery alone.[71] In part, this practice pattern may reflect the influence of data from a group from Van Nuys, California. These investigators have argued that not all subsets of patients with DCIS benefit from irradiation. In 1995 Silverstein and colleagues[72] developed the Van Nuys Prognostic Index (VNPI) (Table 15-6) with the hope of defining the optimal treatment strategy according to clinical and pathologic characteristics of the disease. The classification was based on retrospective analysis of 333 patients treated at two institutions between 1979 and 1995. The VNPI incorporated tumor grade and the presence or absence of necrosis (combined into one category), tumor size, and margin status. The 8-year local recurrence–free survival results for patients treated either with surgery alone or with surgery and

TABLE 15-6

The Van Nuys Prognostic Index for Ductal Carcinoma In Situ of the Breast*

Score Components	Definitions
MARGINS	
1	≥ 10 mm
2	1-9 mm
3	< 1 mm
HISTOLOGIC SUBTYPE	
1	Grade 1-2, no necrosis
2	Grade 1-2, necrosis present
3	Grade 3
SIZE	
1	≤ 1.5 cm
2	1.6-4 cm
3	> 4 cm

Modified from Silverstein MJ, Lagios MD, Craig PH, et al. *Cancer* 1996;77:2267-2274.

*One point is given for each category, for a total score ranging from 3 to 9.

TABLE 15-7

Eight-Year Local Recurrence Rates for Patients Treated at the Van Nuys Breast Center According to the Van Nuys Prognostic Index Score

Van Nuys Prognostic Index Score	Treatment	Number of Patients	Breast Recurrence Rate (%)	P Value
3-4	Radiation	25	0	NS
	No radiation	76	3	
5-7	Radiation	103	15	0.017
	No radiation	106	32	
8-9	Radiation	10	60	0.03
	No radiation	13	100	

Data from Silverstein MJ, Lagios MD, Craig PH, et al. *Cancer* 1996;77:2267-2274.
NS, Not significant.

radiation therapy for VNPI scores of 3 to 4, 5 to 7, and 8 to 9 are shown in Table 15-7.[72] These data suggest that radiation therapy benefits only individuals with a VNPI score of 5 to 7, and for those with a VNPI score of 8 to 9, the failure rate with BCT is unacceptably high. On the basis of these data, the authors advocated breast-conserving surgery alone for VNPI scores of 3 to 4, breast-conserving surgery with radiation therapy for VNPI scores of 5 to 7, and mastectomy for VNPI scores of 8 to 9.[72]

Although the Van Nuys data were a significant contribution to the literature concerning DCIS, they must be interpreted within the limitations of the study. Unlike the data from the B-17 trial, the Van Nuys data were generated from two institutions that used special pathologic handling that is not routine in all United States hospitals. Specifically, ocular micrometry was used to measure tumor size and margin distances, serial sectioning at 2- to 3-mm intervals was performed through the entire specimen, and serial sections were incorporated in the tumor size calculations. Assignment of patients to radiation therapy was not random and therefore was subject to physician and temporal biases. Finally, as seen in Table 15-7,[72] the patient numbers in the comparative subcategories of patients were as small as 10, so the confidence intervals for the data, particularly for the VNPI 3 to 4 and VNPI 8 to 9 categories, were large.

Margin status. The importance of margin status was further highlighted in a subsequent report from Silverstein and colleagues.[73] In this analysis of 469 patients with DCIS treated with breast-conserving surgery with or without radiation therapy, margin status was highly predictive of outcome. For patients with a margin width of 10 mm or more, the local recurrence rate at 8 years was only 4% for the 40 patients who received radiation therapy and 3% for the 93 patients treated with surgery alone. Closer margin significantly increased the risk of recurrence both for irradiated patients and for patients treated with surgery alone. The 8-year probability of recurrence for women treated with surgery alone was 20% when margin width was 1 to 10 mm and 58% when margins were less than 1 mm. When radiation was used, the recurrence rates were 12% and 30%, respectively.[73]

Like the Van Nuys study, this retrospective study had limitations that must be recognized. The numbers of patients in the radiation and no-radiation subgroups for each of the margin widths were relatively small compared with the numbers of patients treated in the NSABP B-17 and EORTC 10853 trials. Also, in the Silverstein report, assignment to radiation therapy was not random, and decisions concerning radiation therapy were likely biased by characteristics such as tumor size and era of treatment.

Role of Tamoxifen

After the B-17 trial, the NSABP began the B-24 trial to investigate the role of tamoxifen therapy for patients with DCIS.[74] Patients eligible for this trial were women who had undergone breast-conserving surgery for DCIS. Unlike the B-17 trial, the B-24 trial included patients with involved surgical margins and patients with suspicious scattered calcifications. Approximately 25% of the patients entered into the study had positive or unknown margin status. All women received radiation therapy consisting of 50 Gy to the breast. More than 1800 patients were then randomly assigned to receive tamoxifen or placebo for 5 years. The primary endpoint of the trial was breast events, which included the development of invasive and noninvasive ipsilateral and contralateral disease. The 5-year results of the study indicated that the tamoxifen-treated patients had fewer breast cancer events (8.2% vs. 13.4%, P = 0.0009). The difference in the rate of development of invasive breast cancer was also reduced in the tamoxifen-treated patients.[74]

The results of this important trial are likely to have a significant impact on the management of DCIS in the United States. In women with DCIS, tamoxifen can be considered both a therapeutic agent and a chemoprevention agent. However, with respect to tamoxifen's therapeutic value in women with DCIS, the inclusion of patients with unknown or positive margins after surgery makes the results of the B-24 trial less relevant for patients with negative surgical margins. In the subset of women with negative surgical margins, tamoxifen treatment prevented or delayed the onset of only 2 recurrences in the ipsilateral breast over a 5-year period for every 100 women treated. In addition, over this same period, tamoxifen prevented or delayed the onset of 1.4 cases of contralateral breast cancer. Therefore fewer than 3.5% of DCIS patients with negative surgical margins would be predicted to benefit from tamoxifen use. Because the clinical benefit seems to be low, the use of tamoxifen for women with DCIS and negative margins remains controversial.

RADIATION THERAPY FOR EARLY-STAGE BREAST CANCER

Several revolutionary changes over the past 3 decades have significantly improved the management of early-stage (stage I and II) breast cancer. The increased use of mammographic screening and heightened efforts in public education about breast cancer have dramatically increased the percentage of cases of breast cancer diagnosed at noninvasive or early stages of disease.[13] Simultaneously, treatment options for early-stage breast cancer have changed significantly. Limited breast surgery followed by radiation therapy has been shown to result in outcomes equivalent to outcomes after modified radical mastectomy for the majority of women with early-stage disease. This organ-preserving approach to treatment has had a profound impact on patient well-being and quality of life.[75] In addition, recent advances in radiation techniques and axillary surgery have reduced the morbidity of treatment of axillary lymph nodes. Perhaps even more important than these advances in local–regional therapies has been the introduction of systemic treatment for the majority of women with early-stage breast cancer. It is now clear that treatment with chemotherapy or hormonal therapy or both modalities reduces the odds of cancer recurrence for all women with invasive breast tumors larger than 1 cm in diameter, independent of lymph node status.[76,77]

This section of the chapter addresses several clinically relevant questions concerning the management of early-stage breast cancer. Some of these questions have been answered through well-conducted clinical trials, whereas others remain subjects of controversy. The questions to be addressed include: Is BCT an equivalent local–regional treatment to modified radical mastectomy? Do all patients treated with BCT require radiation therapy? What are the patient, tumor, and treatment characteristics that influence outcome with BCT? Can the morbidity of breast-conserving surgery be further decreased? Do all patients with early-stage disease benefit from chemotherapy or hormonal therapy? What is the optimal sequencing of surgery, chemotherapy, and radiation therapy?

Equivalence of Breast Conservation Therapy and Modified Radical Mastectomy

After single-institution reports of the successful use of breast-conserving surgery and radiation therapy as an alternative to mastectomy for early-stage breast cancer, several phase III clinical trials were developed and conducted to directly compare these two approaches for the management of local–regional disease. Between 1976 and 1984, the NSABP conducted the largest of these trials, the B-06 trial. In this trial, a total of 1600 women were randomly assigned to one of three local–regional treatments: modified radical mastectomy, lumpectomy plus axillary dissection plus breast irradiation, or lumpectomy plus axillary dissection alone.[21] All patients treated with breast-conserving surgery were required to have negative surgical margins after lumpectomy, defined in this study as no tumor present at the inked margin of resection. Breast irradiation consisted of 50 Gy in 2-Gy fractions delivered to the whole breast with no tumor bed boost. The trial was open to women with primary tumors up to 4 cm. Women with positive lymph nodes were treated with chemotherapy, whereas women with negative lymph nodes did not receive systemic treatment. The 12-year outcome data conclusively demonstrated that treatment with lumpectomy and radiation therapy was equivalent to modified radical mastectomy in terms of disease-free and overall survival. In this trial, recurrences in the ipsilateral breast after BCT that were successfully salvaged with mastectomy were not considered events for the purposes of calculating disease-free survival or local–regional recurrences. At 8 years, the local recurrence rates were 1.1% for the lumpectomy and radiation group and 8.8% for the modified radical mastectomy group.[78] The 8-year actuarial rate of recurrence in the ipsilateral breast was 10% for the lumpectomy and radiation group. These data indicate that lumpectomy and radiation therapy not only produces disease-free and overall survival rates comparable to those with mastectomy but also achieves statistically equivalent rates of recurrence in local–regional sites.

The data from NSABP B-06 plus six other randomized trials comparing modified radical mastectomy to breast-conserving surgery plus radiation therapy for early-stage breast cancer were compiled by the Early Breast Cancer Trialists' Collaborative Group (EBCTCG). Their analysis of these data from 3100 women revealed no difference in overall survival according to treatment type, with both treatment groups having a 10-year survival rate of 71%.[79] A second meta-analysis by a different group that focused only on the outcome of breast-conserving surgery and radiation therapy vs. modified radical mastectomy for lymph node–positive patients again found the two treatments to be equivalent with respect to overall survival.[80] The interesting finding from this second meta-analysis was that BCT offered a survival advantage over mastectomy in the combined analysis of trials in which postmastectomy radiation was not used (odds ratio favoring BCT of 0.69). In the studies that compared BCT against modified radical mastectomy with postoperative irradiation, the two treatments achieved equivalent outcomes. These data suggest that radiation therapy should be a component of care for women with high-risk lymph node–positive breast cancer.

Role of Radiation Therapy in Breast Conservation Therapy

Once it was established that limited breast surgery combined with a course of breast irradiation achieved an outcome equivalent to treatment with mastectomy, several trials studied whether radiation therapy is needed as a component of BCT. In the NSABP B-06 trial, patients treated with lumpectomy and axillary dissection alone were found to have a significantly higher rate of recurrence in the ipsilateral breast than those treated with lumpectomy, axillary dissection, and irradiation.[21] The 12-year actuarial local recurrence data from this trial revealed an ipsilateral breast recurrence rate of 35% in the lumpectomy-alone group compared with 10% in the lumpectomy–plus–radiation therapy group ($P < 0.001$). These data were again included and confirmed in the meta-analysis compiled by the EBCTCG. In their analysis of more than 2200 women treated in randomized clinical trials, breast irradiation reduced the chance of tumor recurrence within the breast after 20 years from 30.3% to 10.6%.[79] Despite the reduction in local recurrence, no difference in overall survival was evident between patients who received radiation therapy and those who did not. In part, this is because some of the determinants of local–regional recurrence simultaneously affect the risk of distant recurrence. In addition, the equivalent survival may also reflect the high successful salvage rate with mastectomy after recurrence in the ipsilateral breast.

The NSABP and EORTC trials showed that radiation therapy is beneficial for most patients treated with breast-conserving surgery for early-stage breast cancer. Additional randomized trials are have proven the value of radiation therapy for subgroups of patients with early-stage breast cancer with a favorable prognosis. Whether radiation therapy is needed after excision of a small tumor with widely negative margins was in part addressed by a trial from Milan, Italy. This study included only women with tumors 2.5 cm or smaller and compared quadrantectomy and axillary dissection to quadrantectomy and axillary dissection plus breast irradiation. In this trial, only tumors recurring within 2 cm of the surgical scars were considered to be local recurrences. Despite the extensive surgical procedure and the narrow definition of local recurrence, after 5 years the patients treated with radiation had a lower local recurrence rate than those treated with surgery alone (0.5% vs. 8.8%, $P = 0.001$).[22]

A randomized trial from Sweden specifically addressed whether patients with stage I disease require radiation therapy after breast-conserving surgery. Again, the local recurrence rate for the 197 patients treated with surgery alone was higher than that for the 184 patients randomly assigned to radiation therapy (18.4% vs. 2.3%, respectively, at 5 years, $P < 0.0001$).[81]

The question of whether systemic treatment with either chemotherapy or tamoxifen obviates the need for breast irradiation has also been partially addressed in the available clinical trials. The results of these trials are shown in Table 15-8.[21,82,83] In the NSABP B-06 trial, chemotherapy was used only for patients with lymph node–positive disease; patients with negative lymph nodes were not given systemic treatment.[21] In the

TABLE 15-8

Effects of Systemic Therapy and Radiation Therapy on Breast Recurrence Rates

Trial	Postsurgical Treatment	Breast Recurrence Rate
NSABP B-06[21]	Chemotherapy plus radiation	5% at 12 years
	Radiation alone	12% at 12 years
	Chemotherapy alone	41% at 12 years
	None	32% at 12 years
Scottish trial[82]	Systemic therapy plus radiation	6% at 6 years
	Systemic therapy alone	25% at 6 years
NSABP B-21[83]*	Tamoxifen plus radiation	3% at 5 years
	Radiation alone	6.5% at 5 years
	Tamoxifen alone	13.1% at 5 years

NSABP, National Surgical Adjuvant Breast and Bowel Project.
*Based on annual rates of events provided in the abstract.

randomized trial from Scotland, all patients underwent systemic treatment, with approximately 75% of the 589 enrolled patients receiving tamoxifen as the sole systemic treatment.[82] Finally, in the NSABP B-21 trial, women with lymph node–negative breast tumors measuring less than 1.0 cm that were treated with lumpectomy and axillary lymph node dissection were randomly assigned to receive tamoxifen alone, radiation therapy alone, or tamoxifen and irradiation.[83] It is clear from the data in Table 15-8[21,82,83] that systemic treatments should not be considered alternatives to radiation therapy but may have synergistic effects with radiation therapy in further reducing the rate of ipsilateral breast recurrences.

The issue of whether radiation is needed in all subcategories of patients with favorable early-stage breast cancer treated with BCT was also addressed by the Joint Center for Radiation Therapy (JCRT). These investigators conducted a single-arm prospective trial investigating the omission of radiation therapy in patients with unicentric clinical T1 disease with pathologically negative lymph nodes.[84] All patients in this trial were required to have undergone a wide local excision that achieved negative margins of at least 1 cm. The median tumor size in this study was 0.9 cm, and the median age of the patients was 67 years. The local recurrence rate reached the rate defined in the predefined stopping rules, and the trial was closed before full, planned accrual. With a median follow-up time of 56 months, 16% of the patients had experienced a local recurrence.[84]

Finally, an Intergroup trial has recently been completed in the United States to further determine whether radiation therapy is needed in elderly patients with favorable disease features. Patients eligible for this trial included women age 60 and older with tumors less than 3 cm, estrogen receptor– and progesterone receptor– positive disease, and wide negative margins. Patients were randomly assigned to receive breast-conserving surgery plus tamoxifen or breast-conserving surgery, tamoxifen, and breast irradiation. This trial closed to accrual in 1999 so the results are not yet available.

In conclusion, all of the clinical studies to date have indicated that breast irradiation reduces the risk of local recurrences after breast-conserving surgery and therefore should be considered a standard component of treatment for all women with early-stage invasive disease. Thus far, all attempts to define subsets of breast cancer patients with favorable early-stage disease who may not require radiation therapy have been unsuccessful.

Trends in the Use of Breast Conservation Therapy

It is currently estimated that each year, 100,000 patients with stage 0 to II breast cancer are treated in the United States with BCT. It is clear that not every patient prefers to be treated with BCT, and some patients with early-stage disease are not suitable candidates for breast preservation. Therefore a reasonable benchmark for the use of BCT is that 60% of patients with stage 0 to II disease should be treated with this approach. Figure 15-7 shows how estimates of the frequency of BCT in 1995 compared against this benchmark.[71,85] Although significant

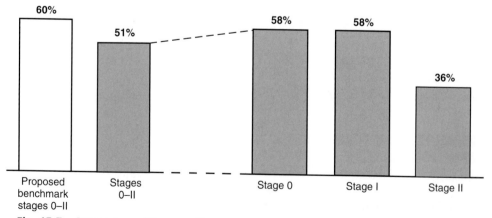

Fig. 15-7 Comparison of the use of breast conservation therapy (BCT) with and without axillary dissection in the United States in 1995 against a benchmark representing use of BCT in 60% of all early-stage breast cancer cases. The benchmark is based on assumptions that 74% of stage 0 through II patients are eligible for BCT and 81% of those would opt for the procedure. (From The Health Care Advisory Board: *Innovations in Breast Cancer Care: A Summary of an Annual Oncology Roundtable* [pt II]. Washington, DC: The Advisory Board; 1999.)

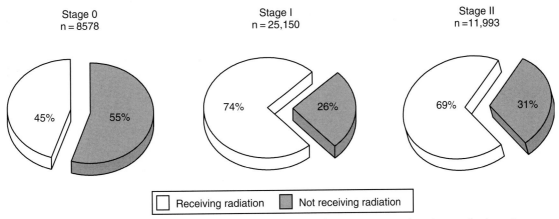

Fig. 15-8 Use of radiation therapy as a component of breast conservation therapy for breast cancer in the United States in 1995. (From The Health Care Advisory Board: *Innovations in Breast Cancer Care: a Summary of an Annual Oncology Roundtable* [pt II]. Washington, DC: The Advisory Board; 1999.)

improvements in both patient and physician education concerning BCT are still needed, these data indicate that BCT is being appropriately used in many regions of the United States.

Despite the proven efficacy of radiation therapy as a component of BCT, this important treatment modality remains underused. Figure 15-8 shows an estimate of the use of radiation therapy in cases treated with BCT in the United States in 1995.[71,84] The data displayed in Figure 15-8,[85] from a study of more than 40,000 cases from the National Cancer Database, show that 28% of patients with early-stage breast cancer did not receive radiation therapy as a component of BCT. The most common reason for the omission of radiation therapy in these cases was a failure to refer the patient for treatment, with only 15% of patients not receiving radiation therapy because of patient refusal.

The underuse of irradiation in the more elderly population is even more distressing. In a study of 27,399 women with early-stage breast cancer treated with breast-conserving surgery who were enrolled in the Surveillance Epidemiology and End Results program, the use of radiation therapy after surgery was highly dependent on patient age ($P < 0.001$). Rates of use of radiation therapy by age group were as follows: 70 to 74 years, 69%; 75 to 79 years, 57%; 80 to 84 years, 36.5%; and 85+ years, 13.9%.[86] A similar trend was seen in a study of 1174 women age 50 and older in Quebec, Canada.[87] In this study, only 55% of women age 70 and older treated with breast-conserving surgery received radiation therapy. These data indicate that an urgent need remains for physician and public education about the value of radiation therapy as a component of BCT in the treatment of early-stage breast cancer.

Contraindications for Breast Conservation Therapy

Not all patients with early-stage breast cancer are suitable for BCT. BCT is contraindicated when the primary tumor cannot successfully be removed with less than a mastectomy. Examples of such patients include women with mammographic diffuse suspicious microcalcifications throughout the breast and women in whom repeated attempts at breast-conserving surgery fail to achieve negative surgical margins.

BCT is also contraindicated when a more optimal aesthetic result can be achieved with mastectomy and breast reconstruction (e.g., if the ratio of the primary tumor size to the breast size is large or if a central segmentectomy with resection of the nipple-areola complex is required to achieve negative margins).

Finally, BCT is contraindicated for patients in whom the potential for severe injury from radiation therapy is high. Specific examples of this category of patients are women who are pregnant and women with certain connective tissue diseases. For women early in the course of their pregnancy, internal radiation scatter from irradiation of the intact breast can reach lethal and teratogenic dose levels.[88] For these reasons, it is critical that all women of child-bearing age be counseled against becoming pregnant during the course of radiation therapy. Women with connective tissue disorders may be at increased risk for significant late radiation complications, including significant breast fibrosis and pain, chest wall necrosis, and brachial plexopathy. The collagen vascular diseases associated with the greatest risk for radiation injury are systemic scleroderma, lupus erythematosus, polymyositis or dermatomyositis, and mixed connective tissue disorders. In a study of 209 patients from

Massachusetts General Hospital in Boston, 131 patients with rheumatoid arthritis seemed not to have elevated rates of late toxic effects.[89] Therefore use of BCT is a reasonable option for patients with rheumatoid arthritis.

Factors Affecting the Outcome of Breast Conservation Therapy

Several patient, tumor, and treatment-related factors have been found to influence local recurrence rates after BCT. These factors are described briefly in the following paragraphs.

Patient Factors

Age. The clearest example of a patient factor that influences both local and distant recurrence rates after BCT is patient age. Several single-institution studies have reported that young patient age, usually defined as age less than 30, 35, or 40 years, is associated with an increased risk of distant metastases and reduced disease-specific survival.[90-92] In addition, young age has been shown to increase the risk of recurrence in the ipsilateral breast after BCT. Table 15-9 presents the rates of local recurrence as a function of patient age in selected modern series.[92-97]

Because age may also affect local recurrence rates after mastectomy, investigators from the M.D. Anderson Cancer Center performed a retrospective study of breast cancer patients less than 35 years old in which 79 patients treated with BCT were matched according to tumor stage, nodal status, and follow-up time, with 79 patients treated with modified radical mastectomy. No statistically significant difference was evident between the patients treated with BCT and the patients treated with modified radical mastectomy in the 5-year recurrence rate (12% and 18.8%, respectively) or the 10-year recurrence rate (7.4% and 11.8%, respectively) (P = 0.236).[98]

An increasing trend is evident in the United States to think of breast cancer as an indolent disease in the elderly population. As indicated earlier in this chapter in the section on "Trends in the Use of Breast Conservation Therapy," use of radiation therapy and systemic treatment after BCT decreases as patient age increases. Data reported by Solin and colleagues[99] suggest that breast cancer is not an indolent disease in the elderly population and that decisions concerning treatment recommendations should not be based on the patient's chronologic age. These authors compared the 10-year outcomes of BCT in women at least 65 years old and women 50 to 65 years old and reported that the two groups had equally virulent disease (as determined by stage and prognostic factors) and equivalent rates of breast cancer deaths.[99]

Race. Data are limited regarding the influence of race on the success of BCT. The data that do exist mostly concern African-American women; virtually no data are available concerning Hispanics, Asian Americans, and other ethnic groups. One of the larger series concerning the success of local–regional therapy in African-American breast cancer patients with primary tumors smaller than 5 cm was reported by Newman and colleagues[100] from the M.D. Anderson Cancer Center. In this series, local recurrence rates were similar between the 42 patients treated with BCT (9.8%) and the 168 patients treated with mastectomy (8.9%).[100]

Family history and genetic predisposition. Several retrospective studies have investigated the influence of family history or a genetic predisposition for breast cancer on the success of BCT. Investigators from the JCRT compared local control rates in 29 women age 36 or less who had a first-degree relative with breast cancer before age 50 or a family history of ovarian cancer and 172 women age 36 years or less who did not have these family history criteria.[101] The 5-year crude local recurrence rate was 3% in patients with a positive family history vs. 14% in patients who did not have a family history. In addition, the patients with positive family histories had a 5.7-fold increased risk of developing contralateral breast cancer compared with patients with a negative family history.[101] The impact of family history and young age was also investigated in a series of 1021 patients treated at the University of Pennsylvania.[102] As in the JCRT experience, no difference in local control was found based on family history of breast cancer in young patients. In patients age 40 or younger, the 5-year local failure

TABLE 15-9

Rates of Recurrence in the Breast After Breast-Conserving Surgery and Radiation Therapy as a Function of Patient Age

Study	Patient Age (Years)	Recurrence Rate (%)	Time (Years)	P Value
Fowble et al[92]	≤ 35	24	8	0.001
	36-50	14		
	> 50	12		
Haffty et al[93]	< 36	15	8	< 0.05
	≥ 36	11		
Halverson et al[94]	< 40	12	7	0.13
	≥ 40	12	7	
Kurtz et al[95]	< 40	21	6	< 0.025
	≥ 40	11		
Fisher et al[96]	≤ 35	24	8.6	< 0.01
	> 35	7		
Buchholz et al[97]	< 40	16	10	0.017
	≥ 40	8		

rate was 8% for those with a first-degree relative with breast cancer, 2% for those with a non–first-degree relative with breast cancer, and 12% for those with a negative family history ($P \geq 0.18$).

Data on outcomes of BCT in individuals with known predisposing germline mutations are limited. Investigators from Yale University reported a 15% rate of *BRCA1* or *BRCA2* germline mutations in 52 patients who had previously developed a recurrence in the ipsilateral breast after BCT.[103] Interestingly, the median interval to ipsilateral tumor recurrence was 7.8 years for individuals with a germline *BRCA1* or *BRCA2* mutation compared with 4.7 years for women without either of these mutations. In a second study, Pierce and colleagues[104] reported a 5-year local failure–free survival rate of 98% in 71 women with proven *BRCA1* or *BRCA2* mutations and 96% in 213 matched controls with presumed sporadic breast cancer. These authors also noted no complications from radiation therapy in individuals with *BRCA1* or *BRCA2* germline mutations, which confirmed previously published data from Gaffney and colleagues.[105] Finally, in a recent article from Memorial Sloan-Kettering Cancer Center, the authors reported that *BRCA* mutation status was not an independent predictor of either local or distant recurrence in a group of 329 women of Ashkenazi Jewish heritage.[106] Interestingly, in that study the rate of recurrence in the ipsilateral breast was nearly identical to the rate of new contralateral breast tumors in patients found to have a *BRCA* mutation.

Together, these data indicate that BCT is an appropriate local treatment option for women with a family history of breast cancer or a genetic predisposition to breast cancer. These patients may carry an increased risk of contralateral breast cancer and late local recurrence, possibly because of second primary tumors being present within the treated breast.

Tumor and Pathology Factors

Surgical margins. One of the most important pathologic factors that affects the rate of local control after breast-conserving surgery and radiation therapy is the status of the surgical margins. It is now standard practice to ink surgical specimens and report margin status quantitatively in all cases of invasive breast cancer treated with breast-conserving surgery. In addition, recognition of the importance of margin status in predicting local recurrence has led to increased rates of re-excision to obtain clear surgical margins.

Although margin status is clearly recognized to be predictive for breast tumor recurrence, controversy remains regarding what should be defined as a negative margin. The NSABP B-06 trial defined a *negative margin* as the absence of tumor cells on the ink-defined margin. When a consensus was reached among pathologist reviewers that the surgical margins were involved, resid-

ual disease was found at subsequent mastectomy in 62% of cases.[107] Other groups have defined *surgical margins* more precisely by measuring the total distance from the closest malignant cell to the ink and by further distinguishing *focally positive margins* from margin involvement over a wider area. No consensus is evident regarding the optimal definition of *close margins*. In an analysis of 1021 patients, authors from the University of Pennsylvania reported that local failure rates were not significantly different in patients with negative ($N = 518$), focally close ($N = 96$), focally positive ($N = 124$), or unknown margins ($N = 283$). The rates for these groups at 8 years were as follows: negative, 8%; focally positive, 10%; unknown margin status, 16%; and focally close, 17% ($P = 0.21$).[108] These actuarial curves were nearly identical over the first 4 years and began to separate thereafter. The limited number of patients in this series who had close or positive margins and were followed for more than 5 years leads to uncertainty whether patients with positive or close margins have higher rates of late local recurrence. For this reason, the recommended treatment policy is re-excision for all patients with positive or unknown margin status and to consider re-excision for women younger than 40 years who have close margins (< 2 mm).

For patients with positive margins, the extent of margin involvement likely influences the total risk of recurrence. Wazer and colleagues[109] from New England Medical Center evaluated 105 patients with positive surgical margins after breast-conserving surgery. The 73 patients with focal or minimal margin involvement had a crude local recurrence rate of only 2.8% (median follow-up time of 75 months) compared with a rate of 22.2% in the 27 patients with moderate or extensive margin involvement (median follow-up time of 88 months).[109] The median interval to recurrence in this series was 64 months, and the number of patients at risk at 10 years was very small.

Margin status may also be related to the extent of intraductal disease within or adjacent to invasive carcinoma. In 1990, authors from the JCRT reported that women with tumors that had an *extensive intraductal component (EIC)*, defined as tumors that are predominantly noninvasive or tumors with a DCIS component comprising at least 25% and with DCIS present in surrounding normal breast tissue, are at increased risk of local recurrence.[110] However, in a subsequent analysis, the increased risk associated with an EIC was found to be limited to patients with positive margins. None of the 18 patients with an EIC who had negative, close, or focally positive margins experienced a breast tumor recurrence, whereas six of the 12 patients with more than a focally positive margin and an EIC had a recurrence.[111] These data suggest that an EIC increases the difficulty of achieving negative margins and in selected cases may represent a more diffuse disease process.

However, patients with an EIC in whom negative margins are achieved should be considered appropriate candidates for BCT.

Changes in radiation treatment may not be able to overcome the prognostic importance of margin status. Wazer and colleagues[112] have reported the results of a treatment policy of determining the radiation dose to the tumor bed according to the margin status. After a dose of 50.4 Gy to the breast, the tumor bed was boosted as follows: negative margins after re-excision, 0 Gy; negative margin greater than 5 mm, 10 Gy; negative margin of 2 to 5 mm, 14 Gy; and negative margin less than 2 mm, 20 Gy. For women age 45 or older, this policy resulted in excellent local control. However, for women younger than 45 years, the failure rates remained proportional to the final margin status.[112]

Systemic treatment may also influence the prognostic importance of margin status. In a report of 533 patients treated with conservative surgery and radiation therapy at the JCRT, the prognostic importance of margin status was related to the use of systemic treatment.[113] In this series, among patients with focally positive margins, the crude local recurrence rate at 8 years was 7% in the 45 patients treated with systemic therapy vs. 18% in the 77 patients who did not receive systemic therapy. However, for the patients with more extensive margin involvement, the use of systemic therapy did not reduce the rate of local recurrence (26% vs. 29%).[113] A randomized prospective trial in the United Kingdom reported that women with focally positive margins treated with concurrent chemotherapy (methotrexate and mitoxantrone) and radiation therapy (54 Gy to the breast) had a local recurrence rate of only 1.9% after a median follow-up time of 57 months. The toxicity of this schedule of concurrent chemotherapy and radiation therapy was not reported.[114]

In contrast to these studies, a study from Fox Chase Cancer Center investigating how systemic therapy influenced the rates of local recurrence in patients with close or positive margins suggested that systemic treatment delayed but did not prevent recurrences in the intact breast. For patients with close or positive margins, the rates of local recurrence at 5 years were only 3% for those treated with systemic treatment but 11% in those who did not receive systemic treatment. However, after 10 years, the rates were much more similar (12% with systemic treatment, 16% without systemic treatment) and were higher than local recurrence rates in patients with negative surgical margins (7%).[115]

Taken together, these data suggest that margin status correlates with long-term local control for patients treated with BCT. Recurrences may be delayed with higher radiation dosages and use of systemic therapy. In general, the authors recommend re-excision for patients with positive margins and individualizing treatment recommendations for patients with close margins. The authors also recommend re-excision for young patients with margins of less than 2 mm if re-excision can be done with an acceptable aesthetic outcome. For older women and women in whom re-excision would result in an unacceptable cosmetic outcome, increasing the tumor bed dose to 64 to 66 Gy is a reasonable strategy, particularly if women also receive systemic treatment.

Multicentric and multifocal disease. A second tumor feature associated with an increased recurrence risk after BCT is the presence of *gross multicentric disease*, defined as separate foci of disease in different quadrants of the breast, or *gross multifocal disease*, defined as two or more foci of disease in the same quadrant of the breast. These terms refer to clinically evident disease and do not refer to cases in which pathologic examination reveals two areas of disease separated by an area of normal tissue.

Limited data are available concerning the success of BCT in patients with multicentric or multifocal disease. In one of the largest series, Kurtz and colleagues[116] reported a breast recurrence rate of 25% in 61 patients treated for gross multicentric or multifocal disease compared with a rate of 11% in patients with unifocal disease. Most of these 61 patients had multifocal disease, with only 10 patients requiring a separate incision or a generous partial mastectomy. No increased risk of recurrence was evident for patients with multifocal disease if the disease was detected only on microscopic examination of the specimen, nor was an increased risk evident in the 22 patients in which the final resection margin status was negative. A small series from the JCRT also associated multicentric disease with an increased recurrence risk. In 10 patients with multiple synchronous tumors in one breast, the local failure rate after BCT was 40%.[117] No data concerning the relationship between recurrence and margin status were reported.

The authors recommend mastectomy for women who present with gross multicentric disease that would require separate surgical incisions. For women with multifocal disease within a sphere of 4 cm that is amenable to complete resection with a single segmental mastectomy, the option of BCT is offered, provided that negative surgical margins (> 2 mm) can be achieved. The limited data available for multifocal disease completely resected with adequate margins suggest that patients with such disease are not at increased risk for recurrence.

Tumor stage. Although tumor size and nodal status are powerful prognostic factors for disease-free and overall survival in patients with early-stage breast cancer, these factors have much less impact on local recurrence rates. Among patients in the NSABP B-06 trial who were treated with lumpectomy and radiation therapy, the recurrence rate was 10% for patients with T2 disease and 7% for patients with T1 disease.[21] Even more striking, patients with positive lymph nodes had only a 5% 12-year risk of local recurrence compared with a 12% risk in patients with lymph node–negative disease.[21] These recurrence patterns may have been influenced by the selective use of chemotherapy in patients with lymph node–positive disease.

Histologic subtype. Most of the data concerning the success of BCT were obtained from women with infiltrating ductal carcinoma of the breast. The randomized prospective trials that directly compared BCT and modified radical mastectomy have insufficient data regarding other histologic subtypes of breast cancer. However, several institutions have reported that BCT is an appropriate option for women with invasive lobular carcinoma or the favorable histologic subtypes of medullary, colloid, and tubular carcinoma. Veronesi and colleagues[118] reported that the breast tumor recurrence rate after BCT for 431 cases of lobular cancer was 6% and was equivalent to the rate for infiltrating ductal carcinoma. These data were confirmed by a smaller series from Poen and colleagues,[119] who reported a rate of recurrence in the ipsilateral breast of only 2% in 60 women treated with BCT for lobular carcinoma.

On the basis of currently available data, histologic grade and estrogen and progesterone receptor status do not seem to be independent predictors of local recurrence after BCT. In the NSABP B-06 trial, grade and estrogen and progesterone receptor status affected local recurrence rates for patients treated with lumpectomy alone but had no influence on recurrence patterns for patients treated with lumpectomy and radiation therapy.[120]

More recently, interest has increased with regard to correlating local recurrence risk with newly identified tumor biomarkers. Using case-control methodology, investigators from Yale University retrospectively studied biomarker expression in primary breast tumors from women in whom a local recurrence developed and in matched controls in whom long-term local control was achieved. The investigators found that rates of *Her-2/neu* oncoprotein overexpression and insulin growth factor 1 overexpression were higher in tumors from women with recurrences.[121,122]

Treatment-Related Factors

Systemic therapy. In addition to reducing the probability of development of metastatic disease, systemic therapy has also been shown to reduce the risk of recurrence in the ipsilateral breast. It has been clearly demonstrated in randomized trials that chemotherapy and tamoxifen are not appropriate substitutes for radiation therapy.[21,83,84] However, in patients who are treated with radiation therapy, the use of systemic therapy improves local control. In the NSABP B-06 trial, patients with lymph node–positive disease who were treated with radiation therapy and chemotherapy had an 8-year local recurrence rate of 5% compared with a local recurrence rate of 12% in lymph node–negative patients treated with surgery and radiation therapy alone.[21] In the NSABP B-21 trial, tamoxifen similarly improved local control rates in patients with lymph node–negative breast tumors smaller than 1 cm.[83] The crude rate of breast tumor recurrence was only 3% in women randomly assigned to undergo lumpectomy, radiation therapy, and tamoxifen compared with 7% in women treated with lumpectomy and radiation therapy alone.[83] A retrospective analysis from the M.D. Anderson Cancer Center investigating the impact of systemic therapy on local control after BCT in patients with lymph node–negative breast cancer further confirmed these data.[97] In this study, 277 patients treated with systemic therapy had improved 5-year (97.5% vs. 89.8%) and 10-year (95.6% vs. 85.2%) local control rates compared with 207 patients who received no systemic treatment. No statistically significant difference was evident in local control between patients treated with chemotherapy and those treated with tamoxifen alone ($P = 0.219$). In a Cox regression analysis, the use of systemic therapy was the most powerful clinical, pathologic, or treatment predictor of local control, producing a 3.3-fold reduction in the risk of local recurrence.[97]

Tumor bed boost. The use of a tumor bed boost after irradiation of the intact breast may also influence the risk of local recurrence. The first randomized trial investigating the impact of a 10-Gy boost after 50 Gy of breast irradiation was performed in Lyons, France. The use of a boost led to a small but statistically significant reduction in the rate of local recurrence at 5 years (3.6% vs. 4.5%, $P = 0.04$).[12] The EORTC has subsequently completed a much larger randomized trial investigating the impact of a tumor bed boost. Preliminary findings from this study suggested that a 16-Gy boost reduced the 5-year rate of local recurrence from 6.8% to 4.3% ($P < 0.0001$).[123]

The authors' current policy is to use a tumor bed boost in nearly every patient. A tumor bed boost is routinely used when one or more of the following is present: high-grade disease, vascular or lymphatic invasion, an EIC, margins of 5 mm or less, or a delay of greater than 8 weeks because of healing problems or the use of systemic therapy.

Axillary Treatment

Optimizing the management of the axillary lymph nodes in women with early-stage breast cancer is one of the most active areas of research in the field of BCT.

Traditional Axillary Dissection

Until recently, a level I and II axillary dissection was standard for all women with invasive breast cancer. This procedure effectively treated involved lymph nodes, provided important prognostic information, and provided information that often influenced decisions concerning the use of systemic treatment. However, the positive aspects of axillary dissection are often offset by its associated morbidity. Although serious long-term complications after axillary dissection are rare, the procedure universally has a negative effect on patients' quality of life.

Specifically, all patients undergoing this procedure experience axillary pain and numbness and decreased range of motion in the arm and are at risk for chronic lymphedema. These concerns have led to investigation of a number of alternatives to axillary dissection. Another impetus for the investigation of alternatives to axillary dissection is the increased use of systemic treatment for breast cancer patients with lymph node–negative disease, a trend that makes the prognostic information gained from axillary dissection less important. The two alternative strategies currently in use are nodal irradiation and sentinel lymph node surgery.

Axillary Nodal Irradiation

Whether radiation therapy and surgery have equal efficacy in the therapeutic management of the clinically negative axilla was first studied in the 1970s in the NSABP B-04 trial. This trial was a triple-arm prospective trial in which patients with clinically lymph node–negative disease were randomly assigned to treatment with radical mastectomy, simple mastectomy, or simple mastectomy plus irradiation of the chest wall and regional lymph nodes, including the supraclavicular and infraclavicular areas.[124] As such, this trial directly compared surgical treatment of the axilla with no treatment of the axilla and primary irradiation of the axilla. Thirty percent of the patients with clinically negative lymph nodes who were treated with radical mastectomy had pathologically involved axillary lymph nodes. The lymph node failure rates were 2% for surgery, 18% for no treatment, and 3% for radiation therapy.[124] These results indicated that the rate of pathologic involvement of lymph nodes may be almost double the rate of axillary recurrence without therapy. The results also indicated that radiation therapy and surgery were equivalent in preventing axillary recurrences. The authors did not report a comparison of axillary treatment–related morbidity with the three approaches. Data from this B-04 study also suggested that patients with clinically positive lymph nodes at presentation had lower axillary recurrence rates after surgery than after definitive irradiation.[124]

On the basis of these data, several institutions began to omit axillary dissection in patients for whom knowledge of lymph node status would not affect systemic treatment recommendations. These patients most often were elderly women who would receive tamoxifen as systemic treatment independent of their lymph nodes status. In a prospective single-arm study at New England Medical Center, 73 women age 64 and older with clinically negative lymph nodes were treated with axillary irradiation instead of axillary dissection.[125] Radiation

therapy was delivered with a four-field technique (opposed breast tangents, a matched anterior oblique field to include the remaining axilla and supraclavicular lymph nodes, and a posterior field to supplement the dose to the midaxilla). Only one patient experienced a regional recurrence, which occurred 103 months after treatment.[125] The treatment-related morbidity from the axillary irradiation was minimal. Similar results were obtained at Yale University, where the regional failure rate in 327 women treated with primary irradiation of the breast and regional lymphatics was only 3% at 5 years.[126] The disadvantages of using these comprehensive fields instead of standard breast tangent fields are the increased amount of lung irradiated and the increased risks of arm edema and of fibrosis at the match line of the fields. In an attempt to avoid these disadvantages, the JCRT developed a prospective policy of primary irradiation of the axilla using high tangents. This technique used only two radiation fields (breast tangents) and raised the cranial edge of the treatment field to include the majority of level I and a portion of the level II lymph nodes. In a highly selected population of elderly patients with low-risk disease, only one of 92 patients developed a regional nodal failure, which was also associated with a primary recurrence in the breast.[127]

Sentinel Lymph Node Surgery

A second strategy for minimizing the morbidity of axillary treatment is sentinel lymph node surgery. This strategy attempts to remove only the first-echelon lymph nodes to which the primary tumor drains—the sentinel nodes. The strategy is based on the assumption that the lymphatic drainage of a primary breast tumor progresses first through one or a small number of lymph nodes. Correspondingly, if these lymph nodes do not contain disease, the probability of disease in any other axillary lymph node should be very small. Two strategies are currently used to identify sentinel lymph nodes: injection of blue dye and injection of a radioactive colloid.

Blue-dye and radiocolloid injection techniques. The blue-dye technique involves injection of isosulfan blue dye into the tumor or the dermal lymphatics overlying the tumor bed approximately 3 to 10 minutes before surgery. After massaging the breast, the surgeon makes a small incision in the axilla so that the lymph nodes and lymphatic channels that take up the dye can be visualized. These blue-stained lymph nodes are then excised and examined histologically to determine whether a formal axillary dissection is warranted. This technique is relatively simple and is the least expensive sentinel lymph node technique in that it involves only the breast surgeon and can be done entirely within the operating room.

The second strategy for localizing sentinel lymph nodes is injection of a radioactive colloid such as technetium 99m.

The drainage from the region of the tumor bed to the sentinel lymph node(s) can be imaged preoperatively with lymphoscintigraphy. During the operation, sentinel lymph nodes are identified with a handheld gamma probe, which permits the surgeon to detect and resect radioactive axillary lymph nodes. The radiocolloid technique offers the advantage of preoperative assessment of lymphatic drainage and allows identification of secondary or primary drainage to the internal mammary lymph node chain. The primary disadvantage of the radiocolloid localization technique is the added schedule coordination and cost. In addition, the radioactivity from the primary tumor can mask that of a sentinel lymph node.

Both blue dye injection and radiocolloid injection are currently accepted as standard methods for sentinel lymph node surgery. In addition, a number of institutions believe that the best results are obtained by using the blue dye and radiocolloid techniques in combination.

Results. Several centers have reported the results of sentinel lymph node surgery followed by formal axillary dissection. These initial studies were performed to judge the effectiveness of sentinel lymph node procedures in identifying sentinel lymph nodes and the rate of false-negative results (the probability of having a positive nonsentinel lymph node when the sentinel lymph node is negative). In these reports, the success rate in identifying a sentinel lymph node ranged from 91% to 99% and seemed to be independent of the localization technique used.[128-130] These studies also reported that in 67% to 93% of patients, a single sentinel lymph node was identified, and fewer than 10% of patients had three or more sentinel nodes identified. The false-negative rates (determined using all patients with identified sentinel lymph nodes who had histologically confirmed lymph node metastases as the denominator) ranged from 0% to 11.4%.[128-130] In an important contribution, Krag and colleagues[129] reported the results from a series of community surgeons. They reported that the false-negative rate depended in part on the skill and experience of the surgeon and could range as high as 29%. It is currently recommended that all surgeons, before performing sentinel lymph node surgery as a sole modality of axillary treatment, first establish their personal sentinel lymph node identification rate and false-negative rate by performing sentinel lymph node surgery followed by axillary dissection.

In addition to minimizing the morbidity of axillary treatment, sentinel lymph node surgery may permit a more thorough investigation for nodal pathology. As the sentinel lymph nodes are believed to represent the primary echelon of nodes at risk, it is more feasible for the pathologist to serially section these lymph nodes and more carefully examine them for micrometastases. In addition, the sentinel nodes can be stained with a nonspecific epithelial marker, cytokeratin, which has greater sensitivity than routine histopathologic examination in the detection of metastases. The prognostic significance of lymph node metastases detected with immunostaining alone has yet to be determined.

A current area of controversy is how to treat patients with positive sentinel lymph nodes. The current standard is to perform a standard level I and II axillary dissection. Veronesi and colleagues[130] reported that 60% of patients with positive sentinel lymph nodes had additional disease found at the time of axillary dissection. Chu and colleagues[131] have demonstrated that the rate of additional positive lymph nodes depends on the degree of sentinel lymph node involvement. In their series, none of the 33 patients with metastases detected solely with cytokeratin staining had additional nodal disease, whereas 14% of the 36 patients with sentinel lymph node disease measuring less than 2 mm and 55% of the 88 patients with disease measuring 2 mm or more had additional nodal disease.[131] An ongoing national trial run by the American College of Surgeons is investigating the optimal management of patients with positive sentinel lymph nodes. In this trial, patients with positive sentinel lymph nodes are randomly assigned to axillary dissection or no further axillary treatment.

Radiation therapy. Radiation therapy complements sentinel lymph node surgery. With careful design of the tangential breast fields, most level I and II axillary nodes will be included in the radiation field. In theory, axillary recurrence rates in cases with false-negative results on sentinel lymph node surgery should be very low when proper axillary radiation therapy is delivered. However, tangential irradiation alone may be inadequate for patients with extensive sentinel lymph node disease. For patients who undergo axillary dissection, it is currently standard to add a third radiation field to cover the supraclavicular fossa and axillary apex for all patients with four or more positive lymph nodes. In the series described by Krag and colleagues,[129] the rate of having four or more positive lymph nodes after axillary dissection was 16% for patients with a single involved sentinel lymph node, 30% for patients with two involved sentinel lymph nodes, and 60% for patients with three involved sentinel lymph nodes.

Systemic Therapy

Several randomized clinical trials have clearly shown that systemic therapy can improve outcomes for both women with lymph node–positive breast cancer and women with lymph node–negative breast cancer. The EBCTCG has performed important meta-analyses of all the phase III trials of polychemotherapy and hormonal therapy for breast cancer. The analysis of chemotherapy trials included data on 18,000 women treated in 47 randomized controlled trials that compared chemotherapy vs. no chemotherapy; 6000 women treated in trials that investigated the optimal duration of chemotherapy; and 6000 women treated in trials that compared anthracycline-containing chemotherapy vs. cyclophosphamide, methotrexate, and 5-fluorouracil (CMF).[76] For the trials that compared chemotherapy with no treatment, the meta-analysis indicated that chemotherapy reduced recurrences and improved survival for all women under 70 years of age, with the greatest absolute reduction in recurrence rates seen in women younger than 50 years and women with lymph node–positive disease. The proportional risk reduction produced by chemotherapy was similar for all tumor stages (in general, chemotherapy reduced the risk of recurrence by approximately one third). The greatest risk reduction was seen in women under age 50. The absolute improvement in 10-year survival was 5.7% for lymph node–negative patients younger than 50 years ($P = 0.02$) and 12.4% for lymph node–positive patients younger than 50 years ($P < 0.00001$). A modest gain appeared to occur with the use of anthracycline-containing regimens instead of CMF, with a 3.2% absolute decrease in recurrence at 5 years ($P = 0.006$) and a 2.7% absolute increase in overall survival at 5 years ($P = 0.02$). The benefits of chemotherapy were complementary with rather than competitive with the benefits of tamoxifen.

In an overview of tamoxifen trials, the EBCTCG analyzed data on 37,000 women treated in 55 trials.[77] The benefit of tamoxifen in 8000 women with negative estrogen receptor status was clinically insignificant. For the remaining patients, tamoxifen improved overall survival. Five years of tamoxifen use was found to offer an advantage over 1 to 2 years of tamoxifen therapy. In trials that used 5 years of tamoxifen, the absolute benefit in 10-year survival was 10.9% for lymph node–positive patients ($P < 0.00001$) and 5.6% for lymph node–negative patients ($P < 0.00001$). The benefit was present for both premenopausal and postmenopausal women. Again, the benefits of tamoxifen appeared to complement those of chemotherapy.

The degree of benefit from systemic treatment depends on the risk of metastatic disease. For patients at very low risk of metastatic disease, the incremental benefit from additional treatment reaches a level that is not clinically meaningful. In these patients, the risks and expenses of systemic treatment outweigh the small benefits. Currently, women whose tumors are smaller than 1 cm in diameter who have negative axillary lymph nodes and women with tumors of low metastatic potential (tubular, mucinous, or colloid histologic subtype) smaller than 2 cm who have negative axillary lymph nodes are not advised to receive systemic therapy.[132] The benefit of adjuvant tamoxifen as a chemopreventive agent remains controversial.

Sequencing of Radiation Therapy and Chemotherapy

With the increasing use of systemic therapy in patients with early-stage breast cancer, the integration of this treatment with surgery and radiation therapy has become an important clinical question. Initial retrospective series evaluating treatment sequencing suggested that a delay in the onset of radiation therapy to permit delivery of chemotherapy increased local recurrence rates.[133,134] These data led the JCRT to investigate the sequencing of radiation therapy and chemotherapy in a randomized prospective clinical trial. In this trial, women treated with breast-conserving surgery were randomly assigned to either four cycles of doxorubicin-based combination chemotherapy followed by radiation therapy or radiation therapy followed by four cycles of the same chemotherapy.[135] Patients who received chemotherapy first had a significantly lower rate of distant metastasis than patients who received radiation first (25% vs. 36% at 5 years, $P = 0.05$). A higher percentage of patients treated with chemotherapy first experienced local recurrence within the breast, but the difference did not reach statistical significance (14% vs. 5% at 5 years, $P = 0.07$). The conclusion of this trial was that patients treated with breast-conserving surgery who are to receive radiation and doxorubicin chemotherapy for high-risk breast cancer benefit from early administration of chemotherapy. In a subgroup analysis, the benefit of early chemotherapy administration was seen only in the women with four or more positive axillary lymph nodes, and the increased local failure rate with radiation delay was seen only in the women with close or positive surgical margins.[135]

Although the JCRT study provided important data concerning treatment sequencing, this study predominantly focused on patients with lymph node–positive disease. Recently, investigators from the M.D. Anderson Cancer Center performed a retrospective analysis of sequencing of chemotherapy and radiation in 124 patients with lymph node–negative disease treated with BCT. In this series, 79% of the patients had negative margins. The 5-year actuarial rates of local control were 100% for the chemotherapy-first group (most commonly 6 cycles of doxorubicin-based chemotherapy) and 94% for the radiation-first group ($P = 0.351$). The 5-year recurrence-free survival rates for the chemotherapy-first and radiation-first groups were 92% and 77% ($P = 0.083$), respectively.[136] These data again support an adjuvant-therapy schedule in which chemotherapy is delivered first. The median delays in radiation delivery were 6.7 months in the M.D. Anderson Cancer Center series and 16 weeks in the JCRT series. It is not known whether increased rates of local recurrence will be found with the longer delay required to give four cycles of anthracycline-based treatment followed by four cycles of a taxane (the M.D. Anderson Cancer Center approach).

The concept that earlier administration of chemotherapy can decrease rates of distant metastasis has led to enthusiasm for neoadjuvant chemotherapy for early-stage breast cancer. This strategy moves the treatments against micrometastatic disease into the earliest possible time frame and also allows oncologists to assess the response of gross disease to chemotherapy. A potential disadvantage of this approach is the risk that the primary tumor may continue to seed metastatic deposits during the course of therapy. To investigate these issues, the NSABP conducted the B-18 trial to directly compare the sequencing of chemotherapy and surgery in patients with operable breast cancer.[137] In that study, 1523 patients were randomly assigned to four cycles of doxorubicin and cyclophosphamide given before surgery or the identical chemotherapy given after surgery. After 5 years, no differences in disease-free or distant disease-free survival were evident. The NSABP has adopted neoadjuvant chemotherapy as its standard for future trials because of this equivalence and because neoadjuvant chemotherapy appeared to increase the percentage of women who received BCT.

POSTMASTECTOMY RADIATION THERAPY

The history of postmastectomy radiation therapy can be characterized as one of conflicting data and passionate debate. When few or no systemic-therapy options were available for the treatment of localized breast cancer, radiation therapy was used alone or as an adjunct to surgery to prevent local–regional recurrence.[138-143] Radiation therapy alone was associated with excessive morbidity.[144] Mastectomy followed by radiation therapy alone could result in long-term control of disease, even in patients with locally advanced breast cancer.[145] However, although multiple studies showed that postmastectomy irradiation could decrease the risk of local–regional recurrence, these studies failed to show clear improvements in survival. After the publication in 1987 of a meta-analysis by Cuzick and colleagues[146] that reported increased mortality in women who had received postmastectomy radiation therapy as a component of their treatment, use of postmastectomy irradiation was intensely challenged. Although these and subsequent meta-analyses were strongly influenced by the results of several early trials that were hampered by poor radiation technique, improper patient selection, and the infrequent use of adjuvant systemic therapy, the attitude toward using radiation in all but the most advanced cases of breast cancer ranged from indifference to opposition. In addition, when effective systemic therapy that showed an unequivocal improvement in overall survival became available, many felt that chemotherapy would make the routine use of radiation therapy unnecessary.

Recent reports from large prospective trials have reversed this former judgment against postmastectomy radiation therapy. These recent reports have shown superior local–regional control, disease-free survival, and overall survival with the use of radiation therapy after mastectomy and chemotherapy. The Danish 82b trial evaluated the use of postoperative radiation therapy in 1708 premenopausal women with node-positive breast cancer treated with mastectomy and methotrexate-based chemotherapy.[143,147] At 10 years, the patients who received radiation therapy to the chest wall and regional lymphatics had a decreased rate of local–regional recurrence (9% vs. 32%) and improved cancer-specific survival (48% vs. 34%) and overall survival rates (54% vs. 45%).[148] This study confirmed that patients with larger tumors or extensive nodal involvement benefited from postmastectomy irradiation, and, surprisingly, it also revealed significant improvements for all other subgroups of patients, including patients with one to three involved nodes. A smaller trial from British Columbia also reported that the addition of radiation therapy after mastectomy and chemotherapy resulted in improved local–regional control (87% vs. 67%) and improved cancer-specific survival (50% vs. 33%) in premenopausal women with lymph node–positive disease.[149] A separate report from the Danish Breast Cancer Cooperative Group demonstrated that postmenopausal women with node-positive breast cancer also benefited from radiation therapy after mastectomy and adjuvant tamoxifen.[150]

Patient Selection

Together, these trials of postmastectomy irradiation have demonstrated that adjuvant radiation therapy can improve overall survival in circumstances in which local–regional failure rates can be substantially reduced. It is therefore imperative to identify the patients at significant risk of recurrence, who are most likely to realize the benefit of adjuvant irradiation.

Postmastectomy irradiation is used to treat subclinical tumor in the remaining tissue of the anterior chest wall and the regional lymphatic basins. Because this subclinical disease is by definition undetectable, the probability of its presence and its likely distribution must be inferred from a variety of data sources. These include histologic data from surgical specimens, pattern-of-failure analyses, and prospective trials in which defined groups of patients (e.g., those with lymph node–positive disease) or specific target volumes are allotted to treatment vs. observation.

In the United States the standard procedure for modified radical mastectomy is the procedure described by Madden and colleagues.[151,152] This procedure generally consists of removal of all visible breast tissue along with a complete level I and II axillary dissection. All of the axillary tissue is removed in a single piece, to the level of the pectoralis minor muscle. In contrast to the classic Halsted mastectomy, the skin flaps are not completely undermined, and both pectoral muscles are spared.

Given the presumption that only patients with residual subclinical disease in the remaining tissue will obtain any advantage from radiation therapy, only patients assessed as having an intermediate to high risk of persistent disease after mastectomy should be considered for irradiation. At the M.D. Anderson Cancer Center, postmastectomy radiation therapy is not routinely offered to patients unless their cumulative (lifetime) risk of local–regional recurrence exceeds 20%. The problem is defining which clinical parameters will accurately predict this level of risk.

Most authors would agree that patients with locally advanced primary breast cancer, extensive lymph node involvement,[153] or incomplete surgery[154] fit this description. The lower end of this risk range is less well defined.

Evidence from Clinical Trials

Few studies have been published concerning patterns of failure in patients treated with modified radical mastectomy and modern chemotherapy. The only large series reported to date included patients treated with various CMF-related regimens.[133,155] Because evidence is growing that anthracycline-based chemotherapy is superior for women with lymph node–positive breast cancer,[156] data about outcomes after anthracycline-containing regimens would be more relevant to current practice. However, only a few small series have reported local–regional recurrence rates after mastectomy and anthracycline-containing regimens.[156-161] These studies are discussed in the following paragraphs.

British Columbia trial. The British Columbia trial[149] included 318 patients with lymph node–positive disease who underwent mastectomy and CMF chemotherapy and were randomly assigned to irradiation vs. observation. The median follow-up time was 150 months. The trial showed that irradiation significantly decreased the local–regional recurrence rate and also resulted in a higher rate of distant metastasis–free survival (51% vs. 34%). local–regional recurrence was reported as the first site of failure for all patients.

Several criticisms of the British Columbia trial have been advanced. First, the patients were treated with CMF chemotherapy, which is now believed by many authors to be less effective than doxorubicin- or taxane-containing regimens (especially in *Her-2*–positive patients). Second, the internal mammary chain was treated with cobalt-60 photons with a fairly high dose per fraction, even though the total dose was 35 Gy. Late cardiac toxicity could still develop in this patient group. Third, 44% of patients who had positive nodes had nodes ranging from 2 to 5 cm in size, with an additional 3% of patients

having nodes greater than 5 cm, leading many to speculate that a high proportion of patients may in fact have had N2 (stage III) disease. Fourth, no survival benefit was seen in the group of patients with one to three positive nodes with the addition of radiation therapy unless patients had extranodal extension.[162] Finally, from a statistical standpoint, it should be noted that trials containing approximately 200 to 300 patients have shown trends favoring radiation therapy, but these differences usually have not reached type 1 statistical significance ($P < 0.05$).

Danish Breast Cancer Cooperative Group trials. The Danish Breast Cancer Cooperative Group has done masterful research trials with very large numbers of women with breast cancer treated in a very consistent manner.[143,147,148] The larger randomized trials from Denmark are especially important because each trial showed statistically significant improvement in survival in the combined-modality arms. These trials were directed at premenopausal women treated with CMF (trial 82b) and postmenopausal women treated with tamoxifen (trial 82c). The 82b trial included 1708 women who underwent mastectomy and CMF chemotherapy and were randomly assigned to radiation therapy or observation. The median follow-up time was 114 months. In this group, the median number of nodes examined was seven, with 76% of patients having fewer than 10 lymph nodes removed. Sixty-two percent of the patients had one to three positive lymph nodes, but the size of the largest node and the presence or absence of extranodal extension was not reported. At 10 years, overall survival rates were 54% for the CMF–plus–radiation therapy group and 45% for the CMF-alone group.

Among the major criticisms of this Danish study were the following. First, the chemotherapy regimen was CMF given every 28 days. (Both the British Columbia trial and the Danish Breast Cancer Cooperative Group 82b trial sandwiched the irradiation between courses of CMF.) Second, the limited axillary sampling was the source of significant concern, particularly because the local recurrence rate in the chemotherapy-alone group was much higher than that reported in most other trials and almost half of these recurrences occurred in the axilla, which is quite unusual. At the 1999 meeting of the Gilbert A. Fletcher Society, patients with T1 or T2 tumors and three positive lymph nodes out of 10 nodes sampled were reported to have an 80% to 85% chance of having additional positive nodes if the axillary dissection was completed. In other words, many critics of the Danish trial believe that the group of patients with one to three positive nodes actually would have included patients with four or more positive nodes if patients had undergone a more complete axillary dissection. Although Overgaard did subsequently re-analyze the subset of 409 patients with 10 or more nodes removed and found a similar outcome, the above argument still holds because patients were not stratified at protocol entry by number of lymph nodes.

The M.D. Anderson Cancer Center studies. The relevant M.D. Anderson Cancer Center studies of outcomes after mastectomy and chemotherapy have been performed in a cohort of 1031 patients who were treated with mastectomy and doxorubicin-based chemotherapy but without irradiation in five prospective clinical trials over a 20-year span. The median follow-up time was nearly 10 years.[163,164] In the M.D. Anderson Cancer Center studies, only patients with four or more involved nodes were consistently found to have local–regional recurrence rates in excess of 20% (Table 15-10).[163] Among patients with one to three involved nodes, patients who had tumors measuring 4 cm or larger, gross extranodal extension, or inadequate axillary dissection had higher rates of recurrence than did patients without these factors. Most patients in the authors' practice with stage II breast cancer and one to three involved nodes have had a substantially lower risk of recurrence than the risk seen in the Danish and British Columbia trials, so it is unclear whether these patients with one to three positive nodes would have benefited from radiation therapy.

The pattern of local–regional recurrence is also instructive. The vast majority of local–regional recurrences in published series have a chest wall component. The second most common location for recurrences is the anterior structures of the undissected (level III) axilla, infraclavicular fossa, and supraclavicular fossa. In the M.D. Anderson Cancer Center studies, consistent with numerous other reports (Tables 15-11 and 15-12),[143,155,163,165-170] failure in the dissected portion of the axilla (levels I and II) was rare (3%). Because the risk of failure in the midaxilla at

---

TABLE 15-10

Ten-Year Risk of Local–Regional Recurrence After Mastectomy and Doxorubicin-Containing Chemotherapy at the M.D. Anderson Cancer Center According to Tumor Stage and Number of Involved Lymph Nodes

Tumor Stage	RISK OF LOCAL–REGIONAL RECURRENCE (%)*			
	0 Nodes Involved	1-3 Nodes Involved	4-9 Nodes Involved	≥ 10 Nodes Involved
ISOLATED LOCAL–REGIONAL RECURRENCE*				
T1	6	7	9	17
T2	11	12	23	17
T3	29	9	31	29
CUMULATIVE LOCAL–REGIONAL RECURRENCE*				
T1	11	9	17	17
T2	14	16	27	34
T3	29	23	40	29

Modified from Katz A, Strom EA, Buchholz TA, et al. *J Clin Oncol* 2000;18:2817-2827.
*Isolated local–regional recurrence indicates local–regional recurrence alone as the first site of failure; cumulative local–regional recurrence indicates local–regional recurrence occurring at any time.

TABLE 15-11

Patterns of Local–Regional Recurrence After Mastectomy and Doxorubicin-Containing Chemotherapy at the M.D. Anderson Cancer Center*

Location of Recurrence	ISOLATED LOCAL–REGIONAL RECURRENCE†		CUMULATIVE LOCAL–REGIONAL RECURRENCE	
	Number	Percent	Number	Percent
Chest wall	122	98	122	68
Supraclavicular nodes	41	33	71	40
Axilla	21	17	25	14
Infraclavicular nodes	10	8	12	7
Internal mammary chain	—	—	15	8
Any site	124	100	179	100

Modified from Katz A, Strom EA, Buchholz TA, et al. *J Clin Oncol* 2000;18:2817-2827.
*Some patients experienced more than one site of failure, resulting in cumulative percentages greater than 100%.
†Isolated local–regional recurrence indicates recurrence alone as the first site of failure; cumulative local–regional recurrence indicates local–regional recurrence at any time.

TABLE 15-12

Local–Regional Recurrence Patterns After Mastectomy by Site

Study	Number of Patients	SITE OF RECURRENCE*			
		Chest Wall	Clavicular Nodes	Internal Mammary Glands	Axilla
University Hospital of Cleveland[†169]	209	142 (68)	52+ (25)	NS	15 (7)
M.D. Anderson Cancer Center[168†]	148	89 (60)	19+ (13)	5+ (3)	11+ (7)
Mallinckrodt[165]	129	77 (60)	42 (33)	14 (11)	23 (18)
University of Pennsylvania[167]	128	106 (83)	30 (24)	4 (3)	14 (11)
Institut Jules Bordet[170]	128	99 (77)	32 (25)	NS	13 (10)
Mt. Sinai-Miami[166]	124	95 (77)	14 (11)	10 (8)	26 (21)
ECOG[155]	70	37 (53)	17+ (24)	NS	8+ (11)
DBCG[143]	214	137 (64)	15 (7)	NS	73 (34)

NS, Not stated; *ECOG*, Easter Cooperative Oncology Group; *DBCG*, Danish Breast Cancer Cooperative Group.
*Values are number (percentages), unless otherwise indicated. Because of inclusion of patients with multiple failure sites, totals for some studies may be greater than 100%.
†Details regarding multiple regional sites were not provided.

the M.D. Anderson Cancer Center is not significantly higher for patients with increasing numbers of involved nodes or increasing percentage of involved nodes,[164] it is likely that specific irradiation of the axilla is rarely indicated if the axilla has been adequately dissected.

Current Practice at the M.D. Anderson Cancer Center

Because this institution's findings conflict with the results of both the Danish and British Columbia trials but are consistent with past United States experience, the current practice at the M.D. Anderson Cancer Center for patients with one to three positive lymph nodes is to enroll them in the ongoing Intergroup postmastectomy irradiation trial. Patients with stage II breast cancer who are found to have one to three positive lymph nodes are eligible. Patients must have undergone modified radical mastectomy sparing the pectoralis minor muscle with level I and II axillary dissection. A minimum of 10 nodes must be present in the specimen and examined. Patients with clinically matted nodes, evident residual disease, or gross extranodal extension are excluded. Radiation therapy must begin within 8 months of mastectomy and within 6 weeks of the completion of systemic chemotherapy. Patients are stratified by type and duration of systemic chemotherapy. Patients are then randomly assigned to comprehensive irradiation of the chest wall and regional lymphatics, including the internal mammary chain, or observation. A total of 2500 patients are expected to be enrolled in this trial, which is sponsored by the Southwest Oncology Group and opened in most of the National Cancer Institute–supported cooperative groups (available at: http://www.swog.org).

Treatment of the Internal Mammary Chain

Whether the internal mammary chain should be treated as part of postmastectomy radiation therapy continues to be hotly debated. This controversy arises because the available data are confusing and seem to conflict with one another. In patients with axillary-node–positive breast cancer, histologic sampling of the internal mammary chain reveals occult disease in 20% to 50% of cases (Table 15-13).[8,171-173] In contrast, clinical recurrence in the internal mammary chain is rare. Only one prospective trial has been reported that assessed the value of various forms of treatment of the internal mammary chain.[174,175] Between 1958 and 1978, patients with histologically positive axillary nodes undergoing mastectomy for operable breast cancer were prospectively treated by one of four methods: internal mammary chain dissection, internal mammary chain irradiation, both, or neither. A total of 1159 women were included in the analysis. Eligibility criteria included age younger than 70 years, tumor size less than 7 cm, and histologically positive nodes. Patients with T4 lesions were excluded. From 1958 to 1963 and from 1968 to 1972, all patients with histologic evidence of axillary node metastasis, regardless of tumor site, were treated with internal mammary chain dissection and postoperative radiation therapy. In addition, some patients with medial-quadrant lesions and negative axillae underwent both internal mammary chain dissection and radiation therapy. From 1963 to 1968, internal mammary chain dissection without postoperative irradiation was performed according to randomization in a multicenter trial. From 1972 to 1978, lymph node–positive patients were randomly assigned to peripheral lymphatic irradiation or no further treatment. The 10-year risk of death

TABLE 15-13

Probability of Pathologically Involved Internal Mammary Nodes in Patients with Positive Axillary Nodes

Reference	Number of Patients	PROBABILITY OF INVOLVED INTERNAL MAMMARY NODES		
		Outer Quadrant Tumors (%)	Inner Quadrant Tumors (%)	Any Quadrant Tumors (%)
Urban and Marjani[8]	341	42	53	
Bucalossi et al[171]	553			29%
Handley[172]	535	21	48	
Ki and Shen[173]	635	25	35	

TABLE 15-14

Radiation Sites and Doses in Selected Trials of Postmastectomy Radiation Therapy

Trial	Dose per Fraction	Chest Wall	Subclavicular Nodes	Axillary Nodes	IMC Supplement
DBCG[148]	2.0 Gy	Electrons 50 Gy	Photons ≥ 50 Gy	Selected patients	Electrons 50 Gy
British Columbia[149]	2.34 Gy	Tangents 27.5 Gy	Photons ≥ 35 Gy	Yes 35 Gy	Photons 35 Gy
Stockholm[177]	1.8-2.0 Gy	Electrons or tangents > 45 Gy	Photons 45 Gy	Yes 45 Gy	Electrons or wide tangents 45 Gy
Oslo[178]	2.5 Gy	Not treated	Photons 50 Gy	Not treated	Photons 50 Gy
Dana-Farber[160]	1.8 Gy	Tangents 43 Gy	Photons 45 Gy	Selected patients	Not treated

DBCG, Danish Breast Cancer Cooperative Group; *IMC*, internal mammary chain.

from all causes was decreased ($P = 0.06$) for all patients who received internal mammary chain treatment of any kind vs. those who did not, but statistically significant benefit was seen only in patients with medial-quadrant lesions who had improved survival ($P = 0.001$) and lowered risk of metastasis ($P = 0.005$).[174,175]

Further complicating this apparent paradox, the randomized trials showing survival advantages for postmastectomy irradiation included the internal mammary chain in their intended treatment volume. Although a more complete exploration of this issue has been published elsewhere,[176] the basic philosophy at the M.D. Anderson Cancer Center is to attempt to include the internal mammary chain in the treatment volume, provided that doing so does not compromise other aspects of treatment. This philosophy is consistent with the approaches used in the more recent randomized trials evaluating postmastectomy irradiation (Table 15-14).* Currently, the EORTC is conducting a trial (trial 22922) to assess the role of internal mammary and medial supraclavicular lymph node chain irradiation in stage I to III breast cancer.

*References 8, 148, 149, 160, 171-173, 177, 178.

Target Volume Considerations

At the M.D. Anderson Cancer Center, the choice of treatment techniques and volumes for postmastectomy irradiation is the result of the synthesis of the authors' own experience with important studies from other institutions. A substantial portion of the patient population has locally advanced breast cancer, which clearly has an impact on the authors' perceptions about the disease and, in particular, the techniques used for postmastectomy irradiation in patients with intermediate-stage disease. In the authors' practice, metastases to the internal mammary chain, interpectoral region, and supraclavicular nodes are common. This results in a treatment philosophy that tends to be inclusive of all local–regional volumes at risk, even if encompassing these regions is technically difficult. Multiple adjacent fields are commonly used to optimize treatment and minimize irradiation of uninvolved adjacent structures. Detailed treatment techniques are discussed later in this chapter in the section on "Radiation Techniques and Treatment Planning."

One of the keys to the successful treatment of intermediate-stage and locally advanced breast cancer is obtaining a detailed and accurate definition of the extent of disease before initiation of therapy. Because most patients with intermediate-stage and locally advanced breast cancer will be treated with neoadjuvant (preoperative) chemotherapy, the initial pathologic description of the disease (extent of disease in the breast and the lymph nodes) will not be helpful to the radiation oncologist in the subsequent decision-making process. Therefore the decision whether radiation therapy is appropriate may be based on the initial breast examination. Subtle skin involvement, attachment of the tumor to the underlying chest wall structures, and the presence of satellite lesions and multicentric tumors can affect local recurrence rates

and determine whether BCT is possible if the tumor responds well. Radiologic or clinical evidence of tumor in the internal mammary, axillary apical, or supraclavicular nodal basins is important for correctly staging the disease and for planning local therapy (Fig. 15-9). Areas of putative disease extent that are identified on radiologic studies but will not be surgically addressed (e.g., internal mammary chain or infraclavicular nodes) should be subjected to needle biopsy before initiation of therapy. The systemic staging evaluation for patients with intermediate-stage and locally advanced breast cancer is similar to that for patients with early-stage disease except that a bone scan

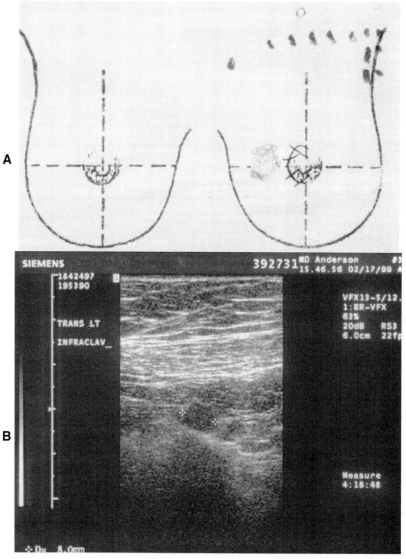

Fig. 15-9 **A,** Diagram and **B,** sonogram of regional lymphatics demonstrating extensive infraclavicular disease. Areas of disease that are unlikely to be resected during a standard mastectomy should be confirmed with needle biopsy before the initiation of systemic therapy. Sonography can be used to establish the presence of residual disease at the time of radiation treatment planning and to visualize the depth of the identified node.

and abdominal CT or sonography is performed even in the absence of clinical symptoms or biochemical abnormalities.

RADIATION THERAPY IN BREAST CONSERVATION THERAPY FOR ADVANCED PRESENTATIONS

One of the most exciting developments in breast cancer treatment in recent years is the use of combined-modality therapy with initial chemotherapy to offer BCT to patients with advanced disease at presentation.[179-183] Patients with T2 tumors larger than 4 cm (stage IIA disease) and patients with T3 tumors without fixed or matted axillary nodes (stage IIB and IIIA disease) are technically operable by classic criteria. Although total mastectomy with axillary lymph node dissection may be an acceptable initial treatment choice for patients with significant comorbid diseases, neoadjuvant doxorubicin-based or taxane-based chemotherapy is the preferred option for initial treatment. This permits observation for tumor responsiveness to the chosen regimen and allows some patients to subsequently undergo BCT. When BCT is being considered, it is important to percutaneously insert radio-opaque markers in the tumor bed (typically under sonographic guidance) to facilitate future surgical resection.[184] For patients treated initially with mastectomy, adjuvant therapy with a doxorubicin-based or paclitaxel-based regimen before local–regional irradiation is recommended for all patients who are medically fit.

Patients being considered for BCT after neoadjuvant systemic therapy are first assessed by a multidisciplinary team that includes the surgeon, the medical oncologist, the diagnostic radiologist, and the radiation oncologist. Although most patients have objective responses to neoadjuvant chemotherapy, only one quarter of patients with advanced disease at the M.D. Anderson Cancer Center have become candidates for BCT on the basis of the following objective criteria[185]: complete resolution of skin edema, residual tumor size of less than 5 cm, and absence of known tumor multicentricity or extensive intramammary lymphatic invasion.

If the response of the tumor to neoadjuvant chemotherapy is sufficient to fulfill these criteria for BCT, the surgeon attempts a wide local excision of the residual abnormality and an axillary dissection. Removal of all mammographically abnormal tissue (although not necessarily the initial extent of disease) and histologically clear margins are required. After surgery, patients undergo the remainder of their chemotherapy followed by radiation therapy to the breast and regional lymphatics.

The radiotherapeutic technique used for BCT in the context of locally advanced breast cancer can be challenging. In contrast to the target volume for early breast cancer, the target volume extends beyond the intact breast to include the regional lymphatics. These may include the axillary, interpectoral, and supraclavicular and internal mammary chain lymph nodes. Classically, treatment of the target volume requires the use of multiple adjacent fields, resulting in greater complexity of set-up and reproducibility. Imprecise matching of adjacent fields can result in an underdose in this region or in areas of dose excess with resulting normal tissue complications. Ideally, noncoplanar beams with precise matching techniques such as those recommended by Chu and colleagues[186] are used when photon fields abut one another. Use of adjacent electron beam fields with shaped, matching field edges may be useful when part of the target area, such as the internal mammary chain, can be adequately covered with electrons. An example of a typical field arrangement is seen in Figure 15-10. Typically, the breast and undissected lymphatics will be treated to a dose of 50 Gy in 25 fractions over 5 weeks, followed by a 10-Gy boost to the tumor bed.[187]

An analysis of the first patients treated at the M.D. Anderson Cancer Center in this manner has revealed encouraging results.[188] Between 1982 and 1994, a total of 93 patients underwent BCT after initial chemotherapy. The stage distribution of these patients at presentation was as follows: IIA, 24%; IIB, 28%; IIIA, 33%; IIIB, 12%; and IV (supraclavicular node involvement only), 3%. The majority of patients (93%) had invasive ductal carcinoma, not otherwise specified. With a median follow-up time of 59 months, the crude local recurrence rate was 7.5%, and the distant metastasis–free rate was 94%. The overall survival rate in the group at 5 years was 89%. The local control and survival rates for this highly selected patient group are very encouraging and warrant further study of BCT after neoadjuvant chemotherapy for large primary tumors and locally advanced breast cancer.

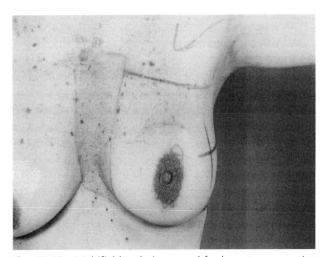

Fig. 15-10 Multifield technique used for breast conservation therapy after tumor downstaging with induction chemotherapy. The internal mammary chain electron field must be tilted to match the tangent fields.

RADIATION THERAPY FOR ADENOCARCINOMA IN AXILLARY NODES WITH UNKNOWN PRIMARY TUMOR

Although adenocarcinoma presenting in axillary lymph nodes without an identifiable primary tumor site is an uncommon clinical entity, the oncologist must be aware of its predictable clinical course. This presentation is usually the result of an occult primary breast tumor, although carcinomas of the thyroid, lung, stomach, and colorectum may also metastasize to axillary nodes. The true incidence of this rare phenomenon is unknown. Reports from major referral centers indicate that it accounts for 0.3% to 1% of breast cancer cases.[189-191]

Initial Evaluation

In most female patients, the source of the tumor seems to be the ipsilateral breast,[192] but it is difficult to determine how extensive the investigation of other possible tumor sites should be. Reviews by Patel and colleagues[193] and Fortunato and colleagues[194] have asserted that exhaustive investigations are unlikely to yield additional information. Consequently, the following tests are probably adequate for the initial evaluation: a full history and physical examination, hemogram, biochemical profile, bilateral mammography, chest radiography, and bone scan. Sonography of the breast and regional lymphatics may help delineate disease extent or detect mammographically occult lesions. Nonetheless, mammography remains the gold standard for assessing the breast in this context. Other investigational tools that may be helpful in the search for an occult primary tumor include magnetic resonance imaging (MRI)[195,196] and color Doppler sonography,[197] but neither tool has yet proven useful on a routine basis. If mammography, breast sonography, and breast MRI fail to disclose an obvious primary lesion, the subsequent therapeutic plan is based on the assumption that a microscopic cancer is present in the ipsilateral breast.

Treatment

Ever since Halsted[198] observed that three of his patients with adenocarcinoma in axillary nodes with an unknown primary tumor subsequently manifested an overt primary breast tumor, the classic treatment for patients with this presentation has included ipsilateral mastectomy. Careful evaluation of the mastectomy specimen often reveals a primary lesion in the breast, with the large range of specimen positivity (8% to 67%)[190,193,199-203] reflecting variation in pathologists' diligence in examining specimens[190,193,200-204] (Table 15-15). Tumors, when found, are usually no larger than a few millimeters.

In most cases, axillary lymph nodes must reach a substantial size before the patient notices any abnormality, and thus the most common disease stage at presentation is T0 N2 (stage IIIA). After careful assessment of the extent and distribution of the regional disease—usually with a combination of physical and sonographic examinations of the axilla, infraclavicular fossa, and supraclavicular fossa—treatment is initiated in a manner consistent with the treatment of any other stage III breast tumor. Neoadjuvant chemotherapy is the norm, and typically six to eight cycles are given preoperatively.

Today, local–regional therapy for most patients with adenocarcinoma in axillary nodes with an unknown primary tumor consists of surgical excision of all gross disease, followed by radiation therapy to the breast and regional lymphatics. (A few studies have investigated simple observation of the ipsilateral breast, but the existing data suggest that this approach is associated with a high probability of local failure in the observed breast,

TABLE 15-15

Results of Mammography and Pathologic Evaluation of the Breast in Patients with Axillary Adenocarcinoma with Unknown Primary Tumor

Institution and Study	Year of Publication	Number of Patients	Normal Mammograms/ Total Mammograms	Tumor Identified in Mastectomy Specimen/Breasts Examined
Roswell Park (Patel[193])	1981	29	9/17	16/29
City of Hope (Kemeny[201])	1986	20	19/20	5/11
Rush Presbyterian-St. Luke's (Bhatia[202])	1987	11	11/11	11/11
M.D. Anderson Cancer Center (Ellerbroek[200])	1990	42	37/40	2/17
Memorial Sloan-Kettering (Knapper[190])	1991	35	23/32	22/32
Milan (Merson[203])	1991	56	55/55	27/33
TOTALS		193	154/175	83/133 (62%)

which often necessitates salvage mastectomy [Table 15-16].[200,203,205-208]) In most cases, surgical removal of the apparently normal breast has no therapeutic advantage because in any case, comprehensive irradiation will be required. Definitive irradiation of the breast at the same time as adjuvant irradiation of the regional nodes is a logical combination. Whillis and colleagues[191] treated 12 patients with radiation therapy to the breast and lymphatics and reported no local recurrences with follow-up times ranging from four to 89 months. Campana and colleagues[209] also used conservative treatment; in their series of 30 patients, eight local–regional recurrences were evident, four in the breast and four in the axilla, with a median time to recurrence of 112 months in the breast and 23 months in the axilla. The survival rate at 10 years was 71%. These results are very similar to the ones obtained in the M.D. Anderson Cancer Center series. All of these studies also show that long follow-up times are necessary to determine the true local control rates because many relapses may not occur until several years after treatment. Evidently, local control rates approximating 85% are possible from using radiation therapy to the breast. Most patients can retain their breasts (Table 15-17),[191,203,209,210] and those few patients in whom BCT fails can usually be successfully treated with salvage mastectomy at the time of recurrence. If regional nodes are irradiated without the breast being treated, it is difficult to irradiate the breast (or the chest wall if a salvage mastectomy is needed) because of uncertainties regarding junctions and overlap into the previously treated fields.

In a recent analysis of 27 patients with adenocarcinoma in axillary nodes with an unknown primary tumor and treated with BCT at the M.D. Anderson Cancer Center, high rates of local and regional control were achieved.[210] The 5-year actuarial local control rate in the breast was 100%, and the regional control rate at 5 years was 92.6%.

The ipsilateral breast is treated with tangential fields of megavoltage photons to a dose of 50 Gy in 25 fractions. The supraclavicular fossa and axillary apex are also treated to 50 Gy in 25 fractions, and because most patients have N2 disease, the midaxilla is often supplemented using a posterior field to a dose of 40 to 50 Gy, depending on the pathologic extent of disease.

TABLE 15-16

Axillary Adenocarcinoma with Unknown Primary Tumor: Results of Breast Observation

Institution and Study	Year of Publication	Axillary Treatment*	Breast Failures/ Breasts Observed	Average Follow-up Period (Years)
Nottingham (Griffith[205])	1987	Dissection	2/4	NS
M.D. Anderson Cancer Center (Ellerbroek[200])	1990	Biopsy and dissection	7/13	NS
Milan (Merson[203])	1992	Biopsy and dissection	9/17	6
Rotterdam (van Ooijen[206])	1993	Dissection and biopsy	2/15	7.7
University of Mississippi (Jackson[207])	1995	Dissection	7/8	3.5
Netherlands (van de Weijer[208])	1995	Dissection	1/5	2.2
TOTALS			28/62 (45%)	

NS, Not stated.

*In each study, some patients were treated with lymphatic irradiation, and others were not.

TABLE 15-17

Axillary Adenocarcinoma with Unknown Primary Tumor: Results of Breast Conservation Therapy

Institution and Study	Year of Publication	Treatment	Breast Failures/Breasts Treated	Disease-Free Survival Rate (%)
Insitut Curie (Campana[209])	1989	Ax Diss + RT RT alone	6/30	76
Western General Edinburgh (Whillis[191])	1990	Ax Diss + RT	3/20	66
Milan (Merson[203])	1996	Ax Bx + RT Ax Diss + RT	2/6	NS
M.D. Anderson Cancer Center (Read[210])	1996	Ax Bx + RT Ax Diss + RT	2/27	69
TOTALS			13/83	16

Ax Diss, Axillary dissection; *RT,* radiation therapy to breast and lymphatics; *Ax Bx,* axillary biopsy; *NS,* not stated.

RADIATION THERAPY FOR INFLAMMATORY BREAST CANCER

Inflammatory breast cancer is a rare but virulent form of breast cancer, accounting for approximately 3% of all breast cancer cases.[211] It is characterized by a clinical triad of ridging (distended lines in the breast), peau d' orange (orange-peel appearance of the breast), and diffuse erythema of the skin. Rapid onset of symptoms (within 3 months) is used to distinguish inflammatory breast cancer from locally advanced breast cancer that has secondarily involved the skin. The latter is a more indolent disease and is typically associated with longer survival.[212,213]

The skin changes associated with inflammatory breast cancer result from extensive involvement of dermal lymphatics, and a skin biopsy is usually positive for dermal lymphatic invasion, although positive findings on skin biopsy are not considered necessary to establish the diagnosis.[63,214-216] Those rare patients who present without the clinical triad of symptoms but with dermal lymphatic invasion seen only on biopsy also appear to have a poor prognosis, although a slightly better prognosis than that of patients with more obvious diffuse breast involvement.[217-221]

Staging

The AJCC TNM staging system designates inflammatory breast cancer as a T4 breast carcinoma, automatically placing localized disease in the stage IIIB category. In the United States, Haagensen and Stout[63] in 1943 described inflammatory breast cancer as involving more than one third of the breast, and this description is still what is characteristically used at the M.D. Anderson Cancer Center. The Institut Gustave-Roussy in France, however, has developed a different staging system called the *Poussee evolutive (PEV)*.[222] This system includes tumor growth characteristics and signs of inflammation. The categories are as follows:

PEV0: A tumor without a recent increase in volume and without inflammatory signs

PEV1: A tumor showing a marked increase in volume for at least 2 months but without inflammatory signs

PEV2: A tumor in which the overlying breast tissue, particularly the skin, is affected by subacute inflammation and edema involving less than half of the breast

PEV3: A tumor with acute or subacute inflammation and edema involving more than half of the breast surface

In the Institut Gustave-Roussy system, inflammatory breast cancer may be classified as PEV2 or PEV3. A rapid growth history is not required, and therefore a number of patients classified as having inflammatory breast cancer according to the Institut Gustave-Roussy system may have secondary inflammation, which would explain differences in results among inflammatory breast cancer studies in the literature.

Physical Examination

On physical examination of patients with inflammatory breast cancer, one sees a swollen tender breast that is warm to the touch and often associated with ipsilateral axillary and even supraclavicular lymphadenopathy. Approximately one quarter of these patients present with distant metastases, and therefore a careful staging work-up is mandatory. The authors recommend that photographs of the involved breast be taken at the time of diagnosis, not only to aid physicians in monitoring clinical response but also to help the radiation oncologist plan field placement because the skin erythema can often extend even beyond the posterior axillary line.

At the M.D. Anderson Cancer Center, half of the patients with inflammatory breast cancer present with a dominant mass, known as *common presentation*; the remaining patients have no visible or palpable discrete mass, known as *classic presentation*.[223] Often, patients without a well-defined tumor mass have been treated with antibiotics for several weeks before the appropriate diagnosis is established.[224] Because conventional imaging such as mammography may not be helpful in establishing the diagnosis, the role of MRI is being investigated.[225,226] Compared with other breast tumors, inflammatory breast tumors tend to be poorly differentiated, are more often estrogen receptor and progesterone receptor negative, and also are more likely to have *Her-2/neu* overexpression, *p53* mutations, and a high thymidine-labeling index.[213,227-230]

Early Treatments

Before the availability of systemic chemotherapy combinations, inflammatory breast cancer was almost uniformly fatal. Local treatment with surgery, radiation therapy, or both modalities produced 5-year survival rates of 5% or less and a median survival time of less than 15 months.[231] Local recurrence rates with surgical treatment alone were approximately 50%.[54,232-235] Therefore from the late 1940s until the mid-1970s, radiation therapy alone was the treatment modality used for most cases of inflammatory breast cancer. Even with this approach, however, local–regional failure rates remained at approximately 50%. In 1972 the M.D. Anderson Cancer Center began investigating accelerated hyperfractionation in an attempt to counteract the rapid growth rate and repair of sublethal damage in the tumor. The twice-daily fractionation scheme was 51 Gy to the breast and regional nodes in 40 fractions over 4 weeks, with a 6-hour interfraction interval. The breast and any residual nodal masses were treated with boost doses of an additional 15 to 20 Gy, also twice daily. local–regional control improved from 54% in patients treated with standard fractionation to 73% in those treated with the twice-daily regimen.[232] Similar results were also reported by Chu and colleagues,[236] who reported a 66% local–regional control rate with twice-daily treatment compared with 31% with conventional fractionation.

Multimodality Therapy

After doxorubicin-based chemotherapy was introduced into clinical practice in 1974, significant improvement in survival was noted, with 5-year overall survival rates improving to 30% to 40%,[237,238] but the local–regional failure rate decreased by only 1%.[216] Because these local–regional recurrence rates were still quite high, in 1977 mastectomy was added in patients who were deemed to have become operable after neoadjuvant chemotherapy. With the addition of mastectomy, the twice-daily fractionation scheme was altered to 45 Gy over a period of 3 weeks, with a 15-Gy boost to the chest wall. A retrospective analysis of outcomes of this approach in 61 patients with clinically diagnosed inflammatory breast cancer treated at the M.D. Anderson Cancer Center with multimodality therapy between September 1977 and September 1985 was published in 1989.[223]

The planned course of treatment for all patients was three courses of doxorubicin-based chemotherapy followed by mastectomy, further chemotherapy, and postoperative irradiation. The minimum follow-up time was 36 months. Ten patients (16%) had a complete response—either complete resolution of the clinical signs of inflammatory breast cancer (four patients) or no evidence of tumor in the mastectomy specimen (six patients). Twenty-seven patients (45%) had a partial response, defined as a greater than 50% reduction in the clinical signs of inflammatory breast cancer. Twenty-four patients (39%) had either no response or disease progression. Fifty-six patients underwent mastectomy before irradiation, and five patients whose disease was not resectable underwent preoperative irradiation. Nine patients underwent postoperative irradiation immediately after mastectomy and before resumption of chemotherapy because of positive margins at surgery; of these, five had local failure. Radiation therapy was delivered to the chest wall and regional lymphatics using either standard fractionation (2 Gy per day) to 50 Gy (14 patients) or accelerated hyperfractionation (1.5 Gy twice daily) to 45 Gy (32 patients), with a boost to the chest wall to a maximum dose of 60 Gy. Forty-six patients completed chemotherapy, surgery, and radiation therapy as originally planned without tumor progression while being treated. Six patients had local or regional failure before irradiation, and nine patients developed distant spread before irradiation.

Outcomes

Outcomes were analyzed according to response to neoadjuvant chemotherapy. The 5-year actuarial disease-free survival rate was 70% for the complete response group vs. 35% for the partial response group. All patients with no response had recurrence by 34 months. The actuarial 5-year disease-free survival rate for the entire group was 27%. The 5-year actuarial local–regional control rate was 89% in the complete response group, 68% in the partial response group, 33% in the no response group, and 58% for all patients. (Note, however, that if these numbers are reported as crude failure rates and analyzed as first site of failure, as in previous publications, the local–regional control rate for all patients was 75%.) Most recurrences were on the chest wall within the irradiated volume. However, three nodal failures were evident, although none occurred in the dissected axilla.

The local–regional control rate and actuarial 5-year disease-free survival for the entire group were not significantly improved when mastectomy was done, although if patients with complete and partial response were analyzed separately from patients with no response, local–regional control was significantly better, as shown in Figure 15-11.[239] The authors concluded that surgery should be done in patients who respond adequately to chemotherapy so that late sequelae of high-dose irradiation can be minimized. Also, the authors were unable to detect any difference in local control between the two irradiation schedules, with three (21%) of 14 patients in the standard fractionation arm and seven (22%) of 32 patients in the twice-daily fractionation arm having local failure. However, fewer complications were found in the accelerated treatment arm (13% vs. 29%), and it was believed that in the twice-daily fractionation arm, a dose escalation study should be performed. On the basis of

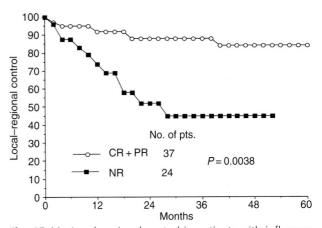

Fig. 15-11 Local–regional control in patients with inflammatory breast cancer by response to chemotherapy. *CR*, Complete response; *PR*, partial response; *NR*, no response. (From Kuske RR. *Semin Radiat Oncol* 1994;4:270-282.)

these results, the twice-daily regimen was changed to 51 Gy in 34 fractions over 3.5 weeks to the chest wall and supraclavicular, infraclavicular, and internal mammary nodes, followed by a 15-Gy boost to the chest wall over 1 week. The dose to the midaxilla continued to be limited to 40 Gy because no failures were evident in that region.

A comparison of the two different dose regimens was recently published.[240] Sixty-one patients treated between September 1977 and September 1985 received a maximum dose of 60 Gy to the chest wall and 45 to 50 Gy to the regional lymph nodes. Twenty-two patients were treated once a day, and 35 were treated twice daily, of whom 32 had radiation therapy after mastectomy and completion of all chemotherapy, two had radiation therapy immediately after mastectomy, and one developed distant metastases during twice-daily irradiation and had radiation treatment stopped. Four additional patients received preoperative radiation therapy with standard fractionation. From January 1986 to December 1993, 39 patients were treated twice daily to 51 Gy after mastectomy and chemotherapy, and eight additional patients had twice-daily preoperative irradiation, also to 51 Gy. Another seven patients were treated using standard daily doses of 2 Gy per fraction to a total dose of 60 Gy, in most cases because the patient's work schedule did not accommodate the twice-daily regimen. The median follow-up time was 5.7 years (range of 1.8 to 17.6 years).

For the entire patient group, the 5- and 10-year local control rates were 73.2% and 67.1%, respectively. The 5- and 10-year disease-free survival rates were 32.0% and 28.8%, respectively, and the 5- and 10-year overall survival rates for the entire group were 40.5% and 31.3%, respectively. A specific comparison was performed of the 32 patients who completed twice-daily radiation therapy to 60 Gy after mastectomy and chemotherapy and the 39 patients who completed a similar course of chemotherapy and surgery but received twice-daily treatment to 66 Gy. The 66-Gy treatment significantly improved the rate of local–regional control at 5 years (84.3% vs. 57.8%) and at 10 years (77.0% vs. 57.8%) ($P = 0.028$). Results are summarized in Table 15-18.[240] Long-term complications of radiation therapy were similar in the two groups, indicating that the dose escalation did not result in increased morbidity. Comparison of overall survival and disease-free survival also showed a trend that favored the patients who received the higher dose of radiation.

Breast Conservation Therapy

Several attempts at BCT have been made for patients with inflammatory breast cancer who have a complete response to chemotherapy. Swain and Lippman[241] reported local recurrence rates of 30% in such patients

TABLE 15-18

Inflammatory Breast Cancer: Effect of Dose Escalation in Twice-Daily Postmastectomy Radiation Therapy

Outcome	5-YEAR FOLLOW-UP		10-YEAR FOLLOW-UP	
	60 Gy	66 Gy	60 Gy	66 Gy
Local–regional control (%)	62.8	91.7	62.8	83.9
Disease-free survival (%)	20.8	49.5	20.8	44.3
Overall survival (%)	40.1	60.7	26.6	47.8

Data from Liao Z, Strom EA, Buzdar AU, et al. *Int J Radiat Oncol Biol Phys* 2000;47:1191-1200.

despite multiple biopsies before irradiation. Brun and colleagues[214] reported local failures in seven of 13 patients who underwent attempted BCT. Chevallier and colleagues[242] similarly noted failure in 20 of 33 patients judged to have had a complete response after chemotherapy and irradiation. Arthur and colleagues[243] recently reported on the use of chemotherapy and an accelerated radiation therapy regimen similar to the one in use at the M.D. Anderson Cancer Center but that treated the involved areas, including the intact breast, to 63 to 66 Gy. At a median follow-up time of 23.9 months, the breast preservation rate and ultimate control rate was 74%. Although these numbers are promising, the short median follow-up time does not allow long-term assessment of either recurrence rates or late complications of higher doses of irradiation. One concern is that most patients judged to have a clinical and mammographic complete response have been found to have residual tumor at mastectomy, with the incidence ranging from 33% to 100%.[215,223,242,244] Moreover, when these patients have a recurrence in the irradiated breast, the recurrent disease tends to be inflammatory, inoperable disease. Because the patients with a clinical complete response are the most potentially curable, their lives should not be put at risk by attempts at breast conservation, at least until better methods of detecting residual tumor become available.

Many institutions deliver concomitant chemotherapy and radiation therapy for the treatment of inflammatory breast cancer. The authors have been reluctant to do this in the past because of radiosensitization of the skin by some drugs, possibly resulting in treatment interruptions or decreased doses of chemotherapy, neither of which is desirable. However, future efforts will aim to develop a regimen that allows less delay of local–regional treatment if possible. For example, Gurney and colleagues[245] have been using hyperfractionated irradiation sandwiched between courses of chemotherapy with encouraging results. The use of angiogenesis inhibitors may also hold promise in this type of breast cancer.

Despite the strides made in improving local–regional control, the majority of patients with inflammatory breast cancer still succumb to systemic disease,[246] and better systemic therapy is still needed. High-dose chemotherapy and stem cell support have been shown to improve response rates but have not as yet been shown to improve survival.[247-251]

RADIATION THERAPY FOR LOCAL–REGIONAL RECURRENCE AFTER MASTECTOMY

Local–regional recurrence of breast cancer after mastectomy represents a heterogeneous mix of entities resulting from a variety of causes, including inadequate initial treatment and virulent tumor biology. Patients with an isolated chest wall nodule after a long disease-free interval have a different prognosis from that of patients with an extensive, inflammatory-type recurrence involving the entire chest wall. Despite the wide variety of presentations of local–regional recurrence after mastectomy, a few basic principles may be commonly applied in the evaluation and treatment of this phenomenon:

- Treat with curative intent using aggressive local and systemic therapy.
- Use initial chemotherapy or surgical excision to achieve resolution of gross disease.
- Use large-field radiation techniques to include the site of the recurrence, the entire chest wall, and undissected regional lymphatics.
- Treat to doses of at least 66 Gy in the boost volume.

The most important principle is the first one—patients with local–regional recurrence should be treated with curative intent, not automatically treated with palliative intent as though they had visceral metastases. Although up to half of patients with local–regional recurrence will also manifest visceral metastases at presentation, a subgroup of patients who are free of documented metastasis can be long-term survivors when treated with curative intent.

Treatment of local or regionally recurrent breast cancer after initial mastectomy has evolved from simple surgical excision and localized irradiation to comprehensive multimodality therapy. Complete surgical excision, comprehensive irradiation, and systemic chemotherapy is now considered the standard of care by many authors.[252-254] Occasionally, the recurrent disease can initially be completely resected with clear margins. In these circumstances, systemic therapy and local–regional irradiation can both be delivered in the adjuvant setting. More commonly, induction chemotherapy is required to render the disease resectable, and radiation therapy is delivered after surgery. Overall 5-year

survival rates in the range of 35% to 50% have been reported,[165-167,253,255,256] although 5-year disease-free survival is generally only 25%.[166,167,256] Local–regional control rates ranging from 42% to 57% have been reported with the use of modern surgical and radiotherapeutic techniques.[165]

The need for radiation therapy after adequate surgical excision is well supported by clinical experience: recurrence rates after surgical excision alone range from 67% to 76%.[165,257,258] Early studies determined the importance of radiation therapy technique in the treatment of local–regionally recurrent disease.[165,166,259] In 1981, Bedwinek and colleagues[165] reported the following local control rates: surgical excision alone, 24%; radiation therapy alone, 38%; and surgical excision plus radiation therapy, 40%. When the radiation therapy results were analyzed, adequate irradiation in combination with surgical excision was found to produce local control rates of 72% compared with 28% when inadequate irradiation was used.[165] That study established the criteria for optimal irradiation of local–regional-recurrent disease after initial mastectomy, including both dose and volume recommendations that have continued to hold true to this day.

It is consistently noted that the chest wall is the most common site of local–regional recurrence after mastectomy (see Table 15-12). To prevent uncontrolled local–regional disease, which severely reduces the quality of life of individuals with recurrence, all sites of potential disease should be treated. At a minimum, the anatomic site or sites of disease and the entire ipsilateral chest wall and undissected lymphatic basins should be included within the target volume. Another reason that local–regional disease control is so important is the suggestion that improved local–regional control may improve overall survival rates.[167,252,259] This is inferred from the survival improvement noted after the use of postmastectomy radiation therapy, as discussed earlier in this chapter. Schwaibold and colleagues[167] reported a 5-year survival rate of 64% in patients with locally controlled disease compared with 35% in patients with locally uncontrolled disease ($P = 0.001$). The influence of local control on overall survival was highly significant in the authors' series.[252]

Although the increased complexity of treatment has improved long-term survival in the case of local–regional recurrence after mastectomy, rates of disease-free survival and local–regional control of recurrent disease have changed little in more than a decade. The local–regional control rates of 68% and 55% at 5 and 10 years, respectively, reported in the authors' series of patients treated with combined-modality therapy[168] are consistent with those of previous studies[167,253,255,256] and represent, for reasons outlined above, the benchmarks for local–regional control at the M.D. Anderson Cancer Center. Factors that predict for a poor outcome have been defined, especially a short interval between initial mastectomy and recurrence and the presence of residual gross disease, but more aggressive local therapy beyond comprehensive irradiation after complete surgical excision of the recurrence has done little to improve outcome. Specifically, in an M.D. Anderson Cancer Center study, hyperfractionated-accelerated radiation therapy[168] did not seem to substantially improve local control rates, as it has for inflammatory breast cancer.[239]

Patients with locally recurrent disease that does not respond to initial chemotherapy have a particularly guarded prognosis. Treatment of macroscopic recurrences with radiation therapy alone is unlikely to be successful. In the authors' series of patients treated with multimodal therapy, the presence of gross disease at initiation of radiation therapy was associated with a 36% local–regional control rate. Inevitably, these individuals also developed distant metastases. Because of the typically massive amount of tumor present, it is not surprising that reasonable doses of radiation failed to control the disease. Although dose escalation may have some value with this population, concurrent chemotherapy and radiation therapy as an alternative is currently being investigated.

Local–regional-recurrent breast cancer after mastectomy is a challenging yet potentially curable condition. Adequate local–regional control is a prerequisite for improved overall survival. The appropriate treatment volume for these patients is similar to that in the postmastectomy setting. The entire chest wall and the undissected lymphatics of the axillary apex and supraclavicular fossa comprise the minimum treatment volume. Commonly, the internal mammary chain and the midaxilla will also be treated. Because of the substantial number of treatment failures seen with the use of doses comparable with those used in the postmastectomy setting, a 10% dose escalation (as compared with the dose in other postmastectomy settings) is used when treating local–regional-recurrent disease. All areas treated prophylactically are treated to 54 Gy in 27 fractions, and all areas to be boosted because of microscopic disease receive an additional 12 Gy in 6 fractions.

RADIATION THERAPY FOR PALLIATION

Radiation therapy is an effective palliative tool for patients with symptomatic breast cancer. The two main indications for palliative radiation therapy are relief of symptoms such as pain and malodorous discharge and control of local tumor growth to prevent complications resulting from increasing pressure or structural compromise. Examples of such complications are paralysis from spinal cord infringement and fractures resulting from extensive cortical destruction of weight-bearing bones.

Optimal palliation is achieved by balancing the potential benefits of palliative treatment with the side effects, costs, and inconvenience that the patient must bear. Various radiation therapy schemes are used depending on the volume to be irradiated, the tolerance of the surrounding tissues, and comorbid conditions. Generally, higher cumulative doses and smaller fraction sizes are used for patients with a relatively good long-term outlook, whereas ultrarapid schedules are preferred in patients with rapidly evolving disease.

Bone metastases respond particularly well to radiation therapy. Relief of pain and reversal of disability can be expected in most patients with bone metastases. Although some pain relief can be expected during the radiation therapy course, most of the benefit occurs after completion of treatment. After treatment, restoration of bone can be expected, but normalization of radiographs is uncommon. It is important to keep patients physically active even though they have metastases. Effective use of nonsteroidal antiinflammatory agents, narcotic analgesics, and physical therapy support are crucial to good long-term function.

Because breast cancer patients with bone-only disease are likely to live for years or even decades, treatment must be designed to minimize late effects, and the possibility of future courses of radiation therapy must be anticipated. The careful selection of field borders and the use of an appropriate fractionation scheme are both factors that contribute to these goals. Typically, 30 Gy is delivered in 10 fractions over 2 weeks, although higher doses may be appropriate for patients with indolent disease and 8 Gy in a single fraction can be used for patients with limited life expectancy.

Patients with extensive soft-tissue disease involving the breast, chest wall, or brachial plexus often require intensive radiation therapy to minimize pain, neuropathy, and wound-care problems. In patients with unresectable disease that is unresponsive to systemic agents, radiation therapy may provide substantial palliation. Because of the large volume of disease, high doses are required to achieve the desired effect. At a minimum, the region is treated to 45 Gy in 15 fractions with vigorous use of bolus doses over cutaneous nodules. Because it is common to see confluent moist desquamation and exfoliation of thin layers of normal skin overlying bulk tumor, a treatment break is usually required after this initial treatment course. After this break, an additional 15 to 30 Gy can be delivered to any residual tumor, provided that no dose-limiting structures are located in the boost volume. Recent pilot studies of radiation therapy delivered concurrently with chemosensitizing agents such as paclitaxel, docetaxel, and capecitabine have produced encouraging response rates. Additional study is required, however, before this approach can be recommended for general use.

The development of brain metastases usually represents the beginning of an accelerated phase of breast cancer. Whenever possible, symptomatic brain lesions should be excised to achieve the most rapid response. Although whole-brain irradiation is probably effective in controlling microscopic and small-volume macroscopic disease, these benefits must be balanced against the potential late morbid effects on normal brain parenchyma. Both total dose and fraction size contribute to the risk of late effects in this setting. Fractions of 2 or 2.5 Gy are preferable to larger fractions. A dose of 30 Gy is commonly delivered to the whole brain, and boost doses may be directed at individual tumor nodules using either reduced-field or radiosurgical techniques.

Spinal cord compression represents a true radiotherapeutic emergency. In patients with symptomatic compression of the cord by tumor, after initiation of high-dose steroids, radiation therapy should be delivered as quickly as possible to prevent irreversible myelopathy. The diagnostic dilemma is to differentiate this clinical scenario from cord impingement by retropulsed bony fragments from a collapsed vertebra. In this latter setting, surgical intervention is preferred because radiation therapy cannot reverse the mechanical abnormality. Typically, 30 to 45 Gy is delivered in 3-Gy fractions using parallel opposed fields.

RADIATION TECHNIQUES AND TREATMENT PLANNING

The objective of radiation therapy in the management of breast cancer is to minimize the risk of local–regional recurrence while simultaneously minimizing the risk of treatment-related normal tissue injury. To accomplish this goal, careful treatment planning is critical. Principles of radiation biology, radiation physics, mathematics, and physical and radiographic anatomy all must be understood for optimal treatment to be delivered. Radiation fields used for the treatment of breast cancer are relatively standard, but each field must be individualized according to patient anatomy, volumes at risk, and the acceptable risk of normal tissue injury. The description of treatment fields provided in this chapter is not an adequate substitute for the experience and careful attention to detail that are required for optimal patient care.

Treatment Fields
Intact Breast

The intact breast is most commonly irradiated using opposed tangential fields. These two matched fields travel obliquely across the thorax on the side of the affected breast and include the entire ipsilateral breast but the smallest possible volume of the lung and heart. Several equally effective techniques are available for designing tangential radiation fields. Patients are usually treated in a supine position with their ipsilateral arm abducted and externally rotated. For patients with very large breasts, a prone radiation technique can be considered. Immobilization devices such as a vacuum-sealed beaded cradle that conforms to the patient's individual anatomy are effective methods for precisely reproducing the patient position for daily treatments.

When tangential fields are designed with a conventional fluoroscopic simulator, the next step is to mark the estimated medial, lateral, cranial, and caudal field borders with radio-opaque wires. The gantry of the simulator is rotated to the point where the medial and lateral field-border estimates are superimposed under fluoroscopic visualization. Once the medial and lateral field borders are aligned, these borders can be adjusted to optimize breast coverage and minimize irradiation of normal tissue volumes. Typically, coverage of both the medial and lateral extent of breast tissue as it wraps around the ipsilateral thorax requires inclusion of 1.5 to 2 cm of underlying lung. During the adjustment of the medial and lateral borders, the radiation oncologist should confirm that adequate margins are included in the fields. This step of treatment planning is easier when radio-opaque clips have been placed around the tumor bed at the time of surgery.

It is critical to design the tangential fields with a nondivergent deep (intrathoracic) field border. This can be accomplished with additional gantry rotation to compensate for the beam divergence or with the use of a half-beam block. The angle of additional gantry rotation can be calculated with simple geometric formulas or visually determined by superimposing the deep field edge and the radio-opaque metal wires at the medial and lateral field borders. The tangential fields are also collimated to match the slope of the chest wall.

For cancer of the left breast, care should be taken to avoid irradiation of the heart, particularly the coronary arteries. Unfortunately, the left anterior descending artery often lies very close to the deep edge of the tangential radiation fields. Figure 15-12 shows the relationship between tangential fields used to treat a left breast after segmental mastectomy and the left anterior descending coronary artery.

The isocenter should be placed in the breast near the center of the treatment field. Many radiation oncologists place the isocenter exactly at the center of the fields—that is, at the point equal to half of the field width and length and at the point of midseparation of the axial central plane. At the M.D. Anderson Cancer Center, we emphasize placing the isocenter at a reproducible point rather than at the center of the field. Placing the isocenter in an area of the breast or chest wall with significant slope should be avoided. During simulation, fluoroscopy is used to visually verify that the isocenter is in the center of the field. With this technique, the process of simulation is considerably faster, and the daily reproducibility of the set-up is improved. As the isocenter may be off-center, differential weighting of treatment fields is used to compensate for the

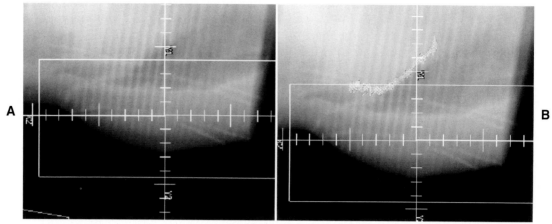

Fig. 15-12   **A,** Digitally reconstructed radiograph of a medial tangent field (outlined by the rectangular box) used for treatment of a tumor of the left breast. To include the entire breast, it was necessary to include 2 cm of underlying left lung. The shadow of the cardiac silhouette appears to indicate that a minimal amount of heart is within the radiation field. **B,** The identical field displaying the position of the left anterior descending coronary artery. The anatomic position of this artery often leads to its inclusion in the radiation fields used for left-sided breast tumors.

possibility that the isocenter is not in the midseparation point.

The use of CT simulations in designing radiation fields for breast cancer is becoming increasingly common. This technology permits physicians to design breast tangential fields virtually on the basis of CT data sets from individual patients. Because the breast volume is difficult to distinguish from the surrounding connective tissue on CT, it is imperative that the results of physical examination also be taken into account in the design of treatment fields. At the M.D. Anderson Cancer Center the practice is to mark the anatomic borders of the breast tissue with a thin radio-opaque wire before scanning. After acquisition of the CT data, a field isocenter is placed, and the patient is marked. The fields are then designed with treatment-planning software using the three-dimensional anatomic display available from the scans and verified with reconstructed radiographs. The CT simulation enhances estimates of the extent of lung and heart volume in the treatment fields.

Most tangential fields include the low axilla and the breast. For patients at risk of having residual disease in axillary lymph nodes, the deep and cranial corner of the tangential field should remain within the thorax to ensure inclusion of axillary tissue at risk. A greater percentage of the axilla can be treated within the tangential fields by increasing the cranial edge of the field and making this field edge nondivergent, a technique often referred to as the *high tangent technique.* To accomplish this technique, the treatment couch is rotated such that the feet of the patient are moved away from the gantry. Mathematical formulas can be used to calculate the required rotation of the couch, but a simpler method is to use a device known as a *rod and chain.* This device consists of a radio-opaque rod, which is placed at the nondivergent cranial edge of the tangent fields, and a chain that hangs freely at a 90-degree angle from the end of the rod just below the abducted ipsilateral arm.[186] Under fluoroscopy, the couch is rotated until the rod and chain are superimposed. As the couch is rotated, the gantry and collimator angles are readjusted to assure alignment of the medial and lateral edge wires and proper coverage of the chest wall. The couch, gantry, and collimator can be rotated simultaneously under fluoroscopic visualization. Areas of the treatment field cranial to the rod and chain are then excluded with a customized mounted cerrobend block. The high tangent technique is also an effective strategy for treatment of tumors located high in the breast or tail of Spence.

Selected patients with stage II disease treated with breast-conserving surgery should also be treated with irradiation of the axillary apex and supraclavicular fossa. In these patients, this region is treated with a third field that is exactly matched to be cranial to the breast tangential fields. This third field is indicated for patients with four or more axillary lymph nodes. The use of a third field for patients with one to three positive nodes who have undergone an adequate axillary lymph node dissection (more than 15 lymph nodes examined) is controversial because the failure rate in the supraclavicular fossa is low.[260] The recommendations are individualized for these patients on the basis of their age, the presence and degree of extracapsular extension of disease (with ≥ 2 mm considered an indication to treat), the size of the lymph node metastasis, and the degree to which the patient is concerned about arm lymphedema.

The technique for matching an axillary apex–supraclavicular fossa field to the tangents is described below.

Chest Wall

Postmastectomy irradiation always includes treatment of the chest wall. Tangential 6-MV photons or, occasionally, photons of higher energy are most commonly used. An adjacent, matching electron beam field is routinely added to treat the most medial portion of the chest wall and encompass the lymph nodes of the ipsilateral internal mammary chain. In addition to covering both targets, this treatment plan gives the added benefit of broad coverage of the chest wall while avoiding irradiation of excessive amounts of the intrathoracic contents. With this technique, the left ventricle can be completely excluded from the treatment volume for cancer of the left breast. Generally, inclusion of a maximum of 2 to 3 cm of lung is acceptable (Fig. 15-13).

Alternatively, electrons can be used to treat the chest wall and internal mammary nodes. Although this technique has the advantage of improved conformation of the treatment volume to the target volume, a greater risk exists for geographic miss of tumor or excess transmission into lung. Variations in tissue thickness make treatment planning difficult, particularly in patients with irregular surface contours.

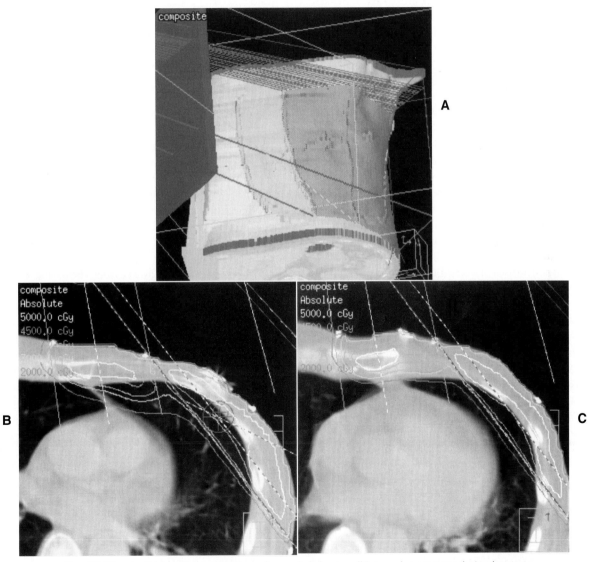

Fig. 15-13 **A,** Skin-surface rendering of a medial chest wall/internal mammary chain electron field (light gray) matched to a pair of opposed tangential lateral chest photon beams for postmastectomy treatment of a tumor of the left breast. **B** and **C,** Axial planes and dose distributions of these fields at a slice in the center of the field (**B**) and at a more caudal slice near the heart (**C**). The dose contours nicely around the chest wall and largely avoids the heart.

Regardless of the technique employed, the entire mastectomy flaps must be included in the treatment volume. This includes the entire length of the mastectomy scar and any clips and drain sites. Typically, the fields extend from midsternum to at least the midaxillary line. Depending on the extent of original disease and patient anatomy, the fields may need to extend even to the posterior axillary line. A common error in treatment planning is to skimp on the inferior border. This should be placed approximately 2 cm caudad to the previous location of the inframammary sulcus.

The superior border of the chest wall fields abuts the supraclavicular field. To avoid junctional hot spots, one of several techniques must be employed to eliminate a divergent edge. The authors routinely use the rod-and-chain technique.[186] This technique has several advantages: the border can be placed in any desired orientation, the full length of the tangential beam is used, and the match line can be confirmed visually during treatment. The other alternative, use of a monoisocentric technique, has the disadvantage of permitting use of only half the available beam length (usually 20 cm) for chest wall treatment. In patients with long torsos, this results in an excessively large supraclavicular field, and, as a consequence, a larger volume of lung is treated.

CT-based treatment planning is important because it permits precise visualization of the intrathoracic contents encompassed by the proposed treatment fields. Treatment of any cardiac volume should be actively avoided because such treatment is associated with late morbidity and mortality. Although most reports evaluating the cardiac morbidity of breast irradiation have studied the portion of myocardium treated, it is likely that the sensitive target structures are the epicardial vessels. The implication is that no safe volume of heart can be included in the high-dose volume.

Tissue heterogeneity correction is routinely used in the planning process to minimize the hot spots caused by increased lung transmission. The dose of 50 Gy in 25 fractions is specified at an isodose that encompasses the entire target and thus represents the target minimum dose. Moderate bolus schedules permit the completion of treatment without interruption. Typically, 3-mm or 5-mm bolus is used every other day for the first two to three weeks. Additional bolus can be used during the boost if the patient's skin reaction permits. Moderate erythema and dry desquamation are the desired end results.

All patients receive a boost to the chest wall flaps. These fields are only slightly smaller than the initial chest wall fields; treatment is delivered using electrons (two fields are often required). The skin and subcutaneous tissues are the primary targets and are included within the distal 90% line. For patients with negative margins, 10 Gy in five fractions is given. For patients with close or positive margins, 14 to 16 Gy is the usual boost dose. Electron doses are all specified at the 100% isodose line, consistent with the recommendations of the International Commission on Radiation Units and Measurements.[261]

Supraclavicular Fossa

The second obligate treatment target for postmastectomy radiation therapy and a component of treatment for selected patients after breast-conserving surgery is the lymphatics of the supraclavicular fossa and undissected axillary apex. After a classic level I and II axillary dissection, the undissected portion of the axillary apex lies directly beneath the pectoralis major muscle. Therefore the supraclavicular field extends from the jugular groove medially to the lateral edge of the pectoralis major muscle. Careful placement of the inferior border, which is also the superior border of the chest wall fields, to be as cephalad as possible can substantially reduce the volume of lung included in the aggregate treatment fields. Although photons are most commonly used to treat the supraclavicular and axillary apical nodes, the use of electrons may be considered in thin patients because all the structures are anterior. The dose for microscopic disease is 50 Gy in 25 fractions.

To ensure a geometric match of this third field with the tangents, the tangential fields must have a nondivergent superior edge. Also, collimator rotation of the tangential fields leads to an angled cranial edge relative to the matched third field, and this angle must be corrected. The use of a rod and chain (see the subsection on "Intact Breast" under "Radiation Techniques and Treatment Planning") and a mounted block of the tissue above the rod and chain corrects both the divergence and angulation problems. A half-beam block is used for the caudal edge of the supraclavicular fossa–axillary apex field to eliminate divergence into the tangential fields. The supraclavicular fossa–axillary apex field is anterior in its orientation; a 15-degree gantry rotation is used to exclude the spinal cord while including the supraclavicular fossa. The upper border of the supraclavicular field should be above the acromioclavicular joint. The medial border should be set on the pedicles of the vertebral bodies. The lateral border can be set at the coracoid process of the scapula to exclude the dissected axilla or lateral to the humeral head to include a portion of the dissected axilla. The targeted lymph node chain lateral to the coracoid becomes progressively deeper from the anterior surface, ending at a point deeper than the supraclavicular lymph nodes. Rarely, a posterior field that covers only the axilla above the rod and chain is added to supplement the dosage to this deeper anatomic region. Because axillary recurrences are rare after level I and II axillary dissection and because increases in dose to the axilla elevate the risk of arm edema, the use of these fields (often called posterior axillary boost fields) is now less common. A posterior axillary boost field is currently used only when concern exists as to the adequacy of the axillary dissection or when foci of disease are present in the axillary soft tissues.

Axilla

Specific radiation treatment of the dissected axilla is rarely required. When irradiation of the axilla is desired, most of the axillary dose is delivered through the anterior supraclavicular field, using photons. It is important to verify that all operative clips left by the surgeon in the axilla are included in either the chest wall fields or the lateral portion of the supraclavicular field. In the typical patient, delivering 50 Gy to the supraclavicular fossa–axillary apical field results in 35 to 37 Gy at the midline axillary structures. A posterior photon field is then used to supplement the midaxilla to the desired target dose. Because of the morbidity of axillary irradiation and the infrequency of axillary failure, the usual dose is 40 Gy. Higher doses are employed only in patients with extensive axillary soft tissue disease or an undissected axilla.

Internal Mammary Lymph Nodes

When the decision has been made to treat the internal mammary nodes, either of two techniques can be used. The preferred technique is to use a separate electron beam field on the most medial chest wall. Because the nodes typically lie 3 to 3.5 cm from the midline, this field must extend even further laterally to compensate for beam constriction. The usual field extends 5 to 6 cm away from the midline and is shaped to precisely match the edge of the tangent fields. A small lateral tilt often results in better field matching at depth. CT-based treatment planning with heterogeneity correction is mandatory to ensure selection of an electron beam that covers the nodes without excess exit into the lung. Ideally, the nodes will be located within the distal 90% line, and the dose of 50 Gy in 25 fractions is specified at the 100% isodose line.

Some patients have anatomic conformations that are not well suited to the use of a separate electron beam field to treat the internal mammary nodes. This is especially true in obese patients, patients with an intact breast, and patients who have undergone breast reconstruction after mastectomy. The use of a half-wide tangent field can be considered in these cases. The tangent fields are made extra deep at the superior border to encompass the first three intercostal spaces. Additional field blocking is placed on the lower portion of the tangents, similar to the field blocking used in a standard conformation. This technique has a number of disadvantages. The volume of lung treated is substantially larger than the volume treated with other techniques. In addition, the upper field edges often extend well beyond the midline, resulting in treatment of a part of the contralateral breast. For these reasons, immediate reconstruction is strongly discouraged if postoperative irradiation is to be delivered.

Dose Prescriptions

Even though breast cancer is one of the most common types of cancer treated with radiation in both the private and academic sectors, no consistent dose prescriptions are evident across centers in the United States. At the M.D. Anderson Cancer Center the standard dosage for the initial fields is 50 Gy in 25 fractions over 5 weeks. This dose is typically prescribed two thirds of the way through the intact breast. For patients treated after breast-conserving surgery, the tumor bed is then boosted an additional 10 Gy (in patients with negative margins), 14 Gy (in patients with margins with ≤ 2 mm), or 16 Gy (in patients with focally positive margins) using electrons. CT planning is performed to assure that the targeted boost volume is encompassed by the 90% isodose curve. The design of the boost fields is often aided by fluoroscopic visualization of tumor bed clips or with virtual CT treatment planning. For patients treated with chest wall tangents after mastectomy, a similar prescription point is chosen just anterior to the pectoralis major muscle. After the initial 50 Gy is delivered, most of the chest wall is then given a boost with electron fields to a total dose of 60 Gy. All electron fields are prescribed to the D-max point and an electron beam energy is chosen with CT planning to assure that 90% of the dose is delivered to the deep portion of the pectoralis major muscle.

Dosimetry

Careful dosimetry is a critical component of effective radiation therapy for breast cancer. A three-dimensional treatment planning system calculates the dose in off-axis planes and incorporates the contribution of scatter into the dose calculation algorithm. The goal of treatment planning is to achieve the most homogeneous distribution of dose throughout the target volume. To achieve this, two-dimensional treatment field wedges, differential field weighting, and various beam energies are used to customize the treatment according to the patient's anatomy. Initially, the radiation dose distribution on an axial plane in the center of the treatment volume is examined. The amount of lung tissue within the treated volume significantly affects the radiation dose at the medial and lateral corners of the axial planes. To account for this, heterogeneity correction factors are used in the dose calculation algorithm.

The initial goal of treatment planning is to use wedging and weighting to achieve a central-plane dose distribution that has three equivalent-size regions of increased dose (hot spots) that are located in the medial corner, the lateral corner, and the breast apex, respectively. An example of a dose distribution and a comparison distribution without tissue heterogeneity corrections is shown in Figure 15-14. Once the correct distribution pattern is achieved, changes in wedging or weighting cannot significantly decrease the dose inhomogeneity. The dose within the hot spots is compared with the dose at the central base of the breast to determine if the plan is acceptable. Ideally, the dose at the hot spots should be no more than 105% of the dose at the prescription point located in the central deep breast. The most common reason for higher doses at hot spots is

that the patient has a large separation size (the length of tissue the beam traverses in traveling through the field) and a beam energy of 6 MV is insufficient. In these situations, compromises must be made. One compromise would be to normalize the dose to a point closer to the breast apex, thereby reducing the hot spots relative to the dose at the normalization point to a value of 105% or less. This comes at the expense of a lower dose in the deep central portion of the breast. Alternatively, a higher-energy beam could be used, which would decrease the dose at the hot spots relative to the deep central dose. However, increased beam energy comes at

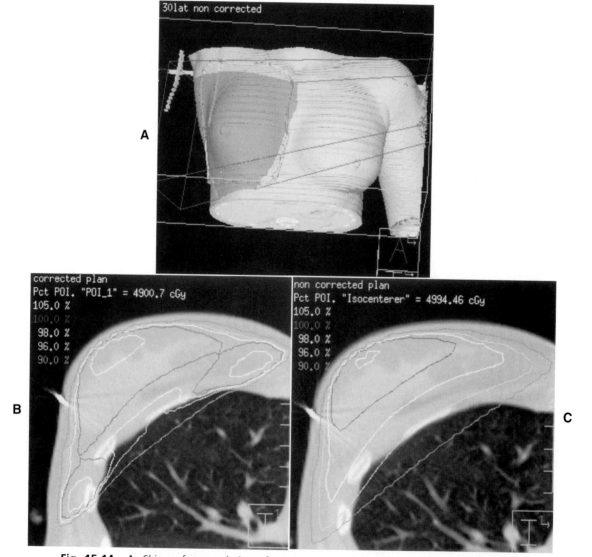

Fig. 15-14 **A,** Skin-surface rendering of opposed tangential photon fields used to treat a tumor of the right breast. **B,** Central plane dosimetry plan for this case using tissue heterogeneity corrections. The hot-spot regions shown in the white contoured volumes are equally distributed in the deep medial and lateral corners and the breast apex. **C,** Identical plan calculated without tissue heterogeneity corrections.

the expense of a lower dose to the superficial regions of the breast. It is important to individualize these choices on the basis of the location of the tumor bed and the specifics of the individual case.

Interest is increasing in optimizing the dose distribution in off-axis and central planes through static intensity-modulated radiation beams. With this technique, beams are modulated by dynamic multileaf collimators that can selectively attenuate dosages to small areas of the field with respect to each other. The precision of this beam attenuation requires that the position of the breast be reproduced exactly on a daily basis and that small movements during normal respiration be accounted for. These concerns, in part, have limited the widespread use of this technology to date. However, continued advances in treatment planning, online portal imaging, and gated radiation delivery will most likely continue to improve the delivery of radiation therapy for breast cancer patients.

REFERENCES

1. Haagensen C. *Disease of the Breast.* 2nd ed. Philadelphia, Pa: WB Saunders; 1971:576-584.
2. Donegan WL. Diagnosis of mammary cancer. *Major Probl Clin Surg* 1967;5:34-69.
3. Osborne MP, Kinne DW. Breast development and anatomy. In: Harris JR, Hellman S, Henderson KC, eds. *Breast Disease.* Philadelphia, Pa: JB Lippincott; 1987:1-14.
4. Veronesi U. Rationale and indications for limited surgery in breast cancer: current data. *World J Surg* 1987;11:493-498.
5. Rosen PP, Lesser ML, Kinne DW, et al. Discontinuous or "skip" metastases in breast carcinoma. Analysis of 1228 axillary dissections. *Ann Surg* 1983;197:276-283.
6. Larson D, Weinstein M, Goldberg I, et al. Edema of the arm as a function of the extent of axillary surgery in patients with stage I-II carcinoma of the breast treated with primary radiotherapy. *Int J Radiat Oncol Biol Phys* 1986;12:1575-1582.
7. Clarke D, Martinez A, Cox RS. Analysis of cosmetic results and complications in patients with stage I and II breast cancer treated by biopsy and irradiation. *Int J Radiat Oncol Biol Phys* 1983;9:1807-1813.
8. Urban JA, Marjani MA. Significance of internal mammary lymph node metastases in breast cancer. *Am J Roentgenol Radium Ther Nucl Med* 1971;111:130-136.
9. Taylor GW, Meltzer A. Inflammatory carcinoma of the breast. *Am J Cancer* 1995;33:33-49.
10. Wazer DE, DiPetrillo T, Schmidt-Ullrich R, et al. Factors influencing cosmetic outcome and complication risk after conservative surgery and radiotherapy for early-stage breast carcinoma. *J Clin Oncol* 1992;10:356-363.
11. Rose MA, Olivotto I, Cady B, et al. Conservative surgery and radiation therapy for early breast cancer. Long-term cosmetic results. *Arch Surg* 1989;124:153-157.
12. Romestaing P, Lehingue Y, Carrie C, et al. Role of a 10-Gy boost in the conservative treatment of early breast cancer. *J Clin Oncol* 1997;15:963-968.
13. Van Limbergen E, Rijnders A, van der Schueren E, et al. Cosmetic evaluation of breast conserving treatment for mammary cancer. 2. A quantitative analysis of the influence of radiation dose, fractionation schedules and surgical treatment techniques on cosmetic results. *Radiother Oncol* 1989;15:545-550.
14. Schnitt S, Connolly J, Harris J, et al. Radiation-induced changes in the breast. *Hum Pathol* 1984;15:545-550.
15. Tralins AH. Lactation after conservative breast surgery combined with radiation therapy. *Am J Clin Oncol* 1995;18:40-43.
16. Tokunaga M, Land CE, Tokuoka S, et al. Incidence of female breast cancer among atomic bomb survivors, 1950-1985. *Radiat Res* 1994;138:209-233.
17. Hildreth N, Shore R, Dvoretsky P. The risk of breast cancer after irradiation of the thymus in infancy. *N Engl J Med* 1989;321:1281-1284.
18. Hrubec Z, Boice J, Monson R, et al. Breast cancer after multiple chest flouroscopies: second follow-up of Massachusetts women with tuberculosis. *Cancer Res* 1989;49:229-234.
19. Bhatia S, Robison LJ, Oberlin O, et al. Breast cancer and other second neoplasms after childhood Hodgkin's disease. *N Engl J Med* 1996;334:745-751.
20. Boice JD Jr, Harvey EB, Blettner M, et al. Cancer in the contralateral breast after radiotherapy for breast cancer. *N Engl J Med* 1992;326:781-785.
21. Fisher B, Anderson S, Redmond CK, et al. Reanalysis and results after 12 years of follow-up in a randomized clinical trial comparing total mastectomy with lumpectomy with or without irradiation in the treatment of breast cancer. *N Engl J Med* 1995;333:1456-1461.
22. Veronesi U, Luini A, Del Vecchio M, et al. Radiotherapy after breast-preserving surgery in women with localized cancer of the breast. *N Engl J Med* 1993;328:1587-1591.
23. Magrini SM, Papi MG, Bagnoli R, et al. Late sequelae involving the breast after radiotherapy for lung metastasis of Wilms' tumor. Experience of the Florence Radiotherapy and analysis of the literature. *Radiol Med* (Torino) 1995;89:865-869.
24. Greenlee RT, Hill-Harmon MB, Murray T, et al. Cancer statistics, 2001. *CA Cancer J Clin* 2001;51:15-36.
25. American Cancer Society. *Breast Cancer Facts and Figures 1999-2000.* Atlanta, Ga: American Cancer Society; 2000.
26. Lambe M, Hsieh C, Tsaih S, et al. Maternal risk of breast cancer following multiple births: a nationwide study in Sweden [published erratum appears in *Cancer Causes Control* 1997;8:260]. *Cancer Causes Control* 1996;7:533-538.
27. Breast cancer and hormone replacement therapy: collaborative reanalysis of data from 51 epidemiological studies of 52,705 women with breast cancer and 108,411 women without breast cancer. Collaborative Group on Hormonal Factors in Breast Cancer. *Lancet* 1997;350:1047-1059.
28. Schairer C, Lubin J, Troisi R, et al. Menopausal estrogen and estrogen-progestin replacement therapy and breast cancer risk. *JAMA* 2000;283:485-491.
29. Schairer C, Lubin J, Troisi R, et al. Estrogen-progestin replacement and risk of breast cancer. *JAMA* 2000;284:691-694.
30. Hankinson SE, Colditz GA, Manson JE, et al. A prospective study of oral contraceptive use and risk of breast cancer (Nurses' Health Study, United States). *Cancer Causes Control* 1997;8:65-72.
31. Guzman RC, Yang J, Rajkumar L, et al. Hormonal prevention of breast cancer: mimicking the protective effect of pregnancy. *Proc Natl Acad Sci U S A* 1999;96:2520-2525.
32. Burke W, Daly M, Garber J, et al. Recommendations for follow-up care of individuals with an inherited predisposition to cancer. II. *BRCA1* and *BRCA2.* Cancer Genetics Studies Consortium. *JAMA* 1997;277:997-1003.
33. Holmes MD, Hunter DJ, Colditz GA, et al. Association of dietary intake of fat and fatty acids with risk of breast cancer. *JAMA* 1999;281:914-920.
34. Smith-Warner SA, Spiegelman D, Yaun SS, et al. Alcohol and breast cancer in women: a pooled analysis of cohort studies. *JAMA* 1998;279:535-540.
35. Carpenter CL, Ross RK, Paganini-Hill A, et al. Lifetime exercise activity and breast cancer risk among post-menopausal women. *Br J Cancer* 1999;80:1852-1858.

36. Shoff SM, Newcomb PA, Trentham-Dietz A, et al. Early-life physical activity and postmenopausal breast cancer: effect of body size and weight change. *Cancer Epidemiol Biomarkers Prev* 2000;9: 591-595.

37. Kumar NB, Cantor A, Allen K, et al. Android obesity at diagnosis and breast carcinoma survival: evaluation of the effects of anthropometric variables at diagnosis, including body composition and body fat distribution and weight gain during life span, and survival from breast carcinoma. *Cancer* 2000;88:2751-2757.

38. Newcomb PA, Egan KM, Titus-Ernstoff L, et al. Lactation in relation to postmenopausal breast cancer. *Am J Epidemiol* 1999;150:174-182.

39. Benichou J, Gail MH, Mulvihill JJ. Graphs to estimate an individualized risk of breast cancer. *J Clin Oncol* 1996;14:103-110.

40. Gail MH, Brinton LA, Byar DP, et al. Projecting individualized probabilities of developing breast cancer for white females who are being examined annually. *J Natl Cancer Inst* 1989;81: 1879-1886.

41. Malkin D, Li FP, Strong LC, et al. Germ line *p53* mutations in a familial syndrome of breast cancer, sarcomas, and other neoplasms. *Science* 1990;250:1233-1238.

42. Velculescu VE, El-Deiry WS. Biological and clinical importance of the *p53* tumor suppressor gene. *Clin Chem* 1996;42:858-868.

43. Miyashita T, Krajewski S, Krajewska M, et al. Tumor suppressor *p53* is a regulator of *bcl-2* and *bax* gene expression in vitro and in vivo. *Oncogene* 1994;9:1799-1805.

44. Hollstein M, Soussi T, Thomas G, et al. *p53* gene alterations in human tumors: perspectives for cancer control. *Recent Results Cancer Res* 1997;143:369-389.

45. Hall JM, Lee MK, Newman B, et al. Linkage of early-onset familial breast cancer to chromosome 17q21. *Science* 1990;250: 1684-1689.

46. Wooster R, Bignell G, Lancaster J, et al. Identification of the breast cancer susceptibility gene *BRCA2* [published erratum appears in *Nature* 1996;379:749]. *Nature* 1995;378:789-792.

47. Scully R, Chen J, Plug A, et al. Association of *BRCA1* with *Rad51* in mitotic and meiotic cells. *Cell* 1997;88:265-275.

48. Sharan SK, Morimatsu M, Albrecht U, et al. Embryonic lethality and radiation hypersensitivity mediated by *Rad51* in mice lacking *BRCA2*. *Nature* 1997;386:804-810.

49. Gowen LC, Avrutskaya AV, Latour AM, et al. *BRCA1* required for transcription-coupled repair of oxidative DNA damage. *Science* 1998;281:1009-1012.

50. Zhong Q, Chen CF, Li S, et al. Association of *BRCA1* with the *hRad50-hMre11-p95* complex and the DNA damage response. *Science* 1999;285:747-750.

51. Ford D, Easton DF, Bishop DT, et al. Risks of cancer in *BRCA1*-mutation carriers. Breast Cancer Linkage Consortium. *Lancet* 1994;343:692-695.

52. Struewing JP, Hartge P, Wacholder S, et al. The risk of cancer associated with specific mutations of *BRCA1* and *BRCA2* among Ashkenazi Jews. *N Engl J Med* 1997;336:1401-1408.

53. Friedman LS, Gayther SA, Kurosaki T, et al. Mutation analysis of *BRCA1* and *BRCA2* in a male breast cancer population. *Am J Hum Genet* 1997;60:313-319.

54. Mavraki E, Gray IC, Bishop DT, et al. Germline *BRCA2* mutations in men with breast cancer. *Br J Cancer* 1997;76:1428-1431.

55. Shattuck-Eidens D, Oliphant A, McClure M, et al. *BRCA1* sequence analysis in women at high risk for susceptibility mutations. Risk factor analysis and implications for genetic testing. *JAMA* 1997;278:1242-1250.

56. Burke W, Culver JO, Bowen D, et al. Genetic counseling for women with an intermediate family history of breast cancer. *Am J Med Genet* 2000;90:361-368.

57. Statement of the American Society of Clinical Oncology: genetic testing for cancer susceptibility, Adopted on February 20, 1996. *J Clin Oncol* 1996;14:1730-1736.

58. Fisher B, Costantino J, Redmond C, et al. A randomized clinical trial evaluating tamoxifen in the treatment of patients with node-negative breast cancer who have estrogen-receptor-positive tumors. *N Engl J Med* 1989;320:479-484.

59. Adjuvant tamoxifen in the management of operable breast cancer: the Scottish Trial. Report from the Breast Cancer Trials Committee, Scottish Cancer Trials Office (MRC), Edinburgh. *Lancet* 1987;2:171-175.

60. Fornander T, Rutqvist LE, Cedermark B, et al. Adjuvant tamoxifen in early breast cancer: occurrence of new primary cancers. *Lancet* 1989;1:117-120.

61. Fisher B, Costantino JP, Wickerham DL, et al. Tamoxifen for prevention of breast cancer: report of the National Surgical Adjuvant Breast and Bowel Project P-1 Study. *J Natl Cancer Inst* 1998;90:1371-1388.

62. Hartmann LC, Schaid DJ, Woods JE, et al. Efficacy of bilateral prophylactic mastectomy in women with a family history of breast cancer. *N Engl J Med* 1999;340:77-84.

63. Haagensen CD, Stout AP. Carcinoma of the breast: criteria of operability. *Ann Surg* 1943;118:859-870, 1032-1051.

64. Fleming I, Cooper JS, Henson DE, et al, eds. *AJCC Cancer Staging Manual*, 5th ed. Philadelphia, Pa: Lippincott Williams and Wilkins; 1997:171-180.

65. Danforth DN Jr, Findlay PA, McDonald HD, et al. Complete axillary lymph node dissection for stage I-II carcinoma of the breast. *J Clin Oncol* 1986;4:655-662.

66. Consensus conference on the classification of ductal carcinoma in situ [editorial]. *Hum Pathol* 1997;28:1221-1225.

67. Fisher ER, Leeming R, Anderson S, et al. Conservative management of intraductal carcinoma (DCIS) of the breast. Collaborating NSABP investigators. *J Surg Oncol* 1991;47:139-147.

68. Fisher B, Dignam J, Wolmark N, et al. Lumpectomy and radiation therapy for the treatment of intraductal breast cancer: findings from National Surgical Adjuvant Breast and Bowel Project B-17. *J Clin Oncol* 1998;16:441-452.

69. Fisher ER, Dignam J, Tan-Chiu E, et al. Pathologic findings from the National Surgical Adjuvant Breast Project (NSABP) eight-year update of Protocol B-17: intraductal carcinoma. *Cancer* 1999;86:429-438.

70. Julien JP, Bijker N, Fentiman IS, et al. Radiotherapy in breast-conserving treatment for ductal carcinoma in situ: first results of the EORTC randomised phase III trial 10853. EORTC Breast Cancer Cooperative Group and EORTC Radiotherapy Group. *Lancet* 2000;355:528-533.

71. Bland KI, Menck HR, Scott-Conner CE, et al. The National Cancer Data Base 10-year survey of breast carcinoma treatment at hospitals in the United States. *Cancer* 1998;83:1262-1273.

72. Silverstein MJ, Lagios MD, Craig PH, et al. A prognostic index for ductal carcinoma in situ of the breast. *Cancer* 1996;77: 2267-2274.

73. Silverstein MJ, Lagios MD, Groshen S, et al. The influence of margin width on local control of ductal carcinoma in situ of the breast. *N Engl J Med* 1999;340:1455-1461.

74. Fisher B, Dignam J, Wolmark N, et al. Tamoxifen in treatment of intraductal breast cancer: National Surgical Adjuvant Breast and Bowel Project B-24 randomised controlled trial. *Lancet* 1999;353:1993-2000.

75. Keibert GM, de Haes JCJM, van den Velde CJH, et al. The impact of breast-conserving treatment and mastectomy on the quality of life of early-stage breast cancer patients: a review. *J Clin Oncol* 1991;9:1059-1070.

76. Polychemotherapy for early breast cancer: an overview of the randomised trials. Early Breast Cancer Trialists' Collaborative Group. *Lancet* 1998;352:930-942.

77. Tamoxifen for early breast cancer: an overview of the randomised trials. Early Breast Cancer Trialists' Collaborative Group. *Lancet* 1998;351:1451-1467.

78. Fisher B, Redmond C, Poisson R, et al. Eight-year results of a randomized clinical trial comparing total mastectomy and lumpectomy with or without irradiation in the treatment of breast cancer [published erratum appears in *N Engl J Med* 1994; 330:1467]. *N Engl J Med* 1989;320:822-828.

79. Favourable and unfavourable effects on long-term survival of radiotherapy for early breast cancer: an overview of the randomised trials. Early Breast Cancer Trialists' Collaborative Group. *Lancet* 2000;355:1757-1770.

80. Morris AD, Morris RD, Wilson JF, et al. Breast-conserving therapy vs mastectomy in early-stage breast cancer: a meta-analysis of 10-year survival. *Cancer J Sci Am* 1997;3:6-12.

81. Liljegren G, Lindgren A, Bergh J, et al. Risk factors for local recurrence after conservative treatment in stage I breast cancer. Definition of a subgroup not requiring radiotherapy. *Ann Oncol* 1997;8:235-241.

82. Forrest AP, Stewart HJ, Everington D, et al. Randomised controlled trial of conservation therapy for breast cancer: 6-year analysis of the Scottish trial. Scottish Cancer Trials Breast Group. *Lancet* 1996;348:708-713.

83. Wollmark N, Dignam J, Margolese R, et al. The role of radiotherapy in the management of node negative invasive breast cancer < 1.0 cm treated with lumpectomy: preliminary results of NSABP Protocol B-21 [abstract]. *Proc Am Soc Clin Oncol* 2000;19:271. Abstract 70.

84. Schnitt SJ, Hayman J, Gelman R, et al. A prospective study of conservative surgery alone in the treatment of selected patients with stage I breast cancer. *Cancer* 1996;77:1094-1100.

85. From The Health Care Advisory Board: *Innovations in Breast Cancer Care: A Summary of an Annual Oncology Roundtable* (pt II). Washington, DC: The Advisory Board Company; 1999.

86. Joslyn SA. Radiation therapy and patient age in the survival from early-stage breast cancer. *Int J Radiat Oncol Biol Phys* 1999;44:821-826.

87. Hebert-Croteau N, Brisson J, Latreille J, et al. Compliance with consensus recommendations for the treatment of early-stage breast carcinoma in elderly women. *Cancer* 1999;85:1104-1113.

88. Stovall M, Blackwell CR, Cundiff J, et al. Fetal dose from radiotherapy with photon beams. Report of AAPM Radiation Therapy Committee Task Group No. 36. *Med Phys* 1995;22:63-82.

89. Morris MM, Powell SN. Irradiation in the setting of collagen vascular disease: acute and late complications. *J Clin Oncol* 1997;15:2728-2735.

90. Lee CG, McCormick B, Mazumdar M, et al. Infiltrating breast carcinoma in patients age 30 years and younger: long-term outcome for life, relapse, and second primary tumors. *Int J Radiat Oncol Biol Phys* 1992;23:969-975.

91. Nixon AJ, Neuberg D, Hayes DF, et al. Relationship of patient age to pathologic features of the tumor and prognosis for patients with stage I or II breast cancer. *J Clin Oncol* 1994;12:888-894.

92. Fowble BL, Schultz DJ, Overmoyer B, et al. The influence of young age on outcome in early-stage breast cancer. *Int J Radiat Oncol Biol Phys* 1994;30:23-33.

93. Haffty BG, Fischer D, Rose M, et al. Prognostic factors for local recurrence in the conservatively treated breast cancer patient: a cautious interpretation of the data. *J Clin Oncol* 1991;9:997-1003.

94. Halverson KJ, Perez CA, Taylor ME, et al. Age as a prognostic factor for breast and regional nodal recurrence following breast conserving surgery and irradiation in stage I and II breast cancer. *Int J Radiat Oncol Biol Phys* 1993;27:1045-1050.

95. Kurtz JM, Jacquemier J, Amalric R, et al. Why are local recurrences after breast-conserving therapy more frequent in younger patients? *J Clin Oncol* 1990;8:591-598.

96. Fisher ER, Anderson S, Redmond C, et al. Ipsilateral breast tumor recurrence and survival following lumpectomy and irradiation. *Semin Surg Oncol* 1992;8:161-166.

97. Buchholz TA, Tucker SL, Mathur D, et al. Impact of systemic treatment on local control for lymph node–negative breast cancer patients treated with breast-conservation therapy. *J Clin Oncol* 2001;19:2240-2246.

98. Bouvet M, Babiera GV, Tucker SL, et al. Does breast conservation therapy in young women with breast cancer adversely affect local disease control and survival rate? The M.D. Anderson Cancer Center experience. *Br J Radiol* 1997;3:169-175.

99. Solin LJ, Schultz DJ, Fowble BL, et al. Ten-year results of the treatment of early-stage breast carcinoma in elderly women using breast-conserving surgery and definitive breast irradiation. *Int J Radiat Oncol Biol Phys* 1995;33:45-51.

100. Newman LA, Kuerer HM, Hunt KK, et al. Local recurrence and survival among black women with early-stage breast cancer treated with breast-conservation therapy or mastectomy. *Ann Surg Oncol* 1999;6:241-248.

101. Chabner E, Nixon A, Gelman R, et al. Family history and treatment outcome in young women after breast-conserving surgery and radiation therapy for early-stage cancer. *J Clin Oncol* 1998;16:2045-2051.

102. Haas JA, Schulta DJ, Peterson ME, et al. An analysis of age and family history on outcome after breast-conservation treatment: the University of Pennsylvania experience. *Cancer J* 1998;4:308-315.

103. Turner BC, Harrold E, Matloff E, et al. BRCA1/BRCA2 germline mutations in locally recurrent breast cancer patients after lumpectomy and radiation therapy: implications for breast-conserving management in patients with *BRCA1/BRCA2* mutations. *J Clin Oncol* 1999;17:3017-3024.

104. Pierce L, Strawderman M, Narod S, et al. Effect of radiotherapy after breast-conserving treatment in women with breast cancer and germline *BRCA1/2* mutations. *J Clin Oncol* 2000;18:3360-3369.

105. Gaffney DK, Brohet RM, Lewis CM, et al. A response to radiation therapy and prognosis in breast cancer patients with *BRCA1* and *BRCA2* mutations. *Radiother Oncol* 1998;47:129-136.

106. Robson M, Levin D, Federici M, et al. Breast conservation therapy for invasive breast cancer in Ashkenazi women with *BRCA* gene founder mutations. *J Natl Cancer Inst* 1999;91:2112-2117.

107. Fisher ER. Lumpectomy margins and much more. *Cancer* 1994;74:1453-1458.

108. Peterson ME, Schultz DJ, Reynolds C, et al. Outcomes in breast cancer patients relative to margin status after treatment with breast-conserving surgery and radiation therapy: the University of Pennsylvania experience. *Int J Radiat Oncol Biol Phys* 1999;43:1029-1035.

109. Wazer DE, Jabro G, Ruthazer R, et al. Extent of margin positivity as a predictor for local recurrence after breast conserving irradiation. *Radiat Oncol Investig* 1999;7:111-117.

110. Boyages J, Recht A, Connolly JL, et al. Early breast cancer: predictors of breast recurrence for patients treated with conservative surgery and radiation therapy. *Radiother Oncol* 1990;19:29-41.

111. Schnitt SJ, Abner A, Gelman R, et al. The relationship between microscopic margins of resection and the risk of local recurrence in patients with breast cancer treated with breast-conserving surgery and radiation therapy. *Cancer* 1994;74:1746-1751.

112. Wazer DE, Schmidt-Ullrich RK, Ruthazer R, et al. Factors determining outcome for breast-conserving irradiation with margin-directed dose escalation to the tumor bed. *Int J Radiat Oncol Biol Phys* 1998;40:851-858.

113. Park CC, Mitsumori M, Nixon A, et al. Outcome at 8 years after breast-conserving surgery and radiation therapy for invasive breast cancer: influence of margin status and systemic therapy on local recurrence. *J Clin Oncol* 2000;18:1668-1675.

114. Assersohn L, Powles TJ, Ashley S, et al. Local relapse in primary breast cancer patients with unexcised positive surgical margins after lumpectomy, radiotherapy and chemoendocrine therapy. *Ann Oncol* 1999;10:1451-1455.

115. Freedman G, Fowble B, Hanlon A, et al. Patients with early-stage invasive cancer with close or positive margins treated with conservative surgery and radiation have an increased risk of breast recurrence that is delayed by adjuvant systemic therapy. *Int J Radiat Oncol Biol Phys* 1999;44:1005-1015.

116. Kurtz JM, Jacquemier J, Amalric R, et al. Breast-conserving therapy for macroscopically multiple cancers. *Ann Surg* 1990;212:38-44.

117. Leopold KA, Recht A, Schnitt SJ, et al. Results of conservative surgery and radiation therapy for multiple synchronous cancers of one breast. *Int J Radiat Oncol Biol Phys* 1989;16:11-16.

118. Veronesi U, Salvadori B, Luini A, et al. Conservative treatment of early breast cancer. Long-term results of 1232 cases treated with quadrantectomy, axillary dissection, and radiotherapy. *Ann Surg* 1990;211:250-259.

119. Poen JC, Tran L, Juillard G, et al. Conservation therapy for invasive lobular carcinoma of the breast. *Cancer* 1992;69:2789-2795.

120. Fisher ER, Sass R, Fisher B, et al. Pathologic findings from the National Surgical Adjuvant Breast Project (protocol 6). I. Intraductal carcinoma (DCIS). *Cancer* 1986;57:197-208.

121. Haffty BG, Brown F, Carter D, et al. Evaluation of Her-2/neu oncoprotein expression as a prognostic indicator of local recurrence in conservatively treated breast cancer: a case-control study. *Int J Radiat Oncol Biol Phys* 1996;35:751-757.

122. Turner BC, Haffty BG, Narayanan L, et al. Insulin-like growth factor-I receptor overexpression mediates cellular radioresistance and local breast cancer recurrence after lumpectomy and radiation. *Cancer Res* 1997;57:3079-3083.

123. Bartelink H, Collette L, Fourquest A, et al. Impact of a boost of 16 Gy on local control and cosmesis in patients with early breast cancer: the EORTC "boost versus no boost" trial [abstract]. *Int J Radiat Oncol Biol Phys* 2000;48:111.

124. Fisher B, Montague E, Redmond C, et al. Findings from NSABP Protocol No. B-04—comparison of radical mastectomy with alternative treatments for primary breast cancer. I. Radiation compliance and its relation to treatment outcome. *Cancer* 1980;46:1-13.

125. Wazer DE, Erban JK, Robert NJ, et al. Breast conservation in elderly women for clinically negative axillary lymph nodes without axillary dissection. *Cancer* 1994;74:878-883.

126. Haffty BG, McKhann C, Beinfield M, et al. Breast conservation therapy without axillary dissection. A rational treatment strategy in selected patients. *Arch Surg* 1993;128:1315-1319.

127. Wong JS, Recht A, Beard CJ, et al. Treatment outcome after tangential radiation therapy without axillary dissection in patients with early-stage breast cancer and clinically negative axillary nodes. *Int J Radiat Oncol Biol Phys* 1997;39:915-920.

128. Giuliano AE, Jones RC, Brennan M, et al. Sentinel lymphadenectomy in breast cancer. *J Clin Oncol* 1997;15:2345-2350.

129. Krag D, Weaver D, Ashikaga T, et al. The sentinel node in breast cancer—a multicenter validation study. *N Engl J Med* 1998;339:941-946.

130. Veronesi U, Paganelli G, Viale G, et al. Sentinel lymph node biopsy and axillary dissection in breast cancer: results in a large series. *J Natl Cancer Inst* 1999;91:368-373.

131. Chu KU, Turner RR, Hansen NM, et al. Do all patients with sentinel node metastasis from breast carcinoma need complete axillary node dissection? *Ann Surg* 1999;229:536-541.

132. Goldhirsch A, Glick JH, Gelber RD, et al. Meeting highlights: International Consensus Panel on the Treatment of Primary Breast Cancer. *J Natl Cancer Inst* 1998;90:1601-1608.

133. Recht A, Come SE, Gelman RS, et al. Integration of conservative surgery, radiotherapy, and chemotherapy for the treatment of early-stage, node-positive breast cancer: sequencing, timing, and outcome. *J Clin Oncol* 1991;9:1662-1667.

134. Buchholz TA, Austin-Seymour MM, Moe RE, et al. Effect of delay in radiation in the combined modality treatment of breast cancer. *Int J Radiat Oncol Biol Phys* 1993;26:23-35.

135. Recht A, Come SE, Henderson IC, et al. The sequencing of chemotherapy and radiation therapy after conservative surgery for early-stage breast cancer. *N Engl J Med* 1996;334:1356-1361.

136. Buchholz TA, Hunt KK, Amosson CM, et al. Sequencing of chemotherapy and radiation in lymph node-negative breast cancer. *Cancer J Sci Am* 1999;5:159-164.

137. Fisher B, Bryant J, Wolmark N, et al. Effect of preoperative chemotherapy on the outcome of women with operable breast cancer. *J Clin Oncol* 1998;16:2672-2685.

138. Effects of radiotherapy and surgery in early breast cancer. An overview of the randomized trials. Early Breast Cancer Trialists' Collaborative Group. *N Engl J Med* 1995;333:1444-1455.

139. McArdle CS, Crawford D, Dykes EH, et al. Adjuvant radiotherapy and chemotherapy in breast cancer. *Br J Surg* 1986;73:264-266.

140. Velez-Garcia E, Carpenter JT Jr, Moore M, et al. Postsurgical adjuvant chemotherapy with or without radiotherapy in women with breast cancer and positive axillary nodes: a South-Eastern Cancer Study Group (SEG) Trial. *Eur J Cancer* 1992;28A:1833-1837.

141. Host H, Brennhovd IO, Loeb M. Postoperative radiotherapy in breast cancer—long-term results from the Oslo study. *Int J Radiat Oncol Biol Phys* 1986;12:727-732.

142. Rutqvist LE, Cedermark B, Glas U, et al. Radiotherapy, chemotherapy, and tamoxifen as adjuncts to surgery in early breast cancer: a summary of three randomized trials. *Int J Radiat Oncol Biol Phys* 1989;16:629-639.

143. Overgaard M, Christensen JJ, Johansen H, et al. Postmastectomy irradiation in high-risk breast cancer patients. Present status of the Danish Breast Cancer Cooperative Group trials. *Acta Oncol* 1988;27:707-714.

144. Spanos WJ, Montague ED, Fletcher GH. Late complications of radiation only for advanced breast cancer. *Int J Radiat Oncol Biol Phys* 1980;6:1473-1476.

145. Strom EA, McNeese MD, Fletcher GH, et al. Results of mastectomy and postoperative irradiation in the management of locoregionally advanced carcinoma of the breast. *Int J Radiat Oncol Biol Phys* 1991;21:319-323.

146. Cuzick J, Stewart H, Peto R, et al. Overview of randomized trials of postoperative adjuvant radiotherapy in breast cancer. *Cancer Treatment Reports* 1987;71:15-29.

147. Overgaard M, Christensen JJ, Johansen H, et al. Evaluation of radiotherapy in high-risk breast cancer patients: report from the Danish Breast Cancer Cooperative Group (DBCG 82) Trial. *Int J Radiat Oncol Biol Phys* 1990;19:1121-1124.

148. Overgaard M, Hansen PS, Overgaard J, et al. Postoperative radiotherapy in high-risk premenopausal women with breast cancer who receive adjuvant chemotherapy. Danish Breast Cancer Cooperative Group 82b Trial. *N Engl J Med* 1997;337:949-955.

149. Ragaz J, Jackson SM, Le N, et al. Adjuvant radiotherapy and chemotherapy in node-positive premenopausal women with breast cancer. *N Engl J Med* 1997;337:956-962.

150. Overgaard M. Overview of randomized trials in high risk breast cancer patients treated with adjuvant systemic therapy with or without postmastectomy irradiation. *Semin Radiat Oncol* 1999;9:292-299.

151. Madden JL. Modified radical mastectomy. *Surg Gynecol Obstet* 1965;121:1221-1230.

152. Madden JL, Kandalaft S, Bourque RA. Modified radical mastectomy. *Ann Surg* 1972;175:624-634.

153. Pierce LJ, Oberman HA, Strawderman MH, et al. Microscopic extracapsular extension in the axilla: is this an indication for axillary radiotherapy? *Int J Radiat Oncol Biol Phys* 1995;33:253-259.

154. Harris JR, Halpin-Murphy P, McNeese M, et al. Consensus statement on postmastectomy radiation therapy. *Int J Radiat Oncol Biol Phys* 1999;44:989-990.

155. Fowble B, Gray R, Gilchrist K, et al. Identification of a subgroup of patients with breast cancer and histologically positive axillary

nodes receiving adjuvant chemotherapy who may benefit from postoperative radiotherapy. *J Clin Oncol* 1988;6:1107-1117.

156. Levine MN, Bramwell VH, Pritchard KI, et al. Randomized trial of intensive cyclophosphamide, epirubicin, and fluorouracil chemotherapy compared with cyclophosphamide, methotrexate, and fluorouracil in premenopausal women with node-positive breast cancer. National Cancer Institute of Canada Clinical Trials Group. *J Clin Oncol* 1998;16:2651-2658.

157. Buzdar AU, Blumenschein GR, Smith TL, et al. Adjuvant chemotherapy with fluorouracil, doxorubicin, and cyclophosphamide, with or without bacillus Calmette-Guerin and with or without irradiation in operable breast cancer. A prospective randomized trial. *Cancer* 1984;53:384-389.

158. Blomqvist C, Tiusanen K, Elomaa I, et al. The combination of radiotherapy, adjuvant chemotherapy (cyclophosphamide-doxorubicin-ftorafur) and tamoxifen in stage II breast cancer. Long-term follow-up results of a randomised trial. *Br J Cancer* 1992;66:1171-1176.

159. Buzzoni R, Bonadonna G, Valagussa P, et al. Adjuvant chemotherapy with doxorubicin plus cyclophosphamide, methotrexate, and fluorouracil in the treatment of resectable breast cancer with more than three positive axillary nodes. *J Clin Oncol* 1991;9:2134-2140.

160. Griem KL, Henderson IC, Gelman R, et al. The 5-year results of a randomized trial of adjuvant radiation therapy after chemotherapy in breast cancer patients treated with mastectomy. *J Clin Oncol* 1987;5:1546-1555.

161. Fisher B, Redmond C, Wickerham DL, et al. Doxorubicin-containing regimens for the treatment of stage II breast cancer: the National Surgical Adjuvant Breast and Bowel Project experience. *J Clin Oncol* 1989;7:572-582.

162. Overgaard M. Evaluation of radiotherapy in high-risk breast cancer patients given adjuvant systemic therapy. *Rays* 2000; 25:325-330.

163. Katz A, Strom EA, Buchholz TA, et al. Locoregional recurrence patterns after mastectomy and doxorubicin-based chemotherapy: implications for postoperative irradiation. *J Clin Oncol* 2000; 18:2817-2827.

164. Katz A, Strom EA, Buchholz TA, et al. The influence of pathologic tumor characteristics on locoregional recurrence rates following mastectomy. *Int J Radiat Oncol Biol Phys* 2001;50:735-742.

165. Bedwinek JM, Lee J, Fineberg B, et al. Prognostic indicators in patients with isolated local-regional recurrence of breast cancer. *Cancer* 1981;47:2232-2235.

166. Toonkel LM, Fix I, Jacobson LH, et al. The significance of local recurrence of carcinoma of the breast. *Int J Radiat Oncol Biol Phys* 1983;9:33-39.

167. Schwaibold F, Fowble BL, Solin LJ, et al. The results of radiation therapy for isolated local regional recurrence after mastectomy. *Int J Radiat Oncol Biol Phys* 1991;21:299-310.

168. Ballo MT, Strom EA, Prost H, et al. Local-regional control of recurrent breast carcinoma after mastectomy: does hyperfractionated accelerated radiotherapy improve local control? *Int J Radiat Oncol Biol Phys* 1999;44:105-112.

169. Crowe JP Jr, Gordon NH, Antunez AR, et al. Local-regional breast cancer recurrence following mastectomy. *Arch Surg* 1991;126:429-432.

170. Andry G, Suciu S, Vico P, et al. Locoregional recurrences after 649 modified radical mastectomies: incidence and significance. *Eur J Surg Oncol* 1989;15:476-485.

171. Bucalossi P, Veronesi U, Zingo L, et al. Enlarged mastectomy for breast cancer. Review of 1,213 cases. *Am J Roentgenol Radium Ther Nucl Med* 1971;111:119-122.

172. Handley RS. Carcinoma of the breast. *Ann R Coll Surg Engl* 1975;57:59-66.

173. Ki KY, Shen ZZ. An analysis of 1242 cases of extended radical mastectomy. *Breast* 1984;10:10-19.

174. Arriagada R, Le MG, Mouriesse H, et al. Long-term effect of internal mammary chain treatment. Results of a multivariate analysis of 1195 patients with operable breast cancer and positive axillary nodes. *Radiother Oncol* 1988;11:213-222.

175. Lê MG, Arriagada R, de Vathaire F, et al. Can internal mammary chain treatment decrease the risk of death for patients with medial breast cancers and positive axillary lymph nodes? *Cancer* 1990;66:2313-2318.

176. Strom EA, McNeese MD. Postmastectomy irradiation: rationale for treatment field selection. *Semin Radiat Oncol* 1999;9:247-253.

177. Rutqvist LE, Lax I, Fornander T, et al. Cardiovascular mortality in a randomized trial of adjuvant radiation therapy versus surgery alone in primary breast cancer. *Int J Radiat Oncol Biol Phys* 1992;22:887-896.

178. Auquier A, Rutqvist LE, Host H, et al. Post-mastectomy megavoltage radiotherapy: the Oslo and Stockholm trials. *Eur J Cancer* 1992;28:433-437.

179. Jacquillat C, Weil M, Baillet F, et al. Results of neoadjuvant chemotherapy and radiation therapy in the breast-conserving treatment of 250 patients with all stages of infiltrative breast cancer. *Cancer* 1990;66:119-129.

180. Lippman ME, Sorace RA, Bagley CS, et al. Treatment of locally advanced breast cancer using primary induction chemotherapy with hormonal synchronization followed by radiation therapy with or without debulking surgery. *NCI Monogr* 1986;1:153-159.

181. Mauriac L, MacGrogan G, Avril A, et al. Neoadjuvant chemotherapy for operable breast carcinoma larger than 3 cm: a unicentre randomized trial with a 124-month median follow-up. Institut Bergonie Bordeaux Groupe Sein (IBBGS). *Ann Oncol* 1999;10:47-52.

182. Hortobagyi GN, Ames FC, Buzdar AU, et al. Management of stage III primary breast cancer with primary chemotherapy, surgery, and radiation therapy. *Cancer* 1988;62:2507-2516.

183. Hortobagyi GN, Buzdar AU, Strom EA, et al. Primary chemotherapy for early and advanced breast cancer. *Cancer Lett* 1995;90:103-109.

184. Edeiken BS, Fornage BD, Bedi DG, et al. US-guided implantation of metallic markers for permanent localization of the tumor bed in patients with breast cancer who undergo preoperative chemotherapy. *Radiology* 1999;213:895-900.

185. Singletary SE, McNeese MD, Hortobagyi GN. Feasibility of breast-conservation surgery after induction chemotherapy for locally advanced breast carcinoma. *Cancer* 1992;69:2849-2852.

186. Chu JC, Solin LJ, Hwang CC, et al. A nondivergent three field matching technique for breast irradiation. *Int J Radiat Oncol Biol Phys* 1990;19:1037-1040.

187. Strom EA, McNeese MD, Fletcher GH. Treatment of the peripheral lymphatics: rationale, indications, and techniques. In: Levitt GH, ed. *Medical Radiology in Non-Disseminated Breast Cancer—Controversial Issues in Management.* Berlin, Germany: Springer-Verlag; 1993:57-72.

188. Vlastos G, Mirza NQ, Lenert JT, et al. The feasibility of minimally invasive surgery for stage IIA, IIB, and IIIA breast carcinoma patients after tumor downstaging with induction chemotherapy. *Cancer* 2000;88:1417-1424.

189. Vezzoni P, Balestrazzi A, Bignami P, et al. Axillary lymph node metastases from occult carcinoma of the breast. *Tumori* 1979;65:87-91.

190. Knapper WH. Management of occult breast cancer presenting as an axillary metastasis. *Semin Surg Oncol* 1991;7:311-313.

191. Whillis D, Brown PW, Rodger A. Adenocarcinoma from an unknown primary presenting in women with an axillary mass. *Clin Oncol (R Coll Radiol)* 1990;2:189-192.

192. Copeland EM, McBride CM. Axillary metastases from unknown primary sites. *Ann Surg* 1973;178:25-27.

193. Patel J, Nemoto T, Rosner D, et al. Axillary lymph node metastasis from an occult breast cancer. *Cancer* 1981;47:2923-2927.

194. Fortunato L, Sorrento JJ, Golub RA, et al. Occult breast cancer. A case report and review of the literature. *N Y State J Med* 1992;92:555-557.

195. Davis PL, Julian TB, Staiger M, et al. Magnetic resonance imaging detection and wire localization of an 'occult' breast cancer. *Breast Cancer Res Treat* 1994;32:327-330.

196. Orel SG, Schnall MD, Powell CM, et al. Staging of suspected breast cancer: effect of MR imaging and MR-guided biopsy. *Radiology* 1995;196:115-122.

197. Lee WJ, Chu JS, Chung MF, et al. The use of color Doppler in the diagnosis of occult breast cancer. *J Clin Ultrasound* 1995;23:192-194.

198. Halsted WS. The results of radical operations for the cure of carcinoma of the breast. *Ann Surg* 1907;46:1-19.

199. Baron PL, Moore MP, Kinne DW, et al. Occult breast cancer presenting with axillary metastases. Updated management. *Arch Surg* 1990;125:210-214.

200. Ellerbroek N, Holmes F, Singletary E, et al. Treatment of patients with isolated axillary nodal metastases from an occult primary carcinoma consistent with breast origin. *Cancer* 1990;66:1461-1467.

201. Kemeny MM. Mastectomy: is it necessary for occult breast cancer? *N Y State J Med* 1992;92:516-517.

202. Bhatia SK, Saclarides TJ, Witt TR, et al. Hormone receptor studies in axillary metastases from occult breast cancers. *Cancer* 1987;59:1170-1172.

203. Merson M, Andreola S, Galimberti V, et al. Breast carcinoma presenting as axillary metastases without evidence of a primary tumor. *Cancer* 1992;70:504-508.

204. Rosen PP. Occult carcinoma presenting with axillary lymph node metastases [abstract]. Paper presented at: 12th Annual International Breast Cancer Conference; March 16-18, 1995; Ann Arbor, Mich.

205. Griffith CD, Christmas TJ, Elston CW, et al. Axillary lymph node metastases from clinically occult breast carcinoma. *J R Coll Surg Edinb* 1987;32:237-238.

206. van Ooijen B, Bontenbal M, Henzen-Logmans SC, et al. Axillary nodal metastases from an occult primary consistent with breast carcinoma. *Br J Surg* 1993;80:1299-1300.

207. Jackson B, Scott-Conner C, Moulder J. Axillary metastasis from occult breast carcinoma: diagnosis and management. *Am Surg* 1995;61:431-434.

208. van de Weijer GH, van Ooijen B, Hesp WL, et al. Expectant management concerning the breast in 5 patients with occult breast carcinoma. *Ned Tijdschr Geneeskd* 1995;139:1648-1650.

209. Campana F, Fourquet A, Ashby MA, et al. Presentation of axillary lymphadenopathy without detectable breast primary (T0 N1b breast cancer): experience at Institut Curie. *Radiother Oncol* 1989;15:321-325.

210. Read NE, Strom EA, McNeese MD. Carcinoma in axillary nodes in women with unknown primary site—results of breast-conserving therapy. *Breast Journal* 1996;2:403-409.

211. A randomized study of tumor resection versus mastectomy in breast cancer. 2. 6-year results of the DBCG-82TM (Danish Breast Cancer Cooperative Group) protocol [in Danish]. *Ugeskr Laeger* 1991;153:2272-2276.

212. Rubens R, Armitage P, Winter P, et al. Prognosis in inoperable stage III carcinoma of the breast. *Eur J Cancer* 1977;13:805-811.

213. Kokal WA, Hill LR, Porudominsky D, et al. Inflammatory breast carcinoma: a distinct entity? *J Surg Oncol* 1985;30:152-155.

214. Brun B, Otmezguine Y, Feuilhade F, et al. Treatment of inflammatory breast cancer with combination chemotherapy and mastectomy versus breast conservation. *Cancer* 1988;61:1096-1103.

215. Fastenberg NA, Martin RG, Buzdar AU, et al. Management of inflammatory carcinoma of the breast. A combined modality approach. *Am J Clin Oncol* 1985;8:134-141.

216. Barker JL, Montague ED, Peters LJ. Clinical experience with irradiation of inflammatory carcinoma of the breast with and without elective chemotherapy. *Cancer* 1980;45:625-629.

217. Lucas FV, Perez-Mesa C. Inflammatory carcinoma of the breast. *Cancer* 1978;41:1595-1605.

218. Rao D, Bedwinek J, Perez C, et al. Prognostic indicators in stage III and localized stage IV breast cancer. *Cancer* 1982;50:2037-2043.

219. Bonnier P, Charpin C, Lejeune C, et al. Inflammatory carcinomas of the breast: a clinical, pathological, or a clinical and pathological definition? *Int J Cancer* 1995;62:382-385.

220. Ellis DL, Teitelbaum SL. Inflammatory carcinoma of the breast. A pathologic definition. *Cancer* 1974;33:1045-1047.

221. Fields JN, Perez CA, Kuske RR, et al. Inflammatory carcinoma of the breast: treatment results on 107 patients. *Int J Radiat Oncol Biol Phys* 1989;17:249-255.

222. Rouesse J, Friedman S, Mouriesse H, et al. Therapeutic strategies in inflammatory breast carcinoma based on prognostic factors. *Breast Cancer Res Treat* 1990;16:15-22.

223. Thoms WW Jr, McNeese MD, Fletcher GH, et al. Multimodal treatment for inflammatory breast cancer. *Int J Radiat Oncol Biol Phys* 1989;17:739-745.

224. Dahlbeck SW, Donnelly JF, Theriault RL. Differentiating inflammatory breast cancer from acute mastitis. *Am Fam Physician* 1995;52:929-934.

225. Yasumura K, Ogawa K, Ishikawa H, et al. Inflammatory carcinoma of the breast: characteristic findings of MR imaging. *Breast Cancer* 1997;4:161-169.

226. Bock E, Palazzoni G, Marcelli G, et al. Radiological and ultrasonographical diagnosis of inflammatory breast cancer. *Rays* 1988;13:53-57.

227. Harvey HA, Lipton A, Lawrence BV, et al. Estrogen receptor status in inflammatory breast carcinoma. *J Surg Oncol* 1982;21:42-44.

228. Paradiso A, Tommasi S, Brandi M, et al. Cell kinetics and hormonal receptor status in inflammatory breast carcinoma. Comparison with locally advanced disease. *Cancer* 1989;64:1922-1927.

229. Guerin M, Gabillot M, Mathieu MC, et al. Structure and expression of *c-erbB-2* and *EGF* receptor genes in inflammatory and non-inflammatory breast cancer: prognostic significance. *Int J Cancer* 1989;43:201-208.

230. Riou G, Le MG, Travagli JP, et al. Poor prognosis of *p53* gene mutation and nuclear overexpression of *p53* protein in inflammatory breast carcinoma. *J Natl Cancer Inst* 1993;85:1765-1767.

231. Bozzetti F, Saccozzi R, De Lena M, et al. Inflammatory cancer of the breast: analysis of 114 cases. *J Surg Oncol* 1981;18:355-361.

232. Barker JL, Nelson AJ, Montague ED. Inflammatory carcinoma of the breast. *Radiology* 1976;121:173-176.

233. Wang CC, Griscom NT. Radiotherapy for inflammatory carcinoma of the breast. *Male Nurses J* 1966;110:13-14.

234. Rosen P. Inflammatory carcinoma of the breast. *Rocky Mt Med J* 1970;67:35-36.

235. Zucali R, Uslenghi C, Kenda R, et al. Natural history and survival of inoperable breast cancer treated with radiotherapy and radiotherapy followed by radical mastectomy. *Cancer* 1976;37:1422-1431.

236. Chu AM, Cope O, Russo R, et al. Treatment of early-stage breast cancer by limited surgery and radical irradiation. *Int J Radiat Oncol Biol Phys* 1980;6:25-30.

237. Fields JN, Kuske RR, Perez CA, et al. Prognostic factors in inflammatory breast cancer. *Cancer* 1989;63:1225-1232.

238. Krutchik AN, Buzdar AU, Blumenschein GR, et al. Combined chemoimmunotherapy and radiation therapy of inflammatory breast carcinoma. *J Surg Oncol* 1979;11:325-332.

239. Kuske RR. Diagnosis and management of inflammatory breast cancer. *Semin Radiat Oncol* 1994;4:270-282.

240. Liao Z, Strom EA, Buzdar AU, et al. Locoregional irradiation for inflammatory breast cancer: effectiveness of dose escalation in decreasing recurrence. *Int J Radiat Oncol Biol Phys* 2000;47: 1191-1200.

241. Swain SM, Lippman ME. Treatment of patients with inflammatory breast cancer. *Important Adv Oncol* 1989:129-150.

242. Chevallier B, Asselain B, Kunlin A, et al. Inflammatory breast cancer. Determination of prognostic factors by univariate and multivariate analysis. *Cancer* 1987;60:897-902.

243. Arthur DW, Schmidt-Ullrich RK, Friedman RB, et al. Accelerated superfractionated radiotherapy for inflammatory breast carcinoma: complete response predicts outcome and allows for breast conservation. *Int J Radiat Oncol Biol Phys* 1999;44:289-296.

244. Knight CJ, Martin JJ, Welch JS, et al. Surgical considerations after chemotherapy and radiation therapy for inflammatory breast cancer. *Surgery* 1986;99:385-391.

245. Gurney H, Harnett P, Kefford R, et al. Inflammatory breast cancer: enhanced local control with hyperfractionated radiotherapy and infusional vincristine, ifosfamide and epirubicin. *Aust N Z J Med* 1998;28:400-402.

246. Ueno NT, Buzdar AU, Singletary SE, et al. Combined-modality treatment of inflammatory breast carcinoma: twenty years of experience at M.D. Anderson Cancer Center. *Cancer Chemother Pharmacol* 1997;40:321-329.

247. Arun B, Slack R, Gehan E, et al. Survival after autologous hematopoietic stem cell transplantation for patients with inflammatory breast carcinoma. *Cancer* 1999;85:93-99.

248. Ragaz J. Biologic aspects, classification, surgery, and radiotherapy of stage III breast cancer. *Curr Opin Oncol* 1990;2:1053-1067.

249. Viens P, Penault-Llorca F, Jacquemier J, et al. High-dose chemotherapy and haematopoietic stem cell transplantation for inflammatory breast cancer: pathologic response and outcome. *Bone Marrow Transplant* 1998;21:249-254.

250. Viens P, Palangie T, Janvier M, et al. First-line high-dose sequential chemotherapy with rG-CSF and repeated blood stem cell transplantation in untreated inflammatory breast cancer: toxicity and response (PEGASE 02 trial). *Br J Cancer* 1999;81: 449-456.

251. Cagnoni PJ, Nieto Y, Shpall EJ, et al. High-dose chemotherapy with autologous hematopoietic progenitor-cell support as part of combined modality therapy in patients with inflammatory breast cancer. *J Clin Oncol* 1998;16:1661-1668.

252. Janjan NA, McNeese MD, Buzdar AU, et al. Management of locoregional recurrent breast cancer. *Cancer* 1986;58:1552-1556.

253. Aberizk WJ, Silver B, Henderson IC, et al. The use of radiotherapy for treatment of isolated locoregional recurrence of breast carcinoma after mastectomy. *Cancer* 1986;58:1214-1218.

254. Ames FC, Balch CM. Management of local and regional recurrence after mastectomy or breast-conserving treatment. *Surg Clin North Am* 1990;70:1115-1124.

255. Deutsch M, Parsons JA, Mittal BB. Radiation therapy for local-regional recurrent breast carcinoma. *Int J Radiat Oncol Biol Phys* 1986;12:2061-2065.

256. Halverson KJ, Perez CA, Kuske RR, et al. Isolated local-regional recurrence of breast cancer following mastectomy: radiotherapeutic management. *Int J Radiat Oncol Biol Phys* 1990;19:851-858.

257. Beck TM, Hart NE, Woodard DA, et al. Local or regionally recurrent carcinoma of the breast: results of therapy in 121 patients. *J Clin Oncol* 1983;1:400-405.

258. Dahlstrom KK, Andersson AP, Andersen M, et al. Wide local excision of recurrent breast cancer in the thoracic wall. *Cancer* 1993;72:774-777.

259. Chen KK, Montague ED, Oswald MJ. Results of irradiation in the treatment of locoregional breast cancer recurrence. *Cancer* 1985;56:1269-1273.

260. Taylor ME, Perez CA, Halverson KJ, et al. Factors influencing cosmetic results after conservation therapy for breast cancer. *Int J Radiat Oncol Biol Phys* 1995;4:753-764.

261. International Commission on Radiation Units and Measurements. *Prescribing, Recording, and Reporting Photon Beam Therapy.* Bethesda, Md: International Commission on Radiation Units and Measurements, 1993. ICRU Report 50.

PART V

Thorax

CHAPTER 16

The Blood Vessels and Heart

Roger W. Byhardt and William T. Moss

BLOOD VESSELS

In every part of the body, cellular viability and organ function depend on the integrity of blood vessels. Thus radiation oncologists must be aware of the effects of irradiation on the vascular system. The acute reactions to radiation in highly radiosensitive tissues, such as hematopoietic tissue and the intestine, are initiated before radiation-induced vascular changes become apparent. By contrast, the late radiation reactions in the brain and myocardium may be almost entirely due to radiation-induced changes in the vasculature.

The vascular system is the most important system in the body in terms of regulation of cellular radiosensitivity. Irradiation damages blood vessels of all sizes, leading to impairment of circulation. An impaired blood supply leads quickly to local changes in nutrition, electrolyte concentrations, and tissue oxygenation, and these changes, in turn, decrease the ability of tissues to respond to other types of injury.

Radiation-induced effects on blood vessels can be either acute or chronic and depend on vessel size and location; associated vascular disease; the dose of radiation, the time over which radiation is delivered, and the volume irradiated; and finally, the stresses to which the irradiated volume is subjected. The use of small fraction sizes (up to 2 Gy/fraction) is generally associated with an improved therapeutic ratio. Such small fractions result in relative sparing of small blood vessels with no decrease in the rate of cancer control.

Anatomy

Walls of blood vessels consists of three concentric layers (tunicae). The inner layer (intima) consists of endothelium; the outer layer (adventitia) is made up of connective tissue, bracketing a middle layer (media) consisting of smooth muscle.

Small Blood Vessels
Acute Vascular Changes

Erythema. The first and most noticeable gross vascular change after irradiation is cutaneous or mucosal erythema. The intensity of the erythema increases in direct proportion to the radiation dose and the area irradiated. Erythema of the skin appears in waves that occur at predictable times during the course of radiation therapy—on the first day, during the second or third week, and at the end of the first month.

The mechanism of radiation-induced erythema is not known, but the first period of erythema is thought to be a vascular response to local extracapillary cell injury, whereas the later periods of erythema are presumed to be caused by direct capillary damage.[1] Radiation-induced erythema is not a result of nerve injury. It has been suggested that a histamine-like substance is produced by the radiation injury and that this substance diffuses through tissues to produce erythema within and slightly beyond the margins of the irradiated volume. However, this mechanism is questionable because radiation-induced erythema is not decreased by administration of antihistamines. Moreover, during the first period of erythema, the vessels maintain their ability to constrict in response to a scratch test, and histamine does not produce wheal formation.

Skin temperature rises several degrees with the onset of radiation-induced erythema, suggesting that vasodilation and not merely vasocongestion occurs. Local administration of epinephrine or acetylcholine reduces but does not eliminate vasoconstrictive and vasocongestive responses. Direct observation of radiation-induced changes in arterioles and capillaries in bats' wings, the webs of frogs' feet, human nail folds, and through experimentally placed transparent "windows" confirms that acute radiation-induced damage to small blood vessels is nonspecific.

During the acute phase of erythema, damage of the vessel endothelium is not striking. With radiation doses used clinically, however, some endothelial cells are killed, and thrombi form and narrow or obliterate the vessel lumen.

Increased vessel permeability and vessel dilation. The functions of small blood vessels are to deliver oxygen and nutrients to cells and to carry waste products away from cells. These functions depend not only on blood flow rates but also on transmission and transport of nutrients and waste products through the capillary wall. The relative contributions of the two layers of the capillary wall—the endothelium and the basement membrane—to capillary permeability remain uncertain. A few hours to a few weeks after treatment with moderate doses of radiation, the permeability of the capillary wall increases, as manifested by associated edema. As might be expected, the rapidly proliferating endothelial cells of newly developing capillaries are more sensitive to radiation than are endothelial cells in older capillaries.[2,3] This fact explains some of the inhibitory effects of irradiation on wound healing.

One of the most consistent early effects seen in the capillaries and prearterioles after irradiation is dilation of the vessel. This can be accompanied by endothelial cell swelling, degeneration, and necrosis and the presence of a cellular inflammatory infiltrate. Increased vascular permeability with resulting tissue edema is a common early manifestation (Fig. 16-1).

The pathogenesis of radiation-induced vascular dilation and increased capillary permeability is not clear. Endothelial cell damage can be minimal or absent even in the case of severe edema. It is possible that irradiation interferes, at least temporarily, with vasomotor regulatory mechanisms and results in hemodynamic alterations conducive to tissue edema.

Increased capillary permeability manifested as local edema can be seen after doses of 5 Gy or more. Various substances, including labeled plasma, erythrocytes, Evans blue dye, and colloidal gold, permeate the capillary walls more rapidly after irradiation. The peak change develops 2 weeks after a single exposure. The contribution of thrombi and vasodilation to the increased permeability is unknown. The capillaries exhibit increased fragility. Bleeding occurs more readily even though the clotting mechanism is normal. The combination of thrombus formation, vasodilation, and increased capillary fragility and bleeding resemble an inflammatory response.[4] As with an inflammatory response, they subside as the chronic vascular changes become manifest.

Chronic Vascular Changes

After the acute reaction to radiation subsides and before major narrowing of the vessel lumen develops, diffusion of material through capillary walls decreases. The vessel wall may not appear to be seriously damaged; however, the ultrafiltration ability of the endothelial lining is decreased.[4] Furthermore, the basement membrane of the capillary wall is thickened, and this thickening is presumed to contribute to decreased capillary permeability. The connective-tissue barrier between the capillaries and the dependent tissues becomes thicker as a result of extracapillary fibrosis. The cause of this extracapillary fibrosis is unknown, although Rubin and Casarett[5] related it to a connective-tissue reaction after "leakage" of plasma constituents from capillaries.

Still later, the number of small vessels is decreased through the process of vessel occlusion (Fig. 16-2). Arteriolar capillary intimal hyalinosis proceeds as a discontinuous process. Tumoricidal doses of radiation inhibit capillary sprouting and vascular remodeling,[6] which probably contributes to delays in wound healing after irradiation. However, vascular endothelium seems to recover rapidly, and it is possible that migrating unirradiated endothelial cells account for this apparently rapid recovery.

The most common chronic radiation-induced changes seen in vessels of small and medium caliber are swelling and vacuolation of the endothelial cells of the tunica intima vasorum. Later, proliferation of endothelial cells and lipid deposits may occur. These lesions resemble atheromatous plaques but differ in their location because atheromatous plaques rarely occur spontaneously in small arteries. These lesions are not specific

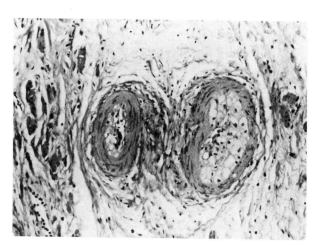

Fig. 16-1 Arteries from a 34-year-old woman irradiated 5 months previously with 65 Gy for carcinoma of the cervix. Fatty deposits in the intima have caused great narrowing of the lumina. Note the edema surrounding the blood vessels.

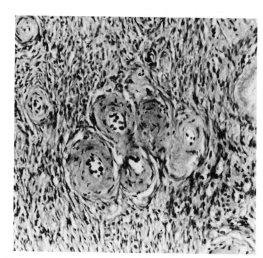

Fig. 16-2 Small blood vessels 5 months after irradiation with 65 Gy in 7 weeks. The vessels have strikingly thickened walls and narrowed lumina.

for radiation damage; any physical or chemical damage to the vessel, especially the tunica adventitia vasorum (adventitia), results in similar lesions. This is particularly true in experimental situations in which animals are rendered hyperlipemic by dietary means. In humans no evidence has been found of any relationship between serum cholesterol levels and development of the foamy lesions in the intima after irradiation. These lesions can be seen a few days after radiation therapy and can persist for many years.

Concomitant with these changes in the intima, vacuolation and degeneration of the smooth muscle cells of the tunica media vasorum may occur. Repair with fibrosis of the tunica media is seen in chronic lesions. Narrowing of the lumen occurs mainly as a result of concentric fibrosis and loss of vascular elasticity, but thrombosis and intimal proliferation also play important roles. In the superficial part of the cutis, extensive dilation of capillaries, recognized as telangiectasia, is usually seen after radiation therapy. The telangiectatic vessels arise from existing capillaries and are presumed to be a result of greater blood flow through the few remaining damaged small blood vessels. The sequelae of small blood vessel obliteration vary with the organ in question. The vasculoconnective tissue of the skin can tolerate extensive damage before necrosis occurs. On the other hand, rather minor defects in the vasculature of the brain, myocardium, kidney, or lungs may result in seriously limited function.

In addition to the changes in small blood vessels that occur as a direct result of irradiation, changes secondary to tumor shrinkage also can be seen. Quantitative studies show improved vascular filling after irradiation. Also, after irradiation, the appearance of vessels in large tumors reverts to the appearance of vessels in small tumors.[7,8] These vascular changes are fundamental to the process of radiation-induced reoxygenation of the tumor.

The popularity of radiation doses of about 60 Gy in 6 weeks is a recognition of the tolerance of most normal vasculoconnective tissues. The incidence of necrosis of normal tissues increases rapidly with increasing dose when doses higher than 60 Gy in 6 weeks (or the equivalent) are delivered to large volumes. A variety of factors modify the response of small vessels to radiation, including tissue oxygen concentration, associated inflammatory reactions, sclerotic changes in aged patients, hypertension, associated trauma such as surgery, and fractionation schedule. The recognition of these factors and the exploitation of the advantages of increased fractionation are the basis for individualization of radiation therapy techniques.

Large Blood Vessels

In large blood vessels, high doses of radiation produce little recognizable acute change. Veins are little affected, and the changes affecting large, elastic arteries usually occur as late manifestations.

Mechanism of Radiation-Induced Injury

The mechanisms of chronic radiation injury to large blood vessels are not known. Although a direct effect of radiation on the cellular elements of the tunica media cannot be excluded, the changes seen are similar to those observed after damage of the adventitial vessels nourishing most of the vascular wall—changes that also can be produced experimentally by burning or freezing the adventitia. Extensive dissection around the vessels with destruction of their blood supply is likely to be a predisposing factor but is by no means a prerequisite for such radiation-induced changes.

The changes themselves basically consist of degeneration of muscle cells of the tunica media. The muscle-cell degeneration can be a patchy, localized process or can present as a wide zone of cystic medionecrosis. Weakening of the vessel wall may lead to rupture, but more often, fibrosis of the tunica media is observed. The intima overlying the areas of medial degeneration usually develops changes indistinguishable from those of ordinary atherosclerosis.[8] Again, similar changes can be produced experimentally by damaging the adventitia by chemical or physical means.

The pathogenesis of these experimental lesions seems to be interference with nutrition of the arterial wall through damage of the adventitial vasa vasorum. It seems likely that a similar mechanism operates in radiation-induced damage to large arteries, that is, this damage is mediated through narrowing and occlusion of the vasa vasorum caused by irradiation. In clinical situations, the presence of tumor cells and the tissue reactions they may elicit also may contribute to the decreased blood supply of the vessels.

The decreased strength of the vessel walls after irradiation has unusual importance when radical neck dissection is performed after high doses have been given to the carotid arteries; in this situation, rupture of the carotid arteries may occur.[9]

Arteriosclerosis and atherosclerosis. After irradiation, changes within the vessel lumen are more obvious than changes in the vessel walls. Single large doses of 15 to 20 Gy produce arteriosclerosis and atherosclerosis within 30 to 40 weeks. This sclerosis is confined to the irradiated zone.[8] Fractionated doses of 30 to 50 Gy produce less severe changes than large single doses.

Hypertensive vascular damage. Asscher[10] found that radiation sensitizes blood vessels to hypertension. Hypertension from any cause produces early profound hypertensive vascular damage in irradiated blood vessels, whereas unirradiated blood vessels subjected to the same hypertension may appear relatively normal for months.[10] When hypertension develops years after high-dose irradiation, the patient can develop a localized vascular insufficiency leading to necrosis of the irradiated volume.

Radiation-Induced Carotid Artery Disease

Silverberg and colleagues[11] compared a variety of variables in nine patients with atherosclerotic carotid artery disease associated with neck irradiation and 40 unirradiated control patients. The nine irradiated patients with occlusive carotid artery disease were younger than the controls, were less likely to have peripheral vascular disease and coronary artery disease, and were less likely to have hyperlipemia or hypercholesterolemia.[11] These findings support the recognition of radiation-induced carotid artery disease as a clinical entity. Reconstructive carotid surgery in patients with carotid artery damage resulting from radiation therapy should be approached as if radiation were not a factor even though there may be some periarterial fibrosis and increased difficulty in separating the plaques from the tunica media.[11]

Arrest of Growth of Vessel Diameter

During childhood, the aorta and other large vessels grow in proportion to increasing body surface area and not in relation to chronologic age.[12] In children, doses of 25 to 28 Gy given to large vessels over 2 to 3 weeks arrest growth in vessel diameter.[13] The inhibitory effect of irradiation on the growth of vessel diameter is greatest with irradiation delivered during infancy and decreases with increasing age at irradiation.

THE HEART

Various amounts of cardiac tissue are included in the radiation field during treatment of the chest wall and internal mammary nodes in patients with breast cancer and during treatment of the mediastinum in patients with lung cancer, esophageal cancer, lymphoma, or seminoma. The variety of radiation doses and dose distributions used to treat each tumor type have provided useful clinical data regarding dose-effect relationships for cardiac irradiation, including fraction size effects. The most useful data on late effects of cardiac irradiation come from studies of patients with breast cancer, Hodgkin's disease, and seminoma, which include large numbers of patients with long-term survival. In general, because of the poor survival after definitive irradiation of inoperable lung cancer, follow-up data from lung cancer studies, even prospective studies, contribute little to the understanding of late cardiac effects.

Clinical observations through the early 1970s suggested that the heart was relatively unaffected by conventionally fractionated radiation therapy. However, animal experiments in the early 1970s showed significant cardiac changes after irradiation of the heart. Since that time, as the clinical effects of cardiac irradiation

have been more rigorously studied, especially through tests of cardiac function, subclinical effects have been demonstrated after commonly used radiation therapy techniques. Using animal models and multifraction techniques similar to those used in clinical practice, investigators have shown that late cardiac radiation injury mainly consists of damage to the cardiac microvasculature.[14,15] Other components of the heart are also affected, but at a lower frequency and with less severe consequences.

When both the heart and the lung are included in the irradiated volume, there is a complex interplay of cardiac and pulmonary effects of radiation therapy. In general, radiation-induced cardiac effects depend on the total dose, fraction size, volume of heart irradiated, and presence or absence of mediastinal tumor. Numerous clinical studies[8,16-26] have shown a relationship between cardiac irradiation and both accelerated coronary vessel atherosclerosis and increased risk of ischemic coronary artery disease, which in turn increases the risk of myocardial infarction. These effects, however, depend on dose and volume and are not inevitable.

Anatomy

The wall of the heart is composed of three layers: the epicardium (visceral layer of the pericardium), the myocardium, and the endocardium. The epicardium and pericardium are thin, relatively avascular layers that function to minimize friction and provide damping of cardiac contractions. These layers are particularly susceptible to radiation damage, and the response is not unlike that produced by an infection. The myocardium varies in thickness according to the site within the heart wall. The endocardium is continuous with the intima of the blood vessels, and the two layers seem to respond to irradiation in similar ways.

Radiation-induced injuries of the heart trigger a dose-related thickening of one or more layers of the heart wall. The heart valves and conduction system also may show dose-related radiation effects. In addition, both the microvasculature and the larger blood vessels of the heart, such as the coronary arteries, may undergo dose-related radiation changes. The effects of radiation on the microvasculature of the heart often form the basis for radiation injury of the cardiac components. Irradiation of the coronary arteries may lead to the most serious side effects.

Methods of Assessing Radiation-Induced Cardiac Effects

A spectrum of tests are now available to evaluate potential radiation-induced heart damage. Many tests are capable of detecting subtle, subclinical changes in cardiac function. Electrocardiography can reveal conduction abnormalities. Echocardiography can reveal changes in the thickness of the myocardium. Radionuclide angio-cardiography can reveal changes in myocardial perfusion and also can assess cardiac output changes by measurement of left ventricular ejection fraction. Exercise treadmill or bicycle ergometer testing using ^{201}Tl scintigraphy can demonstrate subclinical changes in cardiac output. Various radiographic imaging techniques, including computed tomography and magnetic resonance imaging, can identify thickening of the pericardium and pericardial effusion.

Radiation Factors Related to Cardiac Injury

Factors that influence the risk of cardiac injury resulting from radiation therapy include total dose and fraction size.

Total Dose

Stewart[27] performed a probit analysis of 318 patients treated with radiation therapy for Hodgkin's disease and derived a sigmoid dose-response curve for radiation-induced heart disease, as shown in Figure 16-3. The curve shows a steep rise in radiation-induced cardiac injury above a total dose of 40 Gy. Stewart's findings have since been confirmed by other clinical and animal studies.[14,28-32]

The dose-response curve also depends on the volume of heart irradiated. When large cardiac volumes are irradiated, as takes place in the treatment of Hodgkin's disease, doses lower than 40 Gy given over 4 weeks may induce cardiac injury. However, when small cardiac volumes are treated, as is the case in postoperative

treatment of breast cancer, doses above 40 Gy in 4 weeks may be well tolerated.[33] Thus the *tolerance dose*, the total dose causing an incidence of radiation-related cardiac injury of 5% or less, varies with the volume of heart irradiated. Small heart volumes may tolerate 60 Gy given at 1.8 to 2.0 Gy/day 5 days/week, whereas large volumes may tolerate only 40 Gy at 1.8 to 2.0 Gy/day.

Fraction Size

Fraction size is also an important determinant of the risk of radiation-induced cardiac injury. Larger doses per fraction tend to cause more cardiac damage.[33] For example, some of the highest rates of pericarditis were reported in a study of patients with Hodgkin's disease treated with anteriorly weighted fields.[28] In that study, the anterior cardiac structures received a larger dose per fraction than the midline tumor.[28] Equally weighted fields, lower total doses, and treatment of each field daily, along with the use of cardiac shielding whenever possible, have reduced the risk of cardiac damage in patients with Hodgkin's disease.[27]

Analyses of the effect of fraction size on radiation-induced heart damage are complicated because of the recent trends toward lower total dose and lower dose per fraction. Nevertheless, reviews of the available clinical data and observations of cardiac injury after fractionated irradiation of canine hearts confirm a fraction-size effect.[3,34] In a rat model assessing the effect of fractionated irradiation on the number of adrenergic receptors, myocardial norepinephrine concentration, and cardiac function, Wondergem and colleagues[29] showed a dependence of radiation-induced cardiac damage on radiation fraction size.

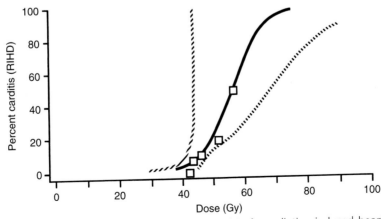

Fig. 16-3 Probit analysis of dose-response relationship for radiation-induced heart disease. The curve is derived by replotting by probit of the analysis of 318 determinant cases of Hodgkin's disease. *Squares*, Data points; *solid line*, fitted probit curve; *dashed lines*, 95% confidence limits. LD$_5$ (dose causing heart disease in 5% of patients), 43.3 Gy (95% confidence interval, 40.3 to 46.4 Gy). (From Stewart JR. *Front Radiat Ther Oncol* 1989;23:302-309.)

Effects of Irradiation on the Pericardium
Acute Pericardial Changes

Radiation-induced acute pericarditis may appear a few weeks or several years after irradiation. If pericarditis is clinically overt, the patient may present with fever, tachycardia, substernal pain, and pericardial friction rub. Pericardial effusion is common, and cardiac tamponade may develop as the effusion increases. The cardiac silhouette is widened. The echocardiogram may show inversion and flattening of the T waves, elevation of the ST segment, and decrease of the QRS segment. The course of acute pericarditis is variable. The condition is self-limited in about half of the patients who present with clinical symptoms; the remaining patients have recurrence or progression to chronic constrictive pericarditis.

The dose-time relationship for acute pericarditis has been clarified by Stewart and Fajardo.[35] Most patients with symptoms of acute pericarditis have received at least 40 Gy in 4 weeks to a major portion of the heart, yet the disease is not common even after 50 Gy given in 5 to 6 weeks.[35] This observation has led to investigation of possible contributing factors. Cardiac venous and lymphatic pathways drain to the mediastinal lymphatics, and tumor-related changes in these pathways may contribute to the formation of pericardial effusion. This may partially account for the correlation between larger mediastinal tumor size and higher risk of pericardial effusion after radiation therapy to the chest. The incidence of pericardial effusion increases rapidly with increasing dose above 50 Gy in 5 weeks.[30,36]

Some cases of postirradiation pericardial effusion are linked to myxedema, which may develop after thyroid irradiation. Rogoway and colleagues[37] suggested that prolonged high iodide levels after lymphangiography provoke thyroid hyperplasia and thus increase the radiosensitivity of the thyroid gland. Therefore, in patients with pericardial effusion, thyroid function should be evaluated before the effusion is attributed solely to the effects of radiation on the heart. However, studies in humans and in animal models confirm that most cardiac effects of radiation are a result of direct cellular damage to the pericardium, the epicardium, and the blood vessels of these layers and are not due to indirect mechanisms.

Chronic Constrictive Pericarditis

Chronic constrictive pericarditis usually manifests as chronic constrictive changes associated with myocardial and endocardial fibrosis or with varying degrees of effusion. The latent period from the beginning of radiation therapy to the onset of chronic pericarditis varies from 6 months to several years. Chronic pericarditis may or may not be preceded by acute pericarditis.

Symptoms and signs of chronic pericarditis may include dyspnea, chest pain, venous distention, and pleural effusion. Paradoxical pulse and fever may be present. The electrocardiogram may show a decreased QRS voltage, flat or inverted T waves, and elevation of the ST segment. The cardiac silhouette is enlarged. The morphologic changes are not specific for radiation damage. The pericardium is thickened as a result of deposition of collagen. The myocardium and endocardium are often fused or adherent to each other, with a fibrinous exudate. The pericardium may be adherent to the heart and pleura. The blood vessels in the pericardium show characteristic subendothelial connective-tissue proliferation. The underlying myocardium usually appears to be normal on gross examination but may not be microscopically or functionally normal.

Although the etiology of chronic constrictive pericarditis is the same as that of acute pericarditis, fewer than half of patients with chronic constrictive pericarditis have a history of previous acute pericarditis. Overall, about 5% of patients who receive more than 40 Gy to at least 50% of the heart will develop chronic pericarditis.[38] The treatment of chronic constrictive pericarditis depends on the severity of the condition and consists of antipyretics in the case of fever, pericardiocentesis in the case of tamponade, and pericardiectomy in the case of severe constrictive symptoms.

Effects of Irradiation on the Myocardium

Three components of the myocardium are important in the response of the myocardium to irradiation: the vascular component, the connective tissue component, and the muscle component.[2,3] Gillette and colleagues[2,3] found that the vasculature of the heart was diminished by all fractionation schedules with a variety of total doses of radiation. The higher the fraction size and the higher the total dose, the greater the decrease in vasculature. The amount of connective tissue in the heart, which is distributed between the muscle bundles throughout the heart, increases with increasing dose up to a maximum of about 44 Gy at 4 Gy/fraction, after which further increases in dose produce smaller increases in connective tissue, both at 3 months and at 6 months after irradiation. Subsequent studies of fractionated irradiation of the beagle heart confirmed early and late myocardial damage, which was manifested as increased heart rates, increased heart wall thickness, and conduction abnormalities (early effects) and thinning of the cardiac wall and fibrosis with functional abnormalities (late effects).[34]

Cardiac and pulmonary function are highly interdependent. When both the heart and the lung are included in the radiation field, subclinical levels of radiation-induced myocardial injury may become clinically manifest as a consequence of radiation-induced changes in the pulmonary vasculature. Studies in rat and canine models have shown radiation-induced reduction of pulmonary capillary volume, which causes an increase in pulmonary artery pressure.[14,39] The radiation-damaged heart may not be able to overcome this increased resistance. Thus some of the volume effects previously noted[38] (see the section on "Total Dose" earlier in this chapter) may be partially related to the amount of lung irradiated at the same time as the heart.

Studies in rat models[15,39] using autoradiography with tritium-labeled thymidine have shown that radiation also damages the myocardial capillary network, with this damage followed by compensatory proliferation after a latent period of 6 to 8 months. These changes precede myocardial degeneration, but the findings cannot be linked to hypoxia or radiation-induced mitotic death of endothelial cells alone.

Early reductions in α- and β-adrenergic receptors followed by up-regulation of the receptors, which are located in endothelial cells, have been observed.[15,40] In the early period after radiation therapy, catecholamines may be released from sympathetic nerve endings, leading to depletion of catecholamines and down-regulation of the receptors. The subsequent up-regulation of α- and β-adrenergic receptors seen in later stages may be caused by prolonged decrease in sympathetic stimulation. The release of catecholamines could be due to a direct effect of radiation on the sympathetic nerve endings or could be mediated by radiation damage to the capillary network and resultant local hypoxia. The relationships between the vasculature, connective tissue, and muscle of the myocardium at various times after irradiation are quite complex, and additional sequential studies are necessary to better understand the mechanism of radiation-induced myocardial injury.

The lack of mitotic activity in the cardiac muscle makes the myocardium one of the more radioresistant tissues and suggests that most of the changes seen in heavily irradiated myocardium result from radiation-induced vascular changes. Direct radiation injury of the muscle fiber is presumed to be a minor factor, but the degree of fibrosis between the muscle bundles does change with dose and with fractionation.[3,34] This connective tissue that forms in response to radiation is diffuse in distribution and does not resemble the fibrosis seen after an infarct. This radiation-induced fibrosis may not necessarily be secondary to small vessel occlusion and may not parallel the severity of vascular occlusion.

After total body irradiation in the rhesus monkey, high plasma levels of atrial natriuretic peptide were associated with a change in cardiac dimensions and predicted cardiac damage.[41] Serial measurements of atrial natriuretic peptide levels after cardiac radiation exposure in humans may serve as a surrogate marker for cardiac toxicity. Procollagen I and III levels also may become elevated about 6 months after heart irradiation, corresponding to the appearance of fibrosis in myocardial connective tissue.[42]

Radiation-induced cardiac effects presenting as overt clinical syndromes were initially used to estimate the incidence of radiation-induced heart damage and dose-response relationships. When more accurate assessment of cardiac function became possible, mild, occult abnormalities of heart function could be detected, suggesting that radiation-induced cardiac injury is not a threshold phenomenon. In one early study, left ventricular ejection fraction (LVEF) was reduced to 50% in clinically asymptomatic patients who received more than 35 Gy to the heart during mediastinal irradiation for Hodgkin's disease.[31] Gottdiener and colleagues[32] observed decreased systolic left ventricular function and reserve at rest in asymptomatic patients 5 to 15 years after irradiation for Hodgkin's disease in which an anteriorly weighted mediastinal field was used to deliver 50 to 55 Gy to the midheart. Abnormalities on radionuclide angiography were found in 24% of patients 25 to 35 years old with Hodgkin's disease who were treated with 40 Gy in 4 weeks with a mantle field.[16] Gyenes and colleagues,[43] using bicycle ergometry stress testing with Tc 99m sestamibi scintigraphy, found radiation-induced microvascular myocardial damage in some breast cancer patients who received left-sided internal mammary node irradiation. Several authors have described subtle, clinically silent T-wave changes on electrocardiography after left-sided internal mammary irradiation for breast cancer.[44,45] It should be emphasized that, although the incidence of abnormalities detected by electrocardiography was high, the functional effect at the radiation dose levels used was negligible.

In patients previously treated with doxorubicin (Adriamycin), radiation can worsen the drug's cardiac side effects. The cardiac effects of doxorubicin, which are expressed in some patients but not others, appear about 6 months after treatment and consist of a diffuse cardiomyopathy that can lead to congestive heart failure. The cardiac vessels are usually normal. The myocardium shows profound degeneration of the muscle cells, combined with interstitial edema and fibrosis. These effects can be worsened by radiation therapy. Care should be taken to limit the cardiac dose and the volume irradiated after doxorubicin has been given.

Effects of Irradiation on the Conduction System and Heart Valves

Conduction abnormalities, such as AV block, occur in up to 5% of patients after mediastinal irradiation that includes the heart; these abnormalities are thought to be related to late myocardial fibrosis.[38,46]

Valvular defects, often subclinical, may be found in 15% to 20% of patients who undergo mediastinal irradiation that includes the heart. Autopsy studies of hearts exhibiting radiation injury (e.g., after mediastinal irradiation for Hodgkin's disease) have shown that any of the four heart valves may be affected, but clinical evidence of valvular dysfunction is evident in only about half of the valves, with damage identified at autopsy.[47] Successful replacement of radiation-damaged valves is possible.[48] As is the case for radiation-induced injury to the other components of the heart, valvular radiation damage is related to dose and is rarely seen below doses of 30 Gy.

Effects of Irradiation on the Coronary Arteries

The effects of irradiation on the cardiac blood vessels are the same as the effects of irradiation on blood vessels elsewhere in the body (see the previous section on "Blood Vessels"). However, radiation-induced injury of cardiac vessels is more serious than radiation-induced vascular injury in most other sites and is therefore worthy of special attention. No specific vessels are affected more often than others. The consequence of radiation-induced vessel occlusion is the same as vessel occlusion from other causes. The incidence of infarction after conventional doses of radiation is poorly defined but has become better elucidated over the past several years. The clinical experience with the consequences of coronary irradiation is reviewed here.

Our understanding of the relationship between coronary artery disease and prior cardiac irradiation continues to evolve. Although the issue remains somewhat controversial, several recent studies[32,43,49,50] that used sophisticated cardiac function testing to assess the effects of incidental cardiac irradiation in large groups of patients have clarified the risk of coronary vessel damage when modern radiation therapy techniques are used. Early reviews summarized case reports of precocious coronary artery disease in long-term survivors who had undergone mediastinal irradiation for Hodgkin's disease and other malignancies.[17,18] The number of affected patients was small, and many long-term survivors were without apparent coronary artery disease. However, reproducible postirradiation coronary artery disease had been observed in animals,[17,39] and thus investigators realized that the risk of coronary artery disease in humans might be discovered to be higher with longer-term follow-up.

The early case reports showed that the mechanism of coronary artery disease was accelerated coronary atherosclerosis and fibrosis. Some of the cases of coronary artery disease after chest irradiation occurred in older patients with predisposing metabolic factors or familial risk for coronary disease. However, some cases occurred in young patients with no predisposing risk factors. Angiographic and pathologic findings suggested a localized process limited to the portion of the heart included in the radiation field. Concern was expressed that these occult early effects would predispose patients to earlier or more severe coronary artery disease.

Reviews of long-term follow-up information on patients who underwent irradiation of the mediastinum for treatment of Hodgkin's disease, breast cancer, or seminoma have reported on the risk of coronary artery disease and death resulting from acute myocardial infarction. Several factors make interpretation and comparison of these reports difficult. In some of these studies, the risk of coronary artery disease was compared to the risk in a control population that did not receive mediastinal irradiation. Some studies reported the total number of deaths from acute myocardial infarction in the treated population, whereas others reported the percentage of total deaths attributable to acute myocardial infarction. The risk of subclinical or nonfatal coronary artery disease could not always be discerned from the reviews. Further, some reviews were based on information gleaned from death certificates, which may be misleading. These studies of radiation-induced coronary artery disease are reviewed in the following sections.

Irradiation for Breast Cancer

In older series, postmastectomy radiation therapy for treatment of tumors of the left breast was associated with an increased risk of death resulting from heart disease.[19,20] Much of this experience was based on radiation given after radical mastectomy. A recent meta-analysis of the effects of such postmastectomy irradiation showed a significantly increased risk of death resulting from heart disease in patients who survived at least 10 years after the treatment ended.[21]

A population-based tumor-registry analysis of 55,000 Swedish breast cancer patients also suggested an association between death resulting from heart disease and irradiation of the left breast.[19] However, no information about radiation therapy was present in the registry data, and the authors simply assumed that, because about 50% of the patients who underwent mastectomy were irradiated, the higher risk of cardiac mortality in patients with tumors of the left breast was caused by irradiation. Similar problems with study design leave in question the association between non–breast-cancer deaths and radiation therapy reported in a recent overview of randomized clinical trials.[22] The review conclusions were limited because the authors were not able to analyze specifically for cardiac death and for inclusion of postmastectomy irradiation techniques that included much larger volumes of the heart than are included with breast irradiation after breast-conserving surgery, which seems to be associated with a lower risk of cardiac injury.

The volume of heart included in the radiation field is directly related to the radiation technique used. Several investigators have shown that modern techniques of breast irradiation, especially techniques used after conservative breast surgery, result in significant volume sparing that reduces the risk of cardiac injury.[51] Cowen and colleagues[49] used angioscintigraphy to evaluate the effect on late myocardial damage of mixed-beam (photons and electrons) irradiation of left-sided internal mammary nodes and found no perfusion defects. In a series of 231 patients treated with conservative surgery and postoperative irradiation of the left or right breast, Hardenbergh and colleagues[52] reported no cardiac events at a median follow-up time of 53 months, even in the subset of patients treated with adjuvant doxorubicin-containing chemotherapy. In a 12-year follow-up study of 1624 patients with early-stage breast cancer treated with conservative surgery and breast irradiation using modern techniques, the risk of death resulting from heart disease was not increased in patients with primary tumors of the left breast.[23]

Irradiation for Hodgkin's Disease

Compared with radiation therapy for breast cancer, radiation therapy for Hodgkin's disease typically involves a somewhat lower cardiac dose (35 to 45 Gy in 4 to 5 weeks) but often includes a larger cardiac volume. In older reports of radiation therapy using anteriorly weighted fields, the cardiac doses often exceeded 50 Gy. With modern techniques using partial transmission block shielding of the heart, shrinking field technique, or interrupted therapy, the volume of heart exposed can be high, but the actual or biological dose can be low. As is true for breast cancer, more recent analyses reflecting the use of newer radiation therapy techniques suggest a lower incidence of cardiac injury.

Boivin and colleagues[24] documented relative risks of cardiac death and myocardial infarction of 1.87 and 2.56, respectively, in 4665 patients treated with radiation therapy for Hodgkin's disease.[24] Various radiation techniques were used, and the determinant information was provided by death certificates. The observations in this study were in contrast to the findings in an earlier study by Boivin and Hutchinson[25] based on 900 patients, which showed no increase in the risk of acute myocardial infarction. No other factors, including age, changed the risk, except for treatment with older techniques that did not spare the heart instead of newer techniques that did spare the heart. A review of 2232 Hodgkin's disease patients treated at Stanford disclosed a relative risk of death from heart disease of 3.1.[26] Cosset and colleagues[53] reviewed 499 patients with Hodgkin's disease treated with 25-MeV photons and 138 patients with Hodgkin's disease treated without mediastinal irradiation and found a 10-year cumulative incidence of acute myocardial infarcts of 3.9% in the irradiation group, compared with no myocardial infarcts in the no-irradiation group ($P < 0.05$).

More recent studies do not confirm these findings. In a review of 145 patients with early-stage Hodgkin's disease, only some of whom had undergone mediastinal irradiation, no significant difference in the incidence of coronary artery disease was found between the irradiated and nonirradiated groups.[54] To assess myocardial perfusion in asymptomatic patients who were long-term survivors after treatment with radiation therapy for early-stage Hodgkin's disease, Constine and colleagues[50] performed radionuclide angiography and measured LVEF, among other variables. Among the 50 patients assessed, the median cardiac dose was 35 Gy (range, 18.5 to 47.5 Gy). No significant impairment of LVEF or myocardial perfusion was found, although modest abnormalities of uncertain significance were identified. Patients treated to the entire cardiac volume demonstrated reduced but normal LVEF compared with patients treated to subtotal cardiac volumes. No physiologic or clinical impacts were associated with these effects in repeat measurements up to 3 years. The authors noted that longer follow-up was warranted.

Irradiation for Seminoma

Lederman and colleagues[55] reported a 3.4% incidence of death resulting from acute myocardial infarction in a group of 58 patients with seminoma treated with mediastinal irradiation to 24 Gy, compared with no cases of infarction in 61 patients with seminoma treated to the abdomen only. The relative risk of infarction was 1.97 ($P = 0.019$); however, this risk was not different from the risk in their large Framingham normal population study.[56] Although the findings of Peckham and McElwain[57] tend to support these findings, the reports of Willan and McGowan[58] do not.

Summary of Studies

In summary, some older series show a modest but significant increase in the risk of acute myocardial infarction after mediastinal irradiation, a risk that may be related to dose and volume. Newer reviews report lower risk levels of cardiac damage and less frequent functional effects among patients treated for breast cancer and Hodgkin's disease. For Hodgkin's disease, it seems that the previously reported increased risk of death resulting from heart disease may relate to use of older radiation therapy techniques involving higher total doses and no cardiac shielding. The use of death certificates to determine endpoints and the absence of clear information about radiation techniques render these findings inconclusive. Treatment with adequate heart sparing yields minor subclinical functional effects. Because acute myocardial infarction has been reported at doses below 40 Gy, consideration of reducing the cardiac dose or the volume irradiated should be a routine part of treatment planning for all patients receiving mediastinal irradiation—especially young patients with a good probability of long-term survival.

Coronary Irradiation to Prevent Restenosis

An in-depth discussion of coronary irradiation to prevent restenosis is beyond the scope of this chapter. However, the recent emergence of endovascular brachytherapy and external-beam irradiation as effective means of reducing the risk of coronary artery restenosis after angioplasty or stenting for atherosclerotic narrowing of the coronary arteries warrants discussion here of the relevant radiobiological mechanisms of action. It is somewhat ironic that incidental fractionated irradiation of the coronary arteries in doses used for treatment of chest malignancy can cause coronary stenosis by accelerating the atherosclerotic process, whereas modest single fractions of radiation can prevent the response to angioplasty that causes restenosis.

Findings from animal studies suggest that there is no reason to believe that irradiation reverses established coronary stenosis; however, irradiation is thought to prevent the overexuberant healing response associated with balloon injury or stent implantation. Studies in animal models suggest that the activated adventitial macrophages or monocytes are responsible for initiating the arterial neointimal hyperplasia and vascular remodeling that occur after angioplasty.[59] This reaction is the prerequisite for the initiation and perpetuation of atheromatous thickening, whether incited by balloon injury or occurring as a natural process. A cytokine cascade, including platelet-derived growth factor, is likely responsible for initiating the macrophage response.[60] Smooth muscle cells also are stimulated to migrate and proliferate. Irradiation delivered immediately after balloon injury is most likely effective because the macrophage population is very radiosensitive; irradiation short-circuits this process.

Because macrophages are quite radiosensitive, large radiation doses are not necessary. For example, in the Scripps Coronary Radiation Trial to Inhibit Proliferation Post Stenting, a placebo-controlled randomized trial, a 69% reduction in the restenosis rate was reported at 6 months of follow-up.[61] At the time of angioplasty, ^{192}Ir seeds were temporarily inserted into the dilated coronary vessel site through a catheter and held in position until the protocol-specified dose was delivered. The average minimal dose to the leading edge of the intima was 7.3 Gy; the average maximal dose was 26.5 Gy. For a more detailed discussion of this topic, the interested reader is directed to the list of additional readings at the end of this chapter.

Intravascular brachytherapy also may be used to prevent restenosis after angioplasty for atherosclerotic peripheral vascular disease and to prevent stenosis of peripheral vascular access vessels.[62,63]

Prevention of Radiation-Induced Heart Damage

Over the past two decades, technical innovations in the delivery of radiation therapy have permitted significant reduction of the volume of heart exposed to radiation during treatment of intrathoracic, breast, and chest wall tumors. In turn, the incidence of radiation-induced heart damage with treatment of these tumors has been substantially reduced.[23,49,50,52,54] For example, in postoperative radiation therapy for breast cancer, the use of tangential chest wall fields instead of anteroposterior fields to encompass the internal mammary nodes reduces the volume of heart exposed to radiation and is associated with no increase in cardiac damage.[23] Three-dimensional treatment planning, noncoplanar field arrangements, and intensity-modulated radiation therapy also have been shown to reduce both the cardiac radiation dose and the volume treated.[64,65] Chen and colleagues[66] showed that simple respiratory maneuvers, such as inspiration during radiation delivery, can reduce the volume of heart included within radiation fields by up to 40%. Cardioprotection with an antioxidant regimen or with amifostine, an aminothiol, seems promising in preliminary clinical trials.[67,68] It is likely that techniques such as these will significantly improve our ability to spare the heart during radiation therapy and further reduce the incidence and severity of cardiac damage.

Management Strategies for Patients at Risk for Radiation-Induced Heart Damage

In view of the subtle functional effects of irradiation on the heart that can occur after conventional radiation doses, techniques to limit the dose to the heart and the volume of heart irradiated are especially important in patients expected to have long-term survival (e.g., patients with Hodgkin's disease or breast cancer). Careful follow-up of patients who undergo cardiac irradiation in any form is mandatory. The evaluation should include a careful clinical history, with special attention to signs and symptoms that may be transient and illusory, and attention to cardiac diameter and silhouette on follow-up chest radiography, electrocardiography, echocardiography, and periodic radionuclide angiography. In the case of transient episodes of overt pericardial effusion, pericardiocentesis and treatment with an anti-inflammatory agent may be sufficient. However, chronic recurrent effusions, especially with the development of constrictive changes and tamponade, may require therapeutic pericardiectomy.[69,70]

REFERENCES

1. Fajardo LF. *Pathology of Radiation Injury*. New York, NY: Masson; 1982:186-200.

2. Gillette EL, Maurer GD, Severin GA. Endothelial repair of radiation damage following beta irradiation. *Radiology* 1975;116:175-177.

3. Gillette EL, McChesney SL, Hoopes PJ. Isoeffect curves for radiation-induced cardiomyopathy in the dog. *Int J Radiat Oncol Biol Phys* 1985;11:2091-2097.

4. Reinhold HS, Keyeux A, Dunjic A, et al. The influence of radiation on blood vessels and circulation. XII. Discussion and conclusions. *Curr Top Radiat Res Q* 1974 Jun;10:185-198.

5. Rubin P, Casarett GW. *Clinical Radiation Pathology.* Philadelphia, Pa: WB Saunders; 1968.

6. Van den Brenk HAS. The effect of ionizing radiations on capillary sprouting and vascular remodeling in the regenerating repair blastema observed in the rabbit ear chamber. *Radiology* 1959;81:859-884.

7. Hilmas DE, Gillette EL. Tumor microvasculature following fractionated x irradiation. *Radiology* 1975;116:165-169.

8. Lindsay S, Kohn HI, Dakin RL, et al. Arteriosclerosis due to roentgen radiation. *Circ Res* 1962;10:51-60.

9. Roscher AA, Steele BC, Woodward JS. Carotid artery rupture after irradiation of the larynx. *Arch Otolaryngol* 1966;83:472-476.

10. Asscher AW. The delayed effects of renal irradiation. *Clin Radiol* 1964;15:320-325.

11. Silverberg GD, Britt RH, Goffinet DR. Radiation-induced carotid artery disease. *Cancer* 1978;41:130-137.

12. Taber P, Kosobkin MT, Gooding LT, et al. Growth of the abdominal aorta and renal arteries in childhood. *Radiology* 1972;102:129-134.

13. Colguhoun J. Hypoplasia of the abdominal aorta following therapeutic irradiation in infancy. *Radiology* 1966;86:454-456.

14. McChesney SL, Gillette EL, Powers BE, et al. Early radiation response of the canine heart and lung. *Radiat Res* 1991;125:34-40.

15. Lauk S, Trott KR. Endothelial cell proliferation in the rat heart following local heart irradiation. *Int J Radiat Biol* 1990;57:1017-1030.

16. Morgan G, Freeman A, McLean R, et al. Late cardiac, thyroid, and pulmonary sequelae of mantle radiotherapy for Hodgkin's disease. *Int J Radiat Oncol Biol Phys* 1985;11:1925-1931.

17. Fajardo LF. Radiation-induced coronary artery disease. *Chest* 1977;71:563-564.

18. Kopelson G, Herwig KJ: The etiologies of coronary artery disease in cancer patients. *Int J Radiat Oncol Biol Phys* 1978;4:895-906.

19. Rutqvist LE, Lax I, Fornander T, et al. Cardiovascular mortality in a randomized trial of adjuvant radiation therapy versus surgery alone in primary breast cancer. *Int J Radiat Oncol Biol Phys* 1992;22:887-896.

20. Host H, Brennhovd IO, Loeb M. Postoperative radiotherapy in breast cancer: long-term results from the Oslo study. *Int J Radiat Oncol Biol Phys* 1986;12:727-732.

21. Cuzick J, Stewart H, Rutqvist L, et al. Cause-specific mortality in long-term survivors of breast cancer who participated in trials of radiotherapy. *J Clin Oncol* 1994;12:447-453.

22. Early Breast Cancer Trialists' Collaborative Group. Effects of radiotherapy and surgery in early breast cancer: an overview of the randomized trials. *N Engl J Med* 1995;333:1444-1455.

23. Nixon AJ, Manola J, Gelman R, et al. No long-term increase in cardiac-related mortality after breast-conserving surgery and radiation therapy using modern techniques. *J Clin Oncol* 1998;16:1374-1379.

24. Boivin JF, Hutchinson GB, Lubin JH, et al. Coronary artery disease mortality in patients treated for Hodgkin's disease. *Cancer* 1992;69:1241-1247.

25. Boivin J, Hutchinson GB. Coronary heart disease mortality after irradiation for Hodgkin's disease. *Cancer* 1982;49:2470-2475.

26. Hancock S, Donaldson S, Hoppe R. Cardiac disease following treatment of Hodgkin's disease in children and adolescents. *J Clin Oncol* 1993;11:1208-1215.

27. Stewart JR. Normal tissue tolerance to irradiation of the cardiovascular system. *Front Radiat Ther Oncol* 1989;23:302-309.

28. Byhardt RW, Brace K, Ruckdeschel JC, et al. Dose and treatment factors in radiation related pericardial effusion associated with a mantle technique for Hodgkin's disease. *Cancer* 1975;35:795-802.

29. Wondergem J, Franken NA, van der Laarse A, et al. Changes in cardiac performance and sympathetic stimulation during and after fractionated radiotherapy in a rat model. *Radiother Oncol* 1996;38:33-40.

30. Mill WB, Baglan RJ, Kurichety P, et al. Symptomatic radiation-induced pericarditis in Hodgkin's disease. *Int J Radiat Oncol Biol Phys* 1984;10:2061-2065.

31. Gomez GA, Park JJ, Panahon AM, et al. Heart size and function after radiation therapy to the mediastinum in patients with Hodgkin's disease. *Cancer Treat Rep* 1983;67:1099-1103.

32. Gottdiener JS, Katin MJ, Borer JS, et al. Late cardiac effects of therapeutic mediastinal irradiation: assessment by echocardiography and radionuclide angiography. *N Engl J Med* 1983;308:569-572.

33. Stewart JR, Fajardo L. Radiation-induced heart disease: an update. *Prog Cardiovasc Dis* 1984;27:173-194.

34. McChesney SL, Gillette EL, Orton EC. Canine cardiomyopathy after whole heart and partial lung irradiation. *Int J Radiat Oncol Biol Phys* 1988;14:1169-1174.

35. Stewart R, Fajardo LF. Dose response in human and experimental radiation-induced heart disease. *Radiology* 1971;99:403-408.

36. Applefeld MM, Cole JF, Pollock SH, et al. The late appearance of chronic pericardial disease in patients treated by radiation therapy for Hodgkin's disease. *Ann Intern Med* 1981;94:338-341.

37. Rogoway WM, Finkelstein S, Rosenberg SA, et al. Myxedema developing after lymphangiography and neck irradiation. *Clin Res* 1966;14:133.

38. Girinsky T, Cosset JM. Pulmonary and cardiac late effects of ionizing radiations alone or combined with chemotherapy. *Cancer Radiother* 1997;1:735-743.

39. Geist BJ, Lauk S, Bornhausen M, et al. Physiologic consequences of local heart irradiation in rats. *Int J Radiat Oncol Biol Phys* 1990;18:1107-1113.

40. Lauk S, Bohm M, Feiler G, et al. Increased number of cardiac adrenergic receptors following local heart irradiation. *Radiat Res* 1989;119:157-165.

41. Wondergem J, Persons K, Zurcher C, et al. Changes in circulating atrial natriuretic peptide in relation to the cardiac status of Rhesus monkeys after total-body irradiation. *Radiother Oncol* 1999;53:67-75.

42. Kruse JJ, Bart CI, Visser A, et al. Changes in transforming growth factor-beta (TGF-beta 1), procollagen types I and II mRNA in the rat heart after irradiation. *Int J Radiat Biol* 1999;75:1429-1436.

43. Gyenes G, Fornander T, Carlens P, et al. Detection of radiation-induced myocardial damage by technetium-99m sestamibi scintigraphy. *Eur J Nucl Med* 1997;24:286-292.

44. Wehr M, Rosskopf BG, Pittner PM, et al. The effect of radiation therapy on the heart in patients with left-sided mammary carcinoma. Presented at: International Association for Breast Cancer Research; March 20, 1983; Denver, Co.

45. Strender L, Lindahl J, Larson L. Incidence of heart disease and functional significance of changes in the electrocardiogram 10 years after radiotherapy for breast cancer. *Cancer* 1986;57:929-934.

46. Kaplan BM, Miller AJ, Bharati S, et al. Complete AV block following mediastinal radiation therapy: electrocardiographic and pathologic correlation and review of the world literature. *J Interv Card Electrophysiol* 1997;1:175-188.

47. Veinot JP, Edwards WD. Pathology of radiation-induced heart disease: a surgical and autopsy study of 27 cases. *Hum Pathol* 1996;27:766-773.

48. Mittal S, Berko B, Bavaria J, et al. Radiation-induced cardiovascular dysfunction. *Am J Cardiol* 1996;78:114-115.

49. Cowen D, Gonzague-Casabianca L, Brenot-Rossi I, et al. Thallium-201 perfusion scintigraphy in the evaluation of late myocardial

damage in left-side breast cancer treated with adjuvant radiotherapy. *Int J Radiat Oncol Biol Phys* 1998;41:809-815.

50. Constine LS, Schwartz RG, Savage DE, et al. Cardiac function, perfusion, and morbidity in irradiated long-term survivors of Hodgkin's disease. *Int J Radiat Oncol Biol Phys* 1997;39:897-906.

51. Fuller SA, Haybittle JL, Smith REA, et al. Cardiac doses in postoperative breast irradiation. *Radiother Oncol* 1992;25:19-24.

52. Hardenbergh PH, Recht A, Gollamudi S, et al. Treatment-related toxicity from a randomized trial of the sequencing of doxorubicin and radiation therapy in patients treated for early stage breast cancer. *Int J Radiat Oncol Biol Phys* 1999;45:69-72.

53. Cosset JM, Henry-Amar M, Pellae-Cosset B, et al. Pericarditis and myocardial infarctions after Hodgkin's disease therapy. *Int J Radiat Oncol Biol Phys* 1991;21:447-449.

54. Vlachaki MT, Ha CS, Hagemeister FB, et al. Long-term outcome of treatment for Ann Arbor stage 1 Hodgkin's disease: patterns of failure, late toxicity and second malignancies. *Int J Radiat Oncol Biol Phys* 1997;39:609-616.

55. Lederman GS, Sheldon TA, Chaffey JT, et al. Cardiac disease after mediastinal irradiation for seminoma. *Cancer* 1987;60: 772-776.

56. Kannel WB, McGee D, Gordon T. A general cardiovascular risk profile: the Framingham study. *Am J Cardiol* 1976;38:46-51.

57. Peckham MJ, McElwain TJ. Radiotherapy of testicular tumors. *Proc R Soc Med* 1974;67:300-303.

58. Willan BD, McGowan DG. Seminoma of the testis: a 22-year experience with radiation therapy. *Int J Radiat Oncol Biol Phys* 1985;11:1769-1775.

59. Rubin P, Williams JP, Riggs PN, et al. Cellular and molecular mechanisms of radiation inhibition of restenosis. Part I: role of the macrophage and platelet-derived growth factor. *Int J Radiat Oncol Biol Phys* 1998;40:929-941.

60. Libby P, Schwartz D, Brogi E, et al. A cascade model for restenosis. A special case of atherosclerosis progression. *Circulation* 1992; 86(suppl III):47-52.

61. Teirstein PS, Massullo V, Jani S, et al. Catheter-based radiotherapy to inhibit restenosis after coronary stenting. *N Engl J Med* 1997; 336:1697-1703.

62. Tripuraneni P, Giap H, Jani S. Endovascular brachytherapy for peripheral vascular disease. *Semin Radiat Oncol* 1999;9:190-202.

63. Parikh S, Nori D. Radiation therapy to prevent stenosis of peripheral vascular accesses. *Semin Radiat Oncol* 1999;9:144-154.

64. Ragazzi G, Cattaneo GM, Fiorino C, et al. Use of dose-volume histograms and biophysical models to compare 2D and 3D irradiation techniques for non-small cell lung cancer. *Br J Radiol* 1999;72:279-288.

65. Smitt MC, Li SD, Shostak CA, et al. Breast conserving radiation therapy: potential of inverse planning with intensity modulation. *Radiology* 1997;203:871-876.

66. Chen MH, Chuang ML, Bornstein BA, et al. Impact of respiratory maneuvers on cardiac volume within left-breast radiation portals. *Circulation* 1997;96:3269-3272.

67. Wagdi P, Fluri M, Aeschbacher B, et al. Cardioprotection in patients undergoing chemo- and/or radiotherapy for neoplastic disease. A pilot study. *Jpn Heart J* 1996;37:353-359.

68. Capizzi RL. The preclinical basis for broad-spectrum selective cytoprotection of normal tissues from cytotoxic therapies by amifostine (Ethyol). *Eur J Cancer* 1996;32A(suppl 4):S5-S16.

69. Morton DL, Glancy DO, Joseph WL. Management of patients with radiation-induced pericarditis with effusion. *Chest* 1973;64:291-297.

70. Steinberg I. Effusive constrictive pericarditis. *Am J Cardiol* 1967;19: 434-439.

ADDITIONAL READINGS

Cohn KE, Stewart JR, Fajardo LF, et al. Heart disease following radiation. *Medicine* 1967;46:281-298.

Crocker I. Radiation therapy to prevent coronary artery restenosis. *Semin Radiat Oncol* 1999;9:134-143.

Eltringham JR, Fajardo LJ, Stewart JR. Adriamycin cardiomyopathy: enhanced cardiac damage in rabbits and combined drug and cardiac irradiation. *Radiology* 1975;115:471-472.

Miller AJ. Some observations concerning pericardial effusions and the relationship to the venous and lymphatic circulation of the heart. *Lymphology* 1970;2:76-78.

Poussin-Rosillo H, Nisce LZ, Lee BJ. Complications of total nodal irradiation of Hodgkin's disease, stages III and IV. *Cancer* 1978;42: 437-441.

Rosen EM, Fan S, Goldberg ID, et al. Biological basis of radiation sensitivity. Part I: factors governing radiation tolerance. *Oncology* 2000; 14:543-550.

Rostock R, Siegelman S, Lenhard R, et al. Thoracic CT scanning for mediastinal Hodgkin's disease: results and therapeutic implications. *Int J Radiat Oncol Biol Phys* 1983;9:1451-1457.

Rubin P, Soni A, Williams JP. The molecular and cellular biologic basis for the radiation treatment of benign proliferative diseases. *Semin Radiat Oncol* 1999;9:203-214.

Stewart JR, Cohn KE, Fajardo LF, et al. Radiation-induced heart disease. *Radiology* 1967;89:302-310.

Stewart R, Fajardo LF. Radiation-induced heart disease. In: Vaeth JM, ed. *Radiation Effect and Tolerance, Human Tissue.* Baltimore, Md: University Park Press; 1972.

CHAPTER 17

The Lung and Thymus

Ritsuko Komaki, Elizabeth L. Travis, and James D. Cox

RESPONSE OF THE TRACHEA AND LUNG TO IRRADIATION

Thoracic irradiation is an important part of the therapy for many types of cancer, including esophageal cancer, breast cancer, and lung cancer. More than 50% of patients with these types of cancer will receive radiation therapy at some point during the management of their disease. Undiseased parts of the lung will, by necessity, receive some exposure as part of these treatments, and the lung is, in fact, the dose-limiting tissue in the treatment of these malignant neoplasms. Optimal treatment planning requires knowledge of the effects of radiation on the normal lung and other normal structures within the treatment field. Although nearly a century has passed since radiation pneumonitis and fibrosis were first described by Evans and Leucutia,[1] these two side effects of pulmonary irradiation remain unable to be circumvented or effectively treated, and they continue to limit the effective treatment of lung cancer.

Normal Lung

The normal lung can be divided into two major functional sections, the non-gas exchange unit and the gas exchange, or respiratory, unit. The first is a system of branching and bifurcating conducting airways, the tracheobronchial tree, which consists of all of the conducting airways from the trachea to the nonconducting bronchioles. The main function of these airways is simply to transport air into and out of the lung. The respiratory unit begins at the ramification of the terminal bronchioles and includes the respiratory bronchioles and the alveolar ducts, which open into the alveolar sacs, each of which bears numerous alveoli, the actual sites of gas exchange. The number of alveoli increases along the whole length of the respiratory unit; thus gas exchange occurs along the entire length of the respiratory unit.

The alveoli are thin-walled structures bound on one side by the alveolar epithelium and on the other by capillaries. The alveolar epithelium consists of two cell types—type I and type II—which together form a continuous surface covering the basement membrane; this surface forms the interface with the air spaces of the lung. Type I cells are squamous, flat, and are normally devoid of organelles. Their attenuated cytoplasmic extensions allow them to cover several adjacent alveoli, providing efficient gas exchange. Type I cells have little capacity to respond to injury; therefore, when they are damaged, they must be replaced by the second surface epithelial cell, the type II cell. Unlike type I cells, which are difficult to identify under the light microscope because of their attenuated cytoplasm, type II cells are easily identified in normal lung tissue by their distinct cuboidal shape, their vacuolated cytoplasm, and their localization at the corners of the alveolar walls. Type II cells synthesize and secrete surfactant, the lipid–protein complex that prevents atelectasis at low lung volumes by reducing surface tension at the air-alveolar interface. In addition to their major functional role in pulmonary function, type II cells are the progenitor cells during normal cell turnover and after injury. The type II cells can divide and differentiate into type I cells or proliferate to replenish their own population, thus restoring normal tissue structure and function. Type II cells are also actively involved in the transport of sodium ions to control fluid balance in the alveolar space. The alveolar epithelium rests on a basement membrane, on the other side of which are the endothelial cells that make up the capillaries of the pulmonary vasculature. Other cell types normally present in the lung are pulmonary macrophages and fibroblasts, both of which are important in pulmonary repair after injury.

Response of the Lung to Irradiation

The lower respiratory tract is composed of many types of tissues, some of which tolerate radiation well and others of which are relatively sensitive. The trachea and bronchi are lined with a ciliated columnar epithelium that is shed only at high radiation doses. This reaction was emphasized when Lacassagne[2] directed a beam sufficient to produce a loss of esophageal epithelium to a rabbit's mediastinum, producing noticeable early macroscopic change in the tracheal lining. Microscopic changes consist of thickening of the epithelium and an increased number of goblet cells. These changes are accompanied by a decrease in ciliary function and a dryness that may result in coughing. Bronchoscopy after therapeutic doses (50 to 60 Gy) reveals a reddened, hyperemic mucosa and thickened secretions that tend to accumulate and obstruct the lumen.

In contrast to the tracheobronchial tree, the lung is relatively radiosensitive to irradiation. Irradiation of the whole lung or a major portion of it results in distinct phases of damage characterized by differences in the time of expression after irradiation and distinct histologic changes, molecular changes, or both. Two of these phases of damage, radiation pneumonitis and fibrosis, have been well characterized,[3] although their pathogenesis remains unclear.

Traditionally the lung's response to irradiation is described as having a latent phase, occurring immediately and up to 3 months after irradiation; an exudative phase, or radiation pneumonitis, occurring from 3 to 6 months after irradiation; and a final fibrotic phase, occurring from 6 months after irradiation onward. Many cell types are involved in this process, but those thought to be the most critical to the process are type II cells, macrophages, and fibroblasts.

During the latent phase of injury, the lung appears histologically and radiographically normal, although it is now clear that the biological processes that culminate in the later outward manifestations of pulmonary irradiation begin during this time. The exudative phase, classical radiation pneumonitis, is characterized by an inflammatory cell infiltrate of macrophages and lymphocytes accompanied by edema in both the air and interstitial spaces (Fig. 17-1). Both type I and type II cells are desquamated into the alveolar spaces, thus removing the barrier between the interstitial capillaries and the air-alveolar wall interface. The loss of type II cells results in alterations in surfactant composition and production by these cells. Alveolar macrophages and proteinaceous materials fill the alveolar spaces, the latter as a result of

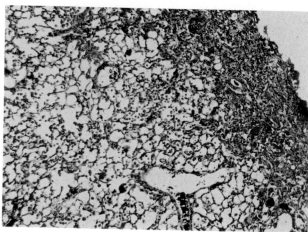

Fig. 17-2 Histologic section from the lung of a C57B1/6J mouse killed 5 months after the administration of 16 Gy to the whole thorax, showing organizing alveolitis and collagen deposition. (See Color Plate 20, after p. 80, for color reproduction.)

capillary leakage from the depopulated alveolar epithelium. The interstitium becomes thickened, further decreasing gas exchange and pulmonary perfusion. As the inflammation wanes, alveolar exudate becomes organized and fibroblasts proliferate.

The incorporation of the fibroproliferative process into the alveolar walls signals the initiation of the fibrotic phase. Interstitial fibrosis, with scarring and altered function of the alveolar unit, occurs in concert with thickening of the alveolar septa and capillary walls. This process leads to airspace and vascular consolidation and obliteration, with remodeling of the pulmonary architecture and attendant loss of pulmonary function (Fig. 17-2). The final phase of pulmonary fibrosis is generally considered chronic, progressive, and irreversible.

Molecular Mechanisms of Lung Damage

The phases of radiation-induced lung damage are a culmination of changes in both the pulmonary parenchyma and vasculature arising from a dynamic interaction among different cell types, including resident cells such as type II cells, endothelial cells, and fibroblasts and nonresident cells, notably macrophages and lymphocytes. However, the idea that killing and depletion of one or more "target cells" is responsible for the later manifestation of pulmonary injury has been replaced by a model in which complex interactions among these cells and the messages produced by them in response to injury culminates months later in the signs and symptoms of radiation pneumonitis and fibrosis.[4,5] It is now well established that at the time of irradiation, events initiated at the molecular level set in motion a persistent cascade of molecular processes that continue and persist through the fibrotic phase. Soluble mediators, or growth factors or cytokines, stimulate cells to overproduce those extracellular matrix

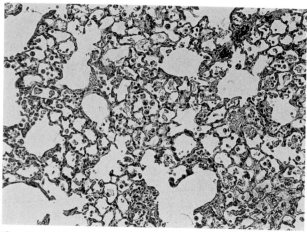

Fig. 17-1 Histologic section from the lung of a C3Hf/Kam mouse irradiated to the whole thorax and killed 4 months later, showing classical radiation pneumonitis, with inflammatory cell infiltrate and edema in the air spaces and interstitium. (See Color Plate 19, after p. 80, for color reproduction.)

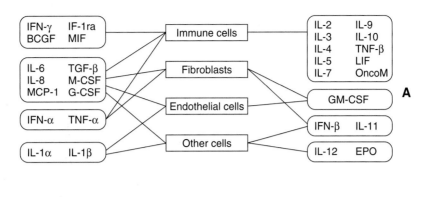

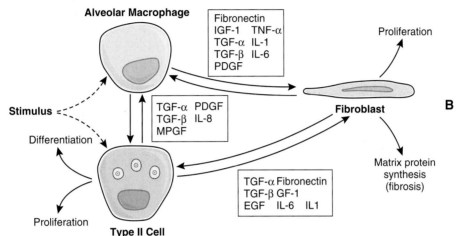

Fig. 17-3 **A,** Schema of cell-to-cell interactions and **B,** control of gene expression by growth factors in lung injury. *IFN,* Interferon; *IL,* interleukin; *BCGF,* B-cell growth factor; *MIF,* macrophage inhibitory factor; *TNF,* tumor necrosis factor; *LIF,* leukocyte inhibitory factor; *TGF,* tumor growth factor; *CSF,* colony-stimulating factor; *GM-CSF,* granulocyte-macrophage colony-stimulating factor; *EPO,* erythropoietin; *PDGF,* platelet-derived growth factor; *MPGF,* macrophage-phagocyte growth factor; *IGF-1,* insulin-like growth factor; *EGF,* endothelial growth factor. (From Rubin P, Johnston CJ, Williams JP, et al. *Int J Radiat Oncol Biol Phys* 1995;33:99-109.)

components that characterize fibrosis. After their initial contact with the cell surface, these molecules activate intracellular signaling pathways, which, in turn, activate the expression of specific genes that determine the phenotype of cells involved in lung injury. Although the factors modulating these events are not completely defined, knowledge of some pathways is beginning to emerge (Fig. 17-3).

Using a rabbit model, it has been shown that immediate damage from irradiation results in either membrane, intracellular, or DNA strand damage that leads to the altered expression and immediate release of such growth factors as transforming growth factor-beta (TGF-β), platelet-derived growth factor (PDGF), and interleukin-1 (IL-1), which in turn activate growth factor receptors, resulting in an activation of collagen genes and an increased production of collagen.[5] These changes are thought to begin and persist throughout the "latent" period, as well as throughout the overt expression of

damage. In addition, it is well accepted that intercellular interactions occur through cytokine pathways that affect changes in the genetic expression of collagen precursors. The intricate pathways that influence fibrocyte and fibroblast maturation are affected in an orderly fashion, resulting in an altered fibrocyte/fibroblast ratio conducive to collagen production and fibrosis.[6]

One cytokine shown to be an important mediator of tissue damage in a variety of conditions characterized by excessive collagen production and accumulation is TGF-β.[7-10] TGF-β is a pleiotropic cytokine that stimulates fibroblast and lymphocyte recruitment to the site of injury, promotes fibroblast proliferation, and stimulates the production of collagen and fibronectin, all of which result in a net increase in extracellular matrix material. In addition to stimulating the overproduction of connective tissue, TGF-β down-regulates the degradation of extracellular matrix, which ultimately results in maturation of the connective tissue to form a scar.

Experimental studies have confirmed the expected increase in TGF-β in postirradiation lung fibrosis.[7-10] However, TGF-β levels also are elevated during the latent phase after irradiation, long before the onset of pneumonitis or fibrosis. In a chemical model of pulmonary fibrosis, elevations in TGF-β have been observed 1 week after bleomycin exposure in mice that develop pulmonary fibrosis 3 weeks later.[11] In addition, antibodies to this cytokine, as well as a receptor antagonist, reduce collagen accumulation in the lung after bleomycin exposure. It is now well accepted that even if this cytokine is not the initial trigger in the fibrotic process, it clearly is a downstream effector in the process. As such, it is an attractive molecular target for interventional strategies in the fibrotic process. Recently, Martin and colleagues[12] suggested that TGF-β has a dual function in the fibrotic process as a master switch for the process and as a specific target for antifibrotic agents. In the latter case, pentoxifylline and vitamin E have been shown to reduce radiation-induced subcutaneous fibrosis both in human patients[13] and in a pig model.[14] These findings challenge the long-held view that tissue fibrosis is irreversible.

A third role for TGF-β in the treatment of lung cancer with radiation is as a predictor of radiation pneumonitis and fibrosis, as previously shown by Anscher and colleagues.[15] More recently, Anscher[16] showed that the plasma level of TGF-β at the end of treatment, combined with the volume of lung irradiated, can be used to reliably predict the outcome of radiation therapy, thus enabling the identification of patients who can tolerate relatively high radiation doses.

Just as the concept that the killing and depletion of a "target" cell might be responsible for radiation pneumonitis and fibrosis is now known to be simplistic, it is likely that TGF-β, although a critical factor in fibrosis, is not the only one involved in the complex fibrotic process. Tumor necrosis factor-α (TNF-α), Fas and Fas ligand, and basic fibroblast growth factor (FGF), to name just a few, have all been suggested as critical to fibrosis.

Volume of Lung Irradiated

An effective method of reducing the damage and morbidity from pulmonary irradiation is to limit the volume of lung irradiated, which is the rationale for the use of techniques such as conformal radiation therapy and intensity-modulated radiation therapy. Radiation oncologists routinely limit the volume of nondiseased tissue irradiated while encompassing all of the tumor volume. However, questions regarding the relationship of volume of lung irradiated and the dose are not clear. For example, is it better to give a large dose to a small volume than a small dose to a large volume?

A large-scale mouse study was undertaken by Liao, Travis, and Tucker[17-19] to define the relationship between dose, volume, and radiation pneumonitis using two assays of total lung function—breathing rate and lethality. In these studies, a range of lung volumes from 20% to 100% was irradiated with a range of doses to produce dose-response curves for each volume. In addition, the effect of location of the irradiated volume in the lung on morbidity was determined by irradiating similar volumes in the base and apex of the lung. These experiments tested the hypothesis that the respiratory unit, the functional subunit in the lung, is randomly and homogeneously distributed throughout the lung.

Figure 17-4 shows the proportion of dead mice after irradiation of two matched volumes in the apex and base of the lung, 50% and 75%.[19a] These data make clear that the base of the lung is more "sensitive" than the apex, at least for these two volumes irradiated. This relationship was subsequently found to hold for any

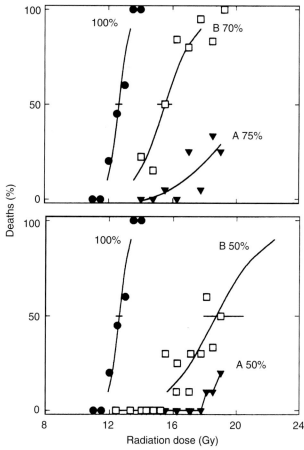

Fig. 17-4 Dose-response curves of lethality from radiation pneumonitis after irradiation of two partial volumes of lung, 75% and 50%, in the apex (*A*) or base (*B*) of C3H mice. Irradiation of 100% of the lung is shown for comparison. These data show a clear volume effect for radiation pneumonitis in the lung and dependence on the location of the partial volume irradiated. (From Travis EL, Komaki R. Treatment-related lung damage. In: Pass HI, Mitchell JB, Johnson DH, et al, eds. *Lung Cancer: Principles and Practice*. 2nd ed. Philadelphia, Pa: Lippincott Williams & Wilkins; 2000.)

volume of lung irradiated (Fig. 17-5); the isoeffect dose calculated from the dose-response curves for lethality resulting from radiation pneumonitis was always lower if the irradiated volume was in the base of the lung rather than the apex. Hence the base of the lung is more sensitive than the apex, at least in this mouse model.

The mechanism of this spatial heterogeneity in the response of the mouse lung to irradiation is unknown. Travis, Liao, and Tucker[17-19] proposed that the heterogeneous distribution of functional units in the lung is a function of pulmonary anatomy, that is, larger portions of the apex and middle regions of the lung are occupied by major conducting airways and fewer gas exchange units than the base of the lung, where the ratio of gas exchange units to conducting airways would be higher. Because the conducting airways are not involved in gas exchange, more of the critical functional units are in the base than in the apex of the lung. Thus a given dose of radiation will have less effect on the same volume irradiated in the apex than in the base of the lung simply because more of the structures critical to lung function are present in this area than in others.

However, it also has been suggested that regional differences in the incidence of pneumonitis could be accounted for by differences in the functionality of cells in the apex and the base.[20] Also, in a series of experiments designed to determine whether factors released by cells in one part of the lung influence the effect in another, Khan and colleagues[21] found that irradiated fibroblasts in the base of the lung sustain more DNA damage than do irradiated fibroblasts residing in the apex of the lung and that this effect is sustained independent of which region is irradiated. This effect disappears when the whole lung is irradiated. Although the mechanism of the regional differences in radiation response is unclear, data from two independent laboratories have shown that the morbidity of lung irradiation is related not only to the volume of lung irradiated but also to the location of this irradiated subvolume in the lung. In addition, the two groups agree that the base is the subvolume most sensitive to radiation.

What remains unanswered by these experiments, however, is the question of whether it is better to irradiate a large volume with a small dose or a small volume with a large dose. Using the findings from the mouse studies, Tucker and colleagues[17-19] calculated the incidence of pneumonitis for subvolumes of the lung irradiated with a fixed dose. As shown in Figure 17-6, the incidence of complications varied from 100% after irradiation of the base to 0% after irradiation of the middle region of the lung, with an intermediate number after irradiation of the apex. These findings indicate that relatively small changes in the location of the irradiated subvolume in the lung may correspond to significantly greater changes in the incidence of pneumonitis than moderate changes in either the dose or the size of the irradiated subvolume.

On the basis of these data, Tucker and colleagues[17-19] found that the risk of pneumonitis after a constant

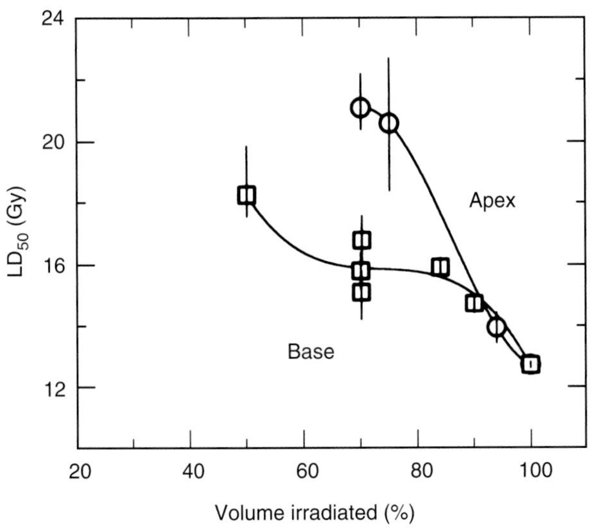

Fig. 17-5 Lethality as measured by the dose causing 50% of experimental subjects to die (LD$_{50}$) from radiation pneumonitis as a function of partial volume irradiated, showing a clear location-dependent response for all partial volumes irradiated. (From Travis EL, Liao Z-X, Tucker SL. *Int J Radiat Oncol Biol Phys* 1997;38:1045-1054.)

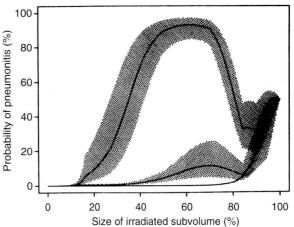

Fig. 17-6 Predicted incidence of pneumonitis in mouse lung as a function of irradiated volume when the integrated dose (dose × volume) is fixed at 12.7 Gy, the single-dose LD$_{50}$. The upper, middle, and lower curves represent volumes in the base, apex, and middle regions of the lung, respectively. In the base, the risk of pneumonitis is greatest after irradiation of an intermediate subvolume with an intermediate dose, whereas in the apex a little radiation to a lot of lung is generally more damaging than a lot to a little. (From Tucker SL, Liao Z-X, Travis EL. *Int J Radiat Oncol Biol Phys* 1997;38:1055-1066.)

integrated dose of 12.7 Gy varied enormously depending on the site of the irradiated subvolume. This analysis of a constant integrated dose (calculated as the product of volume and dose) demonstrated that, for both the apex and the middle region of the lung, a little radiation to a large volume of lung was worse than a lot of radiation to a small volume of lung (i.e., the tails of both curves increased at large volumes). However, in the base of the lung, the peak probability of pneumonitis occurred between irradiated volumes of 50% and 70%; the probability fell off dramatically for volumes outside this range. Although this seems counterintuitive for the large volumes, for which the probability of pneumonitis would be expected to increase with the volume of lung irradiated, this decrease actually reflects use of the constant integrated dose. Thus, as the volume gets larger, the dose necessarily becomes smaller to maintain constancy.

A third factor that can be defined from these curves is the volume below which radiation would be expected to cause no detectable injury even after very high doses (i.e., the threshold volume). Like the radiation doses associated with lethality and complications, the threshold volume depends on the site of irradiation, ranging from 10% in the more sensitive base to 30% to 40% in the more resistant middle region and apex of the lung. Regardless of the parameter examined, these studies indicate that the site of the volume irradiated in the lung is an important consideration when choosing a treatment plan and that the base of the lung is more sensitive than other regions.

Similar findings have been reported in humans. Yamada and colleagues[22] reported that the risk of pneumonitis in patients varied with the location of the irradiated volume. They also found that inclusion of volumes in the lower lung increased the incidence of pneumonitis by 50%, to a 70% incidence from 20% when sites outside the lower lung were included ($P = 0.01$).[22] Multivariate analysis revealed a significant relationship between radiation site and the risk of pneumonitis ($P = 0.0096$). These patient data are consistent with the mouse data and indicate that the risk of pneumonitis is significantly higher when irradiated volumes are in the lower part of the lung than when they are in the upper part of the lung. Thus the site of the irradiated subvolume must be a consideration in treatment planning for all patients with lung cancer.

Clinical Changes

The clinical symptoms related to the effects on the tracheobronchial tree rarely dominate the picture. Excess sputum production may be relieved by agents that shrink the mucosa or decrease secretions; dryness and nonproductive cough may be helped by a cool-mist humidifier.

The clinical manifestations of radiation effects on the lung can be separated into an early degenerative "pneumonitic" phase and a later regenerative phase of scarring or fibrosis. During the degenerative phase, dyspnea and a cough, occasionally productive of a thick, white sputum, may develop. Fever and night sweats may be present. Percussion and auscultation during this phase are often remarkably unrevealing. Usually the symptoms subside in 2 to 3 months and no further symptoms are noticed, despite abnormal radiographic findings. If the volume of lung irradiated to a dose above 25 to 30 Gy is very large, the clinical signs and symptoms of radiation pneumonitis appear in 3 to 6 weeks. The patient may become progressively more dyspneic at rest, febrile, and may develop night sweats and cyanosis. Alveolar-capillary block is the most disabling physiologic change. Symptoms of cough, dyspnea, or fever may range from mild to extreme, depending on the volume of lung irradiated and the dose-fractionation regimen. With careful attention to keeping the high-dose volume as small as possible, symptoms from pulmonary irradiation are the exception rather than the rule.

If the volume of lung irradiated has been extensive, permanent scarring that produces chronic debilitation because of respiratory compromise may develop. Dyspnea and cough may be severe. Clubbing of the fingers may develop. Secondary infection with abscess formation may lead to death from sepsis. Pulmonary hypertension with right-sided heart failure has been reported.[23,24] Arteriovenous shunting may be a major cause of dyspnea and cyanosis; pneumonectomy has rarely proved beneficial in severe cases.[25]

Radiologic Changes

Often the only clinical manifestations of radiation pneumonitis are radiographic changes. An infiltrate may become evident on chest images conforming to the treatment field (Fig. 17-7). In the past, when most treatment fields were square or rectangular, diagnostic radiologists recognized "square pneumonia" as a hallmark of radiation pneumonitis. The phenomenon is now much more subtle because of the use of individualized custom blocks that have irregular, rounded margins defining the treatment portal. In any case, the changes remain confined to the treated volume[26] unless there is a supervening process; no dosimetric or pathophysiologic basis exists for "radiation pneumonitis" to occur in the normal lung outside the treated volume.

Several conditions such as bacterial and viral pneumonias, fungal and protozoal infections, and lymphangitic carcinomatosis can give rise to diffuse pulmonary infiltrates. When such infiltrates follow a course of radiation therapy, they may incorrectly be attributed to radiation pneumonitis. Adult respiratory distress syndrome may sporadically follow thoracic irradiation[27]; diffuse bilateral infiltrates are not confined to the irradiated volume, and rapidly progressive respiratory failure with unresponsive

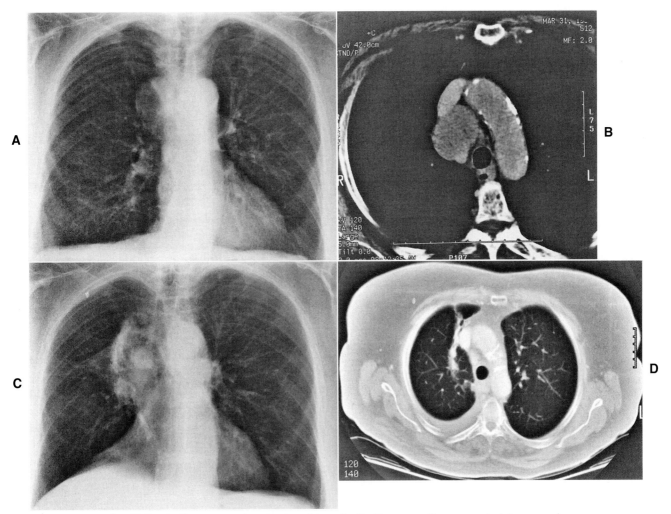

Fig. 17-7 **A,** Posteroanterior chest radiograph. **B,** Corresponding computed tomography (CT) scan in patient with lung cancer. **C,** Chest film 6 months after radiation therapy showing radiation pneumonitis and indeterminate findings relative to the tumor. **D,** CT scan showing that the tumor is no longer evident and linear infiltrates correspond to the radiation.

hypoxemia is seen. Although high-dose corticosteroids are often administered, they probably do not affect outcome,[28] and they may have catastrophic effects if the infiltrates are the result of supervening infection.

It may be difficult to assess the relationship of the distribution of the pulmonary infiltrates to the fields of irradiation with standard posteroanterior and lateral radiographs. Computed tomography (CT) of the thorax usually can provide the answer to the question; if the infiltrates seen on CT scans do not correlate with the irradiated volume and, specifically, if infiltrates appear in portions of the lungs that received no irradiation, radiation pneumonitis can be ruled out and the actual cause can be sought.

Functional Effects

The pathophysiology of radiation pneumonitis and scarring and the associated functional effects are related to vascular, epithelial, and interstitial injury. It is often difficult to determine how much of a given functional outcome is attributable to vascular abnormality and how much is attributable to epithelial and interstitial disease. Carbon monoxide–diffusing capacity decreases strikingly, as one would expect with hyaline membrane formation, interstitial fibrosis of septa, and thrombosis or progressive vascular sclerosis. Compliance is markedly decreased by interstitial sclerosis.[29,30] It follows that lung volumes are diminished. Poor ventilation of the irradiated segment and incomplete oxygenation of the blood contribute to the patient's disability in proportion to the ratio of damage to the normal lung.

Choi and colleagues[31] found the functional changes produced by irradiation for cancer of the lung to vary according to pulmonary reserve before treatment. Patients with less functional compromise (e.g., a forced expiratory volume in less than 1 second [FEV_1] of more than 50% of the predicted value) had significantly lower pulmonary function and higher airway resistance than other patients. Those with an FEV_1 of less than 50% of the predicted value either had improved or minimally reduced pulmonary function. A study by Brady and colleagues[32] confirmed the relative safety of giving effective doses to modest treatment volumes and the hazards of giving high doses to large treatment volumes. The dose-escalation studies of the Radiation Therapy Oncology Group (RTOG) have confirmed the much greater importance of the volume irradiated than the dose given once the radiation is in the therapeutic range (above 50 Gy); increasing the total doses from 60 to 74.4 Gy does not increase the frequency of acute or late pulmonary toxicity.[33-35]

Treatment of Radiation Pneumonitis

Radiation pneumonitis is an inevitable consequence of aggressive therapy for malignant conditions that arise in the thorax. In the great majority of patients, radiographic manifestations of the changes are the first and only evidence of radiation pneumonitis. Usually opacity decreases or disappears without symptoms or treatment.

When symptoms are sufficiently severe to justify treatment, corticosteroids may be of help. About half of patients so treated have early, marked relief.[23,30] Corticosteroids may reverse the symptoms of radiation pneumonitis within hours, but they do not prevent or reverse the fibrotic phase. In addition, they may be contraindicated in disease processes in which they have been shown to have a deleterious effect on outcome, such as carcinoma of the lung.[36] It is important in cases of radiation pneumonitis to withdraw steroids very slowly so as to avoid recrudescence. Unless the symptoms are severe, it is preferable to provide supportive care with bronchodilators, expectorants, antibiotics, bed rest, and oxygen and to avoid the long-term use of corticosteroids.

Prophylactic administration of cortisone to animals irradiated to the entire thorax has been shown to decrease the frequency of severe, acute reactions.[30] However, prophylactic administration of steroids to humans has not been tested. The best prophylaxis is careful treatment planning, minimizing the volume irradiated to high doses.

RADIATION THERAPY FOR LUNG CARCINOMA

Carcinoma of the lung is the most common malignant disease in the United States and several countries in northern and western Europe. It accounts for one of every six new cancer cases diagnosed in the United States, and it is responsible for one of every four cancer deaths. The striking rise in incidence over the past 30 years and the lack of any major improvement

in treatment has led to a steep rise in annual mortality. Not only is lung cancer the most common cause of cancer death among men, it has surpassed cancer of the breast as the number one cause of cancer death among women.

The single most important cause of cancer of the lung is the inhalation of tobacco smoke. Many other agents also have been shown to increase the risk of bronchopulmonary cancer, among them asbestos, iron ore, radioactive ores, and isopropyl oil.[37]

The mainstay of treatment for patients with small, localized carcinomas of the lung continues to be surgical resection. With current imaging procedures, augmented by cervical mediastinoscopy, anterior mediastinotomy, and transtracheal or transbronchial biopsy, only 20% to 25% of all patients are considered candidates for definitive resection. The remaining patients, except for those with distant metastasis, are appropriately treated with radiation alone or, increasingly, with cytotoxic drugs.

It is appropriate to consider therapy according to the different histopathologic types of lung cancer. One classification proposed by the World Health Organization and later modified[38] groups lung cancer as squamous cell carcinoma, small cell carcinoma, adenocarcinoma, large cell carcinoma, and adenosquamous carcinoma. Squamous cell carcinoma is the single most frequent histopathologic type of carcinoma of the lung, but adenocarcinoma is only slightly less frequent.[39] Each constitutes somewhat less than one third of all cases of carcinoma of the lung. Included within adenocarcinoma is bronchioalveolar carcinoma, an infrequent lung cancer but one of the few types not associated with tobacco inhalation. Squamous cell carcinomas and adenocarcinomas are subject to histologic grading, but most of them are moderately to poorly differentiated.

Small cell carcinoma includes the lymphocyte-like type also known as *oat cell carcinoma*. A variant of this, previously thought to represent an intermediate cell type within the small cell grouping, is now recognized as being a mixture of small cell and large cell carcinoma. Large cell carcinoma is quite possibly the most undifferentiated form of adenocarcinoma, and these two cell types have been indistinguishable in a variety of clinicopathologic studies. Giant cell carcinoma and clear cell carcinoma are considered variants of large cell carcinoma.

Carcinoid tumors[40] are relatively indolent, but unquestionably malignant, tumors that occur in younger individuals more often than other carcinomas of the lung; they are unrelated to the inhalation of tobacco smoke. They have neuroendocrine differentiation, and their relationship to small cell carcinomas is controversial. Carcinoid tumors are actually parabronchial tumors that often have a small portion extending into the lumen of the bronchus. Infrequently, they produce vasoactive substances that can cause flushing, diarrhea, and hypotension.

Squamous cell carcinoma has the greatest propensity to remain confined to the thorax, whereas almost every patient with small cell carcinoma will have distant metastasis. Studies of causes of death (Table 17-1)[41] and patterns of failure show that local tumor progression most commonly kills patients with squamous cell carcinoma, whereas widespread dissemination accounts for the majority of deaths in small cell carcinoma. Adenocarcinoma and large cell carcinoma occupy an intermediate place in the spectrum from squamous cell carcinoma to small cell carcinoma; adenocarcinoma and large cell carcinoma have less propensity to cause death because of progression of the intrathoracic tumor than does squamous cell carcinoma, but they both have a greater propensity to spread beyond the thorax.

The lymphatic drainage of the lungs is shown in Figure 17-8.[42,43] In surgical series, one fourth to one half of patients who undergo resection have regional lymph node metastasis (Table 17-2).[44-46] At autopsy, more than 90% of patients are found to have involvement of hilar or mediastinal lymph nodes. However, carcinoma of the lung does not spread in such a predictable manner. Mediastinal lymph nodes and blood vessels are

often involved by the time the diagnosis is established. The highly vascular composition of the lung, with its dual circulation of bronchial and pulmonary vessels, provides a ready anatomic explanation for the high frequency of extrathoracic dissemination.

Small cell carcinoma, adenocarcinoma, and large cell carcinoma all have a notable propensity to spread to the brain (Table 17-3).[39] Even with the relatively high rate of patient survival in small cell carcinoma (because of effective combinations of chemotherapy), 50% to 80% of patients eventually have metastasis to the brain.[47-49] Clinical assessments of the frequency of brain metastasis from adenocarcinoma and large cell carcinoma have confirmed the high rate of involvement found in autopsy studies.[50]

Carcinoma of the lung is most often diagnosed from symptoms resulting from the intrathoracic tumor. Cough, dyspnea, chest pain, and hemoptysis are among the most frequent symptoms and signs. However, a large proportion of patients have unexplained weight loss.

Radiographic studies reveal that squamous cell carcinoma and small cell carcinoma tend to occur as central lesions (Table 17-4),[51] whereas adenocarcinoma and

TABLE 17-1
Cause of Death by Cell Type*

Cancer of Death	NUMBER OF PATIENTS (%) DYING OF THE CANCER				
	Squamous Cell Carcinoma	Small Cell Carcinoma	Adenocarcinoma	Large Cell Carcinoma	Combined
Carcinomatosis	21 (25)	49 (70)	49 (48)	23 (47)	2
Central nervous system metastasis	2 (2)	—	9 (9)	4 (8)	—
Infection	30 (36)	6 (11)	19 (19)	13 (27)	6
Hemorrhage	7 (8)	4 (7)	4 (4)	1 (2)	—
Respiratory failure	5 (6)	2 (3)	7 (7)	4 (8)	—
Heart failure	17 (20)	5 (9)	8 (8)	3 (6)	—
Pulmonary emboli	—	—	4 (4)	1 (2)	—
Other cancer	1 (1)	—	2 (2)	—	

From Cox JD, Yesner RA. *Yale J Biol Med* 1981;54:201-207.
*Taken from 300 consecutive Veterans Administration Lung Group autopsies.

TABLE 17-2
Distribution of Mediastinal and Supraclavicular Lymph Node Metastases by Site of Primary Carcinoma of the Lung

Lobe	DISEASED NODES IN THE REGION (%)				
	Subcarinal	Pararight Tracheal	Supraright Clavicular	Paraleft Tracheal	Supraleft Clavicular
Right upper	32	64	30	4	1
Right lower	46	42	3	12	—
Left upper	42	16	3	42	39
Left lower	50	21	4	29	4

Data from Carlens E. *Chest* 1974;65:442-445; Goldberg EM, Glickman AS, Kahan FR. *Cancer* 1970;25:347-353; Palumbo LT, Sharpe WS. *Arch Surg* 1969;98:90-93.

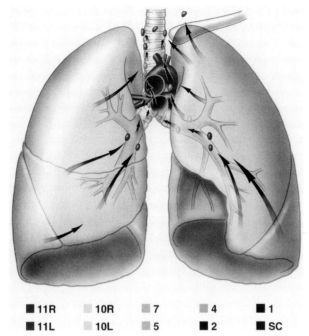

| ■ 11R | ■ 10R | ■ 7 | ■ 4 | ■ 1 |
| ■ 11L | ■ 10L | ■ 5 | ■ 2 | ■ SC |

Fig. 17-8 Lymphatic drainage of the lobes of the lungs related to the schema commonly used for classifying regional lymph nodes. Note crossover from the lingula of the left upper lobe and the superior portion of the left lower lobe to the right paratracheal nodes. Lymph node drainage does not parallel arteries or veins, nor does it remain distinct for each lobe. Node colors correspond to stations in the *AJCC Cancer Staging Manual*. (See Color Plate 21, after p. 80, for color reproduction.) (Modified from Nohl HC. *Thorax* 1956;11:172-185; Fleming I, Cooper JS, Henson DE, et al, eds. *AJCC Cancer Staging Manual*. 5th ed. Philadelphia, Pa: Lippincott Williams & Wilkins; 1997:127-137.)

large cell carcinoma occur more often as peripheral parenchymal tumors. Small cell carcinoma and large cell carcinoma are often found to have mediastinal abnormalities. Any of the histopathologic types of lung carcinoma may occur in the extreme apex of either lung, with

symptoms of shoulder pain, ulnar dysesthesias, Horner's syndrome, and evidence of chest-wall invasion and destruction of the adjacent ribs or vertebrae (Pancoast's syndrome).

Obstruction of the superior vena cava can lead to swelling of the face, neck, and arms and evidence of collateral circulation over the anterior chest wall; approximately 4% of all patients with cancer of the lung present with this syndrome.

Paraneoplastic phenomena include clubbing, ectopic hormone production (adrenocorticotropic hormone, calcitonin, human chorionic gonadotropin, antidiuretic hormone, or parathyroid hormone), and a variety of neuromuscular syndromes. These may disappear with effective treatment of the primary tumor. All but two of the paraneoplastic phenomena are seen more often in patients with small cell carcinoma than in other patients; hypercalcemia and clubbing are rare in small cell carcinoma.

Patients who have cancer of the lung should undergo not only a careful physical examination but also selected laboratory and imaging studies. A complete blood count is always appropriate: anemia or a leukoerythroblastic picture may suggest bone marrow involvement. A biochemical survey, including liver function tests such as alkaline phosphatase and aspartate aminotransferase, can be conducted to help detect hepatic involvement. Carcinoembryonic antigen and lactate dehydrogenase levels may be elevated and may serve as a means of monitoring the effectiveness of therapy.[52]

In addition to plain posteroanterior and lateral chest radiography, CT of the thorax not only contributes to an appreciation of the extent of the primary tumor and regional lymph node metastasis[53] but also performs an important function in treatment planning if radiation therapy is used. CT of the upper abdomen makes a substantial contribution to the search for occult distant metastasis; not only can hepatic metastasis be identified but the more common adrenal metastasis can be seen as well.[54]

TABLE 17-3
Frequency of Brain Metastasis at Autopsy

Primary Tumor (Histopathologic Type)	Number of Patients	Patients with Metastasis Including the Brain (%)	Patients with Brain Metastasis Only (%)
Squamous cell carcinoma	123	13	4
Small cell carcinoma	82	45	6
Adenocarcinoma	129	54	12
Large cell carcinoma	54	52	9
Combined	12	25	0
TOTALS	400	38	8

Modified from Cox JD, Yesner RA. *Am Rev Respir Dis* 1979;120:1025-1029.

TABLE 17-4

Common Abnormalities Observed in Roentgenograms of Various Types of Lung Carcinoma

Mass Characteristics	PROPORTION OF CASES WITH THE ABNORMALITY (%)			
	Squamous Cell Carcinoma (n=263)	Small Cell Carcinoma (n=114)	Adenocarcinoma (n=126)	Large Cell Carcinoma (n=97)
Hilar or perihilar mass	40	78	17	32
Parenchymal mass				
≤ 4 cm	9	21	45	18
> 4 cm	19	8	26	41
Apical mass	3	3	1	4
Consolidation or collapse	53	38	25	33
Mediastinal mass	1	13	2	10
Pleural effusion	3	5	1	2

Modified from Byrd RB, Carr DT, Miller WE. *Thorax* 1969;24:573-575.

In addition, renal and retroperitoneal lymph node metastases are sometimes identified. Finally, CT of the brain is necessary in patients with small cell carcinoma, adenocarcinoma, and large cell carcinoma because as many as 10% of patients without neurologic symptoms or signs may have occult brain metastasis.

Whole-body positron emission tomography (PET) with ^{18}F-fluorodeoxyglucose improves the rate of detection of regional and distant metastasis in patients with non–small cell lung carcinoma (NSCLC). Pieterman and colleagues[55] found PET to be more sensitive than CT (91% vs. 75%) and more specific than CT (86% vs. 66%). In that study, PET identified distant metastases in 11 of 102 patients considered to be free of metastasis by all other pretreatment staging methods. Although PET correctly detected mediastinal lymph node metastasis in 90% of patients with histopathologic evidence of involved lymph nodes, it gave false-positive results for lymph nodes in patients with reactive hyperplasia and silicoanthracosis. PET is complementary to CT for radiation treatment planning.[56]

When the complete clinical evaluation is accomplished, more than half of all patients with lung carcinoma are found to have distant metastasis. Clinical staging classifications for carcinomas of the lung have been used widely for more than 20 years. The current version of the system advocated by the American Joint Committee on Cancer (AJCC)[43] is shown in Box 17-1.

Indications for Radiation Therapy

There are many indications for radiation therapy for cancer of the lung. Radiation therapy can be used as an adjunct to surgery, in place of surgery for patients with small tumors who cannot undergo surgery, with chemotherapy as a cure for unresectable but non-metastatic tumors of all cell types, as prophylactic treatment of subclinical metastasis, and as palliative therapy for distressing symptoms. These indications are described further in the following sections.

Surgical Adjuvant Radiation Therapy

Radiation therapy is indicated only for selected patients with operable carcinoma of the lung. Preoperative irradiation has been studied prospectively and has never been shown to improve results over resection alone.[57] Preoperative irradiation may have conferred no benefit in these studies because, without surgery, physicians cannot identify patients who have the greatest risk of local–regional recurrence. It is curious that preoperative irradiation is still considered by many surgeons and radiation oncologists to be standard treatment in the management of apical sulcus ("Pancoast") tumors.[58]

Studies of postoperative irradiation show that it does not improve results in patients who have no evidence of metastasis to the hilar or mediastinal lymph nodes.[59] In fact, postoperative irradiation might have a net deleterious effect on survival.[59] Shields[60] observed that local recurrence was infrequent in the case of a pathologically complete resection with no evidence of regional lymph node metastasis, so irradiation would accomplish little for such patients. Moreover, radiation therapy may place an additional burden on pulmonary function, especially in patients who have required pneumonectomy. A meta-analysis reiterated the long-recognized potential for adverse effects of radiation therapy when rigorous CT-based treatment planning is not done.[61]

Several retrospective studies[62-64] have suggested that postoperative irradiation can improve outcome when mediastinal nodal metastases are present. An analysis of postoperative radiation therapy in available prospective trials, most of which was not based on CT planning, showed neither a detrimental nor a beneficial effect.[61] On the basis of the striking improvement in local control of squamous cell carcinoma shown by the

---

BOX 17-1 American Joint Committee on Cancer Staging System for Cancer of the Lung

PRIMARY TUMOR (T)

TX Primary tumor cannot be assessed, or tumor proven by the presence of malignant cells in sputum or bronchial washings but not visualized by imaging or bronchoscopy

T0 No evidence of primary tumor

Tis Carcinoma in situ

T1 Tumor 3 cm or less in greatest dimension, surrounded by lung or visceral pleura, without bronchoscopic evidence of invasion more proximal than the lobar bronchus* (i.e., not in the main bronchus)

T2 Tumor with any of the following features of size or extent: more than 3 cm in greatest dimension; involves main bronchus, 2 cm or more distal to the carina; invades the visceral pleura; associated with atelectasis or obstructive pneumonitis that extends to the hilar region but does not involve the entire lung

T3 Tumor of any size that directly invades any of the following: chest wall (including superior sulcus tumors), diaphragm, mediastinal pleura, parietal pericardium; or tumor in the main bronchus less than 2 cm distal to the carina, but without involvement of the carina; or associated atelectasis or obstructive pneumonitis of the entire lung

T4 Tumor of any size that invades any of the following: mediastinum, heart, great vessels, trachea, esophagus, vertebral body, carina; or separate tumor nodules in the same lobe; or tumor with a malignant pleural effusion†

REGIONAL LYMPH NODES (N)

NX Regional lymph nodes cannot be assessed

N0 No regional lymph node metastasis

N1 Metastasis to ipsilateral peribronchial and/or ipsilateral hilar lymph nodes, and intrapulmonary nodes including involvement by direct extension of the primary tumor

N2 Metastasis to ipsilateral mediastinal and/or subcarinal lymph node(s)

N3 Metastasis to contralateral mediastinal, contralateral hilar, ipsilateral or contralateral scalene, or supraclavicular lymph node(s)

DISTANT METASTASIS (M)

MX Distant metastasis cannot be assessed

M0 No distant metastasis

M1 Distant metastasis present‡

STAGE GROUPING

Occult carcinoma	Tx	N0	M0
Stage 0	Tis	N0	M0
Stage IA	T1	N0	M0
Stage IB	T2	N0	M0
Stage IIA	T1	N1	M0
Stage IIB	T2	N1	M0
	T3	N0	M0
Stage IIIA	T1–2	N2	M0
	T3	N1–2	M0
Stage IIIB	Any T	N3	M0
	T4	Any N	M0
Stage IV	Any T	Any N	M1

From Fleming I, Cooper JS, Henson DE, et al, eds. *AJCC Cancer Staging Manual.* 5th ed. Philadelphia, Pa: Lippincott Williams & Wilkins; 1997:127-137.

*NOTE: The uncommon superficial tumor of any size with its invasive component limited to the bronchial wall, which may extend proximal to the main bronchus, is also classified T1.

†NOTE: Most pleural effusions associated with lung cancer are due to tumor. However, there are a few patients in whom multiple cytopathologic examinations of pleural fluid are negative for tumor. In these cases, fluid is non-bloody and is not an exudate. When these elements and clinical judgment dictate that the effusion is not related to the tumor, the effusion should be excluded as a staging element and the patient should be staged T1, T2, or T3.

‡NOTE: M1 includes separate tumor nodule(s) in a different lobe (ipsilateral or contralateral)

Lung Cancer Study Group,[65] the Eastern Cooperative Oncology Group (ECOG) coordinated a large intergroup trial to compare postoperative radiation therapy plus concurrent chemotherapy with cisplatin and etoposide to postoperative radiation therapy alone.[66] In initial results for 373 patients eligible for analysis and a median follow-up of 44 months, the median survival was 42 months for patients given only radiation and 38 months for those given combined-modality treatment ($P = 0.48$). No significant differences were found in failure patterns between the two study groups. Therefore, although postoperative irradiation can clearly reduce the risk of local recurrence in patients

with mediastinal node metastasis,[65,67] its effect on survival (with or without adjuvant chemotherapy) is still under investigation.

Finally, Sawyer and colleagues[68] studied patients with stage IIIA (N2) NSCLC using regression tree analysis to identify patients at low, intermediate, and high risk of local recurrence. Numbers of involved lymph nodes, locations of mediastinal lymph nodes relative to the location of the primary tumor, and T stage were used to identify intermediate-risk and high-risk groups. Excluding the low-risk group, postoperative radiation therapy conferred a highly significant improvement in local recurrence-free and overall survival rates. This approach can form the basis for future studies of the value of postoperative irradiation therapy and chemotherapy.

Controversy continues regarding the most effective treatment for patients with marginally resectable NSCLC. A retrospective review of patients treated at The University of Texas M.D. Anderson Cancer Center[69] confirmed the impression that patients with more favorable disease are selected for surgical intervention. Two small prospective studies[70,71] provided quite similar results suggesting that induction chemotherapy improves survival in patients with resectable NSCLC. The potential advantages of chemotherapy concurrent with radiation therapy delivered preoperatively were studied by the Southwest Oncology Group (SWOG). Albain and colleagues[72] reported the results for 126 patients treated in a phase II trial of cisplatin and etoposide concurrent with radiation therapy (45 Gy at 1.8 Gy/fraction, 5 days/wk). After an interval of 2 to 4 weeks, thoracotomy and resection were attempted. A high resection rate (76%) and a 3-year survival rate of 27% were reported, and the outcome was the same for patients with stage IIIB and IIIA disease. These findings led to initiation of a randomized comparative trial coordinated by the RTOG to determine the role of resection compared with chemotherapy and radiation therapy in patients with confirmed mediastinal node metastasis. Randomization is performed before patients are enrolled in the study, and patients are assigned to undergo either induction chemotherapy and radiation therapy for 5 weeks and then thoracotomy and resection or a continuation of chemoradiation to a total dose of 61.0 Gy in 33 fractions. The study was closed to enrollment in 2001, and results are expected in 2003.

Curative Therapy for Inoperable Non–Small Cell Lung Carcinoma

Curative treatment for inoperable NSCLC was considered so uncommon that attempts at such treatment were not allowed in many developed countries seeking to limit health care resources. But cure is an increasing reality in clinical investigations and standard practice. Two distinct groups of patients can be identified for such treatment—those with stage I or II tumors who cannot undergo surgery because of comorbid medical conditions and those with more advanced, technically unresectable tumors.

The ability of definitive radiation therapy to control small tumors and cure patients when they can undergo surgery is widely recognized. At least 10% of patients with stage I NSCLC cannot undergo surgery for medical reasons. Dosoretz and colleagues[73] reviewed several series showing that 5-year survival rates ranged from 6% to 32% after radiation therapy. Table 17-5[74-77] lists more recent series of patients treated with radiation; although 2-year survival rates range from 34% to 47%, 5-year survival rates fall within the same range as those

TABLE 17-5

Medically Inoperable Stage I Non–Small Cell Lung Cancer Treated by Radiation

Study and Reference	Number of Patients	Dose (Gy)	OVERALL ACTUARIAL SURVIVAL (%)	
			2 Years	5 Years
Morita et al, 1997[74]	149	55-75	34	22
Sibley et al, 1998[75]	141	50-80	39	13
Hayakawa et al, 1999[76]	36	60-81	42 (3 y)	23
M.D. Anderson Cancer Center, 2000[77]	117	20-83.9*	46	18

*Neutrons.

in earlier series. The poor overall survival reflects death from intercurrent disease. In the M.D. Anderson Cancer Center series of 117 patients,[77a] 51% died of intercurrent disease. However, local control was achieved in only one third of patients treated.

Because local control and survival are still far from satisfactory, there is great interest in the use of three-dimensional conformal radiation therapy to deliver higher doses while sparing normal lung for these patients who often have seriously impaired pulmonary reserve. Rosenzweig and colleagues[78] developed dose-escalation studies for such patients. Their preliminary results show the ability to achieve much higher total doses than the usually accepted tolerance dose of 60 to 65 Gy given over 6 weeks. They recognized the volume-related morbidity of pulmonary irradiation and the need to restrict the volume that receives 20 Gy or more to 35%.

One third of all patients with NSCLC have tumors that cannot be resected yet have no demonstrable distant metastasis. The advent of PET scanning for pretreatment evaluation[55] will affect this proportion by detecting extrathoracic metastasis more often than do other imaging studies. PET studies also will amplify the importance of local tumor control in determining outcome for these patients.

The local–regional tumor within the thorax is a major determinant of survival for squamous cell carcinoma in particular and, to a lesser extent, adenocarcinoma and large cell carcinoma of the lung. This concept was suggested by studies of patterns of failure and causes of death (see Table 17-1). Studies of the effect of local control by radiation therapy have confirmed that control of the primary tumor and its regional metastases is associated with much better survival than progression of local–regional disease.[79] This belies the myth that all patients die of distant dissemination regardless of what happens to the primary disease.

The local tumor, if not eradicated, is the actual cause of death in most patients with inoperable NSCLC. Table 17-1[41] clearly shows that death after treatment with palliative irradiation or single-agent chemotherapy is due more often to intrathoracic disease than to extrathoracic metastasis. Saunders and colleagues[80] studied causes of death among patients with localized unresectable NSCLC treated with a few large fractions of irradiation; most were followed until autopsy. These investigators found that 72% of patients died as the result of the intrathoracic tumor and only 15% had extrathoracic metastasis. In a subsequent randomized trial, these investigators showed that continuous hyperfractionated accelerated radiation therapy (1.5 Gy given 3 times/day for 12 consecutive days) improved both local control and survival in patients with inoperable NSCLC compared with standard fractionation radiation therapy (a total dose of 60 Gy given in 2.0 Gy/fraction).[81] Finally, a prospective trial[82] of low-dose cisplatin given concurrently with radiation therapy either daily or weekly as a radiosensitizer improved local control and survival relative to radiation therapy alone. Clonogenic tumor cells evidently continue to proliferate during treatment of NSCLC,[83] which explains the success of the hyperfractionated regimen relative to a 6-week course of irradiation, as well as the value of concurrent chemotherapy.

Techniques of External Irradiation

Radiation therapy is much less effective for carcinoma of the lung than for tumors of similar histopathologic type presenting in other locations. Reasons for this are becoming clearer. Squamous cell carcinomas and adenocarcinomas of the lung may have greater proliferative potential than tumors at other sites, and they may be associated with a greater number of unrecognized extensions of disease. Finally, many tumors in the parenchyma of the lung move in unpredictable directions during respiration.

Careful immobilization of patients is important, and CT planning of therapy is critical. A margin of 1.5 to 2 cm around the intrathoracic tumor, including its movement during respiration, is required. Studies are underway to characterize tumor motion and to stop respiration briefly during treatment to achieve both better tumor coverage and better sparing of normal lung.

Debate continues as to the value of encompassing clinically uninvolved regional lymph node drainage sites. Studies of failure patterns after irradiation of only the demonstrable tumor suggest that failure in the nodes is infrequent.[84] On the other hand, even relatively small tumors not associated with node enlargement on chest CT have been shown to have a high risk of regional node involvement.[68] Preliminary evidence suggests that PET scanning[56] can reveal such subclinical node involvement and thus indicate when lymph nodes must be included or when they can be omitted.

Local control is unacceptably low with standard fractionation and total doses of 60 to 65 Gy. Arriagada and colleagues[85] reported local control in less than 20% of patients who received 65 Gy in 26 fractions over 6½ to 7 weeks. Theirs was the first large study (353 patients) to evaluate local control by fiberoptic bronchoscopy and biopsies of the original tumor site. A total dose of 60 Gy, given in 30 fractions of 2 Gy each, has been the standard in comparative trials of the RTOG for several years. The recent report of a dose-response effect on survival when the radiation dose was between 60 Gy and 69.6 Gy, given in fractions of 1.2 Gy twice daily separated by 4 hours or more, led to a phase III randomized trial of 60 Gy given as 2 Gy/day for 5 days a week, vs. 69.6 Gy given as 1.2 Gy twice daily (with a 6-hour interfraction interval) for 5 days a week. The 69.6-Gy fractionation regimen produced no improvement in short-term survival over the 60-Gy regimen.

The markedly different densities of thoracic tissues and the dose-response relationships for normal tissues and tumors indicate a need for inhomogeneity corrections.[86] Many uncertainties still exist concerning the best way to make such corrections. Advanced treatment planning systems can make corrections automatically; in that case, it is important to anticipate the need to increase total doses. Total doses of 60 Gy or more (without inhomogeneity corrections) are necessary,[87] and much higher total doses may be beneficial. Dose-escalation studies are underway, but they are limited by the fact that larger tumors necessarily require irradiation of larger volumes of normal lung. Treatment planning using three-dimensional systems provides very important information, especially dose-volume histograms. However, advanced treatment planning, even including intensity-modulated radiation therapy, only partially solves the problem. The possibility that proton irradiation could permit dose escalation without increasing the volume of lung treated needs to be explored further.

Chemotherapy and Radiation Therapy for Non–Small Cell Lung Cancer

According to standard staging procedures, half of all patients with NSCLC have evidence of distant metastases. Those without demonstrable extrathoracic spread have a high probability of occult metastasis. Chemotherapy is an important component of treatment for most patients with inoperable NSCLC. Numerous studies have shown the benefit of combining chemotherapy with radiation therapy for inoperable NSCLC.

Induction (neoadjuvant) chemotherapy followed by radiation therapy has many attractive features. Such a plan allows the most immediate treatment of all components of the tumor, both clinically evident and subclinical. The demonstration of response to chemotherapy provides justification for its continuation during or after radiation therapy. Three prospective trials that compared induction chemotherapy and subsequent radiation therapy with high-total-dose radiation therapy alone provide compelling evidence of the value of this combination.

The first of these trials was published by Dillman and colleagues[88] in 1990. The Cancer and Leukemia Group B (CALGB) 8433 trial compared induction therapy with cisplatin and vinblastine for 5 weeks plus radiation therapy (60 Gy given as 2.0 Gy/fraction for 5 days/wk) beginning on day 50 of treatment with immediate radiation therapy but no chemotherapy. Although survival was significantly improved among patients in the induction-chemotherapy group, a high death rate was observed during the first 100 days in the radiation therapy-alone group that was eventually explained by an imbalance in performance status.[89] A replication of the CALGB trial by the RTOG and ECOG studied a much larger number of patients but yielded nearly identical results—induction chemotherapy caused a small but statistically significant improvement in survival (Fig. 17-9).[90]

The third positive trial was reported by Le Chevalier and colleagues.[91] The cooperative group in France enrolled 353 patients in a study that compared induction chemotherapy (three monthly cycles of vindesine, cyclophosphamide, cisplatin, and lomustine followed by radiation therapy [65 Gy given as 2.5 Gy/fraction for 4 days/wk] beginning on day 75 to 80) with radiation therapy given in the same way but beginning on day 1. This group also found that induction chemotherapy improved survival.[92] Perhaps more important, they showed a statistically significant reduction in the incidence of distant metastasis with induction chemotherapy but no improvement in local tumor control.[85] Because of their policy of systematic fiberoptic bronchoscopy and biopsy at the site of the original tumor 3 months after the start of treatment, they were able to show that tumor persisted in more than 80% of patients and that induction chemotherapy conferred no advantage in local control.

The rationale for adding a single chemotherapeutic agent to radiation therapy is to increase local tumor control. Such therapy would be expected to have little if any effect on distant metastasis. An important study from the European Organization for Research and Treatment of Cancer[63] established the value of concurrent chemotherapy, with cisplatin given either daily or weekly at the same time as radiation therapy. Not only did local tumor control improve (Fig. 17-10), but survival was better as well (Fig. 17-11).[82] These findings corroborated the evidence that the intrathoracic tumor is an important determinant of survival and that an improvement in outcome for patients with NSCLC depends on improved local tumor control.

Sause and colleagues[90] reported a small series of patients treated with induction cisplatin and vinblastine followed by radiation therapy with concurrent cisplatin. Komaki and colleagues[89] reported experience with this regimen with larger numbers of patients and found it to be both well tolerated and encouraging with regard to median survival time (15.5 months) and 1-year rate of survival (65%).

The question of whether induction or concurrent chemotherapy is better is a question of whether control of distant metastases is more important than control of local tumor and distant metastases. Two similar trials provide compelling evidence in answer to this question. Furuse and colleagues[93] conducted a phase III trial of induction chemotherapy with cisplatin, vindesine, and mitomycin followed by radiation therapy in which 56 Gy was given in 2.0-Gy fractions for 5 fractions/wk, for 28 fractions starting approximately 7 to 8 weeks after the start of chemotherapy. This regimen was compared with one using the same chemotherapy plus radiation therapy beginning on the second day; the radiation therapy was modified by permitting a 10-day interruption after administration of the first 28 Gy, but the total dose was the same. This trial enrolled 320 patients. The median survival of patients receiving concurrent radiation therapy was 16.5 months, compared with 13.3 months for those receiving sequential treatment. The overall survival rate was significantly better among those given concurrent therapy (P = 0.03998) (Fig. 17-12).[93]

Curran and colleagues[94] reported a study of the RTOG comparing three treatments. The first group was given vinblastine and cisplatin followed by radiation therapy to 60 Gy, given as 2.0 Gy/fraction for 5 fractions/wk beginning on day 50. Patients in the second group were given the same regimen, but with radiation therapy beginning on day 1. A third group was given concurrent cisplatin and etoposide and hyperfractionated irradiation to a total dose of 69.6 Gy, given as 1.2 Gy twice

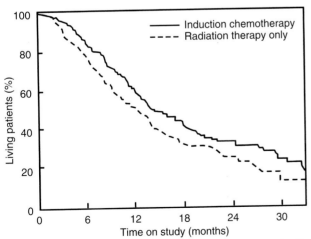

Fig. 17-9 Survival according to treatment group in the Radiation Therapy Oncology Group 88-08 and Eastern Cooperative Oncology Group 4588 trials. Induction chemotherapy plus radiation (*solid line*) resulted in improved outcome over radiation therapy only (*broken line*). (Data from Sause WT, Scott C, Taylor S, et al. *J Natl Cancer Inst* 1995;87:198-205.)

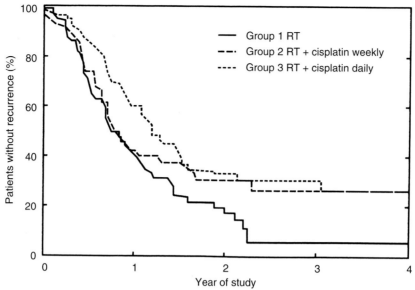

Fig. 17-10 Survival without local recurrence for patients with non–small cell lung cancer. Comparison of treatment group 1 with groups 2 and 3 showed significant differences (*P* = 0.009). (From Schaake-Koning C, van den Bogaert W, Dalesio O, et al. *N Engl J Med* 1992;326:524-530.)

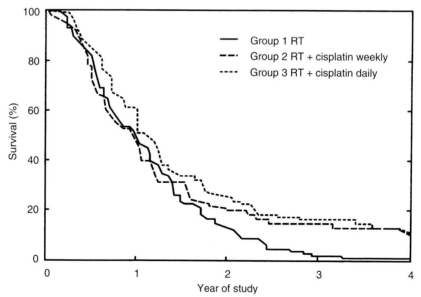

Fig. 17-11 Overall survival for patients with non–small cell lung cancer. Comparison of treatment group 1 with groups 2 and 3 showed significant differences (*P* = 0.04). (From Schaake-Koning C, van den Bogaert W, Dalesio O, et al. *N Engl J Med* 1992;326:524-530.)

daily separated by 6 or more hours. Preliminary results have shown the second treatment to be superior to the first, with median patient survival of 17 months in the former and 14.5 months in the latter. Survival is now statistically superior in cases of concurrent (rather than sequential) chemotherapy and radiation therapy.

The very similar findings of the Furuse and colleagues and RTOG studies[93,94] suggest that concurrent chemoradiation should be considered the standard for unresectable NSCLC as long as the patients have the same favorable performance status and weight loss characteristics of the patients in those trials.

Prophylactic Cranial Irradiation for Non–Small Cell Lung Cancer

Patients with inoperable adenocarcinoma or large cell carcinoma of the lung have a high probability of developing brain metastases (see Table 17-3); the same

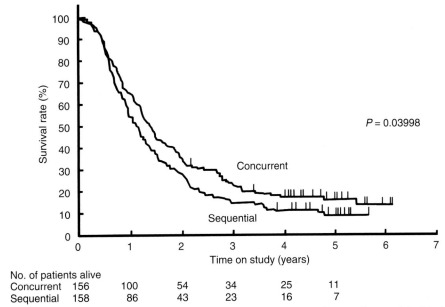

Fig. 17-12 Survival by treatment group in the West Japan Lung Cancer Group trial of induction ("sequential") versus concurrent thoracic irradiation for inoperable non–small cell lung cancer. (From Furuse K, Fukuoka M, Kawahara M, et al. *J Clin Oncol* 1999;17:2692-2699.)

is true of patients with resectable tumors who have metastases to regional lymph nodes.[60] Tables 17-1 and 17-3 show that 8% to 12% of patients who die of these types of cancer of the lung have metastasis only to the brain. Corroborating data come from experiences with patients who have developed clinical brain metastases, have undergone irradiation, and have lived 5 to 10 years with no further evidence of cancer.[50]

In a randomized prospective trial of the Veterans Administration Lung Group, patients with NSCLC received prophylactic cranial irradiation (PCI) to a total dose of 20 Gy, given in 10 fractions over 2 weeks. Brain metastases were present less often in patients with normal brain radionuclide scans before treatment. Although the numbers were too small for correlation with each specific cell type, patients with squamous cell carcinoma, large cell carcinoma, or adenocarcinoma had a statistically significantly lower frequency of brain metastasis (29% vs. 0%, $P < 0.05$).[94a] No difference in survival was found between patients who received cranial irradiation and those who did not.

According to autopsy findings relating to single-organ brain metastasis (see Table 17-3), PCI is likely to affect survival among patients with adenocarcinoma or large cell carcinoma. Russell and colleagues[95] reported results of a phase III study of PCI for patients at high risk of cerebral metastasis. These investigators found a trend toward reduction of intracranial spread with PCI but no effect on survival. They concluded that PCI had no role, even for those with high-risk disease. When local tumor and extracranial metastases can be controlled more consistently, it may be justifiable to study PCI further.

Radiation Therapy for Small Cell Lung Carcinoma

No doubt remains as to the importance of radiation therapy, delivered to the thoracic tumor, for SCLC limited to the chest. Two meta-analyses showed the value of thoracic irradiation in controlling disease within the chest. A small but statistically significant improvement in survival was found as well.[96,97]

The optimal manner of combining chemotherapy and radiation therapy for patients with small cell carcinoma is not yet clear. The use of both modalities simultaneously seems to be associated with a higher complete response rate, but it unquestionably is associated with increased morbidity, especially esophagitis and bone marrow suppression. Administering radiation therapy after the initiation of chemotherapy may permit the most effective use of systemic therapy.

Murray and colleagues[98] in Canada addressed the question of timing in a prospective randomized comparison of early vs. late thoracic irradiation (Fig. 17-13). Cycles of cyclophosphamide, doxorubicin, and vincristine were alternated with cisplatin and etoposide. Thoracic irradiation was given with the cisplatin and etoposide beginning on either week 3 or week 15. The total dose was 40 Gy, given in 15 fractions over 3 weeks. Patients who had a complete response to chemotherapy and thoracic irradiation were offered PCI to 25 Gy, given in 10 fractions over 2 weeks. Survival was significantly better ($P = 0.008$) among patients given early thoracic irradiation (Fig. 17-14).[98] Patients who received early thoracic irradiation also had a significant reduction ($P = 0.006$) in the incidence of brain metastasis.

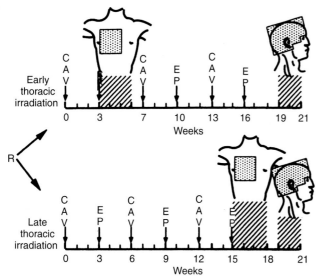

Fig. 17-13 Scheme of the National Cancer Institute of Canada trial of early versus late thoracic irradiation for small cell cancer of the lung. *CAV*, Cyclophosphamide, doxorubicin, and vincristine; *EP*, etoposide and cisplatin. (From Murray N, Coy P, Pater JL, et al. *J Clin Oncol* 1993;11:336-344.)

Another study that addressed the question of timing of thoracic irradiation was conducted by the Japanese Clinical Oncology Group.[99] Investigators randomized 228 patients to receive either induction chemotherapy followed by thoracic irradiation or concurrent treatment. The chemotherapy included cisplatin and etoposide and the total dose of radiation therapy was 45 Gy, given as 1.5 Gy twice daily, 5 days/week, for 3 weeks. The 2-year survival rates favored concurrent (55%) over sequential (35%) treatment ($P = 0.057$).

The fractionation question was approached in two phase II studies. McCracken and colleagues[100] from the SWOG combined intravenous cisplatin, etoposide,

and vincristine in two 4-week cycles with concurrent radiation therapy (45 Gy, given as 1.8 Gy/fraction for 5 days a week); PCI was given with a third cycle of cisplatin and etoposide, and additional chemotherapy including methotrexate, doxorubicin, and cyclophosphamide was given for 12 weeks. Among 154 patients treated, survival rates at 2 and 4 years were 42% and 30%, respectively.

Turrisi and Glover[101] reported the results of 32 patients given cisplatin and etoposide concurrently with accelerated fractionation (45 Gy, given as 1.5 Gy twice daily for 5 days a week). Two cycles of chemotherapy were given at 3-week intervals during irradiation, and six additional cycles alternated cisplatin-etoposide with cyclophosphamide-doxorubicin-vincristine. PCI was given to those who showed complete response after chemotherapy. The 2-year disease-free survival rate was 45%, and no deaths from cancer were observed after 2 years. Long-term results of the combined-modality approach using twice-daily radiation showed 2-year and 4-year survival rates of 54% and 36%, respectively, with 96% local tumor control.[102] An intergroup phase III study coordinated by the ECOG, with participation by the RTOG, compared these two approaches (i.e., once-daily vs. accelerated twice-daily radiation therapy). Both treatment groups involved concurrent administration of cisplatin and etoposide with the radiation. The results, reported by Turrisi and colleagues,[103] showed a significant survival advantage ($P = 0.04$) for the 211 patients treated with twice-a-day irradiation relative to the 208 patients treated once a day (Fig. 17-15). Their 2-year survival rates are the best reported to date in a cooperative group trial (40%). The 5-year survival rates were 28% for patients given accelerated fractionation and 21% for those given once-a-day treatment. Intrathoracic failure rates, nonetheless, were far too high; half of the patients

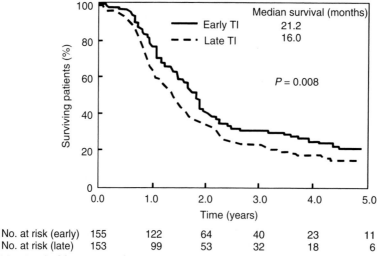

Fig. 17-14 Survival by timing of thoracic irradiation *(TI)* in the National Cancer Institute of Canada trial. (From Murray N, Coy P, Pater JL, et al. *J Clin Oncol* 1993;11:336-344.)

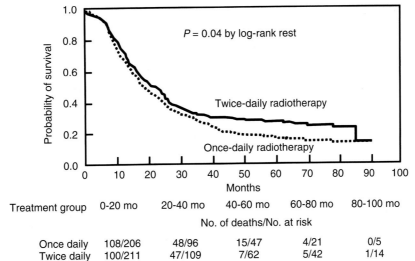

Fig. 17-15 Survival by treatment group: accelerated fractionation (twice-daily radiation therapy) versus standard treatment (once-daily radiation therapy). (From Turrisi AT, Kim K, Blum R, et al. *N Engl J Med* 1999;340:265-271.)

treated once daily and one third of the patients treated twice daily had local recurrence. Efforts are underway to improve local control by increasing the total dose above the 45 Gy used in the ECOG-RTOG intergroup trial, while keeping the overall treatment time as short as possible.

A select group of patients with disseminated disease may benefit from thoracic irradiation. Livingston and colleagues[104] observed a high proportion of patients (29 of 43, or 67%) with disseminated disease that responded completely to chemotherapy but had treatment failure first in the chest without other evidence of disease. Therefore it seems appropriate to consider thoracic irradiation for patients with disseminated disease if the tumor proves to be highly responsive to systemic chemotherapy.

Prophylactic Cranial Irradiation for Small Cell Lung Carcinoma

PCI is an important part of treatment for many patients with SCLC. As with thoracic irradiation, controversy exists about patient selection and the timing of PCI. With effective systemic chemotherapy, the risk of brain metastasis increases at the rate of 2% to 3% per month for 18 to 24 months.[39,105,106] If patients who develop neurologic symptoms and signs and who are found to have brain metastasis could be treated successfully with radiation therapy, PCI would be less important in the overall management plan. In a study of 40 patients with brain metastasis from small cell carcinoma (confirmed by radionuclide scans or CT), 20 died as a direct result of progression of the intracranial tumor.[107] Baglan and Marks[108] reported more successful treatment of patients with overt intracranial metastasis from SCLC, but they eliminated patients who had such rapidly progressive disease that effective treatment could not be instituted; these patients also might have benefited from PCI.

PCI has been considered unnecessary in the treatment of patients with SCLC because it has had no effect on survival in several studies. However, the endpoint analyzed has usually been median survival duration. As is true in evaluations of the effectiveness of thoracic irradiation, this endpoint is relatively meaningless for evaluating PCI. Rosen and colleagues[109] assessed long-term survival rates in three groups of patients given systemic chemotherapy for SCLC at the National Cancer Institute between 1970 and 1980. In group 1, PCI was administered from the first day of treatment; in group 2, PCI was given between the twelfth and twenty-fourth weeks; in group 3, PCI was omitted. These investigators found a significant improvement in long-term survival rates among patients who received PCI; the 30-month survival rate was 27% in group 1, 40% in group 2, and 14% in group 3.

A comparison of two sequential treatment policies at the Memorial Sloan-Kettering Cancer Center by Rosenstein and colleagues[110] also suggested an important role for PCI in long-term survival. Of 36 patients with limited SCLC whose treatment included PCI (from 1979 to 1982), the brain was the first site of failure in 18% of the 22 complete responders. A more recent (1985 to 1989) group of 26 patients treated without PCI had a 45% rate of disease failure in the brain. The 2-year survival rate was 42% for the PCI-treated patients as opposed to 13% for those not receiving PCI; there were no 5-year survivors among those who did not receive PCI, but 38% of patients who were given cranial irradiation were alive 5 years later.

A meta-analysis of seven prospectively randomized clinical trials showed higher rates of disease-free and overall survival in patients who received PCI.[111] However, this analysis can be criticized because more than

TABLE 17-6

Frequency of Brain Metastasis in Small Cell Carcinoma by Treatment Group

Treatment Group	Number of Patients	Number with Brain Metastasis
No PCI	82	21 (26%)
PCI		
30 Gy (10 fractions of 3.0 Gy)	51	5 (10%)
25 Gy (10 fractions of 2.5 Gy)	194	6 (3%)

From Komaki R, Cox JD, Hartz AJ, et al. *Am J Clin Oncol* 1985;8:362-370.
PCI, Prophylactic cranial irradiation.

half the trials had fewer than 100 patients and the dose-fractionation regimens were not consistent. International efforts are underway to address the dose-fractionation question. Another criticism is that the meta-analysis did not address the frequency of late neurotoxicity among patients who did and those who did not receive PCI.

Late neuropsychological sequelae and CT abnormalities have been found in patients given PCI and combination chemotherapy for SCLC.[112,113] The PCI has consistently been implicated, but it is likely that certain chemotherapeutic agents—notably the nitrosoureas, intravenous methotrexate, and the epipodophyllotoxins—interact with cranial radiation to produce late sequelae. In most studies the individual fraction size for PCI has ranged from 3 to 4 Gy. Table 17-6 shows a nonrandomized comparison of the results of 2.5 Gy and 3 Gy/fraction combined with systemic therapy that included cyclophosphamide, doxorubicin, and vincristine. The small fraction size seemed as effective as the larger one.[106] Sufficient long-term follow-up of these patients, with detailed neuropsychological evaluation, was not done. However, the lowest effective fraction size and total dose for PCI are least likely to be associated with late neuropsychological sequelae.

In a prospective study of patients undergoing PCI for SCLC, detailed neuropsychological assessments were performed before and after PCI.[114] The results showed a strikingly high frequency of neurocognitive dysfunction before PCI. Deficits were no greater after PCI. Therefore much of the late neurocognitive deficit after treatment for SCLC may be related to either the disease itself, a paraneoplastic phenomenon, or the chemotherapy.

Apical Sulcus Tumors

As is evident from data given in Table 17-4, any histopathologic type of carcinoma of the lung can occur in the extreme apex or superior sulcus and cause Pancoast's syndrome. Symptoms of shoulder or arm pain are often accompanied by dysesthesia and atrophy along the distribution of the ulnar nerve. Patients also may have Horner's syndrome and radiographic evidence of destruction of ribs or vertebrae. The diagnosis often can be established by percutaneous needle aspiration; sputum cytology studies and bronchoscopy are usually unrevealing.

Preoperative radiation therapy followed by exploratory thoracotomy and resection, if possible, has widely been considered the standard treatment for the past three decades. Although little objective justification was found for this practice other than the results of a small, highly selective series reported by Paulson,[115,116] it was a reasonable approach and no alternative treatment seemed to exist. Several series have now convincingly demonstrated that apical sulcus tumors can be cured with aggressive radiation therapy.[49,117,118] This information, combined with the recognition that split-course radiation therapy is disadvantageous in the local control of cancer of the lung, justifies a completely different approach to patients with potentially resectable carcinoma in the apical sulcus of the lung.

Although tumors that present in the apical sulcus often cannot be diagnosed by bronchoscopy, fine-needle aspiration under CT guidance is nearly always able to yield a diagnosis. Pretreatment evaluation by magnetic resonance imaging (MRI) is essential because it more accurately displays the anatomy of superior sulcus tumors than does CT.[119] A sagittal section obtained by MRI can show extension of such a tumor to the posterior wall of the subclavian artery, the vertebral bodies, and mediastinal lymph nodes. MRI is essential to evaluate the resectability of superior sulcus tumors. MRI of the brain is also important because the propensity of superior sulcus tumors to spread to the brain is greater than that of tumors at other locations in the lung.[120]

Although interest continues with regard to preoperative radiation therapy and, more recently, chemoradiation therapy,[121] this sequence is disadvantageous for the 20% to 50% of patients who prove to have unresectable tumors. It is not possible to pursue a successful course of treatment after an uncontrolled interruption of radiation therapy or chemotherapy because of the operative procedure. If mediastinoscopy shows that no lymph nodes are involved, then thoracotomy can be performed first and some tumors can be resected completely; these patients can be spared all other treatments unless they are participating in an investigational protocol. If the tumors are unresectable, aggressive management using concurrent chemotherapy and radiation therapy can be pursued with curative intent.

Superior Vena Cava Obstruction

Approximately 5% of all patients with cancer of the lung have signs and symptoms suggesting obstruction of the superior vena cava. Currently in the United States, 95%

of patients with these manifestations have a malignant tumor; in three fourths of these patients, it is cancer of the lung. The obstruction is usually the result of extrinsic compression by the tumor, although direct invasion of the vessel wall can occur. Thrombosis can further impede venous return.

Although superior vena cava obstruction is considered a radiation-therapy emergency, the onset of symptoms and signs can be acute or subacute. A histologic or cytologic diagnosis can usually be made by means of sputum cytology tests, fiberoptic bronchoscopy, or percutaneous needle aspiration. If small cell carcinoma is confirmed, it is usually desirable to initiate systemic combination chemotherapy and concomitant thoracic irradiation if the disease is limited to the chest.

The most effective palliation is achieved by radiation therapy involving first large-sized fractions[122] and later more conventional fractionation. Fractions of 3.5 or 4 Gy for the first 3 or 4 days usually relieve the symptoms of dyspnea within a few days; 85% to 90% of patients[123,124] have relief of symptoms and signs within 3 weeks. Addition of corticosteroids is not needed because they have not been shown to contribute to a more rapid relief of symptoms.

PROGNOSIS FOR INOPERABLE CARCINOMA OF THE LUNG

The most important prognostic factors for patients with inoperable carcinoma of the lung, even those who will ultimately die of the disease, are pretreatment performance status[125] and weight loss.[126] Despite the fact that patients with minimal symptoms and no weight loss live longer than those who are more symptomatic, virtually every patient with cancer of the lung who is not effectively treated dies in a relatively short time.

Before the demonstration of the effectiveness of radiation therapy for cancer of the lung and of the dose-response relationships, an argument could be made for withholding treatment from patients who were relatively asymptomatic. It was thought that radiation therapy would have marginal, if any, benefit and might produce symptoms. This idea has persisted into the megavoltage era as a general therapeutic nihilism about lung cancer.[127]

A review of studies conducted by the Veterans Administration Lung Group in which patients with inoperable lung cancer were given placebos and "best-available supportive care" consisting of antibiotics, expectorants, and oxygen showed that only 4% of patients were alive at 2 years.[35] Of the 82 patients who had the highest performance status (80 to 100 score on the Karnofsky scale, meaning they were minimally symptomatic) and who were treated only with supportive measures, none survived 5 years.

Komaki and colleagues[106] reported that 45 of 410 patients (11%) were alive 3 years and 32 (8%) were alive 5 years after therapy for cancer of the lung. The 3-year

TABLE 17-7

Effect of Tumor Extent on 3-Year Survival Rates

Tumor Extent	SURVIVAL RATE (%) DURING THE SPECIFIED TREATMENT PERIOD	
	1971-1975	1975-1978
STAGE		
I	33.3 (36)*	20.8 (48)
II	4.8 (21)	18.2 (33)
III	1.4 (140)	10.6 (132)
NODE INVOLVEMENT		
None	18.2 (72)	8.0 (81)
Hilar	14.3 (21)	15.2 (33)
Mediastinal	1.2 (86)	12.2 (82)
Supraclavicular	5.6 (18)	17.6 (17)

Modified from Komaki R, Cox JD, Hartz AJ, et al. *Am J Clin Oncol* 1985;8:362-370.
*Numbers in parentheses are numbers of patients.

TABLE 17-8

Effect of Pretreatment Status on 3-Year Survival Rates

Status	Survival Rate (%)
PERFORMANCE STATUS (KARNOFSKY SCALE)	
80	0.0 (193)*
80-89	6.6 (76)
90-99	25.5 (131)
100	70.0 (10)
TUMOR HISTOLOGY	
Squamous cell	9.6 (228)
Small cell	9.0 (67)
Adenocarcinoma	16.2 (37)
Large cell	28.6 (35)
Adenosquamous	10.0 (5)
Unspecified	0.0 (38)

Modified from Komaki R, Cox JD, Hartz AJ, et al. *Am J Clin Oncol* 1985;8:362-370.
*Numbers in parentheses are numbers of patients.

survival rate for 197 patients treated between 1971 and 1975 was 7%, compared with 14% for patients treated from 1975 through 1978. The improvement in survival was not because of selecting more favorable stages for treatment, but because of the more effective treatment of patients with advanced-stage cancer, especially those with metastases to the mediastinal and supraclavicular lymph nodes (Table 17-7).[106] All long-term survivors had a performance status score of 80 or above on the Karnofsky scale (Table 17-8). Of the patients who were alive at 36 months, 80% lived 5 or more years, and two-thirds lived 10 years.

The observation that large cell carcinoma is associated with the greatest probability of long-term survival prompted a subsequent study of more recently treated patients.[128] In that study, large cell carcinoma and adenocarcinoma were combined because failure pattern analyses had not shown any differences between these two groups. When compared with the squamous cell carcinoma group, the adenocarcinoma/large cell carcinoma group had a higher probability of long-term survival.[128]

PALLIATIVE IRRADIATION

Tumors that recur postoperatively in the bronchial stump or mediastinum can be reduced by radiation, although long-term control is rare. Postirradiation recurrences that have an endobronchial component may benefit from brachytherapy. Remote afterloading of bronchoscopically placed catheters with radioactive sources, usually ^{192}Ir, can be used to relieve symptoms and reverse atelectasis.[129]

The majority of patients with cancer of the lung develop distant metastases that produce distressing symptoms and eventually threaten life. Radiation is the most effective means of alleviating symptoms when they are clearly localized. The most common sites of distant metastasis are the liver, adrenal glands, bones, and brain.[38] The only symptom from hepatic metastases that can be relieved by radiation therapy is pain.[130] Adrenal metastasis also can cause pain in the back, flank, or upper abdomen, and irradiation usually confers rather prompt relief.

Prospective studies of radiation therapy for skeletal metastasis have been carried out by the RTOG.[131] The patients treated in these trials had metastases from many primary sites, but cancer of the lung was common. The results of treatment of approximately 1000 patients showed that 90% experienced some relief, and more than half had complete disappearance of pain.

Similarly, the RTOG conducted prospective trials of the palliative treatment of metastasis to the brain.[132] The frequency with which symptoms were relieved was related to the types of neurologic symptoms and signs. Complete relief was achieved in 35% to 72% of patients, and some benefit was observed in 65% to 85%. Seizures, both major motor and focal in type, and headache are the symptoms most consistently relieved (in 60% to 70% of cases). Symptoms disappear completely less often in patients with impaired mentation, cerebellar dysfunction, motor loss, and cranial nerve abnormalities than in patients without these impairments, but fully two thirds of them experience some benefit.

Back pain and neurologic symptoms and signs may herald the onset of paraplegia caused by metastases from cancer of the lung, especially small cell carcinoma. Myelography or MRI can demonstrate the level of the block, and CT or MRI usually shows whether the spinal cord is being impinged on as the result of an extradural tumor or vertebral collapse with mechanical compromise. Widening of the spinal cord may represent intramedullary metastasis.[133] It is important to identify the cause as quickly as possible; the sooner dexamethasone is started and palliative irradiation is begun, the greater the probability of stabilizing or reversing symptoms and signs.

THE THYMUS

The thymus plays a critical role in the development of cell-mediated immunity. It acts on primitive cells that originate in the bone marrow to render them immunologically competent. Surgical removal of the thymus in the newborn decreases circulating lymphocytes and severely impairs cellular immunity. Thymectomy in older children and adults does not result in immune deficiencies, although the circulating lymphocytes may still decrease. Similarly, irradiation of the adult thymus may decrease the number of circulating lymphocytes; however, vast experience with incidental irradiation of the thymus during treatment of Hodgkin's disease, malignant lymphoma, and cancer of the breast, lung, and esophagus has not led to evidence of immune alteration independent of the diseases themselves.

Thymomas

Tumors of the thymus are uncommon, and most are benign. Limited experiences, therefore, have led to disparate views of the natural history and treatment of invasive thymus neoplasms. Thymomas are neoplasms of the thymic epithelial cells; tumors that were grouped with them in the past, namely, "granulomatous thymomas," are discussed with tumors of hematopoietic tissues (Chapter 33) and are now properly identified as Hodgkin's disease with nodular sclerosis. Seminomas and related tumors are discussed along with extragonadal malignant germinal tumors so that they can be compared and contrasted with their gonadal counterparts in Chapters 26 and 31.

Thymomas account for at least 10% of all mediastinal tumors.[37] They arise in the anterior mediastinum, although they may rarely be found in the posterior mediastinum or in the neck.[134] Although the median patient age at the time of diagnosis is 50 years, thymomas can occur at any age. They constitute about 10% of mediastinal tumors in children and are seen with equal frequency in males and females.

Thymomas have been grouped according to their histopathologic features. Most authors recognize predominantly epithelial, predominantly lymphoid, and spindle cell types. Little correlation exists between natural history and subtype. In fact, the correlation is poor between microscopic criteria for malignancy and the behavior of these neoplasms. Suster and Rosai[135] studied histologic material in which they found malignant cytologic features that justified the designation *thymic carcinoma* from 60 patients, 48 of whom had undergone resection. They found that patients who had high-grade tumors that were poorly circumscribed, lacked lobular growth patterns, and had a high mitotic index had a rapidly fatal outcome. In general, however, the terms *benign* and *malignant* can be quite misleading when referring to thymomas. Pollack and colleagues[136] performed flow cytometric analysis of paraffin-imbedded tissues from 25 patients with thymomas, specifically excluding thymic carcinomas; they found no relationship between the percentage of cells in S phase and patient outcome, but survival was significantly better for the 16 patients with diploid tumors than for the 9 patients whose tumors were aneuploid ($P = 0.002$).

Even tumors that are considered relatively benign have a propensity to recur locally, but distant metastasis is uncommon. Metastasis, however, has been reported in 5% of all thymomas.[137,138] At least one fourth of patients with invasive thymomas develop metastases, usually to supraclavicular lymph nodes, liver, or bone.

The most important features that determine treatment and outcome are whether a thymoma is encapsulated or invasive and whether myasthenia gravis is present. One third to one half of all thymomas are invasive. Although only 15% of all patients with myasthenia gravis have a thymic tumor, one third to one half of all patients with thymomas have myasthenia gravis.

A useful staging classification, based on surgical and pathologic findings, was originally proposed by Bergh and colleagues[139] and modified by Masaoka and colleagues[140]:

Stage I   Macroscopically completely encapsulated; no microscopic capsular invasion

Stage II   Microscopic invasion into capsule; macroscopic invasion into surrounding fatty tissue or mediastinal pleura

Stage III   Macroscopic invasion into neighboring organs

Stage IVA   Pleural or pericardial implants

Stage IVB   Lymphogenous or hematogenous metastasis

Treatment

Complete resection of the tumor should be accomplished if at all possible. Encapsulated (stage I) and minimally invasive (stage II) thymomas are virtually always resectable unless there are medical contraindications to thoracotomy. At least 20% of obviously invasive (stage III) thymomas are unresectable.[140,141] Contemporary imaging procedures, primarily high-resolution CT with intravenous contrast or MRI, can provide information to suggest that a tumor is unresectable.

A stage I thymoma that is completely resected can recur locally or by pleural implantation. Whether

TABLE 17-9

Invasive Thymoma Recurrence After Complete Resection by Treatment Group (Number of Recurrences in Number of Patients Treated)*

Study and Reference	No Postoperative Irradiation	Postoperative Irradiation
Nordstrom et al[142]	1 in 1	9 in 19
Cohen et al[143]	4 in 5	5 in 8
Batata et al[141]	8 in 8	6 in 11
Ariaratnam et al[144]	—	3 in 8
Gerein et al[145]	—	2 in 6
Penn and Hope-Stone[146]	1 in 1	0 in 3
Monden et al[147]	9 in 21	14 in 68
Marks et al[148]	—	0 in 3
Arriagada et al[149]	—	1 in 6
Pollack et al[150]	1 in 3	1 in 6
Krueger et al[151]	—	0 in 1
Urgesis et al[152]	—	3 in 33
Curran et al[153]	8 in 19	0 in 5
TOTALS	32 in 58 (57%)	44 in 177 (25%)

*Recurrence indicates a new manifestation at any site, local or distant.

radiation therapy also should be given for encapsulated tumors is unsettled. No evidence supports the systematic use of postoperative irradiation for completely resected stage I tumors.

If total gross removal can be achieved and the tumor proves to be invasive, postoperative irradiation is well justified. Batata and colleagues,[141] reporting the experience from Memorial Hospital in New York City, found that no patient with invasive thymoma was cured by resection alone. A review of the very limited data available (Table 17-9)[141-153] strongly suggests that surgical adjuvant radiation therapy reduces the probability of tumor recurrence in patients who have invasive thymomas. (Notably, these data were based on all recurrences, not just recurrence within the irradiated volume.)

It is possible to increase the resectability of invasive thymomas. Unresectable thymomas can be made resectable by preoperative radiation therapy. However, encouraging results with chemotherapy[154] have led us to pursue initial chemotherapy for unresectable thymomas, reserving radiation therapy for use postoperatively or as definitive therapy if unresectability persists. Our current regimen consists of a combination of cyclophosphamide, doxorubicin, cisplatin, and prednisone.[155]

For every patient with an invasive thymoma that cannot be completely resected, definitive radiation therapy is necessary. Such tumors have a considerable propensity to disseminate within the pleural cavity and to spread beyond the thorax.

The entire mediastinum and both hila should be encompassed within the irradiated volume, as well as

TABLE 17-10

Local Control of Unresectable Invasive Thymoma According to Total Radiation Dose*

Study and Reference	TOTAL DOSE (Gy)		
	≤ 48	49-59	≥ 60
Gerein et al[145]	2 in 9	—	1 in 2
Marks et al[148]	6 in 6	—	—
Chahinian et al[157]	—	0 in 3	—
Ariaratnam et al[144]	6 in 10	1 in 1	—
Arriagada et al[149]	7 in 12	11 in 17	3 in 3
Kersh et al[158]	1 in 1	5 in 8	—
Krueger et al[151]	1 in 3	6 in 8	—
TOTAL	23 in 47 (49%)	26 in 41 (63%)	4 in 5 (80%)

*Number of cases controlled in the number of cases treated.

any sites of pleural implantation identified by the thoracic surgeon. The supraclavicular region also should be included if adenopathy is present. Prophylactic irradiation of one or both supraclavicular fossae can be recommended, but its contribution to survival remains to be measured. Similarly, it might be desirable to irradiate the entire hemithorax if pleural implantation has been documented, although experience with this approach is limited.[156]

The dose required to control invasive thymoma is not clear. In the series studied by Gerein and colleagues[145] and Marks and colleagues,[148] patients treated to a total dose of 45 Gy or less after complete tumor resection had recurrent disease, whereas those who received a higher total dose remained free of cancer. When only a partial resection or biopsy is performed, higher total doses are advisable. Available data concerning the dose response of unresectable thymoma are summarized in Table 17-10.* Although the published experience is not sufficient to indicate what the control rate might be at total doses of 60 Gy and above, the substantial failure rate at lower doses suggests that the total dose should be as high as can be tolerated by the surrounding normal tissues.

Results

Myasthenia gravis has long been considered to have an unfavorable effect on the prognosis of patients with

*References 144, 145, 148, 149, 151, 157, 158.

thymoma. However, the studies of Shamji and colleagues,[159] Verley and Hollmann,[160] Wilkins and Castleman,[161] Maggi and colleagues,[162] and Urgesi and colleagues[152] have shown that myasthenia does not adversely affect prognosis.

The role of radiation therapy for invasive thymoma is clearly established, although many uncertainties still exist as to the optimal treatment volume and dose-time relationships. Of 24 patients reported by Batata and colleagues,[141] 5 (21%) were alive and well 5 years after irradiation, 7 (29%) were alive with disease, and 12 (50%) were dead of disease. No patient who underwent only surgical tumor resection was cured. Nordstrom and colleagues[142] reported on 20 patients with stage III thymoma, all but one of whom received radiation therapy: no patients were alive and well 5 or more years after treatment. Kersh and colleagues[158] reviewed 10 cases of invasive thymoma in which no complete resection was performed; local control was achieved in six patients, but three of them died of distant metastatic disease. Arriagada and colleagues [149] reported a retrospective study of 56 cases from four hospitals in or near Paris; 6 patients underwent complete tumor resection, 22 had incomplete resections, and 28 had only biopsies. All received radiation therapy. The local recurrence rate at 2 years was 31%, and 21 patients (37.5%) developed metastasis beyond the thorax. The actuarial survival rate at 5 years was 46%. With more systematic use of radiation therapy as soon as the diagnosis of invasive thymoma is established, the prognosis for these patients might be substantially improved.

The initial stage of the tumor is an important prognostic factor. Stage is closely related to the achievement of complete resection. Thus patients with stage I or II completely resected tumors have an excellent outlook.[153] Patients who have complete or subtotal resection and then postoperative radiation have a far more favorable prognosis if their cancer can be classified as stage III rather than stage IV.[152]

REFERENCES

1. Evans WA, Leucutia T. Intrathoracic changes induced by heavy radiation. *Am J Roentgenol* 1925;13:203-220.
2. Lacassagne A. Action des rayons du radium sur les muqueuses de l'oesophage et de la trachee chez le lapin. *CR Soc Biol* 1921; 84:26-27.
3. Fajardo LF, Berthrong M, Anderson RE. Respiratory tract. In: *Radiation Pathology*. New York, NY: Oxford University Press; 2001:198-208.
4. King RJ, Jones MB, Minoo P. Regulation of lung cell proliferation by polypeptide growth factors. *Am J Physiol* 1989;257:23-38.
5. Rubin P, Johnston CJ, Williams JP, et al. A perpetual cascade of cytokines postirradiation leads to pulmonary fibrosis. *Int J Radiat Oncol Biol Phys* 1995;33:99-109.
6. Rodemann HP, Binder A, Burger A, et al. The underlying cellular mechanism of fibrosis. *Int J Radiat Oncol Biol Phys* 1996;54: S32-S36.

7. Franklin TJ. Therapeutic approaches to organ fibrosis. *Int J Biochem Cell Biol* 1997;29:79-89.

8. Grande JP. Role of transforming growth factor-β in tissue injury and repair. *Proc Soc Exp Biol Med* 1997;214:27-40.

9. Anscher MS, Murase T, Prescott DM, et al. Changes in plasma TGFβ levels during pulmonary radiotherapy as a predictor of the risk of developing radiation pneumonitis. *Int J Radiat Oncol Biol Phys* 1994;30:671-676.

10. Beck LS, DeGuzman L, Lee WP, et al. One systemic administration of transforming growth factor-β1 reverses age- or glucocorticoid-impaired wound healing. *J Clin Invest* 1993; 92:2841-2849.

11. Finkelstein JN, Johnston CJ, Baggs R, et al. Early alterations in extracellular matrix and transforming growth factor beta gene expression in mouse lung indicative of late radiation fibrosis. *Int J Radiat Oncol Biol Phys* 1994;28:621-631.

12. Martin M, Lefaix J, Delanian S. TGF-beta1 and radiation fibrosis: a master switch and a specific therapeutic target? *Int J Radiat Oncol Biol Phys* 2000;47:277-290.

13. Delanian S. Striking regression of radiation-induced fibrosis by a combination of pentoxifylline and tocopherol. *Br J Radiol* 1998;71:892-894.

14. Piguet PF, Rosen H, Vesin C, et al. Effective treatment of the pulmonary fibrosis elicited in mice by bleomycin or silica with anti-CD-11 antibodies. *Am Rev Respir Dis* 1993;147: 435-441.

15. Anscher MS, Kong F-M, Andrews K, et al. Plasma transforming growth factor β1 as a predictor of radiation pneumonitis. *Int J Radiat Oncol Biol Phys* 1998;41:1029-1035.

16. Fu XL, Huang H, Benkl G, et al. Predicting the risk of symptomatic radiation-induced lung injury using both the physical and biological parameters V30 and transforming growth factor β. *Int J Radiat Oncol Biol Phys* 2001;50:899-908.

17. Liao Z-X, Travis EL, Tucker SL. Damage and morbidity from pneumonitis after irradiation of partial volumes of mouse lung. *Int J Radiat Oncol Biol Phys* 1995;32:1359-1370.

18. Tucker SL, Liao Z-X, Travis EL. Estimation of the spatial distribution of target cells in mouse lung. *Int J Radiat Oncol Biol Phys* 1997;38:1055-1066.

19. Travis EL, Liao Z-X, Tucker SL. Spatial heterogeneity of the volume effect for radiation pneumonitis in mouse lung. *Int J Radiat Oncol Biol Phys* 1997;38:1045-1054.

19a. Travis EL, Komaki R. Treatment-related lung damage. In: Pass HI et al, eds. *Lung Cancer: Principles and Practice.* 2nd ed. Philadelphia, Pa.: Lippincott Williams & Wilkins; 2000.

20. Boersma LJ, Theuws JCM, Kwa SLS, et al. Regional variation in functional subunit density in the lung: regarding Liao et al IJROBP 32(5):1359-1370; 1995. *Int J Radiat Oncol Biol Phys* 1996;34:1187-1188.

21. Khan MA, Hill RP, Van Dyk J. Partial volume rat lung irradiation: an evaluation of early DNA damage. *Int J Radiat Oncol Biol Phys* 1998;40:467-476.

22. Yamada M, Kudoh S, Hirata K, et al. Risk factors of pneumonitis following chemoradiotherapy for lung cancer. *Eur J Cancer* 1998;34:71-75.

23. Whitfield AGW, Bond WM, Kunkler PB. Radiation damage to thoracic tissues. *Thorax* 1963;18:371-380.

24. Stone DJ, Schwarz MJ, Green RA. Fatal pulmonary insufficiency due to radiation effect upon the lung. *Am J Med* 1956;21: 211-226.

25. Bergmann M, Graham EA. Pneumonectomy for severe irradiation damage. *J Thorac Surg* 1951;22:549-564.

26. Lipshitz HI, Shuman LS. Radiation-induced pulmonary change: CT findings. *J Comput Assist Tomogr* 1984;8:15-19.

27. Byhardt RW, Abrams R, Almagro U. The association of adult respiratory distress syndrome (ARDS) with thoracic irradiation (RT). *Int J Radiat Oncol Biol Phys* 1988;15:1441-1446.

28. Bernard GR, Luce JM, Sprung CL. High-dose corticosteroids in patients with the adult respiratory distress syndrome. *N Engl J Med* 1987;317:1565-1570.

29. Sweany SK, Moss WT, Haddy FJ. The effects of chest irradiation on pulmonary function. *J Clin Invest* 1959;38:587-593.

30. Moss WT, Haddy FJ, Sweany SK. Some factors altering the severity of acute radiation pneumonitis: variation with cortisone, heparin, and antibiotics. *Radiology* 1960;75:50-54.

31. Choi NC, Kanarek DJ, Kazemi H. Physiologic changes in pulmonary function after thoracic radiotherapy for patients with lung cancer and role of regional pulmonary function studies in predicting postradiotherapy pulmonary function before radiotherapy. *Cancer Treat Symp* 1985;2:119.

32. Brady LW, Germon PA, Cander L. The effects of radiation therapy on pulmonary function in carcinoma of the lung. *Radiology* 1965;85:130-134.

33. Cox JD. Fractionation: a paradigm for clinical research in radiation oncology. *Int J Radiat Oncol Biol Phys* 1987;13:1271-1281.

34. Cox JD, Azarnia N, Byhardt RW, et al. A randomized phase I/II trial of hyperfractionated radiation therapy with total doses of 60.0 Gy to 79.2 Gy: possible survival benefit with ≥ 69.6 Gy in favorable patients with Radiation Therapy Oncology Group stage III non-small-cell lung carcinoma: report of Radiation Therapy Oncology Group 83-11. *J Clin Oncol* 1990;8: 1543-1555.

35. Cox JD, Komaki K, Byhardt RW. Is immediate chest radiotherapy obligatory for any or all patients with limited-stage non-small cell carcinoma of the lung? Yes. *Cancer Treat Rep* 1983; 67:327-331.

36. Wolf J, Spear P, Yesner R. Nitrogen mustard and the steroid hormones in the treatment of inoperable bronchogenic carcinoma. *Am J Med* 1960;29:1008-1016.

37. Del Regato JA, Spjut HJ, Cox JD. *Cancer: Diagnosis, Treatment and Prognosis.* 6th ed. St Louis, Mo.: Mosby; 1985.

38. Yesner R, Carter D. Pathology of carcinoma of the lung: changing patterns. *Clin Chest Med* 1982;3:257-289.

39. Cox JD, Yesner RA. Adenocarcinoma of the lung: recent results from the Veterans Administration Lung Group. *Am Rev Respir Dis* 1979;120:1025-1029.

40. Kuhn C III, Askin FB. Lung and mediastinum. In: Kissane JM, ed. *Anderson's Pathology.* 9th ed. St. Louis, Mo: Mosby; 1990: 920-1046.

41. Cox JD, Yesner RA. Causes of treatment failure and death in carcinoma of the lung. *Yale J Biol Med* 1981;54:201-207.

42. Nohl HC. Investigation into lymphatic and vascular spread of carcinoma of bronchus. *Thorax* 1956;11:172-185.

43. Fleming I, Cooper JS, Henson DE, et al, eds. *AJCC Cancer Staging Manual.* 5th ed. Philadelphia, Pa: Lippincott Williams & Wilkins; 1997:127-137.

44. Carlens E. Appraisal of choice and results of treatment for bronchogenic carcinoma. *Chest* 1974;65:442-445.

45. Goldberg EM, Glickman AS, Kahan FR. Mediastinoscopy for assessing mediastinal spread in clinical staging of carcinoma of lung. *Cancer* 1970;25:347-353.

46. Palumbo LT, Sharpe WS. Scalene node biopsy: correlation with other diagnostic procedures in 550 cases. *Arch Surg* 1969;98:90-93.

47. Nugent J, Bunn P, Matthews M, et al. CNS metastases in small cell bronchogenic carcinoma: increasing frequency and changing pattern with lengthening survival. *Cancer* 1979;44:1885-1893.

48. Komaki R, Cox JD, Whitson W. Risk of brain metastasis from small cell carcinoma of the lung related to length of survival and prophylactic irradiation. *Cancer Treat Rep* 1981;65:811-814.

49. Komaki R, Roh J, Cox JD, et al. Superior sulcus tumors: results of irradiation of 36 patients. *Cancer* 1981;48:1563-1568.

50. Komaki R, Cox JD, Stark R. Frequency of brain metastasis in adenocarcinoma and large cell carcinoma of the lung: correlation with survival. *Int J Radiat Oncol Biol Phys* 1983;9:1467-1470.

51. Byrd RB, Carr DT, Miller WE. Radiographic abnormalities in carcinoma of the lung as related to histological type. *Thorax* 1969;24:573-575.

52. Byhardt RW, Hartz A, Libnoch JA, et al. Prognostic influence of TNM staging and LDH levels in small cell carcinoma of the lung (SCCL). *Int J Radiat Oncol Biol Phys* 1986;12:771-777.

53. McLoud TC, Bourgouin PM, Greenberg RW, et al. Bronchogenic carcinoma: analysis of staging in the mediastinum with CT by correlative lymph node mapping and sampling. *Radiology* 1992;182:319-323.

54. Norlund JD, Byhardt RW, Foley WD, et al. Computed tomography in the staging of small lung cancer: implications for combined modality therapy. *Int J Radiat Oncol Biol Phys* 1985;11:1081-1084.

55. Pieterman RM, van Putten JWG, Meuzelaar JJ, et al. Preoperative staging of non-small cell lung cancer with positron emission tomography. *N Engl J Med* 2000;343:254-261.

56. Mac Manus MP. Influence of PET scanning on radiotherapeutic management of NSCLC. *Lung Cancer* 2000;29:180-181.

57. Komaki R. Preoperative and postoperative irradiation for cancer of the lung. *J Belge Radiol* 1985;68:195-198.

58. Komaki R. Preoperative radiation therapy for superior sulcus lesions. *Chest Surg Clin N Am* 1991;1:13-35.

59. van Houtte P. Postoperative radiotherapy for lung cancer. *Lung Cancer* 1991;7:57-64.

60. Shields TW. Treatment failures after surgical resection of thoracic tumors. *Cancer Treat Symp* 1983;2:69.

61. PORT Meta-analysis Trialists Group. Postoperative radiotherapy in non-small-cell lung cancer: systematic review and meta-analysis of individual patient data from nine randomized controlled trials. *Lancet* 1998;352:257-263.

62. Chung CK, Stryker JA, O'Neill MJ. Evaluation of adjuvant postoperative radiotherapy for lung cancer. *Int J Radiat Oncol Biol Phys* 1982;8:1877-1880.

63. Green N, Kurohara SS, George FWI. Postresection irradiation for primary lung cancer. *Radiology* 1975;116:405-407.

64. Kirsh MM, Prior M, Gago O. The effect of histological cell type on the prognosis of patients with bronchogenic carcinoma. *Ann Thorac Surg* 1972;13:303-310.

65. The Lung Cancer Study Group: Effects of postoperative mediastinal radiation on completely resected stage II and stage III epidermoid cancer of the lung. *N Engl J Med* 1986;315:1377-1381.

66. Keller SM, Adak S, Wagner H, et al. A randomized trial of postoperative adjuvant therapy in patients with completely resected stage II or IIIA non-small-cell lung cancer. *N Engl J Med* 2000;343:1217-1222.

67. Stephens RJ, Girling DJ, Bellehen NM, et al. The role of postoperative radiotherapy in non-small cell lung cancer: a multicentre randomised trial in patients with pathologically staged T_{1-2}, N_{1-2}, M_0 disease. *Br J Cancer* 1996;74:632-639.

68. Sawyer TE, Bonner JA, Gould PM, et al. Effectiveness of postoperative irradiation in stage IIIA non-small cell lung cancer according to regression tree analyses of recurrence risks. *Ann Thorac Surg* 1997;64:1402-1408.

69. Durci ML, Komaki R, Oswald MJ. Comparison of surgery and radiation therapy for non-small cell carcinoma of the lung with mediastinal metastasis. *Int J Radiat Oncol Biol Phys* 1991;21:629-636.

70. Rossell R, Gomez-Codina J, Camps C. Preresectional chemotherapy in stage IIIA non-small cell lung cancer: a 7-year assessment of a randomized controlled trial. *Lung Cancer* 1999;26:7-14.

71. Roth J, Fossella F, Komaki R, et al. A randomized trial comparing peri-operative chemotherapy and surgery with surgery alone in resectable stage IIIA non-small cell lung cancer. *J Natl Cancer Inst* 1994;86:650-651.

72. Albain J, Rusch VW, Crowley JJ. Concurrent cisplatin/etoposide plus chest radiotherapy followed by surgery for stages IIIA(N2) and IIIB non-small cell lung cancer: mature results of Southwest Oncology Group phase II study 8805. *J Clin Oncol* 1995;13:1880-1892.

73. Dosoretz DE, Katin MJ, Blitzer PH, et al. Medical inoperable lung carcinoma: the role of radiation therapy. *Semin Radiat Oncol* 1996;6:98-104.

74. Morita K, Fuwa N, Suzuki Y, et al. Radical radiotherapy for medically inoperable non-small cell lung cancer in clinical stage I: a retrospective analysis of 149 patients. *Radiother Oncol* 1997;42:31-36.

75. Sibley GS, Jamieson TA, Marks LB, et al. Radiotherapy alone for medically inoperable stage I non-small-cell lung cancer: the Duke experience. *Int J Radiat Oncol Biol Phys* 1998;40:149-154.

76. Hayakawa K, Mitsuhashi N, Saito Y, et al. Limited field irradiation for medically inoperable patients with peripheral stage I non-small cell lung cancer. *Lung Cancer* 1999;26:137-142.

77. Arzu JY, Komaki RU, Allen P, et al. Outcomes of patients with medically inoperable stage I non-small cell lung cancer (NSCLC) treated by radiation therapy (RT) alone. In: Proceedings of the 86th Scientific Assembly and Annual Meeting of the Radiological Society of North America, November 2000; Chicago, Ill. Abstract 261.

77a. Komaki R, Arzu IY, Allen P, et al. Radiation therapy for clinical stage I non-small cell lung cancer. *Lung Cancer* 2000;29(suppl 2):153-154.

78. Rosenzweig KE, Mychalczak B, Fuks Z, et al. Final report of the 70.2 Gy and 75.6 Gy dose levels of a phase I dose escalation study using three-dimensional conformal radiotherapy in the treatment of inoperable non-small cell lung cancer. *Cancer J* 2000;6:82-87.

79. Eisert DR, Cox JD, Komaki R. Irradiation for bronchial carcinoma: reasons for failure. I. Analysis as a function of dose-time-fractionation. *Cancer* 1976;37:2665-2670.

80. Saunders MI, Bennett MH, Dische S, et al. Primary tumor control after radiotherapy for carcinoma of the bronchus. *Int J Radiat Oncol Biol Phys* 1984;10:499-501.

81. Saunders MI. The implications of the CHART trial for the treatment of non-small cell lung cancer. *Lung Cancer* 2000;2:177-178.

82. Schaake-Koning C, van den Bogaert W, Dalesio O, et al. Effects of concomitant cisplatin and radiotherapy on inoperable non-small cell lung cancer. *N Engl J Med* 1992;326:524-530.

83. Cox JD, Pajak TF, Marcial VA, et al. Interruptions adversely affect local control and survival with hyperfractionated radiation therapy of carcinomas of the respiratory/digestive tracts: new evidence for accelerated proliferation from RTOG Protocol 83-13. *Cancer* 1992;69:2744-2748.

84. Graham MV. Conformal 3-dimensional radiation therapy for early lung cancer [abstract]. *Lung Cancer* 2000;29 (suppl 2):179.

85. Arriagada R, Le Chevalier T, Quoix E, et al. ASTRO plenary: effect of chemotherapy on locally advanced non-small cell lung carcinoma: a randomized study of 353 patients. *Int J Radiat Oncol Biol Phys* 1991;20:1183-1190.

86. Mah K, van Dyk J. On the impact of tissue inhomogeneity corrections in clinical thoracic radiation therapy. *Int J Radiat Oncol Biol Phys* 1991;21:1257-1267.

87. Perez CA, Stanley K, Grundy G. Impact of irradiation technique and tumor extent in tumor control and survival of patients with unresectable non-oat cell carcinoma of the lung. *Cancer* 1982;50:1091-1099.

88. Dillman RO, Seagren SL, Propert KJ, et al. A randomized trial of induction chemotherapy plus high-dose radiation versus radiation alone in stage III non-small-cell lung cancer. *N Engl J Med* 1990;323:940-945.

89. Komaki R, Pajak TF, Byhardt RW, et al. Analysis of early and late deaths on RTOG non-small cell carcinoma of the lung trials: comparison with CALGB 8433. *Lung* 1993;10:189-197.

90. Sause WT, Scott C, Taylor S, et al. Radiation Therapy Oncology Group (RTOG) 88-08 and Eastern Cooperative Oncology Group (ECOG) 4588: preliminary results of a phase III trial in regionally advanced, unresectable non-small cell lung cancer. *J Natl Cancer Inst* 1995;87:198-205.

91. Le Chevalier T, Arriagada R, Quoix E. Radiotherapy alone versus combined chemotherapy and radiotherapy in nonresectable non-small cell lung cancer. First analysis of a randomized trial in 353 patients. *J Natl Cancer Inst* 1991;83:417-423.

92. Le Chevalier T, Arriagada R, Tarayre M. Significant effect of adjuvant chemotherapy on survival in locally advanced non-small-cell lung carcinoma. *J Natl Cancer Inst* 1992;84:58.

93. Furuse K, Fukuoka M, Kawahara M, et al. Phase III study of concurrent versus sequential thoracic radiotherapy in combination with mitomycin, vindesine, and cisplatin in unresectable stage III non-small-cell lung cancer. *J Clin Oncol* 1999;17:2692-2699.

94. Curran WJ, Scott C, Langer C, et al. Phase III comparison of sequential vs. concurrent chemoradiation for PTS with unresected stage III non-small cell lung cancer (NSCLC): initial report of Radiation Therapy Oncology Group (RTOG) 9410. *Proc Am Soc Clin Oncol* 2000;19:484a.

94a. Cox JD, Stanley K, Petrovich Z, et al. Cranial irradiation for cancer of the lung of all cell types. *JAMA* 1981;245:469-472.

95. Russell AH, Pajak TE, Selim HM, et al. Prophylactic cranial irradiation for lung cancer patients at high risk for development of cerebral metastasis: results of a prospective randomized trial conducted by the Radiation Therapy Oncology Group. *Int J Radiat Oncol Biol Phys* 1991;21:637-643.

96. Pignon JP, Arriagada R, Ihde DC, et al. A meta-analysis of thoracic radiotherapy for small cell lung cancer. *N Engl J Med* 1992;327:1618-1624.

97. Warde P, Payne D. Does thoracic irradiation improve survival and local control in limited-stage small cell carcinoma of the lung? *J Clin Oncol* 1992;10:890-895.

98. Murray N, Coy P, Pater JL, et al. Importance of timing for thoracic irradiation in the combined modality treatment of limited-stage small-cell lung cancer. *J Clin Oncol* 1993;11:336-344.

99. Goto K, Nishiwaki Y, Takada M, et al. Final results of a phase III study of concurrent versus sequential thoracic radiotherapy (TRT) in combination with cisplatin (P) and etoposide (E) for limited-stage small cell lung cancer (LD-SCLC): the Japan Clinical Oncology Group (JCOG) study. *Proc Am Soc Clin Oncol* 1999;18:468a.

100. McCracken JD, Janaki LM, Crowley JJ, et al. Concurrent chemotherapy/radiotherapy for limited small cell lung carcinoma: a Southwest Oncology Group study. *J Clin Oncol* 1990; 8:892-898.

101. Turrisi AT, Glover D. Thoracic radiotherapy variables: influences on local control in small cell lung cancer limited disease. *Int J Radiat Oncol Biol Phys* 1990;19:1473.

102. Turrisi ATI, Glover DJ, Mason B. Long-term results of platinum etoposide (PE) thoracic radiotherapy (TRT) for limited small cell lung cancer: results on 32 patients with 48 month minimum follow-up. *Proc Am Soc Clin Oncol* 1992;11:975.

103. Turrisi AT, Kim K, Blum R, et al. Twice-daily compared with once-daily thoracic radiotherapy in limited small-cell lung cancer treated concurrently with cisplatin and etoposide. *N Engl J Med* 1999;340:265-271.

104. Livingston RB, Mira JG, Chen TT, et al. Combined modality treatment of extensive small cell lung cancer: a Southwest Oncology Group study. *J Clin Oncol* 1984;2:585-590.

105. Komaki R, Byhardt R, Anderson T, et al. What is the lowest effective biologic dose for prophylactic cranial irradiation? *Am J Clin Oncol* 1985;8:523-527.

106. Komaki R, Cox JD, Hartz AJ, et al. Characteristics of long-term survivors after treatment of inoperable carcinoma of the lung. *Am J Clin Oncol* 1985;8:362-370.

107. Cox JD, Komaki R, Byhardt RW, et al. Results of whole-brain irradiation for metastases from small cell carcinoma of the lung. *Cancer Treat Rep* 1980;64:957-961.

108. Baglan RJ, Marks JE. Comparison of symptomatic and prophylactic irradiation of brain metastases from oat cell carcinoma of the lung. *Cancer* 1981;47:41-45.

109. Rosen ST, Makuch RW, Lichter AS. Role of prophylactic cranial irradiation in prevention of central nervous system metastasis in small cell lung cancer: potential benefit restricted to patients with complete response. *Am J Med* 1983;74: 615-624.

110. Rosenstein M, Armstrong J, Kris M. A reappraisal of the role of prophylactic cranial irradiation in limited small cell lung cancer. *Int J Radiat Oncol Biol Phys* 1992;24:43-48.

111. Auperin A, Arriagada R, Pignon J-P. Prophylactic cranial irradiation for patients with small cell lung cancer in complete remission. *N Engl J Med* 1999;341:476-484.

112. Johnson BE, Becker B, Goff WBI. Neurologic, neuropsychologic, and computed cranial tomography scan abnormalities in 2- to 10-year survivors of small-cell lung cancer. *J Clin Oncol* 1985; 3:1659-1667.

113. Chak LY, Zatz LM, Wasserstein PD. Neurologic dysfunction in patients treated for small cell carcinoma of the lung: a clinical and radiological study. *Int J Radiat Oncol Biol Phys* 1986;12: 385-389.

114. Komaki R, Meyers CA, Shin DM, et al. Evaluation of cognitive function in patients with limited small cell lung cancer prior to and shortly following prophylactic cranial irradiation. *Int J Radiat Oncol Biol Phys* 1995;33:179-182.

115. Paulson DL. Carcinoma of the superior pulmonary sulcus. *Ann Thorac Surg* 1979;28:3-4.

116. Paulson DL. The survival rate in superior sulcus tumors treated by presurgical irradiation. *JAMA* 1966;196:342.

117. van Houtte P, MacLennan I, Poulter C. External radiation in the management of superior sulcus tumor. *Cancer* 1984;54:223-227.

118. Ahmad K, Fayos JV, Kirsh MM. Apical lung carcinoma. *Cancer* 1984:913-917.

119. Heelan RT, Demas BE, Caravelli JF. Superior sulcus tumor: CT and MR imaging. *Radiology* 1989;170:637-641.

120. Komaki R, Derus SB, Perez-Tamayo C, et al. Brain metastasis in patients with superior sulcus tumors. *Cancer* 1987;59:1649-1653.

121. Kraut MJ, Rusch VW, Crowley JJ. Induction chemoradiation plus surgical resection is a feasible and highly effective treatment for pancoast tumors: initial results of SWOG 9416 (Intergroup 0160) trial. *Proc Am Soc Clin Oncol* 2000;19:487a.

122. Scarantino C, Salazar OM, Rubin P, et al. The optimum radiation schedule in treatment of superior vena caval obstruction: importance of 99mTc scintiangiograms. *Int J Radiat Oncol Biol Phys* 1979;5:1987-1995.

123. Slawson RG, Scott RM. Radiation therapy in bronchogenic carcinoma. *Radiology* 1979;132:175-176.

124. Davenport D, Ferree CL, Blake D. Response of superior vena caval syndrome to radiation therapy. *Cancer* 1976;38:1577-1580.

125. Karnofsky DA, Burchenal JH. The clinical evaluation of chemotherapeutic agents in cancer. In: Macleod CM, ed. *Evaluation of Chemotherapeutic Agents.* New York, NY: Columbia University Press; 1949:191-205.

126. Bauer M, Birch R, Pajak TF. Prognostic factors in cancer of the lung. In: Cox JD, ed. *Lung Cancer: A Categorical Course in Radiation Therapy.* Oak Brook, Ill: Radiological Society of North America; 1985:87-112.

127. Cohen M. Is immediate radiation therapy indicated for patients with unresectable "non-small cell" cancer? *Cancer Treat Rep* 1983;67:333-336.

128. Cox JD, Barber-Derus S, Hartz AJ, et al. Is adenocarcinoma/large cell carcinoma the most radiocurable type of cancer of the lung? *Int J Radiat Oncol Biol Phys* 1986;12:1801-1805.

129. Komaki R, Garden AS, Cundiff JH. *Endobronchial Radiotherapy.* Cambridge, Mass: Blackwell Scientific Publications; 1993.

130. Leibel SA, Guse C, Order SE. Accelerated fractionation radiation therapy for liver metastases: selection of an optimal patient population for the evaluation of late hepatic injury in RTOG studies. *Int J Radiat Oncol Biol Phys* 1990;18:523-528.

131. Tong D, Gillick L, Henrickson FR. The palliation of symptomatic osseous metastases: final results of the study by the Radiation Therapy Oncology Group. *Cancer* 1982;50:893-899.

132. Borgelt B, Gelber R, Kramer S, et al. The palliation of brain metastases: final result of the first two studies by the Radiation Therapy Oncology Group. *Int J Radiat Oncol Biol Phys* 1980; 6:1-9.

133. Holoye PY, Samuels ML, Lanzotti VC. Combination chemotherapy and radiation therapy for small cell carcinoma. *JAMA* 1977;237:1221-1224.

134. Salyer WR, Eggleston JC. Thymoma: a clinical and pathological study of 65 cases. *Cancer* 1976;37:229-249.

135. Suster S, Rosai J. Thymic carcinoma: a clinicopathologic study of 60 cases. *Cancer* 1991;67:1025-1032.

136. Pollack A, el-Naggar AK, Cox JD, et al. Thymoma. The prognostic significance of flow cytometric DNA analysis. *Cancer* 1992; 69:1702-1709.

137. Jose B, Yu AT, Morgan TF. Malignant thymoma with extrathoracic metastasis: a case report and review of literature. *J Surg Oncol* 1980;15:259-263.

138. Wick MR, Weiland LH, Schetthauer BW. Primary thymic carcinomas. *Am J Surg Pathol* 1982;6:613-630.

139. Bergh NP, Gatzinsky P, Larsson S. Tumors of the thymus and thymic region. I. Clinicopathological studies on thymomas. *Ann Thorac Surg* 1978;25:91-98.

140. Masaoka A, Monden Y, Nakahara K. Followup study of thymomas with special reference to their clinical stage. *Cancer* 1981; 41:2485-2492.

141. Batata MA, Martini N, Huvos AG. Thymomas: clinicopathologic features, therapy, and prognosis. *Cancer* 1974;34: 389-396.

142. Nordstrom DG, Tewfik HH, Latourette HB. Thymoma: therapy and prognosis as related to operative staging. *Int J Radiat Oncol Biol Phys* 1979;5:2059-2062.

143. Cohen DJ, Ronnigen LD, Graeber GM. Management of patients with malignant thymoma. *J Thorac Cardiovasc Surg* 1984;87: 301-307.

144. Ariaratnam LS, Kalnicki S, Mincer F. The management of malignant thymoma with radiation therapy. *Int J Radiat Oncol Biol Phys* 1979;5:77-80.

145. Gerein AN, Srivastava SP, Burgess J. Thymoma: a ten year review. *Am J Surg* 1979:49-53.

146. Penn CRH, Hope-Stone HF. The role of radiotherapy in the management of malignant thymoma. *Br J Surg* 1972;59:533-539.

147. Monden Y, Nakahara K, Nanjo S. Invasive thymoma with myasthenia gravis. *Cancer* 1984;54:2513-2518.

148. Marks RDJ, Wallace KM, Pettit HS. Radiation therapy control of nine patients with malignant thymoma. *Cancer* 1978;41: 117-119.

149. Arriagada R, Bretel JJ, Caillaud JM. Invasive carcinoma of the thymus: a multicenter retrospective review of 56 cases. *Eur J Cancer Clin Oncol* 1984;20:69-74.

150. Pollack A, Komaki R, Cox JD, et al. Thymoma: treatment and prognosis. *Int J Radiat Oncol Biol Phys* 1992;23:1037-1043.

151. Krueger JB, Sagerman RH, King GA. Stage III thymoma: results of postoperative radiation therapy. *Radiology* 1988;186:855-858.

152. Urgesi A, Monetti U, Rossi G. Role of radiation therapy in locally advanced thymoma. *Radiother Oncol* 1990;19:273-280.

153. Curran WJ, Kornstein MJ, Brooks JJ. Invasive thymoma: the role of mediastinal irradiation following complete or incomplete surgical resection. *J Clin Oncol* 1988;6:1722-1727.

154. Goldel N, Boning L, Fredrik A. Chemotherapy of invasive thymoma: a retrospective study of 22 cases. *Cancer* 1989;63: 1493-1500.

155. Shin DM, El-Naggar AK, Putnam JB. Pathologic remission of invasive thymoma after induction chemotherapy. *Cancer Bull* 1992;44:346-348.

156. Uematsu M, Kondo M. A proposal for treatment of invasive thymoma. *Cancer* 1986;58:1979-1984.

157. Chahinian AP, Bhardwa JS, Meyer RJ. Treatment of invasive or metastatic thymoma: report of eleven cases. *Cancer* 1981;47: 1752-1761.

158. Kersh CR, Eisert DR, Hazra TA. Malignant thymoma: role of radiation therapy in management. *Radiology* 1985;256: 207-209.

159. Shamji F, Pearson FG, Todd TRI. Results of surgical treatment for thymoma. *J Thorac Cardiovasc Surg* 1984;87:43-47.

160. Verley JM, Hollmann KH. Thymoma: a comparative study of clinical stages, histologic features and survival in 200 cases. *Cancer* 1985;55:1074-1086.

161. Wilkins EWJ, Castleman B. Thymoma: a continuing survey at the Massachusetts General Hospital. *Ann Thorac Surg* 1979;28: 252-256.

162. Maggi G, Giaccone G, Donadio M. Thymomas: a review of 169 cases, with particular reference to results of surgical treatment. *Cancer* 1986;58:765-776.

PART VI

Gastrointestinal Tract

CHAPTER 18

The Esophagus

Ritsuko Komaki and James D. Cox

ANATOMY

The esophagus is a hollow, muscular tube, approximately 25 cm in length, that extends from the lower border of the cricoid cartilage at the level of vertebra C7 to the stomach. The esophagogastric junction is near the lower border of vertebra T11. The esophagus is divided anatomically into three parts: the cervical part, the thoracic part, and the abdominal part. Locations within the esophagus are often described in terms of their endoscopic distance from the upper incisor teeth. The esophagus begins approximately 18 cm from the upper incisors, the thoracic part of the esophagus relates to the tracheal bifurcation approximately 24 cm from the upper incisors, and the esophagogastric junction is approximately 40 cm from the upper incisors (Fig. 18-1). The anterior surface of the esophagus is immediately adjacent to the trachea along its entire length. The esophagus relates to the azygos vein on the right and the pleura on the left and is adjacent to the recurrent laryngeal nerve, common carotid artery, and subclavian artery. The cross-sectional anatomy of the esophagus as seen on computed tomography (CT) is shown in Figure 18-2.

The lymphatic networks that extend from the submucosal and muscular layers of the esophagus form three groups: the upper, middle, and lower lymphatic trunks. All three groups of lymphatics drain to the paraesophageal lymph nodes located immediately adjacent to the esophagus (Fig. 18-3). In addition, the upper lymphatic trunks, which drain the esophagus above the aortic arch, drain to the cervical and supraclavicular lymph nodes; the middle lymphatic trunks end in the posteromediastinal and retrotracheal lymph nodes; and the lower lymphatic trunks drain to the lymph nodes along the gastric cardia and the lesser curvature of the stomach. Extensive communication takes place between the submucosal and muscular lymphatic networks. This is most marked and most complex in the midthoracic part of the esophagus. Drainage from the thoracic part of the esophagus may occur in a superior direction but usually occurs in a caudal direction (see Fig. 18-1).

RESPONSE OF THE NORMAL ESOPHAGUS TO IRRADIATION

The esophagus is lined with nonkeratinizing stratified squamous epithelium. This epithelium, the thin submucous layer, and the muscular layer of the tunica mucosa form longitudinal folds. No serosal layer exists, and the esophageal wall is less than 5 mm thick. The epithelium of the esophagus has a moderate sensitivity to irradiation, similar to the sensitivity of the oral cavity and oropharynx.[1] The timing of onset of symptoms from irradiation is predictable, and the duration of symptoms varies with the intensity of the irradiation.

Acute Effects

The acute reaction of the esophagus to irradiation consists of pseudomembranous inflammation. In rats,

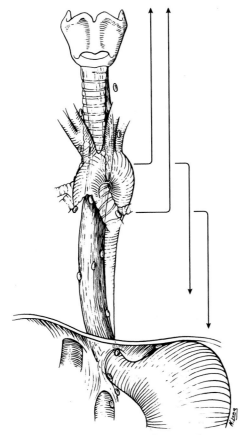

Fig. 18-1 Relationships between the esophagus and surrounding structures. *Arrows* indicate directions of lymphatic drainage by location within the thorax.

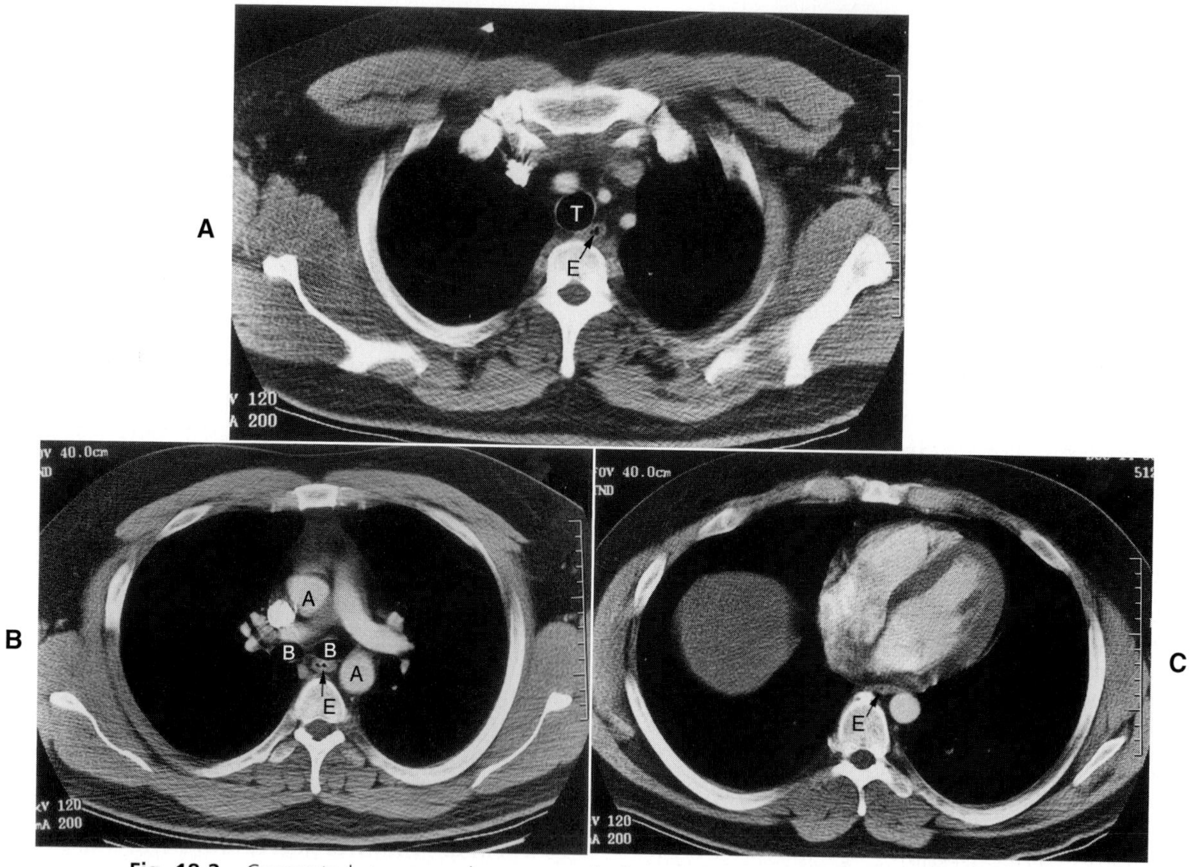

Fig. 18-2 Computed tomography scans of the esophagus and surrounding normal structures. **A,** Upper thoracic structures (approximately 15 cm from the upper incisors). **B,** Midthoracic structures at the level of the carina (approximately 25 cm from the upper incisors). **C,** Lower thoracic structures (approximately 36 cm from the upper incisors). (Courtesy Ronelle A. DuBrow, M.D.; Houston, Tex.)

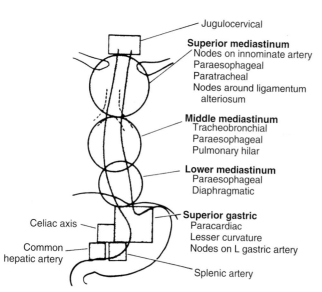

Fig. 18-3 Lymph node groups that drain the esophagus. (From Thompson WM. *Int J Radiat Oncol Biol Phys* 1983; 9:1533-1565, after Akiyama H, Tsurumaru M, Kawamura T, et al. *Ann Surg* 1981;194:438-446.)

a single dose of 30 Gy produces submucosal edema at 4 days, basal epithelial cell death at 6 days, and denudation of the mucosa with a pseudomembrane consisting of necrotic debris by 10 days. Re-epithelialization begins by 14 days, and complete regeneration of the epithelium is usually seen by 20 days.

In humans, the response of the esophagus to irradiation follows a similar time course: odynophagia begins between 10 and 12 days after the first treatment, the severity of the odynophagia peaks at 12 to 14 days, and then symptoms lessen over the next week. This decrease in symptoms while the treatment continues is an excellent example of accelerated proliferation in response to irradiation.

Administration of cytotoxic chemotherapy concurrently with irradiation can slightly accelerate the onset of the esophageal reaction and may profoundly increase its magnitude. Esophageal reactions are the most important dose-limiting side effects in patients treated with combinations of chemotherapy and radiation therapy for cancer of the lung.[2]

Late Effects

The acute effects of esophageal irradiation usually resolve completely, and prolonged reactions leading to permanent effects are rare. Berthrong and Fajardo[3] found complete epithelial regeneration 3 months to 2 years after irradiation. Late effects that may be observed include thickening of the epithelium, telangiectasis underlying an intact epithelium, and thickening of the tunica mucosa and surrounding connective tissue. Narrowing of the lumen resulting from submucosal scarring is uncommon.

EPIDEMIOLOGY OF ESOPHAGEAL CANCER

The incidence of cancer of the esophagus varies widely by geographic region, but throughout the world, esophageal cancer is among the 10 most common forms of cancer.[4] The highest incidences are seen in northern Turkey, northern and eastern China, and Zimbabwe. In the United States, cancer of the esophagus accounts for fewer than 2% of all new cancer cases, although it causes 3% of cancer deaths in men.

The two forms of esophageal cancer are squamous carcinoma of the esophagus and adenocarcinoma of the esophagus. In the United States, the incidence of adenocarcinoma of the esophagus has risen steadily, whereas the incidence of squamous cell carcinoma has remained relatively constant or decreased slightly. Most adenocarcinomas of the esophagus present in the lower third. A high proportion of the population of the United States has symptomatic gastroesophageal reflux, and the relationship between that condition and adenocarcinoma of the esophagus is strong enough to constitute presumptive evidence that gastroesophageal reflux is a causative factor in this neoplastic disease.[5] Long-standing gastroesophageal reflux leads to Barrett's esophagus, a form of columnar epithelial metaplasia in which the squamous epithelium of the distal esophagus is gradually replaced by columnar epithelium like that in the lining of the stomach. Barrett's esophagus is considered a major contributor to the rising incidence of esophageal adenocarcinoma. At present, the incidences of squamous cell carcinoma and adenocarcinoma of the esophagus are nearly equal in North America.[6]

In the United States the incidence and mortality rates for squamous carcinoma of the esophagus are markedly higher in black men than in white men (Fig. 18-4),[7] whereas the incidence of adenocarcinoma is lower in black men than in white men. In addition to having a higher frequency of squamous cell carcinoma, black patients also present with larger tumors and more weight loss.[8]

Esophageal cancer is far more common in men than in women in the United States.[4] The proportion of women with esophageal cancer is much higher in Scandinavia.[9]

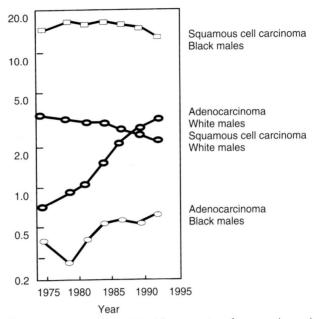

Fig. 18-4 Age-adjusted incidence rates for esophageal cancer among men in the United States according to race and tumor type. (From Devesa SS, Blot WJ, Fraumeni JF Jr. *Cancer* 1998;83:2049-2053.)

The major etiologic factors for squamous cell carcinoma appear to be alcohol consumption, especially consumption of whiskey and drinks with high concentrations of spirits, and tobacco use; hot drinks may also contribute.[10] In addition, the Plummer-Vinson syndrome has been associated with increased risk of squamous cell carcinoma of the esophagus; the proposed mechanism is deficiency of iron and vitamins.[9]

CLINICAL EVOLUTION

Carcinoma of the esophagus usually presents with obstruction caused by a fungating mass that obliterates the lumen. Less often, diffusely infiltrating tumors may cause stenosis. A compensatory dilatation proximal to the obstructing tumor is common. Because the esophagus lacks a serosa, tumors may readily spread into the adjacent mediastinum. Tumors of the middle third of the esophagus may invade the left main stem bronchus, the thoracic duct, and even the aortic arch. Tumors of the lower third of the esophagus may invade the pericardium and descending aorta.

The rich interconnecting lymphatic network contributes to extension of disease superiorly and inferiorly well beyond the gross tumor. Although tumors of the upper third of the esophagus may spread to lymph nodes in the anterior jugular chain or the supraclavicular region, tumors of the middle and lower third preferentially spread to the subdiaphragmatic lymph nodes. Distant metastases are found in more than half of patients at autopsy, most commonly in the lung and liver but also in the adrenal glands, bones, and brain.

Progressive dysphagia is the most common early symptom, and weight loss is almost inevitable. Pain in the chest or abdomen is present in approximately half of all patients. More advanced disease can result in cough, sialorrhea, and laryngeal paralysis from involvement of the recurrent laryngeal nerve. Progression of any symptom as reflected by deteriorating performance status scores and weight loss is associated with a worse prognosis.

Carcinoma of the esophagus has a propensity to spread regionally and distantly. Table 18-1[11] shows a typical distribution of metastases to regional and distant sites. The pattern of distribution differs according to the level of the esophagus at which the carcinoma originated. In the case of carcinomas of the upper third of the esophagus, metastasis is most commonly to the paratracheal and paraesophageal lymph nodes; metastasis to the liver and lungs is less frequent. Middle-third lesions tend to spread to mediastinal and abdominal lymph nodes and more often involve the liver. Tumors arising in the lower third of the esophagus also have a high probability of spread to mediastinal and abdominal lymph nodes but involve the liver more often than the more proximal lesions. Involvement of the lungs and pleura occurs with similar frequency regardless of the site of origin within the esophagus.

Advanced cancer of the esophagus causes death through complications associated with the local–regional tumor—pneumonia associated with inanition, tracheoesophageal fistula formation, or erosion of the aorta. More effective control of local–regional tumors may be associated with a higher risk of death from distant metastasis. Failure-pattern studies show approximately equal risks of local failure and distant metastasis regardless of whether the primary treatment is surgery[6] or radiation therapy and chemotherapy.[12]

PRETREATMENT EVALUATION

In patients with esophageal cancer, a complete medical history and a physical examination with associated hematologic and biochemical studies are essential. Chest radiographs, CT of the chest and upper abdomen, barium contrast imaging of the upper gastrointestinal tract, and endoscopic sonography contribute to the evaluation of the extent of disease. Esophagoscopy with biopsy is essential. Bronchoscopy is required for tumors of the upper third of the esophagus.

Esophagography

Double-contrast esophagography with fluoroscopy is important in localizing a suspected tumor and characterizing its intraluminal growth pattern (Fig. 18-5). It may be difficult to determine the length of the tumor by contrast esophagography because of the variable degree of obstruction.

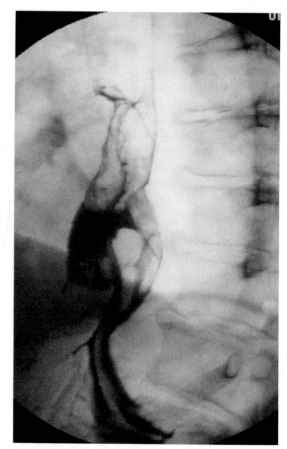

Fig. 18-5 Esophagram showing typical fungating mass obliterating the lumen and proximal esophageal dilatation. (Courtesy Ronelle A. DuBrow, M.D.; Houston, Tex.)

TABLE 18-1		
Anatomic Sites of Metastases from Esophageal Carcinoma in 67 Male Patients with Metastasis Disease		
Site	Number of Patients	Percentage (%)
Lymph nodes	58	73
Lung	41	52
Liver	37	47
Adrenals	16	20
Thyroid	5	6
Gastrointestinal serosa	5	6
Aorta	4	5
Peritoneum	4	5

Modified from Anderson LL, Lad TE. *Cancer* 1982;50:1587-1590.

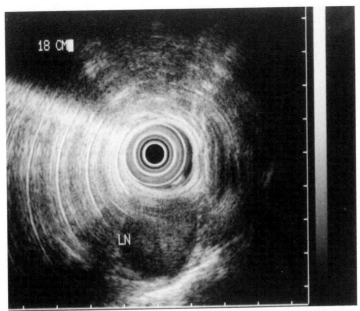

Fig. 18-6 Endoscopic sonogram showing thickened esophageal wall and adjacent enlarged lymph node *(LN)*. (Courtesy Ronelle A. DuBrow, M.D.; Houston, Tex.)

Endoscopic Sonography

Endoscopic sonography contributes to the evaluation of the endoluminal tumor, the area of involvement on the wall of the esophagus, and the immediately adjacent paraesophageal lymph nodes (Fig 18-6). However, in approximately one third of patients, the transducer cannot be passed into the esophagus at the level of the tumor. Endoscopic sonography is superior to any imaging study currently available for determining the depth of penetration of the tumor into or through the wall of the esophagus. Endoscopic sonography is also superior to other imaging modalities in identifying enlarged lymph nodes immediately adjacent to the esophagus.

Computed Tomography and Positron Emission Tomography

CT of the thorax is important to establish the degree of extra-esophageal extension of the tumor (Fig. 18-7). CT is more effective than endoscopic sonography in detecting more distant involved mediastinal lymph nodes, enlarged nodes in the celiac axis, and hepatic metastases. Endoscopic sonography and CT are clearly complementary in assessing the local and regional extensions of esophageal cancer. Positron emission tomography (PET) is currently being compared with the imaging techniques mentioned above. The role of PET scanning in the assessment of local–regional disease is unclear. No evidence yet suggests an improvement in assessment of local–regional tumor with PET. However, PET can improve the detection of unsuspected distant metastases.[13]

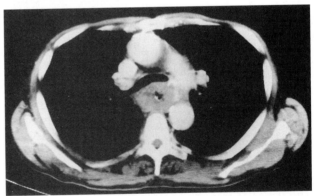

Fig. 18-7 Computed tomography scan of esophageal squamous cell carcinoma. The patient later developed a fistula between the esophagus and the left main stem of the bronchus during radiation therapy.

Bronchoscopy

Bronchoscopy is important as an adjunct to careful examination of the upper aerodigestive tract because the risk of second primary malignant tumors associated with esophageal cancer is relatively high. In addition, thoracic esophageal tumors may involve the tracheal bronchial tree directly, and such involvement can lead to the ominous complication of fistula formation.

STAGE CLASSIFICATION

Earlier classifications of esophageal cancer were based on surgical findings alone. In contrast, the 1997 classification by the American Joint Committee on Cancer (AJCC) was designed to reflect all regions of the esophagus

---

BOX 18-1   American Joint Comittee on Cancer Staging System for Esophageal Cancer

PRIMARY TUMOR (T)

TX	Primary tumor cannot be assessed
T0	No evidence of primary tumor
Tis	Carcinoma in situ
T1	Tumor invades lamina propria or submucosa
T2	Tumor invades muscularis propria
T3	Tumor invades adventitia
T4	Tumor invades adjacent structures

REGIONAL LYMPH NODES (N)

NX	Regional lymph nodes cannot be assessed
N0	No regional lymph node metastasis
N1	Regional lymph node metastasis

DISTANT METASTASIS (M)

MX	Distant metastasis cannot be assessed
M0	No distant metastasis
M1	Distant metastasis

Tumors of the lower thoracic esophagus:

M1a	Metastasis in celiac lymph nodes
M1b	Other distant metastasis

Tumors of the midthoracic esophagus:

M1a	Not applicable
M1b	Nonregional lymph nodes and/or other distant metastasis

Tumors of the upper thoracic esophagus:

M1a	Metastasis in cervical nodes
M1b	Other distant metastasis

STAGE GROUPING

Stage 0	Tis	N0	M0
Stage I	T1	N0	M0
Stage IIA	T2	N0	M0
	T3	N0	M0
Stage IIB	T1	N1	M0
	T2	N1	M0
Stage III	T3	N1	M0
	T4	Any N	M0
Stage IV	Any T	Any N	M1
Stage IVA	Any T	Any N	M1a
Stage IVB	Any T	Any N	M1b

From Fleming I, Cooper JS, Henson DE, et al, eds. *AJCC Cancer Staging Manual*, 5th ed. Philadelphia, Pa: Lippincott Williams & Wilkins; 1997:65-69.

---

and both clinical and pathologic findings. The clinical findings include findings on endoscopic sonography and CT. Pathologic staging is based on examination of the resected specimen. The 1997 AJCC tumor–nodes–metastasis classification is shown in Box 18-1.[14] Although the stage classification is considered essential in reporting results of clinical investigations, another important prognostic factor is weight loss. Patients who have lost more than 10% of their body weight are significantly more likely to die whether treatment is by surgical resection[6] or nonsurgical means. Ellis and colleagues[15] also found that tumor stage profoundly affected the outcome after surgical resection for esophageal cancer; they also found that the number of involved lymph nodes (0, 1 to 4, or 5 or more) also greatly influenced prognosis.

TREATMENT

Until the early 1980s, the literature on treatment for esophageal cancer dealt predominantly with squamous cell carcinoma. When other histopathologic types were considered, they were often denoted as anaplastic rather than being identified as adenocarcinomas. Although many reports are in the literature on adenocarcinoma of the esophagogastric junction, these tumors are most appropriately considered synonymous with distal esophageal adenocarcinomas unless they arise in the gastric cardia.[16]

Surgery

Surgical resection continues to be the mainstay of treatment for carcinoma of the esophagus. An extensive review of the surgical literature before 1980 by Earlam and Cunha-Melo[17] concluded that the mortality rate for esophageal resection (29%) was the highest of the mortality rates for frequently performed surgical procedures. The authors surveyed 122 reports including 83,783 patients. The techniques of esophageal surgery have changed since that 1980 report, and a national Intergroup trial published in 1998 involving institutions throughout the United States and southern Canada revealed an operative mortality rate of only 6%.[6] The operative procedures currently in use include transhiatal esophagectomy; the Ivor-Lewis esophagectomy, which includes a right thoracotomy and a celiotomy; and left thoracotomy, which also may be combined with a celiotomy (Table 18-2).[18]

The transhiatal esophagectomy has been popularized and widely used by Orringer.[18] This procedure permits a subtotal esophagectomy with anastomosis in the cervical region and avoids the need for thoracotomy in most patients. Although Orringer's indications for transhiatal esophagectomy include tumors of the entire esophagus and gastric cardia,[18,19] many surgeons consider the transhiatal esophagectomy to be most applicable for lesions located below the carina.

Thoracoabdominal approaches are preferred by many thoracic surgeons. Left thoracoabdominal approaches are used most often for distal esophageal lesions. If Barrett's (intestinal) metaplasia extending superiorly into the middle third of the esophagus is evident, the Ivor-Lewis procedure is usually preferred. In the large Intergroup study reported by Kelsen and colleagues,[6] in which the specific operative procedure performed was left to the discretion of the participating surgeon, the overall operative mortality rate was 6%. The relative advantages and disadvantages of these various operative procedures have been summarized by Whyte and Orringer.[19]

Although long-term survival rates in selected patients have ranged from 10%[17,20] to 40%,[20] the large North American Intergroup trial[6] showed a median survival of 17 months and a 3-year survival rate of 26%. These results seem representative of the current state of the art with surgical resection alone.

Less than satisfactory results with resection have led to waning enthusiasm in many quarters for the use of surgical resection alone. Although some studies have not shown improvement from the use of preoperative chemotherapy (Fig. 18-8),[6] considerable interest has

TABLE 18-2
Techniques of Esophagectomy

Approach	Location of Tumor	Location of Anastomosis	Advantages	Disadvantages
Transhiatal esophagectomy	Entire esophagus and gastric cardia	Cervical region	Low-morbidity cervical anastomosis, few respiratory side effects	Lack of exposure of midesophagus
Right thoracotomy (Ivor-Lewis procedure)	Mid to upper esophagus	Thoracic or cervical region	Good exposure of midesophagus	Intrathoracic anastomosis, thoracotomy
Left thoracotomy	Lower third of esophagus or gastric cardia	Low to mid thoracic region	Good exposure of lower esophagus	Intrathoracic anastomosis, thoracotomy
Radical (en bloc) resection	Entire esophagus and gastric cardia	Cervical or thoracic region	More extensive lymphadenectomy, potentially better survival	Increased operative risk with no proven increase in survival

From Whyte RI, Orringer MB. *Semin Radiat Oncol* 1994;4:146-156.

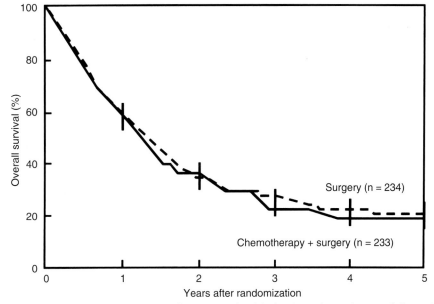

Fig. 18-8 Survival outcomes in a phase III trial of induction chemotherapy followed by surgery compared with surgery alone for esophageal carcinoma. (From Kelsen DP, Ginsberg R, Pajak TF, et al. *N Engl J Med* 1998;339:1979-1984.)

risen in using chemotherapy plus radiation therapy as an adjuvant to surgical treatment.

Radiation Therapy
Radiation Therapy Alone

The comprehensive and critical review by Earlam and Cunha-Melo[17] of 8500 patients with esophageal cancer treated with radiation therapy alone revealed a 5-year survival rate of 5%. Although patients with small (< 5-cm) tumors might be candidates for resection, radiation therapy for some of these patients can also provide favorable results. For example, Yang and colleagues[21] analyzed 1136 patients in China who lived 5 years or longer after radiation therapy. These investigators found a higher proportion of long-term survivors among patients with tumors less than 5 cm in diameter. However, for those with larger tumors, particularly tumors considered unresectable, the results with radiation therapy alone are less favorable. Long-term results of the radiation therapy arm in an Intergroup trial conducted by the Radiation Therapy Oncology Group (RTOG)[12] showed that none of 60 such patients treated with radiation therapy alone lived beyond 3 years.

Postoperative Radiation Therapy

Because 20% to 25% of recurrences after surgical treatment consist of local recurrence alone,[6] postoperative irradiation theoretically could improve outcome. Postoperative irradiation has not been studied in comparative trials in the United States. However, three separate prospective comparative trials throughout the world showed no improvement in long-term survival with the addition of postoperative irradiation.[22-24]

Preoperative Radiation Therapy

Preoperative radiation therapy has not been investigated in prospective comparative trials in the United States. In principle, this approach could improve resectability, decrease the risk of regional or distant metastasis, and improve survival in patients with operable carcinoma of the esophagus. The most useful data come from trials conducted in other countries. The trials tend to have unusual fractionation schemes compared with those widely used in the United States.

An early trial[25] from France enrolled a total of 124 patients, who were randomly assigned to preoperative radiation therapy with 39 to 45 Gy (average 40 Gy) in 8 to 12 days or to immediate surgical exploration and resection if possible. The results showed no between-group difference in resectability or operative mortality, which was 23% within 30 days in both groups. The median survival was 12 months for the 57 patients who had surgery alone compared with 11 months for the 67 patients who had preoperative irradiation. No difference in 5-year survival rates was evident, which were 11.5% for patients who had immediate operation and 9.5% for patients who underwent preoperative irradiation.

Investigators from the European Organization for Research and Treatment of Cancer[26] also used a rapid fractionation approach. A total dose of 33 Gy in 10 fractions over 12 days was followed by exploration and esophagectomy 8 days later. A total of 229 patients with potentially resectable esophageal carcinomas were randomly assigned to preoperative irradiation or immediate exploration and resection. Two hundred eight patients were evaluable. Five of the 102 irradiated patients were not operated on; the operative mortality rate for the other 97 was 25%. The operative mortality rate among the 106 patients who had immediate exploration was 18%. The median survival was 11 months in both arms of the study, and no difference was found between the study arms in the 5-year survival rate (10%).

A third trial was reported by Wang and colleagues[27] from China. Patients were randomly assigned to preoperative irradiation with 40 Gy in eight fractions or immediate resection. No difference was found in the local failure rate between the two treatment groups (50%). The 5-year survival rate was 30% for the preoperative irradiation group and 35% for the immediate surgery group.

More conventional fractionation was studied in two other trials. Arnott and colleagues[28] reported a randomized study of preoperative irradiation with 20 Gy in 10 fractions over 2 weeks compared with surgical resection alone. Only 129 of the 176 patients who were randomized underwent radical resection. The 5-year survival rate for the 62 patients randomized to immediate surgery was 17% as compared with 9% for the 67 patients who received preoperative irradiation. (The overall operative mortality rate for the 129 patients was 14%, with no difference between the two groups.) The only trial to show an advantage for preoperative irradiation came from Scandinavia.[29] Patients were randomly assigned to either preoperative irradiation with 35 Gy in 20 fractions or surgery alone. The 3-year survival rate for the 41 patients who had surgery alone was 9% compared with 21% for the 48 patients who had preoperative radiation therapy ($P = 0.08$). This study included two additional treatment arms: preoperative chemotherapy followed by surgery, and chemotherapy plus concurrent irradiation (for more details on this approach, see the section on "Definitive Radiation Therapy with Concurrent Chemotherapy" later in this chapter). The 3-year survival rate was 19% for patients who received any radiation therapy vs. 6% for patients who received none ($P = 0.0009$). Taken together, these studies do not suggest a benefit for preoperative irradiation as the only adjuvant to surgery.

Preoperative Radiation Therapy with Concurrent Chemotherapy

As has been the case with all single- and multiple-modality treatments for esophageal cancer studied to date, single-institution studies that have not included concurrent control groups have suggested benefit from concurrent chemotherapy and radiation therapy (chemoradiation) before surgical resection.

Urba and colleagues[30] reported a randomized trial from the University of Michigan that included both squamous cell carcinoma (25% of patients) and adenocarcinoma (75% of patients). A total of 100 patients were equally divided between surgery alone (transhiatal esophagectomy) and chemoradiation before surgery (cisplatin, vinblastine, and fluorouracil [5-FU] plus radiation therapy with 1.5 Gy twice daily, 5 days per week for 3 weeks). The median survival was 17 months in both groups. A significant reduction in the rate of local failure occurred in the chemoradiation arm (19% vs. 39% in the surgery-alone arm; P = 0.039). The 3-year survival rate was 32% for the combined-modality arm compared with 15% for the surgery-alone arm.

Two other small studies that each included fewer than 100 patients provide no support for the use of chemoradiation before surgical resection. Nygaard and colleagues[29] randomly assigned patients with squamous cell carcinoma to cisplatin, bleomycin, and concurrent irradiation (35 Gy in 20 fractions) followed by resection or immediate resection alone. The 41 patients who had surgery alone had a 3-year survival rate of 9% compared with 21% for the 47 patients who had the combined-modality treatment (P = 0.3). Le Prise and colleagues[31] randomly assigned 86 patients with squamous cell carcinoma of the esophagus to immediate resection or to preoperative cisplatin and 5-FU plus 20 Gy in 10 fractions over 2 weeks. The median survival was 12 months

in both groups, and the 3-year survival rates were similar (19% for combined-modality therapy and 14% for surgery).

The two largest studies reported to date of preoperative chemoradiation produced conflicting results. Walsh and colleagues from Ireland[32] randomly assigned 113 patients with adenocarcinoma of the esophagus to surgical resection alone or preoperative 5-FU for 5 days beginning on day 1, cisplatin on day 7, and radiation therapy (40 Gy in 15 fractions) beginning on day 1. The chemotherapy was repeated during week 6, and surgery was carried out 8 weeks after the start of treatment. CT was performed in some patients but the selection was not done systematically. Abdominal sonography was performed in all patients. The median survival in the patients treated with multiple modalities was 16 months, compared with 11 months in the patients who had resection alone. In an intent-to-treat analysis, the 3-year survival rates were 32% for induction chemoradiation and 6% for resection alone (P = 0.01) (Fig. 18-9). A much larger study was conducted by a group of French investigators led by Bosset with support from the European Organization for Research and Treatment of Cancer Data Center in Brussels.[33] These investigators randomly assigned 282 patients with squamous cell carcinoma of the thoracic esophagus to receive either immediate resection or induction chemoradiation followed by resection. Although esophageal sonography was not available, patients were evaluated with CT of the chest and upper abdomen plus sonography of the liver. The chemotherapy consisted of cisplatin alone 0 to 2 days before each course of irradiation. Two courses of

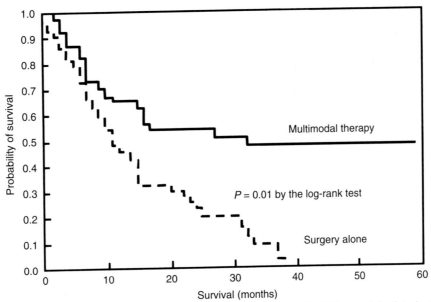

Fig. 18-9 Survival according to treatment (intent-to-treat analysis) in a trial of induction radiation therapy, cisplatin, and fluorouracil followed by surgery compared with surgery alone for adenocarcinoma of the esophagus. (From Walsh TN, Noonan N, Hollywood D, et al. *N Engl J Med* 1996;335:462-467.)

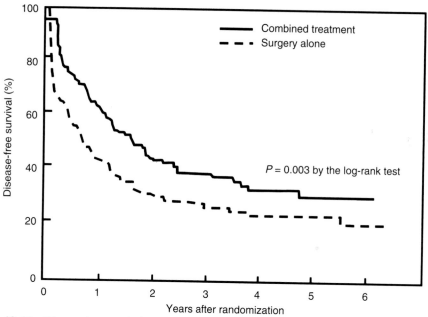

Fig. 18-10   Disease-free survival among patients with squamous cell carcinoma of the esophagus treated with induction radiation therapy and concurrent cisplatin followed by surgery or with surgery alone. Overall survival rates did not differ in the two treatment groups. (From Bosset J-F, Gignou M, Triboulet J-P, et al. *N Engl J Med* 1997;337:161-167.)

irradiation were administered, each consisting of 18.5 Gy in five fractions in 1 week, separated by 2 weeks. Thus the total dose of irradiation was 37 Gy in 10 fractions in 4 weeks with a 2-week interruption. The median survival for both treatment groups was 18.6 months, and more long-term survival outcomes did not differ between the groups. However, local tumor control was significantly better ($P = 0.01$) in the combined-modality arm, as was disease-free survival ($P = 0.003$) (Fig. 18-10). Important differences between this study and that of Walsh and colleagues[32] are the large number of patients, the much better survival in the surgical control arm, the use of a split-course regimen rather than continuous irradiation, and the use of single-agent cisplatin rather than cisplatin and 5-FU. The fact that there was a significant difference in disease-free survival in the French trial supports the possible benefit of induction chemoradiation.

Brachytherapy

Intraluminal insertion of radioactive isotopes for the treatment of esophageal cancer has a long history. Interest in this approach continues to be considerable, especially in countries such as Japan, where a high index of suspicion for this relatively common disease often leads to detection of superficial esophageal cancer at early stages.

Larger and more infiltrating carcinomas cannot be adequately treated with brachytherapy alone but may be treated with brachytherapy in conjunction with external irradiation.[34] However, some risk exists. The RTOG

conducted a study of esophageal brachytherapy[35] combined with external irradiation and concurrent chemotherapy with cisplatin and 5-FU. The chemotherapy was given during weeks 1, 5, 8, and 11. The external irradiation dose was 50 Gy given in 25 fractions over 5 weeks beginning at the same time as the first chemotherapy administration. Two weeks after completion of external irradiation, esophageal brachytherapy was administered—either high-dose-rate therapy with 5 Gy delivered in weeks 8, 9, and 10 for a total dose of 15 Gy or low-dose-rate therapy with 20 Gy delivered during week 8. More than 90% of the 49 patients treated had squamous cell carcinoma. Five patients (10%) died of complications of treatment, and another 12 patients (24%) experienced life-threatening toxic effects. Esophageal fistulas seemingly related to treatment occurred in 6 patients (12%) within 7 months of brachytherapy. Therefore, although brachytherapy may be indicated as the sole treatment in the unusual patient with superficial esophageal cancer, great caution must be exercised when esophageal brachytherapy is combined with external irradiation and concurrent chemotherapy.

Definitive Radiation Therapy with Concurrent Chemotherapy

The standard of care for patients with inoperable carcinoma of the esophagus is concurrent radiation therapy and chemotherapy. The most appropriate chemotherapy regimen is 5-FU and cisplatin unless contraindications to the use of either of these drugs are evident.

The basis for this treatment standard is a relatively small but highly significant Intergroup trial conducted by the RTOG (protocol 85-01). The rationale for this trial was the suggestion of improvement in local tumor control and survival in several studies of concurrent radiation therapy and chemotherapy reported in the early 1980s.[36-38] The RTOG trial was designed to compare radiation therapy alone (total dose of 64 Gy in 32 fractions, five fractions per week for 6.5 weeks) with concurrent chemotherapy and radiation therapy using a total dose of 50 Gy in 25 fractions, five fractions per week. The chemotherapy consisted of 75 mg/m^2 cisplatin given intravenously on the first day and 1 g/m^2 5-FU given by continuous infusion for the first 4 days of weeks 1, 5, 8, and 11. Although 150 patients were to be enrolled in this study, a planned interim analysis was conducted when 90 patients were evaluable. This analysis showed a marked improvement in survival in the combined-modality arm ($P = 0.005$) and led to cessation of randomization. Subsequently enrolled patients were allocated only to the combined-modality arm. The original report[12] included only the randomized patients (Fig. 18-11). It was evident that combined-modality therapy produced improvement in both local control and freedom from distant metastasis. The rate of local tumor persistence or recurrence was reduced from 67% to 50%. The long-term results[39,40] showed that 26% of patients treated with combined-modality therapy lived 5 years. The outcomes for the 69 nonrandomized patients enrolled in the combined-modality arm were quite similar to those of the 61 patients treated on the randomized combined-modality arm (Fig. 18-12).[39]

thus providing corroboration of the results. None of the patients in the randomized combined-modality arm had died of esophageal cancer after 5 years, indicating that these patients with esophageal cancer were actually cured.[40] Although the number of patients with adenocarcinoma treated with combined-modality therapy in this series was small (23 of 130, or 18%), no significant difference was evident in outcome between these patients and those with squamous cell carcinoma.

Several additional studies support the value of definitive radiation therapy and concurrent chemotherapy for patients with esophageal cancer. Results of a study begun in 1980 at the Fox Chase Cancer Center that used concurrent 5-FU, mitomycin C, and radiation therapy with 60 Gy in 6 to 7 weeks were similar to those of the RTOG study. Coia and colleagues[38,41] reported 3- and 5-year survival rates of 29% and 18%, respectively, for 57 patients with clinical stage I and II tumors.

On the basis of the Fox Chase Cancer Center study, the Eastern Cooperative Oncology Group conducted a randomized trial between 1982 and 1988.[42] In this trial, patients were randomly assigned to concurrent 5-FU, mitomycin, and radiation therapy with 60 Gy in 6 to 7 weeks or radiation therapy alone. An option for esophagectomy after a total dose of 40 Gy was available. Survival for the 59 evaluable patients treated with combined modalities was superior to that for the 60 patients who received radiation therapy alone (median survival, 14.8 months vs. 9.2 months; 2-year survival, 27% vs. 12%), but the uncontrolled use of resection confounds interpretation of the results (Fig. 18-13). No difference was evident in median survival between the

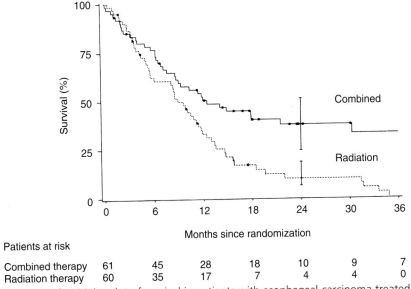

Patients at risk						
Combined therapy	61	45	28	18	10	9	7
Radiation therapy	60	35	17	7	4	4	0

Fig. 18-11 Kaplan-Meier plot of survival in patients with esophageal carcinoma treated with radiation therapy alone or with radiation therapy and chemotherapy combined. Bars indicate 95% confidence intervals at 24 months. (From Herskovic A, Martz K, Al-Sarraf M, et al. *N Engl J Med* 1992;326:1593-1598.)

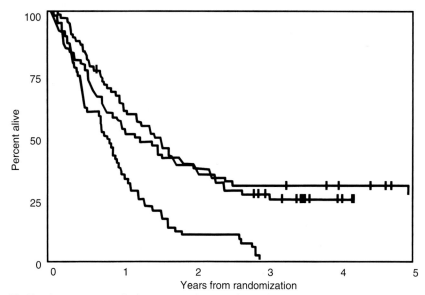

Fig. 18-12 Long-term survival among patients with esophageal cancer treated with radiation therapy alone (line at bottom of graph; median survival 9.3 months) or radiation therapy with concurrent cisplatin and fluorouracil. When an interim analysis showed a marked improvement in survival in the patients randomized to receive chemoradiation (line at top of graph; median survival 17.2 months), all of the remaining patients enrolled in the trial were treated with the combined-modality therapy (middle line; median survival 14.1 months). (Modified from Al-Sarraf M, Martz K, Herskovic A, et al. *J Clin Oncol* 1997;1:277-284.)

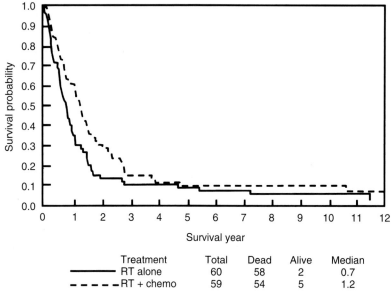

Treatment	Total	Dead	Alive	Median
—— RT alone	60	58	2	0.7
– – – RT + chemo	59	54	5	1.2

Fig. 18-13 Survival in Eastern Cooperative Oncology Group trial EST-1282 according to assigned treatment group (radiation therapy alone vs. radiation therapy and concurrent mitomycin C and fluorouracil). These data represent eligible patients only. (From Smith TJ, Ryan LM, Douglass HOJ, et al. *Int J Radiat Oncol Biol Phys* 1998;42:269-276.)

patients who underwent resection and those who received chemotherapy and radiation therapy without esophagectomy.

Richmond and colleagues[43] also provided information about the contribution of esophagectomy to outcome after chemotherapy and radiation therapy. They reported a nonrandomized comparison of radiation therapy alone vs. concurrent radiation therapy, 5-FU, and cisplatin with or without surgical resection. No patient treated with radiation therapy alone lived for 2 years, whereas 37% of patients treated with combined modalities lived for 2 years. No significant difference was evident in survival between patients treated with chemotherapy and radiation therapy and patients treated with chemotherapy, radiation therapy, and resection.

These studies suggested that outcome in patients with esophageal cancer could be improved further, either by adding induction chemotherapy before the chemoradiation in an effort to further reduce the incidence of distant metastasis or by increasing the total dose of radiation therapy to greater than 50 Gy in an effort to reduce the incidence of local failure. The former approach was studied in Intergroup trial 0122 (Eastern Cooperative Oncology Group trial PE-289; RTOG trial 90-12).[44] Patients received three monthly cycles of cisplatin (day 1) and 5-FU (days 1 to 5) followed by concurrent cisplatin, 5-FU, and radiation therapy. The results in the 38 evaluable patients did not suggest improvement over concurrent chemoradiation alone, and 9% of patients died of complications of treatment. A randomized Intergroup trial (INT 0123) comparing a higher total dose of radiation therapy (64 Gy) to the now standard total dose of 50 Gy with concurrent cisplatin and 5-FU was terminated early when it became evident that no improvement was provided by the higher total dose.[45]

It may be concluded that concurrent chemotherapy and radiation therapy is unquestionably superior to radiation therapy alone. The important question of whether concurrent therapy is equal to or better than surgery is likely to go unanswered. It may be possible to study concurrent chemotherapy and radiation therapy with or without esophagectomy. A trial of such design is being conducted in the Intergroup setting (RTOG 93-09, INT 0139) for carcinomas of the lung with proven mediastinal nodal involvement.

PALLIATION

Rapid and long-term palliation of dysphagia can be expected with concurrent chemotherapy and radiation therapy for esophageal carcinoma. Whether undertaken as a preoperative measure or as definitive treatment, concurrent therapy achieves symptomatic benefit in most patients. Coia and colleagues[38,41] reported improvement in swallowing for 90% of patients treated in their pilot study. Patients had improvement within 2 weeks. Moreover, patients with stage I and II tumors had durable palliation. Of the 25 patients who were disease-free more than 1 year after treatment, 68% were asymptomatic, 25% had dysphagia only with solid foods, and 12% had some dysphagia with soft foods.

Most patients with esophageal carcinoma have distressing symptoms ranging from slight to marked dysphagia and odynophagia to complete obstruction of the esophagus with inability to handle natural secretions or intractable cough from tracheoesophageal fistula.

The most common treatment in the past was dilatation and placement of an intraluminal tube (a Celestin tube or Atkinson tube). Among patients who are to be treated with curative intent, the definitive treatment, whether esophagectomy or concurrent radiation therapy and chemotherapy, also produces palliation.

Among patients for whom definitive treatment with curative intent is not possible, palliation can be achieved with radiation therapy in approximately 75% of patients.[46] Although a wide variety of procedures, including surgical resection, dilatation, laser debulking, intraluminal stent or tube placement, and endoesophageal brachytherapy, may achieve relief of symptoms,[47] external radiation therapy is the least invasive and usually produces some benefit within 2 weeks. It is better to pursue immediate irradiation for palliation than to await the development of more severe symptoms because immediate irradiation produces a greater and more lasting palliation. The single relative contraindication to external irradiation is fistula formation between the esophagus and the tracheobronchial tree. Irradiation can increase symptoms from fistulae by tumor regression leading to a larger communication between the esophagus and respiratory structures. Placement of an intraluminal tube followed by external irradiation may permit healing, but results are not predictable.

TECHNIQUES OF IRRADIATION

Although successful irradiation of patients with cancer of the esophagus can be accomplished with ^{60}Co teletherapy, modern linear accelerators with a source to axial distance of 100 cm permit more successful avoidance of normal lung, heart, and, especially, spinal cord. Cervical esophageal carcinomas can be treated with the patient in a supine position similar to that used for irradiation of hypopharyngeal cancer. If the lesion is located at or near the esophagogastric junction, it is also important to limit irradiation of the heart and liver. In the case of lesions of the mid- and lower esophagus, positioning the patient in the prone position usually permits a greater distance between the spinal cord and the planning target volume (PTV). CT with the patient in either the prone or the supine position facilitates treatment planning with anterior-posterior and oblique fields.

The propensity of carcinoma of the esophagus to extend along the mucosa and submucosa and the richly interconnecting lymphatics mandates that the superior and inferior margins of the field be well beyond the visible tumor. To determine the gross tumor volume (GTV), it is important to use all information from CT and findings on endoscopy. Endoscopic sonography helps define the thickness of the lesion and any adjacent enlarged lymph nodes. Second (skip) lesions may be identified and must be included. An initial PTV that encompasses the entire esophagus from the thoracic inlet to the gastroesophageal junction is appropriate for large lesions, especially those of the thoracic esophagus. Margins of 5 cm or more are recommended for small tumors and for the reduced PTV. Tumors of the upper and middle thirds of the esophagus require treatment of the supraclavicular regions. Irradiation of the celiac lymph node region is appropriate for tumors of the lower third of the esophagus. A minimal field width for the PTV is usually 2 cm beyond the GTV, but the most appropriate radial margin around tumors of various locations and sizes is not known. Esophagography with thin-barium swallowing during simulation and associated CT helps determine the most appropriate radial margin. It is also common to begin the treatment with anterior-posterior parallel-opposed fields while oblique fields are being planned.

Fractions of 1.8 Gy or 2.0 Gy are appropriate for treatment with curative intent. Larger fractions may be indicated if palliation is the only goal. Although total doses of 60 to 70 Gy are indicated if radiation therapy is the only treatment, a total dose of 50 Gy in 5 weeks is appropriate if concurrent chemotherapy is used. To date, no data support higher total doses of radiation therapy with concurrent chemotherapy. With or without chemotherapy, the total dose to the spinal cord should be limited to 45 Gy. The dose to the normal lungs and heart should be limited to 20 Gy and 40 Gy, respectively. Advanced treatment planning with systems that provide dose-volume histograms permits the most judicious balance of dose to the clinical target volume and to the surrounding normal tissues. It is never appropriate to place a posterior spinal cord block that simultaneously blocks the clinical target volume. An example of an appropriate field arrangement for carcinoma of the thoracic esophagus is shown in Color Plate 22, after p. 80. Although total doses of 50 Gy in 5 or 6 weeks are considered necessary to control subclinical extensions of disease, lower total doses may be used with concurrent chemotherapy. In the chemotherapy arm of RTOG protocol 85-01,[12] a total dose of 30 Gy was used for the initial large field; the smaller "boost" field that still had a minimal margin of 5 cm above and below the gross tumor received an additional 20 Gy for a total dose of 50 Gy to the known tumor.

SUMMARY

In the last decade, outcomes after treatment of patients with cancer of the esophagus have improved greatly. Palliation of dysphagia and odynophagia can be achieved with radiation therapy alone, but palliation may be more consistent and durable if irradiation is combined with chemotherapy. Patients with inoperable tumors can be cured with concurrent chemotherapy and moderate-dose radiation therapy. The addition of esophageal brachytherapy to external irradiation and concurrent chemotherapy is associated with a high risk of complications. Surgical techniques and support have improved such that mortality rates after esophagectomy have decreased dramatically. However, results of surgical treatment for esophageal cancer remain disappointing. It may be advantageous to use concurrent chemotherapy and radiation therapy before esophageal resection, but further studies are needed. As results of nonsurgical combined-modality therapy improve, the need to compare chemotherapy and radiation therapy with and without esophageal resection is becoming more compelling.

REFERENCES

1. Fajardo LF, Berthrong M, Anderson RE. Esophagus. In: *Radiation Pathology.* New York, NY: Oxford University Press; 2001: 214-220.
2. Komaki R, Scott C, Ettinger D, et al. Randomized study of chemotherapy/radiation therapy combinations for favorable patients with locally advanced inoperable nonsmall cell lung cancer: Radiation Therapy Oncology Group (RTOG) 9204. *Int J Radiat Oncol Biol Phys* 1997;38:149-155.
3. Berthrong M, Fajardo LF. Radiation injury in surgical pathology. II. Alimentary tract. *Am J Surg Pathol* 1981;5:153-178.
4. Munoz N, Day NE. Esophageal cancer. In: Schottenfeld D, Fraumeni J Jr, eds. *Cancer Epidemiology and Prevention.* 2nd ed. New York, NY: Oxford University Press; 1996:681-706.
5. Lagergren J, Bergstrom R, Lindgren A, et al. Symptomatic gastroesophageal reflux as a risk factor for esophageal adenocarcinoma. *N Engl J Med* 1999;340:825-831.
6. Kelsen DP, Ginsberg R, Pajak TF, et al. Chemotherapy followed by surgery compared with surgery alone for localized esophageal cancer. *N Engl J Med* 1998;339:1979-1984.
7. Devesa SS, Blot WJ, Fraumeni JF Jr. Changing patterns in the incidence of esophageal and gastric carcinoma in the United States. *Cancer* 1998;83:2049-2053.
8. Streeter OE Jr, Martz KL, Gaspar LE, et al. Does race influence survival for esophageal cancer patients treated on the radiation and chemotherapy arm of RTOG #85-01? *Int J Radiat Oncol Biol Phys* 1999;44:1047-1052.
9. Appelqvist P. Carcinoma of the oesophagus and gastric cardia. A retrospective study based on statistical and clinical material from Finland. *Acta Chir Scand Suppl* 1972;430:1-92.
10. Greenlee RT, Hill-Harmon MB, Murray T, et al. Cancer statistics, 2001. *CA Cancer J Clin* 2001;51:15-36.
11. Anderson LL, Lad TE. Autopsy findings in squamous cell carcinoma of the esophagus. *Cancer* 1982;50:1587-1590.
12. Herskovic A, Martz K, Al-Sarraf M, et al. Combined chemotherapy and radiotherapy compared with radiotherapy alone in patients with cancer of the esophagus. *N Engl J Med* 1992;326: 1593-1598.
13. Block MI, Patterson GA, Sundaresan RS, et al. Improvement in staging of esophageal cancer with the addition of positron emission tomography. *Ann Thorac Surg* 1997;64:770-777.
14. Fleming I, Cooper JS, Henson DE, et al, eds. *AJCC Cancer Staging Manual,* 5th ed. Philadelphia, Pa: Lippincott Williams & Wilkins; 1997:65-69.
15. Ellis FHJ, Heatley GJ, Krasna MJ, et al. Esophagogastrectomy for carcinoma of the esophagus and cardia: a comparison of findings and results after standard resection in three consecutive eight-year intervals with improved staging criteria. *J Thorac Cardiovasc Surg* 1997;113:836-846.

16. Swisher SG, Pisters PWT, Komaki R. Gastroesophageal junction adenocarcinoma. *Curr Treat Opt Oncol* 2000;1:387-398.

17. Earlam R, Cunha-Melo JR. Oesophageal squamous cell carcinoma. I. A critical review of surgery. *Br J Surg* 1980;67:381-390.

18. Orringer MB. Resection of the esophagus. In: Shields TW, LoCicero JI, Ponn RB, eds. *General Thoracic Surgery*. 5th ed. Philadelphia, Pa: Lippincott Williams & Wilkins; 2000:1697-1722.

19. Whyte RI, Orringer MB. Surgery for carcinoma of the esophagus: the case for transhiatal esophagectomy. *Semin Radiat Oncol* 1994; 4:146-156.

20. Whittington R. Controversies in the management of adenocarcinoma of the esophagus and esophagogastric junction. *Semin Radiat Oncol* 1994;4:170-178.

21. Yang ZY, Gu XZ, Zhao S. Long-term survival of radiotherapy for esophageal cancer: analysis of 1136 patients surviving for more than 5 years. *Int J Radiat Oncol Biol Phys* 1983;9:1769-1773.

22. Teniere P, Hay JM, Fingerhut A, et al. Postoperative radiation therapy does not increase survival after curative resection for squamous cell carcinoma of the middle and lower esophagus as shown by a multicenter controlled trial. *Surg Gynecol Obstet* 1991;173:123-130.

23. Fok M, Sham JS, Choy D, et al. Postoperative radiotherapy for carcinoma of the esophagus: a prospective, randomized controlled study. *Surgery* 1993;113:138-147.

24. Zieren HU, Muller JM, Jacobi CA, et al. Adjuvant postoperative radiation therapy after curative resection of squamous cell carcinoma of the thoracic esophagus: a prospective randomized study. *World J Surg* 1995;19:444-449.

25. Launois B, Delarue D, Campion JP, et al. Preoperative radiotherapy for carcinoma of the esophagus. *Surg Gynecol Obstet* 1981;153:690-692.

26. Gignoux M, Roussel A, Paillot B, et al. The value of preoperative radiotherapy in esophageal cancer: results of a study of the E.O.R.T.C. *World J Surg* 1987;11:426-432.

27. Wang M, Gu XZ, Yin WB, et al. Randomized clinical trial on the combination of preoperative irradiation and surgery in the treatment of esophageal carcinoma: report on 206 patients. *Int J Radiat Oncol Biol Phys* 1989;16:325-327.

28. Arnott SJ, Duncan W, Kerr GR, et al. Low dose preoperative radiotherapy for carcinoma of the oesophagus: results of a randomized clinical trial. *Radiother Oncol* 1992;24:108-113.

29. Nygaard K, Hagen S, Hansen HS, et al. Pre-operative radiotherapy prolongs survival in operable esophageal carcinoma: a randomized, multicenter study of pre-operative radiotherapy and chemotherapy. The second Scandinavian trial in esophageal cancer. *World J Surg* 1992;16:1104-1110.

30. Urba S, Orringer M, Turrisi A. A randomized trial comparing surgery (S) to preoperative concomitant chemoradiation plus surgery in patients (pts) with resectable esophageal cancer (CA): updated analysis [abstract]. *Proc Am Soc Clin Oncol* 1997;16:983.

31. Le Prise E, Etienne PL, Meunier B, et al. A randomized study of chemotherapy, radiation therapy, and surgery versus surgery for localized squamous cell carcinoma of the esophagus. *Cancer* 1994;73:1779-1784.

32. Walsh TN, Noonan N, Hollywood D, et al. A comparison of multimodal therapy and surgery for esophageal adenocarcinoma. *N Engl J Med* 1996;335:462-467.

33. Bosset J-F, Gignou M, Triboulet J-P, et al. Chemoradiotherapy followed by surgery compared with surgery alone in squamous-cell cancer of the esophagus. *N Engl J Med* 1997;337: 161-167.

34. Sur RK, Singh DP, Sharma SC, et al. Radiation therapy of esophageal cancer: role of high dose rate brachytherapy. *Int J Radiat Oncol Biol Phys* 1992;22:1043-1046.

35. Gaspar LE, Winter K, Kocha WI, et al. A phase I/II study of external beam radiation, brachytherapy, and concurrent chemotherapy for patients with localized carcinoma of the esophagus (RTOG 9207): final report. *Cancer* 2000;88:988-995.

36. Kelsen DP, Bains M, Hilaris B, et al. Combination chemotherapy of esophageal carcinoma using cisplatin, vindesine, and bleomycin. *Cancer* 1982;49:1174-1177.

37. Leichman L, Steiger Z, Seydel HG, et al. Combined preoperative chemotherapy and radiation therapy for cancer of the esophagus: the Wayne State University, Southwest Oncology group and Radiation Therapy Oncology Group experience. *Semin Oncol* 1984;11:178-185.

38. Coia LR, Engstrom PF, Paul A, et al. A pilot study of combined radiotherapy and chemotherapy for esophageal carcinoma. *Am J Clin Oncol* 1984;7:653-659.

39. Al-Sarraf M, Martz K, Herskovic A, et al. Progress report of combined chemoradiotherapy versus radiotherapy alone in patients with esophageal cancer: an intergroup study. *J Clin Oncol* 1997;1:277-284.

40. Cooper JS, Guo MD, Herskovic A, et al. Chemoradiotherapy of locally advanced esophageal cancer: long-term follow-up of a prospective randomized trial (RTOG 85–01). *JAMA* 1999;281: 1623-1627.

41. Coia LR, Engstrom PF, Paul AR, et al. Long-term results of infusional 5-FU, mitomycin-C and radiation as primary management of esophageal carcinoma. *Int J Radiat Oncol Biol Phys* 1991; 20:29-36.

42. Smith TJ, Ryan LM, Douglass HOJ, et al. Combined chemoradiotherapy vs. radiotherapy alone for early stage squamous cell carcinoma of the esophagus: a study of the Eastern Cooperative Oncology Group. *Int J Radiat Oncol Biol Phys* 1998;42: 269-276.

43. Richmond J, Seydel HG, Bae Y, et al. Comparison of three treatment strategies for esophageal cancer within a single institution. *Int J Radiat Oncol Biol Phys* 1987;13:1617-1620.

44. Minsky BD, Neuberg D, Kelsen DP. Final report of intergroup trial 0122 (ECOG PE-289, RTOG 90–12): phase II trial of neoadjuvant chemotherapy plus concurrent chemotherapy and high-dose radiation for squamous cell carcinoma of the esophagus. *Int J Radiat Oncol Biol Phys* 1999;43:517-523.

45. Minsky B, Berkey B, Kelsen D. Preliminary results of intergroup INT 0123 randomized trial of combined modality therapy (CMT) for esophageal cancer: conventional vs. high dose radiation therapy [abstract]. *Proc Am Soc Clin Oncol* 2000;19:239.

46. Caspers RJ, Welvaart K, Verkes RJ, et al. The effect of radiotherapy on dysphagia and survival in patients with esophageal cancer. *Radiother Oncol* 1988;12:15-23.

47. Bown SG. Palliation of malignant dysphagia: surgery, radiotherapy, laser, intubation alone or in combination? *Gut* 1991;32: 841-844.

CHAPTER 19

The Stomach and Small Intestine

Christopher H. Crane and Nora A. Janjan

THE STOMACH
Normal Anatomy and Histology

The stomach is divided into four major anatomic regions: the cardia, fundus, body, and pylorus (Fig. 19-1). The gastroesophageal junction is located just to the left of midline at the level of the 11th thoracic vertebral body, and the pylorus is located to the right of midline at the level of the first lumbar vertebral body. The pylorus empties into the first portion of the duodenum. The greater and lesser curvatures form attachments with the greater omentum and lesser omentum, respectively. The undistended stomach relaxes into longitudinal folds known as rugae, which flatten out when the stomach is filled with food.

The stomach has three histologically distinct regions: the cardia, body/fundus, and pyloric regions. Throughout the stomach, the mucosa consists of surface epithelium that invaginates to various degrees into the lamina propria to form gastric pits, which end blindly in glands with neck and base regions (see Fig. 19-1). The undifferentiated cells of the neck region of the glands migrate either to the surface to form mucus-producing cells or deeper into the glands to differentiate into mucous neck cells, parietal cells, enterendocrine cells, or chief cells. The structure of the pits is distinct in each region of the stomach. In the cardia region, mucus-producing glands predominate, whereas the fundus and body are rich in parietal and chief cells. Parietal cells are eosinophilic and tend to be pyramidal. They produce and secrete hydrochloric acid and intrinsic factor, the latter of which is essential for vitamin B_{12} absorption. The chief cells secrete pepsinogen, which is a proteolytic proenzyme contained in characteristic zymogen granules. The antrum is rich in gastrin-secreting G cells and somatostatin-secreting D cells, which have stimulatory and inhibitory effects, respectively, on gastric acid secretion.

Acute Reactions to Radiation Therapy

Before modern pharmacology, radiation therapy was used to treat peptic ulcer disease. The rationale for treatment was based on the empiric observation that radiation therapy reduces gastric acid secretion. This practice stimulated investigations of the physiologic effects of gastric irradiation.[1] Important observations were recorded that allowed insight into the acute reactions of the stomach to radiation therapy. To understand the histologic changes that occur with irradiation, Goldgraber and colleagues[2] conducted serial biopsies in three patients treated with 1500 rad (15 Gy) in 10 equal fractions to the entire stomach through anteroposterior-posteroanterior portals with 250-kV x-rays. The biopsies showed a loss of cytoplasmic detail and a disappearance of cytoplasmic granules in the parietal and chief cells as early as 8 days after initial radiation treatment. The cytoplasm became glassy and eosinophilic, and the nuclei of these cells became elongated and pyknotic. These changes were termed *coagulation necrosis* and occurred with a relative sparing of the mucosal surface. By day 16 after initiation of irradiation, the architecture of the mucosal epithelium began to change. The glandular pits began to deepen and many of the parietal and chief cells sloughed into the gastric lumen while cells at the glandular neck started to proliferate. At this point, other than some cuboidal change, changes in the surface columnar epithelium were still minimal. Three weeks after initiation of therapy, marked architectural disorganization, a patchy loss of glandular architecture, and an overall loss of mucosal thickness were seen. At this point, the surface epithelial cells varied in appearance from flat to columnar (Fig. 19-2).[2] Regeneration began in the glandular neck cells. At 5 weeks, the mucosal and glandular architecture began to revert to normal. By week 6, nearly all radiation changes had resolved, with only focal areas of glandular coagulation necrosis being evident. Although the same dose was used in each of the three patients treated, the time of onset of the earliest changes varied between 5 and 16 days. The severity and duration of the changes also varied.

Palmer and Templeton[3] studied the gastric secretory response in 88 patients treated at the University of Chicago with 1800 rad (18 Gy, a relatively low dose of radiation) in 10 equal fractions for peptic ulcer disease. Both basal gastric acid production and histamine-induced gastric acid response were measured. Achlorhydria was documented in 35 patients and varied in duration from a few days to 6 months. Unable to find a correlation of the inhibitor effect with either sex or body weight, the authors hypothesized the existence of differences in parietal cell radiation sensitivity among

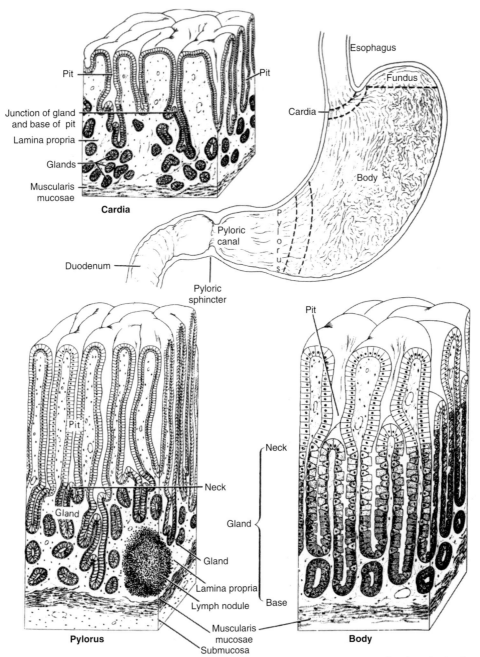

Fig. 19-1 The 4 major anatomic regions of the stomach are the cardia, the fundus, the body, and the pylorus (antrum). The structure of the gastric pits is distinct in each region as shown.

individuals. Overall, 1500 patients were given similar doses in the University of Chicago series, and 40% experienced a 50% reduction in gastric acid secretion that lasted for a year or more.[4] Gastric secretory function tended to parallel the observed glandular changes. Gastric acid was present at fasting concentrations 2 days after the start of therapy but undetectable thereafter. Secretory studies using histamine showed achlorhydria at 2 weeks and an attenuated induction of the peak response of gastric acid by histamine at 12 weeks, although by then the mucosa had reverted to normal.[2]

The critical structures in a typical radiation field for gastric carcinoma include the stomach, small intestine, liver, kidneys, and spinal cord. The acute reactions that occur with irradiation of these structures include gastritis (epigastric pain), nausea, anorexia, diarrhea, abdominal cramping, fatigue, and hematologic suppression. Most patients experience some degree of nausea and fatigue and a moderate to severe amount of hematologic suppression depending on the type of concurrent chemotherapy used. Acute reactions usually peak during the fourth week of treatment and subside 1 to 2 weeks after completion of a 5-week course of treatment.

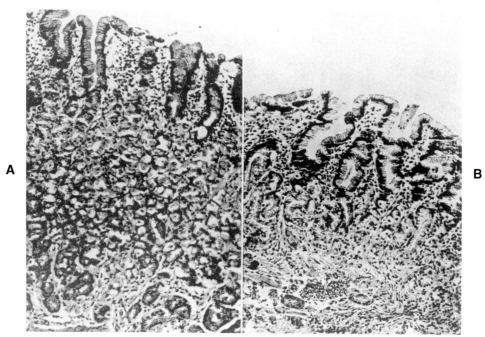

Fig. 19-2   **A,** Endoscopic biopsy sample of normal gastric mucosa. (×110) **B,** Sample of gastric mucosa 3 weeks after treatment with 15 Gy given over 10 days. (×100) (From Goldgraber M, Rubin C, Palmer W, et al. *Gastroenterology* 1954;27:1-20.)

Late Effects of Radiation Therapy

The effects of fractionated radiation therapy (up to 60 Gy) on the canine stomach have been demonstrated. Perforating gastric ulcers are seen within 4 weeks of irradiation.[5] In humans, gastritis, ulceration, and obstruction are unusual at doses of less than 40 Gy but have been documented with a sharp increase in incidence above 45 Gy in patients irradiated for gastric ulcer using low-energy photons and suboptimal technique. At Walter Reed Army Medical Center, 35 (14%) of 256 patients who underwent prophylactic irradiation for malignant germ cell tumor experienced gastric ulceration 2 to 3 months after completion of treatment.[6] The rates of ulceration, perforation, or obstruction in this setting have been observed to be 25% to 50% at 55 Gy and 63% at doses between 55 and 64 Gy, with perforation occurring in one fourth of the patients. Most of these patients were treated with 200-kV to 1-MV photons, short source-to-skin distances, large fractions, and only one field per day. Although these data illustrate the sensitivity of the upper abdomen to irradiation, they should be interpreted in the context of these technical inadequacies. The use of modern linear accelerators and techniques has produced a very low risk of gastric injury with doses of less than 50 Gy.[1,7-11] A dose-response relationship does seem to exist for radiation injury between 50 and 60 Gy. Morbidity risks of less than 10% are expected for 50 to 55 Gy and 5% to 15% for doses in excess of 60 Gy.[7,8,12-23] For those complications that do not require gastrectomy,[24] healing of radiation-induced lesions is characterized by re-epithelialization with fibrosis and contraction in 2 to 3 years.[21]

The other critical structures in the region include the kidneys, liver, small intestine, and spinal cord. Mean decreases in creatinine clearance of 10% and 24% have been observed in patients when 50% and 90% to 100%, respectively, of a single kidney is irradiated with doses higher than 26 Gy.[25] However, clinically relevant compromise of kidney function rarely develops if at least one kidney is spared from the field.

Radiation-induced liver disease, often called *radiation hepatitis*, is characterized by the development of anicteric ascites approximately 2 weeks to 4 months after hepatic irradiation.[26] The whole liver has been treated safely to doses of more than 20 Gy in patients with pancreatic cancer,[27] but whole-liver doses of more than 35 Gy have resulted in a significant risk of radiation hepatitis.[28] Although the risk of radiation hepatitis can be predicted from dose and volume considerations,[29,30] it is now clear that limited volumes can tolerate high doses of irradiation.[31] Radiation effects on the small bowel are discussed in the section on "Small Intestine" in this chapter; effects on the spinal cord are discussed in Chapter 32.

EPIDEMIOLOGY OF GASTRIC CANCER

Since the 1930s, when gastric cancer was the leading cause of cancer-specific mortality among men in the

United States,[32] the overall incidence rates have dropped dramatically, and the location of presenting lesions has changed from noncardia to cardia sites.[33] In 2001, 21,700 people in the United States will be diagnosed with gastric cancer, with a slight male predominance.[34] Currently, blacks, hispanics, and Native Americans are 1.5 to 2.5 times more likely to develop gastric cancer than are whites in the United States.[35] Although the same trend of declining incidence is seen throughout the world, gastric cancer is still the second leading cause of cancer-specific mortality worldwide.[36] It is the most common malignancy in Japan and is also common in China, South America, and Eastern Europe.[37]

The decline in incidence of gastric cancer from 1930 to 1976 has paralleled a decline in the incidence of distal gastric lesions. This phenomenon lags 20 to 30 years behind the widespread availability of refrigeration, and this factor has been proposed to account for the sharp decline in gastric carcinoma.[38-40] Since 1976, however, the incidence of proximal cardia and gastroesophageal junction adenocarcinoma in the United States and Europe have increased at a rate that exceeds that of any other malignancy.[41] The rise in incidence of gastroesophageal junction and cardia lesions suggests a common pathogenesis distinct from that of distal gastric lesions, but the cause remains unclear.

Gastric cancer occurs in two general histologic types—an intestinal type in which cells are closely adherent and tend to form glands and a diffuse type that tends to infiltrate and thicken the gastric wall without forming a discrete mass.[42] The intestinal type is more common, is more often distal, and predominates in endemic areas. The diffuse type has a worse prognosis, tends to occur in younger patients, and can occur anywhere in the stomach but is most common in the cardia.[43,44] A separate, similar classification, Borrman's classification, distinguishes five types. The first three types are analogous to the intestinal type with increasing degrees of ulceration, the fourth is diffusely infiltrating, and the fifth is unclassifiable.[45]

ETIOLOGY

The shift in anatomic site of origin in gastric cancer has stimulated much epidemiologic research. Chronic atrophic gastritis and the resulting intestinal metaplasia seem to be precursor conditions to the intestinal type of gastric cancer.[46] Mucosal changes brought about by a variety of environmental insults can eventually lead to atrophic gastritis. Environmental, host-related, and infectious causes may all play roles.

Environmental Factors

Environmental factors, especially early in life, probably determine the risk of stomach cancer.[47,48] As noted previously, the widespread availability of refrigeration has paralleled the reduction in the incidence of gastric carcinoma.[38] Refrigeration may have resulted in reduced exposure to various carcinogens such as nitrates and nitrites used to prevent bacterial and fungal contamination of food. Another possibility is that refrigeration allowed the possibility of an increase in dietary intake of fresh fruit and a reduction in the consumption of smoked, cured, and salted foods. These dietary factors have correlated with lower gastric carcinoma rates in epidemiologic studies.[39,49-61] In a prospective study of Japanese residents of Hawaii, consumption of pickled, processed, or salted foods was not associated with gastric cancer, but frequent consumption of fresh fruit and raw vegetables was inversely related to the incidence of gastric cancer.[62] Serum vitamin C levels did not correlate with gastric cancer in a multicenter study,[63] although high or low intake of other micronutrients (e.g., beta-carotene, ascorbic acid, methionine, ferritin) could play a role.[64,65] Dietary diversity, especially with regard to fruits and vegetables, has been reported to be protective.[66] A positive correlation with the extent of cooking red meat has also been reported in gastric cancer patients interviewed for food preparation preference.[67] Another study found no relationship between nitrate concentrations in drinking water and the incidence of stomach or esophageal cancer.[68]

An interaction between dietary methionine and salt has also been suggested.[69] Other environmental factors such as smoking[54,55,63,70] and industrial dust exposure[70] may have an association, but convincing evidence is still lacking to demonstrate a role for alcohol.[50,58,62,70-74] The most compelling evidence for an environmental cause of the intestinal type of gastric cancer comes from studies of migrating populations.[74] Japanese,[75] South American,[47] and Eastern European migrants assume a lower risk of developing gastric cancer after two to three generations spent in a lower-risk environment with a lower-risk diet.[47,74,75]

Host-Related Factors

Host factors such as low serum ferritin levels[76] and pernicious anemia are associated with a twofold to threefold excess risk of gastric cancer.[77-79] An association is evident between gastric ulcer and an increase in the risk of gastric cancer.[80] Medically treated peptic ulcer disease does not seem to be associated with an increased risk, but patients who have undergone distal gastrectomy for benign peptic ulcer disease have been reported to have up to a fivefold increase in risk after a long latency period.[81-83] An association between adenomatous polyps and gastric cancer has been suggested,[84] and clear associations exist between Barrett's esophagus and adenocarcinoma of the distal esophagus and gastric cardia,[85,86] with the risk estimated to be 0.8% per annum. Evidence is also clear for a heritable risk of gastric cancer in a small proportion of patients. Familial predisposition[74,75,87-89] seems to be independent of environmental factors.[89] Controlling for dietary risk, patients with hereditary nonpolyposis colorectal cancer but not those with familial adenomatous polyposis are at increased risk of gastric cancer.[90]

Infectious Factors

Although an association between *Helicobacter pylori* infection and gastric cancer has been reported in epidemiologic studies,[91] no reduction in risk after treatment of *H. pylori* infection has been demonstrated. Prospective serologic studies have shown that patients with *H. pylori* infection have a threefold to fivefold higher risk.[92-94] Recent evidence points to a specific strain, cytotoxin-associated gene A–positive *H. pylori*,[95,96] and infection early in life.[97] The increased risk has been reported to be for noncardia lesions only.[98] A recent analysis concluded that screening is substantially more cost effective in endemic areas (outside the United States).[99] A cohort study looking at stored serum suggests that chronic Epstein-Barr virus (EBV) infection may play an etiologic role in a subset of patients.[100] Because only a small proportion of patients infected with either *H. pylori* or EBV develop malignancy, undoubtedly additional environmental cofactors contribute to the carcinogenic process.[101,102]

SCREENING

Countries in which gastric cancer is endemic have implemented endoscopic screening programs. Japan, in particular, has successfully increased detection of early-stage disease, and some have suggested that such programs have reduced gastric cancer–specific mortality rates.[103] Widespread implementation of screening programs has resulted in 34.5% of cases being diagnosed while disease is confined to the mucosa.[103,104] The Cancer Institute Hospital of Tokyo has also reported an increase in the rate of curative resections from 48% in the 1940s to 98% during the 1980s.[105] Without prospective evaluation, however, this contention cannot be confirmed because of confounding environmental variables that have also changed, such as westernization of the diet. Validation of a role for screening radiography is also lacking. A case-control study evaluating the value of screening radiography in Venezuela failed to demonstrate a positive effect.[106]

PATTERN OF SPREAD

Gastric cancer can spread by direct extension, lymphatic or hematologic invasion, or transperitoneal dissemination. Critical organs such as the pancreas, diaphragm, transverse colon, duodenum, spleen, jejunum, liver, left kidney, left adrenal gland, and the celiac axis are in close proximity and are frequently involved. Lymphatic spread initially occurs to the perigastric nodes along the lesser and greater curvatures and then to lymphatics that accompany the branches of the celiac axis (hepatic, subpyloric, gastroduodenal, and pancreatosplenic). Remote lymphatic spread can occur to the hepatoduodenal, peripancreatic, superior mesenteric, and paraaortic nodal chains. Similar to cancer of the esophagus and duodenum, clinically occult spread of gastric cancer beyond the gross lesion can occur through the abundant subserosal and submucosal lymphatics. Distant metastasis occurs most commonly through portal venous drainage to the liver. Systemic spread occurs less commonly to the lungs and even less often to other sites. Lesions of the gastroesophageal junction have a stronger tendency to spread to the lungs. Transperitoneal spread occurs in 23% to 43% of patients who have undergone gastrectomy.[107-110]

Clinical,[108,110] reoperative,[109] and autopsy series[111-115] have been used to define the pattern of failure in gastric cancer. The report of Gunderson and Sosin[109] on Wangensteen's second-look laparotomy series[116] defined the pattern of failure for surgically treated gastric cancer. At 1 year after the initial surgical treatment, failures were seen in the anastamoses, gastric bed, gastric remnant, duodenal stump, and regional nodes; the isolated local–regional failure rate was 29%, and a local–regional component of failure was present in 88% of patients with initially localized disease[109] (Fig. 19-3). A similar pattern of failure was reported in surgically treated patients from the Massachusetts General Hospital, with local–regional component of relapse in 38% of these patients and isolated local–regional relapse in 16%.[108] The true incidence of failure was probably underestimated owing to the limitations of imaging disease in the gastric bed, regional nodes, and peritoneum and the lack of uniformity in restaging relapsed disease. Autopsy studies have correlated well with these findings.[111-115]

In summary, surgically treated gastric cancer is associated with a significant isolated local–regional component of failure. Effective adjuvant or neoadjuvant therapy thus could be significantly beneficial.

PRESENTATION AND WORK-UP

The most common presenting symptoms of gastric cancer are upper abdominal discomfort, weakness from anemia, and weight loss.[117] Early satiety, hematemesis, or melena occur less commonly. Obstructing lesions in the antrum or cardia can cause vomiting or dysphagia, respectively. Typically, presenting symptoms are nonspecific and unfortunately do not usually occur with superficially invasive disease; rather, disease usually has progressed to the point of transmural invasion or distant metastasis at the time of presentation. Palpable disease is usually indicative of advanced disease.

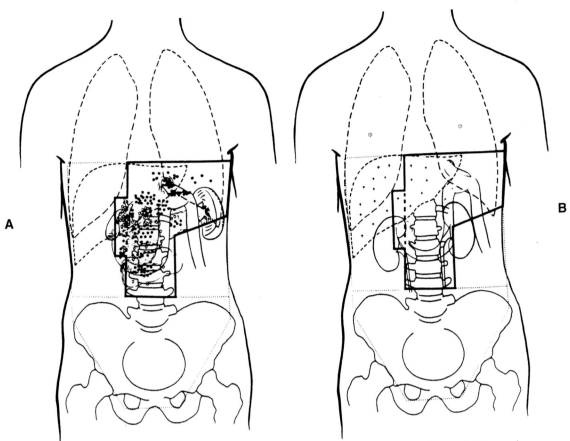

Fig. 19-3 Patterns of failure in gastric cancer as documented in a landmark report of second-look laparotomy 1 year after surgical treatment. Isolated local–regional failure was found in 29% of patients and a local–regional component of failure was found in 88% of patients. A hypothetical radiation therapy field is included in the figure, but it was not intended to be used as a standard radiotherapy port. (**A,** Local–regional disease; **B,** distant disease). •, local failures in surrounding organs or tissues; o, lymph node failures; *, lung metastases; +, liver metastases. (From Gunderson LL, Sosin H. *Int J Radiat Oncol Biol Phys* 1982;8:1-11.)

Careful physical examination can detect metastases in the left supraclavicular fossa or those forming a Blumer's (rectal) shelf indicative of peritoneal dissemination.

Initial work-up usually includes a double-contrast upper gastrointestinal study, chest x-ray, and blood work that includes tests of liver enzymes and a differential blood count. Upper endoscopy is sensitive[118-120] and allows tissues to be sampled but is invasive and costly. Biopsies should be multiple and deep,[120] and fresh tissue samples should undergo flow cytometric analysis if lymphoma is suspected. When the diagnosis of gastric cancer is established, computed tomography (CT) scans of the abdomen with intravenous phase-contrast medium are indicated. Evaluation of CT findings in comparison with those of laparotomy reveal many limitations for CT, including poor characterization of primary disease and a lack of sensitivity in detecting peritoneal or liver metastases.[121,122] Staging laparoscopy and endoscopic ultrasonography have sometimes been used to improve identification of patients who can benefit from curative therapies.[123,124] Accuracy rates for

tumor staging of between 80% and 85% have been reported for endoscopic ultrasonography.[125,126] In comparing modern and historical series, it is crucial to realize the selection bias introduced by improvements in preoperative imaging, the use of peritoneal staging, and the increased use of endoscopic sonography.

STAGING

Gastric cancer staging is based on the tumor-nodes-metastasis (TNM) system (Box 19-1).[127] Although pathologic staging has traditionally been used, clinical staging has become more common with the use of endoscopic sonography and laparoscopic peritoneal exploration for patients undergoing neoadjuvant treatment.

PATHOLOGY

Between 90% and 95% of malignant gastric tumors are adenocarcinomas, with non-Hodgkin's lymphoma, leiomyosarcoma, carcinoid, adenocanthoma, squamous

---

BOX 19-1   American Joint Committee on Cancer Staging System for Carcinoma of the Stomach

PRIMARY TUMOR (T)

TX   Primary tumor cannot be assessed

T0   No evidence of primary tumor

Tis   Carcinoma in situ; intraepithelial tumor without invasion of the lamina propria

T1   Tumor invades lamina propria or submucosa

T2   Tumor invades muscularis propria or subserosa*

T3   Tumor penetrates serosa (visceral peritoneum) without invasion of adjacent structures[†,‡]

T4   Tumor invades adjacent structures[†,‡]

REGIONAL LYMPH NODES (N)

NX   Regional lymph node(s) cannot be assessed

N0   No regional lymph node metastasis

N1   Metastasis in 1 to 6 regional lymph nodes

N2   Metastasis in 7 to 15 regional lymph nodes

N3   Metastasis in more than 15 regional lymph nodes

DISTANT METASTASIS (M)

MX   Distant metastasis cannot be assessed

M0   No distant metastasis

M1   Distant metastasis

STAGE GROUPING

Stage 0	Tis	N0	M0
Stage IA	T1	N0	M0
Stage IB	T1	N1	M0
	T2	N0	M0
Stage II	T1	N2	M0
	T2	N1	M0
	T3	N0	M0
Stage IIIA	T2	N2	M0
	T3	N1	M0
	T4	N0	M0
Stage IIIB	T3	N2	M0
Stage IV	T4	N1	M0
	T1	N3	M0
	T2	N3	M0
	T3	N3	M0
	T4	N2	M0
	T4	N3	M0
	Any T	Any N	M1

From Fleming I, Cooper JS, Henson DE, et al, eds. *AJCC Cancer Staging Manual*, 5th ed. Philadelphia, Pa: Lippincott Williams & Wilkins; 1997:71-76.

*A tumor may penetrate the muscularis propria with extension into the gastrocolic or gastrohepatic ligaments, or into the greater or lesser omentum without perforation of the visceral peritoneum covering these structures. If there is perforation of the visceral peritoneum covering the gastric ligaments or the omentum, the tumor should be classified T3.

†The adjacent structures of the stomach include the spleen, transverse colon, liver, diaphragm, pancreas, abdominal wall, adrenal gland, kidney, small intestine, and retroperitoneum.

‡Intramural extension to the duodenum or esophagus is classified by the depth of greatest invasion in any of these sites, including stomach.

---

cell, and neuoendocrine undifferentiated tumors also occasionally occurring. Tumor cells may contain mucin vacuoles that may distend the cell and compress the nucleus, creating the characteristic signet-ring appearance. Diffusely infiltrative tumors often stimulate a marked desmoplastic response, leading to a diffusely thickened gastric wall; this particular form of infiltrative tumor is termed linitis plastica.

PROGNOSTIC FACTORS

The most important prognostic factor for patients with gastric cancer is the TNM stage.[128,129] Gross hematogenous or transperitoneal disease is incurable. The degree of transmural penetration beyond the gastric wall[109,128,130-135] and the presence, number, and location of lymph node involvement correlate with survival.[128,130-136] Patients with both transmural penetration and nodal involvement have a particularly poor prognosis.[109,131,134,136]

Peritoneal cytology analysis has shown evidence of disease in 16% to 35% of patients at the time of resection.[137-139] Such results have been consistently reported to have a negative influence on survival in univariate analyses,[137-143] but not all patients with cytologic evidence of disease will develop peritoneal carcinomatosis.[137,138,143]

Intestinal-type lesions are associated with a better prognosis than diffusely infiltrative lesions.[42-44] Patients with linitis plastica have an extremely poor prognosis.[16,17,144,145]

The presence of receptors for estrogen[146] on tumor cells is associated with higher rates of tumor infiltration, poorer differentiation, and a worse prognosis.

SURGICAL THERAPY

Since Theodore Billroth successfully performed the first gastrectomy for gastric cancer in 1881, surgery has been the cornerstone of curative therapy for this disease. The initial surgical approach for malignant disease was a partial gastrectomy that was not radically different from gastric surgery for benign disease. A more aggressive approach involving resection of the entire stomach, spleen, and distal pancreas followed a landmark autopsy series from Memorial Sloan-Kettering Cancer Center published in

1951, which reported 80% local failure and 50% involvement of the gastric remnant.[107] Wangensteen's initial findings at second-look laparotomy[116] also prompted extensive lymphanedectomy. A prospective, randomized study from France comparing total and subtotal gastrectomy found no survival difference and similar perioperative morbidity for the two procedures.[147] The optimal surgical procedure has not been defined and remains controversial. For lesions arising in the gastric body and antrum, a radical subtotal gastrectomy is preferred. In this procedure, 80% of the stomach with the perigastric lymphatics, the gastrohepatic and gastrocolic omenta, and the first portion of the duodenum are resected. Retrospective studies from Memorial Sloan-Kettering and Japan have not shown a survival benefit from the addition of splenectomy.[148-151] More proximal lesions require a total gastrectomy. Rates of positive margins vary from 30% with a 2-cm margin to 0% with a 4- to 6-cm margin beyond the gross lesion.[152] Mucosal margins should be at least 5 to 6 cm. Overall, the reported frequency of positive margins in patients undergoing curative resection is approximately 25%.[153-157] Although this rate is similar to those reported for anastomotic and gastric remnant failures,[108,109] anastomotic failure has been reported to occur in only 23% of patients with positive margins.[152]

Extensive lymph node dissection has been advocated by some Japanese investigators and has been reported to improve survival.[110,158-160] Other investigators have found no improvement in local–regional control or survival.[109,158] The impressive results in the Japanese studies, even in patients with advanced disease, seem to be improving with time and have stimulated much debate in the literature. Extended lymphadenectomy has not been embraced by western surgeons largely because of the lack of a clear benefit and high morbidity associated with the procedure.[161-166] A recently reported Dutch randomized trial showed a survival disadvantage for more extensive lymphadenectomy.[163] Part of the explanation for a difference in morbidity rates lies in the epidemic rates of morbid obesity in the United States compared with Japan; such obesity increases operative risk and creates a more technically demanding operation. The high morbidity rates likely obscure any benefit. Another explanation for the apparent difference in results could lie in the concept of stage migration. More extensive lymphadenectomies and more compulsive pathologic evaluation give rise to an apparent improvement in stage-specific survival without an overall benefit. The overall operative mortality in the United States has been reported to be as high as 7% in some centers[117] but is typically 1% to 3% in more experienced hands.[164]

Modern surgery is highly successful in patients with early-stage disease, with 5-year survival rates of 80% to 90% for T1 disease and 50% to 60% for T2 disease.[103,128,129,167] Unfortunately, in the United States fewer than 5% of patients have T1 or T2 disease. Potentially curative resection is possible in only 25% to 40% of cases that are judged to be resectable by clinical staging.[168] Complete gross resection without adjuvant therapy has resulted in median survival durations of 15 to 18 months and 5-year survival rates of 20% to 30% in western populations.[117,128,130,169-171]

ADJUVANT THERAPY
Historical Perspective

With the advent of modern surgical techniques and the recognition of surgery's limitations, adjuvant therapies began to be evaluated. Radiation therapy was a key component of initial investigations. Unfortunately, during that early era, adequate technique, technology, and especially supportive care were either not available or not used. This led to widespread toxic effects and consequent failure to define a role for radiation therapy in gastric cancer. This left an opportunity for the investigation of adjuvant chemotherapy. Over the next decade, adjuvant chemotherapy was exhaustively evaluated. From that experience, substantial toxicity was demonstrated with intensive chemotherapy, but a survival benefit could not be established. This has led some centers to evaluate induction (neoadjuvant) chemotherapy over the past decade. With intensive and toxic regimens, single-arm prospective studies have shown modest response rates and unimpressive pathologic complete response rates. This has most recently led to the inclusion of radiation, the single most active agent in gastric cancer, in the most recent single-arm prospective studies. With vital supportive care, very large radiation fields with potent concurrent radiosensitizers are actually very well tolerated, and a substantial increase in the pathologic complete response rate has been observed. In the future, phase III studies are imperative, but the relevant questions will be under considerable debate. Clearly, the relative roles of neoadjuvant chemotherapy and concurrent chemoradiation must be established.

Postoperative Chemotherapy, Radiation Therapy, or Chemoradiation Therapy

The patterns of failure discussed previously (see Fig. 19-3) served as the rational basis for the use of postoperative radiation therapy in gastric cancer. Several single-institutional experiences suggest that postoperative radiation confers an advantage with or without concurrent chemotherapy.[154,157,172-174] One randomized study from Japan[175] showed that intraoperative radiation therapy with 28 to 35 Gy conferred a survival advantage in stage II to IV gastric cancer but not in stage I gastric cancer. Although methodologically flawed, this study offered proof of principle for intraoperative radiation therapy in cancer treatment. A smaller subsequent study also showed that intraoperative radiation conferred significant local control advantage.[176] However, results of another trial by the British Stomach Cancer Group shifted the direction of subsequent investigations toward the use of chemotherapy for gastric cancer. In that phase III trial, 436 patients were stratified by age, symptom duration, and stage and then randomized to undergo surgery alone, surgery followed by chemotherapy (with agents such as 5-fluorouracil [5-FU], doxorubicin, or mitomycin), or surgery followed by radiation therapy (45 Gy in 25 fractions with or without a 5-Gy boost).[171,177] A local–regional control advantage was demonstrated in the radiation therapy group (90% vs. 73% for surgery alone and 81% for surgery followed by chemotherapy, $P < 0.01$), but cause-specific and overall survival rates were not statistically different among the groups. Despite several confounding factors and flaws in study design (e.g., one third of patients had residual disease, 18% had positive margins, and one third received 40 Gy or less) and despite the lack of inclusion of a chemoradiation arm, the results of this trial influenced subsequent investigations of strategies that did not include radiation therapy for gastric cancer.

The use of postoperative 5-FU–based chemoradiation has been investigated since the 1960s. In one trial,[10] patients were randomized to undergo resection with or without postoperative chemoradiation (37.5 Gy with bolus 5-FU at 15 mg/kg for 3 days). Patients were not stratified for known prognostic factors, and 10 of 39 patients refused adjuvant therapy after randomization. An overall and relapse-free survival advantage was seen in the adjuvant therapy arm (23% vs. 4%, $P = 0.05$). The local–regional recurrence rate was also diminished (39% vs. 54%). The overall survival rate was highest (30%) in the group who refused treatment after randomization to chemoradiation. However, when the results were analyzed by treatment actually received, survival was not statistically different between groups. The survival difference seen was therefore the result of an imbalance of prognostic features between the treatment groups.[10] These results illustrate the problems that can arise from using small numbers of patients in clinical trials, the importance of stratification for known prognostic variables, and the importance of obtaining consent for treatment before randomization.

Preliminary results are available from the recently completed INT-0116 trial, a well-designed and conducted trial evaluating the role of postoperative chemoradiation with bolus 5-FU and 45 to 55.8 Gy.[178] This trial showed an 11% absolute (28% relative) survival advantage (52% vs. 41%) for postoperative chemoradiation compared with surgery alone for patients with completely resected gastric cancer. It was estimated that approximately 10% of cases had potentially life-threatening technical errors in radiation therapy that were corrected by a centralized quality assurance effort. Despite significant gastrointestinal and hematologic toxic effects, the results of this trial established

postoperative adjuvant 5-FU–based chemoradiation as the standard of care for resected gastric cancer. Chemoradiation led to a significant reduction in local–regional failure, but the 19% local–regional failure rate still leaves room for further improvement.

Postoperative (Adjuvant) Chemotherapy

After initial trials failed to establish a role for radiation therapy in resected gastric cancer, adjuvant chemotherapy was evaluated for its role after curative resection. The results of two small trials suggested a survival benefit,[170,179] but numerous other studies have not.[177,180-183] Authors of a meta-analysis[184] concluded that despite a probable publication bias in favor of positive trials, chemotherapy after curative surgery does not offer a survival benefit. No basis for the routine recommendation of adjuvant chemotherapy is evident at this time.

Preoperative (Neoadjuvant or Induction) Chemotherapy

Neoadjuvant chemotherapy has been investigated in patients with potentially resectable gastric cancer.[185-190] Although the criteria for resectability have been variable and sometimes not stated, this approach has been reported to increase the rate of curative resection. Analysis of a series of patients treated at The University of Texas M.D. Anderson Cancer Center on separate single-arm, prospective studies of intensive chemotherapy regimens revealed overall response rates of 24% to 38%, a resectability rate of 72%, a modest pathologic complete response rate of 4%, and high rates of toxic effects (40% of patients required hospitalization).[188] The median survival time of 15 months is comparable to that for historical surgical controls, but such a comparison is biased in favor of the surgical series because such series report only patients who underwent resection. A multivariate analysis found that response to induction chemotherapy was the only independent prognostic factor. Limitations of the preoperative chemotherapy approach are the high rates of local–regional and peritoneal failure. To address these shortcomings, postoperative and preoperative radiation therapy were added to a recently completed multi-institutional trial.[190]

Preoperative Chemotherapy, Radiation Therapy, and Chemoradiation Therapy

Preoperative radiation therapy, with or without chemotherapy, has been reported in single-arm, single-institutional experiences to improve outcome.[191-195] Prospective, randomized trials conducted in Russia[196-198] have shown improvements in resectability and survival without increased morbidity from the use of suboptimal radiation doses without concurrent chemotherapy. A phase II trial at the M.D. Anderson Cancer Center has been completed evaluating preoperative irradiation (45 Gy) with concurrent protracted venous infusion of 5-FU (300 mg/m^2/day, 5 days/week) and intraoperative radiation therapy (10 Gy). After clinical staging with CT, endoscopic sonography, and exploratory laparoscopy, 82% of the patients had T3 or T4 disease. Two patients refused surgery, 32 (73%) underwent resection, and nine (20%) were found to have metastases on restaging. The 4-year disease-specific survival rate was more than 60% among patients who underwent resection.[199] These data support the hypothesis that preoperative chemoradiation is both safe and effective in gastric cancer. Prospective studies of this hypothesis are ongoing in the United States.

Preoperative (Neoadjuvant) Chemotherapy Followed by Concurrent Chemoradiation

Neoadjuvant chemotherapy followed by concurrent chemoradiation for gastric cancer is currently being investigated at the M.D. Anderson Cancer Center. Current practice involves clinical staging by CT scanning and endoscopic sonography, as well as laparoscopic peritoneal staging, which includes visual inspection and cytologic evaluation of washings. A jejunostomy feeding tube is placed at the time of laparoscopy and plays a critical role in the supportive care of patients during neoadjuvant therapy and in preparation for and recovery from surgery. One phase II trial has been completed that involved preoperative chemotherapy (5-FU, cisplatin, and folinic acid) for two cycles followed by 45 Gy and concurrent continuous infusion of 5-FU (300 mg/m^2). A current phase II trial, also at the M.D. Anderson Cancer Center, is evaluating 5-FU, cisplatin, and paclitaxel followed by 45 Gy and concurrent continuous infusion of 5-FU (300 mg/m^2) followed by weekly paclitaxel (45 mg/m^2). A similar phase II study (trial 99-04) is currently being conducted by the Radiation Therapy Oncology Group (RTOG). Another phase II study is under way at the University of Cincinnati evaluating the combination of neoadjuvant gemcitabine and paclitaxel followed by chemoradiation with 5-FU and cisplatin for resectable proximal gastric and esophageal carcinomas. Because the findings from these trials are preliminary, the possible benefit from the addition of neoadjuvant chemotherapy to subsequent concurrent chemoradiation remains to be established.

Chemoradiation for Unresectable Gastric Cancer

Studies of unresectable or partially resected gastric cancer indicate that chemoradiation can be curative in a small percentage of patients.[10,16,17,200] Initial strategies for the nonoperative management of gastric cancer demonstrated an advantage for combining 5-FU with radiation. A randomized trial was conducted at Mayo Clinic that involved 35 to 40 Gy with and without bolus 5-FU for 3 days for a variety of unresected gastrointestinal malignancies.[10] A small group of gastric cancer patients were found to have superior 5-year survival after combination treatment (12% vs. 0% without chemotherapy), thus verifying the efficacy of a combination that has endured for three decades. Further evidence of the importance of 5-FU administration came from a randomized study conducted by the European Organization for Research and Treatment of Cancer[153] that showed a survival advantage for patients treated with chemoradiation compared with those who were treated with radiation alone to 55.5 Gy. The few patients who had residual disease and who remained free of progressive disease for at least 19 months after treatment had been given both concurrent chemoradiation and long-term (18 months) treatment with 5-FU thereafter.[153]

In a trial conducted by the Gastrointestinal Tumor Study Group with patients with incompletely resected gastric cancer, chemotherapy with 5-FU and methyl-lomustine was compared with a split course of radiation total dose of 50 Gy and bolus 5-FU given at the beginning of each course of radiation therapy.[200] The trial was discontinued early because of at least six treatment-related deaths and six disease-related deaths in the combined-modality group within the first 6 months of therapy. Nevertheless, a statistically significant survival benefit was seen in the combined-therapy group at 5 years (20% vs. 6%, $P < 0.01$). Modern supportive care, conventional treatment planning, and infusional chemotherapy schedules would have enhanced the difference in favor of the combined-modality group. Seeking to confirm these results, the Study Group designed a second trial[201] with similar entry criteria comparing 5-FU, methyl-lomustine, and doxorubicin with a schedule of the same chemotherapy followed on day 57 by chemoradiation (43.2 Gy with bolus 5-FU). Unfortunately, the trial was not well designed (radiation doses were low and delayed) and problems were encountered with patient accrual and compliance (11 of the 59 patients in the radiation group did not receive the prescribed dose, 7 of whom received no radiation at all). These difficulties may explain why no survival difference was found between treatment groups.

Supportive Care

The importance of aggressive supportive care, as illustrated by the experience of the Gastrointestinal Tumor Study Group in the previous paragraph,[200,201] cannot be overemphasized. Although the outcome of the chemoradiation group was better than that of the chemotherapy group, six of the 45 patients in that group died of sepsis or nutritional inadequacy. In using radiation for gastric cancer, the routine use of prophylactic antiemetics and jejunostomy-tube feeding vastly improves treatment tolerance. Feeding tubes can obviate the need for intravenous fluid replacement or hyperalimentation and reduce the incidence of hospitalization for acute reactions. Nutritionists can monitor patients' energy intake and weight, provide energy-intake goals, and serve as a resource for other nutrition-related issues.

Palliative Radiation Therapy

Radiation effectively relieves the symptoms associated with locally advanced gastric cancer. Several series have indicated that between 50% and 75% of patients experience improvement of bleeding, gastric outlet obstruction, and pain.[7,202-204]

Palliative Chemotherapy

The single agents most active in gastric cancer are 5-FU, mitomycin, and doxorubicin.[11,205-207] Randomized studies that have compared multiagent chemotherapy with supportive care have consistently shown a median survival advantage for chemotherapy, but no long-term survival.[208-210] The advantage of multiagent regimens over single-agent treatment has not been established.[211] The median survival duration is relatively short (5 to 7 months) in most studies. A phase III trial recently reported from Europe[212] evaluated high-dose methotrexate, 5-FU, and doxorubicin vs. etoposide, leucovorin, and 5-FU vs. infusional 5-FU and cisplatin for advanced gastric cancer. The most remarkable finding in that trial was the lack of efficacy of any of the three treatments. The authors concluded that none of these regimens should be considered standard for advanced or metastatic gastric cancer.[212] Because of the high morbidity, cost, and lack of an established benefit for multiagent regimens, patients should be offered participation in clinical trials that evaluate new agents or new combinations.

RADIATION TECHNIQUES
Techniques

Typical anteroposterior and lateral simulation films are shown in Color Plate 23, after p. 80. Simulation films should be obtained when patients have an empty stomach (nothing by mouth for 3 hours), and patients should be treated in the morning before eating to minimize organ motion resulting from stomach distention. Oral contrast medium should be given 15 to 30 minutes before simulation, and arm-elevation and stabilization devices should be used. CT-based dosimetry is helpful in planning field arrangements. Patients can be treated with either a four-field technique or through opposed

anterior and posterior portals. The use of four or more irradiation fields can significantly reduce the incidence of grade 4 or 5 toxicity compared with two fields.[213] However, lateral fields are not always advisable in patients with an intact stomach because the gastric fundus often extends too far posteriorly. In such instances, the kidneys and spinal cord cannot be shielded without shielding the target, and opposed fields are preferred. To keep the spinal cord dose below 45 Gy, the anterior field can be more heavily weighted (usually 3:2) or an off-cord boost can be delivered with oblique fields after the initial 39.6 Gy. If preoperative imaging or fluoroscopy indicates that the tumor is located anteriorly, lateral fields can be used with beam weighting that limits their contribution to 20 Gy. Customized blocking is used to shield the critical structures in the field, including the small bowel, liver, spinal cord, and kidneys. CT-based treatment planning and dose-volume histograms can help objectively evaluate various technical treatment options for individual patients.

The target volume should include the entire stomach or gastric bed and the draining lymphatics in most cases. All available imaging (CT and barium swallowing) findings, endoscopic findings, and intraoperative findings should be reviewed and correlated before simulation. According to the surgical data discussed in the previous section on "Surgical Therapy," surgical margins greater than 4 to 6 cm are associated with a low recurrence rate in the gastric remnant in patients undergoing partial gastrectomy. By analogy, radiation therapy fields could be limited to a partial gastric volume if the gross tumor volume is well defined by endoscopy. When designing radiation fields for patients with an intact stomach, it is important to examine the CT scans for evidence of perigastric extension, which will not be apparent when viewing the contrast-filled stomach at the time of simulation. Endoscopic and surgical reports should also be correlated with imaging findings. Anterior and posterior fields should include the gastric, gastro-omental, celiac, hepatic, subpyloric, gastroduodenal, pancreatosplenic, and retropancreaticoduodenal nodes. The splenic hilum, porta hepatis, and celiac trunk can be located on CT scans. The celiac axis usually arises at the bottom of the T12 vertebra, and the porta hepatis is 4 to 5 cm to the right of the T11 and L1 vertebral bodies. The remaining nodal tissue can be encompassed by treating the stomach and the medial portion of the C-loop of the duodenum or the stomach and duodenal bed. The lower border usually extends to the inferior aspect of L3 to encompass the entire C-loop.

For proximal lesions involving the cardia or gastroesophageal junction (as defined by endoscopy, upper gastrointestinal radiography, or CT), the paraesophageal nodes should be included and a 5-cm margin should be included in the cephalad field margin. For distal lesions at or near the gastroduodenal junction, a 5-cm margin of duodenum should be included.

Future Investigations
Altered Fractionation

The safe administration of conventionally fractionated radiation is limited by the tolerance of surrounding organs and of the stomach itself. Pilot studies evaluating the tolerance of hyperfractionated radiation have demonstrated the feasibility of this approach.[214-216] Small fractions sizes seem to be better tolerated.

New Radiosensitizing Agents

Radiosensitizers such as irinotecan (CPT-11) and paclitaxel are currently being investigated in combination with radiation therapy at the M.D. Anderson Cancer Center for advanced, unresectable gastric cancer. Preliminary experience indicates that the concurrent administration of these agents with radiation therapy is well tolerated when appropriate supportive care is given. Future investigations center on optimizing the dose, timing, and scheduling of these agents in combination with radiation therapy. Such new strategies should be evaluated in comparative trials to establish their superiority over 5-FU–based chemoradiation.

Conformal Therapy

The current technical limitations of conformal therapy in gastric cancer include the ability to identify gross tumor and problems associated with organ motion (respiratory motion and gastric distention). The RTOG is beginning to assess the feasibility of conformal therapy in its emerging gastric cancer protocols. Charged particle therapy with helium ions or protons also offers improved dose distribution but has limitations similar to those of conformal therapy. Several ways of addressing respiratory motion are currently being addressed, including active and passive respiratory gating. These techniques must be refined to fully realize the potential of conformal therapy for tumors in the upper abdomen.

Neutron Therapy

Evaluations of the toxicity and efficacy of neutron therapy for gastric cancer have indicated that this treatment holds little promise. Severe late effects indicate a narrow therapeutic index,[217] which is referable to the lack of an opportunity for sublethal damage repair between fractions. In the stomach, an organ with limited radiotolerance, the use of neutrons eliminates the most important radiotherapeutic advantage.

Hepatic and Peritoneal-Directed Approaches

Liver and peritoneal disease represents a significant problem in gastric cancer.[108,109,204,218] Prospective evaluations of regimens that address peritoneal failure have been conducted by the University of Southern California[186] and Memorial Sloan-Kettering.[219] Both involved preoperative chemotherapy followed by postoperative intraperitoneal chemotherapy in patients undergoing curative resection. Although the median survival times were not drastically different from those of studies that did not include intraperitoneal chemotherapy, the peritoneal failure rate in the Memorial Sloan-Kettering study[219] (16%) was lower than expected. Intraperitoneal chemotherapy combined with hyperthermia also has documented activity.[220-222] Although intraperitoneal chemotherapy is conceptually provocative, controlled validation of these approaches is lacking at this time.

Whole-abdomen radiation therapy has been investigated for ovarian and endometrial cancer. However, the maximum tolerated dose of whole-abdomen irradiation is limited to 20 to 25 Gy, which makes this approach unlikely to be of benefit in gastric cancer. The role of prophylactic hepatic irradiation in pancreatic cancer has been evaluated by the RTOG,[27] at the M.D. Anderson Cancer Center,[223] and at Johns Hopkins University.[224] All studies used at least 23.4 Gy to the whole liver. The first site of failure was the liver in 13% of patients in the first study.[27] The M.D. Anderson Cancer Center study was closed early because of toxicity after only 11 patients had been treated,[223] and no survival benefit was detected in the Johns Hopkins study.[224] Although extended-field irradiation could hypothetically reduce hepatic or peritoneal failure, it does not currently have a role in the treatment of gastric cancer.

SMALL INTESTINE
Anatomy and Histology

The small bowel extends from the gastric pylorus to the iliocecal valve and is divided into three parts: the duodenum, jejunum, and ileum. Although its length varies, the average small bowel is 6 to 7 m long. The first section of small bowel, the duodenum, is about 12 fingerbreadths long and forms a C-shaped loop around the head of the pancreas. The ampulla of Vater is located in the second or descending portion of the duodenum. The jejunum and ileum compose the remainder of the small bowel and are attached to the posterior abdominal wall by a fan-shaped mesentery. The root of this mesentery runs obliquely from the left upper abdominal quadrant to the right lower abdominal quadrant.

The processes of digestion are completed and the products of digestion are absorbed in the small intestine. Plicae circulares, longitudinal folds that are often visible on radiographs, innumerable intestinal villi (0.5 to 1.5 mm in length), and microvilli greatly increase the luminal surface area for absorption. Intestinal crypts are found between the villi.

Undifferentiated cells normally migrate and differentiate upward from the lower half of the crypts to the tips of the villi as they mature. Most will form absorptive cells, but others become mucus-secreting goblet cells or enteroendocrine cells. All three cell types live only 3 to 6 days.

Acute Effects of Radiation

The acute effects of radiation on the small intestine reflect the sensitivity of the rapidly dividing undifferentiated intestinal crypt cells. These immature cells are the most sensitive to radiation and thus are preferentially lost after treatment with radiation, resulting in an eventual loss of mature replacement cells at the surface of the villi. The mature mucosal cells then become denuded and a loss of absorptive function follows. This loss of function results in fluid and nutrient wasting, diarrhea, and sometimes dehydration.[225] Re-epithelialization typically occurs within 96 hours in a murine model, starting with the recovery of the rapidly dividing crypt cells.[226]

The clinical symptoms of acute small bowel radiation injury are diarrhea, cramps with abdominal pain, and sometimes nausea. The incidence and severity of small bowel injury are related to the dose, volume, and dose rate of radiation delivery.[227] These acute effects can be managed with appropriate supportive care such as dietary modification, antimotility agents, narcotics, and antiemetic agents. Diets low in fiber can decrease transit time and increase absorption in patients with acute radiation enteritis. The liberal use of antimotility agents such as diphenoxylate hydrochloride and atropine (Lomotil) or loperamide and the judicious use of narcotics will alleviate most cases of radiation-induced diarrhea.

Late Effects of Radiation Therapy

Possible late manifestations of radiation therapy include chronic diarrhea, abdominal cramping, nausea, vomiting, malabsorption with weight loss, and chronic blood loss. Progressive fibrosis, shortening, constriction, and stenosis of the irradiated portion of bowel can occur in radiation-injured patients. Adhesions related to surgical and radiation injury can form between loops of bowel. Predisposing conditions to small bowel injury include fixation of the bowel at the time of treatment, pelvic inflammatory disease, diabetes, hypertension, and thin body habitus. Irradiation of the small bowel to a dose of 45 Gy given in 25 fractions would be expected to produce less than a 5% risk of late complications. In freely mobile sections of small intestine, a boost dose of 5.4 Gy in three fractions is routinely given safely. The dose to any segment of small bowel should not exceed 50.4 Gy, although boost doses are often delivered if the small bowel can be completely excluded from the treatment field.

EPIDEMIOLOGY AND ETIOLOGY OF SMALL BOWEL CANCER

Primary small bowel malignancies are exceedingly rare, representing 1% to 3% of all gastrointestinal malignancies.[228,229] Approximately 2100 to 2400 new cases are diagnosed each year in the United States.[230] Most small bowel tumors occur in the duodenum or proximal jejunum.[231] Several hypotheses have been proposed to explain the low incidence of small bowel malignancies. Transit time is shorter in the small bowel than in the large bowel, the large volume of secretions in the small bowel dilutes potential carcinogens, and the small bowel is colonized with fewer and comparatively more inert bacteria.[232] The liquid contents of the small bowel are also less mechanically irritating than are feces in the large bowel. Many lymphocytes and B cells secrete immunoglobulin A in the distal ileum. Immunodeficient patients are more prone to develop small bowel lymphoma than are immunocompetent patients. Adenocarcinomas occur predominately in the proximal small bowel, correlating well with the duration of contact of bile salts and pancreatic enzymes with the mucosa.[233] In animal studies, biliary diversion has been shown to decrease the incidence of experimentally induced small bowel malignancy.[234] The risk of small bowel cancer has been reported to be increased with consumption of red meat and salt-cured food.[235] The per capita consumption of dietary fat in different countries correlates well with small bowel cancer risk.[231] Patients with a history of large bowel cancer also have an increased risk of developing small bowel cancer, indicating some overlap in predisposing factors.[228,236]

Patients with Crohn's disease,[237-240] celiac disease,[241] Peutz-Jeghers syndrome, and von Recklinghausen's disease (neurofibromatosis type 1)[242] have been reported to have a higher incidence of small bowel malignancy.

STAGING

Because primary cancer of the small bowel is rare, a staging system has been published only recently by the American Joint Committee on Cancer (Box 19-2).[243] The primary tumor is staged according to its depth of penetration and the involvement of adjacent structures or distant sites. Lateral spread within the duodenum, jejunum, or ileum is not considered in this classification.

THE ROLE OF RADIATION THERAPY
Adenocarcinomas

Radiation therapy can be used as an adjuvant to surgery or as primary palliative treatment of small bowel adenocarcinoma. Anatomic constraints and the intrinsic sensitivity of the normal small bowel to radiation limit the role of radiation as a local–regional treatment. Localized

BOX 19-2   American Joint Committee on Cancer Staging System for Carcinoma of the Small Intestine

PRIMARY TUMOR (T)

TX   Primary tumor cannot be assessed
T0   No evidence of primary tumor
Tis   Carcinoma in situ
T1   Tumor invades lamina propria or submucosa
T2   Tumor invades muscularis propria
T3   Tumor invades through muscularis propria into the subserosa or into the nonperitonealized perimuscular tissue (mesentery or retroperitoneum) with extension 2 cm or less*
T4   Tumor invades the visceral peritoneum, or directly invades other organs or structures (includes other loops of small intestine, mesentery, or retroperitoneum more than 2 cm, and abdominal wall by way of serosa; for duodenum only, invasion of pancreas)

REGIONAL LYMPH NODES (N)

NX   Regional lymph nodes cannot be assessed
N0   No regional lymph node metastasis
N1   Regional lymph node metastasis

DISTANT METASTASIS (M)

MX   Distant metastasis cannot be assessed
M0   No distant metastasis
M1   Distant metastasis

STAGE GROUPING

Stage 0	Tis	N0	M0
Stage I	T1	N0	M0
	T2	N0	M0
Stage II	T3	N0	M0
	T4	N0	M0
Stage III	Any T	N1	M0
Stage IV	Any T	Any N	M1

From Fleming I, Cooper JS, Henson DE, et al, eds. *AJCC Cancer Staging Manual*, 5th ed. Philadelphia, Pa: Lippincott Williams & Wilkins; 1997:77-79.
*The nonperitonealized perimuscular tissue is, for jejunum and ileum, part of the mesentery and, for duodenum in areas where serosa is lacking, part of the retroperitoneum.

segments of the small bowel can tolerate doses of 45 to 50 Gy with conventional fractionation of 1.8 to 2.0 Gy per fraction; however, tolerance to radiation is significantly less when large volumes of bowel are in the radiation field. Because the small bowel and surrounding mesenteric lymphatics are mobile, regional treatment for malignancies of the jejunum and ileum would have to include very large fields. The tolerance of the whole abdomen to radiation[244] is less than the dose that would reliably sterilize microscopic disease. Because most of the small intestine is suspended by mesentery, surgical resection is usually adequate local therapy for adenocarcinoma of the small bowel. Given these limitations and the rarity of these tumors, the role of adjuvant radiation has not been clearly defined for adenocarcinoma of the small bowel. For lesions that involve contiguous structures, either preoperative or postoperative radiation can theoretically improve resectability and local control over results that can be achieved by surgical resection alone.

Forty-five percent of small bowel adenocarcinomas arise in the duodenum[245-249]; for these tumors, the treatment is surgical resection. For lesions arising in the first and second portions of the duodenum, pancreaticoduodenectomy is usually required, but for more distal lesions a segmental duodenectomy is often possible. The 5-year survival rates after surgery alone range from 20% to 60%.[245,248-255] Johns Hopkins and Memorial Sloan-Kettering have reported 5-year survival rates of 60%[256] and 53%,[255] respectively, in patients who have undergone resection.

In duodenal cancer, regional lymphatics are often involved, and the competing risk of distant failure is modest.[245-249] The spread pattern provides a rationale for either preoperative or postoperative chemoradiation. Although some investigators have not found adjuvant therapy to be beneficial in small groups of patients,[255] no study conducted as yet has included enough patients to adequately detect even large differences in survival according to type of therapy. The role of adjuvant therapy has therefore not yet been defined. In pancreatic cancer, which also has a significant local–regional pattern of spread, a survival benefit has been demonstrated with postoperative adjuvant therapy.[257]

The primary tumor site and regional lymphatic drainage can be safely treated with 45 to 50 Gy, a dose that reliably eliminates microscopic residual disease. Radiation portals should cover the entire duodenum and the hepatoduodenal, pancreatic, superior mesenteric, periportal, subpyloric, pyloric, and para-aortic nodal chains. Mucosal margins of at least 5 cm proximally and distally are recommended because of the potential for submucosal spread. Localized boost doses of 10 Gy at most to areas believed to be at highest risk can be given with external-beam or intraoperative radiation therapy. The risk of duodenal ulceration or perforation increases sharply at total doses higher than 55 Gy. Extrapolation from treating pancreatic cancer suggests that preoperative therapy is likely to be better tolerated.[258]

Palliative radiation can be beneficial in cases of unresectable or recurrent tumors. When the goal is palliation, tumor regression and symptomatic improvement can be achieved with 30 Gy, given in 10 fractions. Goals of palliative radiation include controlling blood loss, decreasing pain, and relieving obstructive symptoms.

Sarcoma

Similar principles can be applied for evaluating the role of radiation in treating sarcomas of the small bowel. Experience with extremity sarcoma suggest that preoperative or postoperative radiation therapy may reduce the risk of local recurrence if wide surgical margins cannot be obtained. When locally advanced disease is recognized at staging, preoperative therapy to a dose of 45 to 50 Gy is preferred.

Carcinoid Tumors

The specific indications for radiation therapy of small bowel carcinoid tumors are lacking, given the rarity of this clinical presentation. However, radiation has been shown to be beneficial in palliation of unresected disease with perhaps less benefit for patients with carcinoid syndrome.[259]

Radiation techniques. The choice of radiation techniques for tumors of the small bowel depends on the tumor location and individual anatomic variations. For duodenal primary tumors, a four-field technique is usually preferred. The dose contribution from the lateral fields should be limited to 20 Gy and appropriate shielding should be used wherever possible to limit the dose to critical adjacent structures such as the liver, kidneys, stomach, spinal cord, and uninvolved small bowel.

SUMMARY

The role of radiation therapy in the treatment of small bowel tumors is largely undefined, owing to the rarity of these tumors, anatomic constraints, and the wide range of clinical presentations. Problems specific to irradiation of the small bowel include the mobility of the primary tumor and the limited radiation tolerance of uninvolved tissues. Although a role for adjuvant therapy has yet to be defined, radiation therapy remains an important modality for selected cases in the adjuvant setting and for palliation of small bowel tumors of all histologic types.

REFERENCES

1. Fajardo LF, Berthrong M, Anderson RE. Stomach. In: *Radiation Pathology*. New York, NY: Oxford University Press; 2001: 221-227.
2. Goldgraber M, Rubin C, Palmer W, et al. The early gastric response to irradiation, a serial biopsy study. *Gastroenterology* 1954;27:1-20.
3. Palmer WL, Templeton F. The effect of radiation therapy on gastric secretion. *JAMA* 1939;112:1429-1434.
4. Palmer W. *Gastric Irradiation in Peptic Ulcer*. Chicago, Ill: University of Chicago Press; 1974.
5. Hueper WC, DeCarvajal-Forero J. The effects of repeated irradiation of the gastric region with small doses of roentgen rays upon the stomach and blood of dogs. *AJR Am J Roentgenol* 1944; 40:1938.
6. Hamilton F. Gastric ulcer following radiation. *Arch Surg* 1947; 55:394-399.
7. Klaassen DJ, MacIntyre JM, Catton GE, et al. Treatment of locally unresectable cancer of the stomach and pancreas: a randomized comparison of 5-fluorouracil alone with radiation plus concurrent and maintenance 5-fluorouracil—an Eastern Cooperative Oncology Group study. *J Clin Oncol* 1985;3:373-378.
8. Caudry M, Escarmant P, Maire JP, et al. Radiotherapy of gastric cancer with a three-field combination: feasibility, tolerance, and survival. *Int J Radiat Oncol Biol Phys* 1987;13:1821-1827.
9. Haas CD, Mansfield CM, Leichman LP, et al. Combined nonsimultaneous radiation therapy and chemotherapy with 5-FU, doxorubicin, and mitomycin for residual localized gastric adenocarcinoma: a Southwest Oncology Group pilot study. *Cancer Treatment Reports* 1983;67:421-424.
10. Moertel CG, Childs DS Jr, Reitemeier RJ, et al. Combined 5-fluorouracil and supervoltage radiation therapy of locally unresectable gastrointestinal cancer. *Lancet* 1969;2:865-867.
11. Schein PS, Smith FP, Woolley PV, et al. Current management of advanced and locally unresectable gastric carcinoma. *Cancer* 1982;50:2590-2596.
12. Brookland RK, Rubin S, Danoff BF. Extended field irradiation in the treatment of patients with cervical carcinoma involving biopsy proven para-aortic nodes. *Int J Radiat Oncol Biol Phys* 1984;10:1875-1879.
13. Ballon SC, Berman ML, Lagasse LD, et al. Survival after extraperitoneal pelvic and paraaortic lymphadenectomy and radiation therapy in cervical carcinoma. *Obstet Gynecol* 1981;57:90-95.
14. Hughes RR, Brewington KC, Hanjani P, et al. Extended field irradiation for cervical cancer based on surgical staging. *Gynecol Oncol* 1980;9:153-161.
15. Fletcher GH, Rutledge FN. Extended field technique in the management of the cancers of the uterine cervix. *Am J Roentgenol Radium Ther Nucl Med* 1972;114:116-122.
16. Asakawa H, Otawa H, Yamada S, et al. Combination therapy of gastric carcinoma with radiation and chemotherapy. *Tohoku J Exp Med* 1982;137:445-452.
17. Asakawa H, Takeda T. High energy x-ray therapy of gastric carcinoma. *Nippon Gan Chiryo Gakkai Shi—J Japan Society Cancer Ther* 1973;8:362-371.
18. Emami B, Watring WG, Tak W, et al. Para-aortic lymph node radiation in advanced cervical cancer. *Int J Radiat Oncol Biol Phys* 1980;6:1237-1241.
19. Macdonald JS, Schnall SF. Adjuvant treatment of gastric cancer. *World J Surg* 1995;19:221-225.
20. Roswit B, Malsky SJ, Reid CB. Severe radiation injuries of the stomach, small intestine, colon and rectum. *Am J Roentgenol Radium Ther Nucl Med* 1972;114:460-475.
21. Roswitt B, Malsky S, Reid C. Radiation tolerance of the gastrointestinal tract. *Front Radiat Ther Oncol* 1971;5:160-180.
22. Rubin SC, Brookland R, Mikuta JJ, et al. Para-aortic nodal metastases in early cervical carcinoma: long-term survival following extended-field radiotherapy. *Gynecol Oncol* 1984;18:213-217.
23. Welander CE, Pierce VK, Nori D, et al. Pretreatment laparotomy in carcinoma of the cervix. *Gynecol Oncol* 1981;12:336-347.
24. Bowers R, Brick I. Surgery in radiation injury of the stomach. *Surgery* 1947;22:20-40.

25. Willett CG, Tepper JE, Orlow EL, et al. Renal complications secondary to radiation treatment of upper abdominal malignancies. *Int J Radiat Oncol Biol Phys* 1986;12:1601-1604.

26. Lawrence TS, Robertson JM, Anscher MS, et al. Hepatic toxicity resulting from cancer treatment. *Int J Radiat Oncol Biol Phys* 1995;31:1237-1248.

27. Komaki R, Wadler S, Peters T, et al. High-dose local irradiation plus prophylactic hepatic irradiation and chemotherapy for inoperable adenocarcinoma of the pancreas. A preliminary report of a multi-institutional trial (Radiation Therapy Oncology Group Protocol 8801). *Cancer* 1992;69:2807-2812.

28. Ingold J, Reed G, Kaplan H, et al. Radiation hepatitis. *AJR Am J Roentgenol* 1965;93:200-208.

29. Lawrence TS, Ten Haken RK, Kessler ML, et al. The use of 3-D dose volume analysis to predict radiation hepatitis. *Int J Radiat Oncol Biol Phys* 1992;23:781-788.

30. McGinn CJ, Ten Haken RK, Ensminger WD, et al. Treatment of intrahepatic cancers with radiation doses based on a normal tissue complication probability model. *J Clin Oncol* 1998;16:2246-2252.

31. Dawson LA, McGinn CJ, Normolle D, et al. Escalated focal liver radiation and concurrent hepatic artery fluorodeoxyuridine for unresectable intrahepatic malignancies. *J Clin Oncol* 2000;18:2210-2218.

32. Haenszel W. Variation in incidence of and mortality from stomach cancer, with particular reference to the United States. *J Natl Cancer Inst* 1958;21:213-262.

33. Devesa SS, Blot WJ, Fraumeni JF Jr. Changing patterns in the incidence of esophageal and gastric carcinoma in the United States. *Cancer* 1998;83:2049-2053.

34. Greenlee RT, Hill-Harmon MB, Murray T, et al. Cancer statistics, 2001. *CA Cancer J Clin* 2001;51:15-36.

35. Wiggins CL, Becker TM, Key CR, et al. Stomach cancer among New Mexico's American Indians, Hispanic whites, and non-Hispanic whites. *Cancer Res* 1989;49:1595-1599.

36. Pisani P, Parkin DM, Bray F, et al. Estimates of the world-wide mortality from 25 cancers in 1990. *Int J Cancer* 1999;83:18-29.

37. Parkin DM, Pisani P, Ferlay J. Global cancer statistics. *CA Cancer J Clin* 1999;49:33-64.

38. La Vecchia C, Negri E, D'Avanzo B, et al. Electric refrigerator use and gastric cancer risk. *Br J Cancer* 1990;62:136-137.

39. Coggon D, Barker DJ, Cole RB, et al. Stomach cancer and food storage. *J Natl Cancer Inst* 1989;81:1178-1182.

40. Howson CP, Hiyama T, Wynder EL. The decline in gastric cancer: epidemiology of an unplanned triumph. *Epidemiol Rev* 1986;8:1-27.

41. Blot WJ, Devesa SS, Kneller RW, et al. Rising incidence of adenocarcinoma of the esophagus and gastric cardia. *JAMA* 1991;265:1287-1289.

42. Lauren P. The two histological main types of gastric carcinoma: diffuse and so-called intestinal-type carcinoma. *Acta Pathol Microbiol Scand* 1965;64:31-49.

43. Lauren PA, Nevalainen TJ. Epidemiology of intestinal and diffuse types of gastric carcinoma. A time-trend study in Finland with comparison between studies from high- and low-risk areas. *Cancer* 1993;71:2926-2933.

44. Munoz N, Asvall J. Time trends of intestinal and diffuse types of gastric cancer in Norway. *Int J Cancer* 1971;8:144-157.

45. Borrmann R. Geschwulste des Mangens and Duodenums. In: Henke F, Lanbarsch O, eds. *Handbuch der Speziellen Pathologischen Anatomie and Histologie.* Vol. 4. Berlin, Germany: Julius Springer; 1926.

46. Morson B. Carcinoma arising from areas of intestinal metaplasia in the gastric mucosa. *Br J Cancer* 1955;9:377-385.

47. Correa P, Cuello C, Duque E, et al. Gastric cancer in Colombia. III. Natural history of precursor lesions. *J Natl Cancer Inst* 1976;57:1027-1035.

48. Coggon D, Osmond C, Barker DJ. Stomach cancer and migration within England and Wales. *Br J Cancer* 1990;61:573-574.

49. Buiatti E, Palli D, Decarli A, et al. A case-control study of gastric cancer and diet in Italy: II. Association with nutrients. *Int J Cancer* 1990;45:896-901.

50. Chyou PH, Nomura AM, Hankin JH, et al. A case-cohort study of diet and stomach cancer. *Cancer Res* 1990;50:7501-7504.

51. Boeing H, Frentzel-Beyme R, Berger M, et al. Case-control study on stomach cancer in Germany. *Int J Cancer* 1991;47:858-864.

52. Correa P, Fontham E, Pickle LW, et al. Dietary determinants of gastric cancer in south Louisiana inhabitants. *J Natl Cancer Inst* 1985;75:645-654.

53. Demirer T, Icli F, Uzunalimoglu O, et al. Diet and stomach cancer incidence. A case-control study in Turkey. *Cancer* 1990;65:2344-2348.

54. Gonzalez CA, Sanz JM, Marcos G, et al. Dietary factors and stomach cancer in Spain: a multi-centre case-control study. *Int J Cancer* 1991;49:513-519.

55. Nomura A, Grove JS, Stemmermann GN, et al. Cigarette smoking and stomach cancer [letter]. *Cancer Res* 1990;50:7084.

56. Ramon JM, Serra L, Cerdo C, et al. Dietary factors and gastric cancer risk. A case-control study in Spain. *Cancer* 1993;71:1731-1735.

57. Risch HA, Jain M, Choi NW, et al. Dietary factors and the incidence of cancer of the stomach. *Am J Epidemiol* 1985;122:947-959.

58. Trichopoulos D, Ouranos G, Day NE, et al. Diet and cancer of the stomach: a case-control study in Greece. *Int J Cancer* 1985;36:291-297.

59. Wu-Williams AH, Yu MC, Mack TM. Life-style, workplace, and stomach cancer by subsite in young men of Los Angeles County. *Cancer Res* 1990;50:2569-2576.

60. You WC, Chang YS, Yang ZT, et al. Etiological research on gastric cancer and its precursor lesions in Shandong, China. *IARC Sci Publ* 1991:33-38.

61. Gonzalez CA, Riboli E, Badosa J, et al. Nutritional factors and gastric cancer in Spain. *Am J Epidemiol* 1994;139:466-473.

62. Galanis DJ, Kolonel LN, Lee J, et al. Intakes of selected foods and beverages and the incidence of gastric cancer among the Japanese residents of Hawaii: a prospective study. *Int J Epidemiol* 1998;27:173-180.

63. Webb PM, Bates CJ, Palli D, et al. Gastric cancer, gastritis and plasma vitamin C: results from an international correlation and cross-sectional study. The Eurogast Study Group. *Int J Cancer* 1997;73:684-689.

64. La Vecchia C, Ferraroni M, D'Avanzo B, et al. Selected micronutrient intake and the risk of gastric cancer. *Cancer Epidemiol Biomarkers Prev* 1994;3:393-398.

65. Zhang L, Blot WJ, You WC, et al. Serum micronutrients in relation to pre-cancerous gastric lesions. *Int J Cancer* 1994;56:650-654.

66. La Vecchia C, Munoz SE, Braga C, et al. Diet diversity and gastric cancer. *Int J Cancer* 1997;72:255-257.

67. Ward MH, Sinha R, Heineman EF, et al. Risk of adenocarcinoma of the stomach and esophagus with meat cooking method and doneness preference. *Int J Cancer* 1997;71:14-19.

68. Barrett JH, Parslow RC, McKinney PA, et al. Nitrate in drinking water and the incidence of gastric, esophageal, and brain cancer in Yorkshire, England. *Cancer Causes Control* 1998;9:153-159.

69. La Vecchia C, Negri E, Franceschi S, et al. Case-control study on influence of methionine, nitrite, and salt on gastric carcinogenesis in northern Italy. *Nutr Cancer* 1997;27:65-68.

70. Coggon D, Barker DJ, Cole RB. Stomach cancer and work in dusty industries. *Br J Industr Med* 1990;47:298-301.

71. Nomura A, Grove JS, Stemmermann GN, et al. A prospective study of stomach cancer and its relation to diet, cigarettes, and alcohol consumption. *Cancer Res* 1990;50:627-631.

72. Kneller RW, McLaughlin JK, Bjelke E, et al. A cohort study of stomach cancer in a high-risk American population. *Cancer* 1991;68:672-678.

73. Jedrychowski W, Boeing H, Wahrendorf J, et al. Vodka consumption, tobacco smoking and risk of gastric cancer in Poland. *Int J Epidemiol* 1993;22:606-613.

74. Staszewski J. Migrant studies in alimentary tract cancer. *Recent Results Cancer Res* 1972;39:85-97.

75. Haenszel W, Kurihara M, Locke FB, et al. Stomach cancer in Japan. *J Natl Cancer Inst* 1976;56:265-274.

76. Nomura A, Chyou PH, Stemmermann GN. Association of serum ferritin levels with the risk of stomach cancer. *Cancer Epidemiol Biomarkers Prev* 1992;1:547-550.

77. Blackburn EK, Callender ST, Dacie JV, et al. Possible association between pernicious anaemia and leukaemia: a prospective study of 1,625 patients with a note on the very high incidence of stomach cancer. *Int J Cancer* 1968;3:163-170.

78. Brinton LA, Gridley G, Hrubec Z, et al. Cancer risk following pernicious anaemia. *Br J Cancer* 1989;59:810-813.

79. Hsing AW, Hansson LE, McLaughlin JK, et al. Pernicious anemia and subsequent cancer. A population-based cohort study. *Cancer* 1993;71:745-750.

80. La Vecchia C, Braga C, Negri E, et al. Risk of stomach cancer in patients with gastric or duodenal ulcer. *Eur J Cancer Prev* 1997;6:20-23.

81. Stalnikowicz R, Benbassat J. Risk of gastric cancer after gastric surgery for benign disorders. *Arch Intern Med* 1990;150:2022-2026.

82. Tersmette AC, Offerhaus GJ, Tersmette KW, et al. Meta-analysis of the risk of gastric stump cancer: detection of high risk patient subsets for stomach cancer after remote partial gastrectomy for benign conditions. *Cancer Res* 1990;50:6486-6489.

83. Dubrow R. Gastric cancer following peptic ulcer surgery [editorial]. *J Natl Cancer Inst* 1993;85:1268-1270.

84. Nakamura T, Nakano G. Histopathological classification and malignant change in gastric polyps. *J Clin Pathol* 1985;38:754-764.

85. Spechler SJ. The role of gastric carditis in metaplasia and neoplasia at the gastroesophageal junction. *Gastroenterology* 1999;117:218-228.

86. Spechler SJ. Barrett's esophagus. *Gastroenterologist* 1994;2:273-284.

87. La Vecchia C, Negri E, Franceschi S, et al. Family history and the risk of stomach and colorectal cancer. *Cancer* 1992;70:50-55.

88. Barker DJ, Coggon D, Osmond C, et al. Poor housing in childhood and high rates of stomach cancer in England and Wales. *Br J Cancer* 1990;61:575-578.

89. Munoz SE, Ferraroni M, La Vecchia C, et al. Gastric cancer risk factors in subjects with family history. *Cancer Epidemiol Biomarkers Prev* 1997;6:137-140.

90. Offerhaus GJ, Giardiello FM, Krush AJ, et al. The risk of upper gastrointestinal cancer in familial adenomatous polyposis. *Gastroenterology* 1992;102:1980-1982.

91. Zhang L, Blot WJ, You WC, et al. *Helicobacter pylori* antibodies in relation to precancerous gastric lesions in a high-risk Chinese population. *Cancer Epidemiol Biomarkers Prev* 1996;5:627-630.

92. Nomura A, Stemmermann GN, Chyou PH, et al. *Helicobacter pylori* infection and gastric carcinoma among Japanese Americans in Hawaii. *N Engl J Med* 1991;325:1132-1136.

93. Parsonnet J, Harris RA, Hack HM, et al. Should we treat *H. pylori* infection to prevent gastric cancer? *Gastroenterology* 1997;112:1044-1045.

94. Forman D, Newell DG, Fullerton F, et al. Association between infection with *Helicobacter pylori* and risk of gastric cancer: evidence from a prospective investigation. *BMJ* 1991;302:1302-1305.

95. Webb PM, Crabtree JE, Forman D. Gastric cancer, cytotoxin-associated gene A-positive *Helicobacter pylori*, and serum pepsinogens: an international study. The Eurogast Study Group. *Gastroenterology* 1999;116:269-276.

96. Blaser MJ, Perez-Perez GI, Kleanthous H, et al. Infection with *Helicobacter pylori* strains possessing *cagA* is associated with an increased risk of developing adenocarcinoma of the stomach. *Cancer Res* 1995;55:2111-2115.

97. Blaser MJ, Chyou PH, Nomura A. Age at establishment of *Helicobacter pylori* infection and gastric carcinoma, gastric ulcer, and duodenal ulcer risk. *Cancer Res* 1995;55:562-565.

98. Chow WH, Blaser MJ, Blot WJ, et al. An inverse relation between *cagA*+ strains of *Helicobacter pylori* infection and risk of esophageal and gastric cardia adenocarcinoma. *Cancer Res* 1998;58:588-590.

99. Harris RA, Owens DK, Witherell H, et al. *Helicobacter pylori* and gastric cancer: what are the benefits of screening only for the *cagA* phenotype of *H. pylori*? *Helicobacter* 1999;4:69-76.

100. Levine PH, Stemmermann G, Lennette ET, et al. Elevated antibody titers to Epstein-Barr virus prior to the diagnosis of Epstein-Barr-virus–associated gastric adenocarcinoma. *Int J Cancer* 1995;60:642-644.

101. Forman D. *Helicobacter pylori* infection and cancer. *Br Med Bull* 1998;54:71-78.

102. Forman D. *Helicobacter pylori*: the gastric cancer problem. *Gut* 1998;43:S33-S34.

103. Maruyama K, Okabayashi K, Kinoshita T. Progress in gastric cancer surgery in Japan and its limits of radicality. *World J Surg* 1987;11:418-425.

104. Prolla JC, Kobayashi S, Kirsner JB. Gastric cancer. Some recent improvements in diagnosis based upon the Japanese experience. *Arch Intern Med* 1969;124:238-246.

105. Nakajima T, Nishi M, Kajitani T. Improvement in treatment results of gastric cancer with surgery and chemotherapy: experience of 9,700 cases in the Cancer Institute Hospital, Tokyo. *Semin Surg Oncol* 1991;7:365-372.

106. Pisani P, Oliver WE, Parkin DM, et al. Case-control study of gastric cancer screening in Venezuela. *Br J Cancer* 1994;69:1102-1105.

107. McNeer G, Vandenberg H Jr, Donn F, et al. A critical evaluation of sub-total gastrectomy for cure of cancer of the stomach. *Ann Surgery* 1951;134:2-7.

108. Landry J, Tepper JE, Wood WC, et al. Patterns of failure following curative resection of gastric carcinoma. *Int J Radiat Oncol Biol Phys* 1990;19:1357-1362.

109. Gunderson LL, Sosin H. Adenocarcinoma of the stomach: areas of failure in a re-operation series (second or symptomatic look) clinicopathologic correlation and implications for adjuvant therapy. *Int J Radiat Oncol Biol Phys* 1982;8:1-11.

110. Papachristou DN, Fortner JG. Local recurrence of gastric adenocarcinomas after gastrectomy. *J Surg Oncol* 1981;18:47-53.

111. Horn R. Carcinoma of the stomach. Autopsy findings in untreated cases. *Gastroenterology* 1955;29:515-525.

112. McNeer G, Vandenberg H, Donn F, et al. A critical evaluation of subtotal gastrectomy for the cure of cancer of the stomach. *Arch Surg* 1957;134:2-7.

113. Stout A. Pathology of carcinoma of the stomach. *Arch Surg* 1943;46:807-822.

114. Thomson F, Robbins R. Local recurrence following subtotal resection for gastric carcinoma. *Surg Gynecol Obstet* 1952;95:341-344.

115. Wisbeck WM, Becher EM, Russell AH. Adenocarcinoma of the stomach: autopsy observations with therapeutic implications for the radiation oncologist. *Radiother Oncol* 1986;7:13-18.

116. Wangensteen OH, Lewis F, Arhelger S, et al. An interim report upon the "second look" procedure for cancer of the stomach, colon, and rectum and for "limited intraperitoneal carcinomatosis." *Surg Gynecol Obstet* 1954;99:257-267.

117. Wanebo HJ, Kennedy BJ, Chmiel J, et al. Cancer of the stomach. A patient care study by the American College of Surgeons. *Ann Surg* 1993;218:583-592.

118. Kurihara M, Shirakabe H, Yarita T, et al. Diagnosis of small early gastric cancer by x-ray, endoscopy, and biopsy. *Cancer Detect Prev* 1981;4:377-383.

119. Kurtz RC, Sherlock P. The diagnosis of gastric cancer. *Semin Oncol* 1985;12:11-18.

120. Graham DY, Schwartz JT, Cain GD, et al. Prospective evaluation of biopsy number in the diagnosis of esophageal and gastric carcinoma. *Gastroenterology* 1982;82:228-231.

121. Cook AO, Levine BA, Sirinek KR, et al. Evaluation of gastric adenocarcinoma. Abdominal computed tomography does not replace celiotomy. *Arch Surg* 1986;121:603-606.

122. Sussman SK, Halvorsen RA Jr, Illescas FF, et al. Gastric adenocarcinoma: CT versus surgical staging. *Radiology* 1988;167:335-340.

123. Ajani JA, Mansfield PF, Ota DM. Potentially resectable gastric carcinoma: current approaches to staging and preoperative therapy. *World J Surg* 1995;19:216-220.

124. Smith JW, Brennan MF, Botet JF, et al. Preoperative endoscopic ultrasound can predict the risk of recurrence after operation for gastric carcinoma. *J Clin Oncol* 1993;11:2380-2385.

125. Botet JF, Lightdale CJ, Zauber AG, et al. Preoperative staging of esophageal cancer: comparison of endoscopic US and dynamic CT. *Radiology* 1991;181:419-425.

126. Tio LT, Blank LE, Wijers OB, et al. Staging and prognosis using endosonography in patients with inoperable esophageal carcinoma treated with combined intraluminal and external irradiation. *Gastrointest Endosc* 1994;40:304-310.

127. Fleming I, Cooper JS, Henson DE, et al, eds. *AJCC Cancer Staging Manual.* 5th ed. Philadelphia, Pa: Lippincott Williams & Wilkins; 1997:71-76.

128. Shiu MH, Perrotti M, Brennan MF. Adenocarcinoma of the stomach: a multivariate analysis of clinical, pathologic and treatment factors. *Hepatogastroenterology* 1989;36:7-12.

129. Baba H, Korenaga D, Okamura T, et al. Prognostic factors in gastric cancer with serosal invasion. Univariate and multivariate analyses. *Arch Surg* 1989;124:1061-1064.

130. Serlin O, Keehn RJ, Higgins GA Jr, et al. Factors related to survival following resection for gastric carcinoma: analysis of 903 cases. *Cancer* 1977;40:1318-1329.

131. Hartley LC, Evans E, Windsor CJ. Factors influencing prognosis in gastric cancer. *Aust NZ J Surg* 1987;57:5-9.

132. Kennedy BJ. TNM classification for stomach cancer. *Cancer* 1970;26:971-983.

133. Bedikian AY, Chen TT, Khankhanian N, et al. The natural history of gastric cancer and prognostic factors influencing survival. *J Clin Oncol* 1984;2:305-310.

134. Dockerty MB. Pathologic aspects of primary malignant neoplasms of the stomach. In: ReMine W, Priestly J, Berkson J, eds. *Cancer of the Stomach.* Philadelphia, Pa: WB Saunders; 1964:173.

135. Baba H, Korenaga D, Haraguchi M, et al. Width of serosal invasion and prognosis in advanced human gastric cancer with special reference to the mode of tumor invasion. *Cancer* 1989;64:2482-2486.

136. Nagatomo T, Murakami E, Kondo K. Histologic criteria of serosal rupture and prognosis in gastric carcinoma. *Cancer* 1972;29:180-190.

137. Hayes N, Wayman J, Wadehra V, et al. Peritoneal cytology in the surgical evaluation of gastric carcinoma. *Br J Cancer* 1999;79:520-524.

138. Benevolo M, Mottolese M, Cosimelli M, et al. Diagnostic and prognostic value of peritoneal immunocytology in gastric cancer. *J Clin Oncol* 1998;16:3406-3411.

139. Nakajima T, Harashima S, Hirata M, et al. Prognostic and therapeutic values of peritoneal cytology in gastric cancer. *Acta Cytol* 1978;22:225-229.

140. Kitamura M, Arai K, Iwasaki Y. Evaluation of intraoperative peritoneal cytology and intraperitoneal chemotherapy using CDDP combined with MMC for gastric carcinomatous peritonitis [in Japanese]. *Gan To Kagaku Ryoho* 1995;22:1523-1526.

141. Shirakawa T, Onda M, Tokunaga A, et al. Role of peritoneal lavage smears and gastric wall brushing smears in gastric cancer surgery [in Japanese]. *Gan To Kagaku Ryoho* 1996;23:1472-1475.

142. Teramoto T, Onda M, Tokunaga A, et al. Prognostic evaluation of peritoneal lavage smears and gastric wall brushing smears in gastric cancer surgery [in Japanese]. *Gan To Kagaku Ryoho* 1995;22:1606-1609.

143. Koga S, Kaibara N, Iitsuka Y, et al. Prognostic significance of intraperitoneal free cancer cells in gastric cancer patients. *J Cancer Res Clin Oncol* 1984;108:236-238.

144. MacComb WS. Planned combination of surgery and radiation in treatment of advanced primary head and neck cancer. *AJR Am J Roentgenol* 1957;77.

145. Maruta K, Shida H. Some factors which influence prognosis after surgery for advanced gastric cancer. *Ann Surg* 1968;167:313-318.

146. Harrison JD, Morris DL, Ellis IO, et al. The effect of tamoxifen and estrogen receptor status on survival in gastric carcinoma. *Cancer* 1989;64:1007-1010.

147. Gouzi JL, Huguier M, Fagniez PL, et al. Total gastrectomy versus partial gastrectomy of adenocarcinoma of the antrum. A French prospective controlled study [in French]. *Ann Chir* 1989;43:356-360.

148. Sugimachi K, Kodama Y, Kumashiro R, et al. Critical evaluation of prophylactic splenectomy in total gastrectomy for the stomach cancer. *Gann* 1980;71:704-709.

149. Brady MS, Rogatko A, Dent LL, et al. Effect of splenectomy on morbidity and survival following curative gastrectomy for carcinoma. *Arch Surg* 1991;126:359-364.

150. Otsuji E, Yamaguchi T, Sawai K, et al. Total gastrectomy with simultaneous pancreaticosplenectomy or splenectomy in patients with advanced gastric carcinoma. *Br J Cancer* 1999;79:1789-1793.

151. Otsuji E, Yamaguchi T, Sawai K, et al. End results of simultaneous pancreatectomy, splenectomy and total gastrectomy for patients with gastric carcinoma. *Br J Cancer* 1997;75:1219-1223.

152. Papachristou DN, Agnanti N, D'Agostino H, et al. Histologically positive esophageal margin in the surgical treatment of gastric cancer. *Am J Surg* 1980;139:711-713.

153. Bleiberg H, Goffin JC, Dalesio O, et al. Adjuvant radiotherapy and chemotherapy in resectable gastric cancer. A randomized trial of the gastro-intestinal tract cancer cooperative group of the EORTC. *Eur J Surg Oncol* 1989;15:535-543.

154. Slot A, Meerwaldt JH, van Putten WL, et al. Adjuvant postoperative radiotherapy for gastric carcinoma with poor prognostic signs. *Radiother Oncol* 1989;16:269-274.

155. Allum WH, Hallissey MT, Ward LC, et al. A controlled, prospective, randomised trial of adjuvant chemotherapy or radiotherapy in resectable gastric cancer: interim report. British Stomach Cancer Group. *Br J Cancer* 1989;60:739-744.

156. Gill PG, Jamieson GG, Denham J, et al. Treatment of adenocarcinoma of the cardia with synchronous chemotherapy and radiotherapy. *Br J Surg* 1990;77:1020-1023.

157. Gez E, Sulkes A, Yablonsky-Peretz T, et al. Combined 5-fluorouracil (5-FU) and radiation therapy following resection of locally advanced gastric carcinoma. *J Surg Oncol* 1986;31:139-142.

158. Kern KA. Gastric cancer: a neoplastic enigma. *J Surg Oncol Suppl* 1989;1:34-39.

159. Kodama Y, Sugimachi K, Soejima K, et al. Evaluation of extensive lymph node dissection for carcinoma of the stomach. *World J Surg* 1981;5:241-248.

160. Okajima K. Surgical treatment of gastric cancer with special reference to lymph node removal. *Acta Med Okayama* 1977;31:369-382.

161. Bonenkamp JJ, Songun I, Hermans J, et al. Randomised comparison of morbidity after D1 and D2 dissection for gastric cancer in 996 Dutch patients. *Lancet* 1995;345:745-748.

162. Bonenkamp JJ, van de Velde CJ, Sasako M, et al. R2 compared with R1 resection for gastric cancer: morbidity and mortality in a prospective, randomised trial. *Eur J Surg* 1992;158:413-418.

163. Bonenkamp JJ, Hermans J, Sasako M, et al. Extended lymph-node dissection for gastric cancer. Dutch Gastric Cancer Group. *N Engl J Med* 1999;340:908-914.

164. Smith JW, Shiu MH, Kelsey L, et al. Morbidity of radical lym-phadenectomy in the curative resection of gastric carcinoma. *Arch Surg* 1991;126:1469-1473.

165. Robertson CS, Chung SC, Woods SD, et al. A prospective randomized trial comparing R1 subtotal gastrectomy with R3 total gastrectomy for antral cancer. *Ann Surg* 1994;220: 176-182.

166. Dent DM, Madden MV, Price SK. Randomized comparison of R1 and R2 gastrectomy for gastric carcinoma. *Br J Surg* 1988; 75:110-112.

167. Noguchi Y, Imada T, Matsumoto A, et al. Radical surgery for gastric cancer. A review of the Japanese experience. *Cancer* 1989; 64:2053-2062.

168. Adashek K, Sanger J, Longmire WP Jr. Cancer of the stomach. Review of consecutive ten-year intervals. *Ann Surg* 1979;189:6-10.

169. Buchholtz TW, Welch CE, Malt RA. Clinical correlates of resectability and survival in gastric carcinoma. *Ann Surg* 1978; 188:711-715.

170. Controlled trial of adjuvant chemotherapy following curative resection for gastric cancer. Gastrointestinal Tumor Study Group. *Cancer* 1982;49:1116-1122.

171. Allum WH, Hallissey MT, Kelly KA. Adjuvant chemotherapy in operable gastric cancer. 5 year follow-up of first British Stomach Cancer Group trial. *Lancet* 1989;1:571-574.

172. Robinson E, Cohen Y. The combination of surgery, radiother-apy, and chemotherapy in the treatment of gastric cancer. *Recent Results Cancer Res* 1977:177-180.

173. Regine WF, Mohiuddin M. Impact of adjuvant therapy on locally advanced adenocarcinoma of the stomach. *Int J Radiat Oncol Biol Phys* 1992;24:921-927.

174. Martinez-Monge R, Calvo FA, Azinovic I, et al. Patterns of fail-ure and long-term results in high-risk resected gastric cancer treated with postoperative radiotherapy with or without intra-operative electron boost. *J Surg Oncol* 1997;66:24-29.

175. Takahashi M, Abe M. Intra-operative radiotherapy for carci-noma of the stomach. *Eur J Surg Oncol* 1986;12:247-250.

176. Sindelar WF, Kinsella TJ, Tepper JE, et al. Randomized trial of intraoperative radiotherapy in carcinoma of the stomach. *Am J Surg* 1993;165:178-186.

177. Hallissey MT, Dunn JA, Ward LC, et al. The second British Stomach Cancer Group trial of adjuvant radiotherapy or chemotherapy in resectable gastric cancer: five-year follow-up. *Lancet* 1994;343:1309-1312.

178. MacDonald J, Smalley S, Benedetti J, et al. Postoperative com-bined radiation and chemotherapy improves disease-free and overall survival in resected adenocarcinoma of the stomach and GE junction [abstract 1]. *Proc Am Soc Clin Oncol* 2000;19:1a.

179. Alcobendas F, Milla A, Estape J, et al. Mitomycin C as an adju-vant in resected gastric cancer. *Ann Surg* 1983;198:13-17.

180. Engstrom PF, Lavin PT, Douglass HO Jr, et al. Postoperative adjuvant 5-fluorouracil plus methyl-CCNU therapy for gastric cancer patients. Eastern Cooperative Oncology Group Study (EST 3275). *Cancer* 1985;55:1868-1873.

181. Higgins GA, Humphrey EW, Dwight RW, et al. Preoperative radiation and surgery for cancer of the rectum. Veterans Administration Surgical Oncology Group Trial II. *Cancer* 1986;58:352-359.

182. Coombes RC, Schein PS, Chilvers CE, et al. A randomized trial comparing adjuvant fluorouracil, doxorubicin, and mitomycin with no treatment in operable gastric cancer. International Collaborative Cancer Group. *J Clin Oncol* 1990;8:1362-1369.

183. Krook JE, O'Connell MJ, Wieand HS, et al. A prospective, ran-domized evaluation of intensive-course 5-fluorouracil plus doxorubicin as surgical adjuvant chemotherapy for resected gastric cancer. *Cancer* 1991;67:2454-2458.

184. Hermans J, Bonenkamp JJ, Boon MC, et al. Adjuvant therapy after curative resection for gastric cancer: meta-analysis of ran-domized trials. *J Clin Oncol* 1993;11:1441-1447.

185. Ajani JA, Ota DM, Jessup JM, et al. Resectable gastric carcinoma. An evaluation of preoperative and postoperative chemotherapy. *Cancer* 1991;68:1501-1506.

186. Leichman L, Silberman H, Leichman CG, et al. Preoperative systemic chemotherapy followed by adjuvant postoperative intraperitoneal therapy for gastric cancer: a University of Southern California pilot program. *J Clin Oncol* 1992;10:1933-1942.

187. Lowy AM, Mansfield PF, Leach SD, et al. Response to neoadju-vant chemotherapy best predicts survival after curative resection of gastric cancer. *Ann Surg* 1999;229:303-308.

188. Lerner A, Gonin R, Steele GD Jr, et al. Etoposide, doxorubicin, and cisplatin chemotherapy for advanced gastric adenocarci-noma: results of a phase II trial. *J Clin Oncol* 1992;10:536-540.

189. Plukker JT, Mulder NH, Sleijfer DT, et al. Chemotherapy and surgery for locally advanced cancer of the cardia and fundus: phase II study with methotrexate and 5-fluorouracil. *Br J Surg* 1991;78:955-958.

190. Groves LK, Rodriguez-Antunez A. Treatment of carcinoma of the esophagus and gastric cardia with concentrated preoperative irradiation followed by early operation. A progress report. *Ann Thoracic Surg* 1973;15:333-338.

191. Hoshi H. Histologic study on the effect of preoperative irradia-tion of gastric cancer. *Tohoku J Exp Med* 1968;96:293-311.

192. Kamimura S, Mikuriya S, Hara O, et al. Preoperative radiother-apy of carcinoma of the stomach and breast [in Japanese]. *Gan To Kagaku Ryoho* 1987;14:1558-1563.

193. Mikuriya S, Oh'ami H. Radiotherapy and cellular infiltration of tumor nests. *Radiat Med* 1983;1:248-254.

194. Stoliarov VI, Volkov ON, Kanaev SV, et al. Comparative evalua-tion of surgical and combined treatment of cancer of the proximal region of the stomach [in Russian]. *Vopr Onkol* 1984;30:31-35.

195. Kosse VA. Combined treatment of gastric cancer using hypoxic radiotherapy [in Russian]. *Vopr Onkol* 1990;36:1349-1353.

196. Shchepotin IB, Evans SR, Chorny V, et al. Intensive preoperative radiotherapy with local hyperthermia for the treatment of gas-tric carcinoma. *Surg Oncol* 1994;3:37-44.

197. Talaev MI, Starinskii VV, Kovalev BN, et al. Results of combined treatment of cancer of the gastric antrum and gastric body [in Russian]. *Vopr Onkol* 1990;36:1485-1488.

198. Mansfield P, Lowy A, Feig B, et al. Pre-operative chemoradi-ation for potentially resectable gastric cancer. *Proc Am Soc Clin Oncol* 2000;19:246a [abstract 955].

199. Wieland C, Hymmen U. Mega-volt therapy of malignant stom-ach neoplasms [in German]. *Strahlentherapie* 1970;140:20-26.

200. A comparison of combination chemotherapy and combined modality therapy for locally advanced gastric carcinoma. Gastrointestinal Tumor Study Group. *Cancer* 1982;49: 1771-1777.

201. The concept of locally advanced gastric cancer. Effect of treat-ment on outcome. Gastrointestinal Tumor Study Group. *Cancer* 1990;66:2324-2330.

202. Buffet C, Turner K, Pelletier G, et al. Palliative radiotherapy [letter]. *Br J Surg* 1983;70:131.

203. Falkson G, van Eden EB. A controlled clinical trial of fluo-rouracil plus imidazole carboxamide dimethyl triazeno plus vincristine plus bis-chloroethyl nitrosourea plus radiotherapy in stomach cancer. *Med Pediatr Oncol* 1976;2:111-117.

204. Gunderson LL, Hoskins RB, Cohen AC, et al. Combined modal-ity treatment of gastric cancer. *Int J Radiat Oncol Biol Phys* 1983;9:965-975.

205. Phase II-III chemotherapy studies in advanced gastric cancer. Gastrointestinal Tumor Study Group. *Cancer Treatment Reports* 1979;63:1871-1876.

206. Comis RL, Carter SK. A review of chemotherapy in gastric cancer. *Cancer* 1974;34:1576-1586.

207. Moertel CG. Chemotherapy of gastrointestinal cancer. *Clin Gastroenterol* 1976;5:777-793.

208. Pyrhonen S, Kuitunen T, Nyandoto P, et al. Randomised comparison of fluorouracil, epidoxorubicin and methotrexate (FEMTX) plus supportive care with supportive care alone in patients with non-resectable gastric cancer. *Br J Cancer* 1995;71:587-591.

209. Glimelius B, Ekstrom K, Hoffman K, et al. Randomized comparison between chemotherapy plus best supportive care with best supportive care in advanced gastric cancer. *Ann Oncol* 1997;8:163-168.

210. Murad AM, Santiago FF, Petroianu A, et al. Modified therapy with 5-fluorouracil, doxorubicin, and methotrexate in advanced gastric cancer. *Cancer* 1993;72:37-41.

211. Cullinan SA, Moertel CG, Fleming TR, et al. A comparison of three chemotherapeutic regimens in the treatment of advanced pancreatic and gastric carcinoma. Fluorouracil vs fluorouracil and doxorubicin vs fluorouracil, doxorubicin, and mitomycin. *JAMA* 1985;253:2061-2067.

212. Vanhoefer U, Rougier P, Wilke H, et al. Final results of a randomized phase III trial of sequential high-dose methotrexate, fluorouracil, and doxorubicin versus etoposide, leucovorin, and fluorouracil versus infusional fluorouracial and cisplatin in advanced gastric cancer: a trial of the European Organization for Research and Treatment of Cancer Gastrointestinal Tract Cancer Cooperative Group. *J Clin Oncol* 2000;18:2648-2657.

213. Henning GT, Schild SE, Stafford SL, et al. Results of irradiation or chemoirradiation following resection of gastric adenocarcinoma. *Int J Radiat Oncol Biol Phys* 2000;46:589-598.

214. Schuster-Uitterhoeve AL, Gonzalez Gonzalez D, Blank LE. Radiotherapy with multiple fractions per day in pancreatic and bile duct cancer. *Radiother Oncol* 1986;7:205-213.

215. Seydel HG, Stablein DM, Leichman LP, et al. Hyperfractionated radiation and chemotherapy for unresectable localized adenocarcinoma of the pancreas. Gastrointestinal Tumor Study Group. *Cancer* 1990;65:1478-1482.

216. O'Connell MJ, Gunderson LL, Moertel CG, et al. A pilot study to determine clinical tolerability of intensive combined modality therapy for locally unresectable gastric cancer. *Int J Radiat Oncol Biol Phys* 1985;11:1827-1831.

217. Ellis F, Weatherburn H. RBE and clinical response in radiotherapy with neutron beams. *Br J Radiol* 1984;57:817-822.

218. Galandiuk S, Wieand HS, Moertel CG, et al. Patterns of recurrence after curative resection of carcinoma of the colon and rectum. *Surg Gynecol Obstet* 1992;174:27-32.

219. Kelsen D, Karpeh M, Schwartz G, et al. Neoadjuvant therapy of high-risk gastric cancer: a phase II trial of preoperative FAMTX and postoperative intraperitoneal fluorouracil-cisplatin plus intravenous fluorouracil. *J Clin Oncol* 1996;14:1818-1828.

220. Fujimoto S, Shrestha RD, Kokubun M, et al. Intraperitoneal hyperthermic perfusion combined with surgery effective for gastric cancer patients with peritoneal seeding. *Ann Surg* 1988; 208:36-41.

221. Fujimoto S, Shrestha RD, Kobayashi K, et al. Combined treatment with surgery and intraperitoneal hyperthermic perfusion (IPHP) for far-advanced gastrointestinal cancer with peritoneal seeding. *Acta Med Austriaca* 1989;16:76-80.

222. Koga S, Hamazoe R, Maeta M, et al. Prophylactic therapy for peritoneal recurrence of gastric cancer by continuous hyperthermic peritoneal perfusion with mitomycin C. *Cancer* 1988; 61:232-237.

223. Evans DB, Abbruzzese JL, Cleary KR, et al. Preoperative chemoradiation for adenocarcinoma of the pancreas: excessive toxicity of prophylactic hepatic irradiation. *Int J Radiat Oncol Biol Phys* 1995;33:913-918.

224. Abrams RA, Grochow LB, Chakravarthy A, et al. Intensified adjuvant therapy for pancreatic and periampullary adenocarcinoma: survival results and observations regarding patterns of failure, radiotherapy dose and CA19–9 levels. *Int J Radiat Oncol Biol Phys* 1999;44:1039-1046.

225. Fajardo LF, Berthrong M, Anderson RE. Small intestine. In: *Radiation Pathology*. New York, NY: Oxford University Press; 2001:228-229.

226. Montagna W. Cytologic study of intestinal epithelium of mouse after total body x-irradiation. *J Natl Cancer Inst* 1955;15: 1703-1736.

227. Kinsella TJ, Bloomer WD. Tolerance of the intestine to radiation therapy. *Surg Gynecol Obstet* 1980;151:273-284.

228. Neugut AI, Jacobson JS, Suh S, et al. The epidemiology of cancer of the small bowel. *Cancer Epidemiol Biomarkers Prev* 1998;7: 243-251.

229. Ellis H. Tumours of the small intestine. *Semin Surg Oncol* 1987;3:12-21.

230. Ciccarelli O, Welch JP, Kent GG. Primary malignant tumors of the small bowel. The Hartford Hospital experience, 1969–1983. *Am J Surg* 1987;153:350-354.

231. Lowenfels AB, Sonni A. Distribution of small bowel tumors. *Cancer Lett* 1977;3:83-86.

232. Lowenfels AB. Why are small-bowel tumours so rare? *Lancet* 1973;1:24-26.

233. Ross RK, Hartnett NM, Bernstein L, et al. Epidemiology of adenocarcinomas of the small intestine: is bile a small bowel carcinogen? *Br J Cancer* 1991;63:143-145.

234. Scudamore CH, Freeman HJ. Effects of small bowel transection, resection, or bypass in 1,2-dimethylhydrazine-induced rat intestinal neoplasia. *Gastroenterology* 1983;84:725-731.

235. Chow WH, Linet MS, McLaughlin JK, et al. Risk factors for small intestine cancer. *Cancer Causes Control* 1993;4:163-169.

236. Neugut AI, Santos J. The association between cancers of the small and large bowel. *Cancer Epidemiol Biomarkers Prev* 1993; 2:551-553.

237. Frank JD, Shorey BA. Adenocarcinoma of the small bowel as a complication of Crohn's disease. *Gut* 1973;14:120-124.

238. Hawker PC, Gyde SN, Thompson H, et al. Adenocarcinoma of the small intestine complicating Crohn's disease. *Gut* 1982; 23:188-193.

239. Morowitz DA, Block GE, Kirsner JB. Adenocarcinoma of the ileum complicating chronic regional enteritis. *Gastroenterology* 1968;55:397-402.

240. Michelassi F, Testa G, Pomidor WJ, et al. Adenocarcinoma complicating Crohn's disease. *Dis Colon Rectum* 1993;36:654-661.

241. Swinson CM, Slavin G, Coles EC, et al. Coeliac disease and malignancy. *Lancet* 1983;1:111-115.

242. Hochberg FH, Dasilva AB, Galdabini J, et al. Gastrointestinal involvement in von Recklinghausen's neurofibromatosis. *Neurology* 1974;24:1144-1151.

243. Fleming I, Cooper JS, Henson DE, et al, eds. *AJCC Cancer Staging Manual.* 5th ed. Philadelphia, Pa: Lippincott Williams & Wilkins; 1997:77-79.

244. Whelan TJ, Dembo AJ, Bush RS, et al. Complications of whole abdominal and pelvic radiotherapy following chemotherapy for advanced ovarian cancer. *Int J Radiat Oncol Biol Phys* 1992;22: 853-858.

245. Lai EC, Doty JE, Irving C, et al. Primary adenocarcinoma of the duodenum: analysis of survival. *World J Surg* 1988;12: 695-699.

246. Kerremans RP, Lerut J, Penninckx FM. Primary malignant duodenal tumors. *Ann Surg* 1979;190:179-182.

247. Spira IA, Ghazi A, Wolff WI. Primary adenocarcinoma of the duodenum. *Cancer* 1977;39:1721-1726.

248. Joesting DR, Beart RW Jr, van Heerden JA, et al. Improving survival in adenocarcinoma of the duodenum. *Am J Surg* 1981;141:228-231.

249. Alwmark A, Andersson A, Lasson A. Primary carcinoma of the duodenum. *Ann Surg* 1980;191:13-18.

250. Lillemoe K, Imbembo AL. Malignant neoplasms of the duodenum. *Surg Gynecol Obstet* 1980;150:822-826.

251. Lillemoe KD. Primary duodenal adenocarcinoma: role for aggressive resection [editorial]. *J Am Coll Surg* 1996;183:155-156.

252. Cohen JR, Kuchta N, Geller N, et al. Pancreaticoduodenectomy. A 40-year experience. *Ann Surg* 1982;195:608-617.

253. Herter FP, Cooperman AM, Ahlborn TN, et al. Surgical experience with pancreatic and periampullary cancer. *Ann Surg* 1982;195:274-281.

254. Williamson RC, Welch CE, Malt RA. Adenocarcinoma and lymphoma of the small intestine. Distribution and etiologic associations. *Ann Surg* 1983;197:172-178.

255. Sohn TA, Lillemoe KD, Cameron JL, et al. Adenocarcinoma of the duodenum: factors influencing long-term survival. *J Gastrointest Surg* 1998;2:79-87.

256. Rose DM, Hochwald SN, Klimstra DS, et al. Primary duodenal adenocarcinoma: a ten-year experience with 79 patients. *J Am Coll Surg* 1996;183:89-96.

257. Further evidence of effective adjuvant combined radiation and chemotherapy following curative resection of pancreatic cancer. Gastrointestinal Tumor Study Group. *Cancer* 1987;59:2006-2010.

258. Spitz FR, Abbruzzese JL, Lee JE, et al. Preoperative and postoperative chemoradiation strategies in patients treated with pancreaticoduodenectomy for adenocarcinoma of the pancreas. *J Clin Oncol* 1997;15:928–937.

259. Order SE, Donaldson SS. Carcinoids. In: Order SE, Donaldson SS, eds. *Radiation Therapy of Benign Diseases.* Berlin, Germany: Springer-Verlag; 1998:66-68.

CHAPTER 20

The Pancreas

Christopher H. Crane, Douglas B. Evans, Robert A. Wolff,
James L. Abbruzzese, Peter W.T. Pisters, and Nora A. Janjan

ANATOMY

The pancreas is located in the retroperitoneum at the level of the first two lumbar vertebrae and is intimately surrounded by critical organs and vessels. Among the radiosensitive critical structures in close proximity to the pancreas are the stomach, liver, kidneys, spleen, jejunum, and duodenum. The pancreas consists of four parts: the head, neck, body, and tail. The tail is located superior to the head and abuts the hilum of the spleen. The head and neck are located anterior and lateral to the superior mesenteric artery, and the uncinate process extends around posterior to this artery. The anterior surface of the pancreas is covered with peritoneum, but the posterior surface is not; the posterior surface is in direct contact with the preaortic soft tissues and in close proximity to the superior mesenteric artery and splenic vein. Early tumor invasion often occurs by direct extension from the primary tumor to surrounding critical vessels, such as the superior mesenteric vessels, the portal vein, and the celiac artery and its branches. The presence or absence of invasion of these critical vascular structures determines the resectability of the tumor.

The pancreas is drained by an abundant supply of lymphatics. Primary drainage is to the pancreaticoduodenal, suprapancreatic, pyloric, and pancreaticosplenic nodal regions, which all drain to the celiac lymph nodes and the superior mesenteric nodes. Nodes in the porta hepatis region also can be involved, especially in advanced disease.

The pancreatic duct and common bile duct are in close proximity to one another because they both travel through the head of the pancreas on their way to the ampulla of Vater. Invasion or compression of the common bile duct and main pancreatic duct is responsible for the presenting symptoms of jaundice and exocrine pancreatic insufficiency.

The divisions of the vagus and splanchnic nerves form the celiac and superior mesenteric plexuses. Nerve fibers reach the pancreas and other abdominal organs by traveling along the celiac and superior mesenteric artery and their branches. Arterial resection and repair with an arterial graft often results in denervation of the midgut and subsequently in disabling diarrhea. Direct extension of tumor posteriorly to the first and second celiac ganglia leads to characteristic sharp pain that is perceived as back pain.

ACUTE EFFECTS OF IRRADIATION

The acute effects of irradiation to the upper abdomen result from depletion of the rapidly dividing mucosal lining of the stomach (or, in postoperatively treated patients, gastric remnant), which can lead to nausea and vomiting. Severe acute reactions can involve ulceration of the stomach or duodenum. Nausea also can result when large volumes of the liver are irradiated. Diarrhea is less common because the volume of jejunum that is typically in the radiation field is relatively small. Antiemetics and either a proton pump inhibitor or an H2 blocker should be routinely used for prophylaxis in patients undergoing upper-abdominal radiation therapy.

LATE EFFECTS OF IRRADIATION

With regard to late effects, the dose-limiting structures surrounding the pancreas include the stomach, small bowel (particularly the duodenum), kidneys, spinal cord, and liver. The dose of conventional external-beam radiation that can safely be used in the upper abdomen depends on the tolerance of surrounding organs; these doses have been established for patients given radiation therapy either alone[1-4] or in combination with 5-fluorouracil (5-FU).[5,6] Doses up to 50 Gy, given in 2-Gy fractions, are well tolerated even when large volumes of tissue are irradiated. When conventional treatment planning is used, radiation doses of between 50 Gy and 60 Gy seem to injure the gastric and duodenal mucosa if large volumes of tissue are treated. Doses up to 68 Gy are well tolerated with or without 5-FU–based chemotherapy if care is taken to limit the volume of mucosa irradiated.[7]

The most common late radiation injury is ulceration of the mucosal surface; perforation is rare. Usually these complications can be managed medically. With regard to kidney function, mean decreases in creatinine clearance of 10% and 24% have been observed in patients when 50% and 90% to 100%, respectively, of a single kidney is irradiated with doses greater than 26 Gy.[8] Despite these physiologic changes, clinically relevant compromise of kidney function rarely develops if at least one kidney is spared from the field. Radiation-induced liver disease, often called *radiation hepatitis*, is characterized by the development of anicteric ascites approximately 2 weeks to 4 months after hepatic irradiation.[9] In patients with pancreatic cancer, the whole liver has been treated safely to doses greater than 20 Gy,[10] but whole-liver doses greater than 35 Gy carry a significant risk of radiation hepatitis.[11] Although the risk of radiation hepatitis can be predicted on the basis of dose and volume considerations,[12,13] it is now clear that limited volumes of liver can tolerate high doses of irradiation.[4]

EPIDEMIOLOGY OF PANCREATIC CANCER

Pancreatic cancer is currently the ninth most common malignancy in women and the tenth most common malignancy in men in the United States but is the fourth most common cause of cancer death.[14] The incidence of and absolute mortality from pancreatic cancer increased dramatically from 1920 to 1970.[15] Pancreatic cancer is found primarily in western countries, paralleling the epidemiology of colorectal cancer.[16] Since 1970, the incidence has decreased among white men and increased in women and black men,[17] resulting in a stabilization of rates overall.

ETIOLOGY

The cause or causes of pancreatic cancer remain somewhat enigmatic. On balance, the evidence suggests a causative relationship between pancreatic cancer and smoking.[18,19] The relative risk of developing pancreatic cancer is 1.6 to 3.1 times higher for smokers than for nonsmokers. Although some investigators have proposed an association with alcohol and coffee consumption, the evidence there is not as strong.[20] Studies evaluating dietary factors indicate that consumption of fruits and vegetables may be protective, but diets high in animal fat may increase risk.[21,22] Exposure to toxic chemicals such as dichlorodiphenyltrichloroethane (DDT) and some petroleum derivatives also may increase risk.[23,24] Ionizing radiation[16] and chemotherapy,[25] both known carcinogens, probably account for a small number of cases. The relationship between pancreatic cancer and diabetes mellitus is unclear. Although results from a 1995 meta-analysis[26] suggested an association, results from a more recent study showed that the association was weaker if patients with recent-onset diabetes were excluded.[27] Chronic pancreatitis also has been implicated, but this too remains controversial.[28] A very small proportion (about 3%) of cases of pancreatic cancer seem to be clustered in some families, suggesting a genetic predisposition.[29,30]

PRESENTING SYMPTOMS

The most common presenting symptoms of pancreatic cancer are jaundice, weight loss caused by anorexia and exocrine insufficiency, and abdominal pain. Jaundice is usually a presenting symptom in pancreatic head lesions. Patients with lesions arising in the body or tail of the pancreas more often present with pain, typically described as sharp and knife-like, in the mid-epigastric region radiating to the back. Pain is a symptom of locally advanced disease and often indicates unresectable disease.

DIAGNOSIS AND MANAGEMENT

The initial goals in the evaluation and treatment of the symptomatic patient are to determine the resectability of the disease, to establish a histologic diagnosis, and to reestablish biliary-tract outflow. Diagnosis, clinical evaluation, and management of pancreatic cancer differ among centers in the United States. Hence the definition of resectability after clinical evaluation also varies from center to center and from surgeon to surgeon. Various diagnostic approaches may include preoperative imaging, laparoscopy, or laparotomy with attempted resection. Among diagnostic imaging techniques, abdominal computed tomography (CT) scanning is the most common for confirming suspected pancreatic malignancy. However, standard CT techniques are relatively insensitive for the assessment of resectability, although vascular involvement and liver metastases can be assessed with newer techniques.[31]

Helical CT is capable of rapid scanning at thin-slice collimation at various phases after intravenous contrast administration. The timing of contrast administration is critical for detecting small pancreatic masses and liver metastases. This technique improves the ability to both detect the lesion and define its relationship to the adjacent vessels for accurate staging before treatment.

Magnetic resonance imaging (MRI) was initially limited by long scanning times that resulted in the introduction of artifact caused by organ motion. Dynamic MRI with rapid scanning sequences and bolus intravenous contrast enhancement, however, is reported to have sensitivity and specificity comparable to those for helical CT.[32]

Histologic confirmation historically has been most commonly obtained by means of percutaneous CT-guided fine-needle aspiration. This method is operator-dependent and is not possible if the lesion is not visible on CT. Brushings during endoscopic retrograde cholangiopancreatography have a relatively low yield.[33] Although some clinicians advocate laparoscopic exploration as a means of identifying patients who might benefit from pancreatic dissection, its role in screening patients with pancreatic cancer remains to be established.

Endoscopy of the upper gastrointestinal tract is the most valuable initial step in the management of disease in patients who present with obstructive jaundice from a pancreatic head mass. With this procedure, biliary outflow can be easily reestablished with the placement of an endobiliary stent, and endoscopic ultrasound can be performed. A rapidly evolving modality, endoscopic ultrasound adds sensitivity and specificity to lesion detection,[34] and endoscopic ultrasound-directed fine-needle biopsy of the pancreas is rapidly becoming the procedure of choice for the diagnosis of pancreatic malignancy at many centers. The use of endobiliary stents is replacing the more traditional palliative surgical bypass; however, because biliary-tract patency with stents is less durable than a bypass, patients with potentially resectable disease who are found to have unresectable or metastatic disease at surgical exploration are best treated with a palliative surgical bypass.

Tumor markers such as carcinoembryonic antigen (CEA) and CA19-9 are complementary to a complete work-up. Because these tests lack sensitivity and specificity, they have no role as screening tests for pancreatic cancer. However, elevated CA19-9 or CEA in combination with positive results on imaging studies increases the positive predictive value of the diagnosis of pancreatic cancer.[35]

TREATMENT
Pancreaticoduodenectomy

Whipple and colleagues[36] first described pancreaticoduodenectomy in 1935. More than 65 years later, this procedure remains the mainstay of curative treatment for pancreatic cancer. Nevertheless, 80% to 95% of tumors, depending on the series, are unresectable at diagnosis because of local or regional extension or metastatic spread. Of the 5% to 20% of patients with resectable disease, obtaining margins free of disease is possible for only 16% to 30%. Unfortunately, patients with positive margins after surgery[37-39] and patients treated with chemoradiation alone[5,40-45] have a similar median survival time of only 9 to 11 months. Thus preoperative radiographic assessment of resectability is critical in order to avoid incomplete resections.

As noted earlier, lesions of the pancreatic body and tail often present with signs and symptoms referable to invasion of surrounding structures, and most are inoperable because of arterial encasement or distant metastasis. By contrast, tumors arising in the pancreatic head often produce painless jaundice and symptoms referable to exocrine pancreatic insufficiency; these symptoms more often lead to the disease being diagnosed when it is still resectable. The best surgical series report 5-year survival rates of 20% to 25%.[46-48] The use of modern surgical techniques by experienced surgeons can produce operative mortality rates of less than 5% for patients who undergo pancreaticoduodenectomy.[46,47]

Staging

The American Joint Committee on Cancer (AJCC) staging system for pancreatic cancer[49] (Box 20-1) does not correlate well with resectability. Another classification system[50] that is more applicable to clinical practice

---

BOX 20-1 American Joint Committee on Cancer Staging System for Pancreatic Cancer

PRIMARY TUMOR (T)

TX	Primary tumor cannot be assessed
T0	No evidence of primary tumor
Tis	In situ carcinoma
T1	Tumor limited to the pancreas 2 cm or less in greatest dimension
T2	Tumor limited to the pancreas more than 2 cm in greatest dimension
T3	Tumor extends directly into any of the following: duodenum, bile duct, peripancreatic tissues
T4	Tumor extends directly into any of the following: stomach, spleen, colon, adjacent large vessels

REGIONAL LYMPH NODES (N)

NX	Regional lymph node(s) cannot be assessed
N0	No regional lymph node metastasis
N1	Regional lymph node metastasis
	pN1a Metastasis in a single regional lymph node
	pN1b Metastasis in multiple regional lymph nodes

DISTANT METASTASIS (M)

MX	Distant metastasis cannot be assessed
M0	No distant metastasis
M1	Distant metastasis

STAGE GROUPING

Stage 0	Tis	N0	M0
Stage I	T1	N0	M0
	T2	N0	M0
Stage II	T3	N0	M0
Stage III	T1	N1	M0
	T2	N1	M0
	T3	N1	M0
Stage IVA	T4	Any N	M0
Stage IVB	Any T	Any N	M1

From Fleming I, Cooper JS, Henson DE, et al, eds. *AJCC Cancer Staging Manual.* 5th ed. Philadelphia, Pa: Lippincott Williams & Wilkins; 1997:121-126.

groups tumors as resectable, locally advanced (unresectable), or metastatic. Three criteria are necessary for tumors to be considered resectable: (1) no metastasis, (2) no encasement of the celiac artery or superior mesenteric artery, and (3) patency of the superior mesenteric and portal veins.

Prognostic Factors

Tumor size (< 2 cm), the presence or absence of perineural invasion, and lymph node status have been reported to be significant prognostic pathologic variables.[51-53] Treatment-related variables include obtainment of microscopically negative margins at resection, the lack of need for intraoperative transfusion,[54] and the use of adjuvant chemoradiation.[55]

Pattern of Failure

For patients who undergo surgery but not postoperative adjuvant therapy, the pattern of failure is both local and distant. Local failure occurs 50% to 80% of the time.[39,56,57] The most common distant sites of failure are the liver and peritoneum[57]; the lungs and bone are less commonly involved.

Radiation Therapy Techniques
Postoperative Adjuvant Radiation Therapy

Patients given postoperative radiation therapy are typically treated to 50.4 Gy, given in 1.8-Gy fractions. Field reductions are often made after 45 Gy. A four-field technique using anterior, posterior, and opposed lateral fields allows sparing of critical tissues such as the liver, kidneys, stomach, spinal cord, and small bowel. Fields are weighted so that the dose contribution from the lateral fields is restricted to 20 Gy. This can be accomplished by weighting the anteroposterior–posteroanterior fields at twice that of the lateral fields. This approach prevents the liver and kidney tissue in the lateral fields that are not also in the anteroposterior and posteroanterior fields from receiving doses beyond their tolerance.

Simulation films are taken while the patient lies supine in a treatment device that stabilizes the arms overhead. Barium is given, the films are obtained, and the preoperative tumor volume, duodenum, and kidneys are drawn on all of the films. CT-based treatment plans with dose-volume histograms can help verify the dose to be delivered to the target and limit the dose to critical structures.

For lesions located in the pancreatic head, the anteroposterior–posteroanterior fields typically cover the T11 through L3 vertebrae (see Color Plate 24, after p. 80). The celiac trunk, which is typically located at T12, should be covered with a 2-cm margin superiorly. Inferiorly,

the goal is to cover the tumor bed and the duodenal bed with a 2-cm margin. The left border is located 2 cm to the left of the vertebral-body edge, as long as coverage of the preoperative tumor volume is adequate. The preoperative tumor volume and preoperative location of the duodenum define the right field border and the anterior extent of the lateral fields. The porta hepatis should be identified on the planning CT scans and covered. This usually means that the upper right border of the field is located 4 to 5 cm to the right of the vertebral-body edge and the anterior aspect of the lateral field is 5 to 6 cm from the anterior vertebral-body edge. A cerrobend block is placed over the inferior pole of the right kidney in the anteroposterior–posteroanterior fields, bisecting the vertebral bodies in the lateral fields. Corner blocks can be placed in lateral fields as well. Care should be taken not to block the preoperative tumor volume or porta hepatis.

For lesions of the pancreatic body and tail, similar fields are used except that the splenic hilum is covered and the porta hepatis and duodenal bed are not covered. The right field border is typically located 2 cm from the right vertebral-body edge.

Radiation Therapy Technique for Patients with an Intact Pancreas

The guidelines described previously for postoperative irradiation also apply to patients with an intact pancreas. In the case of an intact pancreas, the use of simulation illuminates the duodenal C-loop on the simulation film. The biliary stent also can be visualized, facilitating coverage of the porta hepatis (Fig. 20-1). Some investigators reduce the treatment volume in patients with locally advanced disease who are receiving potent radiosensitizers such as gemcitabine.[58] This approach is reasonable because the toxicity arises from in-field gastrointestinal effects that are related to treatment volume.

Three-Dimensional Conformal Radiation Therapy

The role of three-dimensional conformal therapy in pancreatic cancer is currently undefined, although its feasibility has been investigated. In a study using a simulated tumor model in a cylindrical phantom, the dose to surrounding tissues delivered by conformal irradiation was significantly less than that delivered through conventional treatment planning.[59] No clinical data have been published analyzing the clinical effect of this or any other improved dose distribution in pancreatic cancer, although it stands to reason that three-dimensional conformal therapy may have a role in safely escalating the radiation dose or reducing the toxicity of concurrent chemoradiation. The significant toxicity of radiation with concurrent gemcitabine or paclitaxel, for example, results from damage to normal tissue in the

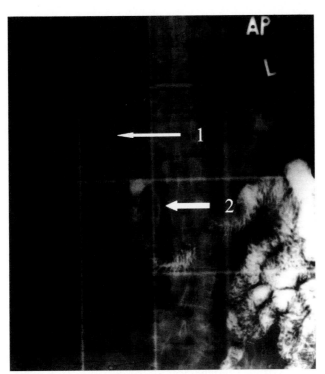

Fig. 20-1 Typical anteroposterior simulation film for the treatment of intact pancreatic head. Contrast medium fills the duodenal "C-loop." Blocking is placed to shield the right kidney. *Arrow 1* indicates refluxed contrast in the biliary system, demonstrating the location of the porta hepatis. *Arrow 2* indicates an endobiliary stent in the intrapancreatic portion of the common bile duct.

field of irradiation. A reduction in the volume of normal tissue that is irradiated can only improve the therapeutic ratio by reducing this toxicity. Prospective studies are ongoing.

Dose escalation using three-dimensional conformal therapy is limited only by the proximity of dose-limiting structures and by the uncertainty created by organ motion such as that associated with free breathing. Respiratory motion must either be accounted for and minimized[60] or controlled through the use of a gating technique (see Chapter 2) to optimize the benefit of conformal therapy. Respiratory gating strategies are currently being developed and evaluated.[61]

Chemoradiation

Nearly 20 years ago, external-beam radiation therapy and concomitant chemotherapy with 5-FU were shown in a landmark randomized trial conducted by the Gastrointestinal Tumor Study Group (GITSG) to prolong survival in patients with locally advanced adenocarcinoma of the pancreas.[5,41] In this trial, use of a split course of radiation therapy with bolus 5-FU prolonged the median survival time over that after radiation alone. However, no survival benefit was found for groups given concurrent 5-FU with high-dose (60 Gy) radiation

relative to those given low-dose (40 Gy) radiation.[5] Because this study was conducted before CT scanning was available, the pattern of failure could not be documented. Nevertheless, local disease was a component of the first clinical site of failure in more of the patients treated with 40 Gy than those treated with 60 Gy. This suggestion of improved local control with the 60-Gy dose over that of the 40-Gy dose was offset by the problem of competing risk of distant failure.

Somewhat different results were seen in an Eastern Cooperative Oncology Group study that randomly allocated patients to therapy with 5-FU alone (600 mg/m^2 in a weekly intravenous bolus) or to radiation therapy (40 Gy) with concurrent 5-FU (600 mg/m^2, days 1 to 3) followed by maintenance 5-FU (600 mg/m^2). No difference was found between groups in median survival, which could be explained either by inadequacies in the chemoradiation dose or schedule or by the fact that 22% of patients did not follow the protocol or could not be evaluated.[45] Nevertheless, additional randomized studies from the Mayo Clinic and the GITSG support the superiority of combined-modality therapy[42-44] over either radiation or chemotherapy alone, as do other single-institution studies.[40]

Radiation Dose-Response Relationship in Locally Advanced Pancreatic Cancer

Single-institution studies have addressed the role of radiation dose escalation in an attempt to improve local disease control in patients with unresectable pancreatic cancer. Intraoperative brachytherapy and electron-beam boosts after preoperative radiation have been investigated for this purpose. Use of an intraoperative boost substantially improved local control but only modestly improved median survival times.[62-66] The use of brachytherapy by means of implants has produced similar results with regard to enhanced local control.[67,68] Although selection bias is probably responsible for the improvement in median survival, a radiation dose response does seem to exist for local tumor control.

Even if improved local control does improve median survival somewhat, high rates of intra-abdominal failure in unirradiated areas continue to prevent significant improvements in long-term survival. The poor results with systemic therapy in patients with measurable metastatic disease and the inability to prevent the development of distant metastatic disease with adjuvant chemotherapy have led to the investigation of new systemic agents in pancreatic cancer. Radiosensitizers such as gemcitabine are being investigated for their possible systemic effect. Effective local control in patients with unresectable pancreatic cancer is an important issue from the standpoint of symptomatic palliation as well as being a prerequisite to the development of curative therapies.

Adjuvant Chemoradiation in Potentially Resectable Disease

Postoperative Chemoradiation

The superiority of the combination of 5-FU and radiation in the GITSG trial for patients with locally advanced pancreatic cancer[5,41] prompted investigations of the role of chemoradiation for patients who had undergone resection for their disease. The same GITSG group initiated a prospective randomized study of postoperative adjuvant chemoradiation that eventually accrued 49 patients over 8 years. Disease in all patients was surgically staged; only patients with disease confined to the pancreas and peripancreatic organs, regional lymph nodes, and regional peritoneum were eligible for the study. After pancreaticoduodenectomy, radiation therapy was delivered to the primary site of disease and regional lymphatics in a split course of 40 Gy given over 6 weeks with concurrent 5-FU ($500 \text{ mg/m}^2\text{/day}$) as an intravenous bolus on days 1 to 3 of the beginning of each 2-week course of radiation).

Despite the use of what is now considered to be suboptimal chemotherapy (dose and schedule) as well as inadequate radiation (dose, equipment [supervoltage], and schedule [split course]), that trial also demonstrated a survival advantage from multimodality therapy relative to resection alone (43% vs. 18% at 2 years, and 14% vs. 5% at 5 years, $P < 0.05$).[69] An additional 30 patients were subsequently entered in the experimental group, and the results were duplicated (Table 20-1).[69-73] Approximately 50% of patients undergoing postoperative therapy experienced local recurrence, which indicates that the results might have been more striking if improved chemoradiation doses and techniques had been used.

Similar findings were reported recently by the European Organization for Research and Treatment of Cancer.[70] Between 1987 and 1995, 218 patients who had undergone pancreaticoduodenectomy for adenocarcinoma of the pancreas or periampullary region were randomly assigned to receive either chemoradiation (40 Gy in a split course of external-beam radiation therapy and 5-FU given as a continuous infusion at a dose of 25 mg/kg/day during radiation) or no further treatment. Because of incomplete resection of extensive local disease, 11 patients were deemed ineligible for analysis. Of the remaining 207 patients, 114 (55%) had cancer of the pancreas. The median survival duration for the entire group was 24.5 months for patients given adjuvant therapy and 19 months for patients given surgery alone (log-rank test, $P = 0.21$). For patients with pancreatic cancer, the median survival was 17.1 months for those given adjuvant therapy and 12.6 months for those given surgery alone ($P = 0.099$).[70]

As was true in the GITSG trial, patients in the European trial were considered for enrollment after they had recovered from pancreaticoduodenectomy. Even so, 21 (20%) of 104 evaluable patients assigned to undergo chemoradiation did not receive the intended therapy because of patient refusal, comorbid medical conditions, or rapid tumor progression. In this intent-to-treat analysis, the low level of compliance could have been responsible for the lack of a clear benefit. In addition to these randomized studies, single-institution reports also have shown that postoperative chemoradiation improves overall survival (see Table 20-1).[72-74]

The Radiation Therapy Oncology Group is currently conducting a randomized trial (RTOG 9704) in which patients who have undergone pancreaticoduodenectomy are given systemic therapy consisting of either gemcitabine or 5-FU (250 mg/m^2) in a protracted infusion, followed by concurrent chemoradiation (in which both groups receive 50.4 Gy in 28 fractions to regional fields plus concurrent 5-FU [$250 \text{ mg/m}^2\text{/day}$]) followed again by either gemcitabine or 5-FU. The accrual goal of 518 patients was met by July 2002.

TABLE 20-1

Postoperative Adjuvant Chemoradiation Studies in Patients with Resectable Pancreatic Cancer

Study and Reference	Number of Patients*	EBRT Dose (Gy)	Chemotherapy Agent	Median Survival (Months)
RANDOMIZED TRIALS				
Kalser and Ellenberg, 1985[69]	21	40	5-FU	20
Surgery alone	22	—	—	11
Klinkenbijl et al, 1999[70]	60	40	5-FU	17.1
Surgery alone	54	—	—	12.6
NONRANDOMIZED TRIALS				
GITSG, 1987[71]	30	40	5-FU	18
Foo et al, 1993[72]	29	45+	±5-FU	22.8
Yeo et al, 1997[73]	120	>45	5-FU	20
Surgery alone	53	—	—	14

EBRT, External-beam radiation therapy; *GITSG*, Gastrointestinal Tumor Study Group; *5-FU*, 5-fluorouracil.
*All patients underwent pancreatectomy with curative intent.

The controversial recently reported interim results of the European Study Group of Pancreatic Cancer (ESPAC)-1 study put the benefit of radiation therapy into question.[75] The ESPAC-1 trial was a four-arm study with a 2 × 2 factorial design that compared the effects of adjuvant chemoradiation (40 Gy in a split course with concurrent 5-FU), adjuvant chemotherapy (5-FU and leucovorin), chemoradiation followed by chemotherapy, and observation alone after pancreaticoduodenectomy for pancreatic or periampullary carcinoma. Accrual for this study began in 1994, and medical centers in 11 countries have enrolled 530 patients. Most patients have been entered into the randomized 2 × 2 factorial design. However, either because of lack of access to radiation therapy or because of specific institutional bias, 188 patients were randomly assigned to receive only chemotherapy or no chemotherapy, and 68 patients were randomly assigned to receive either chemoradiation or no chemoradiation. In the latter two nonfactorial groups, patients could receive nonstandard therapy at the discretion of their treating physicians. For example, patients who were assigned in the nonfactorial design to chemotherapy or no chemotherapy could receive radiation therapy. Moreover, the nonrandom treatments were not standardized, and 25% of living patients had less than 1 month of follow-up. Preliminary analysis of all patients suggests no benefit from being given postoperative chemoradiation but a survival benefit from receiving adjuvant 5-FU and leucovorin chemotherapy. In fact, data from the 2 × 2 factorial analysis suggested that chemoradiation had a harmful effect.[75]

The nonfactorial and 2 × 2 factorial arms of the study produced contradictory results. Improved survival that did not reach statistical significance was seen for the 33 patients who were randomized to undergo postoperative adjuvant chemoradiation in the nonfactorial arm, but survival was worse in the 2 × 2 factorial arm. Inadequacies in follow-up, supportive care, or radiation therapy dose or technique could explain the inferior results suggested in the chemoradiation arm of the 2 × 2 factorial arm. In addition, for the 285 patients randomized in the 2 × 2 factorial design, postoperative chemotherapy showed no survival benefit over surgery alone, but improved survival was found in the 92 patients who received chemotherapy in the nonfactorial arm. The finding of improved survival from systemic therapy that is known to have minimal activity in metastatic disease was surprising. Because no attempt at quality assurance of radiation was made, technique cannot be assessed. These inconsistencies and apparent deficiencies in study design make accurate analysis of the findings quite difficult.

In general, in the postoperative setting, pathologic examination of the surgical specimen clarifies the indication for postoperative therapy. Treating patients who have already undergone surgical staging does generate a more uniform study population, but it also introduces a significant selection bias—only rapidly recovering patients with more favorable disease are generally included in such trials and series. Comparison of these findings with those from clinically staged patients treated with preoperative therapy must take this bias into account.

Preoperative Chemoradiation

The use of preoperative chemoradiation for pancreatic cancer requires a safe and accurate means of establishing a diagnosis, a reliable, noninvasive means of relieving biliary obstruction, and an accurate means of determining resectability. Historically, patients with a pancreatic mass have routinely undergone surgical exploration without a tissue diagnosis. The use of neoadjuvant therapy makes establishing a tissue diagnosis much more important. CT-guided fine-needle aspiration is possible for most patients, and endoscopic ultrasound-guided fine-needle aspiration is rapidly becoming the "gold standard" procedure for diagnosis. Endobiliary stents have reduced the need for percutaneous drains and palliative biliary-bypass procedures.

Preoperative chemoradiation has been used to improve tumor control rates in patients who have clearly resectable tumors and, less commonly, as a means of down-staging disease in patients who have unresectable disease. Several accepted theoretical advantages of preoperative therapy apply to pancreatic cancer: (1) reduced treatment-related toxicity; (2) better oxygenation and drug delivery, leading to enhancement of treatment efficacy; (3) increased potential for resection with negative margins; and (4) reduced risk of intraoperative tumor seeding. Because pancreatic cancer is an aggressive disease and patients often tolerate cytotoxic and surgical treatment poorly, several additional advantages of preoperative therapy also apply, namely that (1) more, if not all, patients are candidates for adjuvant treatment; (2) selection of patients for surgery is improved; and (3) the surgery may be better tolerated.

Pancreaticoduodenectomy requires complete reconstruction of the upper gastrointestinal tract, including reanastomosis of the pancreas, bile duct, and stomach. The associated morbidity often results in a lengthy recovery period. For instance, in the GITSG study, 5 (24%) of the 21 patients in the adjuvant chemoradiation group could not begin chemoradiation until more than 10 weeks after pancreaticoduodenectomy because of prolonged recovery time, despite the fact that the patients likely to be considered for the protocol were those who recovered rapidly from surgery and had good performance status. The number of patients whose recovery from surgery was delayed and therefore were not considered for postoperative adjuvant therapy is unknown. Judging from the slow accrual rate for this study (only 49 patients over 9 years), many patients must have been ineligible because of prolonged postoperative recovery. Data from The University of Texas M.D. Anderson Cancer Center[6] and Johns Hopkins University[73] suggest that at least 25% of patients who undergo pancreatico-duodenectomy do not receive the intended postoperative therapy. Also common are delays in implementation of therapy, which may allow repopulation of microscopic disease. Most, if not all, patients are eligible for preoperative therapy.

Unfortunately, most patients have incurable systemic micrometastatic disease at presentation. At the M.D. Anderson Cancer Center, 25% of patients given preoperative 5-FU–based chemoradiation for clinically resectable disease localized to the pancreas had radiographically definable liver metastases on CT scans at restaging, before surgery.[6] These patients had a median survival of 7 months and obviously would not have benefited from surgery as an initial treatment. Thus a strategy for sequencing preoperative treatments would spare such patients the morbidity and risk of mortality associated with pancreaticoduo-denectomy.

Leakage of the pancreaticojejunal anastomosis is the most common complication after pancreaticoduodenectomy. In a multivariate analysis of 120 patients enrolled in a randomized trial at the M.D. Anderson Cancer Center, receipt of preoperative chemoradiation was associated with a reduced risk of anastomotic leakage.[76] This reduction in leak rate may have been related to radiation-related glandular fibrosis and decreased exocrine output.

These results suggest that it is possible to deliver potentially beneficial adjuvant therapy to more patients, to identify patients who would be most likely to benefit from surgery by eliminating those likely to rapidly develop disseminated disease, and to minimize surgical complications through the use of a preoperative strategy.

Spitz and colleagues[6] from the M.D. Anderson Cancer Center reported a study of 142 consecutive patients with localized adenocarcinoma of the pancreatic head for whom disease was deemed resectable on the basis of pretreatment radiographic imaging. Outcome for a subset of 41 patients who completed protocol-based preoperative chemoradiation and pancreaticoduode-nectomy (standard-fractionation chemoradiation with 50.4 Gy for 27 patients and rapid-fractionation chemoradiation with 30 Gy for 14 patients) was compared with outcome for 19 patients who underwent pancreati-coduodenectomy and postoperative adjuvant chemoradiation. The overall median follow-up time for these 60 patients was 19 months.

No patient who received preoperative chemoradiation experienced a delay in surgery because of chemoradiation toxicity, but 6 (24%) of 25 eligible patients did not receive the intended postoperative chemoradiation because of delayed recovery after surgery. No significant differences in effects from chemoradiation were observed between the groups. No patient given preoperative chemoradiation and pancreaticoduodenectomy experienced local recurrence, but 10% experienced

peritoneal (regional) recurrence. Local or regional recurrence occurred in 21% of patients given pancreaticoduo-denectomy and postoperative chemoradiation. Reports of preoperative standard-fractionation chemoradiation (50.4 Gy over 5.5 weeks with concomitant 5-FU) from the M.D. Anderson Cancer Center[77] and from the Eastern Cooperative Oncology Group[78] have documented that acute gastrointestinal toxicity that leads to hospitalization occurs in up to one third of patients.

More recent data from the M.D. Anderson Cancer Center regarding 132 consecutive patients who underwent preoperative chemoradiation and pancreaticoduo-denectomy for adenocarcinoma of the pancreas also supported the use of rapid-fractionation chemoradia-tion.[79] Of these patients, 44 were given 45 to 50 Gy in 25 to 28 fractions, and 88 patients were given 30 Gy in 10 fractions. Thirty-six patients (27%) had undergone an unsuccessful attempt at tumor resection before referral, and 57 (43%) required vascular resection and reconstruction at the time of pancreaticoduodenectomy. Concurrent chemotherapy consisted of 5-FU or pacli-taxel. Seventy-four patients received intraoperative radiation therapy. Of the 129 patients evaluable for local failure (another three patients had not undergone imaging before they died), 79 had recurrences; the first site of failure in most (73%) was distant metastasis. None of the 25 patients given 45 or 50.4 Gy and intra-operative radiation therapy had local recurrence as the first site of recurrence. The overall median survival from the time of tissue diagnosis was 21 months.

In that study, survival duration was not affected by the dose of preoperative external-beam radiation, the chemotherapy agent used, or the use of intraoperative radiation. Univariate and multivariate analyses revealed superior survival times among patients who had no pathologic evidence of lymph node metastasis ($P = 0.03$). These findings suggest that in combination with pan-creaticoduodenectomy, short-course chemoradiation (30 Gy given in 10 fractions) for patients with accurately staged disease may produce survival equivalent to that of standard-fractionation chemoradiation (45 to 50 Gy in 25 to 28 fractions).

RADIOSENSITIZER INVESTIGATIONS

Preclinical evidence of the radiosensitizing and systemic activities of agents such as paclitaxel and gemcitabine has led to their evaluation in pancreatic cancer. Because the risk of systemic failure in this type of cancer is so high, the addition of any radiosensitizing agent must provide radiosensitization without significantly compromising systemic activity. The toxicity of paclitaxel and gemcitabine in combination with radiation has been established in single-institution studies, and both drugs are currently being investigated in multi-institutional trials.

Gemcitabine-based Chemoradiation

Gemcitabine, a nucleoside analogue, has been shown in preclinical and clinical studies to be active against a variety of solid tumors, including pancreatic cancer. Responses to systemic gemcitabine in patients with pancreatic adenocarcinoma have been documented in phase I and phase II clinical settings.[80,81] A recent randomized trial comparing gemcitabine and 5-FU as first-line therapy for advanced pancreatic adenocarcinoma showed a modest survival benefit for gemcitabine (median 5.65 vs. 4.41 months, $P = 0.0025$).[82] Gemcitabine also has been shown to improve cancer-related symptoms and performance status, as assessed by a quantitative clinical benefit scale, in untreated or previously treated metastatic pancreatic adenocarcinoma.[82,83] These results led the U.S. Food and Drug Administration to approve gemcitabine as first-line therapy for advanced adenocarcinoma of the pancreas.

In addition to its antitumor properties, gemcitabine is also a potent radiosensitizer.[84-88] Several phase I studies have been conducted to evaluate gemcitabine in combination with radiation (Table 20-2).[58,89-100] Although many of these studies, particularly the clinical ones, have been empirical and their findings preliminary, similarities in their overall approaches allow some generalizations to be made regarding the safety and efficacy of this combination in pancreatic cancer. Variables that have emerged as being important include the schedule, timing, dose, and infusion rate of gemcitabine when used in combination with radiation, as well as the field size and dose of radiation. Studies supporting these observations are reviewed briefly below.

Preclinical Studies

As a nucleoside analogue, gemcitabine inhibits cellular repair and repopulation, induces apoptosis, delays tumor growth, and enhances radiation-induced growth delay.[85] Studies of the kinetics of cellular recovery from gemcitabine-induced damage showed that normal tissues seem to recover more quickly than do tumor tissues.[101] Investigations at the M.D. Anderson Cancer Center indicate that gemcitabine inhibits the repair of radiation-induced DNA damage in a dose-dependent manner and that this inhibition remains apparent 24 to 48 hours after the last dose of gemcitabine.[102] Milas and colleagues[84] and Hittelman and colleagues[101] confirmed these findings in a mouse model, showing that gemcitabine produced a time-dependent inhibition of DNA synthesis and a dose-dependent radioenhancement when delivered to tumor-bearing mice at a dose of 50 mg/kg at various times before and after radiation. The greatest enhancement of tumor radioresponse in terms of tumor cure (dose modification factor, 1.54) occurred when gemcitabine was given 24 hours before irradiation. These findings indicate that the optimal combination of gemcitabine and radiation

in terms of therapeutic gain will depend on the timing and the schedule of administration of both agents.

Schedule effects have been reported by investigators at the M.D. Anderson Cancer Center[85] and the University of Michigan.[103] Both studies involved delivery of radiation to mice over 5-day periods. In the M.D. Anderson Cancer Center study,[85] gemcitabine was given once (before the radiation), twice weekly (before the first and third radiation doses), or daily (before each radiation dose). Although all of the schedules produced similar therapeutic gains, the normal tissue (the jejunum in that model) was spared only when the gemcitabine was given once. These investigators concluded that the best therapeutic ratio in that model was obtained by weekly gemcitabine dosing.[85] The University of Michigan group,[103] however, reached a different conclusion. Using a different mouse model, they compared weekly vs. biweekly dosing of gemcitabine first by identifying the equitoxic doses of gemcitabine given with fractionated irradiation to the oral mucosa, and then comparing the response of those combinations in a xenograft model. These investigators concluded that twice-weekly gemcitabine had a better therapeutic index than once-weekly gemcitabine when combined with daily radiation therapy.[103] Further work is needed to clarify this complex issue.

Clinical Studies

As noted earlier in this section, most clinical data on gemcitabine-based chemoradiation come from phase I dose-escalation studies, many of which have been published only in abstract form. Assessments of the toxicity and maximum tolerated doses of gemcitabine given with radiation are reviewed briefly below.

Dose limitations for the use of concurrent gemcitabine and radiation arise mostly from profound effects on normal tissue in the field of irradiation; in one study conducted at the M.D. Anderson Cancer Center, these effects included nausea, anorexia, abdominal pain, gastrointestinal bleeding, and dehydration.[89] Nonhematologic toxic effects were also significant and included fatigue, anorexia, nausea, vomiting, and dehydration. In the M.D. Anderson Cancer Center study, 44% of patients required admission to the hospital for management of treatment-related nausea, vomiting, and dehydration. The risk of hospitalization seemed to be dose-related; all three of the patients given weekly 500 mg/m^2 gemcitabine (the highest dose) required admission during treatment. Similar chemoradiation-related toxic effects have been reported in unresectable pancreatic cancer treated with paclitaxel, another potent radiosensitizer.[104]

Drug Infusion Rate

The rate at which the radiosensitizing agent is infused also seems to affect outcome in pancreatic cancer, indicating that the intracellular utilization may be limited by the intracellular phosphorylation of gemcitabine.

TABLE 20-2

Selected Phases I and II Studies of Gemcitabine, Radiation, and Other Agents for Pancreatic Cancer

Study and Reference	Institution or Group	Number of Patients	Radiation Dose (Field)	MTD and Schedule of Gemcitabine	Duration of Therapy (weeks)	Other Agents
Fuchs et al, 1999[91]	Dana Farber	10	50.4 Gy in 28 fx (field not stated)	Ongoing escalation	5	5-FU, 200 mg/m^2*
Safar et al, 1999[93]	Beth Israel, Boston	6	50.4 Gy in 25 fx (tumor)	Ongoing escalation	≥ 5	Cisplatin, 20 mg/m^2
Wilkowski et al, 2000[90]	Munich, Germany	13	45 Gy in 25 fx (regional)	300 (weekly)	17	5-FU, 350 mg/m^2*
Brunner et al, 2000[92]	University of Erlangen, Germany	26	55.8 Gy in 28 fx (regional)	400 (weekly)	6	Cisplatin, 20 mg/m^2 (days 1-5, 29-33)
Harris et al, 2000[94]	Emory University	29	49.5 Gy (hyperfractionated) (regional)	175 (days 1-5)	12	5-FU, 600 mg/m^2 Cisplatin, 20 mg/m^2 (days 1-5)
Wolff et al, 2001[89]	M.D. Anderson Cancer Center	18	30 Gy in 10 fx (regional)	350 (weekly)	7	
Epelbaum et al, 2000[95]	Israeli Cooperative Group	30	50.4 Gy in 28 fx (regional)	400 (weekly)	12+	
Abad et al, 1998[96]	Spanish Cooperative Group	6	45 Gy in 25 fx + 22.5 Gy (regional)	200 (weekly)	12	
McGinn et al, 1999[58]	University of Michigan	22	42 Gy in 15 fx (to gross disease)	1000[†]	7	
Hoffman et al, 1999[97]	Fox Chase Cancer Center	18	50.4 Gy in 28 fx (to gross disease)	700[‡] (weekly)	23	
Blackstock et al, 1999[98]	Wake Forest University	19	50.4 Gy in 28 fx (to the pancreas)	40 (twice weekly)	5	
Wong et al, 2000[99]	Princess Margaret Hospital	23	52.5 Gy in 20 fx, split course [†§]	40 (twice weekly)	7	
Kudrimoti et al, 1999[100]	University of Kentucky	18	40 Gy in 20 fx	125 (weekly)[‖]	5	

MTD, Maximum tolerated dose; *fx*, fractions; *5-FU*, 5-fluorouracil.

*Given as a protracted venous infusion.

[†]Gemcitabine dose was fixed and radiation dose was escalated.

[‡]Radiation dose was fixed and gemcitabine dose was escalated.

[§]Radiation schedule consisted of 20 fractions split by a 2-week rest period, after which the radiation dose per fraction was escalated.

[‖]Gemcitabine was given as a 24-hour infusion on the first day of each week of radiation (except for week 4).

In a randomized phase II trial of patients with metastatic pancreatic cancer in which the infusion rates of gemcitabine were compared,[105] the objective response rate (16.6% vs. 2.3%, verified by CT scanning), median survival duration, and overall survival rate (23% vs. 0% at 1 year) were better in patients treated with a lower dose (1500 mg/m^2, given at 10 mg/min) than those given a higher dose (2200 mg/m^2, given over 30 minutes).

These findings seem to indicate that lower doses of gemcitabine, given more slowly than in the typical 30-minute infusion, are used more efficiently than higher doses, perhaps because of the rate-limiting effects of intracellular phosphorylation of this drug. Most of the clinical studies that have been conducted to date have infused gemcitabine over 30-minute periods; no studies have evaluated higher doses given at 10 mg/min with radiation. This issue, unfortunately, further confounds interpretation of preliminary clinical data.

Radiation Field Size and Dose

The studies listed in Table 20-2[58,89-100] offer some insight as to the radiation doses and field sizes that can be used with gemcitabine. Confining fields to the tumor alone have allowed the use of weekly gemcitabine doses

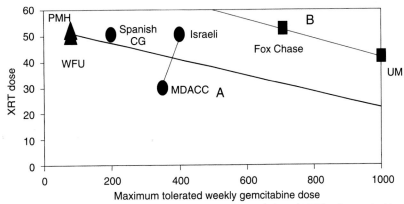

Fig. 20-2 Phase I preliminary results: maximum tolerated dose (*MTD*) of gemcitabine versus radiation therapy (*XRT*) doses. The MTD of gemcitabine is inversely proportional to the radiation field size (*A* vs. *B*), and the radiation dose (note the negative slope of both *A* and *B*). The MTD is substantially lower with biweekly dosing than with weekly dosing (*A* or *B*). *Squares* indicate small radiation fields; *ovals*, large fields; and *triangles*, biweekly gemcitabine dosing. (See Table 20-2 for data references.) *PMH*, Princess Margaret Hospital; *Spanish CG*, Spanish Cooperative Group; *Israeli*, Israeli Cooperative Group; *WFU*, Wake Forest University; *MDACC*, M.D. Anderson Cancer Center; *UM*, University of Michigan.

that are 2 to 3 times higher than doses tolerated with regional-field irradiation (Fig. 20-2). Because the gemcitabine dose limitation is attributable predominantly to gastrointestinal toxicity in the radiation field, radiation field size is a critical variable. Regardless of the drug-infusion rate, weekly doses in the range of 200 to 400 mg/m^2 are tolerated when given when radiation fields encompass the primary tumor and regional lymphatics; in contrast, doses in the range of 700 to 1000 mg/m^2 can be given when radiation is given to smaller fields. In all of the phase I trials conducted to date, either the gemcitabine dose is escalated while the radiation dose is fixed or the radiation dose is escalated while the gemcitabine dose is fixed. The dose combinations in these trials are illustrated in Figure 20-2. These preliminary prospective clinical data suggest that the maximum tolerated dose of gemcitabine seems to be linearly and inversely related to the radiation dose used.

Chemoradiation with Gemcitabine and Other Agents

Several groups have begun to investigate novel combinations of other radiosensitizing agents with radiation (see Table 20-2). Combinations studied have included regional radiation with continuous-infusion 5-FU and gemcitabine,[90,91] cisplatin and radiation with escalated doses of weekly gemcitabine,[92,93] and a combination of 5-FU, cisplatin and gemcitabine.[94] Preliminary evidence suggests that such combinations are feasible, and further studies, including multicenter trials, are ongoing.

Theoretically, normal tissue can be protected from the effects of chemoradiation by adding a pharmacologic radioprotector or using specialized techniques to ensure more accurate delivery of radiation. This concept

is appealing for gemcitabine-based chemoradiation because the effects on normal tissue are so profound. The addition of amifostine to twice-weekly gemcitabine protocols has recently been reported to allow the gemcitabine dose in a twice-weekly gemcitabine-based chemoradiation schedule to be escalated from 60 mg/m^2 to 120 mg/m^2.[106] These promising results should be investigated further. Another recent phase I dose-escalation trial at the M.D. Anderson Cancer Center attempted to evaluate whether dynamic intensity-modulated radiation would allow escalation of either chemotherapy or radiation dose (unpublished data). The trial was closed, however, because of excessive gastrointestinal and hematologic toxicity, findings that could have resulted from increased dose heterogeneity from organ motion or an increased integral dose to the spleen or circulating hematologic elements. Although these findings are hardly definitive, they at least affirmed that dynamic intensity-modulated radiation does not necessarily improve the therapeutic ratio when used with toxic combinations of chemotherapy and radiation. Although dynamic intensity-modulated radiation has been abandoned for this purpose at the M.D. Anderson Cancer Center, static-field intensity-modulated radiation should perhaps be investigated.

Summary

Important observations from the phase I clinical data are that the amount of acute toxicity from gemcitabine-based chemoradiation is strongly related to the dose and administration schedule of gemcitabine as well as the radiation field size. The maximum tolerated gemcitabine dose seems to be inversely and linearly related to the radiation dose that is used. Preclinical evidence suggests that the timing of administration is also important, but this issue has yet to be confirmed by clinical findings. Also important, but less clear, is the effect of infusion rate on the systemic efficacy of gemcitabine. The addition of other agents to gemcitabine and radiation seems feasible. Finally, the addition of radioprotectors may enable chemotherapy dose escalation, but safe escalation of the radiation dose with newer techniques has not been established.

Encouraging findings with regard to the emergence of pathologic complete response with acceptable treatment-related toxicity from several institutions (authors' unpublished observations) provide evidence of gemcitabine's potential as a radiosensitizer. As the results of these preliminary experiences mature, treatment efficacy can be examined through comparative, multi-institutional trials. Only then will we be able to draw conclusions about important issues such as the optimal dose, schedule, and combination of agents to use with radiation therapy in pancreatic cancer.

DOWN-STAGING INITIALLY UNRESECTABLE DISEASE

The interpretation of down-staging is limited by nonuniform definitions and inadequate preoperative assessment of resectability. Chemoradiation based on 5-FU is unlikely to produce meaningful down-staging in more than a very few patients. Whether true "down-staging," that is, conversion of unresectable disease to resectable disease, actually occurs is controversial and impossible to prove in the absence of defined criteria for resectability that actually show change on standardized imaging. Because current surgical definitions of resectability differ widely and are often subjective, studies that include unresectable or "potentially resectable" patients who subsequently undergo resection after neoadjuvant therapy must use defined and reproducible criteria for resection if the issue of down-staging is to be addressed.

Chemoradiation has been administered to patients with locally advanced, unresectable pancreatic cancer in an effort to improve survival and, more recently, to down-stage the disease so as to allow surgical resection. Because surgical resection of the primary tumor remains the only potentially curative treatment for pancreatic cancer, preoperative chemoradiation has been studied for its ability to convert locally unresectable pancreatic cancer to resectable disease (Table 20-3).[107-116]

Early studies used 5-FU–based chemoradiation, and subsequently, various combinations of agents have been used. Newer radiosensitizers such as paclitaxel and gemcitabine have been tested. Review of the available literature suggests that only 8% to 16% of patients with clinically unresectable disease treated with 5-FU–based or paclitaxel-based chemoradiation are able to eventually undergo margin-negative resection. Preliminary reports in abstract form indicate that the margin-negative resectability rate could be as high as 40% to 50% in selected unresectable patients treated with gemcitabine-based chemoradiation (see Table 20-3). These studies suggest that the combination of multiple, more effective radiosensitizers with radiation therapy may result in significant local tumor response.

However, as the definition of locally advanced pancreatic cancer is broadened, results will appear more promising. Thus all studies of novel chemoradiation regimens should adhere to a strict CT-based definition of locally advanced pancreatic cancer that includes arterial involvement (low-density tumor inseparable from the superior mesenteric artery or celiac axis on contrast-enhanced CT) or venous occlusion. A multi-institutional randomized phase II study, to be conducted by the Eastern Cooperative and Radiation Therapy Oncology Groups, is planned with the goal of increasing resectability of locally advanced disease.

PROPHYLACTIC HEPATIC IRRADIATION

Two single institutions and the Radiation Therapy Oncology Group have prospectively evaluated prophylactic hepatic irradiation. At the M.D. Anderson Cancer Center, a phase I trial of preoperative radiation therapy for patients with resectable disease used 50.4 Gy to the pancreatic head and regional lymphatics and 23.4 Gy to the whole liver with concurrent continuous infusion of 5-FU (300 mg/m^2/day, Monday to Friday). The study was abandoned after two early treatment-related deaths among 11 patients.[117]

At Johns Hopkins University, a prospective study of patients who had undergone resection evaluated 50.4 to 57.6 Gy of external-beam radiation to the operative bed and regional lymphatics and 23.4 to 27.0 Gy to the whole liver with concurrent continuous-infusion 5-FU (200 mg/m^2/day) and leucovorin (5 mg/m^2) both given Monday through Friday. That treatment was followed by four cycles of the same chemotherapy 1 month after completion of the radiation. Although the toxicity of this regimen was judged acceptable, the site of first failure was the liver in 9 of the 21 patients so treated.[74]

In a study by the Radiation Therapy Oncology Group of localized, unresectable pancreatic cancer, 61.2 Gy was delivered to the primary disease site and 23.4 Gy to the whole liver with a concurrent 5-day continuous infusion of 5-FU (1000 mg/m^2/day) on days 1 and 30, followed by a weekly bolus of 600 mg/m^2 for 6 months beginning 3 weeks after the completion of therapy. More than half of the patients had grade 3 or greater acute reactions, and the median survival time was only 8.4 months. The first site of failure was the liver in 13% of the patients, which is less than what would be expected from historical controls; however, survival remained poor because of local failure and intra-abdominal metastasis.[10]

TABLE 20-3

Experience with Neoadjuvant Chemoradiation to Allow Eventual Surgical Resection in Patients with Locally Advanced Pancreatic Cancer

Study and Reference	Number of Patients	EBRT Dose (Gy)	Chemotherapy	Number Showing Radiographic Response	Number Undergoing Surgical Resection	Percent with Margin-Negative Resections	Median Survival (months)
5-FU–BASED CHEMORADIATION							
Kornek et al, 2000[107]	38	55	5-FU + LV + cisplatin	4 CR 14 PR	3	8	14
Bajetta et al, 1999[108]	32	50	5-DFUR	7 PR	5	16	9
White et al, 1999[109]	25	45	5-FU + Mito (12) or cisplatin (10)	6 of 22 showed shrinkage of >1 cm	5[*] (1 CR[†])	8	NS
Todd et al, 1998[110]	38	0	5-FU + LV + Mito + dipyridamole	1 CR 14 PR	4 (1 CR[†])	11	15.5
Kamthan et al, 1997[111]	35	54	5-FU + STZ + cisplatin	6 CR 9 PR	5 (2 CR[†])	14	15
Jessup et al, 1993[112]	16	45	5-FU	NS	2	13	9.6[‡]
Jeekel and Treurniet-Donker, 1991[113]	20	50 (split course)	5-FU	NS	2	10	10
PACLITAXEL-BASED CHEMORADIATION							
DiPetrillo, 2000[114]	40	50.4	Paclitaxel	PR, 11 of 38 (29%)	3	8	8.5
Safran et al, 1999[115]	24	50.4	Paclitaxel	PR, 6 of 18	2	8	NS
GEMCITABINE-BASED CHEMORADIATION							
McGinn et al, 2000[116]	22	24-50.4	Gem	8	5	23	NS
Brunner et al, 2000[92]	24	55.8	Gem + cisplatin	NS	7 of 13	54	NS
Epelbaum et al, 2000[95]	20	50.4	Gem	PR, 4	2	10	12
Wilkowski et al, 2000[90]	10	45	Gem + 5-FU	7	5[§]	40	NS

EBRT, External-beam radiation therapy; *5-FU,* 5-fluorouracil; *LV,* leucovorin; *CR,* complete response; *PR,* partial response; *5-DFUR,* doxifluridine; *Mito,* mitomycin C; *STZ,* streptozocin; *NS,* not stated; *Gem,* gemcitabine.
[*]Three of five had positive resection margins.
[†]Histologic complete response.
[‡]Mean.
[§]One of five had positive resection margins.

ADJUVANT THERAPY FOR AMPULLARY CARCINOMAS

The reported 5-year survival rate for patients with ampullary carcinomas is 2 to 3 times greater than for patients with lesions arising in the pancreas. A significant regional spread pattern was documented at Johns Hopkins; in a recent report, regional nodal involvement was found in 20 (43%) of the 46 patients who underwent resection.[118] The recognition that resection can carry a better prognosis has led some investigators to not recommend postoperative therapy. The same investigators at Johns Hopkins subsequently reported a disease-free survival rate of 90% in patients with periampullary tumors treated with postoperative therapy.[119] These results are by no means definitive, but with longer follow-up this series could provide important evidence that the use of adjuvant therapy improves outcome in this population. Although the role of adjuvant chemoradiation has not been defined for ampullary carcinomas, early results regarding the pattern of spread suggest that it may confer benefit.

REFERENCES

1. Coia LR, Myerson RJ, Tepper JE. Late effects of radiation therapy on the gastrointestinal tract. *Int J Radiat Oncol Biol Phys* 1995; 31:1213-1236.
2. Goldgraber M, Rubin C, Palmer W, et al. The early gastric response to irradiation, a serial biopsy study. *Gastroenterology* 1954;27:1-20.
3. Roswitt B, Malsky S, Reid C. Radiation tolerance of the gastrointestinal tract. *Front Radiat Ther Oncol* 1971;5:160-180.
4. Hamilton F. Gastric ulcer following radiation. *Arch Surg* 1947; 55:394-399.
5. Moertel CG, Frytak S, Hahn RG, et al. Therapy of locally unresectable pancreatic carcinoma: a randomized comparison of high dose (6000 rads) radiation alone, moderate dose radiation (4000 rads + 5-fluorouracil), and high dose radiation + 5-fluorouracil: the Gastrointestinal Tumor Study Group. *Cancer* 1981;48:1705-1710.
6. Spitz FR, Abbruzzese JL, Lee JE, et al. Preoperative and postoperative chemoradiation strategies in patients treated with pancreaticoduodenectomy for adenocarcinoma of the pancreas. *J Clin Oncol* 1997;15:928-937.
7. Dawson LA, McGinn CJ, Normolle D, et al. Escalated focal liver radiation and concurrent hepatic artery fluorodeoxyuridine for unresectable intrahepatic malignancies. *J Clin Oncol* 2000;18: 2210-2218.
8. Willett CG, Tepper JE, Orlow EL, et al. Renal complications secondary to radiation treatment of upper abdominal malignancies. *Int J Radiat Oncol Biol Phys* 1986;12:1601-1604.
9. Lawrence TS, Robertson JM, Anscher MS, et al. Hepatic toxicity resulting from cancer treatment. *Int J Radiat Oncol Biol Phys* 1995; 31:1237-1248.
10. Komaki R, Wadler S, Peters T, et al. High-dose local irradiation plus prophylactic hepatic irradiation and chemotherapy for inoperable adenocarcinoma of the pancreas. A preliminary report of a multi-institutional trial (Radiation Therapy Oncology Group Protocol 8801). *Cancer* 1992;69:2807-2812.
11. Ingold J, Reed G, Kaplan H, et al. Radiation hepatitis. *AJR Am J Roentgenol* 1965;93:200-208.
12. Lawrence TS, Ten Haken RK, Kessler ML, et al. The use of 3-D dose volume analysis to predict radiation hepatitis. *Int J Radiat Oncol Biol Phys* 1992;23:781-788.
13. McGinn CJ, Ten Haken RK, Ensminger WD, et al. Treatment of intrahepatic cancers with radiation doses based on a normal tissue complication probability model. *J Clin Oncol* 1998;16:2246-2252.
14. Greenlee RT, Hill-Harmon MB, Murray T, et al. Cancer statistics, 2001. *CA Cancer J Clin* 2001; 51:15-36.
15. Gordis L, Gold EB. Epidemiology of pancreatic cancer. *World J Surg* 1984;8:808-821.
16. Ahlgren JD. Epidemiology and risk factors in pancreatic cancer. *Semin Oncol* 1996;23:241-250.
17. Howe GR. Pancreatic cancer. *Cancer Surv* 1994;19-20:139-158.
18. Whittemore AS, Paffenbarger RS Jr, Anderson K, et al. Early precursors of pancreatic cancer in college men. *J Chronic Dis* 1983; 36:251-256.
19. Best EW, Walker CB, Baker PM, et al. Summary of a Canadian study of smoking and health. *CMAJ* 1967;96:1104-1108.
20. Velema JP, Walker AM, Gold EB. Alcohol and pancreatic cancer. Insufficient epidemiologic evidence for a causal relationship. *Epidemiol Rev* 1986;8:28-41.
21. Howe GR, Burch JD. Nutrition and pancreatic cancer. *Cancer Causes Control* 1996;7:69-82.
22. Gold EB. Epidemiology of and risk factors for pancreatic cancer. *Surg Clin North Am* 1995;75:819-843.
23. Garabrant DH, Held J, Langholz B, et al. DDT and related compounds and risk of pancreatic cancer. *J Natl Cancer Inst* 1992; 84:764-771.
24. Mancuso TF, el-Attar AA. Cohort study of workers exposed to betanaphthylamine and benzidine. *J Occup Med* 1967;9: 277-285.
25. Krause JR, Ayuyang HQ, Ellis LD. Secondary non-hematopoietic cancers arising following treatment of hematopoietic disorders. *Cancer* 1985;55:512-515.
26. Everhart J, Wright D. Diabetes mellitus as a risk factor for pancreatic cancer. A meta-analysis. *JAMA* 1995;273:1605-1609.
27. Gullo L, Pezzilli R, Morselli-Labate AM. Diabetes and the risk of pancreatic cancer. Italian Pancreatic Cancer Study Group. *N Engl J Med* 1994;331:81-84.
28. Gold EB, Cameron JL. Chronic pancreatitis and pancreatic cancer. *N Engl J Med* 1993;328:1485-1486.
29. Hruban RH, Petersen GM, Goggins M, et al. Familial pancreatic cancer. *Ann Oncol* 1999;10(suppl 4):69-73.
30. Fernandez E, La Vecchia C, D'Avanzo B, et al. Family history and the risk of liver, gallbladder, and pancreatic cancer. *Cancer Epidemiol Biomarkers Prev* 1994;3(3):209-212.
31. Fuhrman G, Charnsagavej C, Abbruzzese J, et al. Thin-section contrast-enhanced computed tomography accurately predicts resectability of malignant pancreatic neoplasms. *Am J Surg* 1994; 167:104-113.
32. Ichikawa T, Haradome H, Hachiya J, et al. Pancreatic ductal adenocarcinoma: preoperative assessment with helical CT versus dynamic MR imaging. *Radiology* 1997;202:655-662.
33. Ferrari AP Jr, Lichtenstein DR, Slivka A, et al. Brush cytology during ERCP for the diagnosis of biliary and pancreatic malignancies. *Gastrointest Endosc* 1994;40:140-145.
34. Rosch T, Lorenz R, Braig C, et al. Endoscopic ultrasonography in diagnosis and staging of pancreatic and biliary tumors. *Endoscopy* 1992;24(suppl 1):304-308.
35. Ritts RE Jr, Nagorney DM, Jacobsen DJ, et al. Comparison of preoperative serum CA19-9 levels with results of diagnostic imaging modalities in patients undergoing laparotomy for suspected pancreatic or gallbladder disease. *Pancreas* 1994;9: 707-716.
36. Whipple A, Parson W, Mullin C. Treatment of carcinoma of the ampulla of Vater. *Ann Surg* 1935;763-779.
37. Makary MA, Warshaw AL, Centeno BA, et al. Implications of peritoneal cytology for pancreatic cancer management. *Arch Surg* 1998;133:361-365.
38. Yeo CJ, Cameron JL, Lillemoe KD, et al. Pancreaticoduodenectomy for cancer of the head of the pancreas. 201 patients. *Ann Surg* 1995; 221:721-731.
39. Willett CG, Lewandrowski K, Warshaw AL, et al. Resection margins in carcinoma of the head of the pancreas. Implications for radiation therapy. *Ann Surg* 1993;217:144-148.
40. Mohiuddin M, Cantor RJ, Biermann W, et al. Combined modality treatment of localized unresectable adenocarcinoma of the pancreas. *Int J Radiat Oncol Biol Phys* 1988;14:79-84.
41. A multi-institutional comparative trial of radiation therapy alone and in combination with 5-fluorouracil for locally unresectable pancreatic carcinoma. The Gastrointestinal Tumor Study Group. *Ann Surg* 1979;189:205-208.
42. Radiation therapy combined with Adriamycin or 5-fluorouracil for the treatment of locally unresectable pancreatic carcinoma. Gastrointestinal Tumor Study Group. *Cancer* 1985;56:2563-2568.
43. Treatment of locally unresectable carcinoma of the pancreas: comparison of combined-modality therapy (chemotherapy plus radiotherapy) to chemotherapy alone. Gastrointestinal Tumor Study Group. *J Natl Cancer Inst* 1988;80:751-755.

44. Moertel CG, Childs DS Jr, Reitemeier RJ, et al. Combined 5-fluorouracil and supervoltage radiation therapy of locally unresectable gastrointestinal cancer. *Lancet* 1969;2:865-867.

45. Klaassen DJ, MacIntyre JM, Catton GE, et al. Treatment of locally unresectable cancer of the stomach and pancreas: a randomized comparison of 5-fluorouracil alone with radiation plus concurrent and maintenance 5-fluorouracil—an Eastern Cooperative Oncology Group study. *J Clin Oncol* 1985;3:373-378.

46. Warshaw AL, Fernandez-del Castillo C. Pancreatic carcinoma. *N Engl J Med* 1992;326:455-465.

47. Trede M. The surgical treatment of pancreatic carcinoma. *Surgery* 1985;97:28-35.

48. Yeo CJ, Cameron JL, Sohn TA, et al. Six hundred fifty consecutive pancreaticoduodenectomies in the 1990s: pathology, complications, and outcomes. *Ann Surg* 1997;226:248-257.

49. Fleming I, Cooper JS, Henson DE, et al, eds. *AJCC Cancer Staging Manual.* 5th ed. Philadelphia, Pa: Lippincott Williams & Wilkins; 1997;121-126.

50. Kawarada Y, Isaji S. Stage classifications of pancreatic cancer: comparison of the Japanese and UICC classifications and proposal for a new staging system. Union Internationale Contre le Cancer. *Pancreas* 1998;16:255-264.

51. Takeuchi M, Kondo S, Sugiura H, et al. Pre-operative predictors of short-term survival after pancreatic cancer resection. *Hepatogastroenterology* 1998;45:2399-2403.

52. Ozaki H, Hiraoka T, Mizumoto R, et al. The prognostic significance of lymph node metastasis and intrapancreatic perineural invasion in pancreatic cancer after curative resection. *Surg Today* 1999;29:16-22.

53. Birk D, Fortnagel G, Formentini A, et al. Small carcinoma of the pancreas. Factors of prognostic relevance. *J Hepatobiliary Pancreat Surg* 1998;5:450-454.

54. Millikan KW, Deziel DJ, Silverstein JC, et al. Prognostic factors associated with resectable adenocarcinoma of the head of the pancreas. *Am Surg* 1999;65:618-623; discussion 623-624.

55. Yeo CJ, Cameron JL. Prognostic factors in ductal pancreatic cancer. *Langenbecks Arch Surg* 1998;383:129-133.

56. Westerdahl J, Andren-Sandberg A, Ihse I. Recurrence of exocrine pancreatic cancer—local or hepatic? *Hepatogastroenterology* 1993;40:384-387.

57. Griffin JF, Smalley SR, Jewell W, et al. Patterns of failure after curative resection of pancreatic carcinoma. *Cancer* 1990;66:56-61.

58. McGinn C, Shureiqi J, Robertson J, et al. A phase I trial of radiation dose escalation with full dose gemcitabine in patients with pancreatic cancer [abstract]. *Proc Am Soc Clin Oncol* 1999;18:274a.

59. Higgins PD, Sohn JW, Fine RM, et al. Three-dimensional conformal pancreas treatment: comparison of four- to six-field techniques. *Int J Radiat Oncol Biol Phys* 1995;31:605-609.

60. Balter JM, Lam KL, McGinn CJ, et al. Improvement of CT-based treatment-planning models of abdominal targets using static exhale imaging. *Int J Radiat Oncol Biol Phys* 1998;41:939-943.

61. Ramsey CR, Scaperoth D, Arwood D, et al. Clinical efficacy of respiratory gated conformal radiation therapy. *Med Dosim* 1999;24:115-119.

62. Roldan GE, Gunderson LL, Nagorney DM, et al. External beam versus intraoperative and external beam irradiation for locally advanced pancreatic cancer. *Cancer* 1988;61:1110-1116.

63. Gunderson LL, Martin JK, Kvols LK, et al. Intraoperative and external beam irradiation +/- 5-FU for locally advanced pancreatic cancer. *Int J Radiat Oncol Biol Phys* 1987;13:319-329.

64. Mohiuddin M, Regine WF, Stevens J, et al. Combined intraoperative radiation and perioperative chemotherapy for unresectable cancers of the pancreas. *J Clin Oncol* 1995;13:2764-2768.

65. Garton GR, Gunderson LL, Nagorney DM, et al. High-dose preoperative external beam and intraoperative irradiation for locally advanced pancreatic cancer. *Int J Radiat Oncol Biol Phys* 1993;27:1153-1157.

66. Shipley WU, Tepper JE, Warshaw AL, et al. Intraoperative radiation therapy for patients with pancreatic carcinoma. *World J Surg* 1984;8:929-934.

67. Mohiuddin M, Rosato F, Barbot D, et al. Long-term results of combined modality treatment with I-125 implantation for carcinoma of the pancreas. *Int J Radiat Oncol Biol Phys* 1992;23:305-311.

68. Shipley WU, Nardi GL, Cohen AM, et al. Iodine-125 implant and external beam irradiation in patients with localized pancreatic carcinoma: a comparative study to surgical resection. *Cancer* 1980;45:709-714.

69. Kalser MH, Ellenberg SS. Pancreatic cancer. Adjuvant combined radiation and chemotherapy following curative resection [published erratum in Arch Surg 1986; 121:1045]. *Arch Surg* 1985;120:899-903.

70. Klinkenbijl JH, Jeekel J, Sahmoud T, et al. Adjuvant radiotherapy and 5-fluorouracil after curative resection of cancer of the pancreas and periampullary region: phase III trial of the EORTC Gastrointestinal Tract Cancer Cooperative group. *Ann Surg* 1999;230:776-782; discussion 782-784.

71. Further evidence of effective adjuvant combined radiation and chemotherapy following curative resection of pancreatic cancer. Gastrointestinal Tumor Study Group. *Cancer* 1987;59:2006-2010.

72. Foo ML, Gunderson LL, Nagorney DM, et al. Patterns of failure in grossly resected pancreatic ductal adenocarcinoma treated with adjuvant irradiation +/- 5 fluorouracil. *Int J Radiat Oncol Biol Phys* 1993;26:483-489.

73. Yeo CJ, Abrams RA, Grochow LB, et al. Pancreaticoduodenectomy for pancreatic adenocarcinoma: postoperative adjuvant chemoradiation improves survival: a prospective, single-institution experience. *Ann Surg* 1997;225:621-633; discussion 633-636.

74. Abrams RA, Grochow LB, Chakravarthy A, et al. Intensified adjuvant therapy for pancreatic and periampullary adenocarcinoma: survival results and observations regarding patterns of failure, radiotherapy dose and CA19-9 levels. *Int J Radiat Oncol Biol Phys* 1999;44:1039-1046.

75. Neoptolemos JP, Dunn JA, Stocken DD, et al. Adjuvant chemoradiotherapy and chemotherapy in resectable pancreatic cancer: a randomised controlled trial. *Lancet* 2002;358:1576-1585.

76. Lowy AM, Lee JE, Pisters PW, et al. Prospective, randomized trial of octreotide to prevent pancreatic fistula after pancreaticoduodenectomy for malignant disease. *Ann Surg* 1997;226:632-641.

77. Evans DB, Rich TA, Byrd DR, et al. Preoperative chemoradiation and pancreaticoduodenectomy for adenocarcinoma of the pancreas. *Arch Surg* 1992;127:1335-1339.

78. Hoffman JP, Lipsitz S, Pisansky T, et al. Phase II trial of preoperative radiation therapy and chemotherapy for patients with localized, resectable adenocarcinoma of the pancreas: an Eastern Cooperative Oncology Group Study. *J Clin Oncol* 1998;16:317-323.

79. Breslin TM, Hess KR, Harbison DB, et al. Neoadjuvant chemoradiation for adenocarcinoma of the pancreas: treatment variables and survival duration. *Ann Surg Oncol* 2001;8:123-132.

80. Casper ES, Green MR, Kelsen DP, et al. Phase II trial of gemcitabine (2,2'-difluorodeoxycytidine) in patients with adenocarcinoma of the pancreas. *Invest New Drugs* 1994;12:29-34.

81. Abbruzzese JL, Grunewald R, Weeks EA, et al. A phase I clinical, plasma, and cellular pharmacology study of gemcitabine. *J Clin Oncol* 1991;9:491-498.

82. Burris HA III, Moore MJ, Andersen J, et al. Improvements in survival and clinical benefit with gemcitabine as first-line therapy for patients with advanced pancreas cancer: a randomized trial. *J Clin Oncol* 1997;15:2403–2413.

83. Rothenberg ML, Burris HA III, Anderson JS, et al. Gemcitabine: effective palliative therapy for pancreas cancer patients failing 5-FU [abstract]. *Proc Am Soc Clin Oncol* 1995;14:198a.

84. Milas L, Fujii T, Hunter N, et al. Enhancement of tumor radioresponse in vivo by gemcitabine. *Cancer Res* 1999;59:107-114.

85. Mason KA, Milas L, Hunter NR, et al. Maximizing therapeutic gain with gemcitabine and fractionated radiation. *Int J Radiat Oncol Biol Phys* 1999;44:1125-1135.

86. Joschko M, Webster L, Groves J, et al. Radioenhancement by gemcitabine with accelerated fractionated radiotherapy in a human tumor xenograft model. *Radiat Oncol Investig* 1997;5:62-71.

87. Lawrence TS, Chang EY, Hahn TM, et al. Radiosensitization of pancreatic cancer cells by 2',2'-difluoro-2'-deoxycytidine. *Int J Radiat Oncol Biol Phys* 1996;34:867-872.

88. Lawrence T, Eisbruch A, Shewach D. Gemcitabine-mediated radiosensitization. *Semin Oncol* 1997;24:S724-S728.

89. Wolff RA, Evans DB, Gravel DM, et al. Phase I trial of gemcitabine combined with radiation for the treatment of locally advanced pancreatic adenocarcinoma. *Clin Cancer Res* 2001; 7:2246-2253.

90. Wilkowski R, Heinemann V, Rau H. Radiochemotherapy including gemcitabine and 5-fluorouracil for treatment of locally advanced pancreatic cancer [abstract]. *Proc Am Soc Clin Oncol* 2000;19:1078a.

91. Fuchs C, Clark JW, Berg DT, et al. Phase I trial of concurrent gemcitabine, infusional 5-FU, and radiation therapy in patients with localized, unresectable pancreatic cancer [abstract]. *Proc Am Soc Clinl Oncol* 1999;18:1091a.

92. Brunner T, Grabenbauer G, Kasti S, et al. A phase I trial of simultaneous gemcitabine/cisplatin and radiotherapy for patients with locally advanced pancreatic cancer [abstract]. *Proc Am Soc Clin Oncol* 2000;19:1109a.

93. Safar A, Altamira P, Recht A, et al. Phase I trial of gemcitabine, cisplatin, and external beam radiation therapy [abstract]. *Proc Am Soc Clin Oncol* 1999;18:227a.

94. Harris W, Landry J, Staley C, et al. A phase I study of gemcitabine, cisplatin, and 5-fluorouracil with radiation for patients with advanced GI malignancies [abstract 87U]. *Proc Am Soc Clin Oncol* 2000;19:1205.

95. Epelbaum R, Rosenblatt E, Nasrallah S, et al. Phase II study of gemcitabine combined with radiation therapy in localized, unresectable pancreatic cancer [abstract]. *Proc Am Soc Clin Oncol* 2000;19:1029a.

96. Abad A, Arellano A, Brunet J, et al. Gemcitabine plus radiotherapy in stage II-III pancreatic cancer: a phase I trial [abstract]. *Proc 23rd Congress Eur Soc Med Oncol* 1998:253a.

97. Hoffman J, McGinn C, Ross E, et al. A phase I trial of preoperative gemcitabine and radiotherapy followed by postoperative gemcitabine for patients with localized, resectable, pancreatic adenocarcinoma. *Cancer Invest* 1999;17:30-32.

98. Blackstock A, Bernard S, Richards F, et al. Phase I trial of twice-weekly gemcitabine and concurrent radiation in patients with advanced pancreatic cancer. *J Clin Oncol* 1999;17:2208-2212.

99. Wong S, Oza A, Brierley J, et al. Phase I trial of gemcitabine and escalating dose radiation therapy in patients with pancreatic carcinoma [abstract]. *Proc Am Soc Clin Oncol* 2000;19:1041a.

100. Kudrimoti M, Regine W, Hanna N, et al. Concurrent gemcitabine and radiation in the treatment of advanced unresectable GI malignancy: a phase I/II study [abstract 928]. *Proc Am Soc Clin Oncol* 1999;18:242a.

101. Hittelman W, Fujii T, Hunter N, et al. Identification of a window of therapeutic opportunity for the combination of gemcitabine and radiation [abstract]. *Proc Annu Meet Am Assoc Cancer Res* 1996;37:A1973.

102. Huang N, Hittelman W. Transient inhibition of chromosome damage repair after ionizing radiation by gemcitabine [abstract A3643]. *Proc Annu Meet Am Assoc Cancer Res* 1995;36:612.

103. Fields MT, Eisbruch A, Normolle D, et al. Radiosensitization produced in vivo by once- vs. twice-weekly 2'2'-difluoro-2'-deoxycytidine (gemcitabine). *Int J Radiat Oncol Biol Phys* 2000; 47:785-791.

104. Safran H, Cioffi W, Iannitti D, et al. Paclitaxel and concurrent radiation for locally advanced pancreatic carcinoma. *Front Biosci* 1998;3:E204-E206.

105. Tempero M, Plunkett W, Ruiz V, et al. Randomized phase II trial of dose intense gemcitabine by standard infusion vs. fixed dose rate in metastatic pancreatic adenocarcinoma [abstract]. *Proc Am Soc Clin Oncol* 1999;18:1048a.

106. Yavuz A, Aydin F, Yavuz M, et al. A Phase I trial of radiation therapy plus concurrent fixed dose amifostine with escalating doses of twice-weekly gemcitabine in advanced pancreatic cancer [abstract]. *Proc Am Soc Clin Oncol* 2000;19:1105a.

107. Kornek GV, Schratter-Sehn A, Marczell A, et al. Treatment of unresectable, locally advanced pancreatic adenocarcinoma with combined radiochemotherapy with 5-fluorouracil, leucovorin and cisplatin. *Br J Cancer* 2000;82:98-103.

108. Bajetta E, Di Bartolomeo M, Stani SC, et al. Chemoradiotherapy as preoperative treatment in locally advanced unresectable pancreatic cancer patients: results of a feasibility study. *Int J Radiat Oncol Biol Phys* 1999;45:285-289.

109. White R, Lee C, Anscher M, et al. Preoperative chemoradiation for patients with locally advanced adenocarcinoma of the pancreas. *Ann Surg Oncol* 1999;6:38-45.

110. Todd KE, Gloor B, Lane JS, et al. Resection of locally advanced pancreatic cancer after downstaging with continuous-infusion 5-fluorouracil, mitomycin-C, leucovorin, and dipyridamole. *J Gastrointest Surg* 1998;2:159-166.

111. Kamthan AG, Morris JC, Dalton J, et al. Combined modality therapy for stage II and stage III pancreatic carcinoma. *J Clin Oncol* 1997;15:2920-2927.

112. Jessup JM, Steele G Jr, Mayer RJ, et al. Neoadjuvant therapy for unresectable pancreatic adenocarcinoma. *Arch Surg* 1993; 128:559-564.

113. Jeekel J, Treurniet-Donker AD. Treatment perspectives in locally advanced unresectable pancreatic cancer. *Br J Surg* 1991; 78:1332-1334.

114. DiPetrillo T. Paclitaxel and concurrent radiation for locally advanced pancreatic cancer [abstract 1152]. *Proc Am Soc Clin Oncol* 2000;19:294.

115. Safran H, Akerman P, Cioffi W, et al. Paclitaxel and concurrent radiation therapy for locally advanced adenocarcinomas of the pancreas, stomach, and gastroesophageal junction. *Semin Radiat Oncol* 1999;9:53-57.

116. McGinn CJ, Shureiqi I, Eckhauser FI, et al. Surgical resection following concurrent gemcitabine/radiation therapy in patients with previously unresectable pancreatic cancer. *Radiother Oncol* 2000;56:S57.

117. Evans DB, Abbruzzese JL, Cleary KR, et al. Preoperative chemoradiation for adenocarcinoma of the pancreas: excessive toxicity of prophylactic hepatic irradiation. *Int J Radiat Oncol Biol Phys* 1995;33:913-918.

118. Yeo CJ, Sohn TA, Cameron JL, et al. Periampullary adenocarcinoma: analysis of 5-year survivors. *Ann Surg* 1998; 227:821-831.

119. Chakravarthy A, Abrams R, Yeo C, et al. Intensified adjuvant combined modality therapy for resected periampullary adenocarcinoma: acceptable toxicity and suggestion of improved 1-year disease-free survival. *Int J Radiat Oncol Biol Phys* 2000; 48:1089-1096.

CHAPTER 21

The Liver and Biliary System

Kenneth R. Stevens, Jr.

TOLERANCE OF THE LIVER TO RADIATION

Liver tolerance depends on both the radiation dose and the relative volume of liver that is irradiated. Whole-liver irradiation, with doses ranging from 13 Gy in 18 days to 51 Gy in 40 days, produces no immediate evidence of liver dysfunction or injury. However, 2 to 6 weeks after the completion of such irradiation, one third of patients have evidence of liver abnormalities such as enlarged liver, ascites, or elevated serum alkaline phosphatase. The threshold tolerance dose for irradiating the entire liver in normal adults is 30 Gy; 75% of patients given more than 40 Gy develop liver dysfunction. Histologic acute abnormalities occur primarily in the centrilobular region and consist of sinusoidal congestion, hyperemia or hemorrhage, some atrophy of the central hepatic cells, and mild dilatation of central veins. Late changes are variable, although atrophy of the centrilobular hepatic cords and thickening of the central vein wall have been seen. Fajardo and Colby[1] proposed that radiation hepatitis is characterized by endothelial lesions with fibrinous deposits that trap erythrocytes. Collagen condenses and replaces the fibrin, leading to venous obstruction.[2]

When radiation fields are limited to the biliary tumor bed and adjacent nodal areas, radiation-induced hepatic dysfunction has been rare. Kopelson and colleagues[3] have reported asymptomatic, nonobstructing biliary fibrosis after 60 Gy of external irradiation. Gastrointestinal bleeding has been reported to occur in 25% to 30% of patients given external irradiation plus transluminal therapy with [192]Ir.

The Hepatic Normal-Tissue Complication Probability Model

Preirradiation estimates of liver radiation tolerance are difficult when liver function is damaged or when the total liver volume has been reduced by cancer, chemotherapy, or previous disease. No accurate measure of liver reserve exists, although liver function tests coupled with computed tomography (CT) or isotope scanning, angiography, and sonography are extremely helpful. The challenge for radiation oncologists is in balancing the severity of parenchymal destruction produced in irradiating a volume of liver against the degree of functional restoration that is likely to be achieved. Maintaining this balance becomes increasingly difficult as the volume to be subjected to high-dose radiation increases in size. In critical situations, the guides are to keep the high-dose volume as small as practical by using multiple portals and by using reduced fields for the final one third of the treatment. If high doses are given to a segment of the liver, then that segment will cease to function after a few weeks.

In their attempts to safely escalate the radiation dose for intrahepatic cancer, researchers at the University of Michigan Department of Radiation Oncology developed a hepatic normal-tissue complication probability model.[4,5] This model uses volume and radiation dose parameters calculated from previous patient data to prescribe a dose that subjects each patient to a 10% risk of hepatic complications. In this method, conformal three-dimensional radiation treatment is planned to treat the tumor volume plus a 1.5-cm margin. Dose-volume histograms are generated for the plans, and these histograms are used to calculate the portion of the whole normal liver volume receiving 50% of the effective volume (V_{eff}). This is the portion of the liver volume that if treated uniformly to the prescribed isocenter dose would be predicted to produce the same risk of complications as did the nonuniform irradiation that was actually given. Once the V_{eff} has been determined, the point at which that value intersects the 10% isocomplication probability contour is used to determine the isocenter prescribed dose (Fig. 21-1; see also Color Plate 25, after p. 80).[4]

Using this model, McGinn and colleagues have been able to safely escalate the dose of radiation for patients with intrahepatic cancer. In one study,[6] 21 patients were treated with radiation, given in 1.5-Gy fractions at 11 fractions per week, and concurrent fluorodeoxyuridine for up to a maximum of 14 days' continuous infusion to the hepatic artery. The total radiation dose was delivered in two parts, with a 2-week break between treatment blocks. The prescribed dose ranged from 40.5 Gy (for a V_{eff} of 0.831) to 81 Gy (for a V_{eff} of 0.224). Radiation-induced liver disease occurred in the sole patient with the V_{eff} of 0.831. This patient's liver injury manifested by a seven-fold elevation of alkaline phosphatase and ascites that lasted for 1 month; however, that patient did well until the tumor progressed 6 months after treatment.

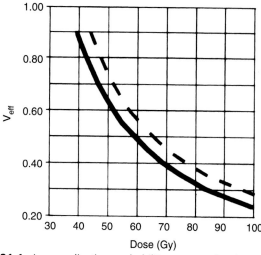

Fig. 21-1 Isocomplication probability contours for the normal tissue complication probability model based on prior clinical data; solid line, 10%; dashed line, 20%. Once the effective dose was determined, the point at which that value intersected the 10% isocomplication probability contour was used to determine the dose prescribed. (From McGinn CJ, Ten Haken RK, Ensminger WD, et al. *J Clin Oncol* 1998;16:2246-2252.)

This model for liver tolerance, which is based on three-dimensional volume and irradiation dose, is still being refined as more patients are treated and evaluated. Focal radiation doses as high as 90 Gy to small portions of the liver have been given. In another University of Michigan experience treating 36 patients with unresectable liver malignancies,[7] the median in-radiation-field progression-free survival duration was 10.8 months among patients treated with a median dose of 58.5 Gy (28.5 to 90 Gy).

As three-dimensional conformal treatment planning and delivery become increasingly used, isocomplication probability curves should become more precise. As radiation doses intended for small hepatic volumes are escalated, consideration should also be given to the radiation tolerance of other adjacent organs such as the kidney, stomach, duodenum, jejunum, and spinal cord.

Tolerance of the liver to irradiation is modified by chemotherapy. Fatal hepatopathy has been reported after a dose of 24 Gy given in 17 fractions over 28 days to the whole liver with preceding and concurrent doxorubicin therapy.[8] Liver complications have been evaluated in patients with lymphoma treated with combination chemotherapy and whole- or upper-abdomen irradiation.[9] In that study, the right liver lobe received 20 Gy in all patients, and the left lobe received 20 Gy in three patients, 25 Gy in 10 patients, and 30 to 40 Gy in seven patients. Doxorubicin was given to 16 patients. The rate of hepatic complications was higher in patients given 30 to 40 Gy to the left lobe, with subclinical liver damage evident in two patients and clinical damage in four patients. Chemotherapy potentiates the effect of radiation, and the tolerance of

liver may be reduced to 20 to 25 Gy when high-dose doxorubicin is given weeks before radiation therapy.[9]

ETIOLOGY, PATHOLOGIC FEATURES, AND PROGNOSIS OF HEPATOBILIARY CANCER

An estimated 16,200 new cases of liver and intrahepatic bile-duct cancer are expected to occur in the United States in 2001.[10] Hepatocellular carcinoma is particularly common in sub-Saharan Africa and Southeast Asia. Hepatocellular carcinoma is often associated with a history of cirrhosis and hepatitis B or C infection. The highest risk occurs in patients with hepatitis, cirrhosis, and elevated alpha-fetoprotein (AFP) levels.

Carcinoma of the gallbladder is associated with cholelithiasis, with an estimated incidence of carcinoma of 50% in patients with a calcified gallbladder. However, the incidence of carcinoma in patients with asymptomatic cholelithiasis is insufficient to warrant removal of the gallbladder. In Asia, liver fluke infection is associated with bile duct carcinoma. Patients with ulcerative colitis have an increased incidence of sclerosing cholangitis and bile duct carcinoma. The development of carcinoma of the bile duct in patients with sclerosing cholangitis results in difficulty in radiographically distinguishing between the two conditions. The prognosis of these hepatobiliary tumors is very poor, with a median survival of 6 to 12 months and a 5-year survival rate of approximately 5%.

EVALUATION AND STAGING

Primary hepatocellular carcinoma arising in the cirrhotic liver manifests as a rapid deterioration of hepatic function with a median survival of 2 months. Serum AFP levels of more than 400 mg/ml and a diagnostic angiogram or liver scan are probably equivalent to tissue diagnosis. However, benign and malignant neoplasms of the hepatobiliary system have similar symptoms; abnormalities of hepatic function and biliary obstruction cause jaundice and right upper quadrant pain.

In addition to physical examination and liver function tests, evaluation should include sonography, serum AFP measurement, percutaneous transhepatic cholangiography, and endoscopic retrograde cholangiopancreatography. Sonography is accurate in identifying dilated bile ducts and is the most sensitive noninvasive test for distinguishing between obstructive and nonobstructive jaundice. Transhepatic cholangiography, sonography, and CT are most accurate in identifying the presence and extent of extrahepatic biliary carcinoma. Endoscopic sonography provides high-resolution images of the biliary duct and provides guidance in biopsy of suspected abnormalities.[11]

Percutaneous transhepatic cholangiography usually defines the site and nature of the obstruction; endoscopic retrograde cholangiopancreatography may also define the area of obstruction or at least the distal extent of the biliary obstruction and permit placement of a stent to relieve obstruction. Transhepatic internal biliary drainage is possible by passing a perforated drainage tube from the dilated ducts through the obstructing lesion into the duodenum. However, if internal biliary-enteric anastomosis is planned, it should precede percutaneous biliary drainage because the anastomosis is easier with dilated ducts. Many patients have contiguous involvement of more than one duct. Cholangiocarcinoma can be very difficult to distinguish from cholangitis because of the desmoplastic reaction that produces fibrotic tissue with a few clumps of malignant cells. Cancer antigen (CA) 19-9 levels of more than 100 U/ml are highly accurate for diagnosing cholangiocarcinoma.[12]

In 1997 the American Joint Committee on Cancer revised its staging classification for cancer of the liver, gallbladder, and extrahepatic bile ducts (Boxes 21-1 to 21-3).[13-15]

BILIARY CARCINOMA
Treatments and Results
Surgery

Curative resection alone for extrahepatic biliary carcinoma fails 64% of the time. In their study of 16 patients with recurrent or residual tumor, Kopelson and colleagues[16] reported that regional failure occurred in

13 patients (81%) and distant failure occurred in nine patients (56%). Penetration of tumor through the ductal wall was more predictive of the risk of local–regional recurrence than was tumor grade, lymph node status, or perineural-lymphatic-venous invasion. Autopsy analysis of patients who died of recurrent cancer of the main hepatic duct junction after extensive initial resection showed that 93% of recurrences are in the liver hilum. Nodal recurrences occurred in 29%, peritoneal spread was found in 14%, and 57% of patients had spread to distant sites. Cancer cells infiltrating and remaining in the connective tissue of the hepatoduodenal ligament may be the main reason for the frequent failure in the liver hilum.[17]

Complete surgical resection with negative margins results in the best chance for long-term survival and ultimate cure from biliary duct or gallbladder carcinoma. Radiation therapy with or without chemotherapy has been used for patients with unresectable tumors and as adjuvant therapy for patients with resected tumors.

Miyazaki and colleagues[18] reported on 76 patients with hilar cholangiocarcinoma treated with surgery only. Curative resection was obtained in five of 11 patients undergoing local resection and in 49 of 65 patients undergoing hepatic resection. Five-year survival rates were 26% for all resections, 40% for curative resections,

---

BOX 21-1 American Joint Committee on Cancer Staging System for Cancer of the Liver, Including Intrahepatic Bile Ducts

PRIMARY TUMOR (T)

TX Primary tumor cannot be assessed
T0 No evidence of primary tumor
T1 Solitary tumor 2 cm or less in greatest dimension without vascular invasion
T2 Solitary tumor 2 cm or less in greatest dimension with vascular invasion, or multiple tumors limited to one lobe, none more than 2 cm in greatest dimension without vascular invasion, or a solitary tumor more than 2 cm in greatest dimension without vascular invasion
T3 Solitary tumor more than 2 cm in greatest dimension with vascular invasion, or multiple tumors limited to one lobe, none more than 2 cm in greatest dimension, with vascular invasion, or multiple tumors limited to one lobe, any more than 2 cm in greatest dimension, with or without vascular invasion
T4 Multiple tumors in more than one lobe, or tumor(s) involve(s) a major ranch of the portal or hepatic vein(s) or invasion of adjacent organs other than the gallbladder or perforation of the visceral peritoneum

REGIONAL LYMPH NODES (N)

NX Regional lymph nodes cannot be assessed
N0 No regional lymph node metastasis
N1 Regional lymph node metastasis

DISTANT METASTASIS (M)

MX Distant metastasis cannot be assessed
M0 No distant metastasis
MI Distant metastasis

STAGE GROUPING

Stage I	T1	N0	M0
Stage II	T2	N0	M0
Stage IIIA	T3	N0	M0
Stage IIIB	T1	N1	M0
	T2	N1	M0
	T3	N1	M0
Stage IVA	T4	Any N	M0
Stage IVB	Any T	Any N	M1

From Fleming I, Cooper JS, Henson DE, et al, eds. *AJCC Cancer Staging Manual.* 5th ed. Philadelphia, Pa: Lippincott Williams &Wilkins; 1997:97-101.

BOX 21-2   American Joint Committee on Cancer Staging System for Cancer of the Gallbladder

PRIMARY TUMOR (T)

TX	Primary tumor cannot be assessed
T0	No evidence of primary tumor
Tis	Carcinoma in situ
T1	Tumor invades lamina propria or muscle layer
	T1a Tumor invades lamina propria
	T1b Tumor invades muscle layer
T2	Tumor invades perimuscular connective tissue; no extension beyond serosa or into liver
T3	Tumor perforates the serosa (visceral peritoneum) or directly invades one adjacent organ, or both (extension 2 cm or less into the liver)
T4	Tumor extends more than 2 cm into the liver, and/or into two or more adjacent organs (stomach, duodenum, colon, pancreas, omentum, extrahepatic bile ducts, any involvement of liver)

REGIONAL LYMPH NODES (N)

NX	Regional lymph nodes cannot be assessed
N0	No regional lymph node metastasis
N1	Metastasis in cystic duct, pericholedochal, and/or hilar lymph nodes (i.e., in the hepatoduodenal ligament)
N2	Metastasis in peripancreatic (head only), periduodenal, periportal, celiac, and/or superior mesenteric lymph nodes

DISTANT METASTASIS (M)

MX	Distant metastasis cannot be assessed
M0	No distant metastasis
M1	Distant metastasis

STAGE GROUPING

Stage 0	Tis	N0	M0
Stage I	T1	N0	M0
Stage II	T2	N0	M0
Stage III	T1	N1	M0
	T2	N1	M0
	T3	N0	M0
	T3	N1	M0
Stage IVA	T4	N0	M0
	T4	N1	M0
Stage IVB	Any T	N2	M0
	Any T	Any N	M1

From Fleming I, Cooper JS, Henson DE, et al, eds. *AJCC Cancer Staging Manual.* 5th ed. Philadelphia, Pa: Lippincott Williams & Wilkins; 1997:103-105.

BOX 21-3   American Joint Committee on Cancer Staging System for Cancer of the Extrahepatic Bile Ducts

PRIMARY TUMOR (T)

TX	Primary tumor cannot be assessed
T0	No evidence of primary tumor
Tis	Carcinoma in situ
T1	Tumor invades subepithelial connective tissue or fibromuscular layer
	T1a Tumor invades subepithelial connective tissue
	T1b Tumor invades fibromuscular layer
T2	Tumor invades the perifibromuscular connective tissue
T3	Tumor invades adjacent structures: liver, pancreas, duodenum, gallbladder, colon, stomach

REGIONAL LYMPH NODES (N)

NX	Regional lymph nodes cannot be assessed
N0	No regional lymph node metastasis
N1	Metastasis in cystic duct, pericholedochal and/or hilar lymph nodes (i.e., in the hepatoduodenal ligament)
N2	Metastasis in peripancreatic (head only), periduodenal, periportal, celiac, and/or superior mesenteric and/or posterior pancreaticoduodenal lymph nodes

DISTANT METASTASIS (M)

MX	Distant metastasis cannot be assessed
M0	No distant metastasis
M1	Distant metastasis

STAGE GROUPING

Stage 0	Tis	N0	M0
Stage I	T1	N0	M0
Stage II	T2	N0	M0
Stage III	T1	N1	M0
	T1	N2	M0
	T2	N1	M0
	T2	N2	M0
Stage IVA	T3	Any N	M0
Stage IVB	Any T	Any N	M1

From Fleming I, Cooper JS, Henson DE, et al, eds. *AJCC Cancer Staging Manual.* 5th ed. Philadelphia, Pa: Lippincott Williams & Wilkins; 1997:109-111.

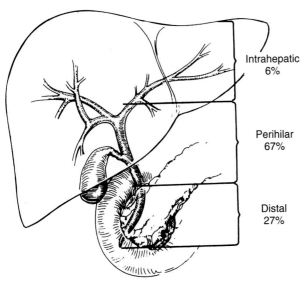

Fig. 21-2 Distribution of 294 cholangiocarcinomas into intrahepatic, perihilar, and distal subgroups. (From Nakeeb A, Pitt HA, Sohn TA, et al. *Ann Surg* 1996;224:463-475.)

Labels on figure:
Intrahepatic 6%
Perihilar 67%
Distal 27%

and 0% for noncurative resections. These authors stressed the importance of aggressive surgical approaches to obtain curative resection.

A review of 294 patients with cholangiocarcinoma who underwent surgical exploration at Johns Hopkins Hospital found that 6% had intrahepatic tumors, 67% had perihilar tumors, and 27% had distal tumors (Fig. 21-2).[19] The resectability rates were 50% for intrahepatic, 56% for perihilar tumors, and 91% for distal tumors. The respective 5-year actuarial survival rates for the 191 patients with resected intrahepatic, perihilar, and distal tumors were 44%, 11%, and 28%, and the median survival rates were 26, 19, and 22 months. Patients with negative surgical margins had 5-year actuarial survival rates of 57% for intrahepatic tumors, 19% for perihilar tumors, and 29% for distal tumors. Patients with positive lymph nodes or with poorly differentiated tumors had a shortened survival duration. Survival curves were similar for patients with resected tumors who did or did not undergo radiation therapy, but the details comparing the characteristics of the tumors of those who did or did not receive irradiation were not given. The median survival duration for patients with nonresected tumors was 8 months.

Valverde and colleagues[20] analyzed results of aggressive surgery for intrahepatic cholangiocarcinoma in 42 patients, 30 of whom underwent resection with curative intent. Of these 30 patients, nine patients were given external beam irradiation plus chemotherapy, and six patients given chemotherapy. Overall and disease-free survival rates were adversely affected by the presence of satellite nodules and by lymph node invasion. Vascular and biliary invasion and adjuvant therapy had no influence on survival. Of the 28 patients who survived

curative resection, 22% were alive at 3 years; median survival duration was 28 months.

Treatment in the Absence of a Histologic Diagnosis

Histologic proof of tumor is always preferred; however, the diagnosis may be based on clinical radiographic evidence, particularly for Klatskin's tumors (carcinoma arising in the bifurcation of the right and left hepatic ducts). Veeze-Kuijpers and colleagues[21] treated 42 patients with bile duct tumors and obtained no histologic proof of cancer in seven patients. Minsky and colleagues[22] found no histologic proof in three of 10 treated patients with extrahepatic bile duct cancer; Flickinger and colleagues[23] had no histologic proof in nine of 55 treated patients. These histologically unproven tumors were primarily Klatskin's tumors.

Radiation Therapy Techniques

The external radiation volume should include the tumor bed as identified by cholangiography, surgical description and clips, and CT images; regional nodes in the porta hepatis and celiac axis should also be included for biliary tumors. Three-dimensional treatment planning provides greater precision in identifying and treating the appropriate tumor volume. The movement of the liver with respiration needs to be considered in planning the radiation volume. Techniques being developed to reduce this movement include the use of a stereotactic frame with an upper abdominal compression plate.[24]

Conformal irradiation of intrahepatic tumors should include the tumor volume plus a 1.5-cm margin in cross-sectional directions and a 1.5- to 3-cm margin in the cephalocaudad direction to account for diaphragm movement during treatment. The volume for cholangiocarcinoma should extend 3 to 5 cm along the intrahepatic length of the bile ducts.

Four-field (anteroposterior, posteroanterior, and lateral) techniques allow doses of 45 to 60 Gy, given at 1.8 to 2 Gy/day, to be well tolerated. Doses greater than 50 Gy should be limited to the area of the tumor bed. The position of the spinal cord and kidneys relative to the radiation volume should be identified. When four-field external beam irradiation is used, the spinal cord and most of the kidney volume should be posterior to the lateral radiation beams. It is important that most of the liver in the volume does not receive more than 25 to 30 Gy. Transhepatic or internal biliary drainage should be maintained during radiation therapy. Innovative nonaxial convergent beams may allow greater sparing of the kidney and other normal structures.

Intraluminal irradiation with a linear arrangement of ^{192}Ir can be given through percutaneous transhepatic biliary drainage tubes that traverse the tumor. Such radiation is most effective when combined with 50 Gy of external irradiation. With rapid decrease in radiation dose at increasing distance from the line of sources, the effectively irradiated cylindric volume is small. The usual radiation dose from the implant is 20 to 30 Gy at 1 cm from the axis of the central-source line. To prevent the radioactive strand from going through the side-hole perforations in the biliary drainage tube, an internal catheter without side holes is first placed over a guidewire within the biliary tube, and the radioactive strand is placed within the internal catheter. Placement of the ^{192}Ir strand is performed under fluoroscopic

guidance with the source crossing the biliary-jejunal anastomosis. This technique is illustrated in Figure 21-3.

Intracatheter hyperthermia with ^{192}Ir has been evaluated for the treatment of bile duct carcinoma.[25] For tumors of the lower biliary tract, radiation doses can be boosted with intraoperative electron beam irradiation so as to give 20 to 25 Gy in a single treatment. Intrahepatic tumors, however, cannot be treated effectively with this technique.

Radiation and Chemotherapy

The true effect of radiation treatment on patients with bile duct carcinoma remains difficult to know. Because

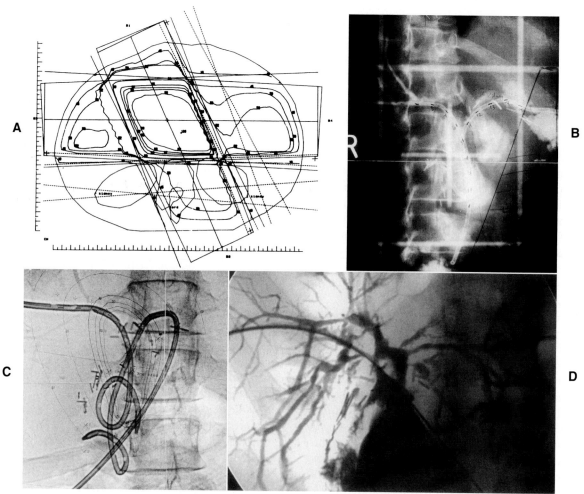

Fig. 21-3 Postoperative radiation for cholangiocarcinoma at the bifurcation of hepatic ducts with positive hepatic surgical margin after central hepatic resection and right and left hepaticojejunostomy. **A,** Isodose plan of four-field (right anterior oblique–left posterior oblique, right and left lateral) radiation technique, total external dose 50.4 Gy in 28 fractions. **B,** Simulation film of right anterior oblique radiation field shows preliminary plan for ^{192}Ir seeds to be placed in the right and left hepatic duct catheters, which extend from skin to hepaticojejunostomy. **C,** Anteroposterior radiograph of intraluminal ^{192}Ir seeds, with 10 seeds in the right catheter and five seeds in left catheter. The total activity was 234 mg radium equivalent, duration 44 hours, for an implant dose of 25 Gy at 1 cm from axis of ^{192}Ir strands. **D,** Cholangiogram 3.5 years after treatment shows some narrowing of hepatic ducts. The patient was alive 4.5 years after that treatment.

of the low incidence of this cancer, most reported series involve small numbers of patients. No randomized studies have been conducted to compare patients with similar tumor characteristics who have or have not been treated with radiation. In most reported treatment series comparing surgery alone to surgery plus radiation therapy with or without chemotherapy, the radiation is usually given to the patients with adverse prognostic factors such as positive surgical margins or lymph node or portal vein involvement. These reports then compare the survival results of patients who did or did not undergo irradiation. In such comparisons, if the survival rates were similar among the irradiated and nonirradiated groups, the authors typically report no benefit from radiation therapy (with or without chemotherapy) despite the fact that, in most reports, the adjuvant therapy was given to patients with the worse prognosis. Moreover, most series report survival data, and only a few reports provide information on local–regional control. Considering the ongoing discussion of whether adjuvant radiation affects survival in patients with more common tumors (e.g., breast or rectal cancer), it is understandable why credible information is still lacking regarding the effect of radiation therapy on survival of patients with biliary carcinoma.

After curative, as opposed to palliative, radiation therapy is given, peritoneal spread seems to be a significant cause of failure. The risk of this type of spread is higher when the tumor has penetrated through the gallbladder wall, the distended gallbladder has been surgically decompressed before removal, any ductal tumors have been surgically transected, or ducts have been through dilatation and curettage with a probe.

After analyzing 65 published studies on the results of using radiation therapy and chemotherapy for biliary cancer, Hejna and colleagues[26] reported that "despite widespread use of both chemotherapy and radiation, there is no standard therapy for advanced biliary cancer ... the benefit of adjuvant treatment remains largely unproven."

Mahe and colleagues[27] reported a median survival duration of 22 months for 26 patients with extrahepatic bile-duct carcinoma who were given radiation therapy with curative intent (27.5 months after complete gross resection and 13 months after incomplete gross resection). Treatment was external irradiation alone (42 to 48 Gy) in 14 patients, combined external and intraluminal brachytherapy (external 40 to 48 Gy, intraluminal 10 to 15 Gy) in nine patients, and intraluminal brachytherapy alone (50 to 60 Gy) in three patients.

Alden and colleagues[28] reported treatment results in a study of 56 patients with proximal or midduct cholangiocarcinoma and 25 patients with distal duct (included ampulla of Vater) cholangiocarcinoma. Of the 56 patients with proximal or midduct tumors, seven had resection without irradiation, six had surgery and

postoperative irradiation, 28 had irradiation without surgery, and 15 were given chemotherapy or palliative measures without irradiation. Chemotherapy was given to 20 of the 34 irradiated patients and to seven of the 22 nonirradiated patients. Median survival duration of patients with proximal bile duct cancer was more than twice as long after radiation therapy (17 months) than without irradiation (6 months). For proximal tumors treated with radiation, no difference in survival was found between patients who did or did not have surgical resection. All of the 25 distal tumors were surgically resected, and 10 of the patients with these tumors underwent adjuvant irradiation. For patients with distal bile duct tumors, median survival was no different between those who were or were not given radiation therapy. Patients with distal tumors given radiation therapy were more likely to have known residual cancer and a higher tumor stage. Although the difference was not statistically significant, the survival rate was higher among irradiated patients who were also given chemotherapy.

Pitt and colleagues[29] prospectively compared 50 patients with perihilar cholangiocarcinoma whose disease was surgically staged at Johns Hopkins Hospital. Of this group, 31 patients underwent complete or partial tumor resection and 19 underwent palliative procedures. Fourteen patients with resected tumors were given external beam irradiation (mean dose, 46 Gy), and eight patients also underwent intraluminal ^{192}Ir (mean dose, 13 Gy). Nine patients with unresectable tumors were given external beam irradiation (mean dose, 50 Gy), and two patients were given additional irradiation with smaller external beams or intraluminal ^{192}Ir. Patient and tumor characteristics were similar between those who were given radiation and those who were not. The actuarial survival curves for patients treated with resection or palliative procedures were not statistically different for irradiated (14 months) or nonirradiated patients (15 months). However, the survival curve beyond 3 years for patients with resected tumors was better among patients who had undergone irradiation. Mean survival duration was longer for patients who underwent resection (20 months) than for those who underwent palliative procedures (11 months). This study did not analyze the survival of irradiated versus nonirradiated patients with resected tumors on the basis of positive or negative surgical margins. Surgical margins were positive in 71% of resected tumors.

Roayaie and colleagues[30] reported on 26 patients who underwent exploratory surgery for intrahepatic cholangiocarcinoma (excluding perihilar tumors). Resection was accomplished in 16 patients, for whom the median survival time was 43 months and the 5-year actuarial survival rate was 44%. Adjuvant radiation therapy and chemotherapy was given to five patients with positive margins, to one patient with nodal invasion, and to one patient with right portal vein involvement. No significant difference in survival was found between those who received adjuvant therapy and those who did not. However, the patients who underwent adjuvant treatment had worse prognostic factors.

Urego and colleagues[31] reported on 61 patients with cholangiocarcinoma seen and treated in the Radiation Oncology Department at the University of Pittsburgh. Of these patients, 23 had complete resections (including 17 with orthotopic liver transplant), four had partial resections, and 34 had biopsy only. All patients underwent preoperative or postoperative external beam irradiation (median dose, 49.5 Gy). Thirty patients also were given chemotherapy with 5-fluorouracil (5-FU), leucovorin, and interferon-alpha ($N = 27$) or paclitaxel ($N = 3$). The median survival duration was 20 months, and the 5-year actuarial survival rate was 24 months. Patients who had undergone complete resections had a 5-year actuarial survival rate of 53%, an improvement over other reports and the department's prior experience. These authors concluded that complete surgical resection with negative surgical margins was the most important factor for achieving cure or long-term survival in cholangiocarcinoma.

McMasters and colleagues[32] used preoperative chemoradiation (45 to 50.4 Gy or equivalent, with continuous-infusion 5-FU) to treat nine patients with extrahepatic cholangiocarcinoma. Three patients had a complete pathologic response. However, among a total of 40 resected tumors, no difference in survival was found among patients who underwent no radiation, those who underwent preoperative chemoradiation, or those who underwent postoperative chemoradiation.

Researchers from the Mayo Clinic[33] recently reported impressive early results from an aggressive protocol involving adjuvant preoperative chemoradiation and orthotopic liver transplantation for patients with unresectable early-stage cholangiocarcinoma above the cystic duct without intrahepatic or extrahepatic metastases. To date, 19 patients have been enrolled and given initial external beam radiation at 40.5 to 45 Gy, given in 30 fractions over 3 weeks, with bolus 5-FU. This treatment was followed by transcatheter ^{192}Ir to give an additional 20 to 30 Gy at a 1-cm radius, plus protracted continuous-infusion 5-FU. After irradiation, patients underwent an exploratory laparotomy to exclude metastatic disease. Eight patients did not have the liver transplantation, six because of metastasis at the time of the exploratory laparotomy, one because of development of malignant ascites, and one because of death from intrahepatic biliary sepsis. Eleven patients completed the protocol with a successful orthotopic liver transplantation. All but one patient had early-stage disease in the liver. At the time of the report, all patients who had undergone liver transplantation were alive; three patients were at risk at 12 months or less, and the other eight patients had a median follow-up of 44 months

(range, 17 to 83 months; seven of nine patients had a follow-up of more than 36 months). Only one patient had developed tumor relapse. This is a very encouraging, albeit aggressive, treatment option for highly selected patients with cholangiocarcinoma. The authors reported that only 2% of the total population of patients with cholangiocarcinoma seen at the Mayo Clinic were even potential candidates for this treatment study.

Iwatsuki and colleagues[34] from the University of Pittsburgh reported on 72 patients with hilar cholangiocarcinoma treated with hepatic resection ($N = 34$) or transplantation ($N = 38$) with curative intent. Forty-four patients received adjuvant preoperative or postoperative external beam irradiation. When patients who died within 3 months of surgery were excluded from analysis, adjuvant radiation therapy did not significantly improve survival. However, eight of the 10 patients who survived for 5 or more years had been given radiation.

Schoenthaler and colleagues[35] evaluated treatment outcome in 129 patients with extrahepatic bile-duct adenocarcinoma. For patients treated with curative attempt, no significant difference was found in median survival time between patients treated with surgery alone (16 months), surgery with conventional irradiation (16 months), or surgery with charged helium or neon particles (23 months). Patients with microscopic negative margins had a survival advantage over those with positive surgical margins. Patients with microscopic or gross residual tumor had improved survival times when they were treated with adjuvant irradiation (Table 21-1).[35]

Special Radiation Therapy Techniques

Gunderson and colleagues[36] reviewed many series involving dose-intensification techniques such as external beam plus intraluminal, intraoperative, or conformal radiation. Such techniques may improve local control and survival over what would be expected after lower-dose external beam radiation.

Sixteen eligible patients with unresected, resected with residual, or locally recurrent biliary duct cancer were studied by the Radiation Therapy Oncology Group (RTOG) in a protocol involving external radiation (45 to 50 Gy) and intraoperative radiation therapy (IORT) (14 to 22 Gy).[37] Eight patients completed the protocol; at a median follow-up of 10.5 months, two of those eight patients were alive. All patients with residual disease larger than 2 cm at the time of IORT died of disease.

Buskirk and colleagues[38] documented local failure in 9 of 17 patients treated with external radiation (45 to 60 Gy) alone or with 5-FU, in three of 10 patients given an ^{192}Ir transcatheter boost, and in two of six patients given an IORT boost with curative intent. Median survival time was 12 months. The only patients surviving longer than 18 months had gross total or subtotal resection before external irradiation or had been given ^{192}Ir or IORT boosts.

TABLE 21-1

Survival After Surgery and Adjuvant Radiation for Extrahepatic Bile-Duct Carcinoma

| | MEDIAN ACTUARIAL SURVIVAL DURATION (IN MONTHS) | | | |
| | TREATMENT TYPE | | | |
Margin Status	S (N = 62)	S + X (N = 45)	S + CP (N = 22)	Overall (N = 120)
Microscopic negative	39	—	—	39
Microscopic positive	11	21.5	61	19
P value (relative to S)		0.0109	0.0005	
Gross residual	5	9	10	7
P value (relative to S)		0.05	0.0423	

Modified from Schoenthaler R, Phillips TL, Castro J, et al. *Ann Surg* 1994;219:267–274.

S, Surgery; S + X, surgery plus conventional x-ray; S + CP, surgery plus charged-particle helium or neon radiation therapy.

TABLE 21-2

Survival in Patients with Stage IVA Klatskin's Tumor After Intraoperative or Postoperative Radiation Therapy

Treatment	5-Year Survival Rate (%)	Median Survival Duration (Months)	Local–Regional Control Rate (%)
Resection alone (N = 21)	13.5	10	31
Resection + RT (N = 42)		32	79
Resection + PORT (N = 8)	0		
Resection + IORT (N = 34)	17		
Resection + IORT and PORT (N = 22)	39		

Data from Todoroki T, Ohara K, Kawamoto T, et al. *Int J Radiat Oncol Biol Phys* 2000;46:581-587.

RT, Radiation therapy; PORT, postoperative (external) radiation therapy; IORT, intraoperative (electron-beam) radiation therapy.

Intraoperative Irradiation

Kurosaki and colleagues[39] suggested that IORT and external beam radiation are useful in patients with bile duct cancer who undergo a noncurative resection or who have lymph node metastases, but they may not extend survival in patients who undergo a curative resection and do not have lymph node metastases.

Todoroki and colleagues[40] reported that intraoperative and postoperative radiation therapy improve survival in patients with locally advanced Klatskin's tumors with microscopically positive surgical margins and no macroscopic malignancies. Only the combination of the intraoperative and postoperative radiation was beneficial for survival (Table 21-2). Survival curves comparing resection alone with resection followed by intraoperative and postoperative radiation for microscopic residual tumor are shown in Figure 21-4. Todoroki and colleagues[40] recommend that IORT be given as a 20-Gy dose of less than 8 MeV electrons in a cone of less than 6 cm in diameter. The challenge in determining whether to give IORT lies in the fact that the pathologic status of the surgical margin may not be known at surgery. Todoroki and

colleagues[41] have also reported results of IORT for patients with gallbladder cancer (as described in the section on "Gallbladder Cancer" later in this chapter).

Intraluminal Irradiation

Fields and Emami[42] showed improved median survival time for patients with extrahepatic biliary carcinoma treated with external radiation plus a ^{192}Ir implant (15 months) as compared with that for patients treated with external irradiation only (7 months).

In another study, evaluation of radiation therapy in the treatment of 55 patients with carcinoma of the extrahepatic bile ducts showed a median survival of 9 months; by comparison, eight patients with carcinoma of the gallbladder had a median survival of only 3 months. The only long-term survivors were those treated with liver transplantation and irradiation (22% 4-year actuarial survival). In that study, 51 patients received external beam irradiation alone (54 to 62 Gy), nine received external beam (26 to 60 Gy) plus intraluminal brachytherapy (14 to 45 Gy to a 0.5-cm depth), and three received intraluminal brachytherapy alone (28, 30, and 55 Gy at a 0.5-cm depth).[43] Endoluminal sonography can be useful for

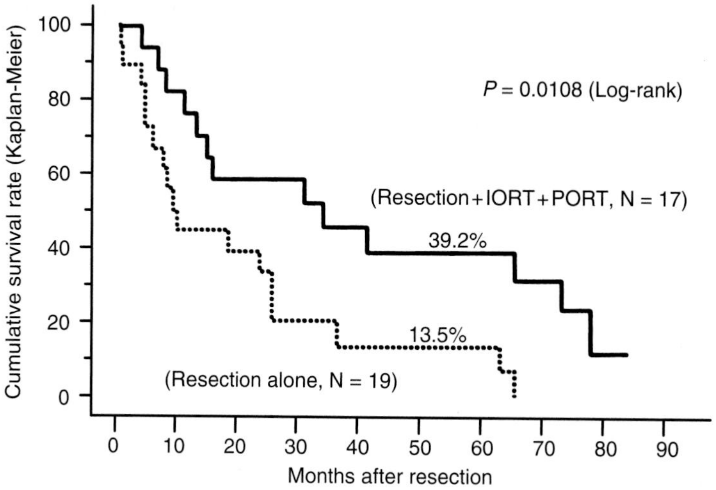

Fig. 21-4 Survival curves for patients with stage IVA Klatskin's tumor after resection followed by intraoperative (IORT) and postoperative (PORT) adjuvant radiation therapy for microscopic residue. (From Todoroki T, Ohara K, Kawamoto T, et al. *Int J Radiat Oncol Biol Phys* 2000; 46:581-587.)

determining tumor volume and response to endoluminal brachytherapy.[44]

Morganti and colleagues[45] reported on 20 patients with unresectable or residual nonmetastatic extrahepatic bile tumors (eight in the common bile duct, 11 Klatskin's tumors, and one gallbladder tumor) treated with 39.6 to 50.4 Gy external irradiation. Nineteen patients were also given 5-FU at 1000 mg/m^2/day during days 1 to 4, and 12 others were given an intraluminal ^{192}Ir wire boost to 30 to 50 Gy at 1 cm from the source axis. Median survival time for all patients was 21 months; distant metastases occurred in 50% of all patients. Two patients with unresectable disease survived for 5 years.

Alden and Mohiuddin[46] reported that increasing the radiation dose had a favorable effect on survival. In that study, irradiation of 24 patients with cancer of the extrahepatic bile ducts produced 2-year survival rates of 40% for 13 patients treated with external beam and intraluminal irradiation with or without chemotherapy, 25% for eight patients treated with external beam irradiation and chemotherapy, 29% for seven patients treated with chemotherapy only, 0% for three patients treated with intraluminal brachytherapy, 17% for 6 patients treated with surgery only, and 9% for 11 patients who were not treated. The median survival duration according to radiation dose given was 4.5 months for less than 45 Gy, 9 months for 45 to 54 Gy, 18 months for 55 to 65 Gy, 25 months for 66 to 70 Gy, and 24 months for more than 70 Gy. These authors recommended 44 to 46 Gy of external irradiation plus 25 Gy at 1 cm from intraluminal ^{192}Ir as an effective and well-tolerated treatment.

Gonzalez Gonzalez and colleagues[47] analyzed results obtained with radiation therapy for proximal cholangiocarcinoma. Of 71 patients who underwent tumor resection, postoperative radiation was given to 52 patients and preoperative plus postoperative radiation was given to 19 patients. Of these patients, 41 were given a boost of 10 Gy to the bilioanastomosis by means of intraluminal brachytherapy. Another 38 patients in that study underwent external irradiation for unresectable tumor, 19 of whom were also given a brachytherapy boost (22 to 25 Gy) through a nasobiliary catheter. Among the 71 patients who underwent resection, the mean survival duration was 24 months and the 5-year survival rate was 24%. Among the 38 patients who did not undergo resection, the mean survival duration was 10 months and the 2-year survival was 10%. The brachytherapy boost did not influence survival for either group; in fact, a total dose of more than 55 Gy had a significant negative influence on survival.

Bowling and colleagues[48] compared survival among 56 patients with nonresectable cholangiocarcinoma treated with endoscopic biliary stenting alone or with stenting followed by external beam irradiation and intraluminal ^{192}Ir brachytherapy. The median overall survival time was 7 months (range, 1 to 29 months) in the group that underwent only stenting and 10 months (range, 4 to 75 months) in the group that underwent radiation therapy. The survival advantage from radiation therapy was seen only in the first 10 months after diagnosis. Given the costs associated with radiation therapy and increased hospitalization time, the authors expressed doubts over the routine use of radiation therapy in the management of nonresectable cholangiocarcinoma.

Eschelman and colleagues[49] evaluated the effect of combined-modality therapy (including intraluminal ^{192}Ir) on stent patency and survival in 22 patients with malignant biliary obstruction treated with Gianturco stents. Eleven of these patients had cholangiocarcinoma and 11 had secondary extrahepatic bile duct malignancies. All patients were given intraluminal ^{192}Ir brachytherapy, with a mean dose of 25 Gy at a 1-cm radius. Of the 11 patients with cholangiocarcinoma, 8 were also given external beam radiation to a mean dose of 45 Gy. In the 11 patients with cholangiocarcinoma, the mean duration of stent patency was 19.5 months, and the mean survival time was 22.6 months.

Leung and colleagues[50] reported results of treating 16 cases of bile duct carcinoma with intraluminal ^{192}Ir. Prior treatment included complete resection in three patients, partial resection in one, bypass procedures in eight, endoscopic stents in five, external biliary drainage in 15, and external irradiation in one patient. Median survival time was 23 months, and 61% of patients survived 1 year. The most common acute complication was cholangitis in four patients; the most common late complications were duodenal ulcer, seen in two patients, and cholangitis, also seen in two patients.

Kuvshinoff and colleagues[51] treated 12 patients with unresectable or recurrent hilar cholangiocarcinoma with internal biliary drainage followed by intraluminal ^{192}Ir and external beam irradiation. Jaundice was relieved in 10 patients. All patients survived at least 6 months, and five patients were still alive 16 to 36 months after treatment.

Foo and colleagues[52] reviewed 24 patients (22 with locally unresectable and two with residual carcinoma) with extrahepatic bile duct carcinoma treated with external beam irradiation and transcatheter ^{192}Ir. Median survival time was 12.8 months. The overall survival rates were 19% at 2 years and 14% at 5 years. Three patients survived free of disease for 5 or more years. Two of nine patients who were also given 5-FU survived for 5 or more years. A trend toward improved survival was noted among the patients given 5-FU in addition to radiation.

GALLBLADDER CANCER
Treatments and Results
Surgery

A review of 724 patients with gallbladder cancer treated surgically showed that the projected 5-year survival rate correlated with tumor stage, being 93% for Tis tumors, 18% for T1, and 10% for T2. No patient with T3 or T4 tumors survived for 3 years; indeed, only 10% of those patients survived for 1 year or more.[53]

The value of a complete resection with negative surgical margins is exemplified in a review[54] of 162 patients with carcinoma of the gallbladder, of whom 109 underwent surgical therapy. Complete resection was possible in 36 patients, 44 patients had pathologically involved margins, and 29 either underwent resection that left gross residual disease or had a palliative surgical procedure. Patients with no residual disease after resection had a median survival time of 67 months as compared with 9 months for those with microscopic residual disease

and 4 months for those with gross residual disease after surgery. Although 41 patients were treated with chemotherapy with or without radiation therapy, the effect of that treatment was not analyzed in this series.

Radiation

Mahe and colleagues[55] treated 19 patients with gallbladder cancer with postoperative external radiation therapy. Of these patients, 11 had a complete resection, six an incomplete gross resection, and two only percutaneous transhepatic biliary drainage. The radiation dose ranged from 30 to 50 Gy. For the 11 patients who had undergone complete resection, the overall survival rates at 4 and 5 years were 55% and 36%. When the report was written, three of those 11 patients were alive at 54, 65, and 76 months after surgery and the other eight had died of cancer 8 to 114 months after surgery. Local control was achieved after complete resection and postoperative irradiation in all six patients with T1 or T2 disease.

A review of data from six reports collected by Houry and colleagues,[56] involving a total of 28 patients with gallbladder cancer given postoperative irradiation after curative surgery, indicates 2-year and 5-year survival rates of 79% (11 of 14) and 55% (6 of 11), respectively, for patients who had tumors without lymph-node or liver-bed involvement. For patients given postoperative irradiation after curative surgery for gallbladder tumors involving the lymph nodes or liver bed, the 2-year survival rate was 33% (3 of 9), with no 5-year survivors. Median survival was 8 months, with the longest being 15 months, among patients with gallbladder cancer who underwent postoperative irradiation after palliative resection; median survival was 3 months, with the longest being 11 months, for those who underwent irradiation with no prior resection.

Intraoperative irradiation. In a study of the effect of IORT for stage IV gallbladder carcinoma,[42] 46 patients underwent resection with adjuvant radiation therapy; 37 were given IORT, and 19 of these 37 patients also underwent postoperative external beam radiation therapy. The mean single IORT dose was 20.9 Gy, and the mean external radiation dose was 40 Gy. The average 5-year survival rate for patients with stage IV disease who underwent resection and radiation therapy was 9%. In contrast, no patient treated with resection alone survived for more than 26 months after surgery. IORT did not significantly affect survival when macroscopic tumor residue was left behind. However, IORT significantly prolonged survival in patients with microscopic residual tumor; the median survival time for these patients was 415 ± 76 days, and the 5-year survival rate was 19%.

Laparoscopic Port-Site Recurrence

Tumor recurrence in port sites after laparoscopic and thorascopic procedures in malignancy are a recognized complication of these procedures. Johnstone and colleagues[57] identified 15 cases from the literature of port-site recurrences after laparoscopic procedures for unsuspected gallbladder cancer. In 14 of these cases, the interval to recurrence was 5 months or less. Such recurrences carry a poor prognosis. The role of irradiation in primary or adjuvant treatment of this condition is unclear. We have treated only one such patient; although local control was achieved, the patient died of cancer 2 years later.

Summary of Biliary Tract Treatment Results

A review of the current literature suggests the following. Cholangiocarcinoma and gallbladder cancer have a poor prognosis. The most curative treatment is complete surgical resection, which may require a liver transplant. Unresectable tumors may benefit from radiation therapy with or without chemotherapy.

The role for adjuvant chemoradiation therapy after resection is controversial, but a survival benefit is evident for patients with microscopically positive margins treated with specialized boost radiation techniques. Although it is difficult to show a difference in survival curves for the first 3 years between patients who do or do not receive adjuvant irradiation, a few studies indicate that those who undergo irradiation are more likely to be among the few that survive beyond 3 or 5 years.

Consensus does not exist regarding whether to use radiation therapy or chemotherapy for patients with cholangiocarcinoma. The use of these treatment modalities needs to continue being investigated, and studies need to be performed that will provide credible information regarding their role for patients with biliary carcinoma.

HEPATOCELLULAR CARCINOMA
Treatments and Results

Surgical resection is the only potentially curative therapy for hepatocellular carcinoma. However, centrally located tumors, involvement of both lobes or the portal or hepatic vein, or the presence of cirrhosis and inadequate hepatic reserve reduce the number of potential candidates for subtotal hepatic resection to only 20% to 30%. Liver transplantation has been performed for many years, and some series report survival results similar to those after subtotal resection for stage I and II tumors.

The extremely poor response rate of nonresectable hepatocellular carcinoma to systemic chemotherapy has prompted exploration of innovative treatment techniques. The RTOG[58] treated patients with nonresectable hepatocellular carcinoma in a prospective trial of induction external radiation (21 Gy in 3-Gy fractions) integrated with doxorubicin and 5-FU followed by random

administration of either further full-dose doxorubicin and 5-FU or ^{131}I antiferritin with or without lesser amounts of doxorubicin and 5-FU. If tumor progression occurred, patients were permitted to receive the other therapy. Induction irradiation and chemotherapy produced a partial response rate of 15%, stable disease in 46%, and progressive disease in 39%. A partial response was obtained in 28% of patients treated with full-dose chemotherapy and in 22% of patients treated with ^{131}I antiferritin. Median survival duration (6 months) was similar between those two treatment groups. Median survival was 5 months for patients with measurable AFP titers and 10 months for those without measurable AFP. Seven of 11 AFP-negative patients for whom chemotherapy had failed achieved remission with ^{131}I antiferritin, and three of these patients underwent surgical resection.

In a French multicenter phase II trial,[59] intrahepatic artery injection of ^{131}I lipiodol resulted in a 44% partial response rate in patients with unresectable hepatocellular carcinoma.

A prospective randomized trial in which patients with hepatocellular carcinoma were given postoperative adjuvant intraarterial iodized oil (^{131}I lipiodol) (1850 MBq) showed fewer recurrences (29% vs. 59%) and improved median disease-free survival (57 months vs. 14 months) compared with patients who had not undergone adjuvant treatment.[60]

Researchers from Johns Hopkins Hospital[61] treated 76 patients with unresectable hepatoma with external beam radiation therapy (21 Gy given in 7 fractions over 10 days) and cisplatin (50 mg/m^2) followed by monthly intrahepatic-artery injections of cisplatin. Disease in 32% of these patients progressed during induction. The overall objective response rate was 43%. Results were better in patients who had no elevation in AFP titer or early-stage tumors.

A Korean study treated 30 patients with unresectable hepatocellular carcinoma by transcatheter arterial chemoembolization (with lipiodol, doxorubicin, and gelatin [Gelfoam]) followed 1 week later by local irradiation (mean dose, 44 Gy). The objective response rate (assessed by CT scanning) was 63%, and the median survival duration was 17 months; six patients survived for more than 3 years.[62]

This same group identified 27 patients for whom this chemoembolization procedure produced incomplete tumor filling.[63] Those patients were treated with local irradiation (mean dose, 52 Gy) that was started 1 to 2 weeks after the last chemoembolization. An objective response was observed in 67% (16) of 24 evaluable patients, including one complete response. The median survival duration was 14 months, and the 3-year survival rate was 21%.[63]

Radiation therapy is only one of several techniques used to treat patients with unresectable liver tumors.

These techniques include chemoembolization, intra-arterial infusion of chemotherapy, isolated hepatic chemotherapy infusion, cryotherapy, interstitial laser photocoagulation, microwave tissue coagulation, and injection therapy of alcohol. The best technique is yet to be determined, and the number of techniques being explored indicates the importance of and difficulty in treating unresectable hepatoma.[64]

HEPATOBLASTOMA

Few children with hepatoblastoma have been treated with radiation therapy. In a study at the Institut Gustave-Roussy in which 11 children with hepatoblastoma were treated,[65] one child with an initially unresectable tumor underwent preoperative radiation therapy and chemotherapy before subsequent resection of a completely microscopically necrotic tumor; that child was alive with no evidence of disease 68 months later. Seven other children underwent postoperative irradiation and chemotherapy after incomplete resection, six of whom remained free of disease 22 to 98 months after completion of radiation therapy. One child with unresectable tumor was alive without disease at 33 months after radiation therapy and chemotherapy. Two other patients with pulmonary metastases were given chemotherapy and whole-lung irradiation; one was living free of disease 58 months later, and the other had pulmonary metastases 20 months after diagnosis. These investigators recommended limited radiation fields of 35 to 40 Gy to the liver for microscopic residual disease and 45 Gy for gross residual disease.

METASTASES TO LIVER

The success of surgical resection of colorectal carcinoma metastatic to the liver depends on several factors. A large study from France[66] found that 2-year and 5-year survival rates after resection were affected by age (younger or older than 60 years), tumor size (smaller or larger than 5 cm), number of metastases (1 to 3 vs. 4 or more), surgical margin (larger or smaller than 1 cm), interval since the appearance of the primary tumor (2 years or more vs. less than 2 years), and the absence or presence of lymphatic spread or extension into serosa. Giving one point to each factor, they identified three risk groups as having different 2-year survival rates: those with up to two factors had a survival rate of 79%; those with three to four factors had 60%; and those with five to seven factors had 43%.

As stated in the previous section on "Hepatocellular Cancer," radiation therapy is only one of several techniques used to treat unresectable liver tumors, particularly tumors that metastasize to the liver. As is the case for hepatocellular cancer, the best technique for treating unresectable metastatic tumors in the liver is yet to be determined, and the number of techniques being tested underscores the difficulty and importance of this endeavor.[65,67,68]

Cryotherapy or radiofrequency thermoablation are being evaluated for treatment of unresectable primary or metastatic tumors in the liver. Complete response at the treated site of liver metastasis is reported to range from 60% to 90% for these locally ablative techniques, with most recurrences occurring away from the treated lesion.[69]

The German Cooperative Group on Liver Metastases[70] recently reported results of a prospective, multicenter, randomized study involving the following three treatment arms: 5-FU and leucovorin administered intravenously, 5-FU and leucovorin administered by infusion into the hepatic artery, or fluorodeoxyuridine administered by infusion into the hepatic artery. Median times to disease progression and median survival times were 6.6 months and 17.6 months for the intravenous 5-FU and leucovorin, 9.2 months and 18.7 months for the hepatic-arterial 5-FU and leucovorin, and 5.9 months and 12.7 months for the hepatic-arterial fluorodeoxyuridine. No significant differences in survival rates were found among the three treatment groups.

Irradiation of hepatic metastases probably has little significant effect on longevity, but it often relieves symptoms. The RTOG[71] reported that liver irradiation produced complete relief of the following signs and symptoms: abdominal pain (24% of patients treated), nausea and vomiting (34%), fever and night sweats (27%), ascites (29%), anorexia (9%), abdominal distension (10%), jaundice (17%), and weakness and fatigue (7%). Irradiation doses ranged from 20 Gy in 10 fractions to 30 Gy in 15 fractions with a 20 Gy boost dose to solitary metastases.

Another RTOG study[72] reported that the patients most likely to benefit from irradiation of hepatic metastases are those with a Karnofsky performance score of more than 80, a colorectal primary tumor, no extrahepatic metastases, and a bilirubin level of less than 1.5 mg/dl. Whole-liver irradiation with 21 Gy given in seven fractions was effective in decreasing abdominal pain in 80% of symptomatic patients (median response duration, 13 weeks) with complete relief of pain in 54% of patients. Patients with primary carcinoma of the colon and an initial Karnofsky performance score of 80 or more had a median survival of 5.8 months.

An RTOG[73] dose-escalating protocol showed no survival advantage for whole-liver irradiation with 27, 30, or 33 Gy (given in 1.5-Gy fractions twice daily) over whole-liver treatment with 21 Gy in seven fractions of 3 Gy. Moreover, although none of the 122 patients assigned to receive 27 or 30 Gy had clinical or biochemical evidence of radiation hepatitis, five of the 51 patients assigned to receive 33 Gy developed grade 3 radiation hepatitis.[73]

Using conformal hepatic radiation therapy (given in 1.5- to 1.65-Gy fractions twice daily) and concurrent hepatic-arterial fluorodeoxyuridine chemotherapy (with a 2-week break between 1- or 2-week infusions), physicians at the University of Michigan[74] treated 22 patients with colorectal liver metastases. Eleven patients were treated with 48 to 52.8 Gy and 11 patients were given 66 to 72.6 Gy. Two patients achieved a complete response, nine had a partial response, and 11 had stable disease. Disease progressed in the volume that received the full dose of radiation in 5 patients, elsewhere in the liver in six patients, and at both sites in two patients. Actuarial freedom from hepatic progression was 25% at 1 year. The overall median survival time was 20 months. The combination of conformal high-dose radiation and fluoropyrimidines may result in improved results in both primary and metastatic intrahepatic tumors.[6]

Mohiuddin and colleagues[75] reported improved palliation of symptoms and prolonged survival when patients received a boost dose (total dose, 33 to 60 Gy) to the area of dominant disease in addition to whole-liver irradiation (8 to 31 Gy).

Internal hepatic radiation techniques have been developed to selectively irradiate primary or metastatic tumors. Techniques involving (1) interstitial irradiation and direct intratumoral injection of ^{90}Y microspheres, (2) intraarterial infusion of ^{131}I lipiodol, (3) intraarterial infusion of ^{90}Y microspheres, and (4) parenteral administration of radiolabeled monoclonal antibodies were recently reviewed by Ho and colleagues.[76] In another study,[77] ^{125}I intraoperative liver brachytherapy for colorectal adenocarcinoma metastatic to the liver has resulted in 1-year and 5-year actuarial control rates of liver disease of 41% and 23%; the 5-year actuarial control of liver disease was 39% for solitary metastases and 9% for multiple metastases.[77]

In a randomized study,[78] the addition of hepatic irradiation (25.5 Gy) to intraarterial 5-FU produced no benefit in response or survival. In another study, hepatic-arterial infusion of 5-fluorodeoxyuridine and hyperfractionated irradiation (33 Gy given in 1.5-Gy fractions twice daily) to the whole liver with boost irradiation to tumor resulted in partial response in 48% and stable disease in 45% of patients who had cancer metastatic to the liver.[79]

Hartley and colleagues[80] reported that irradiation of patients with obstruction of the inferior vena cava caused by malignant hepatic enlargement produced a complete response in seven patients, a partial response in eight patients, and no response in three patients who completed local irradiation with 30 to 45 Gy. However, an additional 14 patients were unable to complete the radiation therapy because of marked deterioration or death. Radiation fields in that study were 10 to 12 cm wide and extended the length of the obstruction in the inferior vena cava.

SUMMARY

Hepatobiliary tumors continue to carry a very poor prognosis. Adequacy of surgical margins is a prime prognostic factor for resected tumors. Further studies analyzing the role of radiation therapy and chemotherapy as adjuvant therapy for resectable tumors and as primary treatment for unresectable tumors are needed. Innovative three-dimensional focused radiation techniques seem to allow high doses to be delivered to small liver volumes.

REFERENCES

1. Fajardo LF, Colby TV. Pathogenesis of venoocclusive liver disease after radiation. *Arch Pathol Lab Med* 1980;104:584-588.
2. Fajardo LF, Berthrong M, Anderson RE. Liver. In: *Radiation Pathology*. New York, NY: Oxford University Press; 2001:249-258.
3. Kopelson G, Harisiadis L, Tretter P, et al. The role of radiation therapy in cancer of extrahepatic biliary system: an analysis of 13 patients and a review of the literature of the effectiveness of surgery, chemotherapy, and radiotherapy. *Int J Radiat Oncol Biol Phys* 1977;2:883-894.
4. McGinn CJ, Ten Haken RK, Ensminger WD, et al. Treatment of intrahepatic cancers with radiation doses based on a normal tissue complication probability model. *J Clin Oncol* 1998;16:2246-2252.
5. Ten Haken TK, Hayman J, McGinn C, et al. The use of DVHs and NTCP models in guiding radiation therapy in the treatment of liver and lung cancer. Presented at: 41st Annual Meeting of the American Society for Therapeutic Radiology and Oncology, San Antonio, Texas, October 31, 1999.
6. McGinn CJ, Lawrence TS. Clinical results of the combination of radiation and fluoropyrimidines in the treatment of intrahepatic cancer. *Semin Radiat Oncol* 1997;4:313-323.
7. Dawson LA, McGinn CJ, Normolle D, et al. Escalated focal liver radiation and concurrent hepatic artery fluorodeoxyuridine for unresectable intrahepatic malignancies. *J Clin Oncol* 2000;18:2210-2218.
8. Kun LE, Camitta BM. Hepatopathy following irradiation and adriamycin. *Cancer* 1978;42:81-84.
9. Haddad E, LeBourgeois JP, Kuentz M, et al. Liver complications in lymphomas treated with a combination of chemotherapy and radiotherapy: preliminary results. *Int J Radiat Oncol Biol Phys* 1983;9:1313-1319.
10. American Cancer Society. *Cancer Facts and Figures, 2001*. Atlanta, Ga: American Cancer Society; 2001.
11. Brugge WR, Van Dam J. Pancreatic and biliary endoscopy. *N Engl J Med* 1999;341:1808-1816.
12. de Groen PC, Gores GJ, LaRusso, et al. Biliary tract cancers. *N Engl J Med* 1999;341:1368-1378.
13. Fleming I, Cooper JS, Henson DE, et al, eds. *AJCC Cancer Staging Manual*. 5th ed. Philadelphia, Pa: Lippincott Williams & Wilkins; 1997:97-101.
14. Fleming I, Cooper JS, Henson DE, et al, eds. *AJCC Cancer Staging Manual*. 5th ed. Philadelphia, Pa: Lippincott Williams & Wilkins; 1997:103-105.
15. Fleming I, Cooper JS, Henson DE, et al, eds. *AJCC Cancer Staging Manual*. 5th ed. Philadelphia, Pa: Lippincott Williams & Wilkins; 1997:109-111.
16. Kopelson G, Galdabini J, Warshaw AL, et al. Patterns of failure after curative surgery for extrahepatic biliary tract carcinoma: implications for adjuvant therapy. *Int J Radiat Oncol Biol Phys* 1981;7:413-417.
17. Tsuzuki T, Kuramochi S, Sugioka A, et al. Postresection autopsy findings in patients with cancer of the main hepatic duct junction. *Cancer* 1991;67:3010-3013.

18. Miyazaki M, Ito H, Nakagawa K, et al. Aggressive surgical approaches to hilar cholangiocarcinoma: hepatic or local resection? *Surgery* 1998;123:131-136.
19. Nakeeb A, Pitt HA, Sohn TA, et al. Cholangiocarcinoma, a spectrum of intrahepatic, perihilar, and distal tumors. *Ann Surg* 1996;224:463-475.
20. Valverde A, Bonhomme N, Farges O, et al. Resection of intrahepatic cholangiocarcinoma: a Western experience. *J Hepatobiliary Pancreat Surg* 1999;6:122-127.
21. Veeze-Kuijpers B, Meerwaldt JH, Lameris JS, et al. The role of radiotherapy in the treatment of bile duct carcinoma. *Int J Radiat Oncol Biol Phys* 1990;18:63-67.
22. Minsky BD, Kemeny N, Armstrong JG, et al. Extra-hepatic biliary system cancer: an update of a combined modality approach. *Am J Clin Oncol* 1991;14:433-437.
23. Flickinger JC, Epstein AH, Iwatsuki S, et al. Radiation therapy for primary carcinoma of the extrahepatic biliary system. *Cancer* 1991;68:289-294.
24. Herforth KK, Dedus J, Lohr F, et al. Extracranial stereotactic radiation therapy: set-up accuracy of patients treated for liver metastases. *Int J Radiat Oncol Biol Phys* 2000;46:329-335.
25. Wong JYC, Vora NL, Chon CK, et al. Intracatheter hyperthermia and iridium-192 radiotherapy in the treatment of bile duct carcinoma. *Int J Radiat Oncol Biol Phys* 1988;14:353-359.
26. Hejna M, Pruckmayer M, Raderer M. The role of chemotherapy and radiation in the management of biliary cancer: a review of the literature. *Eur J Cancer* 1998;34:977-986.
27. Mahe M, Romestaing P, Talon B, et al. Radiation therapy in extrahepatic bile duct carcinoma. *Radiother Oncol* 1991;21:121-127.
28. Alden ME, Waterman FM, Topham AK, et al. Cholangiocarcinoma: clinical significance of tumor location along the extrahepatic bile duct. *Radiology* 1995;197:511-516.
29. Pitt HA, Nakeeb A, Abrams RA, et al. Perihilar cholangiocarcinoma. Postoperative radiotherapy does not improve survival. *Ann Surg* 1995;221:788-798.
30. Roayaie S, Guarrera JV, Ye MQ, et al. Aggressive surgical treatment of intrahepatic cholangiocarcinoma: predictors of outcomes. *J Am Coll Surg* 1998;187:365-372.
31. Urego M, Flickinger JC, Carr BI. Radiotherapy and multimodality management of cholangiocarcinoma. *Int J Radiat Oncol Biol Phys* 1999;44:121-126.
32. McMasters KM, Tuttle TM, Leach SD, et al. Neoadjuvant chemoradiation for extrahepatic cholangiocarcinoma. *Am J Surg* 1997;174:605-609.
33. De Vreede I, Steers JL, Burch PA, et al. Prolonged disease-free survival after orthotopic liver transplantation plus adjuvant chemoirradiation for cholangiocarcinoma. *Liver Transpl* 2000;6:309-316.
34. Iwatsuki S, Todo S, Marsh JW, et al. Treatment of hilar cholangiocarcinoma (Klatskin tumors) with hepatic resection or transplantation. *J Am Coll Surg* 1998;187:358-364.
35. Schoenthaler R, Phillips TL, Castro J, et al. Carcinoma of the extrahepatic bile ducts: the University of California at San Francisco experience. *Ann Surg* 1994;219:267-274.
36. Gunderson LL, Haddock MG, Foo ML, et al. Conformal irradiation for hepatobiliary malignancies. *Ann Oncol* 1999;10:S221-S225.
37. Wolkov HB, Graves GM, Won M, et al. Intraoperative radiation therapy of extrahepatic biliary carcinoma: a report of RTOG-8605. *Am J Clin Oncol* 1992;15:323-327.
38. Buskirk SJ, Gunderson LL, Adson MA, et al. Analysis of failure following curative irradiation of gallbladder and extrahepatic bile duct carcinoma. *Int J Radiat Oncol Biol Phys* 1984;10:2013-2023.
39. Kurosaki H, Karasawa K, Kaizu T, et al. Intraoperative radiotherapy for resectable extrahepatic bile duct cancer. *Int J Radiat Oncol Biol Phys* 1999;45:635-638.
40. Todoroki T, Ohara K, Kawamoto T, et al. Benefits of adjuvant radiotherapy after radical resection of locally advanced main hepatic duct carcinoma. *Int J Radiat Oncol Biol Phys* 2000; 46:581-587.
41. Todoroki T, Kawamoto T, Otsuka M, et al. IORT combined with resection for stage IV gallbladder carcinoma. *Front Radiat Ther Oncol* 1997;31:165-172.
42. Fields JN, Emani B. Carcinoma of the extrahepatic biliary system: results of primary and adjuvant radiotherapy. *Int J Radiat Oncol Biol Phys* 1987;13:331-338.
43. Flickinger JC, Epstein AH, Iwatsuki S, et al. Radiation therapy for primary carcinoma of the extrahepatic biliary system. *Cancer* 1991;68:289-294.
44. Minsky B, Botet J, Gerdes H, et al. Ultrasound-directed extrahepatic bile duct intraluminal brachytherapy. *Int J Radiat Oncol Biol Phys* 1992;23:165-167.
45. Morganti AG, Trodella L, Valentini V, et al. Combined modality treatment in unresectable extrahepatic biliary carcinoma. *Int J Radiat Oncol Biol Phys* 2000;46:913-919.
46. Alden ME, Mohiuddin M. The impact of radiation dose in combined external beam and intraluminal Ir-192 brachytherapy for bile duct cancer. *Int J Radiat Oncol Biol Phys* 1994;28:945-951.
47. Gonzalez Gonzalez DG, Gouma DJ, Rauws EA, et al. Role of radiotherapy, in particular intraluminal brachytherapy, in the treatment of proximal bile duct carcinoma. *Ann Oncol* 1999; 10:S215-S220.
48. Bowling TE, Galbraith SM, Hatfield ARW, et al. A retrospective comparison of endoscopic stenting alone with stenting and radiotherapy in non-resectable cholangiocarcinoma. *Gut* 1996; 9:852-855.
49. Eschelman DJ, Shapiro MJ, Bonn J, et al. Malignant biliary duct obstruction: long-term experience with Gianturco stents and combined-modality radiation therapy. *Radiology* 1996;200:717-724.
50. Leung J, Guiney M, Das R. Intraluminal brachytherapy in bile duct carcinomas. *Aust N Z J Surg* 1996;66:74-77.
51. Kuvshinoff BW, Armstrong JG, Fong Y, et al. Palliation of irresectable hilar cholangiocarcinoma with biliary drainage and radiotherapy. *Br J Surg* 1995;82:1522-1525.
52. Foo ML, Gunderson LL, Bender CE, et al. External radiation therapy and transcatheter iridium in the treatment of extrahepatic bile duct carcinoma. *Int J Radiat Oncol Biol Phys* 1997;39:929-935.
53. Cubertafond P, Mathonnet M, Gainant A, et al. Radical surgery for gallbladder cancer. Results of the French Surgical Association survey. *Hepatogastroenterol* 1999;46:1567-1571.
54. North Jr JH, Pack MS, Hong C, et al. Prognostic factors for adenocarcinoma of the gallbladder: an analysis of 162 cases. *Am Surg* 1998;64:437-440.
55. Mahe M, Stampfli C, Romestaing P, et al. Primary carcinoma of the gall-bladder: potential for external radiation therapy. *Radiother Oncol* 1999;33:204-208.
56. Houry S, Haccart V, Huguier M, et al. Gallbladder cancer: role of radiation therapy. *Hepatogastroenterology* 1999;46:1578-1584.
57. Johnstone PAS, Rohde DC, Swartz SE, et al. Port site recurrences after laparoscopic and thorascopic procedures in malignancy. *J Clin Oncol* 1996;14:1950-1956.
58. Order S, Pajak T, Leibel S, et al. A randomized prospective trial comparing full dose chemotherapy to ^{131}I antiferritin: an RTOG study. *Int J Radiat Oncol Biol Phys* 1991;20:953-963.
59. Raoul JI, Bretagne JF, Caucanas JP, et al. Internal radiation therapy for hepatocellular carcinoma. *Cancer* 1992;69:346-352.
60. Lau WY, Leung TWT, Ho SKW, et al. Adjuvant intra-arterial iodine-131-labelled lipiodol for resectable hepatocellular carcinoma: a prospective randomized trial. *Lancet* 1999;353:797-801.
61. Abrams RA, Cardinale RM, Enger C, et al. Influence of prognostic groupings and treatment results in the management of unresectable hepatoma: experience with cis-platinum-based

chemoradiotherapy in 76 patients. *Int J Radiat Oncol Biol Phys* 1997;39:1077-1085.

62. Seong J, Keum KC, Han KH, et al. Combined transcatheter arterial chemoembolization and local radiotherapy of unresectable hepatocellular carcinoma. *Int J Radiat Oncol Biol Phys* 1999; 43:393-397.

63. Seong J, Park HC, Han KH, et al. Local radiotherapy for unresectable hepatocellular carcinoma patients who failed with transcatheter arterial chemoembolization. *Int J Radiat Oncol Biol Phys* 2000;47:1331-1335.

64. Alexander HR, Bartlett DL, Fraker DL, et al. Regional treatment strategies for unresectable primary or metastatic cancer confined to the liver. *Updates Prin Pract Oncol* 1996;10(8):1-19.

65. Habrand JL, Nehme D, Kalifa C, et al. Is there a place for radiation therapy in the management of hepatoblastomas and hepatocellular carcinomas in children? *Int J Radiat Oncol Biol Phys* 1992;23:525-531.

66. Nordlinger B, Guiguet M, Vaillant J-C, et al. Surgical resection of colorectal carcinoma metastases to the liver. A prognostic scoring system to improve case selection, based on 1568 patients. *Cancer* 1996;77:1254-1262.

67. Cascinu S, Catalano V, Baldelli AM, et al. Locoregional treatments of unresectable liver metastases from colorectal cancer. *Cancer Treat Rev* 1998;24:3-14.

68. Geoghegan JG, Scheele J. Treatment of colorectal liver metastases. *Br J Surg* 1999;86:158-169.

69. Ravikumar TS, Kaleya R, Kishinevsky A. Surgical ablative therapy of liver tumors. *Updates Prin Pract Oncol* 2000;14(3): 1-12.

70. Lorenz M, Muller H-H. Randomized, multicenter trial of fluorouracil plus leucovorin administered either via hepatic arterial or intravenous infusion versus fluorodeoxyuridine administered via hepatic arterial infusion in patients with nonresectable liver metastases from colorectal carcinoma. *J Clin Oncol* 2000;18: 243-254.

71. Borgelt BB, Gelber R, Brady LW, et al. The palliation of hepatic metastases: results of the RTOG pilot study. *Int J Radiat Oncol Biol Phys* 1981;7:587-591.

72. Leibel SA, Pajak TF, Massullo V, et al. A comparison of misonidazole sensitized radiation therapy to radiation therapy alone for the palliation of hepatic metastases: results of an RTOG randomized prospective protocol. *Int J Radiat Oncol Biol Phys* 1987;13: 1057-1064.

73. Russell AH, Clyde C, Wasserman TH, et al. Accelerated hyperfractionated hepatic irradiation in the management of patients with liver metastases: results of the RTOG dose escalating protocol. *Int J Radiat Oncol Biol Phys* 1993;27:117-123.

74. Robertson JN, Lawrence TS, Walker S, et al. The treatment of colorectal liver metastases with conformal radiation therapy and regional chemotherapy. *Int J Radiat Oncol Biol Phys* 1995;32: 445-450.

75. Mohiuddin M, Chen E, Ahmad N. Combined liver radiation and chemotherapy for palliation of hepatic metastases from colorectal cancer. *J Clin Oncol* 1996;14:722-728.

76. Ho S, Lau WY, Leung TW, et al. Internal radiation therapy for patients with primary or metastatic hepatic cancer: a review. *Cancer* 1998;83:1894-1907.

77. Martinez-Monge R, Nag S, Nieroda CA, et al. Iodine-125 brachytherapy in the treatment of colorectal adenocarcinoma metastatic to the liver. *Cancer* 1999;85:1218-1225.

78. Wiley AL, Wirtanen GW, Stephenson JA, et al. Combined hepatic artery 5-FU and irradiation of liver metastases: a randomized study. *Cancer* 1989;64:1783-1789.

79. Lawrence TS, Dworzanin LM, Walker-Andrews SC, et al. Treatment of cancers involving the liver and porta hepatis with external beam irradiation and intraarterial hepatic fluorodeoxyuridine. *Int J Radiat Oncol Biol Phys* 1991;20:555-561.

80. Hartley JW, Awrich AE, Wong J, et al. Diagnosis and treatment of the inferior vena cava syndrome in advanced malignant disease. *Am J Surg* 1986;152:70-74.

CHAPTER **22**

The Colon and Rectum

Nora A. Janjan, Marc E. Delclos, Matthew T. Ballo, and
Christopher H. Crane

ANATOMY

The large intestine originates at the cecum in the right
iliac fossa and continues in the retroperitoneum as the
ascending colon. At the hepatic flexure, it becomes
intraperitoneal and crosses the abdomen to again
become retroperitoneal at the splenic flexure. In the left
iliac fossa, it again becomes intraperitoneal, curving on
itself as the sigmoid colon. The rectum begins at the
sacrum with the anterior portion covered by the peritoneum and terminates at the anus. Given the close
proximity of the sigmoid colon and rectum to the uterus
and prostate, these structures are especially subject to
acute and late effects of radiation treatment.

TOLERANCE OF THE COLON AND RECTUM TO IRRADIATION

The rectum and rectosigmoid colon are usually considered more tolerant of radiation than the small intestine.
However, the fixation of these structures in the pelvis
and the high radiation doses often delivered in curative
treatment of carcinomas arising in pelvic structures
might be expected to lead to more consistent adverse
effects than are usually reported. Studies of prostate carcinoma suggest that the volume of rectum irradiated is
as important as the total doses received.[1,2] Two factors
are important in establishing the radiation tolerance
dose: the rate of repair of nonlethally injured cells
between fraction doses, and the rate of regeneration and
maturation of the remaining undifferentiated cells in
the crypt bases.[3] Small portions of the colon and rectum
can tolerate total doses in excess of 70 Gy if delivered in
fractions of 1.8 to 2.0 Gy or at low dose rates (less than
1.0 Gy per hour). However, large fractions (10 Gy) can
produce severe effects even if the total dose is as low as
30 Gy.[4]

Acute Effects

Although the threshold dose for early colorectal injury
seems to be 10 to 20 Gy (given in daily fractions of 1.5 to
2.0 Gy, 5 days a week),[3] doses as small as 5 Gy can produce significant changes in the epithelial ultrastructure of
the small bowel.[5] Extending the dose period to 25 days
(0.2 Gy per day) allows changes in the villous entero-
cytes, goblet cells and lamina propria to return to
normal by 3 days after the irradiation was terminated.[5]
The pathogenesis of early lesions consists of direct injury
to the rapidly responding mucosal cells. Mast cell hyperplasia is characteristic of both inflammatory and fibrotic
intestinal radiation injury. Mast cells have been shown
to allow transforming growth factor-β to stimulate a
fibrotic reaction.[6] Serving to protect the intestinal
mucosa during the early phase of radiation enteropathy,
mast cells promote intestinal fibrosis after breakdown of
the mucosal barrier, a process that begins with early
lesions and continues throughout the appearance of
delayed complications.[3]

Radiation also produces a dose-dependent decrease
in absorption of water and sodium/chloride ions and a
twofold increase in the secretion of potassium 4 days
after exposure.[7] Acute effects of radiation on the bowel
wall have included reductions of 40% to 70% in tensile
strength 3 days after surgery when 10 to 25 Gy was given
to a colonic anastomosis in a rat model.[8] Although the
anastomosis remained patent 7 days after surgery, the
adjacent area of colon was at increased risk of perforation. Therefore anastomotic regions seem to be at
increased risk during the acute period after intraoperative radiation.

Late Effects

Late radiation effects on the colon have also been evaluated. The threshold dose for delayed lesions is about
50 Gy, given in 1.5- to 2.0-Gy fractions.[3] In a mouse
model, a dose of 32 Gy given to various lengths of the
colorectum produced a threshold effect at a length of 10
to 15 mm.[9] Re-epithelization resulting from the proliferation of epithelial cells outside the crypt on the mucosal
surface was complete after 32 Gy when the irradiated
length of colorectum was less than 20 mm. When the
irradiated length was more than 20 mm, obstruction
resulting from secondary fibrosis occurred. However, a
single dose of 10 Gy to 20 Gy, administered as an intraoperative dose of radiation to the distal limb of a bowel

anastomosis, did not threaten anastomotic integrity or bowel function, but dose-related changes, like fibrosis, were observed between 6 and 12 months after surgery.[10]

COLORECTAL CANCER

Colorectal cancer is the third most commonly diagnosed cancer in the United States, with 98,200 new cases of colon cancer and more than 37,200 new cases of rectal cancer expected in 2001.[11] The incidence rates for colorectal cancer began to decrease by an average of 1.8% per year after 1985[12]; rates have leveled off since the early 1990s.[13] Epidemiologically, colorectal cancer has been linked to specific genetic syndromes, breast and ovarian cancer, and dietary consumption patterns. Widespread screening for colorectal cancer is based on a defined risk that benign lesions will be transformed into cancerous ones. Clarification of the influence of these and other possible risk factors will help establish guidelines for early detection.

Etiology and Risk Factors

Colorectal cancer generally arises from adenomatous polyps that form in a field of epithelial cell hyperproliferation and crypt dysplasia. The multistep process that occurs involves several suppressor genes that result in abnormalities of cell regulation. Results from the National Polyp Study demonstrated that two thirds of all polyps removed were adenomatous with the potential for malignant transformation.[14] That study also indicated that the transformation of a polyp into a cancer, termed the *adenoma-adenocarcinoma' sequence,* took about 5.5 years for an adenomatous polyp larger than 1 cm and that smaller polyps took about 10 years for malignant transformation. Removing polyps sharply decreased the expected incidence of colorectal cancer.[14]

Known risk factors for colorectal tumors include a family history of such tumors, consumption of meat, smoking, and consumption of alcohol. Inverse associations have been noted between risk and consumption of a high-fiber diet, use of nonsteroidal anti-inflammatory drugs (NSAIDs), hormone replacement therapy, and physical activity. Incidence rates for colorectal cancer vary by a factor of 20 around the world.[15] The risk of colorectal cancer is highly reflective of the environment; incidence rates among immigrants and their descendants can reach those of the country in which they reside within a single generation. This effect is particularly evident among the Hawaiian Japanese, who have the highest rates of colon cancer in the world, even though the rates of colon cancer in Japan are among the lowest.

Age, race, and sex were found to be independent risk factors for both proximal and distal colorectal cancer in a study of 38,931 cases of colorectal cancer in Illinois.[16] In that study, whites were more likely to develop distal colorectal cancer than blacks, and blacks were more likely to develop proximal colorectal cancer than whites.[16] A similar study of three geographical areas indicated that age had a greater effect on the development of proximal rather than distal colorectal cancer.[17] Many factors, including socioeconomic issues, contribute to the generally poorer survival rates among blacks than whites with colorectal cancer. In a study conducted by the National Surgical Adjuvant Breast and Bowel Project (NSABP), disease stage, number of involved lymph nodes, rate of local recurrence, and other factors were similar between blacks and whites, but blacks had a 21% higher mortality rate.[18]

According to data from the Surveillance Epidemiology and End Results program and the National Cancer Data Base, most cases of colorectal cancer arise in the proximal colon; the distribution across anatomic sites in 1997 was 15% in the cecum/appendix, 14% in the ascending colon/hepatic flexure, 14% in the transverse colon/splenic flexure and descending colon, 24% in the sigmoid, and 28% in the rectosigmoid and rectum.[19] The anatomic distribution of adenomatous polyps differs somewhat, totaling 40% in the proximal colon, 45% in the distal colon, and 15% in the rectum. Approximately 45% of the adenomatous polyps in the colon (but only 12% of those in the rectum) are at least 1 cm in size. Although 30% to 50% of individuals have adenomatous polyps, only 6% develop clinically diagnosed colorectal cancer.[20] Studies of the genetic and molecular basis of colorectal cancer are beginning to reveal why only some polyps undergo malignant transformation.

Genetic and Molecular Basis

Colorectal cancer has provided a model for studying genetically based types of cancer. As a group, familial cancer syndromes make up only about 5% of all types of cancer. A small proportion of common types of cancer such as colorectal, breast, ovarian, and endometrial cancer are caused by highly penetrant autosomal dominant genes.[21] Ethnic differences in cancer incidence and mortality are the result of genetic and environmental factors, as germline mutations in cancer susceptibility genes have been identified in individuals of all races and ethnic groups. The differences in cancer risk among ethnic groups are thought to be the result of founder mutations within cancer-predisposing genes; studies of these genes are expected to help create novel therapies that are based on specific mutations.[22]

Several molecular pathways exist by which colorectal cancer could develop. Among them are the adenomatous polyposis coli (APC)-β-catenin–T-cell factor (Tcf, a transcriptional activator) pathway and pathways that involve abnormalities of deoxyribonucleic acid (DNA) mismatch repair.[15] Expression of key genes in any of these pathways can be lost through acquired mutation or hypermethylation, which would account for sporadic cases, or through inheritance, as seems to be the case in inherited syndromes such as familial adenomatous polyposis and hereditary nonpolyposis colorectal cancer (HNPCC). In a study at the Hereditary Cancer Institute at Creighton University, among 316 family members of patients with HNPCC, the mutation was present in 123; among 79 family members of patients with APC, the mutation was present in 39.[23]

A distinct autosomal dominant syndrome caused by defective mismatch repair genes, HNPCC accounts for 5% of the total number of cases of colorectal cancer. The median age at diagnosis is 45 years. HNPCC is characterized by right-sided lesions, excess synchronous and metachronous lesions, and an increased risk of extracolonic neoplasms.[24] Risk is also increased for the formation of lesions of the endometrium, small bowel, stomach, renal pelvis and ureter, ovary, and skin; skin lesions such as sebaceous adenomas, carcinomas, and keratoacanthomas are common among patients with HNPCC. However, at the present time, no specific histopathologic characteristics have been identified that can distinguish HNPCC from sporadic colorectal cancer, with the possible exception of tumors of right-sided, undifferentiated, or signet ring cell type occurring in young people.

Several risk factors are known to be associated with the molecular mechanisms underlying colorectal cancer. Mutations in APC have been identified in up to 80% of families of patients with familial adenomatous polyposis. On the other hand, HNPCC mutations are found in only about half of patients with colorectal cancer who meet the Amsterdam Criteria (i.e., having three relatives with colon cancer, two of whom must be first-degree relatives of the third; the presence of colon cancer that spans two generations; and one case in which colon cancer was diagnosed before 50 years of age).[25] However, the HNPCC mutation is present in only 8% of families that have a strong positive history of colon cancer but who do not meet the Amsterdam criteria. The presence of microsatellite instability, an indicator of frequent genetic mutations throughout the genome, may be an effective alternative for identifying individuals at risk of developing HNPCC, because it is found in virtually all patients with HNPCC but in only 15% of patients with sporadic disease. However, because patients with HNPCC contribute only about 15% to 20% of the total number of colorectal cancer cases,[24] assessment of microsatellite instability in all colorectal tumors would not be cost-effective. Hence, a working group convened by the National Cancer Institute in 1996 created the Bethesda Guidelines (Box 22-1),[24] an expansion of the Amsterdam criteria, with the goal of identifying clinicopathologic criteria that could aid in early identification of additional patients with HNPCC.

BOX 22-1   The Bethesda Guidelines*

1. Individuals who meet the Amsterdam Criteria
2. Individuals with two HNPCC-related cancerous tumors, including synchronous and metachronous colorectal cancer or associated extracolonic cancer (e.g., endometrial, ovarian, gastric, hepatobiliary, small-bowel, or transitional cell cancer of the renal pelvis or ureter)
3. Individuals with colorectal cancer and a first-degree relative with colorectal cancer and/or HNPCC-related extracolonic cancer and/or a colorectal adenoma
   a. One of the cancers was diagnosed at < 45 years
   b. One of the adenomas was diagnosed at < 40 years
4. Individuals with colorectal cancer or endometrial cancer diagnosed at < 45 years
5. Individuals with right-sided colorectal cancer with an undifferentiated histopathologic pattern diagnosed at < 45 years
6. Individuals with a signet-ring-cell-type colorectal cancer (i.e., tumor consists of at least 50% signet ring cells) diagnosed at age < 45 years
7. Individuals with adenomas diagnosed at age < 40 years

Modified from Rodriguez-Bigas MA, Boland CR, Hamilton SR, et al. *J Natl Cancer Inst* 1997;89:1758-1762.
HNPCC, Hereditary nonpolyposis colorectal cancer.
*Tumors from individuals who meet these criteria should be tested for microsatellite instability.

Other Etiologic Associations
Cyclooxygenases

A variety of other etiologic associations for colorectal cancer have been identified; among them is the finding that the gene for cyclooxygenase-2 (COX-2) is overexpressed in some cases of sporadic and HNPCC-type colonic adenomas.[26,27] The cyclooxygenase enzymes participate in the synthesis of prostaglandins from arachidonic acid; their peroxidase activity also catalyzes the conversion of procarcinogens to proximate carcinogens.[28] The increased production of prostaglandins in inflammation, and possibly by tumor cells as well, are due in part to cytokine-mediated induction of COX-2.

Use of NSAIDs has been reported to decrease the risk of developing colorectal cancer through the inhibition of COX-2.[27] However, NSAIDs also have deleterious effects on the small bowel and colonic mucosa, including ulceration and strictures of the jejunum, ileum, and colon. Clinically, NSAIDs can cause diarrhea, abdominal pain, blood and protein loss, colitis, and perforation,[29] and thus NSAIDs should not be used for patients with ulcerative colitis or Crohn's disease.

Hormone Replacement Therapy

The use of hormone replacement therapy seems to be associated with a reduced risk of colon cancer.[15,30,31] A meta-analysis of 18 epidemiologic studies of hormone replacement therapy in postmenopausal women showed a 20% reduction in the risk of colorectal cancer.[30] Several hypotheses have been proposed to explain this effect. Issa and colleagues[32] found that colon tumors had abnormal methylation patterns in the estrogen receptor gene and postulated that hypermethylation of and a reduction in expression of that gene, both of which increase with age, result in deregulated growth of the colonic mucosa.[32] Alternatively, exogenous estrogens also decrease bile acid synthesis by up to 15%; this is important because bile acids, which are absorbed in the proximal colon, are thought to promote malignant changes in the colonic epithelium. High fecal bile acid concentrations have been linked to recurrence of colon polyps; according to one study, bile acid concentrations in the upper quartile were associated with a threefold increase in risk of polyp formation.[30] Estrogen may also reduce levels of the mitogen insulin-like growth factor-1,[15] which is required by some cells to progress from G_1 to S phase.

Dietary Factors

Evidence from both case-control and cohort studies has supported strong links between diet and risk of colorectal cancer.[15] In a case-controlled study of 402 cases of colorectal cancer and 668 controls, high intake of total fat and saturated fat and low intake of dietary fiber, especially from vegetable sources, calcium, and vitamins A and E were associated with the development of colorectal cancer.[33] Results from the Australian Polyp Prevention Project and other studies have shown that wheat bran fiber, which reduces fecal bile acid concentrations, reduces the incidence of large colorectal adenomas, which is thought to be a critical step in the development of malignancies.[34-36] In another study, dietary changes involving increased intake of calcium and decreased consumption of fat produced reductions in colonic epithelial cell proliferation and the size of the proliferative compartment, and it restored markers of normal cellular differentiation such as acidic mucin, cytokeratin AE1 distribution, and nuclear size.[37] Vitamins A and D, fatty acids, and zinc may affect colon cancer progression through their direct effects on gene transcription.[38]

Nitrosamines and heterocyclic amines, bloodborne carcinogens from tobacco smoke and meat, have been linked to mutations in *APC* or *K-ras*.[15] Consumption of alcohol may contribute to carcinogenesis by reducing folate levels, which can result in DNA damage. Consumption of vegetables has a protective effect, because vegetables are a source of folate, antioxidants, and inducers of detoxifying enzymes.[15,39] Folate is important for DNA integrity, antioxidants reduce DNA damage, and fiber affects short-chain fatty acids, which themselves influence apoptosis. It is also possible that polymorphisms in the genes coding for methylene-tetrahydrofolate reductase and N-acetyltransferases -1 and -2 affect the metabolism of folate and heterocyclic amines.[15]

Prior Irradiation

Previous radiation exposure can increase the risk of developing colorectal cancer. Among men treated with radiation for prostate cancer, the overall risk of a second malignancy was 1:290, and that risk increased to 1:70 for those surviving at least 10 years.[40] The increase in relative risk in that study was 15% at 5 or more years and 34% among those who survived 10 years or longer.[40]

The risk of colorectal cancer is increased and the radiation tolerance level is reduced among patients with inflammatory bowel disease. Ulcerative colitis and Crohn's disease have been linked to abnormalities in chromosomes 3, 6, 7, 12, and 16 that result in a dysregulated mucosal response that leads to chronic mucosal inflammation. These disease entities are part of a larger group of autoimmune diseases. Ulcerative colitis causes superficial inflammation of the mucosa that can cause ulcer formation in the colon. Most commonly, ulcerative colitis affects the rectal and sigmoid areas and progresses proximally.[41] Pathologically, ulcerative colitis is characterized by acute inflammatory events with neutrophils and crypt abscesses.

In contrast, Crohn's disease can occur anywhere in the gastrointestinal tract, but it is particularly common in the terminal ileum and ascending colon.[41] Often Crohn's disease affects discontinuous areas, with areas of inflammation dispersed between normal mucosa throughout the gastrointestinal tract. Lymphocytes and macrophages accumulate within the intestinal crypt and protogranulomas are seen. Crohn's disease produces transmural inflammation of the bowel resulting in the formation of strictures, fistulas, and abscesses. Crohn's disease affects about 400,000 people in the United States.

Screening

Screening procedures have had a significant effect on the detection of colorectal cancer. Over the second half of the 1900s, the incidence of colon cancer rose sharply, especially among males and blacks. Trends in the rates of colorectal cancer were specifically evaluated between 1975 and 1994 from more than 220,000 cases of colorectal cancer in the United States using data from the U.S. Surveillance, Epidemiology, and End Results program. In the late 1970s, the incidence of metastatic disease at diagnosis began to decline among whites; 10 years later, declines were also seen in the incidence of regional disease.[42] These trends correlated with increased rates of screening for colorectal cancer during the mid-1980s.

The numbers of cases of cancer found in the distal colon and rectum decreased more significantly because screening initiatives focused on the use of the least invasive techniques.[15,42] Consequently, numbers of proximal colon cancer cases were higher than distal colon and rectal cancer cases throughout the study period.[42] Most cases of cancer arose in the proximal colon (39%), followed by the distal colon (30%) and rectum (29%). Localized disease was diagnosed in 37%, regional disease in 37%, and distant disease in 20%. More commonly, localized disease was diagnosed in the distal colon and rectum, and regional disease was found in proximal colon tumors. The incidence of cancer in the proximal colon was significantly higher among blacks than whites (Fig. 22-1).[13]

Despite its success in cancer detection, screening, especially genetic testing, is fraught with difficulties, including patients' concerns about insurability, employment discrimination, denial, and fear.[23] In a study of 208 members of four extended families with HNPCC, 43% elected to undergo testing and 57% declined. Of the 139 subjects (67%) who consented to a telephone interview, 55 (40%) did not wish to receive their test results. Among the 84 people who did accept the test results, 35 (42%) found out that they had HNPCC-associated mutations.[43] Those who wished to receive the test information were better educated and were more likely to have participated in a previous genetic linkage study than those who declined to receive their test results. The presence of depressive symptoms resulted in a fourfold decrease in acceptance of test results among women and

a slight decrease among men, although equal numbers of men and women underwent the testing.[43]

A survey among first-degree relatives of patients with colorectal cancer revealed that perceived barriers to screening included lack of public awareness, lack of physician recommendation for screening procedures, questionable efficacy of the screening procedures, fear of positive results, embarrassment, and discomfort and uncleanliness associated with the test.[44] For these reasons, only 14% of those individuals had ever been tested for fecal occult blood; 59% had never had a digital rectal exam, 73% had never had a flexible sigmoidoscopy, and 64% had never had a colonoscopy. Nevertheless, this survey group understood that screening would reduce the chance of dying from colorectal cancer and that undergoing screening procedures would reassure them of being cancer-free.

In another study, 199 family members of patients with HNPCC underwent genetic testing for the presence of known mutations.[26] Before their mutation status was disclosed, subjects were asked about prior screening tests; only 55% had undergone at least one colonoscopy, and 47% had undergone at least one other screening test for colon cancer.[26] After their mutation status was revealed, 95% of those who carried the mutation were willing to undergo lifelong surveillance (annual or semiannual colonoscopy beginning at age 20 years),[45] and 70% were willing to undergo prophylactic colectomy.

A cross-sectional study of 98 patients with colorectal cancer showed that 61% reported being worried about their relatives having colorectal cancer, and 64% were

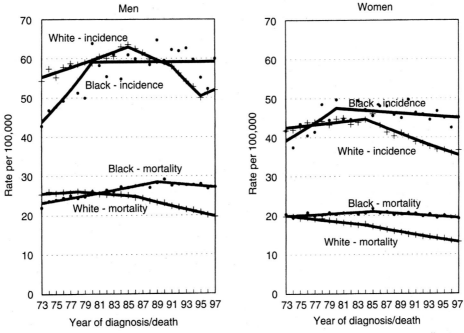

Fig. 22-1 Cancer incidence by sex and ethnic origin. (From Ries LAG, Wingo PA, Miller DS, et al. *Cancer* 2000;88:2398-2424.)

concerned about the risk of genetic transmission.[46] Although 81% were unaware that genetic testing for colorectal cancer was available, 72% reported being willing to take such a test if it were available to them.[46]

From the physician's point of view, the difficulties associated with screening for inherited cancer can be classified in terms of confidentiality, coordination, and communication. It is often difficult for physicians to distinguish between cases that are sporadic, familial (at least one relative but no clear Mendelian pattern or known mutation), or inherited (a single gene mutation playing a causative role).[47] However, if an inherited syndrome is suspected, referral should be made to a center for genetic assessment. Another resource is the Online Mendelian Inheritance in Man (OMIM) Database, which can be accessed at http://www3.ncbi.nim.nih.gov/Omim/searchomim.html.[48] Of the 35 familial cancer-predisposing disorders identified to date,[49] tumors of the colon or rectum have been reported in six: familial adenomatous polyposis, Bloom's syndrome, breast/ovarian cancer (*BRCA1*), breast cancer/other (*BRCA2*), HNPCC, and Peutz-Jeghers syndrome. Moreover, at least 10 types of hereditary colon cancer have been identified.[48]

Obligation to Inform

All of the physicians involved in the care of a patient assume the responsibility of documenting that the possibility of a genetic link to the disease was discussed with that patient.[50] Without this knowledge, patients cannot inform family members regarding their potential risk and the need to seek medical evaluation. Various court cases involving familial cases of breast, ovarian, and colon cancer have set precedents regarding the obligation to inform. The legal precedents are based on the experience with multiple endocrine neoplasia (MEN) type II syndrome, in which identification of the *RET* proto-oncogene can lead to a precise diagnosis of susceptibility to medullary thyroid carcinoma. It is now considered mandatory to offer testing to at-risk family members, including children as young as age 3, so that they can undergo prophylactic thyroidectomy.[23]

Risk-reduction strategies can yield great improvements in life expectancy for people with colorectal cancer. One decision-analysis model[51] suggested that prophylactic proctocolectomy at age 25 increased life expectancy by 14 years over that of no intervention; however, colectomy performed at the time of cancer diagnosis produced only minimal benefit. As the age of the patient increased, surveillance proved as beneficial as colectomy. However, when health-related quality of life was considered, surveillance led to the greatest quality-adjusted life expectancy benefit.[51]

Screening Procedures

Procedures currently in use for colorectal cancer screening include the fecal occult blood test, colonoscopy, sigmoidoscopy, and proctoscopy. Each technique has advantages and disadvantages; for example, fecal occult blood tests are the least invasive, but their sensitivity and specificity are questionable. Endoscopic procedures are invasive, require preparation, and are often costly. Proctoscopy, although beneficial for detecting rectal tumors, cannot detect tumors in the colon. Sigmoidoscopy allows examination of a larger portion of the colon than does proctoscopy, but results from one prospective trial of 114 patients indicated that sigmoidoscopy detected abnormalities identified in only 28% of patients, although 41% of these patients were found to have a proximal adenoma.[52] Computed tomography (CT) scanning of the colon, or virtual colonoscopy, may be an alternative to endoscopic colonoscopy, but the procedure still involves insufflation of air and the attendant discomfort. More experience is needed with the technique to resolve issues regarding accuracy.[53,54]

The need to educate primary care physicians in cancer screening is critical. In a recent survey, 168 internal medicine residents in four accredited programs completed questionnaires regarding colorectal cancer screening and the use of fecal occult blood tests. Seventy-one percent of those surveyed correctly identified 50 years as the age at which an asymptomatic patient at average risk should begin colorectal cancer screening as recommended in national guidelines.[55] Only 64% routinely performed fecal occult blood testing at outpatient clinic visits, 79% performed a digital rectal exam, and only 29% recommended colonoscopy to evaluate the appearance of blood in the feces. The residents' level of training influenced their use of annual fecal occult blood tests and flexible sigmoidoscopy (58% among those in their first or second year of training vs. 80% among those in their third or fourth years of training) and the practice of following a positive fecal occult blood test with colonoscopy (19% vs. 48%, respectively).

The Minnesota Colon Cancer Control Study saw a decrease in mortality over a 13-year period that was attributed to early detection of colorectal cancer.[56] In that study, patients underwent an expanded version of the annual fecal occult blood test each year during that 13-year period. In that test, two fecal samples from each of three consecutive stools were placed on a test card. If any one sample was positive, a diagnostic work-up that included a colonoscopy was performed. The sensitivity of this procedure was found to be about 90%; it produced a cure rate for early colorectal cancer of about 90%, and it reduced the mortality from colorectal cancer by one third among patients older than 50 years. Because the incidence of colorectal cancer did not change over the 13-year study period, the decrease in mortality was attributed to its early detection. Finally, the number of slides that were positive among the six slides in the set was linked to the presence of polyps and colorectal cancer.[56]

Screening also benefits patients with known colorectal abnormalities. In another study, 204 patients with a history of adenomatous polyps underwent screening and two follow-up colonoscopies.[57] During the median total surveillance period of 55 months, 493 adenomas and one cancer were detected. The first follow-up colonoscopy was normal in 91 patients (45%); among these patients, the second colonoscopy was also normal in 57 (63%), but adenomas were identified in 34 (37%). Of the 113 patients (55%) who were found to have adenomas on the first follow-up colonoscopy, only 46 (40%) had a subsequent normal colonoscopy; the other 67 (60%) had adenomas on the second follow-up colonoscopy. The risk of subsequent adenomas was significantly reduced if the findings at interim colonoscopy were normal; at 3 years, only 15% of those whose interim colonoscopy was normal had adenomas vs. 40% of those for whom the interim colonoscopy was positive. However, by 4 years of follow-up, the risk of adenoma was the same regardless of the findings from the interim colonoscopy. Adenomas found after a normal colonscopy were dispersed throughout the colon in 28 cases and limited to the rectosigmoid in only 6 cases. A significant reduction in the risk of a subsequent diagnosis of colon cancer was seen when the follow-up colonoscopy was normal. These results led the authors of this study to recommend surveillance colonoscopy at 4- to 5-year intervals.

The importance of screening for colorectal cancer in asymptomatic individuals cannot be overemphasized. An autopsy series of 1105 cases between 1986 and 1995 revealed 250 cases of cancer, of which 111 tumors in 100 patients had either been undiagnosed or misdiagnosed.[58] The immediate cause of death was attributable to the cancer in 57 patients. In this study, as in other reports, the discordance between clinical and autopsy diagnoses of cancer was 44%. Of the undiagnosed tumors, only 33% were clinically suspected, and 23% of undiagnosed cancerous tumors were in the gastrointestinal tract. Another study in which 186 premenopausal women with iron-deficiency anemia underwent colonic endoscopy,[59] a "clinically important" lesion was found in 23 cases, of which six were colon cancer.[59] Independent predictors for having a gastrointestinal lesion identified by endoscopy included having positive findings on the fecal occult blood test, a hemoglobin level of less than 10 g/dl, and abdominal symptoms.[59]

Screening Guidelines and Cost Considerations

Evidence-based guidelines[60] recommend that asymptomatic individuals at average risk of colorectal cancer undergo screening beginning at age 50 years and that patients at higher risk undergo more intensive screening and follow-up. Adopting these principles could reduce the mortality from colorectal cancer by more than 50%.

In the Minnesota trial mentioned earlier in this section, annual fecal occult blood testing found 260 of the first 281 cancer cases, for a sensitivity rate of 92.5%.[61] Reductions in mortality rates have been attributed in part to the use of colonoscopy to evaluate positive findings from fecal occult blood tests; only 20% of the observed benefit resulted from colonoscopy after false-positive screening tests.[61]

As for the question of sigmoidoscopy vs. colonoscopy, cohort and case-control studies have shown that use of flexible sigmoidoscopy as the only screening procedure reduces the risk of death from distal colorectal cancer by about 70%.[61] Although the "miss" rate for flexible sigmoidoscopy can be as high as 50% owing to incomplete bowel preparations and technical limitations, combining this test with fecal occult blood testing overcomes many of the limitations of both tests used separately.[61]

The estimated cost of fecal occult blood testing and flexible sigmoidoscopy in the United States has been estimated at almost $1 billion over 7 years.[61] However, this expense is considered cost-effective because of the corresponding savings in the cost of treating cancer. In the University of Minnesota study, the cost of screening was calculated to be between $15,000 to $25,000 per year of life saved; this cost is well below the $40,000 considered by the Federal government to be cost-effective. (By way of comparison, the cost of screening mammography is about $30,000 per year of life saved.) Following screening guidelines could lead to an estimated 35,000 lives being saved each year.

The cost of treating colorectal cancer is second only to that of breast cancer, totaling more than $6.5 billion per year. The overall cost of cancer care in the United States is more than $40 billion, which is more than 12% of the total expenditures for health care.[62] The average cost for treatment of colorectal cancer is about $50,000 per patient. As the results of screening initiatives become more mature, cost-effectiveness analysis, particularly for the more invasive screening procedures, will become increasingly important.

The American College of Gastroenterology recently updated the Agency for Health Care Policy and Research Guidelines for colorectal cancer screening. For the average-risk individual, defined as 50 years of age and older with no risk factors for colorectal cancer except for age, the preferred screening strategy is a colonoscopy every 10 years.[25] Colonoscopy confers several advantages over flexible sigmoidoscopy, in particular the ability to evaluate the entire colon and the ability to remove adenomas during the same procedure. Roughly half of all patents with colon cancer have disease proximal to the splenic flexure, and the incidence of proximal colon cancer has increased over the past 30 years.[63] Nevertheless, when resources are limited, the recommendation is to use flexible sigmoidoscopy every 5 years with annual fecal occult blood testing. However, patients whose fecal occult blood test results are positive should undergo colonoscopy. Although reports of virtual (CT-based) colonoscopy have indicated that polyps as small as 6 mm can be detected with this technique, more experience is needed before virtual colonoscopy can be recommended as an alternative to colonoscopy.

Individuals considered to be at high risk of developing colorectal cancer include those with familial adenomatous polyposis, HNPCC, or a family history of colon polyps or cancer that does not meet the clinical criteria for these syndromes. (According to the American College of Gastroenterology, about 10% of people in the United States will eventually have an immediate family member with colon cancer, and having a family history of colon cancer doubles one's risk of this cancer.[25]) Other groups at high risk include those with a history of adenomatous polyps, ulcerative colitis, or Crohn's disease. Screening for familial adenomatous polyposis should begin in childhood, with a sigmoidoscopy every 1 to 2 years beginning at 10 to 12 years of age. Once polyps appear, a colectomy should be planned. Individuals diagnosed at a later age and unscreened individuals and relatives should have a full colonoscopy; screening should continue until 40 years of age, when standard-risk screening procedures can begin. Even if the criteria for HNPCC are not met, individuals with a strong family history of colon polyps or cancer should begin screening either at age 40 or at 10 years earlier than the age of the youngest affected relative, whichever is first. Colonoscopy should be performed every 10 years if a single first-degree relative with colorectal cancer is diagnosed at or after 60 years of age. If the first-degree relative was younger than 60 at diagnosis, then colonoscopy should be performed every 3 to 5 years.

Surveillance Guidelines

Screening strategies have also been adapted for surveillance purposes after colorectal cancer has been diagnosed and treated. Recommendations for surveillance depend on the anatomic location and natural history of the disease; colon cancer generally metastasizes to the liver first, but rectal cancer can spread through paravertebral venous and lymphatic channels to the lungs without involving the liver. Most recurrences appear within 3 years of surgery, and almost all appear within 5 years.

The American Society of Clinical Oncology used evidence-based criteria to create the Guidelines for Colorectal Cancer Surveillance.[64] Standard follow-up includes a regular history, physical examination, and diagnostic studies (complete blood count, liver function studies, carcinoembryonic antigen [CEA] levels, and fecal occult blood tests). Intensive evaluations comprise standard follow-up tests and yearly radiography of the chest, CT scans of the liver, and colonoscopy. The rationale for including the imaging studies was that about 30% of recurrent tumors do not produce CEA and that a false-negative CEA level is common in poorly differentiated tumors. Although one report suggested that routine CEA testing can detect metastatic disease an average of 5 months before it becomes apparent on routine clinical evaluations,[65] the clinical significance of this finding is unknown given the limited options available for treating metastatic disease.

Little consensus exists regarding the usefulness of the various components of follow-up evaluations. In a large cooperative group trial of 1247 patients with colon cancer,[66] 548 patients had recurrent disease; salvage surgery was attempted in 222 of these patients and another 109 underwent surgery with curative intent.[66] Among those for whom salvage was attempted, surgery was prompted because of abnormal CEA test results (38%), symptoms (25%), or abnormalities found on CT scanning (33%) or other tests (5%). Only 5% of these patients were free of disease 5 years after the recurrence. Among the 109 patients who underwent curative-attempt surgery (20% of those with recurrent disease), the presence of a solitary lesion at recurrence was the most favorable prognostic factor. At a median follow-up period exceeding 5 years, the estimated 5-year disease-free survival rate among those treated with curative intent was 23%. The limited potential for benefit must be balanced with the substantial morbidity associated with progressive disease; the authors of this report concluded that follow-up testing and early evaluation of symptoms can often prompt surgery, which in turn can extend disease-free survival.

In another study, intensive vs. limited follow-up was evaluated prospectively among 216 patients who had undergone resection of rectal cancer. Reoperation was attempted in 30% of both intensive and limited follow-up groups; the median survival of 19 months in the intensive group was not statistically different than the 8-month median survival for the limited follow-up group.[67] Median survival duration for both asymptomatic and symptomatic patients was 15 months, even though 44% of asymptomatic patients vs. 27% of symptomatic patients underwent reoperation.

With regard to laboratory studies, of 8749 total laboratory values obtained in follow-up among 105 patients with colorectal cancer,[68] 5894 values (67%) were normal. Of the 2004 (23%) values that were low, 5% elicited a therapeutic response.[68] Of the 851 (10%) values that were high, 2.5% elicited a response. These findings led the authors of this study to recommend that laboratory tests be conducted for patients with coexisting medical problems such as diabetes and cardiovascular disease requiring potassium supplementation, patients for whom laboratory values were likely to be abnormal.

Imaging Modalities

The usefulness of routine CT scanning for surveillance is considered unproven. Results from an Italian study suggest that even when liver metastases can be identified in asymptomatic patients, less than one third of cases are resectable and less than 10% of patients are alive 2 years later.[67] Moreover, a retrospective study of CT scans from patients with colorectal cancer concluded that although metastatic disease was common (present in 34% [1040] of the 3073 CT scans reviewed), pelvic metastases from colon tumors were rare.[69] Hence, although the false-negative rate and the cost of CT scanning are low, the diagnostic yield is low, and the absolute benefit is also low because the chances of undergoing resection and improving survival are very limited.

Magnetic resonance imaging (MRI) may be better able than CT to visualize the extent of disease in the peritoneum, bowel, and mesentery. In one study, MRI was able to identify 90% of 154 surgically confirmed extrahepatic tumor sites, whereas CT revealed only 66%.[70] Because the additional information from the MRI did affect the therapeutic recommendations in that study, the authors concluded that MRI may be beneficial for identifying resectable disease in some patients.

Whole-body positron emission tomography (PET) scanning has been used to identify recurrent disease before it becomes evident on other imaging studies. In this technique, a glucose analog labeled with ^{18}F (2-fluoro-2-deoxy-D-glucose [FDG]) is used to detect malignancy by making visible the increase in glucose uptake and metabolism by cancer cells. The agent is transported into cells by epithelial glucose-transporter proteins; because FDG cannot be converted to the fructose analog, it accumulates in the cells.[71,72] In a recent Belgian study,[71] a discordance rate of 10% was found between FDG-PET and conventional diagnostic imaging, but FDG-PET was determined to have additional diagnostic value in 14 of 16 local–regional, six of seven hepatic, seven of eight abdominal, and eight of nine extraabdominal recurrences. In a patient-based analysis, FDG-PET was shown to have additional diagnostic value in terms of defining resectability in 20% of patients. Another analysis at the Mallinckrodt Institute of Radiology showed that FDG-PET had a positive predictive value of 89% and a negative predictive value of 100% among patients with rising CEA levels after surgery for colorectal cancer.[73] Yet another group found the sensitivity and specificity of FDG-PET to be 93% and 98%, compared with 69% and 98% for CT scans, for detecting recurrent colorectal cancer.[74] In the latter study, the potential savings resulting from demonstration of unresectable disease by FDG-PET was calculated as being more than $3000 per preoperative study.

FDG-PET has been especially useful in evaluating the retroperitoneum for adenopathy because PET can detect very small lesions and lesions in postoperative surgical fields that are difficult to assess with CT.[75] In terms of histologic features, the cellularity and amount of mucin in the tumor mass were predictive of FDG-PET results, with FDG-PET being of limited value for evaluating mucinous tumors, particularly hypocellular lesions with abundant mucin.[76]

In general, good data on which to base recommendations for surveillance after therapy for rectal cancer are lacking. The nonrandomized studies in which patients are found to have recurrent disease at routine diagnostic testing are prone to bias[77]; however, ethical concerns make randomized studies extremely difficult to perform. Future studies should target screening modalities that are most likely to have the greatest influence on survival. Nevertheless, because the morbidity of progressive symptoms is substantial, close clinical follow-up is necessary, and diagnostic studies should be undertaken promptly when symptoms appear to determine their etiology and to initiate appropriate measures for their control. Because treatment-related effects and intercurrent medical problems like infection and inflammation can also produce symptoms and other diagnostic abnormalities, scanning can provide important information regarding treatable causes of intercurrent disease.[78]

STAGING CONSIDERATIONS

The tumor-nodes-metastasis (TNM) system from the American Joint Committee on Cancer (AJCC), used for staging tumors of the colon and rectum, is outlined in Box 22-2.[79] T stage is determined by a combination of physical examination, including proctoscopy, and imaging by transrectal ultrasonography, CT, or MRI with an intrarectal coil. Patients with T2 or higher tumors should also undergo chest radiography and CT scanning of the abdomen and pelvis to exclude the presence of occult metastases. Specialized techniques for the administration of contrast agents and scan time should be used in CT scanning so as to increase its sensitivity and specificity for detecting liver metastases.

Although CT and MRI are more than 90% accurate for identifying metastatic spread before treatment, both are limited with respect to their ability to reveal local disease extension. The ability of CT to visualize a primary tumor depends on the size and location of the tumor; in one study of 158 patients, CT identified the primary tumor in only 75% of cases.[80] The sensitivity and specificity of CT in detecting perirectal fat involvement range from about 50% to 75%; tumors in the lower rectum are difficult to evaluate with CT because of the paucity of fat in this region.[81,82] The accuracy of transrectal MRI for detecting tumor involvement of the perirectal fat has been greater than 85% in several series.[81] The success rate of CT and MRI for identifying perirectal lymph node involvement is about 60%.[82]

BOX 22-2   American Joint Committee on Cancer Staging System for Cancer of the Colon and Rectum

PRIMARY TUMOR (T)

TX	Primary tumor cannot be assessed
T0	No evidence of primary tumor
Tis	Carcinoma in situ: intraepithelial or invasion of lamina propria*
T1	Tumor invades submucosa
T2	Tumor invades muscularis propria
T3	Tumor invades through the muscularis propria into the subserosa or into nonperitonealized pericolic or perirectal tissues
T4	Tumor directly invades other organs or structures and/or perforates visceral peritoneum†

REGIONAL LYMPH NODES (N)

NX	Regional lymph nodes cannot be assessed
N0	No regional lymph node metastasis
N1	Metastasis in 1 to 3 regional lymph nodes
N2	Metastasis in 4 or more regional lymph nodes

DISTANT METASTASIS (M)

MX	Distant metastasis cannot be assessed
M0	No distant metastasis
M1	Distant metastasis

STAGE GROUPING

AJCC/UICC				Dukes‡
Stage 0	Tis	N0	M0	—
Stage I	T1	N0	M0	A
	T2	N0	M0	—
Stage II	T3	N0	M0	B
	T4	N0	M0	—
Stage III	Any T	N1	M0	C
	Any T	N2	M0	—
Stage IV	Any T	Any N	M1	—

From Fleming I, Cooper JS, Henson DE, et al, eds. *AJCC Cancer Staging Manual.* 5th ed. Philadelphia, Pa: Lippincott Williams & Wilkins; 1997:83-90.

AJCC, American Joint Committee on Cancer; *UICC,* International Union Against Cancer.

*Tis includes cancer cells confined within the glandular basement membrane (intraepithelial) or lamina propria (intramucosal) with no extension through the muscularis mucosae into the submucosa.

†Direct invasion in T4 includes invasion of other segments of the colorectum by way of the serosa (e.g., invasion of the sigmoid colon by a carcinoma of the cecum).

‡Dukes B is a composite of better (T3 N0 M0) and worse (T4 N0 M0) prognostic groups, as is Dukes C (any T N1 M0 and Any T N2 M0)

Endorectal Sonography

Endorectal sonography can be useful for accurately staging primary rectal tumors before surgery or preoperative chemoradiation. Preparations for the procedure are minimal, requiring only an enema. The normal rectal wall appears as concentric alternating hyperechoic and hypoechoic bands (Fig. 22-2). Drawbacks of this technique are its inability to visualize normal perirectal lymph nodes, which are less than 3 mm in diameter, and the ease with which lesions at or near the anal verge can be missed because the balloon on the transducer tip will not pass through a normal sphincter without being deflated. In the latter situation, replacing the balloon with a hard plastic cap improves the resolution of the images.[83]

Because the choice of surgical technique is determined by whether tumor involves the sphincteric muscles, other sonographic techniques should be used to evaluate muscle involvement. In women, transvaginal sonography is one such option. For detecting internal sphincter defects, the sensitivity of this technique is 44%, and its specificity is 96%; for external sphincter defects, the corresponding rates are 48% and 88%.[84] Transperineal sonography of the rectum also can be useful for evaluating the distal anorectum, particularly when tumors in the distal rectum render that region stenotic and painful.[85]

Lymph nodes that are visible on endorectal sonography may contain metastatic disease or they may be inflamed. The sonographic criteria for distinguishing the two conditions overlap somewhat,[83] but metastatic disease generally is characterized by the appearance of discrete margins and are of either uniform hypoechogenicity or the same echotexture as the primary tumor.

The overall rate of accuracy of endorectal sonography was reported in one study[86] to be 70%, with a positive predictive value of 67% and a negative predictive value of 75%. Overstaging of the primary tumor occurred in only 11% of patients who had not undergone irradiation, but overstaging occurred in 21% of patients who had undergone preoperative radiation therapy because of fibrosis in the tumor bed. Estimation of lymph node involvement in this study was accurate in 71% of patients, with a positive predictive value of 47% and a negative predictive value of 76%. No false-positive results were obtained in unirradiated patients, but eight of 54 patients who underwent preoperative radiation had false-positive results. False-negative results occurred in six of 36 unirradiated patients and in 12 of 54 patients who underwent preoperative radiation.[86]

The overall accuracy of endorectal sonography in determining the depth of penetration of the pelvic wall

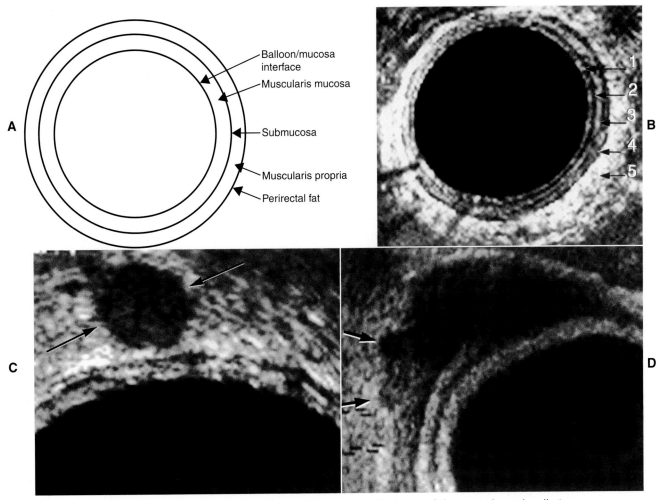

Fig. 22-2 Endorectal sonographic images. **A** and **B,** The layers of the normal rectal wall. *1,* balloon/mucosa interface; *2,* muscularis mucosa; *3,* submucosa; *4,* muscularis propria; *5,* perirectal fat. **C,** Perirectal lymph node involvement is indicated by a hypoechoic lesion outside the rectal wall. **D,** A tumor extending through the bowel wall into the perirectal fat.

during preoperative staging ranges from 72% to 97%, with up to 12% of tumors overstaged and 9% understaged.[83] The lack of specific imaging criteria are reflected in the rates of accuracy of predicting perirectal lymph node invasion, which range from 60% to 85% with sensitivity of 59% to 89% and specificity of 64% to 87%. Other sources of error in endorectal sonographic staging include tumor location and stenosis, peritumoral inflammation, changes after biopsy or surgery, hemorrhage, and pedunculated or villous tumors.[83]

Sonographic staging after preoperative chemoradiation should be done before surgery. In one study,[87] endorectal sonography was performed 6 to 8 weeks after completion of chemoradiation therapy to assess the residual fibrosis that had replaced the original tumor. The depth of penetration in the bowel wall from the fibrotic reaction was often easier to evaluate than that arising from the original tumor. Also, the residual tumor depth could be assessed directly because the residual tumor always appeared within the fibrotic region.[87]

When used to evaluate tumor recurrence after completion of all therapy, sonography compares favorably with other follow-up techniques. A German group[88] used sonography to prospectively follow 338 patients with rectal cancer, 116 of whom developed recurrent disease. Among the follow-up tests performed, the accuracy of tumor markers was 58% (sensitivity 36%, specificity 88%), the accuracy of digital examination was 23% (sensitivity 21%, specificity 99%), the accuracy of proctoscopy was 35% (sensitivity 31%, specificity 98%), and the accuracy of endorectal sonography was 79% (sensitivity 79%, specificity 100%).[88] Thus in this study, follow-up endorectal sonography had the highest rates of sensitivity and specificity and had a positive predictive value of 100% and a negative predictive value of 90%. In contrast, the positive predictive value for tumor markers was 62% and that for a digital examination with proctoscopy was 90%; the negative predictive value for these procedures was 70%. The authors of this study concluded that assessment of local recurrence may be best evaluated by the cost-effective option of endorectal sonography.[88]

TREATMENT STRATEGIES: RECTAL CANCER

The anatomic location of and the structures involved by tumors in the rectal area often determine therapeutic recommendations. The rectum is classically divided into three levels: the low rectum, midrectum, and upper or proximal rectum (Fig. 22-3). Variations in anatomy and body habitus make it difficult to precisely delineate each of these segments. The American College of Surgeons considers tumors located from the anal verge to 15 cm proximally to be rectal tumors; others contend that tumors located 12 to 15 cm proximal to the anal verge act more like colon cancer than rectal cancer. A more stringent definition of rectal tumors includes those tumors found during rigid proctoscopy, with the patient in the left lateral Sims position, to be within 12 cm of the anal verge.

Surgical Approaches

The success of combined-modality therapy (described in further detail later in this section) has meant that abdominoperineal resection is now reserved for tumors located within 5 to 6 cm from the anal verge, or from the distal aspect of the coccyx to the levator ani muscles

(discussed further in Chapter 23). Surgical procedures in current use are local excision, standard low-anterior resection, low-anterior resection with coloanal anastomosis, and low-anterior resection or coloanal anastomosis with the creation of a J-pouch colonic reservoir. Success rates and outcomes after each type of surgery are discussed in the remainder of this section.

The surgical management of colorectal cancer has 4 goals. The first goal is cure, defined as the prevention of systemic spread; the second is local control; the third is preservation of the anal sphincter or anorectal function; and the fourth is the preservation of sexual and urinary functions by preserving the integrity of the autonomic nervous system.[89] In one study,[90] resection of rectal cancer that spared the pelvic autonomic nerves and included lateral lymph node dissection resulted in local control rates of 100% in patients with Dukes stage A or B disease at a median follow-up of 53 months. In that same study, the 5-year survival rate for patients with Dukes stage A disease was 96%, that for patients with stage B disease was 84%, and that for those with stage C disease was 67%.[90] Urinary function was preserved in 94% of patients undergoing dissection of the unilateral pelvic plexus. When the complete pelvic plexus was preserved, sexual function could be preserved in 70% of men; if the hypogastric nerves had to be removed but the pelvic plexus could be preserved, 67% of men could maintain the ability to have an erection and intercourse without normal ejaculation.[90]

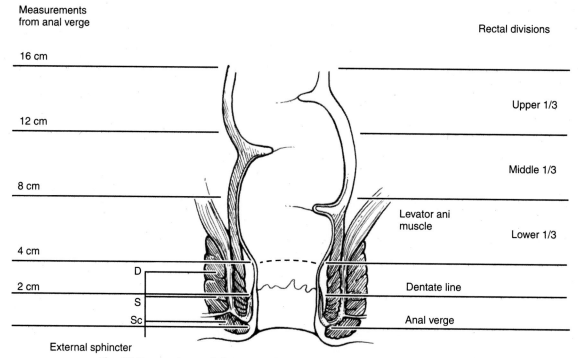

Fig. 22-3 Anatomy of the rectum. *D,* Deep; *S,* superficial; *Sc,* subcutaneous.

The Importance of Mesorectal Resection

Critical for achieving local control is complete resection of the mesorectum. Incomplete resection of the mesorectal fat consistently results in local failure rates as high as 90% within 18 months because of residual tumor in the lymph nodes attached to the pelvic sidewall.[89] The visceral fascia covers the rectum and the mesorectum. The parietal fascia covers the musculoskeletal and vascular structures of the pelvic sidewalls, including the pelvic autonomic plexus. When the mesorectal lymph nodes are positive, one third of patients will also have lateral nodal involvement. Lateral lymph node involvement is also associated with transmural and extraperitoneal disease, so lateral lymph node dissection is performed in the event of perirectal penetration (T3) or mesorectal lymph node involvement. For patients treated with surgery only, the overall recurrence rates are 65% when the lateral pelvic lymph nodes are positive versus 38% when those nodes are negative; the corresponding local recurrence rates are 26% and 10%, and the corresponding 5-year overall survival rates are 49% and 74%. In contrast, the addition of pelvic radiation and concurrent chemotherapy to surgical treatment can clear residual microscopic tumor in pelvic lymph nodes. Combined-modality therapy that includes surgical resection with total mesorectal excision can produce local control rates in excess of 90% for locally advanced rectal cancer.

Another detailed study involved assessing the local depth of invasion of colon cancer in terms of the site and extent of regional lymph node metastases.[91] A total of 12,496 lymph nodes from 164 patients (about 76 nodes per patient) were evaluated, and metastatic involvement of the mesenteric lymph nodes was documented in 59% of cases. Of these 724 metastatic lymph nodes, 33% had tumor deposits that were less than 4 mm in diameter. The pattern and extent of pericolonic lymph node spread led the authors to suggest that proximal and distal margins of at least 7 cm, with excision of the regional mesentery and both intermediate and central lymph nodes, were needed to prevent recurrence.[91]

Further information regarding the effect of nodal involvement is available from a study of 1664 patients with T3, T4, or node-positive rectal cancer treated with radiation and chemotherapy.[92] In that study, the number of nodes examined in the pathologic specimen correlated with relapse and survival rates among patients who were considered node-negative after therapy. Among node-negative patients who had up to four nodes examined, the 5-year relapse and survival rates were 27% and 68%; the corresponding rates for patients who had five to eight nodes examined were 34% and 73%: for patients who had nine to 13 nodes examined, 26% and 72%; and for patients who had 14 or more nodes examined, 19% and 82%.[92] No such associations were found among patients with node-positive disease.

Advances in surgical technique have greatly improved local control of rectal cancer, as demonstrated in a retrospective review of 1581 patients who underwent curative resection for rectal cancer between 1974 and 1991.[93] (Total mesorectal excision was introduced in 1985.) The median follow-up time for this study was 13 years; none of these patients were given adjuvant chemotherapy or radiation therapy.[93] The local recurrence rate decreased from 39% to 10% during the study period, and the observed 5-year survival rate increased from 50% to 71%. The overall survival rate was significantly lower among the 306 patients who experienced local recurrence. Distant disease developed in 275 of 1285 patients who had no local recurrence, 8% of whom had stage I disease, 16% stage II disease, and 40% stage III disease. Because the type of the surgery had no effect on the development of distant metastases, the authors concluded that improvements in surgical technique independently improved survival by improving local control of the disease.[93]

Sphincter Preservation

The three major types of sphincter-preserving operations are a standard low-anterior resection, a low-anterior resection with coloanal anastomosis, and a low-anterior resection or coloanal anastomosis with the creation of a J-pouch colonic reservoir. All low-anterior resections involve resection and an anastomosis between a serosalized colon and the extraperitoneal nonserosalized rectum. The standard low-anterior resection involves an intrapelvic anastomosis within the sacral hollow; the length of the remaining distal segment of rectum is variable.[94,95] By comparison, a coloanal anastomosis is an extrapelvic anastomosis at the apex of the anal canal or at the dentate line, and no distal rectum remains. A J-pouch reconstruction can be combined with either a low-anterior resection or a coloanal resection; the reconstruction recreates the reservoir function of the rectum and improves long-term bowel function. Extensive experience with this technique has confirmed excellent rates of tumor control and functional outcome, including fecal continence.[96,97]

Other innovations in rectal surgery include intersphincteric resection, with excision of the internal anal sphincter, after preoperative radiation therapy.[98] Early results with this technique suggest that it produces rates of local control and continence that are comparable to those of other techniques,[98] but additional experience is necessary to confirm these findings.

At the other end of the surgical spectrum is the use of limited resection and organ preservation for disease that has infiltrated adjacent organs. Often the bladder can be spared during resection of a locally advanced rectal cancer without sacrificing local control. In one study,[99] partial resection of the bladder led to obtainment of negative pathologic margins in 94% of cases. Moreover, the incidence of postoperative urinary complications and the rates of local control (about 85%) and survival at 3 years (about 45%) were the same for those who underwent bladder-sparing surgery as for those who underwent standard total pelvic exenteration.

Therapeutic recommendations must be linked to the experience of the treating physicians and also to patient factors. Considerable variability has been shown among surgeons and between institutions in the rates of local–regional recurrence and survival.[100] The variability among seven institutions for local recurrence ranged between 10% and 37%, and the cancer-related survival rate ranged between 54% and 75%. Local recurrence rates among 14 surgeons ranged between 4% and 55%, with a mean of 23% among surgeons who performed colorectal cancer surgery infrequently. Cancer-specific survival rates for those surgeons ranged from 73% to 85%, with a mean of 69% for those who performed colorectal surgery infrequently. A clear correlation was apparent between local recurrence and survival.[100] In another study,[101] the only factors related to local recurrence rate were the length of the resection specimen obtained and the surgeon specializing in colorectal surgery; the local recurrence rate in that study was 3.42 times higher if general surgeons did the resection instead of colorectal surgeons. Advanced disease stage, the presence of vascular invasion, and having a surgeon who had not specialized in colorectal surgery were independent predictive factors for local and overall recurrence.

Independent predictors of major perioperative complications after resection, with or without preoperative chemoradiation, have been evaluated in several studies.[102,103] Some predictors of perioperative complications include the American Society of Anesthesiologists score for operative complications, the use of a temporary ileostomy, the type of surgical procedure, the preoperative hemoglobin level, and extent of intraoperative blood loss; the failure to use a temporary diverting stoma was especially important in this regard.[103] Importantly, the use of preoperative chemoradiation does not influence the risk of perioperative complications when the surgeons are experienced[102]; rather, length of hospital stay, readmission rates, and mortality are related to the severity of the illness rather than to any preoperative treatment.[104]

Local Excision

Local excision, although technically a type of sphincter-preserving operation, can cure only those tumors confined to the bowel wall because it does not include a mesorectal resection. The risk of lymph node involvement in rectal cancer is linked to the tumor stage; for T1 tumors, the risk is 0% to 12%; for T2 tumors, 12% to 28%; and for T3 and T4 tumors, the risk ranges from 36% to 79%.[105] Thus local failure rates among patients who undergo local excision would be expected to be higher than those among patients who undergo more comprehensive surgery, particularly for patients with higher-stage tumors. A group at the University of Minnesota compared outcome between 108 patients with T1 or T2 tumors who underwent transanal excision and 153 patients with similar characteristics who were treated with standard radical surgery. The local recurrence rate was higher in the transanal excision group (28% vs. 4% in the radical-surgery group).[105] Moreover, this effect was stage-dependent: 18% of T1 and 47% of T2 tumors removed by transanal excision recurred as compared with 0% of T1 and 6% of T2 tumors removed by comprehensive surgical resection. This increase in local recurrence rate also resulted in an increased overall recurrence rate of 21% for T1 tumors and 47% for T2 tumors in the local–excision group vs. 9% and 16%, respectively, in the radical-surgery group. The 5-year survival rate also was lower among those undergoing transanal excision (72% for those with T1 tumors and 65% for those with T2 tumors) than among those undergoing radical surgery (80% for those with T1 tumors and 81% for those with T2 tumors).[105]

Other series involving local excision have produced similar results. A 1998 review revealed that the local recurrence rates for 234 T1 or T2 tumors treated by local excision was 27% and the overall survival rate at 5 years was 65%.[106] In 404 such cases at 2 to 3 years of follow-up, the local recurrence rate was 5% and the overall survival rate 97% for those with T1 tumors, with corresponding rates of 18% and 92% for those with T2 tumors and 22% and 80% for those with T3 tumors. The addition of postoperative radiation improved outcome despite the radiation group having had more adverse features such as higher T stage (T2 tumors were present in 15% of those treated with local excision vs. 70% in those treated with local excision plus radiation). In another study,[107] the 5-year actuarial results among 52 cases of local excision vs. 47 cases of local excision plus radiation showed better local control rates (72% vs. 90%) and better relapse-free survival rates (66% vs. 74%) among those given postoperative radiation. Adverse findings on pathology examination such as poor differentiation and the presence of lymphovascular invasion were associated with higher rates of local recurrence after local excision without radiation.[107]

The only prospective multi-institutional trial performed to date evaluating the use of local excision for T1 or T2 rectal tumors was conducted by the Cancer and Leukemia Group B.[108] This group studied 59 patients with T1 tumors and 51 with T2 tumors; the tumors had to be smaller than 4 cm, encompass less than 40% of the bowel wall circumference, and be located less than 10 cm from the dentate line (see Fig. 22-3). T1 tumors were treated with local excision only, and T2 tumors were treated with local excision followed by postoperative radiation with 54 Gy (given in 30 fractions) and chemotherapy (an intermittent infusion of 500 mg/m^2 5-fluorouracil [5-FU]).[108] Significantly, of the 161 patients for whom a full-thickness local excision was attempted, 51 either had positive margins or the tumor stage was higher than T2 or lower than T1. Among the 59 patients with T1 disease, four had a local recurrence and three of these four patients died with disseminated disease. Among the 51 patients with T2 disease, 20% had a local recurrence at a median follow-up of 4 years; moreover, half of these local recurrences also involved distant disease and could not be treated with salvage surgery. The four conclusions provided by this study were as follows: (1) Sphincter preservation was not easy to accomplish in a uniformly defined manner; 51% of the patients evaluated proved to be ineligible after surgical resection. (2) Sphincter-preserving surgery was associated with less morbidity than was radical surgery. (3) Because of the few recurrences, predictors of outcome were not available. (4) The effectiveness of salvage therapy remains to be determined.[108]

At this point, the role of local excision in the treatment of rectal cancer depends on stage and other tumor characteristics and is still largely undefined.[109] Attempts to maximize sphincter preservation must not be compromised by inferior rates of tumor control or functional outcome.

Combined-Modality Therapy for Locally Advanced Disease

The concept that chemotherapy can improve the therapeutic ratio of radiation therapy was first demonstrated in studies of these modalities for rectal cancer. These seminal studies provided a model for combined-modality therapy for cancer at other sites as well. As described at length in Chapter 4 of this volume, radiosensitization is generally accomplished by limiting tumor-cell repopulation and reducing the efficiency of radiation repair during treatment.[110-112] The benefit of adjuvant radiation and chemotherapy for locally advanced rectal cancer (T3 or T4 tumors, with or without positive regional lymph nodes) has been clearly demonstrated in several prospective randomized trials.[113-118] Treatment with only surgery produces an overall 5-year disease-free survival rate of about 55%. The local failure rate after surgery ranges from 35% to 50%; this rate is reduced to 10% to 20% by the addition of postoperative radiation.[119,120] However, in the absence of systemic therapy, the risk of distant metastasis after surgery plus radiation is approximately 20% in stage II disease and 40% to

60% in stage III disease. Without chemotherapy, the 5-year survival rates are approximately 70% to 90% for stage II disease, 40% for T3 N1 disease, and 15% to 20% for T4 N1 disease.

Several prospective randomized studies have been conducted to specifically evaluate the influence of adjuvant chemotherapy and radiation therapy for rectal cancer. In the late 1980s, the NSABP compared outcome among patients treated with surgery only, surgery plus postoperative radiation, and surgery plus postoperative chemotherapy.[118] The radiation dose was 46 Gy in 25 fractions; however, only 86% of the patients received the total prescribed dose. The group given surgery plus postoperative radiation had a lower local recurrence rate than the other groups, but this difference did not affect survival (Table 22-1).[118] The addition of adjuvant chemotherapy to surgery significantly improved disease-free and overall survival rates over those for the surgery-only group, but the rates of local failure and distant metastasis were no different.

Two other randomized studies, one conducted by the Gastrointestinal Tumor Study Group (GITSG) and the other by the Mayo/North Central Cancer Treatment Group (NCCTG), also showed reductions in local recurrence rates and improvements in disease-free and overall survival rates when postoperative radiation and chemotherapy were administered to patients with Dukes stage B2 or C rectal cancer. The GITSG trial compared four treatments: surgery alone, surgery plus postoperative radiation (40 to 48 Gy), surgery plus postoperative chemotherapy, and surgery plus postoperative radiation (40 to 48 Gy) plus chemotherapy. The addition of any form of adjuvant therapy improved local control, disease-free, and overall survival rates over those produced by surgery only (Table 22-2).[115-117] The addition of radiation therapy decreased the incidence of local failure as

TABLE 22-1

Combined-Modality Treatment for Colorectal Cancer: the NSABPR01 Trial*

Treatment Group	OUTCOME MEASURES AT 5 YEARS (%)		
	Overall Survival Rate	Disease-Free Survival Rate	Local Failure Rate
Surgery	43	30	25
Surgery + chemotherapy	53	42	21
Surgery + radiation therapy	39	34	16

Data from Fisher B, Wolmark N, Rockette H, et al. *J Natl Cancer Inst* 1988;80:21-29.
*The trial included 528 patients; the total radiation dose was 46 to 47 Gy; and chemotherapy consisted of fluorouracil, semustine, and vincristine.

TABLE 22-2

Combined-Modality Treatment for Colorectal Cancer: the GITSG7175 Trial*

Treatment Group	OUTCOME MEASURES (%)			
	10-Year Overall Survival Rate	10-Year Disease-Free Survival Rate	Recurrence Rate	Local Failure Rate
Surgery	26	44	55	25
Surgery + chemotherapy	41	51	46	27
Surgery + radiation therapy	33	50	46	20
Surgery + chemoradiation	45	65	35	10

Data from Gastrointestinal Tumor Study Group. *N Engl J Med* 1985;312:1465-1472; Thomas PR, Lindblad AS. *Radiother Oncol* 1988;13: 245-252.

*The trial included 202 patients; the total radiation dose was 40 to 48 Gy; and chemotherapy consisted of fluorouracil and semustine.

the initial form of disease recurrence and, in combination with chemotherapy, reduced the risk of local failure to 10%. The addition of chemotherapy to surgery did not improve the risk of local recurrence (see Table 22-2).[115-117,121] The Mayo/NCCTG trial,[113] which compared outcome after postoperative radiation (50.4 Gy in 28 fractions) with or without chemotherapy (5-FU and semustine), also showed an advantage for combined-modality therapy. The addition of chemotherapy reduced the rate of local failure from 25% to 13.5% and reduced the rate of distant metastasis from 46% to 29%. These reductions resulted in improvements in both disease-free survival rate (from 37% to 59%) and overall survival rate (from 48% to 58%). In short, the combined-modality treatment reduced local and distant recurrences by 34%, and the overall death rate was reduced by 29%.[113] On the basis of these findings, the National Cancer Institute announced in 1991 that adjuvant radiation and chemotherapy was to be the standard of care for locally advanced rectal cancer.[122]

Changes in Treatment Trends over Time

Analysis of the National Cancer Data Base revealed the following four trends in the patterns of care for rectal adenocarcinoma between 1985 and 1995.[123] First, stage I disease was diagnosed at decreasing frequencies over time, being found in only one third of cases at the end of the study period. Second, local excision was being performed with increasing frequency for stage I disease over time. Third, stage for stage, a decline in the use of abdominoperineal resection occurred over time. Finally, multimodal treatments were being used with greater frequency, especially for stage II and III disease, over the course of the study period.[123] In 1985, the combination of radiation, chemotherapy, and surgery was used for less than 1% of patients with stage I disease, 6% of patients with stage II disease, 13% of patients with stage III disease, and 8% of patients with stage IV disease; by 1995, the corresponding percentages had increased to

11%, 40%, 52%, and 15%, respectively. For patients diagnosed with stage II disease in 1989 to 1990, survival rates at 5 years were 62% for those treated with chemotherapy and surgery, with or without radiation, as compared with 55% for those treated with surgery alone or in combination with radiation.[118] For those with stage III rectal cancer, the 5-year survival rates were 42% for those treated with chemotherapy and surgery, with or without radiation, 39% for those treated with surgery and radiation, and 31% for those treated with surgery alone.[118]

The influence of the National Cancer Institute statement was evident in a Patterns of Care study[124] in which treatment of rectal cancer at 57 institutions in the United States between 1992 and 1994 was evaluated. Radiation was given postoperatively to 75% of the patients, preoperatively to 22%, and both preoperatively and postoperatively to 2%. Among the 507 patients in this study, 243 had T3 or N1-N2 M0 disease. Although only 7% of those with locally advanced disease were enrolled in clinical trials, 90% were given chemotherapy, which lasted a median of 21 weeks. With regard to surgery, 54% of those with locally advanced disease underwent a low-anterior resection and 46% had an abdominoperineal resection. Modern radiation techniques with high-energy photons were used for most patients, and 93% were treated with three or four radiation portals.[124] In short, 90% of the patients treated in the United States in 1992 to 1994 were given combined-modality therapy.

Long-term follow-up analysis of patients treated in a Patterns of Care study performed between 1988 and 1989 confirmed that only stage and use of chemotherapy were significant with regard to survival.[125] The 5-year survival rate among those treated with postoperative chemoradiation was 69% as compared with 50% for those treated with postoperative radiation. Preoperative radiation resulted in a higher survival rate, 85% at 5 years, than did postoperative radiation (50%)

but not postoperative chemoradiation (69%).[125] Survival also depended on disease stage; 5-year overall survival rates were 85% for those with stage I disease, 69% for stage II disease, and 54% for stage III disease.[125] The 5-year survival rate also dropped from 89% for those with Dukes stage C1 disease to 48% for those with stage C2 or C3 disease.[125]

Chemotherapy Agents

The type, dose, means of administration, and timing of the various components of combined-modality therapy are critical issues in optimizing treatment. A comprehensive review of the antitumor effect and toxicity of 5-FU–based chemotherapy regimens, for example, supported the idea that 5-FU can be considered two distinct chemotherapeutic agents on the basis of its mode of delivery—bolus vs. continuous infusion.[126] (A third mode, oral delivery, is discussed later in this chapter in the section "Other Treatment Approaches"). First, the two modes of intravenous (IV) delivery produce different toxic effects; bolus schedules cause leukopenia, mucositis, and diarrhea, whereas continuous-infusion schedules cause stomatitis and dermatitis.[126] Second, continuous infusion of 5-FU allows much higher dose-intensities to be achieved (1625 to 2875 mg/m²/week) than are possible with bolus dosing (500 to 750 mg/m²/week). Moreover, in most North American trials, bolus 5-FU is given over a 1- to 2-minute period, a practice that produces severe mucositis or diarrhea in about 30% of patients treated. In European trials, where bolus 5-FU is administered over a 15-minute period, these effects occurred in only 10% of patients.[126]

The effectiveness of biomodulation of 5-FU with other agents (e.g., leucovorin, semustine, or irradiation) also depends on the schedule of administration.[126] In a large trial of 1696 patients with rectal cancer, the effectiveness and toxicity of three types of chemotherapy were compared: bolus 5-FU alone, 5-FU with leucovorin or levamisole, or 5-FU with both leucovorin and levamisole. All patients were to be given two cycles of chemotherapy followed by pelvic irradiation with chemotherapy and two more cycles of chemotherapy.[127] At a median follow-up time of 48 months, no advantage was apparent from the use of biomodulation; however, more gastrointestinal toxicity was experienced in the group that took all three drugs than in the group that took only bolus 5-FU.[127]

Differences in effectiveness and toxicity between bolus and infusional 5-FU were also evaluated in a study of 660 patients with stage II or stage III rectal cancer.[128] Adjuvant 5-FU was given at a dose of 500 mg/m² on days 1 to 5 and days 36 to 40, and 450 mg/m² was given on days 134 to 138 and 169 to 173. During pelvic irradiation, which began on day 64, patients received either 500 mg/m² bolus 5-FU for 3 consecutive days during weeks 1 and 5 of irradiation or infusional 5-FU given at a rate of 225 mg/m², 7 days per week.[128] The infusional 5-FU schedule produced significant improvements in the time to relapse and overall survival rates over those of bolus 5-FU, and local control rates were similar in the two treatment groups. The improvements in time to relapse and overall survival rate were attributed to the systemic effect of 5-FU during radiation therapy. The average dose of 5-FU during radiation was 6546 mg/m² when given by infusion and 2499 mg/m² when given by bolus technique. The higher total doses and the more prolonged exposure to 5-FU were thought to enhance cytotoxicity. The toxicity profiles were also different; bolus 5-FU was associated with more hematologic effects, and infusional 5-FU was associated with more gastrointestinal effects.[128]

Outcomes based on schedule of chemotherapy administration were evaluated by meta-analysis among 1219 patients given 5-FU either by bolus or continuous infusion. The tumor response and overall survival rates were significantly higher among patients who received the drug by continuous infusion.[129] Only performance status and the type of 5-FU administration predicted tumor response; these factors, plus the primary tumor site (rectum vs. colon) predicted survival. Grade 3 or 4 hematologic toxicity occurred more often in the bolus-infusion group than in the infusion group (31% vs. 4%). In contrast, hand-foot syndrome occurred more often with infusional 5-FU (34% of the infusion group vs. 13% in the bolus group).

In summary, combined-modality therapy has significantly improved the rates of local and distant disease control and is now the standard of care for locally advanced rectal cancer. However, the challenge remains as to how best to optimize the components of therapy.

Radiation Therapy

Radiation therapy has three general roles in rectal cancer management. First, radiation is used to enhance local–regional control by eliminating microscopic residual disease around the primary tumor and in the draining lymphatics. Second, significant tumor regression can result when radiation is administered preoperatively to locally advanced primary tumors. In cases such as these, an inoperable lesion can become resectable or amenable to a more conservative surgical approach that involves sphincter preservation. Third, radiation therapy can be used to palliate symptoms arising from the infiltration of pelvic structures or metastatic disease.

Prognostic factors that have been identified for rectal cancer treated by surgery alone reflect the risk of residual microscopic disease; these factors include stage, tumor location, and the presence of serosal, lymphatic, and neurovascular invasion.[130,131] Adjuvant radiation eradicates microscopic residual tumor and eliminates local recurrence in approximately 90% of patients with adverse prognostic factors. Extension of tumor into the perirectal fat or adjacent viscera (stage II; T3-T4 N0) raises the rate of local recurrence to approximately 30% and tumor in the regional lymphatics to more than 50% in patients treated with surgery only. Adjuvant radiation can reduce these recurrence rates substantially.

Adjuvant radiation can be administered either preoperatively or postoperatively. Regardless of the sequence, the primary goal is to improve local–regional control by eradicating microscopic residual disease. Each approach has specific advantages and disadvantages. Prospective randomized assessment of preoperative vs. postoperative adjuvant radiation has been attempted, but because of low patient accrual such studies had to be closed before they were completed. Emphasis has shifted to other issues like the combination of newer systemic agents with radiation and studies of fractionation schedules.[111] The remainder of this section reviews radiation techniques and goes on to describe available information on the use of radiation with surgery, with or without chemotherapy, for the treatment of rectal cancer.

Radiation-Field Arrangement

Careful attention to radiation technique is important regardless of whether the radiation is delivered before or after surgery. Whenever possible, the small bowel should be displaced from the treatment portal because the volume of small bowel in the radiation portal correlates directly with radiation toxicity.[132]

Use of a belly board to displace the small bowel from the radiation portal helps reduce gastrointestinal side effects (Fig. 22-4).[121] Comparisons of CT treatment plans made when the patient is supine vs. those made when the patient is prone and the belly board is used have shown the median reduction in exposed small-bowel volume to be 54% and that of the bladder to be 62%.[133] The corresponding median doses to the small bowel were 24 Gy (supine) and 15 Gy prone with the belly board. When the belly board cannot be used because of the size of the patient or extension of the tumor to anterior structures, treatment while the patient is prone is still preferred over having the patient supine. Another study showed that the belly board could reduce the irradiated small-bowel volume by as much as 70%, regardless of the patient's weight, age, or sex or whether the radiation was given preoperatively or postoperatively.[134]

Exclusion of small bowel from the radiation field is particularly important because diarrhea can result from either radiation or chemotherapy. Two of the chemotherapeutic agents used in the treatment of rectal cancer, 5-FU and irinotecan, cause diarrhea. Maximizing the doses of radiation and chemotherapy that can be given without treatment interruption requires as much small bowel to be excluded as possible and aggressive supportive care to be provided during treatment.

In most cases, the radiation treatment portals encompass the entire pelvis through a posterior and a right and left lateral treatment portal. High-energy photons (e.g., 18 MV) should be used to reduce the integral dose. Unlike the treatment of other pelvic malignancies, the external iliac lymph node chain need not be routinely included in the treatment portal.[135] Anterior fields should be considered when disease extends anteriorly to the urogenital regions. In some cases, anterior-posterior fields or a four-field arrangement may prove necessary because of tumor extension or anatomic constraints. Adequate coverage of the tumor volume should be confirmed with treatment-planning imaging. If an anterior portal is used, the dose to the small bowel must be determined. The volume of small bowel in the field can be determined either by using contrast at the time of the simulation or by CT-based treatment planning.

Even in cases of distal rectal involvement, including infiltration of the anal canal, the risk of inguinal node involvement is limited and radiation treatment portals need not include the inguinal region. The risk of recurrence in the inguinal region for distal rectal tumors is less than 5%.[136] However, radiation techniques should be modified if inguinal lymph nodes are evident clinically and confirmed pathologically to be involved with metastatic disease. Metastatic involvement of these nodes portends an especially poor prognosis with regard to dissemination of disease.[137]

The superior border of the radiation field, in general, should be placed at the L5-S1 interspace. However, if the rectosigmoid is involved, individual anatomy may dictate that the superior border be placed at the L4-L5 interspace (Fig. 22-5). The inferior border of the field is dictated by the inferior extent of the tumor; generally the inferior aspect of the field should be placed 2 cm inferior to the lowest aspect of the tumor. The anus may need to be included in the treatment field in some cases when the tumor is located in the distal rectum. Whenever possible, however, the anus should be blocked from the radiation portal to reduce treatment-related morbidity. For tumors located in the mid- and proximal rectum, the inferior border of the radiation field is placed at the bottom of the obturator foramen. The lateral border should include the sacroiliac joints, and a 2-cm margin should be placed around the pelvic brim to include the internal iliac lymph node chains in the posterior treatment portal.

For the lateral treatment fields, the superior and inferior borders should be consistent with the posterior portal. In routine simulations, contrast should be placed in the rectum to ensure that margins around the primary tumor are adequate. The anterior aspect of the field should be placed 2 cm in front of the most anterior aspect of the sacral promontory and anterior to the femoral heads to include the obturator (internal iliac) nodes. Every effort should be made to exclude small

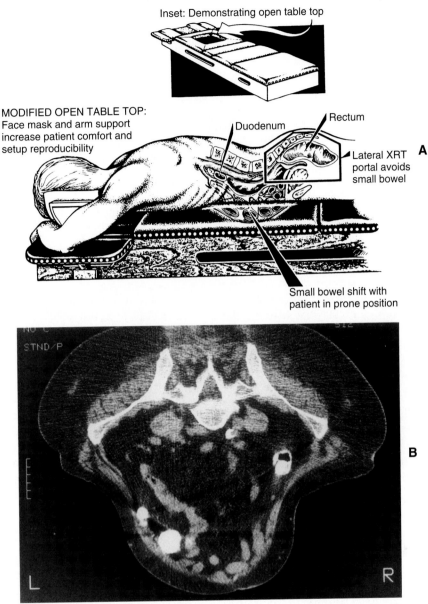

Inset: Demonstrating open table top

MODIFIED OPEN TABLE TOP:
Face mask and arm support
increase patient comfort and
setup reproducibility

Duodenum

Rectum

A

Lateral XRT
portal avoids
small bowel

Small bowel shift with
patient in prone position

B

Fig. 22-4 Use of a belly board in the treatment of colorectal cancer, **A,** The patient lies prone on a modified table top. **B,** A treatment planning computed tomography scan confirms displacement of the small bowel. (**A** From Rich T, Ajani JA, Morrison WH, et al. *Radiother Oncol* 1993;27:209-215.)

bowel. To reduce morbidity to the genitalia, a block should be placed anterior to the femur. Posteriorly, the entire sacrum should be included. This is important to avoid the penumbra of the beam and ensure the adequacy of the radiation dose to the radial margin of resection in the presacral region. Care should also be taken to exclude chemotherapy infusion pumps, if any, from the radiation field.[138]

Endocavitary Radiation and Brachytherapy

Brachytherapy and endocavitary radiation can be used alone or more commonly in conjunction with external beam radiation to treat rectal cancer. The delivery of high doses of radiation directly to well-defined, circumscribed volumes can be effective for local control. Indeed, these approaches are most often used for patients who cannot undergo surgical resection.

Endocavitary treatment. In contact or endocavitary radiation, soft (50-kV) x-rays are produced by a generator that delivers radiation through a tube containing an anode and ring filament.[139] Of the two types of aluminum filters available, the 0.5-cm filter is used for most applications. Using this filter at a focal distance of 4 cm, an output of 0.2 Gy per minute, and a 3-cm circular field, the percentage depth doses are 100% at 0 mm depth, 44% at 5 mm, 23% at 10 mm, and 9% at 20 mm.

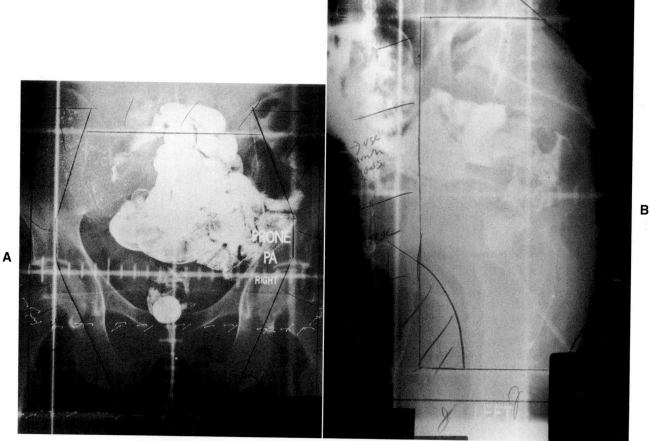

Fig. 22-5 Routine radiation portals for rectal cancer. **A,** Posterior field. **B,** Lateral fields showing displacement of the bowel.

This depth distribution precludes the use of contact therapy to treat highly infiltrative tumors. The tumor must be within 12 cm of the anal verge and accessible; posterior wall tumors can occasionally be difficult to localize with the cone.

The typical dose in the first contact treatment is between 30 and 40 Gy, given in 2 to 4 minutes with a 0.5-mm aluminum filter. One to two weeks later, a second application of contact radiation is given. Three weeks after the initiation of therapy, the third contact application is given; at this time a smaller (2-cm) cone is generally used to account for tumor regression. For 3-cm or larger tumors, 90 to 120 Gy is given in 4 to 5 fractions over 5 to 8 weeks. For tumors smaller than 2 cm that regress completely after two sessions, a total dose of 80 Gy in four fractions (30 Gy on day 1, 20 Gy on day 7, 15 Gy on day 21, and 15 Gy on day 36) is sufficient.[139] The normal mucosa of the rectal wall should not receive more than 15 to 20 Gy.

As is true for local excision, patient selection is critical for the success of contact therapy. Patients with lymph node involvement are not candidates for contact therapy.[139] Factors that increase the risk of lymph node involvement such as high histologic grade, perineural or lymphovascular invasion, or ulceration generally are contraindications for contact therapy. The response to contact therapy also is predictive of therapeutic success. The probability of local control is good if the tumor regresses by more than 80% of its original volume by 2 weeks after the second contact session.[139]

Endocavitary therapy can produce complete response rates of more than 90% in carefully selected patients.[140] Although the local failure rate can be as high as 28%, the addition of external-beam radiation in cases involving poor prognostic factors (e.g., tumors larger than 3 cm and tumors that are partially fixed to the pelvic sidewall) can improve local control. In one study of patients so treated,[140] the local control rate (after salvage therapy) was 82%, and sphincter preservation was possible in 82% of patients. The incidence of severe late effects was 4%.

Brachytherapy. The choice of brachytherapy technique depends on anatomic considerations. The four techniques available involve the use of metallic needles through a perineal template, an iridium "fork," a plastic loop, or a remote afterloading device.[139] To localize the radiation dose to the lesion and to avoid irradiating the opposite rectal wall, obturators are often used with the implants to distend the rectum.

Lesions smaller than 3 cm can be treated with brachytherapy alone, but external beam radiation should be added for larger tumors. Using this approach, local control rates of 90% can be achieved without significant complications.[141] Although continuous low-dose-rate brachytherapy is usually used, pulsed low-dose-rate brachytherapy results in similar late effects and can be considered as an alternative approach.[142]

Endocavitary therapy and brachytherapy can be effective means of administering localized radiation, especially for patients with limited treatment options. Further integration of these techniques should be considered for use with conservative surgical approaches.

Postoperative Radiation

The advantages of administering radiation postoperatively include the ability to plan treatment on the basis of the pathologic response of the primary tumor and, theoretically, a reduction in perioperative morbidity because surgery is performed in an unirradiated field. Pathologic tumor staging can confirm the need for adjuvant radiation and allows precise definition of the regions that are to be included in the radiation portal.[143] For tumors of the mid- to proximal rectum, postoperative radiation is often used because sphincter-preserving surgery can be performed routinely in such cases without the need for tumor downstaging. Prompt surgical intervention and postoperative radiation are also indicated in cases that involve significant bleeding or risk of obstruction.

The disadvantages of postoperative radiation include the relative hypoxic state within the operative bed and the associated potential for growth of residual disease during postoperative healing. Hypoxia enhances resistance to radiation; approximately three times the radiation dose is required to kill hypoxic tumor cells as to kill the same number of well-oxygenated cells. Therefore the total dose of radiation is generally higher when the radiation is given after surgery (53 to 55 Gy) as opposed to before surgery (45 to 50 Gy). However, the risk of both short- and long-term gastrointestinal toxicity increases precipitously as the total dose of radiation increases.[144] The potential risk of radiation morbidity from postoperative radiation also increases because the small bowel is less mobile, owing to the formation of adhesions after surgery.

Preoperative Radiation

The key advantage of preoperative radiation is the potential for shrinking the tumor, thereby improving the chance that a sphincter-preserving surgical procedure can be used. This advantage is especially important

for lesions located in the distal rectum. Preoperative radiation also offers the opportunity for sterilizing potential sites of residual disease, such as the radial surgical margin and regional lymphatics.[145-148] Another advantage is that the effects of preoperative radiation and chemotherapy may be enhanced because the blood supply in the affected area has not been disrupted by surgery. Thus a lower total dose of radiation can be given, which in turn reduces the risk of radiation morbidity. That risk is also less after preoperative radiation than postoperative radiation because the small bowel is more mobile before surgery, allowing it to be more easily displaced from the radiation field.[149] The ability to assess response to induction chemotherapy and radiation also may have prognostic implications.

The disadvantages of preoperative radiation include not having information from pathologic tumor staging,[145,146] the need for particular surgical expertise to minimize the perioperative morbidity associated with resecting an irradiated field,[102,150] and the need for a two-stage surgical approach (resection with fecal diversion followed by reestablishment of intestinal continuity) to allow the anastomosis to heal. A recent meta-analysis of 14 randomized controlled trials of preoperative radiation therapy for resectable rectal cancer (6426 patients) indicated that preoperative radiation did not increase postoperative mortality, although it did increase morbidity in some studies.[151] Moreover, preoperative radiation was found to reduce the 5-year overall mortality rate, cancer-related mortality rate, and local recurrence rate, but no reduction was seen in the incidence of distant metastases.[151]

Local Control and Survival

Among the three randomized trials that evaluated the use of postoperative radiation without chemotherapy (conducted by the NSABP,[118] the GITSG,[115] and the NCCTG[113]), only the NSABP trial showed a modest improvement in the rates of local failure over surgery alone (see Table 22-1).[118] However, the total doses of radiation used were different in these trials; the NSABP trial involved doses of 46 to 47 Gy,[118] the GITSG trial 40 or 48 Gy,[115] and the Mayo/NCCTG trial 45 to 50.4 Gy.[113] Furthermore, the NSABP trial was the only one in which the radiation was given as a continuous course and using modern techniques.[143] The GITSG[115] NCCTG[113] studies both demonstrated a benefit for combined-modality therapy over surgery only, surgery plus radiation, or surgery plus chemotherapy. The results of the treatment arms for these studies are shown in Table 22-3.[113,115,128,152]

The effect of adjuvant radiation on local control and survival was also evaluated in the Uppsala and the Swedish Rectal Cancer Trials. In those trials, the addition of radiation to surgery decreased the risk of local failure over the risk conferred by treatment with surgery only.[153-155] The use of preoperative radiation was found to improve survival rates over those conferred by surgery

TABLE 22-3

Outcomes in Three Large Trials of Treatment for Colorectal Cancer

Trial and Treatment Regimen	Local Relapse Rate (%)	Distant Relapse Rate (%)	Disease-Free Survival Rate (%)	Overall Survival Rate (%)	P Value
GITSG (N = 202)[115]					
Surgery	24	34	45	32	0.005
Surgery + chemotherapy*	27	27	54	48	
Surgery + radiation	20	30	52	45	
Surgery + radiation + chemotherapy*	11	26	67	57	
NCCTG (N = 204)[†113]					
Surgery + radiation	25	46	38	38	0.025
Surgery + radiation + chemotherapy*	14	29	58	53	
INT (N = 660)[‡128]					
Surgery + radiation + bolus fluorouracil	NS	NS	53	60	0.01
Surgery + radiation + PVI fluorouracil	NS	NS	63	70	

From Vaughn DJ, Haller DG. *Cancer Invest* 1997;15:435-447.
GITSG, Gastrointestinal Tumor Study Group; *NCCTG*, North Central Cancer Treatment Group; *INT*, intergroup; *NS*, not stated; *PVI*, protracted venous infusion.
*Chemotherapy is with fluorouracil and semustine.
[†]7-Year follow-up.
[‡]4-Year follow-up.

only.[154] Comparisons of preoperative and postoperative radiation were difficult to interpret because of significant differences in the fractionation schedules used.[156,157] Further, the issue of whether sphincter preservation could be used after preoperative radiation was not addressed because not enough time was allowed for downstaging between the completion of radiation and surgery.

A prospective randomized trial by the Stockholm Colorectal Cancer Study Group compared the use of preoperative radiation with surgery for 285 patients with rectal cancer at any stage.[153,155] Local recurrence occurred in 16% of the group given preoperative radiation and in 30% who underwent surgery only (P < 0.001). The advantage was confined to patients with Dukes stage B disease, although this may have been true for patients with Dukes stage C disease as well (P = 0.068). At a median follow-up of 50 months, the rate of distant metastases was 19% after preoperative radiation and surgery and 26% after surgery alone (P = 0.02), a difference that translated into a survival advantage for irradiated patients (P = 0.02). Although the disease-free interval was initially longer in the group given preoperative radiation, the lower rate of distant metastases and overall survival advantage after preoperative radiation did not last when the follow-up extended to 107

months. This loss in survival advantage, however, was accounted for by the higher perioperative mortality rate in the preoperative radiation group, because the radiation continued to confer an advantage in terms of disease-specific survival (P < 0.01).

Advantages of preoperative radiation were then shown in the Swedish Rectal Cancer Trial in which patients were randomized to undergo surgery only or preoperative radiation followed by surgery.[154] Consistent with the previously reported Stockholm experience,[155] preoperative therapy totaled 25 Gy, given in five fractions over 1 week followed by surgery within 1 week afterward. After 5 years of follow-up, the local recurrence rate was 11% among those given preoperative radiation and 27% among those given surgery only (P < 0.001).[154] Improvements in local control were observed for all stages of disease. The overall survival rate at 5 years was also significantly improved by the addition of preoperative radiation (58% vs. 48%, P = 0.004). The cancer-specific survival rates at 9 years was 74% for the preoperative radiation group and 65% for the surgery-only group (P = 0.002).

Outcomes after preoperative or postoperative radiation were compared in a trial conducted at Uppsala University.[156] In that study, 471 patients with resectable rectal cancer were assigned to undergo either a short course of preoperative radiation or, for those who had Dukes 2 or 3 disease, high-dose postoperative radiation. For the 236 patients given preoperative radiation, radiation was delivered in five 5.1-Gy fractions (total dose 25.5 Gy) over 5 to 7 days, and resection was performed 1 week later. For the 235 patients given postoperative radiation, radiation treatment was initiated 4 to 6 weeks after surgery. Patients were given 40 Gy in 2-Gy fractions over a period of 4 weeks; at that point, the radiation was discontinued for 10 to 14 days after which an additional 10 Gy was administered to the entire pelvis and another 10 Gy was administered to a reduced treatment volume. (In this regimen, the pelvis was treated to 50 Gy and the tumor bed to 60 Gy.) Only those patients who had evidence of transmural extension of disease or positive pelvic nodes at resection received postoperative chemotherapy. Although the radiation doses and the effective biological doses were substantially different among treatment groups in this trial, a local control benefit was observed for preoperative radiation over postoperative radiation; local failure rates at 5 years were 13% vs. 22%, respectively. No difference was evident in survival rate between the groups.

Toxicity

In the trials described above, moderate to mild acute radiation effects were observed in virtually all patients given postoperative radiation; in contrast, preoperative radiation led only infrequently to acute radiation effects such as diarrhea and cystitis.[156-158] Perioperative complications included small bowel obstruction, diagnosed radiographically and requiring surgical intervention, in 6% after surgery only, 5% after preoperative therapy, and 11% after postoperative radiation. However, perioperative complications were more common after preoperative therapy. For example, perineal wound sepsis occurred after abdominoperineal resection in 33% of those given preoperative radiation and in 18% of those given postoperative radiation.[156-158] However, because of perioperative complications, half of the patients in the postoperative group could not start radiation therapy within the recommended 6 weeks after surgery.

Although the Stockholm trials did identify advantages for combined-modality therapy, significant late morbidity was also observed. Peripheral nerves are relatively resistant to the late effects of radiation, but lumbosacral plexopathy occurred after the preoperative radiation regimen used in that trial.[156] Other late adverse effects of that preoperative radiation regimen included thromboembolism ($P = 0.01$), femoral neck and pelvic fractures ($P = 0.03$), intestinal obstruction ($P = 0.02$), and postoperative fistulae ($P = 0.01$). No difference in genitourinary complications was observed between groups.

The radiation techniques that were used significantly influenced the risk of complications and mortality. The incidence of complications resulting from small bowel toxicity was high because the superior border was placed at L2 in many of the studies rather than at the L5-S1 interspace.[156-158] Mortality rates were higher among patients treated with anterior-posterior opposed portals than among those treated with three- or four-field techniques (15% vs. 3%; $P < 0.001$). Because of these complications, the overall mortality rates were the same for those treated with surgery only and those treated with preoperative radiation. Although the addition of radiation therapy significantly improved the local control and disease-specific survival rates, the substantial morbidity of radiation therapy was enough to negate the effect of these improvements.

In another experience,[159] giving hypofractionated preoperative radiation to 83 patients did not result in significant treatment-related morbidity. The dose given was similar to those given in the Swedish trials[154] (25 Gy in five fractions over 1 week followed immediately by surgery), but anterior-posterior portals were avoided and the superior border of the radiation field was limited to the L5-S1 interspace. At a mean follow-up of about 5 years, the actuarial local control rate was 95% and the disease-specific survival rate was 77%.[159] The incidence of grade 3 or higher perioperative or late toxic reactions was only 13%; the incidence of bowel obstruction was 3.5%. No significant difference in toxic reactions was noted among the 16 patients who were also given chemotherapy during the irradiation.

Although not a prospective randomized trial, results from a 1988–1989 Patterns of Care study[125] allow comparison of survival on the basis of whether radiation was given preoperatively or postoperatively and whether chemotherapy was given during radiation. Local failure rates were approximately 10% for all stages of disease and in all treatment groups. Survival rates were significantly higher after preoperative radiation or postoperative chemoradiation than after postoperative radiation only.[125] At 5 years, the overall survival rates were 50% in the postoperative radiation group, 85% in the preoperative radiation group, and 69% in the postoperative chemoradiation group.[125]

These studies demonstrate the benefit of radiation therapy in terms of reducing the risk of local failure and possibly affecting overall survival. Variations in radiation techniques and in whether chemotherapy was administered significantly affect morbidity and outcome. Although it is difficult to interpret outcome when radiation is given with planned treatment interruptions, the treatment interruptions may have improved tolerance to therapy. Some trials included chemotherapy agents that provided no benefit but may have contributed to the overall toxicity of therapy. The routes and schedules of administration of chemotherapy also significantly influence the patterns of failure. No direct comparisons have been made for preoperative vs. postoperative conventional radiation schedules given with standardized chemotherapy. Therefore the relative advantages and disadvantages of preoperative and postoperative chemoradiation remain theoretical. Nevertheless, preoperative therapy can confer the substantial advantage of tumor downstaging, which may allow the use of sphincter-sparing surgical procedures. This topic is discussed further in the following section.

Sphincter Preservation

Sphincter preservation is a major goal of preoperative radiation therapy. The current use of preoperative chemoradiation builds on the experience with postoperative combined-modality therapy and the data that demonstrate the efficacy of preoperative radiation alone.[160,161] Tumors located less than 6 cm from the anal verge generally require an abdominoperineal resection. However, variation exists in surgical practices regardless of whether preoperative radiation is used. Among 18,695 cases of operable rectal cancer in Ontario, wide geographic variations were demonstrated in rates of abdominoperineal resection and referrals for postoperative radiation.[162] Sphincter preservation rates after preoperative radiation or chemoradiation also vary, ranging between 65% and 85%.[145,146,163] These variations probably are related to details of the clinical presentation, including tumor size, circumference, and extent of invasion of the sphincter muscles. However, an interim analysis of the NASBP R-03 trial showed that preoperative therapy allowed only 27% of patients to undergo a sphincter-preserving procedure rather than an abdominoperineal resection.[164] The reasons for this were unclear.

With the goals of preserving sphincter function, minimizing the total radiation dose, and maximizing tumor oxygenation, many centers have evaluated the use of preoperative radiation therapy, with the most recent series also using chemotherapy in conjunction with that radiation. The results of several of these series are summarized in Table 22-4.[102,165-173] Preoperative radiation produces pathologic complete response rates of about 15%. The addition of bolus or infusional 5-FU during the first and last week of radiation increases that rate to about 20%, and use of a continuous infusion of 5-FU throughout the course of preoperative radiation further increases that rate to 27%.[102] Tumor regression or downstaging is evident in about 65% of cases. Sphincter preservation after preoperative chemoradiation is possible in more than two thirds of patients with low rectal cancer.[102]

Factors that can increase tumor regression and the possibility of performing sphincter-sparing surgery include allowing an appropriate interval between completion of radiation therapy and surgery to maximize tumor regression, administration of higher radiation doses, and the administration of chemotherapy. Issues specific to chemotherapy during preoperative radiation include the type of agent and the schedule of infusion.

Radiation–surgery interval. The interval between completion of preoperative radiation and surgery is critical for allowing maximal tumor regression. In one study, when the interval between preoperative radiation (39 Gy in 3 weeks) and surgery was increased from 2 weeks to 6 to 8 weeks, the downstaging rate increased from 10% to 26%.[174] Although it was intended that surgery be performed within 10 days of completion of radiation in the Swedish Rectal Cancer Trial, the interval between radiation and surgery varied widely (5 to 155 days).[150] In that trial, the downstaging rate was found to be only 4% among patients who underwent resection within 10 days of completing therapy; in contrast, the downstaging rate was 45% when more than 10 days elapsed between completion of radiation and surgery. Another trial specifically evaluated the interval between completion of radiation (39 Gy in 13 fractions) and pathologic downstaging after surgery among 201 patients.[175] Pathologic evidence of downstaging was evident in only 11% when surgery was performed within 2 weeks of completing radiation therapy, but that rate increased to 26% when the interval after radiation was extended to 6 to 8 weeks.[175]

Radiation doses. A possible disadvantage of increasing the total preoperative radiation dose is the possible increase in treatment-related toxicity. Although this was not reported in a dose-escalation trial that included an intermittent infusion of 5-FU during irradiation, no significant improvements in the rates of pathologic complete response, downstaging, or sphincter preservation were observed.[171] In another study, a dose-response relationship for downstaging with preoperative radiation was identified at 44 Gy, given in conventional fractions.[174] However, this relationship held for Dukes stage A and B but not stage C disease.

Administration of chemotherapy. The influence of combined-modality therapy for locally advanced rectal cancer was evaluated by comparing the types of surgical procedures performed between 1975 and 1990 vs. between 1991 and 1997 at the University of Florida. Of the 328 patients who underwent preoperative radiation therapy, 219 were treated in the early period vs. 109 in the late period; none of the patients in the early era but 64 in the late era were given preoperative chemotherapy.[176] The rate at which sphincter-sparing procedures were performed increased from 13% to 52%, and the rate of pathologic tumor downstaging increased from 42% to 58%. However, the incidence of lymph node metastases and 5-year local recurrence rates remained similar between groups. Adjustments for other independent prognostic factors such as T stage, nodal status, and age led to significant improvement in the overall 5-year survival rate among the group treated in the late period (87% vs. 58% for those treated in the

TABLE 22-4

Preoperative Radiation Therapy and Sphincter Preservation, Pathologic Response, and Tumor Downstaging in Colorectal Cancer

Study and Reference	Number of Patients	Preoperative Radiation Dose	Chemotherapy During Radiation	Time Between Radiation and Surgery	Complete Response Rate (%)	Downstaging Rate (%)	Sphincter Preservation Rate (%)
Janjan et al, 2000[166]	42	45 Gy to pelvis + 7.5-Gy CB	CI 5-FU 300 mg/m^2 5 days/week during pelvic irradiation	4-6 weeks	31	86	79
Bosset et al, 2000[167]	60	45 Gy	Bolus 5-FU week 1, 350-450 mg/m^2 week 5, 350-370 mg/m^2	3 weeks (range, 13-111 days)	15.6	30	58
Pucciarelli et al, 2000[168]	51	45 Gy	5-day 5-FU infusion 350 mg/m^2 days 1–5 and days 29–33	4-5 weeks (range, 19-53 days)	15.7	59	84
Valentini et al, 1999[169]	40	45 Gy to pelvis + 5.4-Gy boost	5-day 5-FU infusion 1000 mg/m^2 days 1-4 and days 29-32; cisplatin 60 mg/m^2 days 1, 29	6-8 weeks	23	68	85
Movsas et al, 1998[171]	23	45 Gy to pelvis + hyperfx boost to total doses of 54.6, 57, or 61.8 Gy	5-day 5-FU infusion 1000 mg/m^2 days 1-4 and days 29-32	4-6 weeks	17.4	57	30
Janjan et al, 1998[102]	117	45 Gy to pelvis	CI 5-FU 300 mg/m^2; 5 days/week during pelvic XRT	4-6 weeks	27	62	59
Wagman et al, 1998[172]	35	46.8 Gy to pelvis + 3.6-Gy boost	No	4-5 weeks	14	63	77
Mohiuddin et al, 1998[173]	70	40 to 45 Gy +10- to 15-Gy boost	No	5-10 weeks	NR	30	86

CI, Continuous infusion; *CB*, concomitant boost; *hyperfx*, hyperfractionated; *XRT*, radiation therapy; *NR*, not reported.

early period).[176] Therefore in this study, the addition of chemotherapy to radiation significantly improved local control and overall survival.

Administration of 5-FU as a continuous infusion rather than a bolus during radiation seems to confer benefit in terms of disease-free and overall survival. This benefit has been shown in studies of postoperative chemoradiation[128] and indirectly in studies of preoperative radiation using conventional fractionation and a concomitant boost.[102,166,177,178] Using a lower total dose of preoperative radiation (45 Gy) with continuous-infusion 5-FU produced downstaging comparable with higher total radiation doses.[179] When accelerated fractionation (concomitant boost) was used to deliver a total radiation dose of 52.5 Gy with a continuous infusion of 5-FU, the pathologic complete response rates were nearly twice those of other series using the same or higher doses of radiation and bolus or intermittent infusion of 5-FU.[166] The pathologic downstaging rates were approximately 20% higher than those achieved with other series that used bolus or intermittent infusion of 5-FU.[166]

Aside from its potential influence on sphincter preservation, tumor response to preoperative therapy may also be of prognostic importance. The level of response to preoperative radiation for locally advanced rectal cancer has been reported to influence survival rates, with improved survival rates observed among patients who showed pathologic evidence of downstaging.[174] The 5-year overall survival rate after preoperative radiation was 92% for patients whose tumors were downstaged to Dukes stage A; the corresponding 5-year survival rate for Dukes B disease was 67% and that for Dukes C disease was 26%. The corresponding disease-free survival rates were 87%, 56%, and 28%.[174]

In another study, patients who had pathologic evidence of tumor downstaging after preoperative radiation and bolus 5-FU had much higher cancer-specific survival rates (100%) than those whose tumors did not respond (45%).[180] In that same study, the corresponding 5-year recurrence-free survival rates were 94% and 50%.[180] A similar relationship was seen when 5-FU was given as a continuous infusion in combination with preoperative radiation.[181] Any response to preoperative chemoradiation resulted in a reduced risk of distant metastases and in improved disease-free survival.

Higher rates of tumor regression have been observed for tumors that shrink and have higher Ki-67 levels and higher mitotic activity in response to irradiation.[182] In that same study, having tumors that had elevated proliferative activity after preoperative irradiation strongly correlated with improved survival.[182] FDG-PET, which allows imaging of tumor function, is now being used in investigational settings to evaluate response to preoperative chemoradiation.[183]

In another study, the risk of pelvic relapses was evaluated as a function of total radiation dose and overall treatment time. After adjustments were made for the overall duration of radiation, the dose-response curves were found to be steep.[184] The time-related displacement of these dose-response curves was consistent with a median tumor doubling time of about 4 to 5 days. This doubling time was more rapid than that for the primary tumor at diagnosis. The authors of this study concluded that growth of subclinical tumor deposits in the pelvis accelerated rapidly during preoperative radiation and thus strategies that shorten overall treatment time or provide uninterrupted administration of antineoplastic therapy should be investigated.[184]

Other Treatment Approaches
Radiation with Oral Fluoropyrimidine Analogs

The possibility of using oral chemotherapy confers several advantages over the use of intravenous chemotherapy; among them are ease of administration and avoidance of the inconvenience, discomfort and cost associated with intravenous 5-FU.[183,185,186] Some of the newer agents may also become concentrated in tumor cells to a greater extent than infused 5-FU does. Although oral agents can produce severe diarrhea,[187-189] they produce less mucositis, neutropenia, and hand-foot syndrome than does infused 5-FU.[190]

With these advantages, however, come concerns regarding optimization of dose for the greatest efficacy with the least toxicity, the pharmacokinetics of the various available agents, and patient compliance.[65,191] Some oral fluoropyrimidines completely inactivate dihydropyrimidine dehydrogenase activity.[192] The time at which the oral formulation should be taken relative to the radiation schedule also remains unclear. Because most studies done to date have focused on the use of oral fluoropyrimidines in chemotherapy regimens, information on their use in combination with radiation is extremely limited.

A review of clinical trials conducted to date has shown objective response rates of about 40% among patients with colorectal cancer given uracil-tegafur (ftorafur) in combination with leucovorin[187]; response rates tended to be lower (about 25%) when the oral agent was given alone or with lower leucovorin doses.[187] The highest dose-intensities have been achieved with 28-day schedules of the drug.

Early experience with oral agents given during preoperative radiation has included a dose-escalation trial to establish the maximum tolerated dose. The maximum tolerated dose for oral uracil and tegafur was found in one study to be 350 mg/m^2/day when leucovorin was given at 90 mg/day, 5 days a week, concurrent with radiation.[193] These results were comparable with those involving use of infusional 5-FU. Sphincter-preserving surgery was performed in 12 of 14 patients and produced a pathologic complete response in three cases.[193]

Many issues need to be resolved before oral fluoropyrimidines become the new standard of care during radiation therapy. Given the differences among the various agents, each will require clinical assessment with radiation therapy. The activity of other chemotherapy agents such as irinotecan and oxaliplatin in combination with oral fluoropyrimidines will also need to be considered.[194]

Radiation with Local Excision

As part of the trend to maintain sphincter function whenever possible, radiation therapy has been used in combination with local excision of early-stage tumors that involve the distal rectum. The Radiation Therapy Oncology Group (RTOG) was among the first to report using such an approach.[195] In that trial, 65 patients who had undergone local excision were either observed or given adjuvant treatment with 5-FU and one of two radiation dose levels according to tumor size and stage, tumor grade, and surgical margins.[195] The 14 patients who were followed with observation had microscopic confirmation of a total excision, a well- or moderately well-differentiated T1 tumor that was smaller than 3 cm, and no evidence of vascular or lymphatic permeation on pathologic examination. At a median follow-up of 5 years, 11 of 65 patients had recurrent tumor. The incidence of local failure correlated with T stage, with tumors recurring among 4% of T1 cases, 16% of T2 cases, and 23% of T3 cases. Other factors that affected local failure were the extent of circumferential involvement; local failure rate was only 6% for tumors with less than 20% circumferential involvement but was 18% when 20% to 40% of the circumference was involved.

Selection of patients is extremely important in deciding whether to perform a local excision. Because lymph nodes are not resected in this procedure, local excision is contraindicated for patients with evident lymph node metastases.[196] The depth of tumor penetration and the tumor grade are directly related to the risk of perirectal node involvement. The risk of lymph node involvement for a low-grade T2 tumor is about 12%, but the risk is 55% for a high-grade T2 tumor.[197] Other studies have shown that tumor ulceration and histologic evidence of lymphatic, vascular, or perineural invasion are also associated with an increased risk of nodal metastases.[196,197] Tumors that are to be locally excised should be 3 cm or smaller and involve less than half of the rectal circumference. Fewer complications are associated with a transanal approach than with a Kraske approach to local excision and postoperative radiation.[198]

Radiation therapy after local excision is unnecessary for T1 tumors with favorable clinical and histologic characteristics because the risk of local failure is less than 10%.[163] Postoperative radiation is recommended for T1 tumors with unfavorable characteristics or for T2 tumors because the risk of local failure is about 20%.[163,197-199] A complete surgical resection with mesorectal excision is recommended for patients with T3 tumors; in one study, the local recurrence rate was approximately 30% among patients with T3 tumors treated with local excision and chemoradiation.[163]

Techniques for delivering radiation in association with local excision are similar to those used for postoperative therapy.[197] The entire pelvis is treated to 45 Gy, with the boost volume treated to a total dose of 54 to 65 Gy depending on the resection margins and the presence of aggressive histologic features.[197] Small bowel must be excluded from the radiation boost volume.

The use of preoperative chemoradiation followed by local excision for patients with T1 rectal tumors, especially those tumors with favorable characteristics, is controversial because no information on tumor pathology is available and thus such patients may be able to avoid radiation. Preoperative chemoradiation or radiation followed by local excision traditionally has been used for patients who decline or are medically unfit for a radical resection.[200] The opportunity for pathologic downstaging and the theoretical advantages of preoperative chemoradiation have led to this approach being judiciously applied in a broader population of patients with rectal cancer.

MANAGEMENT OF TREATMENT-RELATED SIDE EFFECTS

Attempts to minimize the hematologic toxic effects of chemotherapy have included prolonging the infusion of 5-FU so that higher total doses can be administered with fewer hematologic side effects.[128] Although the use of protracted infusions or alternative agents (e.g., irinotecan) can improve disease-free and overall survival rates, they carry the risk of gastrointestinal side effects, including profound diarrhea, and other toxic effects such as mucositis and hand-foot syndrome.[201] The possibility of superinfection, especially with candida species, must be closely monitored; clinical signs such as fever and blood in the stool may suggest underlying sepsis and should initiate prompt evaluation.[201] The occasional occurrence of mild nausea dictates evaluation of nutritional and fluid balance as needed. Gastrointestinal symptoms that occur during the first 2 weeks of radiation are generally attributable to chemotherapy. However, management of treatment-related diarrhea is the same regardless of whether it is caused by the radiation or the chemotherapy.

Controlling Treatment-Related Diarrhea
The Three-Step Bowel Management Program

The University of Texas M.D. Anderson Cancer Center has instituted a three-step bowel management program for controlling diarrhea associated with chemoradiation for locally advanced rectal cancer. Preliminary results of a prospective evaluation of this program have shown no difference between the presenting symptoms and the symptoms reported at the completion of chemoradiation.[202]

The goal of the three-step program is to prevent rather than treat symptoms such as frequent stooling (defined as more than three bowel movements per day), fluid and electrolyte imbalances, and skin irritation. All patients are given written instructions at the treatment simulation session and a prescription for an antidiarrheal agent (e.g., loperamide) and an antiemetic agent. The strategy underlying the program is proactive; at the first sign of symptoms, the patient should proceed to the next step in the program.[202]

In step 1, initial symptoms, which usually occur in the third week of therapy, are treated with loperamide as needed. When that need exceeds two tablets per day, the patient proceeds to step 2, in which loperamide is administered according to a schedule (usually four times a day, 30 minutes before meals and before bedtime) so as to prevent frequent stooling. Should that procedure fail to control symptoms, the patient proceeds to step 3, in which opioid analgesics are added to relieve the abdominal cramping and provide a constipating effect. The doses of analgesic are titrated to effect in accordance with established principles for pain management; the doses of opioids required in step 3 are usually modest. Because the treatment-related changes in the bowel do not resolve while therapy continues, sustained-release analgesics are preferred in step 3 to avoid the need for multiple drug doses during the day and the possible development of cyclical symptoms. The use of fentanyl patches should be avoided because of the difficulty in titrating the dose and because the need for analgesic does not remain stable over the course of radiation therapy. Immediate-release analgesics can be used as well for breakthrough abdominal cramping or bleeding.

Skin reactions are generally restricted to the perianal region. At the first signs of dry desquamation, a barrier-emollient cream (e.g., Skin Protectant, Lantiseptic, Marietta, Ga.), is applied and used consistently except during the irradiation. Use of such a cream can ease the irritation and discomfort arising from dry desquamation of the perianal skin; it can also help prevent moist desquamation and the attendant risk of secondary infections from fecal bacteria, a particular concern when chemotherapy is given with radiation. Patients who develop candidiasis in the perianal region can benefit significantly from use of a mixture of creams or ointments containing zinc oxide (e.g., Desitin), nystatin, and lidocaine. Patients who develop localized moist desquamation in the perianal area during treatment of distal rectal tumors can maintain hygiene and relieve symptoms by using sitz baths or warm compresses with an aluminum acetate solution such as Domeboro (Bayer Corporation, Pittsburgh, Pa.).

Other Approaches

Other approaches to treating chemotherapy-induced diarrhea have included varying the dose-intensity of the chemotherapy agent. In one such study, pharmacokinetic evaluations showed broad variation in the metabolism of 5-FU among patients; acute toxic effects correlated with blood 5-FU levels that were higher than 3000 μg/L but not with the 5-FU dose given.[203] Because metabolism of most cytotoxic drugs will vary considerably among patients, at least one group has proposed basing chemotherapy dose calculations on body surface area.[204]

An alternative strategy for controlling secretory diarrhea is the use of loperamide with an enkephalinase inhibitor such as acetorphan to treat the secretory diarrhea induced by irinotecan. Octreotide, a somatostatin analog that prolongs intestinal transit time, promotes absorption of electrolytes in the intestine, decreases mesenteric blood flow, and decreases the secretion of fluids and electrolytes, is also effective against secretory diarrhea. Octreotide has been used to treat diarrhea associated with 5-FU or bone marrow transplants.[201,205] The optimal dose and route of administration of octreotide are currently unknown.[201] Assessments of the cost-effectiveness of octreotide or alternative strategies should reflect the cost of preventing hospitalization or infusional therapies for treatment-related complications.

Late Effects

The success of sphincter-preserving strategies is defined largely in terms of late treatment-related complications. One such complication, proctitis, may represent a continuum of symptoms. Despite the radiobiological dissociation between acute and late toxic effects, acute proctitis has been linked in at least one study[206] to three other late symptoms (tenesmus, frequency, and diarrhea) and the late morbidity score on a scale developed by the European Organization for the Research and Treatment of Cancer and the RTOG. Although rectal bleeding and discharge greatly affected the late morbidity score, tenesmus and bleeding had the greatest effect on daily living.[206] Moreover, concordance was low between the patient's assessment of symptoms and the late morbidity score.[206]

In a different study of 386 patients, a relationship was also observed between the development of symptomatic acute enteritis and chronic bowel injury.[207] Only 13 patients developed acute radiation-induced enteritis; three of these patients also experienced chronic bowel injury. A total of 18 patients developed chronic treatment-related symptoms, and reoperation was required in 17 of these cases.[207] Chronic proctitis had developed in 19% of the men in this study at 5 years. Factors related to an increased risk of complications were transanal excision, high radiation dose, and old age.

Other quality-of-life issues relate to fertility. Given the risk of sexual dysfunctions such as retrograde ejaculation associated with surgical treatment of rectal cancer, men can consider preoperative sperm preservation. According to one cost-effectiveness analysis, the cost of sperm preservation was 2.2 to 5 times higher than the cost of one microsurgical epididymal sperm-aspiration procedure.[208] Because the prostate is included in the radiation portal for rectal cancer, men undergoing radiation therapy for rectal cancer should consider sperm preservation.

Assessments of quality of life should include consideration of not only how the intervention will affect survival but also how it will affect the health-related quality of that life. Factors to be considered in such analyses of rectal cancer treatment include the risk of local recurrence, having to live with a permanent colostomy, the acute and late side effects of treatment, and the costs associated with the recommended therapies.[209] Moreover, long-term follow-up is required to account for the completion of therapy, especially for locally advanced rectal cancer. Combined-modality therapy can involve 1 to 2 months of radiation, approximately 1 month between radiation and surgery, and about 4 months of adjuvant chemotherapy after recovery from surgery. If a sphincter-sparing procedure is performed, a second operation is necessary to remove the temporary ileostomy. Hence the total treatment time can be as long as 8 to 12 months. Quality of life ratings predictably improve after 3 years of follow-up, and bowel function is closely linked to quality of life.[210-213]

RECURRENT RECTAL CANCER

Recurrent rectal cancer can vary significantly in its clinical presentation, and it requires a broad range of therapeutic approaches. When a recurrence is identified early, the patient is usually asymptomatic and resection is possible. Regrettably, recurrent rectal cancer is often diagnosed in the course of evaluating progressive symptoms, and at that time the disease is often inoperable. Given the profound morbidity associated with recurrent disease, aggressive therapeutic attempts are often undertaken to achieve local–regional control.

Reirradiation

Management of recurrent disease in patients who have previously been treated with radiation poses significant challenges. Approaches have included reirradiation with external-beam and intraoperative radiation therapy. The dose of external-beam radiation given to such patients varies, especially when given in conjunction with intraoperative radiation. In one study, reirradiation relieved bleeding in 100% of cases, pain in 65%, and mass effect in 24% of cases; moreover, for most responding patients, palliation lasted until death.[214,215] Acute grade 3 toxicity appeared in 31% of cases and late grade 3 and 4 toxicity in 23% and 10% of cases, including small bowel obstruction in 17%. The only factor that reduced late toxicity was hyperfractionation; however, factors that influenced median survival were Karnofsky Performance Score, initial stage of disease, and the reirradiation dose, with up to 30.6 Gy leading to median survival of 22 months versus more than 30.6 Gy leading to median survival of 9.5 months.[214]

A Danish study showed that the risk of pelvic recurrence after the diagnosis of recurrent rectal cancer was no different for patients initially treated with an abdominoperineal resection (18%) than for those treated with a low-anterior resection (24%).[216] Of the 175 patients evaluated, 25 had a pelvic recurrence without evidence of distant metastasis[216]; among those patients, those given radiation therapy survived longer (15.9 months) than those given surgery or analgesics (2.4 months).

Among 519 patients treated with radiation for locally recurrent rectal cancer at the Princess Margaret Hospital in Toronto, 326 had undergone an abdominoperineal resection; 151, a low anterior resection; and 42, a local excision. None had been given radiation as part of the initial treatment.[217] The mean time between the initial surgery and salvage radiation was 18 months (range of 3 to 138 months). The relapse was confined to the pelvis in 355 patients, but distant metastases were found with local recurrence in 164 cases (32%). The median survival time was 14 months, and the median time to local disease progression was 5 months; the pelvic disease progression-free rate was 7%, and the 5-year survival rate was 5%.[217] Multivariate analysis showed that overall survival was associated with the performance status (measured on an Eastern Cooperative Oncology Group [ECOG] scale), absence of extrapelvic metastases, a long interval between the initial surgery and salvage radiation, total radiation dose, and absence of obstructive uropathy.[217]

No dose-response relationship between radiation and recurrent rectal cancer was found in a review of the available retrospective series in the literature.[218] No significant differences were observed in initial response or durability of the response to therapy.[218] However, a dose-response relationship may have been present when patients with primary untreated cancer and postoperative residual disease were evaluated separately.[218]

At the Peter MacCallum Cancer Institute, three dose regimens were used to treat incompletely resected, locally recurrent rectal cancer[219,220]: radical radiation (50 to 60 Gy), high-dose radiation (45 Gy, given in conventional fractionation), and palliative radiation (less than 45 Gy). No significant difference was observed in symptomatic relief between the radical and high-dose groups (about 80%), but only 33% of those given palliative therapy achieved even partial relief of symptoms.[219,220] The estimated median survival was 16 months for all patients; for patients in the radical-radiation group, the median survival was 26 months, and for those in the high-dose group, it was 16 months. Survival was compromised when macroscopic residual disease was present; the median survival in that case was 14 months versus 31 months if only microscopic residual tumor was present.

Intraoperative Radiation

Intraoperative radiation has been used either as a supplement to external-beam radiation or as the only therapy when further external-beam radiation is not possible. Outcome after such therapy was evaluated among 73 patients with recurrent rectal cancer, 86% of whom had locally recurrent disease without metastasis.[221] External-beam radiation had been given previously to 52% of these cases, and the recurrences were located in the presacral region (radial margin) in 55%. Surgical resection resulted in complete macroscopic resection of disease in 57% of cases; partial resection with gross residual disease was performed in 29%, and no resection was performed in 14% of the recurrences. Intraoperative radiation dose ranged from 10 Gy to 25 Gy; 30 patients also received either preoperative or postoperative external-beam radiation. Actuarial overall survival rates were 72% at 1 year, 45% at 2 years, and 31% at 3 years; comparable actuarial local control rates were 71%, 48%, and 31%, and actuarial disease-free survival rates were 58%, 27%, and 18%.

Controlling symptoms of recurrent disease is a critical factor for quality of life, given the relatively long survival times that can be achieved. In the study described above,[221] actuarial survival rates were improved after either complete or partial resection. Among the 21 instances of local failure, eight appeared in the intraoperative radiation field, eight in the external-beam radiation field, and three in areas that received both intraoperative and external-beam radiation. For patients in whom the recurrence appeared in the intraoperative radiation field, local control rates were 87% at 1 year, 72% at 2 years, and 65% at 3 years. At 3 years, actuarial local control rates in the intraoperative radiation field were better for those without gross residual disease (77%) than for those with gross residual disease (51%). Among patients with an isolated local recurrence who underwent partial or complete resection, the local control rates at 3 years were 61% for those given intraoperative and external-beam radiation and 0% for those given only intraoperative radiation. Of the four cases of long-term morbidity, one involved sciatic plexopathy that resolved with further follow-up (in a person given 12 Gy intraoperatively plus 45 Gy postoperatively), two involved the appearance of sacral necrosis at 6 months (in a person given 39 Gy preoperatively plus 25 Gy intraoperatively) and at 13 months (in a person given 40 Gy preoperatively plus 20 Gy intraoperatively), and one involved necrosis of the L5 vertebra after 51 months of follow-up (in a person given 28 Gy preoperatively plus 15 Gy intraoperatively).[221]

In contrast to this study, which showed that adding external-beam radiation to intraoperative radiation therapy conferred an advantage,[221] another study showed that the advantage resulted from the addition of intraoperative radiation to external-beam radiation for locally advanced or recurrent rectal cancer.[222] Again, local control depended on the amount of residual disease; for all patients, the 2-year actuarial local control rates were 77% (64% among those with recurrent disease) if no gross disease remained vs. 10% if gross residual disease was present after surgery. For all patients, the overall survival rate was improved if no gross disease remained after surgery (88% vs. 46% for those with gross residual disease). The 2-year actuarial risk of major complications attributable to intraoperative radiation was 16%. In sum, intraoperative radiation therapy seems to be feasible in all clinical settings and adds less than 1 hour to the surgical procedure.[223]

Chemoradiation and surgery can improve resectability, local control, and survival in patients with recurrent rectal cancer. In a study of 47 such patients given a preoperative dose of 45 Gy with concomitant 5-FU and mitomycin chemotherapy,[170] more than half showed an objective response and 45% were able to undergo radical resection. Pain relief was accomplished in 86%, with higher radiation doses producing better pain control. After radical resection, the overall 5-year survival and local control rates were 22% and 32%; when intraoperative radiation was added, the corresponding 5-year rates were 79% and 41%. A modified Suzuki classification system, based on the extent to which the recurrence was fixated along the pelvic sidewall, was found to be useful for predicting level of pain, disease-free survival, and overall survival.[170]

A comparison of three intraoperative radiation approaches for recurrent colorectal cancer (intraoperative radiation therapy, high-dose-rate brachytherapy, and intraoperative placement of ^{125}I seeds) showed no difference in local control rate among treatment groups; at 5 years, the overall 5-year local control rate in that study was 26%.[224] Although patients with tumors in the para-aortic region had better rates of local control than did patients with tumors in the pelvis (65% vs. 19% at 5 years), this difference did not lead to an improvement in overall survival rate. The 5-year overall survival rate in that study[224] was 4%; only the presence of residual disease (30% for those with microscopic disease and 7% for those with macroscopic disease at 3 years) and the use of postoperative external-beam radiation (48% vs. 12% at 3 years and 24% vs. 0% at 5 years) influenced overall survival rates. Given the difficulty of identifying residual disease, radioimmunoguided surgery has been advocated by some[225] as a way of identifying occult tumor deposits.

Combined-modality therapy that includes intraoperative radiation for recurrent colorectal cancer can produce problems in the healing of wounds in 46% to 65% of patients so treated; however, the introduction of unirradiated tissue by means of myocutaneous flap reconstruction has reduced the risk of major complications to 12%.[226,227]

Regardless of whether intraoperative radiation is used, resection of recurrent disease often requires extensive surgery for tumor clearance, a situation that is often complicated by previous irradiation. In one study of 131 patients, resection of recurrent disease was possible among 103 (79%), and this resulted in a 5-year survival rate of 31%. Favorable prognostic factors included having a normal CEA level before surgery and the recurrent tumor being limited to the bowel wall.[228] Aggressive surgical resection, including abdominosacral resection for fixed tumors, can also produce long-term survival rates of about 31%.[229] These aggressive surgical approaches are possible with reconstruction procedures that include placement of a myocutaneous graft.

In summary, long-term survival is possible among patients with recurrent disease if the disease is detected early and if total surgical resection is possible. Radiation therapy is needed to clear potential nests of residual microscopic tumor. Prior therapies like surgery and radiation may have created hypoxic regions that require higher radiation doses for sterilization of residual tumor. Reirradiation, especially with hyperfractionated treatment schedules, can be well tolerated.

PALLIATIVE RADIATION

Achieving local–regional control is important in the management of rectal cancer regardless of stage. Local–regional failure, occurring in approximately 75% of all patients who die of rectal cancer, often produces significant symptoms such as pain, bleeding, and obstruction that are difficult to control.[230-232] Although palliative radiation can relieve pain and bleeding in about 70% of cases, high-grade obstructive symptoms may require a diverting colostomy. Occasionally, urinary diversion may also be necessary. Palliative radiation relieves symptoms by causing partial regression of the tumor. The goal is to provide palliation of symptoms for the duration of the patient's life.

At the Princess Margaret Hospital, the radiation schedule most often used for palliation involves giving 50 Gy in 20 fractions over 4 weeks in a four-field technique. The 5-year survival rate after such treatment depends on the extent of the tumor; 48% of patients with mobile tumors, 27% with partially fixed tumors, and only 4% of patients with fixed tumors were alive at 5 years.[233,234] Tumor extent also predicted response to radiation; 50% of those with mobile tumors, 30% of those with partially fixed tumors, and only 9% of those with fixed tumors (Fig. 22-6) achieved a complete clinical response to radiation. The rate of tumor regression was slow; only 60% achieved a complete response by 4 months, and 9 months was required for 90% of those who had a complete response. Of the complete responders, approximately half of those with mobile or partially fixed tumors and more than 70% of those with fixed tumors developed progressive disease. However, salvage surgery to relieve symptoms was accomplished without significant complications in

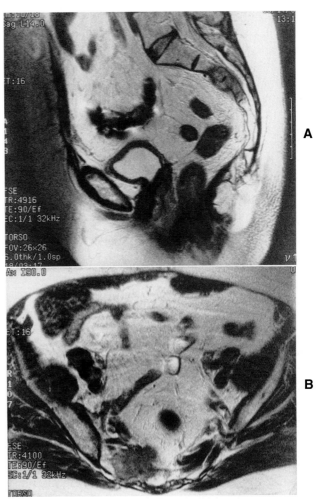

Fig. 22-6 A, Magnetic resonance imaging scan demonstrating a presacral recurrence infiltrating into the bone. B, Axial section showing extensive infiltration of the fixed tumor into the sacrum and nerve roots.

more than 90% of patients who developed progressive or recurrent disease.[233,234]

At the M.D. Anderson Cancer Center, hypofractionated radiation with concurrent chemotherapy produced symptomatic relief in 75 of 80 patients with locally advanced rectal cancer presenting with synchronous metastases.[165,235] The hypofractionated regimen in that study consisted of 35 Gy, given in 2.5-Gy fractions; when the tumor extended anteriorly, an anterior-posterior treatment portal was used. When a belly board could be used, 30 Gy was given in six fractions over 3 weeks. These treatments produced endoscopic evidence of complete response in 36% of patients.[165,235] Twenty-five patients underwent primary tumor resection. Although the 2-year survival rate was greater in the group that underwent resection than in those who did not (46% vs. 11%), the colostomy-free survival rate was higher in the group that did not undergo surgery (79% vs. 51%). Predictors of worse prognosis included pelvic pain at presentation, biological equivalent dose of less than 35 Gy at 2 Gy per fraction, and poorly differentiated tumor histology. By way of comparison, the median survival time in another study of patients with locally advanced rectal cancer who had liver metastases at presentation was 17 months when treated with palliative radiation, with or without chemotherapy.[236]

Radiation is often given when tumors are inoperable because of extensive infiltration. Radiation may produce sufficient tumor regression to render such disease operable and thereby offer the patient a chance to be free of disease. In one such study,[237] 29 patients with inoperative locally advanced tumors were given preoperative radiation totaling 54 Gy and continuous-infusion 5-FU. Resection was undertaken in 23 of these cases, 18 of which were done with curative intent (13 abdominoperineal resections, three low-anterior resections and two local excisions). Pathologic findings included a complete response rate of 13% and a tumor downstaging rate of 90%. At a median follow-up of 28 months, 15 patients were free of disease. The authors of this study concluded that an aggressive surgical approach can render patients free of disease and may improve overall survival. Another group found that multivisceral resection for patients with locally advanced rectal cancer resulted in approximately a 50% survival rate at 5 years.[238]

Tumor infiltration that leads to acute colonic obstruction can be relieved through placement of a stent; in addition to relief of symptoms, this procedure can facilitate the administration of radiation therapy or cleansing of the colon before surgery.[231,239,240] Stent placement relieves bowel obstruction in up to 96% of cases, with a risk of colonic perforation of less than 5%. Moreover, such stents can remain patent for long periods; in one study, 91% of stents were patent 6 months after their placement.[239]

When surgical resection of extensively infiltrating tumors is undertaken, radiation therapy must be administered because of the high risk of microscopic residual disease and subsequent recurrence—a risk that can exceed 80% after pelvic exenteration if radiation therapy is not administered.[241] This risk is substantially higher than the risk of local recurrence for locally advanced, but operable, rectal cancer. Thus radiation-based approaches have included the use of intraoperative radiation therapy in conjunction with external-beam therapy. In the Mayo Clinic experience, for example, factors related to improvements in overall survival were the use of preoperative external-beam radiation with chemotherapy plus intraoperative radiation.[242] The presence of gross residual disease after maximum tumor resection resulted in a 25% risk of progressive disease; gross total excision and the use of preoperative chemoradiation also decreased the risk of distant metastases.[242]

The addition of intraoperative radiation can also improve local control rates among patients who present with inoperable rectal cancer. In one such study, the addition of intraoperative radiation improved the local control rate after preoperative external-beam therapy from 33% to 92%.[226] Others have found that surgery preceded and followed by chemoradiation (the sandwich technique) improved 4-year local failure rates over the use of preoperative chemoradiation followed by surgery (0% and 23%, respectively).[243] The distant failure rate in this study decreased from 47% for those in the preoperative protocol to 28% for those in the sandwich protocol, which corresponded to overall survival rates of 41% and 72%.[243]

The use of continuous, chronobiologically shaped 5-FU infusions with radiation (45 or 55.8 Gy) has also reportedly improved the response of initially unresectable tumors (pathologic complete response rates of 28%[244] vs. 11% for preoperative radiation with 50.4 Gy and bolus 5-FU with leucovorin[245]). Another sandwich protocol involving preoperative and postoperative 5-FU with leucovorin for patients with unresectable disease produced a local failure rate of 30% and a distant metastasis rate of 40%,[246] with an actuarial disease-free survival rate at 4 years of 67% and an overall survival rate of 76%.[245]

In summary, substantial progress has been made in the therapy of rectal cancer, especially with the advent of combined-modality therapy. Each component treatment contributes to the local and systemic control of disease, and, in combination, they have allowed the development of function-preserving surgical approaches.[247]

PROXIMAL COLON CANCER

In contrast to its role in rectal cancer, the role of chemoradiation in colon cancer is controversial. By the early 1990s, the benefit of adjuvant 5-FU chemotherapy for stage III colon cancer was well established, and no benefit had been observed from the addition of levamisole to 5-FU and leucovorin. Other questions remain, however, regarding the treatment of colon cancer. First, it is unclear whether adjuvant chemotherapy is of benefit in stage II disease. Second, the role of new agents, like oral fluorinated pyrimidines, irinotecan, or oxaliplatin, has yet to be established, although these agents have shown some activity in metastatic disease.[248] Third, a role for adjuvant radiation, based on principles established in the treatment of rectal cancer, needs to be determined.[249]

As is true for other forms of cancer, ability to achieve complete resection is important for local control and survival. When primary colon cancer invades other viscera such as the pancreas or duodenum, en bloc resection can improve overall survival without increasing perioperative morbidity.[250] In that study, perioperative morbidity occurred among 28% of 5853 cases after colectomy for colon cancer. Preoperative factors that predicted a high risk of mortality included ascites, serum sodium level of more than 145 mg/dl, low albumin level, and high American Society of Anesthesiologists score for operative complications (classes III, IV, or V).[251]

Adjuvant Radiation

The use of adjuvant postoperative radiation was evaluated among 78 cases of locally advanced (Dukes stage B2 to C) colon cancer.[252] In that study, no patients were lost to follow-up and all were followed for a minimum of 3 years. The overall local control rate was 88%. Multivariate analysis showed that the postoperative radiation dose was the only factor that influenced local control rates; the 5-year local control rate was 96% when the dose was 50 to 55 Gy but that rate decreased to 76% when the postoperative dose was less than 45 Gy.[252] These improvements in local control were achieved without significant radiation-induced morbidity. Only 50% of stage C3 tumors, as compared with 75% of stage C2 and B2 tumors, were locally controlled by 45 Gy.[249,252] Disease stage was the only factor that influenced cause-specific survival.[252]

The efficacy of radiation in node-positive colon cancer was demonstrated in a pilot trial of 14 patients conducted by the ECOG. In that trial, 45 Gy was delivered to the tumor bed and periaortic lymph nodes and 30 Gy to the liver; the 10-year survival rate was 58%.[253]

A retrospective analysis of 152 patients with T4 N0 or T4 N1 colon cancer who were given postoperative radiation showed improved actuarial rates of local control (88%) and recurrence-free survival (58%).[254] The local control rate decreased to 66% and the recurrence-free survival rate decreased to 27% among patients with T4 N2-N3 disease. Disease could not be controlled in any patient with four or more positive nodes. Given the variability in the use of concurrent and adjuvant chemotherapy in this series, no benefit could be identified by the addition of 5-FU during radiation.[254]

Adjuvant Chemotherapy

Adjuvant chemotherapy has an established role in the treatment of colon cancer. In one study of 317 patients with high-risk stage II or stage III colon cancer, six cycles of 5-FU (425 mg/m^2) and leucovorin (20 mg/m^2) administered postoperatively for 5 consecutive days every 4 to 5 weeks[255] significantly improved time to relapse and overall survival relative to surgery only.[255]

An analysis of randomized trials of adjuvant chemotherapy for colorectal cancer demonstrated that use of 5-FU and leucovorin improved disease-free and overall survival rates over those produced after surgery only.[256] Disease-free survival rates ranged from 71% to 77% after adjuvant chemotherapy vs. 58% to 64% after surgery only; corresponding overall survival rates were 75% to 84% vs. 63% to 77% with surgery only.[256]

The International Union Against Cancer compared the efficacy of adjuvant chemotherapy with 5-FU and leucovorin or 5-FU and levamisole among 680 patients with curatively resected stage III colon cancer.[257] In that trial, biomodulation with leucovorin significantly improved disease-free and overall survival rates over those produced by 5-FU and levamisole.[257] The NSABP C-04 trial also found no improvement from the addition of levamisole to 5-FU alone or in combination with leucovorin in any aspect of outcome.[258]

The comparative efficacy of adjuvant chemotherapy was evaluated among four NSABP trials (C-01, C-02, C-03, and C-04). In all four studies, adjuvant chemotherapy improved the overall, disease-free, and recurrence-free survival rates improved among patients with Dukes stage B or C disease.[259] In combined analyses, the mortality reduction was 30% for patients with Dukes stage B disease and 18% for those with Dukes stage C, regardless of adverse prognostic factors.

Several other agents also have been developed for the treatment of colorectal cancer. Although 5-FU remains the primary chemotherapeutic agent, other agents are being considered as evidence mounts regarding their efficacy in the treatment of metastatic disease. Irinotecan and oxaliplatin have shown considerable therapeutic activity in the treatment of 5-FU-refractory disease owing to their unique mechanisms of action.[260-262] Among 387 patients with metastatic disease who had never undergone chemotherapy, the response rate after irinotecan was much higher (49%) than that after 5-FU (31%); irinotecan also produced improvements in the time to progression and overall survival.[263] Irinotecan, a radiosensitizer, has been incorporated into adjuvant therapy for colon cancer[264] and for locally advanced rectal cancer.[265,266]

SUMMARY

Optimal treatment of colorectal cancer requires a multimodality approach. For maximum therapeutic benefit, the biological basis of all therapeutic components—in all treatment disciplines—should be understood and exploited. Adjuvant chemotherapy has significantly improved disease-free and overall survival rates, and adjuvant radiation has provided tremendous benefit by improving local-control rates and avoiding the morbidity associated with recurrent disease. Tumor regression in response to preoperative chemoradiation has allowed the increasing use of sphincter-preserving surgical procedures with excellent functional outcome, even for locally advanced tumors of the distal rectum. Sphincter preservation may be possible in even more cases as the ability to clear microscopic disease improves, especially disease in the mesorectum. Newer chemotherapeutic agents hold promise for further improvements through their increased systemic activity and their synergistic effects with radiation.

REFERENCES

1. Michalski JM, Purdy JA, Winter K, et al. Preliminary report of toxicity following 3D radiation therapy for prostate cancer on 3DOG/RTOG 9406. *Int J Radiat Oncol Biol Phys* 2000;46:391-402.
2. Pollack A, Zagars GK, Starkschall G, et al. Conventional vs. conformal radiotherapy for prostate cancer: preliminary results of dosimetry and acute toxicity. *Int J Radiat Oncol Biol Phys* 1996;34:555-564.
3. Fajardo LF, Berthrong M, Anderson RE. Large intestine and anal canal. In: *Radiation Pathology*. New York, NY: Oxford University Press; 2001:239-247.
4. Spanos WJ Jr, Wasserman T, Meoz R, et al. Palliation of advanced pelvic malignant disease with large fraction pelvic radiation and misonidazole: final report of RTOG phase I/II study. *Int J Radiat Oncol Biol Phys* 1987;13:1479-1482.
5. Brennan PC, Carr KE, Seed T, et al. Acute and protracted radiation effects on small intestinal morphological parameters. *Int J Radiat Biol* 1998;73:691-698.
6. Zheng H, Wang J, Hauer-Jensen M. Role of mast cells in early and delayed radiation injury in rat intestine. *Radiat Res* 2000;153:533-539.
7. Dublineau I, Ksas B, Griffiths NM. Functional changes in the rat distal colon after whole-body irradiation: dose-response and temporal relationships. *Radiat Res* 2000;154:187-195.
8. Hendricks T, Wobbes T, deMan BM, et al. Moderate doses of intraoperative radiation severely suppress early strength of anatomoses in the rat colon. *Radiat Res* 1998;150:431-435.
9. Skwarchuk MW, Travis EL. Volume effects and epithelial regeneration in irradiated mouse colorectum. *Radiat Res* 1998;149:1-10.
10. Seifert WF, Biert J, Wobbes T, et al. Late effects of intraoperative radiation therapy in anastomotic rat colon. *Int J Radiat Oncol Biol Phys* 1998;42:623-629.
11. American Cancer Society. *Cancer Facts and Figures, 2001*. Atlanta, Ga: American Cancer Society; 2001.
12. Greenlee RT, Hill-Harmon MB, Murray T, et al. Cancer statistics, 2001. *CA Cancer J Clin* 2001;51:15-36.
13. Ries LAG, Wingo PA, Miller DS, et al. The annual report to the nation on the status of cancer, 1973-1997, with a special section on colorectal cancer. *Cancer* 2000;88:2398-2424.
14. Winawer SJ. Natural history of colorectal cancer. *Am J Med* 1999;106:3S-6S.
15. Potter JD. Colorectal cancer: molecules and populations. *J Natl Cancer Inst* 1999;91:916-932.
16. Nelson RL, Dollear T, Freels S, et al. The relation of age, race, and gender to the subsite location of colorectal carcinoma. *Cancer* 1997;80:193-197.
17. Slattery ML, Friedman GD, Potter JD, et al. A description of age, sex, and site distributions of colon carcinoma in three geographic areas. *Cancer* 1996;78:1666-1670.
18. Dignam JJ, Colangelo L, Tian W, et al. Outcomes among African-Americans and Caucasians in colon cancer adjuvant therapy trials: findings from the National Surgical Adjuvant Breast and Bowel Project. *J Natl Cancer Inst* 1999;91:1933-1940.
19. Mettlin CJ, Menck HR, Winchester DP, et al. A comparison of breast, colorectal, lung, and prostate cancers reported to the National Cancer Data Base and the Surveillance, Epidemiology, and End Results Program. *Cancer* 1997;79:2052-2061.
20. Ikeda Y, Mori M, Yoshizumi T, et al. Cancer and adenomatous polyp distribution in the colorectum. *Am J Gastroenterol* 1999;94:191-193.
21. Weitzel JN. Genetic cancer risk assessment—putting it all together. *Cancer* 1999;86:2483-2492.
22. Neuhausen SL. Ethnic differences in cancer risk resulting from genetic variation. *Cancer* 1999;86:2575-2582.
23. Lynch HT, Watson P, Shaw TG, et al. Clinical impact of molecular genetic diagnosis, genetic counseling, and management of hereditary cancer, I: Studies of cancer in families. *Cancer* 1999;86:2449-2456.
24. Rodriguez-Bigas MA, Boland CR, Hamilton SR, et al. A National Cancer Institute Workshop on Hereditary Nonpolyposis Colorectal Cancer Syndrome: meeting highlights and Bethesda guidelines. *J Natl Cancer Inst* 1997;89:1758-1762.
25. Rex DK, Johnson DA, Lieberman DA, et al. Colorectal cancer prevention 2000: screening recommendations of the American College of Gastroenterology. *Am J Gastroenterol* 2000;95:868-877.
26. Lynch HT, Watson P, Shaw TG, et al. Clinical impact of molecular genetic diagnosis, genetic counseling, and management of hereditary cancer, II: Hereditary nonpolyposis colorectal carcinoma as a model. *Cancer* 1999;86:2457-2463.
27. Hawk E, Lubet R, Limburg P. Chemoprevention in hereditary colorectal cancer syndromes. *Cancer* 1999;86:2551-2563.
28. Dannenberg AJ, Zakim D. Chemoprevention of colorectal cancer through inhibition of cyclooxygenase-2. *Semin Oncol* 1999;26:499-504.
29. Felder JB, Korelitz BI, Rajapakse R, et al. Effects of nonsteroidal anti-inflammatory drugs on inflammatory bowel disease: a case-control study. *Am J Gastroenterol* 2000;95:1949-1954.
30. Grodstein F, Newcomb PA, Stampfer MJ. Postmenopausal hormone therapy and the risk of colorectal cancer: a review and meta-analysis. *Am J Med* 1999;106:574-582.
31. Paganini-Hill A. Estrogen replacement therapy and colorectal cancer risk in elderly women. *Dis Colon Rectum* 1999;42:1300-1305.
32. Issa JP, Ottaviano YL, Celano P, et al. Methylation of the oestrogen receptor CpG island linking ageing and neoplasia in human colon. *Nat Genet* 1994;7:536-540.
33. Ghadirian P, Lacroix A, Maisonneuve P, et al. Nutritional factors and colon carcinoma—a case-control study involving French Canadians in Montreal, Quebec, Canada. *Cancer* 1997;80:858-864.
34. Macrae F. Wheat bran fiber and development of adenomatous polyps: evidence from randomized, controlled clinical trials. *Am J Med* 1999;106:38S-42S.
35. Earnest DL, Einspahr JG, Alberts DS. Protective role of wheat bran fiber: data from marker trials. *Am J Med* 1999;106:32S-37S.
36. Reddy BS. Role of dietary fiber in colon cancer: an overview. *Am J Med* 1999;106:16S-19S.
37. Holt PR, Atillasoy EO, Gilman J, et al. Modulation of abnormal colonic epithelial cell proliferation and differentiation by low-fat dairy foods—a randomized controlled trial. *JAMA* 1998;280:1074-1079.
38. Cousins RJ. Nutritional regulation of gene expression. *Am J Med* 1999;106:20S-23S.
39. Shike M. Diet and lifestyle in the prevention of colorectal cancer: an overview. *Am J Med* 1999;106:11S-15S.
40. Brenner DJ, Curtis RE, Hall EJ, et al. Second malignancies in prostate carcinoma patients after radiotherapy compared with surgery. *Cancer* 2000;88:398-406.
41. Strober W, Ludviksson BR, Fuss IJ. The pathogenesis of mucosal inflammation in murine models of inflammatory bowel disease and Crohn's disease. *Ann Intern Med* 1998;128:848-856.
42. Troisi RJ, Freedman AN, Devesa SS. Incidence of colorectal carcinoma in the U.S.—an update of trends by gender, race, age, subsite, and stage, 1975-1994. *Cancer* 1999;85:1670-1676.
43. Lerman C, Hughes C, Trock BJ, et al. Genetic testing in families with hereditary nonpolyposis colon cancer. *JAMA* 1999;17:1618-1622.
44. Rawl SM, Menon U, Champion RL, et al. Colorectal cancer screening beliefs—focus groups with first-degree relatives. *Cancer Practice* 2000;8:32-37.
45. Lynch PM. Clinical challenges in management of familial adenomatous polyposis and hereditary nonpolyposis colorectal cancer. *Cancer* 1999;86:2533-2550.
46. Kinney AY, Choi YA, DeVellis B, et al. Attitudes toward genetic testing in patients with colorectal cancer. *Cancer Practice* 2000;8:178-186.

47. Worthen HG. Inherited cancer and the primary care physician-barriers and strategies. *Cancer* 1999;86:2583-2588.

48. Lynch HT, Smyrk TC. Hereditary colorectal cancer. *Semin Oncol* 1999;26:478-484.

49. Lindor NM, Greene MH. The concise handbook of family cancer syndromes. Mayo Familial Cancer Program. *J Natl Cancer Inst* 1998;90:1039-1071.

50. Severin MJ. Genetic susceptibility for specific cancers—medical liability of the clinician. *Cancer* 1999;86:2564-2569.

51. Syngal S, Weeks JC, Schrag D, et al. Benefits of colonoscopic surveillance and prophylactic colectomy in patients with hereditary nonpolyposis colorectal cancer mutations. *Ann Intern Med* 1998;129:787-796.

52. Stern MA, Fendrick AM, McDonnell WM, et al. A randomized, controlled trial to assess a novel colorectal cancer screening strategy: the conversion strategy—a comparison of sequential sigmoidoscopy and colonoscopy with immediate conversion from sigmoidoscopy to colonoscopy in patients with an abnormal screening sigmoidoscopy. *Am J Gastroenterol* 2000;95:2074-2079.

53. Karadi C, Beaulieu CF, Jeffrey RB, et al. Display modes for CT colonography, I: synthesis and insertion of polyps into patient CT data. *Radiology* 1999;212:195-201.

54. Schwartz LH. Advances in cross-sectional imaging of colorectal cancer. *Semin Oncol* 1999;26:569-576.

55. Sharma VK, Corder FA, Raufman JP, et al. Survey of internal medicine residents' use of the fecal occult blood test and their understanding of colorectal cancer screening and surveillance. *Am J Gastroenterol* 2000;95:2068-2073.

56. Church TR, Ederer F, Mandel JS. Fecal occult blood screening in the Minnesota study: sensitivity of the screening test. *J Natl Cancer Inst* 1997;89:1440-1448.

57. Blumberg D, Opelka FG, Hicks TC, et al. Significance of a normal surveillance colonoscopy in patients with a history of adenomatous polyps. *Dis Colon Rectum* 2000;43:1084-1092.

58. Burton EC, Troxclair DA, Newman WP. Autopsy diagnoses of malignant neoplasms—how often are clinical diagnoses incorrect? *JAMA* 1998;280:1245-1248.

59. Bini EJ, Micale PL, Weinshel EH. Evaluation of the gastrointestinal tract in premenopausal women with iron deficiency anemia. *Am J Med* 1998;105:281-286.

60. Markowitz AJ, Winawer SJ. Screening and surveillance for colorectal cancer. *Semin Oncol* 1999;26:485-498.

61. Bond JH. Screening guidelines for colorectal cancer. *Am J Med* 1999;106:7S-10S.

62. Schrag D, Weeks J. Costs and cost-effectiveness of colorectal cancer prevention and therapy. *Semin Oncol* 1999;26:561-568.

63. Nelson RL, Persky V, Turyk M. Time trends in distal colorectal cancer subsite location related to age and how it affects choice of screening modality. *J Surg Oncol* 1998;69:235-238.

64. Desch CE, Benson AB, Smith TJ, et al. Recommended colorectal cancer surveillance guidelines by the American Society of Clinical Oncology. *J Clin Oncol* 1999;17:1312-1321.

65. Macdonald JS. Carcinoembryonic antigen screening: pros and cons. *Semin Oncol* 1999;26:556-560.

66. Goldberg RM, Fleming TR, Tangen CM, et al. Surgery for recurrent colon cancer: strategies for identifying resectable recurrence and success rates after resection. *Ann Intern Med* 1998;129:27-35.

67. Secco GB, Fardelli R, Rovida S, et al. Is intensive follow-up really able to improve prognosis of patients with local recurrence after curative surgery for rectal cancer? *Ann Surg Oncol* 2000;7:32-37.

68. Skenderis BS, Rodriguez-Bigas M, Weber TK, et al. Utility of routine postoperative laboratory studies in patients undergoing potentially curative resection for adenocarcinoma of the colon and rectum. *Cancer Invest* 1999;17:102-109.

69. Giess CS, Schwartz LH, Bach AM, et al. Patterns of neoplastic spread in colorectal cancer: implications for surveillance CT studies. *AJR Am J Roentgenol* 1998;170:987-991.

70. Low RN, Semelka RC, Worawattanakul S, et al. Extrahepatic abdominal imaging in patients with malignancy: comparison of MR imaging and helical CT with subsequent surgical correlation. *Radiology* 1999;210:625-632.

71. Flamen P, Stroobants S, Van Cutsem E, et al. Additional value of whole-body positron emission tomography with fluorine-18-2-fluoro-2-deoxy-D-glucose in recurrent colorectal cancer. *J Clin Oncol* 1999;17:894-901.

72. Akhurst T, Larson SM. Positron emission tomography and imaging of colorectal cancer. *Semin Oncol* 1999;26:577-583.

73. Flanagan FL, Dehdashti F, Ogunbiyi O, et al. Utility of FDG-PET for investigating unexplained plasma CEA elevation in patients with colorectal cancer. *Ann Surg* 1998;227:319-323.

74. Valk PE, Abella-Columna E, Haseman MK, et al. Whole-body PET imaging with (^{18}F) fluorodeoxygluocse in management of recurrent colorectal cancer. *Arch Surg* 1999;134:503-511.

75. Vesselle HJ, Miraldi FD. FDG PET of the retroperitoneum: normal anatomy, variants, pathologic conditions, and strategies to avoid diagnostic pitfalls. *Radiographics* 1998;18:805-823.

76. Berger KL, Nicholson SA, Dehdashti F, et al. FDG PET evaluation of mucinous neoplasms: correlation of FDG uptake with histopathologic features. *AJR Am J Roentgenol* 2000;174:1005-1008.

77. Weiss NS, Cook LS. Evaluating the efficacy of screening for recurrence of cancer. *J Natl Cancer Inst* 1998;90:1870-1872.

78. Kawamoto S, Soyer PA, Fishman EK, et al. Nonneoplastic liver disease: evaluation with CT and MR imaging. *Radiographics* 1998;18:827-848.

79. Fleming I, Cooper JS, Henson DE, et al, eds. *AJCC Cancer Staging Manual.* 5th ed. Philadelphia, Pa: Lippincott Williams & Wilkins; 1997:83-90.

80. Horton KM, Abrams RA, Fishman EK. Spiral CT of colon cancer: imaging features and role in management. *Radiographics* 2000;20:419-430.

81. Vogl TJ, Pegios W, Mack MG, et al. Accuracy of staging rectal tumors with contrast-enhanced transrectal MR imaging. *AJR Am J Roentgenol* 1997;168:1427-1434.

82. Zerhouni EA, Rutter C, Hamilton SR, et al. CT and MR imaging in the staging of colorectal carcinoma: report of the Radiology Diagnostic Oncology Group II. *Radiology* 1996;200:443-451.

83. Kruskal JB, Kane RA, Sentovich SM, et al. Pitfalls and sources of error in staging rectal cancer with endorectal US. *Radiographics* 1997;17:609-626.

84. Frudinger A, Bartram CI, Kamm MA. Transvaginal versus anal endosonography for detecting damage to the anal sphincter. *AJR Am J Roentgenol* 1997;168:1435-1438.

85. Rubens DJ, Strang JG, Bogineni-Misra S, et al. Transperineal sonography of the rectum: anatomy and pathology revealed by sonography compared with CT and MR imaging. *AJR Am J Roentgenol* 1998;170:637-642.

86. Lindmark GE, Kraaz WG, Elvin PAB, et al. Rectal cancer: evaluation of staging with endosonography. *Radiology* 1997;204:533-538.

87. Gavioli M, Bagni A, Piccagli I, et al. Usefulness of endorectal ultrasound after preoperative radiotherapy in rectal cancer—comparison between sonographic and histopathologic changes. *Dis Colon Rectum* 2000;43:1075-1083.

88. Lohnert MSS, Doniec JM, Henne-Bruns D. Effectiveness of endoluminal sonography in the identification of occult local rectal cancer recurrences. *Dis Colon Rectum* 2000;43:483-491.

89. Enker WE. Designing the optimal surgery for rectal carcinoma. *Cancer* 1996;78:1847-1850.

90. Sugihara K, Moriya Y, Akasu T, et al. Pelvic autonomic nerve preservation for patients with rectal carcinoma. Oncologic and functional outcome. *Cancer* 1996;78:1871-1880.

91. Hida J, Yasutomi M, Maruyama T, et al. The extent of lymph node dissection for colon carcinoma: the potential impact on laparoscopic surgery. *Cancer* 1997;80:188-192.

92. Tepper JE, O'Connell MJ, Niedzwiecki D, et al. Impact on number of nodes retrieved on outcome in patients with rectal cancer. *J Clin Oncol* 2001;19:157-163.

93. Kockerling F, Reymond MA, Altendorf-Hofmann A, et al. Influence of surgery on metachronous distant metastases and survival in rectal cancer. *J Clin Oncol* 1988;16:324-329.

94. Enker WE. Sphincter-preserving operations for rectal cancer. *Oncology* 1996;10:1673-1689.

95. Paty PB, Cohen AM. Technical considerations for coloanal anastomosis and J-pouch. *Semin Radiat Oncol* 1998;8:48-53.

96. Berger A, Tiret E, Cunningham C, et al. Rectal excision and colonic pouch—anal anastomosis for rectal cancer-oncologic results at five years. *Dis Colon Rectum* 1999;42:1265-1271.

97. Renner K, Rosen HR, Novi G, et al. Quality of life after surgery for rectal cancer—do we still need a permanent colostomy? *Dis Colon Rectum* 1999;42:1160-1167.

98. Rullier E, Zerbib F, Laurent C, et al. Intersphincteric resection with excision of internal anal sphincter for conservative treatment of very low rectal cancer. *Dis Colon Rectum* 1999;42: 1168-1175.

99. Balbay MD, Slaton JW, Trane N, et al. Rationale for bladder-sparing surgery in patients with locally advanced colorectal carcinoma. *Cancer* 1999;86:2212-2216.

100. Hermanek P. Impact of surgeon's technique on outcome after treatment of rectal carcinoma. *Dis Colon Rectum* 1999;42:559-562.

101. Dorrance HR, Docherty GM, O'Dwyer PJ. Effect of surgeon specialty interest on patient outcome after potentially curative colorectal cancer surgery. *Dis Colon Rectum* 2000;43:492-498.

102. Janjan NA, Khoo VS, Rich TA, et al. Locally advanced rectal cancer: surgical complications after infusional chemotherapy and radiation therapy. *Radiology* 1998;206:131-136.

103. Pucciarelli S, Toppan P, Friso ML, et al. Preoperative combined radiotherapy and chemotherapy for rectal cancer does not affect early postoperative morbidity and mortality in low anterior resection. *Dis Colon Rectum* 1999;42:1276-1284.

104. Gorksi T, Rosen L, Lawrence S, et al. Usefulness of a state-legislated comparative database to evaluate quality in colorectal surgery. *Dis Colon Rectum* 1999;42:1381-1387.

105. Mellgren A, Sirivongs P, Rothenberger DA, et al. Is local excision adequate therapy for early rectal cancer? *Dis Colon Rectum* 2000;43:2064-2074.

106. Weber TK, Petrelli NJ. Local excision for rectal cancer: an uncertain future. *Oncology* 1998;12:933-943.

107. Chakravarti A, Compton CC, Shellito PC, et al. Long-term follow-up of patients with rectal cancer managed by local excision with and without adjuvant irradiation. *Ann Surg* 1999; 230:49-54.

108. Steele GD, Herndon JE, Bleday R, et al. Sphincter-sparing treatment for distal rectal adenocarcinoma. *Ann Surg Oncol* 1999;6: 433-441.

109. Petrelli NJ, Weber TK. Sphincter preservation for distal rectal cancer: paradise lost? *Ann Surg Oncol* 1999;6:413-415.

110. Kinsella TJ. An approach to the radiosensitization of human tumors. *Cancer J Sci Am* 1996;2:184-193.

111. Milas L. Chemoradiation interactions: potential of newer chemotherapeutic agents. In: *American Society of Clinical Oncology Educational Handbook.* Alexandria, Va: American Society of Clinical Oncology; 2000:207-213.

112. Koutcher JA, Alfieri AA, Thaler H, et al. Radiation enhancement by biochemical modulation and 5-fluorouracil. *Int J Radiat Oncol Biol Phys* 1997;39:1145-1152.

113. Krook JE, Moertel CG, Gunderson LL, et al. Effective surgical adjuvant therapy for high-risk rectal carcinoma. *N Engl J Med* 1991;324:709-715.

114. Douglas HO, Moertel CG, Mayer RJ, et al. Survival after postoperative combination treatment of rectal cancer. *N Engl J Med* 1986;315:1294-1295.

115. Gastrointestinal Tumor Study Group. Prolongation of the disease-free interval in surgically treated rectal carcinoma. *N Engl J Med* 1985;312:1465-1472.

116. Douglass HO Jr, Moertel CG, Mayer RJ, et al. Survival after postoperative combination treatment of rectal cancer [letter]. *N Engl J Med* 1986;315:1294-1295.

117. Thomas PR, Lindblad AS. Adjuvant postoperative radiotherapy and chemotherapy in rectal carcinoma: a review of the Gastrointestinal Tumor Study Group experience. *Radiother Oncol* 1988;13:245-252.

118. Fisher B, Wolmark N, Rockette H, et al. Postoperative adjuvant chemotherapy or radiation therapy for rectal cancer: results from NSABP R-01. *J Natl Cancer Inst* 1988;80:21-29.

119. Freedman GM, Coia LR. Adjuvant and neoadjuvant treatment of rectal cancer. *Semin Oncol* 1995;22:611-624.

120. Gunderson LL, Martenson JA. Postoperative adjuvant irradiation with or without chemotherapy for rectal carcinoma. *Semin Radiat Oncol* 1993;3:55-63.

121. Rich T, Ajani JA, Morrison WH, et al. Chemoradiation therapy for anal cancer. Radiation plus continuous infusion of 5-fluorouracil with or without cisplatin. *Radiother Oncol* 1993;27: 209-215.

122. *Adjuvant Therapy of Rectal Cancer.* Bethesda, Md: National Cancer Institute; 1991.

123. Jessup JM, Stewart AK, Menck HR. The National Cancer Data Base Report on patterns of care for adenocarcinoma of the rectum, 1985-1995. *Cancer* 1998;83:2408-2418.

124. Minsky BD, Coia L, Haller DG, et al. Radiation therapy for rectosigmoid and rectal cancer: results of the 1992-1994 Patterns of Care Process Survey. *J Clin Oncol* 1998;16:2542-2547.

125. Coia LR, Gunderson LL, Haller D, et al. Outcomes of patients receiving radiation for carcinoma of the rectum. *Cancer* 1999;86:1952-1958.

126. Sobrero AF, Aschele C, Bertino JR. Fluorouracil in colorectal cancer—a tale of two drugs: implications for biochemical modulation. *J Clin Oncol* 1997;15:368-381.

127. Tepper JE, O'Connell MJ, Petroni GR, et al. Adjuvant postoperative fluorouracil modulated chemotherapy combined with pelvic radiation therapy for rectal cancer: initial results of intergroup 0114. *J Clin Oncol* 1997;15:2030-2039.

128. O'Connell MJ, Martenson JA, Wieand HS, et al. Improving adjuvant therapy for rectal cancer by combining protracted-infusion fluorouracil with radiation therapy after curative surgery. *N Engl J Med* 1994;331:502-507.

129. Meta-Analysis Group in Cancer. Efficacy of intravenous continuous infusion of fluorouracil compared with bolus administration in advanced colorectal cancer. *J Clin Oncol* 1998;16:301-308.

130. Tominaga T, Sakabe T, Koyama Y, et al. Prognostic factors for patients with colon or rectal carcinoma treated with resection only—five year followup report. *Cancer* 1996;78:403-408.

131. Phillips RKS, Hittinger R, Blesovsky L, et al. Local recurrence following "curative" surgery for large bowel cancer. 1. The overall picture. *Br J Surg* 1984;71:12-16.

132. Minsky BD, Conti JA, Huang Y, et al. Relationship of acute gastrointestinal toxicity and the volume of irradiated small bowel in patients receiving combined modality therapy for rectal cancer. *J Clin Oncol* 1995;13:1409-1416.

133. Koelbl O, Richter S, Flentje M. Influence of patient positioning on dose-volume histogram and normal tissue complication probability for small bowel and bladder in patients receiving pelvic irradiation: a prospective study using a 3D planning system and a radiobiological model. *Int J Radiat Oncol Biol Phys* 1999;45:1193-1198.

134. Das IJ, Lanciano RM, Movsas B, et al. Efficacy of a belly board device with CT-simulation in reducing small bowel volume within pelvic irradiation fields. *Int J Radiat Oncol Biol Phys* 1997;39:67-76.

135. Chun M, Timmerman RD, Mayer R, et al. Radiation therapy of external iliac lymph nodes with lateral pelvic portals: identification of patients at risk for inadequate regional coverage. *Radiology* 1995;194:147-150.

136. Taylor N, Crane C, Skibber J, et al. Elective groin irradiation is not indicated among patients with adenocarcinoma of the rectum extending to the anal canal. *Radiology* 2000;(suppl):352. Abstract 628.

137. Tocchi A, Lepre L, Costa G, et al. Rectal cancer and inguinal metastases-prognostic role and therapeutic indications. *Dis Colon Rectum* 1999;42:1464-1466.

138. Lacerna MD, Sharpe MB, Robertson JM. The effect of radiation on an ambulatory chemotherapy infusion pump. *Cancer* 1999;86:2150-2153.

139. Gerard JP, Romestaing P, Ardiet JM, et al. Endocavitary radiation therapy. *Semin Radiat Oncol* 1998;8:13-23.

140. Maingon P, Guerif S, Darsouni R, et al. Conservative management of rectal adenocarcinoma by radiotherapy. *Int J Radiat Oncol Biol Phys* 1998;40:1077-1085.

141. Salembier C, Battermann JJ. Interstitial brachytherapy in the conservative treatment of anal and rectal cancers. *Endocurietherapy/Hyperthermia Oncology* 1996;12:183-189.

142. Armour EP, White JR, Armin AR, et al. Pulsed low dose rate brachytherapy in a rat model: dependence of late rectal injury on radiation pulse size. *Int J Radiat Oncol Biol Phys* 1997;38:825-834.

143. Minsky BD. Multidisciplinary management of resectable rectal cancer. *Oncology* 1996;10:1701-1714.

144. Minsky BD, Cohen AM, Enker WE, et al. Efficacy of postoperative 5-FU, high-dose leucovorin, and sequential radiation therapy for clinically resectable rectal cancer. *Cancer Invest* 1995;13:1-7.

145. Minsky BD. Adjuvant therapy of rectal cancer. *Semin Oncol* 1999;26:540-544.

146. Minsky BD. Preoperative radiation therapy followed by low anterior resection with coloanal anastomosis. *Semin Radiat Oncol* 1998;8:30-35.

147. Bosset JF, Pelissier EP, Manion G, et al. Plea for a preoperative adjuvant approach in the management of rectal cancer. *Int J Radiat Oncol Biol Phys* 1994;29:205-208.

148. Rich TA. Adjuvant radiotherapy for rectal cancer: more on pre- or postoperative therapy. *Int J Radiat Oncol Biol Phys* 1995;32:547-548.

149. Coucke PA, Sartorelli B, Cuttat JF, et al. The rationale to switch from postoperative hyperfractionated accelerated radiotherapy to preoperative hyperfractionated accelerated radiotherapy in rectal cancer. *Int J Radiat Oncol Biol Phys* 1995;32:181-188.

150. No authors listed. Improved survival with preoperative radiotherapy in resectable rectal cancer. Swedish Rectal Cancer Trial. *N Engl J Med* 1997;336:980-987.

151. Camma C, Giunta M, Fiorica F, et al. Preoperative radiotherapy for resectable rectal cancer: a meta-analysis. *JAMA* 2000;284:1008-1015.

152. Vaughn DJ, Haller DG. Adjuvant therapy for colorectal cancer: past accomplishments, future directions. *Cancer Invest* 1997;15:435-447.

153. Cedermark B, Johansson H, Rutqvist LE, et al. The Stockholm I trial of preoperative short term radiotherapy in operable rectal carcinoma: a prospective randomized trial. *Cancer* 1995;75:2269-2275.

154. Swedish Rectal Cancer Trial. Improved survival with preoperative radiotherapy in resectable rectal cancer. *N Engl J Med* 1997;336:980-987.

155. Stockholm Colorectal Cancer Study Group. Randomized study on preoperative radiotherapy in rectal carcinoma. *Ann Surg Oncol* 1996;3:423-430.

156. Frykholm GJ, Glimelius B, Pahlman L. Preoperative or postoperative irradiation in adenocarcinoma of the rectum: final treatment results of a randomized trial and an evaluation of late secondary effects. *Dis Colon Rectum* 1993;36:564-572.

157. Pahlman L, Glimelius B. Pre- or postoperative radiotherapy in rectal and rectosigmoid carcinoma: a report from a randomized multicenter trial. *Ann Surg* 1990;211:187-195.

158. Frykholm GJ, Isacsson U, Nygard K, et al. Preoperative radiotherapy in rectal carcinoma—aspects of acute adverse effects and radiation technique. *Int J Radiat Oncol Biol Phys* 1996;35:1039-1048.

159. Myerson RJ, Genovesi D, Lockett MA, et al. Five fractions of preoperative radiotherapy for selected cases of rectal carcinoma: long-term tumor control and tolerance to treatment. *Int J Radiat Oncol Biol Phys* 1999;43:537-543.

160. Minsky BD, Cohen AM, Enker WE, et al. Sphincter preservation with preoperative radiation therapy and coloanal anastomosis. *Int J Radiat Oncol Biol Phys* 1995;31:553-559.

161. Marks G, Mohiuddin M, Masoni L, et al. High-dose preoperative radiation therapy as the key to extending sphincter-preservation surgery for cancer of the distal rectum. *Surg Oncol Clin North Am* 1992;1:71-86.

162. Paszat LF, Brundage MD, Groome PA, et al. A population-based study of rectal cancer: permanent colostomy as an outcome. *Int J Radiat Oncol Biol Phys* 1999;45:1185-1191.

163. Ng AK, Recht A, Busse PM. Sphincter preservation therapy for distal rectal carcinoma: a review. *Cancer* 1997;79:671-683.

164. Hyams DM, Mamounas EP, Petrelli N, et al. A clinical trial to evaluate the worth of preoperative multimodal therapy in patients with operable carcinoma of the rectum: a progress report of the National Surgical Adjuvant Breast and Bowel Project protocol R-03. *Dis Colon Rectum* 1997;40:131-139.

165. Janjan NA, Breslin T, Lenzi R, et al. Avoidance of colostomy placement in advanced colorectal cancer with twice weekly hypofractionated radiation plus continuous infusion 5-fluorouracil. *J Pain Symptom Manage* 2000;20:266-272.

166. Janjan NA, Crane CH, Feig BW, et al. Prospective trial of preoperative concomitant boost radiotherapy with continuous infusion 5-fluorouracil for locally advanced rectal cancer. *Int J Radiat Oncol Biol Phys* 2000;47:713-718.

167. Bosset JF, Magnin V, Maingon P, et al. Preoperative radiochemotherapy in rectal cancer: long-term results of a phase II trial. *Int J Radiat Oncol Biol Phys* 2000;46:323-327.

168. Pucciarelli S, Friso ML, Toppan P, et al. Preoperative combined radiotherapy and chemotherapy for middle and lower rectal cancer: preliminary results. *Ann Surg Oncol* 2000;7:38-44.

169. Valentini V, Coco C, Cellini N, et al. Preoperative chemoradiation with cisplatin and 5-fluorouracil for extraperitoneal T3 rectal cancer: acute toxicity, tumor response, sphincter preservation. *Int J Radiat Oncol Biol Phys* 1999;45:1175-1184.

170. Valentini V, Morganti AG, De Franco A, et al. Chemoradiation with or without intraoperative radiation therapy in patients with locally recurrent rectal carcinoma—prognostic factors and long term outcome. *Cancer* 1999;86:2612-2624.

171. Movsas J, Hanlon AL, Lanciano R, et al. Phase I dose escalating trial of hyperfractionated pre-operative chemoradiation for locally advanced rectal cancer. *Int J Radiat Oncol Biol Phys* 1998;42:43-50.

172. Wagman R, Minsky BD, Cohen AM, et al. Sphincter preservation in rectal cancer with preoperative radiation therapy and coloanal anastomosis: long term follow-up. *Int J Radiat Oncol Biol Physics* 1998;42:51-57.

173. Mohiuddin M, Regine WF, Marks GJ, et al. High-dose preoperative radiation and the challenge of sphincter-preservation surgery for cancer of the distal 2 cm of the rectum. *Int J Radiat Oncol Biol Phys* 1998;40:569-574.

174. Berger C, deMuret A, Garaud P, et al. Preoperative radiotherapy [RT] for rectal cancer: predictive factors of tumor downstaging and residual tumor cell density (RTCD): prognostic implications. *Int J Radiat Oncol Biol Phys* 1997;37:619-627.

175. Francois Y, Nemoz CJ, Baulieux J, et al. Influence of the interval between preoperative radiation therapy and surgery on downstaging and on the rate of sphincter-sparing surgery for rectal cancer: the Lyon R90-01 randomized trial. *J Clin Oncol* 1999;17:2396-2402.

176. Vauthey JN, Marsh RW, Zlotecki RA, et al. Recent advances in the treatment and outcome of locally advanced rectal cancer. *Ann Surg* 1999;229:745-752.

177. Rich TA, Skibber JM, Ajani JA, et al. Preoperative infusional chemoradiation therapy for stage T3 rectal cancer. *Int J Radiat Oncol Biol Phys* 1995;32:1025-1029.

178. Weinstein GD, Rich TA, Shumate CR, et al. Preoperative infusional chemoradiation and surgery with or without an electron beam intraoperative boost for advanced primary rectal cancer. *Int J Radiat Oncol Biol Phys* 1995;32:197-204.

179. Janjan NA, Khoo VS, Abbruzzese J, et al. Tumor downstaging and sphincter preservation with preoperative chemoradiation in locally advanced rectal cancer: the M.D. Anderson Cancer Center experience. *Int J Radiat Oncol Biol Phys* 1999;44:1027-1038.

180. Kaminsky-Forrett MC, Conroy T, Luporsi E, et al. Prognostic implications of downstaging following preoperative radiation therapy for operable T3-T4 rectal cancer. *Int J Radiat Oncol Biol Phys* 1998;42:935-941.

181. Janjan NA, Abbruzzese J, Pazdur R, et al. Prognostic implications of response to preoperative infusional chemoradiation in locally advanced rectal cancer. *Radiother Oncol* 1999;51:153-160.

182. Willett CG, Warland G, Hagan MP, et al. Tumor proliferation in rectal cancer following preoperative irradiation. *J Clin Oncol* 1995;13:1417-1424.

183. DeMario MD, Ratain MJ. Oral chemotherapy: rationale and future directions. *J Clin Oncol* 1998;16:2557-2567.

184. Suwinski R, Taylor JMG, Withers HR. Rapid growth of microscopic rectal cancer as a determinant of response to preoperative radiation therapy. *Int J Radiat Oncol Biol Phys* 1998;42:943-951.

185. Hoff PM, Lassere Y, Pazdur R, et al. Preoperative UFT and calcium folinate and radiotherapy in rectal cancer. *Oncology* 1999;13(suppl 3):129-131.

186. Sharma S, Saltz LB. Oral chemotherapeutic agents for colorectal cancer. *Oncologist* 2000;5:99-107.

187. Sulkes A, Benner SE, Canetta RM. Uracil-Ftorafur: an oral fluoropyrimidine active in colorectal cancer. *J Clin Oncol* 1998;16:3461-3475.

188. Mani S, Hochster H, Beck T, et al. Multicenter phase II study to evaluate a 28-day regimen of oral fluorouracil plus eniluracil in the treatment of patients with previously untreated metastatic colorectal cancer. *J Clin Oncol* 2000;18:2894-2901.

189. Van Cutsem E, Findlay M, Osterwalder B, et al. Capecitabine, an oral fluoropyrimidine carbamate with substantial activity in advanced colorectal cancer: results of a randomized phase II study. *J Clin Oncol* 2000;18:1337-1345.

190. Pazdur R, Lassere Y, Diaz-Canton E, et al. Phase I trial of uracil-tegafur (UFT) plus oral leucovorin: 28-day schedule. *Cancer Invest* 1998;16:145-151.

191. Budman DR, Meropol NJ, Reigner B, et al. Preliminary studies of a novel oral fluoropyrimidine carbamate: capecitabine. *J Clin Oncol* 1998;16:1795-1802.

192. Ahmed FY, Johnston SJ, Cassidy J, et al. Eniluracil treatment completely inactivates dihydropyrimidine dehydrogenase in colorectal tumors. *J Clin Oncol* 1999;17:2439-2445.

193. Hoff PM, Saad ED, Janjan N, et al. A phase I study. Preoperative UFT/leucovorin and radiation therapy in rectal cancer. *Oncology* 2000;14:56-58.

194. Punt CJA. New drugs in the treatment of colorectal carcinoma. *Cancer* 1998;83:679-689.

195. Russell AH, Harris J, Rosenberg PJ, et al. Anal sphincter conservation for patients with adenocarcinoma of the distal rectum: long-term results of Radiation Therapy Oncology Group Protocol 89-02. *Int J Radiat Oncol Biol Phys* 2000;46:313-322.

196. Johnson DE, Hoffman JP. Surgical considerations for local excision. *Semin Radiat Oncol* 1998;8:39-47.

197. Willett CG. Local excision followed by postoperative radiation therapy. *Semin Radiat Oncol* 1998;8:24-29.

198. Bouvet M, Milas M, Giacco GG, et al. Predictors of recurrence after local excision and postoperative chemoradiation therapy of adenocarcinoma of the rectum. *Ann Surg Oncol* 1999;6:26-32.

199. Jessup JM, Loda M, Bleday R. Clinical and molecular prognostic factors in sphincter-preserving surgery for rectal cancer. *Semin Radiat Oncol* 1998;8:54-69.

200. Ahmad NR, Nagle DA. Preoperative radiation therapy followed by local excision. *Semin Radiat Oncol* 1998;8:36-38.

201. Wadler S, Benson AB, Engelking C, et al. Recommended guidelines for the treatment of chemotherapy-induced diarrhea. *J Clin Oncol* 1998;16:3169-3178.

202. Callister M, Janjan N, Crane C, et al. Effective management of symptoms during preoperative chemoradiation for locally advanced rectal cancer. *Int J Radiat Oncol Biol Phys* 2000;48(suppl):177. Abstract 60.

203. Gamelin EC, Danquechin-Dorval EM, Dumesnil YF, et al. Relationship between 5-fluorouracil (5-FU) dose intensity and therapeutic response in patients with advanced colorectal cancer receiving infusional therapy containing 5-FU. *Cancer* 1996;77:441-451.

204. Gurney H. Dose calculation of anticancer drugs: a review of the current practice and introduction of an alternative. *J Clin Oncol* 1996;14:2590-2611.

205. Kornblau S, Benson AB, Catalano R, et al. Management of cancer treatment related diarrhea: issues and therapeutic strategies. *J Pain Symptom Manage* 2000;19:118-129.

206. Denham JW, O'Brien PC, Dunstan RH, et al. Is there more than one late radiation proctitis syndrome? *Radiother Oncol* 1999;51:43-53.

207. Miller AR, Martenson JA, Nelson H, et al. The incidence and clinical consequences of treatment-related bowel injury. *Int J Radiat Oncol Biol Phys* 1999;43:817-825.

208. Van Duijvendijk P, Slors JFM, Taat CW, et al. What is the benefit of preoperative sperm preservation for patients who undergo restorative proctocolectomy for benign disease? *Dis Colon Rectum* 2000;43:838-842.

209. Porter GA, Skibber JM. Outcomes research in surgical oncology. *Ann Surg Oncol* 2000;7:367-375.

210. Ramsey SD, Andersen MR, Etzioni R, et al. Quality of life in survivors of colorectal carcinoma. *Cancer* 2000;88:1294-1303.

211. Ko CY, Rusin LC, Schoetz DJ, et al. Does better functional result equate with better quality of life? Implications for surgical treatment in familial adenomatous polyposis. *Dis Colon Rectum* 2000;43:829-837.

212. Soffer EE, Hull T. Fecal incontinence: a practical approach to evaluation and treatment. *Am J Gastroenterol* 2000;95:1873-1880.

213. Ulander K, Jeppsson B, Grahn G. Quality of life and independence in activities of daily living preoperatively and at follow-up in patients with colorectal cancer. *Support Care Cancer* 1997;8:402-409.

214. Lingareddy V, Ahmad NR, Mohiuddin M. Palliative reirradiation for recurrent rectal cancer. *Int J Radiat Oncol Biol Phys* 1997;38:785-790.

215. Mohiuddin M, Marks GM, Lingareddy V, et al. Curative surgical resection following reirradiation for recurrent rectal cancer. *Int J Radiat Oncol Biol Phys* 1997;39:643-649.

216. Nymann T, Jess P, Christiansen J. Rate and treatment of pelvic recurrence after abdominoperineal resection and low anterior resection for rectal cancer. *Dis Colon Rectum* 1995;38: 799-802.

217. Wong CS, Cummings BJ, Brierley JD, et al. Treatment of locally recurrent rectal carcinoma—results and prognostic factors. *Int J Radiat Oncol Biol Phys* 1998;40:427-435.

218. Wong R, Thomas G, Cummings B, et al. In search of a dose-response relationship with radiotherapy in the management of recurrent rectal carcinoma in the pelvis: a systematic review. *Int J Radiat Oncol Biol Phys* 1998;40:437-446.

219. Guiney MJ, Smith JG, Worotniuk V, et al. Results of external beam radiotherapy alone for incompletely resected carcinoma of rectosigmoid or rectum: Peter MacCallum Cancer Institute Experience 1981-1990. *Int J Radiat Oncol Biol Phys* 1999;43: 531-536.

220. Guiney MJ, Smith JG, Worotniuk V, et al. Radiotherapy treatment for isolated loco-regional recurrence of rectosigmoid cancer following definitive surgery: Peter MacCallum Cancer Institute experience, 1981-1990. *Int J Radiat Oncol Biol Phys* 1997;38:1019-1025.

221. Bussieres E, Gilly FN, Rouanet P, et al. Recurrences of rectal cancers: results of a mutlimodal approach with intraoperative radiation therapy. *Int J Radiat Oncol Biol Phys* 1996;34:49-56.

222. Lanciano RM, Calkins AR, Wolkov HB, et al. A phase I/II study of intraoperative radiotherapy in advanced unresectable or recurrent carcinoma of the rectum: a Radiation Therapy Oncology Group (RTOG) study. *J Surg Oncol* 1993;53:20-29.

223. Sofo L, Ratto C, Doglietto GB, et al. Intraoperative radiation therapy in integrated treatment of rectal cancers—results of a phase II study. *Dis Colon Rectum* 1996;39:1396-1403.

224. Martinez-Monge R, Nag S, Martin EW. Three different intraoperative radiation modalities (electron beam, high-dose-rate brachytherapy, and Iodine-125 brachytherapy) in the adjuvant treatment of patients with recurrent colorectal adenocarcinoma. *Cancer* 1999;86:236-247.

225. Schneebaum S, Papo J, Fraif M, et al. Radioimmunoguided surgery benefits for recurrent colorectal cancer. *Ann Surg Oncol* 1997;4:371-376.

226. Kim HK, Jessup JM, Beard CJ, et al. Locally advanced rectal carcinoma: pelvic control and morbidity following preoperative radiation therapy, resection, and intraoperative radiation therapy. *Int J Radiat Oncol Biol Physics* 1997;38:777-783.

227. Shibata D, Hyland W, Busse P, et al. Immediate reconstruction of the perineal wound with gracilis muscle flaps following abdominoperineal resections and intraoperative radiation therapy for recurrent carcinoma of the rectum. *Ann Surg Oncol* 1999;6:33-37.

228. Salo JC, Paty PB, Guillem J, et al. Surgical salvage of recurrent rectal carcinoma after curative resection: a 10-year experience. *Ann Surg Oncol* 1999;6:171-177.

229. Wanebo HJ, Antoniuk P, Koness RJ, et al. Pelvic resection of recurrent rectal cancer—technical considerations and outcomes. *Dis Colon Rectum* 1999;42:1438-1448.

230. Wesselmann U, Burnett AL, Heinberg LJ. The urogenital and rectal pain syndromes. *Pain* 1997;73:269-294.

231. Mancini I, Bruera E. Constipation in advanced cancer patients. *Support Care Cancer* 1998;6:356-364.

232. Rousseau P. Management of malignant bowel obstruction in advanced cancer: a brief review. *J Palliat Med* 1998;1:65-72.

233. Wong CS, Brierley JD. External beam radiation therapy alone. *Semin Radiat Oncol* 1998;8:3-12.

234. Brierley JD, Cummings BJ, Wong CS, et al. Adenocarcinoma of the rectum treated by radical external radiation therapy. *Int J Radiat Oncol Biol Phys* 1995;31:255-259.

235. Crane CH, Janjan NA, Abbruzzese JL, et al. Effective pelvic symptom control using initial chemoradiation without colostomy in metastatic rectal cancer. *Int J Radiat Oncol Biol Phys* 2001;49:107-116.

236. Scoggins CR, Meszoely IM, Blanke CD, et al. Nonoperative management of primary colorectal cancer in patients with stage IV disease. *Ann Surg Oncol* 1999;6:651-657.

237. Videtic GM, Fisher BJ, Perera FE, et al. Preoperative radiation with concurrent 5-fluorouracil continuous infusion for locally advanced unresectable rectal cancer. *Int J Radiat Oncol Biol Phys* 1998;42:319-324.

238. Rowe VL, Frost DB, Huang S. Extended resection for locally advanced colorectal carcinoma. *Ann Surg Oncol* 1997;4:131-136.

239. Camunez F, Echenagusia A, Simo G, et al. Malignant colorectal obstruction treated by means of self-expanding metallic stents: effectiveness before surgery and in palliation. *Radiology* 2000;216:492-497.

240. Binkert CA, Ledermann H, Jost R, et al. Acute colonic obstruction: clinical aspects and cost-effectiveness of preoperative and palliative treatment with self-expanding metallic stents—a preliminary report. *Radiology* 1998;206:199-204.

241. Luna-Perez P, Delgado S, Labastida S, et al. Patterns of recurrence following pelvic exenteration and external radiotherapy for locally advanced primary rectal adenocarcinoma. *Ann Surg Oncol* 1996;3:526-533.

242. Gunderson LL, Nelson H, Martenson JA, et al. Locally advanced primary colorectal cancer: intraoperative electron beam and external beam irradiation +/- 5-FU. *Int J Radiat Oncol Biol Phys* 1997;37:601-614.

243. Chan AKP, Wong AO, Langevin JM, et al. "Sandwich" preoperative and postoperative combined chemotherapy and radiation in tethered and fixed rectal cancer: impact of treatment intensity on local control and survival. *Int J Radiat Oncol Biol Phys* 1997;37:629-637.

244. Marsh RD, Chu NM, Vauthey JN, et al. Preoperative treatment of patients with locally advanced unresectable rectal adenocarcinoma utilizing continuous chronobiologically shaped 5-fluorouracil infusion and radiation therapy. *Cancer* 1996;78:217-225.

245. Minsky BD, Cohen AM, Enker WE, et al. Preoperative 5-FU, low-dose leucovorin, and radiation therapy for locally advanced and unresectable rectal cancer. *Int J Radiat Oncol Biol Phys* 1997;37: 289-295.

246. Minsky BD, Cohen AM, Enker WE, et al. Preoperative 5-FU, low dose leucovorin, and concurrent radiation therapy for rectal cancer. *Cancer* 1993;73:273-278.

247. Ky AJ, Sung MW, Milsom JW. Research in colon and rectal cancer, with an emphasis on surgical progress. *Dis Colon Rectum* 1999;42:1369-1380.

248. Moore HCF, Haller DG. Adjuvant therapy of colon cancer. *Semin Oncol* 1999;26:545-555.

249. Janjan NA. Postoperative radiotherapy for locally advanced colon cancer. *Ann Surg Oncol* 1996;3:421-422.

250. Koea JB, Conlon K, Paty PB, et al. Pancreatic or duodenal resection or both for advanced carcinoma of the right colon—is it justified? *Dis Colon Rectum* 2000;43:460-465.

251. Longo WE, Virgo KS, Johnson FE, et al. Risk factors for morbidity and mortality after colectomy for colon cancer. *Dis Colon Rectum* 2000;43:83-91.

252. Amos EH, Mendenhall WM, McCarty PJ, et al. Postoperative radiotherapy for locally advanced colon cancer. *Ann Surg Oncol* 1996;3:431-436.

253. Merrick HW, Turner SS, Dobelbower RR, et al. Large-field external beam irradiation as a surgical adjuvant for node-positive colon carcinoma: an Eastern Cooperative Oncology Group Pilot Study (PA285). *Am J Clin Oncol* 2000;23: 337-340.

254. Willett CG, Goldberg S, Shellito PC, et al. Does postoperative irradiation play a role in the adjuvant therapy of T4 colon cancer? *Cancer J Sci Am* 1999;5:242-247.

255. O'Connell MJ, Mailliard JA, Kahn MJ, et al. Controlled trial of fluorouracil and low-dose leucovorin given for 6 months as postoperative adjuvant therapy for colon cancer. *J Clin Oncol* 1997;15:246-250.

256. Zaniboni A. Adjuvant chemotherapy in colorectal cancer with high-dose leucovorin and fluorouracil: impact on disease-free survival and overall survival. *J Clin Oncol* 1997;15:2432-2441.

257. Porschen R, Bermann A, Loffler T, et al. Fluorouracil plus leucovorin as effective adjuvant chemotherapy in curatively resected stage III colon cancer: results of the trial adjCCA-01. *J Clin Oncol* 2001;19:1787-1794.

258. Wolmark N, Rockette H, Mamounas E, et al. Clinical trial to assess the relative efficacy of fluorouracil and leucovorin, fluorouracil and levamisole, and fluorouracil, leucovorin, and levamisole in patients with Dukes B and C carcinoma of the colon: results from National Surgical Adjuvant Breast and Bowel Project C-04. *J Clin Oncol* 1999;17:3553-3559.

259. Mamounas E, Wieand S, Wolmark N, et al. Comparative efficacy of adjuvant chemotherapy in patients with Dukes B versus Dukes C colon cancer: results from four National Adjuvant Breast and Bowel Project Adjuvant Studies (C-01, C-02, C-03, and C-04). *J Clin Oncol* 1999;17:1349-1355.

260. Royce ME, Medgyesy D, Zukowski TH, et al. Colorectal cancer: chemotherapy treatment overview. *Oncology* 2000;14:40-46.

261. Mayer RJ. Newer cytotoxic agents for advanced colon cancer. In: *American Society of Clinical Oncology Educational Handbook.* Alexandria, Va: American Society of Clinical Oncology; 2000:625-629.

262. Henderson CA. Therapeutic options for the treatment of colorectal cancer following 5-fluorouracil failure. *Semin Oncol* 1998;25:29-38.

263. Douillard JY, Cunningham D, Roth AD, et al. Irinotecan combined with fluorouracil compared with fluorouracil alone as first-line treatment for metastatic colorectal cancer: a multicentre randomised trial. *Lancet* 2000;355:1041-1047.

264. Saltz L. Irinotecan-based combinations for the adjuvant treatment of stage III colon cancer. *Oncology* 2000;14:47-50.

265. Mitchell EP. Irinotecan in preoperative combined-modality therapy for locally advanced rectal cancer. *Oncology (Huntingt)* 2000;14:56-59.

266. Omura M, Torigoe S, Kubota N. SN-38, a metabolite of the camptothecin derivative CPT-11, potentiates the cytotoxic effect of radiation in human colon adenocarcinoma cells grown as spheroids. *Radiother Oncol* 1997;43:197-201.

CHAPTER 23

The Anal Region

Nora A. Janjan, Matthew T. Ballo, Marc E. Delclos, and Christopher H. Crane

Although anal cancer is relatively rare, innovations in its treatment have made it a model for the use of organ preservation and combined-modality therapy. Previously, abdominoperineal resection was the only therapeutic option for anal cancer; however, subsequent advances in radiation techniques and seminal studies combining chemotherapy and radiation have led to their use as definitive treatment for anal cancer, reserving surgery for recurrent or persistent disease. Functional outcome and quality of life are key components of anal cancer treatment. Although the total number of patients with anal cancer is small, innovations in the treatment of this disease have led to the establishment of therapeutic principles that have been applied in the treatment of nearly every type of cancer.

ANATOMY

The anatomy of the anal region is shown in Figure 23-1.[1] The anal canal is about 3 to 4 cm long. Tumors that arise around the anus are considered to be of different origin than those that arise in the anal canal, although the demarcation between the anal canal and the anal margin remains a matter of debate. According to one convention, tumors that arise above the pectinate line are considered tumors of the anal canal, and those located below that line are considered tumors of the anal margin. The pectinate or dentate line is a histologic transition zone between squamous and columnar epithelium at the level of the anal valves. The American Joint Commission on Cancer (AJCC) and the Union International Contre le Cancer (UICC) clinical staging guidelines recommend the use of a different definition of the anal canal, one in which the distal end of the anal canal is defined as the level at which the walls come in contact in their normal resting state,[2] at the level of the anorectal ring. The anorectal ring is the palpable muscle bundle formed by the upper portion of the internal sphincter, the deep or subcutaneous part of the external sphincter, the puborectalis muscle, and the distal longitudinal muscle from

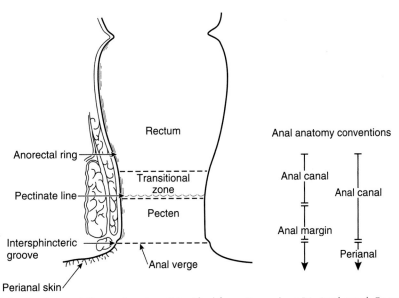

Fig. 23-1 Anatomy of the anal region. (Modified from Cummings BJ. Anal canal. From Perez CA, Brady LW, eds. *Principles and Practice of Radiation Oncology*, 3rd ed. Philadelphia, Pa: Lippincott-Raven; 1998:1511-1524.)

the large bowel.[1,3] In the AJCC system, perianal tumors are those located within a 5- to 6-cm radius from the anal verge in the buttock and perineal region, and those tumors are staged according to the system used for cancer of the skin.

With regard to dissemination, anal cancer can spread hematogenously, although local and lymphatic extension are more common. Blood is supplied to the area above the pectinate line by the superior and middle rectal arteries, which are branches of the inferior mesenteric and hypogastric arteries, respectively. Venous drainage is to the portal system.[3] Below the pectinate line, the arterial supply is to the middle and inferior rectal arteries, and venous drainage is to the inferior rectal vein.

Direct invasion into the sphincteric muscles and perianal connective tissue occurs early in the course of the disease, and about half of patients will present with tumor invasion of the rectum, perianal region, or both.[4,5] Extensive tumors can infiltrate the sacrum or the pelvic sidewalls. Extension to the vagina in women

is common, but invasion of the prostate gland in men is uncommon. Only 10% of patients are found to have distant metastases at the time of diagnosis. When distant metastases occur, they are most commonly found in the liver and lungs. However, local relapse is more common than the development of extrapelvic disease.

With regard to lymphatic drainage, tumors proximal to the pectinate line drain to the perirectal, external iliac, obturator, hypogastric, and para-aortic nodes. At abdominoperineal resection, about 30% of patients with tumors in the anal canal are found to have pelvic lymph node metastases and 16% have inguinal node metastases.[1,4] Tumors in the distal canal drain to the inguinal-femoral node region and the external and common iliac nodal regions. About 15% to 20% of patients have clinical evidence of inguinal lymph node involvement at presentation, and this involvement is usually unilateral.[6] Inguinal node metastases are evident in 30% of superficial and 63% of deeply infiltrating or poorly differentiated tumors.[7]

The inguinal nodes are located in an anatomic region bounded by defined landmarks. The most medial location for the inguinal lymph nodes is 3 cm from the symphysis pubis or midline; from there the inguinal nodes extend to the lateral aspect of the femoral head.[8] The most inferior location is 2.5 cm caudal to the inferior pubic ramus, and the most superior is the superior aspect of the femoral head (Fig. 23-2).

TOLERANCE TO RADIATION

As discussed throughout this chapter, radiation therapy, with or without chemotherapy, provides good tumor control, usually with preservation of anal sphincter function. Radiation has its complications, however,[9] some of which are severe enough to require surgical treatment.

The epithelial cells of the anal canal mucosae are highly radiosensitive; the stromal, vascular, and muscle cells, in contrast, are slow to respond but can give rise to extensive delayed postirradiation disease. Tolerance doses have not been established, in part because of the rarity of the disease. Complication rates after doses of 45 to 50 Gy of external-beam therapy, with a 10- to 12-Gy brachytherapy boost plus chemotherapy with 5-fluorouracil (5-FU) and mitomycin C, have ranged from 10% to nearly 30%.[10-12] Chemoradiation therapy can produce tumor control rates of 74% at 5 years and 71% at 10 years,[11,12] with sphincter control preserved in up to 85% of treated patients.[12] Late complications have included skin or soft tissue necrosis, anal stenosis, anorectal bleeding, diarrhea, bladder bleeding, leg edema, and injury to the small bowel.[9] Colostomies, temporary or permanent, have been necessary in 7% to 9% of irradiated patients, and abdominoperineal resections have been needed in about 3%.[10] Complications

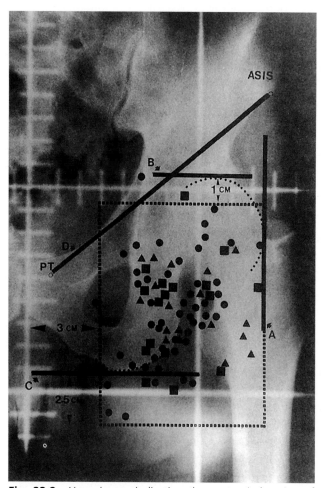

Fig. 23-2 X-ray image indicating the anatomic location of the inguinal nodes; 86% of the lymph nodes lie within the defined rectangle. *PT*, Pubic tubercle; *ASIS*, anterior superior iliac spine.

tend to be more common and severe in patients with higher-grade tumors given fractions of 2.0 Gy or more.[9,10]

Early postirradiation disease results from direct injury to the epithelial and endothelial cells. Delayed injury to fibroblasts and myofibroblasts can lead to stromal fibrosis and intimal vascular lesions. Vascular insufficiency, from both microvasculature injury and arterial and venous occlusive lesions, can contribute to the pathogenesis. Anal sphincter incompetence results from radiation injury to the smooth and striated muscle sphincter apparatus and perhaps from damage to neural controls as well.[9]

EPIDEMIOLOGY

Anal cancer is relatively rare, representing less than 2% of all types of cancer of the digestive tract. However, risk factors for anal cancer share some similarities with those for other types of cancer (Box 23-1), and thus anal cancer tends to be more common in groups that share those factors. For example, high rates of infection with human papillomavirus (HPV) have been observed in cases of cervical cancer, vulvar cancer, and anal cancer. Tissue specimens from more than 85% of patients with anal cancer have been found to contain HPV deoxyribonucleic acid (DNA).[3,13-15] Among women, a history of seropositivity for herpes simplex type 2 or *Chlamydia trachomatis* are associated with an increased risk of anal cancer. Homosexual and bisexual men are at an increased risk for HPV-induced squamous intraepithelial lesions and anal cancer.[16-19] Cost-effectiveness models have shown that screening homosexual and bisexual men every 2 to 3 years would provide life-expectancy benefits comparable to those of other screening procedures.[20]

Regardless of their sexual practices, individuals who are seropositive for the human immunodeficiency virus (HIV) are at increased risk of anal HPV infection. Virus-induced immunosuppression is considered to increase the risk of anal HPV infection and subsequent anal cancer[3,21]; indeed, an inverse relationship has been shown between CD4+ T-cell count and HPV infection.[19] Immunosuppression from other causes, such as organ transplantation, is also associated with a 100-fold increase in the risk of vulvar and anal cancer because of the high prevalence of HPV infection.[22,23] Unlike HPV or HIV infection, however, no direct relationship has been found between the acquired immune deficiency syndrome (AIDS) and the development of anal cancer.[18,24]

Cigarette smoking is strongly associated with both anal cancer and cervical cancer, raising the risk of anal cancer by a factor of 2 to 5.[21] A prior diagnosis of anal cancer also increases the risk of lung cancer by a factor of 2.5.[25-27]

No association has been found between anal cancer and inflammatory bowel disease. Among 9602 patients with Crohn's disease or ulcerative colitis who were followed for up to 18 years, only two cases of anal cancer were identified during 99,229 person-years of observation.[28] Other inflammatory conditions or trauma also have not been found to result in a higher incidence of anal cancer.[29]

PATHOLOGY

The rectum and the anus have separate embryonic origins, and thus different types of cells line the two structures. Glandular mucosa lines the rectum, and hence lieberkuhnian (glandular) adenocarcinoma predominates there; squamous cell mucosa lines the anal canal, and thus squamous epithelial carcinoma predominates in the anus.[30] Between the glandular mucosa of the rectum and the squamous mucosa of the anal region lies the transitional epithelium (see Fig. 23-1), which extends for about 6 to 20 mm and incorporates rectal, urothelial, and squamous elements. Another area of transitional epithelium exists between the squamous epithelium in the anal canal and the skin around the anus; this region, called the *pecten*,[1] is bordered superiorly by the pectinate line (see Fig. 23-1). On the inferior side of the pecten, the perianal region is lined by skin similar to that located elsewhere and contains apocrine glands.

Keratinizing squamous cell carcinoma is the most common type of anal cancer arising distal to the pectinate line; cancer that develops in the transition zone, between the squamous and columnar epithelium around the pectinate line, is usually nonkeratinizing squamous cell carcinoma and is often referred to as *cloacogenic cancer*.[1,3] Squamous cell carcinoma of either histologic type should be treated with definitive chemoradiation.[31] Other histologic types of anal cancer include adenocarcinoma and melanoma.

A National Cancer Data Base report[32] on carcinoma of the anus reflects the substantial improvement achieved in the treatment of anal cancer between 1988 and 1993. At both assessment times, the distribution of histologic

---

BOX 23-1   Risk Factors for Anal Cancer

STRONG SUPPORTING EVIDENCE
Human papillomavirus infection (anogenital warts)
History of receptive anal intercourse
History of sexually transmitted disease
More than 10 sexual partners
History of cervical, vulvar, or vaginal cancer
Immunosuppression after solid-organ transplantation

MODERATELY STRONG SUPPORTING EVIDENCE
Human immunodeficiency virus infection
Long-term use of corticosteroids
Cigarette smoking

subtypes was similar: approximately 75% squamous cell carcinomas and about 19% adenocarcinomas. Among patients with anal squamous cell cancer, 18% were treated with surgery alone in 1988 and 15% in 1993; chemoradiation was given as definitive treatment to 43% of patients in 1988 and 47% in 1993. Of the patients with adenocarcinoma, about 37% were treated with surgery alone at both evaluation times, and only about 8% were treated with definitive chemoradiation (Table 23-1).[32] The patterns of treatment failure among the patients surveyed in this report are shown in Table 23-2.[32] The rates of local and regional recurrence were twice as high for squamous cell tumors as for adenocarcinomas; however, the risk of distant metastasis was twice as high for adeno-

carcinoma as for squamous cell cancer. These findings suggest that more than 25% of patients with anal adenocarcinoma will develop distant metastases.[32]

In a review from the University of Minnesota of 192 cases of anal cancer (119 women and 73 men; median age 58 years),[33] squamous cell carcinoma accounted for 74%, adenocarcinoma for 19%, and melanoma for 4% of all tumors. The remaining 3% were neuroendocrine tumors (two cases), carcinoid (one case), Kaposi's sarcoma (one case), leiomyosarcoma (one case), and lymphoma (one case). In terms of T stage, 3% of patients had T1 disease, 46% had T2, 28% had T3, and 12% had T4 disease. The 5-year survival rates according to tumor histology were 57% for patients with

TABLE 23-1

National Cancer Data Base Comparison of Treatment Modalities for Anal Cancer

| | YEARS SURVEYED | | | |
| | 1988 | | 1993 | |
	Number of Cases	Percentage (%)	Number of Cases	Percentage (%)
ALL CASES				
Surgery only	252	24.0	258	20.0
Radiation therapy only	40	3.8	61	4.7
Chemotherapy only	22	2.1	11	0.9
Surgery and radiation therapy	104	9.9	64	5.0
Surgery and chemotherapy	17	1.6	14	1.1
Radiation and chemotherapy	357	34.0	511	39.6
Surgery, radiation, and chemotherapy	207	19.7	299	23.2
No treatment	34	3.3	52	4.0
Unknown	17	1.6	19	1.5
TOTAL	1050	100.0	1289	100.0
EPIDERMOID CARCINOMA				
Surgery only	141	18.1	157	15.4
Radiation therapy only	27	3.5	53	5.2
Chemotherapy only	18	2.3	9	0.9
Surgery and radiation therapy	48	6.2	44	4.3
Surgery and chemotherapy	12	1.5	4	0.4
Radiation and chemotherapy	336	43.1	483	47.4
Surgery, radiation, and chemotherapy	174	22.3	230	22.5
No treatment	15	1.9	25	2.5
Unknown	9	1.2	15	1.5
TOTAL	780	100.0	1020	100.0
ADENOCARCINOMA				
Surgery only	89	38.7	78	36.8
Radiation therapy only	13	5.7	8	3.8
Chemotherapy only	3	1.3	0	0.0
Surgery and radiation therapy	53	23.0	19	9.0
Surgery and chemotherapy	4	1.7	8	3.8
Radiation and chemotherapy	17	7.4	19	9.0
Surgery, radiation, and chemotherapy	30	13.0	59	27.8
No treatment	14	6.1	19	9.0
Unknown	7	3.0	2	0.9
TOTAL	230	100.0	212	100.0

From Myerson RJ, Karnell LH, Menck HR. *Cancer* 1997;80:805-815.

TABLE 23-2

Tumor Recurrences According to Histologic Type and Disease Stage

	TYPE OF RECURRENCE (%)*			No Recurrence (%)*	Never Disease-Free (%)*	Total (%)	Total Number of Cases
	Local	Regional	Distant				
All cases	9.2	6.4	16.4	48.7	19.3	100.0	347
Histology							
Epidermoid carcinoma	10.5	7.7	11.8	51.8	18.2	100.0	247
Adenocarcinoma	5.6	3.4	28.1	41.6	21.3	100.0	89
Stage†							
I	9.8	3.3	8.2	68.9	9.8	100.0	61
II	9.8	16.4	16.4	42.6	14.8	100.0	61
III	4.5	11.1	33.3	20.0	31.1	100.0	45
IV	3.2	0.0	16.1	42.0	38.7	100.0	31

From Myerson RJ, Karnell LH, Menck HR. *Cancer* 1997;80:805-815.

*Recurrence status was unknown for 703 cases, reducing the total number of cases from 1050 to 347.

†Pathologic stage, augmented by clinical stage when pathologic stage was not available.

squamous cell carcinoma, 63% for those with adenocarcinoma, and 33% for those with melanoma. The 5-year survival rates according to T stage were 62% for those with T1 disease, 57% for T2 disease, 45% for T3 disease, and 17% for T4 disease.[32] Although anal adenocarcinoma is generally considered to be more aggressive than squamous cell carcinoma, the outcome for the 36 patients with adenocarcinoma in the University of Minnesota series[33] was comparable to that for patients with squamous cell carcinoma. Of those patients, 22 (61%) underwent surgery and the other 14 (39%) underwent surgery and adjuvant chemoradiation. The 5-year survival rate was 63% and the recurrence rate was 21%, rates similar to those among patients with squamous cell carcinoma (who had been treated with either surgery or chemoradiation). Chemoradiation therapy also provided good local–regional control in another smaller study of anal adenocarcinoma at the Peter MacCallum Cancer Institute in Melbourne, Australia.[34] In that study, all six of the patients given chemoradiation or radiation therapy with curative intent achieved local–regional control; none of the nine patients treated with palliative intent survived the disease.

CLINICAL PRESENTATION

Bleeding and anal discomfort are the most common symptoms of anal cancer, occurring in about half of the patients with this disease. Other less common symptoms include the sensation of a mass in the anus, pruritis, and anal discharge.[1] Proximal tumors can cause obstructive symptoms, but distal tumors rarely do. Fewer than 5% of patients have sphincteric destruction resulting in fecal incontinence. Vaginal or other fistulas are uncommon.

In metastatic disease, metastases involve primarily the lymph nodes, liver, and lung. In one study of 19 cases of metastatic anal cancer,[35] six were considered synchronous and 13 metachronous. Nodal metastases involved the para-aortic nodes in five cases, the iliac region in four cases, and the inguinal nodes in two cases; nine of these cases involved solitary metastases. Metastases to the liver were documented in 10 cases (of which seven were solitary) and metastases to the lung in three cases. With local and systemic therapy, the median survival time was 35 months.[35]

STAGING

The AJCC staging system (Box 23-2)[2] is the most commonly used scheme for staging carcinomas of the anal canal. Like colorectal tumors, anal canal tumors are staged largely according to their size and local extension.[2,3] As noted earlier in this chapter, tumors that arise in the anal margin are staged according to the system used for skin cancer.

PROGNOSTIC FACTORS

Tumor size and state of differentiation and nodal status are the most significant prognostic factors in anal cancer. Among 132 patients who underwent abdominoperineal resection for anal cancer, the 5-year survival rates were 78% for those with 1- to 2-cm tumors, 55% for those with 3- to 5-cm tumors, and 40% for 6-cm or larger tumors.[7] The relationship between tumor size and survival rate also holds regardless of whether the treatment is radiation alone[10] or chemoradiation.[36,37] In another study, patients with poorly differentiated tumors had a 5-year survival rate of only 24% as compared with 75% for those with well-differentiated tumors.[38] The presence of nodal disease also influences survival, with another study showing 5-year survival rates of 44% among node-positive patients and 74% among node-negative patients.[7]

BOX 23-2   American Joint Committee on Cancer Staging System for Cancer of the Anal Canal

PRIMARY TUMOR (T)

TX	Primary tumor cannot be assessed
T0	No evidence of primary tumor
Tis	Carcinoma in situ
T1	Tumor 2 cm or less in greatest dimension
T2	Tumor more than 2 cm but not more than 5 cm in greatest dimension
T3	Tumor more than 5 cm in greatest dimension
T4	Tumor of any size that invades adjacent organ(s), e.g., vagina, urethra, bladder (involvement of the sphincter muscle[s] alone is not classified as T4)

REGIONAL LYMPH NODES (N)

NX	Regional lymph nodes cannot be assessed
N0	No regional lymph node metastasis
N1	Metastasis in perirectal lymph node(s)
N2	Metastasis in unilateral internal iliac and/or inguinal lymph node(s)
N3	Metastasis in perirectal and inguinal lymph nodes and/or bilateral internal iliac and/or inguinal lymph nodes

DISTANT METASTASIS (M)

MX	Distant metastasis cannot be assessed
M0	No distant metastasis
M1	Distant metastasis

STAGE GROUPING

Stage 0	Tis	N0	M0
Stage I	T1	N0	M0
Stage II	T2	N0	M0
	T3	N0	M0
Stage IIIA	T1	N1	M0
	T2	N1	M0
	T3	N1	M0
	T4	N0	M0
Stage IIIB	T4	N1	M0
	Any T	N2	M0
	Any T	N3	M0
Stage IV	Any T	Any N	M1

From Fleming I, Cooper JS, Henson DE, et al, eds. *AJCC Cancer Staging Manual.* 5th ed. Philadelphia, Pa: Lippincott Williams & Wilkins; 1997:91-95.

Disease stage at presentation is also predictive of outcome. Among patients with T1 or T2 disease, disease-free and colostomy-free survival rates were significantly better (87% and 94%, respectively) than those among patients who presented with T3 or T4 disease (59% disease-free survival and 73% colostomy-free survival). Patients who were node-negative at presentation also had significantly better cancer-related survival rates (85%, as compared with 58% among node-positive patients) and disease-free survival rates (80%, as compared with 53% among node-positive patients).[39]

Molecular Characteristics

Efforts are currently under way to assess possible associations between molecular characteristics and clinical outcome. Overexpression of *p53* was evaluated in terms of outcome among patients treated in trial 87-04 of the Radiation Therapy Oncology Group (RTOG), which prospectively randomized patients to receive radiation with 5-FU or radiation with 5-FU and mitomycin C. *p53* was overexpressed in 48% of the entire group. Although *p53* overexpression seemed to be associated with less favorable outcome, no statistical differences were found.[40] Specifically, local control rates were 52% among those whose tumors overexpressed *p53* and 72% among those with normal *p53* expression; the corresponding disease-free survival rates were 52% and 68%, and the corresponding overall survival rates were 58%

and 78%. Patients given combination therapy that included mitomycin C also had no differences in local control or survival rates according to *p53* expression. At present, the value of *p53* as a prognostic factor remains limited.

TUMORS OF THE ANAL CANAL
Combined-Modality Therapy

The superiority of radiation or chemoradiation treatment over surgery alone in terms of preserving anorectal function without sacrificing local control or survival has focused attention on combined-modality treatments for anal cancer. The use of radiation alone (to total doses of 60 to 65 Gy) has produced local control rates of about 70% and 5-year survival rates of about 60%.[36,41] However, these rates have varied considerably among studies, ranging from 56% to 100% for local control and from 50% to 94% for 5-year overall survival.[41,42]

Exploration of combined-modality therapy for anal cancer began in 1974, when Nigro and colleagues[43] gave three patients radiation in combination with 5-FU and mitomycin C before abdominoperineal resection. Pathologic examination of surgical specimens from two of these patients revealed complete response with no evidence of residual tumor; the third patient declined surgery and remained disease-free. Subsequent trials conducted by the United Kingdom Coordinating Committee for Cancer Research[44] and the European

TABLE 23-3

Randomized Phase III Trials of Radiation and Chemotherapy for Anal Cancer

Study Sponsors	Treatment Groups	Radiation Dose	Chemotherapy	Number of Eligible Patients	Colostomy-Free Survival Rates	Local Recurrence Rates	Overall Survival Rates
EORTC[45,46]	Radiation alone	45 Gy + 15-20 Gy boost if CR/PR	None	51	56%	42%	56% (all patients)
	Radiation + 5-FU + Mito C	45 Gy + 15-20 Gy boost if CR/PR	5-FU, 750 mg/m^2 on days 1-5 and 29-33; Mito C, 15 mg/m^2 on day 1	52	70% ($P = 0.002$)	31% ($P = 0.02$)	56% (all patients)
UKCCCR[44]	Radiation alone	45 Gy + 15-25 Gy boost if CR/PR	None	279	N/A	59%	58% (3-year)
	Radiation + 5-FU + Mito C	45 Gy + 15-25 Gy boost if CR/PR	5-FU, 1000 mg/m^2 on days 1-4 and 29-32 or 750 mg/m^2 on days 1-5 and 29-33 Mito C, 12 mg/m^2 on day 1	283	N/A	36% ($P < 0.0001$)	65% ($P = 0.25$) (3-year)
RTOG/ ECOG[47]	Radiation + 5-FU	45 Gy	5-FU, 1000 mg/m^2 on days 1-4 and 28-31	145	78%	NR	67%
	Radiation + 5-FU + Mito C	45 Gy	5-FU, 1000 mg/m^2 on days 1-4 and 28-31 Mito C 10 mg/m^2 on days 1 and 29	146	91% ($P = 0.002$) (4-year)	NR	76% ($P = 0.31$) (4-year)

Modified from Chawla AK, Willett CG. *Hematol Oncol Clin North Am* 2001;15:321-344.
EORTC, European Organization for research and Treatment of Cancer; *CR/PR*, complete response/partial response; *5-FU*, 5-fluorouracil; *Mito C*, mitomycin C; *UKCCCR*, United Kingdom Coordinating Committee for Cancer Research; *RTOG*, Radiation Therapy Oncology Group; *ECOG*, Eastern Cooperative Oncology Group; *NR*, not reported.

Organization for Research and Treatment of Cancer[45,46] have shown significant improvements from the addition of chemotherapy to irradiation in terms of primary-tumor control and colostomy-free survival rate but not in terms of overall survival rate (Table 23-3).[3,44-47] These trials are described in further detail in the following paragraphs.

Radiation Therapy vs. Chemoradiation with 5-Fluorouracil and Mitomycin C

In a trial conducted by the United Kingdom Coordinating Committee for Cancer Research,[44] 577 patients were randomized to receive radiation alone or combined-modality therapy. In all cases, the total radiation dose was 45 Gy, given in 20 to 25 fractions over 4 or 5 weeks. The combined-modality group was given radiation in combination with 5-FU (1000 mg/m^2 for 4 days

or 750 mg/m^2 for 5 days) and mitomycin C (12 mg/m^2 as an intravenous bolus injection) on the first day of each course of chemotherapy (see Table 23-3).[44] If the tumor had not regressed by at least 50% at 6 weeks after the completion of chemoradiation, then surgery or further irradiation (15 Gy given in six fractions to a perineal field or an interstitial implant of 25 Gy over 2 to 3 days) was considered. The local recurrence rates were 36% in the combined-modality group and 59% in the radiation-only group (see Table 23-3). Except for hematologic effects, which were more common in the combined-modality group, the side effects of treatment were comparable among the groups.

Another comparison of radiation alone versus chemoradiation by the European Organization for Research on the Treatment of Cancer[45,46] included 103 patients and was of similar design to the United Kingdom trial. Radiation was given to a total dose of 45 Gy over 5 weeks; chemotherapy included 5-FU (750 mg/m^2 for 5 days), given as a continuous infusion during the first and fifth weeks of radiation, and mitomycin C (15 mg/m^2), given as an intravenous bolus on the first day of each course of chemotherapy. After 6 weeks, a boost dose of radiation, either by external beam or interstitial techniques, was given depending on the level of the response; 15 Gy was given if the response was complete and 20 Gy was given if the response was partial. These studies that showed the benefit of combined-modality therapy over radiation alone are summarized in Table 23-3. Tumor regression rates were significantly higher for the combined-modality arm.[45,46] The colostomy-free survival rate at 5 years was 70% for combined-modality therapy and only 52% for the group treated with radiation alone (P = 0.002). As was true in the United Kingdom study, combined-modality treatment resulted in better local-control and colostomy-free survival rates but did not affect overall survival rate (see Table 23-3).

Chemoradiation Protocols with 5-Fluorouracil and Mitomycin C

Several other trials have shown combinations of radiation plus chemotherapy with 5-FU and mitomycin C to be effective in anal cancer. In one such study, the Eastern Cooperative Oncology Group (ECOG)[48] treated 50 patients with 40 Gy to the pelvis and a 10- to 13-Gy boost to the tumor; 5-FU and mitomycin C were given on days 1 and 28 of radiation. An abdominoperineal resection was performed if a biopsy conducted 6 to 8 weeks after the completion of the chemoradiation protocol showed signs of disease. This protocol produced a 74% complete response rate and a 24% partial response rate; the local control rate was 80% and the overall survival rate was 58%. However, this protocol was found to be highly toxic; 37% of patients experienced severe toxic effects, including life-threatening hematologic toxicity in 4%.

In another trial of chemoradiation,[49] the RTOG evaluated 79 patients who had been treated between 1983 and 1987. The radiation dose to the pelvis and perineum was 40.8 Gy (given in 24 fractions over 35 days), and chemotherapy again consisted of 5-FU (1000 mg/m^2/hr as a continuous intravenous infusion on days 2 through 5 and 28 through 31 of radiation) and mitomycin C (given as a bolus dose of 10 mg/m^2 on the first day of radiation). In that study, the colostomy-free survival rate was 90% and the local control and survival rates at 3 years were 71% and 73%. Acute toxic effects of the treatment included mild to moderate diarrhea in 67% of patients, skin reactions in 86%, moist desquamation in 19%, and neutropenia in 18% (severe in 3%). Late toxic effects were uncommon.

A group at Memorial Sloan-Kettering Cancer Center treated 42 patients with one cycle of 5-FU and mitomycin C and a 30-Gy dose of radiation.[50] This protocol produced

a 5-year survival rate of 82%; moreover, only half of the 18 patients in whom disease persisted after therapy had progressive disease.[50] The conclusion from this study was that evidence of disease at biopsy shortly after completing chemoradiation does not represent clinically viable tumor nor should it prompt an abdominoperineal resection.

Issues of toxicity and biopsy confirmation after combination chemotherapy were also addressed in a joint RTOG/ECOG study in which chemoradiation was prospectively compared with 5-FU alone or in combination with mitomycin C.[47] Radiation consisted of 45 Gy given in 25 fractions or 50.4 Gy given in 28 fractions over 5 weeks. In all cases, 5-FU (1000 mg/m^2) was given as a continuous infusion over 4 days on the first and fifth week of radiation. One group was given mitomycin C (10 mg/m^2) on the first day of each course of chemotherapy. Grade 4 or 5 toxic effects were experienced by 23% of the patients given combined-modality therapy, as compared with 7% of those given radiation alone. Mitomycin C was associated with more severe hematologic toxic effects, with fatal neutropenia occurring in 2% of cases. At 4 years of follow-up, the combination-chemotherapy group showed better colostomy rates (9% vs. 23%), colostomy-free survival rates (71% vs. 59%), and disease-free survival rates (73% vs. 51%) relative to the radiation-plus-5-FU–only group.[47] However, no difference was found in terms of overall survival between the two groups (see Table 23-3). These findings are consistent with the results of a subsequent retrospective review of 287 cases of anal cancer treated with radiation either alone or in combination with chemotherapy. In that review, the 5-year overall survival rate with combined-modality therapy was 78% and with radiation alone was 60%.[51]

Other aspects of the RTOG/ECOG study[47] that must be considered involved the timing of biopsies and the use of salvage therapy. Biopsies were required 6 weeks after the completion of the irradiation. Patients with positive biopsy findings (15% in the radiation-plus-5-FU–only group vs. 8% in the radiation-plus-combination-chemotherapy group) were given an additional 9 Gy of irradiation (in five fractions) with a 4-day infusion of 5-FU (1000 mg/m^2) and a single injection of cisplatin (100 mg/m^2). Of the 24 patients who underwent salvage therapy, 12 were rendered disease free. However, in light of the Memorial Sloan-Kettering findings,[50] it is unclear how many of these patients actually derived benefit from the additional chemoradiation. Moreover, repeated biopsies traumatize irradiated tissues, increasing the risk of infection and delayed wound healing.

Despite many trials having been conducted on the topic (Table 23-4),[5,43,49,52-56] the optimal radiation dose and schedule for radiation given in combination with 5-FU and mitomycin C remain unknown. Local

TABLE 23-4

Selected Studies of Mitomycin C and 5-Flourouracil for Anal Cancer

Study and Reference	5-FU*	Mitomycin C	Irradiation (Dose/Number of Fractions/ Time)	Primary Tumor Control		Serious Complications†	5-Year Survival Rate
Leichman et al, 1985[52]	1000 mg/m² 24 hr IVI D1-4, D29-32	15 mg/m² IVB D1	30 Gy/15/ D1-21	31/34 (91%) (≤ 5 cm)	7/10 (70%) (> 5 cm)	NS	80% (crude)
Sischy et al, 1989[49]	1000 mg/m² 24 hr IVI D2-5, D28-31	10 mg/m² IVB D1	40.8 Gy/24/ D1-35	22/26 (85%) (< 3 cm)	32/50 (85%) (≥ 3 cm)	2/79 (3%)	73% (3-year actuarial)
Cummings et al, 1991[42]	1000 mg/m² 24 hr IVI D1-4, D43-46	10 mg/m² IVB D1 and D43	48 Gy/24/ D1-58 (split course)	15/17 (88%) (≤ 5 cm)	13/16 (81%) (> 5 cm or T4)	1/33 (3%)	65% (actuarial)
Cummings et al, 1984,[5,42]	1000 mg/m² 24 hr IVI D1-4, D43-46	10 mg/m² IVB D1 and D43	50 Gy/20/ D1-56 (split course)	10/10 (≤ 5 cm)	3/4 (> 5 cm or T4)	5/14 (36%)	65% (actuarial)
Schneider et al, 1992[53]	1000 mg/m² 24 hr IVI D1-4, D29-32	10 mg/m² IVB D1 and D29	50 Gy/25-28/ D1-35± boost	21/22 (95%) (≤ 5 cm)	14/19 (74%) (> 5 cm or T4)	3/41 (7%)	77% (actuarial)
Tanum et al, 1991[54]	1000 mg/m² 24 hr IVI D1-4	10-15 mg/ m² IVB D1	50-54 Gy/ 25-27/ D1-35	28/30 (93%) (≤ 5 cm)	42/56 (75%) (> 5 cm or T4)	14/89 (16%)	72% (actuarial)
Cummings et al, 1984[5,42]	1000 mg/m² 24 hr IVI D1-4	10 mg/m² IVB D1	50 Gy/20/ D1-28	3/3 (≤ 5 cm)	11/13 (85%) (> 5 cm or T4)	10/16 (63%)	75% (actuarial)
Doci et al, 1996[55]	750 mg/m² 24 hr IVI (120 hr) D1-5, D43-47, D85-89	15 mg/m² IVB D1, D43, D85	54-60 Gy/ 30-33/D1-53 (split course)	28/38 (74%) (≤ 5 cm)	9/17 (53%) (> 5 cm)	2/56 (4%)	81% (actuarial)
Papillon et al, 1987[56]	600 mg/m² 24 hr IVI (120 hr) D1-5	12 mg/m² IVB D1	42 Gy/10/ D1-19 DPF + interstitial boost 20 Gy D78	—	57/70 (81%) (≥ 4 cm)	< 5%	NS

From Cummings BJ. Anal canal. In: Perez CW, Brady LW, eds. *Principles and Practice of Radiation Oncology*, 3rd ed. Philadelphia, Pa: Lippincott-Raven; 1998:1511-1524.
IVI, Continuous intravenous infusion; *IVB*, intravenous bolus injection; *NS*, not stated; *T4*, invading adjacent organs; *DPF*, direct perineal field (all other series used pelvic fields tangential to perineum).
*All infusions were for 96 hours except where shown.
†Serious complications required surgery or were grade 3 or greater.

control rates have ranged between 70% and 95%, and the incidence of treatment-related complications leading to colostomy have ranged from 5% to 10%. For treating tumors up to about 3 cm in size, schedules that give 30 Gy in 15 fractions over 3 weeks or 40.8 Gy in 24 fractions over 5 weeks have shown excellent control rates.[1,49,52] Higher radiation doses are used to treat larger tumors, and generally produce local control rates exceeding 75%.[5,42,49,52-56] The total doses to the pelvis range from 40 to 45 Gy and are given over 5 weeks; additional localized boosts to the area of gross tumor involvement typically bring the total dose to 50 to 65 Gy.

In contrast to the variations in radiation scheduling, the schedule for administering 5-FU and mitomycin C has tended to be more consistent among the trials (see Table 23-4).

Other Drug Combinations

Concerns over the hematologic toxicity of mitomycin C and its long-term effects on the lungs, kidneys, and bone marrow have led to the use of cisplatin with 5-FU for the treatment of anal cancer (Table 23-5).[55,57-63] This combination has been shown to yield complete response rates of 90% to 95% and colostomy-free survival rates of 86% at 3 years.[55,59,60] Moreover, the toxic effects of cisplatin and 5-FU, particularly on the hematologic system, seem to be more limited. For example, early results from the E4292 trial of the ECOG[59] indicated that use of bolus cisplatin with 5-FU led to nine cases of grade 3 leukopenia, one case of grade 3 anemia, one case of grade 4 thrombocytopenia, and no cases of grade 5 hematologic toxicity.[59] In similar studies at the Istituto Nazionale Tumori in Milan[55] and The University of Texas M.D. Anderson Cancer Center,[64] no cases of grade 3 or greater hematologic toxicity were reported, regardless of whether the cisplatin was given as a bolus[55] or an infusion.[64]

A variety of chemotherapeutic schedules involving 5-FU and cisplatin have been explored, including the use of concurrent chemotherapy, induction chemotherapy, and alternating chemotherapy–radiation therapy protocols. In general, the local-control rates in studies of concurrent chemoradiation therapy have been comparable with those in studies of radiation with 5-FU and mitomycin C.

Induction chemotherapy followed by external-beam radiation therapy has been evaluated for toxicity and effectiveness in anal cancer. In one such study conducted in Sweden,[65] induction chemotherapy consisting of carboplatin (300 to 375 mg/m^2, given on days 1, 29, and 57) and 5-FU (given as a 120-hour infusion of 1000 mg/m^2/day on days 1 through 5, 29, and 57), followed by radiation, produced a complete response in 29 of 31 patients.[65] At 5 years, the overall survival rate in this study was 67%, the local control rate was 80%, and the sphincter preservation rate was 69%. Use of bleomycin with radiation by the Swedish National Care Programme for Anal Cancer had no better effect on outcome than did radiation alone.[66] In that study, perineal tumors responded better (5-year survival rate, 90%) than did tumors of the anal canal (5-year survival rate of 68%); however, the 5-year colostomy-free survival rate was only 58%.[66]

Treatment of Patients with Human Immunodeficiency Virus

Tolerance of therapy is a significant consideration among patients with HIV and invasive anal cancer. Excessive mucosal reactions from radiation and significant cytopenia have been reported during treatment, especially when the CD4 count is less than 200 cells per microliter.[67-69] One group reported that a 100% complete response rate with acceptable toxic effects could be achieved for patients with HIV by giving lower doses of radiation (e.g., 30 Gy in 15 fractions) and mitomycin C (e.g., 10 mg/m^2) in combination with standard doses of 5-FU.[69] Another group[70] gave concomitant 5-FU and mitomycin C with radical pelvic radiation to 12 men with HIV (mean CD4 count, 209 cells per microliter, range, 29 to 380). Radiation doses ranged from 38 Gy given in 20 fractions to 51 Gy given in 30 fractions, and most patients underwent a perineal boost of 10 to 18 Gy. The initial complete remission rate was high (nine patients), but two patients experienced relapse within 6 months of diagnosis, and at a median follow-up of almost 5 years, four patients had died (two from anal cancer, one from an opportunistic infection, and one from treatment-related complications).[70] Moreover, grade 3 skin reaction was evident in one case, grade 3 hematologic complications in three, and one case of grade 4 and one case of grade 5 gastrointestinal complications. The actuarial 2-year survival rate was 60%.[70]

Summary

The toxicity of therapy can be profound in anal cancer; however, the consequence of local failure (or colostomy) is also profound. Local control of anal-canal tumors is necessary for three reasons: (1) to eliminate the life-threatening complications of the disease, (2) to decrease the risk of distant metastases, and (3) to preserve sphincter function.[71] Although radiation is effective in achieving local tumor control, the radiation-sensitizing effects of chemotherapy can substantially improve local control rates and reduce the need for aggressive surgical procedures. Although radiation administered with 5-FU and mitomycin C represents the current standard of care, questions remain regarding the optimal chemotherapy agents and schedule and also the radiation dose and schedule for treating anal cancer. With regard to radiation, the total dose necessary to achieve local control probably depends on the clonogenic burden. As for chemotherapy agents, the use of 5-FU alone clearly is not as effective as it is in combination chemotherapeutic regimens; however, it remains unclear whether the addition of mitomycin C to 5-FU has any advantage over the use of cisplatin with 5-FU. Attempts to clarify this issue must consider the toxicity of chemotherapy in addition to local control rates.

TUMORS OF THE ANAL MARGIN

The anal margin, considered by some to be anatomically distinct from the anal canal, involves the anal

TABLE 23-5

Trials of 5-Flourouracil and Cisplatin with Radiation for Anal Cancer

Study and Reference	CHEMOTHERAPY		PRIMARY TUMOR Radiation Therapy (Dose/Number of Fractions/Time)	COMPLETE RESPONSE Rates/Total Number of Patients (%)	Survival Rates
	5-FU	Cisplatin			
CONCURRENT THERAPY					
Wagner et al, 1994[58]	1000 mg/m^2/ 24 hr IVI (96 hr) D1-4	25 mg/m^2 IVB D2-5	42 Gy/10/ D1-19 + interstitial boost D63-64	47/51 (92%)	Approximately 75% (5-year)
Martenson et al, 1996[59]	1000 mg/m^2/ 24 hr IVI (96 h) D43-46	75 mg/m^2 IVB D1, D43	59.4 Gy/33/ D1-59 (split after 36 Gy)	14/17 (82%)	Not stated
Rich et al, 1993[60]	300 mg/m^2/ 24 hr IVI 5 days (120 hr)/wk D1-42	4 mg/m^2 IVI D1-42, 5 days/wk	45-54 Gy/ 25-30/ D1-42	20/21 (95%)	91% (2-year actuarial)
INDUCTION THERAPY					
Brunet et al, 1990[61]	1000 mg/m^2/ 24 hr IVI (120 hr) D2-6; repeat cycles D22, D43	100 mg/m^2 IVB D1, D22, D43	45 Gy/25/ D64-69+ boost	17/19 (89%)	No cancer deaths, 10-40 months
Svensson et al, 1993[62]	1000 mg/m^2/ 24 hr IVI (120 hr) D1-5; repeat cycles D29, D57	Carboplatin 300-350 mg/m^2 IVB D1, D29, D57	66 Gy/33/ D79-125	6/6 (100%)	No recurrences 8-21 months
ALTERNATING THERAPY					
Roca et al, 1990[63]	750 mg/m^2/ 24 hr IVI (120 hr) D2-7, D23-28	50 mg/m^2 IVB D1-2, D22-23	20 Gy/10/ D8-21, D29-42 + boost	18/25 (72%)	87% (5-year actuarial)

From Cummings BJ. Anal canal. In: Perez CW, Brady, LW, eds. *Principles and Practice of Radiation Oncology.* 3rd ed. Philadelphia, Pa: Lippincott-Raven; 1998:1511-1524.

5-FU, 5-Fluorouracil; *IVI,* continuous intravenous infusion; *IVB,* intravenous bolus injection.

verge and includes the perianal tissues around the anal canal. Squamous cell carcinomas in this region are staged like other tumors of the skin and generally have a good prognosis.[3] Most are well-differentiated and keratinized. Visceral metastases are rare, and inguinal-node metastases are uncommon. Disease management depends on tumor location and extent and patient factors.

Anal margin tumors can be treated by local excision or radiation; abdominoperineal resection should be reserved for patients in whom fecal incontinence is present at diagnosis or for those with locally recurrent disease. Local excision is sufficient for T1 lesions, but pelvic and inguinal-node irradiation is indicated for T2 lesions. Chemotherapy should be included with radiation for T3 and T4 tumors.[12,72]

RADIATION THERAPY TECHNIQUES

Radiation therapy approaches for anal cancer vary among centers, but some basic principles are common to all reported techniques. First, a dose-response relationship based on clonogenic burden has been demonstrated.[31,73] Second, computed tomography (CT)–based treatment planning is imperative, particularly given the presence of significant anatomic variation in the depth of the inguinal nodes. These principles are discussed in further detail in the following paragraphs.

As noted in the previous section on "Combined-Modality Therapy," larger tumor volumes should be treated with higher total doses of radiation. Tumors smaller than 3 cm can be treated with total radiation doses of 30 Gy (given in 15 fractions) to 40.8 Gy (given in 24 fractions).[1] Tumors larger than about 3 cm should be treated with 40 to 45 Gy to the pelvis with a localized boost that raises the dose to the gross tumor volume to between 50 and 65 Gy.[1] Potential improvements in local control rates and disease-free and overall survival rates from increasing the dose of radiation[31,73] must be balanced against the increased risk of toxic effects from higher radiation doses. Reductions in treatment portals and adjustments in dose over the course of the irradiation have also been explored[59] and offer indirect evidence of a dose-response relationship. Generally, the initial radiation fields used in primary treatment of anal canal cancer include the primary tumor, with an adequate margin, and the regional lymph nodes (Fig. 23-3, A). Then, after 30 Gy is given (in conventional fractions), the superior border of the radiation volume is shifted down from the L5-S1 interspace to the inferior aspect of the sacroiliac joint (see Fig. 23-3, B). The fields are reduced a third time to cover the anterior fields so that uninvolved inguinal nodes would receive a total radiation dose of 36 Gy (see Fig. 23-3, C).

Experience from the M.D. Anderson Cancer Center suggests that 30 Gy, given in conventional fractionation schedules, may be sufficient to control microscopic disease.[74,75] In the authors' experience, the local failure rate

for patients with clinically uninvolved inguinal nodes given this dose is less than 5%.[74,75] Another group at Memorial Sloan-Kettering also achieved excellent local control rates when 30 to 34 Gy was given after gross tumor removal by excisional biopsy.[76]

On the basis of the existing evidence and in an attempt to minimize treatment-related toxicity, the irradiation technique used at the M.D. Anderson Cancer Center involves first administering 30.6 Gy, in 1.8-Gy fractions, through anteroposterior-posteroanterior portals that include the inguinal region (Fig. 23-4).[60] The patient is placed in the prone position so as to displace the small bowel superiorly by compression of the abdominal cavity. After that, a 3-field technique, including the use of a "belly board," is used to deliver an additional 19.8 Gy to the pelvis. The treatment portals are weighted (posteroanterior 2:right lateral 1:left lateral 1), and the radiation dose is prescribed to the 95% isodose curve (Fig. 23-5). The fields are then reduced so that the superior border of the radiation portal is now at the inferior aspect of the sacroiliac joints (see Fig. 23-3, A [dashed line]). A supplemental boost to a total dose of 55 Gy is given to clinically involved inguinal nodes. The electron energy is selected from CT-based treatment plans. The contribution to the inguinal region when the three-field belly-board technique is used is usually 5 to 7 Gy, and conventional fractionation (1.8 to 2 Gy) is used for the electron-beam radiation that is directed to the inguinal region. A localized boost to the primary tumor (4.6 Gy, given in two fractions) is then administered with the three-field technique. Typical simulation films are shown in Figure 23-6. A total dose of 30 Gy is given to the volume between L5-S1 interspace and the inferior aspect of the sacroiliac joints and to the inguinal region in patients without gross adenopathy. A more limited field to the pelvis receives 50.4 Gy and the primary tumor and involved inguinal nodes receive 55 Gy. Cisplatin (4 mg/m^2/day) and 5-FU (250 mg/m^2/day) are given as a continuous infusion, 5 days each week throughout the radiation course.

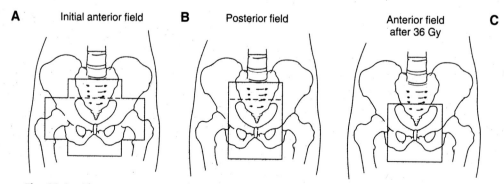

A   Initial anterior field   **B**   Posterior field   Anterior field after 36 Gy   **C**

Fig. 23-3 The treatment portals used for high-dose radiation therapy in the Radiation Therapy Oncology Group trials. (Modified from Martenson JA, Lipsitz SR, Wagner H, et al. *Int J Radiat Oncol Biol Phys* 1996;35:745-749.)

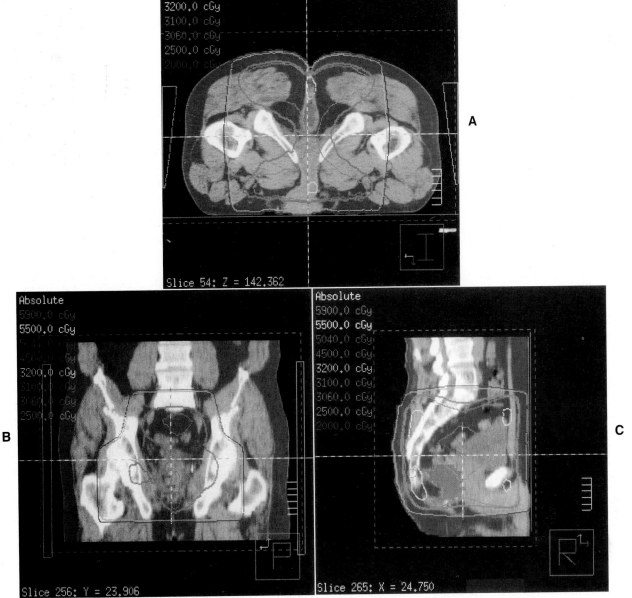

Fig. 23-4 In this technique, which is used at the M.D. Anderson Cancer Center, the initial 30.6 Gy is administered via anteroposterior-posteroanterior portals **(A)** while the patient is prone; these fields include the inguinal regions. The radiation dose to the bladder and bowel is higher if the belly board technique is not used after 30.6 Gy **(B** and **C)**.

Balancing Efficacy with Toxicity: Dose-Time Considerations

The timing of radiation delivery, in addition to total dose, significantly affects the response to therapy for anal cancer. Higher radiation doses given in an uninterrupted course are considered necessary to improve local control rates, but concern exists about treatment-related toxic effects.[5,42,77] Results of sequential studies are shown in Table 23-4. In early RTOG protocols involving the use of 5-FU, mitomycin C, and a 59.4-Gy radiation dose, instituting a planned 2-week treatment interruption after

36 Gy of radiation had been administered, produced toxic effects similar to those of previous protocols but led to unacceptably high rates (23%) of local failure and colostomy.[77] When the planned 2-week interruption was eliminated, the local failure rate dropped to 11%, but the appearance of toxic reactions mandated treatment interruptions (median duration, 11 days) for half of the patients so treated. Investigators at the Princess Margaret Hospital in Toronto reported a similar experience. Early protocols in which radiation (50 Gy in 20 fractions without interruption) was given with 5-FU and mitomycin C

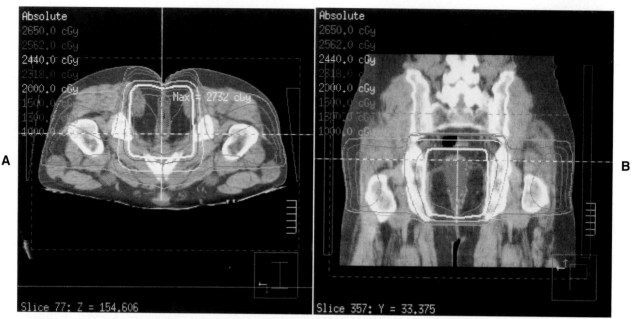

Fig. 23-5 **A** and **B,** In the technique used at the M.D. Anderson Cancer Center, an additional 19.8 Gy is given to the pelvis, for a total dose of 50.4 Gy, in a three-field approach that includes a belly board to displace the small bowel. The boost volume to the primary tumor is 4.6 Gy, given in two fractions.

produced good local-control rates but also produced high rates of acute and late toxicity.[5] Reduction of the dose per fraction to 2 Gy and splitting the course of therapy significantly decreased treatment-related toxic effects without appearing to affect local control rates.[42] An attempt to minimize hematologic complications by omitting mitomycin C from the chemotherapy was successful in that regard but compromised local-control rates.[42] Another study of time-dose considerations[73] verified that local-control rates were improved when radiation doses were 54 Gy or more and when overall treatment time was less than 40 days.[73] Multivariate analyses in that study showed that radiation dose and hemoglobin level independently influenced local control; that radiation dose influenced disease-free survival; and that radiation dose, hemoglobin level, T stage, and HIV status all influenced overall survival.[73] Therefore outcomes depend on optimizing the radiation dose and chemotherapy regimen and minimizing the treatment-related toxicity.

Toxicity in the Elderly

Special concerns exist about treatment-related toxic effects among the elderly. In a Swiss study[78] of patients age 75 years or more, 21 were given radiation therapy and 21 were given radiation therapy with chemotherapy. The total dose of radiation to the pelvis equaled 39.6 Gy; after a median treatment interruption of 43 days, a boost dose (median, 20 Gy) was given by

brachytherapy or perineal external-beam therapy. Chemotherapy consisted of mitomycin C (9.5 mg/m^2) and a 96-hour infusion of 5-FU (600 mg/m^2/day). Of the 40 patients able to complete therapy (95%), acute toxic effects led to reduction in the total radiation dose administered to two patients (one in the radiation-only group and one in the chemoradiation group) and led to interruptions in treatment for 11 patients (four in the radiation-only group and seven in the chemoradiation group). Grade 3 toxic effects were noted in 54% of patients (32% in the radiation-only group and 68% in the chemoradiation group). Among the chemoradiation group, grade 2 to 3 effects were leukopenia (observed in 25% of patients) and fatigue (58% of patients). At 5 years, the overall survival rate was 54% (49% for the radiation group and 59% for the chemoradiation group) and the actuarial local control rate was 79% (73% for the radiation group and 83% for the chemoradiation group). The authors of this study emphasized that particular attention be paid to acute reactions so as to avoid treatment interruptions.[78]

External-Beam Radiation Therapy with an Interstitial Implant

Other attempts to reduce treatment-related morbidity have included the use of lower-dose external-beam radiation therapy with interstitial [192]I implants. One report of such an approach[79] involved giving 40 Gy by

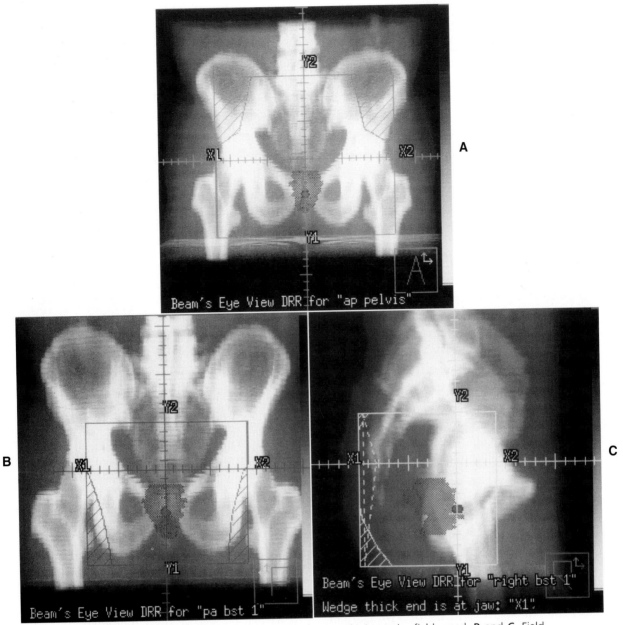

Fig. 23-6 Radiation treatment portals. **A,** The anterior/posterior fields used. **B** and **C,** Field reductions used with the three-field belly board technique. The superior border of the field now is at the inferior aspect of the sacroiliac joint. **C,** Lateral fields used during the belly board technique.   *Continued*

external-beam therapy plus 20 Gy by means of an implant to 69 patients; 45 of these patients were also given 5-FU and mitomycin C. This approach resulted in a complete response rate of 81% despite relatively low actuarial local control rates at 2 years (65%) and 5 years (59%).[79] However, the colostomy-free survival rates were 61% at 2 years, 47% at 5 years, and 37% at 10 years.

External-beam radiation therapy administered with 5-FU and cisplatin and an interstitial implant also has

been effective. In a long-term study conducted in France,[80] this strategy resulted in colostomy-free survival rates of 71% at 5 years and 67% at 8 years; the corresponding overall response rates were 84% and 77%. Among the 78 patients whose sphincters were preserved surgically, sphincter function was judged excellent or good in 72 (92%).[80] Careful assessment of pararectal lymph node involvement at staging is imperative; the 5-year overall survival rate in the French study was 76% among node-positive patients as compared

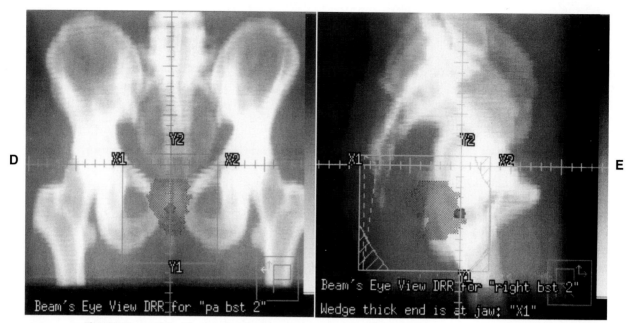

Fig. 23-6, cont'd   The last 4.6 Gy (given in two fractions) are given to a localized boost field using posteroanterior (**D**) and lateral (**E**) fields.

with 88% among node-negative patients.[80] Results from a German study suggest that the success rate of interstitial implants can be further improved by using sonography for three-dimensional tumor reconstruction and brachytherapy simulation.[81]

Results of a retrospective review at the Beatson Oncology Centre in Glasgow, Scotland show that external-beam radiation used with interstitial implants but without chemotherapy can achieve excellent local control for small tumors (100% for T1 tumors and 90% for T2 tumors).[82] In that study, the dose of external-beam radiation was 40 to 50 Gy, given at 2 Gy per fraction, and about 25 Gy was administered through the implant.[82] Citing an increased risk for acute toxicity and a 1% to 2% incidence of chemotherapy-related death from the use of 5-FU and mitomycin C, Mitchell and colleagues at the University of Florida also advocate the use of radiation alone for T1 and T2 tumors.[83]

MEDICAL MANAGEMENT OF TREATMENT-RELATED TOXIC EFFECTS

Expert medical management and an aggressive approach are needed to control the side effects of chemoradiation for anal cancer. Adverse effects that can be prevented and treated include those on the skin (desquamation), blood counts, fluid and electrolyte levels, pain, nutritional status, and fatigue. Supportive care measures can help prevent treatment interruption and thereby improve therapeutic outcome;

however, aggressive supportive care is required during and after the completion of therapy regardless of whether that therapy is given in a continuous or interrupted protocol.

With attentive medical management, fewer than 5% of patients at the M.D. Anderson Cancer Center have needed treatment interruption because of adverse effects.[64] At the first signs of dry desquamation, which generally occur during the end of the second week of radiation, emollient ointments such as Aquaphor (Beiersdorf AG) should be used in the inguinal region, and barrier creams (e.g., Lantiseptic's Skin Protectant; Marietta, Ga.) should be used in the perianal region. The barrier cream is especially important for preventing secondary infection from fecal bacteria. Moist desquamation often occurs in the intergluteal region and along the inguinal folds. Products that act as a skin, like the hydrogel sheet dressing from Vigilon (Bard, Murray Hill, N.J.), can be placed over the area to prevent secondary infection and trauma and to provide a soothing, protective dressing. Secondary infections, especially those from candida, can occur and must be treated. Difficulties with hygiene can be addressed by using sitz baths with Domeboro (Bayer Corporation, Pittsburgh, Pa.), an aluminum acetate solution; such products should also be used to clean and soak the inguinal region. Pain during urination from the contact of the acidic urine with the skin can be minimized by using barrier creams and spraying warm water over the perineum during urination.

Significant pain from perianal and inguinal skin reactions can manifest during urination, defecation, and movement. Opioid analgesics can be helpful in controlling both pain and, through their constipating effect, the frequent stooling often experienced as a result of pelvic irradiation and chemotherapy.

Bowel management programs have been established to address frequent stooling and pain associated with treatment for colorectal or anal cancer. The three-step program used at the M.D. Anderson Cancer Center involves the use of antidiarrheal agents such as diphenoxylate with atropine (Lomotil) or loperamide hydrochloride (Imodium) and opioid analgesics. The goal of this program (described in further detail in Chapter 22) is to maintain the number of stools produced at no more than three per day so as to avoid fluid and electrolyte imbalances and reduce trauma and possible infection in the perianal region.[84,85] Initial symptoms, which usually occur in the third week of therapy, are treated with antidiarrheal agents as needed. When that need reaches three times per day, the agents are then given according to a schedule (one to two tablets three or four times a day). If symptoms persist, opioid analgesics are given; a long-acting preparation is preferred, both for the convenience of the patient and for avoiding episodic diarrhea. Pain-management principles dictate that the analgesics be titrated to effect and that short-acting analgesics be made available until the appropriate dose of long-acting analgesic is identified. In general, the use of analgesics that contain acetaminophen should be avoided in patients undergoing chemotherapy; not only must the dose of such agents be limited to avoid potential toxicity to the kidneys and liver, but their antipyretic properties could mask the presence of an infection.

Blood counts and perhaps cytokine levels should be closely monitored, especially if mitomycin C is given, to avoid the need to interrupt treatment because of toxic effects. Administration of cisplatin also warrants close monitoring of magnesium levels; in the event of magnesium wasting, supplemental magnesium is required. The profound fatigue occasionally experienced during chemoradiation can also contribute to poor oral intake and thus lead to nutritional and electrolytic imbalance. Fatigue can improve with correction of anemia, fluid, and nutritional status.

Close follow-up is necessary after treatment until re-epithelialization of the anal region is complete. During this time, symptoms, evidence of infection, blood counts, and fluid and electrolyte status must be evaluated and treated as necessary. Response to therapy can also be monitored during this time, but biopsy of a residual abnormality is discouraged when tumor regression remains evident. Fatigue can be present for several months after completion of therapy; treatable causes such as anemia and hypothyroidism should be sought, treated, or ruled out as appropriate. Long-term bowel-management strategies, especially the scheduled use of antidiarrheal agents and fluid management, should be pursued to optimize bowel control and improve quality of life.

Excellent functional outcomes can be achieved after definitive chemoradiation therapy, particularly among patients who had limited symptoms at presentation and are rendered free of disease. In a long-term study in Geneva,[86] quality of life was assessed, in terms of symptoms and functioning, among 41 disease-free patients (35 women and six men with a median age of 71 years) who had completed treatment for anal cancer at least 3 years before. The median follow-up time was 116 months. In terms of function (the best score being 100), the global quality of life rating was 71, the role-function score was 85, and the body image score was 74. As for symptoms (the best score being 0), the scores were 28 for persistent diarrhea and 66 for sexual dysfunction among men. Patients who presented with anal dysfunction resulting from extensive tumor involvement had poorer scores and poorer outcomes in general.[86]

Types of long-term morbidity related to the use of chemoradiation therapy for anal cancer in a study of 34 patients is illustrated in Table 23-6.[87] In that study, only four patients (12%) experienced treatment toxicity of grade 3 or 4[87]; no long-term sequelae were identified

TABLE 23-6

Incidence of Late Toxic Effects in 34 Patients with Anal Cancer After Chemoradiation*

Site of Toxic Effect	Grade 0	Grade 1	Grade 2	Grade 3	Grade 4
Small or large bowel	17 (50%)	9 (26%)	7 (20%)	1 (3%)	0
Skin	24 (70%)	4 (12%)	3 (9%)	1 (3%)	2 (6%)
Anal canal	18 (53%)	5 (15%)	10 (29%)	1 (3%)	0
Worst cytotoxicity (per patient)	10 (29%)	10 (29%)	10 (29%)	2 (6%)	2 (6%)

From John M, Flam M, Palma N. *Int J Radiat Oncol Biol Phys* 1996;34:65-69.
*Late was defined as an effect occurring more than 90 days after treatment was begun; all incidents were included, even those that were transient and resolved spontaneously.

in 29%, and 58% experienced either grade 1 or 2 effects. Authors of a study of anorectal dysfunction after pelvic irradiation for cervical cancer attributed the late proctitis to sensory and motor abnormalities caused by the irradiation.[88]

SURGERY AS SALVAGE TREATMENT

Abdominoperineal resection remains essential as a salvage treatment for recurrent anal cancer. About half of patients with isolated disease recurrence can be rendered disease-free after this procedure, as demonstrated in a subset of 42 patients who developed local recurrence among 185 consecutive cases of anal cancer.[89] Of these 42 patients, 27 had only local failure and the other 15 had regional or distant disease in addition to local failure. Supportive care was given to 16 patients (38%) and curative resection was undertaken in 26 patients (local excision in three and abdominoperineal resection in 23). At a median follow-up of about 22 months, all 11 patients given supportive care had died, and 11 of the 26 patients that had undergone resection were free of disease. The survival rate for the entire group after the diagnosis of local failure was 28% but that for the resected group was nearly 45%.[89]

In another series,[33] outcome among 192 patients was evaluated in terms of primary tumor histology, primary therapy, and salvage surgery. Among the 143 cases of squamous cell cancer, an abdominoperineal resection was performed as the primary therapy in 21 cases; at 5 years, the survival rate in this subgroup was 60% and the recurrence rate was 23%.[33] Among the 122 patients undergoing chemoradiation as the definitive treatment, the 5-year survival and recurrence rates were 55% and 34%. Forty-two patients experienced recurrent disease after chemoradiation; 13 underwent salvage surgery, and eight (62%) of them were alive at a mean follow-up of 32 months.

Another group evaluated outcome after abdominoperineal resection as salvage treatment for residual disease (21 patients, 11 of whom had evidence of disease on biopsy within 6 months of completing chemoradiation) or recurrent disease (10 patients, in all of whom recurrence appeared more than 6 months after completing therapy [mean, 15 months, range, 9 to 41 months]).[90] No patient had evidence of nodal or distant metastases at diagnosis or at abdominoperineal resection, although lymph node metastases were found at pathologic evaluation in two cases. Of the 11 patients who lived, nine were disease-free at a mean follow-up of 40 months. The overall survival rate at 3 years after salvage treatment was 58%. Overall survival rates at 3 years for patients with residual disease was 72% versus 29% for those with recurrent disease; at 5 years the corresponding survival rates for these groups were 60% and 0% ($P = 0.06$).[90]

SUMMARY

Significant advances have been made in the treatment of anal cancer. Anal sphincter function can be preserved in most patients through the use of chemoradiation as definitive treatment. Close clinical follow-up is imperative for supportive care and assessment of response. Salvage surgery should not be pursued unless clinical evidence of disease progression is shown. Routine biopsies are discouraged, because positive findings on biopsy after chemoradiation in the absence of clinical evidence of disease progression are not predictive of persistent disease.

A dose-response relationship has been observed for radiation and chemotherapy. However, treatment-related toxic effects can be significant, and toxic effects that mandate interruptions in treatment can compromise local control. Aggressive supportive care and clinical strategies that further reduce treatment-related toxic effects are necessary for further therapeutic advances. Strategies are under investigation to minimize toxic effects and improve rates of local control. These strategies include the development of therapeutic approaches that are specific for tumor stage and optimize the effectiveness of chemoradiation therapy.

REFERENCES

1. Cummings BJ. Anal canal. In: Perez CW, Brady, LW, eds. *Principles and Practice of Radiation Oncology*, 3rd ed. Philadelphia, Pa: Lippincott-Raven; 1998:1511-1524.
2. Fleming I, Cooper JS, Henson DE, et al, eds. *AJCC Cancer Staging Manual*. 5th ed. Philadelphia, Pa: Lippincott Williams & Wilkins; 1997:91-95.
3. Chawla AK, Willett CG. Squamous cell carcinoma of the anal canal and anal margin. *Hematol Oncol Clin North Am* 2001;15:321-344.
4. Boman BM, Moertel CG, O'Connell MJ, et al. Carcinoma of the anal canal. A clinical and pathological study of 188 cases. *Cancer* 1984;54:114-125.
5. Cummings BJ, Keane TJ, Thomas GM, et al. Results and toxicity of the treatment of anal canal carcinoma by radiation therapy or radiation therapy and chemotherapy. *Cancer* 1984;54:2062-2068.
6. Stearns MW Jr, Urmacher C, Sternberg SS, et al. Cancer of the anal canal. *Curr Probl Cancer* 1980;4:1-44.
7. Frost DB, Richards PC, Montague ED, et al. Epidermoid cancer of the anorectum. *Cancer* 1984;53:1285-1293.
8. Wang CJ, Chin YY, Leung SW, et al. Topographic distribution of inguinal lymph nodes metastasis: significance in determination of treatment margin for elective inguinal lymph nodes irradiation of low pelvic tumors. *Int J Radiat Oncol Biol Phys* 1996;35:133-136.
9. Fajardo LF, Berthrong M, Anderson RE. Large intestine and anal canal. In: *Radiation Pathology*. New York, NY: Oxford University Press; 2001:239-247.
10. Touboul E, Schlienger M, Buffat L, et al. Epidermoid carcinoma of the anal canal. Results of curative intent radiation therapy in a series of 270 patients. *Cancer* 1994;173:1569-1579.
11. Martenson JA Jr, Gunderson LL. External radiation therapy without chemotherapy in the management of anal cancer. *Cancer* 1993;71;1736-1740.
12. Peiffert D, Bey P, Pernot M, et al. Conservative treatment by irradiation of epidermoid carcinomas of the anal margin. *Int J Radiat Oncol Biol Phys* 1997;39:57-66.

13. Frisch M, Glimelius B, van den Brule AJ, et al. Sexually transmitted infection as a cause of anal cancer. *N Engl J Med* 1997;337: 1350-1358.

14. Palefsky JM, Holly EA, Gonzales J, et al. Detection of human papillomavirus DNA in anal intraepithelial neoplasia and anal cancer. *Cancer Res* 1991;51:1014-1019.

15. Zaki SR, Judd R, Coffield LM, et al. Human papillomavirus infection and anal carcinoma. Retrospective analysis by in situ hybridization and the polymerase chain reaction. *Am J Pathol* 1992;140:1345-1355.

16. Daling JR, Weiss NS, Hislop TG, et al. Sexual practices, sexually transmitted diseases, and the incidence of anal cancer. *N Engl J Med* 1987;317:973-977.

17. Daling JR, Weiss NS, Klopfenstein LL, et al. Correlates of homosexual behavior and the incidence of anal cancer. *JAMA* 1982;247:1988-1990.

18. Frisch M, Melbye M, Moller H. Trends in incidence of anal cancer in Denmark. *Br Med J* 1993;306:419-422.

19. Palefsky JM, Holly EA, Ralston ML, et al. Anal squamous intraepithelial lesions in HIV-positive and HIV-negative homosexual and bisexual men: prevalence and risk factors. *J Acquir Immune Defic Syndr Hum Retrovirol* 1998;17:320-326.

20. Goldie SJ, Kuntz KM, Weinstein MC, et al. Cost-effectiveness of screening for anal squamous intraepithelial lesions and anal cancer in human immunodeficiency virus-negative homosexual and bisexual men. *Am J Med* 2000;108:634-641.

21. Ryan DP, Compton CC, Mayer RJ. Carcinoma of the anal canal. *N Engl J Med* 2000;342:792-800.

22. Penn I. Cancers of the anogenital region in renal transplant recipients. Analysis of 65 cases. *Cancer* 1986;58:611-616.

23. Arends MJ, Benton EC, McLaren KM, et al. Renal allograft recipients with high susceptibility to cutaneous malignancy have an increased prevalence of human papillomavirus DNA in skin tumours and a greater risk of anogenital malignancy. *Br J Cancer* 1997;75:722-728.

24. Biggar RJ, Horm J, Goedert JJ, et al. Cancer in a group at risk of acquired immunodeficiency syndrome (AIDS) through 1984. *Am J Epidemiol* 1987;126:578-586.

25. Daling JR, Sherman KJ, Hislop TG, et al. Cigarette smoking and the risk of anogenital cancer. *Am J Epidemiol* 1992;135:180-189.

26. Rabkin CS, Biggar RJ, Melbye M, et al. Second primary cancers following anal and cervical carcinoma: evidence of shared etiologic factors. *Am J Epidemiol* 1992;136:54-58.

27. Winkelstein W Jr. Smoking and cervical cancer—current status: a review. *Am J Epidemiol* 1990;131:945-957.

28. Frisch M, Johansen C. Anal carcinoma in inflammatory bowel disease. *Br J Cancer* 2000;83:89-90.

29. Frisch M, Olsen JH, Bautz, et al. Benign anal lesions and the risk of anal cancer. *N Engl J Med* 1994;331:300-302.

30. Godlewski G, Prudhomme M. Embryology and anatomy of the anorectum. Basis of surgery. *Surg Clin North Am* 2000;80:319-343.

31. Hughes LL, Rich TA, Delclos L, et al. Radiotherapy for anal cancer: experience from 1979-1987. *Int J Radiat Oncol Biol Phys* 1989;17: 1153-1160.

32. Myerson RJ, Karnell LH, Menck HR. The National Cancer Data Base report on carcinoma of the anus. *Cancer* 1997;80:805-815.

33. Klas JV, Rothenberger DA, Wong WD, et al. Malignant tumors of the anal canal: the spectrum of disease, treatment, and outcomes. *Cancer* 1999;85:1686-1693.

34. Joon DL, Chao MWT, Ngan SYK, et al. Primary adenocarcinoma of the anus: a retrospective analysis. *Int J Radiat Oncol Biol Phys* 1999;45:1199-1205.

35. Faivre C, Rougier P, Ducreux M, et al. 5-fluorouracile and cisplatinum combination chemotherapy for metastatic squamous-cell anal cancer. *Bull Cancer* 1999;86:861-865.

36. Touboul E, Schlienger M, Buffat L, et al. Conservative versus nonconservative treatment of epidermoid carcinoma of the anal canal

for tumors longer than or equal to 5 centimeters. A retrospective comparison. *Cancer* 1995;75:786-793.

37. Zelnick RS, Haas PA, Ajlouni M, et al. Results of abdominoperineal resections for failures after combination chemotherapy and radiation therapy for anal canal cancers. *Dis Colon Rectum* 1992; 35:574-577.

38. Goldman S, Auer G, Erhardt K, et al. Prognostic significance of clinical stage, histologic grade, and nuclear DNA content in squamous cell carcinoma of the anus. *Dis Colon Rectum* 1987;30: 444-448.

39. Grabenbauer GG, Matzel KE, Schneider IH, et al. Sphincter preservation with chemoradiation in anal canal carcinoma: abdominoperineal resection in selected cases? *Dis Colon Rectum* 1998;41:441-450.

40. Bonin SR, Pajak TF, Russell AH, et al. Overexpression of *p53* protein and outcome of patients treated with chemoradiation for carcinoma of the anal canal: a report of randomized trial [Radiation Therapy Oncology Group] RTOG 87-04. *Cancer* 1999;85:1226-1233.

41. Salmon RJ, Fenton J, Asselain B, et al. Treatment of epidermoid anal canal cancer. *Am J Surg* 1984;147:43-48.

42. Cummings BJ, Keane TJ, O'Sullivan B, et al. Epidermoid anal cancer: treatment by radiation alone or by radiation and 5-fluorouracil with and without mitomycin-c. *Int J Radiat Oncol Biol Phys* 1991;21:1115-1125.

43. Nigro N, Vaitkevicius V, Considine B. Combined therapy for cancer of the anal canal: a preliminary report. *Dis Colon Rectum* 1974;15:354-356.

44. Epidermoid anal cancer: results from the [UK Co-ordinating Committee on Cancer Research] UKCCCR [Anal Cancer Trial Working Party] randomized trial of radiotherapy alone versus radiotherapy, 5-fluorouracil, and mitomycin. *Lancet* 1996;348: 1049-1054.

45. Roelofsen F, Bosset JF, Eschwege F, et al. Concomitant radiotherapy and chemotherapy are superior to radiotherapy alone in the treatment of locally advanced anal cancer: results of a phase III randomized trial of the EORTC Radiotherapy and Gastrointestinal Cooperative Group [abstract]. *Proc Am Soc Clin Oncol* 1995;14:194.

46. Bartelink H, Roelofsen F, Eschwege F, et al. Concomitant radiotherapy and chemotherapy is superior to radiotherapy alone in the treatment of locally advanced anal cancer: results of a phase III randomized trial of the European Organization for Research and Treatment of Cancer Radiotherapy and Gastrointestinal Cooperative Groups. *J Clin Oncol* 1997;15:2040-2049.

47. Flam M, John M, Pajak TF, et al. Role of mitomycin in combination with fluorouracil and radiotherapy and of salvage chemoradiation in the definitive non-surgical treatment of epidermoid carcinoma of the anal canal: results of a phase III randomized intergroup study. *J Clin Oncol* 1996;14:2527-2539.

48. Martenson JA, Lipsitz SR, Lefkopoulou M, et al. Results of combined modality therapy for patients with anal cancer (E7283): an Eastern Cooperative Oncology Group study. *Cancer* 1995;76:1731-1736.

49. Sischy B, Doggett RL, Krall JM, et al. Definitive irradiation and chemotherapy for radiosensitization in management of anal carcinoma: interim report on Radiation Therapy Oncology Group study no. 8314. *J Natl Cancer Inst* 1989;81:850-856.

50. Miller EJ, Quan SH, Thaler T. Treatment of squamous cell carcinoma of the anal canal. *Cancer* 1991;67:2038-2041.

51. Gerard JP, Morignat E, Romestaing P, et al. Radiotherapy of cancer of the anal canal. 15 years experience at the Lyon civil hospices and brief review of the literature. *Ann Chir* 1998;52:17-23.

52. Leichman L, Nigro N, Vaitkevicius VK, et al. Cancer of the anal canal. Model for preoperative adjuvant combined modality therapy. *Am J Med* 1985;78:211-215.

53. Schneider IHF, Grabenbauer GG, Reck T, et al. Combined radiation and chemotherapy for epidermoid carcinoma of the anal canal. *Int J Colorectal Dis* 1992;7:192-196.

54. Tanum G, Tveit K, Karlsen KO, et al. Chemoradiotherapy and radiation therapy for anal carcinoma. Survival and late morbidity. *Cancer* 1991;67:2462-2466.

55. Doci R, Zucali R, LaMonica G, et al. Primary chemoradiation therapy with fluorouracil and cisplatin for cancer of the anus. Results in 35 consecutive patients. *J Clin Oncol* 1996;14:3121-3125.

56. Papillon J, Montbarbon JF. Epidermoid carcinoma of the anal canal. A series of 276 cases. *Dis Colon Rectum* 1987;30:324-333.

57. Gerard JP. Chemotherapy in the treatment of cancer of the anal canal. *Cancer Radiother* 1998;2:708-712.

58. Wagner JP, Mahe MA, Romestaing P, et al. Radiation therapy in the conservative treatment of carcinoma of the anal canal. *Int J Radiat Oncol Biol Phys* 1994;29:17-23.

59. Martenson JA, Lipsitz SR, Wagner H, et al. Initial results of a phase II trial of high dose radiation therapy, 5-fluorouracil and cisplatin for patients with anal cancer (E4292): an Eastern Cooperative Oncology Group study. *Int J Radiat Oncol Biol Phys* 1996;35:745-749.

60. Rich T, Ajani JA, Morrison WH, et al. Chemoradiation therapy for anal cancer. Radiation plus continuous infusion of 5-fluorouracil with or without cisplatin. *Radiother Oncol* 1993;27:209-215.

61. Brunet R, Becouarn Y, Pigneux J, et al. Cisplatine et fluorouracile en chimiotherapie neoadjuvante des carcinomas epidemoides du canal anal [in French]. *Lyon Chirurgical* 1990;87:77.

62. Svensson C, Goldman S, Friberg B. Radiation treatment of epidermoid cancer of the anus. *Int J Radiat Oncol Biol Phys* 1993;27:67-73.

63. Roca E, De Simone G, Barugel M, et al. A phase II study of alternating chemoradiotherapy including cisplatin in anal canal carcinoma [abstract]. *Proc Am Soc Clin Oncol* 1990;9:128.

64. Paleologo F, Goswitz M, Rich TA, et al. Results of radiation and concomitant continuous infusion 5-fluorouracil and cisplatin for anal cancer [abstract]. *Int J Radiat Oncol Biol Phys* 1997;39(suppl):202. Abstract 135.

65. Svensson C, Goldman S, Friberg B, et al. Induction chemotherapy and radiotherapy in loco-regionally advanced epidermoid carcinoma of the anal canal. *Int J Radiat Oncol Biol Phys* 1998;41:863-867.

66. Friberg B, Svensson C, Goldman S, et al. The Swedish National Care Programme for Anal Carcinoma: implementation and overall results. *Acta Oncol* 1998;37:25-32.

67. Hoffman R, Welton ML, Klencke B, et al. The significance of pretreatment CD4 count on the outcome and treatment tolerance of HIV-positive patients with anal cancer. *Int J Radiat Oncol Biol Phys* 1999;44:127-131.

68. Chadha M, Rosenblatt EA, Malamud S, et al. Squamous-cell carcinoma of the anus in HIV-positive patients. *Dis Colon Rectum* 1994;37:861-865.

69. Peddada AV, Smith DE, Rao AR, et al. Chemotherapy and low-dose radiotherapy in the treatment of HIV-infected patients with carcinoma of the anal canal. *Int J Radiat Oncol Biol Phys* 1997;37:1101-1105.

70. Cleator S, Fife K, Nelson M, et al. Treatment of HIV-associated invasive anal cancer with combined chemoradiation. *Eur J Cancer* 2000;36:754-758.

71. Cox JD. Chemoradiation for malignant epithelial tumors. *Cancer Radiother* 1998;2:7-11.

72. Mendenhall WM, Zlotecki RA, Vauthey JN, et al. Squamous cell carcinoma of the anal margin. *Oncology* 1996;10:1843-1854.

73. Constantinou EC, Daly W, Fung CY, et al. Time-dose considerations in the treatment of anal cancer. *Int J Radiat Oncol Biol Phys* 1997;39:651-657.

74. Janjan NA, Crane CH, Ajani J, et al. 30 Gy is a sufficient dose to control micrometastases from anal cancer-dosimetric evaluation of N0 patients undergoing chemoradiation [abstract]. *Cancer J* 1999;5:117. Abstract 11.

75. Hung AV, Ballo MT, Crane C, et al. Platinum-based combined modality therapy for anal carcinoma [abstract]. *Proc Am Soc Clin Oncol* 2001;19:A679.

76. Hu K, Minsky BD, Cohen AM, et al. 30 Gy may be an adequate dose in patients with anal cancer treated with excisional biopsy followed by combined-modality therapy. *J Surg Oncol* 1999;70:71-77.

77. John M, Pajak TJ, Flam MS, et al. Dose escalation in chemoradiation for anal cancer. Preliminary results of RTOG 92-08. *Cancer J Sci Am* 1996;2:205-211.

78. Allal AS, Obradovic M, Laurencet F, et al. Treatment of anal carcinoma in the elderly: feasibility and outcome of radical radiotherapy with or without concomitant chemotherapy. *Cancer* 1999;85:26-31.

79. Berger C, Felix-Faure C, Chauvet B, et al. Conservative treatment of anal canal carcinoma with external radiotherapy and interstitial brachytherapy, with or without chemotherapy: long-term results. *Cancer Radiother* 1999;3:461-467.

80. Gerard JP, Ayzac L, Hun D, et al. Treatment of anal canal carcinoma with high dose radiation therapy and concomitant fluorouracil-cisplatinum. Long term results in 95 patients. *Radiother Oncol* 1998;46:249-256.

81. Lohnert M, Doniec JM, Kovacs G, et al. New method of radiotherapy for anal cancer with three-dimensional tumor reconstruction based on endoanal ultrasound and ultrasound-guided afterloading therapy. *Dis Colon Rectum* 1998;41:169-176.

82. Sandhu AP, Symonds RP, Robertson AG, et al. Interstitial iridium-192 implantation combined with external radiotherapy in anal cancer: ten years experience. *Int J Radiat Oncol Biol Phys* 1998;40:575-581.

83. Mitchell SE, Mendenhall WM, Zlotecki RA, et al. Squamous cell carcinoma of the anal canal. *Int J Radiat Oncol Biol Phys* 2001;49:1007-1013.

84. Callister M, Janjan N, Brown T, et al. Effective management of treatment-related enteritis during preoperative chemoradiation for locally advanced rectal cancer (abstract). *Int J Radiat Oncol Biol Phys* 1997;48(suppl):225. Abstract 228.

85. Throckmorton T, Janjan NA, Bisanz A, et al. Development of a bowel function assessment tool to measure bowel function in patients receiving radiation and/or chemotherapy [abstract]. *Int J Radiat Oncol Biol Phys* 1997;39(suppl):235. Abstract 1040.

86. Allal AS, Sprangers MA, Laurencet F, et al. Assessment of long-term quality of life in patients with anal carcinomas treated by radiotherapy with or without chemotherapy. *Br J Cancer* 1999;80:1588-1594.

87. John M, Flam M, Palma N. Ten-year results of chemoradiation for anal cancer: focus on late morbidity. *Int J Radiat Oncol Biol Phys* 1996;34:65-69.

88. Kim GE, Lim JJ, Park W, et al. Sensory and motor dysfunction assessed by anorectal manometry in uterine cervical carcinoma patients with radiation induced late rectal complications. *Int J Radiat Oncol Biol Phys* 1998;41:835-841.

89. Allal AS, Laurencet FM, Reymond MA, et al. Effectiveness of surgical salvage therapy for patients with locally uncontrolled anal carcinoma after sphincter-conserving treatment. *Cancer* 1999;86:405-409.

90. Pocard M, Tiret E, Nugent K, et al. Results of salvage abdominoperineal resection for anal cancer after radiotherapy. *Dis Colon Rectum* 1998;41:1488-1493.

PART VII

Urinary Tract

CHAPTER 24

The Kidney

Lewis G. Smith III and Harper D. Pearse

At present, radiation therapy has a relatively small role in the management of renal cancer in adults. However, renal tolerance is very important in cancer treatment, especially treatment that involves abdominal irradiation. The kidney is unavoidably irradiated during therapy for many abdominal and retroperitoneal malignancies, and knowledge of the early and late effects of radiation is essential for proper treatment planning.

ANATOMY

The kidneys are retroperitoneal structures surrounded by fat and enclosed within Gerota's fascia. Each kidney is 11 to 12 cm long (3 to 4.4 times the height of the L2 vertebra).[1] The renal axis is parallel to the lateral margin of the greater psoas muscle. The right kidney is usually 1 to 2 cm lower than the left kidney and is close to the liver, the duodenum, and the hepatic flexure of the

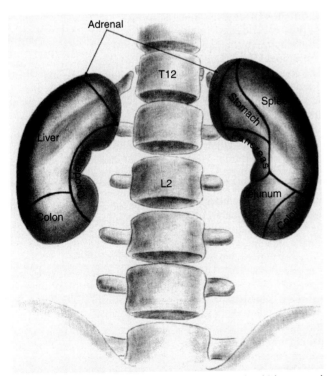

Fig. 24-1 Anatomic relationships between the kidneys and the abdominal viscera. The proximity of the kidneys to multiple dose-limiting intraperitoneal structures is evident.

TABLE 24-1	
Tolerance Doses for Late-Responding Tissues Affected by Abdominal and Retroperitoneal Irradiation	
Tissue	**Dose (Gy)**
Kidney	23 (whole-abdomen irradiation)
Liver	35 (whole-abdomen irradiation)
Spinal cord	45
Bowel	50
Ureter	75

Data from Roswit B, Malsky SJ, Reid CB. *Front Radiat Ther Oncol* 1972;6:160-181; Withers HR. *Int J Radiat Oncol Biol Phys* 1986;12:693-698; Rubin P, Casarett GW. *Clinical Radiation Pathology*. Philadelphia, Pa: WB Saunders; 1968.
*1.8- to 2-Gy fractions of megavoltage irradiation.

colon. The left kidney is immediately adjacent to portions of the spleen, stomach, pancreas, jejunum, and colon (Fig. 24-1). These consistent anatomic relationships are of prime importance in the planning of abdominal and retroperitoneal irradiation because they limit the dose that can be given safely (Table 24-1).[2,3]

Each kidney contains roughly one million glomeruli, small knots of blood vessels that facilitate the excretion of fluid from the blood. Selective reabsorption of the fluid takes place in the complex renal tubule system. The glomeruli and tubules are the most important structures of the kidney from the perspective of radiation effects.

The renal vein is the most anterior structure in the renal hilum. The renal artery is posterior to the renal vein, and the renal pelvis is posterior to the renal artery. The lymphatic drainage of the kidney and renal pelvis is along the vessels in the renal hilum to the periaortic nodes. The blood supply and lymph node drainage of the ureter are segmental and diffuse, with abundant subadventitial interconnections making precise drainage patterns difficult to predict.

RESPONSE OF THE NORMAL KIDNEY TO IRRADIATION

Radiation-induced renal damage is a slowly progressive, noninflammatory disease, the severity of which depends on the volume of renal parenchyma irradiated, the total dose and fractionation schedule, the age of the patient, associated conditions such as hypertension and diabetes mellitus, and interactions with nephrotoxic or radiomimetic chemotherapeutic agents. Because of the lack of inflammation, *radiation nephropathy* is probably a better term than *radiation nephritis* to describe this clinical-pathologic entity.

Gassman observed radiation nephropathy in 1899, and Baermann and Linser described it in 1904.[4] Domagk accurately documented the clinical presentation and histopathologic findings in 1927.[5,6] The classic studies (1948 to 1962) by Kunkler and colleagues[7,11] and Luxton[8-10] provided guidelines regarding the human kidney's tolerance of fractionated irradiation. The findings of these and more recent studies are discussed in the following paragraphs.

Acute Radiation Nephropathy

The common qualitative studies of renal function (e.g., blood urea nitrogen or creatinine clearance levels) fail to show any consistent early or late changes after fractionated renal doses of 10 to 20 Gy; however, Avioli and colleagues[12] found measurable decreases in renal function at all doses above 4 Gy. These studies were performed in 10 patients before, during, and after abdominal irradiation for cancer. Before irradiation, all patients had normal renal function. Total renal doses of 20 to 24 Gy were given in 3 to 4 weeks. A subtle but progressive decrease in renal plasma flow proved to be the most sensitive and consistent index of radiation-induced renal damage.

The pathogenesis of the acute phase of renal damage has proved difficult to elucidate by histologic examination; however, initial changes appear to be most extensive in the capillary endothelium (where slight swelling is seen) and in the proximal tubular epithelial cells.[13,14] Additional evidence of early tubular injury is the decrease in neprilysin (kidney brush-border enzyme) activity and the increase in lysosomal activity that are seen after irradiation.[6] Between 30 and 60 days after irradiation, capillary endothelial and tubular epithelial cells show vacuolation and patchy degeneration and in places separate from their basement membrane. In the 1950s, Flanagan found that after a single dose of 28 Gy to the rabbit kidney, tubular damage—from both a histologic and a functional standpoint—reaches its peak in 4 weeks. Slow, incomplete recovery follows (Fig. 24-2).

The clinical manifestations of acute radiation nephropathy appear 6 to 12 months after exposure to radiation and consist of hypertension, edema, proteinuria, anemia, and uremia. Histologic manifestations include segmental glomerular sclerosis, tubular atrophy, and vascular injury. Arteriolar intimal thickening, fibrin deposition, thrombosis, fibrinoid necrosis, and cellular proliferation similar to that seen in malignant hypertension are apparent. This important tissue response to radiation injury seems to begin when vascular endothelial and tubular epithelial cells start to replicate, that is, 2 to 3 months after the radiation insult.[15,16]

Historically, doses in excess of 23 Gy in 5 weeks have produced acute radiation nephropathy in about half of treated patients.[8,10] Hypertension is the most important prognostic sign in patients with this condition. Although

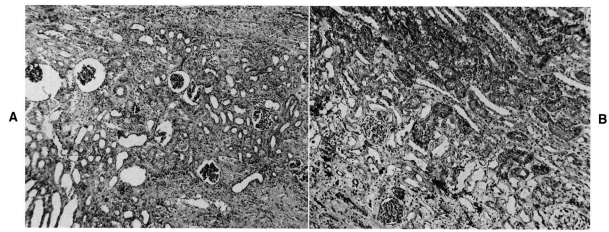

Fig. 24-2 Microscopic changes after a single dose of 28 Gy to the exteriorized rabbit's kidney (220 kV; half-value layer, 1.2 mm Cu; target-to-skin distance, 52 cm). **A,** One month after irradiation. Every glomerulus shows extensive changes. Widespread tubular necrosis and atrophy are evident. Round cells have infiltrated interstitial tissues. Vascular damage is not evident except in the glomeruli. **B,** Five months after irradiation. Incomplete recovery of all elements has occurred. Some glomeruli have recovered strikingly. Tubular damage is still severe, although noticeable recovery has occurred. The initial infiltration has decreased. Associated studies revealed some recovery of function. (Courtesy Dr. C.L. Flanagan.)

hypertension may disappear and the kidneys may recover, this is not usually the case. Of the 20 patients with acute radiation nephropathy on whom Luxton[10] reported, 10 died.

Within several months after the onset of acute radiation nephropathy, the so-called chronic or late changes begin to appear, and survivors will have some degree of chronic nephropathy. Among the 10 subjects who died in the Luxton series,[10] six died of malignant hypertension within 12 months and three died of renal failure 7 to 11 years after the onset of the nephropathy.

Chronic (Late) Radiation Nephropathy

The changes associated with late radiation nephropathy are closely related to the changes associated with acute nephropathy. These late changes develop several months to years after irradiation and can result in death years later. A history of clinical acute radiation nephropathy is not a prerequisite for chronic radiation nephropathy.

Pathogenesis

Vascular and parenchymal cell damage contribute in a complex, interrelated way to the time course and progression of radiation nephropathy. During the chronic phase of radiation nephropathy, the earliest change seen on light microscopy is tubular atrophy.[14] This is followed by more severe tubular loss, interstitial fibrosis, and hyalinization of some glomeruli (Fig. 24-3).[1] Characteristic postirradiation vascular changes (proliferation of subendothelial fibrous connective tissue in the medium and smaller arteries) also appear, but the degree of vascular narrowing at this point is trivial in comparison with the tubular changes.[5,6] Experimental studies

confirm the early vulnerability of the tubules, whose atrophy and loss are independent of vascular changes.

Because the glomerular efferent vessels subdivide to form the microvasculature of the tubules, damage to the glomerular circulation also affects the blood supply of the tubules.[17] This direct effect of vascular damage could account for the atrophy of kidneys seen after doses of radiation sufficient to affect the small renal vessels.

Understanding of the pathogenesis of radiation-induced hypertension and the late effects of irradiation in all areas of the body owes much to the work of Asscher and others.[15] The higher the renal dose and the higher the dose per fraction, the earlier the hypertension secondary to renal irradiation appears. Furthermore, the severity of hypertension depends not so much on the absolute amount of renal tissue irradiated as on the proportion of the total renal mass irradiated. Hypertension from any cause produces profound vascular damage in irradiated blood vessels, whereas nonirradiated vessels subjected to the same hypertension may appear normal for months. In other words, irradiation sensitizes the blood vessels to hypertensive changes.

In the kidney, this sensitization of vessels to hypertensive damage has serious implications because hypertension is an expected sequela of high renal radiation doses. However, the sensitization of vessels to hypertensive damage is not confined to the kidney; it develops in all irradiated tissues. Asscher and Anson[18] pointed out that a patient who previously had vital tissues irradiated (brain, spinal cord, bowel, or lung) could, because of hypertension, develop vascular necrosis leading to sequelae that could not be explained if the history of irradiation were not taken into account. These laboratory findings must be kept in mind when one weighs the

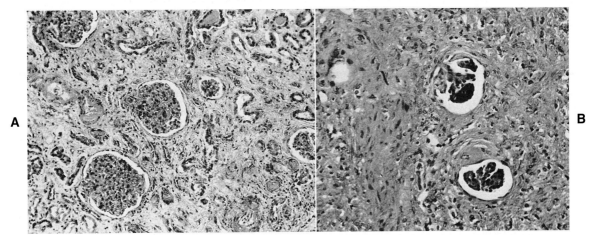

Fig. 24-3 Chronic radiation nephropathy. **A,** Thirteen months after delivery of a calculated minimum of 30 Gy to the left kidney. Glomerular changes are moderately severe, and tubular damage is very severe. Interstitial edema, round cell infiltration, and fibrosis are striking. **B,** Findings in a patient who was irradiated repeatedly for upper abdominal Hodgkin's disease and died of radiation nephritis. The dose-time relationship is not known. The glomeruli are almost completely destroyed, and no tubules are left. (Courtesy Dr. L.V. Ackerman.)

radiation tolerances in hypertensive patients or the causes of necrosis in patients who have recently become hypertensive.

As Asscher[19] demonstrated, the pathogenesis of radiation-induced hypertension from renal irradiation can be summarized as follows. In rats, renal arteries manifest their sensitization within 60 days after a single dose of 12 Gy given to both kidneys. About 90 days after renal irradiation, hypergranulation of the juxtaglomerular cells appears. This is one of the first morphologic changes related to subsequent hypertension, and it is apparently a consequence of decreased renal blood flow, even though at this point the vessels appear normal. About 5 months after irradiation, hypertension is well developed, and necrosis of the sensitized arteries develops.

Time Course

Recently, functional endpoints measured using noninvasive scintigraphic and biochemical assays have been used to document the time course of radiation nephropathy. Dewit and colleagues[20] prospectively analyzed glomerular function (with ^{99m}Tc pentetic acid renography and measurement of creatinine clearance and β-2 microglobulin level) and tubular function (with ^{99m}Tc dimercaptosuccinic acid scintigraphy and measurement of urine β-2 microglobulin level, alanine aminopeptidase level, and urine concentration) in 26 patients undergoing renal irradiation for abdominal cancer (lymphoma, ovarian carcinoma, and testicular seminoma). In patients who received 40 Gy in $5\frac{1}{2}$ weeks to the entire left kidney, split glomerular and tubular function as assessed by scintigraphy decreased to 30% to 40% of pretreatment values after 3 to 5 years. Overall glomerular function (creatinine clearance) decreased by 20% after 3 to 5 years. Functional impairment was reduced by half if a part of the kidney was shielded. No changes were noted after bilateral renal irradiation to 18 Gy in $3\frac{1}{2}$ weeks. Dewit's group stressed that radiation nephropathy progresses slowly and that long-term follow-up is essential in accurately assessing functional impairment.

Limits of Renal Radiation Tolerance

Clinical assessment of renal tolerance after irradiation has been determined in great part by historical studies that used orthovoltage techniques and large doses per fraction and in many cases did not treat each field each day. Precise determination of renal tolerance with high-energy photons and conventional fractionation is incomplete.

In their excellent analysis, Kunkler and colleagues[7] defined the limit of renal radiation tolerance in human beings. They studied patients with testicular seminoma and ovarian cancer who had sites of probable abdominal metastases irradiated through large ports, with the kidneys included in the treated volume. When a dose of 25 to 32.5 Gy in 3 to 6 weeks was delivered to the whole of both kidneys in 55 patients, 22 developed renal damage, and 7 died of radiation-induced renal failure. Luxton[10] and Kunkler[11] later reported further clinical developments in this same group of 55 patients. Of 24 patients with chronic radiation nephropathy, 9 were normotensive for 8 years. The other 15 patients developed the clinical picture of chronic glomerular nephritis (hypertension, proteinuria, anemia, casts in the urine, and uremia). As might be expected, the kidneys became small and fibrotic.

Historical studies[21] suggest that renal irradiation to 23 Gy is associated with a 5% incidence of radiation-induced renal failure at 5 years; after 28 Gy, the rate of renal failure increases to 50%. Therefore, on those rare occasions when both kidneys must be included in the irradiated volume, the maximum fractionated dose delivered to the kidneys should not exceed 20 Gy or its biological equivalent unless the risk of late renal damage is justified.

In the treatment of upper abdominal malignancies, irradiation of 50% or more of a single kidney with 25 to 40 Gy with conventional fractionation has been associated with a limited risk of clinical nephropathy. However, in adults, creatinine clearances are depressed 10% to 24% depending on the volume irradiated.[22] Decreases in creatinine clearance are not likely to occur in children.[23] In a recent study of unilateral renal irradiation incident to treatment of gastric lymphoma, 27 patients received irradiation to the left kidney. In 13 of these patients, the entire left kidney was irradiated to total doses ranging from 24 to 40 Gy; all of these patients had undergone previous combination chemotherapy. At a median follow-up of 40 months, renal length was reduced by 2 to 3 cm, but no changes were evident in blood urea nitrogen or creatinine levels, and only one patient developed hypertension (blood pressure of 150/90). The other 14 patients whose kidneys were only partially irradiated had little or no evidence of late effects.[24]

It is important to realize that irradiation of a single kidney can produce malignant hypertension that may disappear after nephrectomy. Therefore, any patient who develops hypertension after upper abdominal irradiation should be examined to rule out the possibility of radiation-induced renal damage.

Effect of Chemotherapy

A variety of chemotherapeutic agents can damage the kidneys, and many patients receiving cytotoxic chemotherapy have had or will have abdominal radiation therapy. The radiation oncologist should be aware that these patients may have reduced renal radiation tolerance.

Chemotherapeutic agents associated with nephrotoxicity are shown in Box 24-1. Various histologic changes have been observed, and in almost every case the initial

From Vogelzang NJ. *Oncology (Huntingt)* 1991;5:97-102, 105.

BOX 24-1 Chemotherapeutic Agents Associated with Nephrotoxicity

ALKYLATING AGENTS
Nitrosoureas
Cisplatin and analogues
Ifosfamide
Diaziquone

ANTIMETABOLITES
Methotrexate
Azacitidine

GALLIUM NITRATE

toxic insult is acute tubular damage at high drug concentrations. (The exception is mitomycin C, which initially produces vascular damage.) Even nitrosourea-induced interstitial nephritis is associated with tubular loss.[25]

Treatment with chemotherapeutic agents that are not nephrotoxic by themselves may increase the sensitivity of the kidney to radiation. In children, radiation nephropathy has been seen after 15 to 20 Gy when radiation therapy is delivered in combination with dactinomycin.[26] Total-body irradiation with concomitant cyclophosphamide has been associated with nephrotoxicity.[27]

Experimentally, doxorubicin potentiates radiation.[28] It may be possible to reduce the sensitivity of the kidney to radiation in patients treated with doxorubicin by using glutathione, cysteine, or a low-protein diet.[16,29]

The most common drug interaction resulting in renal toxicity is the interaction between cisplatin and aminoglycoside antibiotics. These two classes of compounds are commonly used in today's cancer patient and when given within 3 months of each other have been associated with enhanced nephrotoxicity.

RECOMMENDATIONS FOR MINIMIZING RADIATION-INDUCED RENAL DAMAGE

The precautions necessary to prevent radiation-induced renal failure are obvious. Renal irradiation should be avoided whenever possible. This necessitates accurate definition of tumor extent and recognition of any congenital abnormalities and the position of the kidneys. At a minimum, contrast-enhanced computed tomography (CT) should be available to meet these needs. When renal irradiation is judged unavoidable, as much renal tissue as possible should be shielded, and the dose should be limited to 20 Gy in 2 to 3 weeks. In rare instances (e.g., massive involvement of the periaortic lymph nodes by lymphoma or seminoma), this can be accomplished by redefining the tumor volume after the

initial dose. The possibility of autotransplanting the kidney to the iliac fossa should be considered if doses greater than the tolerance level of the kidney are necessary. When neither of these alternatives is possible and chronic renal insufficiency is an accepted sequela of treatment, consideration of dialysis or kidney transplantation is not unreasonable if cure by irradiation is obtainable. Such a circumstance could develop in a child with bilateral Wilms' tumor.

RENAL CELL CARCINOMA
Epidemiology and Risk Factors

Renal tumors account for approximately 3% of new cases of cancer and cancer-related deaths in the United States and are 1.5 times more common in men than in women.[30] The average age at diagnosis is 55 to 60 years, and 30% of patients have evidence of metastatic disease at diagnosis. Of renal tumors found in adults, 90% are renal cell carcinomas.

Risk factors for renal cell carcinoma include exposure to urban environmental toxins, tobacco use, von Hippel-Lindau disease, acquired cystic disease of the kidney associated with renal failure, and possibly dietary fat and obesity.

A variety of industrial and environmental toxins have been linked to renal cell carcinoma in humans. These include cadmium, asbestos, and various petrochemicals.[31] Cigarette smoking has been implicated as a risk factor in several studies; these studies suggest that increased duration of smoking and increased number of cigarettes smoked per day are correlated with higher risk.[32,33]

Von Hippel-Lindau disease is an autosomal dominant inherited disorder in which individuals have a predisposition to develop multiple benign and malignant tumors, including retinal angioma, central nervous system hemangioblastoma, pheochromocytoma, pancreatic tumors, and renal cell carcinoma. Renal cell carcinoma in patients with von Hippel-Lindau disease occurs at an earlier age than sporadic renal cell carcinoma and often involves multiple tumors and bilateral disease.[34] Loss or translocation of DNA on the short arm of chromosome 3 is common in patients with von Hippel-Lindau disease, suggesting that a gene at this location functions as a tumor suppressor gene for renal cell carcinoma.[34-37]

An association between acquired cystic disease of the kidney and chronic renal failure was first noted in 1977.[38] Acquired cystic disease seems to be a premalignant condition associated with renal changes ranging from hyperplasia and adenoma to renal cell carcinoma. The reported incidence of renal cell carcinoma in patients with acquired cystic disease is 4% to 9%.[31] The actual incidence is probably lower; however, renal ultrasonography is now recommended for these patients at the initiation of dialysis and every 2 years thereafter.

In patients with acquired cystic disease and an enlarging solid renal mass, nephrectomy should be considered.

Animal studies in Syrian hamsters showed that diethylstilbestrol induces hormonally dependent renal adenocarcinomas similar to human renal adenocarcinomas.[39,40] These animal studies formed the basis for attempts at hormonal manipulation in the treatment of patients with metastatic renal cell carcinoma. Of historical interest is the induction of tumors of the kidney and renal pelvis by the radioactive contrast agent thorium oxide.[41]

Pathology and Staging

Renal cell carcinoma is an adenocarcinoma of proximal tubular origin.[42] Clear cell carcinoma (glycogen-rich, few organelles) is the most common cell type; granular cell carcinoma (glycogen-poor, abundant organelles) is less common.[43] Its location and clear cell features led to renal cell carcinoma being termed *hypernephroma.* Sarcomas of the kidney are rare, constituting 1% of all malignant renal tumors.[44] They are a histologically diverse group of tumors, with leiomyosarcoma being the most common subtype, accounting for 20% to 60% of renal sarcomas. Sarcomas of the kidney are usually large and locally advanced at diagnosis. Local recurrence of renal sarcoma

is common after surgical resection, and they have a propensity for hematogenous dissemination.

The stage of the tumor at diagnosis is the most important prognostic factor, with extrarenal extension and lymph node involvement being more important than renal vein invasion. The American Joint Committee on Cancer (AJCC) 1997 tumor-nodes-metastasis (TNM) classification for cancer of the kidney is shown in Box 24-2.[45]

The histopathologic types are as follows: renal cell carcinoma, other adenocarcinoma, renal papillary adenocarcinoma, tubular carcinoma, granular cell carcinoma, and clear cell carcinoma (hypernephroma). The predominant type is adenocarcinoma; subtypes of adenocarcinoma are clear cell and granular cell carcinoma.

Clinical Features and Diagnosis

Patients with renal cell carcinoma have varied signs and symptoms. Hematuria is noted in at least 60%, an abdominal or flank mass is noted in 45%, and pain is noted in 40%.[46] The classic triad of hematuria, a mass, and pain is noted in fewer than 10% of patients. Several paraneoplastic syndromes are associated with renal cell carcinoma, including nonmetastatic hepatic

---

Box 24-2 American Joint Committee on Cancer Staging System for Cancer of the Kidney

PRIMARY TUMOR (T)

TX	Primary tumor cannot be assessed
T0	No evidence of primary tumor
T1	Tumor 7 cm or less in greatest dimension limited to the kidney
T2	Tumor more than 7 cm in greatest dimension limited to the kidney
T3	Tumor extends into major veins or invades the adrenal gland or perinephric tissues, but not beyond Gerota's fascia
	T3a Tumor invades the adrenal gland or perinephric tissues but not beyond Gerota's fascia
	T3b Tumor grossly extends into the renal vein(s) or vena cava below the diaphragm
	T3c Tumor grossly extends into the renal vein(s) or vena cava above the diaphragm
T4	Tumor invades beyond Gerota's fascia

REGIONAL LYMPH NODES (N)*

NX	Regional lymph nodes cannot be assessed
N0	No regional lymph node metastases
N1	Metastases in a single regional lymph node
N2	Metastases in more than one regional lymph node

DISTANT METASTASIS (M)

MX	Distant metastasis cannot be assessed
M0	No distant metastasis
M1	Distant metastasis

STAGE GROUPING

Stage I	T1	N0	M0
Stage II	T2	N0	M0
Stage III	T1	N1	M0
	T2	N1	M0
	T3a	N0	M0
	T3a	N1	M0
	T3b	N0	M0
	T3b	N1	M0
	T3c	N0	M0
	T3c	N1	M0
Stage IV	T4	N0	M0
	T4	N1	M0
	Any T	N2	M1
	Any T	Any N	M1

From Fleming I, Cooper JS, Henson DE, et al, eds. *AJCC Cancer Staging Manual.* 5th ed. Philadelphia, Pa: Lippincott Williams & Wilkins; 1997:231-234.

*Note: Laterality does not affect the N classification.

dysfunction, hypercalcemia, fever of unknown origin, hypertension, and erythrocytosis (although anemia is more common).[47,48]

The diagnosis of renal cell carcinoma is established radiographically in 95% of cases, with intravenous pyelography, angiography, CT, or magnetic resonance imaging demonstrating the characteristic solid, hypervascular intrarenal mass (Fig. 24-4).

Treatment of Localized Disease
Surgery

Surgery is the only treatment modality recognized to have the potential to cure localized renal cell carcinoma.

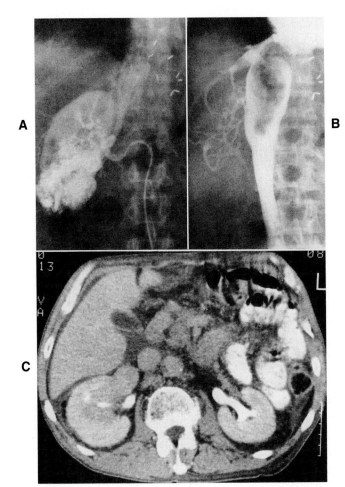

Fig. 24-4 Radiographic studies in renal cell carcinoma. **A,** Selective right renal angiogram showing a characteristic hypervascular renal cell carcinoma with inferior capsular extension. The linear opacification in the vena cava adjacent to the upper pole of the kidney suggests new vessel formation in a tumor thrombus. Note the characteristic origin of the renal artery at the inferior border of the L1 vertebra. **B,** The caval tumor thrombus is well demonstrated as a filling defect on the venacavogram. **C,** Computed tomography scan documenting the solid right renal mass with extension into the renal vein. The left kidney and opacified renal pelvis are normal. (Courtesy Dr. B. Kozak.)

Treatment for patients with localized renal cell carcinoma consists of radical nephrectomy—removal of the kidney and adrenal gland with surrounding perinephric fat and the intact Gerota's fascia. This procedure requires early clamping or ligation of the renal artery and vein. A limited lymph node dissection is usually included, although it has not been conclusively shown to improve patient survival.[49]

In patients with stage I or stage II disease, radical nephrectomy with lymph node dissection results in 5-year survival rates of about 80% and 65%, respectively.[50-52] In patients with lymph node metastases (stage III disease), radical nephrectomy results in a 5-year survival rate of approximately 40%.

Radiation Therapy

Moderately high doses of radiation can be delivered to the renal tubular epithelium before physiologic or morphologic injury becomes obvious. Thus it is not surprising that renal cell carcinoma, which arises from these same cells, has a similar or greater radiation tolerance.

Preoperative irradiation has been used as an adjuvant to facilitate resection, to sterilize well-oxygenated peripheral extensions of tumor that might be transected during nephrectomy, and to decrease the chance of dissemination at the time of nephrectomy. No studies show a consistent survival benefit, although improvement in resectability has been noted.[53-57] Preoperative irradiation to 20 to 30 Gy in 3 weeks produces few significant gross or microscopic changes.[58]

Postoperative irradiation has been used for patients with perinephric, lymphatic, or venous involvement. Several series demonstrate improved local disease control but with inconsistent effects on survival (Table 24-2).[46,58-66] For example, Rafla[64] noted a survival

		TABLE 24-2

Five-Year Survival Rates in Patients with Renal Cell Carcinoma Treated with Nephrectomy or Nephrectomy and Irradiation

	5-YEAR SURVIVAL (%)	
Authors and Reference	Nephrectomy	Irradiation
Bratherton[59]	29	43
Fugitt et al[60]	44	36
Flocks and Kadesky[58]	48	52
Kjaer et al[61]	62*	38
Mantyla et al[62]	57	56
Peeling et al[63]	52	25
Rafla[64]	37	56
Riches et al[65,66]	30	49
Skinner et al[44]	57	50

*Estimated.

advantage only for patients with capsular invasion and no other adverse prognostic factors. We suggest that this selected group of patients with extensive local disease should be considered for postoperative irradiation. The chance of local recurrence is significant, and the risk of dissemination is not so great as in patients with lymph node involvement. Studies have indicated that doses of 45 to 50 Gy can be given with acceptable bowel and hepatic complications; however, a dose of 50 Gy is suggested as the tolerance limit for the upper abdominal gastrointestinal tract.[27,67]

Two studies[61,68] have called attention to the problem of complications. Kjaer and colleagues[61] reported excessive bowel and hepatic complications in 12 of 27 patients and an irradiation-related mortality rate of 19% in a prospective clinical trial in which patients received 2.5 Gy four times a week to large fields. In this study, the poor outcomes are explained in part by the fractionation scheme. Feh and colleagues[68] noted four radiation-related deaths in 29 patients treated with postoperative irradiation. They have since become more selective in choosing patients for adjuvant irradiation and have noted fewer complications and no increase in the local failure rate. In a recent study by Stein and colleagues,[69] postnephrectomy irradiation reduced the rate of local recurrence in 67 patients with stage T3 tumors from 37% (11 of 30 nonirradiated patients) to 11% (4 of 37 irradiated patients). No benefit was noted in patients with earlier-stage disease.

Irradiation portals (Fig. 24-5) should initially encompass the renal fossa and primary hilar and periaortic nodal drainage areas. Opposed anteroposterior or oblique portals are used with a shrinking field technique, which reduces exposure to dose-limiting adjacent structures (spinal cord, bowel, and liver).[57] Figure 24-6 shows bowel filling the left renal fossa after nephrectomy for renal cell carcinoma. This underscores the importance of careful treatment planning to avoid gastrointestinal injuries. Intraoperative irradiation has the advantage of precise retroperitoneal localization with the ability to exclude intraperitoneal structures from the treatment field. This initial boost is then supplemented with moderate-dose external irradiation to the larger volume at risk.

In the rare case of local recurrence in the renal fossa as the only site of failure, aggressive therapy may result in long-term disease-free survival.[70] We have used brachytherapy after surgical excision in this situation.

Adjuvant Systemic Therapy

Adjuvant systemic therapy has not been found to be beneficial in the treatment of nonmetastatic renal cell carcinoma. No published randomized trials of adjuvant chemotherapy for localized renal cell carcinoma have been done, and few nonrandomized trials are available for review. Masuda and colleagues[71] reported a series of

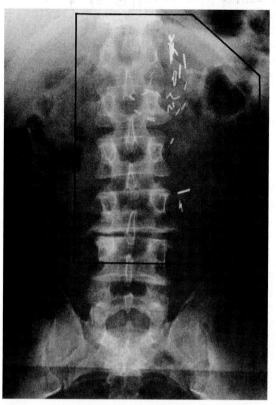

Fig. 24-5 Initial postoperative irradiation portals designed to encompass the renal fossa and primary lymphatic drainage.

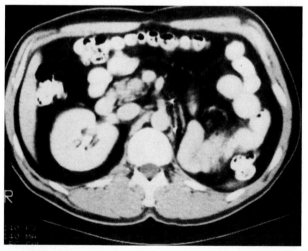

Fig. 24-6 Computed tomography scan showing the left renal fossa occupied by bowel after left radical nephrectomy for renal cell carcinoma. Careful treatment planning is necessary to avoid radiation-induced gastrointestinal injuries.

31 patients who received vinblastine, doxorubicin, and tegafur in a postoperative setting. The results from this trial were promising—the 1-year survival rate was 100%, and the 3- and 5-year survival rates were 96%—but no subsequent studies have been designed to confirm these findings. In addition, three randomized trials have

TABLE 24-3

Relationship between Tumor-Node-Metastasis Stage and Survival in Patients with Renal Cell Carcinoma

Stage/Grade	5-YEAR SURVIVAL (%)	
	Bassil*	Literature†
T1	100	55-85
T2	90	—
T3	58	8-70
T3a	72	—
T3b	56	—
T3c	29	—
T4	25	0-20
N+	7	5-30
M+	18	0-10
Solitary metastasis	—	20-35
Grade 1	—	80
Grade 2	—	60
Grade 3	—	40

*Data from Bassil B, Dosoretz DE, Prout GR Jr. *J Urol* 1985;134:450-454.
†Data from McDonald MW. *J Urol* 1982;127:211-217.

examined the use of interferon-? in an adjuvant setting, but none of these trials showed a delay in time to relapse or an improvement in overall survival.[72-74]

Results

The TNM staging system accurately indicates prognosis in patients with renal cell carcinoma (Table 24-3).[75,76] Local extension, lymph node involvement, extensive vena caval extension, and distant metastases are strong predictors of worse prognosis. However, the wide variety of results of therapy reported in the literature makes it difficult to predict outcomes after treatment. This variety is in great part the result of differences between the various staging systems (e.g., some old systems do not distinguish renal vein extension and lymph node involvement) and the unpredictable natural history of renal cell carcinoma.

Treatment of Disseminated Disease

Most patients with renal cell carcinoma will either have at diagnosis (30%) or subsequently develop (50%) disseminated disease. The most common metastatic sites, in descending order of frequency, are lung, lymph nodes, liver, bone, adrenal glands, opposite kidney, brain, and soft tissue. The outcome for patients with metastatic disease (stage IV disease) after radical nephrectomy is dismal, with 5-year survival rates of less than 10%. Rarely, distant metastases have regressed after nephrectomy, but response of metastases is not considered justification for nephrectomy.

TABLE 24-4

Rates of Response of Renal Cell Tumors to Single-Agent Chemotherapy

Agent	Number of Patients	Number of Responders	Response Rate (%)
Cisplatin	54	0	0
Cyclophosphamide	66	2	3
Epirubicin	39	0	0
Fluorouracil	138	7	5
Isofosfamide	46	3	6
Vinblastine	135	9	7

Modified from Hartmann JT, Bokemeyer C. *Anticancer Res* 1999;19:1541-1543.

Cytotoxic Chemotherapy

Renal cell carcinoma is believed to be highly resistant to systemic chemotherapy, and no agent is considered to be standard in the treatment of this disease. Commonly used agents produce only marginal response rates, and no clear survival benefit has been demonstrated.[77] For single agents, response rates of 4% to 6% are commonly seen, which are similar to response rates in patients not receiving chemotherapy[78] (Table 24-4). As Amato[78] has noted, most trials of single-agent therapy did not have adequate control groups, and therefore the response rates are difficult to assess.

Only two agents have shown more than minimal antitumor activity. A 1984 trial with 19 patients treated with vinblastine (4 to 6 mg/m^2/wk) reported a response rate of 16%.[79] However, no complete responses were obtained, and only 3 of 19 patients had a partial response. Furthermore, subsequent trials have failed to replicate these findings and have yielded results more in line with other reported rates of response to chemotherapy—about 5%.[80] The other single agent that has produced more than minimal response is floxuridine. Hrushesky and colleagues,[81] in a trial with 63 patients, noted a complete response in four patients and a partial response in another seven patients, for an overall response rate of 20%. Unfortunately, as was true for vinblastine, floxuridine has in subsequent trials failed to measure up to initial expectations.

Combinations of chemotherapeutic agents also have been tried—most often combinations including vinblastine—but to date none has consistently or significantly shown improvement in the survival of patients with disseminated renal cell carcinoma (Table 24-5). A recent study by Childs and colleagues,[82] using high-dose cyclophosphamide and fludarabine followed by allogenic peripheral stem-cell transplantation in 19 patients with metastatic renal cell carcinoma, showed promising results, with complete responses in three patients and partial responses in seven patients, for an overall response rate of 53%. This represents one of the best

TABLE 24-5

Rates of Response of Renal Cell Tumors to Multiagent Chemotherapy

Agents	Number of Patients	Number of Responders	Responmse Rate (%)
Vinblastine+ floxuridine	11	2	18
Vinblastine+ doxorubicin	28	4	14
Vinblastine+ hydroxyurea	14	2	14
Cyclophosphamide+ metronidazole	31	1	3

From Hartmann JT, Bokemeyer C. *Anticancer Res* 1999;19: 1541-1543.

TABLE 24-6

Results of Combination Therapy with Multidrug Resistance Modulators in Renal Cell Carcinoma

Agents	Number of Patients	Response Rate and Study Reference
Vinblastine+ interferon	40	42%[a]
	56	16%[b]
	42	14%[c]
Fluorouracil+ interferon	21	24%[d]
	31	23%[e]
Floxuridine+ interferon	20	0%[f]
	15	33%[g]

[a]Data from Bergerat JP, Herbrecht R, Dufour P, et al. *Cancer* 1988;62:2320-2324.
[b]Data from Schornagel JH, Verweij J, ten Bokkel Huinink WN, et al. *J Urol* 1989;142:253-256.
[c]Massidda B, Migliari R, Padovani A, et al. *J Chemother* 1991;3:387-389.
[d]Schuth J, Goldschmidtt JW, Tunn UV. *Eur J Cancer* 1993;29:234.
[e]Haarstad H, Jacobsen AB, Schjolseth SA, et al. *Ann Oncol* 1994;5:245-248.
[f]Stadler WM, Vogelzang NJ, Vokes EE, et al. *Cancer Chemother Pharmacol* 1992;31:213-216.
[g]Falcone A, Cianci C, Ricci S, et al. *Cancer* 1993;72:564-568.

response rates reported to date in renal cell carcinoma and indicates that this treatment strategy deserves further investigation.

The failure of single-agent and multiagent chemotherapy to improve survival in patients with disseminated renal cell carcinoma is believed to be due in part to the phenomenon of multidrug resistance (MDR). MDR has been associated with the *MDR1* gene and its product, p-glycoprotein 170.[83] RNA for *MDR1* and its product have been found in 80% of renal tumors.[84] Thus chemotherapy alone would not be expected to have much success in renal cell carcinoma. Understanding of the process of MDR has resulted in attempts being made to overcome drug resistance by using modulators of MDR. Although in vitro studies with MDR modulators such as cyclosporin A, dipyridamole, nifedipine, and tamoxifen in combination with either vinblastine or floxuridine showed increased activity, in vivo studies failed to confirm these findings[85-87] (Table 24-6). Thus combination therapy with MDR modulators has, like chemotherapy, failed to significantly improve survival in disseminated renal cell carcinoma. These findings have led to the realization that MDR is a multifactorial process in renal cell carcinoma. Accordingly, although chemotherapy may still offer some degree of improvement in survival, investigational options should be offered to patients whose disease does not respond to conventional therapy.

Immunotherapy

In addition to chemotherapy, immunoresponsive therapies have been proposed in the treatment of renal cell carcinoma. Immunotherapy is based on enhancing the immune response against the tumor. This strategy relies on a variety of immune-response modifiers, including interferons, tumor necrosis factor, and interleukins. Interferon-? and interleukin-2 have been extensively studied in metastatic renal cell carcinoma and have produced response rates up to 20%.[88] Interferons act

by activating mononuclear cells to increase expression of major histocompatibility complex molecules. Two possible mechanisms of action are antiproliferation and antiangiogenesis.[88] Interleukins seem to work by activating cytotoxic lymphocytes of the natural killer and thymic subsets.[89]

The initial single-institution phase II trials of interferon showed response rates greater than the 5% typically seen with chemotherapy. However, results from multicenter studies have not been so promising. The Medical Research Council multicenter phase III trial in which interferon-α was delivered at daily doses of 10×10^6 U/m^2 for at least 3 months resulted in a maximal response rate of 14%.[90] From the various studies, no clear dose-response effect or optimal duration of therapy has been established. Side effects do seem to be dose-related, with nausea, diarrhea, anorexia, liver dysfunction, thrombocytopenia, and leukopenia seen at higher doses.[91] Recent results from a randomized trial by the Southwest Oncology Group[91a] indicate that nephrectomy followed by subcutaneous therapy with interferon-α-2b conferred a survival benefit relative to treatment with interferon-α-2b alone for patients with metastatic renal cell cancer (median survival duration 11.1 months vs. 8.1 months, $P = 0.05$). This difference was independent of performance status, metastatic site, and the presence or absence of a measurable metastatic lesion.[91a]

The principal interleukin used in the treatment of renal cell carcinoma has been interleukin-2. Multiple dosing regimens have been proposed and tested in phase II trials. A National Cancer Institute trial tested the efficacy of high-dose bolus, continuous-infusion therapy, and subcutaneous administration.[92] An interim analysis showed similar response rates in the three study arms (11.3% for high-dose bolus, 10.9% for continuous infusion, and 14.7% for subcutaneous administration). The high-dose bolus arm did have a longer durability of response, but completion of the trial is needed before a complete analysis can be done.[93,94]

Adjuvant Nephrectomy

On rare but well-publicized occasions, renal cell carcinoma has been associated with the spontaneous regression of metastases (usually pulmonary and many times not histologically documented).[39] Adjuvant nephrectomy has been suggested in an attempt to induce regression of metastases. Present evidence does not support nephrectomy in this situation. However, nephrectomy and angiographic infarction or placement of radioactive sources (see the next section) are options for the patient with severe hemorrhage or intractable pain.

Radiation Therapy

Although renal cell carcinoma has been regarded as a relatively radioresistant neoplasm, irradiation is the most consistent method of palliation in patients with symptomatic metastases. Doses of 45 to 50 Gy in 4 to 5 weeks are effective in more than 65% of patients with painful bone and soft tissue metastases. Irradiation of central nervous system metastases has been less successful.[54,94-96]

Aggressive therapy in patients with apparently solitary metastatic lesions seems warranted, with several series reporting 5-year survival rates of 30%.[76,97,98] Surgical resection and irradiation both can be effective in treating isolated metastases. Kjaer[99] recently updated a series of 25 patients treated primarily with irradiation (45 to 50 Gy). Bone and lung were the two most common metastatic sites, and the 5- and 10-year survival rates were 36% and 16%, with women faring noticeably better than men. However, many of these patients died of disseminated disease after 5 years.

UROTHELIAL TUMORS OF THE RENAL PELVIS AND URETER
Epidemiology and Risk Factors

Tumors of the renal pelvis and ureter account for 8% to 10% of renal tumors and fewer than 1% of all genitourinary neoplasms. Tumors of the renal pelvis and ureter are 3 times as common in men as in women, and the peak incidence is in the sixth and seventh decades.[100] These tumors are associated with exposure to occupational and environmental toxins and cigarette smoking.[101] Analgesic abuse,[1,102,103] Balkan nephropathy,[104,105] cyclophosphamide chemotherapy,[106] and exposure to thorium dioxide contrast agent[41] (withdrawn from use in the 1950s) also are associated with increased risk.

Pathology and Staging

Among tumors of the renal pelvis and ureter, 85% to 90% are transitional cell carcinomas, and two thirds of these are papillary tumors with the same histologic features and propensity for multicentricity and recurrence as transitional cell carcinomas of the urinary bladder. A patient with a transitional cell carcinoma of the upper urinary tract has a 30% to 50% chance of having or developing an associated bladder tumor.[107-110] Tumors of the renal pelvis are 3 times as common as ureteral tumors. The majority of ureteral tumors occur in the lower third of the ureter.[111]

No universally accepted staging system exists for tumors of the renal pelvis and ureter. We favor a system similar to the bladder tumor staging system, which recognizes the prognostic significance of depth of invasion and histologic grade and the correlation between these two factors and the presence of lymph node involvement and propensity for dissemination. The AJCC TNM classification for cancer of the renal pelvis and ureter is shown in Box 24-3.[45]

One in 10 patients have squamous cell carcinomas, which are often associated with urinary tract obstruction, infection, and kidney stones. In contrast to many transitional cell tumors, squamous cell carcinomas are likely to be asymptomatic, solitary, sessile, invasive, and associated with a poor prognosis.[100,112] Squamous cell carcinomas account for 30% to 50% of the upper urinary tract tumors found in patients who abuse analgesics.

The histologic types are as follows: transitional cell carcinoma, papillary carcinoma, squamous cell carcinoma, epidermoid carcinoma, adenocarcinoma, and urothelial carcinoma.

Clinical Features and Diagnosis

Patients with tumors of the renal pelvis and ureter present with hematuria (60% to 75%) and sometimes pain (20% to 40%).[113] Only 5% to 15% have a palpable abdominal or flank mass.[114] Intravenous or retrograde pyelography (the most definitive radiographic study) demonstrates a nonopaque filling defect in the renal pelvis or ureter. The differential diagnosis includes tumor, uric acid stone, a sloughed renal papilla, blood clot, or air. The diagnosis is established with cytologic evaluation or endoscopic biopsy.

Treatment of Localized Disease
Surgery

The classic treatment for tumors of the renal pelvis and ureter has been nephroureterectomy including a cuff of bladder, although local resection is becoming more popular as accurate in situ staging allows better selection of patients. Because of the high local tumor

---

Box 24-3   American Joint Committee on Cancer Staging System for Cancer of the Renal Pelvis and Ureter

PRIMARY TUMOR (T)

TX	Primary tumor cannot be assessed
T0	No evidence of primary tumor
Ta	Papillary noninvasive carcinoma
Tis	Carcinoma in situ
T1	Tumor invades subepithelial connective tissue
T2	Tumor invades the muscularis
T3	(For renal pelvis only) Tumor invades beyond muscularis into peripelvic fat or the renal parenchyma
T3	(For ureter only) Tumor invades beyond muscularis into periureteric fat
T4	Tumor invades adjacent organs, or through the kidney into the perinephric fat

REGIONAL LYMPH NODES (N)*

NX	Regional lymph nodes cannot be assessed
N0	No regional lymph node metastasis
N1	Metastasis in a single lymph node, 2 cm or less in greatest dimension
N2	Metastasis in a single lymph node, more than 2 cm but not more than 5 cm in greatest dimension; or

multiple lymph nodes, none more than 5 cm in greatest dimension

N3	Metastasis in a lymph node more than 5 cm in greatest dimension

DISTANT METASTASIS (M)

MX	Distant metastasis cannot be assessed
M0	No distant metastasis
M1	Distant metastasis

STAGE GROUPING

Stage 0a	Ta	N0	M0
Stage 0is	Tis	N0	M0
Stage I	T1	N0	M0
Stage II	T2	N0	M0
Stage III	T3	N0	M0
Stage IV	T4	N0	M0
	Any T	N1	M0
	Any T	N2	M0
	Any T	N3	M0
	Any T	Any N	M1

From Fleming I, Cooper JS, Henson DE, et al, eds. *AJCC Cancer Staging Manual.* 5th ed. Philadelphia, Pa: Lippincott Williams & Wilkins; 1997:235-237.

---

recurrence rate (20% to 40%) after failure to remove the entire ureter, the high frequency of ipsilateral multicentricity (50%), and the possibility of bilateral tumors (2% to 4%), local resection is indicated only in patients with solitary, low-grade, noninvasive tumors, in patients with bilateral tumors, and in patients in whom preservation of renal function is mandatory.[100,108,113-115]

Radiation Therapy

The overall survival rate of less than 30% in patients with poor risk factors (muscle invasion, high-grade tumors, nodal involvement) has prompted consideration of adjuvant irradiation in an attempt to increase local tumor control and improve survival. Brookland and Richter[116] identified 23 such patients and administered postoperative irradiation (50 Gy in 5 weeks) to 11 of them. Only one local treatment failure was noted, and it was associated with systemic disease. In contrast, five local treatment failures occurred in the control group of 12 patients not treated with radiation therapy. This experience suggests that postoperative irradiation reduced the local failure rate. However, survival was only marginally improved, which indicates the need for effective systemic therapy. A report by Cozad and colleagues[117] supports the value of radiation therapy in patients with advanced (T3 and T4) tumors of the renal pelvis and ureter: local failure occurred in 9 of 17 patients who had resection alone but in only 1 of 9

patients who received adjuvant radiation therapy. Multivariate analysis revealed the grade of the tumor and the use of radiation therapy to be significant predictors of local recurrence. Radiation therapy did not alter distant metastasis and survival rates. Babaian and colleagues[118] were more apt to use postoperative irradiation in patients with invasive ureteral tumors than in those with tumors of the renal pelvis. These different approaches to tumors of the renal pelvis and the ureter are based on the perceived difference in the natural history of the two tumors. In patients with tumors of the renal pelvis, systemic metastasis is more common than local treatment failure, whereas patients with ureteral tumors are more apt to have symptomatic local disease recurrences (pain, edema).

Although adjuvant irradiation has no clearly defined role in the treatment of tumors of the renal pelvis and ureter, we favor consideration of postoperative irradiation and chemotherapy after surgical resection in patients having positive tumor margins, local tumor extension, residual gross disease, or limited nodal involvement.

In patients who undergo nephroureterectomy for tumors of the renal pelvis and ureter, postoperative irradiation portals may encompass not only the renal fossa but the entire ureteral bed and ipsilateral trigone, the extent being dictated by clinical information obtained at the time of surgery and from pathologic analysis of the resected specimen. Trials are needed to assess the use of

TABLE 24-7

Relationship Between Grade and Stage and Survival in Urothelial Tumors of the Renal Pelvis

Classification	5-Year Survival (%)
GRADE	
1	80
2	50
3	20
STAGE	
T1-T2	80
T3-T4	20
POSITIVE LYMPH NODES	**10**
METASTASES	**0**

Data from Kakizoe T, Fujita J, Murase T, et al. *J Urol* 1980;124:17-19; Williams CB, Mitchell JP. *Br J Urol* 1973;45:370-376; Nativ O, Reiman HM, LieberMM, et al. *Cancer* 1991;68:2575-2578; Cummungs KB. *Urol Clin North Am* 1980;7:569-578; Latham HS, Kay S. *Surg Gynecol Obstet* 1974;138:613-622; Rubenstein MA, Walz BJ, Bucy JG. *J Urol* 1978;119:594-597.

adjuvant irradiation and chemotherapy with seemingly effective agents such as methotrexate, vinblastine, doxorubicin, and cisplatin in patients at high risk for local and systemic treatment failure after surgical resection.

Results

Two thirds of patients with tumors of the renal pelvis are diagnosed with invasive (stage T2 to T4) or metastatic disease, and the reported overall 5-year survival rate of 20% to 50% reflects this.[113] However, as is true for transitional cell carcinoma of the bladder, prognosis depends on and treatment is dictated by the depth of invasion and the histopathologic grade of the tumor (Table 24-7).[100,110,113,119-121]

Treatment of Disseminated Disease

Tumors of the renal pelvis and ureter are similar to the urothelial tumors of the bladder, and irradiation of specific symptomatic sites, as well as combination chemotherapy with methotrexate, vinblastine, doxorubicin, and cisplatin, should be considered in patients with advanced disease.

SUMMARY

The kidney is unavoidably irradiated during therapy for many abdominal and retroperitoneal malignancies, and knowledge of the early and late effects of irradiation is essential for proper treatment planning. When significant portions of both kidneys are included within the therapy field, the total dose should be kept under 20 Gy at usual

fractionation to avoid the risk of progressive radiation nephropathy. When more than half of one kidney receives 26 Gy or more, clinical radiation nephropathy is rare, but measurable functional changes do occur.

Renal cell carcinoma is the predominant renal tumor in adults and is an adenocarcinoma of proximal tubular origin. Patients usually have hematuria. The stage of the neoplasm at the time of initial therapy is the most important prognostic factor. Radical nephrectomy is the treatment of choice in patients with localized disease. The clinical course in these patients is unpredictable, with metastatic disease sometimes appearing after 10 to 20 years of apparently disease-free status. Routine adjuvant irradiation, either preoperative or postoperative, has no well-defined role in the management of patients with renal cell carcinoma, and no effective systemic therapy has been found. We favor postoperative irradiation, 45 to 50 Gy at 1.8 Gy/fraction, to shrinking fields covering the resected renal fossa and hilar nodal drainage areas in patients with perinephric invasion or limited nodal involvement. Aggressive therapy in patients with solitary metastases is associated with an expected 5-year survival rate of 30% after surgery or irradiation.

Tumors of the renal pelvis and ureter are epithelial carcinomas having their origin in the transitional epithelium lining the renal pelvis and ureter. Like urinary bladder tumors, they range from superficial, well-differentiated papillary tumors with a tendency for multicentricity and recurrence to sessile, invasive lesions with early metastatic potential. The majority of patients have hematuria as the initial sign, and the diagnosis is made using endoscopy, pyelography, and cytologic examination. Classic treatment has been nephroureterectomy including a cuff of bladder, although local resection is applicable in selected patients with solitary, well-differentiated tumors. Prognosis is dependent on the histologic grade of the tumor and the depth of invasion, which accurately predict the probability of nodal involvement and dissemination. Although adjuvant irradiation has no strictly defined role, we favor consideration of postoperative irradiation and chemotherapy in patients having positive tumor margins, local tumor extension, residual gross disease, or limited nodal involvement. Combination chemotherapy with methotrexate, vinblastine, doxorubicin, and cisplatin has demonstrated activity in metastatic disease. Because of the high incidence of multiple and recurrent tumors in patients with transitional cell carcinoma of the renal pelvis and ureter, careful long-term follow-up is mandatory.

REFERENCES

1. Simon AL. Normal renal size: an absolute criterion. *Am J Roentgenol* 1964;92:270-273.
2. Roswit B, Malsky SJ, Reid CB. Radiation tolerance of the gastrointestinal tract. *Front Radiat Ther Oncol* 1972;6:160-181.
3. Withers HR. Predicting late normal tissue responses. *Int J Radiat Oncol Biol Phys* 1986;12:693-698.

4. Zuelzer WW, Palmer HD, Newton WA Jr. Unusual glomerulo-nephritis in young children is probably radiation nephritis. *Am J Pathol* 1950;26:1019-1039.

5. Bennett WM, Elzinga LW, Porter GA. Tubulointerstitial disease and toxic nephropathy. In: Brenner BM, Rector FC, eds. *The Kidney.* Vol 2. 4th ed. Philadelphia, Pa: WB Saunders; 1991: 1430-1496.

6. Heptinstall RH. Irradiation injury and effects of heavy metals. In: Heptinstall RH, ed. *Pathology of the Kidney.* Vol 3. 4th ed. Boston, Mass: Little-Brown; 1992:2085-2111.

7. Kunkler PB, Farr RF, Luxton RW, et al. The limit of renal tolerance to x-rays: an investigation into renal damage occurring following the treatment of tumors of the testis by abdominal baths. *Br J Radiol* 1952;25:190-201.

8. Luxton RW. Radiation nephritis. *Q J Med* 1953;22:215-242.

9. Luxton RW. Radiation nephritis: a long-term study of 54 patients. *Lancet* 1961;2:1221-1224.

10. Luxton RW. The clinical and pathological effects of renal irradiation. *Progress in Radiation Therapy* 1962;2:15-34.

11. Kunkler PB. The significance of radiosensitivity of the kidney. *Progress in Radiation Therapy* 1962;2:35-41.

12. Avioli LV, Lazor MZ, Cotlove E. Early effects of radiation on renal function in man. *Am J Med* 1963;34:329-337.

13. Madrazo AA, Churg J. Radiation nephritis. Chronic changes following moderate doses of radiation. *Lab Invest* 1976;34:283-290.

14. Mostofi FK. Radiation effects on the kidney. In: Mostofi FK, Smith DE, eds. *The Kidney* (International Academy of Pathology monograph no. 6). Baltimore, Md: Williams & Wilkins; 1966:338-363.

15. Ives HE, Daniel TO. Vascular diseases of the kidney. In: Brenner BM, Rector FC, eds. *The Kidney.* Vol 2. 4th ed. Philadelphia, Pa: WB Saunders; 1991:1497-1550.

16. Maher JF. Radiation nephropathy. In: Massrey SG, Glassock RJ, eds. *Textbook of Nephrology.* Baltimore, Md: Williams & Wilkins; 1989:860-862.

17. White DC. *An Atlas of Radiation Histopathology.* Washington, DC: United States Energy and Research Administration; 1975.

18. Asscher AW, Anson SC. Arterial hypertension and irradiation damage to the nervous system. *Lancet* 1962;2:1343-1346.

19. Asscher AW. The delayed effects of renal irradiation. *Clin Radiol* 1964;15:320-325.

20. Dewit L, Anninga JK, Hoefnagel CA, et al. Radiation injury in the human kidney: a prospective analysis using specific scintigraphic and biochemical endpoints. *Int J Radiat Oncol Biol Phys* 1990; 19:977-983.

21. Rubin P. The law and order of radiation sensitivity, absolute and relative. In: Vaeth JM, Meyer JL, eds. *Radiation Tolerance of Normal Tissues.* Vol. 23. Basel, Switzerland: Karger; 1989:7-40.

22. Willett CG, Tepper JE, Orlow EL, et al. Renal complications secondary to radiation treatment of upper abdominal malignancies. *Int J Radiat Oncol Biol Phys* 1986;12:1601-1604.

23. Donaldson SS, Moskowitz PS, Canty EL, et al. Radiation-induced inhibition of compensatory renal growth in the weanling mouse kidney. *Radiology* 1978;128:491-495.

24. Maor MH, North LB, Cabanillas FF, et al. Outcomes of high-dose unilateral kidney irradiation in patients with gastric lymphoma. *Int J Radiat Oncol Biol Phys* 1998;41:647-650.

25. Vogelzang NJ. Nephrotoxicity from chemotherapy: prevention and management. *Oncology (Huntingt)* 1991;5:97-102.

26. Phillips TL, Fu KK. Quantification of combined radiation therapy and chemotherapy effects on critical normal tissues. *Cancer* 1976;37:1186-1200.

27. Bergstein J, Andreoli SP, Provisor AJ, et al. Radiation nephritis following total-body irradiation and cyclophosphamide in preparation for bone marrow transplantation. *Transplantation* 1986;41:63-66.

28. Donaldson SS, Moskowitz PS, Canty EL, et al. Combination radiation-Adriamycin therapy: reniprival growth, functional and structural effects in the immature mouse. *Int J Radiat Oncol Biol Phys* 1980;6:851-859.

29. Yatvin MB, Oberley TD, Mahler PA. The beneficial effect of dietary protein restriction on radiation nephropathy. *Strahlentherapie* 1984;160:707-714.

30. Greenlee RT, Hill-Harmon MB, Murray T, et al. Cancer statistics, 2001. *CA Cancer J Clin* 2001;51:15-36.

31. McLaughlin JK, Blot WJ, Devesa SS. Renal cancer. In: Schotterfeld T, Fraumeni JFJ, eds. *Cancer Epidemiology and Prevention.* 2nd ed. New York, NY: Oxford University Press; 1996:1142-1155.

32. Bennington JL, Ferguson BR, Campbell PB. Epidemiologic studies of carcinoma of the kidney. II. Association of renal adenoma with smoking. *Cancer* 1968;22:821-823.

33. Moul JW. Renal cell carcinoma. *Probl Urol* 1990;4:225-275.

34. Keeler LL III, Klauber GT. Von Hippel-Lindau disease and renal cell carcinoma in a 16-year-old boy. *J Urol* 1992;147:1588-1591.

35. Christoferson LA, Gustafson MB, Petersen AG. Von Hippel-Lindau's disease. *JAMA* 1961;178:280-282.

36. Goodman MD, Goodman BK, Lubin MB, et al. Cytogenetic characterization of renal cell carcinoma in von Hippel-Lindau syndrome. *Cancer* 1990;65:1150-1154.

37. Glenn GM, Choyke PL, Zbar B. Von Hippel-Lindau disease: clinical review and molecular genetics. *Probl Urol* 1990;4: 312-330.

38. Dunnill MS, Millard PR, Oliver D. Acquired cystic disease of the kidneys: a hazard of long-term intermittent maintenance haemodialysis. *J Clin Pathol* 1977;30:868-877.

39. Bloom HJG, Dukes CE, Mitchelen BCV. Hormone dependent tumors of the kidney—the estrogen induced renal tumor in the Syrian hamster: hormone treatment and possible relationship to carcinoma of the kidney in man. *Br J Cancer* 1963;17: 611-645.

40. Bloom HJ. Proceedings: Hormone-induced and spontaneous regression of metastatic renal cancer. *Cancer* 1973;32:1066-1071.

41. Almgard LE, Ahlgren L, Boeryd B, et al. Thorotrast-induced renal tumours after retrograde pyelogram. *Eur Urol* 1977;3:69-72.

42. Oberling C, Riviere M, Haguenau F. Ultrastructure of the clear cells in renal carcinomas and its importance of the demonstration of their renal origins. *Nature* 1960;186:402-403.

43. Ericsson JLE, Seljeled R, Orrenius S. Comparative light and electron microscopic observations of the cytoplasmic matrix in renal carcinomas. *Virchows Arch* 1966;341:204-223.

44. Krueger RP. Sarcomas of the kidney. *Probl Urol* 1990;4:296-311.

45. Fleming I, Cooper JS, Henson DE, et al, eds. *AJCC Cancer Staging Manual.* 5th ed. Philadelphia, Pa: Lippincott Williams & Wilkins; 1997:231-234.

46. Skinner DG, Colvin RB, Vermillion CD, et al. Diagnosis and management of renal cell carcinoma. A clinical and pathologic study of 309 cases. *Cancer* 1971;28:1165-1177.

47. Cronin RE, Kaehny WD, Miller PD, et al. Renal cell carcinoma: unusual systemic manifestations. *Medicine (Baltimore)* 1976;55:291-311.

48. Sufrin G, Chasan S, Golio A, et al. Paraneoplastic and serologic syndromes of renal adenocarcinoma. *Semin Urol* 1989;7:158-171.

49. Herrlinger A, Schrott KM, Schott G, et al. What are the benefits of extended dissection of the regional renal lymph nodes in the therapy of renal cell carcinoma. *J Urol* 1991;146:1224-1227.

50. Guinan PD, Vogelzang NJ, Fremgen AM, et al. Renal cell carcinoma: tumor size, stage and survival. Members of the Cancer Incidence and End Results Committee. *J Urol* 1995;153:901-903.

51. Dinney CP, Awad SA, Gajewski JB, et al. Analysis of imaging modalities, staging systems, and prognostic indicators for renal cell carcinoma. *Urology* 1992;39:122-129.

52. Golimbu M, Joshi P, Sperber A, et al. Renal cell carcinoma: survival and prognostic factors. *Urology* 1986;27:291-301.

53. Brady LW, Jr. Carcinoma of the kidney—the role for radiation therapy. *Semin Oncol* 1983;10:417-421.

54. Cox CE, Lacy SS, Montgomery WG, et al. Renal adenocarcinoma: 28-year review, with emphasis on rationale and feasibility of preoperative radiotherapy. *J Urol* 1970;104:53-61.

55. Rost A, Brosig W. Preoperative irradiation of renal cell carcinoma. *Urology* 1977;10:414-417.

56. Rubin P, Keller B, Cox C, et al. Preoperative irradiation in renal cancer. Evaluation of radiation treatment plans. *Am J Roentgenol Radium Ther Nucl Med* 1975;123:114-121.

57. Van der Werf-Messing B. Carcinoma of the kidney. *Cancer* 1973;32:1056-1061.

58. Flocks RH, Kadesky MC. Malignant neoplasms of kidney. *J Urol* 1958;79:196-201.

59. Bratherton DG. Tumors of kidneys and suprarenals: place of radiotherapy in treatment of hypernephroma. *Br J Radiol* 1964;37:141-146.

60. Fugitt RB, Wu GS, Martinelli LC. An evaluation of postoperative radiotherapy in hypernephroma treatment: a clinical trial. *Cancer* 1973;32:1332-1340.

61. Kjaer M, Frederiksen PL, Engelholm SA. Postoperative radiotherapy in stage II and III renal adenocarcinoma. A randomized trial by the Copenhagen Renal Cancer Study Group. *Int J Radiat Oncol Biol Phys* 1987;13:665-672.

62. Mantyla M, Nordman E, Minkkinen J. Postoperative radiotherapy of renal adenocarcinoma. *Ann Clin Res* 1977;9:252-256.

63. Peeling WB, Mantell BS, Shepheard BG. Post-operative irradiation in the treatment of renal cell carcinoma. *Br J Urol* 1969;41:23-31.

64. Rafla S. Renal cell carcinoma. Natural history and results of treatment. *Cancer* 1970;25:26-40.

65. Riches EW, Griffiths IH, Thackray AC. New growths of the kidney and ureter. *Br J Urol* 1951;23:297-356.

66. Riches E. The place of radiotherapy in the management of parenchymal carcinoma of the kidney. *J Urol* 1966;95:313-317.

67. Rubin P, Casarett GW. *Clinical Radiation Pathology*. Philadelphia, Pa: WB Saunders; 1968.

68. Feh M, Pinter J, Szokoly V. Problems of the indications of radiotherapy in renal tumours after radical nephrectomy. *Int Urol Nephrol* 1984;16:29-32.

69. Stein M, Kuten A, Halpern J, et al. The value of postoperative irradiation in renal cell cancer. *Radiother Oncol* 1992;24:41-44.

70. Esrig D, Ahlering TE, Lieskovsky G, et al. Experience with fossa recurrence of renal cell carcinoma. *J Urol* 1992;147:1491-1494.

71. Masuda F, Nakada J, Kondo I, et al. Adjuvant chemotherapy with vinblastine, Adriamycin, and UFT for renal-cell carcinoma. *Cancer Chemother Pharmacol* 1992;30:477-479.

72. Sandock DS, Seftel AD, Resnick MI. A new protocol for the follow-up of renal cell carcinoma based on pathological stage. *J Urol* 1995;154:28-31.

73. Rabinovitch RA, Zelefsky MJ, Gaynor JJ, et al. Patterns of failure following surgical resection of renal cell carcinoma: implications for adjuvant local and systemic therapy. *J Clin Oncol* 1994;12:206-212.

74. Levy DA, Slaton JW, Swanson DA, et al. Stage specific guidelines for surveillance after radical nephrectomy for local renal cell carcinoma. *J Urol* 1998;159:1163-1167.

75. Bassil B, Dosoretz DE, Prout GR Jr. Validation of the tumor, nodes, and metastasis classification of renal cell carcinoma. *J Urol* 1985;134:450-454.

76. McDonald MW. Current therapy for renal cell carcinoma. *J Urol* 1982;127:211-217.

77. Hartmann JT, Bokemeyer C. Chemotherapy for renal cell carcinoma. *Anticancer Res* 1999;19:1541-1543.

78. Amato RJ. Chemotherapy for renal cell carcinoma. *Semin Oncol* 2000;27:177-186.

79. Kuebler JP, Hogan TF, Trump DL, et al. Phase II study of continuous 5-day vinblastine infusion in renal adenocarcinoma. *Cancer Treat Rep* 1984;68:925-926.

80. Fossa SD, Droz JP, Pavone-Macaluso MM. Vinblastine in metastatic renal cell carcinoma: EORTC phase II trial 30882. *Eur J Cancer* 1992;28A:878.

81. Hrushesky WJ, von Roemeling R, Lanning RM, et al. Circadian-shaped infusions of floxuridine for progressive metastatic renal cell carcinoma. *J Clin Oncol* 1990;8:1504-1513.

82. Childs R, Chernoff A, Contentin N. Regression of metastatic renal cell carcinoma after nonmyeloablative allogeneic peripheral blood stem-cell transplantation. *N Engl J Med* 2000;343:750-758.

83. Fojo AT, Shen DW, Mickley LA. Intrinsic drug resistance in human kidney cancer is associated with expression of a human multidrug-resistance gene. *J Clin Oncol* 1987;5:1922-1927.

84. Goldstein LJ, Galski H, Fojo A. Expression of multidrug resistance gene in human cancers. *J Natl Cancer Inst* 1989;81:116-124.

85. Samuels BL, Trump DL, Rosner G, et al. Multidrug resistance modulator in renal cell carcinoma using cyclosporine-A or tamoxifen. *Proc Am Soc Clin Oncol* 1994;13:252.

86. Rodenburg CJ, Nooter K, Herewijer H. Phase II study of combining vinblastine and cyclosporine-A to circumvent multidrug resistance in renal cell cancer. *Ann Oncol* 1991;2:305-306.

87. Stadler WM, Vogelzang NJ, Vokes EE. Continuous infusion fluorodeoxyuridine with leucovorin and high-dose interferon: a phase II study in metastatic renal-cell cancer. *Cancer Chemother Pharmacol* 1992;31:213-216.

88. Vuky J, Motzer RJ. Cytokine therapy in renal cell cancer. *Urol Oncol* 2000;5:249.

89. Margolin KA. Interleukin-2 in the treatment of renal cancer. *Semin Oncol* 2000;27:194-203.

90. Interferon-alpha and survival in metastatic renal carcinoma: early results of a randomised controlled trial. Medical Research Council Renal Cancer Collaborators. *Lancet* 1999;353:14.

91. Pyhonen SO, Salminen E, Ruutu M. Prospective randomized trial of interferon alpha-2a plus vinblastine versus vinblastine alone in patients with advanced renal cell cancer. *J Clin Oncol* 1999;17:2859-2867.

91a. Flanigan RC, Salmon SE, Blumenstein BA, et al. Nephrectomy followed by interferon-alfa-2b compared with interferon alfa-2b alone for metastatic renal-cell cancer. *N Engl J Med* 2001;345:1655-1659.

92. Yang JC, Topalian SL, Parkinson D. Randomized comparison of high-dose and low-dose intravenous interleukin-2 for the therapy of metastatic renal cell carcinoma: an interim report. *J Clin Oncol* 1994;12:1572-1576.

93. Yang JC, Rosenberg SA. An ongoing prospective randomized comparison of interleukin-2 regimens for the treatment of metastatic renal cell cancer. *Cancer J Sci Am* 1997;3:S79-S84.

94. Halperin EC, Harisiadis L. The role of radiation therapy in the management of metastatic renal cell carcinoma. *Cancer* 1983;51:614-617.

95. Onufrey V, Mohiuddin M. Radiation therapy in the treatment of metastatic renal cell carcinoma. *Int J Radiat Oncol Biol Phys* 1985;11:2007-2009.

96. Van der Werf-Messing BH. Radiotherapeutic treatment of metastasized urological malignancies. *Prog Clin Biol Res* 1984;153:577-583.

97. Flanigan RC. Role of surgery in metastatic renal cell carcinoma. *Semin Urol* 1989;7:191-194.

98. Forman JD. The role of radiation therapy in the management of carcinoma of the kidney. *Semin Urol* 1989;7:195-198.

99. Kjaer M. The treatment and prognosis of patients with renal adenocarcinoma with solitary metastasis. 10-year survival results. *Int J Radiat Oncol Biol Phys* 1987;13:619-621.

100. Pearse HD. Nephroureterectomy. In: Johnson DE, Boileau MA, eds. *Genitourinary Tumors: Fundamental Principles and Surgical Techniques*. New York, NY: Grune & Stratton; 1982:371-378.

101. Morrison AS. Advances in the etiology of urothelial cancer. *Urol Clin North Am* 1984;11:557-566.

102. Gonwa TA, Corbett WT, Schey HM, et al. Analgesic-associated nephropathy and transitional cell carcinoma of the urinary tract. *Ann Intern Med* 1980;93:249-252.

103. McCredie M, Stewart JH, Ford JM. Analgesics and tobacco as risk factors for cancer of the ureter and renal pelvis. *J Urol* 1983;130:28-30.

104. Hall PW, Dammin GJ. Balkan nephropathy. *Nephron* 1978;22:281-300.

105. Petkovic SD. Epidemiology and treatment of renal pelvic and ureteral tumors. *J Urol* 1975;114:858-865.

106. Fuchs EF, Kay R, Poole R, et al. Uroepithelial carcinoma in association with cyclophosphamide ingestion. *J Urol* 1981;126:544-545.

107. Kakizoe T, Fujita J, Murase T, et al. Transitional cell carcinoma of the bladder in patients with renal pelvic and ureteral cancer. *J Urol* 1980;124:17-19.

108. Kinder CH, Wallace DM. Recurrent carcinoma of ureteric stump. *Br J Surg* 1962;50:202-205.

109. Strong DW, Pearse HD. Recurrent urothelial tumors following surgery for transitional cell carcinoma of the upper urinary tract. *Cancer* 1976;38:2173-2183.

110. Williams CB, Mitchell JP. Carcinoma of the renal pelvis: a review of 43 cases. *Br J Urol* 1973;45:370-376.

111. Williams CB, Mitchell JP. Carcinoma of the ureter—a review of 54 cases. *Br J Urol* 1973;45:377-387.

112. Nativ O, Reiman HM, Lieber MM, et al. Treatment of primary squamous cell carcinoma of the upper urinary tract. *Cancer* 1991;68:2575-2578.

113. Johnson DE. Renal pelvic and ureteral tumors: overview. In: Johnson DE, Boileau MA, eds. *Genitourinary Tumors: Fundamental Principles and Surgical Techniques.* New York, NY: Grune & Stratton; 1982:353-370.

114. Gittes RF. Management of transitional cell carcinoma of the upper tract: case for conservative local excision. *Urol Clin North Am* 1980;7:559-568.

115. Kimball FN, Ferris HW. Papillomatous tumor of the renal pelvis associated with similar tumors of the ureter and bladder. *J Urol* 1934;31:257-304.

116. Brookland RK, Richter MP. The postoperative irradiation of transitional cell carcinoma of the renal pelvis and ureter. *J Urol* 1985;133:952-955.

117. Cozad SC, Smalley SR, Austenfeld M, et al. Adjuvant radiotherapy in high stage transitional cell carcinoma of the renal pelvis and ureter. *Int J Radiat Oncol Biol Phys* 1992;24:743-745.

118. Babaian RJ, Johnson DE, Chan RC. Combination nephroureterectomy and postoperative radiotherapy for infiltrative ureteral carcinoma. *Int J Radiat Oncol Biol Phys* 1980;6:1229-1232.

119. Cummings KB. Nephroureterectomy: rationale in the management of transitional cell carcinoma of the upper urinary tract. *Urol Clin North Am* 1980;7:569-578.

120. Latham HS, Kay S. Malignant tumors of the renal pelvis. *Surg Gynecol Obstet* 1974;138:613-622.

121. Rubenstein MA, Walz BJ, Bucy JG. Transitional cell carcinoma of the kidney 25-year experience. *J Urol* 1978;119:594-597.

CHAPTER 25

The Urinary Bladder

Michael F. Milosevic and Mary K. Gospodarowicz

EFFECTS OF RADIATION ON THE NORMAL URINARY BLADDER

The urinary bladder, by virtue of its central location in the pelvis and its relative radiosensitivity, strongly influences the radiation dose that can safely be used to treat pelvic malignancies. Irradiation of tumors arising in the bladder itself or in adjacent pelvic organs, including the prostate, cervix, uterus, and rectum, may result in the delivery of doses to the normal bladder or portions of the bladder that are sufficient to produce side effects. Therefore, adequate treatment planning requires a detailed understanding of the normal bladder's response to radiation.

The histologic changes that occur in the bladder after irradiation are similar to the changes seen in many other normal tissues and have been well described.[1-3] They are broadly classified as acute (during or immediately after irradiation) or chronic (6 months to many years after irradiation).

Information about the radiation response of the normal bladder has largely been derived from animal studies and from the treatment of patients with bladder, cervix, and prostate cancer. The patient data are more relevant to clinical practice but have limited applicability, mainly because it is difficult to accurately determine the dose to the bladder during a course of fractionated radiation therapy.

The bladder dose can be easily and reliably calculated when the entire organ is irradiated. However, in most clinical situations, especially those in which the cervix or prostate is being irradiated, the dose to the bladder is heterogeneous. Techniques for estimating dose as a function of the irradiated bladder-wall volume and correlating the estimated dose with the development of side effects have only recently become available.[4] Historically, bladder dose estimates were based on the calculated or measured dose to a single point near the trigone. For example, the International Commission on Radiological Units and Measurements reference bladder dose for the intracavitary treatment of gynecologic malignancies is specified at a point along the posterior surface of a Foley-catheter balloon that is inflated in the bladder and pulled tight against the urethra.[5] Point dose calculations of this type, though they may provide an indication of the maximum dose to the bladder and the dose to an anatomic region important in normal bladder function, do not reflect the wide variation in bladder wall dose that often occurs. Computer-based dose-volume histogram techniques have the potential to provide more comprehensive estimates of the dose delivered to the bladder during a course of radiation therapy and therefore more clinically relevant estimates of bladder radiation tolerance.

Other problems that may cloud the interpretation of historical data on the radiation tolerance of the bladder include variation in the clinical definitions of radiation-induced side effects and their severity, underreporting of less severe but nevertheless clinically important side effects, and the now-abandoned practice of treating only one radiation field per day.

Acute Effects

The bladder is lined by transitional epithelium, which is characterized by proliferating basal cells and more superficial differentiated cells. The acute effects of radiation on the normal bladder are generally believed to arise from injury to the rapidly dividing basal cells, as is the case in other tissues such as skin.[1] Irradiation of the bladder produces cellular changes—including cellular swelling, vacuolization of the cytoplasm, and alterations in the appearance of the plasma membrane—that are often seen within hours to days after irradiation. Cellular and nuclear pleomorphism may result. Epithelial desquamation leading to focal ulceration is common. Irradiation of the bladder also causes early hyperemia and interstitial edema, which appear as focal or generalized erythema on cytoscopy. These histologic changes correlate with reduced bladder capacity and symptoms of acute radiation cystitis, including dysuria, nocturia, urinary frequency, and microscopic or gross hematuria.

Chronic Effects

The interval between irradiation and the onset of late bladder complications is typically 2 to 3 years, although it may be substantially longer. Bladder complications generally occur later than rectosigmoid complications.[6]

Late radiation-induced bladder injury is a result of changes in the vasculature of the bladder wall that lead to ischemia. Irradiation of the bladder may produce dilation of vessels, followed by endothelial cell swelling and vacuolization. Dilated vessels are often visible cystoscopically after irradiation and may spontaneously rupture, leading to microscopic or gross hematuria. Later vascular changes may include endothelial cell proliferation and collagenous hyalinization. Thickening of the vessel media may develop, leading to narrowing or complete occlusion of the vessel lumen. The end result of this process in extreme cases is a fibrotic, thickened, relatively avascular bladder wall. Chronic bladder contracture results, with symptoms of dysuria, hematuria, and urinary frequency. In severe cases, fistulas may arise between the bladder and adjacent organs.

Mechanism of Radiation-Induced Normal Tissue Injury

The acute and late effects of irradiation on the bladder are mediated principally by epithelial and endothelial cell damage that leads to cell death. However, irradiation also may produce changes in gene and protein expression that may contribute to the development of symptoms. At least one recent study in rodents has suggested that the early changes in bladder capacity that manifest clinically as urinary frequency and nocturia may be due not only to denudation of the transitional cell epithelium but also to local changes in prostaglandin metabolism.[7] Disruption of tight epithelial cell junctions and loss of the polysaccharide mucosal lining also may contribute to the development of acute bladder symptoms by compromising the normal barrier between the hypertonic urine and the isotonic bladder wall tissues.[6] Irradiation of the bladder probably causes increased expression of a variety of proteins that mediate vascular and fibrotic responses long after the completion of radiation therapy.

Evidence is also mounting from both animal and clinical studies that the severity of acute radiation-induced bladder reactions correlates with the severity of late reactions.[8-11] This suggests that early pathophysiologic changes in the bladder wall, which are at least partly responsible for the acute reaction to radiation, also may have long-term consequences and play a role in the development of late bladder side effects.

Role of Dose and Irradiated Volume

Numerous studies of adjuvant pelvic radiation therapy for endometrial cancer and rectal cancer[12,13] have described severe acute cystitis in fewer than 5% of patients after whole-pelvis doses of 45 to 50 Gy in 1.8- to 2-Gy daily fractions. Recently, more detailed analyses of the effects of partial bladder irradiation have been reported. These analyses are largely based on patients with prostate cancer treated with high-dose conformal radiation therapy. Storey and colleagues[14] described severe irritative voiding symptoms or bleeding in approximately 20% of patients who received 70 Gy or more to at least 30% of the bladder but in only 5% of patients who received 70 Gy or more to at least 15% of the bladder. Michalski and colleagues[4] reported a twofold increase in the risk of acute bladder effects when 65 Gy or more was administered to at least 30% of the bladder wall. These studies were limited by relatively small numbers of patients in some of the dose-volume strata, and further investigation is therefore required to refine the risk estimates.

The dose-volume relationship for late radiation-induced bladder complications was reviewed by Emami and colleagues,[15] with symptomatic bladder contracture and volume loss as the endpoint. These authors estimated that 65 Gy in 1.8- to 2-Gy fractions to the entire bladder resulted in a 5% risk of complications. They further estimated that a total dose of 80 Gy was tolerable if only two thirds of the bladder was irradiated. Marks and colleagues,[6] in a separate thorough review of the clinical literature, estimated the whole-bladder tolerance dose for late effects to be lower, at 45 Gy. A dose of 67 Gy to less than 30% of the bladder volume also was believed to be tolerable, as was a dose of 75 Gy to less than 10% of the bladder.[6] A more recent report showed that the proportion of the bladder irradiated to greater than 65 Gy correlated with the risk of late side effects in patients who underwent conformal radiation therapy for prostate cancer.[4] However, at least two other contemporary studies have failed to identify any relationship between dose-volume histogram parameters and late bladder side effects in patients with prostate cancer.[14,16]

The discrepancies among these studies probably arise from many factors, including differences in the toxicity endpoints; differences in the way that the irradiated bladder volume was defined (solid organ vs. bladder wall only); variation in the position and size of the bladder during a course of fractionated radiation therapy; and low numbers of late bladder complications, which render the risk estimates of bladder toxicity as a function of dose and bladder volume unreliable. Overall, the available data suggest that a radiation dose of 50 to 60 Gy in 1.8- to 2-Gy daily fractions to the entire bladder is well tolerated in most patients and that smaller bladder volumes will tolerate higher doses, in the range of 65 to 70 Gy. More detailed studies will be required to better define the late partial-organ radiation tolerance of the bladder.

Role of Fraction Size

The estimates of bladder radiation tolerance have largely been derived from series of patients who received pelvic radiation therapy in daily fractions of 1.8 to 2.5 Gy. The fraction delivered to the bladder or a portion of the bladder may actually have been smaller than 1.8 to 2.5 Gy in many of the patients in these studies, depending on the anatomic relationship of the bladder to the treatment fields and the irradiated volume. Fraction size is probably a fundamental determinant of late radiation side effects in the bladder as in most other normal tissues,[6,17] although perhaps to a lesser extent. Animal studies have suggested that the α/β ratio for late bladder toxicity may be in the range of 5 to 7 Gy,[9,18,19] compared to 2 to 3 Gy for most normal tissues.[17] This raises the possibility that the influence of fraction size on late bladder complications may be less than that for other tissues. Future studies of late bladder complications should consider the effect of both fractional and total radiation dose.

Role of Patient and Tumor Factors

Several patient- and tumor-related factors may increase the risk of both early and late side effects in patients receiving pelvic radiation therapy. Preexisting bladder symptoms arising from coexisting infection or long-standing outflow obstruction may be aggravated by irradiation. Multiple prior transurethral resections may lead to bladder wall fibrosis, decreased bladder compliance, and irritative voiding symptoms that similarly may worsen with irradiation.[20] Systemic chemotherapy with high-dose cyclophosphamide can cause hemorrhagic cystitis and late bladder contracture[21] and may reduce the bladder's tolerance of subsequent irradiation.[22] There is no evidence that cisplatin administered before, during, or after pelvic radiation therapy increases the risk of late radiation-induced bladder complications.[23]

Management of Radiation-Induced Side Effects

The management of radiation-induced side effects in the bladder is primarily aimed at controlling symptoms. Urinary infections should be treated. Bladder spasms may be relieved with topical anesthetics or anticholinergic agents. Acute irritative voiding symptoms usually resolve within 1 month after the completion of radiation therapy. Patients who present with voiding symptoms or hematuria months to years after completing pelvic radiation therapy should be examined to exclude tumor recurrence either in the bladder or at other sites in the pelvis, which may be clinically indistinguishable from late radiation-induced side effects.

Cystoscopic coagulation of bleeding vessels may help alleviate hematuria caused by radiation-induced vascular dilation and fragility. Patients with persistent hematuria may benefit from treatment with hyperbaric oxygen.[24,25] Late bladder symptoms will resolve within 2 to 3 years of onset in 70% to 80% of patients.[11] In extreme cases, cystectomy may be necessary to alleviate severe, persistent, or disabling bladder symptoms. It is unclear whether early aggressive management of acute radiation-induced side effects in the bladder will reduce the risk of severe late reactions.

BLADDER CANCER
Epidemiology and Risk Factors

Malignant tumors of the urinary bladder are common and cause significant morbidity and mortality. It is estimated that in the United States in 2001, 54,300 new cases will be diagnosed, and 12,400 men and women will die of the disease.[26] The incidence has been relatively constant over the past 20 years, at 20 to 25 cases/100,000, adjusted for age. Men are affected 3 times as often as women. Bladder cancer is the fourth most common malignancy in men, after prostate cancer, lung cancer, and colorectal cancer. Prostate cancer is the eighth most common cancer in women.[25] Most cases are diagnosed in people 50 to 80 years of age. The incidence is lower in blacks than in whites, Hispanics, and people of Japanese and Indian descent.[27]

The strongest risk factor for the development of carcinoma of the bladder is a history of cigarette smoking, and the incidence of this disease generally parallels the incidence of lung cancer and other smoking-related illnesses. Between 50% and 80% of all cases of bladder cancer have been attributed to smoking.[28] Brennan and colleagues,[29] in a meta-analysis of 11 case-controlled studies, found a linear relationship among men between smoking duration and the risk of developing bladder cancer. The relative risk compared with the risk in nonsmokers increased from 2.0 after 20 years of smoking to 5.6 after 60 years. The risk of bladder cancer also was related to the number of cigarettes smoked per day.[29] People who stopped smoking realized a 30% reduction in their risk of bladder cancer within 1 to 4 years and a 60% reduction by 25 years. However, the risk of bladder cancer never returned to the lower level of lifelong nonsmokers.[29] Bladder cancer patients who are current or former smokers also may have other serious medical problems, such as heart or vascular disease, and a limited capacity to tolerate aggressive therapies, including surgery.

Several studies have suggested a link between occupational exposure to agents such as aromatic amines and heavy metals and development of bladder cancer.[27,30-33] Aniline dyes, which are used in the textile and rubber industries, have been strongly linked to the development of bladder cancer. In one study, individuals exposed to paints or dyes, herbicides, or other chemicals had a risk of developing bladder cancer that was 2 to 5 times higher than the risk in unexposed controls.[33] Occupational exposure is estimated to account for only about 25% of cases of bladder cancer,[34] and the latency interval from exposure to manifestation of the disease usually exceeds 15 years. Studies of occupational exposure are often difficult to interpret, in part because of the confounding effect of cigarette smoking, which is a stronger risk factor for bladder cancer development.

Long-term use of the analgesic phenacetin and exposure to high-dose cyclophosphamide contribute to the development of bladder cancer in a minority of cases.[34] Recurrent urinary tract infections may increase the risk of squamous cell bladder cancer, especially in paraplegics who have permanent indwelling catheters.[35,36] The pathogenesis of bladder cancer arising in this setting is not known but may relate to nitrate production by bacteria.[37] Recent studies have suggested that bladder cancer is more common in individuals who consume a diet high in fat and low in fruits and vegetables.[38,39] Urinary schistosomiasis is an important etiologic factor in areas of Africa and the Eastern Mediterranean where bladder cancer is endemic. The infective agent, *Schistosoma haematobium*, is a waterborne fluke that deposits ova in the bladder wall. The ova incite a chronic inflammatory reaction that leads to transitional cell dysplasia and the development of frank malignancy. Approximately 70% of schistosomiasis-associated tumors are squamous cell carcinomas, and the rest are transitional cell carcinomas.[28]

Pathology

The histologic subtypes of primary tumors of the urinary bladder are summarized in Box 25-1. Most tumors are of epithelial origin, and only 5% develop from the mesenchymal components of the bladder wall.[28] Of the epithelial tumors, 90% are transitional cell carcinomas that arise from the transitional epithelium of the bladder mucosa. The remainder are squamous cell carcinomas, adenocarcinomas, neuroendocrine tumors, and mixed tumors. Adenocarcinomas may be either urachal or nonurachal in origin, but both tumor types express a unique colonic epithelial epitope, suggesting a common

---

BOX 25-1   Histologic Subtypes of Primary Bladder Cancer

Urothelial (transitional cell) tumor
   Papilloma
   Transitional cell carcinoma in situ
   Transitional cell carcinoma, grade 1-3
Squamous cell carcinoma
Adenocarcinoma
Mixed carcinoma
Sarcoma
Carcinosarcoma
Lymphoma

---

underlying developmental pathway.[40] Transitional cell carcinomas of the bladder may be broadly classified as superficial or muscle invasive.

Superficial Transitional Cell Carcinoma

Superficial transitional cell carcinomas account for about 75% of all cases and typically are characterized by well-differentiated to moderately differentiated papillary tumors with minimal cellular and nuclear pleomorphism. They may be confined to the epithelial layer of the bladder wall or invade the lamina propria. Carcinoma in situ (CIS), characterized by full-thickness dysplasia of the transitional cell epithelium, may be present focally or diffusely in the bladder in association with superficial transitional cell carcinoma. In CIS, there is reduced cohesion among the dysplastic cells, which may be sloughed from the mucosa into the urine. Full-thickness epithelial denudation occurs often with CIS; when this finding is seen in biopsy specimens, it implies the existence of CIS. Contact between urine and the denuded mucosa leads to inflammation and a characteristic velvety red appearance at cystoscopy.

Multiple superficial tumors may be present in the bladder at diagnosis, and a pattern of repeated recurrence or new superficial tumor development despite treatment is common. This pattern of synchronous and metachronous tumor development throughout the urothelium implies a generalized, probably genetic, predisposition affecting the entire mucosa. Risk factors for recurrence of superficial bladder cancer after initial diagnosis and treatment include high histologic grade, involvement of the tunica muscularis, multifocality, and associated CIS.[41] Superficial bladder tumors rarely metastasize to lymph nodes or distant sites. About 15% of cases of superficial disease will eventually progress to muscle invasion,[27] most commonly poorly differentiated, sessile, T1 tumors with diffuse CIS.

Muscle-Invasive Transitional Cell Carcinoma

Only about 25% of bladder cancer cases involve the lamina propria mucosae. In most cases, no prior history of bladder cancer was found, and the muscle-invasive tumor is the index lesion. These tumors are usually poorly differentiated and may be either papillary or sessile in appearance. Most are solitary, but multiple invasive tumors may be present, particularly in the setting of prior or coexisting superficial disease and CIS. The natural history of muscle-invasive tumors is progressive extension through the muscular and serosal layers of the bladder wall to involve perivesical fat. Adjacent organs and tissues, including the prostate, uterus, vagina, rectum, and pelvic bones, may be invaded. Tumors arising in the region of the trigone may occlude the ureteric orifices, leading to hydronephrosis. Lymph node metastases and distant metastases often develop, making muscle-invasive bladder cancer a life-threatening illness.

Associated Genetic Changes

Bladder cancer is characterized by a variety of acquired genetic changes that are promoted at least in part by exposure to environmental carcinogens. The progression from normal bladder mucosa to intraepithelial malignancy to invasive bladder cancer requires a series of molecular changes that involve the activation of specific proto-oncogenes and the inactivation of tumor suppressor genes. These acquired genetic changes lead to alterations in important processes that determine the balance between cell proliferation and cell death, including signaling, cell cycle regulation, and apoptosis.

Numeric and structural abnormalities of chromosomes 9, 11, and 17 are seen often.[27] Complete or partial deletions of chromosome 9 occur in a large percentage of patients with both superficial and muscle-invasive bladder cancer and are the most common cytogenetic abnormality. Deletions involving the short arm of chromosome 9 lead to inactivation of the *p16* tumor suppressor gene, which is an important cell cycle regulator.[42] Other tumor suppressor genes often inactivated include the *p53* and *pRB* (retinoblastoma) genes. Several studies have associated altered *p53* and *pRB* expression with clinical and histopathologic indicators of aggressive disease and an increased risk of progression from superficial to muscle-invasive cancer.[43-48] Alterations in these genes also may predict decreased survival in patients with muscle-invasive tumors undergoing cystectomy,[49] although this is controversial.[50-52] The apparent differences in the predictive value of gene expression from study to study probably stem from the relatively small number of patients, nonstandard assay procedures, and the use of immunohistochemical techniques rather than DNA sequencing to document alterations in gene function.[53,54]

Screening

The impact of population screening on bladder cancer mortality has never been evaluated in a randomized study. However, single-arm studies have suggested that bladder cancer screening in healthy men 50 years of age and older with repeated home hematuria testing may be a cost-effective means of significantly decreasing bladder cancer morbidity and mortality.[55,56] Screening with urine cytology may be useful in high-risk populations, such as those with known industrial exposure to urinary-tract carcinogens. Urine cytology identifies 50% to 80% of poorly differentiated urothelial cancer but only 20% of well-differentiated tumors.[57] In general, early detection of bladder cancer depends on prompt evaluation of patients who develop new urinary symptoms.

Presentation, Natural History, and Staging

Patients with bladder cancer typically present with hematuria with or without irritative urinary symptoms. Urinary frequency, nocturia, and dysuria are common as a result of reduced bladder-wall compliance, reduced capacity, outflow obstruction, or superimposed infection. Hematuria may be grossly evident or detectable only by microscopic examination of the urine. Superficial tumors rarely produce symptoms beyond the bladder. However, patients with advanced muscle-invasive tumors often have symptoms that reflect the pattern of disease spread. Ureteric obstruction may result in costovertebral angle pain, particularly if the obstruction develops rapidly, and places patients at risk of urinary sepsis. Direct extension of tumor to adjacent pelvic organs may produce pain, change in bowel habits, rectal bleeding, or vaginal bleeding. Extensive pelvic lymphadenopathy is a cause of leg edema. Distant metastases most often involve liver, lung, and bone.

All patients with a suspected or confirmed new diagnosis of bladder cancer should undergo a thorough history and physical examination, cystoscopy, and examination under anesthesia. Transurethral resection or a deep biopsy of the bladder tumor is required to establish the diagnosis and determine important prognostic characteristics, including histologic subtype, grade, and the presence or absence of muscle invasion. The rest of the bladder also should be examined, and abnormal areas should be biopsied. In addition, random biopsies of normal-appearing mucosa are required to exclude CIS.[58] The location, size, mobility, and extravesical extension of palpable disease should be carefully evaluated. Patients with muscle-invasive disease require chest radiography, computed tomography (CT) of the abdomen and pelvis, and bone scan to exclude lymph node and distant metastases.

The 1997 American Joint Committee on Cancer and Union Internationale Contre le Cancer tumor-nodes-metastasis (TNM) staging system for bladder cancer is outlined in Box 25-2.[59,60] The T categories reflect the progressively worsening prognosis associated with penetration of tumor through the anatomic layers of the bladder wall into the perivesical tissues and organs. Detailed pathologic information is essential to properly categorize the primary tumor using this system. Tissue may be obtained during transurethral resection of the primary tumor (clinical staging) or at cystectomy (pathologic staging). The 1978 TNM classification was based on the absence (clinical T2 [cT2]) or presence (cT3a) of induration in the bladder wall after complete transurethral resection of an intravesical tumor or the presence of a mobile mass after transurethral resection (cT3b).[61] The prognostic value of clinical stage has been demonstrated in many radiation therapy series.[62-64] However, clinical stage determined by physical examination, imaging, and transurethral biopsy alone usually underestimates the

---

BOX 25-2   American Joint Committee on Cancer Staging System for Bladder Cancer

PRIMARY TUMOR (T)

TX   Primary tumor cannot be assessed
T0   No evidence of primary tumor
Ta   Noninvasive papillary carcinoma
Tis   Carcinoma in situ: "flat tumor"
T1   Tumor invades subepithelial connective tissue
T2   Tumor invades muscle
    T2a   Tumor invades superficial muscle (inner half)
    T2b   Tumor invades deep muscle (outer half)
T3   Tumor invades perivesical tissue
    T3a   microscopically
    T3b   macroscopically (extravesical mass)
T4   Tumor invades any of the following: prostate, uterus, vagina, pelvic wall, abdominal wall
    T4a   Tumor invades prostate, uterus, vagina
    T4b   Tumor invades pelvic wall, abdominal wall

REGIONAL LYMPH NODES (N)*

NX   Regional lymph nodes cannot be assessed
N0   No regional lymph node metastasis
N1   Metastasis in a single lymph node, 2 cm or less in greatest dimension
N2   Metastasis in a single lymph node, more than 2 cm but not more than 5 cm in greatest dimension; or multiple lymph nodes, none more than 5 cm in greatest dimension
N3   Metastasis in a lymph node more than 5 cm in greatest dimension

DISTANT METASTASIS (M)

MX   Distant metastasis cannot be assessed
M0   No distant metastasis
M1   Distant metastasis

STAGE GROUPING

Stage 0a	Ta	N0	M0
Stage 0is	Tis	N0	M0
Stage I	T1	N0	M0
Stage II	T2a	N0	M0
	T2b	N0	M0
Stage III	T3a	N0	M0
	T3b	N0	M0
	T4a	N0	M0
Stage IV	T4b	N0	M0
	Any T	N1-3	M0
	Any T	Any N	M1

From Fleming I, Cooper JS, Henson DE, et al, eds. *AJCC Cancer Staging Manual.* 5th ed. Philadelphia, Pa: Lippincott Williams & Wilkins; 1997:241-246.
*Regional lymph nodes are those within the true pelvis; all others are distant lymph nodes.

---

true extent of disease,[65] which precludes a direct comparison of the results of treatment with cystectomy versus radiation therapy.

In patients undergoing definitive radiation therapy, the primary tumor should be staged according to the current TNM classification, with all available clinical, radiographic, and pathologic information taken into account. Magnetic resonance imaging (MRI) provides a more accurate indication of anatomic disease extent than does clinical evaluation alone.[66] MRI also may provide valuable information about the extent of local disease that can be used to plan surgery or radiation therapy. A midsagittal MRI scan of a patient with a tumor arising from the anterior wall of the bladder is shown in Figure 25-1.

In men, bladder cancer may involve the prostate gland. Tumor that extends directly from the bladder into the prostate carries a worse prognosis than a separate focus of transitional cell bladder carcinoma in the prostate or superficial involvement of the mucosa of the prostatic urethra by bladder cancer.[67,68] The latter two situations reflect the generally more favorable prognosis associated with primary transitional cell carcinoma of the prostate. Patients with tumor involving the bladder neck should undergo random biopsies of the prostatic

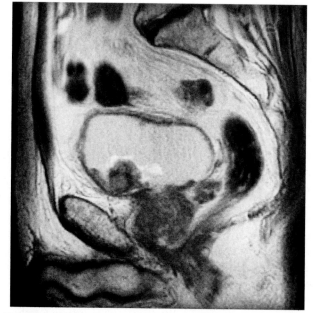

Fig. 25-1 Midsagittal magnetic resonance imaging scan of a T3b bladder tumor.

urethra as a component of routine staging. It is important to exclude occult CIS of the prostatic urethra, particularly if continent urinary diversion with an ortho-topic bladder, which involves conservation of a portion of the urethra, is contemplated.[69]

The lymphatic drainage of the bladder begins in a network of lymphatic channels that permeate the lamina propria and lamina muscularis of the bladder wall. These lymphatic channels terminate in collecting ducts that emerge from the bladder near the trigone and along the anterior and posterior walls. Small lymph nodes are present in the perivesical fat. Drainage is pre-dominantly to the external iliac nodes, but the internal iliac and common iliac nodes are also commonly involved.[70] Reports of patients undergoing thorough pelvic lymph node dissection at the time of cystectomy have shown an overall risk of nodal metastases in the range of 20% to 30%. The risk is less than 10% in patients with superficial bladder cancer, 15% to 20% in patients with muscle-invasive disease confined to the bladder wall, and 30% to 50% in the setting of extraves-ical disease.[71-74] CT and MRI are inaccurate in the detec-tion of metastases in nodes measuring 5 to 10 mm in size,[75,76] which may contribute to apparent differences in outcome between patients treated surgically (in whom pathologic information about nodal involve-ment is usually available) and patients treated with definitive radiation therapy. The role of laparoscopic or extraperitoneal pelvic lymphadenectomy before radia-tion therapy should be investigated as a means of improving the accuracy of lymph node staging.

Management of Superficial Bladder Cancer

Superficial bladder cancer is typically managed with complete transurethral resection of intravesical disease. Careful pathologic examination of the resected tissue is required to exclude invasion of the muscularis propria. Given the high likelihood of recurrence or new tumor development, patients should be examined at regular intervals (every 4 to 6 months for 5 years) after resection with urine cytology and cystoscopy. Persistently abnor-mal findings on urine cytology after normal findings on cystoscopy should prompt evaluation of the prostatic urethra in men, and the upper urinary tract in both men and women.[77-79]

Intravesical chemotherapy and immunotherapy are used to treat superficial bladder cancer in two settings: primary treatment of existing intravesical disease that is too extensive to be completely resected, including exten-sive CIS; and adjuvant therapy after complete trans-urethral resection with the aim of preventing disease recurrence and progression to muscle invasion. The agents that have been used include bacillus Calmette-Guérin (BCG), thiotepa, doxorubicin, and mitomycin C.

Cumulative evidence from several studies suggests that BCG is the most effective form of intravesical therapy.[80]

BCG is typically administered into the bladder weekly for 6 weeks and incites an intense inflammatory response in the bladder wall that is responsible for the therapeutic effect. Complete regression of existing superficial disease may occur in up to 70% of patients treated with BCG, including those with extensive CIS.[80,81] However, recur-rence rates are high, and patients therefore require ongo-ing surveillance with urine cytology and cystoscopy.

Adjuvant BCG after complete transurethral resection was shown in a randomized study to significantly reduce the rate of local tumor recurrence in the bladder and the development of invasive or metastatic disease and to enhance disease-free survival.[82] The 10-year pro-gression-free rate in this trial was 62% in patients treated with BCG and 37% in those treated with transurethral surgery alone. The corresponding 10-year disease-free survival figures were 75% and 55%, respectively. This result strongly supports the use of intravesical BCG after transurethral resection in patients who are at high risk for recurrence or progression.

Cystectomy
Radical Cystectomy

Radical cystectomy is the most common treatment for patients with bladder cancer that invades the muscu-laris propria. Radical cystectomy also should be consid-ered in patients with extensive recurrent superficial disease that is refractory to intravesical BCG and in patients who have disease progression in the bladder after radiation therapy.[83] In men, radical cystectomy involves the en bloc removal of the bladder, perivesical tissues, prostate, and seminal vesicles; in women, the procedure involves the en bloc removal of the bladder, uterus, fallopian tubes, ovaries, anterior vaginal wall, and urethra.[84] Bilateral pelvic lymph node dissection is usually performed at the same time. Lymph node dis-section provides important prognostic information in addition to being of therapeutic benefit in patients with limited lymph node involvement. Lymph nodes in the common iliac, external iliac, and internal iliac chains are typically removed. Urinary diversion is required. This was traditionally accomplished with an ileal conduit; however, continent urinary diversion based on stomal or orthotopic neobladders eliminates the need for an external appliance and is now standard practice.

Advances in surgical technique and perioperative care have resulted in reduced operative morbidity and mor-tality. The major complication rate after radical cystec-tomy is typically less than 20%, and operative mortality is less than 5%.[65,85] Radical cystoprostatectomy with preservation of sexual function can be performed in some men.

Most radical cystectomy series comprise patients accumulated over many years at a single institution. These series may not account for changes over time in patient selection, surgical technique, and perioperative management. Although these studies must be interpreted cautiously, they provide important information about outcome after radical cystectomy on which to base treatment decisions.

The major prognostic factors for survival after cystectomy are pathologic tumor stage and the presence or absence of pelvic lymph node metastases. Local recurrence is expected in fewer than 10% of patients with primary tumors confined to the bladder wall (pathologic T2 [pT2] or pT3a) but in 30% to 50% of patients with extravesical disease extension (pT3b or pT4a).[72,86] Overall 5-year survival rates are in the range of 60% to 80% for patients with pT2 disease and in the range of 20% to 40% for patients with pT3b or pT4 disease.[83]

Pelvic lymphadenectomy provides important prognostic information in patients with bladder cancer. Survival is significantly lower in the setting of involved lymph nodes, and patients with involved nodes should therefore be considered for adjuvant chemotherapy. The therapeutic benefit of pelvic lymphadenectomy has never been tested in a randomized study. However, several retrospective series have suggested that the combination of cystectomy and bilateral pelvic lymph node dissection cures between 15% and 30% of patients with nodal metastases.[71-74,87-89]

The likelihood of cure depends on the extent of nodal involvement.[71,87,89] Lerner and colleagues[71] reported a 5-year survival rate of 29% in 132 patients with lymph node metastases identified at the time of lymphadenectomy. Survival rates were 35% among patients with one to five involved nodes and 17% among patients with six or more involved nodes. Lymph node dissection also may contribute to the cure of patients with small-bulk gross pelvic lymph node involvement identified at the time of surgery.[90]

Partial Cystectomy

Partial cystectomy plays a limited role in the management of bladder cancer. It is appropriate only in patients with small, solitary tumors that are situated near the dome and well separated from the trigone and bladder neck. Fewer than 5% of patients have this presentation. Low-dose preoperative external-beam radiation therapy and postoperative brachytherapy have been used in conjunction with partial cystectomy to reduce the risk of recurrence in the abdominal scar and bladder, respectively.

Radiation Therapy

The goal of definitive radiation therapy for bladder cancer is to permanently eradicate the local tumor in the bladder and preserve normal bladder function. Optimal delivery of definitive radiation therapy requires a detailed understanding of the multiple biological and treatment parameters that influence both local tumor control and the development of radiation-induced side effects.

Any decision to treat initially with radiation therapy in hopes of maintaining normal bladder function must be part of a larger treatment plan that includes salvage cystectomy in the case of persistent or residual tumor after radiation therapy. Many patients referred for definitive radiation therapy have bulky unresectable tumors and a high risk of occult micrometastases or have concurrent medical problems that make them unsuitable for initial surgery. These patients often are not considered for salvage cystectomy for the same reasons. However, in the setting of local failure after radiation therapy, surgery remains the only option for prolonged survival, and a higher risk of complications may therefore be acceptable in some circumstances. In general, all patients with residual or recurrent bladder cancer after radiation therapy should be evaluated for cystectomy.

Extensive experience, dating back to the early 1900s, has been documented regarding the use of radiation therapy alone to treat bladder cancer.[91] However, the published series are often difficult to interpret. Most are retrospective single-institution reports of patients treated over several decades, and many studies do not consider differences over time in patient assessment, imaging, stage classification, radiation therapy technique, and supportive treatment. Management strategies, including the criteria for salvage cystectomy, vary from institution to institution, making comparison of results problematic. In addition, these factors, together with differences in patient selection, make it impossible to meaningfully compare the results of primary treatment with radiation therapy and primary treatment with surgery. Nevertheless, it is evident from the accumulated experience that a significant proportion of patients, particularly those who present with small tumors, are cured and maintain normal bladder function after definitive radiation therapy.

Treatment of Superficial Bladder Cancer

Because of the availability of other minimally invasive and effective management options, radiation therapy is not commonly used to treat superficial bladder cancer. However, radiation therapy has been used in the setting of rapidly recurrent or extensive superficial disease that is not amenable to transurethral resection and in cases in which the risk of progression to muscle-invasive disease is deemed to be high.

The limited data available for patients with superficial disease suggest that irradiation is of minimal benefit in this setting. The complete response rate of superficial tumors to radiation therapy is in the range of 40% to 60%,[63,92,93] possibly reflecting the difficulty of distinguishing residual disease at the site of the original tumor from the development of new tumors shortly after completion of treatment. No evidence has shown that radiation therapy reduces the likelihood of new tumor development, especially in patients with an established pattern of recurrence, and no evidence has shown that radiation is more likely than other treatments to result in long-term bladder preservation.

The ability of radiation therapy to control CIS concurrent with superficial bladder cancer is probably also limited (see the discussion in the next section). Perhaps the only situation in which radiation therapy may be appropriate in the treatment of superficial bladder cancer is in the setting of disease that is likely to progress to muscle invasion. Radiation therapy for poorly differentiated tumors that invade the lamina propria (T1, grade 3) leads to complete tumor regression in 65% to 75% of cases and long-term survival rates of 55% to 65%.[93,94] However, the success of radiation therapy in this setting may be adversely influenced by the presence of coexisting CIS.[95] Radiation therapy for T1 disease has never been compared in a randomized study to more conservative therapy with transurethral resection and intravesical BCG. Given the effectiveness and convenience for the patient of the surgery-immunotherapy approach, it remains standard management in this situation.

Treatment of Muscle-Invasive Bladder Cancer

The response of muscle-invasive bladder cancer to radiation therapy is strongly influenced by the volume of local disease, as indicated by factors such as T category, tumor size, and the presence or absence of an extravesical mass or ureteric obstruction.[62-64,96-98] Overall, approximately 50% of patients treated with external-beam radiation therapy—50% to 70% of those with T2 or T3a disease and 40% to 50% of those with T3 or T4a tumors—have complete regression of disease.[63,64,96,98-101] Sustained local control (complete disease regression without subsequent recurrence in the bladder) can be expected in 30% to 50% of patients with T2 disease and 20% to 30% of patients with T3 disease.[63,96,102] It has been demonstrated that local control is more likely in patients who undergo complete transurethral resection before radiation therapy.[103] However, not all reports concur with this observation,[98,101,104] and it is possible that the apparent benefit of transurethral resection relates mainly to patient selection. Nevertheless, because tumor size is a strong predictor of local control, the possible benefit of preradiation debulking should not be dismissed.

Several factors in addition to tumor volume may influence disease progression in the bladder. When present in association with muscle-invasive bladder cancer, CIS indicates a reduced likelihood of sustained local tumor control after irradiation because CIS predisposes to the development of new tumors.[63,105,106] Wolf and colleagues[106] reported the development of a new bladder cancer after radiation therapy in 58% of patients with dysplasia or CIS at initial presentation but in none of the patients without concomitant CIS. Nevertheless, CIS is not an absolute contraindication to the use of radiation therapy in patients with muscle-invasive disease, and the presence of CIS in these patients should be considered in the context of other tumor and patient factors when treatment choices are being made. Patients with recurrent CIS after radiation therapy can be treated effectively with intravesical BCG[107,108] providing that BCG was not used to manage previous superficial disease.

Local control may be more likely with solitary nonpapillary tumors.[63,109] Anemia at presentation (hemoglobin concentration < 120 to 130 g/L) was an independent adverse prognostic factor with respect to local control in at least two studies,[63,110] particularly in patients with bulky disease. Our results also suggest that anemic patients may be more likely to develop distant metastases and be more likely to die of disease.[63] One explanation is that anemia contributes to the development of local tumor hypoxia and, in turn, to radioresistance and the emergence of more aggressive metastatic phenotypes.[111-113] Oxygen tension has not been measured directly in bladder cancer patients treated with radiation therapy, and no randomized studies of the effect of transfusion on outcome have been done. Pollack and colleagues[114,115] described a relationship between altered expression of the *pRB* and *bcl-2* genes and local response to preoperative radiation therapy. These genes are important in cell cycle regulation, DNA repair, and control of spontaneous and radiation-induced apoptosis. Other studies have suggested that pretreatment apoptotic index may be an independent prognostic factor for local control in bladder cancer.[116,117] Further study of biological prognostic factors is essential to advancing the role of radiation therapy in the management of muscle-invasive disease.

The prognostic factors for survival in patients with muscle-invasive disease are similar to those for local control and generally reflect primary tumor bulk. In addition, histologic grade and age at diagnosis may be important predictors of death from bladder cancer.[63] Overexpression of the *p53* tumor suppressor gene has been associated with an increased risk of distant metastases and death after preoperative radiation therapy for bladder cancer.[118] However, *p53* seems to have little effect on local tumor control.[117,118] Expression of *p21* also may be an independent predictor of survival in patients who undergo preoperative radiation therapy.[119]

The overall 5-year survival rate of patients with muscle-invasive bladder cancer varies from 25% to 30% (Tables 25-1 and 25-2).[62,64,96-102,109,120-124] Patients with T2 tumors have an expected survival rate of 30% to 50%, and those with T3 disease have a survival rate of 15% to 35%.* Patients with muscle-invasive disease are

---

*References 62-64, 96, 100-104, 109, 120-123, 125.

TABLE 25-1

Effectiveness of Radiation Therapy Alone for Muscle-Invasive Bladder Cancer

Outcome	T2	T3	Overall
Complete response rate	50% to 70%	40% to 50%	50%
Sustained local control rate	30% to 50%	20% to 30%	30%
Distant metastasis rate			> 50%
5-Year overall survival rate	30% to 50%	15% to 35%	25% to 30%
5-Year overall survival rate after salvage cystectomy			40% to 60%

See Table 25-2 and text for references.

often elderly and suffer from other medical problems. The rate of death from intercurrent illness is high and may approach 30% by 5 years.[126] Bladder cancer cause-specific survival after radiation therapy is typically in the range of 25% to 45%.[62,63,121] Distant metastases are common and in the Princess Margaret Hospital series accounted for 57% of all deaths.[63] About 50% of these patients had recurrence only at distant sites. The remaining patients either had documented local as well as

distant recurrence or developed metastases before the response of the primary tumor to radiation therapy could be assessed.

An area of concern in current radiation therapy practice that may affect the survival of patients with muscle-invasive bladder cancer is management of the pelvic lymph nodes. Depending on primary tumor extent, 10% to 50% of patients have lymph node metastases at diagnosis.[71-74] In many cases, the nodal metastases are microscopic and not reliably detected by CT or MRI. These subclinical metastases may consist of a single malignant cell or a nodule near the threshold of radiographic detection containing 10^8 or more cells. The radiation therapy dose that can safely be delivered to nodal areas is limited to 45 to 50 Gy, which is insufficient to reliably eradicate the larger metastases in the subclinical range. Therefore, it is likely that in a large proportion of patients, especially those with bulky primary tumors, the pelvic lymph nodes are inadequately treated with conventional radiation therapy. This is important because several surgical series have suggested a survival advantage from thorough pelvic lymph node dissection.[71-74,87-89] In addition, because patients with pelvic lymph node metastases are at high risk for distant recurrence, adjuvant chemotherapy is often recommended. Patients receiving radiation therapy usually do not undergo pelvic lymph node dissection and evaluation and therefore may not be offered the opportunity to benefit from chemotherapy.

TABLE 25-2

Survival by Tumor Extent after Radiation Therapy Alone for Muscle-Invasive Bladder Cancer

Study and Reference	Number of Patients	5-YEAR SURVIVAL BY T CATEGORY (%)			
		T2	T3 (T3a/T3b)	T4 (T4a/T4)	Overall
Goffinet et al, 1975[122]	384	35-42	20	—	—
Yu et al, 1985[123]	356	42	(35/23)	—	—
Goodman et al, 1981[124]	470	—	—	—	38
Duncan et al, 1986[64]	963	40	26	12	30
Blandy et al, 1988[99]	614	27	38	9	—
Jenkins et al, 1988*[100]	182	46	35	—	40
Gospodarowicz et al, 1991*[62]	355	50	(38/280)	—	46
Jahnson et al, 1991*[102]	319	31	16	6	28
Davidson et al, 1990*[121]	709	49	28	2	25
Greven et al, 1990[96]	116	59	10	0	—
Smaaland et al, 1991[101]	146	26	10†	—	—
Fossa et al, 1993[120]	308	38‡	14§	—	24
Vale, 1993[98]	60	38	12	—	—
Pollack et al, 1994[97]	135	42	20	0	26
Moonen et al, 1998[109]	379	25	17	—	22

*Cause-specific survival.
†T3/T4.
‡T2/T3a.
§T3b/T4.

The use of pelvic lymph node dissection before radiation therapy should be investigated in patients with bladder cancer who have no gross lymphadenopathy seen on CT or MRI. Pelvic lymph node dissection seems to be an effective means of controlling microscopic lymph node metastases and, if done properly, should not interfere with radiation therapy aimed at preserving normal bladder function. An extraperitoneal approach to the pelvic lymph nodes probably does not significantly increase the risk of late radiation complications. Laparoscopic lymphadenectomy also might be useful. Surgical management of the lymph nodes in this way would facilitate escalation of the dose to the primary tumor through the use of small-field conformal or intensity-modulated radiation therapy, with the expectation of enhanced local control. Adjuvant chemotherapy could be administered selectively to patients with lymph node metastases, who are at highest risk of distant recurrence.

Management of Local Recurrence After Radiation Therapy

Three situations are treated as "local recurrence" after radical radiation therapy: development of a new superficial or invasive bladder tumor; residual or recurrent CIS; and failure of radiation therapy to control the index tumor. New invasive tumors and failure to control the index tumor generally require prompt salvage cystectomy. However, some patients with local recurrence after radical radiation therapy can be treated without immediate cystectomy. A new superficial transitional cell tumor, for example, may be managed with transurethral resection with or without intravesical chemotherapy. Local recurrence that presents as CIS alone can be managed with intravesical BCG.[107,108] However, in cases in which the original muscle-invasive tumor developed against a background of BCG-resistant superficial disease, recurrence with CIS is an indication for salvage cystectomy. In all patients with muscle-invasive bladder cancer treated with radical radiation therapy, careful follow-up is essential to detect local failure and implement further treatment at an early stage and thereby maximize overall survival.

Salvage cystectomy for progressive muscle-invasive bladder cancer present after radiation therapy—either index tumor not controlled by irradiation or a new primary tumor—has historically been undertaken in only 20% to 30% of patients.[63,96,120,127] This reflects the generally poor prognosis of patients treated with radiation, who often have relative contraindications to surgery. Quilty and colleagues[127] reported a long-term local control rate of 86% in 111 patients who underwent salvage cystectomy, and long-term survival in several series has ranged from 40% to 60%.[63,127-134] The strongest predictor of survival after salvage cystectomy is the extent of tumor at the time of the procedure

(Ta/Tis vs. T1/T2 vs. T3).[127,130-132,135] Postoperative morbidity rates in the range of 25% to 35% and mortality rates between 5% and 8% have been described, but these rates are probably highly dependent on radiation fraction size and operative technique.[128,130,133] Other reports have suggested that salvage cystectomy can be performed safely, with a risk of complications that is not significantly different from the risk associated with cystectomy alone or planned preoperative radiation therapy and cystectomy.[63,134,136] Previous high-dose pelvic radiation therapy does not preclude continent urinary diversion at the time of cystectomy.[136,137]

Hayter and colleagues[126] reported the results of a population-based study of 1372 patients with bladder cancer who were treated with radical radiation therapy in Ontario, Canada, between 1982 and 1994. The 5-year overall survival, cause-specific survival, and cystectomy-free survival rates were 28%, 41%, and 25%, respectively. Radiation therapy was the sole treatment in 57% of patients, whereas 31% underwent transurethral resection for recurrence at some point after the completion of radiation therapy, and 12% underwent salvage cystectomy at a median interval of 10 months after the start of radiation therapy. The 5-year overall survival rate after cystectomy was 28%, and the cause-specific survival rate was 36%. Most deaths were due to bladder cancer.

Treatment Planning and Delivery

Patient selection. The goal of definitive radiation therapy for bladder cancer is cure with maintenance of normal bladder function. The criteria for selection of patients include a high probability of durable local control, an ability to deliver treatment in a reproducible fashion, and a low risk of serious complications. Bladder cancer is a heterogeneous disease, and in an unselected population, the outcome is influenced more by clinical and pathologic prognostic factors than by therapy. Although many powerful prognostic factors have been identified, the response to radiation therapy and the relative risks and benefits cannot be predicted accurately for an individual patient.

All patients with bladder cancer in whom definitive radiation therapy is being contemplated should be thoroughly examined to document the location and size of the tumor in the bladder, the degree of muscle invasion, the presence and extent of coexisting CIS, and the presence or absence of lymph node or distant metastases. Intravesical tumors should be completely resected to facilitate clinical staging and to improve the likelihood of achieving a complete response to radiation therapy.[103] Large residual tumor masses greater than 5 cm in maximal size that involve extravesical tissues or organs are unlikely to be controlled with radiation therapy. Gross pelvic lymphadenopathy also implies a low probability of success with irradiation. Patients with these presentations are probably better treated with cystectomy, if they are candidates for surgery, in combination with chemotherapy. Patients with extensive bladder CIS are at high risk for tumor recurrence after radiation therapy and the development of new bladder tumors and should be considered for cystectomy.[63] However, the presence of CIS does not absolutely preclude the use of radiation therapy because recurrent CIS after irradiation can be managed effectively with intravesical BCG.[107,108] Before radiation therapy is begun, urinary infection should be treated, and significant bladder outflow obstruction should be corrected.

The benefit of definitive radiation therapy is limited in the settings of irreversible severe impairment of bladder function, anatomic and technical factors that limit the accuracy and reproducibility of treatment delivery, and high risk of intolerable acute and late complications. Patients with severe irritable bladder symptoms at presentation as a result of factors such as long-standing outflow obstruction, chronic infection, or prior transurethral resection often have aggravation of symptoms during treatment and chronic impairment of bladder function and are thus better served by cystectomy. Pelvic radiation therapy is not appropriate for patients with active inflammatory bowel disease, previous pelvic irradiation, extensive prior pelvic surgery, or chronic pelvic infections because of a high risk of serious late bowel complications. Definitive radiation therapy also should be questioned in patients with large bladder diverticula or atonic bladders. In these patients, treatment reproducibility is likely to be poor, which may increase the risk of local tumor recurrence, and larger than normal fields may be required, which may increase the risk of serious late radiation complications.

Overall, ideal candidates for definitive radiation therapy and bladder preservation have a small cT2 tumor with no associated CIS, no significant bladder symptoms, no other serious medical problems, a desire to maintain normal bladder function, and a willingness to commit to both a prolonged course of therapy and regular follow-up cystoscopy afterwards. In these patients, the probability of long-term local control with an intact bladder is at least 50%.[63]

Volume definition. The successful treatment of bladder cancer with radiation requires accurate and reproducible delivery of multiple radiation fractions to the gross tumor and regions of subclinical disease extension. Microscopic infiltrative tumor is likely to be present in the lamina propria, lamina muscularis, and lymphovascular spaces adjacent to the primary tumor, although the degree of extension beyond gross disease has not been studied and is likely highly variable. Disease also may extend into paravesical tissues. The benefit of including radiographically uninvolved pelvic lymph nodes in the clinical target volume has not been extensively studied, but in light of surgical data suggesting a survival advantage with treatment of lymph nodes,

inclusion of radiographically uninvolved pelvic nodes should be considered, particularly in patients with bulky primary tumors, who are at high risk of harboring occult lymph node metastases.[71-74,87-89] Irradiation of pelvic nodes is generally well tolerated and does not significantly increase the risk of serious late radiation complications. It is common practice in many centers, but should be used with caution in elderly patients, who may have less physiologic reserve and less capacity to tolerate aggressive therapy. Future studies should evaluate the role of pelvic lymphadenectomy before radiation therapy in patients with bladder cancer.

Definitive radiation therapy for bladder cancer usually involves a two-phase technique. First, a dose aimed at controlling microscopic disease (45 to 50 Gy in 1.8- to 2-Gy daily fractions) is delivered to an initial clinical target volume that encompasses the entire bladder and paravesical tissues at a minimum and also may include the pelvic lymph nodes. This is followed by a boost dose to a reduced volume encompassing the primary tumor alone. No data exist regarding the effect of partial bladder irradiation alone on local tumor control.

Accurate definition of the gross tumor volume and knowledge of tumor and bladder movement during a course of fractionated radiation therapy are the basic requirements for accurate and reproducible treatment delivery. Information about gross tumor location and extent is available from diagnostic and staging investigations, including cystoscopy, examination under anesthesia, pelvic CT, and pelvic MRI. This information should be integrated with findings on CT imaging of the patient in the treatment position and used to develop a three-dimensional radiation therapy plan. CT-based treatment planning is more accurate than conventional planning techniques based on cystography alone, in part because CT allows delineation of the entire thickness of the tumor and bladder wall—not just the inner surface.[138-140] However, significant interobserver variability probably exists in the definition of gross tumor using CT.[141] This may be improved in the future with the use of planning MRI and registration of the CT and MRI scans. Cystography at the time of simulation is useful as a means of confirming the final treatment plan.

The bladder varies in size and position with differences in the volume of urine. To minimize this variability, patients are asked to completely empty their bladders immediately before any imaging done for treatment planning purposes and before delivery of each radiation fraction. However, significant changes in bladder volume may be present depending on the interval between voiding and treatment delivery and on other factors, such as the patient's state of hydration, use of diuretic medications, and ingestion of diuretic beverages, including coffee and soft drinks. Movement also may be influenced by extrinsic pressure, such as might arise from differences in rectal filling,[142] and by the characteristics of the tumor, including size and degree of extravesical extension. Turner and colleagues[142] demonstrated interfraction bladder wall movement of at least 1.5 cm in 18 of 30 patients, with the greatest movement being seen in those with large initial bladder volumes. Bladder movement resulted in inadequate coverage of the clinical target volume in 10 patients. A planning target volume (PTV) of 2 cm around the gross tumor has been recommended to account for random internal movement.[142,143] The development of equipment and techniques that allow daily verification of the treatment fields relative to the gross tumor volume, such as tomotherapy and the use of fiducial markers, may allow narrower margins to be used in the future.

It is likely that inadequate treatment planning and delivery, with underdosing of the gross tumor, have historically contributed to an excess number of local treatment failures in patients with bladder cancer. In theory, more accurate and reproducible treatment should improve tumor control and patient survival, although this has not been demonstrated in a prospective study. In addition, careful three-dimensional treatment planning may contribute to lower small bowel and rectal doses and thus reduced toxicity.

Field arrangement. The study protocols of the Radiation Therapy Oncology Group (RTOG) provide useful benchmarks for radiation treatment planning for bladder cancer.[144,145] Radiation is typically delivered using an isocentric technique, with anterior, posterior, right lateral, and left lateral 10- to 25-MV fields. To minimize both the volume of small bowel irradiated and interfraction differences in the size and position of the bladder, simulation and treatment are done while the patient has an empty bladder.

When internal and external iliac lymph nodes are encompassed in the first phase of treatment, the cranial aspect of the PTV is usually positioned at the level of the midsacrum, the caudal aspect is usually positioned at the lower pole of the obturator foramen, and the lateral aspects are usually positioned at least 1 cm beyond the bony margins of the true pelvis at its widest point. The anterior aspect of the PTV is usually dictated by the bladder wall, which often extends 1 to 2 cm anterior to the pubic symphysis in patients who are treated in the supine position. The anterior bladder wall is best determined on planning CT and by the position of the bladder air bubble on air contrast cystography. The PTV is 1 cm anterior to the bladder and at least at the anterior aspect of the symphysis. Posteriorly, the PTV is 1.5 cm behind the most posterior aspect of the bladder or bladder tumor. Shielding may be used in the corners of the fields to exclude small bowel and the femoral heads. The field arrangement for the first phase of a typical bladder treatment plan that includes pelvic lymph nodes is shown in Figure 25-2. When the first phase of treatment includes only the bladder, the PTV is 1.5 cm beyond the gross bladder volume (including the thickness of the bladder wall) as determined by CT and cystography.

The PTV for the boost phase of treatment encompasses the bladder tumor alone with a 1.5-cm margin. Digitally reconstructed radiographs illustrating typical bladder boost fields are shown in Figure 25-3. In the future, once the problem of internal bladder motion has been overcome, conformal and intensity-modulated radiation therapy techniques based on multiple fields or continuous rotations may be used to deliver a boost to the primary tumor and minimize the dose to adjacent bowel.

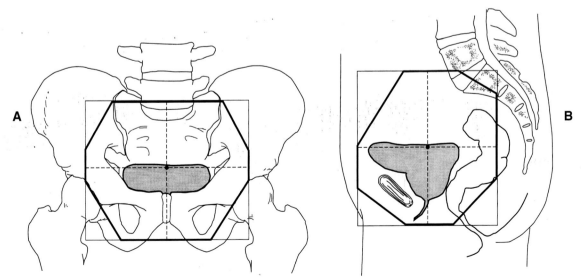

Fig. 25-2 Arrangement of fields for the initial phase of radiation therapy, encompassing the bladder and pelvic lymph nodes. **A,** Anterior view; **B,** lateral view.

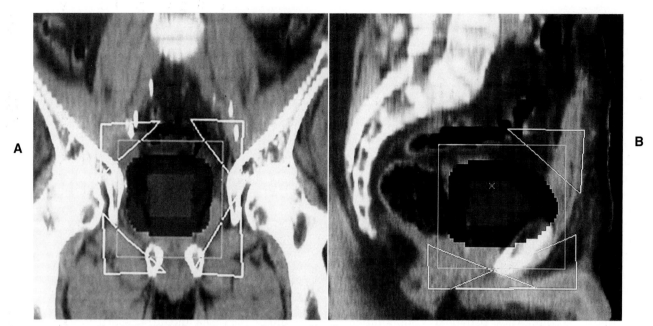

Fig. 25-3 Digitally reconstructed radiographs illustrating typical radiation therapy fields for the boost phase of treatment, encompassing the primary tumor and a 2-cm margin of normal tissue. **A,** Anterior view; **B,** lateral view.

Conventional radiation dose and fractionation. Definitive radiation therapy for bladder cancer has been administered using a variety of doses and fractionation schemes. In North America, the dose to the primary bladder tumor is typically 60 to 65 Gy in 1.8- to 2-Gy daily fractions over 6 to 7 weeks. The dose-response relationship for bladder cancer is poorly defined. Doses in the range of 55 to 60 Gy have been reported to produce higher local control rates than lower doses.[146] However, this apparent effect of dose on outcome may be explained by unrecognized differences in the distribution of important prognostic factors. Dose escalation beyond 60 to 65 Gy is probably not feasible with conventional treatment techniques and fractionation because of an unacceptably high risk of serious late radiation complications.

Complications. The risk and severity of radiation-induced side effects during and after treatment of bladder cancer depend on the condition of the bladder and other normal tissues before radiation therapy is begun, the location and extent of the tumor, the volume of normal bowel and bladder within the irradiated volume, treatment technique, dose and fraction size, concurrent medical problems, and individual intrinsic radiosensitivity. Most patients treated with external-beam radiation therapy experience acute gastrointestinal and lower urinary tract side effects. Abdominal cramping, diarrhea, and general rectal and bladder irritation are common and are usually easily controlled with dietary modification and medications. Attention should be paid to the diagnosis and eradication of

urinary tract infections, which may be clinically indistinguishable from acute radiation cystitis. Urinary tract infection is known to occur in a significant proportion of patients undergoing radiation therapy for bladder cancer.[147] Severe bowel or bladder symptoms before radiation therapy is begun would be predictive of a difficult course during treatment.

Late complications of radiation therapy for bladder cancer primarily affect the bowel and normal bladder and typically arise 1 to 4 years after treatment is completed. Approximately 75% of late complications are present by 3 years.[64,102] Symptoms of severe bladder damage include urinary frequency, dysuria, and intermittent hematuria. In severe cases, uncontrollable bleeding or a severely contracted bladder with little useful functional capacity may arise. Estimates of the risk of severe late bladder side effects range from 8% to 15%.[64,102,148] Treatment with large doses per fraction and a history of multiple prior transurethral bladder resections or intravesical chemotherapy may increase the risk.[6,20] Mounting evidence indicates that severe bladder side effects during radiation therapy may predispose to the development of late side effects.[8-11] Severe intestinal damage is manifested by persistent diarrhea, rectal bleeding, bowel obstruction, or fistula formation and has been reported in 6% to 17% of patients.[64,102] Large dose per fraction and rotational treatment techniques using ^{60}Co historically contributed to unacceptably high rates of gastrointestinal side effects.[98] Although data on quality of life are sparse, general quality of life appears to be preserved after radiation therapy for bladder cancer.[149-151] Sexual function remains normal in 30% to 40% of patients.[149,152]

The median survival time of patients with locally advanced bladder cancer is short, and many patients do not live long enough to manifest late side effects. Nevertheless, recognition of the factors that contribute to the development of side effects and careful attention to radiation treatment planning and delivery are essential for all patients. Current practice should result in a rate of serious late bladder and gastrointestinal complications of less than 5% with doses in the range of 60 to 65 Gy in 1.8- to 2-Gy daily fractions. Patients who develop bladder or bowel symptoms after radiation therapy need to be carefully examined to distinguish tumor recurrence from radiation-related side effects.

Evaluation of treatment response after radiation therapy. Traditionally, treatment response was evaluated 4 to 6 months after the completion of radiation therapy. This had the effect of assuring maximal disease regression but also delayed salvage cystectomy in patients with residual or locally progressive disease. The effect of such delays on long-term patient survival is unknown. However, salvage cystectomy is now generally performed within 3 months after completion of radiation therapy, and there is a trend towards even earlier evaluation.

The RTOG conducted a phase II study in which local tumor response was assessed cystoscopically 2 weeks after an initial dose of 40 Gy in 2-Gy daily fractions with concurrent cisplatin chemotherapy. Complete responders received a further 24 Gy, and patients with residual tumor were considered for immediate cystectomy. Overall, 66% of patients had a complete response after the initial 4 weeks of therapy. The overall actuarial survival rate was 60% at 4 years.[153,154] This approach, which introduces a 2-week treatment split for complete responders, has not been compared in a randomized fashion with more conventional continuous-course radiation therapy with later cystoscopy and salvage cystectomy for patients with disease progression. Follow-up cystoscopy should be performed at 6-month intervals for 3 years after a complete response is achieved and then annually.

Combined Treatment with Radiation Therapy and Chemotherapy

Radiation therapy alone for bladder cancer has been reported to produce long-term overall survival rates of 25% to 30% (see Table 25-1) and cause-specific survival rates of 25% to 45%. An incomplete response to radiation therapy or local recurrence after initial complete regression of disease occurs in more than 50% of patients. In addition, distant metastases arise in a large proportion of patients within 2 years after the completion of treatment. Improving the local effectiveness of

radiation therapy and treating occult distant metastases that are present at initial diagnosis are especially important. Combined treatment with radiation therapy and chemotherapy is one approach that has been investigated towards this end.

Cisplatin is the most active single agent in the treatment of urothelial carcinoma.[155] In addition, cisplatin has been shown in preclinical studies to enhance the cytotoxic effects of radiation under both oxic and hypoxic conditions. The precise mechanism of this sensitization is unknown but may relate to deficiencies in cellular repair processes. In general, radiation and cisplatin have nonoverlapping side effects. No evidence exists to indicate that cisplatin exacerbates the effects of radiation on normal tissues.[23,156]

Other drugs that are active against urothelial carcinoma include methotrexate, vinblastine, doxorubicin, fluorouracil, paclitaxel, and gemcitabine.[155,157-160] Gemcitabine has been shown in preclinical studies to be a potent radiation sensitizer and is presently being tested in phase I and II clinical trials to confirm this effect.[161] Experience in patients with metastatic bladder cancer has shown that combinations of chemotherapy agents are more effective than any of the agents individually but also are more toxic.[162]

Chemotherapy may be administered before definitive radiation therapy (neoadjuvant chemotherapy), at the same time as radiation therapy (concurrent chemotherapy) or after radiation therapy (adjuvant chemotherapy). Each approach has advantages and disadvantages.

Neoadjuvant chemotherapy has the potential to reduce the size of the primary tumor before delivery of radiation, thereby reducing the number of clonogenic cells that need to be killed by radiation. A reduction in tumor size may be associated with improved oxygenation, making the remaining clonogenic cells more sensitive to radiation. Neoadjuvant chemotherapy also offers the important advantage of early treatment of occult metastatic disease. A potential disadvantage is the delay of several weeks before the start of definitive radiation therapy, during which the primary tumor may progress. Induction chemotherapy also may worsen the side effects of radiation therapy.

Chemotherapy administered concurrently with radiation therapy may increase local tumor control by sensitizing cells to radiation, killing cells that are resistant to radiation, and off-setting the adverse affect of tumor proliferation during treatment. As is true for neoadjuvant chemotherapy, however, concurrent chemotherapy has the potential to increase the side effects of radiation therapy.

Adjuvant chemotherapy, administered after radiation therapy has been completed, may overcome the problem of increased side effects. However, with this approach, a complementary effect of radiation and chemotherapy with respect to control of the primary tumor is less likely, and the treatment of occult metastases is delayed. The optimal method of sequencing radiation therapy and chemotherapy in the treatment of bladder cancer and the optimal drug or drug combination have not been defined.

Trials of Neoadjuvant Chemotherapy

Neoadjuvant chemotherapy before definitive radiation therapy for bladder cancer has been the focus of several clinical trials. Initial phase II studies suggested increased local control, prolonged survival, and minimal toxicity.[145,163,164] However, the early enthusiasm for neoadjuvant chemotherapy has diminished in light of the results of several phase III clinical studies that have recently been reported.[23,165-167] These are summarized in Table 25-3.

The largest of these studies included 976 patients with T2 to T4, N0 or NX, M0 transitional cell carcinoma of the bladder who were randomly assigned to receive either cystectomy or radiation therapy alone or three cycles of neoadjuvant chemotherapy with cisplatin, methotrexate, and vinblastine (CMV) followed by radical radiation therapy.[23] A total of 485 patients underwent cystectomy alone, 415 were treated with radiation therapy alone, and 76 were treated with preoperative radiation therapy followed by cystectomy. No difference in overall survival rates at 5 years was noted between the chemotherapy and no-chemotherapy arms of the study

(55.5% and 50%, respectively). Local control was not affected by chemotherapy, although a suggestion was made that chemotherapy delayed the development of metastases. Side effects were similar in the chemotherapy and no-chemotherapy arms.

In a similar study, the RTOG randomly assigned 123 patients to receive radiation therapy with concurrent cisplatin followed by either further radiation therapy or cystectomy or the same treatment preceded by two cycles of CMV chemotherapy.[165] The study was closed prematurely because of an unexpectedly high rate of severe neutropenic sepsis and death in the neoadjuvant-chemotherapy arm. Again, no difference in 5-year overall survival rates was noted between the concurrent-chemotherapy and neoadjuvant-chemotherapy groups (49% and 48%, respectively) and no difference in local or distant control. Approximately 40% of patients in both arms of the study were alive with an intact bladder 5 years after diagnosis. These studies indicate that the benefit of combination chemotherapy before radiation therapy in patients with bladder cancer is small at best and probably of minimal clinical relevance.

Studies of chemotherapy before cystectomy have shown improved resectability and delayed progression of disease.[168-170] In the Nordic Cystectomy Trial I, 311 patients were randomly assigned to receive two cycles of cisplatin and doxorubicin followed by cystectomy or cystectomy alone. Preoperative radiation therapy

---

TABLE 25-3

Randomized Studies of Combination Chemotherapy and Radiation Therapy in Patients with Bladder Cancer

Study and Reference	Number of Patients	Disease Stage	Chemotherapy Regimen	Control Group	3-Year vs. 5-Year Survival Rates
NEOADJUVANT					
Shearer et al, 1988[167]	376	T3	Methotrexate	RT alone or PreRT + cyst	39% vs. 37%, NS
Wallace et al, 1991[166]	255	T2-T4	Cisplatin	RT	NS
Shipley et al, 1998[165] (RTOG 89-03)	123	T2-T4	CMV	RT + cisplatin ± cyst	48% vs. 49%, NS
Ghersi et al, 1999[23] (EORTC)	976	T2-T4	CMV	RT or cyst	55% vs. 50%, NS
CONCURRENT					
Coppin et al, 1996*[156]	99	T2-T4	Cisplatin	RT alone or PreRT + cyst	47% vs. 33%, NS
ADJUVANT					
Richards et al, 1982[174]	129	T3	Doxorubicin Fluorouracil	RT	NS

Cyst, Cystectomy; *CMV*, cisplatin, methotrexate, and vinblastine; *EORTC*, European Organization for Research and Treatment of Cancer; *NS*, not significant; *PreRT*, planned preoperative radiation therapy; *RTOG*, Radiation Therapy Oncology Group.
*Improved pelvic control.

consisting of 20 Gy in five daily fractions was administered to all patients. A significant improvement occurred in overall survival associated with the use of chemotherapy.[170] However, a recent meta-analysis of both surgery and radiation therapy studies showed no survival advantage with chemotherapy.[171] The authors concluded that neoadjuvant chemotherapy should not be used in routine clinical practice and that future trials should include a "no chemotherapy" control arm.

Trials of Concurrent Chemotherapy

The only phase III clinical study of concurrent chemotherapy and radiation therapy in patients with bladder cancer was conducted by the National Cancer Institute of Canada.[156] Patients with T2 to T4b transitional cell carcinoma of the bladder were randomly assigned to receive local–regional therapy (definitive radiation therapy or preoperative radiation therapy and cystectomy) with or without concurrent cisplatin. Cisplatin was administered at a dose of 100 mg/m^2 every 2 weeks for three cycles during radiation therapy. No difference was found in overall survival or distant relapse-free survival between the treatment groups. However, patients who received concurrent chemotherapy had a significantly lower rate of pelvic recurrence than patients treated with radiation alone. No difference in the risk of serious side effects was noted. This study supports the use of cisplatin concurrently with radiation therapy in patients with bladder cancer as a means of enhancing local tumor control and minimizing the likelihood of future tumor-related morbidity. However, several questions remain about how best to combine these two modalities.

Eapen and colleagues[172,173] reported excellent results using concurrent intraarterial cisplatin in patients with T3 or T4 bladder cancer. Complete clearance of pelvic tumor was seen in 96% of patients, and the 2-year actuarial survival rate was 90%. However, 46% of patients developed sacral sensory neuropathy. The risk of neuropathy was significantly lower in a subsequent cohort of patients who received a lower dose of cisplatin. Future studies will need to address the issue of optimal dose and delivery of chemotherapy in combination with radiation therapy in the current practice environment, in which new potentially useful drugs are constantly emerging and radiation therapy practice is evolving, driven by improvements in technology.

Trials of Adjuvant Chemotherapy

Only one phase III clinical study of adjuvant chemotherapy after radiation therapy in patients with high-risk bladder cancer has been conducted. This study is from the precisplatin era and showed no difference in overall survival.[174] In contrast, several randomized studies of chemotherapy after cystectomy in patients with either locally extensive primary tumors or involved pelvic lymph nodes have been conducted.[175-178] The chemotherapy in these studies typically consisted of two to four cycles of cisplatin, either alone or in combination with other drugs. In general, the results showed improved disease-free survival with adjuvant chemotherapy but no difference in overall survival. This may in part reflect that chemotherapy administered at the time of recurrence was associated with a high likelihood of response, particularly in chemotherapy-naïve patients, so that the beneficial effect of adjuvant treatment on overall survival was diminished. Nevertheless, it is reasonable to offer high-risk patients chemotherapy after cystectomy with the aim of delaying tumor progression and minimizing overall morbidity. The benefits of adjuvant chemotherapy also may be attainable in patients undergoing radiation therapy. However, the indications for adjuvant chemotherapy after radiation therapy are less well defined, mainly because the detailed surgicopathologic prognostic information provided by cystectomy and pelvic lymphadenectomy is not usually available. In general, further study is needed to identify clinical, surgicopathologic, microenvironmental, and molecular factors predictive of disease recurrence after radiation therapy to aid in selecting patients for additional treatment.

Preoperative Radiation Therapy

The rationale for planned preoperative radiation therapy in the management of bladder cancer is enhancement of tumor control in the pelvis. Preoperative radiation therapy may enable complete resection of disease in a proportion of patients who would otherwise be left with residual disease after resection. In addition, preoperative radiation therapy may reduce the clonogenic viability of cancer cells that are disseminated at the time of surgery and provide early treatment of microscopic pelvic lymph node metastases. The disadvantages of preoperative radiation therapy include the possibility of problems in interpreting the pathologic findings in cystectomy and lymphadenectomy specimens and the possibility of side effects as a result of operating on previously irradiated tissues.

The patients most likely to benefit from preoperative radiation therapy are those who would have a high risk of pelvic recurrence after cystectomy alone. Primary tumors that are confined to the bladder wall (pT2 or pT3a) can usually be completely resected, carry a low risk of pelvic lymph node involvement, and are associated with a pelvic recurrence rate of less than 10%.[72,86,179] Preoperative radiation therapy is unlikely to be beneficial in these cases. In contrast, 30% to 50% of patients with extravesical extension of the primary tumor (pT3b or pT4) will have involved pelvic lymph nodes, and a similar proportion will develop a pelvic recurrence after cystectomy. Preoperative radiation therapy has the potential to reduce the rate of pelvic recurrence and overall morbidity in these high-risk patients. However, it is unlikely to yield a significant improvement in overall survival because the clinical and surgicopathologic prognostic factors that predict local recurrence also strongly predict distant recurrence.

The largest experience with preoperative radiation therapy for bladder cancer is from The University of Texas M.D. Anderson Cancer Center.[125] Between 1960 and 1983, 338 patients with T2 to T4 bladder cancer were treated with planned preoperative radiation therapy consisting of 50 Gy in 25 daily fractions. This was followed 4 to 6 weeks later by radical cystectomy and dissection of clinically suspicious pelvic lymph nodes. Preoperative radiation therapy resulted in pathologic downstaging in 65% of patients, and no tumor was found in the surgical specimen in 42%. The overall survival rate at 5 years was 44%. The pelvic and distant recurrence rates (at a median follow-up of 90 months for living patients) were 16% and 43%, respectively. Tumor size and response to preoperative radiation therapy were important independent predictors of disease-free survival. Comparison with a more recent cohort of patients who underwent cystectomy alone revealed no improvement in local control with preoperative radiation therapy for patients with cT2 or cT3a disease.[179] However, local control was significantly improved in patients with cT3b tumors (91% for preoperative radiation therapy vs. 72% for cystectomy alone). No difference was found in overall survival.

Several randomized comparisons of planned preoperative radiation therapy plus cystectomy vs. either cystectomy alone or radical radiation therapy alone with cystectomy for salvage have been conducted (Table 25-4).[148,180-183] Many of these studies included patients who had early-stage disease and thus were unlikely to benefit from preoperative irradiation. Other problems include the use of relatively low doses of radiation and infrequent reporting of local control, which is the endpoint most likely to be affected by preoperative treatment.

Pathologic downstaging as a result of preoperative radiation therapy was described in many of the studies, as was a correlation between response to radiation therapy and overall treatment outcome.[180,181] Only one of the studies showed a survival advantage in favor of preoperative radiation therapy, and that study contained a high proportion of patients with schistosomiasis.[183] The results of this study may or may not be generalizable to the broader population of patients with bladder cancer. A recent meta-analysis based on four of the studies listed in Table 25-4 showed no effect of preoperative radiation therapy on survival.[184]

Planned preoperative radiation therapy and early cystectomy does not increase the risk of significant surgical morbidity or mortality.[148,183] This probably reflects the fact that surgery is usually performed within 4 to 8 weeks of the completion of radiation therapy, after resolution of the acute radiation-induced inflammatory response but before the onset of the normal tissue vascular and fibrotic changes that are important in the development of late radiation complications.

Overall, the indications for planned preoperative radiation therapy in the management of bladder cancer are probably limited. Patients with early-stage tumors confined to the bladder wall are unlikely to benefit from pelvic irradiation. On the other hand, patients with locally extensive tumors are at high risk of pelvic recurrence but also at high risk of distant recurrence, which is likely to dominate the clinical course in most cases. These high-risk patients are probably better treated with cystectomy and pelvic lymph node dissection followed by adjuvant systemic chemotherapy. It is not known whether radiation therapy and chemotherapy are equivalent in their potential to reduce pelvic recurrence or, alternatively, if irradiation contributes to local control beyond that attainable with chemotherapy alone. Therefore, preoperative radiation therapy may play a role in selected patients who are deemed to be at particularly high risk of developing locally progressive disease and patients who are not candidates for systemic

TABLE 25-4

Randomized Studies of Planned Preoperative Radiation Therapy and Cystectomy in Patients with Bladder Cancer

Study and Reference	Number of Patients	Disease Stage	Radiation Dose	Control Group	3-Year vs. 5-Year Survival Rates
Bloom et al, 1982[181]	189	T3	40 Gy	RT	38% vs. 29%, NS
Anderstrom et al, 1983[180]	44	T1-T3		Cystectomy	75% vs. 61%
Ghoneim et al, 1985*[183]	92		20 Gy	Cystectomy	
Sell et al, 1991[148]	183	T2-T4a	40 Gy	RT	NS
Smith et al, 1997[182] (SWOG)	140	Tis-T3†	20 Gy	Cystectomy	43% vs. 53%, NS

NS, Not significant; *RT*, radiation therapy; *SWOG*, Southwest Oncology Group.
*High proportion of patients had schistosomiasis.
†64% T3 tumors.

chemotherapy. Reliable preoperative identification of high-risk patients remains a challenge given the limitations of clinical staging based on cystoscopy and examination under anesthesia. However, the development of MRI and positron emission tomography has yielded significant advances in this regard. In addition, cellular and molecular indicators of local tumor aggressiveness, such as apoptotic index and *p53* status, may complement traditional clinical staging investigations as a means of selecting patients for preoperative radiation therapy.[116,118]

Postoperative Radiation Therapy

Postoperative radiation therapy is used in the management of many types of cancer, including prostate, cervix, and endometrial cancer, with the aim of reducing the risk of pelvic recurrence. Postoperative radiation therapy has the advantage over preoperative radiation therapy of allowing treatment to be individualized on the basis of surgicopathologic prognostic factors and administered only to those patients who are most likely to benefit. The major disadvantage of postoperative radiation therapy is the potential for increased toxicity from irradiation of postsurgical tissues.

Postoperative pelvic radiation therapy, similar to preoperative radiation therapy, is most likely to benefit patients who are at high risk of pelvic recurrence. This includes patients with extravesical disease, positive resection margins, or involved pelvic lymph nodes. Postoperative radiation therapy at doses in the range of 40 to 50 Gy appears to reduce the risk of pelvic recurrence in these patients from 30% to 50% to 10% to 20%.[185-187] However, the results in many of the studies are difficult to interpret because patients also often received planned preoperative pelvic radiation therapy.[185,186]

The only randomized study of radical cystectomy alone vs. cystectomy and postoperative irradiation in high-risk bladder cancer was reported by Zaghloul and colleagues[187] and accrued patients with schistosomiasis. The 5-year pelvic recurrence rate was 50% in the cystectomy arm of the study but only 7% with the addition of conventionally fractionated radiation therapy. Radiation therapy also seemed to confer a reduction in the risk of metastases and an improvement in disease-free survival.[187] Notwithstanding these results, which may not necessarily be translatable to patients without schistosomiasis, the factors that predict pelvic recurrence also predict strongly for lymph node and distant recurrence, as previously discussed, and therefore the benefit of pelvic irradiation with respect to overall survival is likely to be small.

Postoperative pelvic radiation therapy might be valuable as a means of reducing potentially morbid pelvic recurrences in patients with high-risk bladder cancer if it were not for the unacceptably high rate of serious late gastrointestinal complications. Several investigators have reported this rate to be in the range of 20% to 40%,[74,185,186,188,189] which is substantially higher than the rate after radical surgery and radiation therapy for other pelvic tumors. Many factors probably contribute to this increased complication rate, but the most important may be the larger volume of small bowel occupying the pelvis after cystectomy. An intact bladder normally displaces small bowel from the pelvis and allows pelvic irradiation at doses necessary for the control of microscopic disease to be administered safely.

Surgical techniques that prevent the small bowel from filling the void left by the bladder after cystectomy may reduce the risk of late complications, as may the use of hyperfractionated radiation therapy.[188] However, further study of these approaches, especially the use of altered fractionation schemes, is necessary to define their role in routine clinical practice. Conformal radiation therapy may allow treatment to be administered postoperatively to focal regions within the pelvis but is unlikely to be helpful in the adjuvant setting, in which large volumes need to be treated. Overall, patients who are identified after cystectomy as being at high risk of recurrence are probably better treated with chemotherapy, which affects both local and distant relapse and is usually well tolerated in otherwise healthy patients.

Altered Radiation Fractionation

Radiation fractionation schemes that deviate from the norm of 1.8 to 2 Gy/day have been investigated in bladder cancer as a means of enhancing local tumor control. Substantial clinical and laboratory evidence indicates that tumors and normal tissues have different capacities to repair radiation-induced DNA damage in the clinically relevant dose range of 1 to 3 Gy/fraction.[17] This is reflected in α/β ratios of approximately 10 for radiation killing of tumor cells vs. 2 to 4 for the development of late normal tissue side effects.[17] Fractionated radiation therapy exploits this difference and allows the administration of tumoricidal doses with relative sparing of normal tissues.

Hyperfractionated radiation therapy, defined as the delivery of a larger number of smaller fractions with no increase in overall treatment time, has been examined in patients with bladder cancer as a means of further exploiting the biological differences between the tumor and the surrounding normal tissues. In theory, hyperfractionated radiation therapy should allow an increase in radiation dose leading to a greater likelihood of tumor control with no increase in the risk of late radiation complications.

A meta-analysis was recently reported of randomized hyperfractionated radiation therapy trials involving a variety of human tumors.[190] The pooled results from two bladder cancer studies indicated a significant improvement in overall survival with hyperfractionated treatment. One of the studies included in the meta-analysis included 168 patients with T2 to T4 bladder cancer who were randomly assigned to receive hyper-fractionated radiation therapy consisting of 84 Gy in 1-Gy fractions administered 3 times a day or 64 Gy in 2-Gy daily fractions.[191] Both treatment regimens were administered in two 3-week sessions separated by a 2-week rest period to minimize acute side effects. The hyperfractionation was associated with improved local control and improved overall survival. A trend towards a higher rate of serious bowel complications was noted with hyperfractionated therapy, although this did not reach statistical significance. At present, evidence is insufficient to support the routine use of hyperfractionated radiation therapy in the management of bladder cancer. However, the existing evidence is sufficiently intriguing to warrant further investigation.

Hypofractionated radiation schedules, based on larger daily doses, in the range of 2.5 to 5 Gy, also have been used to treat patients with bladder cancer, usually in the palliative setting. The larger fraction size increases the potential for late radiation complications, and the total dose needs to be decreased in comparison to the dose used in standard fractionation schemes to ensure patient safety. Salminen[192] reported late side effects affecting the bladder, small bowel, or rectum in 29% of patients after 30 Gy in six fractions over 3 weeks. Scholten and colleagues,[193] in a similar study of 36 Gy in six fractions over 3 weeks, found a 33% rate of late complication and a 9% rate of severe complications. These results imply that the benefit of hypofractionated radiation therapy in terms of patient convenience must be balanced against the possibility of increased side effects. Careful attention must be given to treatment planning, with the aim of excluding as much bladder, small bowel, and rectum as possible from the high-dose volume. Conformal radiation therapy techniques may be helpful in achieving this goal.

Laboratory and clinical studies have shown that tumor growth may increase during a course of fractionated radiation therapy as a result of changes in the balance between cellular proliferation and cell loss.[17] Several indicators of cell proliferation, including labeling index, potential doubling time, Ki-67 level, and proliferating cell nuclear antigen level, are being evaluated as predictors of accelerated population during radiation.[194-197] Labeling index and potential doubling time have been estimated in bladder cancer and appear to correlate with histologic grade.[195-197] In poorly differentiated transitional cell carcinoma, the labeling index and potential doubling time have been estimated to be 22% and 3 days, respectively, similar to the values in carcinoma of the cervix, in which overall treatment time is known to be an important determinant of outcome.[198]

At least one study has demonstrated an inferior result in patients with bladder cancer who receive radiation over a prolonged interval.[199] These results suggest that accelerated radiation therapy regimens, which are designed to deliver the same total dose of radiation therapy in a shorter interval, have the potential to improve the outcome of patients with bladder cancer. Sufficient time must be allowed between fractions to ensure complete repair of sublethal radiation damage and minimize the risk of severe late radiation side effects.

Horwich and colleagues[200] recently reported the results of a prospective study in which 229 patients with bladder cancer were randomly assigned to receive accelerated radiation therapy consisting of 60.8 Gy in 32 fractions over 26 days or conventional radiation therapy with 64 Gy in 32 fractions over 45 days. No difference was found in local control, time to metastasis, or overall survival between the groups, but patients in the accelerated arm of the study had a significantly higher rate of bowel complications.

Interstitial Radiation Therapy

Interstitial radiation therapy for bladder cancer has been practiced in some parts of Europe for many years, with the first reports dating to the early twentieth century.[201] This approach allows a high dose of radiation to be delivered focally to a small area of the bladder with relative sparing of surrounding normal tissues. Several techniques have been described that involve the permanent implantation of radon or gold seeds[202,203] or the temporary placement of radium or cesium needles.[204,205] Afterloading techniques that employ low-dose-rate iridium wire are now commonly used to minimize the radiation exposure of medical and nursing personnel.[206-209] Pulsed-dose-rate radiation therapy also has been described; with this approach, a single iridium source is sequentially moved from position to position in the implant to simulate low-dose-rate treatment.[206] At least one report of high-dose-rate brachytherapy for bladder cancer using a similar stepped technique with a high-activity iridium source has been presented.[210]

Only selected bladder tumors are suitable for treatment with interstitial radiation therapy.[205,206,208,211-213] Tumors should be solitary, less than 5 cm in diameter, and preferably confined to the bladder wall (pT1 or pT2) with no extravesical extension. Random biopsies of uninvolved bladder mucosa should be negative for CIS. The patient must be medically fit for surgery. These criteria are similar to the selection criteria for partial cystectomy, and interstitial radiation therapy often has been used in conjunction with partial cystectomy to minimize the risk of local recurrence.

The technique used for interstitial bladder irradiation consists of initial thorough clinical, radiographic, and cystoscopic examination to ensure that the eligibility criteria are met. A suprapubic surgical approach is commonly used to visualize the bladder and position the interstitial catheters. Early experience with this technique identified a high rate of disease recurrence at the operative site, presumably as a result of tumor cell dissemination during surgery. It was later demonstrated that recurrence could be prevented by short-course preoperative external-beam radiation therapy.[204]

Preoperative radiation therapy typically consists of 10.5 Gy in three daily fractions to the pelvis, although higher doses in the range of 30 to 40 Gy also have been used.[205,206,212,213] Preoperative radiation therapy is followed as soon as possible by surgery that may include transurethral resection of visible tumor, laparotomy, pelvic lymphadenectomy, partial cystectomy, and placement of plastic catheters to form a single-plane implant. Interstitial radiation therapy is begun 1 to 7 days after surgery (earlier treatment has been associated with a higher risk of acute radiation side effects in some series).[207] The interstitial radiation dose is in the range of 50 Gy if low-dose preoperative external-beam radiation therapy is used and 30 to 35 Gy after high-dose preoperative radiation therapy.[205-208]

The largest experience with interstitial radiation therapy for bladder cancer was described by Rozan and colleagues[208] and was based on 205 patients treated at eight radiation therapy centers in France. Most patients had solitary T1 or T2 tumors, and the median tumor size was 2.9 cm. Of these patients, 58% underwent partial cystectomy before interstitial radiation therapy. Tumor recurred locally in 17% of patients, and often this was the only site of recurrence. The long-term overall survival rate was 67%, which is higher than in most series of cystectomy and external-beam irradiation, probably reflecting the generally more favorable characteristics of patients who are candidates for interstitial treatment. Moderate to severe late side effects (persistent hematuria, chronic cystitis, or fistula formation) were seen in 14% of patients. Other authors have described chronic mucosal ulceration in 15% to 30% of patients, although this is usually asymptomatic and heals spontaneously.[206,207,213]

The limited clinical evidence suggests that interstitial radiation therapy may contribute to enhanced pelvic control and bladder preservation in selected patients. However, no phase III clinical studies have been conducted comparing interstitial radiation therapy with conservative surgery alone, external-beam radiation therapy, or—particularly important—modern three-dimensional conformal treatment approaches. The role of interstitial radiation therapy in routine clinical practice therefore remains unclear.

Palliative Treatment

It is important to place palliative radiation therapy for bladder cancer in the context of overall palliative care. The Canadian Palliative Care Standards Task Force defined palliative care as "the combination of active and compassionate therapies intended to comfort and support the patient and family who are living with a life-threatening illness."[214] Unlike definitive treatment, the objective of which is long-term tumor control, palliative therapy has as its goals symptom relief and preservation of quality of life. The endpoints for evaluating the success of palliative therapy should reflect these goals.

Radiation Therapy

In bladder cancer, palliative irradiation may be used to relieve or prevent symptoms caused by either local tumor progression in the pelvis or metastatic disease. Both types of disease may result in significant morbidity and impairment of quality of life. Uncontrolled bladder tumor often results in intractable hematuria, pelvic pain, and irritative voiding symptoms that are incapacitating. Box 25-3 lists indications for palliative radiation therapy.

Palliative radiation therapy for locally progressive bladder cancer may be considered in the setting of extensive, symptomatic disease in the bladder in a patient who, because of either the characteristics of the disease or associated medical problems, is not suitable for radical treatment administered with curative intent. The commonly used fractionation schemes for palliative radiation therapy include 30 Gy in 10 daily fractions, 35 Gy in 10 daily fractions, and 20 Gy in 5 daily fractions.

Retrospective studies of palliative radiation therapy administered for local bladder symptoms have documented significant improvement in hematuria but less improvement in urinary frequency, urgency, and nocturia.[215] Salminen[192] reported the Australian experience with palliative bladder irradiation in 94 patients treated with 30 Gy in six fractions given twice a week over 3 weeks. Reduced hematuria and relief of pelvic pain were seen in more than 60% of patients, and urgency was

---

BOX 25-3 Indications for Palliative Radiation Therapy in Patients with Bladder Cancer

LOCAL DISEASE
Hematuria
Pelvic pain
Dysuria
Urinary frequency
Urgency

METASTATIC DISEASE
Spinal cord compression
Bone pain
Nerve entrapment
Nodal metastases causing pain or lymphedema
Brain metastases
Bronchial obstruction or hemoptysis

improved in 50%. The irradiated pelvic volume was not described in detail, but this hypofractionated-radiation-therapy protocol was associated with considerable side effects, as previously discussed in the section on "Altered Fractionation."

Holmang and Borghede[216] reported the results of palliative radiation therapy in 96 patients with locally advanced bladder cancer treated with 21 Gy given in three fractions on alternate days. Improvement in hematuria was observed in the majority of patients, but no improvement was noted in urgency, dysuria, or urinary frequency. Five treatment-related deaths were noted, and severe gastrointestinal complications occurred in 26% of patients. Wijkstrom and colleagues[217] reported the results of palliative radiation therapy in 162 patients with locally advanced, incurable bladder cancer unfit for radical therapy who received 21 Gy in three fractions of 7 Gy given every other day over 5 days. Improvement in symptoms was observed in 46% of patients. However, 40% of patients developed significant acute complications, and two patients required colostomy because of late gastrointestinal complications.

The Medical Research Council in the United Kingdom recently completed a prospective randomized trial of two dose prescriptions for palliative radiation therapy in bladder cancer, comparing 35 Gy in 10 fractions over 2 weeks to 21 Gy in 3 fractions given every second day over 5 days.[218] The study accrued 500 patients, but only 272 were fully assessable 3 months after completing radiation therapy, reflecting the high mortality rate in this population. No differences in symptom relief or side effects were noted between the two arms of the study. Overall, symptom improvement was observed in 68% of patients. Hematuria improved in 88% of patients, dysuria improved in 72%, urinary frequency improved in 82%, and nocturia improved in 64%.

These studies point out several issues that need to be considered in prescribing palliative pelvic radiation therapy for patients with bladder cancer. The goals of treatment should be clear. In the series just discussed, short palliative fractionation schemes were used to relieve symptoms in lieu of conventional fractionation. Although treatment duration was short, toxicity was high and counter to the goal of palliation. Therefore, if local tumor control (not just palliation of symptoms) is the desired objective, a higher, more conventional radiation dose with smaller daily fractions should be prescribed. If palliation is the goal, short-course treatment appears beneficial and will temporarily alleviate hematuria and pain. However, symptoms will probably recur given sufficient time. Short-course treatment is therefore most appropriate for patients with pelvic pain or hematuria from bladder cancer, who also have rapidly worsening performance status, metastases, or limited life expectancy for other reasons. Severe urinary symptoms are rarely adequately controlled with radiation therapy,

and urinary diversion may be more appropriate in such cases.

Chemotherapy

A large proportion of patients with bladder cancer either present with lymph node or distant metastases or develop metastatic disease during the course of their illness. Although small-bulk pelvic nodal disease may be managed effectively with lymphadenectomy and adjuvant chemotherapy, paraaortic lymphadenopathy is associated with a poor prognosis, and patients with such disease are less likely to benefit from aggressive surgery. Overall, the survival of patients with untreated metastatic bladder cancer is usually less than 6 months,[155] and patients may develop a variety of disabling symptoms during this interval that disrupt quality of life. Chemotherapy may be effective in ameliorating these symptoms.

Transitional cell carcinoma is very sensitive to chemotherapy. Cisplatin is the most active single agent, and response rates in the range of 15% to 30% have been documented in a number of studies.[155] Cisplatin has been combined with other active agents to yield regimens with higher response rates, usually at the expense of greater toxicity. Currently, the most commonly used regimens are CMV and CMV plus doxorubicin (M-VAC, methotrexate, vinblastine, doxorubicin [Adriamycin], and cisplatin). M-VAC was compared to cisplatin alone in a cooperative-group randomized study and was found to produce a higher overall response rate (39% vs. 12%), enhanced progression-free survival, and enhanced overall survival. However, only 3.7% of patients randomly assigned to receive M-VAC were alive at 6 years. Good performance status at the time of treatment, transitional cell histologic subtype, and the presence of nodal or soft issue metastases only (no visceral metastases) were associated with prolonged survival. Patients receiving M-VAC experienced greater nausea and vomiting, mucositis, and hematologic toxicity, and 4% died of drug-related complications.[162,219] Other randomized studies have demonstrated M-VAC to be superior to the combination of cyclophosphamide, doxorubicin, and cisplatin and have demonstrated CMV to be superior to methotrexate and vinblastine alone.[220,221] None of these studies adequately addressed the important issues of symptom improvement and changes in quality of life.

M-VAC and CMV, although yielding improved survival compared to expectant management or treatment with cisplatin alone, also are associated with significant toxicity that may detract from the goal of palliation in patients with metastatic disease. Therefore, other regimens comprising active agents with nonoverlapping toxicities are currently being investigated with the aim of enhancing the therapeutic ratio. These include combinations of cisplatin with gemcitabine[159] or paclitaxel.[160] The results of a large international randomized study that compared M-VAC to gemcitabine plus cisplatin in patients with metastatic bladder cancer were recently reported.[157] No significant differences were noted between the M-VAC and gemcitabine-cisplatin groups in response rate (46% vs. 49%), overall survival (median 14.8 vs. 13.8 months), or quality of life. However, gemcitabine plus cisplatin was significantly less toxic: more patients completed the full course of treatment, fewer had significant neutropenia or sepsis, and the rate of death from side effects was lower. The authors argued that the more favorable benefit-risk ratio of gemcitabine plus cisplatin justified a change in the standard management of these cases.

REFERENCES

1. Rubin P, Casarett GW. *Clinical Radiation Pathology*. Philadelphia, Pa: WB Saunders; 1968.
2. Mettler FA, Upton AC. *Medical Effects of Ionizing Radiation*. Philadelphia, Pa: WB Saunders; 1995.
3. Fajardo LF, Berthrong M, Anderson RE. Ureters and urinary bladder. In: *Radiation Pathology*. New York, NY: Oxford University Press; 2001:281-287.
4. Michalski JM, Purdy JA, Winter K, et al. Preliminary report of toxicity following 3D radiation therapy for prostate cancer on 3DOG/RTOG 9406. *Int J Radiat Oncol Biol Phys* 2000;46: 391-402.
5. International Commission on Radiological Units and Measurements. ICRU report 38. *Dose and Volume Specifications for Reporting Intracavitary Therapy in Gynecology*. Bethesda, Md: ICRU; 1985.
6. Marks LB, Carroll PR, Dugan TC, et al. The response of the urinary bladder, urethra and ureter to radiation and chemotherapy. *Int J Radiat Oncol Biol Phys* 1995;31:1257-1280.
7. Dorr W, Eckhardt M, Ehme A, et al. Pathogenesis of acute radiation effects in the urinary bladder. Experimental results. *Strahlenther Onkol* 1998;174(suppl):93-95.
8. Dorr W, Beck-Bornholdt HP. Radiation-induced impairment of urinary bladder function in mice: fine structure of the acute response and consequences on late effects. *Radiat Res* 1999; 151:461-467.
9. Dorr W, Bentzen SM. Late functional response of the mouse urinary bladder to fractionated x-irradiation. *Int J Radiat Biol* 1999;75:1307-1315.
10. Schultheiss TE, Lee WR, Hunt MA, et al. Late GI and GU complications in the treatment of prostate cancer. *Int J Radiat Oncol Biol Phys* 1997;37:3-11.
11. Zelefsky MJ, Cowen D, Fuks Z, et al. Long-term tolerance of high-dose three-dimensional conformal radiotherapy in patients with localized prostate carcinoma. *Cancer* 1999;85:2460-2468.
12. Greven KM, Lanciano RM, Herbert SH, et al. Analysis of complications in patients with endometrial carcinoma receiving adjuvant irradiation. *Int J Radiat Oncol Biol Phys* 1991;21:919-923.
13. Minsky BD. Primary treatment of rectal cancer: present and future. *Crit Rev Oncol Hematol* 1999;32:19-30.
14. Storey MR, Pollack A, Zagars G, et al. Complications from radiotherapy dose escalation in prostate cancer: preliminary results of a randomized trial. *Int J Radiat Oncol Biol Phys* 2000;48: 635-642.
15. Emami B, Lyman J, Brown A, et al. Tolerance of normal tissue to therapeutic radiation. *Int J Radiat Oncol Biol Phys* 1991;21: 109-122.
16. Boersma LJ, Brink MVD, Bruce AM, et al. Estimation of the incidence of late bladder and rectum complications after high-dose
(70-78 Gy) conformal radiotherapy for prostate cancer, using dose-volume histograms. *Int J Radiat Oncol Biol Phys* 1998;41: 83-92.
17. Thames HD, Hendry JH. *Fractionation in Radiotherapy*. London, England: Taylor and Francis Inc; 1987.
18. Stewart FA, Randhawa VS, Michael BD. Multifraction irradiation of mouse bladders. *Radiother Oncol* 1984;2:131-140.
19. Bentzen SM, Lundbeck F, Christensen LL, et al. Fractionation sensitivity and latency of late irradiation injury to the mouse urinary bladder. *Radiother Oncol* 1992;25:301-307.
20. Kagan AR. Bladder, testicle, and prostate irradiation injury. In: Vaeth JM, Meyer JL, eds. *Radiation Tolerance of Normal Tissues. Frontiers in Radiation Therapy and Oncology*. Basel, Switzerland: Karger; 1989.
21. Levine L, Richie JP. Urological complications of cyclophosphamide. *J Urol* 1989;141:1063-1069.
22. Edrees G, Luts A, Stewart F. Bladder damage in mice after combined treatment with cyclophosphamide and x-rays. The influence of timing and sequence. *Radiother Oncol* 1988;11:349-360.
23. Ghersi D, Stewart LA, Parmar MKB, et al. Neoadjuvant cisplatin, methotrexate, and vinblastine chemotherapy for muscle-invasive bladder cancer: a randomised controlled trial. *Lancet* 1999;354: 533-540.
24. Pizzo JJD, Chew BH, Jacobs SC, et al. Treatment of radiation induced hemorrhagic cystitis with hyperbaric oxygen: long-term results. *J Urol* 1998;160:731-733.
25. Mathews R, Rajan N, Josefson L, et al. Hyperbaric oxygen therapy for radiation induced hemorrhagic cystitis. *J Urol* 1999;161:435-437.
26. Greenlee RT, Hill-Harmon MB, Murray T, et al. Cancer statistics, 2001. *CA Cancer J Clin* 2001;51:15-36.
27. Brauers A, Jakse G. Epidemiology and biology of human urinary bladder cancer. *J Cancer Res Clin Oncol* 2000;126:575-583.
28. Cottran RS, Kumar V, Collins T. *Pathologic Basis of Disease*. Philadelphia, Pa: WB Saunders; 1999.
29. Brennan P, Bogillot O, Cordier S, et al. Cigarette smoking and bladder cancer in men: a pooled analysis of 11 case-controlled studies. *Int J Cancer* 2000;86:289-294.
30. Sellers C, Markowitz S. Reevaluating the carcinogenicity of ortho-toluidine: a new conclusion and its implication. *Regul Toxicol Pharmacol* 1992;16:301-317.
31. Ward E, Carpenter A, Markowitz S, et al. Excess number of bladder cancers in workers exposed to ortho-toluidine and aniline. *J Natl Cancer Inst* 1991;83:501-506.
32. Sadetzki S, Bensal D, Blumstein T, et al. Selected risk factors for transitional cell bladder cancer. *Med Oncol* 2000;17:179-182.
33. la Vecchia C, Negri E, D'Avanzo B, et al. Occupation and the risk of bladder cancer. *Int J Epidemiol* 1990;19:264-268.
34. Wynder EL, Goldsmith R. The epidemiology of bladder cancer: a second look. *Cancer* 1977;40:1246-1268.
35. Locke JR, Hill DE, Walzer Y. Incidence of squamous cell carcinoma in patients with long-term catheter drainage. *J Urol* 1985;133:1034-1035.
36. Dolin PJ, Darby SC, Beral V. Paraplegia and squamous cell carcinoma of the bladder in young women: findings from a case-control study. *Br J Cancer* 1994;70:167-168.
37. Stickler DJ, Chawla JC, Tricker AR, et al. N-nitrosamine generation by urinary tract infections in spine injured patients. *Paraplegia* 1992;30:855-863.
38. Steinmaus CM, Nunez S, Smith AH. Diet and bladder cancer: a meta-analysis of six dietary variables. *Am J Epidemiol* 2000; 151:693-702.
39. Nagano J, Kono S, Preston DL, et al. Bladder-cancer incidence in relation to vegetable and fruit consumption: a prospective study of atomic bomb survivors. *Int J Cancer* 2000;86:132-138.
40. Pantuck AJ, Bancila E, Das KM, et al. Adenocarcinoma of the urachus and bladder expresses a unique colonic epithelial epitope: an immunohistochemical study. *J Urol* 1997;158:1722-1727.

41. Millan-Rodriguez F, Chechile-Toniolo G, Salvador-Bayarri J, et al. Primary superficial bladder cancer risk groups according to progression, mortality and recurrence. *J Urol* 2000;164:680-684.

42. Nobori T, Miura K, Wu DJ, et al. Deletions of the cyclin-dependent kinase-4 inhibitor gene in multiple human tumors. *Nature* 1994;368:753-756.

43. Fujimoto K, Yamada Y, Okajima E, et al. Frequent association of *p53* gene mutation in invasive bladder cancer. *Cancer Res* 1992; 52:1393-1398.

44. Sidransky D, Eschenbach AV, Tsai YC, et al. Identification of *p53* gene mutations in bladder cancers and urine samples. *Science* 1991;252:706-709.

45. Sarkis AS, Dalbagni G, Cordon-Cardo C, et al. Nuclear overexpression of *p53* protein in transitional cell bladder carcinoma: a marker for disease progression. *J Natl Cancer Inst* 1993;85: 53-59.

46. Sarkis AS, Dalbagni G, Cordon-Cardo C, et al. Association of *p53* nuclear overexpression and tumor progression in carcinoma in situ of the bladder. *J Urol* 1994;152:388-392.

47. Sarkis A, Bajorin D, Reuter V, et al. Prognostic value of *p53* nuclear overexpression in patients with invasive bladder cancer treated with neoadjuvant MVAC. *J Clin Oncol* 1995;13:1384-1390.

48. Grossman HB, Liebert M, Antelo M, et al. *p53* and RB expression predict progression in T1 bladder cancer. *Clin Cancer Res* 1998; 4:829-834.

49. Esrig D, Elmajian D, Groshen S, et al. Accumulation of nuclear *p53* and tumor progression in bladder cancer. *N Engl J Med* 1994; 331:1259-1263.

50. Jahnson S, Karlsson MG. Predictive value of *p53* and pRB immunostaining in locally advanced bladder cancer treated with cystectomy. *J Urol* 1998;160:1291-1296.

51. Glick SH, Howell LP, White RW. Relationship of *p53* and *bcl-2* to prognosis in muscle-invasive transitional cell carcinoma of the bladder. *J Urol* 1996;155:1754-1757.

52. Fleshner N, Kapusta L, Ezer D, et al. *p53* nuclear accumulation is not associated with decreased disease-free survival in patients with node positive transitional cell carcinoma of the bladder. *J Urol* 2000;164:1177-1182.

53. Gospodarowicz MK, Warde P, Bristow RG. Radiotherapy for bladder cancer. In: Hall RR, ed. *Clinical Management of Bladder Cancer.* London, England: Arnold Publishing; 1999.

54. Schmitz-Drager BJ, Goebell PJ, Ebert T, et al. *p53* immunohistochemistry as a prognostic marker in bladder cancer. Playground for urologic scientists? *Eur Urol* 2000;38:691-700.

55. Messing EM, Young TB, Hunt VB, et al. Home screening for hematuria: results of a multiclinic study. *J Urol* 1992;148:289-292.

56. Messing EM, Young TB, Hunt VB, et al. Comparison of bladder cancer outcome in men undergoing hematuria home screening versus those with standard clinical presentations. *Urology* 1995;45:387-396.

57. Brown FM. Urine cytology: is it still the gold standard for screening? *Urol Clin North Am* 2000;27:25-37.

58. Quilty PM, Hargreave TB, Smith G, et al. Do normal mucosal biopsies predict prognosis in patients with transitional cell carcinoma of bladder treated by radical radiotherapy? *Br J Urol* 1987;59:242-247.

59. Sobin LH, Wiitekind CH. *TNM Classification of Malignant Tumors.* 5th ed. Union Internationale Contre le Cancer. New York, NY; Wiley-Liss; 1997.

60. Fleming I, Cooper JS, Henson DE, et al, eds. *AJCC Cancer Staging Manual.* 5th ed. Philadelphia, Pa: Lippincott Williams & Wilkins; 1997:241-246.

61. Prout GR. Bladder carcinoma and a TNM system of classification. *J Urol* 1977;117:583-590.

62. Gospodarowicz MK, Rider WD, Keen CW, et al. Bladder cancer: long term follow-up results of patients treated with radical radiation. *Clin Oncol* 1991;3:155-161.

63. Gospodarowicz MK, Hawkins NV, Rawlings GA, et al. Radical radiotherapy for the muscle invasive transitional cell carcinoma of the bladder: failure analysis. *J Urol* 1989;142:1448-1454.

64. Duncan W, Quilty PM. The results of a series of 963 patients with transitional cell carcinoma of the urinary bladder primarily treated by radical megavoltage x-ray therapy. *Radiother Oncol* 1986;7:299-310.

65. Pagano F, Bassi P, Galetti TP, et al. Results of contemporary radical cystectomy for invasive bladder cancer: a clinicopathological study with an emphasis on the inadequacy of the tumor, nodes and metastases classification. *J Urol* 1991;145:45-50.

66. Cheng D, Tempany CM. MR imaging of the prostate and bladder. *Semin Ultrasound CT MR* 1998;19:67-89.

67. Pagano F, Bassi P, Ferrante GL, et al. Is stage pT4a (D1) reliable in assessing transitional cell carcinoma involvement of the prostate in patients with a concurrent bladder cancer? A necessary distinction for contiguous or noncontiguous involvement. *J Urol* 1996;155:244-247.

68. Esrig D, Freeman JA, Elmajian DA, et al. Transitional cell carcinoma involving the prostate with a proposed staging classification for stromal invasion. *J Urol* 1996;156:1071-1076.

69. Freeman JA, Esrig D, Stein JP, et al. Management of the patient with bladder cancer. Urethral recurrence. *Urol Clin North Am* 1994;21:645-651.

70. Williams PL. *Gray's Anatomy.* New York, NY: Churchill Livingstone; 1995.

71. Lerner SP, Skinner DG, Lieskovsky G, et al. The rationale for en bloc pelvic lymph node dissection for bladder cancer patients with nodal metastases: long-term results. *J Urol* 1993;149: 758-764.

72. Frazier HA, Robertson JE, Dodge RK, et al. The value of pathologic factors in predicting cancer-specific survival among patients treated with radical cystectomy for transitional cell carcinoma of the bladder and prostate. *Cancer* 1993;71:3993-4001.

73. Bassi P, Ferrante GD, Piazza N, et al. Prognostic factors of outcome after radical cystectomy for bladder cancer: a retrospective study of a homogeneous patient cohort. *J Urol* 1999;161:1494-1497.

74. Skinner DG, Tift JP, Kaufman JJ. High dose, short course preoperative radiation therapy and immediate single stage radical cystectomy with pelvic node dissection in the management of bladder cancer. *J Urol* 1982;127:671-674.

75. Barentsz JO, Witjes JA, Ruijs JH. What is new in bladder cancer imaging. *Urol Clin North Am* 1997;24:583-602.

76. Roy C, Bras YL, Mangold L, et al. Small pelvic lymph node metastases: evaluation with MR imaging. *Clin Radiol* 1997;52: 437-440.

77. Rabbani F, Perrotti M, Russo P, et al. Upper-tract tumors after an initial diagnosis of bladder cancer: argument for long-term surveillance. *J Clin Oncol* 2001;19:94-100.

78. Herr HW, Cookson MS, Soloway SM. Upper tract tumors in patients with primary bladder cancer followed for 15 years. *J Urol* 1996;156:1286-1287.

79. Schwalb DM, Herr HW, Fair WR. The management of clinically unconfirmed positive urinary cytology. *J Urol* 1993;150:1751-1756.

80. Herr HW, Laudone VP, Whitmore WF. An overview of intravesical therapy for superficial bladder tumors. *J Urol* 1987;138:1363-1368.

81. Herr HW, Pinsky CM, Whitmore WF, et al. Long-term effect of intravesical bacillus Calmette-Guerin on flat carcinoma in situ of the bladder. *J Urol* 1986;135:265-267.

82. Herr HW, Schwalb DM, Zhang ZF, et al. Intravesical bacillus Calmette-Guérin therapy prevents tumor progression and death from superficial bladder cancer: ten-year follow-up of a prospective randomized trial. *J Clin Oncol* 1995;13:1404-1408.

83. Lerner SP, Skinner DG. Radical cystectomy for bladder cancer. In: Vogelzang NJ, Shipley WU, Scardino PT, et al, eds. *Comprehensive Textbook of Genitourinary Oncology.* Philadelphia, Pa: Lippincott Williams & Wilkins; 2000:442-463.

84. Richie JP. Surgery for invasive bladder cancer. *Hematol Oncol Clin North Am* 1992;6:129-145.

85. Amling CL, Thrasher JB, Frazier HA, et al. Radical cystectomy for stages Ta, Tis and T1 transitional cell carcinoma of the bladder. *J Urol* 1994;151:31-36.

86. Greven KM, Spera JA, Solin LJ, et al. Local recurrence after cystectomy alone for bladder carcinoma. *Cancer* 1992;69: 2767-2770.

87. Vieweg J, Gschwend JE, Herr HW, et al. Pelvic lymph node dissection can be curative in patients with node positive bladder cancer. *J Urol* 1999;161:449-454.

88. Poulsen AL, Horn T, Steven K. Radical cystectomy: extending the limits of pelvic lymph node dissection improves survival for patients with bladder cancer confined to the bladder wall. *J Urol* 1998;160:2015-2019.

89. Bretheau D, Ponthieu A. Results of radical cystectomy and pelvic lymphadenectomy for bladder cancer with pelvic node metastases. *Urol Int* 1996;57:27-31.

90. Herr HW, Donat SM. Outcome of patients with grossly node positive bladder cancer after pelvic lymph node dissection and radical cystectomy. *J Urol* 2001;165:62-64.

91. Paschkis R. Radiumbehandling von Blasengeschwulsten. *Wienner Klinische Wochenschrift* 1911;24:1962.

92. Sawchuk IS, Olsson CA, deVere White R. The limited usefulness of external beam radiotherapy in the control of superficial bladder cancer. *Br J Urol* 1988;61:330-332.

93. Quilty PM, Duncan W. Treatment of superficial (T1) tumours of the bladder by radical radiotherapy. *Br J Urol* 1986;58:147-152.

94. Jenkins BJ, Nauth-Misir RR, Martin J, et al. The fate of G3pT1 bladder cancer. *Br J Urol* 1989;64:608-610.

95. Vicente J, Laguna MP, Duarte D, et al. Carcinoma in situ as a prognostic factor for G3pT1 bladder tumours. *Br J Urol* 1991; 68:380-382.

96. Greven KM, Solin LJ, Hanks GE. Prognostic factors in patients with bladder carcinoma treated with definitive irradiation. *Cancer* 1990;65:908-912.

97. Pollack A, Zagars GK, Swanson DA. Muscle-invasive bladder cancer treated with external beam radiotherapy: prognostic factors. *Int J Radiat Oncol Biol Phys* 1994;30:267-277.

98. Vale JA, A'Hern RP, Liu K, et al. Predicting the outcome of radical radiotherapy for invasive bladder cancer. *Eur Urol* 1993;24:48-51.

99. Blandy JP, Jenkins BJ, Fowler CG, et al. Radical radiotherapy and salvage cystectomy for T2/3 cancer of the bladder. *Prog Clin Biol Res* 1988;260:447-451.

100. Jenkins BJ, Caulfield MJ, Fowler CG, et al. Reappraisal of the role of radical radiotherapy and salvage cystectomy in the treatment of invasive (T2/T3) bladder cancer. *Br J Urol* 1988;62:342-346.

101. Smaaland R, Akslen L, Tonder B, et al. Radical radiation treatment of invasive and locally advanced bladder cancer in elderly patients. *Br J Urol* 1991;67:61-69.

102. Jahnson S, Pedersen J, Westman G. Bladder carcinoma—a 20-year review of radical irradiation therapy. *Radiother Oncol* 1991; 22:111-117.

103. Shipley WU, Prout GR, Kaufman SD, et al. Invasive bladder carcinoma. The importance of initial transurethral surgery and other significant prognostic factors for improved survival with full-dose irradiation. *Cancer* 1987;60:514-520.

104. Timmer PR, Harlief HA, Hooijkaas JA. Bladder cancer: pattern of recurrence in 142 patients. *Int J Radiat Oncol Biol Phys* 1985; 11:899-905.

105. Fung CY, Shipley WU, Young RH, et al. Prognostic factors in invasive bladder carcinoma in a prospective trial of preoperative adjuvant chemotherapy and radiotherapy. *J Clin Oncol* 1991; 9:1533-1542.

106. Wolf H, Olsen PR, Hojgaard K. Urothelial dysplasia concomitant with bladder tumours: a determinant for future new occurrences in patients treated by full-course radiotherapy. *Lancet* 1985;1:1005-1008.

107. Pisters LL, Tykochinsky G, Wajsman Z. Intravesical bacillus Calmette-Guérin or mitomycin C in the treatment of carcinoma in situ of the bladder following prior pelvic radiation therapy. *J Urol* 1991;146:1514-1517.

108. Palou J, Sanchez-Martin FM, Rosales A, et al. Intravesical bacille Calmette-Guérin in the treatment of carcinoma in situ or high-grade superficial bladder carcinoma after radiotherapy for bladder carcinoma. *BJU Int* 1999;83:429-431.

109. Moonen L, vd Voet H, de Nijs R, et al. Muscle-invasive bladder cancer treated with external beam radiotherapy: pretreatment prognostic factors and the predictive value of cystoscopic re-evaluation during treatment. *Radiother Oncol* 1998;49:149-155.

110. Quilty PM, Duncan W. The influence of hemoglobin level on the regression and long term control of transitional cell carcinoma of the bladder following photon irradiation. *Int J Radiat Oncol Biol Phys* 1986;12:1735-1742.

111. Graeber TG, Osmanian C, Jacks T, et al. Hypoxia-mediated selection of cells with diminished apoptotic potential in solid tumours. *Nature* 1996;379:88-91.

112. Dachs GU, Chaplin DJ. Microenvironmental control of gene expression: implications for tumor angiogenesis, progression and metastasis. *Semin Radiat Oncol* 1998;8:208-216.

113. Sutherland RM, Ausserer WA, Murphy BJ, et al. Tumor hypoxia and heterogeneity: challenges and opportunities for the future. *Semin Radiat Oncol* 1996;6:59-70.

114. Pollack A, Wu CS, Czerniak B, et al. Abnormal *bcl-2* and *pRb* expression are independent correlates of radiation response in muscle-invasive bladder cancer. *Clin Cancer Res* 1997;3: 1823-1829.

115. Pollack A, Czerniak B, Zagars GK, et al. Retinoblastoma protein expression and radiation response in muscle-invasive bladder cancer. *Int J Radiat Oncol Biol Phys* 1997;39:687-695.

116. Chyle V, Pollack A, Czerniak B, et al. Apoptosis and downstaging after preoperative radiotherapy for muscle-invasive bladder cancer. *Int J Radiat Oncol Biol Phys* 1996;35:281-287.

117. Rodel C, Grabenbauer GG, Rodel F, et al. Apoptosis, *p53*, *bcl-2*, and *KI-67* in invasive bladder carcinoma: possible predictors for response to radiochemotherapy and successful bladder preservation. *Int J Radiat Oncol Biol Phys* 2000;46:1213-1221.

118. Wu CS, Pollack A, Czerniak B, et al. Prognostic value of *p53* in muscle-invasive bladder cancer treated with preoperative radiotherapy. *Urology* 1996;47:305-310.

119. Osen I, Fossa SD, Majak B, et al. Prognostic factors in muscle-invasive bladder cancer treated with radiotherapy: an immuno-histochemical study. *Br J Urol* 1998;81:862-869.

120. Fossa SD, Waehre H, Aass N, et al. Bladder cancer definitive radiation therapy of muscle-invasive bladder cancer. A retrospective analysis of 317 patients. *Cancer* 1993;72:3036-3043.

121. Davidson SE, Symonds RP, Snee MP, et al. Assessment of factors influencing the outcome of radiotherapy for bladder cancer. *Br J Urol* 1990;66:288-293.

122. Goffinet DR, Schneider MJ, Glatstein EJ, et al. Bladder cancer: results of radiation therapy in 384 patients. *Radiology* 1975; 117:149-153.

123. Yu WS, Sagerman RH, Chung CT, et al. Bladder carcinoma. Experience with radical and preoperative radiotherapy in 421 patients. *Cancer* 1985;56:1293-1299.

124. Goodman GB, Hislop TG, Elwood JM, et al. Conservation of bladder function in patients with invasive bladder cancer treated by definitive irradiation and selective cystectomy. *Int J Radiat Oncol Biol Phys* 1981;7:569-573.

125. Pollack A, Zagars GK, Dinney CP, et al. Preoperative radiotherapy for muscle-invasive bladder carcinoma. Long term follow-up and prognostic factors for 338 patients. *Cancer* 1994; 74:2819-2827.

126. Hayter CRR, Paszat LF, Groome PA, et al. A population-based study of the use and outcome of radical radiotherapy for invasive bladder cancer. *Int J Radiat Oncol Biol Phys* 1999;45: 1239-1245.

127. Quilty PM, Duncan W, Chisholm GD, et al. Results of surgery following radical radiotherapy for invasive bladder cancer. *Br J Urol* 1986;58:396-405.

128. Abratt RP, Wilson JA, Pontin AR, et al. Salvage cystectomy after radical irradiation for bladder cancer—prognostic factors and complications. *Br J Urol* 1993;72:756-760.

129. Blandy JP, England HR, Evans SJ, et al. T3 bladder cancer—the case for salvage cystectomy. *Br J Urol* 1980;52:506-510.

130. Crawford ED, Skinner DG. Salvage cystectomy after irradiation failure. *J Urol* 1980;123:32-34.

131. Konnak JW, Grossman HB. Salvage cystectomy following failed definitive radiation therapy for transitional cell carcinoma of bladder. *Urology* 1985;26:550-553.

132. Nurmi M, Valavaara R, Puntala P, et al. Single-stage salvage cystectomy: results and complications in 20 patients. *Eur Urol* 1989;16:89-91.

133. Smith JA, Whitmore WF. Salvage cystectomy for bladder cancer after failure of definitive irradiation. *J Urol* 1981;125:643-645.

134. Swanson DA, Eschenbach AC, Bracken RB, et al. Salvage cystectomy for bladder carcinoma. *Cancer* 1981;47:2275-2279.

135. Osborn DE, Honan RP, Palmer MK, et al. Factors influencing salvage cystectomy results. *Br J Urol* 1982;54:122-125.

136. Bochner BH, Figueroa AJ, Skinner EC, et al. Salvage radical cystoprostatectomy and orthotopic urinary diversion following radiation failure. *J Urol* 1998;160:29-33.

137. Mannel RS, Manetta A, Buller RE, et al. Use of ileocecal continent urinary reservoir in patients with previous pelvic irradiation. *Gynecol Oncol* 1995;59:376-378.

138. Larsen LE, Engelholm SA. The value of three-dimensional radiotherapy planning in advanced carcinoma of the urinary bladder based on computed tomography. *Acta Oncol* 1994;33:655-659.

139. Bentzen SM, Jessen KA, Jorgensen J, et al. Impact of CT-based treatment planning on radiation therapy of carcinoma of the bladder. *Acta Radiol Oncol* 1984;23:199-203.

140. Rothwell RI, Ash DV, Jones WG. Radiation treatment planning for bladder cancer: a comparison of cystogram localisation with computed tomography. *Clin Radiol* 1983;34:103-111.

141. Logue JP, Sharrock CL, Cowan RA, et al. Clinical variability of target volume description in conformal radiotherapy planning. *Int J Radiat Oncol Biol Phys* 1998;41:929-931.

142. Turner SL, Swindell SL, Bowl N, et al. Bladder movement during radiation therapy for bladder cancer: implications for treatment planning. *Int J Radiat Oncol Biol Phys* 1997;39:355-360.

143. Miralbell R, Nouet P, Rouzaud M, et al. Radiotherapy of bladder cancer: relevance of bladder volume changes in planning boost treatment. *Int J Radiat Oncol Biol Phys* 1998;41:741-746.

144. Kaufman DS, Winter KA, Shipley WU, et al. The initial results in muscle-invading bladder cancer of RTOG 95-06: phase I/II trial of transurethral surgery plus radiation therapy with concurrent cisplatin and 5-fluorouracil followed by selective bladder preservation or cystectomy depending on the initial response. *Oncologist* 2000;5:471-476.

145. Tester W, Caplan R, Heaney J, et al. Neoadjuvant combined modality program with selective organ preservation for invasive bladder cancer: results of Radiation Therapy Oncology Group phase II trial 8802. *J Clin Oncol* 1996;14:119-126.

146. Moonen L, vd Voet H, de Nijs R, et al. Muscle-invasive bladder cancer treated with external beam radiation: influence of total dose, overall treatment time, and treatment interruption on local control. *Int J Radiat Oncol Biol Phys* 1998;42:525-530.

147. Bialas I, Bessell E, Sokal M, et al. A prospective study of urinary tract infection during pelvic radiotherapy. *Radiother Oncol* 1989;16:305-309.

148. Sell A, Jakobsen A, Nerstrom B, et al. Treatment of advanced bladder cancer category T2, T3 and T4a. *Scand J Urol Nephrol* 1991;138:193-201.

149. Mommsen S, Jakobsen A, Sell A. Quality of life in patients with advanced bladder cancer. A randomized study comparing cystectomy and irradiation—the Danish Bladder Cancer Study Group (DAVECA protocol 8201). *Scand J Urol Nephrol* 1989; 125:115-120.

150. Lynch WJ, Jenkins BJ, Fowler CG, et al. The quality of life after radical radiotherapy for bladder cancer. *Br J Urol* 1992;70: 519-521.

151. Caffo O, Fellin G, Graffer U, et al. Assessment of quality of life after cystectomy or conservative therapy for patients with infiltrating bladder carcinoma. A survey by a self-administered questionnaire. *Cancer* 1996;78:1089-1097.

152. Little FA, Howard GC. Sexual function following radical radiotherapy for bladder cancer. *Radiother Oncol* 1998;49:157-161.

153. Tester W, Porter A, Asbell S, et al. Combined modality program with possible organ preservation for invasive bladder carcinoma: results of RTOG protocol 85-12. *Int J Radiat Oncol Biol Phys* 1993;25:783-790.

154. Shipley WU, Kaufman DS, Heney NM, et al. An update of combined modality therapy for patients with muscle invading bladder cancer using selective bladder preservation or cystectomy. *J Urol* 1999;162:445-450.

155. Raghaven D. Systemic chemotherapy for metastatic cancer of the uro-epithelial tract. In: Hall RR, ed. *Clinical Management of Bladder Cancer*. London, England: Arnold Publishing; 1999.

156. Coppin C, Gospodarowicz M, James K, et al. The NCI-Canada trial of concurrent cisplatin and radiotherapy for muscle invasive bladder cancer. *J Clin Oncol* 1996;14:2901-2907.

157. von der Maase H, Hansen SW, Roberts JT, et al. Gemcitabine and cisplatin versus methotrexate, vinblastine, doxorubicin, and cisplatin in advanced or metastatic bladder cancer: results of a large, randomized, multinational, multicenter, phase III study. *J Clin Oncol* 2000;18:3068-3077.

158. Moore MJ, Tannock IF, Ernst DS, et al. Gemcitabine: a promising new agent in the treatment of advanced urothelial carcinoma. *J Clin Oncol* 1997;15:3441-3445.

159. Moore MJ, Winquist EW, Murray N, et al. Gemcitabine plus cisplatin, an active regimen in advanced urothelial cancer: a phase II trial of the National Cancer Institute of Canada Clinical Trials Group. *J Clin Oncol* 1999;17:2876-2881.

160. Bajorin DF. Paclitaxel in the treatment of advanced urothelial cancer. *Oncology* 2000;14:43-52.

161. Lawrence TS, Eisbruch A, Shewach DS. Gemcitabine-mediated radiosensitization. *Semin Oncol* 1997;24(suppl):S7-S24.

162. Loehrer PJ, Einhorn LH, Elson PJ, et al. A randomized comparison of cisplatin alone or in combination with methotrexate, vinblastine, and doxorubicin in patients with metastatic urothelial carcinoma: a cooperative group study. *J Clin Oncol* 1992;10: 1066-1073.

163. Farah R, Chodak GW, Vogelzang NJ, et al. Curative radiotherapy following chemotherapy for invasive bladder carcinoma (a preliminary report). *Int J Radiat Oncol Biol Phys* 1991;20:413-417.

164. Wajsman Z, Marino R, Parsons J, et al. Bladder-sparing approach in the treatment of invasive bladder cancer. *Semin Urol* 1990; 8:210-215.

165. Shipley WU, Winter KA, Kaufman DS, et al. Phase III trial of neoadjuvant chemotherapy in patients with invasive bladder cancer treated with selective bladder preservation by combined radiation therapy and chemotherapy: initial results of Radiation Therapy Oncology Group 89-03. *J Clin Oncol* 1998;16: 3576-3583.

166. Wallace DMA, Raghavan D, Kelly KA, et al. Neo-adjuvant (preemptive) cisplatin therapy in invasive transitional cell carcinoma of the bladder. *Br J Urol* 1991;67:608-615.

167. Shearer RJ, Chilvers CED, Bloom HJG, et al. Adjuvant chemotherapy in T3 carcinoma of the bladder. A prospective trial and preliminary report. *Br J Urol* 1988;62:558-564.

168. Martinez-Pineiro JA, Martin MG, Arocena F, et al. Neoadjuvant cisplatin chemotherapy before radical cystectomy in invasive transitional cell carcinoma of the bladder: a prospective randomized phase III trial. *J Urol* 1995;153:964-973.

169. Logothetis C, Swanson D, Amato R, et al. Optimal delivery of perioperative chemotherapy: preliminary results of a randomized, prospective, comparative trial of preoperative and postoperative chemotherapy for invasive bladder cancer. *J Urol* 1996; 155:1241-1245.

170. Rintala E, Hannisdahl E, Fossa SD, et al. Neoadjuvant chemotherapy in bladder cancer: a randomized study. Nordic Cystectomy Trial I. *Scand J Urol Nephrol* 1993;27:355-362.

171. Ghersi D, Stewart LA, Parmar MKB, et al. Does neoadjuvant cisplatin-based chemotherapy improve the survival of patients with locally advanced bladder cancer: a meta-analysis of individual patient data from randomized clinical trials. *Br J Urol* 1995;75:206-213.

172. Eapen L, Stewart D, Danjoux C, et al. Intraarterial cisplatin and concurrent radiation for locally advanced bladder cancer. *J Clin Oncol* 1989;7:230-235.

173. Eapen L, Stewart D, Crook J, et al. Intraarterial cisplatin and concurrent pelvic radiation in the management of muscle invasive bladder cancer. *Int J Radiat Oncol Biol Phys* 1992;24(suppl 1):211.

174. Richards B, Bastable JRG, Freedman L, et al. Adjuvant chemotherapy with doxorubicin (Adriamycin) and 5-fluorouracil in T3, NX, M0 bladder cancer treated with radiotherapy. *Br J Urol* 1982;55:386-391.

175. Skinner DG, Daniels JR, Russell CA, et al. The role of adjuvant chemotherapy following cystectomy for invasive bladder cancer: a prospective comparative trial. *J Urol* 1991;145:459-464.

176. Freiha F, Reese J, Torti FM. A randomized trial of radical cystectomy versus radical cystectomy plus cisplatin, vinblastine and methotrexate chemotherapy for muscle invasive bladder cancer. *J Urol* 1996;155:495-499.

177. Stockle M, Meyenburg W, Wellek S, et al. Adjuvant polychemotherapy of nonorgan-confined bladder cancer after radical cystectomy revisited: long-term results of a controlled prospective study and further clinical experience. *J Urol* 1995; 153:47-52.

178. Studer UE, Bacchi M, Biedermann C, et al. Adjuvant cisplatin chemotherapy following cystectomy for bladder cancer: results of a prospective randomized trial. *J Urol* 1994;152:81-84.

179. Cole CJ, Pollack A, Zagars GK, et al. Local control of muscle-invasive bladder cancer: preoperative radiotherapy and cystectomy versus cystectomy alone. *Int J Radiat Oncol Biol Phys* 1995;32:331-340.

180. Anderstrom C, Johansson S, Nilsson S, et al. A prospective randomized study of preoperative irradiation with cystectomy or cystectomy alone for invasive bladder carcinoma. *Eur Urol* 1983;9:142-147.

181. Bloom HJ, Hendry WF, Wallace DM, et al. Treatment of T3 bladder cancer: controlled trial of pre-operative radiotherapy and radical cystectomy versus radical radiotherapy. *Br J Urol* 1982;54:136-151.

182. Smith J, Crawford E, Paradelo J, et al. Treatment of advanced bladder cancer with combined preoperative irradiation and radical cystectomy versus radical cystectomy alone: a phase III intergroup study. *J Urol* 1997;157:805-808.

183. Ghoneim MA, Ashamallah AK, Awaad HK, et al. Randomized trial of cystectomy with or without preoperative radiotherapy for carcinoma of the bilharzial bladder. *J Urol* 1985;134:266-268.

184. Huncharek M, Muscat J, Geschwind JF. Planned preoperative radiation therapy in muscle invasive bladder cancer: results of a meta-analysis. *Anticancer Res* 1998;18:1931-1934.

185. Spera JA, Whittington R, Littman P, et al. A comparison of preoperative radiotherapy regimens for bladder carcinoma: the University of Pennsylvania experience. *Cancer* 1988;61:255-262.

186. Reisinger SA, Mohiuddin M, Mulholland SG. Combined pre- and postoperative adjuvant radiation therapy for bladder cancer—a ten year experience. *Int J Radiat Oncol Biol Phys* 1992;24:463-468.

187. Zaghloul MS, Awwad HK, Akoush HH, et al. Postoperative radiotherapy of carcinoma in bilharzial bladder: improved disease free survival through improving local control. *Int J Radiat Oncol Biol Phys* 1992;23:511-517.

188. Zaghloul MS. Radiation as adjunctive therapy to cystectomy for bladder cancer: is there a difference for bilharzial association? [letter]. *Int J Radiat Oncol Biol Phys* 1994;28:783.

189. Kopelson G, Heaney JA. Postoperative radiation therapy for muscle-invading bladder carcinoma. *J Surg Oncol* 1983;23: 263-268.

190. Stuschke M, Thames HD. Hyperfractionated radiotherapy of human tumors: overview of the randomized clinical trials. *Int J Radiat Oncol Biol Phys* 1997;37:259-267.

191. Naslund I, Nilsson B, Littbrand B. Hyperfractionated radiotherapy of bladder cancer. A ten-year follow-up of a randomized clinical trial. *Acta Oncol* 1994;33:397-402.

192. Salminen E. Unconventional fractionation for palliative radiotherapy of urinary bladder cancer. A retrospective review of 94 patients. *Acta Oncol* 1992;31:449-454.

193. Scholten AN, Leer JW, Collins CD, et al. Hypofractionated radiotherapy for invasive bladder cancer. *Radiother Oncol* 1997; 43:163-169.

194. Bush C, Price P, Norton J, et al. Proliferation in human bladder carcinoma measured by Ki-67 antibody labelling: its potential clinical importance. *Br J Cancer* 1991;64:357-360.

195. Trott KR, Kummermehr J. What is known about tumour proliferation rates to choose between accelerated fractionation or hyperfractionation. *Radiother Oncol* 1985;3:1-9.

196. Hainau B, Dombernowsky P. Histology and cell proliferation in human bladder tumors. *Cancer* 1974;33:115-126.

197. Rew DA, Thomas DJ, Coptcoat M, et al. Measurement of in vivo urological tumour cell kinetics using multiplanar flow cytometry. Preliminary study. *Br J Urol* 1991;68:44-48.

198. Fyles A, Keane TJ, Barton M, et al. The effect of treatment duration in the local control of cervix cancer. *Radiother Oncol* 1992; 25:273-279.

199. De Neve W, Lybeert ML, Goor C, et al. Radiotherapy for T2 and T3 carcinoma of the bladder: the influence of overall treatment time. *Radiother Oncol* 1995;36:183-188.

200. Horwich A, Dearnaley D, Huddart R, et al. A trial of accelerated fractionation (AF) in T2/3 bladder cancer [abstract]. *Eur J Cancer* 1999;35(suppl 4):S342.

201. Braasch WF, Scholl AJ. Preoperative treatment by radium of malignant tumors of the bladder. *Arch Surg* 1922;5:334-347.

202. Barringer BS. Twenty-five years of radon treatment of cancer of the bladder. *JAMA* 1947;135:616-618.

203. Munro AI. The results of using radioactive gold grains in the treatment of bladder growths. *Br J Urol* 1964;36:541-548.

204. van der Werf-Messing BHP. Cancer of the urinary bladder treated by interstitial radium implant. *Int J Radiat Oncol Biol Phys* 1978;4:373-378.

205. De Neve W, Lybeert ML, Goor C, et al. T1 and T2 carcinoma of the urinary bladder: long term results with external, preoperative, or interstitial radiotherapy. *Int J Radiat Oncol Biol Phys* 1992;23:299-304.

206. Wijnmaalen A, Helle PA, Koper PCM, et al. Muscle invasive bladder cancer treated by transurethral resection, followed by external beam radiation and interstitial iridium-192. *Int J Radiat Oncol Biol Phys* 1997;39:1043-1052.

207. Pernot M, Hubert J, Guillemin F, et al. Combined surgery and brachytherapy in the treatment of some cancers of the bladder

(partial cystectomy and interstitial iridium-192). *Radiother Oncol* 1996;38:115-120.

208. Rozan R, Albuisson E, Donnarieix D, et al. Interstitial iridium-192 for bladder cancer (a multicentric survey: 205 patients). *Int J Radiat Oncol Biol Phys* 1992;24:469-477.

209. Van Poppel H, Lievens Y, Limbergen EV, et al. Brachytherapy with iridium-192 for bladder cancer. *Eur Urol* 2000;37: 605-608.

210. Soete G, Coen V, Verellen D, et al. A feasibility study of high dose rate brachytherapy in solitary urinary bladder cancer. *Int J Radiat Oncol Biol Phys* 1997;38:743-747.

211. van der Werf-Messing BHP, Hop WCL. Carcinoma of the urinary bladder (category T1 NX M0) treated either by radium implant or by transurethral resection only. *Int J Radiat Oncol Biol Phys* 1981;7:299-303.

212. van der Werf-Messing B, Menon RS, Hop WCJ. Cancer of the urinary bladder category T2, T3, (NXM0) treated by interstitial radium implant: second report. *Int J Radiat Oncol Biol Phys* 1983;9:481-485.

213. Moonen LM, Horenblas S, van der Voet JC, et al. Bladder conservation in selected T1G3 and muscle-invasive T2-T3a bladder carcinoma using combination therapy of surgery and iridium-192 implantation. *Br J Urol* 1994;74:322-327.

214. Mackillop WJ. The principles of palliative radiotherapy: a radiation oncologist's perspective. *Can J Oncol* 1996;6(suppl):5-11.

215. Fossa SD, Hosbach G. Short-term moderate-dose pelvic radiotherapy of advanced bladder carcinoma. A questionnaire-based evaluation of its symptomatic effect. *Acta Oncol* 1991;30: 735-738.

216. Holmang S, Borghede G. Early complications and survival following short-term palliative radiotherapy in invasive bladder carcinoma. *J Urol* 1996;155:100-102.

217. Wijkstrom H, Naslund I, Ekman P, et al. Short-term radiotherapy as palliative treatment in patients with transitional cell bladder cancer. *Br J Urol* 1991;67:74-78.

218. Duchesne GM, Bolger JJ, Griffiths GO, et al. A randomized trial of hypofractionated schedules of palliative radiotherapy in the management of bladder carcinoma: results of medical research council trial BA09. *Int J Radiat Oncol Biol Phys* 2000;47:379-388.

219. Saxman SB, Propert KJ, Einhorn LH, et al. Long-term follow-up of a phase III intergroup study of cisplatin alone or in combination with methotrexate, vinblastine, and doxorubicin in patients with metastatic urothelial carcinoma: a cooperative group study. *J Clin Oncol* 1997;15:2564-2569.

220. Mead GM, Russel M, Clark P, et al. A randomized trial comparing methotrexate and vinblastine (MV) with cisplatin, methotrexate and vinblastine (CMV) in advanced transitional cell carcinoma: results and a report on prognostic factors in a Medical Research Council study. MRC Advanced Bladder Cancer Working Party. *Br J Cancer* 1998;78:1067-1075.

221. Logothetis CJ, Dexus FH, Finn L, et al. A prospective randomized trial comparing MVAC and CISCA chemotherapy for patients with metastatic urothelial tumors. *J Clin Oncol* 1990;8:1050-1056.

PART VIII

Male Genital Tract

CHAPTER 26

The Testicle

David H. Hussey and Marvin L. Meistrich

RESPONSE OF THE NORMAL TESTICLE TO IRRADIATION

The testis has long been an important area of study for radiation biologists. This is not only because it is an important organ but also because it is readily accessible for irradiation and is composed of a variety of cell types with a wide range of radiosensitivities. The radiobiology of the testis has been studied from a variety of perspectives.[1] Histologic, hormonal, genetic, and fertility studies have all contributed to current understanding of the radiation response of this organ.

Initial information regarding the radiosensitivity of the cells that make up the testis came from studies of experimental animals. Data regarding the effects of irradiation on the human were limited because the testis is rarely directly irradiated in the clinical setting. However, the testicles receive a significant amount of scatter radiation when the pelvis is irradiated, and this may be sufficient to cause infertility. Measurements of the functional response of the testis to measured levels of scattered dose have also provided information regarding the radiation response of the human testis.

ANATOMY

An ovoid gland measuring $4.5 \times 3 \times 2.5$ cm (Fig. 26-1), the testis is surrounded by a thick fibrous capsule, the tunica albuginea. The tunica albuginea is enclosed in the tunica vaginalis, a double layer of peritoneum, the layers of which slide freely on one another, enabling the testis to move easily within the scrotal sac.

The testis is composed of a mass of coiled tubules, the convoluted seminiferous tubules. These are arranged in wedge-shaped compartments or lobules that are formed by incomplete connective tissue septae. At the apex of the lobules, the seminiferous tubules unite to form the straight tubules that anastomose to form a network, the rete testis. The rete testis is located in the hilum or posterior part of the testicle. In this region, 12 to 15 efferent

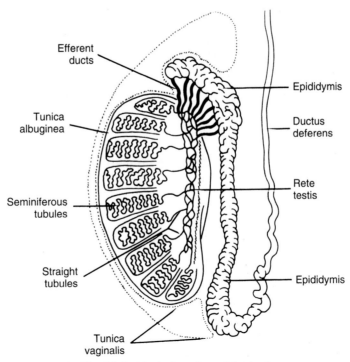

Fig. 26-1 Vertical section of the testis.

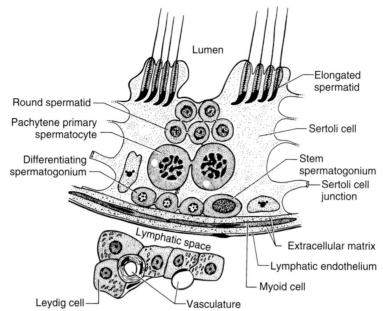

Fig. 26-2 Diagram of a normal seminiferous tubule containing five different generations of germ cells at various stages of spermatogenesis. (From Meistrich ML. *Br J Cancer* 1986; 53:89-101.)

ducts from the rete testis perforate the tunica albuginea to carry spermatozoa and secreted fluid to the epididymis. The efferent ducts join to form the duct of the epididymis, which abruptly bends cranially at the tail of the epididymis and continues as the vas deferens (see Fig. 26-1).

The seminiferous tubules are 35 to 70 cm long and 170 µm in diameter. They are lined by multiple layers of spermatogenic cells (Fig. 26-2).[2] Interspersed among the spermatogenic cells at fairly regular intervals are the Sertoli cells, which serve nutritional, paracrine regulatory, and supportive functions for developing spermatozoa. The seminiferous tubules lie within a stroma of connective tissue containing clumps of irregularly shaped polyhedral cells, the Leydig cells, which are responsible for the production of testosterone.

SPERMATOGENESIS

Spermatogenesis is a complex process that begins with the stem cells or primitive spermatogonia lying next to the basement membrane of the seminiferous tubule (see Fig. 26-2).[1a,2] The spermatogonia are the source of spermatocytes, which divide to become spermatids (Fig. 26-3).[3] The spermatids in turn transform into spermatozoa, which are released into the lumen of the tubule.

The stem cells are type A spermatogonia and consist of two populations in primates.[4] The type A dark spermatogonia, which under normal conditions are in a resting, nondividing phase, are considered reserve stem cells. The type A pale spermatogonia, which are slowly

proliferating, are normally considered to be the self-renewing stem cells of the testis.[5] When the population of the latter cells is diminished, however, the type A dark spermatogonia can replenish the supply of type A pale spermatogonia. These type A pale cells divide and their daughter cells either remain as type A pale spermatogonia or divide again to become type B spermatogonia.

In rodents, no nonproliferative population of stem cells equivalent to the type A dark cells of primates is evident. Instead, the stem cells are isolated, undifferentiated type A spermatogonia that proliferate slowly.[5,6] These cells are self-renewing; some of their daughters remain as isolated stem cells, but others are committed to differentiation when they form pairs and eventually chains of type A spermatogonia. These chains of spermatogonia morphologically differentiate into type A_1 spermatogonia, which undergo five cell divisions, producing type A_{2-4}, intermediate, and then type B spermatogonia.

In humans and rodents, the type B spermatogonia undergo one more amplification division to give rise to primary spermatocytes, which replicate their deoxyribonucleic acid (DNA), leave the basement membrane, move toward the lumen of the seminiferous tubule, and grow. During this period of growth, the DNA in the primary spermatocytes undergoes genetic recombination as the cells prepare for the meiotic divisions. In the first meiotic division, secondary spermatocytes having a haploid chromosome number and a diploid DNA content are formed. This is soon followed by a second meiotic division, which produces spermatids having both a

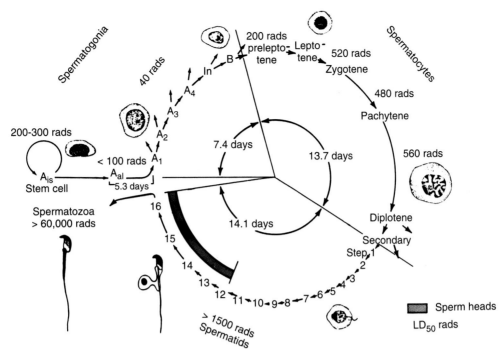

Fig. 26-3 Kinetics and radiation sensitivities of spermatogenic cells in the mouse. Radiation sensitivity is given for most cells as the median lethal dose (LD$_{50}$) value for cell loss; the value for the stem cells is the threshold dose (D$_0$) on the linear high-dose part of the survival curve. (Modified from Meistrich ML, Hunter N, Suzuki N, et al. *Radiat Res* 1978;74:349-362.)

haploid chromosome number and a haploid DNA content. The spermatids then undergo a process of metamorphosis, in which the nuclear material condenses and elongates and the tail forms, to yield mature spermatozoa. The spermatozoa then pass through the rete testis, efferent ducts, epididymis, and vas deferens, where they are stored for ejaculation.

In a human male, the time required for type A spermatogonia to develop into mature spermatozoa in the ejaculate is about 67 days.[7] Type B spermatogonia require 58 to 67 days to become spermatozoa, spermatocytes between 34 and 58 days, and spermatids between 12 and 34 days.[8]

Effects of Irradiation on Spermatogenesis
Radiosensitivity of Germ Cells

The sensitivity of germ cells to a given dose of radiation is related to the stage they are in at the time they are irradiated (see Fig. 26-3).[3,9] In both rodents and humans, type B spermatogonia are the most radiosensitive, type A spermatogonia are somewhat less sensitive, and primary and secondary spermatocytes and spermatids are much less sensitive than either of the spermatogonial cell types.[9,10] Except for the fact that primitive type A spermatogonia are more resistant than the latter, more proliferative type A, intermediate, and type B spermatogonia, radiosensitivity

diminishes as the cells progress along the maturation pathway.[3]

In mice, the majority of the stem spermatogonia have a threshold dose (D$_0$) of about 2 Gy, whereas type A$_{2-4}$, intermediate, and type B spermatogonia have a median lethal dose (LD$_{50}$) ranging from 0.21 to 1 Gy.[11,12] The extreme radiosensitivity of these spermatogonia now appears to be a result of their sensitivity to radiation-induced apoptosis.[13,14]

Study of the effects of single-dose irradiation of human testis[9] showed that spermatogonia are the most radiosensitive cells; they display morphologic and quantitative signs of injury after single doses as low as 0.1 Gy. Spermatocytes had no visible signs of injury even after single doses of 2 to 3 Gy, but they did suffer damage because they were unable to complete their meiotic divisions and produce spermatids. Single doses of 4 to 6 Gy did damage spermatocytes morphologically and also affected the ability of spermatids to produce spermatozoa.

Depletion of Germ Cells

Irradiation does not affect the kinetics of differentiation of spermatogenic cells; hence the surviving germ cells differentiate with kinetics identical to those of cells in the normal testis.[15] As a result, sperm production is maintained from surviving, more radioresistant cells until the radiosensitive cells would have become sperm.

Thus the sperm counts of mice[16] and men[17] are not at first (until 30 and 50 days, respectively) affected by single doses of about 1 Gy, which will kill many of the differentiating spermatogonia but few of the other germ cells. Higher doses of radiation (more than 4 Gy) will kill germ cells at later stages and thus deplete sperm earlier.

The size of the decline in sperm count is related to radiation dose. Single doses of less than 0.1 Gy do not significantly decrease sperm count,[10,18] whereas doses between 0.1 and 0.7 Gy produce oligospermia. Minimum sperm counts are about 15 million per ml after 0.15 Gy and 2 million per ml after 0.5 Gy. Total azoospermia occurs at doses of 0.78 Gy and higher.

Similar results have been reported after radiation given over 3- to 7-week periods during fractionated radiation therapy.[19] Doses to the testis of less than 0.15 Gy have little effect on sperm count. Oligospermia is generally induced at doses between 0.15 and 0.35 Gy, although 50% of men may experience transient azoospermia after 0.35 Gy.[20] Almost all men become azoospermic after 1 Gy to the testis.

Recovery of Spermatogenesis

Recovery of spermatogenesis after irradiation involves regeneration of the stem cell compartment and repopulation of the seminiferous tubules with maturing cells. In the mouse, stem cell number recovers with a 5-day doubling time,[3] but differentiation begins almost immediately,[21] resulting in increases in sperm count within 6 weeks after irradiation.[16] Sperm count recovers to 80% of control values within 20 weeks after 6 Gy. Thus in the mouse, both regeneration of stem cell numbers and their differentiation proceed after irradiation, even at doses of up to 16 Gy.

In certain strains of rat, the process is quite different. Doses as low as 3.5 Gy produce azoospermia lasting more than 1 year.[22] In this situation, stem cells survive, but the ability to support their differentiation is progressively lost. The stem cells proliferate and divide but are lost by apoptosis, apparently as a result of the production of an apoptotic factor or the absence of a factor required for their differentiation. Transient suppression of testosterone results in the restoration of spermatogenic differentiation, recovery of sperm production, and restoration of fertility by a mechanism that is as yet unknown.[23]

The delay in recovery of spermatogenesis in the human male is more like that in rats than in mice. After single doses of radiation, the numbers of stem and differentiated cells progressively decrease for 7 months after doses of 1 to 6 Gy,[10] after which recovery of germ cell numbers begins.[18,20] Although sperm may be found in the semen of some men at 7 months after irradiation with 1 Gy, 24 months are required for the appearance of sperm after 6 Gy, indicating that differentiation of spermatogenic cells into spermatozoa is blocked for a while.

The causes of this block and the trigger for the apparently spontaneous recovery of spermatogenesis at long times after moderate doses of radiation are not known. There is no proof that the delay is a result of the need to first replenish the stem cell pool before differentiation can proceed. Whether testosterone inhibits the recovery in humans, as is the case in the rat, still remains to be tested. Nevertheless, the azoospermia produced by doses of up to 6 Gy was temporary because recovery eventually occurred in all cases. The single dose required for permanent sterilization in normal human males is not clearly established, but estimates of 6 to 9.5 Gy were reported in the older literature.[17]

After gonadal doses of fractionated irradiation of less than 1 Gy, recovery to maximal counts generally occurs between 1 and 2 years, although some individuals show even more gradual recovery. After doses between 1 and 2 Gy, 2 to 6 years are required for full recovery.[19,24] After higher doses of fractionated irradiation, recovery is sporadic, but based on results observed after chemotherapy, rare instances of recovery may even be possible after 10 years.[25]

Generally, the sperm count recovers, at least after lower doses, to normospermic levels (more than 20 million/ml) or to the level of the patient's sperm count before irradiation. However, after higher doses, it is possible that the count will reach only severely oligospermic levels (less than 1 million/ml), as has been observed in cases of recovery after chemotherapy.[25] Although no absolute boundary of sperm count (except azoospermia) separates fertile from infertile men, the risk of infertility in the general population progressively increases as sperm counts progressively decline below 20 million per ml.[26] However, some men whose sperm counts remain as low as 1 million per ml remain fertile, likely because sperm quality, including sperm morphology and motility, return to normal or preexposure levels concomitant with the recovery of sperm count.[19,27]

Effects of Fractionation

Spermatogenesis has long been known to be more sensitive to fractionated irradiation than to single doses, even though the cumulative dose for fractionated treatment is the same as or lower than the single dose. This seemingly paradoxical observation was first noted by Regaud in his classic study on rams' testicles.[28] In that study, radon needles were inserted into the testicles and the effects of irradiation on spermatogenesis and scrotal skin were monitored. Regaud found that suppression of spermatogenesis was more severe when the radiation dose was delivered over 28 days than when similar or even greater doses were given over 30 to 42 hours. However, the more fractionated schedule resulted in less damage to scrotal skin, as is typical of all other tissues. Regaud repeated these studies using fractionated x-rays and obtained similar results.[29]

Similar findings have been observed in other species. For example, single doses as large as 1000 roentgen (R) failed to sterilize canine testicles, whereas a total cumulative dose as low as 475 R caused complete and permanent azoospermia in dogs when delivered in fractions of 3 R/day, 5 days/wk.[17] The recovery of spermatogenesis from surviving stem cells in some strains of mice is lower when the same dose is delivered in two daily fractions as opposed to a single fraction.[30]

Spermatogenesis in man also appears to be more sensitive to fractionated irradiation than it is to single doses.[20] Rowley and colleagues[10] found that sperm production recovered 2 years after a single dose of 6 Gy to normal males. However, azoospermia lasting at least 2 to 5 years can occur in patients who have received doses in the range of 2.3 to 3.0 Gy given in courses fractionated over periods of 3 to 7 weeks.[31,32] The upper dose limit given in these fractionation regimens, above which permanent azoospermia is probable, is generally considered to be about 2.5 Gy.[20]

However, it has recently been observed that recovery of spermatogenesis occurs in about 15% of men who received either a 10-Gy single dose total-body exposure (testicular dose of 8 Gy) or 12- to 16-Gy exposures (testicular doses of 10 to 13 Gy) fractionated over 6 or 7 days, with a median follow-up time of 5 years.[33,34] It seems that recovery after both single doses and 6 or 7 daily fractions occurs after higher doses than when the dose is fractionated over 3 to 7 weeks, but no indication is shown of greater sensitivity of the testis to fractionation over 6 or 7 days than to single-dose irradiation.

The mechanism of the sensitizing effect of fractionation is still not completely known. During fractionated irradiation, spermatogonial stem cells may be recruited into a more radiosensitive phase, although radiosensitivity appears to actually be inversely related to the proliferative state of these cells.[35] The sensitizing effect of fractionation must exceed the capacity for repair of sublethal damage[30,35] and repopulation.[3,12]

Doses from Radiotherapeutic Procedures

In the typical patient being treated with megavoltage irradiation using a "hockey-stick" field to irradiate the periaortic and ipsilateral iliac lymph nodes for pure seminoma, the dose to the remaining testis, outside the radiation field, is in the range of 0.3 to 1.8 Gy,[32] although a more recent report indicates doses at the lower end of this range can be achieved.[36] An even greater dose may be delivered to the contralateral testis if the hemiscrotum is irradiated. In the treatment of Hodgkin's disease, periaortic-spleen or abdominal fields result in doses of 0.9 to 3.5 Gy to the testes.[19,36] Doses from pelvic fields are about 2 Gy.[37]

Whenever possible, a testicular shield should be used in men undergoing pelvic irradiation (Fig. 26-4).[38] This apparatus works principally by shielding the testicles

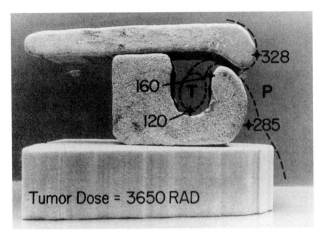

Fig. 26-4 Individually designed Cerrobend testicular shield with balanced lid to prevent pinching of scrotum as it drops over the lip of the base. Total testicular dose was 120 to 160 cGy for a total dose of 3650 cGy to the midpelvis and inguinal nodes. Doses measured on the perineum outside the scrotal shield were 328 cGy and 285 cGy. (Courtesy Million RR. The lymphomatous diseases. In Fletcher GH, ed. *Textbook of Radiotherapy*. 3rd ed. Philadelphia, Pa: Lea & Febiger; 1980.)

from radiation scattered from within the patient. The use of such shielding devices can reduce testicular exposure to approximately 1% of the dose delivered to the midpelvis. In addition, when hemiscrotal irradiation is used, a device to position and shield the remaining testicle should be used.[39]

GENETIC EFFECTS

Anyone using irradiation should be aware that ionizing radiation produces genetic mutations in germ cells of experimental animals and in somatic cells in humans. The frequency of the mutations depends on the radiation dose delivered, and the relationship is often a straight line without a threshold. Radiation-induced mutations are almost always harmful. Although there are no conclusive data showing heritable mutations induced in human germ cells by radiation,[40] it is most likely that such mutations are produced, but the frequency falls below the level that can be detected in epidemiologic studies with present techniques.

In male rodents, although meiotic and postmeiotic cells are resistant to killing by radiation, they are susceptible to induction of mutations. In fact, the induction of mutations, which can be transmitted to embryos and offspring, is higher in later stage germ cells than in stem spermatogonia.[41] Because they are eliminated through the differentiation and maturation processes, mutations induced in spermatocytes and spermatids only produce mutation-carrying sperm for a brief time. However, mutations induced in stem cells may result in the production of abnormal spermatozoa for a long time. Fortunately, the frequency of transmissible mutations is much lower in spermatozoa arising from these stem cells. Patients should also be advised against having children from the start of radiation therapy treatments (especially during the first 2 months, when fertility is likely to be maintained) until 6 months after the end of all cytotoxic therapy. By then, the body has eliminated spermatozoa derived from cells that were beyond the stem cell stage during radiation therapy. At present, no evidence exists to suggest any significant increase in birth defects or other genetically related abnormalities in offspring conceived 6 months or more after radiation therapy.

ENDOCRINE EFFECTS

Sertoli cells are directly involved in the support of spermatogenesis and secretion of various factors. The Leydig cells are the major source of testosterone. Their functions are regulated by paracrine and endocrine mechanisms.

Sertoli Cells

Sertoli cells provide nutrients to developing spermatocytes and spermatids, isolate them from bloodborne molecules, and facilitate their movement toward the lumen of the seminiferous tubule. Optimal Sertoli cell function depends on the action of testosterone and follicle-stimulating hormone from the pituitary. Sertoli cells also produce and secrete androgen-binding protein, which acts as a reservoir and transport molecule for testosterone; inhibin, which suppresses the release of follicle-stimulating hormone; and stem cell factor, which stimulates spermatogenesis.

Although Sertoli cells do not seem to be killed in the adult by radiation doses of up to 20 Gy, their function may be altered. The alterations in Sertoli cell function are manifest by increased follicle-stimulating hormone levels, which are a consequence of decreased inhibin production both in rat and in human, and by decreased androgen-binding protein levels in the rat. Prolonged alterations in these measures of Sertoli cell function were observed at doses of 0.75 and 5 Gy and above in man and rat, respectively.[10,42] However, it is not possible to determine from in vivo studies whether any of these alterations in Sertoli cell function are a result of direct damage to the Sertoli cell because Sertoli cell function is dramatically influenced by paracrine and juxtacrine interactions from the germ cells. Hence the changes in question can result from the depletion of all germ cells produced by these doses. In vitro, Sertoli cell secretion of a cytokine, interleukin-6, is indeed enhanced by radiation doses as low as 3 Gy.[43]

Leydig Cells

Luteinizing hormone (LH) from the anterior pituitary stimulates Leydig cells to form testosterone, which diffuses into the general circulation and into the seminiferous tubules to stimulate spermatogenesis. High testosterone levels suppress LH release through a negative feedback mechanism.

Increased serum LH, sometimes accompanied by decreased serum testosterone, has been observed in humans and rats after doses of 2 and 5 Gy, respectively.[42,44] Although such increases in LH have been considered to be measures of Leydig cell dysfunction after irradiation, that belief is not necessarily valid. The radiation doses used cause germinal aplasia, which reduces testis size, and a concomitant reduction in testicular blood flow.[45] With reduced blood flow, less testosterone is distributed into the circulation (note that intratesticular testosterone concentration is elevated after irradiation[23]). Because testosterone in the serum inhibits LH secretion by the pituitary, LH increases. In addition, the reduced blood flow lessens Leydig cell exposure to LH, and more LH is required to maintain a certain level of testosterone production. These alterations in the pituitary-gonadal feedback loop could elevate the levels of serum LH necessary to maintain serum testosterone in the normal range even in the absence of any Leydig cell injury. Radiation therapy may lower testosterone levels to the low-normal range in some men[46]; some of these men with low testosterone levels might benefit from androgen therapy.

High doses of radiation (20 to 30 Gy), such as are used in treatment of or prophylaxis for leukemia in the testis or for testicular carcinoma in situ, damage Leydig cells and markedly reduce testosterone levels even in adult men.[47] In rats the Leydig cells are much more sensitive to irradiation during puberty than during adulthood.[48] Similarly, an inverse age dependence of Leydig cell damage is evident in humans; in boys, doses as low as 12 Gy cause a high incidence of failure of testicular function to normally progress through puberty and subsequently extremely low testosterone levels.[49,50]

CANCER OF THE TESTICLE

Significant changes in the treatment of cancer of the testis have occurred over the last several decades. These changes are mainly the result of the development of effective chemotherapy regimens for nonseminomatous cancer and new imaging techniques and tumor markers for cancer detection and staging. These advances have made testicular cancer one of the most curable of all cancer types, with disease-specific 5-year survival rates in excess of 90%.[51]

The discovery of effective chemotherapeutic agents for germ cell tumors has also affected the indications for radiation therapy in the management of cancer of the testis. Although radiation therapy still plays a major role in the treatment of patients with pure seminoma, its role in the management of patients with nonseminomatous tumors has diminished considerably. The focus of this chapter is on the current status of radiation therapy in the management of the primary tumors of the testis, including seminomas, nonseminomas, stromal cell tumors, and lymphomas.

Incidence

Testicular cancer is a relatively rare tumor, with only about 7000 new cases diagnosed each year in the United States.[51] The number of new cases, however, has increased significantly over the last 20 years, from 3.2 cases per 100,000 in 1976 to 4.6 cases per 100,000 in 1996. Testis cancer is the most common cancer in males between the ages of 15 and 35. However, the incidence peaks somewhat later for seminomas (35 to 40 years) than for nonseminomas (25 to 30 years).[52] Testis cancer is much more common in whites (5.4 cases per 100,000 per year) than in blacks (0.9 cases per 100,000 per year).[51]

Considerable variation is evident in the incidence of testis cancer geographically. The Scandinavian countries, for example, report almost 10 times as many new cases per capita as do Japan or Puerto Rico. The populations that have the highest incidence of seminoma also have the highest incidence of nonseminoma, and vice versa.[53] A slight familial predilection is evident for this disease; testicular cancer is somewhat more common in identical twins or family members of a patient with a testis tumor than it is in men without a family history of this disease.

Approximately 10% of testicular cancer patients have a history of cryptorchidism,[54,55] and patients with cryptorchidism have about 35 times the risk of testicular cancer as patients with normally descended testicles.[56] The risk of cancer in a cryptorchid testis is directly related to the degree of maldescent. The incidence is approximately one in 20 if the testis is located intraabdominally and one in 80 if it is located in the inguinal canal. Testicular cancer is slightly more common in the right testis than the left, and this differential correlates with the increased incidence of cryptorchidism in the right testis.[57]

Most investigators believe that the high incidence of germ cell malignancies in patients with cryptorchidism is related to a developmental defect.[58] Evidence for this opinion includes the observations that a significant percentage (5% to 10%) of the cases of cancer associated with cryptorchidism occur in the contralateral, normally descended testis and that approximately one fourth of patients who have a testicular cancer in a cryptorchid testis have carcinoma in situ in the other testis.[59]

Overall, approximately 1% to 3% of testicular cancer cases are bilateral, and more than half of patients with bilateral tumors have a history of cryptorchidism.[60] Approximately 5% of patients with germ cell tumors of the testis have carcinoma in situ in the contralateral testis,

and in many of them invasive cancer eventually develops in the second testis.[61,62] Bilateral testicular cancer may occur synchronously or metachronously, with the second cancer usually appearing within 2 years of the original diagnosis. However, cancer in the second testis has been noted up to 15 years after the first.

Pathology

About 95% of cases of primary cancer of the testis are germ cell tumors. These are usually divided into seminomas and nonseminomatous categories for the purpose of treatment decisions. Of these, approximately one third are seminomas and two thirds are nonseminomatous tumors. Less than 5% of testicular malignancies originate from the gonadal stroma (e.g., Sertoli cell tumors, Leydig cell tumors, gonadoblastomas). Sertoli cell tumors and Leydig cell tumors are usually benign and are most often treated surgically. Other tumors that can originate in the testis include lymphomas (usually diffuse large cell lymphomas), melanomas, and rhabdomyosarcomas. The tumors that are of the most interest to radiation oncologists are the germ cell tumors and, to a lesser extent, lymphomas and rhabdomyosarcomas.

Histopathologic Classification

The histopathologic classifications of germ cell tumors differ in Great Britain and the United States. Each is based on a theory of germ cell tumor development, and several theories focus on the histogenesis of germ cell tumors. The British histopathologic classification is based on the model of Willis,[63] who proposed that all nonseminomatous tumors are teratomas that have descended from displaced blastomeres.

The classification used in the United States is based on the model proposed by Friedman and Moore,[64] Dixon and Moore,[65] and Mostofi[66] (Fig. 26-5). These investigators proposed that primordial germ cells divide into two groups of cells when they are fertilized: extraembryonic or trophoblastic cells and embryonic or somatic cells (see Fig. 26-5). The trophoblastic cells can implant into the uterus just as the placenta does during normal development. The embryonic cells, however, may take one of several paths: one cell becomes identifiable as the germ cell early in embryogenesis and the others differentiate into somatic cells (i.e., ectoderm, mesoderm, and endoderm), which form the various organs of the embryo. Thus primordial germ cells have the potential to differentiate into aggressive cells (trophoblasts) or into somatic cells, which will later develop into mature tissues and organs.

Germ cell tumors are believed to be able to develop anywhere along this pathway. Seminomas are thought to originate from the germinal epithelium of the seminiferous tubules. Evidence that supports this hypothesis

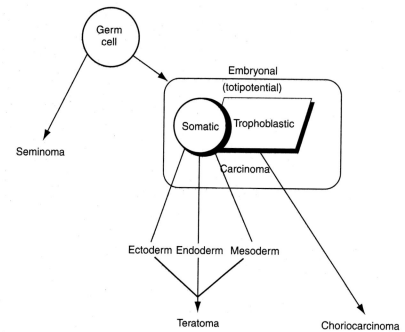

Fig. 26-5 Diagram illustrating the histogenesis of the germ cell tumors of the testis.

includes the observation that seminoma cells are morphologically similar to spermatogonia and that carcinoma in situ is often found within the seminiferous vessels in the early stage of development of a seminoma.

According to this theory, nonseminomatous germ cell tumors arise from the primordial cells or their progeny.[67,68] Embryonal carcinomas are believed to originate from totipotential primordial germ cells, whereas the other germ cell tumors are thought to develop further along the pathway (see Fig. 26-5). If the embryonal cells develop intraembryonically along somatic lines, teratomas or teratocarcinomas may develop, and if they develop along extraembryonic pathways, choriocarcinomas or yolk sac tumors may be formed.

In general, the U.S. and British histopathologic classification systems are not easily compared. Seminomas and spermatocytic seminomas are identical in the two classifications, but differences exist in the way the nonseminomatous germ cell tumors are organized.

Seminoma (Dixon-Moore Category I)

Seminomas make up 35% of all germ cell tumors of the testis. They tend to occur in a slightly older age group than do the nonseminomatous tumors. Grossly, seminomas present as pale gray to yellow nodules of a uniform or slightly lobulated consistency. Three histologic subtypes have been described: classic, anaplastic, and spermatocytic.

Classic seminomas. Classic seminomas are composed of a monotonous sheet of seminoma cells. Seminoma cells are large cells containing a clear cytoplasm and a hyperchromatic nucleus. Syncytiotrophoblasts or foreign body giant cells may be seen, but mitoses are infrequent. The syncytiotrophoblastic elements are seen in 10% to 15% of cases, an incidence that corresponds with the incidence of β-human chorionic gonadotropin (β-HCG) elevations in seminomas. Approximately 85% of pure seminomas have a classic pattern.

Anaplastic seminomas. Anaplastic seminomas are characterized by marked nuclear pleomorphism and a higher mitotic rate than classic seminomas. The diagnosis is made by finding three or more mitotic figures per high power field. The radiosensitivity of anaplastic seminomas is similar to that of classic seminomas, but patients with anaplastic seminomas usually present with disease of a higher clinical stage.[69] Approximately 10% to 12% of seminomas are anaplastic.

Spermatocytic seminomas. Spermatocytic seminomas contain cells resembling secondary spermatocytes and spermatids. They tend to occur in elderly men and are characterized by an excellent prognosis. Spermatocytic seminomas account for 4% to 5% of all seminomas.

Embryonal Carcinoma (Dixon-Moore Category II)

Embryonal carcinomas have a grayish-white, slightly variegated appearance with areas of hemorrhage and necrosis. Histologically, they contain cells that resemble malignant epithelial cells, with considerable pleomorphism. The nuclei are variable in shape, and mitotic figures are common. The infantile variety is known as *orchioblastoma, yolk sac tumor,* or *endodermal sinus tumor.* Approximately 20% of germ cell tumors of the testis are embryonal carcinomas.

Teratoma (Dixon-Moore Category III)

Teratomas contain more than one germ cell layer in various stages of maturation. Grossly, they may contain cysts filled with clear gelatinous or mucinous material along with various amounts of solid tissue. They may contain squamous or neuronal tissue of ectodermal origin; gastrointestinal or respiratory tissue of endodermal origin; and cartilage, muscle, or bone of mesodermal origin. Teratomas are benign in infants, but they may metastasize in adults. They account for approximately 5% of all germ cell tumors.

Choriocarcinoma (Dixon-Moore Category V)

Choriocarcinomas are highly malignant tumors that tend to metastasize early in the course of the disease. They are composed entirely of syncytiotrophoblasts and cytotrophoblasts, as compared with mixed tumors with foci of choriocarcinoma, which have only scattered syncytiotrophoblasts. Choriocarcinomas are extremely rare, making up less than 1% of all germ cell tumors.

Mixed Tumors

Almost 40% of germ cell tumors contain more than one histopathologic type. The most common type of mixed tumor is teratocarcinoma (Dixon-Moore Category IV), which is a combination of teratoma and embryonal carcinoma, with or without seminoma.[65]

Routes of Spread
Local Extension

A testicular cancer usually presents as a painless mass within the testis. It may spread locally to the rete testis, epididymis, and spermatic cord. However, this occurs in only 10% to 15% of patients.[70] Testis cancer can also extend through the tunica albuginea into the scrotum, but this is even more uncommon (less than 5%) because the tunica albuginea forms a natural barrier to direct extension.[70,71] This is important with regard to management, because the scrotum rarely requires treatment.

Differential Diagnosis

The differential diagnosis of a testis tumor includes epididymitis, hydrocele, spermatocele, hematocele, granulomatous orchitis, and varicocele. Epididymitis usually presents as an enlarged tender epididymis, which is clearly separable from the testis, and usually with an acute onset of symptoms such as fever and urethral discharge. It is usually identifiable on ultrasonography. A hydrocele can usually be transilluminated and is easily distinguished as a fluid-filled mass on scrotal sonography.

Lymphatic Metastasis

Embryologically, the testes originate from the genital ridge near the second lumbar vertebra before migrating into the scrotum. As they do so, they carry along their own vascular and lymphatic supply. The primary collecting lymphatic trunks follow the internal spermatic vessels to the periaortic area (Fig. 26-6).[72] The channels swing out wide laterally, particularly on the left (Fig. 26-7).

The primary drainage from the right and left testis differs. The lymphatics from the right testis tend to drain to lymph nodes located along the inferior vena cava from L2 to L5. However, these vessels can cross over directly to terminate in the contralateral left periaortic lymph

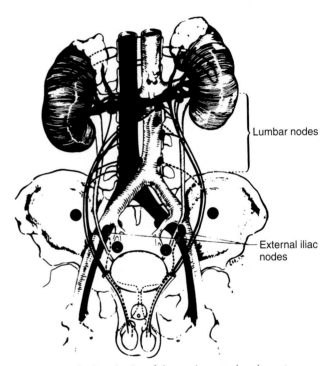

Fig. 26-6 The lymphatics of the testis ascend and anastomose along the spermatic cord. The majority of the collecting trunks accompany the internal spermatic artery and vein to the point where these blood vessels cross the ureter and then separate from the internal spermatic vessels by turning medially to terminate in the lumbar lymph nodes. The nodal connections differ on the right and left. On the right, the majority of these channels end in the lateral aortic, precaval, or preaortic nodes situated between the renal vein and the aortic bifurcation. In about 10% of patients, some of the trunks end in a node situated at the junction of the renal vein and inferior vena cava. On the left, the majority of the collecting trunks drain into the lateral aortic nodes situated below the left renal vein, usually terminating in the superior nodes of this group. However, they may also end in the preaortic nodes or in nodes situated at the level of the aortic bifurcation. On both sides, some of the lymphatic channels abandon the spermatic vessels after they reach the vesical peritoneum, ending in nodes lying along the external iliac vein. (From Weiss L, Gilbert HA, Ballon SC, eds. *Lymphatic System Metastasis.* Vol III, Boston, Mass: GK Hall; 1980.)

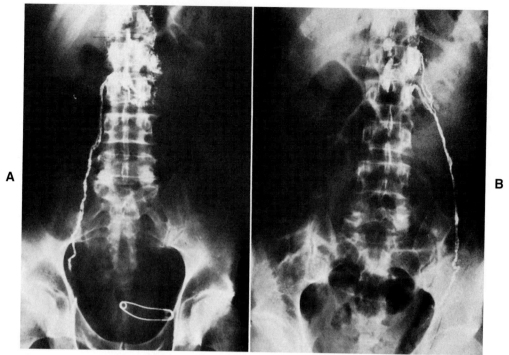

Fig. 26-7 Direct filling of periaortic lymph nodes draining the testicle, demonstrated by testicular lymphangiograms of the **(A)** right and **(B)** left sides. The iliac nodes are bypassed. (Courtesy Dr. F.M. Busch.)

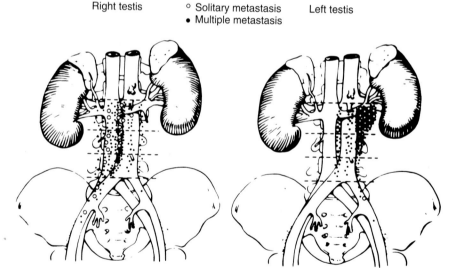

Right testis   ○ Solitary metastasis   Left testis
                ● Multiple metastasis

Fig. 26-8 Distribution of lymph node metastases found at lymphadenectomy for nonseminomatous tumors. (From tabular data supplied by Ray B, Hajdu S, Whitmore W. *Cancer* 1974; 33:340-348.)

nodes. The lymphatics from the left testis tend to drain to nodes located just below the renal vein (Fig. 26-8).[73] However, they can also drain to lymph nodes located elsewhere in the left periaortic area. Unlike the lymphatic vessels from the right testis, the vessels from the left testis do not cross over directly to the contralateral side. The lymphatics from either testis can extend to

periaortic nodes located above the renal hila or to nodes situated at the level of the aortic bifurcation.

On both sides, some of the lymphatic channels abandon the spermatic vessels after they reach the vesicle peritoneum, ending in nodes lying along the external iliac vein (see Fig. 26-6). This lymphatic drainage is usually ipsilateral unless the patient has had groin surgery or extensive retroperitoneal metastasis leading to retrograde spread.

Metastasis to the lymph nodes above the diaphragm is rare in the absence of involvement of the periaortic lymph nodes. However, supraclavicular metastasis may occur in the absence of mediastinal disease because the main route of lymphatic spread from the periaortic area is through the thoracic duct. Supraclavicular metastases are usually located on the left side, near the junction of the thoracic duct and the left subclavian vein.

Hematogenous Metastasis

The regional lymph nodes are almost always the first site of metastasis for a pure seminoma, and hematogenous metastasis is very uncommon with this disease. Embryonal carcinomas and teratocarcinomas also tend to spread to the lymph nodes first, but in those tumors, hematogenous metastasis is not uncommon. On the other hand, choriocarcinomas almost always have hematogenous metastasis by the time the diagnosis is established. The lungs are usually the first site of hematogenous spread from a testicular tumor.

Staging

The results achieved with radiation therapy are reported in terms of clinical staging because the pathologic status of the retroperitoneal lymph nodes is not known in those cases. In general, the results are better stage for stage when a series is reported in terms of pathologic staging than when they are reported in terms of clinical staging. This is true for both stage I and stage II cancer because patients whose disease is clinically stage I but pathologically stage II have less extensive retroperitoneal disease than those who have both clinically and pathologically stage II disease. These differences must be considered when comparing the results of surgical series with those obtained with radiation therapy.

A variety of staging systems have been used for testis cancer. The classification that was used for testis cancer for many years was first proposed by Boden and Gibb.[74] A modification of this classification is shown below:

Stage I	Tumor clinically limited to the testis and spermatic cord
Stage II	Clinical or radiographic evidence of tumor spread beyond the testis but limited to the regional nodes below the diaphragm
Stage IIA	Moderate-size retroperitoneal metastasis
Stage IIB	Massive retroperitoneal metastasis
Stage III	Extension above the diaphragm
Stage IIIA	Extension above the diaphragm but still confined to the mediastinal or supraclavicular lymphatics
Stage IIIB	Extranodal metastasis

The stage distributions for seminomas and nonseminomas differ because the patterns of spread are different (Box 26-1).[75-77] In a series of patients seen at The University of Texas M.D. Anderson Cancer Center, 32% of patients with nonseminomatous tumors had clinical evidence of hematogenous spread (Royal Marsden stage IIIB) at the time of diagnosis, compared with only 6% of those with pure seminomas.[75] However, the percentage of patients with bulky retroperitoneal disease (Royal Marsden stage IID) was significantly greater for those with pure seminomas than it was for those with nonseminomas (16% vs. 6%). This is because nonseminomatous tumors are more likely to have metastasized hematogenously by the time the retroperitoneal disease becomes large.

Several other staging systems have been proposed in recent years.[76,77] These staging systems describe the extent of the tumor at the primary site, in the regional lymphatics, and in distant organs in more detail. The two most widely used staging systems today are the American Joint Committee on Cancer (AJCC) and Royal Marsden Hospital systems. The AJCC system uses the tumor-nodes-metastasis notation, whereas the Royal Marsden system closely resembles the original Boden and Gibb classification. The AJCC and Royal Marsden classifications are compared in Box 26-1.

The Royal Marsden classification is used in this chapter whenever possible. This staging system was selected because it subdivides stage II into four subcategories on the basis of the size of the retroperitoneal lymph node metastases (smaller than 2 cm, 2 to 5 cm, 5 to 10 cm, and larger than 10 cm). This makes it easy to convert to other staging systems that may use different size criteria to differentiate between moderate-size and bulky disease in the regional lymph nodes. For pure seminomas, 10 cm is usually used to distinguish between moderately advanced and massive retroperitoneal metastasis, whereas 5 cm is usually used to differentiate between moderately advanced and massive retroperitoneal disease for nonseminomatous testicular cancer.[77,78]

Pretreatment Evaluation

Clinical evaluation of a patient suspected of having a testicular tumor should begin with a complete history and physical examination. This should include careful palpation of both testicles and transillumination to differentiate a solid mass from a hydrocele or spermatocele. The abdomen should be examined carefully to evaluate for retroperitoneal lymphadenopathy and hepatosplenomegaly. The neck should be palpated because the supraclavicular area is the most likely site of lymphatic spread above the diaphragm. The breasts should be evaluated for gynecomastia, which is commonly seen with choriocarcinomas.

The initial laboratory studies should include a complete blood count, urinalysis, liver function studies, and

BOX 26-1 Staging Classification Systems for Germ Cell Tumors of the Testis

American Joint Committee on Cancer Tumor-Nodes-Metastasis Staging System*	Royal Marsden Staging System†

PRIMARY TUMOR (T)

pTx   Primary tumor cannot be assessed (if no radical orchiectomy has been performed, TX is used)

pT0   No evidence of primary tumor (e.g., histologic scar in testis)

pTis   Intratubular germ cell neoplasia (CIS)

pT1   Tumor limited to the testis and epididymis without vascular/lymphatic invasion; tumor may invade into the tunica albuginea but not the tunica vaginalis

pT2   Tumor limited to the testis and epididymis with vascular/lymphatic invasion, or tumor extending through the tunica albuginea with involvement of the tunica vaginalis

pT3   Tumor invades the spermatic cord with or without vascular/lymphatic invasion

pT4   Tumor invades the scrotum with or without vascular/lymphatic invasion

REGIONAL LYMPH NODES (N) (CLINICAL)

NX   Regional lymph nodes cannot be assessed

N0   No regional lymph node metastasis

N1   Metastasis with a lymph node mass 2 cm or less in greatest dimension; or multiple lymph nodes, none more than 2 cm in greatest dimension

N2   Metastasis with a lymph node mass more than 2 cm but not more than 5 cm in greatest dimension; or multiple lymph nodes, any one mass greater than 2 cm but not more than 5 cm in greatest dimension

N3   Metastasis with a lymph node mass more than 5 cm in greatest dimension

DISTANT METASTASIS (M)

MX   Distant metastasis cannot be assessed

M0   No distant metastasis

M1   Distant metastasis

   M1a   Nonregional nodal or pulmonary metastasis

   M1b   Distant metastasis other than to nonregional lymph nodes and lungs

---

Royal Marsden Staging System†

I   Tumor confined to the testis and spermatic cord

II   Metastasis to lymph nodes below the diaphragm

   IIA   Maximum diameter < 2 cm

   IIB   Maximum diameter 2-5 cm

   IIC   Maximum diameter 5-10 cm

   IID   Maximum diameter > 10 cm

III   Extension to nodes above the diaphragm (abdominal status as listed above: A, B, C, or D)

IV   Extranodal metastasis

From Hussey DH. Testicular cancer. In: Levitt SH, Kahn FM, Potish RA, Perez CA, eds. *Levitt & Tapley's Technological Basis of Radiation Therapy Clinical Applications.* 3rd ed. Philadelphia, Pa: Lippincott Williams & Wilkins; 1998.
*Modified from Fleming I, Cooper JS, Henson DE, et al, eds. *AJCC Cancer Staging Manual.* 5th ed. Philadelphia, Pa: Lippincott Williams & Wilkins; 1997:225-230.
†Modified from Thomas GM. Consensus statement on the investigation and management of testicular seminoma. EORTC Genito-Urinary Group, Monograph 7. In: Newling DW, Jones WG eds. *Prostate Cancer and Testicular Cancer.* New York: Wiley-Liss, 1990.

blood urea nitrogen assay. If a testis tumor is suspected, testicular sonography should be performed and serum markers should be drawn for β-HCG and alpha-fetoprotein (AFP). Semen analysis and sperm banking should be considered when treatment is likely to compromise fertility.

If the initial clinical evaluation remains consistent with testicular tumor, the primary tumor should be removed by a radical orchiectomy through an inguinal incision and the diagnosis confirmed by histopathologic examination. Further studies must then be performed to accurately stage the extent of the disease.

Serum marker measurements should be repeated and compared with the results obtained before orchiectomy. A chest x-ray should be performed to establish whether pulmonary metastases are present. Retroperitoneal lymph nodes should be evaluated by pedal lymphangiography and abdominopelvic computed tomography (CT) scanning.

Abdominal Imaging

Lymphangiography. Pedal lymphangiography is useful for detecting regional lymph node metastasis, as an aid to setting up treatment portals, and for following the response to treatment (the nodes often remain opacified for months after the procedure). Lymphangiography can detect lymph node metastases as small as 5 mm in diameter. These lesions are usually seen as filling defects beneath the capsule of the node. Other findings suggestive of nodal metastasis include deviation or obstruction of the lymph vessels or nonvisualization of a lymph node group. The accuracy of lymphangiography depends on the experience of the diagnostic radiologist, but it is said to have an overall accuracy of 80% in testicular cancer with 15% to 20% false negatives and 5% to 10% false positives.[79,80]

Computed tomography. CT is less sensitive than lymphangiography because the nodes must be 1.5 to 2 cm in size or larger to be detected as abnormal. CT scans have been reported to have an overall accuracy of 76%,[81] but the incidence of false negatives is greater with CT than it is with lymphangiography. However, CT scans are useful for evaluating nodes that do not opacify with pedal lymphangiography, such as the sentinel nodes near the renal hila and those located above the renal pedicles.

Considerable controversy exists as to whether testicular cancer should be staged initially by pedal lymphangiography or by CT. Some oncologists prefer pedal lymphangiography because it is more accurate than CT and has fewer false negatives.[75,82,83] Others recommend CT, particularly if the retroperitoneal nodes are to be irradiated anyway. The argument is that any nodal metastasis from seminoma that is not detectable by CT is small enough to be easily controlled with the radiation therapy doses used electively.[81,84,85] Lymphangiography is not readily available in many institutions, and thus most radiation oncologists rely on CT scans to identify the presence and extent of retroperitoneal spread.

Tumor Markers

The development of tumor markers for germ cell tumors has had a profound effect on the management of testicular cancer. Tumor markers are useful for staging, to monitor the effectiveness of therapy, and to follow patients for the early detection of recurrent cancer. Tumor markers improve the accuracy of clinical staging for patients with testis cancer. Scardino and colleagues,[86] for example, found that the addition of AFP and β-HCG assays to the initial work-up reduced the false-negative rate from 29% to 13% in a series of patients with nonseminomatous testis cancer.

Human chorionic gonadotropin. HCG is a glycoprotein normally secreted by syncytiotrophoblastic cells in the placenta. It is composed of two polypeptide chains, an α- and a β-HCG component. The radioimmune assay for cancer detection is directed to the β-HCG chain because antibodies to the α-HCG chain may cross-react with a variety of other hormones (e.g., LH, follicle-stimulating hormone, and thyroid-stimulating hormone).

β-HCG is found in many patients with germ cell tumors, usually those with trophoblastic elements. Abnormal titers are found in about 40% to 60% of patients with nonseminomatous testicular tumors and in 7% to 10% of patients with pure seminomas.[87,88] However, the elevations seen with pure seminoma are almost always moderate. β-HCG is not found in normal men or boys. However, it can be elevated with a variety of nontesticular malignancies, e.g., breast, stomach, pancreas, and liver cancer.

Alpha-fetoprotein. AFP is a glycoprotein that is normally produced by the fetal yolk sac, liver, and gastrointestinal tract. Abnormal AFP levels can be found in newborns but not in adults. AFP titers may be elevated in patients with hepatomas or other gastrointestinal malignancies or with yolk sac tumors, embryonal carcinomas, or teratocarcinomas of the testis.

Yolk sac tumors tend to produce AFP, just as the normal yolk sac does during fetal development. Approximately 70% of patients with teratocarcinomas or embryonal carcinomas have elevated AFP titers.[87] Elevated AFP values are not found in patients with pure seminomas or choriocarcinomas. Therefore any patient with a histopathologic diagnosis of pure seminoma and an elevated AFP should be considered to have a mixed tumor.

Other markers. Several other markers have been proposed for detecting testicular tumors. Placental alkaline phosphatase and lactate dehydrogenase have been found to be useful in the management of pure seminoma. Placental alkaline phosphatase is the most sensitive for detecting metastatic disease, having a sensitivity of 50% to 55%. However, false positives do occur.[89]

Clinical applications of tumor markers. Tumor markers should be assayed both before and after orchiectomy. However, the postorchiectomy specimen should be obtained after sufficient time has elapsed to allow for metabolism of markers present in the serum at the time of orchiectomy. β-HCG has a metabolic half-life of 24 hours, and AFP has a metabolic half-life of 5 days. If the markers remain elevated after orchiectomy, metastatic disease is present. However, normal findings on postorchiectomy marker studies do not guarantee that metastasis is not present because false-negative results occur in 15% to 30% of cases.[87]

TREATMENT
Controversies Regarding Radiation Therapy for Pure Seminoma

Pure seminomas seem to be ideally suited for treatment with radiation therapy because they are exquisitely radiosensitive and they are characterized by an orderly lymphatic spread. Distant metastasis is rare. A review of the literature shows that the 5-year relapse-free survival rates with orchiectomy and regional lymphatic irradiation were more than 96% for stage I and 82% for stage II tumors (Table 26-1).[55,90-110] In a series reported from the M.D. Anderson Cancer Center,[78,111] the 5-year cause-specific survival rate was 97% for patients with no evidence of metastasis beyond the testis (Royal Marsden stage I) and 95% for patients with small to moderate-size regional lymph node metastasis (nodes smaller than 10 cm in diameter; Royal Marsden stage IIA-C). Even patients with massive nodal disease (measuring more than 10 cm in diameter; Royal Marsden stage IID) had 67% 5-year cause-specific survival. Recurrence within the irradiated area is very rare in any series, even for patients with bulky disease.

In spite of the excellent results achieved with radiation therapy, several controversies, discussed in the following section, have arisen in recent years regarding its use in selected clinical situations.

Elective Irradiation vs. Surveillance for Stage I Tumors

Standard treatment for stage I pure seminoma has been a radical orchiectomy and elective irradiation of the regional lymphatics. However, a number of investigators

---

	STAGE I		STAGE II		
Institution and Reference	**Number of Patients**	**Results (%)**	**Number of Patients**	**Results (%)**	**Endpoints**
Antoni van Leeuwenhoek Hospital[86]	78	95	25	72	3-year RFS
Brooke General Hospital[87]	64	97	—	—	3-year survival
Indiana University[88]	33	94	19	80	2.5-year survival
Johns Hopkins University[89]	42	93	19	89	5-year RFS
Joint Center for Radiation Therapy[90]	79	92	—	—	10-year survival
Institute Gustave Roussy[91]	184	96	—	—	Actuarial 5-year survival
London Cancer Institute[92]	169	97	43	88	2- to 10-year RFS
M.D. Anderson Hospital[93]	282	97	68	84	5-year RFS
Massachusetts General Hospital[94]	135	95	25	84	5-year RFS
Norwegian Radium Hospital[95]	329	94	—	—	10-year survival
Princess Margaret Hospital[96]	338	94	86	74	Actuarial 5-year survival
Rotterdam Institute[97]	153	95	74	82	2-year RFS
Royal Marsden Hospital[53]	121	97	54	81	2-year RFS
Stanford University[98]	71	100	27	85	Actuarial 5-year survival
State University of New York[99]	104	94	—	—	5-year survival
State University of New York[100]	—	—	45	89	5-year RFS
U.S. Naval Hospital San Diego[101]	52	94	—	—	3- to 5-year survival
University of Wisconsin[102]	23	96	11	91	3-year survival
Walter Reed General Hospital[103]	284	97	34	76	Actuarial 10-year survival
Washington University[104]	95	100	—	—	5-year survival
Western General Hospital[105]	185	96	53	90	5-year RFS
Yale University[106]	61	98	18	100	5-year disease-specific survival
TOTALS	2882	96	556	82	

NOTE: Whenever possible, the results were reported in terms of 2- to 5-year relapse-free survival or absolute 5- to 10-year survival rates.
RFS, Relapse-free survival.

in recent years have proposed treating these patients with orchiectomy alone and following them closely for disease progression. The arguments for surveillance in clinical stage I pure seminoma are that (1) only 15% to 20% of these patients actually have retroperitoneal metastasis, and therefore 80% to 85% are being irradiated needlessly; and (2) most patients who experience relapse after treatment with orchiectomy alone can be salvaged with radiation therapy or chemotherapy when the disease becomes apparent clinically.

Surveillance for stage I pure seminoma has been tested in clinical trials in Denmark, Britain, and Canada.[112-115] Each of these studies showed relapse rates in the range of 16% to 20%, which correlates well with the expected incidence of retroperitoneal metastasis in clinical stage I seminoma. Moreover, almost all of the patients who developed recurrent disease were successfully treated with additional therapy, so the ultimate survival rates were not compromised when the patients were followed closely in a protocol situation.

A Danish group,[113] for example, reported a 20% actuarial 4-year relapse rate in 261 patients treated by orchiectomy and close surveillance. Twenty-two percent of 49 patients who relapsed had bulky abdominal disease at the time of progression, and 16% of these patients had metastasis beyond the periaortic area (five in pelvic lymph nodes, two in inguinal lymph nodes, and one in the lungs). Similarly, only four patients (8% of those treated for salvage) relapsed a second time, and only three (1.1 % of the total group) died of seminoma-related events (one of progressive disease and two of complications related to salvage treatment).

A similar relapse rate was reported in the British study from the Royal Marsden Hospital, but the disease was more advanced when it was detected.[116] The authors reported a 16% actuarial 3-year relapse rate in 133 patients treated with surveillance. However, eight of 13 patients in whom progressive disease developed had bulky abdominal disease at relapse, and one had distant metastasis. Thus only a third of the patients who relapsed had early disease when the tumor recurred, and five of the 13 relapsed a second time.

A total of 172 patients were managed by orchiectomy and surveillance in the Canadian study from Princess Margaret Hospital.[114] Twenty-seven of them experienced relapse, for an actuarial 5-year relapse rate of 18%. However, five of the 27 patients who relapsed did so more than 4 years after diagnosis, including one after 9 years. These results support the notion that patients undergoing surveillance for pure seminoma must be followed for a long time because late recurrences are more common with seminomas than they are with nonseminomatous cancer.[117]

These studies show that surveillance is a satisfactory alternative for some patients with clinical stage I disease. However, it is probably not appropriate for most patients because aggressive follow-up is necessary if relapses are to be detected early. In the Canadian study,[114] tumor markers were obtained at 2-month intervals for 2 years, at 4-month intervals for the third year, and at 6-month intervals thereafter. Abdominal CT scans were obtained at 4-month intervals for the first 3 years, at 6-month intervals for years 4 to 7, and at yearly intervals thereafter.

Patients undergoing surveillance must be followed much more closely than patients receiving elective irradiation. Furthermore, not all patients comply with treatment recommendations, and a significant number of those who experience relapse will have bulky disease and require treatment with chemotherapy. For these reasons, most oncologists continue to favor elective irradiation for patients with stage I pure seminoma.

Treatment Portals for Stage I-II Seminoma

The standard treatment portals for stage I-II pure seminoma have in the past been directed toward the periaortic and ipsilateral iliac areas. These fields have usually included the inguinal orchiectomy scar and the hemiscrotum if the tumor has extended through the tunica albuginea. However, inclusion of the inguinal nodes and hemiscrotum results in a significant radiation dose to the contralateral testis, and the risk of tumor seeding in the scrotum and inguinal region is low. Because of this, the International Consensus Conference in Leeds in 1989 recommended that treatment of the inguinal area and scrotum be omitted, even if the orchiectomy incision extends into the scrotum.[77,118]

Several authors have proposed treating an even smaller volume. These investigators have advocated limiting the irradiation to the periaortic region and omitting treatment of the iliac lymph nodes.[119-121] One of the main reasons for limiting the treatment to only the periaortic area is to decrease the risk of second malignancies.

A number of authors[119,122-125] have reported an increased incidence of second cancer in patients with seminomas, and it has been proposed that some of these cases of a second cancer are the result of the abdominal radiation therapy that these patients have received. However, not all of the second primary cancer cases reported have been located in or near the radiation therapy treatment fields, and some authors have noted a greater-than-expected incidence of second malignancies even in testicular cancer patients who received no radiation therapy.[126] Consequently, the high incidence of a second cancer may simply represent a predilection for seminoma patients to develop second primary malignant tumors regardless of the mode of treatment.

Nevertheless, the risk of metastatic disease in the pelvis of patients with clinical stage I seminoma is quite small. Only 15% to 20% of patients with clinical stage I seminoma have occult retroperitoneal metastases, and almost all of these are located in the periaortic area (see Fig. 26-8). Occult metastasis to the pelvic area is much less frequent (about 1% to 3%) because the primary lymphatic drainage is to the periaortic nodes. This projection correlates well with pelvic failure rates when the iliac lymph nodes have not been irradiated. The follow-up for most patients treated with only para-aortic irradiation is still relatively short, but Kiricuta and others[127] reported only a 2.3% incidence of failure in the inguinal-iliac region in a group of patients followed for 1 to 13 years. Similarly, Sedlmayer and colleagues[128] found a 3.5% failure rate in the pelvis in a series of patients followed for a period of 30 to 210 months in Salzburg, Austria.

Elective Irradiation of the Mediastinal and Supraclavicular Nodes

Before 1985, most patients with stage II pure seminoma were treated electively with mediastinal and supraclavicular irradiation. The rationale for this policy was that pure seminomas metastasize in a stepwise fashion, first to the retroperitoneal lymph nodes, then to the mediastinum and supraclavicular nodes, and subsequently to distant organs. The policy was to electively treat the next echelon of uninvolved nodes on the supposition that these areas may harbor occult disease.

Most patients with stage II disease today are not given elective radiation therapy above the diaphragm, mainly because effective chemotherapy for pure seminoma has been developed. The arguments against elective irradiation of the mediastinal and supraclavicular nodes are as follows: (1) that the risk of subclinical disease in these nodes is small if the disease in the retroperitoneal nodes is limited, (2) that elective irradiation of the mediastinum increases the risk of subsequent coronary artery disease, (3) that irradiation of this area would make it more difficult to deliver effective chemotherapy later should progressive disease develop, and (4) that patients with occult metastasis in the mediastinum and supraclavicular area can be treated successfully with further radiation therapy or chemotherapy when the metastases become clinically apparent.

It is generally agreed that elective irradiation to the mediastinum and supraclavicular lymph nodes is not indicated for patients with clinical stage I disease because only 1% to 2% of patients with stage I disease who receive radiation therapy to fields located below the diaphragm have recurrences in the mediastinum or supraclavicular area.[129] This is also true for many patients with stage II pure seminoma. However, elective irradiation above the diaphragm may still have a role in selected patients with stage II disease because a significant number have occult disease in the mediastinal or supraclavicular regions.

Dosmann and Zagars,[97] for example, found a 20% actuarial failure rate in the left supraclavicular area in a group of patients with clinical stage IIA-C disease (Royal

Marsden stage; nodes larger than 10 cm) who did not receive elective irradiation in this area. On the other hand, none of those who received elective supraclavicular irradiation had failures in this area. Similarly, Thomas and colleagues[118] reported a 22% (10 of 46) relapse rate in the lymphatics above the diaphragm in patients with stage IIIB pure seminoma (2- to 5-cm nodes) treated to only the retroperitoneal nodes. However, Hermann and others[129] reported only a 4% incidence of mediastinal and supraclavicular failures in patients with stage IIA disease (smaller than 2-cm nodes), an observation that suggests that elective irradiation is not necessary if the retroperitoneal lesions are smaller than 2 cm.

Speer's group[130] found that the relapse rate in the mediastinum and supraclavicular area correlated well with the volume of disease in the periaortic lymph nodes (Table 26-2). In a review of 35 reports involving 389 patients with stage II disease, they found a 9% failure rate in the mediastinal and supraclavicular areas in stage IIA, 16% in stage IIB, 23% in stage IIC, and 26% in stage IID (Royal Marsden classification).[130]

In view of the limited morbidity associated with supraclavicular irradiation, elective irradiation of the supraclavicular area seems to be appropriate for patients with stage IIB-C disease. However, irradiation of the mediastinum is not advocated because treatment of this area increases the risk of subsequent cardiac disease. In the Dosmann and Zagars series,[97] most relapses above the diaphragm occurred in the supraclavicular area, indicating that tumor emboli follow normal anatomic channels, bypassing the mediastinum by way of the thoracic duct. If mediastinal irradiation is omitted, the risk of cardiac injury and the compromise of subsequent treatment with chemotherapy should be minimized.

Bulky Abdominal Disease

The cure rates with radiation therapy alone for patients with massive retroperitoneal metastasis (stage IID) are

TABLE 26-2

Incidence of Mediastinal or Supraclavicular Failure in Patients with Stage II Disease Who Did Not Undergo Elective Mediastinal and Supraclavicular Irradiation

Royal Marsden Stage	Mediastinal or Supraclavicular Recurrences (%)
IIA (< 2 cm)	9 (2 of 22)
IIB (2-5 cm)	16 (12 of 76)
IIC (> 5 cm or bulky)	23 (38 of 164)
IID (≥ 10 cm or palpable)	16 (33 of 127)

Modified from Speer TW, Sombeck MD, Parsons JT, et al. *Int J Radiat Oncol Biol Phys* 1995;33:89-97.

poorer than they are for patients with small to moderate-size retroperitoneal disease (stage IIA-C). However, most of these failures are the result of distant metastasis. Even massive seminomas can be eradicated with radiation therapy because seminomas are very radiosensitive. Anscher and others[131] reported a 38% relapse rate for patients with bulky intraabdominal disease. However, only 15% had recurrences within the treated area (Table 26-3).[78,92-94,100,110,131-139] Zagars and Babaian[78] also reported a significantly greater relapse rate for patients with bulky retroperitoneal metastasis than for those with less extensive disease, but none of the patients in their series developed in-field recurrences. These results show how exquisitely radiosensitive pure seminomas are, even when they are very large.

Today, most patients with massive retroperitoneal metastases (Royal Marsden stage IID) are treated initially with chemotherapy. These are patients with nodal metastases larger than 10 cm. The use of chemotherapy has led to a modest improvement in survival for stage IID patients. Babaian and Zagars,[78] for example, reported a 78% disease-free survival rate for patients with stage IID disease after treatment with chemotherapy, compared with 68% for patients treated initially with radiation therapy alone.

One reason for not using radiation therapy as the initial treatment for stage IIB is that it can be difficult to detect a relapse in these patients because a residual fibrotic mass is often present. This can also be a problem after treatment with chemotherapy. A greater concern is that it can be difficult to salvage these patients with chemotherapy because of bone marrow suppression after abdominal irradiation. In a review by Anscher and colleagues,[131] only a fourth of the patients who had a relapse after radiation therapy for extensive intra-abdominal metastases were successfully treated with chemotherapy (see Table 26-3).

Recommended Treatment for Pure Seminoma

The recommended treatment policy for pure seminoma is outlined in Figures 26-9 and 26-10.[75] The primary tumor in the testis should be managed by an inguinal orchiectomy with high ligation of the spermatic cord, and the regional lymphatics should be treated with radiation therapy. If an incisional biopsy or scrotal orchiectomy has been performed, the spermatic cord should be resected before proceeding with treatment of the regional lymphatics. In keeping with the recommendations of the Leeds Consensus Conference,[77] the inguinal

---

TABLE 26-3

Patterns of Relapse After Treatment with Radiation Therapy Alone for Stage IIB Pure Seminoma (Bulky Abdominal Disease)

Study and Reference	Number with Relapse	SITES OF RELAPSE		
		Local Only	Local & Distant	Distant Only
Andrews et al[132]	1/4	0	0	1
Ball et al[133]	9/23	2	4	3
Dosoretz et al[98]	4/7	1	2	1
Epstein et al[93]	1/3	0	0	1
Gregory and Peckham[134]	4/14	1	2	1
Hunter and Peschel[110]	0/3	0	0	0
Kellokumpu-Lehtinen and Halme[135]	0/2	0	0	0
Lederman et al[94]	6/9	2	0	4
Lester et al[92]	1/4	0	0	1
Mason and Kearsley[136]	6/24	0	1	5
Sagerman et al[137]	1/11	0	0	1
Thomas et al[100]	24/26	10	0	14
Willan and McGowan[139]	6/14	0	0	6
Zagars and Babain[78]	4/11	2	0	2
TOTALS	67/175 (38%)	18 (10%)	9 (5%)	40 (23%)

Local failure rate = 15%

Distant metastasis rate = 28%

Modified from Anscher MS, Marks LB, Shipley WU. *Oncology* 1992;6:97-108.

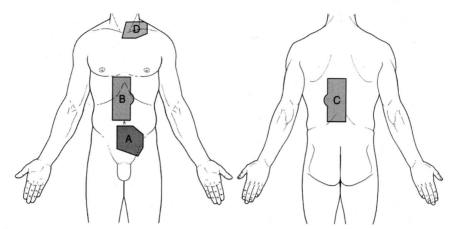

Fig. 26-9   Typical field arrangement for treating a seminoma of the left testis using separate periaortic and iliac fields. (From Hussey DH. Testicular cancer. In: Levitt SH, Kahn FM, Potish RA, et al, eds. *Levitt & Tapley's Technological Basis of Radiation Therapy Clinical Applications.* 3rd ed. Philadelphia, Pa: Lippincott Williams & Wilkins; 1998.)

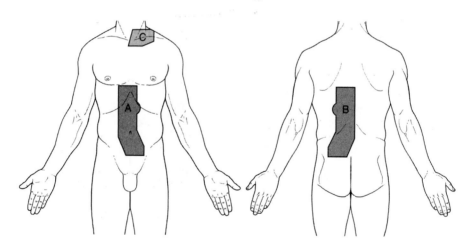

Fig. 26-10   Typical field arrangement for treating a seminoma of the left testis using a hockey-stick–shaped periaortic/iliac field arrangement. (From Hussey DH. Testicular cancer. In: Levitt SH, Kahn FM, Potish RA, et al, eds. *Levitt & Tapley's Technological Basis of Radiation Therapy Clinical Applications.* 3rd ed. Philadelphia, Pa: Lippincott Williams & Wilkins; 1998.)

scar and hemiscrotum do not need to be included in the radiation treatment portals.

Stage I

If the tumor is clinically limited to the testis, the regional lymphatics below the diaphragm should be irradiated electively because 15% to 20% of these patients have occult metastasis in the retroperitoneal lymph nodes. Surveillance after orchiectomy may be used in selected patients, but it is not recommended routinely because patients undergoing surveillance must be followed very closely with CT scans and tumor markers for a long time. The recommended tumor dose is 25 Gy in 15 fractions over 3 weeks. Either periaortic and ipsilateral iliac portals (see Fig. 26-9, *A* to *C*) or periaortic portals only (see Fig. 26-9, *B* and *C*) are appropriate at the present time because the periaortic nodes are the ones that are most likely to be involved. The mediastinum and supraclavicular areas do not need to be irradiated electively in stage I disease because less than 2% of these patients have occult metastasis above the diaphragm.[129]

Stage IIA

In patients with retroperitoneal metastases measuring less than 2 cm in diameter, the periaortic and ipsilateral iliac areas should be treated through portals similar to those used for stage I. A dose of 25 Gy in 15 fractions over 3 weeks is delivered (see Fig. 26-9, A to C), followed by an additional 5 to 10 Gy in two to five fractions through reduced fields directed toward the area initially involved by cancer. Elective irradiation of the mediastinum and supraclavicular area is no longer recommended for stage IIA, because less than 10% of stage IIA patients have occult metastasis in the mediastinal or supraclavicular nodes and most of those who experience relapse in this region can be salvaged with chemotherapy or more irradiation (see Table 26-2).[100,118,130]

Stage IIB-C

In patients with moderate-to-large retroperitoneal metastases (those measuring 2 to 10 cm in diameter), the periaortic and ipsilateral iliac lymph nodes should be irradiated to a basic dose of 25 Gy in 15 fractions over 3 weeks. The fields should then be reduced and the total dose to the initially involved areas taken to 35 to 40 Gy using a shrinking field technique.

Elective irradiation to the left supraclavicular area (see Fig. 26-9, D) is recommended for stage IIB-C disease because approximately 20% of patients with disease at this stage will experience failure in the supraclavicular nodes if this area is not electively treated (see Table 26-2).[97,118,130] The mediastinum is not routinely irradiated because treatment of this area might increase the risk of subsequent coronary artery disease and make it more difficult to deliver effective chemotherapy should the need arise. Supraclavicular irradiation to a dose of 25 Gy given over 3 weeks adds little morbidity, and it should not prolong the treatment because it can be delivered concurrently with the retroperitoneal lymphatic irradiation.

Stage IID

Fifteen years ago, most patients with bulky intra-abdominal disease (stage IID) were treated with radiation therapy. Today, patients with stage IID disease are treated with chemotherapy; radiation therapy is reserved for salvage if chemotherapy fails.

Stage III-IV

Patients with stage III-IV pure seminomas are treated initially with chemotherapy, and radiation therapy is used to eradicate residual disease or to palliate local problems. A significant number of patients with stage III-IV disease can be cured with aggressive treatment.

Treatment Portals

The retroperitoneal lymph nodes can be irradiated through either parallel opposing hockey-stick–shaped portals (see Fig. 26-10) or separate periaortic and iliac fields (see Fig. 26-9). The advantage of using the hockey-stick arrangement is that it avoids a field junction between the periaortic and iliac fields. The advantages of using separate periaortic and iliac fields are that the blocks are smaller and easier to handle, the dose transmitted to the bowel is less, and the periaortic and iliac fields can be weighted differently, which may be appropriate because the iliac nodes are situated anterior to the periaortic nodes.

The periaortic nodes are treated through parallel-opposed, equally weighted anterior and posterior portals, and the tumor dose is assessed at midplane (see Fig. 26-10). The periaortic fields are approximately 10 cm wide and extend from T10 to the L5-S1 junction. The nodes in the renal hila are included, especially on the left where the left spermatic vein joins the left renal vein. The lateral two thirds of the kidney is excluded whenever possible. If separate periaortic and iliac fields are used, the portals are usually matched at the L5-S1 junction. The iliac nodes are usually treated with a single anterior field, and the dose is calculated 3 cm anterior to midplane.

The periaortic and iliac fields are usually treated using 4 to 6 MV x-rays. However, if the patient has a large anteroposterior diameter, 10- to 15-MV x-rays should be employed, and the iliac area should be treated with parallel opposed portals to reduce the risk of subcutaneous fibrosis and other late side effects of irradiation.

The supraclavicular area should also be treated with 4- to 6-MV x-rays. The medial margin of the supraclavicular field should include the sternocleidomastoid muscle with a 1-cm margin, the superior margin should be at the cricoid cartilage, and the inferior margin at the lower edge of the clavicle.

Treatment for Nonseminomatous Testicular Tumors

Radiation therapy played a role in the management of nonseminomatous germ cell tumors of the testis before the development of effective chemotherapy.[55,138] However, it has not been a major part of the treatment of nonseminomas since the early 1980s. Nonseminomatous testicular tumors are not as radiosensitive as pure seminomas, and consequently, 45 Gy or more is required to control them. They also have a greater tendency to spread hematogenously. Therefore nonseminomas are not as easily cured by any form of local–regional treatment.

The recommended treatment policy for nonseminomatous testicular tumors is outlined below. As is true for other testicular tumors, the primary tumor is treated by an inguinal orchiectomy with high ligation of the spermatic cord. Management after this depends on the stage of the disease.

Stage I

Patients with no evidence of metastases are usually treated initially with a retroperitoneal lymphadenectomy. Those who have nodal metastases at surgery or have persistently elevated tumor markers after lymphadenectomy are treated with chemotherapy.

In some institutions, a policy of surveillance is used for selected low-risk patients. At Memorial Sloan-Kettering Cancer Center,[57] patients are considered to be candidates for surveillance if (1) the tumor is confined within the tunica albuginea, (2) no vascular invasion is evident, (3) the tumor marker levels normalize after orchiectomy, (4) radiographic imaging shows no evidence of metastatic disease, and (5) the patient is considered reliable for follow-up. Patients who are being managed by surveillance must be followed closely for at least 3 years. Patients are followed monthly for the first 2 years and bimonthly in the third year. Tumor markers are obtained after each visit, and a chest x-ray and abdominal CT scan is obtained every 3 to 4 months. The majority of relapses of nonseminomatous testicular tumors occur within the first year.

Stage II

Patients with limited stage II disease (nodes smaller than 3 cm) are treated initially with an inguinal orchiectomy and retroperitoneal lymphadenectomy in a manner similar to that described for stage I. However, adjuvant chemotherapy is usually given postoperatively because the rate of recurrence is high when these patients are treated with lymphadenectomy alone.

Patients with moderate-to-bulky retroperitoneal disease (stage IIB-D, nodes larger than 3 cm) are treated with aggressive chemotherapy primarily in a manner similar to those who present with stage III-IV disease. These patients are treated with an orchiectomy followed by primary platinum-based combination chemotherapy. Later resection is required if a residual mass is found on imaging studies. Approximately 20% of these masses will contain residual cancer, usually embryonal carcinoma. In another 40%, the mass will be composed of only teratoma, and in 40%, it will represent only fibrosis. If the tumor marker levels fail to normalize, additional salvage chemotherapy is required.

Stage III-IV

Patients with stage III-IV disease are treated initially with multiagent chemotherapy. Radiation therapy or surgery, or both, may be used if the response to drug therapy is incomplete.

EXTRAGONADAL GERM CELL TUMORS

Approximately 1% of malignant germ cell tumors appear outside the testes.[140] The most common sites are the anterior mediastinum, retroperitoneum, and brain. Less common sites include the prostate, bladder, stomach, and thymus.

Extragonadal germ cell tumors are identical histopathologically to germ cell tumors originating in the testis,[140] and all types of germ cell tumors have been reported in extragonadal sites.[141] They are thought to arise from primordial germ cells that have been displaced during their migration from the yolk sac endoderm to the genital ridge to the testes.[141]

The treatment for an extragonadal germ cell tumor is similar to that used for a testicular tumor of the same histopathologic type. Most patients with extragonadal pure seminomas are treated with radiation therapy alone, with the dose being determined by tumor size.[142] Although Bush and colleagues[143] have suggested that primary mediastinal seminomas require a higher radiation dose than that used for testicular seminomas, few data exist to suggest that extragonadal seminomas are any less radiosensitive than testicular seminomas of a similar size. Nevertheless, multiagent chemotherapy may be indicated if the tumor is massive.[144,145]

For nonseminomatous extragonadal germ cell tumors, chemotherapy similar to that used for nonseminomatous tumors of the testis is recommended. This is usually followed by resection of the residual mass if the tumor mass persists and is technically resectable.

The prognosis for a patient with an extragonadal germ cell tumor is somewhat poorer than it is for a patient with a testicular tumor of the same histopathologic type. For example, disease-free survival rates with radiation therapy for extragonadal seminomas are approximately 65% (range, 40% to 80%).[131] This is probably because many of these tumors are much larger than the typical testicular seminoma. Cure rates in the range of 85% can be expected for patients with small to moderate-size extragonadal seminomas.

The results for nonseminomatous extragonadal germ cell tumors are also poorer than those that can be achieved for testicular cancer of the same histopathologic type. In a review of the literature, Cox[146] found reports of only two patients with embryonal cell carcinomas of the mediastinum who had been cured, and not a single patient with teratocarcinoma or choriocarcinoma of the mediastinum was a long-term survivor. Somewhat higher cure rates have been achieved in recent years with more effective chemotherapy. However, the cure rates for extragonadal tumors are still not as high as those that can be achieved with chemotherapy for nonseminomatous tumors of the testis.[141,145,147]

TUMORS OF THE GONADAL STROMA

A variety of gonadal stromal tumors are found in the testes. These include Leydig cell tumors, Sertoli cell tumors, undifferentiated tumors, and combinations of these histopathologic types. Gonadoblastomas contain a mixture of germ cell and gonadal stromal cell elements. All stromal cell tumors of the testis are quite rare.[73,148]

Leydig cell tumors can occur at any age, but they are most common in men 30 to 50 years of age. The presenting symptoms in children include macrogenitosomia, hirsutism, early musculoskeletal development, and sexual precocity. Adults may have excessive genital development, gynecomastia, or other signs of feminization. Patients with Leydig cell tumors typically have elevated 17-ketosteroid levels in the urine and blood. Estrogen or other steroidal products may also be elevated.

Sertoli cell tumors are very rare neoplasms. About a third of patients with these tumors have gynecomastia, and some of them experience decreased libido. Patients with Sertoli cell tumors may have elevated levels of androgens, estrogens, and pregnanediol in the urine. However, the 17-ketosteroid levels are normal.

Gonadoblastomas occur in patients with an underlying gonadal disorder and abnormal secondary sex characteristics. The typical picture histologically is a mixture of proliferating seminoma-like germ cells, Sertoli cells, granulosal cells, and Leydig cells.

The standard treatment for patients with any of these gonadal stromal tumors is radical orchiectomy. Only about 10% of these tumors are malignant. The most common sites of metastasis from malignant stromal cell tumors are the lymph nodes, liver, and bone. Radiation therapy does not usually play a role in their management.

MALIGNANT LYMPHOMAS

Testicular lymphomas usually occur in older men. They are said to be the most common testicular tumor in men older than 50 years.[58] They account for between 1% and 7% of testicular tumors in various series.[149] Testicular lymphomas are usually diffuse large cell lymphomas, but other varieties of lymphomas can be seen in the testes.[150]

Lymphomas of the testis are usually a manifestation of metastatic disease. However, it is fairly common for one to be the only evidence of disease at the time of presentation. Painless testicular enlargement is the most common presenting symptom. However, patients may have nodal or extranodal disease elsewhere in the body or generalized symptoms such as anorexia, weakness, or weight loss.

A patient diagnosed as having a lymphoma should be carefully evaluated for systemic disease. Special studies that are indicated, besides those usually obtained to evaluate a patient with a testicular malignancy, include a bone marrow biopsy, CT scanning of the head and neck in addition to the chest, abdomen, and pelvis, and lumbar puncture for cytologic examination of the cerebrospinal fluid.[151]

If the disease is confined to the testis, a radical orchiectomy should be performed, and patients should be treated with doxorubicin-based combination chemotherapy, supplemented with intrathecal chemotherapy. The contralateral testis is considered an isolated structure in that it is unlikely to receive the full effect of combination chemotherapy. Thus after combination systemic chemotherapy and intrathecal drug injections, irradiation of the scrotum is recommended. A total dose of 30 Gy, given in 15 to 17 fractions, is considered sufficient to eliminate subclinical lymphoma.

Most patients with testicular lymphoma have systemic disease, even those who have no clinical evidence of tumor elsewhere, and thus the prognosis has been poor. Preliminary results of the treatment policies outlined above suggest an improvement in outcome for what has heretofore been a highly lethal form of testicular cancer.

REFERENCES

1. Fajardo LF, Berthrong M, Anderson RE. Testis. In: *Radiation Pathology*. New York, NY: Oxford University Press; 2001:312-318.
1a. Russell LD, Ettlin RA, Hikim APS, et al. *Histological and Histopathological Evaluation of the Testis*. Clearwater, Fla: Cache River Press; 1990.
2. Meistrich ML. Relationship between spermatogonial stem cell survival and testis function after cytotoxic therapy. *Br J Cancer* 1986;53:89-101.
3. Meistrich ML, Hunter N, Suzuki N, et al. Gradual regeneration of mouse testicular stem cells after ionizing radiation. *Radiat Res* 1978;74:349-362.
4. Clermont Y. Renewal of spermatogonia in man. *Am J Anat* 1996;118:509-524.
5. Meistrich ML, van Beek MEAB. Spermatogonial stem cells. In: *Cell and Molecular Biology of the Testis*. New York, NY: Oxford University Press; 1993.
6. Huckins C. The spermatogonial stem cell population in adult rats. I. Their morphology, proliferation and maturation. *Anat Rec* 1971;169:533-558.
7. Heller CG, Clermont Y. Kinetics of the germinal epithelium in man. *Rec Prog Horm Res* 1964;20:545-575.
8. da Cunha MF, Meistrich ML, Haq MM, et al. Temporary effects of AMSA [4'(9-acridinylamino) methanesulfon-m-anisidide] chemotherapy on spermatogenesis. *Cancer* 1982;49:2459-2462.
9. Oakberg EF. Sensitivity and time of degeneration of spermatogenic cells irradiated in various stages of maturation in the mouse. *Radiat Res* 1955;2:369-391.
10. Rowley MJ, Leach DR, Warner GA, et al. Effect of graded doses of ionizing radiation on the human testis. *Radiat Res* 1974;59:665-678.
11. Oakberg EF. Gamma-ray sensitivity of spermatogonia of the mouse. *J Exp Zool* 1957;134:343-356.
12. Withers HR, Hunter N, Barkley HT, et al. Radiation survival and regeneration characteristics of spermatogenic stem cell of mouse testis. *Radiat Res* 1974;57:88-103.

13. Oakberg EF. Degeneration of spermatogonia of the mouse following exposure to x-rays, and stages in the mitotic cycle at which cell death occurs. *J Morphol* 1955;97:39-54.

14. Hasegawa M, Wilson G, Russell LD, et al. Radiation-induced cell death in the mouse testis: relationship to apoptosis. *Radiat Res* 1997;147:457-467.

15. Edwards RG, Sirlin JL. The effect of 200 R of x-rays on the rate of spermatogenesis and spermiogenesis in the mouse. *Exp Cell Res* 1958;15:522-528.

16. Meistrich ML, Samuels RC. Reduction in sperm levels after testicular irradiation of the mouse. A comparison with man. *Radiat Res* 1985;102:138-147.

17. Lushbaugh CC, Casarett GW. The effects of gonadal irradiation in clinical radiation therapy: a review. *Cancer* 1976;37:1111-1120.

18. Clifton DK, Bremner WJ. The effect of testicular x-irradiation on spermatogenesis in man. A comparison with the mouse. *J Androl* 1983;4:387-392.

19. Dubey P, Wilson G, Mathur KK, et al. Recovery of sperm production following radiation therapy for Hodgkin's disease after induction chemotherapy with mitoxantrone, vincristine, vinblastine and prednisone (NOVP). *Int J Radiat Oncol Biol Phys* 2000;46: 609-617.

20. Meistrich ML, Van Beek MEAB. Radiation sensitivity of the human testis. In: *Advances in Radiation Biology*. Vol 14. New York, NY: Academic Press; 1990.

21. van Beek MEAB, Meistrich ML, de Rooij DG. Probability of self-renewing divisions of spermatogonial stem cells in colonies formed after fission neutron irradiation. *Cell Tissue Kinet* 1990; 23:1-16.

22. Kangasniemi M, Huhtaniemi I, Meistrich ML. Failure of spermatogenesis to recover despite the presence of A spermatogonia in the irradiated $LBNF_1$ rat. *Biol Reprod* 1996;54:1200-1208.

23. Meistrich ML, Kangasniemi M. Hormone treatment after irradiation stimulates recovery of rat spermatogenesis from surviving spermatogonia. *J Androl* 1997;18:80-87.

24. Hansen PV, Trykker H, Svennakjaer IL, et al. Long-term recovery of spermatogenesis after radiotherapy in patients with testicular cancer. *Radiother Oncol* 1990;18:117-125.

25. Meistrich ML, Wilson G, Brown BW, et al. Impact of cyclophosphamide on long-term reduction in sperm count in men treated with combination chemotherapy for Ewing's and soft tissue sarcomas. *Cancer* 1992;70:2703-2712.

26. Meistrich ML, Brown CC. Estimation of the increased risk of human infertility from alterations in semen characteristics. *Fertil Steril* 1983;40:220-230.

27. da Cunha MF, Meistrich ML, Ried HL, et al. Active sperm production after cancer chemotherapy with doxorubicin. *J Urol* 1983; 130:927-930.

28. Regaud C. Influence de la duree d'irradiation sur les effects determines dans le testicule par le radium. *C R Seances Soc Biol Fil* 1922;86:787-790.

29. Ferroux R, Regaud C, Samssonaw N. Effets des rayons de roentgen administres sans fractionement de la dose sur les testicules du rat au point de vue de la sterilisation de l'epithelium seminal. *C R Seances Soc Biol Fil* 128:170-173, 1938.

30. Meistrich ML, Finch M, Lu CC, et al. Strain differences in the response of mouse testicular stem cells to fractionated radiation. *Radiat Res* 1984;97:478-487.

31. Ash P. The influence of radiation on fertility in man. *Br J Radiol* 1980;53:271-278.

32. Hahn EW, Feingold SM, Simpson L, et al. Recovery from aspermia induced by low-dose radiation in seminoma patients. *Cancer* 1982;50:337-340.

33. Sanders JE, Hawley J, Levy W, et al. Pregnancies following high-dose cyclophosphamide with or without high-dose busulfan or total-body irradiation and bone marrow transplantation. *Blood* 1996;87:3045-3052.

34. Jacob A, Barker H, Goodman A, et al. Recovery of spermatogenesis following bone marrow transplantation. *Bone Marrow Transplant* 1998;22:277-279.

35. van der Meer Y, Huiskamp R, Davids JAG, et al. The sensitivity of quiescent and proliferating mouse spermatogonial stem cells to x-irradiation. *Radiat Res* 1992;130:289-295.

36. Jacobsen KD, Olsen DR, Fossa K, et al. External beam abdominal radiotherapy in patients with seminoma stage I: field type, testicular dose, and spermatogenesis. *Int J Radiat Oncol Biol Phys* 1997; 38:95-102.

37. Speiser B, Rubin P, Casarett G, Aspermia following lower truncal irradiation in Hodgkin's disease. *Cancer* 1973;32:692-698.

38. Million RR. The lymphomatous diseases. In Fletcher GH, ed. *Textbook of Radiotherapy*, 3rd ed. Philadelphia, Pa: Lea & Febiger; 1980.

39. Harter DJ, Hussey DH, Delclos L, et al. Device to position the testicle during irradiation. *Int J Radiat Oncol Biol Phys* 1976;1: 361-364.

40. Neel JV, Schull WJ, Awa AA, et al. The children of parents exposed to atomic bombs: estimates of the genetic doubling dose of radiation for humans. *Am J Hum Genet* 1990;46:1053-1072.

41. Joshi DS, Yick J, Murray D, et al. Stage-dependent variation in the radiosensitivity of DNA in developing male germ cells. *Radiat Res* 1990;121:274-281.

42. Delic JI, Hendry JH, Morris ID, et al. Dose and time relationships in the endocrine response of the irradiated adult rat testis. *J Androl* 1986;7:32-41.

43. Guitton N, Brouazin-Jousseaume V, Dupaix A, et al. Radiation effect on rat Sertoli cell function in vitro and in vivo. *Int J Radiat Biol* 1999;75:327-333.

44. Shapiro E, Kinsella TJ, Makuch RW, et al. Effects of fractionated irradiation on endocrine aspects of testicular function. *J Clin Oncol* 1985;3:1232-1239.

45. Wang J, Galil KAA, Setchell BP. Changes in testicular blood flow and testosterone production during aspermatogenesis after irradiation. *J Endocrinol* 1983;98:35-46.

46. Nader S, Schultz PN, Cundiff JH, et al. Endocrine profiles of patients with testicular tumors treated with radiotherapy. *Int J Radiat Oncol Biol Phys* 1983;9:1723-1726.

47. Shalet SM. Effect of irradiation treatment on gonadal function in men treated for germ cell cancer. *Eur Urol* 1993;23:148-151.

48. Delic JI, Hendry JH, Morris ID, et al. Leydig cell function in the pubertal rat following local testicular irradiation. *Radiother Oncol* 1986;5:29-37.

49. Brauner R, Czernichow P, Cramer P, et al. Leydig-cell function in children after direct testicular irradiation for acute lymphoblastic leukemia. *N Engl J Med* 1983;309:25-28.

50. Shalet SM, Tsatsoulis A, Whitehead E, et al. Vulnerability of the human Leydig cell to radiation damage is dependent upon age. *J Endocrinol* 1989;120:161-165.

51. National Cancer Institute. *SEER Cancer Statistics Review, 1973-1996 Tables and Graphs*. Bethesda, Md: NIH Publication No 99-2789; 1999. Available at http://seer.cancer.gov/csr/1973_1999/index.html. Accessed Nov. 11, 2002.

52. Schottenfeld D, Warschauer ME. The epidemiology of testicular cancer in young adults. *Am J Epidemiol* 1980;112: 232-246.

53. Ekbom A, Akre O. Increasing incidence of testicular cancer—birth cohort effects. *APMIS* 1998;106:225-229.

54. Batata MA, Whitmore WF Jr, Chu FC, et al. Cryptorchidism and testicular cancer. *J Urol* 1980;124:382-387.

55. Peckham MJ, McElwain TJ, Hendry WF. Testis and epidydimis. In: Halnan KE, ed. *Treatment of Cancer*, New York, NY: Igaku-Shoin Medical Publishers; 1982.

56. Peckham MJ. Testicular cancer. *Review Oncology* 1988;1:439.

57. Presti JC, Herr HW. Genital tumors. In: Tanagho MOA, McAninch W, eds. *Smith's General Urology*, 13th ed. Norwalk, Conn/San Mateo, Calif: Appleton and Lange; 1992.

58. Mostofi FK, Price EB. *Tumors of the Male Genital System.* Washington, DC: Armed Forces Institute of Pathology; 1973.

59. Skakkebaek NE. Carcinoma in situ of the testis: frequency and relationship of invasive germ cell tumors in infertile men. *Histopathology* 1972;2:157.

60. Sokal M, Peckham MJ, Hendry WF. Bilateral germ cell tumours of the testis. *Br J Urol* 1979;52:158-162.

61. Dieckmann K-P, Loy V. Management of contralateral testicular intraepithelial neoplasia in patients with testicular germ-cell tumor. *World J Urol* 1994;12:131-135.

62. von der Maase H, Giwercman A, Muller J, et al. Management of carcinoma in situ of the testis. *Int J Androl* 1987;10:209-220.

63. Willis RA. *Pathology of Tumors.* New York, NY: Appleton-Century-Crofts; 1967.

64. Friedman NB, Moore RA. Tumors of the testes. *Milit Surg* 1946;99:573-593.

65. Dixon FJ, Moore RA. *Tumors of the Male Sex Organs.* Washington, DC: Armed Forces Institute of Pathology; 1952.

66. Mostofi FK. Testicular tumors: epidemiologic, etiologic, and pathologic factors. *Cancer* 1973;32:1186-1201.

67. Melicow MM. New British classification of testicular tumors: a correlation, analysis and critique. *J Urol* 1965;94:64.

68. Stevens LC. Origin of testicular teratomas from primordial germ cells in mice. *J Natl Cancer Inst* 1967;38:549-552.

69. Johnson DE, Gomez JJ, Ayala AG. Anaplastic seminoma. *J Urol* 1975;114:80-82.

70. Babaian RJ, Zagars GK. Testicular seminoma: the M.D. Anderson experience. An analyis of pathological and patient characteristics, and treatment recommendations. *J Urol* 1988;139:311-314.

71. Sandeman TF, Matthews JP. The staging of testicular tumors. *Cancer* 1979;43:2514-2524.

72. Weiss L, Gilbert HA, Ballon SC, eds. *Lymphatic System Metastasis.* Vol III, Boston, Mass: GK Hall; 1980.

73. Ray B, Hajdu S, Whitmore W. Distribution of retroperitoneal lymph node metastases in testicular germinal tumors. *Cancer* 1974;33:340-348.

74. Boden G, Gibb R. Radiotherapy and testicular neoplasms. *Lancet* 1951;2:1195.

75. Hussey DH. Testicular cancer. In: Levitt SH, Khan FM, Potish RA, et al, eds. *Levitt & Tapley's Technological Basis of Radiation Therapy, Practical Clinical Applications,* 3rd ed. Philadelphia, Pa: Lippincott Williams & Wilkins; 1998.

76. Fleming I, Cooper JS, Henson DE, et al, eds. *AJCC Cancer Staging Manual,* 5th ed. Philadelphia: Lippincott Williams & Wilkins; 1997:225-230.

77. Thomas GM. Consensus statement on the investigation and management of testicular seminoma. EORTC Genito-Urinary Group, Monograph 7. In: Newling DW, Jones WG, eds. *Prostate Cancer and Testicular Cancer.* New York, NY: Wiley-Liss; 1990.

78. Zagars GK, Babain RJ. The role of radiation in stage II testicular seminoma. *Int J Radiat Oncol Biol Phys* 1987;13:163-170.

79. Jing BS, Wallace S, Zornoza J. Metastases to retroperitoneal and pelvic lymph nodes: computed tomography and lymphangiography. *Radiol Clin North Am* 1981;20:511-530.

80. Maier JG, Schamber DT. The role of lymphangiography in the diagnosis and treatment of malignant testicular tumors. *Am J Roentgenol Rad Ther Nucl Med* 1972;114:482-491.

81. Heiken JP, Balfe DM, McClennan BL. Testicular tumors. In: Bragg DG, Rubin P, Youker JE, eds. *Oncologic Imaging,* New York, NY: Pergamon Press; 1985.

82. Cox JD. The testicle. In: Moss WT, Cox JD, eds. *Radiation Oncology Rationale, Technique, Results,* 6th ed. St. Louis, Mo: Mosby; 1989.

83. White RL, Maier JG. Testis tumors. In: Perez CA, Brady LW, eds. *Principles and Practice of Radiation Oncology.* Philadephia, Pa: JB Lippincott; 1987.

84. Marks LB, Anscher MS, Shipley WU. Radiation therapy for testicular seminoma: controversies in the management of early-stage disease. *Oncology* 1992;6:43-48.

85. Zagars GK. Management of stage I seminoma: radiotherapy. In: Horwich A, ed. *Testicular Cancer: Investigation and Management.* Baltimore, Md: Williams & Wilkins; 1991.

86. Scardino PT, Cox HD, Waldmann TA, et al. The value of serum tumor markers in the staging and prognosis of germ cell tumors of the testis. *J Urol* 1977;118:994-999.

87. Javadpour N. The role of biologic markers in testicular cancer. *Cancer* 1980;45:1755-1761.

88. Lange PH, Nochomovitz LE, Rosai J, et al. Serum alpha-fetoprotein and human chorionic gonadotrophin in patients with seminoma. *J Urol* 1980;124:472-478.

89. Weissbach L, Bussar-Maatz R, Mann K. The value of tumor markers in testicular seminomas. Results of a prospective multicenter study. *Eur Urol* 1997;32:16-22.

90. Batterman JJ, et al. Testicular tumors, a retrospective study. *Arch Chir Neelandicurn* 1973;XXV-IV:457.

91. Saxena V. Seminoma of the testis. *Am J Roentgenol* 1973;117:643.

92. Lester SG, Morphis JG II, Hornback NB. Testicular seminoma: Analysis of treatment results and failures. *Int J Radiat Oncol Biol Phys* 1986;12:353-358.

93. Epstein BE, Order SE, Zinreich ES. Staging, treatment and results in testicular seminoma: a 12-year report. *Cancer* 1990;65:405-411.

94. Lederman GS, Herman TS, Jochelson M, et al. Radiation therapy of seminoma: 17 years experience at the Joint Center for Radiation Therapy. *Radiat Oncol* 1989;14:203-208.

95. Giacchetti S, Raoul Y, Wibault P, et al. Treatment of stage I testis seminoma by radiotherapy: long-term results—a 30 year experience. *Int J Radiat Oncol Biol Phys* 1993;27:3-9.

96. Bauman GS, Venkatesan UM, Ago CT, et al. Postoperative radiotherapy for stage I/II seminoma: results for 212 patients. *Int J Radiat Oncol Biol Phys* 1998;42:313-317.

97. Dosmann MA, Zagars GK. Postorchiectomy radiotherapy for stages I and II testicular cancer. *Int J Radiat Oncol Biol Phys* 1993;26:381-390.

98. Dosoretz DE, Shipley WU, Blitzer P, et al. Megavoltage irradiation for pure testicular seminoma. *Cancer* 1981;48:2184-2190.

99. Fossa SD, Aass N, Kaalhus O. Radiotherapy for testicular seminoma stage I: treatment results and long-term post-irradiation morbidity in 365 patients. *Int J Radiat Oncol Biol Phys* 1989;16:383-388.

100. Thomas GM, Rider WD, Dembo AJ. Seminoma of the testis: results of treatment and patterns of failure after radiation therapy. *Int J Radiat Oncol Biol Phys* 1982;8:165-174.

101. Van der Werf-Messing B. Radiotherapeutic treatment of testicular tumors. *Int J Radiat Oncol Biol Phys* 1976;1:235-248.

102. Earle JD, Bagshaw MA, Kaplan HS. Supervoltage radiation therapy of the testicular tumors. *AJR Am J Roentgenol* 1973;117:653-661.

103. van Rooy EM, Sagerman RH. Long-term evaluation of postorchiectomy irradiation for stage I seminomas. *Radiology* 1994;191:852-861.

104. Whipple GL, Sagarman RH, van Rooy EM. Long-term evaluation of postorchiectomy radiotherapy for stage II seminoma. *Am J Clin Oncol* 1997;20:196-201.

105. Kurohara SS, George FW, Dykhuisen RF, et al. Testicular tumors: analysis of 196 cases treated at the U.S. Naval Hospital in San Diego. *Cancer* 1967;20:1089-1098.

106. Kademian MT, Bosch A, Caldwell WL. Seminoma: results of treatment with megavoltage irradiation. *Int J Radiat Oncol Biol Phys* 1976;1:1075-1079.

107. Maier JG, Van Buskirk K. Treatment of testicular germ cell malignancies. *JAMA* 1970;213:97-98.

108. Lai PP, Bernstein MJ, Kim H, et al. Radiation therapy for stage I and IIA testicular seminoma. *Int J Radiat Oncol Biol Phys* 1993;28:373-379.

109. Vallis KA, Howard GCW, Duncan W, et al. Radiotherapy for stages I and II testicular seminoma: results and morbidity in 238 patients. *Br J Radiol* 1995;68:400-405.

110. Hunter M, Peschel RE. Testicular seminoma: results of the Yale University experience, 1964-1984. *Cancer* 1989;64:1608-1611.

111. Zagars GK, Babaian RJ. Stage I testicular seminoma: rationale for postorchiectomy radiation therapy. *Int J Radiat Oncol Biol Phys* 1987;13:155-162.

112. Horwich A, Alsanjari N, A'Hern R, et al. Surveillance following orchidectomy for stage I testicular seminoma. *Br J Cancer* 1992;65:775-778.

113. von der Maase H, Specht L, Jacobsen GK. Surveillance following orchidectomy for stage I seminoma of the testis. *Eur J Cancer* 1993;29:1931-1934.

114. Warde P, Gospodarowicz MK, Panzarella T. Stage I testicular seminoma: results of adjuvant irradiation and surveillance. *J Clin Oncol* 1995;13:2255-2262.

115. Warde PR, Gospodarowicz MK, Goodman PJ. Results of a policy of surveillance in stage I testicular seminoma. *Int J Radiat Oncol Biol Phys* 1993;27:11-15.

116. Duchesne GM, Horwich A, Dearnaley DP, et al. Orchiectomy alone for stage I seminoma of the testis. *Cancer* 1990;65:1115-1118.

117. Whitmore WF. The Marks et al article review. *Oncology* 1992;6:51-52.

118. Thomas GM. Controversies in the management of testicular seminoma. *Cancer* 1985;55:2296-2302.

119. Hanks GE, Peters T, Owen J. Seminoma of the testis: long term beneficial and deleterious results of radiation. *Int J Radiat Oncol Biol Phys* 1992;24:913-919.

120. Read G, Johnston RJ. Short duration radiotherapy in stage I pure seminoma of the testis: preliminary results of a prospective study. *Clin Oncol* 1993;5:364-366.

121. Willich N, Wendt T, Rohlaff R. Radiotherapy of seminoma: small volume irradiation at the stage pT1N0M0—prophylactic irradiation of the mediastinum. *Strahlenther Oncol* 1986;162:735-741.

122. Hay JH, Duncan W, Kerr GR. Subsequent malignancies in patients irradiated for testicular tumours. *Br J Radiol* 1984;57:597-602.

123. Moller H, Mellemgaard A, Jacobsen GK, et al. Incidence of second primary cancer following testicular cancer. *Eur J Cancer* 1993;29A:672-676.

124. Stein ME, Kessel I, Luberan N, et al. Testicular seminoma stage I: treatment results and long-term follow-up (1968-1988). *J Surg Oncol* 1993;53:175-179.

125. van Leeuwen FE, Stiggelbout AM, van den Belt-Dusebout AW. Second cancer risk following testicular cancer: a follow-up study of 1,909 patients. *J Clin Oncol* 1993;11:415-424.

126. Kleinerman RA, Liebermann JV, Li FP. Second cancer following cancer of the male genital system in Connecticut, 1935-82. *Natl Cancer Inst Monogr* 1985;68:139-147.

127. Kiricuta IC, Sauer J, Bohndorf W. Omission of the pelvic irradiation in stage I testicular seminoma: a study of postorchiectomy paraaortic radiotherapy. *Int J Radiat Oncol Biol Phys* 1996;35:293-301.

128. Sedlmayer F, Joos H, Deutschmann H, et al. Long-term tumor control and fertility after para-aortic limited radiotherapy of stage I seminoma. *Strahlenther Onkol* 1999;175:320-324.

129. Herman JG, Sturgeon J, Thomas GM. Mediastinal prophylactic irradiation in seminoma [abstract]. *Proc Am Soc Clin Oncol* 1983;2:133.

130. Speer TW, Sombeck MD, Parsons JT, et al. Testicular seminoma: a failure analysis and literature review. *Int J Radiat Oncol Biol Phys* 1995;33:89-97.

131. Anscher MS, Marks LB, Shipley WU. The role of radiotherapy in patients with advanced seminomatous germ cell tumors. Controversies in management. *Oncology* 1992;6:97-104.

132. Andrews CF, Micaily B, Brady LW. Testicular seminoma: results of a program of megavoltage irradiation. *Am J Clin Oncol* 1987;10:491-495.

133. Ball D, Barrett A, Peckham MJ. The management of metastatic seminoma testis. *Cancer* 1982;50:2289-2294.

134. Gregory C, Peckham MJ. Results of radiotherapy for stage II testicular seminoma. *Radiat Oncol* 1986;6:285-292.

135. Kellokumpu-Lehtinen P, Halme A. Results of treatment in irradiated testicular seminoma patients. *Radiat Oncol* 1990;18:1-8.

136. Mason BR, Kearsley JH. Radiotherapy for stage II testicular seminoma: the prognostic influence of tumor bulk. *J Clin Oncol* 1988;6:1856-1862.

137. Sagerman RH, Kotlove DJ, Regine WIF, et al. Stage II seminoma: results of postorchiectomy irradiation. *Radiology* 1989;172:565-568.

138. Hussey DH, Luk JH, Johnson DE. The role of radiation therapy in the treatment of germinal cell tumors of the testis other than pure seminoma. *Radiology* 1977;123:175-180.

139. Willan BD, McGowan DG. Seminoma of the testis: a 22-year experience with radiation therapy. *Int J Radiat Oncol Biol Phys* 1985;11:1769-1775.

140. Luna MA. Extragonadal germ cell tumors. In: Johnson DE, ed. *Testicular Tumors*. 2nd ed. Flushing, NY: Medical Examination Publishing; 1976.

141. Raghavan D, Boyer MJ. Malignant extragonadal germ cell tumors in adults. In: Horwich A, ed. *Testicular Cancer: Investigation and Management*. Baltimore, Md: Williams & Wilkins; 1991.

142. Buskirk SJ, Evan RG, Farrow GM, et al. Primary retroperitoneal seminoma. *Cancer* 1983;49:1934-1936.

143. Bush SE, Martinez A, Bagshaw MA. Primary mediastinal seminoma. *Cancer* 1981;48:1877-1882.

144. Jain KK, Bosl GJ, Bains MS, et al. The treatment of extragonadal seminoma. *J Clin Oncol* 1984;2:820-827.

145. Logothetis CJ, Samuels ML, Selig DE, et al. Chemotherapy of extragonadal germ cell tumors. *J Clin Oncol* 1985;3:316-315.

146. Cox JD. Primary malignant germinal tumors of the mediastinum: a study of twenty-four cases. *Cancer* 1975;36:1162-1168.

147. Dueland S, Stenwig AE, Heilo A, et al. Treatment and outcome of patients with extragonadal germ cell tumors—the Norwegian Radium Hospital's experience 1979-94. *Br J Cancer* 1998;77:329-335.

148. Donohue JP. Metastatic pathways of nonseminomatous germ cell tumors. *Semin Urol* 1984;11:217-219.

149. Johnson DE, Butler JJ. Malignant lymphoma of the testis. In: Johnson DE, ed. *Testicular Tumors*. 2nd ed. Flushing, NY: Medical Examination Publishing; 1976.

150. Turner RR, Colby TV, MacKintosh FR. Testicular lymphomas: a clinical pathologic study of 35 cases. *Cancer* 1981;48:2095-2102.

151. Touroutoglou N, Dimopoulos MA, Younes A, et al. Testicular lymphoma: late relapses and poor outcome despite doxorubicin-based therapy. *J Clin Oncol* 1995;13:1361-1367.

CHAPTER 27

The Prostate

Alan Pollack

ANATOMY

The prostate is a glandular structure that is bounded superiorly by the bladder, inferiorly by the urogenital diaphragm, anteriorly by the pubic symphysis, and posteriorly by the rectum (Fig. 27-1). Typically the size of a walnut in younger men, the prostate enlarges progressively over time in men over 40 years old. The prostate is somewhat triangular, with the apex inferior at the urogenital diaphragm and the base superior at the urinary bladder neck.

Anatomically, the prostate is divided into the peripheral zone, transition zone, central zone, and anterior fibromuscular stroma (Fig. 27-2).[1,2] The peripheral zone constitutes 70% of the prostate gland and is readily palpated through the rectal wall. The ejaculatory ducts course through the central zone to the verumontanum at the prostatic urethra. The central zone contains 20% to 25% of the prostate glandular tissue. The transition zone consists of two lateral opposing glandular regions around the urethra that tend to enlarge with age because of benign prostatic hypertrophy, causing urinary outlet obstruction. The transition zone normally makes up 5% to 10% of the prostate glandular tissue. The anterior fibromuscular stroma contains very little glandular tissue. The neurovascular bundles that control erectile function[3] are located posterolaterally to the prostate.

Approximately 75% of prostate malignancies originate in the peripheral zone, 20% in the transition zone, and 5% in the central zone. The major routes of disease spread are direct extension, lymphatic drainage, and hematogenous spread. The prostate is encompassed by a capsule except inferiorly at the apex, where it is continuous with the superior fascia of the urogenital diaphragm. Penetration of cancer through the capsule is a prognostic factor and is incorporated into the staging system (category T3). Direct extension to the anterior rectal wall is rare because Denonvilliers' fascia acts as a protective barrier. Lymphatic drainage is primarily to the periprostatic (obturator) and internal and external iliac lymph nodes and, to a lesser degree, the presacral lymph nodes. Hematogenous spread commonly appears first in the axial skeleton (vertebral bodies and ribs). Batson's plexus may have a role in hematogenous spread.

RADIATION EFFECTS ON THE PROSTATE AND SURROUNDING NORMAL TISSUES

The prostate is relatively resistant to radiation. Pelvic irradiation of the prostate in the absence of prostate cancer to doses of 45 to 65 Gy causes a reduction in serum prostate-specific antigen (PSA) to a median level of 0.5 ng/ml.[4,5] Pathologic response to irradiation includes atrophy of glandular tissue, fibrosis, and typical radiation-induced vascular changes.[6-9] Significant prostate shrinkage in response to high-dose radiation is seen in roughly 50% of patients. The prostate also may become firmer because of fibrosis. These changes are

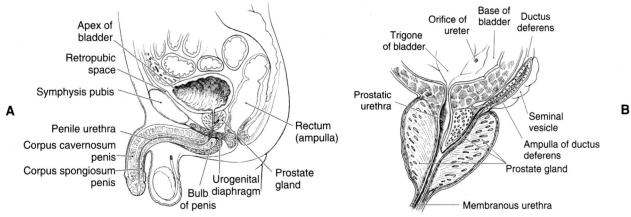

Fig. 27-1 Sagittal section through the pelvis. **A,** The relationship of the prostate to the surrounding pelvic structures. **B,** An enlargement at the region of the prostate and bladder neck.

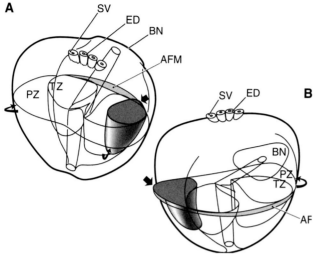

Fig. 27-2 Transparent three-dimensional images of prostate showing the two zones of cancer origin. A representative cancer in each zone is related to a transverse section through the midprostate (*curved arrows*). **A,** Transition zone cancer on left is viewed from the rectal surface and base. Cancer conforms to Z boundary but invades anteriorly into anterior fibromuscular stroma (*arrow*). **B,** Nontransition zone cancer on right is viewed from anterior surface. Cancer conforms to TZ boundary but invades posterolaterally through the capsule (*arrow*) in the region where nerve penetration of capsule is common. *TZ*, Transition zone; *PZ*, peripheral zone; *AFM*, anterior fibromuscular stroma; *BN*, bladder neck; *ED*, ejaculatory duct; *SV*, seminal vesicle. (Redrawn from McNeal JE, Villers AA, Redwine EA, et al. *Am J Surg Pathol* 1990;14:240-247.)

usually not accompanied by significant alteration in urinary function over the long term, although improvement or worsening (possibly requiring a transurethral resection of the prostate [TURP]) may occur. Stricture of the urethra is uncommon and appears mostly in patients who have undergone TURP before radiation therapy.[10,11]

Side effects from high-dose radiation therapy for prostate cancer are primarily related to the bladder and rectum, although the dose to the femoral heads also should be considered in treatment planning. Acute bladder side effects during treatment and for 1 to 6 months afterwards include increased nocturia, urinary frequency, dysuria, hematuria, urgency, bladder spasm, and urinary incontinence. Acute rectal side effects include increased bowel movement frequency, pain on defecation, hematochezia, spasm, and fecal incontinence. Ejaculation during the latter half of radiation therapy is painful. Symptoms lessen considerably by 1 month after external-beam radiation therapy, but chronic symptoms may persist. Urinary symptoms persist for longer periods after brachytherapy, sometimes for more than a year. Acute and late morbidity is traditionally graded on a scale from 0 to 5 using Radiation Therapy Oncology Group criteria[12] or modifications thereof[13,14] (Table 27-1).

Late complications are usually mild to moderate, along the same lines as acute symptoms. Hemorrhagic cystitis or pronounced rectal bleeding from telangiectatic vessels may require coagulation therapy for control. Severe complications such as ulceration and fistula, leading to urinary diversion or colostomy, occur in less than 1 in 1000 cases. The risk of impotence over the long term is about 50%.[15-17] Estimates of normal-tissue complication probabilities have improved considerably as a result of dose-volume histogram (DVH)–based correlates of these complications. These relationships are summarized later in this chapter.

EPIDEMIOLOGY OF PROSTATE CANCER

Except for skin cancer, prostate cancer is the most common malignancy among men in the United States. An estimated 198,100 men will be diagnosed with prostate cancer in 2001, with an estimated 31,500 deaths.[18] Prostate cancer is second to lung cancer as a cause of cancer-related death among men in the United States. African-American men have the highest mortality from prostate cancer worldwide. New developments in screening for prostate cancer such as the use of serum PSA measurements, the free/total PSA ratio, and prostate biopsy guided by transrectal ultrasonography (TRUS) have caused a shift to earlier detection.[19-23]

The introduction of these improvements produced a surge in the number of cases of prostate cancer diagnosed between 1983 and 1991.[24,25] During this period, cases were diagnosed earlier (at lower disease stages), the age at diagnosis dropped, and the use of radical prostatectomy increased dramatically. As a consequence, a unique problem faces physicians treating this disease: the determination of which tumors are clinically relevant and should be treated, as opposed to simply observing those tumors that may be latent. Autopsy studies performed in the pre-PSA era documented that at least 40% of men in their 70s, and higher percentages of men in their 80s, have occult, latent prostate cancer that may not require treatment.[26-29] In more recent series, Sakr and colleagues[30,31] found that more than one third of men in their fifth decade of life harbor malignant cells in their prostates. These astonishing statistics suggest that some cases that are diagnosed by means of aggressive staging may not require treatment.

ETIOLOGY

Numerous theories have been proposed concerning the etiology of prostate cancer, and progress has been made in identifying possible genetic factors. Familial clustering has been documented by several investigators.[32-34] Inherited risk has been linked to loci on the X chromosome[35] and on chromosome 1.[36] Mutations in *BRCA1*

TABLE 27-1

Acute and Delayed Radiation Toxicity Grading Scales

	Grade 1	Grade 2	Grade 3	Grade 4
ACUTE TOXICITY*				
Lower gastrointestinal	Increased frequency or change in quality of bowel habits not needing medication. Rectal discomfort not requiring analgesics.	Diarrhea needing parasympatholytic drugs (e.g. diphenoxylate-atropine [Lomotil]). Mucous discharge infrequently requiring sanitary pads. Rectal pain needing analgesics or occasional narcotics. Mild rectal bleeding.	Diarrhea needing parenteral support. Severe mucous discharge requiring extended use of sanitary pads. Abdominal distention. Rectal pain requiring frequent narcotics. Gastrointestinal bleeding requiring one transfusion.	Acute or subacute obstruction. Fistula or perforation. Gastrointestinal bleeding requiring more than one transfusion. Abdominal pain or tenesmus requiring bowel diversion.
Urinary	Frequency or nocturia twice pretreatment baseline levels. Dysuria not needing medication.	Frequency or nocturia less frequent than hourly. Dysuria, bladder spasm needing local anesthetic (e.g., phenazopyridine hydrochloride [Pyridium]) or occasional narcotics. Infrequent gross hematuria. Temporary catheterization.	Frequency or nocturia hourly or more. Dysuria, pain, or spasm needing frequent narcotics. Gross hematuria requiring one transfusion. Prolonged urinary obstruction caused by prostate inflammation or clots requiring catheterization (including suprapubic).	Hematuria needing more than one transfusion. Hospitalization for sepsis caused by obstruction and/or ulceration, or necrosis of the bladder.
LATE TOXICITY				
Lower gastrointestinal	Excess bowel movements twice baseline level. Slight rectal discharge or blood.	Up to two antidiarrheals/wk. Up to two coagulations for bleeding. Occasional steroids for ulceration. Occasional dilation. Intermittent use of incontinence pads. Regular nonnarcotic or occasional narcotic for pain.	More than two antidiarrheals/day. At least one blood transfusion or more than two coagulations for bleeding. Prolonged steroids for enemas. Hyperbaric oxygen for bleeding or ulceration. Regular dilation. Persistent use of incontinence pads. Regular narcotic for pain.	Dysfunction requiring surgery. Perforation. Life-threatening bleeding.
Urinary	Nocturia twice baseline level. Microscopic hematuria. Slight mucosal atrophy and minor telangiectasia.	Moderate frequency. Nocturia more than twice baseline levels. Generalized telangiectasia. Intermittent macroscopic hematuria. Up to two coagulations. Intermittent use of incontinence pads. Regular nonnarcotic or occasional narcotic for pain.	Severe frequency and dysuria. Nocturia more frequent than once every hour. Reduction in bladder capacity (150 ml). Frequent hematuria requiring at least one transfusion. More than two coagulations for hematuria. Hyperbaric oxygen for bleeding or ulceration. Persistent use of incontinence pads. Regular narcotic for pain.	Severe hemorrhagic cystitis or ulceration requiring urinary diversion, cystectomy, or both.

Modified from Storey MR, Pollack A, Zagars GK, et al. *Int J Radiat Oncol Biol Phys* 2000;48:635-642.
*The acute scale was based on the modified Radiation Therapy Oncology Group criteria.
†The late scale was based on criteria from the Radiation Therapy Oncology Group and the Late Effects Normal Tissue Task Force.

or *BRCA2* also may be involved.[37] However, such genetic factors are believed to account for a relatively small proportion of prostate cancer. Diet, on the other hand, has been said to account for 25% of all cases of prostate cancer. Migration from low-risk, low-fat-intake countries such as Japan to high-risk, high-fat-intake countries such as the United States is associated with a substantial increase in the incidence of prostate cancer.[38,39] Animal studies suggest that the higher risk is not attributable solely to fat intake and that the combination of greater dietary fat intake accompanied by other dietary factors (e.g., fiber intake, protein intake) may contribute. Diet may act by altering circulating hormone levels.[39,40] Another possible etiologic factor is vasectomy; some studies have maintained and others have refuted vasectomy as a causal factor.

Endogenous androgen and estrogen levels have long been hypothesized to influence prostate cancer development and progression. Androgens are responsible for sustaining the equilibrium between cell loss and cell gain in the normal prostate. In rats, when androgen is withdrawn, 90% of the prostate epithelial cells die by apoptosis over a 10-day period.[41,42] Although the administration of androgens to castrated male rats causes prostate cell proliferation, eventually equilibrium is reestablished when cell numbers are replenished. The data concerning endogenous androgen levels and the risk of prostate cancer are not clear, but some relationships have emerged. Serum testosterone concentrations have been higher in patients at the time of prostate cancer diagnosis than in age-matched control subjects in some—but not all—studies. However, African-American men have higher serum testosterone levels until about age 35 years,[43] which may be a predisposing factor for prostate cancer.[44] Findings from Ross and colleagues[45] suggest a relationship between prostate cancer and dihydroxytestosterone metabolites. Androgens do seem to play a role in prostate carcinogenesis. Administration of androgens to rats in vivo causes adenocarcinoma of the prostate.[46,47] Androgens also act as a promoter when administered in conjunction with chemical carcinogens that target the prostate,[48] with cadmium,[49] or with ionizing radiation.[50] The promoter action of androgens may be important in human carcinogenesis.

DETECTION

The use of the PSA assay in the clinic and refinements in TRUS-directed biopsy of the prostate have vastly improved the ability to detect prostate cancer. PSA is a 26-kDa glycoprotein that is produced by epithelial cells in the prostate. A serine protease, PSA has chymotrypsin-like activity and causes liquefaction of semen. Serum PSA level is proportional to prostate volume, both of which increase with age and are strong determinants of outcome.[51-54]

Lepor and colleagues[55] calculated that for every 1 cm^3 of normal prostate epithelium, the amount of PSA in the serum is 0.33 ng/ml. Because about 20% of the prostate consists of epithelial cells,[56] the serum PSA for men with benign prostate tissue is estimated at about 0.066 ng/ml, an amount similar to estimates by Oesterling and colleagues[19] and Collins and colleagues.[57] Serum PSA concentration is elevated in the presence of prostate cancer because of the disruption of the normal glandular pattern by the tumor. Even though high-grade, poorly differentiated tumors are associated with higher serum PSA values, the serum PSA amount contributed per tumor volume is inversely proportional to the Gleason score.[58] Higher-grade tumors are both larger and disrupt more of the gland, thereby compensating for the lower serum PSA per tumor volume such that serum PSA levels are generally higher overall.

Serum PSA level also has been roughly correlated with prostate tumor volume.[51-54] Stamey and colleagues[59] estimated that for every 1 cm^3 of prostate cancer, the serum PSA is elevated by 3.5 ng/ml. As a consequence of the normal changes in prostate volume and increased inflammation with age, Oesterling and colleagues[20] have proposed age-specific PSA cutpoints for the detection of prostate cancer. For example, a serum PSA of more than 4 ng/ml is considered abnormal, but for a 70-year-old man, a better cutpoint may be 6.5 ng/ml, and for a 50-year-old man, the better cutpoint may be 3.5. Modifications to the age-specific reference ranges based on race have been proposed, with lower PSA cutpoints by age proposed for African-American men than for white men.[22,60]

Multiple forms of PSA coexist in the serum, and all but the free PSA form are complexed to protease inhibitors. For unknown reasons, the concentration of free PSA in patients with cancer is reduced. For men older than 50 years, when the free/total PSA ratio is less than 25% and the total PSA level is between 4 and 10 ng/ml, the risk of prostate cancer is increased.[21,61,62] Prostate cancer detection using free PSA measurements may be better than using the age-specific PSA reference ranges.[62] The use of free PSA in screening has gained acceptance and is a valuable aid in the decision to perform a prostate biopsy.

TRUS-guided prostate biopsy for diagnostic purposes has evolved considerably over the past 10 years. At a minimum, sextant (six-core) biopsies should be performed, with additional samples taken from hypoechoic areas. The sextant biopsy scheme, however, is associated with a high rate of subsequent positive biopsy after a negative first sextant biopsy.[63] Repeat sextant biopsies have become common practice for men with a persistently elevated PSA level, a high PSA velocity (rate of PSA rise),[64] or a low free/total PSA ratio. More recent studies have indicated that diagnostic precision is improved by obtaining 8 to 12 biopsy samples. The increase in the number of prostate needle biopsy samples from six was predicated on the finding that cancer was diagnosed in approximately 25% of patients at a second biopsy. Through tumor modeling of radical prostatectomy specimens,[65,66] prostate areas such as the anterior horns, transition zone, and periurethral region have been added to the sampling sites, and their inclusion has reduced the false-negative rate.[23,67,68]

HISTOLOGY

More than 95% of malignant prostatic neoplasms are adenocarcinomas arising from the acinar cells. One of the more common secondary histologic entities is ductal (endometroid) adenocarcinoma, which classically has been described as arising from the large periurethral prostatic ducts or verumontanum. Ductal adenocarcinomas typically display a papillary or cribriform pattern and were initially thought to be less aggressive,[69] although more recent evidence suggests the opposite.[70] Ductal carcinomas are very often associated with acinar adenocarcinomas; they are responsive to androgen ablation (AA), they secrete PSA, and they have been noted in the peripheral zone of the prostate, suggesting that they may actually be variants of acinar adenocarcinoma.[71]

Neuroendocrine cells are prevalent in the prostate, particularly in the prostatic ducts, and are part of the amine precursor uptake and decarboxylation system.[72] The presence of focal neuroendocrine differentiation in prostatic adenocarcinomas is common and of unclear prognostic significance. Small cell carcinomas of the prostate are highly aggressive anaplastic tumors that tend to metastasize early, do not secrete PSA, are rarely associated with paraneoplastic syndromes, and sometimes occur in the setting of acinar carcinoma.[73,74] Other primary prostate cancer variants are very rare and include transitional cell carcinoma, sarcomatoid carcinoma, mucinous adenocarcinoma, signet ring carcinoma, lymphoepithelioma-like carcinoma, squamous and adenosquamous carcinoma, adenocystic (basaloid) carcinoma, and mesenchymal tumors such as rhabdomyosarcomas (in children) and leiomyosarcomas (in adults).[75]

GRADING

The Gleason scoring system[76,77] is the most commonly used grading system for adenocarcinomas of the prostate, although more than 30 other systems have been described.[78] The Gleason score consists of the sum of the major and minor glandular patterns, graded on a 1 to 5 scale. An anaplastic appearance, with the absence of glandular structures, is consistent with a Gleason grade of 5. Discrete glandular formation with slight disorganization is consistent with a Gleason grade of 1. The combined Gleason score ranges from 2 to 10 and has been

shown to correlate strongly with patient outcome in terms of biochemical, clinical, and survival endpoints.

Because the prognostic differences between each of the nine Gleason scoring categories are slight and require large patient numbers to observe, the scores are usually lumped into four or fewer groups. One such four-tier system[79] consists of Gleason scores 2 and 3, 4 to 6, 7, and 8 to 10. A Gleason score of 7 has been established as connoting a significantly worse prognosis than a Gleason score of 6 or less and a significantly better prognosis than a Gleason score of 8 or more. Thus it is common for Gleason 7 to be categorized separately and included in the criteria for classifying intermediate-risk disease. Cases of Gleason 7 disease can be further subdivided according to the major + minor patterns of Gleason 3 + 4 vs. 4 + 3. The latter pattern is associated with a worse outcome,[80] and its presence has been used as a basis for treatment decisions. Along these lines, the proportion of Gleason 4 present in the specimen is of prognostic value.[54,81]

WORK-UP AND STAGING
Role of Rectal Examination and Transrectal Ultrasonography

Fundamental to the staging of prostate cancer is the digital rectal examination, the classification of which has changed minimally since the Whitmore-Jewett system.[82,83] The 1992 version of the American Joint Committee on Cancer (AJCC) staging system[84] (Table 27-2)

TABLE 27-2

Differences Between the 1992 and 1997 American Joint Committee on Cancer Staging Systems with Regard to Tumor Palpability

Tumor Attributes	1992 System	1997 System
NONPALPABLE		
< 5% of resected tissue involved	T1a	T1a
> 5% of resected tissue involved	T1b	T1b
PSA-directed biopsy	T1c	T1c
PALPABLE WITHOUT ECE		
Less than half of one lobe involved	T2a	T2a
More than half of one lobe involved	T2b	T2a
Both lobes involved	T2c	T2b
PALPABLE WITH ECE		
Unilateral involvement	T3a	T3a
Bilateral involvement	T3b	T3a
Seminal vesicle involvement	T3c	T3b

PSA, Prostate-specific antigen; *ECE*, extracapsular extension.

incorporated findings from TRUS, adding a new dimension that clearly has resulted in stage migration. For example, a palpable nodule limited to the prostate on digital rectal examination that would be classified as category T2 could be classified as T3 if the sonographic examination indicated extracapsular extension. The adoption of TRUS for staging may have been premature, because several studies, including significant randomized trials,[85,86] have shown it to be inaccurate in staging prostate cancer.

Prostate tumors are hypoechoic in 65%, isoechoic in 30%, and hyperechoic in 5% of cases.[87] Biopsy sampling of hypoechoic areas does not always yield tumor, and the diagnostic accuracy may be as low as 50%. A classification of T1c assigned by palpation and TRUS implies that the tumor was isoechoic; if hypoechoic or hyperechoic abnormalities were present, the tumor would be classified as T2 or T3. The application of TRUS in this manner has been nonuniform and confusing. The most significant inaccuracy with regard to the use of TRUS for staging comes from the designation of T3 disease on the basis of inhomogeneity to the prostate boundary echo or seminal vesicle invasion.

Although some studies have supported the use of TRUS for the detection of T3 disease,[88-92] others have not.[85,86,93] TRUS is less accurate for detecting seminal vesicle invasion than it is for detecting extracapsular extension.[85,93] Perhaps more important is the lack of clinically relevant correlation of stage—or upstaging or downstaging—as assessed by TRUS with clinical outcome.[94,95] Palpatory staging by digital rectal examination is recommended and should be defined as such in all documentation.

Controversies in Prostate Cancer Staging

Two other aspects of staging are controversial, namely the absence of PSA in the staging criteria and the changes to those criteria that were made between 1992 and 1997. Staging criteria are based on relationships to survival. Although a high PSA level before treatment is the most significant predictor of a rising PSA level and local recurrence after treatment (biochemical failure), the association of pretreatment PSA to survival[79,96,97] has yet to be established. Nonetheless, pretreatment PSA has been shown to be a strong correlate of distant metastasis[98,99] and is always considered in case management along with Gleason score and stage. Eventually, pretreatment PSA will be included in prostate cancer staging systems. The implementation of the 1997 AJCC staging system (Box 27-1)[100] brought about a consolidation of some of the categories, as shown in Table 27-2. However, comparative studies indicate that the 1992 system should not have been abandoned,[81,101-104] and several investigators continue to use it. For this reason, when stage is reported, the year of the AJCC staging system should be designated.

Another drawback of the 1997 staging system lies in its accompanying statement that all available information can be used in the staging process.[100] This statement implies—but does not specify—that biopsy information may be included in the staging; for example, a palpable T2a lesion may be upstaged to T2b if bilateral positive biopsy samples are obtained. The consequent stage migration makes comparisons of results with prior studies that used prior staging systems impossible. Thus use of strict palpable staging criteria is preferable.

Role of Magnetic Resonance Imaging

Endorectal coil magnetic resonance imaging (MRI) is gradually gaining a foothold in staging prostate cancer. The accuracy of endorectal coil MRI in determining extraprostatic extension is far greater than that of TRUS.[85] D'Amico and colleagues[105,106] reported that endorectal coil MRI findings correlate with surgical outcome. Given the improved accuracy of endorectal coil MRI in defining prostate anatomy (e.g., the apex of the prostate[107]) and in identifying suspicious intraprostatic areas,[108] extracapsular extension, and seminal vesicle invasion,[109-111] treatment planning using three-dimensional conformal radiation therapy (CRT) or intensity-modulated radiation therapy (IMRT) should be enhanced. Magnetic resonance spectroscopy permits the visualization of choline-rich areas, which are related to bulky tumor regions identified at pathology examination.[112] "Dose-painting" techniques that use IMRT to focally escalate the dose per fraction in choline-rich areas are being developed.[113,114] Functional imaging methods have tremendous promise in radiation treatment planning for prostate cancer and will undoubtedly become more commonplace over time.

Biopsy Variables

The systematic sampling of six or more regions from the prostate for diagnosis has led to the inspection of biopsy tissue variables. The number of biopsy samples positive for tumor and the proportion of tumor in the samples[115-121] are usually predictive of adverse pathologic features and patient outcome independent of pretreatment PSA level, tumor grade, and disease stage. However, biopsies can give inaccurate or misleading results. For example, the finding of a small amount of tumor in one of six biopsy samples may not equate to a low tumor burden.[122,123] However, the presence of multiple positive tumor cores with extensive tumor involvement is commensurate with a large tumor burden. Caution should be used in basing treatment decisions on biopsy findings, although the predictive value of acquiring more than six core samples may enhance accuracy. Qualitatively, estimates of tumor extent from biopsy samples have been used for years, albeit subjectively, to identify candidates for brachytherapy or other radiation therapy options. Additional studies leading to a consensus as to how to apply such data are needed.

BOX 27-1 1997 American Joint Committee on Cancer Staging System for Prostate Cancer

PRIMARY TUMOR, CLINICAL (T)

TX Primary tumor cannot be assessed
T0 No evidence of primary tumor
T1 Clinically inapparent tumor not palpable nor visible by imaging
　T1a Tumor incidental histologic finding in 5% or less of tissue resected
　T1b Tumor incidental finding in more than 5% of tissue resected
　T1c Tumor identified by needle biopsy (e.g., because of elevated PSA)
T2 Tumor confined within prostate*
　T2a Tumor involves one lobe
　T2b Tumor involves both lobes
T3 Tumor extends through the prostate capsule†
　T3a Extracapsular extension (unilateral or bilateral)
　T3b Tumor invades seminal vesicle(s)
T4 Tumor is fixed or invades adjacent structures other than seminal vesicles: bladder neck, external sphincter, rectum, levator muscles, and/or pelvic wall

PRIMARY TUMOR, PATHOLOGIC (pT)

pT2‡ Organ confined
　pT2a Unilateral
　pT2b Bilateral
pT3 Extraprostatic extension
　pT3a Extraprostatic extension
　pT3b Seminal vesicle invasion
pT4 Invasion of bladder, rectum

REGIONAL LYMPH NODES (N)

NX Regional lymph node(s) cannot be assessed (e.g., previously removed)

N0 No regional lymph node metastasis
N1 Metastasis in regional lymph node or nodes

DISTANT METASTASIS§ (M)

MX Distant metastasis cannot be assessed
M0 No distant metastasis
M1 Distant metastasis
　M1a Nonregional lymph node(s)
　M1b Bone(s)
　M1c Other site(s)

HISTOPATHOLOGIC GRADE (G)

GX Grade cannot be assessed
G1 Well differentiated (slight anaplasia)
G2 Moderately differentiated (moderate anaplasia)
G3-4 Poorly differentiated or undifferentiated (marked anaplasia)

STAGE GROUPING

Stage I	T1a	N0	M0	G1
Stage II	T1a	N0	M0	G2-4
	T1b	N0	M0	Any G
	T1c	N0	M0	Any G
	T1	N0	M0	Any G
	T2	N0	M0	Any G
Stage III	T3	N0	M0	Any G
Stage IV	T4	N0	M0	Any G
	Any T	N1	M0	Any G
	Any T	Any N	M1	Any G

From Fleming I, Cooper JS, Henson DE, et al, eds. *AJCC Cancer Staging Manual.* 5th ed. Philadelphia, Pa: Lippincott Williams & Wilkins; 1997:219-224.
*Tumor found in one or both lobes by needle biopsy, but not palpable or reliably visible by imaging, is classified as T1c.
†Invasion into the prostatic apex or into (but not beyond) the prostatic capsule is not classified as T3, but as T2.
‡There is no pathologic T1 classification.
§When more than one site of metastasis is present, the most advanced category is used, pM1c is the most advanced.

Processing and grading of diagnostic material from prostate needle biopsies vary greatly. Because segregation of individual biopsy cores raises cost, biopsy material is occasionally pooled according to the side of the gland it was removed from (right vs. left). In most major cancer treatment centers, each core is processed individually. Segregation of the biopsy specimens allows quantification of the percentage of tumor in each core, the number of positive cores, and the Gleason score of each specimen. The generation of a Gleason score for each biopsy specimen has led to the use of the highest Gleason score as a prognostic variable. Conceptually, however, Gleason score is a composite assessment of all of the tumor tissue obtained. If one biopsy sample shows a focus of Gleason 8 and three samples show substantial Gleason 6 tumor content, then the global Gleason score would be less than Gleason 8. Because the percentage of Gleason grade 4 to 5[54,81] and designation of a tertiary Gleason score may have prognostic value,[124] the scoring of individual biopsy specimens may prove to be important. Few studies have compared the relationship of the highest biopsy Gleason score to the global biopsy Gleason score.[125]

Imaging Studies

The use of the PSA assay in screening and the use of more systematic TRUS-guided prostate biopsy sampling have resulted in a dramatic reduction in the local–regional extent of disease at diagnosis.[81,126,127] As a consequence, the incidence of positive findings on bone scans or pelvic computed tomography (CT) scans has lessened considerably. Detection of metastasis on bone scans is related to pretreatment PSA value, Gleason score, and disease stage.[128] The association with pretreatment PSA is pronounced. Bone scanning is recommended if the PSA value is higher than 10 ng/ml,[19,129] and some would argue that a PSA level of more than 20 ng/ml should be used. Even though pelvic CT scanning is recommended for patients with a high-risk feature, such as a PSA level of more than 20 ng/ml, Gleason score of 8 or more, or category T3 or higher, lymph node enlargement is rarely found.

Another imaging test that has yet to gain wide acceptance is the ProstaScint scan (Cytogen Corp., Princeton, NJ) for imaging the prostate or prostate cancer cells. The test uses an indium 111—labeled antibody (capromab pendetide) to prostate-specific membrane antigen, a transmembrane glycoprotein that is expressed mainly on cells of prostate origin. The ProstaScint scan has been used clinically as an adjunctive test for staging high-risk disease, for identifying lymph node or hematogenous spread, and for characterizing sites of recurrence after definitive therapy.[130-134] Prostate-specific membrane-antigen imaging has been used to visualize lymph node involvement in patients with high-risk disease who are being considered for definitive local therapy; to visualize regional and distant spread in patients who have experienced biochemical failure after radiation therapy and are being considered for salvage prostatectomy or cryosurgery; and to detect isolated recurrences in the prostate bed in patients who show rising PSA levels and are good candidates for salvage radiation therapy. Although the ProstaScint scan has produced generally encouraging results, it does have a significant rate of false-positive findings. Recent improvements in single photon emission CT–CT fusion techniques should reduce such errors.

Lymph Node Dissection

The routine use of lymph node dissection as a staging tool for patients desiring definitive radiation therapy has largely been abandoned. For patients with favorable risk features, the risk of lymph node involvement is less than 5%.[81,101,127,135] Indeed, the incidence of lymph node involvement has dropped in the PSA era.[81,127] For those with intermediate-risk features, the incidence of pelvic lymph node spread is about 10% to 15%. Patients with high-risk features, particularly category T3 disease, have a 40% to 50% risk of regional spread.[135]

Because the standard of care for patients with high-risk prostate cancer is radiation therapy in combination with AA, and because use of this combination seems to be effective in patients with lymph node involvement,[135] a lymph node dissection would be of little benefit. The only justification for performing a lymph node dissection is if the result would alter treatment. Lymph node dissection might influence the decision to use permanent rather than extended temporary AA if lymph nodes are positive. Otherwise, the radiation therapy management of regionally lymph node–positive (stage D1) disease and of clinically defined high-risk disease (PSA > 20 ng/ml, Gleason score 8 or higher, or T3 or higher) is the same.

PROGNOSTIC FACTORS AND MODELS
Biochemical Evidence of Treatment Failure

Ever since the rising PSA profile was identified as a surrogate endpoint, exploration of potential predictors of prostate cancer outcome has expanded rapidly. Pretreatment PSA levels, Gleason score, and disease stage are the three core factors widely considered to be essential in any evaluation of therapeutic options. Terms such as "locally advanced" will always be associated with an increased risk of treatment failure, but such terms describe only the staging portion of risk assessment. The preferred designations of risk assign patients to low-, intermediate-, or high-risk groups on the basis of PSA level, Gleason score, and stage.

Several models have been proposed to approximate the risk of adverse pathologic features after radical prostatectomy as well as the risk of treatment failure after radiation therapy and radical prostatectomy.[98,135-139] Central to such modeling is the use of biochemical failure, that is, rising PSA levels, as an endpoint. Biochemical failure is a harbinger of eventual clinical relapse, with an average delay of 2 to 5 years.[140,141] In most men with a rising PSA level after radiation therapy, biopsy of the prostate indicates residual tumor, suggesting that biochemical failure most often represents local persistence.[142,143] Likewise, intensive biopsy of the vesicourethral anastomosis after prostatectomy when evidence of biochemical failure is present also yields evidence of local persistence in 30% to 50% of cases.[144,145]

The question that remains is whether biochemical failure is a surrogate for eventual distant metastasis and death. Crucial to such determinations is that the follow-up period be long enough to allow disease to progress from local to distant relapse to death for those patients without micrometastatic disease at diagnosis. The relationship between rising PSA levels and the development of distant metastasis is incontrovertible. Pound and colleagues[146] followed a cohort of patients treated solely with radical prostatectomy who did not undergo early salvage treatment after biochemical failure. In that study, 34% of men who experienced biochemical failure developed distant metastasis during the study period. The 8-year actuarial rate of distant metastasis, calculated from the time that the PSA level rose, was 50%. In that study, all patients who developed distant metastasis had biochemical failure first. Many other groups have reported that biochemical failure is a precursor to distant metastasis in all but a few cases.[100,147-149]

Further complicating the use of biochemical failure as an endpoint are inconsistencies in its definition. According to the American Society for Therapeutic Radiology and Oncology consensus guidelines, three consecutive rises in the PSA level constitute treatment failure.[150] Although this definition has helped to standardize research efforts, some situations can lead to misclassification. For example, PSA levels have been observed to transiently rise 1 to 3 years after radiation therapy and then fall back to a stable low level for no apparent reason. This so-called "PSA bounce" phenomenon occurs most often after brachytherapy with permanent radioactive seeds,[151] but it also has been documented after external-beam radiation therapy.[152]

Another consideration in defining biochemical failure is that after AA plus radiation therapy, the PSA level usually reaches a nadir in the undetectable range and then rises, after some delay, after the AA is discontinued. It is not uncommon to see three consecutive rises and then a leveling off, or even a fall, in the PSA level. Characterization of treatment failure in patients treated with AA might best be accomplished by setting a PSA

cutpoint such as 1.5 ng/ml and declaring that PSA levels in excess of this amount indicate biochemical failure.[153]

PSA Nadir Level After Radiation Therapy

Some investigators[154] have advocated using a strict PSA-nadir cutpoint as an indicator of freedom from treatment failure after radiation therapy. The consensus of the American Society for Therapeutic Radiology and Oncology[150] was that nadir PSA level after radiation therapy is not the sole determinant of outcome after radiation therapy, although it can be used, along with pretreatment PSA level, Gleason score, and stage, as a prognostic factor[155-157] (Fig. 27-3). The lower the PSA nadir level after radiation therapy, the lower the likelihood of a rising PSA profile.

The degree of PSA nadir can vary according to the type of radiation therapy administered (brachytherapy vs. external-beam therapy) because of differences in the destruction of normal prostate cells. Usually, more than 3 years are required after radiation therapy to determine PSA nadir level. Nadir PSA levels after radiation therapy are typically grouped as being less or equal to 0.5 ng/ml, from more than 0.5 to 1.0 ng/ml, from more than 1.0 to 2.0 ng/ml, and more than 2.0 ng/ml. As shown in Figure 27-3,

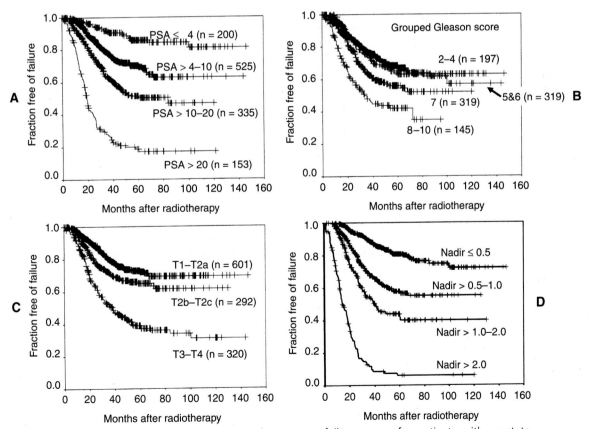

Fig. 27-3 Freedom from biochemical treatment failure curves for patients with prostate cancer treated with definitive radiation therapy, without androgen ablation, according to, **A,** pretreatment prostate-specific antigen (PSA) level; **B,** Gleason score; **C,** clinical stage according to digital rectal examination; and **D,** nadir PSA level after treatment.

the associated 5-year freedom from biochemical failure rates using rising PSA levels are 81%, 58%, 44%, and 6%, respectively.

The earliest and most robust determinant of eventual clinical relapse is a rise in PSA level; the PSA nadir level is a strong posttreatment prognostic factor that is independent of pretreatment PSA, Gleason score, and stage. The nadir PSA measurement approximates the risk of eventual biochemical relapse, but use of this value by itself, without considering other prognostic factors, would result in the misclassification of failure in many patients. More importantly, the nadir PSA level is a research variable and should not be applied clinically. Many patients with nadir PSA levels between 0.5 and 2.0 ng/ml have no biochemical evidence of treatment failure for 5 to 10 years.[158]

PSA Level, Gleason Score, and Clinical Stage

Pretreatment PSA, Gleason score, and clinical stage are independent correlates of treatment success, which for prostate cancer is defined as having no biochemical evidence of disease ("bNED" or "freedom from biochemical failure"). Mathematical modeling that incorporates biochemical (i.e., PSA) evidence of success after radiation therapy has allowed more precise definition of risk groupings.[98,137,139,159-162] Most models assign patients to prognostic "bins" such as those defined by the AJCC staging classification.

Movsas and colleagues[163] compared several of these bin models in a cohort of 421 patients treated at Fox Chase Cancer Center in the PSA era and found that the differences among the models in ability to predict rates of freedom from biochemical failure were minor. The most common prognostic grouping assigns patients to favorable-risk, intermediate-risk, and high-risk groups.[160,161] Patients in the favorable-risk have a pretreatment PSA of 10 ng/ml or less, a Gleason score of less than 7, and category T1 to T2a disease (according to the 1992 AJCC staging system). Patients with a pretreatment PSA level of more than 20 ng/ml, a Gleason score of 8 to 10, or category T3 to T4 disease are considered to be at high risk. Intermediate-risk patients fall between these two groups and include cases without any high-risk features who have a pretreatment PSA level of 10 to 20 ng/ml, a Gleason score of 7 or less, or category T2b to T2c disease. The Kaplan-Meier curves for freedom from biochemical failure among these risk groups in a cohort from The University of Texas M.D. Anderson Cancer Center are shown in Figure 27-4. Refinements to this grouping will certainly be forthcoming, and in the future bin modeling may give way to more precise, continuous-function estimates.

Pretreatment PSA level, Gleason score, and stage are also strong correlates of distant metastasis.[98,99] Gleason score and stage also are predictive of survival. As noted

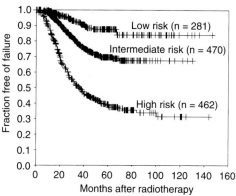

Fig. 27-4 Freedom from biochemical treatment failure curves for 1213 patients with prostate cancer treated at the M.D. Anderson Cancer Center with definitive radiation therapy, without androgen ablation, according to risk level. Patients with favorable (low-risk) disease had a pretreatment PSA level of no more than 10 ng/ml, a Gleason score of no more than 6, and a T1 to T2a tumor according to the 1992 American Joint Committee on Cancer staging system. Intermediate-risk factors were a pretreatment PSA level of more than 10 ng/ml to 20 ng/ml, clinical stage T2b to T2c disease, or a Gleason score of no more than 7, with no high-risk factors. High-risk factors were a pretreatment PSA level of more than 20 ng/ml, a Gleason score of 8 to 10, or clinical stage T3 to T4 disease.

earlier, no association between pretreatment PSA and survival has yet been documented.

TURP for T3 to T4 Disease

Patients with category T3 or T4 disease who have undergone TURP for symptoms of urinary obstruction have been identified as being at greater risk of developing distant metastasis.[164-167] The independence of TURP as a determinant of outcome has been called into question by the results of multivariate analysis.[168,169] The concern about the dissemination of tumor cells from the TURP procedure has diminished considerably, because urinary obstruction can be managed medically in most cases by using 5-α-reductase inhibitors, antiandrogens, luteinizing hormone-releasing hormone agonists, or α-adrenergic blocking agents.

Cell Proliferation and DNA Content Characteristics

The growth rate of prostate cancer is notably slow. Analyses of cell-cycle kinetics have been limited but have produced intriguing findings. The labeling index for prostate tumors, obtained by injecting nucleoside analog tracers into patients, is less than 6%,[170-172] and the potential doubling time (T_{pot}) is more than 24 days. Staining prostate cancer specimens for the proliferation marker Ki-67 with monoclonal antibodies confirmed that only a small proportion of prostate cancer cells are proliferating.[173,174] These findings suggest that most of the tumor cells are in a resting state. The time it takes for the serum PSA concentration to double in patients with prostate cancer is often more than 12 months,[175,176] a number close to estimates of tumor doubling time from measurements of cell-cycle kinetics.[177] Such kinetic attributes have been likened to those of late-reacting tissues and have stimulated interest in the radiobiological characteristics of prostate cancer. Indeed, recent reports suggest that the α/β ratio for prostate cancer seems to be between 1.5 and 5.0,[178-181] suggesting that hypofractionated irradiation may be desirable.[182]

DNA content analysis by either flow cytometry or image analysis supports the findings from cell-cycle kinetics studies. Most malignant prostate tumors are diploid,[183] with fewer than 5% of cells in S phase.[184,185] DNA ploidy has been shown repeatedly to predict outcome after radical prostatectomy.[99] The few studies of patients undergoing radiation therapy also have indicated that DNA ploidy has predictive value for outcome after this treatment as well. DNA diploidy is associated with a more favorable prognosis than is nondiploidy (including tetraploidy and aneuploidy). On the other hand, Khoo and colleagues[173] have suggested that the proliferation marker Ki-67 may be a more significant correlate of biochemical failure than is DNA ploidy. In that study, a low Ki-67 labeling index correlated with improved freedom from biochemical failure. The radiation therapy series that have investigated DNA ploidy and Ki-67 labeling have included few patients, however, and larger prospective studies are needed.

Family History

Family history has been reported by Kupelian and colleagues[186,187] to be a determinant of treatment success after radiation therapy. However, Hanus and colleagues[188] were unable to corroborate these findings. Likewise, Bova and others[189] observed that patients with sporadic and familial prostate cancer who were treated with radical prostatectomy had the same prognosis.

Pretreatment Serum Testosterone Level

Serum testosterone concentration in men with prostate cancer has been associated with outcome. Zagars and Pollack[190] found that a serum testosterone level of more than 500 ng/dl was associated with distant metastasis in patients with clinical T1 to T3, Nx/N0 prostate cancer treated with radiation therapy. Kelly and colleagues[191] reported that similarly high serum testosterone concentrations were predictive of biochemical failure in patients with regionally lymph node–positive (stage D1) disease treated with AA. In contrast, in patients with metastatic

disease, a high serum testosterone concentration has been associated with a better response to AA and prolonged survival.[192-194] The reason for these differences is not clear, but it seems that serum testosterone level affects outcome.

Molecular Markers

The literature on biomarkers for prostate cancer has the same problem as the reports on cell-cycle kinetics and proliferation measurements do—small numbers of patients and promising but inconclusive findings. Some of the markers that have potential as pretreatment predictors of prostate cancer outcome are p53, p21, p27, bcl-2, bax, p16, pRb, and microvessel density.[99]

EXTERNAL-BEAM RADIATION THERAPY: TREATMENT PLANNING AND TECHNIQUES
Evolution of Techniques

Techniques for treating prostate cancer have evolved considerably over the past 5 years. The conventional four-field approach has yielded to more complex conformal arrangements (three-dimensional CRT) and recently to IMRT. Simulations involving fluoroscopy have given way to simulations with CT. The considerations surrounding the application of new technology are complex, and adoption of new methods should be approached systematically. Three-dimensional CRT and the still more precise method of IMRT allow more accurate visualization of the prostate in relation to the surrounding normal structures. The rationale and support for the use of conformal techniques to treat prostate cancer are described in this section. Results from dose-response analyses are described in the subsequent section on radiation therapy results.

Three-Dimensional Treatment Planning and Conformal Radiation Therapy

Three-dimensional CT-based reconstructions of the prostate, bladder, rectum, and pelvic bony anatomy are readily performed with commercial treatment planning systems. An example of a digitally reconstructed radiograph from a pelvic CT scan is shown in Color Plate 26, after p. 80.[195] The fields superimposed on this reconstructed radiograph represent typical conventional anterior–posterior and lateral fields that were used in the past. The prostate and seminal vesicles are shown on both views, with the bladder and rectum in the lateral display. Notably, rather large margins surround the prostate in all dimensions except posteriorly, where a block shields the rectum. Although these fields are generous, they are not considered to be whole-pelvic fields, which would include 1.5 to 2 cm of the pelvic brim.

Three-dimensional treatment planning illustrates the excessiveness of the margins used in conventional treatment planning, except for the posterior (rectal) margin.

Color Plate 27, after p. 80, illustrates examples of oblique three-dimensional CRT fields with 1.5-cm margins from the prostate to the block edge (1.0-cm planning target volume [PTV] margin), except posteriorly, where the margin is 1.0 cm (0.5-cm PTV margin). Three-dimensional treatment planning involves "design" of the gross tumor volume (GTV), the clinical target volume (CTV), and the PTV. In most situations, the CTV is assumed to be the same as the GTV, which is visualized on CT scans as the prostate. The PTV margin around the CTV accounts for uncertainties in set-up and motion of the target. The PTV margin in this example is 1.0 cm in all dimensions except posteriorly, where it is 0.5 cm. Another 0.5 cm from the PTV to the block edge is added for penumbra.

No clear-cut definitions for the CTV in terms of when and how much of the seminal vesicles to include have been determined; the amount depends on the risk of involvement. Common practice is that little if any of the seminal vesicles are included in the CTV for patients with favorable risk features. For patients at intermediate risk, some or all of the seminal vesicles are included for some or all of the treatment duration. For high-risk prostate cancer, most oncologists include the seminal vesicles in their entirety for the duration of treatment. That said, compromises are often made in terms of seminal vesicle coverage because of excessive overlap with the rectum. The seminal vesicles often fall around the rectum when simulations are done while the patients are supine.

The definitions of the bladder and rectum volumes used for DVH analysis also vary among treatment centers. At Memorial Sloan-Kettering Cancer Center, the outline consists of the walls of the bladder and rectum, rather than the walls plus the inner contents.[196] Initially at the M.D. Anderson Cancer Center, the entire rectal contents were outlined, with the length of rectum extending from the ischial tuberosities 11 cm superiorly.[14,195,197] In a dose-escalation trial by the Radiation Therapy Oncology Group (RTOG 94-06),[198] the length of rectum was defined as starting at the ischial tuberosities extending superiorly to the anterior flexion of the rectosigmoid. These differences in structure definition could affect the variables used to determine the adequacy of a plan. Care should be taken to adopt the definitions of structure and DVH variables as specified by the group being emulated.

Conformal field arrangements range widely. At Fox Chase Cancer Center, a four-field technique was used throughout, with a field reduction posteriorly from 1.5 to ≤ 0.5 cm for the last 10 Gy to reduce the risk of rectal bleeding.[199] Others have used six or seven fields[162,197,200,201] from either the beginning of treatment or as a boost after an initial four-field set-up. The six- to seven-field placements include four oblique fields at 30 to 40 degrees above and below the lateral positions, two lateral fields, and in some cases an anterior field for quality assurance (the dose from the anterior field is usually less

than that for the other fields). The lateral fields are classically weighted more heavily to spare more of the rectum.

Assessment of three-dimensional CRT plans relies on examination of isodose lines on transverse CT scan images and DVHs. Visual inspection of the isodose lines on each CT scan slice, taken at 3- to 5-mm intervals, is used to verify that the PTV is covered adequately and that the rectum and bladder are spared from high doses. The DVHs are also essential in determining the suitability of the plan. The DVH variables for determining acceptability vary among treatment centers. At the M.D. Anderson Cancer Center, the proportion of rectum receiving at least 70 Gy strongly correlated with the 5-year actuarial rate of rectal complications of grade 2 or higher.[14]

In a detailed multivariate analysis, Skwarchuk and colleagues[196] found that such factors as a higher maximum dose to the rectum, enclosure of the rectal contour by the 50% isodose line, and a smaller anatomically defined length of rectum were associated with a higher risk of late rectal bleeding. Kupelian and colleagues[202] found in multivariate analysis that absolute rectal volume (15-ml cutpoint), rather than a percentage of rectal volume correlated with late rectal complications. Color Plate 28, *A*, after p. 80, displays the isodose curves for a treatment planned with either the conformal boost technique used in a randomized dose-escalation trial at the M.D. Anderson Cancer Center or with IMRT. The IMRT plan has greater conformality, and the dose fall-off across the rectum is sharper. The dose specification should be to the PTV because the minimum or average dose is more of a determinant of outcome than is the isocenter dose. This recommendation is in accordance with the 1993 specifications of the International Commission on Radiation Units and Measurements.[203]

Intensity-Modulated Radiation Therapy

The fluence of linear accelerator photon beams is even across their length, and that fluence can be modulated to create more ideal dose distributions. Although simply placing a wedge in a beam modulates its intensity, the concept underlying IMRT is that the fluence is altered through the division of the radiation field into multiple beamlets of various intensity, the sum of which constitutes a highly modulated beam. Manually cut transmission blocks or compensating filters have been used, but the procedure is laborious[204] and results can be duplicated or surpassed by using other conceptual IMRT approaches that are available commercially. Systems using tomotherapy or multileaf collimation (MLC) for IMRT are expanding the use of IMRT in community practice, much the way three-dimensional CRT entered into use 5 years ago.

Tomotherapy is the rotational delivery of radiation therapy using multiple, relatively small collimator vanes that open and close during treatment to modulate the intensity of the fan beam.[205] The Peacock apparatus (Nomos Corporation, Sewickley, Pa) delivers dose in a slice-by-slice fashion, via multiple arcs, much as radiation is used in CT scanning to reconstruct three-dimensional images. IMRT delivery using MLC can be static[113,206] or dynamic.[207-209] Recent findings from the M.D. Anderson Cancer Center indicate that identical results in the treatment of prostate cancer can be achieved with tomotherapy (using the Peacock Multileaf intensity-Modulating Collimator, or "MIMiC") and segmental MLC delivery systems.[210]

Rectal DVH analysis of 20 patients with prostate cancer whose treatment was planned by using several methods is shown in Color Plate 28, B. As described in the legend for Color Plate 28, A, these methods (four conformal and two intensity-modulated) include a conformal four-field technique with a field reduction after 46 Gy; a 10-field conformal boost, as was used in the M.D. Anderson Cancer Center randomized dose-escalation trial;[195] a seven-field conformal arrangement throughout with 40% of the dose from the lateral fields; a seven-field conformal arrangement throughout with 50% of the dose from the lateral fields; an IMRT plan using the Peacock MIMiC system; and a 10-field sliding-window MLC plan. The conformal plans used 18-MV photons, whereas the intensity-modulated plans used 6-MV photons. The dose was 75.6 Gy in 42 fractions prescribed to the PTV except in the 10-field plan, in which 78 Gy in 39 fractions was prescribed to the isocenter. The proportion of the rectum that received 70 Gy or more was significantly lower in the IMRT plans. No difference was observed between the Peacock MIMiC and the MLC plans. The benefit from IMRT was apparent despite the choice of favorable-risk patients and very little outlining of the seminal vesicles.

The advantages of IMRT over three-dimensional CRT are seen in two principal areas. First, IMRT allows greater conformality of the radiation beam than does three-dimensional CRT. Second, the dose fall-off from the prescription isodose line is much greater with IMRT than with three-dimensional CRT. Another benefit to the physician is that once the planning parameters are established, the planning process is much faster than that of three-dimensional CRT. There is no need to draw blocks when IMRT is used, and inverse planning methods facilitate planning optimization. As described in Chapter 2 of this volume, inverse planning is a computer planning process wherein the structures of interest and structure dose limits are specified and the computer determines the optimal beam weighting, segmentation, and segment intensity to achieve the stated goals. In tomotherapy, this process is fully automated. In MLC-based IMRT, the number and angles of the beams must be empirically determined first. In the future, the selection of optimal beam angles will be incorporated into commercial MLC inverse-planning software.

Set-up Error and Prostate Movement Considerations

By definition, the PTV is the margin placed around a target organ or site to account for set-up errors and changes in organ position relative to the reference planning CT scan. In treating prostate cancer, the extent to which set-up error can be minimized by immobilization and the best method for immobilization are still somewhat controversial.[211-214] At Memorial Sloan-Kettering Cancer Center, patients are treated while prone, with a thermoplastic body cast used for stabilization.[211] The advantage of this approach is that the prostate and seminal vesicles fall anteriorly away from the rectum, thereby reducing rectal doses. However, this treatment has not been consistently reproducible elsewhere. More recent studies have demonstrated that prostate movement with respiration is more pronounced when thermoplastic abdominopelvic shells are used[215,216]; less respiratory movement is observed when patients are treated while supine, without abdominopelvic casts. At the M.D. Anderson Cancer Center, vacuum-bag immobilization of the legs from the midthigh to below the feet is used for all patients with prostate cancer, leaving the pelvis free to be positioned easily and allowing daily sonographic imaging of the prostate as described below.

Prostate position in the pelvis is affected by rectal and bladder filling; rectal filling seems to have the greater influence. Serial CT scanning during radiation therapy has documented that the changes in prostate position are not inconsequential.[217-226] Positional changes are greatest in the anterior-posterior and superior-inferior directions, probably along the angle of the pubic symphysis. Antolak and colleagues[225] calculated that to include all of the CTV in the PTV 95% of the time, the PTV would have to be 0.7 cm laterally and superior-inferiorly and 1.01 cm in the anterior-posterior direction. Adding 0.5 cm for penumbra would make the posterior margin at the rectum greater than 1.5 cm, which would mean that the entire circumference of the rectum in many patients would be treated to a full dose. Although larger margins may be necessary for some patients, attempting dose escalation to more than 70 Gy using these recommendations would produce unacceptable rectal complications.

Measures to reduce the error associated with changes in prostate position are needed for both three-dimensional CRT and IMRT. Antolak and colleagues[225] found that rectal and bladder volumes were greater on the pretreatment planning CT scans than on subsequent scans obtained during treatment (Fig. 27-5).[225] One way of minimizing the effects of this difference is to prepare another plan after 2 to 3 weeks of treatment; however, this practice is laborious and still does not account for day-to-day deviations. Methods are now available for monitoring

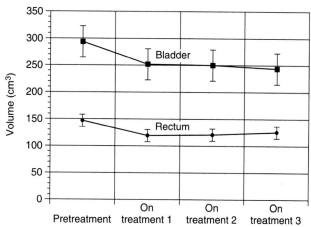

Fig. 27-5 Bladder and rectal volume changes as determined from serial computed tomography scans during radiation therapy. Scans were obtained once before treatment and three times during treatment, with 2- to 3-week intervals between scans. (Redrawn from Antolak JA, Rosen II, Childress CH, et al. *Int J Radiat Oncol Biol Phys* 1998;42:661-672.)

prostate position at each treatment session,[226] methods that will become integral to ensuring that the prostate is centered in the PTV for three-dimensional CRT and IMRT.

The Nomos Corporation has developed the "BAT" system, an ultrasound device that localizes the prostate in three-dimensional space, compares prostate position to that in the pretreatment CT scan, and calculates the shift necessary to place the prostate in the middle of the PTV (Color Plate 29, after p. 80. Lattanzi and colleagues[227] reported that shifts calculated in this way match those derived from daily CT scanning. Prostate position also can be imaged by placing fiducial markers in the prostate before radiation therapy is begun and using those markers to facilitate daily localization by electronic portal imaging.[217] Amorphous silicone detectors are ideal for recording marker position daily and calculating shifts to position the prostate properly within the PTV.

Localization of the Prostate Apex

Use of CT scanning to localize the apex of the prostate is inexact because the apex itself is not visualized; rather, the bulb of the penis, below the urogenital diaphragm, is the best landmark. Retrograde urethrography has been advocated as a means for more precisely determining the position of the prostate apex.[228,229] In this technique, about 10 ml of contrast medium is injected into the urethra, which is then blocked with a Cunningham clamp or a partially inflated Foley (balloon) catheter. The distance from the superior tip of the contrast to the prostate apex is estimated to be about 1.3 cm. However, the manipulations associated with this technique may introduce error. Malone and colleagues[230] found that instilling contrast under pressure displaced the prostate apex superiorly by 5 to 7 mm. Sandler and colleagues[231]

also reported that when radiodense markers were implanted at the prostate apex under sonographic guidance, CT localization of the prostatic apex was more accurate than was retrograde urethrography. The safest approach is to use the bulb of the penis on CT scan as a guide of apex position or to use MRI, which visualizes the apex more clearly.[232]

BRACHYTHERAPY: TREATMENT PLANNING AND TECHNIQUES
Evolution of Techniques

Implantation of permanent radioactive seeds in the prostate (PRSIP) has a long history. The largest series of patients treated in this way with a retropubic approach came from Memorial Sloan-Kettering Cancer Center.[233] These investigators developed a nomogram for the use of ^{125}I, which has a half-life of 60 days, as the primary treatment for prostate cancer. The other isotope commonly used in the past has been ^{198}Au, which has a half-life of 2.7 days and was used in combination with external-beam radiation therapy.[234,235] In these early procedures, an open retropubic approach was used that involved the needles being placed retropubically into the prostate while the prostate was palpated with a finger in the rectum (Fig. 27-6).[234,236] The resultant distribution of seeds in the prostate was uneven and hence the dosimetry was substandard by today's criteria. Local control rates in these early series were very low.[237,238] Scardino and colleagues[239] documented a very high rate of positive biopsy results after therapy with gold seeds and external-beam irradiation, but modern-day ultrasound-guided transperineal approaches have improved the success of PRSIP considerably (Fig. 27-7).[240,241] Techniques for PRSIP continue to evolve with the use of intraoperative treatment planning, as described below.

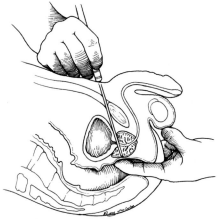

Fig. 27-6 Needle placement for prostate seed implant: open retropubic approach. (Redrawn from Chan RC, Gutierrez AE. *Cancer* 1976;37:2749.)

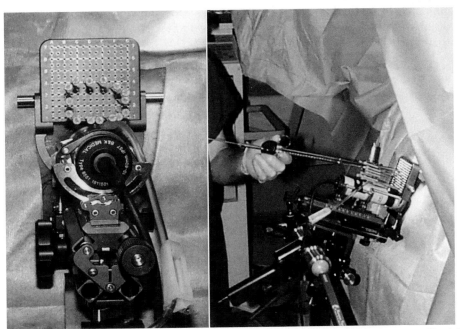

Fig. 27-7 Transperineal implantation of permanent radioactive seeds in the prostate. The *left panel* shows the needles arranged in a peripheral pattern; the *right panel* shows the Mick applicator.

Planning Methods

Two principal methods for brachytherapy treatment planning are in use today. The most common approach involves pretreatment planning with TRUS,[242,243] although intraoperative planning is gaining in popularity.[244,245] Combinations of preplanning and intraoperative planning are also in use. Preplanning involves first acquiring transrectal 0.5-cm step-section sonographic images of the prostate within a month of beginning the treatment. The step-section images are loaded onto a treatment planning computer, and a plan is formulated through an interactive process with the dosimetrist and the attending physician. Inverse planning programs now available have greatly simplified this procedure. The finalized plan designates needle position as well as the location of each seed in each needle.

The seeds are delivered to the predetermined locations in the prostate by one of two primary methods. The first method involves the use of preloaded needles; the seeds are loaded into the needles in locations specified by the plan. The second method involves the Mick applicator system, which allows seeds to be deposited one at a time. The Mick applicator procedure takes longer but offers more control in terms of adjusting seed spacing, which is monitored during the procedure with fluoroscopy.

A drawback of the preplanning approach is that the patient must be placed in precisely the same position as for the preplanning TRUS procedure. Sometimes exact positioning is not possible. Moreover, at surgery, the prostate position, shape, and size may differ slightly from the preplanning images, which can reduce the possibility of achieving acceptable dosimetry. The use of preplanning and preloaded needles requires considerably less operative time than the alternative of real-time intraoperative planning. Use of the Mick applicator system also may involve more of a learning curve than use of preloaded needles.

Intraoperative computer planning provides valuable feedback on the dosimetry as it develops during the implantation procedure. Seed placement is typically monitored with fluoroscopy, and their positions are noted on the planning computer display. The profile that develops is an approximation of the position of the seeds in three-dimensional space. The use of MRI[246] or CT[247] for imaging during implantation allows more precise real-time three-dimensional reconstructions of dose to be generated; however, these procedures take considerably longer than does sonography.

From a clinical standpoint, if more than about 90% of the target volume receives 100% of the dose, it may be difficult to show a difference between three-dimensional intraoperative reconstructions from MRI or CT vs. those from sonography. The same argument can be applied to intraoperative planning; use of intraoperative computer planning techniques requires more time in the operating room, which is costly. If the differences between preplanning reconstructions and intraoperative planning reconstructions are insignificant, then preplanning is probably preferable.

Initial evaluations thus far have favored intraoperative planning in terms of improved dosimetric variables such as the volume of the target that receives 100% of the prescribed dose (V_{100}) and the dose received by 90% of the target volume (D_{90}). Intraoperative planning also may be beneficial in terms of the homogeneity of the dose distribution. On balance, the findings to date support the adoption of intraoperative planning, and there is every indication that this technique will become more standard over time.

Evaluation of the Pretreatment Plan

Development of an acceptable plan through preplanning or intraoperative planning methods requires consideration of possible errors from seed migration and postoperative edema. The goal is to encompass the prostate with the prescription isodose line as uniformly as possible. A 3- to 5-mm margin is recommended, with the tighter margin posteriorly at the rectum. Davis and colleagues[248] and, more recently, Sohayda and colleagues[249] demonstrated that such margins would encompass extracapsular extension in more than 95% of cases of favorable disease treated with brachytherapy.

Evaluation After Treatment

It is customary to obtain a CT scan within 24 hours after the implant and another approximately 1 month later. The postplan evaluation is critical to quality assurance monitoring (Color Plate 30, after p. 80). A CT scan performed immediately after the implant represents the worse-case scenario because edema is pronounced, causing increased spacing of the seeds relative to one another.[250] Much of the swelling is gone by 1 month after the implant, and a CT scan performed 1 to 2 months after the implant, although inconvenient for some patients, provides a better estimate of dosimetry.[250,251]

In either case, postimplant DVH analyses of prostate V_{100} and D_{90} and other similar measures have been shown to correlate with clinical outcome. Color Plate 31, after p. 80 displays four images from a postimplant CT plan and the DVHs for the prostate, bladder, and rectum. Stock and colleagues[252] found that when the D_{90} approximated the prescribed dose of irradiation from ^{125}I, the freedom from biochemical failure rate was significantly better than for cases in which the D_{90} was below this level. The recommendations of the American Brachytherapy Society[253] are that the D_{90} be reported, as well as the D_{80}, D_{100}, V_{80}, V_{90}, V_{100}, V_{150}, and V_{200}.

For definitive prostate cancer treatment, the prescription dose from ^{125}I is 144 Gy and that from [103]Pd is 125 Gy. The prescription dose for prostate boost treatment, when PRSIP is used in conjunction with external-beam radiation therapy, is 110 Gy for ^{125}I and 90 Gy for [103]Pd. Before publication of the American Association of Physicists in Medicine Task Group's report 43,[254] the standard reference dose for ^{125}I prostate implants was 160 Gy. The recommendations of Task Group 43 were based on a new National Institute of Standards and Technology (NIST) air-kerma standard for ^{125}I seeds, which was adjusted by about 10%.[255] The result is that

the prescription dose for ^{125}I implants was reduced to 144 Gy.[256] A similar adjustment has been made for [103]Pd.[257,258] Before the NIST-1999 standard, the prescribed dose for [103]Pd was 115 Gy; that dose should be changed to 125 Gy to achieve the same dosimetry.

Permanent Implantation of ^{125}I or [103]Pd Radioactive Seeds Plus External-Beam Radiation Therapy

Although no standard method has been established for the use of external-beam radiation therapy in combination with PRSIP, most investigators have given external-beam therapy first, followed approximately 2 weeks later with PRSIP. The rationale for substituting [103]Pd for ^{125}I is based on the hypothesis that poorly differentiated prostate tumors have a more rapid proliferation rate and consequently a shortened T_{pot}; hence [103]Pd, with its shorter half-life, would be more effective.[259,260] However, no clinical data exist to suggest that [103]Pd is any better than ^{125}I for the treatment of poorly differentiated or other high-risk forms of prostate cancer.

Critz and colleagues[154] have advocated administering ^{125}I before beginning a protracted course of external-beam radiation therapy given at 1.5 Gy/day during the active decay of the isotope. Others have advocated using [103]Pd and waiting about 2 months after the implant before giving external-beam radiation therapy. The typical sequence, however, is for external-beam therapy to be given first, followed about 2 weeks later by PRSIP.[243,261] The usual external-beam radiation dose is 45 to 50 Gy, given over 5 to 5½ weeks.

Temporary [192]Ir Implants

Temporary implants with high-dose-rate (HDR) [192]Ir are usually combined with external-beam therapy for the treatment of patients with intermediate- to high-risk prostate cancer. The procedure is similar to that for permanent implants, in that temporary afterloading needles are placed transperineally into the prostate under sonographic guidance.[262,263] A pretreatment plan may be used, but real-time planning in the operating room has been used to optimize needle placement.[264] HDR ^{192}Ir implants are more forgiving than are ^{125}I or [103]Pd permanent implants; CT planning in HDR ^{192}Ir is performed before the sources are placed, and the time at which the source dwells at particular points can be adjusted to optimize the dose distribution. The dose of each HDR fraction, the HDR interfraction intervals, and the sequencing with external-beam radiation therapy have varied greatly among investigators. Dosing schemes have ranged from 3.0 to 4.0 Gy in four fractions over 40 hours[262] to 9.5 Gy in two fractions over 2 weeks,[264] and implantation with the HDR ^{192}Ir seeds has been performed before, during, and after the external-beam radiation.[262,264-266]

RADIATION THERAPY RESULTS
Radiation Therapy Alone for Favorable Disease
Treatment Options

Treatment outcome for patients with pretreatment PSA levels of 10 ng/ml or less, a Gleason score of less than 7, and category T1 to T2a disease (according to the 1992 staging system) is very favorable. Outcome after radical prostatectomy, brachytherapy alone, external-beam therapy alone, and the combination of external-beam plus brachytherapy has been comparable. Direct comparisons among single-institution series are complicated by imbalanced prognostic factors and length of follow-up; however, little difference among institutions seems to be found for patients with favorable risk factors. Poorer results are evident if external-beam radiation therapy doses are low.[267-269] In a study of 1213 PSA-era patients treated at the M.D. Anderson Cancer Center with only external-beam irradiation through 1998, the Kaplan-Meier freedom from biochemical failure rates for the 281 patients with favorable risk factors were 88% at 5 years and 84% at 10 years (see Fig. 27-4). The freedom from failure rates for the 713 patients in this study who were treated to more than 67 Gy are shown in Figure 27-8; among the 199 favorable-risk patients in that subgroup, the freedom from failure rate at 5 years was 92%, with no treatment failures observed after 5 years. These results are similar to those of other series evaluating external-beam therapy[163,268,270-272] (Table 27-3), radical prostatectomy (Table 27-4),[101,103,148,273,274] or brachytherapy (Table 27-5)[242,243,271,275-277] for patients with prostate cancer.

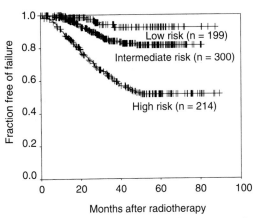

Fig. 27-8 Freedom from biochemical failure rates for 713 patients with prostate cancer treated at the M.D. Anderson Cancer Center with external-beam irradiation to a dose of more than 67 Gy.

Direct comparisons of results from the use of external-beam radiation therapy alone, brachytherapy alone, and radical prostatectomy have been attempted. Zelefsky and colleagues[278] compared patients undergoing external-beam radiation therapy only and those treated with ^{125}I PRSIP at Memorial Sloan-Kettering Cancer Center and found essentially no difference in freedom from biochemical failure rates (88% and 82%, $P = 0.09$). They did note that protracted urinary symptoms of grade 2 or higher were more prevalent in the implantation group. In a study of 2222 men with prostate cancer, Brachman and colleagues[271] found that external-beam radiation therapy produced results similar to those of PRSIP among patients with favorable risk factors. D'Amico and

TABLE 27-3
External-Beam Radiation Series According to Pretreatment Prostate-Specific Antigen Level

Variable	STUDY AND REFERENCE			
	M.D. Anderson Cancer Center, 2000	Hanks et al, 2000[272]	Brachman et al, 2000[271]	Shipley et al, 1999[161]
Number of patients	713*	377†	1527	1765‡
Median follow-up	46 mo	53 mo	41 mo	> 60 mo
Time of analysis	5 yr	5 yr	5 yr	5 yr
Freedom from biochemical failure rates				
All patients	71%	—	—	66%
Patients with PSA§ ≤ 4	88%	—	90%	81%
Patients with PSA > 4-10	80%	—	74%	68%
Patients with PSA > 10-20	63%	~84%	70%	51%
Patients with PSA > 20	32%	~40%	51%	31%
Patients with PSA ≤ 10	81%	~90%	—	78%
Patients with PSA > 10	56%	~52%	—	—

PSA, Prostate-specific antigen.
*Patients treated in the PSA era (i.e., after 1988) were given doses of more than 67 Gy.
†Dose-escalated group.
‡Pooled multi-institutional analysis.
§PSA levels are expressed in ng/ml.

TABLE 27-4

Surgical Series According to Pretreatment Prostate-Specific Antigen Level

	STUDY AND REFERENCE			
Variable	Pound et al, 1997[273]	Kupelian et al, 1996[101]	Dillioglugil et al, 1997[148]	Catalona et al, 1998[274]
Number of patients	1354	337	536	1615
Median follow-up	60 mo	36 mo	24 mo	—*
Time of analysis	5 yr	5 yr	5 yr	5 yr
Freedom from biochemical failure rates				
All patients	80%	61%	78%	—
Patients with PSA[†] ≤ 4	94%	89%	93%	—
Patients with PSA > 4-10	82%	63%	76%	~95%
Patients with PSA > 10-20	72%	57%	69%	~85%
Patients with PSA > 20	54%	27%	46%	—
Patients with PSA ≤ 10	—	71%	—	—
Patients with PSA > 10	—	42%	—	~58%

PSA, Prostate-specific antigen.
*Follow-up for patients with postoperative PSA determinations was not stated.
[†]PSA levels are expressed in ng/ml.

TABLE 27-5

^{125}I Implant Series According to Pretreatment Prostate-Specific Antigen Level

	STUDY AND REFERENCE			
Variable	Blasko et al, 1995[242]	Wallner et al, 1996[275]	Grado et al, 1998[276]	Brachman et al, 2000[271]
Number of patients	197	92	490	695
Median follow-up	36 mo	36 mo	27 mo	51 mo
Time of analysis	4 yr	4 yr	5 yr	5 yr
Freedom from biochemical failure rates				
All patients	93%	63%	79%	—
Patients with PSA* ≤ 4	98%	100%	—	87%
Patients with PSA > 4-10	90%	80%	—	76%
Patients with PSA > 10-20	89%	45%	72%	53%
Patients with PSA > 20	80%	38%	57%	49%
Patients with PSA ≤ 10	—	—	88%	—
Patients with PSA > 10	—	57%	—	—

PSA, Prostate-specific antigen.
*PSA levels are expressed in ng/ml.

colleagues[160] compared outcome among patients from selected institutions who were given external-beam radiation therapy, PRSIP, or radical prostatectomy. At a median follow-up of 38 months, no statistically significant difference in freedom from failure was noted for the favorable-risk patients. Stokes and colleagues[279] reached a similar conclusion. However, when Polascik and colleagues[280] and Ramos and colleagues[281] tried to match their radical prostatectomy patients to the ^{125}I-PRSIP patients described by Ragde and colleagues,[282] the two groups came to different conclusions. Polascik and colleagues[280] found that the 7-year freedom from

biochemical failure rates were 97.8% in the surgery group compared with 79% for the brachytherapy group in the study by Ragde and colleagues,[282] suggesting that surgery was the treatment of choice. Ramos and colleagues,[281] on the other hand, quoted a 7-year freedom from biochemical failure rate of 84% and concluded that surgery and brachytherapy were equally effective. These different conclusions underscore the problems in trying to match patient prognostic factors between institutions. Finally, Keyser and colleagues[270] and Kupelian and colleagues[283] found no difference in outcome between external-beam therapy and radical prostatectomy for favorable-risk patients, despite their later finding of a significant dose-response effect among those patients.[269]

Brachytherapy Alone

The use of brachytherapy in the treatment of prostate cancer has shown a resurgence over the past 15 years, due in large part to the introduction of TRUS for treatment planning and needle placement by a group at the Northwest Prostate Institute in Seattle.[242,243] Several variants of brachytherapy are in use, but most involve the methods described above for permanent radioactive seed–implant monotherapy. [125]I and [103]Pd seeds have been used interchangeably, and no clear-cut evidence has been found that either isotope is more effective than the other. The half-life of [103]Pd is 17 days, which is shorter than the 60-day half-life of [125]I. As noted earlier, some believe that the shorter half-life of [103]Pd is preferable for treating high-grade tumors, which potentially have a shorter doubling time.[259,260] This hypothesis, although seemingly sound, has not been borne out in clinical studies. The T_{pot} of prostate cancer may actually be long enough to favor ^{125}I, even in poorly differentiated tumors.[170-172]

The effectiveness of PRSIP monotherapy has been established in several studies[242,243,271,275-277] (see Table 27-5). This treatment has been shown repeatedly to be most effective for men with a pretreatment serum PSA concentration of no more than 10 ng/ml, a Gleason score of no more than 6, and stage T1 to T2a disease according to the 1992 AJCC staging system. The 1992 AJCC staging system is used here because of the suggested difference between palpable category T2a, T2b, and T2c tumors[81,101,104] (see Fig. 27-3, C). D'Amico and colleagues[160] observed in a retrospective review that the freedom from biochemical failure rates for patients with intermediate- or high-risk prognostic characteristics were significantly lower when treated with PRSIP than when similar patients were treated with external-beam irradiation or radical prostatectomy. Again, no difference between these modalities was observed for patients with favorable prognostic characteristics.

The best results with PRSIP monotherapy have resulted from strict adherence to selection criteria. Most investigators consider such criteria of proportion of biopsy specimens that are positive for tumor, amount of tumor in the specimens, and whether tumor is present bilaterally. These rather subjective criteria are used routinely in the clinic, but they have not been rigorously tested. For example, a patient with otherwise favorable risk factors and a small 1- to 2-mm focus of Gleason grade 7 disease might be considered for PRSIP over someone with three of six biopsy cores containing Gleason 6 disease that involves more than half of each positive core. No distinct guidelines have been developed for the use of biopsy tissue findings such as these, and further work is needed in this area.

The rationale for selecting a treatment strategy on the basis of biopsy findings is that the incidence of extracapsular extension increases as the number of positive biopsy specimens and the extent of tumor in the specimens increase.[117,284,285] The accuracy of the biopsy findings mentioned here depends on the adequacy of the sampling. Sextant biopsies may not be enough to appreciate the extent of disease, particularly if a small focus of Gleason 7 is present. Repeat biopsy in such cases often reveals a larger tumor burden.

Other considerations in the selection of patients for PRSIP are baseline urinary function status, whether the patient has previously undergone TURP, and baseline prostate volume. PRSIP causes significant urinary obstructive symptoms that seem to be greater than those resulting from external-beam radiation therapy. Difficulty emptying the bladder may be experienced for prolonged periods after PRSIP. Urinary side effects tend to resolve 6 to 12 months after the implantation, but improvements may be noted even beyond a year. Alpha-adrenergic blockers such as doxazosin (Cardura), terazosin (Hytrin), or niflumic acid (Flomax) are used liberally during this period to reduce the frequency of nocturia and other symptoms of urinary obstruction.

The American Urological Association symptom index questionnaire or a similar scoring system is useful in identifying patients who may be predisposed to urinary obstruction after PRSIP.[286,287] However, the decision cutpoints on the scale are arbitrary. Certainly a high score, for example, 15 or more, implies additional risk of prolonged urinary obstructive symptoms and the possible need for catheterization or TURP after implantation. Intermediate scores above 10 probably also reflect a higher risk, and clinical judgment through experience is helpful. Consideration should be given to whether the patient is already taking an alpha blocker.

A history of TURP before PRSIP has been associated in the past with an increased risk of urinary incontinence after the implantation,[242,275] which may be related to older, uniform seed distribution methods. Recent studies indicate that peripheral loading techniques can be helpful in avoiding urinary complications in patients who have undergone TURP.[287,288] Another concern is prostate volume and the possibility of interference from the pubic arch. The prostate sits behind the pubic symphysis, and if the gland is large, its lateral aspect may be blocked for needle placement. Placing the patient in an extended lithotomy position minimizes the possibility of pubic arch interference. Although the frequency of pubic arch interference increases as prostate volume exceeds 50 cm^3, TRUS and pelvic CT scanning have been helpful in estimating the risk of this condition before the implant is placed,[289,290] and some patients with large prostates have undergone successful implantation with excellent dosimetry and low morbidity.[291,292] Patients with large prostates, however, are predisposed to experience postimplantation urinary symptoms.[293] The isotope used also can influence the incidence of urinary side effects; urinary morbidity after [103]Pd implantation may not last as long as morbidity after ^{125}I implantation.[294] Late rectal complications after PRSIP may be less than those seen after external-beam therapy.[295] Impotence rates after PRSIP[296-298] do not seem to differ much from those after external-beam therapy (about 50%) overall.[15,16,299] The overall rates of side effects associated with PRSIP, once urinary symptoms resolve, have been low[300] and are comparable to those associated with external-beam radiation therapy.

Radiation Therapy for Intermediate-Risk to High-Risk Disease

Brachytherapy in Combination With External-Beam Radiation Therapy

The options currently available for the treatment of intermediate- to high-risk prostate cancer include an expanding list of techniques that combine external-beam and brachytherapy. These options include PRSIP with ^{125}I or [103]Pd given before or after external-beam therapy,[154,243,261,301] PRSIP with [198]Au plus external-beam therapy (with the implant usually given first[235]), or temporary HDR ^{192}Ir given before, during, or after external-beam therapy.[262,264-266] Each method has technical advantages and disadvantages, and at present comparisons among them are not available. However, results from small retrospective series have been promising. Ragde and colleagues[243] have shown that after long follow-up, the results after PRSIP plus external-beam therapy were slightly, but not significantly, better than results with PRSIP alone, even though the patients treated with PRSIP alone had more favorable risk features.

As has been found for external-beam monotherapy[162,195,269,302,303] and PRSIP monotherapy,[252] a dose-response relationship seems to exist for the combination therapy as well. Martinez and colleagues[264] have gradually escalated the biological equivalent dose from HDR ^{192}Ir implants given during external-beam therapy to 46 Gy. Their preliminary results suggest that the higher biological equivalent doses were associated with improved outcome, but the follow-up period in this study was short.

External-Beam Radiation Therapy Alone: Dose-Response Evaluations

Figure 27-4 displays a Kaplan-Meier analysis of freedom from biochemical failure for patients with favorable-, intermediate-, or high-risk disease treated with external-beam radiation monotherapy at the M.D. Anderson Cancer Center between 1987 and 1998. Those rates at 5 years and 8 years were 70% and 67%, respectively, for the intermediate-risk group and 39% and 34% for the high-risk group.

The evidence in support of three-dimensional CRT and IMRT in the treatment of prostate cancer has been decisive. The margins around the prostate have been reduced, and as a consequence, both the volume of normal tissue that is treated to higher doses and the side effects have been reduced without sacrificing tumor control. These treatment techniques have allowed the dose to be escalated significantly. Patients with intermediate- to high-risk features have benefited greatly from these approaches.

Retrospective dose-response analyses in pre-PSA era studies have been promising. Hanks and colleagues[304,305] and Perez and colleagues[306,307] reported that local control was greater in patients with locally advanced disease when the dose was increased. Conventional radiation techniques were used, although greater side effects were observed when the doses were more than 70 Gy. In a single-institution trial at Massachusetts General Hospital, a proton boost was used to escalate dose from 67.2 Gy to 75.6 Gy.[308] In that trial, the higher dose afforded by the boost did not produce a statistically significant benefit in disease freedom or survival, although the local control rate at 8 years was improved from 19% to 84% ($P = 0.0014$). Freedom-from-disease rates were better in the subset of patients with Gleason 8 to 10 disease who received the higher dose. The patients in this study had locally advanced disease and thus are not representative of patients seen in the PSA era. Nevertheless, several retrospective studies in the PSA era strongly support the conviction that radiation dose is an independent correlate of patient outcome.[162,269,272,302,303]

A positive effect of dose escalation above 70 Gy on freedom from biochemical failure rates has consistently been described for patients with intermediate-risk features such as a PSA level of 10 to 20 ng/ml. Dramatic gains in freedom from biochemical failure can be achieved with a modest elevation in dose (Table 27-6).[162,269,272] The caveat is that dose was raised sequentially in these trials over time, and during that time stage migration was also evident. Randomized comparisons are needed to substantiate observations made in the retrospective analyses.

A randomized dose-escalation trial conducted in the PSA era at the M.D. Anderson Cancer Center was recently reported.[195] Patients were randomly assigned to receive 70 Gy delivered with conventional fields or 78 Gy via a conformal boost technique. Stratification of the 301 evaluable patients was based on pretreatment PSA values. Dose was specified to the isocenter, as was the standard practice at the M.D. Anderson Cancer Center when the trial was begun in 1993. As noted earlier in the section on three-dimensional treatment planning and CRT, the current recommendation is to prescribe to the PTV, which is consistent with the criteria of the International Commission on Radiation Units and Measurements.[203] The freedom from biochemical failure rates for the two treatment groups are illustrated in Figure 27-9.[195]

TABLE 27-6

External-Beam Radiation Therapy: Retrospective Dose-Escalation Studies

Study and Reference	Number of Patients	Risk	PERCENT FREE FROM BIOCHEMICAL FAILURE AT 5 YEARS		
			Dose 1	Dose 2	P Value
Zelefsky et al, 1998[162]*	743	Low	87 (≤ 70 Gy)	96 (≥ 75.6 Gy)	NS
		Intermediate	56 (≤ 70 Gy)	78 (≥ 75.6 Gy)	0.04
		High	37 (≤ 70 Gy)	53 (≥ 75.6 Gy)	0.03
Lyons et al, 2000[269]	738	Low	81 (< 72 Gy)	98 (≥ 72 Gy)	0.02
		High	41 (< 72 Gy)	75 (≥ 72 Gy)	0.001
Hanks et al, 2000[272]	618	Low†	86 (< 70 Gy)	80 (≥ 70 Gy)	NS
		Intermediate	29 (< 71.5 Gy)	66 (≥ 71.5 Gy)	< 0.05
		High	8 (< 71.5 Gy)	29 (≥ 71.5 Gy)	< 0.05
M.D. Anderson Cancer Center Study, 2000	1213	Low	84 (≤ 67 Gy)	91 (> 67-70 Gy)	NS
		Low	91 (> 67-77 Gy)	100 (> 77 Gy)	NS
		Intermediate	55 (≤ 67 Gy)	79 (> 67-70 Gy)	0.0001
		Intermediate	79 (> 67-77 Gy)	89 (> 77 Gy)	NS
		High	27 (≤ 67 Gy)	47 (> 67-77 Gy)	0.0001
		High	47 (> 67-77)	67 (> 77 Gy)	0.016

NS, Not significant.
*4-Year results.
†Based on pretreatment prostate-specific antigen (PSA) level.

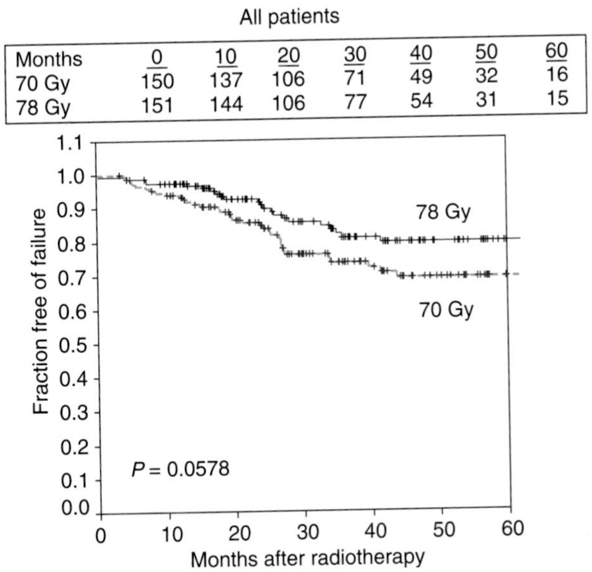

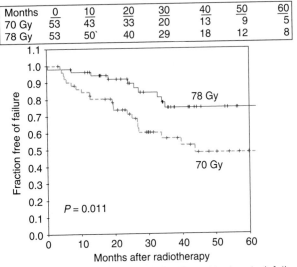

Fig. 27-9 Freedom from biochemical failure rates after external-beam irradiation to 70 Gy (by conventional radiation therapy) or 78 Gy (by conformal boost radiation therapy) in a randomized dose-escalation trial at the M.D. Anderson Cancer Center. The 5-year freedom from biochemical failure rates were 69% in the group treated to 70 Gy and 79% in the group treated to 78 Gy. (From Pollack A, Zagars GK, Smith LG, et al. *J Clin Oncol* 2000;18:3904-3911.)

Fig. 27-10 Differences in freedom from biochemical failure rates after external-beam irradiation to 70 Gy (by conventional radiation therapy) or 78 Gy (by conformal boost radiation therapy) among men with pretreatment prostate-specific antigen levels of more than 10 ng/ml. (From Pollack A, Zagars GK, Smith LG, et al. *J Clin Oncol* 2000;18:3904-3911.)

The apparent difference at 5 years was of borderline statistical significance (79% for the 78-Gy group vs. 69% for the 70-Gy group, $P = 0.06$). The greatest gain was seen for intermediate-risk or high-risk patients who had pretreatment PSA levels of more than 10 ng/ml;

among those subjects, the freedom from failure rates were 75% for the 78-Gy group and 48% for the 70-Gy group ($P = 0.01$; Fig. 27-10).[195] In that trial, however, only 16 patients had pretreatment PSA levels higher than 20 ng/ml, which tends to make this a more intermediate-risk than high-risk group. No difference in freedom from failure rates was found among the relatively favorable-risk subgroup with pretreatment PSA levels of 10 ng/ml or less. Another observation that may be important for future trials was that patients with the relatively favorable but still intermediate-risk features of category T1 to T2 disease and pretreatment PSA level of less than 10 ng/ml demonstrated the greatest difference in freedom from failure rates: 90% for the 78-Gy group vs. 60% for the 70-Gy group ($P = 0.01$). This observation prompted a review of the dose-response relationship among all patients treated in the PSA era (between 1987 and 1997) who had category T1 to T2 disease and pretreatment PSA values of less than 10 ng/ml.[302] The clear dose-response in this subgroup of patients is shown in Figure 27-11.[302]

A prospective randomized trial[309] and several retrospective series have shown that three-dimensional CRT produces fewer side effects than standard techniques do when similar doses are used. Adverse side effects from dose escalation have primarily been rectal. Although significant bladder toxicity has not been reported, longer follow-up may be needed for such effects to become evident. Late rectal bleeding is the most common complication resulting from increasing the radiation dose to the prostate. In the M.D. Anderson Cancer Center randomized trial, the rates of grade 2 or higher rectal reactions at 5 years were 14% in the 70-Gy group and 21% in the 78-Gy group. Although this difference was not statistically significant, the finding that more than 20% of patients in the high-dose group experienced such reactions indicates that 78 Gy to the isocenter is near the limit for this technique.

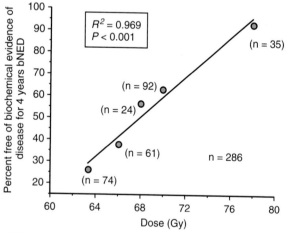

Fig. 27-11 Evidence of a radiation dose-response effect for patients with a pretreatment prostrate-specific antigen (PSA) level of more than 10 ng/ml and category T1-T2 disease treated at the M.D. Anderson Cancer Center with radiation therapy only. Freedom from biochemical failure at 4 years is plotted against the mean dose at five dose levels: ≤ 65 Gy ($N = 74$), 65 to 67 Gy ($N = 61$), > 67 to 69 Gy ($N = 24$), > 69 to 77 Gy ($N = 92$), and > 77 Gy ($N = 35$). A highly significant linear relationship was found between mean dose at each level and freedom from failure. (From Pollack A, Smith LG, von Eschenbach AC. *Int J Radiat Oncol Biol Phys* 2000;48:507-512.)

Rectal reactions have been shown to be a function of dose and volume. The relationship of prescribed dose to the prostate and the incidence of rectal complications of grade 2 or higher is shown in Table 27-7.[14,162,199,308,310] The irradiated volume is also an important determinant of rectal toxicity (Table 27-8).[14,199,309,311,312] For example, Lee and colleagues[199] observed that restricting the dose to the anterior rectal wall to 72 Gy or less reduced the incidence of rectal bleeding from 22% to 7%. In the M.D. Anderson Cancer Center trial, a DVH analysis was performed for patients given the 78-Gy conformal boost treatment to examine possible predictors of rectal bleeding.[14] When more than 25% of the rectum received 70 Gy or more, the 5-year actuarial incidence of grade 2 or higher rectal bleeding was 37%, as opposed to 13% when less than 25% of the rectum received 70 Gy or more (Fig. 27-12).

Risk of Lymph Node Involvement and Whole-Pelvis Treatment

Between 30% and 50% of patients with high-risk prostate cancer have lymph node involvement.[135,136] A key debate that has yet to be resolved has been whether to irradiate the whole pelvis in such patients. Several studies, both randomized and retrospective, have been done, but as yet no conclusive evidence exists to support this practice. RTOG protocol 77-06 examined the use of elective pelvic irradiation for patients with stage A2 or B (T1b or T2) prostatic carcinoma without clinical evidence of lymph node involvement. This population was estimated to have about a 25% risk of nodal involvement. Elective lymph-node treatment did not significantly affect outcome.

With regard to the retrospective data, the reports are about evenly split between those that support this treatment[313-317] and those that do not.[233,318-320] There is

TABLE 27-7

External-Beam Radiation Therapy: Doses that Produce Rectal Reactions of Grade 2 or Higher

Study and Reference	Dose	Incidence of Rectal Toxicity	Time at Analysis
Smit et al, 1990[310]	≤ 70 Gy	22%	2 yr
	70-75 Gy	20%	
	> 75 Gy	60%	
Shipley et al, 1995[308]	67.2 Gy	12%*	10 yr
	75.6 CGE	32%	
Lee et al, 1996[199]	< 72 Gy	7%	1.5 yr
	72-76 Gy	16%	
	> 76 Gy	23%	
Zelefsky et al, 1998[162]	≤ 70.2	6%	5 yr
	> 75.6	17%	
Storey et al, 2000[14]	70 Gy	14%	5 yr
	78 Gy	21%	

CGE, Cobalt Gray equivalent.
*Grade 1 and 2 rectal reactions.

TABLE 27-8

External-Beam Radiation Therapy: Rectal Volume Irradiated and Rectal Reactions of Grade 2 or Higher

Study and Reference	Dose	Rectal Volume Irradiated	Rate of Rectal Toxic Effects
Benk et al, 1993[311]	75 CGE	< 40% ARW	19% (40-month actuarial)*
	75 CGE	≥ 40% ARW	71%
Lee et al, 1996[199]	74-76 Gy	Rectal block	10% (18-month actuarial)
	74-76 Gy	No block	19%
Dearnaley et al, 1999[309]	64 Gy	3-D CRT	8% (5-yr actuarial)
	64 Gy	Conven-RT	18%
Boersma et al, 1998[312]	70 Gy	≤ 30%	0% (crude)†
	70 Gy	> 30%	9%
Storey et al, 2000[14]	70 Gy	≤ 25%	13% (5-yr actuarial)
	70 Gy	> 25%	37%

CGE, Cobalt Gray equivalent; *ARW*, anterior rectal wall; *3-D CRT*, three-dimensional conformal radiation therapy; *Conven-RT*, conventional radiation therapy.
*Any rectal bleeding.
†Severe rectal bleeding.

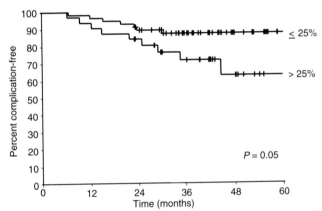

Fig. 27-12 Kaplan-Meier analysis of the incidence of rectal reactions (grade 2 or higher) among patients in the M.D. Anderson Cancer Center dose-escalation trial divided by the percentage of rectum that had been treated to 70 Gy or more. The incidence of rectal side effects was significantly reduced when the amount of rectum receiving 70 Gy or more was less than 25%. (From Storey MR, Pollack A, Zagars GK, et al. *Int J Radiat Oncol Biol Phys* 2000;48:635-642.)

obvious reluctance to limit coverage of areas known to harbor tumor in nearly 40% of patients with prostate cancer. This question is still under investigation by the RTOG in the context of an AA trial (see below), which is more pertinent to the type of therapy that patients with high-risk disease currently receive.

External Beam Radiation Therapy With Androgen Ablation for Clinically High-Risk Disease

The rationale for combining external-beam radiation therapy with AA is that the combination is expected to be more effective in eradicating prostate cancer than would either treatment given separately. Because both modalities cause apoptosis, the suggestion has been made that the combination of the two may result in additive or supra-additive cell killing.[321-323] From an additive perspective, neoadjuvant AA reduces the number of clonogens that must be eradicated by irradiation, and thus the combination should result in improved local control. This hypothesis was initially tested by the RTOG in phase II clinical trials[324,325] and more recently in phase III trials.[326,327]

As summarized in the following paragraphs, the advantage of giving AA before irradiation, as opposed to starting both modalities together, has never been established. Notably, the distinction between neoadjuvant and adjuvant AA is blurred in clinical trials. Neoadjuvant AA is defined as that begun before irradiation, but AA is then continued during the irradiation and for various periods afterward. Adjuvant AA, on the other hand, is that begun during the irradiation; however, when adjuvant AA is started at the beginning of a protracted course of radiation, the tumor shrinks during the irradiation such that fewer clonogens remain at the end of the radiation period. Thus a component of adjuvant AA is in neoadjuvant treatment and vice versa. No evidence has been found to indicate that the results from external-beam radiation therapy preceded by neoadjuvant AA are any different than those achieved with adjuvant AA when the AA is begun at the same time as the irradiation.

Another reason for starting AA before irradiation is to shrink exceptionally large prostates so that the volume of rectum and bladder receiving high doses of radiation is lessened when conformal radiation therapy is applied. This philosophy is espoused by several groups[328-331] (Table 27-9). The prostate shrinks by 30% to 40% in response to 3 months of neoadjuvant AA, and DVH analyses have confirmed significant reductions in the proportions of bladder and rectum that receive 80% to 90% of the prescribed dose. Although these gains will surely translate into reductions in morbidity, the effect

TABLE 27-9

External-Beam Radiation Therapy Given After 3 Months of Androgen Ablation: Effect on Target Volume

Study and Reference	Number of Patients	REDUCTION IN VOLUME (%)		
		Prostate*	Rectum†	Bladder†
Shearer et al, 1992[328]	22	43%	—	—
Yang et al, 1995[329]	7	43%	28 (D_{80})	46 (D_{80})
Forman et al, 1995[330]	20	37%	34 (D_{93})	20 (D_{93})
Zelefsky et al, 1994[331]	22	25%*	25 (D_{95})	50 (D_{95})

*Reduction in target volume.

†Reduction in the percent volume of the rectum or bladder receiving 80% (D_{80}), 93% (D_{93}), or 95% (D_{95}) of the prescribed dose.

of shrinking the PTV with neoadjuvant AA before irradiation in patients with locally advanced disease and extracapsular extension is uncertain. Microscopic foci could be left in the regions where the prostate was originally, regions that after neoadjuvant AA would be filled by rectum or bladder. The published randomized trials that have incorporated neoadjuvant AA[326,327,332-339] (Table 27-10) used whole-pelvis fields initially, with more generous coverage of the periprostatic tissues than can usually be accomplished with three-dimensional CRT.

Interest in combined external-beam radiation therapy and AA has increased in the past several years, primarily in response to encouraging results from randomized trials. Results from published randomized studies, most of which compared external-beam radiation therapy used alone and with AA, are summarized in Table 27-10. Only one trial failed to demonstrate superior rates of freedom from failure (disease or biochemical evidence of disease when available) for treatment with both modalities. A survival advantage also was ascribed to the external-beam radiation therapy plus AA combination in many of these trials. Brief reviews of each trial are given below.

The M.D. Anderson Cancer Center diethylstilbestrol trial. The earliest multi-institutional randomized trial of external-beam radiation therapy with or without AA was championed by Del Regato[340] in the 1960s for locally advanced, category T3 to T4 prostate cancer. AA was accomplished by using diethylstilbestrol, a synthetic estrogen, beginning at the end of the irradiation period. The trial design was to continue the diethylstilbestrol indefinitely. Results from this study were never published in their entirety, but Zagars and colleagues[332] published the results of patients who were randomized and treated at the M.D. Anderson Cancer Center. At a median follow-up of 14.5 years, a highly significant and sustained improvement in freedom from disease was noted for those treated with external-beam irradiation plus AA (see Table 27-10). No survival difference was detected, a finding that may have been attributable to the small number of patients in each

group (approximately 40) and excess intercurrent deaths as a consequence of the diethylstilbestrol. The high dose of diethylstilbestrol (5 mg/day) used when the trial was begun was later reduced in light of evidence that this dose caused increased cardiac mortality from thromboembolic events.[341]

RTOG 86-10. In RTOG protocol 86-10,[326,337] patients in the combined-modality group were given a short course of neoadjuvant AA starting 2 months before external-beam radiation therapy and continuing throughout the irradiation period. Of the 471 patients entered, 456 were evaluable. Eligibility criteria included having local–regionally advanced disease, with T2 to T4 tumors (larger than 25 cm^2 on digital rectal examination). Smaller tumors with evidence of lymph node involvement below the common iliac vessels also were permitted. The median follow-up was 4.5 years. Standard radiation doses were used, with 45 Gy given to the pelvis plus a 20- to 25-Gy boost to the prostate. Extended fields were used to treat the lymph nodes when they were involved. Total AA was accomplished by using goserelin and flutamide. Statistically significant improvements in local control rate and freedom from biochemical failure rate were observed (see Table 27-10), along with a borderline improvement in the rate of freedom from distant metastasis. No difference in overall survival was seen. In a recent update of this trial, these relationships were strengthened and a survival benefit was noted for patients with Gleason 2 to 6 disease.[337]

RTOG 85-31. The RTOG 85-31 protocol[334,339] also involved patients with local–regionally advanced disease, including those who had undergone primary definitive treatment with radiation as well as those who had undergone radical prostatectomy and were identified at pathologic examination as being at high risk. The definitively irradiated patients were men with clinical category T3 (< 25 cm^2) or T1 to T2 disease with radiographic or histologic lymph node involvement (including the para-aortic nodes). Patients were eligible after prostatectomy if capsular penetration with positive margins or seminal vesicle involvement was found. Of 977 patients enrolled,

TABLE 27-10

External-Beam Radiation Therapy Plus Androgen Ablation: Results of Randomized Trials

Study and Reference	Length or Type of Androgen Ablation	Follow-up Period	5-YEAR FREEDOM FROM FAILURE RATE, % (n)		5-YEAR OVERALL SURVIVAL RATE, % (n)		5-YEAR OVERALL SURVIVAL RATE FOR SUBGROUPS, % (n)		
			RT Alone	RT + AA	RT Alone	RT + AA	Subgroup	RT Alone	RT + AA
RTOG 86-10[326,337]	≈4 mo^N	4.5 yr	15 (200)	36 (196)*	~56 (230)	~56 (226)	GL 2-6	52 (NS)	70 (NS)*
Umea University[336]	Perm^N	9.3 yr	39 (46)	69 (45)*	39 (46)	62 (45)*	LN+	0 (20)	50 (19)*
M.D. Anderson Cancer Center[332]	Perm^A	14.5 yr	49 (40)	71 (38)*	68 (40)	73 (38)	—	—	—
MRC[333]	Perm^A	4.5 yr	~30 (88)	~44 (99)	~43 (88)	~58 (99)	—	—	—
RTOG 85-31[334,339]	Perm^A	4.5 yr	20 (429)	53 (438)*	71 (68)	75 (477)	GL 8-10	55 (137)	66 (139)*†
EORTC[335]	3 yr^A	45 mo	48 (208)	85 (207)*	62 (208)	79 (207)*	—	—	—
			RT + AA4	RT + AA28	RT + AA4	RT + AA28		RT + AA4	RT + AA28
RTOG 92-02[327]	4 mo^N vs. 28 mo^N	48 mo	21 (NS)	46 (NS)*	78 (NS)	79 (NS)	GL 8-10	69 (NS)	80 (NS)*
			Early†	Late†	Early†	Late†		Early	Late
MRC[338]	Early vs. late	NS	68 (256)	32 (201)*	37 (469)	43 (465)*	M0	50 (256)	44 (244)*

Modified from Pollack A, Kuban D, Zagars GK. *Urology* 2002;60(suppl 3A):22-30.

RT, Radiation therapy; AA, androgen ablation; RTOG, Radiation Therapy Oncology Group; N, neoadjuvant; GL, Gleason score; NS, not stated; Perm, permanent; LN+, lymph node–positive; A, adjuvant; MRC, Medical Research Council (United Kingdom); EORTC, European Organization for Research and Treatment of Cancer.

*P < 0.05, log-rank test.

†Centrally reviewed Gleason score.

‡Freedom from distant metastasis rate for patients with M0 (nonmetastatic) disease.

945 were evaluable. Conventional radiation therapy techniques were used to deliver a total dose of 65 to 70 Gy, with the whole pelvis (and para-aortic lymph nodes as indicated) treated to 44 to 46 Gy. Radical prostatectomy patients were given a total dose of 65 to 66 Gy. AA was accomplished by monthly injections of goserelin acetate (Zoladex) beginning the last week of radiation therapy. Combined-modality treatment reduced the 5-year rates of local failure (16% vs. 28%), distant metastasis (17% vs. 30%), and biochemical failure (47% vs. 80%). All of these differences were highly statistically significant. No difference was observed in overall survival for the entire cohort; however, the survival rate of patients with Gleason 8 to 10 disease was better among those given combined-modality therapy (see Table 27-10).

Umea trial. In 1986 a trial at Umea University in Sweden was opened to patients with T1 to T4, pN0 to N3 disease. Patients were randomized to receive radiation therapy, given to relatively standard doses, or combined orchiectomy and radiation therapy. AA was started 5 weeks before the start of radiation therapy. The trial was closed early in 1991 when a survival benefit was observed favoring the combined-treatment group. A recent update of this trial,[336] now with a median follow-up of 9.3 years, shows that the combined-modality group continues to have higher rates of freedom from progression and overall survival. The survival benefit was attributed mainly to the effects on men with lymph node–positive disease, where 50% of those treated with radiation and AA remained alive at 10 years compared with no survivors in the group given only radiation. In this trial, early, permanent AA in combination with external-beam radiation therapy had a dramatic effect on survival.

European Organization for Research and Treatment of Cancer trial. Perhaps the most convincing study to document the benefit of combining AA plus radiation comes from the European Organization for Research and Treatment of Cancer. Bolla and colleagues[335] reported the results of this study, in which 415 men with locally advanced disease were randomly assigned to undergo external-beam radiation therapy, either alone or in combination with an extended but temporary course of AA. Most patients had stage T3 to T4 disease, although some had high-grade T1 to T2 disease. AA was accomplished by giving patients goserelin acetate (Zoladex) for 3 years. Cyproterone acetate was given during the first month to counter the surge in androgens that occurs with the first injection of a luteinizing hormone-releasing hormone agonist. The radiation therapy dose was 70 Gy. Median follow-up was 45 months. The local control rates were 97% in the combined-treatment group and 77% in the radiation-only group. Likewise, overall rates of freedom from disease (85% vs. 48%) and survival (79% vs. 62%, see Table 27-10) were significantly higher in the group given radiation therapy plus AA. The finding that overall survival rate was improved with only 45 months of follow-up was surprising. The authors showed that the difference in survival was mainly related to deaths from cancer. A reanalysis of the data in 1999[342] confirmed that the survival advantage from radiation therapy plus AA has been sustained.

RTOG 92-02. The randomized RTOG 92-02 trial[327] compared the efficacy of short-course AA, as was administered in RTOG 86-10, with that of long-course AA, similar in principle to the European study described above. The short-course group received 4 months of AA beginning 2 months before external-beam therapy. The long-course group received the same 4 months of AA before and during irradiation followed by an additional 24 months of AA. There were 1554 patients enrolled and median follow-up was 48 months. Standard radiation doses of 65 to 70 Gy were used, with the pelvic lymph nodes receiving 44 to 50 Gy. The patients had locally advanced T2c to T4 disease, with PSA levels less than 150 ng/ml. The trial was very important, first because it helped to clarify the benefit of long-course AA, and second because it was truly a contemporary PSA-era trial. Long-course AA conferred improvement in every end-point measured except overall survival; improvements were noted in 5-year rates of freedom from biochemical failure (46% vs. 21%; $P = 0.001$), freedom from distant metastasis (89% vs. 83%; $P = 0.001$), and cause-specific survival (92% vs. 87%; $P = 0.07$). In a subset analysis of patients with Gleason 8 to 10 disease, the overall survival rate was higher for those taking long-course AA (80% vs. 69%; $P = 0.02$), demonstrating, as was the case in RTOG protocol 85-10, that patients with high-grade disease require prolonged AA for maximum results.

Androgen ablation alone: the Medical Research Council trials. The need for an AA-alone control cannot be overstated. Except for the Medical Research Council trial, none of the other studies presented in Table 27-10 included such a control group because AA alone is considered palliative treatment and few patients in the United States would agree to participate. However, some evidence suggests that AA alone prolongs survival, which raises the question of what external-beam radiation therapy contributes to AA, especially when long-course AA is used.

The older Veterans Administration studies[341] compared early AA to delayed AA given at relapse. Although most of these studies did not seem to show any survival advantage for early AA, two factors may have played a role. One factor is that diethylstilbestrol, the synthetic estrogen used in most of these studies, predisposes its recipients to thromboembolic and cardiovascular events, resulting in early deaths. Another factor is that intercurrent deaths in older men make it more difficult to detect a survival advantage. When younger men were analyzed separately from older men,[343] early AA was found to confer a survival advantage over delayed AA.

A more recent large multi-institutional study sponsored by the Medical Research Council in the United Kingdom[338] reexamined this question using less toxic

AA methods. Early AA was achieved by either a luteinizing hormone–releasing hormone agonist or orchiectomy. Patients with locally advanced disease (category T2 to T4) or limited asymptomatic metastasis were enrolled. Early AA resulted in lower rates of disease progression and higher survival rates. Mortality was most significantly reduced among patients who had locally advanced disease with no evidence of distant metastasis; these are the patients who are typical of the candidates for the radiation therapy trials summarized in Table 27-10. Such findings emphasize the need for AA-only control groups so that the contribution of each modality toward outcome and survival can be deciphered.

To date, only one randomized trial that examined the utility of external-beam radiation therapy plus AA has included an AA-only group.[333] That trial has been criticized for being underpowered, with only about 90 patients/group, and for not specifying the radiation dose or techniques used. The local and distant failure rates were high (about 70% and 75%, respectively), and the overall survival rate was less than 40% at 7 years. These patients must have had exceedingly advanced disease. That no differences were observed between the AA-only group and the combined-treatment group is not surprising. This trial is not representative of the high-risk patient receiving external-beam radiation therapy plus AA today.

The findings from these Medical Research Council trials force caution in the interpretation of radiation therapy series, particularly because long-course AA suppresses androgens beyond the time of drug administration. Oefelein and colleagues[344] have shown that after a single depot injection, the median time for serum androgen levels to recover to baseline levels is more than 6 months. Still longer androgen-recovery periods have been noted after multiple injections.[345] The survival advantage from long-course AA plus external-beam radiation therapy may be attributable in part to the AA.

Short-course androgen ablation. The concept that short-course AA might be a substitute for radiation in patients with intermediate-risk prostate cancer has been brought to the forefront. In a retrospective analysis, D'Amico and colleagues[346] compared the effects of 6 months of AA plus external-beam irradiation to about 70 Gy to those of external-beam irradiation alone for patients with favorable-, intermediate- and high-risk prostate cancer. The radiation-only group consisted of 1310 patients, and the combined-therapy group had 276 patients. Median follow-up was only 28 months and was calculated from the date of diagnosis; thus follow-up from the completion of treatment was short. These investigators found that among the intermediate- and high-risk patients, combined-modality treatment improved freedom from biochemical failure rates. However, the actual differences in the Kaplan-Meier curves were slight, and very few patients were at risk of failure at 5 years in the combined-modality group. The slight

advantage reported for the short-course AA plus radiation therapy is not as great as the benefit from dose escalation. Moreover, the use of freedom from biochemical failure rates when follow-up is short may be misleading, because AA may delay failure. Substituting short-course AA for radiation dose is not advisable until longer follow-up results are available.

The finding from the RTOG 86-10 trial (see Table 27-10) that patients with Gleason scores of 2 to 6 obtained a survival advantage from external-beam therapy plus AA would suggest that short-course AA is beneficial. However, because the freedom from biochemical failure rates were extremely low, even for patients with more favorable prognostic features, these findings could be explained by slower tumor growth, even after testosterone levels had returned to normal. Animal model experiments have proven that this may occur.[347] Although administering short-course AA with external-beam radiation may be beneficial in that tumor growth is slowed far beyond the time when AA is withdrawn, the main objective is to enhance survival by curing patients of the disease. The other confounding factor is that the subgroup analysis in RTOG 86-10[337] was based on Gleason scores that were centrally reviewed rather than the Gleason scores that were used for stratification. An uneven distribution of prognostic factors in the treatment groups is therefore possible. Multivariate analysis was not reported. Dose escalation will be a necessary component of future trials to determine the role of short-course AA.

RTOG protocol 92-02, in which short-course AA plus external-beam radiation therapy was compared to long-course AA plus external-beam radiation therapy, revealed a survival advantage only for those patients who had Gleason scores of 8 to 10 (see Table 27-10). When considered with the findings described above, these data suggest that patients with Gleason scores of 2 to 6 should not be treated with extended AA plus irradiation, whereas patients with a Gleason score of 8 to 10 should. Although this may be true, longer follow-up would be more convincing. The freedom from biochemical failure and survival results must be examined together to distinguish between a survival advantage from cure vs. a survival advantage from a slowing of tumor growth.

External-Beam Radiation Therapy Plus Androgen Ablation for Lymph Node–Positive Disease

The results of single-modality treatment for regional lymph node–positive (stage D1) disease have been disappointing. The freedom from failure rates at 5 years produced by radiation therapy alone[233,348-353] (Table 27-11) and by radical prostatectomy alone[354-359] (Table 27-12) have been similar at about 20% to 30%. A slightly greater proportion of patients treated with AA alone have been free of failure at 5 years, although few patients remain free of progression by 10 years.[360]

TABLE 27-11

External-Beam Radiation Therapy for Lymph Node–Positive (Stage D1) Disease

Study and Reference	Number of Patients	Follow-Up Period (Months)	5-Year Disease-Free Survival Rate	5-Year Overall Survival Rate
Bagshaw et al, 1984[349]	60	> 60	~15%	~45%
Smith et al, 1984[348]	46	> 60	17%	60%
Gervasi et al, 1989[350]	152	103	22%	65%
Lawton et al,1992[351]	56	108	61%	76%
Hanks et al, 1993[352]	—	—	~30%	64%
Leibel et al, 1994[233]	345	105	~35%*	~70%
Lawton et al, 1997[353]	75	59	11%	65%

*Free of distant metastasis.

TABLE 27-12

Radical Prostatectomy for Lymph Node–Positive (Stage D1) Disease

Study and Reference	Number of Patients	Follow-Up Period (Months)	Disease-Free Survival Rate	Overall Survival Rate
deKernion et al, 1990[354]	35	72	~30%	~55% (5 yr)
Myers et al, 1992[355]	34	54	29%	
Zincke et al, 1992[356]	77	60	24%	71% (10 yr)*
Sgrignoli et al, 1994[357]	113	—	~20%	—
Messing et al, 1999[358]	51	85	—	~58% (10 yr)

*Cause-specific survival rate.

Standard treatment for regional lymph node–positive (stage D1) disease has been (and still is, for the most part) AA. Over the past 10 years, interest has been increasing in adding local therapy to AA to prolong freedom from progression.

Zagars and colleagues[360] found that local failure was the dominant site of progression in patients with lymph node–positive disease, with a median time to local failure of about 8 years. This observation prompted the policy to treat all such patients with permanent AA plus radiation therapy. The preliminary results were positive,[135] and a recent update by Zagars and colleagues[361] revealed that biochemical and clinical failure rates in patients treated with external-beam irradiation plus AA are far lower than those for men treated with AA alone (Fig. 27-13).[360] The AA-alone group consisted of 183 patients (median follow-up, 9.4 years) and the radiation-plus-AA group had 72 patients (median follow-up, 5.9 years). The median radiation dose was 70 Gy, and although generous fields were used, the whole pelvis was not treated. The differences observed between combined vs. AA-only treatment in univariate analyses were sustained in multivariate analyses; combined-modality treatment produced superior rates of freedom from biochemical failure, freedom from distant metastasis, and survival.

Radical prostatectomy may be equally effective at prolonging freedom from failure and survival when combined with AA in lymph node–positive patients.[358,362]

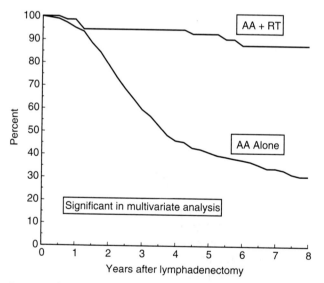

Fig. 27-13 Freedom from relapse or from a rising prostate-specific antigen level among patients with regional lymph node–positive (stage D1) prostate cancer treated with permanent androgen ablation *(AA)* and external-beam radiation therapy *(RT)* vs. AA alone. (From Zagars GK, Sands ME, Pollack A, et al. *J Urol* 1994;151:1330-1333.)

These findings indicate that the addition of a local treatment, such as radiation therapy or radical prostatectomy, to AA improves disease-free and overall survival rates. The RTOG attempted to contrast external-beam radiation therapy plus AA with AA alone in a randomized trial; however, accrual was too slow and the trial was closed. It is doubtful that a randomized trial will be successfully completed. The recommendation is to use radiation therapy plus permanent, or at least extended, AA for the treatment of lymph node–positive disease.

Particle-Beam Therapy

Information available on particle-beam therapy for prostate cancer regards mainly treatment with neutrons and protons. The efficacy of neutron or neutron-photon therapy was reportedly better than the efficacy of photons in two randomized trials, but the side effects of neutrons were significantly greater.[363-365] Some groups continue to use conformal neutrons, and the results remain encouraging.[366,367] It is impossible to assess from existing data the equivalence of neutrons or neutron-photons with dose-escalated photons. Given new data[178,179] indicating that prostate cancer may behave as a late-reacting tissue, interest may be renewed in directly comparing neutrons and photons in the PSA era.

Conformal proton therapy has tremendous potential in the treatment of prostate cancer. The Bragg peak and the similarity in the relative biological effectiveness of protons and photons creates the potential for precipitous dose fall-off beyond the PTV that is much greater for protons than for photons. With photons, the posterior aspect of the rectum usually receives about 50% of the prescribed dose. With protons, the posterior rectum would receive much less proportionally. All of the available results on the dose-volume relationships for rectal morbidity indicates that the complication rates should be lower with protons. A randomized proton boost trial done at Massachusetts General Hospital revealed increased late rectal bleeding in the proton-boost group, which may have been related to the use of a perineal field.[308,311] Results from studies conducted at Loma Linda[368] have been promising, but definitive clinical evidence that protons are superior to photons is still lacking.

Prostate Biopsies After Radiation Therapy

Much debate has ensued over the significance of positive prostate biopsy findings after definitive radiation therapy. Several groups have found high rates of positivity after radiation therapy,[369,370] even in patients with nonrising PSA profiles. The average biopsy positivity rate is about 40%. The assumption that all of these patients will experience treatment failure is unjustified given the findings of Cox and Stoffel[371] and others.[372-375] These investigators found that carcinoma cells are cleared from the prostate over time, suggesting that most of the treated carcinoma cells identified at biopsy eventually die.

In the M.D. Anderson Cancer Center randomized trial of conventional vs. conformal boost dose-escalation therapy,[195] prostate biopsies were performed at 2 years after treatment. A significant proportion of those biopsy samples contained "atypical cells consistent with or suspicious for treated carcinoma" or "carcinoma with treatment effect." The clonogenicity of such cells is unclear. The preliminary analysis of patients in that trial who did not have evidence of biochemical failure at the time of prostate biopsy revealed that the presence of carcinoma cells showing the treatment effect was associated with the same outcome as the presence of frank carcinoma cells.

Investigators at Memorial Sloan-Kettering Cancer Center have advocated that prostate biopsies be taken at 3 years after treatment to allow clearance and the demonstration of a dose response.[162,303] Staining with proliferation markers such as Ki-67 or proliferating-cell nuclear antigen may aid in establishing the true rate of residual cancer clonogenicity. Crook and colleagues[374,375] found that the presence of staining for proliferating-cell nuclear antigen in biopsy samples classified as "indeterminant" correlated with an increased frequency of relapse.

Salvage Procedures After Radiation Therapy

Biochemical failure precedes clinical manifestation of disease by several years, thus allowing much earlier identification of local relapse in the absence of detectable distant spread. Factors associated with slow progression of disease after biochemical failure include a delay in treatment failure of more than 2 years, a PSA doubling time of more than 1 year, and a Gleason score of less than 8.[140,146,376-378] These factors and others such as history or current evidence of extracapsular disease, serum PSA level (the lower the better; salvage therapy when PSA is >10 ng/ml is not advised), DNA ploidy,[379] and possibly the presence of molecular markers[380] should be considered when evaluating patients for salvage procedures. With appropriate selection of patients, salvage procedures are reasonable for young, healthy men with a life expectancy of at least 10 years, although complication rates are invariably high.

Salvage Prostatectomy

All of the reports on salvage prostatectomy suffer from relatively small patient numbers. Careful selection of patients is the key to obtaining 5-year freedom from failure rates of roughly 50% in the PSA era.[379-385] The rates of urinary incontinence and reoperation for complications are high.

Salvage Cryotherapy

Cryotherapy for prostate cancer that recurs after radiation therapy is also associated with high rates of urinary incontinence and severe complications requiring reoperation. Severe complications seem to occur more often and the freedom from failure rates are lower after salvage cryotherapy than after salvage prostatectomy.[386-390] Complications have included urinary incontinence, urinary obstruction, rectal or perineal pain, scrotal edema, hematuria, osteitis pubis, and rectourethral fistulas. Improvements in cryosurgical ablation through better temperature monitoring and control may reduce such side effects. Some groups remain optimistic about this approach; however, at the M.D. Anderson Cancer Center salvage cryosurgery for local radiation treatment failures has been abandoned in favor of salvage prostatectomy.

Salvage Radioactive Seed Implantation After External-Beam Radiation Therapy

Another option for addressing locally persistent prostate cancer after external-beam radiation therapy is brachytherapy by means of PRSIP.[391,392] Although published results in the PSA era have been limited, it seems that PRSIP under these circumstances produces long-term biochemical control in about 30% to 50% of cases. The results may be better with the use of stricter selection criteria. Thus far, the rates of side effects such as urinary incontinence have been lower after PRSIP than those after salvage prostatectomy or salvage cryotherapy. Severe complications have been infrequent.

RADICAL PROSTATECTOMY

Radical prostatectomy was first described more than 140 years ago. The initial perineal approach has given way to the retropubic approach now used by most surgeons. In the late 1970s and early 1980s, Walsh and colleagues[3,393] defined the anatomy of the dorsal vein and periprostatic venous complex and the neurovascular bundles controlling erectile function. These advancements led to nerve-sparing prostatectomy. The nerves that control erectile function are spared in patients for whom the risk of extracapsular extension is thought to be low. Sometimes the neurovascular bundle is sacrificed on one side where the risk of extracapsular extension is deemed to be high. When both nerves are left intact, the risk of impotence is reportedly as low as 15%.[394,395] When one nerve is sacrificed, the potency rate is further reduced by at least half. On average, the incidence of impotence after radical prostatectomy ranges from 40% to 60%,[396-400] with the higher rates typically being reported when questionnaires are used rather than face-to-face interviews.

Overall potency rates for a given population may be related to age, history of diabetes and coronary artery disease, use of medications (e.g., antihypertensives), and other factors. The timing of the assessment is also critical, as erectile function returns gradually after radical prostatectomy.[16] In contrast, erectile function decreases after radiation therapy.[16] Assessment should be made at least 1 year after surgery. In general, impotence rates after radical prostatectomy, when measured beyond 1 year after the surgery, are not much different than those after radiation therapy. Sural nerve grafts may decrease impotence rates after radical prostatectomy.[401]

Urinary incontinence after radical prostatectomy is a major drawback to the procedure. The most objective measure of incontinence is the need for pads after at least 1 year of follow-up. Questionnaire series have shown that rates of incontinence range from 13% to 47%.[398-400] In contrast, the percentage of patients with urinary incontinence requiring pads after radiation therapy is less than 5%.[15,402,403] However, the differences in overall urinary function between men who have undergone radical prostatectomy and those who have undergone radiation therapy are not as great as one would anticipate when urinary incontinence is considered as an isolated factor.[404]

Clinical and Biochemical Endpoints After Radical Prostatectomy

Radical prostatectomy is an effective treatment for prostate cancer. Before the PSA era, clinical local relapse rates were extremely low, suggesting that clinical failure was a consequence of occult regional and distant metastatic disease that had been present at the time of surgery. Although most urologists probably still believe that a detectable PSA level after prostatectomy does not reflect failure to extirpate all prostate cancer cells from the surgical bed, increasing evidence suggests that residual prostate cancer cells remain in the prostatic fossa much more often than previously believed.

Biochemical failure has been shown to occur approximately 3 to 5 years before clinical relapse.[140,141] Even though PSA is secreted in small amounts by nonprostatic tissues,[405] a detectable PSA value of 0.2 to 0.4 ng/ml after prostatectomy is a strong correlate of eventual clinical relapse.[146] This earlier recognition of treatment failure through the use of biochemical criteria has prompted more aggressive biopsies of the prostatic fossa and urethrovesicular anastomosis. In some series, biochemical failure has been associated with the presence of residual prostate cancer cells in the surgical bed in more than 50% of cases.[144,145]

Surgery for Favorable Disease

Most patients undergoing radical prostatectomy in the United States have very favorable pretreatment clinical characteristics, such as a PSA level of 10 ng/ml or less, Gleason score of 6 of less, and a 1992 AJCC clinical T stage of T2a or less. Results from some large studies of outcome after radical prostatectomy are displayed in Table 27-13.[148,273,274,406,407] Because the patients in radical prostatectomy series may have more favorable characteristics on average than those treated with external-beam irradiation, patients should be stratified as much as possible to compare results between modalities. The most important predictor of biochemical failure is

TABLE 27-13

Outcome After Radical Prostatectomy

Study and Reference	Number of Patients	PERCENT SHOWING NO BIOCHEMICAL EVIDENCE OF DISEASE	
		5 Years	10 Years
Trapasso et al, 1994[406]	601	69	47
Catalona et al, 1998[274]	1778	78	65
Dilloglugil et al, 1997[148]	611	78	76
Pound et al, 1997[273]	1623	80	68
Amling et al, 2000[407]	2782	76	60

pretreatment PSA level, which has been the main factor used to compare different treatment modalities. At 5 years, Kaplan-Meier survival estimates of freedom from biochemical failure for patients with a pretreatment PSA level of 10 ng/ml or less are 80% to 90%, estimates similar to those from trials of external-beam radiation or PRSIP (see Tables 27-3 and 27-5).

Comparing patients on the basis of pretreatment PSA may not be sufficient, however, because subtle differences in Gleason score and clinical stage may be present. Other factors that could independently predict outcome also may not have been randomly allocated between groups. The number of pretreatment biopsies involved with cancer and the proportion of cancer in the biopsy specimens, for example, are factors that are considered in recommending radical prostatectomy or PRSIP. Biopsy of the seminal vesicles and extraprostatic tissue may be recommended for patients considered to be at high risk.[408,409] Patients with palpable T2 disease and biopsy-proven extracapsular extension are more often referred for external-beam radiation therapy instead of radical prostatectomy.

A few studies in the PSA era have considered pretreatment PSA level, Gleason score, and T stage in direct comparisons of radical prostatectomy and external-beam radiation therapy.[160,283] The Kaplan-Meier freedom from biochemical failure curves for patients treated with radical prostatectomy or external-beam radiation have been superimposable when patients are grouped according to favorable, intermediate, and unfavorable risk features. These findings are convincing evidence of the equivalence of radical prostatectomy and external-beam therapy across the full range of prostate cancer, at least when disease is localized to the pelvis. The evidence also indicates that PRSIP should be limited to patients with favorable risk features, because the results of radical prostatectomy and external-beam radiation therapy have been found to be superior to those for PRSIP alone among men with intermediate- to high-risk disease characteristics.[160,271]

Surgery for Intermediate-Risk to High-Risk Disease
Radical Prostatectomy Alone

As described previously, patients with intermediate- to high-risk prostate cancer have been shown to fare similarly when treated with radical prostatectomy or external-beam radiation therapy. D'Amico and colleagues[160] and Kupelian and colleagues[283] found that the freedom from biochemical failure rates at 5 years were approximately 60% for patients at intermediate risk and 30% for patients at high risk. Radiation doses in these studies were about 70 Gy, a dose that has recently been shown to be inadequate for this patient group.[161,195,300] There is every reason to believe that because the results after treatment with 70 Gy are similar to those after radical prostatectomy, higher radiation doses will be more efficacious than radical prostatectomy.

Further evidence in support of external-beam radiation therapy is that the freedom from biochemical failure curves after irradiation for patients treated in the PSA era seem to reach a plateau, suggesting a cure fraction. Although the literature is replete with examples of plateaus in Kaplan-Meier survival curves that fall after longer follow-up periods, the maintenance of a plateau with extended follow-up beyond 5 years is convincing. In all but one[148] of the major radical prostatectomy series, freedom from biochemical failure rates have inexorably dropped between 5 and 10 years, with no hint of a plateau. Results of trials of radical prostatectomy[148,273,274,406,407] (see Table 27-13) show a drop between 5 and 10 years of 15% to 20% on average. These data are for all men studied, and the drop is more substantial for those with intermediate- or high-risk features. For example, Amling and colleagues[407] reported a drop in freedom from biochemical failure survival rates from 76% at 5 years to 59% at 10 years for the entire study population; the corresponding rates were 82% and 68% for those confirmed pathologically as having disease confined to the prostate.

The hazard function continued to show a persistent and significant risk of failure at 10 years. The 1-year hazard rates at 9 and 10 years after surgery were on the order of 4 for the entire cohort and 5 to 10 for those with a Gleason score of 8 to 10, cT3 tumors, a PSA level of more than 10 ng/ml, or positive margins. The annual hazard rates changed little between 5 and 10 years. These rates seem to be higher than the annual hazard rates beyond 5 years reported for prostate cancer patients treated definitively with radiation therapy. A group at Fox Chase Cancer Center has described annual hazard rates of less than one between 5 and 10 years.[410,411] Other external-beam radiation therapy series have reported a plateau in freedom from biochemical failure survival curves in patients at risk beyond 5 years. Longer follow-up is needed to establish more conclusively that external-beam radiation therapy results in a lower risk of relapse than radical prostatectomy when follow-up extends into the 10-year range.

Neoadjuvant Androgen Ablation Plus Prostatectomy

Among patients with palpable T2b to T2c disease, the incidence of extracapsular extension approaches 65% and that of margin positivity approaches 50%.[412-419] Although these rates may be declining as a consequence of stage migration, new strategies are needed to reduce the risk of failure after radical prostatectomy. To this end, several randomized studies have investigated the effect of neoadjuvant AA given for 3 months before radical prostatectomy vs. radical prostatectomy alone. Table 27-14[412-420] summarizes the results of these trials, showing that the reduction in margin positivity was nearly 50% when neoadjuvant AA was given for 3 months. Unfortunately, with longer follow-up, no difference was seen in freedom from biochemical failure rates between these groups (Table 27-15).[413,416-423]

Gleave and colleagues[424] hypothesized that extending the duration of neoadjuvant AA to 8 months might affect long-term freedom from biochemical failure rates after radical prostatectomy, because they found two slopes in the PSA response curve to AA, suggesting that the nadir of PSA was maximal at about 8 months. A follow-up report of patients treated in this manner was encouraging,[425] and a phase III trial will investigate this strategy. Other investigators are also examining the effect of prolonging neoadjuvant AA by comparing 3 months and 6 months of such treatment.[426,427] These studies indicate that further reductions in margin positivity and tumor volume can be achieved by extending the duration of neoadjuvant AA from 3 to 6 months.

Adjuvant and Salvage Radiation Therapy
Classification of Adjuvant and Salvage Treatment

The division in the classification of adjuvant vs. salvage radiation therapy after prostatectomy is based on serum PSA level. Adjuvant radiation therapy applies to patients who, in the first month after surgery, develop an undetectable PSA level. Salvage radiation therapy, on the other hand, applies to situations in which PSA levels remain detectable after surgery or rise from undetectable levels at a later time. Although some may consider the administration of radiation therapy for a persistently elevated PSA level to be adjuvant treatment, these patients have a higher risk of regional and distant metastasis and perhaps a greater local residual tumor burden than patients with an undetectable PSA level after prostatectomy. The available data suggest that salvage radiation therapy for a persistently elevated PSA after prostatectomy is slightly less effective than salvage radiation therapy for delayed biochemical failure.[428-431]

The decision to deliver adjuvant external-beam radiation therapy within 6 months of prostatectomy depends on the risk of local recurrence according to adverse pathologic features in the prostatectomy specimen. The hypothesis is that adverse findings are associated with incomplete removal of the tumor, leaving microscopic residual cells behind. Because 1 cm^3 of prostate cancer (10^9 cells) is thought to produce a serum PSA level of 3.5 ng/ml,[59] most current PSA assays would not be able to detect 10^6 to 10^7 residual tumor cells.[432] The correlation between high-risk pathologic features after prostatectomy and biochemical failure is incontrovertible.[54,101,148,273,407]

TABLE 27-14

Neoadjuvant Androgen Ablation Plus Radical Prostatectomy and Margin Status

Study and Reference	Disease Stage	Number of Patients	PERCENT WITH POSITIVE MARGINS		
			Hormones Only	Surgery Only	Hormones + Surgery
Van Poppel et al, 1995[412]	T2b-T3	127	6 wk Estr	47	40
Soloway et al, 1996[413]	T2b	303	3 mo TAB	48	18*
Goldenberg et al, 1996[414]	T1b-T2c	213	12 wk CyA	65	28*
Labrie et al, 1997[415]	T1-T3	161	3 mo TAB	34	8*
Fair et al, 1997[416]	T1-T2	114	3 mo TAB	36	17
Witjes et al, 1997†[417]	T2-T3	354	3 mo TAB	46	26*
Aus et al, 1998[418]	T1b-T3a	122	3 mo TAB	46	24*

Modified from Pollack A, Zagars GK, Rosen I. *Semin Radiat Oncol* 1998;8:95-106; Pollack A. Does radiotherapy add anything to androgen ablation? In: Taylor J, ed. *American Society of Clinical Oncology Spring Educational Book.* Baltimore, Md: Lippincott Williams & Wilkins; 2000: 320-326.

Estr, Estramustine; *TAB,* total androgen blockade; *CyA,* cyproterone acetate.

*$P < 0.05$.

†Benefit in T2 disease was greater than in T3 disease.

TABLE 27-15

Neoadjuvant Androgen Ablation Plus Radical Prostatectomy and Biochemical (Prostate-Specific Antigen) Failure

Study and Reference	Number of Patients	Disease Stage	Follow-Up Period	Hormonal Treatment	PERCENT SHOWING BIOCHEMICAL EVIDENCE OF TREATMENT FAILURE	
					Surgery Only	Hormone + Surgery
Soloway et al, 1996[413]	263	T2b	≥ 12 mo	3 mo TAB	12	16
Fair et al, 1997[416]*	194	T1-3	29 mo	3 mo TAB	11	16
Witjes et al, 1997[417]	215	T2-3	15 mo	3 mo TAB	23	22
Aus et al, 1998[418]	122	T1b-3a	38 mo	3 mo TAB	41	35
Klotz et al, 1999[421]	213	T1b-T2c	36 mo	3 mo CyA	30	40
Baert et al, 1998[422]	161	T2b-T3	40 mo	6 mo Estr	Similar	
Meyer et al, 1999[423]	680	T1-T3	38 mo	≥ 3 mo Mix	36	29

Modified from Pollack A, Zagars GK, Rosen I. *Semin Radiat Oncol* 1998;8:95-106; Pollack A. Does radiotherapy add anything to androgen ablation? In: Taylor J, ed. *American Society of Clinical Oncology Spring Educational Book*. Baltimore, Md: Lippincott Williams & Wilkins; 2000:320-326.

TAB, Total androgen blockade; *CyA*, cyproterone acetate; *Estr*, estramustine; *Mix*, mixed.

*Pooled data from phase II and III studies.

High-Risk Pathologic Features After Prostatectomy

Increased rates of clinical or pathologic failure in patients with clinically organ-confined (cT1 to T2) prostate cancer has been associated with the high-risk pathologic features of extracapsular extension, Gleason score of more than 6, seminal vesicle involvement, margin positivity, and lymph node involvement. Of these factors, lymph node involvement is a strong predictor of distant spread and should be considered separately. Although seminal vesicle involvement also has been associated with a relatively high incidence of regional disease or distant metastasis, modifying factors exist.[433]

A subset of patients with seminal vesicle involvement have a reasonable prognosis; local adjuvant therapy may be beneficial for such patients. The frequency of seminal vesicle involvement and lymph node involvement ranges from 5% to 10% (Table 27-16).* Extracapsular extension is seen in 32% to 61% of patients and margin positivity in 15% to 43%. Stage migration in the PSA era has been considerable; reductions in the proportion of patients presenting with extracapsular extension,[81,126,127] margin positivity,[442] and lymph-node positivity[81,127] have been significant.

A Gleason score of more than 6 is another modifying factor to be considered in assessing the need for adjuvant radiation therapy after radical prostatectomy. An isolated finding of a Gleason score of more than 6 is insufficient grounds for adjuvant radiation therapy. Thus the decision of whether to deliver adjuvant radiation

*References 101, 103, 126, 148, 273, 434-441.

therapy is based primarily on the presence of extracapsular extension and margin positivity. The incidence of failure, however, is clearly higher among patients who have both extracapsular extension and a Gleason score of more than 6.[141,435,442] Moreover, failure rates correlate with the extent of extracapsular extension and margin positivity (focal vs. extensive or single vs. multiple) and are affected by Gleason score.[141,273,435,443]

Another correlate of extracapsular extension and margin positivity is clinical stage. The 1992 AJCC staging system is a better discriminator of the risk of adverse pathologic findings than the 1997 staging system (see Table 27-2). For category cT2a disease (1992 system), Han and colleagues[104] found that the rate of extracapsular extension was 47.1%, that of seminal vesicle involvement was 5.5%, and that of lymph node involvement was 3.5%. The corresponding rates for category cT2b disease were 54.1%, 7.8%, and 11.4%. Other investigators also have reported higher rates of pT3 disease in category cT2b cases than in cT2a tumors.[81,101,103] In contrast, the differences between cT2b and cT2c tumor characteristics were not significant.

As shown in Table 27-17,[141,148,435,441-446] margin positivity is a much stronger determinant of biochemical failure at 5 and 10 years after radical prostatectomy than is extracapsular extension. Approximately half of the patients with margin positivity will experience biochemical failure by 5 years. With longer follow-up, the incidence of failure is higher (see Table 27-17), but not all patients with margin positivity experience biochemical failure. Among the possible explanations for this are that (1) cells may extend to the resection margins but

TABLE 27-16

Adverse Pathologic Features in Prostatectomy Specimens from Patients with cT1 to T2 Disease

Study and Reference	Number of Patients	Extracapsular Extension (%)	Seminal Vesicle Involvement (%)	Lymph Node Involvement (%)	Positive Margins (%)
Ohori et al, 1995[434]	478	43	12	5	16
Kupelian et al, 1996[101]	337	61	18	8	43
Epstein et al, 1996[435]	721	58	7	8	23
Lowe et al, 1997[436]	583	35	4	3	15
Dillioglugil et al, 1997[148]	611	39	11	6	—
Pound et al, 1997[273]	1623	52	6	7	—
Bauer et al, 1998[437]	378	57	—	—	—
Ramos et al, 1999[103]*	1620	32	7	1	24
Gilliland et al, 1999[438]	1395	47	7	3	33
Jhaveri et al, 1999[126]	731	54	—	—	—
Cheng et al, 2000[439]	339	35	14	6	24
Blute et al, 2000[440]	2475	32	15	7	—
Weighted averages		41%	9%	5%	24%

Modified from Pollack A, Smith LG. Adjuvant external beam radiotherapy postprostatectomy. In: D'Amico AV, Carroll P, Kantoff PW, eds. *Prostate Cancer*. Philadelphia, Pa: Lippincott Williams & Wilkins; 2000.
*T1 to T2b (T2c excluded).

TABLE 27-17

Relationships of Extracapsular Extension and Margin Positivity to Freedom from Biochemical Failure

	PERCENT FREEDOM FROM BIOCHEMICAL FAILURE			
	5 YEARS		10 YEARS	
Study and Reference	Extracapsular Extension	Positive Margins	Extracapsular Extension	Positive Margins
Paulson, 1994[141]	—	42	—	38
Zietman et al, 1994[444]	27	26	—	—
Watson et al, 1996[445]	—	66	—	—
Epstein et al, 1996[435,442]	78*†	64	68	55
Dillioglugil et al, 1997[148]	79	—	79	—
Kupelian et al, 1997[443]	~43	~35	—	—
Grossfeld et al, 2000[446]	—	52	—	—

Modified from Pollack A, Smith LG. Adjuvant external beam radiotherapy postprostatectomy. In: D'Amico AV, Carroll P, Kantoff PW, eds. *Prostate Cancer*. Philadelphia, Pa: Lippincott Williams & Wilkins; 2000.
*Confirmed extracapsular extension.
†4-Year rate.

not beyond; (2) a small focus of cells remaining beyond the resection margins may eventually die; (3) the cells could remain dormant; and (4) the follow-up period, even at 10 years, may be too short.

For cancer in nearly every other anatomic site, surgeons would enlist radiation oncologists to assist in reducing the risk of treatment failure when that risk approaches 50%. However, for prostate cancer, other concerns have been raised, not the least of which is that adjuvant radiation therapy has never been shown to prolong survival, perhaps because of the long natural history of the disease and deaths caused by intercurrent illness. Another question is whether the timing of radiation therapy—adjuvant vs. salvage—makes a difference. It is hard to imagine that

leaving tumor behind in more than 50% of patients with high-risk disease after radical prostatectomy would not have an adverse effect on outcome if left untreated until relapse, particularly among younger men with prostate cancer.

Adjuvant Radiation Therapy for High-Risk Pathologic Features After Prostatectomy

Studies done before the PSA era have shown that adjuvant radiation therapy after prostatectomy effectively reduces local failure in the prostatic fossa.[447-452] Differences in local control rates between irradiated and nonirradiated treatment groups are much greater at 10 years than at 5 years, attesting to the prolonged natural history of the disease. Anscher and colleagues[432,450] found that the local control rate at 10 years was 92% for patients given adjuvant radiation vs. 60% for those not given adjuvant radiation. Most series have shown that this local-control effect translates into an overall increase in disease freedom, yet consistent significant reductions in distant metastasis or death rates have not been observed. The argument against adjuvant radiation therapy has centered on these findings and on the belief of some that salvage radiation therapy is as effective.[453,454] Issues in the debate over adjuvant versus salvage radiation therapy are addressed below.

The relationship between local control and distant metastasis (or survival) has never been adequately examined because studies have been small and retrospective, as well as grossly underpowered. If 30 of 100 patients in a cohort are destined to develop local failure in a 10-year period, and if the local failure rate after adjuvant radiation therapy is reduced to 10%, the potential improvement only affects 20 patients of the 100 studied. Even if a high percentage of those 20 men were to develop distant metastasis before dying of intercurrent disease, those men would be mixed in with patients who had distant metastasis without local failure. Thus if 30% of the parent cohort had distant disease at 10 years, and if as many as a third of these cases were attributable to local failure, the numbers would be far too small to detect a difference statistically. Because more than 30,000 men die of prostate cancer every year in the United States, it behooves us to reduce failure rates when possible, particularly among men for whom the life expectancy is at least 10 years because the morbidity of adjuvant treatment is low.

The results of adjuvant postoperative radiation therapy for patients with high-risk pathologic characteristics are displayed in Table 27-18.[429,441,452,455-462] The freedom from biochemical failure rate is about 70% on average, which seems to be higher than the 50% rate for patients treated with radical prostatectomy alone (see Table 27-17). Single-institution comparisons of radical prostatectomy alone vs. radical prostatectomy plus adjuvant radiation therapy are summarized in Table 27-19.* Two of these studies involved matched-pair analyses. In all but one report, the addition of adjuvant radiation therapy significantly improved freedom from biochemical failure rates. The lack of a significant effect in the University of Southern California cohort[461] may be related to the use of lower radiation doses (about 48 Gy); the other studies used doses higher than 60 Gy.

Data on the dose requirements for adjuvant radiation therapy are limited. Valicenti and colleagues[463] found evidence of a dose-response relationship among patients with pT3N0 disease given adjuvant irradiation. The 3-year freedom from biochemical failure rate for patients who received 61.2 Gy or less ($N = 14$) was 64%, as contrasted to 90% ($P = 0.015$) for those who received more than 61.2 Gy ($N = 38$). Small numbers obviated multivariate analysis, making it unclear whether prognostic factors were evenly distributed between the two groups. Nonetheless, these results, combined with the lesser success of Petrovich and colleagues[461] from using 48 Gy, indicate that doses higher than 60 Gy should be used until further information is available.

Seminal vesicle involvement has been equated with distant spread. No doubt exists that involvement of the seminal vesicles is an adverse prognostic factor; patients with this feature are at increased risk of regional and

---

*References 431, 441, 452, 458, 459, 461.

TABLE 27-18

Freedom from Biochemical Failure After Adjuvant External-Beam Radiation Therapy

Study and Reference	Number of Patients	Pathologic Tumor Stage	Positive Margins	Follow-Up Period (Months)	Dose (Gy)	Freedom From Biochemical Failure Rate
Zietman et al, 1993[455]	68*	T3 N0	94%	NS	60-64	64% (5 yr)
Schild et al, 1996[456]	60	T3 N0	82%	32	62	57% (5 yr)
Coetzee et al, 1996[429]	30	T2-T3c	100%	33	66-70	50% (4 yr)
Morris et al, 1997[457]	40	T3 N0	85%	31	60-62	88% (3 yr)
Valicenti et al, 1998[458]	15	T3c N0	20%	~38	64.8	86% (3yr)
Valicenti et al, 1999[459]	52	T3 N0	83%	39	64.8	82% (5 yr)
Vicini et al, 1999[460]	38	T2c-T4	—	49	59.4	67% (5 yr)
Petrovich et al, 1999[461]	201	T3 N0	41%	68	48	67% (5 yr)
Nudell et al, 1999[462]	36	T2-T3	97%	~23	68	~58% (5 yr)
Leibovich et al, 2000[452]	76	T2 N0	100%†	29	63	88%

Modified from Pollack A, Smith LG. Adjuvant external beam radiotherapy postprostatectomy. In: D'Amico AV, Carroll P, Kantoff PW, eds. *Prostate Cancer*. Philadelphia, Pa: Lippincott Williams & Wilkins; 2000.

NS, Not stated.

*Only 27 were confirmed as having undetectable prostate-specific antigen (PSA) levels.

†Single positive margin.

TABLE 27-19

Adjuvant External-Beam Radiation Therapy After Prostatectomy: Recent Comparative Studies

Study and Reference	Number of Patients	Dose (Gy)	Freedom from Biochemical Failure Rate	P Value
Leibovich et al, 2000[452]*	76	None	59% (5 yr)	0.005
	76	63	88% (5 yr)	
Petrovich et al, 1999[461]	40	None	69% (5 yr)	NS
	201	48	68% (5 yr)	
Valicenti et al, 1998[458]*	36	None	66% (3 yr)	NA
	36	64.8	93% (3 yr)	
Schild, 1998[431]	~228	None	40% (5 yr)	0.0003
	~60	60-67	90% (5 yr)	
Valicenti et al, 1999[459]†	20	None	48% (3 yr)	0.01
	15	64.8	86% (3 yr)	

Modified from Pollack A, Smith LG. Adjuvant external beam radiotherapy postprostatectomy. In: D'Amico AV, Carroll P, Kantoff PW, eds. *Prostate Cancer.* Philadelphia, Pa: Lippincott Williams & Wilkins; 2000.
NS, Not significant; *NA*, not available.
*Matched-pair analysis.
†pT3c N0 patients.

distant metastasis, but they are also at increased risk of local failure.[447,464] In the absence of concurrent lymph node involvement, clearly subgroups of patients with seminal vesicle involvement exist that would benefit from adjuvant radiation therapy. Valicenti and colleagues[458] directly addressed this question in 35 men with pT3 cN0 disease who had undetectable PSA levels after prostatectomy. Of these patients, 15 were given adjuvant radiation therapy. The 3-year freedom from biochemical failure rates were 86% for the group given adjuvant radiation and 48% for the observation group.

Salvage External-Beam Radiation Therapy After Prostatectomy

Salvage radiation therapy is given after radical prostatectomy for two distinct indications: a persistently elevated postoperative PSA level and a delayed rise in PSA level 6 months or more after surgery. Differences in prognosis between these groups have not been firmly established, mainly because of small patient numbers, relatively short follow-up, and imbalances in prognostic factors. Although some investigators consider the prognosis to be the same for those two groups,[453] patients with a delay in the appearance of biochemical failure have generally had a better outcome.[428-431]

The success of salvage radiation therapy depends on various patient- and treatment-related factors. Presurgical characteristics such as PSA level, Gleason score, disease stage, and margin status seem to be less important than the PSA level before irradiation. Table 27-20[453,456,457,465-469] illustrates the relationship between preirradiation PSA level and biochemical failure rates, indicating that the earlier treatment is begun the greater the chance for control. Salvage therapy is successful in more than 50% of patients if the PSA level before irradiation is low (e.g., less than 1 ng/ml), whereas the success rate is less than 30% if the

PSA level is high. The relationship between preirradiation PSA level and biochemical failure is probably a continuous function. Younger men with a long life expectancy should be treated as soon as biochemical failure—and the absence of metastasis—are established. Further delay in treatment allows time for the disease to progress.

Ideally, salvage radiation therapy should be considered for cases in which biochemical failure is thought to reflect residual disease in the surgical bed. A history of a positive margin, extracapsular extension, or seminal vesicle involvement provides a rationale for local treatment. Negative results from biopsies of the urethrovesical anastomosis and prostatic bed should not discourage plans for radiation therapy management, because the volume of residual disease may be small. The conundrum comes when there is no identifiable reason to administer local therapy (e.g., organ-confined disease with negative margins) but the PSA level is rising slowly after a delay of several years. In cases such as this, locally persistent disease may well still be present because pathologic assessment of margins is far from perfect. This dilemma should be discussed in detail with the patient, giving the advantages and disadvantages of salvage radiation therapy. A Prosta-Scint scan may be helpful in such cases.

Radiation dose has been shown to be important in several studies of salvage radiation therapy.[431,456,463,468] The best results are obtained when the surgical bed receives more than 65 Gy.

Adjuvant vs. Salvage External-Beam Radiation Therapy: Should Treatment be Delayed?

Younger men with a long life expectancy and high-risk pathologic features after radical prostatectomy should be treated with adjuvant radiation therapy until further data can be generated to support the alternative practice of

TABLE 27-20

Salvage External-Beam Radiation Therapy After Prostatectomy: Importance of Prostate-Specific Antigen Level Before Radiation

Study and Reference	Median Dose, Gy (range)	Number of Patients	PSA Cutpoints	Freedom from Biochemical Failure Rate	P Value
Wu et al, 1995[465]	61.2 (55-66)	53	< 2.5 ng/ml (N = 27)	52% (crude)	0.001
			≥ 2.5 ng/ml (N = 26)	8% (crude)	
Schild et al, 1996[456]	64 (60-67)	46	≤ 1.1 ng/ml (NS)	76% (3 yr)	0.02
			> 1.1 ng/ml (NS)	26% (3 yr)	
Morris et al, 1997[457]	NS (60-64)	48	≤ 1.7 ng/ml (N = 24)	66% (3 yr)	0.03
			> 1.7 ng/ml (N = 24)	29% (3 yr)	
Forman et al, 1997[453]	66 (50-74)	47	≤ 2 ng/ml (N = 29)	44% (4 yr)	0.005
			> 2 ng/ml (N = 18)	13% (4 yr)	
Zelefsky et al, 1997[466]	65 (38-70)	28	≤ 1.0 ng/ml (N = 25)*	75% (2 yr)	0.008
			> 1.0 ng/ml (N = 13)	26% (2 yr)	
Rogers et al, 1998[467]†	70 (61-70)	34	≤ 4 ng/ml (NS)	60% (3.5 yr)	0.03
			> 4 ng/ml (NS)	0% (3.5 yr)	
Anscher et al, 2000[468]	66 (55-70)	89	< 2.5 ng/ml (NS)	4.8 yr (median)	0.03
			≥ 2.5 ng/ml (NS)	1.5 yr (median)	
Pisansky et al, 2000[469]	64 (54-72)	166	≤ 1.0 ng/ml (N = 96)	53% (5 yr)	0.08
			> 1.0 ng/ml (N = 70)	38% (5 yr)	

PSA, Prostate-specific antigen; NS, not stated.
*Includes some patients given adjuvant radiation.
†All had biopsy-confirmed local recurrence.

TABLE 27-21

Adjuvant vs. Salvage External-Beam Radiation Therapy After Prostatectomy: Recent Comparative Studies

Study and Reference	Number of Patients	Treatment Type*	Median Dose, Gy (range)	Freedom from Biochemical Failure Rate	P Value
McCarthy et al, 1994[428]	64	Adj (N = 27)	NS (< 60-65)	66 (3 yr)	0.008
		Salv (N = 22)	NS (< 60-65)	68 (3 yr)	
		Salv (N = 15)†	NS (< 60-65)	32 (3 yr)	
Coetzee et al, 1996[429]	45	Adj (N = 30)	NS (66-70)	50 (5 yr)	NS
		Salv (N = 15)†	NS (66-70)	0 (5 yr)	
Morris et al, 1997[457]	88	Adj (N = 40)	NS (60-64)	81 (3 yr)	0.0006
		Salv (N = 48)	NS (60-64)	48 (3 yr)	
Valicenti et al, 1998[463]	79	Adj (N = 52)	65 (55-70)	93 (3 yr)	< 0.0001
		Salv (N = 27)	65 (55-70)	44 (3 yr)	
Schild, 1998[431]	NS	Adj (NS)	62 (57-68)	90 (5 yr)	NS
		Salv (N = 55)	64 (60-68)	49 (5 yr)	
Vicini et al, 1999[460]	61	Adj (N = 38)	59.4 (50-61)	67 (5 yr)	< 0.001
		Salv (N = 23)	61 (59-68)	16 (5 yr)	

Adj, Adjuvant; Salv, salvage; NS, not stated.
*N, Number per treatment group.
†Persistently elevated prostate-specific antigen level.

watchful waiting and salvage radiation therapy at a later time. The findings presented in Table 27-21* show that salvage radiation therapy produces freedom from biochemical failure rates that are roughly half or less than half of those produced by adjuvant radiation therapy. However, these single-institution analyses are fraught with problems, because they are retrospective, involve small numbers of patients with short follow-up, and have imbalances in the prognostic features of the populations being compared. One must also consider that perhaps 50% of men given adjuvant treatment may never experience relapse. Nonetheless, without conclusive evidence that salvage treatment is equivalent to adjuvant treatment, adjuvant radiation therapy is preferred. Earlier treatment has consistently produced better results

*References 428, 429, 431, 457, 460, 463.

at lower doses for diseases at other anatomic sites. The side effects of adjuvant radiation therapy for prostate cancer are usually mild to moderate, with few severe complications. The side effects can be reduced further by using conformal radiation therapy.

CRYOTHERAPY

TRUS-guided cryotherapy is briefly mentioned here because of a recent resurgence in its use since its introduction in the late 1980s. The procedure involves the percutaneous transperineal placement of multiple cryoprobes and thermosensors to monitor development of the ice ball. Single and double freeze-thaw cycles are used, with the latter more effectively ablating prostate tumors. The urethra is commonly warmed to prevent urethral sloughing. Improvements in the technique have included the use of more cryprobes,[470] miniaturization of the freezing probes,[471] and the use of argon gas.[472] The results of cryosurgery have been preliminary for the most part, with relatively short follow-up. Published series[470,472-475] indicate that long-term failure rates after cryosurgery are higher than those after radical prostatectomy or radiation therapy.

REFERENCES

1. McNeal JE. The zonal anatomy of the prostate. *Prostate* 1981; 2:35-49.
2. McNeal JE, Villers AA, Redwine EA, et al. Capsular penetration in prostate cancer. Significance for natural history and treatment. *Am J Surg Pathol* 1990;14:240-247.
3. Walsh PC, Donker PJ. Impotence following radical prostatectomy: insight into etiology and prevention. *J Urol* 1982;128:492-497.
4. Willett CG, Ooi CJ, Zietman AL, et al. Acute and late toxicity of patients with inflammatory bowel disease undergoing irradiation for abdominal and pelvic neoplasms. *Int J Radiat Oncol Biol Phys* 2000;46:995-998.
5. Zietman AL, Zehr EM, Shipley WU. The long-term effect on PSA values of incidental prostatic irradiation in patients with pelvic malignancies other than prostate cancer. *Int J Radiat Oncol Biol Phys* 1999;43:715-718.
6. Bostwick DG, Egbert BM, Fajardo LF. Radiation injury of the normal and neoplastic prostate. *Am J Surg Pathol* 1982;6:541-551.
7. Sheaff MT, Baithun SI. Effects of radiation on the normal prostate gland. *Histopathology* 1997;30:341-348.
8. Gaudin PB, Zelefsky MJ, Leibel SA, et al. Histopathologic effects of three-dimensional conformal external beam radiation therapy on benign and malignant prostate tissues. *Am J Surg Pathol* 1999;23:1021-1031.
9. Fajardo LF, Berthrong M, Anderson RE. Prostate. In: *Radiation Pathology*. New York, NY: Oxford University Press; 2001: 319-325.
10. Seymore CH, el-Mahdi AM, Schellhammer PF. The effect of prior transurethral resection of the prostate on postradiation urethral strictures and bladder neck contractures. *Int J Radiat Oncol Biol Phys* 1986;12:1597-1600.
11. Sandhu AS, Zelefsky MJ, Lee HJ, et al. Long-term urinary toxicity after 3-dimensional conformal radiotherapy for prostate cancer in patients with prior history of transurethral resection. *Int J Radiat Oncol Biol Phys* 2000;48:643-647.
12. Cox JD, Stetz J, Pajak TF. Toxicity criteria of the Radiation Therapy Oncology Group (RTOG) and the European Organization for Research and Treatment of Cancer (EORTC). *Int J Radiat Oncol Biol Phys* 1995;31:1341-1346.
13. Hanlon AL, Schultheiss TE, Hunt MA, et al. Chronic rectal bleeding after high-dose conformal treatment of prostate cancer warrants modification of existing morbidity scales. *Int J Radiat Oncol Biol Phys* 1997;38:59-63.
14. Storey MR, Pollack A, Zagars GK, et al. Complications from dose escalation in prostate cancer: preliminary results of a randomized trial. *Int J Radiat Oncol Biol Phys* 2000;48:635-642.
15. Nguyen LN, Pollack A, Zagars GK. Late effects after radiotherapy for prostate cancer in a randomized dose-response study: results of a self-assessment questionnaire. *Urology* 1998; 51:991-997.
16. Litwin MS, Flanders SC, Pasta DJ, et al. Sexual function and bother after radical prostatectomy or radiation for prostate cancer: multivariate quality-of-life analysis from CaPSURE. Cancer of the Prostate Strategic Urologic Research Endeavor. *Urology* 1999;54:503-508.
17. Wilder RB, Chou RH, Ryu JK, et al. Potency preservation after three-dimensional conformal radiotherapy for prostate cancer: preliminary results. *Am J Clin Oncol* 2000;23:330-333.
18. Greenlee RT, Hill-Harmon MB, Murray T, et al. Cancer statistics, 2001. *CA Cancer J Clin* 2001;50:15-36.
19. Oesterling JE, Martin SK, Bergstralh EJ, et al. The use of prostate-specific antigen in staging patients with newly diagnosed prostate cancer. *JAMA* 1993;269:57-60.
20. Oesterling JE, Jacobsen SJ, Chute CG, et al. Serum prostate-specific antigen in a community-based population of healthy men. Establishment of age-specific reference ranges. *JAMA* 1993;270:860-864.
21. Catalona WJ, Partin AW, Slawin KM, et al. Use of the percentage of free prostate-specific antigen to enhance differentiation of prostate cancer from benign prostatic disease: a prospective multicenter clinical trial. *JAMA* 1998;279:1542-1547.
22. Morgan TO, Jacobsen SJ, McCarthy WF, et al. Age-specific reference ranges for prostate-specific antigen in black men. *N Engl J Med* 1996;335:304-310.
23. Babaian RJ, Toi A, Kamoi K, et al. A comparative analysis of sextant and an extended 11-core multisite directed biopsy strategy. *J Urol* 2000;163:152-157.
24. Potosky AL, Miller BA, Albertsen PC. The role of increasing detection in the rising incidence of prostate cancer. *JAMA* 1995; 273:548-552.
25. Merrill RM, Potosky AL, Feuer EJ. Changing trends in U.S. prostate cancer incidence rates. *J Natl Cancer Inst* 1996;88:1683-1685.
26. Andrews GS. Latent carcinoma of the prostate. *J Clin Pathol* 1949;2:197-208.
27. Edwards CN, Steinthorsson E, Nicholson D. An autopsy study of latent prostatic cancer. *Cancer* 1953;6:531-554.
28. Franks LM. Latent carcinoma of the prostate. *J Path Bact* 1954;68:603-616.
29. Breslow N, Chan CW, Dhom Q, et al. Latent carcinoma of the prostate at autopsy in seven areas. *Int J Cancer* 1977;20:680-688.
30. Sakr WA, Haas GP, Cassin BF, et al. The frequency of carcinoma and intraepithelial neoplasia of the prostate in young male patients. *J Urol* 1993;150:379-385.
31. Sakr WA, Grignon DJ, Crissman JD, et al. High grade prostatic intraepithelial neoplasia (HGPIN) and prostatic adenocarcinoma between the ages of 20-69: an autopsy study of 249 cases. *In Vivo* 1994;8:439-444.
32. Steinberg GD, Carter BS, Beaty TH, et al. Family history and risk of prostate cancer. *Prostate* 1990;17:337-347.
33. Carter BS, Beaty TH, Steinberg GD, et al. Mendelian inheritance of familial prostate cancer. *Proc Natl Acad Sci U S A* 1992;89: 3367-3371.
34. Shibata A, Whittemore AS. Genetic predisposition to prostate cancer: possible explanation for ethnic differences in risk. *Prostate* 1997;32:65-72.

35. Xu J, Meyers DA, Freije D, et al. Evidence for a prostate cancer susceptibility locus on the X chromosome. *Nat Genet* 1998;20:175-179.

36. Smith JR, Freije D, Carpten JD, et al. Major susceptibility locus for prostate cancer on chromosome 1 suggested by a genome-wide search. *Science* 1996;274:1371-1374.

37. Lehrer S, Fodor F, Stock RG, et al. Absence of 185delAG mutation of the BRCA1 gene and 6174delT mutation of the BRCA2 gene in Ashkenazi Jewish men with prostate cancer. *Br J Cancer* 1998;78:771-773.

38. Bosland MC. The etiopathogenesis of prostate cancer with special reference to environmental factors. *Adv Cancer Res* 1988;51:1-106.

39. Fair WR, Fleshner NE, Heston W. Cancer of the prostate: a nutritional disease? *Urology* 1997;50:840-848.

40. Dorgan JF, Judd JT, Longcope C, et al. Effects of dietary fat and fiber on plasma and urine androgens and estrogens in men: a controlled feeding study. *Am J Clin Nutr* 1996;64:850-855.

41. Kyprianou N, Isaacs JT. Activation of programmed cell death in the rat ventral prostate after castration. *Endocrinology* 1988;122:552-562.

42. English HF, Kyprianou N, Isaacs JT. Relationship between DNA fragmentation and apoptosis in the programmed cell death in the rat prostate following castration. *Prostate* 1989;15:233-250.

43. Ellis L, Nyborg H. Racial/ethnic variations in male testosterone levels: a probable contributor to group differences in health. *Steroids* 1992;57:72-75.

44. Pettaway CA. Racial differences in the androgen/androgen receptor pathway in prostate cancer. *J Natl Med Assoc* 1999;91:653-660.

45. Ross RK, Bernstein L, Lobo RA, et al. 5-Alpha-reductase activity and risk of prostate cancer among Japanese and U. S. white and black males. *Lancet* 1992;339:887-889.

46. Noble RL. Production of Nb rat carcinoma of the dorsal prostate and response of estrogen-dependent transplants to sex hormones and tamoxifen. *Cancer Res* 1980;40:3547-3550.

47. Pollard M, Luckert PH, Schmidt MA. Induction of prostate adenocarcinomas in Lobund Wister rats by testosterone. *Prostate* 1982;3:563-568.

48. Bosland MC. Chemical and hormonal induction of prostate cancer in animal models. *Urol Oncol* 1996;2:103-110.

49. Waalkes MP, Rehm S, Perantoni AO, et al. Cadmium exposure in rats and tumours of the prostate. In: Nordberg GF, Herber RFM, Alessio L, eds. *Cadmium in the Human Environment: Toxicity and Carcinogenicity.* Lyon, France: IARC; 1992:391-400.

50. Takizawa S, Hirose F. Role of testosterone in the development of radiation-induced prostate carcinoma in rats. *Gann* 1978;69:723-726.

51. McNeal JE, Bostwick DG, Kindrachuk RA, et al. Patterns of progression in prostate cancer. *Lancet* 1986;1:60-63.

52. Stamey TA, Freiha FS, McNeal JE, et al. Localized prostate cancer. Relationship of tumor volume to clinical significance for treatment of prostate cancer. *Cancer* 1993;71:933-938.

53. Chan LW, Stamey TA. Calculating prostate cancer volume preoperatively: the D'Amico equation and some other observations. *J Urol* 1998;159:1998-2003.

54. Stamey TA, McNeal JE, Yemoto CM, et al. Biological determinants of cancer progression in men with prostate cancer. *JAMA* 1999;281:1395-1400.

55. Lepor H, Wang B, Shapiro E. Relationship between prostatic epithelial volume and serum prostate-specific antigen levels. *Urology* 1994;44:199-205.

56. Marks LS, Treiger B, Dorey FJ, et al. Morphometry of the prostate: I. Distribution of tissue components in hyperplastic glands. *Urology* 1994;44:486-492.

57. Collins GN, Lee RJ, McKelvie GB, et al. Relationship between prostate specific antigen, prostate volume and age in the benign prostate. *Br J Urol* 1993;71:445-450.

58. Aihara M, Lebovitz RM, Wheeler TM, et al. Prostate specific antigen and Gleason grade: an immunohistochemical study of prostate cancer. *J Urol* 1994;151:1558-1564.

59. Stamey TA, Kabalin JN, McNeal JE, et al. Prostate-specific antigen in the diagnosis and treatment of adenocarcinoma of the prostate. II. Radical prostatectomy treated patients. *J Urol* 1989;141:1076-1083.

60. Weinrich MC, Jacobsen SJ, Weinrich SP, et al. Reference ranges for serum prostate-specific antigen in black and white men without cancer. *Urology* 1998;52:967-973.

61. Catalona WJ, Partin AW, Slawin KM, et al. Percentage of free PSA in black versus white men for detection and staging of prostate cancer: a prospective multicenter clinical trial. *Urology* 2000;55:372-376.

62. Catalona WJ, Southwick PC, Slawin KM, et al. Comparison of percent free PSA, PSA density, and age-specific PSA cutoffs for prostate cancer detection and staging. *Urology* 2000;56:255-260.

63. Fowler JE Jr, Bigler SA, Miles D, et al. Predictors of first repeat biopsy cancer detection with suspected local stage prostate cancer. *J Urol* 2000;163:813-818.

64. Carter HB, Morrell CH, Pearson JD, et al. Estimation of prostatic growth using serial prostate-specific antigen measurements in men with and without prostate disease. *Cancer Res* 1992;52:3323-3328.

65. Chen ME, Troncoso P, Tang K, et al. Comparison of prostate biopsy schemes by computer simulation. *Urology* 1999;53:951-960.

66. Egevad L, Frimmel H, Norberg M, et al. Three-dimensional computer reconstruction of prostate cancer from radical prostatectomy specimens: evaluation of the model by core biopsy simulation. *Urology* 1999;53:192-198.

67. Presti JC Jr, Chang JJ, Bhargava V, et al. The optimal systematic prostate biopsy scheme should include 8 rather than 6 biopsies: results of a prospective clinical trial. *J Urol* 2000;163:163-166.

68. Ravery V, Goldblatt L, Royer B, et al. Extensive biopsy protocol improves the detection rate of prostate cancer. *J Urol* 2000;164:393-396.

69. Sufrin G, Gaeta J, Staubitz WJ, et al. Endometrial carcinoma of prostate. *Urology* 1986;27:18-23.

70. Brinker DA, Potter SR, Epstein JI. Ductal adenocarcinoma of the prostate diagnosed on needle biopsy: correlation with clinical and radical prostatectomy findings and progression. *Am J Surg Pathol* 1999;23:1471-1479.

71. Bock BJ, Bostwick DG. Does prostatic ductal adenocarcinoma exist? *Am J Surg Pathol* 1999;23:781-785.

72. di Sant'Agnese PA, de Mesy Jensen KL, Churukian CJ, et al. Human prostatic endocrine-paracrine (APUD) cells. Distributional analysis with a comparison of serotonin and neuron-specific enolase immunoreactivity and silver stains. *Arch Pathol Lab Med* 1985;109:607-612.

73. Ro JY, Tetu B, Ayala AG, et al. Small cell carcinoma of the prostate. Part II: Immunohistochemical and electron microscopic study of 18 cases. *Cancer* 1987;59:977-982.

74. Oesterling JE, Hauzeur CG, Farrow GM. Small cell anaplastic carcinoma of the prostate: a clinical, pathological and immunohistological study of 27 patients. *J Urol* 1992;147:804-807.

75. Randolph TL, Amin MB, Ro JY, et al. Histologic variants of adenocarcinoma and other carcinomas of prostate: pathologic criteria and clinical significance. *Mod Pathol* 1997;10:612-629.

76. Gleason DF. Classification of prostatic carcinomas. *Cancer Chemother Rep* 1966;50:125-128.

77. Gleason DF. Histologic grading of prostate cancer: a perspective. *Hum Pathol* 1992;23:273-279.

78. Mostofi FK, Sesterhenn IA, Davis CJ Jr. A pathologist's view of prostatic carcinoma. *Cancer* 1993;71:906-932.

79. Zagars GK, Ayala AG, von Eschenbach AC, et al. The prognostic importance of Gleason grade in prostatic adenocarcinoma: a long-term follow-up study of 648 patients treated with radiation therapy. *Int J Radiat Oncol Biol Phys* 1995;31:237-245.

80. Chan TY, Partin AW, Walsh PC, et al. Prognostic significance of Gleason score 3+4 versus Gleason score 4+3 tumor at radical prostatectomy. *Urology* 2000;56:823-827.

81. Stamey TA, Sozen TS, Yemoto CM, et al. Classification of localized untreated prostate cancer based on 791 men treated only with radical prostatectomy: common ground for therapeutic trials and TNM subgroups. *J Urol* 1998;159:2009-2012.

82. Whitmore WF. Hormone therapy in prostatic cancer. *Am J Med* 1956;21:697-713.

83. Jewett HJ. The present status of radical prostatectomy for stages A and B prostatic cancer. *Urol Clin North Am* 1975;2:105-124.

84. American Society for Therapeutic Radiology and Oncology Consensus Panel. Consensus statement: guidelines for PSA following radiation therapy. *Int J Radiat Oncol Biol Phys* 1997;37:1035-1041.

85. Rifkin MD, Zerhouni EA, Gatsonis CA, et al. Comparison of magnetic resonance imaging and ultrasonography in staging early prostate cancer: results of a multi-institutional cooperative trial. *N Engl J Med* 1990;323:621-626.

86. Smith JA, Scardino PT, Resnick MI, et al. Transrectal ultrasound versus digital rectal examination for the staging of carcinoma of the prostate: results of a prospective, multi-institutional trial. *J Urol* 1997;157:902-906.

87. Shinohara K, Wheeler TM, Scardino PT. The appearance of prostate cancer on transrectal ultrasonography: correlation of imaging and pathological examinations. *J Urol* 1989;142:76-82.

88. Pontes JE, Eisenkraft S, Watanabe H. Preoperative evaluation of localized prostatic carcinoma by transrectal ultrasonography. *J Urol* 1985;134:289-291.

89. Perrapato SD, Carothers GG, Maatman TJ, et al. Comparing clinical staging plus transrectal ultrasound with surgical-pathologic staging of prostate cancer. *Urology* 1989;33:103-105.

90. Hamper UM, Sheth S, Walsh PC, et al. Capsular transgression of prostatic carcinoma: evaluation with transrectal US with pathologic correlation. *Radiology* 1991;178:791-795.

91. Vijverberg PM, Giessen MA, Kurth KH, et al. Is preoperative transrectal ultrasonography of value in localized prostatic carcinoma? A blind comparative study between preoperative transrectal ultrasonography and the histopathological radical prostatectomy specimen. *Eur J Surg Oncol* 1992;18:449-455.

92. Vapnek JM, Hricak H, Shinohara K, et al. Staging accuracy of magnetic resonance imaging versus transrectal ultrasound in stages A and B prostatic cancer. *Urol Int* 1994;53:191-195.

93. Ohori M, Egawa S, Shinohara K, et al. Detection of microscopic extracapsular extension prior to radical prostatectomy for clinically localized prostate cancer. *Br J Urol* 1994;74:72-79.

94. Pinover WH, Hanlon A, Lee WR, et al. Prostate carcinoma patients upstaged by imaging and treated with irradiation. *Cancer* 1996;77:1334-1341.

95. Liebross RH, Pollack A, Lankford SP, et al. Transrectal ultrasound for staging prostate cancer prior to radiation therapy: an evaluation based on disease outcome. *Cancer* 1999;85:1577-1585.

96. Jhaveri FM, Zippe CD, Klein EA, et al. Biochemical failure does not predict overall survival after radical prostatectomy for localized prostate cancer: 10-year results. *Urology* 1999;54:884-890.

97. Sandler HM, Dunn RL, McLaughlin PW, et al. Overall survival after prostate-specific-antigen–detected recurrence following conformal radiation therapy. *Int J Radiat Oncol Biol Phys* 2000;48:629-633.

98. Zagars GK, Pollack A, von Eschenbach AC. Prognostic factors for clinically localized prostate carcinoma: analysis of 938 patients irradiated in the prostate specific antigen era. *Cancer* 1997;79:1370-1380.

99. Pollack A, Zagars GK. Pretreatment prognostic factors for prostate cancer patients treated with external beam radiotherapy. In: Greco C, Zelefsky MJ, eds. *Radiotherapy of Prostate Cancer.* Singapore: Harwood Academic Publishers; 2000:113-128.

100. Fleming I, Cooper JS, Henson DE, et al, eds. *AJCC Cancer Staging Manual.* 5th ed. Philadelphia, Pa: Lippincott Williams & Wilkins; 1997:219-224.

101. Kupelian P, Katcher J, Levin H, et al. Correlation of clinical and pathologic factors with rising prostate-specific antigen profiles after radical prostatectomy alone for clinically localized prostate cancer. *Urology* 1996;48:249-260.

102. Iyer RV, Hanlon AL, Pinover WH, et al. Outcome evaluation of the 1997 American Joint Committee on Cancer Staging System for prostate carcinoma treated by radiation therapy. *Cancer* 1999;85:1816-1821.

103. Ramos CG, Carvalhal GF, Smith DS, et al. Clinical and pathological characteristics, and recurrence rates of stage T1C versus T2A or T2B prostate cancer. *J Urol* 1999;161:1212-1215.

104. Han M, Walsh PC, Partin AW, et al. Ability of the 1992 and 1997 American Joint Committee on Cancer staging systems for prostate cancer to predict progression-free survival after radical prostatectomy for stage T2 disease. *J Urol* 2000;164:89-92.

105. D'Amico AV, Whittington R, Malkowicz SB, et al. Combination of the preoperative PSA level, biopsy Gleason score, percentage of positive biopsies, and MRI-T-stage to predict early PSA failure in men with clinically localized prostate cancer. *Urology* 2000b;55:572-577.

106. D'Amico AV, Whittington R, Malkowicz SB, et al. Endorectal magnetic resonance imaging as a predictor of biochemical outcome after radical prostatectomy in men with clinically localized prostate cancer. *J Urol* 2000;164:759-763.

107. Debois M, Oyen R, Maes F, et al. The contribution of magnetic resonance imaging to the three-dimensional treatment planning of localized prostate cancer. *Int J Radiat Oncol Biol Phys* 1999;45:857-865.

108. Perrotti M, Han KR, Epstein RE, et al. Prospective evaluation of endorectal magnetic resonance imaging to detect tumor foci in men with prior negative prostatic biopsy: a pilot study. *J Urol* 1999;162:1314-1317.

109. Scheidler J, Hricak H, Vigneron DB, et al. Prostate cancer: localization with three-dimensional proton MR spectroscopic imaging—clinicopathologic study. *Radiology* 1999;213:473-480.

110. Yu KK, Hricak H, Alagappan R, et al. Detection of extracapsular extension of prostate carcinoma with endorectal and phased-array coil MR imaging: multivariate feature analysis. *Radiology* 1997;202:697-702.

111. Yu KK, Scheidler J, Hricak H, et al. Prostate cancer: prediction of extracapsular extension with endorectal MR imaging and three-dimensional proton MR spectroscopic imaging. *Radiology* 1999;213:481-488.

112. Koutcher JA, Zakian K, Hricak H. Magnetic resonance spectroscopic studies of the prostate. *Mol Urol* 2000;4:143-152.

113. Pickett B, Vigneault E, Kurhanewicz J, et al. Static field intensity modulation to treat a dominant intra-prostatic lesion to 90 Gy compared to seven field 3-dimensional radiotherapy. *Int J Radiat Oncol Biol Phys* 1999;44:921-929.

114. Ling CC, Humm J, Larson S, et al. Towards multidimensional radiotherapy (MD-CRT): biological imaging and biological conformality. *Int J Radiat Oncol Biol Phys* 2000;47:551-560.

115. Ravery V, Boccon-Gibod LA, Dauge-Geffroy MC, et al. Systematic biopsies accurately predict extracapsular extension of prostate cancer and persistent/recurrent detectable PSA after radical prostatectomy. *Urology* 1994;44:371-376.

116. Ravery V, Chastang C, Toublanc M, et al. Is the percentage of cancer biopsy cores predictive of extracapsular disease in T1-T2 prostate carcinoma? *Cancer* 1996;78:1079-1084.

117. Borirakchanyavat S, Bhargava V, Shinohara K, et al. Systematic sextant biopsies in the prediction of extracapsular extension at radical prostatectomy. *Urology* 1997;50:373-378.

118. D'Amico AV, Whittington R, Malkowicz SB, et al. Clinical utility of the percentage of positive prostate biopsies in defining

biochemical outcome after radical prostatectomy for patients with clinically localized prostate cancer. *J Clin Oncol* 2000;18: 1164-1172.

119. D'Amico AV, Whittington R, Malkowicz SB, et al. Clinical utility of percent-positive prostate biopsies in predicting biochemical outcome after radical prostatectomy or external-beam radiation therapy for patients with clinically localized prostate cancer. *Mol Urol* 2000;4:171-176.

120. Gao X, Mohidden N, Flanigan RC, et al. The extent of biopsy involvement as an independent predictor of extraprostatic extension and surgical margin status in low risk prostate cancer: implications for treatment selection. *J Urol* 2000;164:1982-1986.

121. Ravery V, Chastang C, Toublanc M, et al. Percentage of cancer on biopsy cores accurately predicts extracapsular extension and biochemical relapse after radical prostatectomy for T1-T2 prostate cancer. *Eur Urol* 2000;37:449-455.

122. Ravery V, Szabo J, Toublanc M, et al. A single positive prostate biopsy in six does not predict a low-volume prostate tumour. *Br J Urol* 1996;77:724-728.

123. Wang X, Brannigan RE, Rademaker AW, et al. One core positive prostate biopsy is a poor predictor of cancer volume in the radical prostatectomy specimen. *J Urol* 1997;158:1431-1435.

124. Pan CC, Potter SR, Partin AW, et al. The prognostic significance of tertiary Gleason patterns of higher grade in radical prostatectomy specimens: a proposal to modify the Gleason grading system. *Am J Surg Pathol* 2000;24:563-569.

125. Forman JD, DeYoung C, Tekyi-Menash S, et al. The prognostic significance of the worst versus overall Gleason score in patients with multiple positive needle biopsies. *Int J Radiat Oncol Biol Phys* 2000;48(suppl):206.

126. Jhaveri FM, Klein EA, Kupelian PA, et al. Declining rates of extracapsular extension after radical prostatectomy: evidence for continued stage migration. *J Clin Oncol* 1999;17:3167-3172.

127. Amling CL, Blute ML, Lerner SE, et al. Influence of prostate-specific antigen testing on the spectrum of patients with prostate cancer undergoing radical prostatectomy at a large referral practice. *Mayo Clin Proc* 1998;73:401-406.

128. Lee N, Fawaaz R, Olsson CA, et al. Which patients with newly diagnosed prostate cancer need a radionuclide bone scan? An analysis based on 631 patients. *Int J Radiat Oncol Biol Phys* 2000;48:1443-1446.

129. Lee CT, Oesterling JE. Using prostate-specific antigen to eliminate the staging radionuclide bone scan. *Urol Clin North Am* 1997;24:389-394.

130. Polascik TJ, Manyak MJ, Haseman MK, et al. Comparison of clinical staging algorithms and ¹¹¹indium-capromab pendetide immunoscintigraphy in the prediction of lymph node involvement in high risk prostate carcinoma patients. *Cancer* 1999;85:1586-1592.

131. Manyak MJ, Hinkle GH, Olsen JO, et al. Immunoscintigraphy with indium-111-capromab pendetide: evaluation before definitive therapy in patients with prostate cancer. *Urology* 1999;54:1058-1063.

132. Sodee DB, Malguria N, Faulhaber P, et al. Multicenter ProstaScint imaging findings in 2154 patients with prostate cancer. *Urology* 2000;56:988-993.

133. Fang DX, Stock RG, Stone NN, et al. Use of radioimmunoscintigraphy with indium-111–labeled CYT-356 (ProstaScint) scan for evaluation of patients for salvage brachytherapy. *Tech Urol* 2000;6:146-150.

134. Murphy GP, Elgamal AA, Troychak MJ, et al. Follow-up ProstaScint scans verify detection of occult soft-tissue recurrence after failure of primary prostate cancer therapy. *Prostate* 2000;42:315-317.

135. Zagars GK, Pollack A, von Eschenbach AC. Unfavorable local-regional prostate cancer management with radiation and androgen ablation. *Cancer* 1997;80:764-775.

136. Roach M III, Marquez C, You HS, et al. Predicting the risk of lymph node involvement using the pre-treatment prostate specific antigen and Gleason score in men with clinically localized prostate cancer. *Int J Radiat Oncol Biol Phys* 1994;28:33-37.

137. Pisansky TM, Kahn MJ, Rasp GM, et al. A multiple prognostic index predictive of disease outcome following irradiation for clinically localized prostatic carcinoma. *Cancer* 1997;79:337-344.

138. Partin AW, Kattan MW, Subong EN, et al. Combination of prostate specific antigen, clinical stage, and Gleason score to predict pathological stage of localized prostate cancer. A multi-institutional update. *JAMA* 1997;277:1445-1451.

139. Roach M III, Chen A, Song J, et al. Pretreatment prostate-specific antigen and Gleason score predict the risk of extracapsular extension and the risk of failure following radiotherapy in patients with clinically localized prostate cancer. *Semin Urol Oncol* 2000;18:108-114.

140. Pollack A, Zagars GK, Kavadi VS. Prostate specific antigen doubling time and disease relapse after radiotherapy for prostate cancer. *Cancer* 1994;74:670-678.

141. Paulson DF. Impact of radical prostatectomy in the management of clinically localized disease. *J Urol* 1994;152:1826-1830.

142. Zagars GK, Kavadi VS, Pollack A, et al. The source of pretreatment serum prostate-specific antigen in clinically localized prostate cancer—T, N, or M? *Int J Radiat Oncol Biol Phys* 1995;32:21-32.

143. Zagars GK, Pollack A, von Eschenbach AC. Prostate cancer and radiation therapy—the message conveyed by serum prostate-specific antigen. *Int J Radiat Oncol Biol Phys* 1995;33:23-25.

144. Connolly JA, Shinohara K, Presti JC Jr, et al. Local recurrence after radical prostatectomy: characteristics in size, location, and relationship to prostate-specific antigen and surgical margins. *Urology* 1996;47:225-231.

145. Shekarriz B, Upadhyay J, Wood DP Jr, et al. Vesicourethral anastomosis biopsy after radical prostatectomy: predictive value of prostate-specific antigen and pathologic stage. *Urology* 1999; 54:1044–1048.

146. Pound CR, Partin AW, Eisenberger MA, et al. Natural history of progression after PSA elevation following radical prostatectomy. *JAMA* 1999;281:1591-1597.

147. Lee WR, Hanks GE, Hanlon A. Increasing prostate-specific antigen profile following definitive radiation therapy for localized prostate cancer: clinical observations. *J Clin Oncol* 1997;15: 230-238.

148. Dillioglugil O, Leibman BD, Kattan MW, et al. Hazard rates for progression after radical prostatectomy for clinically localized prostate cancer. *Urology* 1997;50:93-99.

149. Smith LG, Pollack A, Zagars GK. Predictors of distant metastasis 7 years after a rising PSA in prostate cancer patients treated with external beam radiotherapy. *Int J Radiat Oncol Biol Phys* 1999;45(suppl):138.

150. American Society for Therapeutic Radiology and Oncology Consensus Panel. Consensus statement: guidelines for PSA following radiation therapy. *Int J Radiat Oncol Biol Phys* 1997;37:1035-1041.

151. Critz FA, Williams WH, Benton JB, et al. Prostate specific antigen bounce after radioactive seed implantation followed by external beam radiation for prostate cancer. *J Urol* 2000;163:1085-1089.

152. Hanlon AL, Pinover WH, Horwitz EM, et al. Patterns and fate of PSA bouncing following 3D-CRT. *Int J Radiat Oncol Biol Phys* 2000;48(suppl):207.

153. Slivjak AM, Pinover WH, Hanlon AL, et al. The ASTRO consensus definition of bNED failure is an inappropriate endpoint for prostate cancer patients receiving conformal radiation therapy and androgen deprivation (CRT+AD). *Int J Radiat Oncol Biol Phys* 1998;42(suppl 1):176.

154. Critz FA, Williams H, Holladay CT, et al. Post-treatment PSA ≤ 0.2 ng/ml defines disease freedom after radiotherapy for

prostate cancer using modern techniques. *Urology* 1999;54: 968-971.

155. Kavadi VS, Zagars GK, Pollack A. Serum prostate-specific antigen after radiation therapy for clinically localized prostate cancer: prognostic implications. *Int J Radiat Oncol Biol Phys* 1994;30:279-287.

156. Lee WR, Hanlon AL, Hanks GE. Prostate specific antigen nadir following external beam radiation therapy for clinically localized prostate cancer: the relationship between nadir level and disease-free survival. *J Urol* 1996;156:450-453.

157. Zietman AL, Tibbs MK, Dallow KC, et al. Use of PSA nadir to predict subsequent biochemical outcome following external beam radiation therapy for T1-2 adenocarcinoma of the prostate. *Radiother Oncol* 1996;40:159-162.

158. Yock TI, Thakral HK, Zietman AL, et al. The durability of PSA failure free survival from 5 years to 13 years following radiotherapy in patients with localized prostate cancer. *Int J Radiat Oncol Biol Phys* 2000;48(suppl):227.

159. D'Amico A, Propert K. Prostate cancer volume adds significantly to prostate specific antigen in the prediction of early biochemical failure after external beam radiation therapy. *Int J Radiat Oncol Biol Phys* 1996;35:273-279.

160. D'Amico AV, Whittington R, Malkowicz SB, et al. Biochemical outcome after radical prostatectomy, external beam radiation therapy, or interstitial radiation therapy for clinically localized prostate cancer. *JAMA* 1998;280:969-974.

161. Shipley WU, Thames HD, Sandler HM, et al. Radiation therapy for clinically localized prostate cancer: a multi-institutional pooled analysis. *JAMA* 1999;281:1598-1604.

162. Zelefsky MJ, Leibel SA, Baudin PB, et al. Dose escalation with three-dimensional conformal radiation therapy affects the outcome in prostate cancer. *Int J Radiat Oncol Biol Phys* 1998;41:491-500.

163. Movsas B, Hanlon AL, Teshima T, et al. Analyzing predictive models following definitive radiotherapy for prostate carcinoma. *Cancer* 1997;80:1093-1102.

164. Hanks GE, Leibel S, Kramer S. The dissemination of cancer by transurethral resection of locally advanced prostate cancer. *J Urol* 1983;129:309-311.

165. Perez CA, Garcia D, Simpson JR, et al. Factors influencing outcome of definitive radiotherapy for localized carcinoma of the prostate. *Radiother Oncol* 1989;16:1-21.

166. Anscher MS, Prosnitz LR. Transurethral resection of prostate prior to definitive irradiation for prostate cancer. *Urology* 1991;38:206-211.

167. Zagars GK, von Eschenbach AC, Ayala AG. Prognostic factors in prostate cancer: analysis of 874 patients treated with radiation therapy. *Cancer* 1993;72:1709-1725.

168. Zelefsky MJ, Whitmore WF Jr, Leibel SA, et al. Impact of transurethral resection on the long-term outcome of patients with prostatic carcinoma. *J Urol* 1993;150:1860-1864.

169. Duncan W, Catton CN, Warde P, et al. The influence of transurethral resection of prostate on prognosis of patients with adenocarcinoma of the prostate treated by radical radiotherapy. *Radiother Oncol* 1994;31:41-50.

170. Nemoto R, Uchida K, Shimazui T, et al. Immunocytochemical demonstration of S phase cells by anti-bromodeoxyuridine monoclonal antibody in human prostate adenocarcinoma. *J Urol* 1989;141:337-340.

171. Haustermans KMG, Hofland I, Poppel HV, et al. Cell kinetic measurements in prostate cancer. *Int J Radiat Oncol Biol Phys* 1997;37:1067-1070.

172. Borre M, Høyer M, Sørensen FB, et al. Association between *in vivo* iododeoxyuridine labeling, MIB-1 expression, malignancy grade and clinical stage in human prostate cancer. *APMIS* 1998;106:389-395.

173. Khoo VS, Pollack A, Cowen D, et al. Relationship of Ki-67 labeling index to DNA-ploidy, S-phase fraction, and outcome in prostate cancer treated with radiotherapy. *Prostate* 1999;41: 166-172.

174. Cowen D, Troncoso P, Khoo VS, et al. Ki-67 staining is an independent correlate of biochemical failure in prostate cancer treated with radiotherapy. *Clin Cancer Res* 2002;8:1148-1154.

175. Schmid HP, McNeal JE, Stamey TA. Observations on the doubling time of prostate cancer: the use of serial prostate-specific antigen in patients with untreated disease as a measure of increasing cancer volume. *Cancer* 1993;71:2031-2040.

176. Hanks GE, Hanlon AL, Lee WR, et al. Pretreatment prostate specific antigen doubling times: clinical utility of this predictor of prostate cancer behavior. *Int J Radiat Oncol Biol Phys* 1996;34:549-553.

177. Berges RR, Vukanovic J, Epstein JI, et al. Implication of cell kinetic changes during progression of human prostatic cancer. *Clin Cancer Res* 1995;1:473-480.

178. Brenner DJ, Hall EJ. Fractionation and protraction for radiotherapy of prostate carcinoma. *Int J Radiat Oncol Biol Phys* 1999;43:1095-1101.

179. Duschesne GM, Peters LJ. What is the α/β ratio for prostate cancer? Rationale for hypofractionated high dose-rate brachytherapy. *Int J Radiat Oncol Biol Phys* 1999;44:747-748.

180. King CR, Mayo CS. Is the α/β ratio of 1.5 from Brenner and Hall a modelling artifact? *Int J Radiat Oncol Biol Phys* 1999;47: 536-538.

181. King CR. What is the Tpot for prostate cancer? Radiobiological implications of the equivalent outcome with ^{125}I or ^{103}Pd. *Int J Radiat Oncol Biol Phys* 2000;47:1165-1167.

182. Mohan DS, Kupelian PA, Willoughby TR. Short-course intensity-modulated radiotherapy for localized prostate cancer with daily transabdominal ultrasound localization of the prostate gland. *Int J Radiat Oncol Biol Phys* 2000;46:575-580.

183. Gauwitz MD, Pollack A, El-Naggar AK, et al. The prognostic significance of DNA ploidy in clinically localized prostate cancer treated with radiation therapy. *Int J Radiat Oncol Biol Phys* 1994;28:821-828.

184. Centeno BA, Zietman AL, Shipley WU, et al. Flow cytometric analysis of DNA ploidy, percent S-phase fraction, and total proliferative fraction as prognostic indicators of local control and survival following radiation therapy for prostate carcinoma. *Int J Radiat Oncol Biol Phys* 1994;30:309-315.

185. Pollack A, Troncoso P, Zagars GK, et al. The significance of DNA-ploidy and S-phase fraction in node-positive (stage D1) prostate cancer treated with androgen ablation. *Prostate* 1997;1:21-28.

186. Kupelian P, Klien EA, Witte JS, et al. Familial prostate cancer: a different disease? *J Urol* 1997;158:2197-2201.

187. Kupelian P, Kupelian VA, Witte JS, et al. Family history of prostate cancer in patients with localized prostate cancer: an independent predictor of treatment outcome. *J Clin Oncol* 1997;15:1478-1480.

188. Hanus MC, Zagars GK, Pollack A. Familial prostate cancer: outcome following radiation therapy with or without adjuvant androgen ablation. *Int J Radiat Oncol Biol Phys* 1999;43:379-383.

189. Bova GS, Isaacs SD, Partin AW, et al. Biological aggressiveness of hereditary prostate cancer (HPC): long term evaluation following radical prostatectomy (RRP) [abstract]. *J Urol* 1995;153:505A.

190. Zagars GK, Pollack A. Serum testosterone levels after external beam radiation for clinically localized prostate cancer. *Int J Radiat Oncol Biol Phys* 1997;39:85-89.

191. Kelly J, Pollack A, Zagars GK. Serum testosterone is not a correlate of prostate cancer lymph node involvement, but does predict biochemical failure for lymph-node-positive disease. *Urol Oncol* 2000;5:78-84.

192. Harper ME, Pierrepoint CG, Griffiths K. Carcinoma of the prostate: relationship of pre-treatment hormone levels to survival. *Eur J Cancer Clin Oncol* 1984;20:477-482.

193. Chodak GW, Vogelzang NJ, Caplan RJ, et al. Independent prognostic factors in patients with metastatic (stage D2) prostate cancer. *JAMA* 1991;265:618-621.

194. Iversen P, Rasmussen F, Christensen IJ. Serum testosterone as a prognostic factor in patients with advanced prostatic carcinoma. *Scand J Urol Nephrol* 1994;157(suppl):41-47.

195. Pollack A, Zagars GK, Smith LG, et al. Preliminary results of a randomized radiotherapy dose-escalation study comparing 70 Gy with 78 Gy for prostate cancer. *J Clin Oncol* 2000;18:3904-3911.

196. Skwarchuk MW, Jackson A, Zelefsky MJ, et al. Late rectal toxicity after conformal radiotherapy of prostate cancer (I): multivariate analysis and dose-response. *Int J Radiat Oncol Biol Phys* 2000;47:103-113.

197. Pollack A, Zagars GK, Starkschall G, et al. Conventional versus conformal radiotherapy for prostate cancer: preliminary results of dosimetry and acute toxicity. *Int J Radiat Oncol Biol Phys* 1996;34:555-564.

198. Michalski JM, Purdy JA, Winter K, et al. Preliminary report of toxicity following 3D radiation therapy for prostate cancer on 3DOG/RTOG 9406. *Int J Radiat Oncol Biol Phys* 2000;46:391-402.

199. Lee WR, Hanks GE, Hanlon AL, et al. Lateral rectal shielding reduces late rectal morbidity following high dose three-dimensional conformal radiation therapy for clinically localized prostate cancer: further evidence for a significant dose effect. *Int J Radiat Oncol Biol Phys* 1996;35:251-257.

200. Pickett B, Roach M III, Horine P, et al. Optimization of the oblique angles in the treatment of prostate cancer during six-field conformal radiotherapy. *Med Dosim* 1994;19:237-254.

201. Perez CA, Michalski JM, Purdy JA, et al. Three-dimensional conformal therapy or standard irradiation in localized carcinoma of prostate: preliminary results of a nonrandomized comparison. *Int J Radiat Oncol Biol Phys* 2000;47:629-637.

202. Kupelian PA, Willoughby TR. Short course intensity modulated radiotherapy (70 Gy at 2.5 Gy per fraction) versus 3D-conformal radiotherapy (78 Gy at 2.0 Gy per fraction) for the treatment of localized prostate cancer: comparable toxicity. *Int J Radiat Oncol Biol Phys* 2000;48(suppl 1):250.

203. ICRU Report 50. Prescribing, recording, and reporting photon beam therapy. International Commission on Radiation Units and Measures, Bethesda, MD. *ICRU Reports* 1993;9:1-72.

204. Sultanem K, Shu H, Xia P, et al. Three-dimensional intensity-modulated radiotherapy in the treatment of nasopharyngeal carcinoma: the University of California-San Francisco experience. *Int J Radiat Oncol Biol Phys* 2000;48:711-722.

205. Mackie TR, Holmes T, Swerdloff S, et al. Tomotherapy: a new concept for the delivery of dynamic conformal radiotherapy. *Med Phys* 1993;20:1709-1719.

206. Verhey LJ. Comparison of three-dimensional conformal radiation therapy and intensity-modulated radiation therapy systems. *Semin Radiat Oncol* 1999;9:78-98.

207. Boyer AL, Yu CX. Intensity-modulated radiation therapy with dynamic multileaf collimators. *Semin Radiat Oncol* 1999;9:48-59.

208. Zelefsky MJ, Fuks Z, Happersett L, et al. Clinical experience with intensity modulated radiation therapy (IMRT) in prostate cancer. *Radiother Oncol* 2000a;55:241-249.

209. Klein EE, Low DA, Sohn JW, et al. Differential dosing of prostate and seminal vesicles using dynamic multileaf collimation. *Int J Radiat Oncol Biol Phys* 2000;48:1447-1456.

210. Dong L, O'Daniel JC, Smith LG, et al. Comparison of 3D conformal and intensity-modulated radiation therapy for early-stage prostate cancer [abstract 2183]. *Int J Radiat Oncol Biol Phys* 51(suppl 1): 320.

211. Zelefsky MJ, Happersett L, Leibel SA, et al. The effect of treatment positioning on normal tissue dose in patients with prostate cancer treated with three-dimensional conformal radiotherapy. *Int J Radiat Oncol Biol Phys* 1997a;37:13-19.

212. Fiorino C, Reni M, Bolognesi A, et al. Set-up error in supine-positioned patients immobilized with two different modalities during conformal radiotherapy of prostate cancer. *Radiother Oncol* 1998;49:133-141.

213. Malone S, Szanto J, Perry G, et al. A prospective comparison of three systems of patient immobilization for prostate radiotherapy. *Int J Radiat Oncol Biol Phys* 2000;48:657-665.

214. Weber DC, Nouet P, Rouzaud M, et al. Patient positioning in prostate radiotherapy: is prone better than supine? *Int J Radiat Oncol Biol Phys* 2000;47:365-371.

215. Dawson LA, Litzenberg DW, Brock KK, et al. A comparison of ventilatory prostate movement in four treatment positions. *Int J Radiat Oncol Biol Phys* 2000;48:319-323.

216. Malone S, Crook JM, Kendal WS, et al. Respiratory-induced prostate motion: quantification and characterization. *Int J Radiat Oncol Biol Phys* 2000;48:105-109.

217. Crook JM, Raymond Y, Salhani D, et al. Prostate motion during standard radiotherapy as assessed by fiducial markers. *Radiother Oncol* 1995;37:35-42.

218. Roeske JC, Forman JD, Mesina CF, et al. Evaluation of changes in the size and location of the prostate, seminal vesicles, bladder, and rectum during a course of external beam radiation therapy. *Int J Radiat Oncol Biol Phys* 1995;33:1321-1329.

219. Rudat V, Schraube P, Oetzel D, et al. Combined error of patient positioning variability and prostate motion uncertainty in 3D conformal radiotherapy of localized prostate cancer. *Int J Radiat Oncol Biol Phys* 1996;35:1027-1034.

220. Van Herk M, Bruce AM, Kroes APG, et al. Quantification of organ motion during conformal radiotherapy of the prostate by three dimensional image registration. *Int J Radiat Oncol Biol Phys* 1995;33:1311-1320.

221. Balter JM, Sandler HM, Lam K, et al. Measurement of prostate movement over the course of routine radiotherapy using implanted markers. *Int J Radiat Oncol Biol Phys* 1995;31:113-118.

222. Althof VG, Hoekstra CJ, te Loo HJ. Variation in prostate position relative to adjacent bony anatomy. *Int J Radiat Oncol Biol Phys* 1996;34:709-715.

223. Melian E, Mageras GS, Fuks Z, et al. Variation in prostate position quantitations and implications for three-dimensional conformal treatment planning. *Int J Radiat Oncol Biol Phys* 1997;38:73-81.

224. Vigneault E, Pouliot J, Laverdiere J, et al. Electronic portal imaging device detection of radioopaque markers for the evaluation of prostate position during megavoltage irradiation: a clinical study. *Int J Radiat Oncol Biol Phys* 1997;37:205-212.

225. Antolak JA, Rosen II, Childress CH, et al. Prostate target volume variations during a course of radiotherapy. *Int J Radiat Oncol Biol Phys* 1998;42:661-672.

226. Zelefsky MJ, Crean D, Mageras GS, et al. Quantification and predictors of prostate position variability in 50 patients evaluated with multiple CT scans during conformal radiotherapy. *Radiother Oncol* 1999;50:225-234.

227. Lattanzi J, McNeeley S, Pinover W, et al. A comparison of daily CT localization to a daily ultrasound-based system in prostate cancer. *Int J Radiat Oncol Biol Phys* 1999;43:719-725.

228. Chen LM, Lubich L, Chiru P, et al. Localization of the prostatic apex for radiotherapy planning: a comparison of two techniques. *Br J Radiol* 1996;69:821-829.

229. Wilder RB, Fone PD, Rademacher DE, et al. Localization of the prostatic apex for radiotherapy treatment planning using urethroscopy. *Int J Radiat Oncol Biol Phys* 1997;38:737-741.

230. Malone S, Donker R, Broader M, et al. Effects of urethrography on prostate position: considerations for radiotherapy treatment planning of prostate carcinoma. *Int J Radiat Oncol Biol Phys* 2000;46:89-93.

231. Sandler HM, Bree BL, McLaughlin PW, et al. Localization of the prostatic apex for radiation therapy using implanted markers. *Int J Radiat Oncol Biol Phys* 1993;27:915-919.

232. Milsosevic M, Voruganti S, Blend R, et al. Magnetic resonance imaging (MRI) for localization of the prostatic apex: comparison to computed tomography (CT) and urethrography. *Radiother Oncol* 1998;47:277-284.

233. Liebel SA, Fuks Z, Zelefsky MJ, et al. The effects of local and regional treatment on the metastatic outcome in prostatic carcinoma with pelvic lymph node involvement. *Int J Radiat Oncol Biol Phys* 1994;28:7-16.

234. Chan RC, Gutierrez AE. Carcinoma of the prostate: its treatment by a combination of radioactive gold-grain implant and external irradiation. *Cancer* 1976;37:2749-2754.

235. Butler EB, Scardino PT, The BS, et al. The Baylor College of Medicine experience with gold seed implantation. *Semin Surg Oncol* 1997;13:406-418.

236. Levitt SH, Tapley N. *Technological Basis of Radiation Therapy: Practical Clinical Applications.* Philadelphia, Pa: Lea & Febiger; 1984.

237. Zelefsky MJ, Whitmore WF Jr. Long-term results of retropubic permanent 125iodine implantation of the prostate for clinically localized prostate cancer. *J Urol* 1997;158:23-29.

238. Eastham JA, Kattan MW, Groshen S, et al. Fifteen-year survival and recurrence rates after radiotherapy for localized prostate cancer. *J Clin Oncol* 1997;15:3214-3222.

239. Scardino PT, Frankel JM, Wheeler TM, et al. The prognostic significance of post-irradiation biopsy results in patients with prostatic cancer. *J Urol* 1986;135:510-516.

240. Prestidge BR, Hoak DC, Grimm PD, et al. Posttreatment biopsy results following interstitial brachytherapy in early-stage prostate cancer. *Int J Radiat Oncol Biol Phys* 1997;37:31-39.

241. Stock RG, Stone NN, Kao J, et al. The effects of disease and treatment-related factors on biopsy results after prostate brachytherapy. *Cancer* 2000;89:1829-1834.

242. Blasko JC, Wallner K, Grimm PD, et al. Prostate specific antigen based disease control following ultrasound guided 125iodine implantation for stage T1/T2 prostatic carcinoma. *J Urol* 1995;154:1096-1099.

243. Ragde H, Korb LJ, Elgamal AA, et al. Modern prostate brachytherapy-prostate specific antigen results in 219 patients with up to 12 years of observed follow-up. *Cancer* 2000;89:135-141.

244. Stock RG, Stone NN, Lo YC. Intraoperative dosimetric representation of the real-time ultrasound-guided prostate implant. *Tech Urol* 2000;6:95-98.

245. Zelefsky MJ, Yamada Y, Cohen G, et al. Postimplantation dosimetric analysis of permanent transperineal prostate implantation: improved dose distributions with an intraoperative computer-optimized conformal planning technique. *Int J Radiat Oncol Biol Phys* 2000b;48:601-608.

246. D'Amico A, Cormack R, Kumar S, et al. Real-time magnetic resonance imaging-guided brachytherapy in the treatment of selected patients with clinically localized prostate cancer. *J Endourol* 2000;14:367-370.

247. Koutrouvelis P, Lailas N, Katz S, et al. High- and low-risk prostate cancer treated with 3D CT-guided brachytherapy: 1- to 5-year follow-up. *J Endourol* 2000;14:357-366.

248. Davis BJ, Pisansky TM, Wilson TM, et al. The radial distance of extraprostatic extension of prostate carcinoma. *Cancer* 1999;85:2630-2637.

249. Sohayda C, Kupelian PA, Levin HS, et al. Extent of extracapsular extension in localized prostate cancer. *Urology* 2000;55:382-386.

250. Prestidge BR, Bice WS, Kiefer EJ, et al. Timing of computed tomography-based postimplant assessment following permanent transperineal prostate brachytherapy. *Int J Radiat Oncol Biol Phys* 1998;40:1111-1115.

251. Yue N, Chen Z, Peschel R, et al. Optimum timing for image-based dose evaluation of 1251 and 103Pd prostate seed implants. *Int J Radiat Oncol Biol Phys* 1999;45:1063-1072.

252. Stock RG, Stone NN, Tabert A, et al. A dose-response study for I-125 prostate implants. *Int J Radiat Oncol Biol Phys* 1998;41:101-108.

253. Nag S, Bice W, DeWyngaert K, et al. The American Brachytherapy Society recommendations for permanent prostate brachytherapy postimplant dosimetric analysis. *Int J Radiat Oncol Biol Phys* 2000;46:221-230.

254. American Association of Physicists in Medicine. AAPM Report No. 43. Dosimetry of interstitial brachytherapy sources: recommendations of the AAPM Radiation Therapy Committee Task Group No. 43. *Med Phys* 1995;22:209-234.

255. Kubo HD, Coursey BM, Hanson WF, et al. Report of the Ad Hoc Committee of the AAPM Radiation Therapy Committee on 125I sealed source dosimetry. *Int J Radiat Oncol Biol Phys* 1998;40:697-702.

256. Bice WS, Prestidge BR, Prete JJ, et al. Clinical impact of implementing the recommendations of AAPM Task Group 43 on permanent prostate brachytherapy using 125I. American Association of Physicists in Medicine. *Int J Radiat Oncol Biol Phys* 1998;40:1237-1241.

257. Beyer D, Nath R, Butler W, et al. American Brachytherapy Society recommendations for clinical implementation of NIST-1999 standards for (103) palladium brachytherapy. The clinical research committee of the American Brachytherapy Society. *Int J Radiat Oncol Biol Phys* 2000;47:273-275.

258. Williamson JF, Coursey BM, DeWerd LA, et al. Recommendations of the American Association of Physicists in Medicine on 103Pd interstitial source calibration and dosimetry: implication for dose specification and prescription. *Med Phys* 2000;27:634-642.

259. Dicker AP, Lin CC, Leeper DB, et al. Isotope selection for permanent prostate implants? An evaluation of 103Pd versus 125I based on radiobiological effectiveness and dosimetry. *Semin Urol Oncol* 2000;18:152-159.

260. Ling CC. Permanent implants using Au-198, Pd-103 and I-125: radiobiological considerations based on the linear quadratic model. *Int J Radiat Oncol Biol Phys* 1992;23:81-87.

261. Dattoli M, Wallner K, Sorace R, et al. 103Pd brachytherapy and external beam irradiation for clinically localized, high-risk prostatic carcinoma. *Int J Radiat Oncol Biol Phys* 1996;35:875-879.

262. Mate TP, Gottesman JE, Hatton J, et al. High dose-rate afterloading 192iridium prostate brachytherapy: feasibility report. *Int J Radiat Oncol Biol Phys* 1998;41:525-533.

263. Vicini FA, Kestin LL, Stromberg JS, et al. Brachytherapy boost techniques for locally advanced prostate cancer. *Oncology* 1999;13:491-509.

264. Martinez AA, Kestin LL, Stromberg JS, et al. Interim report of image-guided conformal high-dose-rate brachytherapy for patients with unfavorable prostate cancer: the William Beaumont phase II dose-escalating trial. *Int J Radiat Oncol Biol Phys* 2000;47:343-352.

265. Borghede G, Hedelin H, Holmäng S, et al. Combined treatment with temporary short-term high dose rate iridium-192 brachytherapy and external beam radiotherapy for irradiation of localized prostatic carcinoma. *Radiother Oncol* 1997;44:237-244.

266. Deger S, Dinges S, Roigas J, et al. High-dose rate iridium192 afterloading therapy in combination with external beam irradiation for localized prostate cancer. *Tech Urol* 1997;3:190-194.

267. Pollack A, Zagars GK. External beam radiotherapy dose response of prostate cancer. *Int J Radiat Oncol Biol Phys* 1997;39:1011-1018.

268. Pinover WH, Hanlon AL, Horwitz EM, et al. Defining the appropriate radiation dose for pretreatment PSA < or = 10 ng/ml prostate cancer. *Int J Radiat Oncol Biol Phys* 2000;47:649-654.

269. Lyons JA, Kupelian PA, Mohan DS, et al. Importance of high radiation doses (72 Gy or greater) in the treatment of stage T1-T3 adenocarcinoma of the prostate. *Urology* 2000;55:85-90.

270. Keyser D, Kupelian PA, Zippe CD, et al. Stage T1–2 prostate cancer with pretreatment prostate-specific antigen level ≤ 10 ng/ml: radiation therapy or surgery? *Int J Radiat Oncol Biol Phys* 1997;38: 723-729.

271. Brachman DG, Thomas T, Hilbe J, et al. Failure-free survival following brachytherapy alone or external beam irradiation alone for T1–2 prostate tumors in 2222 patients: results from a single practice. *Int J Radiat Oncol Biol Phys* 2000;48:111-117.

272. Hanks GE, Hanlon AL, Pinover WH, et al. Dose escalation for prostate cancer patients based on dose comparison and dose response studies. *Int J Radiat Oncol Biol Phys* 2000;46:823-832.

273. Pound CR, Partin AW, Epstein JI, et al. Prostate-specific antigen after anatomic radical retropubic prostatectomy. *Urol Clin North Am* 1997;24:395-406.

274. Catalona WJ, Smith DS. Cancer recurrence and survival rates after anatomic radical retropubic prostatectomy for prostate cancer: intermediate-term results. *J Urol* 1998;160:2428-2434.

275. Wallner K, Roy J, Harrison L. Tumor control and morbidity following transperineal iodine 125 implantation for stage T1/T2 prostate carcinoma. *J Clin Oncol* 1996;14:449-453.

276. Grado GL, Larson TR, Balch CS, et al. Acturial disease-free survival after prostate cancer brachytherapy using interactive techniques with biplane ultrasound and fluoroscopic guidance. *Int J Radiat Oncol Biol Phys* 1998;42:289-298.

277. Stock RG, Stone NN, DeWyngaert JK, et al. Prostate specific antigen findings and biopsy results following interactive ultrasound guided transperineal brachytherapy for early stage prostate carcinoma. *Cancer* 1996;77:2386-2392.

278. Zelefsky MJ, Wallner KE, Ling C, et al. Comparison of the 5-year outcome and morbidity of three-dimensional conformal radiotherapy versus transperineal permanent iodine-125 implantation for early-stage prostatic cancer. *J Clin Oncol* 1999b; 17:517-522.

279. Stokes SH. Comparison of biochemical disease-free survival of patients with localized carcinoma of the prostate undergoing radical prostatectomy, transperineal ultrasound-guided radioactive seed implantation, or definitive external beam irradiation. *Int J Radiat Oncol Biol Phys* 2000;47:129-136.

280. Polascik TJ, Pound CR, De Weese TL, et al. Comparison of radical prostatectomy and iodine 125 interstitial radiotherapy for the treatment of clinically localized prostate cancer: a 7-year biochemical (PSA) progression analysis. *Urology* 1998;51: 884-890.

281. Ramos CG, Carvalhal GF, Smith DS, et al. Retrospective comparison of radical retropubic prostatectomy and ^{125}iodine brachytherapy for localized prostate cancer. *J Urol* 1999;161:1212-1215.

282. Ragde H, Blasko JC, Grimm PD, et al. Interstitial iodine 125 radiation without adjuvant therapy in the treatment of clinically localized prostate carcinoma. *Cancer* 1997;80:442-453.

283. Kupelian P, Katcher J, Levin H, et al. External beam radiotherapy versus radical prostatectomy for clinical stage T1–2 prostate cancer: therapeutic implications of stratification by pretreatment PSA levels and biopsy Gleason scores. *Cancer J Sci Am* 1997;3:78-87.

284. Lee F, Bahn DK, Siders DB, et al. The role of TRUS-guided biopsies for determination of internal and external spread of prostate cancer. *Semin Urol Oncol* 1998;16:129-136.

285. Taneja SS, Penson DF, Epelbaum A, et al. Does site-specific labeling of sextant biopsy cores predict the site of extracapsular extension in radical prostatectomy surgical specimen. *J Urol* 1999;162:1352-1357.

286. Terk MD, Stock RG, Stone NN. Identification of patients at increased risk for prolonged urinary retention following radioactive seed implantation of the prostate. *J Urol* 1998;160:1379-1382.

287. Gelblum DY, Potters L, Ashley R, et al. Urinary morbidity following ultrasound-guided transperineal prostate seed implantation. *Int J Radiat Oncol Biol Phys* 1999;45:59-67.

288. Stone NN, Ratnow ER, Stock RG. Prior transurethral resection does not increase morbidity following real-time ultrasound-guided prostate seed implantation. *Tech Urol* 2000;6:123-127.

289. Bellon J, Wallner K, Ellis W, et al. Use of pelvic CT scanning to evaluate pubic arch interference of transperineal prostate brachytherapy. *Int J Radiat Oncol Biol Phys* 1999;43:579-581.

290. Wallner K, Ellis W, Russell K, et al. Use of TRUS to predict pubic arch interference of prostate brachytherapy. *Int J Radiat Oncol Biol Phys* 1999;43:583-585.

291. Stone NN, Stock RG. Prostate brachytherapy in patients with prostate volumes ≥ 50 cm (3): dosimetric analysis of implant quality. *Int J Radiat Oncol Biol Phys* 2000;46:1199-1204.

292. Wang H, Wallner K, Sutlief S, et al. Transperineal brachytherapy in patients with large prostate glands. *Int J Cancer* 2000;90:199-205.

293. Lee N, Wuu C, Brody R, et al. Factors predicting for postimplantation urinary retention after permanent prostate brachytherapy. *Int J Radiat Oncol Biol Phys* 2000;48:1457-1460.

294. Peschel RE, Chen Z, Roberts K. Long-term complications with prostate implants: iodine-125 vs palladium-103. *Radiat Oncol Investig* 1999;7:278-288.

295. Gelblum DY, Potters L. Rectal complications associated with transperineal interstitial brachytherapy for prostate cancer. *Int J Radiat Oncol Biol Phys* 2000;48:119-124.

296. Sanchez-Ortiz RF, Broderick GA, Rovner ES, et al. Erectile function and quality of life after interstitial radiation therapy for prostate cancer. *Int J Impot Res* 2000;12:S18-24.

297. Zelefsky MJ, Hollister T, Raben A, et al. Five-year biochemical outcome and toxicity with transperineal CT-planned permanent I-125 prostate implantation for patients with localized prostate cancer. *Int J Radiat Oncol Biol Phys* 2000;47:1261-1266.

298. Zelefsky MJ, Wallner KE, Ling CC, et al. Comparison of the 5-year outcome and morbidity of three-dimensional conformal radiotherapy versus transperineal permanent iodine-125 implantation for early-stage prostatic cancer. *J Clin Oncol* 1999; 17:517-522.

299. Wilder RB, Chou RH, Ryu JK, et al. Potency preservation after three-dimensional conformal radiotherapy for prostate cancer: preliminary results. *Am J Clin Oncol* 2000;23:330-333.

300. Brandeis JM, Litwin MS, Burnison CM, et al. Quality of life outcomes after brachytherapy for early stage prostate cancer. *J Urol* 2000;163:851-857.

301. Zeitlin SI, Sherman J, Raboy A, et al. High dose combination radiotherapy for the treatment of localized prostate cancer. *J Urol* 1998;160:91-96.

302. Pollack A, Smith LG, von Eschenbach AC. External beam radiotherapy dose-response characteristics of 1127 men with prostate cancer treated in the PSA era. *Int J Radiat Oncol Biol Phys* 2000;48:507-512.

303. Zelefsky MJ, Fuks Z, Venkatraman ES, et al. Predictors of posttreatment prostatic biopsy outcome after 3-dimensional conformal radiotherapy for patients with clinically localized prostate cancer. *Int J Radiat Oncol Biol Phys* 2000;48(suppl 1):231.

304. Hanks GE, Leibel S, Kramer S. The dissemination of cancer by transurethral resection of locally advanced prostate cancer. *J Urol* 1983;129:309-311.

305. Hanks GE, Martz KL, Diamond JJ. The effect of dose on local control of prostate cancer. *Int J Radiat Oncol Biol Phys* 1988;15:1299-1305.

306. Perez CA, Walz BJ, Zivnuska FR, et al. Irradiation of carcinoma of the prostate localized to the pelvis: analysis of tumor response and prognosis. *Int J Radiat Oncol Biol Phys* 1980;6:555-563.

307. Perez CA, Pilepich MV, Garcia D, et al. Definitive radiation therapy in carcinoma of the prostate localized to the pelvis: experience at the Mallinckrodt Institute of Radiology. *NCI Monogr* 1988;7:85-94.

308. Shipley WU, Verhey LJ, Munzenrider JE, et al. Advanced prostate cancer: the results of a randomized comparative trial of high

dose irradiation boosting with conformal protons compared with conventional dose irradiation using photons alone. *Int J Radiat Oncol Biol Phys* 1995;32:13-20.

309. Dearnaley DP, Khoo VS, Norman AR, et al. Comparison of radiation side-effects of conformal and conventional radiotherapy in prostate cancer: a randomized trial. *Lancet* 1999;353:267-272.

310. Smit WGJM, Helle PA, van Putten WL, et al. Late radiation damage in prostate cancer patients treated by high dose external radiotherapy in relation to rectal dose. *Int J Radiat Oncol Biol Phys* 1990;18:23-29.

311. Benk VA, Adams JA, Shipley WU, et al. Late rectal bleeding following combined x-ray and proton high dose irradiation for patients with stages T3–T4 prostate carcinoma. *Int J Radiat Oncol Biol Phys* 1993;26:551-557.

312. Boersma LJ, van den Brink M, Bruce AM, et al. Estimation of the incidence of late bladder and rectum complications after high-dose (70-78 Gy) conformal radiotherapy for prostate cancer, using dose-volume histograms. *Int J Radiat Oncol Biol Phys* 1998;41:83-92.

313. McGowan DG. The value of extended field radiation therapy in carcinoma of the prostate. *Int J Radiat Oncol Biol Phys* 1981;7:1333-1339.

314. Ploysongsang S, Scott RM, Aron BS, et al. Comparison of whole pelvic versus small-field radiation therapy for carcinoma of the prostate. *Urology* 1986;27:10-16.

315. Lawton CA, Cox JD, Glisch C, et al. Is long-term survival possible with external beam irradiation for stage D1 adenocarcinoma of the prostate? *Cancer* 1992;69:2761-2766.

316. Seaward SA, Weinberg V, Lewis P, et al. Identification of a high-risk clinically localized prostate cancer subgroup receiving maximum benefit from whole-pelvic irradiation. *Cancer J Sci Am* 1998;4:370-377.

317. Seaward SA, Weinberg V, Lewis P, et al. Improved freedom from PSA failure with whole pelvic irradiation for high-risk prostate cancer. *Int J Radiat Oncol Biol Phys* 1998;42:1055-1062.

318. Zagars GK, von Eschenbach AC, Johnson DE, et al. Stage C adenocarcinoma of the prostate. An analysis of 551 patients treated with external beam radiation. *Cancer* 1987;60:1489-1499.

319. Rasp GM, Pisansky TM, Haddock MG, et al. Elective pelvic nodal irradiation in patients with clinically localized prostate cancer at high risk for pelvic nodal involvement (abstract). *Int J Radiat Oncol Biol Phys* 1996;36(suppl):245.

320. Perez CA, Michalski J, Brown KC, et al. Nonrandomized evaluation of pelvic lymph node irradiation in localized carcinoma of the prostate. *Int J Radiat Oncol Biol Phys* 1996;36:573-584.

321. Lim Joon D, Hasegawa M, Sikes C, et al. Supra-additive apoptotic response of R3327-G rat prostate tumors to androgen ablation and radiation. *Int J Radiat Oncol Biol Phys* 1997;38:1071-1077.

322. Zietman AL, Prince E, Nakfoor BM, et al. Androgen deprivation and radiation therapy: sequencing studies using the shionogi in vivo tumor system. *Int J Radiat Oncol Biol Oncol* 1997;38:1067-1070.

323. Pollack A, Ashoori F, Sikess C, et al. The early supra-additive apoptotic response of R3327-G prostate tumors to androgen ablation and radiation is not sustained with multiple fractions. *Int J Radiat Oncol Biol Phys* 1999;46:153-158.

324. Pilepich MV, Krall JM, John MJ, et al. Hormonal cytoreduction in locally advanced carcinoma of the prostate treated with definitive radiotherapy: preliminary results of RTOG 83-07. *Int J Radiat Oncol Biol Phys* 1989;16:813-817.

325. Pilepich MV, John MJ, Krall JM, et al. Phase II Radiation Therapy Oncology Group study of hormonal cytoreduction with Flutamide and Zoladex in locally advanced carcinoma of the prostate treated with definitive radiotherapy. *Am J Clin Oncol* 1990;13:461-464.

326. Pilepich MV, Krall JM, Al-Sarraf M, et al. Androgen deprivation with radiation therapy compared with radiation therapy alone for locally advanced prostatic carcinoma: a randomized comparative trial of the Radiation Therapy Oncology Group. *Urology* 1995;45:616-623.

327. Hanks GE, Lu JD, Machtay M, et al. RTOG protocol 92-02: a phase III trial of the use of long term androgen suppression following neoadjuvant hormonal cytoreduction and radiotherapy in locally advanced carcinoma of the prostate. *Int J Radiat Oncol Biol Phys* 2000;48(suppl):112.

328. Shearer RJ, Davies JH, Gelister JS, et al. Hormonal cytoreduction and radiotherapy for carcinoma of the prostate. *Br J Urol* 1992;69:521-524.

329. Yang FE, Chen GT, Ray P, et al. The potential for normal tissue dose reduction with neoadjuvant hormonal therapy in conformal treatment planning for stage C prostate cancer. *Int J Radiat Oncol Biol Phys* 1995;33:1009-1017.

330. Forman JD, Kumar R, Haas G, et al. Neo-adjuvant hormonal downsizing of localized carcinoma of the prostate: effects on the volume of normal tissue irradiation. *Cancer Invest* 1995;13:132-133.

331. Zelefsky MJ, Leibel SA, Burman CM, et al. Neoadjuvant hormonal therapy improves the therapeutic ratio in patients with bulky prostatic cancer treated with three-dimensional conformal radiation therapy. *Int J Radiat Oncol Biol Phys* 1994;29:755-761.

332. Zagars GK, Johnson DE, von Eschenbach AC, et al. Adjuvant estrogen following radiation therapy for stage C adenocarcinoma of the prostate: long term results of a prospective randomized study. *Int J Radiat Oncol Biol Phys* 1988;14:1085-1091.

333. Fellows GJ, Clark PB, Beynon LL, et al. Treatment of advanced localized prostatic cancer by orchiectomy, radiotherapy, or combined treatment. A Medical Research Council study. *Br J Urol* 1992;70:304-309.

334. Pilepich MV, Caplan R, Byhardt RW, et al. Phase III trial of androgen suppression using goserelin in unfavorable-prognosis carcinoma of the prostate treated with definitive radiotherapy: report of the Radiation Therapy Oncology Group protocol 85-31. *J Clin Oncol* 1997;15:1013-1021.

335. Bolla M, Gonzalez D, Warde P, et al. Improved survival in patients with locally advanced prostate cancer treated with radiotherapy and goserelin. *N Engl J Med* 1997;337:295-300.

336. Granfors T, Modig H, Damber J-E, et al. Combined orchiectomy and external radiotherapy versus radiotherapy alone for non-metastatic prostate cancer with or without pelvic lymph node involvement: a prospective randomized trial. *J Urol* 1998;159:2030-2034.

337. Pilepich MV, Winter K, John MJ, et al. Phase III Radiation Therapy Oncology Group trial 86-10 of androgen deprivation adjuvant to definitive radiotherapy in locally advanced carcinoma of the prostate. *Int J Radiat Oncol Biol Phys* 2001;50:1243-1252.

338. Medical Research Council Prostate Cancer Working Investigators Group. Immediate versus deferred treatment for advanced prostatic cancer: initial results of the Medical Research Council trial. *Br J Urol* 1997;79:235-246.

339. Lawton CA, Winter K, Murray K, et al. Updated results of the phase III Radiation Therapy Oncology Group (RTOG) trial 85-31 evaluating the potential benefit of androgen suppression following standard radiation therapy for unfavorable carcinoma of the prostate. *Int J Radiat Oncol Biol Phys* 2001;49:937-946.

340. Del Regato J. Long term curative results of radiotherapy for patients with inoperable prostatic carcinoma. *Radiology* 1979;131:291-297.

341. Byar DP. The Veterans Administrative Cooperative Research Group's studies of conservative treatment. *Scand J Urol* 1980;55(suppl):99-102.

342. Bolla M, Collette L, Gonzalez D, et al. Long-term results of immediate adjuvant hormonal therapy with goserelin in patients with locally advanced prostate cancer treated with radiotherapy. A phase III EORTC study. *Int J Radiat Oncol Biol Phys* 1999;45(3 suppl):147.

343. Byar DP, Green SB. The choice of treatment for cancer patients based on covariate information: application to prostate cancer. *Bull Cancer* 1988;67:477-490.

344. Oefelein MG, Feng A, Scolieri MJ, et al. Reassessment of the definition of castrate levels of testosterone: implications for clinical decision making. *Urology* 2000;56:1021-1024.

345. Nejat RJ, Rashid HH, Bagiella E, et al. A prospective analysis of time to normalization of serum testosterone after withdrawal of androgen deprivation therapy. *J Urol* 2000;164:1891-1894.

346. D'Amico AV, Schultz D, Loffredo M, et al. Biochemical outcome following external beam radiation therapy with or without androgen suppression therapy for clinically localized prostate cancer. *JAMA* 2000;284:1280-1283.

347. Granfors T, Tomic R, Bergh A, et al. After radiotherapy testosterone stimulation is unable to increase growth in the dunning R3327-PAP prostate tumour. *Urol Res* 1999;27:357-361.

348. Smith JA Jr, Haynes TH, Middleton RG. Impact of external irradiation on local symptoms and survival free of disease in patients with pelvic lymph node metastasis from adenocarcinoma of the prostate. *J Urol* 1984;131:705-707.

349. Bagshaw MA. Radiotherapeutic treatment of prostatic carcinoma with pelvic node involvement. *Urol Clin North Am* 1984;11:297-304.

350. Gervasi LA, Mata J, Easley JD, et al. Prognostic significance of lymph nodal metastases in prostate cancer. *J Urol* 1989;142:332-336.

351. Lawton CA, Cox JD, Glisch C, et al. Is long-term survival possible with external beam irradiation for stage D1 adenocarcinoma of the prostate? *Cancer* 1992;69:2761-2766.

352. Hanks GE. The challenge of treating node-positive prostate cancer. An approach to resolving the questions. *Cancer* 1993;71:1014-1018.

353. Lawton CA, Winter K, Byhardt R, et al. Androgen suppression plus radiation versus radiation alone for patients with D1 (pN+) adenocarcinoma of the prostate (results based on a national prospective randomized trial, RTOG 85-31). Radiation Therapy Oncology Group. *Int J Radiat Oncol Biol Phys* 1997;38:931-939.

354. deKernion JB, Neuwirth H, Stein A, et al. Prognosis of patients with stage D1 prostate carcinoma following radical prostatectomy with and without early endocrine therapy. *J Urol* 1990;144:700-703.

355. Myers RP, Larson-Keller JJ, Bergstralh EJ, et al. Hormonal treatment at time of radical retropubic prostatectomy for stage D1 prostate cancer: results of long-term followup. *J Urol* 1992;147:910-915.

356. Zincke H, Bergstralh EJ, Larson-Keller JJ, et al. Stage D1 prostate cancer treated by radical prostatectomy and adjuvant hormonal treatment: evidence for favorable survival in patients with DNA diploid tumors. *Cancer* 1992;70:311-323.

357. Sgrignoli AR, Walsh PC, Steinberg GD, et al. Prognostic factors in men with stage D1 prostate cancer: identification of patients less likely to have prolonged survival after radical prostatectomy. *J Urol* 1994;152:1077-1081.

358. Messing EM, Manola J, Sarosdy M, et al. Immediate hormonal therapy compared with observation after radical prostatectomy and pelvic lymphadenectomy in men with node-positive prostate cancer. *N Engl J Med* 1999;341:1781-1788.

359. Seay TM, Blute ML, Zincke H. Long-term outcome in patients with pTxN+ adenocarcinoma of prostate treated with radical prostatectomy and early androgen ablation. *J Urol* 1998;159:357-364.

360. Zagars GK, Sands ME, Pollack A, et al. Early androgen ablation for stage D1 (N1-N3, N0) prostate cancer. Prognostic variables and outcome. *J Urol* 1994;151:1330-1333.

361. Zagars G, Pollack A, von Eschenbach A. Addition of radiotherapy to androgen ablation improves outcome for node-positive prostate cancer. *Radiother Oncol* 2000;56:127-128.

362. Ghavamian R, Bergstralh EJ, Blute ML, et al. Radical retropubic prostatectomy plus orchiectomy versus orchiectomy alone for pTxN+ prostate cancer: a matched comparison. *J Urol* 1999;16:1223-1227.

363. Laramore GE, Krall JM, Thomas FJ, et al. Fast neutron radiotherapy for locally advanced prostate cancer. *Am J Clin Oncol* 1993;16:164-167.

364. Russell KJ, Caplan RJ, Laramore GE, et al. Photon versus fast neutron external beam radiotherapy in the treatment of locally advanced prostate cancer: results of a randomized prospective trial. *Int J Radiat Oncol Biol Phys* 1994;28:47-54.

365. Laramore GE. The use of neutrons in cancer therapy: a historical perspective through the modern era. *Semin Oncol* 1997;24:672-685.

366. Lindsley KL, Cho P, Stelzer KJ, et al. Fast neutrons in prostatic adenocarcinomas: worldwide clinical experience. *Recent Results Cancer Res* 1998;150:125-136.

367. Chuba PJ, Maughan R, Forman JD. Three dimensional conformal neutron radiotherapy for prostate cancer. *Strahlenthe Onkol* 1999;175:79-81.

368. Slater JD, Rossi CJ Jr, Yonemoto LT, et al. Conformal proton therapy for early-stage prostate cancer. *Urology* 1999;53:978-984.

369. Kabalin JN, Hodge KK, McNeal JE, et al. Identification of residual cancer in the prostate following radiation therapy: role of transrectal ultrasound guided biopsy and prostate specific antigen. *J Urol* 1989;142:326-331.

370. Babaian RJ, Kohima M, Saitoh M, et al. Detection of residual prostate cancer after external radiotherapy. Role of prostate specific antigen and transrectal ultrasonography. *Cancer* 1995;75:2153-2158.

371. Cox JD, Stoffel TJ. The significance of needle biopsy after irradiation for the stage C adenocarcinoma of the prostate. *Cancer* 1977;40:156-160.

372. Herr HW, Whitmore WF Jr. Significance of prostatic biopsies after radiation therapy for carcinoma of the prostate. *Prostate* 1982;3:339-350.

373. Cox JD, Kline RW. The lack of prognostic significance of biopsies after radiotherapy for prostatic cancer. *Semin Urol* 1983;4:237-242.

374. Crook JM, Perry GA, Robertson S, et al. Routine prostate biopsies following radiotherapy for prostate cancer: results for 226 patients. *Urology* 1995;45:624-632.

375. Crook J, Malone S, Perry G, et al. Postradiotherapy prostate biopsies: what do they really mean? Results for 498 patients. *Int J Radiat Oncol Biol Phys* 2000;48:355-367.

376. Sartor CI, Strawderman MH, Lin XH, et al. Rate of PSA rise predicts metastatic versus local recurrence after definitive radiotherapy. *Int J Radiat Oncol Biol Phys* 1997;38:941-947.

377. Zagars GK, Pollack A. Kinetics of serum prostate-specific antigen after external beam radiation for clinically localized prostate cancer. *Radiother Oncol* 1997;44:213-221.

378. Lee WR, Hanks GE, Hanlon A. Increasing prostate-specific antigen profile following definitive radiation therapy for localized prostate cancer: clinical observations. *J Clin Oncol* 1997;15:230-238.

379. Amling CL, Lerner SE, Martin SK, et al. Deoxyribonucleic acid ploidy and serum prostate specific antigen predict outcome following salvage prostatectomy for radiation refractory prostate cancer. *J Urol* 1999;161:857-862.

380. Cheng L, Lloyd RV, Weaver AL, et al. The cell cycle inhibitors p21WAF1 and p27KIP1 are associated with survival in patients treated by salvage prostatectomy after radiation therapy. *Clin Cancer Res* 2000;6:1896-1899.

381. Rogers E, Ohori M, Kassabian VS, et al. Salvage radical prostatectomy: outcome measured by serum prostate specific antigen levels. *J Urol* 1995;153:104-110.

382. Garzotto M, Wajsman Z. Androgen deprivation with salvage surgery for radiorecurrent prostate cancer: results at 5-year followup. *J Urol* 1998;159:950-954.

383. Gheiler EL, Tefilli MV, Tiguert R, et al. Predictors for maximal outcome in patients undergoing salvage surgery for radio-recurrent prostate cancer. *Urology* 1998;51:789-795.

384. Vaidya A, Soloway MS. Salvage radical prostatectomy for radio-recurrent prostate cancer: morbidity revisited. *J Urol* 2000;164:1998-2001.

385. Pisters LL, English SF, Scott SM, et al. Salvage prostatectomy with continent catheterizable urinary reconstruction: a novel approach to recurrent prostate cancer after radiation therapy. *J Urol* 2000;163:1771-1774.

386. de la Taille A, Hayek O, Benson MC, et al. Salvage cryotherapy for recurrent prostate cancer after radiation therapy: the Columbia experience. *Urology* 2000;55:79-84.

387. Perrotte P, Litwin MS, McGuire EJ, et al. Quality of life after salvage cryotherapy: the impact of treatment parameters. *J Urol* 1999;162:398-402.

388. Pisters LL, von Eschenbach AC, Scott SM, et al. The efficacy and complications of salvage cryotherapy of the prostate. *J Urol* 1997;157:921-925.

389. Lee F, Bahn DK, McHugh TA, et al. Cryosurgery of prostate cancer. Use of adjuvant hormonal therapy and temperature monitoring—a one-year follow-up. *Anticancer Res* 1997;17:1511-1515.

390. Miller RJ Jr, Cohen JK, Shuman B, et al. Percutaneous, transperineal cryosurgery of the prostate as salvage therapy for postradiation recurrence of adenocarcinoma. *Cancer* 1996;77:1510-1514.

391. Beyer DC. Permanent brachytherapy as salvage treatment for recurrent prostate cancer. *Urology* 1999;54:880-883.

392. Grado GL, Collins JM, Kriegshauser JS, et al. Salvage brachytherapy for localized prostate cancer after radiotherapy failure. *Urology* 1999;53:2-10.

393. Reiner WG, Walsh PC. An anatomical approach to the surgical management of the dorsal vein and Santorini's plexus during radical retropubic surgery. *J Urol* 1979;121:198-200.

394. Walsh PC. Radical prostatectomy for localized prostate cancer provides durable cancer control with excellent quality of life: a structured debate. *J Urol* 2000;163:1802-1807.

395. Walsh PC, Marschke P, Ricker D, et al. Patient-reported urinary continence and sexual function after anatomic radical prostatectomy. *Urology* 2000;55:58-61.

396. Catalona WJ, Basler JW. Return of erections and urinary incontinence following nerve sparing radical retropubic prostatectomy. *J Urol* 1993;150:905-907.

397. Benoit RM, Naslund MJ, Cohen JK. Complications after radical retropubic prostatectomy in the Medicare population. *Urology* 2000;56:116-120.

398. Fowler FJ, Roman A, Barry MJ, et al. Patient-reported complications and follow-up treatment after radical prostatectomy, the national Medicare experience: 1988–1990. *Urology* 1993;42:622-629.

399. Jonler M, Messing EM, Rhodes PR, et al. Sequelae of radical prostatectomy. *Br J Urol* 1994;74:352-358.

400. Talcott JA, Rieker P, Propert KJ, et al. Patient-reported impotence and incontinence after nerve-sparing radical prostatectomy. *J Natl Cancer Inst* 1997;89:1117-1123.

401. Kim ED, Scardino PT, Hampel O, et al. Interposition of sural nerve restores function of cavernous nerves resected during radical prostatectomy. *J Urol* 1999;l161:188-192.

402. Jonler M, Ritter MA, Brinkmann R, et al. Sequelae of definitive radiation therapy for prostate cancer localized to the pelvis. *Urology* 1994;44:876-882.

403. Crook J, Esche B, Futter N. Effect of pelvic radiotherapy for prostate cancer on bowel, bladder, and sexual function: the patient's perspective. *Urology* 1996;47:387-394.

404. Litwin MS, Pasta DJ, Yu J, et al. Urinary function and bother after radical prostatectomy or radiation for prostate cancer: a longitudinal, multivariate quality of life analysis from the cancer of the prostate strategic urologic research endeavor. *J Urol* 2000;164:1973-1977.

405. Iwakiri J, Grandbois K, Wehner N, et al. An analysis of urinary prostate specific antigen before and after radical prostatectomy: evidence for secretion of prostate specific antigen by the periurethral glands. *J Urol* 1993;149:783.

406. Trapasso JG, deKernion JB, Smith RB, et al. The incidence and significance of detectable levels of serum prostate specific antigen after radical prostatectomy. *J Urol* 1994;152:1821-1825.

407. Amling CL, Blute ML, Bergstralh EJ, et al. Long-term hazard of progression after radical prostatectomy for clinically localized prostate cancer: continued risk of biochemical failure after 5 years. *J Urol* 2000;164:101-105.

408. Vallancien G, Bochereau G, Wetzel O, et al. Influence of preoperative positive seminal vesicle biopsy on the staging of prostatic cancer. *J Urol* 1994;152:1152-1156.

409. Narayan P, Gajendran V, Taylor SP, et al. The role of transrectal ultrasound-guided biopsy-based staging, preoperative serum prostate-specific antigen, and biopsy Gleason score in prediction of final pathologic diagnosis in prostate cancer. *Urology* 1995;46:205-212.

410. Hanlon AL, Hanks GE. Failure pattern implications following external beam irradiation of prostate cancer: long-term follow-up and indications of cure. *Cancer J Sci Am* 2000;2:S193-197.

411. Hanks GE, Hanlon AL, Pinover WH, et al. Evidence for cure of young men with prostate cancer treated by external beam radiation. *Oncology* 2001;15:563-567.

412. Van Poppel H, De Ridder D, Elgamal AA, et al. Neoadjuvant hormonal therapy before radical prostatectomy decreases the number of positive surgical margins in stage T2 prostate cancer: interim results of a prospective randomized trial. *J Urol* 1995;154:429-434.

413. Soloway MS, Sharifi R, McLeod D, et al. Randomized prospective study—radical prostatectomy alone vs radical prostatectomy preceded by androgen ablation in cT2b prostate cancer—initial results. *J Urol* 1996;155(suppl):555A.

414. Goldenberg SL, Klotz LH, Srigley J, et al. Randomized, prospective, controlled study comparing radical prostatectomy alone and neoadjuvant androgen withdrawal in the treatment of localized prostate cancer. Canadian Urologic Oncology Group. *J Urol* 1996;156:873-877.

415. Labrie F, Cusan L, Gomez JL, et al. Neoadjuvant hormonal therapy: the Canadian experience. *Urology* 1997;49(suppl 3A):56-64.

416. Fair WR, Cookson MS, Stroumbakis N, et al. The indications, rationale, and results of neoadjuvant androgen deprivation in the treatment of prostatic cancer: Memorial Sloan-Kettering Cancer Center results. *Urology* 1997;49(suppl 3A):46-55.

417. Witjes WP, Schulman CC, Frans MJ. Preliminary results of a prospective randomized study comparing radical prostatectomy versus radical prostatectomy associated with neoadjuvant hormonal combination therapy in T2-3 N0 M0 prostatic carcinoma. *Urology* 1997;49(suppl 3A):65-69.

418. Aus G, Abrahamsson PA, Ahlgren G, et al. Hormonal treatment before radical prostatectomy: a 3-year follow-up. *J Urol* 1998;159:2013-2017.

419. Pollack A, Zagars GK, Rosen I. Androgen ablation in addition to radiotherapy for prostate cancer: is there true benefit? *Semin Radiat Oncol* 1998;8:95-106.

420. Pollack A. Does radiotherapy add anything to androgen ablation? In: Taylor J, ed. *American Society of Clinical Oncology Spring*

Educational Book. Baltimore, Md: Lippincott Williams & Wilkins; 2000:320-326.

421. Klotz LH, Goldenberg SL, Jewett M, et al. CUOG randomized trial of neoadjuvant androgen ablation before radical prostatectomy: 36-month post-treatment PSA results. Canadian Urologic Oncology Group. *Urology* 1999;53:757-763.

422. Baert L, Goethuys HJ, De Ridder DJ, et al. Neoadjuvant treatment before radical prostatectomy decreases the number of positive margins in cT2–cT3 but has no impact on PSA progression. *J Urol* 1998;159(suppl):61.

423. Meyer F, Moore L, Bairati I, et al. Neoadjuvant hormonal therapy before radical prostatectomy and risk of prostate specific antigen failure. *J Urol* 1999;162:2024-2028.

424. Gleave ME, Goldenberg SL, Jones EC, et al. Biochemical and pathological effects of 8 months of neoadjuvant androgen withdrawal therapy before radical prostatectomy in patients with clinically confined prostate cancer. *J Urol* 1996;155:213-219.

425. Gleave ME, La Bianca SE, Goldenberg SL, et al. Long-term neoadjuvant hormone therapy prior to radical prostatectomy: evaluation of risk for biochemical recurrence at 5-year follow-up. *Urology* 2000;56:289-294.

426. van der Kwast TH, Tetu B, Candas B, et al. Prolonged neoadjuvant combined androgen blockade leads to a further reduction of prostatic tumor volume: three versus six months of endocrine therapy. *Urology* 1999;53:523-529.

427. Montironi R, Diamanti L, Santinelli A, et al. Effect of total androgen ablation on pathologic stage and resection limit status of prostate cancer. Initial results of the Italian PROSIT study. *Pathol Res Pract* 1999;195:201-208.

428. McCarthy JF, Catalona WJ, Hudson MA, et al. Effect of radiation therapy on detectable serum prostate specific antigen levels following radical prostatectomy: early versus delayed treatment. *J Urol* 1994;1515:1575-1578.

429. Coetzee LJ, Hars V, Paulson DF. Postoperative prostate-specific antigen as a prognostic indicator in patients with margin-positive prostate cancer, undergoing adjuvant radiotherapy after radical prostatectomy. *Urology* 1996;47:232-235.

430. Garg MK, Tekyi-Mensah S, Bolton S, et al. Impact of postprostatectomy prostate-specific antigen nadir on outcomes following salvage radiotherapy. *Urology* 1998;51:998-1002.

431. Schild SE. Radiation therapy after prostatectomy: now or later? *Semin Radiat Oncol* 1998;8:132-139.

432. Anscher MS. Adjuvant therapy for pathologic stage C prostate cancer: a casualty of the PSA revolution? *Int J Radiat Oncol Biol Phys* 1996;34:745-747.

433. Tefilli MV, Gheiler EL, Tiguert R, et al. Prognostic indicators in patients with seminal vesicle involvement following radical prostatectomy for clinically localized prostate cancer. *J Urol* 1998;160:802-806.

434. Ohori M, Wheeler TM, Kattan MW, et al. Prognostic significance of positive surgical margins in radical prostatectomy specimens. *J Urol* 1995;154:1818-1824.

435. Epstein JI, Partin AW, Sauvageot J, et al. Prediction of progression following radical prostatectomy. A multivariate analysis of 721 men with long-term follow-up. *Am J Surg Pathol* 1996;20:286-292.

436. Lowe BA, Lieberman SF. Disease recurrence and progression in untreated pathologic stage T3 prostate cancer: selecting the patient for adjuvant therapy. *J Urol* 1997;158:1452-1456.

437. Bauer JJ, Connelly RR, Seterheinn IA, et al. Biostatistical modeling using traditional preoperative and pathological prognostic variables in the selection of men at high risk for disease recurrence after radical prostatectomy for prostate cancer. *J Urol* 1998;159:929-933.

438. Gilliland FD, Hoffman RM, Hamilton A, et al. Predicting extracapsular extension of prostate cancer in men treated with radical prostatectomy: results from the population based prostate cancer outcomes study. *J Urol* 1999;162:1341-1345.

439. Cheng L, Slezak J, Bergstralh EJ, et al. Preoperative prediction of surgical margin status in patients with prostate cancer treated by radical prostatectomy. *J Clin Oncol* 2000;18:2862-2868.

440. Blute ML, Bergstralh EJ, Partin AW, et al. Validation of Partin tables for predicting pathological stage of clinically localized prostate cancer. *J Urol* 2000;164:1591-1595.

441. Pollack A, Smith LG. Adjuvant external beam radiotherapy. In: D'Amico AV, Carroll P, Kantoff PW, eds. *Prostate Cancer.* Philadelphia, Pa: Lippincott, Williams & Wilkins; 2000:456-463.

442. Epstein JI. Incidence and significance of positive margins in radical prostatectomy specimens. *Urol Clin North Am* 1996;23:651-663.

443. Kupelian PA, Katcher J, Levin HS, et al. Stage T1–2 prostate cancer: a multivariate analysis of factors affecting biochemical and clinical failures after radical prostatectomy. *Int J Radiat Oncol Biol Phys* 1997;37:1043-1052.

444. Zietman AL, Edelstein RA, Coen JJ, et al. Radical prostatectomy for adenocarcinoma of the prostate: the influence of preoperative and pathologic findings on biochemical disease-free outcome. *Urology* 1994;43:828-833.

445. Watson RB, Civantos F, Soloway MS. Positive surgical margins with radical prostatectomy: detailed pathological analysis and prognosis. *Urology* 1996;48:80-90.

446. Grossfeld GD, Tigrani VS, Nudell D, et al. Management of a positive surgical margin after radical prostatectomy: decision analysis. *J Urol* 2000;164:93-100.

447. Gibbons RP, Cole BS, Richardson RG, et al. Adjuvant radiotherapy following radical prostatectomy: results and complications. *J Urol* 1986;135:65-68.

448. Meier R, Mark R, St Royal L, et al. Postoperative radiation therapy after radical prostatectomy for prostate carcinoma. *Cancer* 1992;70:1960-1966.

449. Cheng WS, Frydenberg M, Bergstralh EJ, et al. Radical prostatectomy for pathologic stage C prostate cancer: influence of pathologic variables and adjuvant treatment on disease outcome. *Urology* 1993;42:283.

450. Anscher MS, Robertson CN, Prosnita LR. Adjuvant radiotherapy for pathologic stage T3/4 adenocarcinoma of the prostate: ten-year update. *Int J Radiat Oncol Biol Phys* 1995;33:37-43.

451. Syndikus I, Pickles T, Kostashuk E, et al. Postoperative radiotherapy for stage pT3 carcinoma of the prostate: improved local control. *J Urol* 1996;155:1983-1986.

452. Leibovich BC, Engen DE, Patterson DE, et al. Benefit of adjuvant radiation therapy for localized prostate cancer with a positive surgical margin. *J Urol* 2000;163:1178-1182.

453. Forman JD, Meetze K, Pontes E, et al. Therapeutic irradiation for patients with an elevated post-prostatectomy prostate specific antigen level. *J Urol* 1997;158:1436-1439.

454. Forman JD, Velasco J. Therapeutic radiation in patients with a rising post-prostatectomy PSA level. *Oncology* 1998;12:33-39.

455. Zietman AL, Coen JJ, Shipley WU, et al. Adjuvant irradiation after radical prostatectomy for adenocarcinoma of prostate: analysis of freedom from PSA failure. *Urology* 1993;42:292-299.

456. Schild SE, Buskirk SJ, Wong WW, et al. The use of radiotherapy for patients with isolated elevation of serum prostate specific antigen following radical prostatectomy. *J Urol* 1996;156:1725-1729.

457. Morris MM, Dallow KC, Zietman AL, et al. Adjuvant and salvage irradiation following radical prostatectomy for prostate cancer. *Int J Radiat Oncol Biol Phys* 1997;38:731-736.

458. Valicenti RK, Gomella LG, Ismail M, et al. Pathologic seminal vesicle invasion after radical prostatectomy for patients with prostate carcinoma: effect of early adjuvant radiation therapy on biochemical control. *Cancer* 1998;82:1909-1914.

459. Valicenti RK, Gomella LG, Ismail M, et al. The efficacy of early adjuvant radiation therapy for pT3N0 prostate cancer: a matched-pair analysis. *Int J Radiat Oncol Biol Phys* 1999;45:53-58.

460. Vicini FA, Ziaja EL, Kestin LL, et al. Treatment outcome with adjuvant and salvage irradiation after radical prostatectomy for prostate cancer. *Urology* 1999;54:111-117.

461. Petrovich Z, Lieskovsky G, Langholz B, et al. Comparison of outcomes of radical prostatectomy with and without adjuvant pelvic irradiation in patients with pathologic stage C (T3N0) adenocarcinoma of the prostate. *Am J Clin Oncol* 1999;22:323-331.

462. Nudell DM, Grossfeld GD, Weinberg VK, et al. Radiotherapy after radical prostatectomy: treatment outcomes and failure patterns. *Urology* 1999;54:1049-1057.

463. Valicenti RK, Gomella LG, Ismail M, et al. Durable efficacy of early postoperative radiation therapy for high-risk pT3N0 prostate cancer: the importance of radiation dose. *Urology* 1998;52:1034-1040.

464. Anscher MS, Prosnitz LR. Multivariate analysis of factors predicting local relapse after radical prostatectomy—possible indications for postoperative radiotherapy. *Int J Radiat Oncol Biol Phys* 1991;21:941-947.

465. Wu JJ, King SC, Montana GS, et al. The efficacy of postprostatectomy radiotherapy in patients with an isolated elevation of serum prostate-specific antigen. *Int J Radiat Oncol Biol Phys* 1995;32:317-323.

466. Zelefsky MJ, Aschkenasy E, Kelsen S, et al. Tolerance and early outcome results of postprostatectomy three-dimensional conformal radiotherapy. *Int J Radiat Oncol Biol Phys* 1997;l39:327-333.

467. Rogers R, Grossfeld GD, Roach M III, et al. Radiation therapy for the management of biopsy proved local recurrence after radical prostatectomy. *J Urol* 1998;160:1748-1753.

468. Anscher MS, Clough R, Dodge R. Radiotherapy for a rising prostate-specific antigen after radical prostatectomy: the first 10 years. *Int J Radiat Oncol Biol Phys* 2000;48:369-375.

469. Pisansky TM, Kozelsky TF, Myers RP, et al. Radiotherapy for isolated serum prostate specific antigen elevation after prostatectomy for prostate cancer. *J Urol* 2000;163:845-850.

470. Lee F, Bahn DK, Badalament RA, et al. Cryosurgery for prostate cancer: improved glandular ablation by use of 6 to 8 cryoprobes. *Urology* 1999;54:135-140.

471. Zisman A, Leibovici D, Siegel YI, et al. Prostate cryoablation without an insertion kit using direct transperineal placement of ultrathin freezing probes. *Tech Urol* 2000;6:34-36.

472. De La Taille A, Benson MC, Bagiella E, et al. Cryoablation for clinically localized prostate cancer using an argon-based system: complication rates and biochemical recurrence. *BJU Int* 2000;85:281-286.

473. Long JP, Fallick ML, LaRock DR, et al. Preliminary outcomes following cryosurgical ablation of the prostate in patients with clinically localized prostate carcinoma. *J Urol* 1998;159:477-484.

474. Gould RS. Total cryosurgery of the prostate versus standard cryosurgery versus radical prostatectomy: comparison of early results and the role of transurethral resection in cryosurgery. *J Urol* 1999;62:1653-1657.

475. Koppie TM, Shinohara K, Grossfeld GD, et al. The efficacy of cryosurgical ablation of prostate cancer: the University of California-San Francisco experience. *J Urol* 1999;162:427-432.

PART IX

Female Genital Tract

CHAPTER 28

The Uterine Cervix

Patricia J. Eifel

Radiation therapy plays a central role in the management of invasive carcinoma of the uterine cervix. Because the uterus and vagina tolerate high doses of radiation and form an ideal receptacle for radioactive sources, intracavitary brachytherapy can be exploited to achieve high rates of central disease control. Also, the low frequency of extraregional disease spread at the time of initial diagnosis means that many patients with cervical carcinoma can be cured with a combination of regional external-beam irradiation and brachytherapy. Recent studies demonstrate that the effectiveness of radiation therapy can be even greater when chemotherapy is given concurrently. However, this multidisciplinary treatment requires skill and cooperation. Careful technique is required to minimize the risk of complications in normal structures that are close to the uterus (e.g., the bladder and rectum).

In the United States and other western countries, effective screening has made invasive cervical cancer a relatively rare problem and has contributed to dramatic reductions in cervical cancer mortality rates. The challenge at present is for clinicians to maintain their skills in the specialized techniques that are used to treat cervical cancer.

EFFECTS OF RADIATION ON THE NORMAL CERVIX

Reproductive function is generally not maintained after irradiation of the uterus and cervix. If the ovaries have been transposed and the dose of pelvic radiation is moderate (20 to 40 Gy), spontaneous pregnancy is possible, but few cases have been reported in the literature.[1] In women irradiated during adulthood, these pregnancies may result in normal full-term infants. However, in women who underwent irradiation of the uterus and cervix before menarche, pregnancies often fail in the second trimester, possibly because of incomplete development of the uterine and cervical smooth muscle.[2]

High-dose treatment with external-beam and intracavitary radiation causes an early inflammatory reaction with superficial ulceration.[3] During the first 1 to 3 years after radiation therapy, gradual scarring of the cervix and upper vagina occur with obliteration of the cervical canal. Although the cervix is obstructed, the uterus rarely accumulates enough fluid to cause symptoms. However,

if patients are exposed to cyclical hormones, hematometra may occur. The cervix can usually be treated to very high doses (up to 150 Gy) without untoward effects (aside from loss of reproductive capacity). Minor clinically evident necrosis of the cervix occurs in 5% to 10% of cases, usually within the first 6 months after treatment.[4] This usually heals after 3 to 6 months with conservative local management.

EPIDEMIOLOGY OF CERVICAL CANCER

Worldwide, cervical cancer is the second leading cause of cancer death in women (after breast cancer), with approximately 500,000 new cases diagnosed each year. However, international incidences vary widely, reflecting in part differences in cultural attitudes toward sexual promiscuity and the availability of programs to screen for and treat preinvasive disease. Overall age-adjusted incidence rates in developing countries are approximately twice those in developed countries, with particularly high rates in sub-Saharan Africa, South America, Central America, and southeast Asia. Rates are particularly low in China, North Africa, and the Middle East.

The American Cancer Society estimated that there were 12,800 new cases of cervical cancer and 4600 deaths from cervical cancer in the United States in 2000.[5] This means that deaths from cervical cancer represented less than 2% of cancer deaths in U.S. women in 2000.[6] In part because of the widespread use of cytological screening, incidence rates in the United States have declined steadily since the 1930s.[7] Between 1992 and 1996, rates continued to decrease by an average of about 2.1%/year. However, the incidence in black women (11.2/100,000) was significantly higher than the incidence in white women (7.3/100,000). The incidence in Hispanic and Vietnamese-American women, many of whom are recent immigrants from countries where the incidence of cervical cancer is high, was also higher than the incidence in white women. Although the incidence of squamous carcinoma is clearly decreasing in the United States, the incidence of adenocarcinoma appears to have increased, particularly among women less than 40 years old.[8,9]

Epidemiologic and molecular studies convincingly demonstrate that cervical cancer is a sexually transmitted disease. Increased risk is correlated with young age at first intercourse, high number of sexual partners, a history of sexually transmitted disease, and exposure to sexually promiscuous male partners.[10,11] Today, compelling evidence that genitally transmitted infection with certain strains of human papillomavirus (HPV) plays a causative role in the development of cervical cancer explains, at least in part, the traditional risk factors for this disease. Recent studies have identified HPV DNA in more than 95% of cervical carcinomas.[12] Research suggests that genomic integration of HPV DNA causes persistent transcription of the *E6* and *E7* genes, disrupting cell cycle control mechanisms through functional inactivation of the tumor suppressor genes *p53* and *Rb*, respectively.[13,14] The oncogenicity of various HPV strains is correlated with the ability of their E6 or E7 oncoproteins to bind and inactivate tumor suppressor genes. Strains that are most often associated with cervical cancer in North America include HPV types 16, 18, and, less often, 31 and 33. Types 6 and 11 are associated with benign venereal warts but rarely with cancer.

Epidemiologic evidence suggests that the etiology of cervical cancer is multifactorial. Only a small fraction of women infected with oncogenic strains of HPV develop cancer. Additional genetic alterations, immunologic conditions, or other unknown factors may contribute to the development of a malignant phenotype. Smoking has repeatedly been found to be an independent risk factor for invasive and preinvasive disease,[15-17] and potent carcinogens have been found in the cervical mucus of smokers,[18] suggesting that smoking may play a role. The incidence of cervical cancer may be increased in women who are undergoing immunosuppressive therapy.[19]

In 1993 cervical cancer was added to the list of AIDS-defining illnesses by the U.S. Centers for Disease Control and Prevention. Although analyses of the association between AIDS and cervical cancer incidence have yielded conflicting results,[20,21] several studies have suggested that invasive cervical cancer behaves more aggressively in immunosuppressed patients.[22-24] Maiman and colleagues[22] reported a recurrence rate of 88% in 28 HIV-positive women treated for cervical cancer. Cancer was the immediate cause of death in 95% of these women, underscoring the importance of careful screening and effective treatment of localized disease in this population.[22]

A correlation between prolonged oral contraceptive use and cervical adenocarcinoma has been suggested, but a causative role for oral contraceptives has not been proven.[25,26]

ANATOMY AND PATTERNS OF TUMOR PROGRESSION

The uterus is a flattened, muscular, thick-walled, hollow structure that lies in the true pelvis between the bladder and the rectosigmoid (Fig. 28-1). The uterus is divided by the internal os into two regions—the corpus, or body, and the cervix. The uterus is most commonly anteverted (with its long axis approximately perpendicular to the axis of the vagina) and anteflexed, although it may be axial, retroverted, or retroflexed.

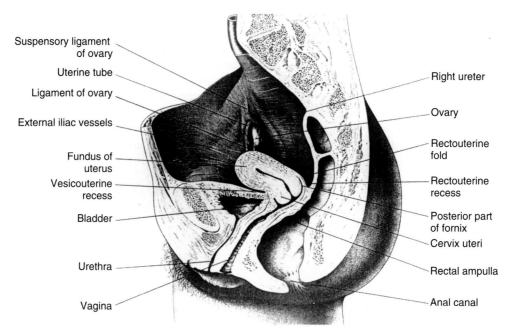

Fig. 28-1 Median sagittal section of the female pelvis. (From *Gray's Anatomy.* Philadelphia, Pa: WB Saunders; 1980.)

The normal cervix is about 2.5 cm long and projects into the anterior wall of the vagina, which divides the cervix into the upper (supravaginal) cervix and the lower (vaginal) cervix, also known as the portio vaginalis cervicis. The external os is visible as a depression on the vaginal cervix. Most cervical carcinomas arise at the junction between the primarily columnar epithelium of the endocervix and the squamous epithelium of the ectocervix. Tumors that penetrate the basement membrane to invade the muscular stroma may remain clinically confined to the cervix until they are quite large, forming an exophytic, cauliflower-shaped mass that protrudes into the vagina or causing an expanded, barrel-shaped cervix. However, they also may infiltrate beyond the cervix into adjacent structures.

Exterior to the smooth muscle of the uterine body and cervix is a layer of visceral pelvic fascia called the *parametrium* (where the fascia surrounds the corpus) or paracervix (where the fascia surrounds the cervix). The uterine fundus is covered by the peritoneum, which extends posteriorly to cover the upper cervix and vaginal fornix and then on to the anterior rectum to form the rectouterine pouch (pouch of Douglas) or cul-de-sac. Although large cervical tumors may erupt into the cul-de-sac, direct invasion of the rectum is extremely rare. Anteriorly, the peritoneum reflects from the fundus onto the posterior bladder at the level of the internal cervical os. The supravaginal cervix is below the peritoneal reflection and is separated from the bladder by only a relatively thin layer of paracervical fascia and cellular connective tissue. This layer may be traversed by deeply invasive cancer, although fewer than 5% of patients with cervical cancer present with cystoscopic evidence of bladder mucosal involvement. Although some clinical texts mistakenly refer to the junction between the cervical stroma and surrounding connective tissue as "serosa," the cervix lacks a true serosal layer except in its posterior supravaginal portion, where the cervix is covered by the peritoneum.

The uterus is connected to surrounding structures by a number of peritoneal folds and ligaments that can serve as conduits for direct extension of cancer from the cervix. The uterus is supported by the cardinal (transverse), uterosacral, and pubocervical ligaments, which are attached peripherally to the lateral pelvic wall, sacrum, and pubis, respectively. These ligaments are formed of dense connective tissue that is continuous with the fibrous tissue of the paracervix. The broad ligaments are formed from peritoneal folds that extend from the sides of the uterus to the lateral pelvic wall. With the uterus, the broad ligaments divide the pelvis into anterior and posterior compartments containing the bladder and rectum, respectively. The uterine arteries pass between the two layers of the broad ligaments at their inferior borders, and the fallopian tubes are located at the upper, free borders of the broad ligaments.

The broad ligaments also enclose the ovarian ligaments and proximal portions of the round ligaments. The cardinal ligaments consist of bands of dense fibroconnective tissue at the base of the broad ligaments; they connect the fascia of the lateral cervix and upper vagina with the fibrous tissue that surrounds the lateral pelvic vessels. The uterosacral ligaments lie within rectouterine peritoneal folds that extend posteriorly from the supravaginal cervix around either side of the rectum. Tumors that penetrate the paracervical fascia can involve the tissues of the broad ligaments or rectouterine spaces by direct extension; tumors also can gain access to these regions by lymphatic extension, particularly to nodes adjacent to the uterine vessels.

The cervical mucosa and stroma are richly supplied with lymphatics that anastomose extensively with those of the lower uterine segment.[27] These lymphatics penetrate the cervical stroma roughly perpendicularly and then spread out in a branching network of flattened lacunae that lie at the junction between the cervix and the surrounding connective tissue (or the peritoneum). The cervical lymphatics eventually merge to form collecting trunks, the most important of which exit laterally from the uterine isthmus in three groups (Fig. 28-2). Upper branches follow the uterine artery and terminate in the uppermost hypogastric nodes. Middle branches drain to deeper hypogastric (obturator) nodes, and the lowest channels course posteriorly to the inferior and superior gluteal, common iliac, and presacral nodes. Other posterior lymphatic channels arising from the posterior lip of the cervix drain to superior rectal nodes or pass through the retrorectal space to subaortic nodes that lie at the level of the sacral promontory. Some anterior channels also parallel the course of the superior vesical arteries to terminate in the internal iliac nodes.

In summary, the primary regional drainage of the cervix includes most of the lymph nodes of the pelvis. Tumors that invade the posterior vaginal wall may involve even the more inferior perirectal nodes, and tumors that invade the lower vagina may involve the inguinal nodes. However, unlike uterine malignancies, which may drain directly to the upper para-aortic lymph nodes (via the tubo-ovarian vessels), cervical cancer nearly always involves pelvic lymph nodes first.

The most common sites of distant metastasis from cervical cancer are the lungs and the secondary (e.g., para-aortic) or other lymph nodes. Less commonly, cervical cancer may spread to liver, bone, and other sites.

PATHOLOGY
Cervical Intraepithelial Neoplasia

It was first suggested more than 90 years ago that invasive cervical cancer arose from pre-existing intraepithelial lesions, subsequently termed *carcinomas in situ*. In the 1940s, Papanicolaou and Traut[28] reported a method of

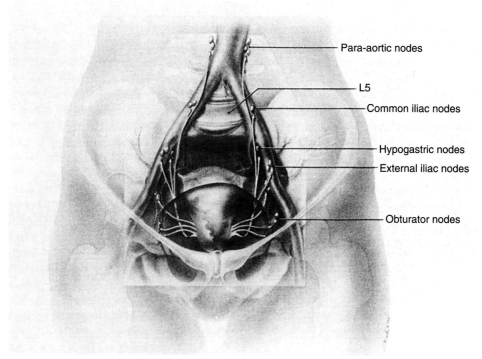

Fig. 28-2 Lymphatic drainage of the uterus and cervix. (From *Gray's Anatomy*. Philadelphia, Pa: WB Saunders; 1980.

screening for these lesions using cytologic samples that could be readily collected from the cervix and vagina. The dramatic reduction in the incidence of invasive cervical cancer that came with successful screening for and treatment of premalignant cervical lesions supported the hypothesis that most invasive malignancies begin with a long preinvasive phase. The fact that the mean age of women with intraepithelial lesions is about 15 years younger than the mean age of women with invasive cancer also suggests that the progression to invasive disease is slow.[29,30] Longitudinal studies of patients followed for untreated preinvasive lesions confirm this but also suggest that fewer than 15% of high-grade preinvasive lesions progress to invasive carcinoma and that approximately half undergo spontaneous regression.[31,32]

Early systems classed atypical lesions as dysplasias of varying degree (classes II to III), carcinoma in situ (class IV), or cancer (class V) (Table 28-1).[15,33] In the 1960s, this method was replaced by the cervical intraepithelial neoplasia system, proposed by Richart and Barron,[33] that more clearly described the spectrum of preinvasive squamous lesions. Although useful, cervical intraepithelial neoplasia grading was subjective and did not make the potentially important distinction between HPV-related koilocytotic atypia and other types of inflammatory change.

In 1988 after a National Institutes of Health consensus conference, the Bethesda System was proposed to reduce ambiguities and improve the clinical relevance of cytologic classification of cervical lesions; with a few more recent modifications,[15] the Bethesda System is now used by most U.S. laboratories. According to this system, pathology reports must include a statement on the adequacy of the specimen; a general categorization to assist with triage (e.g., "within normal limits," "infection or reactive changes," or "epithelial abnormality"); and a descriptive diagnosis. Squamous epithelial abnormalities are divided into four general categories: atypical squamous cells of undetermined significance (ASCUS), low-grade squamous intraepithelial lesions, high-grade squamous intraepithelial lesions (HSIL), and carcinomas. The ASCUS category, introduced to acknowledge limitations in the ability to identify some lesions as reactive or neoplastic with certainty, has now become the most common abnormal Pap test result.[34]

Although most ASCUS lesions are benign, patients with this finding should have a repeat Pap smear within 6 months because about 10% to 15% of cases of ASCUS are associated with underlying HSIL.[35] However, concern about possible false-negative diagnoses has led many clinicians to perform colposcopy on all patients with a diagnosis of ASCUS, significantly increasing the cost of screening and the chance of overtreatment. This has led to the search for better methods of triage. Preliminary studies have suggested that HPV testing of ASCUS smears followed by colposcopy in patients with HPV-positive lesions may provide a highly accurate and cost-effective means of detecting underlying HSIL in equivocal smears.[34]

TABLE 28-1

Comparison of Systems Used to Classify Cervical Cytology

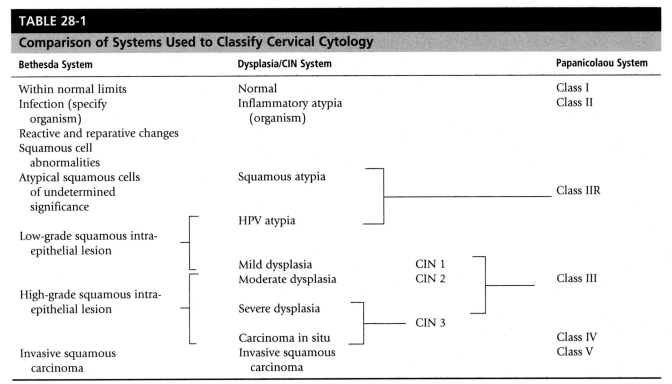

Bethesda System	Dysplasia/CIN System		Papanicolaou System
Within normal limits	Normal		Class I
Infection (specify organism)	Inflammatory atypia (organism)		Class II
Reactive and reparative changes			
Squamous cell abnormalities			
Atypical squamous cells of undetermined significance	Squamous atypia		Class IIR
Low-grade squamous intra-epithelial lesion	HPV atypia		
	Mild dysplasia	CIN 1	Class III
High-grade squamous intra-epithelial lesion	Moderate dysplasia	CIN 2	
	Severe dysplasia	CIN 3	
	Carcinoma in situ		Class IV
Invasive squamous carcinoma	Invasive squamous carcinoma		Class V

From Schiffman MH. *J Natl Cancer Inst* 1992;84:394-398; Richart RM, Barron BA. *Am J Obstet Gynecol* 1969;105:386-393.
CIN, Cervical intraepithelial neoplasia; *HPV,* human papillomavirus.

Adenocarcinoma in situ (AIS) is diagnosed when malignant cells have replaced the normal endocervical glandular epithelium but the normal branching architecture is maintained and the cells do not invade the cervical stroma.[36] High-risk HPV subtypes are often detected in AIS and invasive adenocarcinomas, and HSIL are often found adjacent to areas of AIS. Because AIS is commonly multifocal, residual AIS may remain even after a cone biopsy with negative margins.[37]

Microinvasive Carcinoma

When it occurs, early stromal invasion is usually found close to the transformation zone adjacent to areas of squamous cervical intraepithelial neoplasia. Because the diagnosis of microinvasion is based on a quantitative assessment of the size and depth of the invasive lesion, diagnosis requires a cone biopsy specimen that encompasses the entire lesion and cervical transformation zone. The depth of invasion should be measured from the base of the epithelium to the deepest point of invasion.

Although the International Federation of Gynecology and Obstetrics (FIGO) first included a category for minimally invasive lesions in 1962, the definition was left nonspecific until 1995, when the current definitions of stage IA1 disease (invasion ≤ 3.0 mm deep) and stage IA2 disease (invasion > 3.0 mm and ≤ 5.0 mm deep) were adopted. In the interim, the Society of Gynecologic

Oncologists adopted a different standard that defined microinvasive lesions as those that invaded less than 3 mm into the cervical stroma without evidence of lymphovascular space invasion (LVSI). Today, both definitions are used in the United States, leading to some confusion about the classification of lesions that invade 3.1 to 5 mm and those that invade 3 mm or less with LVSI. These lesions were grouped with "stage IB" in the Society of Gynecologic Oncologists system but would be classed IA1 and IA2, respectively, in the FIGO system. (More detailed information about the FIGO staging system appears in the section "FIGO Staging of Cervical Cancer" later in this chapter.)

Because early invasive adenocarcinomas can arise from deep endocervical glandular epithelium, the depth of invasion may be difficult to determine. For this reason, such lesions are usually classified as FIGO stage IB.

Squamous Carcinoma

More than 75% of cases of cervical cancer are squamous carcinomas. Large-cell nonkeratinizing carcinomas are most common and are characterized by nests of neoplastic cells that may stain for keratin but lack the keratin pearls characteristic of large-cell keratinizing tumors. About 5% of cervical squamous carcinomas are characterized by relatively small cells that demonstrate minimal squamous differentiation, scant cytoplasm, small nucleoli, and abundant mitoses. These tumors have traditionally been termed *small cell squamous cell carcinomas,* but this term should probably be avoided because it is easily confused with *undifferentiated small cell carcinoma,* which is associated with a much poorer prognosis (see the next section). Rare variants of squamous carcinoma include verrucous carcinomas, well-differentiated papillomatous lesions that tend to be locally invasive but rarely metastasize,[38] and papillary squamous cell carcinomas,[39] which form papillae of atypical epithelium with frequent invasion at the base of the tumors.

Adenocarcinoma

Microscopically, adenocarcinomas of the cervix demonstrate a variety of patterns and degrees of histologic differentiation. Mucinous (endocervical) carcinomas are most common, although other müllerian carcinomas (i.e., endometrioid, clear cell, and serous adenocarcinomas) also may originate in the cervix. Mixtures of these cell types also may occur. Adenosquamous carcinomas contain malignant glandular and squamous elements. Reports conflict concerning the relative prognosis of adenocarcinomas and adenosquamous carcinomas of similar grade.

Many rare subtypes of adenocarcinoma have been reported in the cervix. These include signet-ring, glassy cell, adenoid cystic, adenoid basal, and villoglandular carcinomas. Minimal-deviation adenocarcinoma (adenoma malignum) is another rare type of carcinoma, with an extremely well differentiated histologic appearance that can be mistakenly interpreted as benign on the basis of small biopsy specimens. Although early reports suggested that these tumors were associated with a poor prognosis, with frequent local recurrence, more recent studies suggest that early lesions can be cured with local treatment.[40]

Undifferentiated Small Cell Carcinoma

Undifferentiated small cell carcinoma is a rare subtype of cervical cancer but is important because of its aggressive behavior. It is a very poorly differentiated carcinoma with neuroendocrine features, histologically similar to anaplastic small cell carcinoma of the lung.[41] Undifferentiated small cell carcinomas tend to behave very aggressively, with frequent widespread metastasis to multiple sites, including bone, liver, skin, and brain. Efforts to treat these tumors by using approaches typically used for small cell carcinomas of the lung have had mixed results.[42,43] Undifferentiated small cell carcinomas should not be confused with small cell squamous cell carcinomas, which have a better prognosis.

FIGO STAGING OF CERVICAL CANCER

The FIGO clinical staging system[44,45] (Box 28-1) is the internationally accepted method used to classify patients with cervical cancer. The four major stage groupings, designed to reflect the extent of local disease and the feasibility of successful surgical resection, are similar to those set forth in the original 1929 staging system of the League of Nations Health Organization.[46] However, since then FIGO has made many modifications that have altered the compositions of stage groups or defined various substages. Preinvasive lesions were included in stage I until 1950, when they were placed in a new (stage 0) category. Hydronephrosis was first included as a criterion for labeling a tumor "stage III" in 1976. Many different efforts have been made to define a subgroup of patients with more favorable "occult" or microinvasive disease. These descriptions were ambiguous until 1994, when the current definitions of microinvasion (stages IA1 and IA2) were added. All of these changes have created opportunities for stage migration, confounding comparisons between different experiences.

The staging system also has been criticized for not including information about important predictors of outcome such as tumor size and lymph node status. In a significant improvement, FIGO first divided the stage IB category according to cervical diameter in 1994 (see Box 28-1), although substantial size heterogeneity still exists within the IB1 and IB2 groups and other stage groups. Radiographic and surgical assessments of lymph nodes have never been incorporated into the staging system for two important reasons. First, the expense of these studies is often prohibitive in the medically underserved countries where most of the world's cases of cervical cancer occur. Second, the lack of a sensitive, widely accepted method of evaluating the pelvic and aortic lymph nodes has made it difficult to design a staging system that would document regional metastasis in a consistent fashion.

The subjectivity of pelvic examination, the primary method used to define stage groups, also creates hidden biases. Despite admonitions in FIGO's staging notes stressing that equivocal findings should be discounted, clinicians have variable tendencies to overstage tumors. For example, in a large surgical series, approximately two thirds of the cases labeled as "stage IIB" had no evidence of parametrial involvement in the hysterectomy specimens (Fig. 28-3).[47] Comparisons of clinical stage with the findings from carefully sectioned hysterectomy specimens demonstrate dramatic differences between institutions in the tendency to overstage or understage tumors.[47] This is another important source of stage migration that influences the reporting of results.

However, FIGO stage is roughly correlated with outcome, and despite the system's flaws, it is the most consistent language that can currently be used to compare results between institutions. For this reason, the staging system should always be applied strictly according to the rules defined by FIGO (see Box 28-1). When studies that are not used in staging are incorporated into treatment

BOX 28-1 American Joint Committee on Cancer and International Federation of Gynecology and Obstetrics Staging Systems for Cancer of the Uterine Cervix

AJCC TNM Categories	FIGO Stages	
TX	—	Primary tumor cannot be assessed
T0	—	No evidence of primary tumor
Tis	0	Carcinoma in situ
T1	I	Cervical carcinoma confined to uterus (extension to corpus should be disregarded)
T1a	IA	Invasive carcinoma diagnosed only by microscopy. All macroscopically visible lesions—even with superficial invasion—are T1b/IB. Stromal invasion with a maximum depth of 5.0 mm measured from the base of the epithelium and a horizontal spread of 7.0 mm or less. Vascular space invasion, venous or lymphatic, does not affect classification
T1a1	IA1	Measured stromal invasion 3.0 mm or less in depth and 7.0 mm or less in horizontal spread
T1a2	IA2	Measured stromal invasion more than 3.0 mm and not more than 5.0 mm with a horizontal spread 7.0 mm or less
T1b	IB	Clinically visible lesion confined to the cervix or microscopic lesion greater than T1a2/IA2
T1b1	IB1	Clinically visible lesion 4.0 cm or less in greatest dimension
T1b2	IB2	Clinically visible lesion more than 4.0 cm in greatest dimension
T2	II	Cervical carcinoma invades beyond uterus but not to pelvic wall or to the lower third of vagina
T2a	IIA	Tumor without parametrial invasion
T2b	IIB	Tumor with parametrial invasion
T3	III	Tumor extends to the pelvic wall, and/or involves the lower third of the vagina, and/or causes hydronephrosis or nonfunctioning kidney
T3a	IIIA	Tumor involves lower third of the vagina, no extension to pelvic wall
T3b	IIIB	Tumor extends to pelvic wall and/or causes hydronephrosis or nonfunctioning kidney
T4	IVA	Tumor invades mucosa of the bladder or rectum, and/or extends beyond true pelvis (Bullous edema is not sufficient to classify a tumor as T4)
M1	IVB	Distant metastasis

REGIONAL LYMPH NODES (N)
NX   Regional lymph nodes cannot be assessed
N0   No regional lymph node metastasis
N1   Regional lymph node metastasis

DISTANT METASTASIS (M)
MX   Distant metastasis cannot be assessed
M0   No distant metastasis
M1   Distant metastasis

STAGE GROUPING

Stage 0	Tis	N0	M0
Stage IA1	T1a1	N0	M0
Stage IA2	T1a2	N0	M0
Stage IB1	T1b1	N0	M0
Stage IB2	T1b2	N0	M0
Stage IIA	T2a	N0	M0
Stage IIB	T2b	N0	M0
Stage IIIA	T3a	N0	M0
Stage IIIB	T1	N1	M0
	T2	N1	M0
	T3a	N1	M0
	T3b	Any N	M0
Stage IVA	T4	Any N	M0
Stage IVB	Any T	Any N	M1

Continued

BOX 28-1 **American Joint Committee on Cancer and International Federation of Gynecology and Obstetrics Staging Systems for Cancer of the Uterine Cervix—cont'd**

NOTES ABOUT THE STAGING SYSTEM

Stage 0 cases are those with full-thickness involvement of the epithelium with atypical cells but with no signs of invasion into the stroma. (Cases of stage 0 disease should not be included in any therapeutic statistics for invasive carcinoma.)

As a rule, it is impossible to estimate clinically whether a cancer of the cervix has extended to the corpus. Extension to the corpus should therefore be disregarded.

A growth fixed to the pelvic wall by a short and indurated but not nodular parametrium should be assigned stage IIB. It is impossible at clinical examination to decide whether a smooth and indurated parametrium is truly cancerous or only inflammatory, and thus such cases should be classified as stage III only if the parametrium is nodular to the pelvic wall or if the growth itself extends to the pelvic wall.

The presence of hydronephrosis or nonfunctioning kidney caused by stenosis of the ureter by cancer permits a case to be classified as stage III even if, according to the other findings, the case should be classified as stage I or stage II.

The presence of bullous edema, as such, should not permit a case to be classified as stage IV. Ridges and furrows into the bladder wall should be interpreted as signs of submucous involvement of the bladder if they remain fixed to the growth at palposcopy (i.e., examination from the vagina or the rectum during cystoscopy). A finding of malignant cells in cytologic washings from the urinary bladder requires further examination and biopsy from the wall of the bladder.

RULES FOR CLINICAL STAGING

The staging should be based on careful clinical examination and should be performed before any definitive therapy. Ideally, the examination should be performed under anesthesia by an experienced examiner.

The clinical stage must under no circumstances be changed on the basis of subsequent findings.

When doubt exists as to the assignment of stage, the case must be classified as the earlier stage. For staging purposes, the following examination methods are permitted: palpation, inspection, colposcopy, endocervical curettage, hysteroscopy, cystoscopy, proctoscopy, intravenous urography, and x-ray examination of the lungs and skeleton. Suspected bladder or rectal involvement should be confirmed by biopsy and histologic evidence.

Findings on examinations such as lymphangiography, arteriography, venography, laparoscopy, and so forth are valuable for planning therapy, but because such studies are not yet generally available and because interpretation of the results is variable, the findings of such studies should not be the basis for changing the clinical staging.

Infrequently, hysterectomy is performed in the presence of unsuspected extensive invasive cervical carcinoma. Such cases cannot be clinically staged or included in therapeutic statistics, but they should be reported separately.

Only strict observance of the rules for clinical staging will allow meaningful comparison of results between clinics and modes of therapy.

From Fleming I, Cooper JS, Henson DE, et al, eds. *AJCC Cancer Staging Manual*. 5th ed. Philadelphia, Pa: Lippincott Williams & Wilkins; 1997:189-194.

---

planning or patient selection, they should be carefully described in the reports of clinical trials. Only consistent staging and detailed description of methods will improve clinicians' ability to determine the generalizability of studies to their own patients.

The American Joint Committee on Cancer and FIGO suggest a TNM pathologic staging system that may be used to report surgical findings for patients treated with radical hysterectomy and lymph node dissection. This system cannot be applied to patients treated with initial irradiation. Although FIGO and the American Joint Committee on Cancer suggest a method for applying the TNM categories to stage groups, this causes confusion when clinically staged patients are mixed with others who have been classified according to pathologic stage. This inconsistent assignment of stage groupings becomes a particular problem in large epidemiologic studies that use tumor registries or multi-institutional databases to compare treatments according to stage.

CLINICAL EVALUATION

Every patient with cervical cancer should be carefully interviewed to obtain a history of her present illness and any other medical problems. Previous surgical procedures, pelvic infections, medical illnesses, habits (including smoking history), and other conditions that may influence the patient's tolerance of treatment and risk of complications should be documented. The patient's diet and medications and any herbal or complementary health products she is using should be noted because these can interact with treatment to

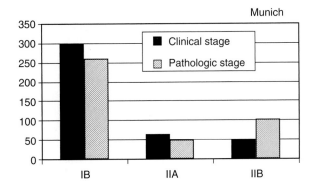

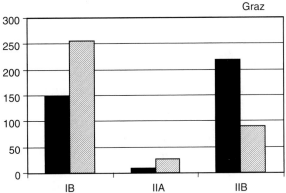

Fig. 28-3 International Federation of Gynecology and Obstetrics (FIGO) clinical and pathologic stages of patients whose radical hysterectomy specimens were reviewed in two regional centers. Similar examination methods were used at the two centers. In Munich, findings on clinical examination predicted parametrial involvement in only about 50% of cases that were judged to be stage IIB on the basis of pathologic findings. In contrast, in Graz, more than half of the cases diagnosed clinically as FIGO stage IIB had no histologic evidence of parametrial involvement. (From Burghardt E, Hofmann HMH, Ebner F, et al. *Cancer* 1992;70:648-655.)

worsen side effects. An early assessment of the patient's social circumstances is particularly important because women with cervical cancer often have distressed finances or young dependents and limited family support. Cultural, educational, and language differences between the patient and her physician can interfere with effective communication. Early recognition of any problems and appropriate intervention can greatly facilitate a patient's ability to comply with the complicated treatment regimens used to treat cervical cancer.

Pelvic Examination

Each patient should have a thorough physical examination, including a detailed pelvic examination. The findings should be documented in a tumor diagram. Pelvic examination should include careful inspection of the external genitalia, vagina, and cervix. The capacity of the vagina should be assessed digitally before a speculum is inserted, and the speculum should be advanced carefully

to minimize trauma to friable tumor. If a histologic diagnosis has not yet been made, a biopsy should be performed. If the lesion is not visible to the naked eye, colposcopy may be helpful. All areas of vaginal mucosa should be systematically visualized as the speculum is withdrawn.

The pelvic examination also should include a thorough digital vaginal examination during which any vaginal abnormalities should be noted and an initial assessment of the size and morphology of the cervical tumor can be made. Again, this should be done with as little trauma to the tumor as possible. With one or two fingers in the vagina in contact with the cervix and the other hand on the suprapubic abdomen, the physician should assess the uterus for its size, shape, mobility, and position in the pelvis. The adnexa should be carefully examined for any masses or tenderness.

A rectovaginal examination should then be performed to determine whether disease is breaking through the paracervix into the broad ligaments or uterosacral ligaments. The mobility of the uterus and any nodularity should be noted. The size of the cervix is evaluated by comparing its diameter with the width of the pelvis (usually about 12 cm at the level of the cervix).

If significant bleeding follows the pelvic examination, a speculum should be reinserted immediately, and Monsel's solution (ferric subsulfate solution) or vaginal packing should be applied to minimize continued blood loss.

Additional Clinical Examinations

Cystoscopy and proctoscopy should be performed if bulky disease or extensive vaginal involvement is present or if the patient has symptoms suggesting possible bladder or rectal pathology. However, the yield is very low for patients with early cervical cancer. Suspected bladder involvement identified on magnetic resonance imaging (MRI) or computed tomography (CT) images must be confirmed with cystoscopy and biopsy before the patient's FIGO stage can be increased (see Box 28-1).[44]

All patients with cervical cancer should have a complete blood count and measurement of serum electrolyte, blood urea nitrogen, and creatinine levels performed at diagnosis. Additional studies may be required depending on the patient's symptoms and any concurrent illnesses.

Radiographic Evaluation

Intravenous pyelography and radiography of the chest and bones are the only radiographic examinations that can be used to determine a patient's FIGO stage (see Box 28-1). However, unless the patient has very early disease (stage IA or IB1), additional radiographic studies are usually required to obtain important information about possible regional involvement.

Today clinicians usually obtain a contrast-enhanced CT scan of the abdomen and pelvis for patients with stage IB2 or greater disease.[48] Lymph nodes larger than 1.0 to 1.5 cm in diameter are suspicious for tumor involvement and should be biopsied. Unfortunately, microscopic metastases are not readily detected with CT, and the inflammation commonly associated with advanced disease may cause enlargement of nodes that do not contain metastases. The sensitivity of MRI in the detection of regional metastases is similar to that of CT. However, MRI provides more detailed images of the cervix and paracervical tissues (Fig. 28-4). Sagittal views are particularly helpful for determining the morphology of the tumor and the position of the uterus. MRI also yields a more objective assessment of tumor diameter than does pelvic examination. However, in medically underserved communities, particularly in developing nations, the cost of MRI may outweigh the benefit. For practical reasons, CT or MRI assessment of the ureters and renal pelvis is often substituted for traditional intravenous pyelography to determine whether a patient has

tumor-related hydronephrosis. Other information gained from these studies should not be used to alter the FIGO stage.

Lymphangiography is more sensitive than CT for assessment of the aortic nodes[49] but does not visualize internal iliac or presacral nodes and is difficult to perform. Positron emission tomography may be more sensitive than more standard radiographic studies in the detection of lymph node involvement but remains investigational.[50]

SURGICAL LYMPH NODE EVALUATION

Although surgical evaluation is the most sensitive method of evaluating whether regional lymph nodes contain metastases, it is invasive and expensive and delays treatment of the patient's primary lesion. Transperitoneal lymphadenectomy, the surgical staging approach most often used in the past, was associated with a high incidence of severe, even fatal, complications in patients treated with radiation therapy. The risk of severe complications seems to be much less when lymphadenectomy is performed using a retroperitoneal approach.[51] Laparoscopic lymph node dissection is associated with a shorter postoperative recovery time and probably less late radiation morbidity than open transperitoneal staging.[52]

The risk of occult para-aortic metastases is greatest in patients with grossly involved pelvic nodes; these patients may be the best candidates for surgical exploration if they have no medical contraindication to the procedure. Several small studies suggest that such patients also may benefit from removal of bulky lymph node metastases, which may be difficult to control with radiation therapy alone.[53,54]

The sensitivity of surgical lymph node evaluation depends on the number of nodes removed and the surgical pathologist's treatment of the specimen. If lymphangiography is performed before surgery, intraoperative abdominal radiographs may be obtained to confirm that the abnormal nodes have been removed.[55] Several investigators are currently exploring the role of intraoperative lymphatic mapping in patients with cervical cancer and other gynecologic malignancies.[56]

PROGNOSTIC FACTORS
Tumor Size and Local Extent

Large tumor size has consistently been demonstrated to be one of the most important predictors of local recurrence and death from cervical cancer. This is true both for patients treated with hysterectomy[47,57,58] (Fig. 28-5) and for patients treated with radiation therapy[59-62] (Fig. 28-6). FIGO stage IB is now divided into two prognostic groups according to tumor size (see Box 28-1); other stage categories act, in part, as surrogates for tumor size.

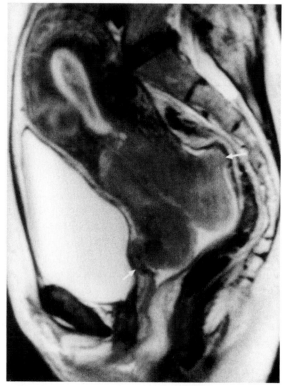

Fig. 28-4 Sagittal magnetic resonance imaging (MRI) scan of a large squamous cell carcinoma of the cervix. On clinical examination, this tumor was estimated to be an exophytic lesion, International Federation of Gynecology and Obstetrics stage IIA, about 8 cm in diameter. MRI demonstrated an 8 × 7 × 7.5 cm tumor with extensive invasion of the vagina, endocervix, and lower uterine segment with bulky pelvic lymphadenopathy. *Arrows* point to areas of vaginal extension.

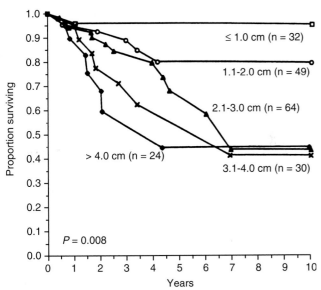

Fig. 28-5 Relationship between tumor diameter and survival for patients treated with radical hysterectomy for cervical cancer. (From Alvarez RD, Potter ME, Soong SJ, et al. *Gynecol Oncol* 1991;43:108-112.)

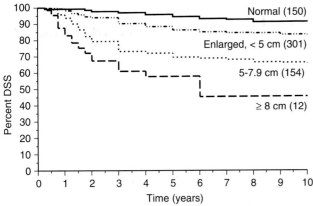

Fig. 28-6 Relationship between tumor diameter and disease-specific survival (DSS) for 1526 patients treated with radiation therapy for International Federation of Gynecology and Obstetrics stage IB squamous carcinoma of the cervix. (Modified from Eifel PJ, Morris M, Wharton JT, et al. *Int J Radiat Oncol Biol Phys* 1994;29:9-16.)

On clinical examination, clinicians may report the size of the visible lesion or the widest diameter of the cervix or palpable cervical lesion. Although the diameter of tumors that infiltrate and are fixed to the pelvis may be difficult to estimate from clinical examination, tumors that are fixed to both pelvic walls tend to be larger and have a poorer prognosis than those with unilateral fixation.[63-65] Before the 1995 revision of the FIGO staging system, surgeons rarely reported clinical diameter; however, various investigators reported measurements from histologic sections of tumor thickness, depth of invasion, diameter, or volume.[47,57,66] Recent

studies have indicated that tomographic imaging methods, particularly MRI, yield more accurate measurements of tumor size than does clinical examination.[67-69] However, results of tomographic imaging cannot be used to assign stage, and guidelines for consistent reporting of these results are needed.

For patients treated with surgery, histologic evidence of extracervical spread is associated with a poorer prognosis. Parametrial extension is associated with a higher rate of lymph node involvement, local recurrence, and death from cancer.[70-73] Paracervical extension occurs with about equal frequency in the right, left, or anterior direction; Landoni and colleagues[74] found evidence of anterior spread through the vesicocervical septa or into the vesicocervical ligaments in 22 of 59 women with paracervical disease. This has important implications for postoperative treatment planning.

Although clinical evidence of vaginal involvement (stage IIA) or parametrial involvement (stage IIB) is associated with a poorer prognosis after radiation therapy, some investigators have found that the predictive power of stage diminishes or is lost when comparisons are corrected for differences in clinical tumor diameter.[75,76] Uterine body involvement is associated with an increased rate of distant metastases in patients treated with radiation therapy or surgery.[77-80]

Lymph Node Involvement

Lymph node involvement is another important independent predictor of outcome. After radical hysterectomy, reported 5-year survival rates are usually about 35% to 40% lower when the pelvic lymph nodes are involved.[57,81,82] However, recent studies suggest that postoperative chemoradiation improves these results.[83] Several authors have reported that survival decreases with increasing size of the largest involved nodes[84,85] and with increasing number of nodes involved.[82,85-87] Survival also decreases with increasing level of regional involvement. Overall, the survival rates for patients with positive para-aortic nodes are about half those of patients who have similar stages of disease without para-aortic lymph node involvement (Fig. 28-7).[88-100] In patients who have para-aortic node metastases from relatively small tumors, cure rates are 40% to 50% with extended-field radiation therapy.

Lymphovascular Space Invasion

LVSI is correlated with an increased risk of recurrence. This reflects in part the strong correlation between LVSI and lymph node involvement. However, a number of recent studies from large series of patients treated with radical hysterectomy have demonstrated LVSI to be an independent predictor of prognosis.[66,82,86,87,101-103] Although LVSI is rarely quantified in these studies,

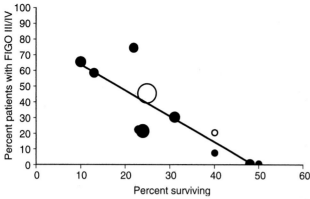

Fig. 28-7 Survival rates of patients treated with radiation for biopsy-confirmed para-aortic node metastases from cervical cancer. Each point represents one series of patients; the area is proportional to the number of patients in the series (ranging from 15 to 98). *Solid* and *open circles* represent series with survival rates calculated at 5 and 3 years, respectively.

Roman and colleagues[104] reported a correlation between the percentage of histopathologic sections containing LVSI and the incidence of lymph node metastases. A strong correlation also exists between LVSI and outcome in patients with adenocarcinoma of the cervix.[105-107]

Histologic Type and Tumor Grade

A number of systems have been developed to subclassify squamous cell carcinomas on the basis of histologic type or tumor grade. Although many of these systems correlate with outcome, no method has been confirmed to independently predict prognosis when other risk factors such as tumor size, depth of invasion, and lymph node status are considered.[66,82,86,108,109]

Investigators who have compared the outcome of patients with adenocarcinomas or squamous carcinomas have reached varying conclusions about the relative prognoses of the two histologic types of cervical cancer. No significant difference was found in several retrospective series of patients treated with radiation.[110-115] However, comparative studies have been confounded by the lack of a consistent definition of stage IA disease (particularly for adenocarcinomas) and by variations in treatment selection for patients with tumors of different histologic type. In a review of 1767 patients with stage IB disease (229 with adenocarcinoma), Eifel and colleagues[116] found that patients with adenocarcinoma had a significantly higher risk of recurrence and death from disease (Table 28-2).[116] This finding was independent of age, tumor size, or tumor morphology. The rate of distant metastasis for patients with bulky (≥ 4 cm) adenocarcinomas was almost twice that for patients with squamous carcinomas (37% vs. 21%; $P < 0.01$).

In contrast, no significant difference was found between patients with adenocarcinoma and those with other subtypes in the rate of pelvic recurrence. Several investigators have reported high recurrence rates after radical hysterectomy for adenocarcinomas that enlarge the cervix, are high grade, or are associated with LVSI.[106,117,118] In one study, Eifel and colleagues[106] reported that in patients with adenocarcinomas 3 to 4 cm in diameter, the rate of pelvic recurrence was 45% after treatment with radical hysterectomy versus 11% after treatment with radiation therapy. This was despite a greater prevalence of adverse prognostic features in the group treated with radiation. However, other investigators have suggested that adenocarcinomas are more effectively treated with hysterectomy or combined treatment than with radiation alone.[119] All of these comparisons are compromised by the relatively small number of patients treated surgically for cervical adenocarcinomas. Although the prognostic significance of histologic grade has been disputed for squamous carcinomas, a clear

---

TABLE 28-2

Risk of Pelvic or Distant Relapse at 5 Years for Patients Treated with Radiation for International Federation of Gynecology and Obstetrics Stage IB Carcinoma of the Cervix

Tumor Size	Histologic Subtype	Number of Patients	ACTUARIAL RISK OF RELAPSE		
			Pelvic*	Distant†	Any Site
< 4 cm	SCC	706	2.6%	7.4%	9.6%
			$P < 0.01$	$P = 0.01$	$P = 0.03$
	AC	113	6.3%	15.2%	16.9%
≥ 4 cm	SCC	797	13.1%	21.2%	26.4%
			$P = 0.16$	$P < 0.01$	$P < 0.01$
	AC	106	16.7%	36.8%	43.6%

From Eifel PJ, Burke TW, Morris M, et al. *Gynecol Oncol* 1995;59:38-44.
SCC, Squamous cell carcinoma; *AC,* adenocarcinoma.
*Progressive or recurrent pelvic disease detected at any time after initial treatment.
†Extrapelvic recurrence detected at any time after initial treatment.

correlation exists between the degree of differentiation and clinical behavior for adenocarcinomas.[106,107,120-122] Anaplastic small cell carcinomas of the cervix have a distinctly poorer prognosis than squamous cell carcinomas, with a tendency to progress rapidly and metastasize widely.[43,44,123]

Other Tumor Factors

Several investigators have reported a correlation between the serum concentration of squamous cell carcinoma antigen and the extent of squamous carcinoma of the cervix, although they disagree about the independent predictive power of the test.[124-126] In one study of 284 patients treated with radical hysterectomy for squamous carcinoma, 65% of the patients with serum squamous cell carcinoma antigen levels above 8 μg/L had lymph node metastases, whereas 86% of the patients with antigen levels below 8 μg/L had no lymph node metastases identified.[125]

A number of other factors have been studied for their prognostic significance in cervical cancer. A strong inflammatory response in the cervical stroma tends to predict a good outcome,[127] whereas increased tumor vascularity has been associated with a relatively poor prognosis.[128,129]

The reported incidence of tumor cells in peritoneal washings varies but is less than 5% in most series.[130-132] Takeshima and colleagues[132] reported a higher rate in patients with adenocarcinomas (11.4%) than in those with squamous carcinomas (1.7%). The finding of tumor cells in peritoneal washings is more common in patients with advanced-stage disease or lymph node metastases; however, the value of this finding as an independent predictor of prognosis or pattern of disease progression is uncertain.

Some authors have reported a correlation between HPV subtype and prognosis.[133,134] Several investigators have reported a higher recurrence rate in patients with histologically negative lymph nodes when a polymerase chain reaction assay of the lymph nodes was strongly positive for HPV DNA.[135,136] Other authors have correlated poor prognosis with the presence of HPV mRNA[137] or HPV-related proteins[138] in the peripheral blood of cervical cancer patients.

Patient-related Factors

The relationship between a patient's age and her outcome is uncertain, with different investigators reporting young age to be a favorable prognostic factor,[108,139] an adverse prognostic factor,[140-142] or not predictive of outcome.[143-145] A number of factors may contribute to these differences. Although most investigators try to correct for potential confounding biases, they often do so incompletely. Studies of patients treated with surgery or radiation therapy may be biased because age is often used to select treatment. For example, patients with small tumors may be more likely to be treated with radiation if they are elderly than if they are young. In some series, older patients may have received less aggressive treatment. It is also possible that cultural or regional differences affect the influence of age on treatment selection or compliance.

Many investigators have reported correlations between a low hemoglobin level before or during treatment and poor prognosis.[65,146-148] These comparisons are striking but are often confounded by the prevalence of other adverse tumor features in anemic patients. Although many investigators have speculated that the poor prognosis of anemic patients is caused in part by hypoxia-induced radiation resistance, only one small 1978 randomized study, conducted at the Princess Margaret Hospital, has tested this hypothesis.[146] In that study, through the use of transfusions, patients' hemoglobin levels were maintained at a level of at least 12 g/dl in one arm of the study whereas hemoglobin levels were allowed to drop to as little as 10 g/dl in the other arm. The 25 patients in the control arm of the study who had hemoglobin levels less than 12 g/dl had a significantly higher local recurrence rate than the patients in the experimental arm who required transfusions to maintain a high hemoglobin level. Larger studies are still needed to confirm this finding.

Unfortunately, other treatment protocols that have been designed to overcome the theoretical radiobiological consequences of intratumoral hypoxia (through the use of hypoxic cell sensitizers, hyperbaric oxygen breathing, or neutron therapy) have not improved the outcome of patients with locally advanced disease.[149-155] Several investigators have correlated low intratumoral oxygen tension levels with poor survival.[156-168] However, these studies have also demonstrated that hypoxic tumors tend to have other adverse features that may explain their greater tendency to recur after treatment.

Although it has been suggested that high platelet count may be associated with poor prognosis, large studies suggest that thrombocytosis may be a marker for more advanced disease but is not an independent predictor of poor prognosis.[159]

Several studies have demonstrated that in the United States, nonwhite women with invasive cervical cancer present with higher-stage disease[160-162] and lower hemoglobin levels[163] than white women. Differences in socioeconomic status may influence minority patients' access to care and ability to comply with treatment recommendations.[164]

In a study of 1304 women treated with radiation for cervical cancer, Kucera and colleagues[169] reported that smokers with cervical cancer had a poorer 5-year survival rate than nonsmokers. This difference was statistically significant for patients with stage III disease (5-year survival 20.3% vs. 33.9%; $P < 0.01$). However, in their analysis, the authors did not analyze the possible influence of smoking-related deaths from causes other than cervical cancer.

TREATMENT OPTIONS

Radiation therapy, surgery, and chemotherapy all play important roles in the curative management of cervical cancer. In recommending treatment for an individual patient, clinicians must consider the characteristics and extent of the cancer, possible side effects of treatment, and the patient's personal needs. Recent studies have led to an expanded role of chemotherapy in the primary treatment of cervical cancer. This has improved the outcome of some patients with local–regionally advanced disease but has also increased the complexity of treatment, which is important because patients with cervical cancer often have severe socioeconomic limitations and little or no experience with health care systems. To achieve the best results, careful counseling and social-services support must be integrated into the treatment plan from its inception.

Stage IA1 Disease

Because the risk of extracervical involvement in patients with stage IA1 disease is low (< 1%), the goal of treatment in these patients is to remove or sterilize disease in the cervix. All patients have a cone biopsy because this is necessary to make the diagnosis of microinvasion and to verify that the paracervical tissues and lymph nodes do not require treatment.

The most conventional treatment for stage IA1 cancer is a type I, simple extrafascial hysterectomy. If the patient is young, the ovaries should be left in place. Stage IA disease also can be treated effectively with radiation therapy. Intracavitary therapy alone is sufficient; it controls disease for more than 10 years in 95% to 100% of patients.[161,162] Patients who want to maintain fertility may be treated with a generous cone biopsy alone if their tumors invade less than 3 mm without LVSI and if the margin of the cone biopsy is negative.[163,164] These patients must be followed closely, but their risk of disease progression seems to be low.[167,168]

Stage IA2 Disease

Small lesions that invade 3 to 5 mm have an average risk of lymph node metastasis of about 5%. This risk is usually considered high enough to justify treatment of the paracervical tissues and pelvic lymph nodes.[72]

Surgical treatment of stage IA2 disease usually includes a type II radical hysterectomy and pelvic lymph node dissection. These tumors also can be treated effectively with radiation therapy. Brachytherapy alone may be used if

there is a contraindication to prolonged treatment, but the risk of pelvic lymph node metastasis, although low, is enough to justify treatment of the pelvic lymph nodes in most cases.

Stage IB1 or Small Stage IIA Disease

Stage IB1 and small (< 3 cm) stage IIA tumors are associated with a significant risk of microscopic paracervical extension or lymph node metastasis. In a prospective Gynecologic Oncology Group (GOG) study of patients treated with radical hysterectomy for stage I disease, lymph node metastases were found in 42 (16%) of 261 patients whose tumors were estimated clinically to have a maximum diameter less than 3 cm.[72] Landoni and colleagues[119] found positive lymph nodes in 28 (25%) of 114 patients treated with radical hysterectomy for stage IB-IIA tumors that measured 4 cm or less on initial clinical examination. This risk is clearly sufficient to necessitate treatment of the paracervical ligaments and pelvic lymph nodes. However, because the probability of extrapelvic spread is low, effective local–regional treatment is curative for most patients.

Radical Radiation Therapy versus Radical Surgery

Radical radiation therapy (external pelvic irradiation) and surgery (type III radical hysterectomy plus bilateral pelvic lymphadenectomy) are acceptable options for most patients. Conventional wisdom suggests that these two alternatives produce approximately equivalent outcomes, with overall 5-year survival rates of approximately 80% reported for each treatment. However, direct comparisons of retrospective reviews may not be appropriate because younger patients and those with more favorable clinical characteristics tend to be selected for treatment with radiation therapy.

Only one prospective randomized trial has directly compared radiation therapy for patients with stage IB versus IIA disease.[119] In that study, patients were randomly assigned to receive treatment with type III radical hysterectomy or radiation therapy. Patients in the surgical arm received postoperative radiation therapy if the tumor involved the parametria, surgical margins, deep stroma, or lymph nodes (Table 28-3).[119] No significant differences were found in the rates of relapse or survival between the two arms of the study, but the overall rate of grade 2 to 3 complications was greater for patients treated with hysterectomy. The dose of radiation therapy received by patients in the radiation therapy arm (76 Gy at point A) was low by conventional standards.

Role of Postoperative Radiation Therapy

The role of postoperative radiation therapy in patients with stage IB or small IIA disease treated with radical

TABLE 28-3

Results of a Randomized Trial Comparing Radical Hysterectomy vs. Radiation Therapy for Stage IB or IIA Carcinoma of the Uterine Cervix

	SURGERY		RADIATION THERAPY	
	Tumor ≤ 4 cm	Tumor > 4 cm	Tumor ≤ 4 cm	Tumor > 4 cm
Number of patients	115	55	113	54
Postoperative RT given	62 (54%)	46 (84%)	—	—
Positive findings on LAG	12 (10%)	12 (22%)	9 (8%)	13 (24%)
Surgically node positive	28 (24%)	17 (31%)	—	—
Clinical stage IIA	8 (7%)	8 (15%)	14 (12%)	9 (17%)
Surgical stage > pT2a	22 (19%)	19 (35%)	—	—
Positive surgical margins	7 (6%)	12 (22%)	—	—
5-Year survival rate	87%	70%	90%	72%
Pelvic relapses	11 (10%)	11 (20%)	12 (11%)	16 (30%)
Distant relapses	12 (10%)	8 (15%)	9 (8%)	7 (13%)
Grade 2-3 side effects	48 (28%)		19 (11%)	

From Landoni F, Maneo A, Colombo A, et al. *Lancet* 1997;350:535-540.
RT, Radiation therapy; *LAG*, lymphangiography.

surgery has been a subject of controversy. However, two recent studies have added valuable information. Most practitioners agree that patients who have more than one positive lymph node, parametrial involvement, or positive margins require postoperative radiation therapy. These patients have significantly lower pelvic recurrence rates with postoperative treatment. In the absence of prospective randomized trials, the impact of such treatment on survival was difficult to determine. However, a recently reported trial[83] in which patients with more than one positive node, parametrial involvement, or positive surgical margins were randomly assigned to receive postoperative radiation therapy and concurrent cisplatin, with or without fluorouracil, demonstrated a significant improvement in survival with chemotherapy plus radiation therapy.

Some patients with negative lymph nodes who have other high-risk features also may benefit from postoperative pelvic irradiation. In a prospective GOG trial,[170] women whose hysterectomy specimens demonstrated various combinations of deep stromal invasion (invasion of more than one third to two thirds of the stroma), LVSI, or large tumor diameter (≥ 4 to 5 cm) were randomly assigned to postoperative radiation therapy or no further therapy. The authors reported a 47% reduction in the risk of recurrence (15% vs. 28%; P = 0.008) when postoperative pelvic irradiation was given (Table 28-4).[170] At the time of the preliminary analysis, an insufficient number of deaths had occurred to permit formal comparison of survival rates; however, 18 deaths had occurred in the radiation therapy group versus 30 in the control (no further treatment) group. Of the 21 recurrences in patients treated with postoperative radiation therapy, 18 (86%) were confined to the pelvis, raising

TABLE 28-4

Recurrences by Treatment Regimen in a Gynecologic Oncology Group Randomized Trial in Selected Patients with Stage IB, Node-Negative Carcinoma of the Cervix Treated with Initial Radical Hysterectomy

Site of Recurrence	Radiation Therapy (N = 137)	No Further Therapy (N = 140)
No recurrence	116 (84.7%)	101 (72.1%)
Recurrence	21 (15.3%)	39 (27.9%)
Local only	18 (13.1%)	27 (19.3%)
Vagina	2	8
Pelvis	15	17
Vagina and pelvis	1	2
Distant	3 (2.2%)	10 (7.1%)
Pelvis and abdomen	0	1
Pelvis and lung	0	2
Abdomen	0	3
Lung	2	2
Lung and brain	0	1
Lymph node	1	1

From Sedlis A, Bundy BN, Rotman MZ, et al. *Gynecol Oncol* 1999; 73:177-183.

questions about the possible benefit of concurrent chemotherapy in selected high-risk cases.

In its 1996 consensus statement, a National Institutes of Health panel concluded that "to minimize morbidity, primary therapy should avoid the routine use of both radical surgery and radiation therapy." If a patient's initial work-up suggests a high likelihood of parametrial invasion, deep stromal invasion, or lymph node metastases, strong consideration should be given to treating the patient with radiation therapy alone or, in selected cases, with chemoradiation. In general, patients who have an enlarged cervix with circumferential tumor involvement or extensive LVSI fall into this category.

Stage IB2 or Minimal Stage IIA Disease

Stage IB2 tumors appear, at least on clinical examination, to be confined to the cervix and are therefore technically resectable. Stage IIA tumors with minimal vaginal involvement may also be resectable. However, bulky stage IB2 and stage IIA tumors are usually deeply invasive and, when treated with initial surgery, often are found to be associated with microscopic paracervical disease or lymph node metastases. The ideal management of stage IB2 and minimal stage IIA tumors is a subject of considerable controversy, and the approach to these tumors differs widely between centers.

Although several investigators continue to advocate initial surgical management for bulky stage IB and even some IIA tumors, most patients who are treated with initial surgery for these tumors require additional treatment with radiation or chemoradiation. In the randomized trial reported by Landoni and colleagues,[119] 84% of surgically treated patients required postoperative radiation therapy, which contributed to a higher complication rate in that arm of the study. Even though the overall survival rates were similar for patients treated with initial surgery and those treated with radiation, the patients in the radiation arm received more protracted, lower-dose treatments than those recommended by most current experts in the field. Recent studies (discussed later in this section) also suggest that chemoradiation should now be considered standard treatment for many of these patients.

To improve the resectability of stage IB2 tumors, some investigators have advocated use of neoadjuvant (preoperative) chemotherapy. Only one prospective trial of this approach has been published so far, although several others are nearing completion. In the published study, reported by Sardi and colleagues,[171] 123 patients with "bulky" tumors ($\geq$ 4 cm) were randomly assigned to treatment with radical hysterectomy with or without neoadjuvant chemotherapy. All patients received postoperative radiation therapy. The patients who received neoadjuvant chemotherapy were more likely to have resectable tumors and had a better survival rate than were patients who had immediate exploration. However, no study has yet reported a comparison between this trimodality treatment and either radiation alone or chemoradiation.

Although primary radiation therapy is effective for many patients with stage IB2 disease, at least 8% to 10% of patients with bulky endocervical tumors treated

with radiation therapy experience central disease recurrences.[59,62,172] This led clinicians to investigate the role of adjuvant extrafascial hysterectomy after radiation therapy. Early retrospective studies from The University of Texas M.D. Anderson Cancer Center[173] suggested that pelvic disease control was improved when adjuvant surgery followed radiation therapy. These results led many clinicians to adopt a combined approach as standard. However, subsequent analyses of the M.D. Anderson Cancer Center experience suggested that the better survival rates observed in patients who received combined treatment reflected, at least in part, clinicians' tendencies to select for this approach patients with smaller, more responsive tumors and those without regional metastases.[76] In 1991, Mendenhall and colleagues[174] reported the outcome of patients treated at the University of Florida before or after clinicians began to add adjuvant hysterectomy to the treatment of bulky (> 6 cm) endocervical tumors. These authors found no difference between the two treatment policies in pelvic disease control or survival rates. A GOG trial completed in 1990 compared treatment using radiation alone or radiation plus extrafascial hysterectomy in 282 patients with stage IB tumors 4 cm or larger. In a 1997 abstract, Keys and colleagues[175] reported no difference in overall survival rates between the two treatment arms, but the final report of this trial has not yet appeared. However, the power of the trial to detect a difference between the two treatments was probably weak: the study included a large number of tumors that were exophytic or less than 5 cm in diameter, for which the margin for improvement with adjuvant surgery in addition to radiation therapy is small. In a review of 1526 patients treated with radiation for squamous carcinoma of the cervix, Eifel and colleagues[59] reported central recurrence rates of only 1% for tumors smaller than 5 cm and 3% for exophytic tumors measuring 5 to 7.9 cm.

In 1999 investigators reported five prospective trials demonstrating improved survival rates when patients treated with radiation for local–regionally advanced cervical cancer also were given concurrent cisplatin chemotherapy (Table 28-5).[83,176-182] Patients with bulky stage IB disease were included in two of these trials. In one trial,[176] patients were treated with radiation or radiation plus weekly cisplatin before brachytherapy and adjuvant hysterectomy (this trial was designed before the results of the Mendenhall study of adjuvant hysterectomy[174] were known to be negative). Patients who received concurrent chemotherapy were more likely to have a complete response in the hysterectomy specimen (52% vs. 41%; $P = 0.04$) and had significantly better progression-free survival ($P < 0.001$) and overall survival ($P = 0.008$). The second trial, Radiation Therapy Oncology Group (RTOG) trial 90-01 (discussed in the next section), included 117 patients with bulky stage IB

TABLE 28-5

Prospective Randomized Trials that Investigated the Role of Concurrent Radiation Therapy and Chemotherapy in Patients with Local–Regionally Advanced Cervical Cancer

Study and Reference	Eligibility	Number of Patients	CT in Investigational Arm	CT in Control Arm	Relative Risk of Recurrence (90% CI)	P Value
Rose et al[178] (GOG)	FIGO IIB–IVA	526	Cisplatin 40 mg/m^2/wk (up to six cycles)	HU 3 g/m^2 (2×/wk)	0.57 (0.42-0.78)	< 0.001
			Cisplatin 50 mg/m^2 5-FU 4 g/m^2/96 hr HU 2 g/m^2 (2×/wk) (two cycles)	HU 3 g/m^2 (2×/wk)	0.55 (0.40-0.75)	< 0.001
Morris et al[177] (RTOG)	FIGO IB–IIA (≥ 5 cm), IIB–IVA or pelvic nodes involved	403	Cisplatin 75 mg/m^2 5-FU 4 g/m^2/96 hr (three cycles)	None*	0.48 (0.35-0.66)	< 0.001
Keys et al[176] (GOG)	FIGO IB (≥ 4 cm)	369	Cisplatin 40 mg/m^2/wk (up to six cycles)	None†	0.51 (0.34-0.75)	0.001
Whitney et al[179] (GOG)	FIGO IIB–IVA	368	Cisplatin 50 mg/m^2 5-FU 4 g/m^2/96 hr (two cycles)	HU 3 g/m^2 (2×/wk)	0.79 (0.62-0.99)	0.03
Peters et al[83] (GOG)	FIGO I–IIA after radical hysterectomy with nodes, margins, or parametrium positive	268	Cisplatin 50 mg/m^2 5-FU 4 g/m^2/96 hr (two cycles)	None	0.50 (0.29-0.84)	0.01
Pearcey et al[181]	FIGO IB–IIA (≥ 5 cm), IIB–IVA or pelvic nodes involved	259	Cisplatin 40 mg/m^2/wk (up to six cycles)	None	0.91 (0.62-1.35)‡	0.43
Wong et al[182]	FIGO IB–IIA (> 4 cm), IIB–III	220	Epirubicin 60 mg/m^2 then 90 mg/m^2 every 4 wk for five more cycles§	None	~ 0.65	0.02
Thomas et al[180]	FIGO IB–IIA (≥ 5 cm), IIB–IVA	234	5-FU 4 g/m^2/96 hr × 2	None‖		NS

CT, Chemotherapy; *CI*, confidence interval; *GOG*, Gynecology Oncology Group; *FIGO*, International Federation of Gynecology and Obstetrics; *5-FU*, 5-fluorouracil; *HU*, hydroxyurea; *RTOG*, Radiation Therapy Oncology Group; *NS*, not significant.
*Patients in the control arm had prophylactic para-aortic irradiation.
†All patients had extrafascial hysterectomy after radiation therapy.
‡Survival.
§Chemotherapy was begun on day 1 and continued every 4 weeks during and after radiation therapy.
‖Patients were also randomly assigned to receive standard or hyperfractionated radiation therapy in a four-arm trial.

or IIA disease (30% of those entered in the trial). These data strongly support the use of concurrent chemoradiation as primary treatment for most patients with bulky (≥ 5 cm diameter) stage IB tumors.

Stage II to III Disease

Although a few surgeons have advocated ultraradical surgical procedures for patients with stage IIB to IIIB disease and for patients with more than minimal vaginal involvement, radiation therapy is usually considered to be the local treatment of choice for these patients. Remarkably, even patients with very large tumors (even tumors measuring 7 cm or more in diameter) have a chance of being cured with radiation therapy alone, particularly if the patient is not found to have extensive regional metastases. Although local control of large tumors continues to be a significant problem, cervical cancer is probably the only epithelial cancer for which control of large tumors with radiation therapy alone is possible. These results reflect the effectiveness of brachytherapy in controlling central disease.

Overall 5-year survival rates for patients with stage IIB disease are usually reported to be between 50% and 75% (Table 28-6).[62,172,183,184] The broad range probably reflects differences in staging, patient selection, and treatment technique between reporting institutions. For patients with stage IIIB disease, reported survival rates range between 30% and 50%. However, both local and distant disease recurrences remain common problems for patients with locally advanced disease. Investigators have tried a number of approaches to improve patients' outcomes—including treatment with neutrons,[153] hyperbaric oxygen,[150] and hypoxic cell sensitizers[151,185,186]—but none of these has significantly improved outcome.

Most recent studies have focused on the use of various combinations of chemotherapy and radiation therapy. Although neoadjuvant chemotherapy produces some impressive tumor responses, randomized trials have repeatedly failed to demonstrate improvements in survival.[187-193] In two trials,[190,192] survival rates were actually poorer when neoadjuvant chemotherapy was added to radiation therapy.

In contrast, trials comparing concurrent chemoradiation with radiation therapy alone have demonstrated consistent improvements in survival with chemoradiation, particularly when cisplatin is included in the chemotherapy regimen. RTOG 90-01[177] and two GOG trials[178,179] evaluated the use of cisplatin-based chemoradiation in patients with stage IIB to IVA disease (RTOG 90-01 also included some patients with bulky stage IB or IIA disease). All three trials demonstrated significant improvements in local disease control, distant metastases, and survival (see Table 28-5). After publication of these results and an associated National Institutes of Health alert, many clinicians considered concurrent cisplatin-based chemoradiation to be a standard treatment for patients with locally advanced cervical cancer.

Although the preliminary findings of RTOG 90-01, published in 1999, demonstrated a highly significant benefit from chemotherapy among patients with stages IB to IIB disease, no significant difference was found in

TABLE 28-6

Results After Low-Dose-Rate Brachytherapy and External-Beam Radiation Therapy

Study and Reference	FIGO Stage	Number of Patients	Pelvic Control (%)	5-Year Survival (%)	Percentage of Tumors ≥ 6 cm
Coia et al, 1990[183]	IB	168	88	74	
	II	243	73	56	
	III	114	49	33	
Barillot et al, 1988[184]	I	218	90*	89	
	IIA	315	86	82	14.5
	IIB	314	78	70	
	IIIB	482	57	49	
Perez et al, 1992[62]	IB	384	94	90	13.5 (≥ 5 cm)
	IIA	128	88	81	39.1 (≥ 5 cm)
	IIB	353	83	77	
	III	293	64	59	
M.D. Anderson Cancer Center (1980-1994) (unpublished study)	IB1	524	98	86	22.8
	IB2	482	81	67	
	IIA	149	84	67	20.5
	IIB	211	81	54	58.8
	III	328	70	47	
Lowrey et al, 1992[172]	IB	130		81	22
	IIA	164		74	5
	IIB	112		64	43

FIGO, International Federation of Gynecology and Obstetrics.
*Pelvic control rates according to personal communication from I. Barillot (from actuarial calculations at 5 years).

overall survival between the two treatments among patients with stages III to IVA disease (63% vs. 57%; $P = 0.44$). Some critics have cited this preliminary result as evidence that chemoradiation is less effective in patients with stage III disease. However, the small number of patients with stage III to IVA disease (117), the incomplete follow-up at the time of the preliminary analysis, and the large confidence intervals on the results suggest that the data were not sufficient to permit sound conclusions about the value of chemotherapy in subgroup analysis. Interestingly, the relapse-free survival rates for chemoradiation and radiation therapy alone were 58% and 38%, respectively ($P = 0.13$) for patients with stage III to IVA disease.

Although concurrent chemotherapy should be considered for patients with stage IIIB disease, some patients cannot be treated with cisplatin because of compromised renal function from tumor-related hydronephrosis. In most cases, the ureters should be decompressed with stents or nephrostomies to optimize renal function before a final determination is made about the feasibility of chemotherapy. If renal compromise prohibits the use of cisplatin, fluorouracil may be given by continuous infusion, although the evidence to support the value of fluorouracil is weaker than that supporting the use of cisplatin (discussed in the section "Chemoradiation" later in this chapter).

Stage IVA Disease

Fewer than 5% of cases of invasive cervical cancer are truly stage IVA (i.e., with biopsy-proven bladder or rectal mucosal involvement). Most of these are classified as IVA because of bladder involvement; rectal involvement is very rarely present at initial diagnosis.

The management of stage IVA disease is particularly challenging because the tumors usually are massive, fixed to pelvic structures, and regionally metastatic. Brachytherapy is often compromised or impossible to perform because vesicovaginal fistulae develop before diagnosis or during treatment (as the tumor responds to radiation). However, at least 10% to 20% of stage IVA tumors are curable with radiation alone.

If the patient has not developed a fistula or if the fistula is small and the urinary stream has been diverted, brachytherapy should be attempted. A small proportion of patients may be curable without brachytherapy with external-beam radiation therapy followed by anterior or total pelvic exenteration.

Only patients who have relatively small, mobile central tumors are likely to be candidates for radical surgical treatment. Although too few patients have been treated with chemoradiation to permit evaluation of the influence of combined treatment, concurrent chemotherapy is usually recommended if the patient's renal function and performance status permit.

Regional Disease

Most patients treated with radical hysterectomy who are found to have lymph node metastases in their lymphadenectomy specimens require postoperative radiation therapy. On the basis of the findings of Peters and colleagues,[83] concurrent chemotherapy is also recommended if no medical contraindications are present. It is sometimes suggested that patients who have only one microscopic focus of regional disease may not require adjuvant treatment. However, because of the small number of women who have this finding and the inconsistent application of postoperative radiation therapy in most of the available series, it is difficult to determine whether adjuvant treatment can be safely omitted.[82,85,86] Patients who are treated with primary radiation therapy for more than microinvasive disease also require treatment of the pelvic lymph nodes.

Because bulky lymph node metastases can be difficult to control with external-beam radiation therapy alone, some investigators have suggested preradiation-therapy resection of nodes that measure more than 1.5 to 2 cm in diameter. Several investigators have reported high local control rates in patients treated with excision of bulky nodes and radiation; however, the numbers of patients in these series were small, and this form of combined regional treatment requires additional study.[53,54] Although it has been difficult to deliver more than 60 Gy of conventional external-beam treatment to lateral pelvic structures, conformal or intensity-modulated radiation therapy may provide a means of delivering a higher dose to well-defined volumes containing bulky regional disease (Fig. 28-8).

Patients who have para-aortic lymph node involvement can be treated effectively with extended-field irradiation. Five-year survival rates range between 25% and 50% (see Fig. 28-7). Because microscopic para-aortic disease may not be detected by routine clinical studies, some investigators have advocated prophylactic irradiation of the aortic nodes for patients with an increased risk of metastases to this region.

The value of prophylactic extended-field irradiation was tested in two randomized trials. In RTOG 79-20,[194] patients with stage IB2 to IIB disease were randomly assigned to receive brachytherapy plus external-beam radiation therapy to the pelvis or to the pelvis and para-aortic nodes (see Fig. 28-8). The absolute 5-year survival rate was significantly better for those who had para-aortic treatment (67% vs. 55%; $P = 0.02$), but no significant difference was found in the disease-free survival rates. The authors' analysis of recurrence patterns in the two groups of patients was difficult to interpret because recurrences that occurred immediately above the pelvic field were not analyzed separately and may have been coded as distant or pelvic failures.

The generalizability of this early study also has been questioned because the initial status of the para-aortic

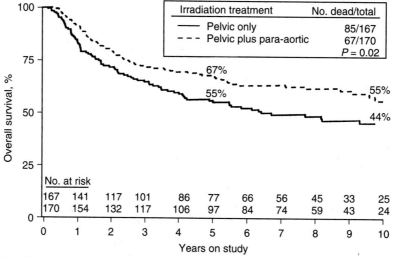

Fig. 28-8   Overall survival of patients treated with pelvic radiation therapy or with extended fields (including both the pelvis and para-aortic nodes) for International Federation of Gynecology and Obstetrics stages IB to IIB cervical cancer in a Radiation Therapy Oncology Group prospective randomized trial. (From Rotman M, Pajak M, Choi K, et al. *JAMA* 1995; 274:387-393.)

region was not evaluated systematically. A concurrent European trial[195] had a similar randomization but included patients with more advanced disease (e.g., with pelvic lymph node metastases or bulky stage IIB or IIIB disease). Patients were required to have negative para-aortic nodes by lymphangiography or surgical staging. No significant difference was found in the 4-year disease-free survival rates between the two arms in this study, but the authors did not compare overall survival rates. The rate of para-aortic node recurrence was significantly higher for patients who did not have that area treated.

In several phase II studies, concurrent chemotherapy has been given with extended-field irradiation. Although side effects are greater when treatment fields are enlarged, combined therapy may be tolerable if careful consideration is given to the chemotherapy regimen, volume of tissue irradiated, and other factors that might increase the risk of serious toxicity. The RTOG combined two cycles of cisplatin (75 mg/m^2) and fluorouracil (4 g/m^2 over 96 hours) with concurrent twice-daily (1 Gy/ fraction) extended-field irradiation in 29 patients with para-aortic node metastases.[196] The authors reported severe acute and late gastrointestinal toxicity with this regimen and an overall survival rate that was not clearly different from that expected with radiation therapy alone. A GOG combination of once-daily extended-field irradiation (1.5 Gy/day to the aortic nodes) with cisplatin (50 mg/m^2) and fluorouracil was better tolerated[197] but resulted in more protracted treatment and used the most conservative cisplatin dose in the randomized trials. Malfetano and Keys[198] reported results of a combination of extended-field irradiation and weekly cisplatin (1 mg/ kg, not to exceed 60 mg) in patients with negative

para-aortic nodes. The dose used in their regimen was similar to the 40 mg/m^2 used by the GOG with pelvic radiation therapy and appeared to be well tolerated.

Although it is tempting to conclude from the impressive results achieved with combinations of pelvic irradiation and chemotherapy that this treatment is appropriate for patients with regional disease, patients should be informed that the cost-benefit ratio of concurrent chemotherapy and extended-field irradiation has not been formally tested.

Locally Recurrent Disease

Selected patients who have a central recurrence of their disease can be cured with radical surgical resection. Only patients with tumors that are mobile and do not involve pelvic lymph nodes are considered candidates for surgery. Patients who have a disease-free interval of less than 1 year tend to have a poor prognosis but are occasionally cured.[199] A total pelvic exenteration is usually required. In rare cases, small recurrences may be treated effectively with radical hysterectomy or anterior exenteration; however, the risk of complications is high when radical hysterectomy follows full-dose radiation therapy. The 5-year survival rate for patients who undergo pelvic exenteration for locally recurrent cervical cancer is usually between 25% and 50%.[199-202] Although several groups have used intraoperative irradiation to treat patients with recurrent pelvic wall disease, patients who have this finding after radical radiation therapy have a very poor prognosis.[203-205]

Patients who have an isolated pelvic recurrence after initial treatment with radical hysterectomy can sometimes

TABLE 28-7

Results of Radiation Therapy for Pelvic Recurrence After Radical Hysterectomy for Cervical Cancer

Authors	Year	Number of Patients	Treatment	Pelvic Control (%)	Survival (%)
Deutsch and Parsons[206]	1974	31	EB ± IC	23	19
Potter et al[207]	1990	28	EB	—	30
Hogan et al[208]	1982	24	EB ± IC	38	22
Jobsen et al[209]	1989	18	EB ± IC	61	44
Thomas et al[210]	1987	17	RT + CT	47	47
Ijaz et al[211]	1998	50	RT ± Brachy ± CT	62	33
No pelvic wall disease		16			69
Pelvic node disease or fixation		34			18

EB, External-beam radiation therapy; *IC*, intracavitary radiation therapy; *CT*, chemotherapy; *Brachy*, brachytherapy.

be cured with radiation therapy (Table 28-7).[206-211] Patients who have isolated central recurrences without pelvic wall fixation or regional metastasis can be cured in up to 60% to 70% of cases by using carefully tailored combinations of external-beam radiation therapy and brachytherapy.[211] The prognosis is much poorer when the pelvic wall is involved; in that case, usually only 10% to 20% of patients survive 5 years after radiation therapy. Intraoperative external-beam therapy or interstitial therapy may contribute to local control in selected patients.[203-205] Salvage rates may be lower for patients with locally recurrent adenocarcinomas.[211,212] Insufficient data are available to permit determination of the benefit of concurrent administration of chemotherapy in patients with locally recurrent cervical cancer.[210]

Inappropriate Simple Hysterectomy for Invasive Cancer

As discussed in the section "Stage IA2 Disease" earlier in this chapter, patients with cervical cancer that invades more than 3 mm should receive treatment that includes the paracervical tissues and pelvic lymph nodes. Although patients should always undergo cytologic screening before undergoing a hysterectomy, deeply invasive cancer is sometimes discovered unexpectedly in a type I hysterectomy specimen.[213] In this situation, the hysterectomy is referred to as an "inappropriate simple hysterectomy" or "cut through hysterectomy"; the latter term may be somewhat misleading because it refers to patients who have various disease extents that may or may not involve the margins of the hysterectomy specimen.

Patients treated with an inappropriate simple hysterectomy have been classified into five groups according to the amount of disease and presentation: (1) microinvasive cancer, (2) tumor confined to the cervix with negative surgical margins, (3) positive surgical margins but no gross residual tumor, (4) gross residual tumor by

clinical examination documented by biopsy, and (5) patients referred for treatment more than 6 months after hysterectomy (usually for recurrent disease).[214]

If the hysterectomy specimen demonstrates more than 3 to 4 mm of invasion, simple hysterectomy is inadequate; however, with postoperative radiation therapy, local control can usually be achieved, and excellent survival rates can be expected in most cases.[215-217]

Roman and colleagues[217] reported survival rates of 79% and 59% after radiation therapy for patients in groups 2 and 3, respectively. However, the survival rate for patients with gross residual or recurrent disease (groups 4 and 5) was only 41%. Patients in groups 4 and 5 were usually treated with external-beam therapy alone to a dose of 65 Gy. Interstitial therapy may be used under laparoscopic guidance to achieve somewhat higher doses if a fairly well defined lesion is found.

The value of chemoradiation is unproven in the setting of inappropriate simple hysterectomy. However, combined treatment is probably reasonable for patients with gross disease because of the relatively high local recurrence rates after radiation therapy alone.

Metastatic Disease (Stage IVB or Recurrent Disease)

Stage IVB disease is rare. This is fortunate because patients with this advanced stage of disease are usually incurable, with 5-year survival rates of less than 10%.[218] Possible rare exceptions include patients who have inguinal metastases from lower vaginal involvement (technically stage IVB disease although the inguinal nodes are part of the primary nodal drainage from the distal vagina). Patients with solitary lung lesions also may be cured in some cases—possibly because they actually have two primary tumors that cannot be distinguished histologically. Most other patients who have stage IVB cervical cancer are treated with palliative intent.

The most active single chemotherapy agent in patients with cervical carcinoma is cisplatin, which produces response rates of 30% to 50% in previously untreated patients. However, the median duration of response tends to be short (4 to 6 months), and complete responses are rare.[219,220] Response rates tend to be lower (10% to 20%) for patients who receive cisplatin for recurrences occurring after pelvic irradiation. Cisplatin analogues (e.g., carboplatin and iproplatin) tend to produce somewhat lower response rates but have been tested less comprehensively. A number of other chemotherapy agents can produce responses in a minority (< 15%) of patients with advanced or recurrent cervical carcinoma. These include doxorubicin, bleomycin, mitomycin C, and fluorouracil.

Many cisplatin-based combinations have been tested in patients with advanced or recurrent cervical carcinoma. High overall response rates have been reported in previously untreated patients, but response rates are poor for tumors that recur within previously irradiated fields. The GOG[221] compared cisplatin alone with cisplatin plus ifosfamide in patients with advanced or recurrent cervical cancer. Although the cisplatin-ifosfamide combination produced a higher response rate than cisplatin alone (33% vs. 19%; $P = 0.02$), the cisplatin-ifosfamide combination also produced significantly more leukopenia, peripheral neuropathy, renal toxicity, and encephalopathy without improving the overall median survival.

Radiation therapy can provide effective pain relief for localized metastases in bone, brain, lymph nodes, or other sites. Hypofractionated pelvic radiation therapy also can relieve pain and reduce bleeding for patients who present with stage IVB disease.[222-224] Effective control of bleeding is of added importance if the patient's treatment plan includes cytotoxic chemotherapy.

RADIATION THERAPY

The goal of radiation therapy for cervical cancer is to deliver adequate doses over an acceptable period without exceeding normal tissue tolerance limits. The required dose varies according to the tumor burden in the cervix, paracervical sites, and regional lymph nodes. Factors that influence the tolerable dose of radiation include the patient's vaginal and uterine anatomy, the degree of tumor-related tissue destruction and infection, and patient characteristics (e.g., body habitus, comorbid illnesses, and smoking habits). The therapeutic ratio is optimized through careful integration of external-beam radiation therapy and brachytherapy, with the dose and intensity of treatment tailored according to estimates of the disease extent and the risk of complications.

External-Beam Radiation Therapy

Microscopic disease in regional lymph nodes can usually be controlled with an external-beam radiation dose of 45 to 50 Gy. However, this dose may not be sufficient to control some areas of heavy microscopic infestation. In particular, the sites of close or positive margins or extracapsular lymph node extension probably require a somewhat higher dose (e.g., 50 to 60 Gy). There is probably also a gradient of risk of metastases within clinically uninvolved paracervical tissues in patients with locally advanced disease. If the uterus has not been removed, the dose gradient from intracavitary (i.e., intravaginal) radiation therapy addresses this risk. Adequate treatment of the paracervical tissues is more difficult after a hysterectomy has been performed because most of the paracervical tissues are no longer within the range of effective intracavitary therapy.

Patients with stage IB to IVA cervical carcinoma require irradiation of the external iliac, internal iliac, common iliac, and presacral nodes. If the posterior vaginal wall is extensively involved, the perirectal nodes also must be treated. If there is cancer in the distal vagina, the inguinal nodes must be irradiated.

External-beam fields also must include the cervix (or operative bed) and paracervical tissues, including the broad ligaments and uterosacral ligaments. Treatment fields must be designed with an understanding that the central pelvic tissues are not static. The positions of the uterus, cervix, and upper vagina can change by 3 cm or more, depending on the filling of the bladder and rectum.

Integration with Brachytherapy

In addition to helping control regional metastasis, external-beam therapy plays an important role in reducing the volume of central disease before intracavitary brachytherapy. Reduction of central disease volume facilitates insertion of brachytherapy applicators and permits delivery of a higher dose to gross disease by reducing the distance between the tumor periphery and intracavitary sources. Although patients are commonly treated with 40 to 45 Gy to the pelvis before brachytherapy, they should be examined regularly during treatment to determine the optimal point at which to begin brachytherapy. Because external-beam therapy tends to cause some contraction of the upper vagina (limiting the size and packing of vaginal applicators), patients who have a narrow vagina should be considered for intracavitary therapy as soon as the cervix is 4 cm or less in diameter. However, when brachytherapy treatments are scheduled in the middle of external-beam therapy, the procedures should be scheduled carefully to avoid more than a 2- or 3-day interruption in treatment of the regional nodes.

Field Arrangements for Treatment of the Whole Pelvis

The most common field arrangement for treatment of the whole pelvis consists of four fields (anteroposterior [AP], posteroanterior [PA], and right and left lateral). When radiation oncologists had only ^{60}Co or 4- to

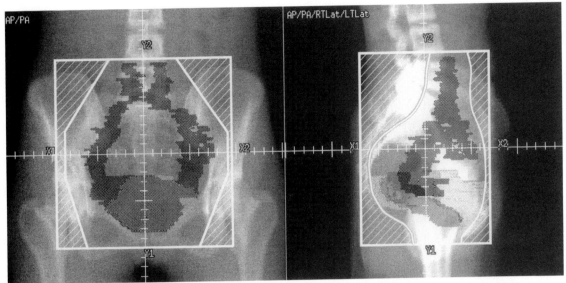

Fig. 28-9   An example of anteroposterior and lateral fields that may be used to treat a patient with cervical cancer. Shading indicates the location of the common, external, and internal iliac lymph nodes and the approximate contour of this patient's 6- to 7-cm endocervical tumor and upper vagina. Lighter shading on the lateral view indicates the contour of the bladder and distal rectum taken from a planning computed tomography scan. When lateral fields are used, blocks must be designed to cover the regional lymph nodes and tumor, taking into account the variable position of the uterus and cervix in the pelvis.

6-MV beams available for external-beam therapy, four fields were needed to avoid delivering an unacceptably high dose to superficial tissues. Today, more penetrating megavoltage beams (≥ 15 MV) are widely available; with these beams, two-field techniques produce relatively homogeneous dose distributions, even when the patient's anterior-posterior separation is 25 cm or more.

However, most clinicians still use a four-field technique (Fig. 28-9) to reduce the dose to the anterior small bowel or rectum.[48] Although in some cases—particularly after hysterectomy—this four-field approach can significantly reduce the dose of radiation to the small bowel, the use of two opposing anterior and posterior fields may be preferred when the patient has local–regionally advanced disease. If the tumor is bulky and lateral fields are used, relatively little of the pelvis can be spared treatment once the tumor, paracervix, and regional nodes are included with a margin (Fig. 28-10). Shielded lateral fields can result in undertreatment if the tumor size or organ motion is underestimated; shielded lateral fields also irradiate additional bone marrow that may be needed when chemoradiation is planned.

Pelvic fields with an upper border at the L4 to L5 interspace are sufficient to cover primary-echelon lymph nodes with a margin. Somewhat smaller fields may be used for patients with small tumors or for patients receiving postoperative radiation therapy if a pelvic lymph node dissection showed no evidence of regional metastasis. However, patients who have common iliac or para-aortic lymph node involvement require treatment with larger fields. In general, the upper border of the radiation field should be at least 4 to 5 cm (or two vertebral bodies) above known disease. However, it is important to recognize that there is a gradient of risk from the primary-echelon nodes to the upper para-aortic nodes. Placement of the upper field border is often based on a qualitative assessment of the risk of microscopic disease versus the added risk of bowel complications from extended fields.

Radiation Dose

Patients who have or are at risk for no more than microscopic regional disease can usually be treated effectively with 45 to 50 Gy of external-beam radiation to the pelvic lymph nodes. If gross lymphadenopathy or extracapsular extension after surgical excision exist, small volumes may be boosted to a total dose of 56 to 66 Gy (including the contribution from intracavitary treatments).

Field Arrangements for Treatment of the Para-aortic Region in Combination with the Pelvis

A variety of techniques can be used to treat the para-aortic region in combination with the pelvis. Although the entire volume can be encompassed in a single large pair of opposing AP and PA fields, this technique usually exposes a large amount of small bowel to the same dose of radiation as the lymph nodes. Alternatively, the

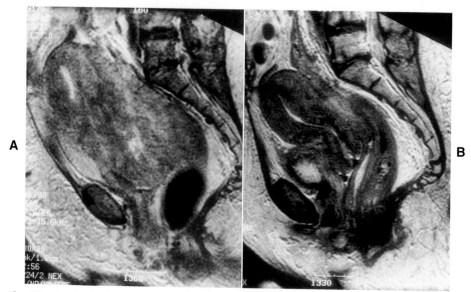

Fig. 28-10 Sagittal magnetic resonance imaging scan demonstrating a large expanding endocervical cancer. **A,** Although this tumor was still clinically confined to the cervix and was mobile on pelvic examination, it nearly filled the pelvis. In this case, little protection of normal tissues would be achieved with lateral pelvic fields. **B,** After 45 Gy of external-beam irradiation and concurrent chemotherapy, there was an excellent partial response of the tumor.

entire volume can be treated with four fields (AP, PA, and two lateral fields), or the pelvis can be treated with AP-PA fields and a different technique can be used for the para-aortic region. If the central axis of the radiation field is placed at the L4 to L5 or L5 to S1 interspace, the upper and lower half of the volume can be treated using different field arrangements without complex matching problems between the fields (Fig. 28-11).

Field Arrangement for Boost to Parametrium or Positive Pelvic Nodes

In the case of lateral involvement of the paracervical tissues or positive pelvic nodes, small anterior and posterior opposing fields can be used to boost the parametria. The goal is to deliver a total dose of 60 to 65 Gy to areas of gross disease or extracapsular extension. The match between the intracavitary system and external fields is complex. In general, boost fields should cover the implants and extend about 0.5 cm lateral to the colpostats (usually at about the 0.5 Gy/hr line). Some clinicians place a midline block during 50% or more of pelvic external-beam treatment, compensating by giving more treatment with intracavitary irradiation. This technique results in a lower total dose of radiation to portions of the bowel and bladder but may undertreat uterosacral disease.[225] When more than half of the pelvic treatment is delivered using a midline block, care should be taken not to overtreat the ureters; if they are included in external-beam fields and are exposed to a higher dose from intracavitary treatment, the risk of ureteral stricture may be increased.[226]

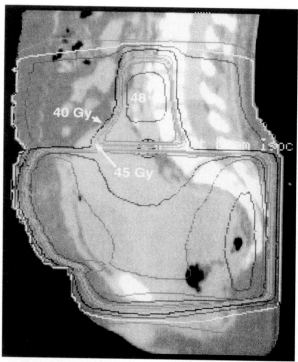

Fig. 28-11 Extended fields can be treated using a split-beam technique that permits the use of different field arrangements above and below the central axis. In this case, very little small bowel was in the pelvis, which was treated using an antero-posterior-posteroanterior (AP-PA) technique that minimized the amount of bone marrow in the field. The para-aortic nodes were treated using AP, PA, and two lateral fields. The match was moved by 0.5 cm twice during treatment (not included in the plan shown).

Treatment of Bulky Lymph Node Disease

In selected cases in which bulky lymph node disease is greater than can be controlled with 60 Gy of radiation, conformal therapy or intensity-modulated radiation therapy can be used to boost a small volume of tissue to a somewhat higher dose. However, tightly conforming fields are usually not used to treat the cervix because of the substantial organ motion that can occur and because brachytherapy usually can be used to deliver even higher doses to the central target volume.

Brachytherapy

The ability to control large cervical tumors with radiation therapy is due in large part to the successful integration of external-beam irradiation and intracavitary brachytherapy. Fortunately, the uterus and vagina are ideal receptacles for intracavitary applicators for several reasons: sources can be placed in the center of the tumor; sources can usually be positioned above and below the tumor (in the fundus and vagina), adding to the lateral dose penetration and improving coverage of the tumor periphery; the distensible vagina can be packed to displace rectum and bladder from intracavitary sources; and the uterus and vagina are relatively resistant to radiation damage.

Traditionally, intracavitary therapy has been delivered at a low dose rate (LDR) using ^{137}Cs, ^{226}Ra, or, occasionally, ^{60}Co sources. Although in recent years some clinicians have moved away from this approach to use remote afterloading high-dose-rate (HDR) systems, LDR systems continue to have a number of advantages. Foremost is the radiobiological advantage achieved when radiation is delivered at a rate of less than 0.6 to 0.8 Gy/hr. At these rates, the recovery of sublethal injury in late-reacting normal tissues is similar to that achieved with external-beam radiation therapy delivered in fractions of 1.8 to 2 Gy.

LDR Therapy for Intact Cervical Tumors

Isotopes for use in gynecologic LDR intracavitary therapy are usually encapsulated in 5- to 30-mg RaEq sources that are 17 to 22 mm long and 3 to 5 mm in diameter. Remote afterloading devices usually contain spherical cesium pellets of approximately 5 mg RaEq each.

Sources are positioned in the uterus and vagina using one of a variety of applicator systems. In early systems, applicators were preloaded with radiation sources before insertion into patients. Modern applicators are positioned in the uterus before the radioactive sources are inserted either manually or remotely. Nearly all applicator types include a hollow tube (tandem) that is inserted in the uterus. Intrauterine tandems may vary somewhat in their length, curvature, and caliber, but the most important variations between applicator systems relate to the arrangement of sources in the vagina. Variations of the Fletcher-Suit-Delclos applicator system are the most common in use in the United States (Fig. 28-12). With this system, vaginal sources are positioned in the center of two cylindrical colpostats; the sources are roughly perpendicular to the axis of the intrauterine line of sources and are 1 to 1.5 cm from the surface of the cervix depending on the diameter of the colpostats (Fig. 28-13, *A*). The anisotropic distribution of dose surrounding the linear sources and shielding in the inferomedial portion of the colpostats reduce the dose of radiation given to the bladder and rectum from the vaginal sources. If the vagina is too narrow to accommodate colpostats or if the lower vagina is involved with cancer, sources are positioned in the vaginal portion of the tandem and are displaced from the vagina with Lucite cylinders (see Fig. 28-13, *B*). Other applicator systems arrange vaginal sources parallel to the tandem (e.g., Henschke applicators) or place the sources perpendicular to the tandem but in closer proximity to the cervix.

Arrangement of vaginal sources, packing of vaginal applicators, and positioning of tandem. A detailed discussion of intracavitary brachytherapy technique is beyond the scope of this chapter, but the most crucial points will be outlined here. In general, sources are positioned to maximize the ratio between the dose to the cervix and paracervical tissues and the dose to the bladder and rectum. Sources in the endocervix deliver a very high dose to central disease; sources in the uterus and vagina expand the dose distribution to cover the periphery of the cervix, increase the dose of radiation to paracervical tissues, and treat the lower uterine segment and vagina.

The arrangement and position of vaginal sources, vaginal packing, and the position of the tandem can be adjusted in several ways to minimize rectal and bladder exposure. The tandem is usually positioned in the mid-sagittal plane of the pelvis about two thirds of the way between the sacrum and pubis. If eccentric involvement of one side of the parametrium is present, the dose to that side can be increased by permitting some lateral deviation of the tandem. The colpostats should be up against the cervix—caudad displacement should be minimized because it reduces the dose to the tumor without decreasing the dose to normal tissues. The colpostats should be centered on the cervix. In most cases, centering them in this manner causes the colpostats to be approximately bisected by the ovoids. Excessive posterior displacement of the ovoids results in an underdosage of the anterior cervical lip and can lead to severe overdosage of rectum draped over the protruding posterior vagina (Fig. 28-14). The vaginal applicators should be carefully packed in place, displacing the vagina (and bladder and rectum) away from the sources. It is particularly important to avoid an anterior dip in the packing

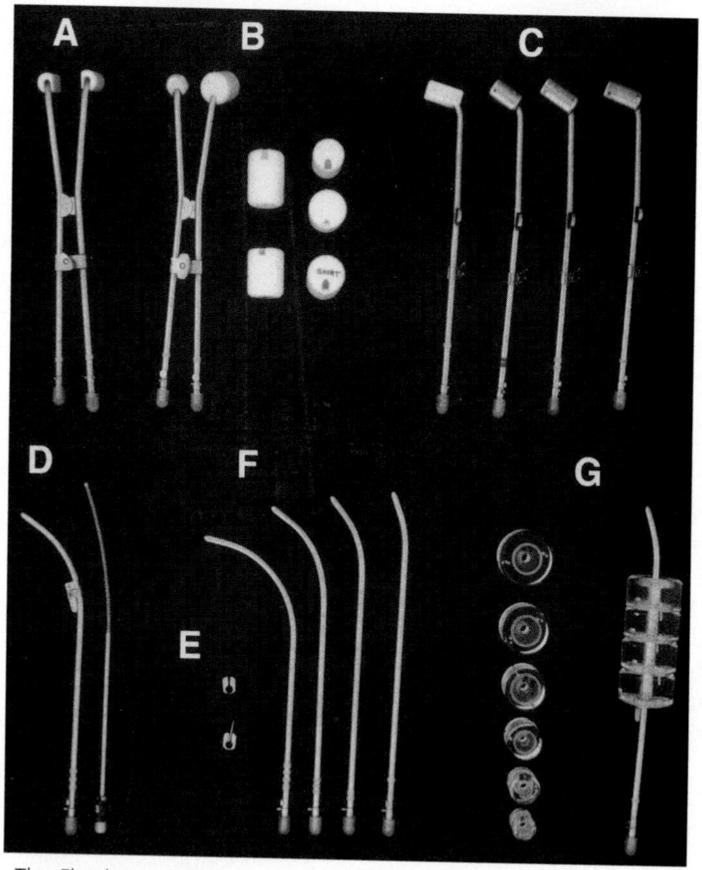

Fig. 28-12 The Fletcher-Suit-Delclos applicator system. **A,** Mini-colpostats. **B,** Small (2-cm) colpostats with various caps used to increase their diameter and length. **C,** Colpostats of varying angles. **D,** Tandem and dummy markers. **E,** Metallic flanges used to set the length of the intrauterine tandem. **F,** Four tandems of varying curvatures. **G,** Lucite cylinders with a central hole to accommodate the central tandem (used for patients who have a narrow vagina or extensive vaginal disease).

caudad to the colpostats; failure to adequately pack this area also exposes the rectum to an unnecessarily high dose. In most cases, the tandem should be placed up against the fundus of the uterus or high enough to permit loading of 6 to 8 cm of intrauterine tandem. If the vagina is sufficiently ample, caps should be placed on the Fletcher-Suit-Delclos colpostats. These facilitate positioning and permit the use of somewhat greater activity in the vaginal applicators, improving the dose to large tumors.

Even the most experienced practitioners occasionally perforate the uterus when they are sounding and dilating a cancerous cervix. The most common site of perforation is the posterior endocervix or lower uterine segment. Although this problem is sometimes appreciated when the sound penetrates beyond 8 cm without reaching a fundus, the findings can be more subtle if the tip of the probe passes into paracervical tissues or rests against the sacrum or other pelvic tissues. Uterine perforation can lead to disastrous secondary complications and underdosage of tumor. Whenever uterine perforation is a possible risk, the position of the tandem should

be verified with CT or sonography. If a perforated uterus is subsequently probed successfully, the tandem can be left in place under antibiotic coverage.[227]

Like any operative technique, optimal intracavitary placement requires skill and experience, whether LDR or HDR equipment is used. Because locally advanced cervical cancer is an uncommon disease in most U.S. communities, radiation oncologists in the United States are not uniformly skilled in brachytherapy procedures. Because brachytherapy is a critical part of cervical cancer treatment, practitioners who treat very few cases of intact cervical cancer should consider referring patients to centers with greater experience.

Selection of sources and calculation of delivered dose. Intracavitary treatments for carcinoma of the cervix are usually reported in terms of the doses to specific pelvic reference points (points A and B) that were initially defined as part of the Paris and Manchester treatment methods.[228] In 1985, the International Commission on Radiation Units and Measurements (ICRU)[229] described the classic Manchester definition of point A as "a point 2 cm lateral to the central canal of the uterus and 2 cm up

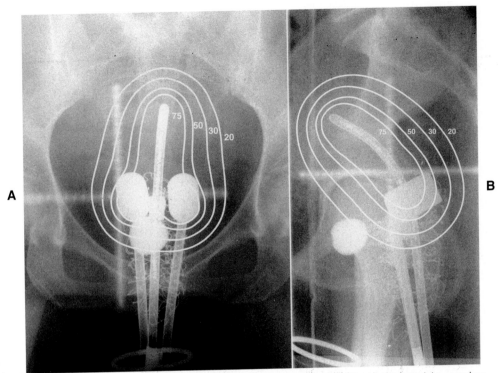

Fig. 28-13 **A,** Anteroposterior and **B,** lateral radiographs of a Fletcher-Suit-Delclos tandem and small (2-cm) colpostats. The tandem bisects the colpostats on the lateral view and is in a roughly central position between the sacrum and bladder. The colpostats are within 0.5 cm of the marker seeds inserted in the anterior and posterior lips of the cervix. The vaginal packing (visible because of a radio-opaque thread in the center of the packing) displaces the vagina away from the vaginal sources. The tandem was loaded with 35 mg RaEq of cesium, and the colpostats each contained 10 mg RaEq of cesium. Contours of the 20, 30, 50, and 75 cGy/hr isodose lines are shown superimposed on the radiographs. The dose rate at *point A* was approximately 50 cGy/hr.

from the mucous membrane of the lateral fornix in the axis of the uterus" (Fig. 28-15). Point B was defined as "being in the transverse axis through points A, 5 cm from the midline." Despite this and other attempts to standardize their definitions, points A and B continue to be calculated in a variety of ways, contributing to discrepancies between reporting institutions. Also, because point A is in a region of the pelvis where the dose of radiation from intracavitary sources is changing rapidly, small inaccuracies in the placement of point A can produce significant differences in the calculated result. In its report, the ICRU suggested an alternative method of reporting that included an estimate of the volume treated to 60 Gy and the reference air kerma. This approach never gained wide acceptance, and most clinicians continue to report their treatments in terms of the dose to point A.

Although the dose to point A can be used as an approximate estimate of dose intensity, the dose to point A must be considered in the context of many other factors in designing treatments. At the M.D. Anderson Cancer Center, the quality of the intracavitary placement is the first consideration.[230] If the applicator position or vaginal packing fails to meet acceptable standards, the applicator is adjusted and repacked. When the position has been optimized, the uterine tandem and vaginal applicators are loaded using relatively standard source combinations that deliver radiation to adjacent tissues at an acceptable rate. Typically, 30 to 40 mg RaEq is distributed in a tandem 6 to 8 cm long using three 10- to 15-mg RaEq sources (spacers may be required). If the tandem is well positioned, its tip may be loaded with 15 mg RaEq to improve the dose to the endocervix and lateral tissues; if the endocervix is expanded, a 15-mg RaEq source also may be used in the mid position to improve the distribution of dose to that region. In general, the distal source should not protrude more than a few millimeters from the external cervical os when colpostats are being used; the use of a protruding source to supplement the dose between widely separated colpostats appears to increase the risk of vaginal fistulae.[231] The loading of vaginal colpostats is usually chosen to give a dose rate of 1 Gy/hr or less at the vaginal surface. Lower dose rates are preferred when unshielded colpostats (i.e., mini-ovoids) or vaginal cylinders are used.

Although most late treatment complications (e.g., anterior rectal ulcers, posterior bladder ulcers, fistulae)

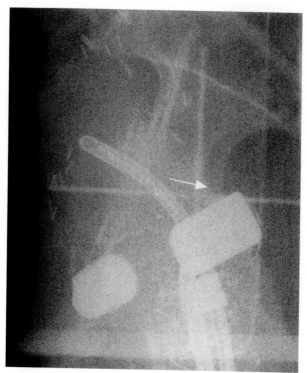

Fig. 28-14 In this case, posterior displacement of the vaginal colpostats would have allowed the rectum to drape over the vaginal sources, producing a high rectal dose cephalad to the vaginal fornix. This problem was identified in the operating room, and the system was repositioned, improving the relationship between the tandem and colpostats.

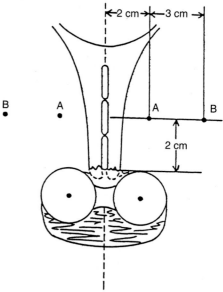

Fig. 28-15 Points *A* and *B*. In the classic Manchester system, point *A* is defined as a point 2 cm lateral to the central canal of the uterus and 2 cm up from the mucous membrane of the lateral fornix. In clinical practice, dose calculations are usually made from radiographs, and point *A* is taken 2 cm up from the flange of the uterine tandem and 2 cm lateral from the central canal.[229] Alternatively, some clinicians use radio-opaque markers in the cervix or a point midway between the surface of the vaginal colpostats to determine the starting point.

are probably the consequence of a high dose delivered to a relatively small volume of tissue, other complications (reduced bladder capacity, severe pelvic fibrosis) may result from a moderately high dose to a large volume. These types of complications are seen when more than 50 to 60 Gy is delivered to a large portion of the pelvis.

Calculations of total reference air kerma or total mg-RaEq hours are used as surrogates for the integral dose to the pelvis from intracavitary radiation. In general, the total mg-RaEq hours of intracavitary treatment is limited to no more than 6000 to 6500 after 40 to 45 Gy to the whole pelvis (or 7500 to 8000 after 20 Gy to the whole pelvis). With typical loadings (usually ≤ 65 mg RaEq), these limits are not exceeded in two 48-hour applications. However, when a capacious vagina or long tandem accommodates more than 65 to 70 mg RaEq, it is usually necessary to reduce the time the implants are left in place or their total activity.

Steep dose gradients, organ motion, and anatomic changes that occur between implant placements make it very difficult to calculate accurate maximum or total organ doses from intracavitary implants. Most clinicians try to calculate doses to normal tissue reference points; these are selected in a wide variety of ways,[232-236] including the method recommended by the ICRU in 1985 (Fig. 28-16).[229]

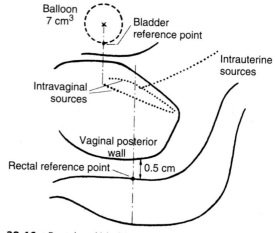

Fig. 28-16 Rectal and bladder reference points according to the International Commission on Radiation Units and Measurements Report 38.[229]

HDR Therapy for Intact Cervical Tumors

In the past, radiation safety requirements prohibited handling of very high activity sources, necessitating the delivery of brachytherapy at relatively low dose rates. It eventually became apparent that LDR treatment had definite radiobiological advantages, and the ability to administer intracavitary radiation at dose rates of 0.4 to

0.6 Gy/hr (to point A) was thought to be a major contributor to the success of cervical cancer treatment. Efforts to shorten the duration of intracavitary radiation therapy by increasing the dose rate by as little as twofold, to 0.8 to 1.0 Gy/hr, have led to increased complication rates even after compensatory dose reductions.[237]

However, in the 1980s and 1990s, the advent of computer-controlled remote-afterloading technology made it possible to accurately deliver brachytherapy treatments at low dose rates or at very high dose rates (> 1 Gy/min) without exposing personnel to ionizing radiation. The possibility that treatment could be delivered entirely within the radiation therapy department without inpatient hospitalization led vendors and investigators to develop methods and protocols for the delivery of HDR intracavitary therapy for patients with cervical cancer. However, although many clinicians now consider HDR brachytherapy to be within the standard of care, it has never been rigorously compared with LDR brachytherapy. Consensus continues to be limited regarding which of the many techniques and fractionation schemes currently being used to treat patients are best.

Two groups have tried to perform randomized trials comparing LDR and HDR brachytherapy.[238,239] Although both concluded that the two approaches were similar with respect to the effectiveness and toxicity of therapy, problems with the methods of treatment allocation, relatively small numbers of patients, and other flaws in the designs of these trials make it impossible to generalize the authors' conclusions about treatment efficacy.

Retrospective experiences also demonstrate that combinations of external-beam irradiation and HDR brachytherapy are curative for a substantial proportion of patients.[240-244] However, differences in the selection of patients, staging of tumors, and reporting of results make it difficult to compare experiences. Although these experiences are encouraging, they would be insufficient to permit detection of moderate differences in outcome after LDR versus after HDR, particularly for subsets of patients with high-risk disease.

Most of the published experiences of HDR brachytherapy are from Asia, Germany, and England.[238,239,242,244-250] Although the use of HDR brachytherapy in the United States has increased during the past decade, few systematic studies of this technique have been conducted, and the experiences that have been reported include few patients. The University of Wisconsin experience is one of the largest.[244] Investigators compared results in 191 patients treated with LDR brachytherapy between 1977 and 1988 and 173 patients treated with HDR brachytherapy after 1988. Although the survival rates with the HDR and LDR approaches were similar for patients with small tumors, the authors reported a significantly lower survival rate for patients with stage IIIB disease who were treated with HDR brachytherapy (Table 28-8).[242,244,245,249,250] Kapp and colleagues[242] also reported encouraging

survival rates for small tumors, but the survival rates for patients with larger tumors were relatively low. Arai and colleagues[245] reported high survival rates for patients with all stages of disease, but the total doses they recommended for HDR or LDR therapy were lower than conventional doses by 30% or more, making it difficult to reconcile their results with other experiences.

Although the radiobiological disadvantages of HDR intracavitary therapy can undoubtedly be overcome if the treatment is divided into a sufficient number of small fractions, doing so may compromise the purported advantages of the technique in terms of patient and physician convenience and cost. Also, although it has often been assumed that the acute complication risk is less with HDR brachytherapy, detailed studies suggest that this may not be true.[227,251] Although HDR brachytherapy is gaining increasing acceptance in the community, its widespread use to treat patients with intact cervical cancer continues to arouse controversy.[247]

Interstitial Therapy for Intact Cervical Tumors

Some radiation oncologists advocate the use of interstitial brachytherapy as an alternative to intracavitary radiation therapy for selected patients with cervical cancer. Although criteria differ, patients with stage III disease or with poor vaginal anatomy are most often considered candidates for interstitial brachytherapy.

To place interstitial implants for the treatment of patients with cervical cancer, most practitioners use a perineal template to guide evenly spaced needles into the cervix and paracervical tissues. An obturator in the vagina helps to determine the direction of needle insertion (Fig. 28-17).

Supporters of interstitial therapy describe as advantages of this method the relatively homogeneous dose, the ease of inserting implants into patients whose uteri are difficult to probe, and the ability to place sources directly into the parametrium. A number of investigators have reported encouraging local control rates, although the follow-up in most series is short.[252-254]

Although interstitial templates have been used to treat cervical cancer for many years, reported series have been small, and patient follow-up has rarely been sufficient to permit calculation of long-term survival rates. In an early series, Syed and colleagues[254] reported a projected 5-year survival rate of 53% for 26 patients with stage IIIB disease. However, survival results from two more recent reports were disappointing. In a review of the combined experiences of Stanford University Medical Center and the Joint Center for Radiation Therapy,[255] Hughes-Davies and colleagues reported 3-year disease-free survival rates for patients with stages IIB and IIIB disease of 36% and 18%, respectively; local control rates were 22% and 44%, respectively, and in patients with local control, the rate of complications requiring

TABLE 28-8

Selected High-Dose-Rate Brachytherapy Regimens and Reported Treatment Outcome

Study	Year	Tumor Description	EBRT DOSE (Gy)			HDR BRACHYTHERAPY SCHEDULE			Number of Patients	5-year DSS (%)
			Whole Pelvis	Parametrum	Dose/ Fraction	Number of Fractions	Frequency	Timing		
Kapp et al[242]	1998	< 3 cm	44-50.4	—	4.7-5.3*	4	2×/wk	After EBRT	29	96
		3-6 cm	30-60					After EBRT	97	66
		> 6 cm	> 60					After EBRT	55	28
Petereit et al[244]	1999	IB nonbulky	0	60	9.1-9.9	5	Weekly		52	85
		IB bulky, IIA	20-30†	30-40	7.2-8.2†	5	Weekly		39	—
		IIB	51†	9	3.7-4.9†	5	Weekly		50	69
		III	60†	—	3.7-4.3†	5	Weekly		50	33
Utley et al[250]	1984	I	20	30	5	8-10	2×/wk	Concurrent	29	89
		II	20-30	50	5	8-10	2×/wk	Concurrent	50	58
		IIIB	20-50	50	5	8-10	2×/wk	Concurrent	43	33
Arai et al[245]	1992	IB	0	45	5.8	5	Weekly	Concurrent	147	82
		II (small)	0	50	5.8	5	Weekly	Concurrent	256	62
		II (large)	20	30	5.75	4	Weekly	Concurrent	—	—
		III (small)	20-30	50	5.75	4	Weekly	Concurrent	515	47
		III (large)	20-30	50	5-6	3-4	Weekly	Concurrent	—	—

EBRT, External-beam radiation therapy; *DSS,* disease-specific survival.

*Schedules evolved during the years covered in this study. These numbers represent the most recent schedules.

†These schedules were changed in the most recent year of the study. Patients now receive 45 to 50 Gy to the whole pelvis and five fractions of HDR brachytherapy of 5.5 to 6 Gy each.[249]

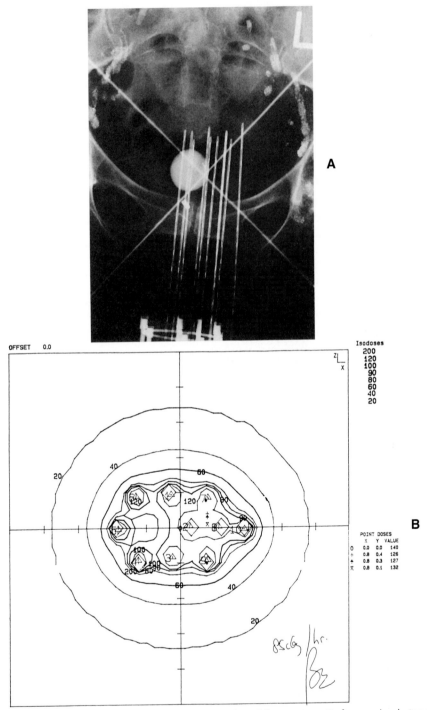

Fig. 28-17 A, Anterior view of a perineal implant placed for treatment of a proximal stage IIB carcinoma of the cervical stump using a perineal template and 10 needles. The screw just inferior to the opacified Foley balloon marks the superior end of the vaginal obturator. B, Dose distribution of the implant seen in A, at the geometric center of the sources.

surgical intervention was high. A report of the University of California Irvine experience described 5-year survival rates of 21% and 29%, respectively, for patients with stage IIB and IIIB disease, also with high complication rates.[256] These survival rates do not appear to improve upon those achieved with combinations of external-beam and intracavitary radiation therapy (55% to 75% for IIB and 40% to 50% for IIIB). More recently, some authors have tried to improve the accuracy of needle placement using laparotomy or ultrasound guidance.[257,258] However, at present, no definite evidence has been found to indicate that interstitial therapy improves the outcome of patients with advanced cervical lesions.

Vaginal Brachytherapy After Hysterectomy

Intracavitary radiation therapy also may be used to treat the vagina in patients with cervical cancer who have had a hysterectomy. Usually vaginal brachytherapy is used to boost the dose to the vaginal apex in women who receive pelvic radiation therapy because of high-risk features in their hysterectomy specimen. The best argument for boosting this region to a higher dose than other tissues potentially at risk for microscopic disease is that the vaginal incision could harbor cells implanted during the surgical procedure. Patients who have disease at the vaginal mucosal margin are particularly good candidates for treatment with vaginal brachytherapy. However, it is important to recognize that most vaginal applicators have very shallow penetration (Fig. 28-18). Deep stromal margins (particularly lateral or anterior paracervical margins) are likely to lie beyond the reach of vaginal intracavitary therapy.

A variety of applicators can be used to treat the vaginal cuff. Two vaginal ovoids may be used, although care must be taken to ensure that the vaginal incision is not packed away from the surface of the ovoids. At the M.D. Anderson Cancer Center, a domed vaginal cylinder is used to deliver LDR irradiation; the applicator is loaded with a single point source of cesium in the center of the hemispherical dome. Depending on the risk of recurrence in the vaginal cuff, a total dose between 30 Gy (prescribed at the vaginal surface) in 48 hours and 50 Gy in 72 hours may be given after 45 Gy of pelvic irradiation.

The vaginal cuff also can be treated using HDR applicators with similar specifications. Many different schedules have been used. At the M.D. Anderson Cancer Center, a relatively conservative fractionation scheme of three fractions of 5 to 6 Gy prescribed at the vaginal surface is favored. When a positive vaginal margin requires delivery of a higher dose, we prefer to use LDR brachytherapy. It should always be remembered that the rectum is approximately 0.5 cm from the surface of the vagina. We prefer not to exceed a dose of 3 Gy/fraction at this depth out of concern that higher doses per fraction could produce an increased risk of rectal injury.

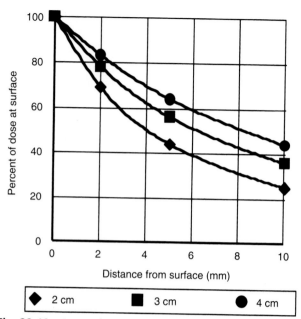

Fig. 28-18 Dose of radiation delivered at various distances from the surface of a Delclos domed vaginal cylinder for cylinders of three different diameters. The rapid fall-off of dose must be considered in planning treatment, particularly when vaginal intracavitary treatment is used to treat gross or recurrent disease.

However, many of the fractionation schemes recommended at other centers do deliver larger doses per fraction to the rectum.

Treatment Duration

Several studies of patients with cervical cancer treated with radiation have demonstrated correlations between longer duration of treatment and decreased pelvic disease control rates.[64,259] Although there may be some tendency for patients with high-risk lesions to have longer treatment courses,[260] the results of these studies and radiobiological principles strongly suggest that protraction of treatment beyond 7 to 8 weeks reduces the probability of pelvic disease control (Fig. 28-19).[259] Results from the Patterns of Care studies[45] and GOG trials[178] suggest that many patients continue to take 10 weeks or more to complete treatment. However, the average duration of treatment at facilities with large reported experiences (e.g., M.D. Anderson Cancer Center and Washington University in St. Louis) tends to be shorter, with few patients requiring more than 8 to 9 weeks to complete their treatment.[260]

To minimize breaks in treatment, intracavitary therapy should begin no more than 1 to 7 days after the completion of whole-pelvic irradiation. Treatments to boost disease in the lateral parametrium or lymph nodes can be given between intracavitary treatments. If holidays or poor compliance protract a course of treatment, patients may be given two treatments, 6 to 8 hours apart, on 1 or 2 days.

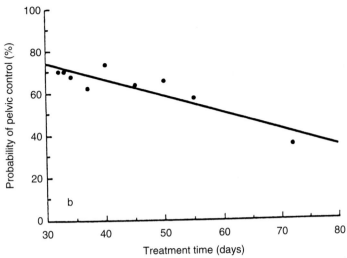

Fig. 28-19 Pelvic control as a function of treatment time for 279 patients with stage III or IVA carcinoma of the cervix treated with curative intent at Princess Margaret Hospital. (From Fyles A, Keane TJ, Barton M, et al. *Radiother Oncol* 1992;25:273-279.)

CHEMORADIATION
Concurrent Chemotherapy and Radiation Therapy

In 1999 and 2000 the results of five prospective randomized trials demonstrated significant improvements in overall survival, disease-free survival, and local control rates when cisplatin-containing chemotherapy was administered concurrently with radiation therapy in patients with local–regionally advanced cervical cancer (see Table 28-5).[83,176-182] These results stimulated an alert from the National Institutes of Health signaling a change in the standard of care for many patients with locally advanced cervical cancer.[261]

In three of these randomized trials,[177-179] the local treatment was radiation therapy alone, whereas the other two trials[83,176] evaluated the role of chemotherapy in patients who received radiation before or after hysterectomy. However, despite differences in the eligibility criteria, the magnitude of the reduction in recurrence risk was remarkably similar across all the studies. For five of the six treatment arms of the study that included concurrent administration of cisplatin and radiation therapy, the risk of recurrence was reduced by 40% to 60% compared with the risk in the control arm (radiation alone or radiation plus hydroxyurea).

In these five trials, two schedules of chemotherapy emerged as superior. The first, which has been adopted as standard by the GOG, is 40 mg/m^2 cisplatin weekly for up to 6 weeks during external-beam irradiation, which reduced the risk of recurrence by about 40%.[178] This regimen was less toxic than a combination of cisplatin, fluorouracil, and hydroxyurea that achieved similar reductions in the risk of recurrence. A regimen of two cycles of cisplatin (50 mg/m^2) and fluorouracil also was

well tolerated but was associated with the least dramatic risk reduction of the five trials. The second chemotherapy regimen that emerged as superior was two to three cycles of cisplatin (75 mg/m^2; each cycle lasted 3 weeks) with fluorouracil, which reduced the risk of recurrence by about 50%.[177] These two regimens have not been compared directly; both can be considered acceptable treatments for patients with locally advanced cervical cancer who meet the eligibility criteria of the randomized trials.

The average total doses of cisplatin delivered with the weekly cisplatin regimen and the cisplatin-and-fluorouracil regimen were similar—approximately 200 mg/m^2. The value of less intensive doses of cisplatin is unknown. A small trial of weekly cisplatin at a dose of 25 mg/m^2 did not demonstrate an improvement over radiation therapy alone.[262]

In the cisplatin-plus-fluorouracil regimen, one cycle of chemotherapy was administered during intracavitary radiation. In contrast, in the weekly cisplatin regimen, cisplatin was administered only during external-beam irradiation. The importance of these factors is unknown. The value of administering fluorouracil with radiation has been well demonstrated in studies of gastrointestinal malignancies. The drug also has produced encouraging results in some smaller studies of patients with cervical cancer.[180,263] Thomas and colleagues[180] have reported encouraging results using a chronic continuous infusion of fluorouracil with radiation in patients with cervical cancer. However, a significant improvement was demonstrated in only one subset of the patients in their trial—patients who had stage I or II disease and who received a single daily fraction as opposed to hyperfractionated irradiation. The GOG is currently completing a trial comparing weekly cisplatin with chronic continuous infusion of fluorouracil. However, no trial has compared cisplatin alone versus cisplatin with fluorouracil.

RTOG 90-01 was the only trial that encouraged the use of chemotherapy during intracavitary radiation therapy.[177] This is an interesting approach, particularly with LDR irradiation, because a high dose of radiation is given over a short time (typically 20 to 25 Gy to point A over 2 days). Although the treatment appeared to be well tolerated, the benefits and risks of giving chemotherapy during brachytherapy have not been studied systematically. HDR intracavitary irradiation was not permitted in any of the five trials discussed above. Although HDR irradiation is currently permitted as an alternative in several prospective randomized trials, the best way to integrate HDR therapy with external-beam irradiation and chemotherapy and the risks of administering chemotherapy concurrently with large fractions of HDR intracavitary irradiation are still incompletely understood.

Recently, the National Cancer Institute of Canada reported preliminary results of a sixth prospective randomized trial that compared pelvic irradiation alone with a combination of weekly cisplatin (40 mg/m^2) and pelvic irradiation (see Table 28-5).[181] In contrast to the other five trials of cisplatin-containing chemotherapy, the National Cancer Institute of Canada trial failed to demonstrate a significant improvement in survival with the addition of chemotherapy (hazard ratio, 1.10; 95% confidence interval, 0.74 to 1.62). This trial was smaller than the earlier ones but had eligibility criteria similar to those of RTOG 90-01. The overall duration of radiation therapy for patients in this trial was 49 days, shorter than that of other studies. The authors argue that this more compact radiation therapy schedule may obviate chemotherapy. However, the 1-year pelvic disease control rates and overall survival rates reported in their abstract are similar to those reported for the control arm

of RTOG 90-01, suggesting that their margin for improvement may have been similar.

Two recent randomized trials have compared radiation therapy alone with radiation plus non-cisplatin-containing regimens.[180,182] In one of those trials, Wong and colleagues[182] randomly assigned 220 patients to receive radiation therapy alone or radiation therapy with epirubicin administered every 4 weeks for five courses. Chemotherapy was begun on the first day of radiation therapy but was continued after radiation therapy until the five courses were completed. The authors reported significantly better disease-free ($P = 0.03$) and overall ($P = 0.04$) survival rates when chemotherapy was given.

Phase II trials of radiation therapy with concurrent mitomycin C and fluorouracil have yielded various conclusions about the efficacy of this combination in patients with cervical cancer. Roberts and colleagues recently reported an interim analysis of a randomized trial (administered by Yale investigators in Venezuela) that compared radiation therapy with or without mitomycin C and fluorouracil. The authors reported a significant improvement in disease free survival ($P = 0.01$) with chemotherapy but a less impressive difference in overall survival ($P = 0.1$). They were most impressed with the improvement for a small subset of patients with stage III disease ($P = 0.03$). However, this report resulted from one of several interim analyses that have been performed on a trial that continues to accrue patients. Further data will be needed to clarify the role of mitomycin C in this disease.

Neoadjuvant Chemotherapy Followed by Radiation Therapy

Although cisplatin-containing chemotherapy produces some impressive responses in patients with cervical

---

TABLE 28-9

Results of Prospective Randomized Trials that Compared Neoadjuvant Chemotherapy Followed by Radiation Therapy with Radiation Therapy Alone in Patients with Locally Advanced Cervical Cancer

Study and Reference	Year	Number of Patients	Stages	Drugs	SURVIVAL RATE (%)			
					CT + RT	RT Alone	P Value	Endpoint
Kumar et al[188]	1994	184	IIB–IVA	BIP	38	43	0.5	OS at 32 mo
Tattersall et al[193]	1992	71	IIB–IVA	PVB	44*	40*	NS	OS at 48 mo
Chauvergne et al[187]	1990	107	IIIB	MtxCVP	47*	50*	NS	OS at 48 mo
Tattersall et al[192]	1995	260	IIB–IVA	EpP	50*	69*	0.02	OS at 36 mo
Sundfør et al[191]	1996	94	IIIB–IVA	PF	34*	37*	0.9	OS at 48 mo
Leborgne et al[189]	1997	96	IB2–IVA	BOP	38	45	0.4	DFS at 60 mo
Souhami et al[190]	1991	107	IIIB	BOMP	23	39	0.02	OS at 60 mo

From Eifel PJ. *Radiat Res* 2000;154:229-236.

CT, Chemotherapy; *RT*, radiation therapy; *B*, bleomycin; *I*, ifosfamide; *P*, cisplatin; *OS*, overall survival; *V*, vinblastine; *NS*, not significant; *Mtx*, methotrexate; *C*, chlorambucil; *Ep*, epirubicin; *F*, fluorouracil; *O*, vincristine; *DFS*, disease-free survival; *M*, mitomycin C.
*Percentages were estimated from survival curves.

cancer, none of the seven randomized trials that have compared radiation therapy with or without neoadjuvant chemotherapy have demonstrated improved survival rates with the neoadjuvant chemotherapy approach (Table 28-9).[187-193,264]

More recently, to permit surgical treatment of patients with bulky lesions who would otherwise be poor candidates for radical hysterectomy, several trials have been initiated to study the role of induction chemotherapy before surgical exploration. In one trial, 205 patients with stage IB cervical cancer underwent surgery with or without an initial course of chemotherapy (cisplatin, vincristine, and bleomycin); all patients also received postoperative radiation therapy.[171] The authors reported that tumors treated with chemotherapy were more often resectable and that the survival rate of patients who had received neoadjuvant chemotherapy was better (81% vs. 66%; $P < 0.05$). Ultimately, this approach may need to be compared with optimized chemoradiation to determine the most effective, least toxic treatment for these patients.

COMPLICATIONS OF RADIATION THERAPY
Acute Side Effects
External-Beam Irradiation

Most patients experience at least some diarrhea during external-beam irradiation; symptoms may be greater when concurrent chemotherapy (particularly fluorouracil) is given. Diarrhea is usually well controlled with oral medications and dietary modifications. Patients with severe diarrhea should have stool cultures done to rule out infection with *Clostridium difficile*.

Less frequently, patients may complain of bladder or urethral irritation. These symptoms may be treated with phenazopyridine hydrochloride (Pyridium) or antispasmodics after urinalysis and urine culture have ruled out a urinary tract complication. Patients with fever or flank pain should be evaluated for possible pyelonephritis. This is most likely to occur in patients with large tumors that have compromised urinary flow.

When radiation fields cover the vulva to treat extensive vaginal involvement, severe skin erythema and even moist desquamation can develop. Treating the patient in an open-leg position can usually dramatically reduce radiation-induced skin reactions. Patients who have unexpectedly severe skin reactions often have an underlying infection with *Candida* organisms; in such cases, treatment with oral or local antifungal agents can dramatically improve symptoms even while radiation treatments continue.

Intracavitary Radiation Therapy

Fatal or life-threatening complications of intracavitary radiation therapy are rare. In 4042 patients who received 7662 LDR intracavitary treatments at the M.D.

Anderson Cancer Center between 1960 and 1992, there were 11 (0.3%) documented or suspected thromboembolic events resulting in four deaths (0.1%).[227] All four deaths were in patients who had extensive pelvic wall disease that may have obstructed flow in pelvic vessels. Today, patients receive low-dose heparin during intracavitary radiation therapy to reduce thromboembolism risk. However, because the number of events was so small before institution of routine heparin prophylaxis, no significant risk reduction has been detectable.

Less serious complications of intracavitary radiation therapy included uterine perforation and vaginal laceration, which occurred in 2.8% and 0.3%, respectively, of patients in the M.D. Anderson Cancer Center series. Both of these complications occurred more often in women who were more than 60 years old. Of patients in that series, 14% had an elevated temperature, usually of uncertain etiology.

Late Complications

Most late complications of radiation therapy involve the rectum, bladder, or small bowel. Although most serious gastrointestinal complications occur within the first 3 years, serious side effects also may occur several decades after treatment (Fig. 28-20). The average time to onset of major urinary tract complications tends to be somewhat longer than that of intestinal complications. The most common serious late complications involve bleeding from the bladder or rectum. In a series of 1784 patients treated for stage IB disease at the M.D. Anderson Cancer Center, the actuarial risks of hematuria or hematochezia severe enough to require transfusion were 2.6% and 0.7%, respectively, at 5 years. The overall risk of developing a gastrointestinal or urinary tract fistula was 1.7% at 5 years, with an increased risk for patients who underwent adjuvant hysterectomy or pretreatment transperitoneal lymphadenectomy.

The risk of small bowel obstruction is strongly correlated with a number of patient characteristics and treatment factors. Several studies have demonstrated threefold to fourfold increases in risk for patients who undergo transperitoneal lymphadenectomy before radiation therapy.[2,51,265] Patients given high doses (> 50 Gy) of external-beam radiation to the central pelvis have a greater risk of all types of complications, including small bowel obstruction.[65] The risk of small bowel obstruction is also greater for patients who are very thin, have a history of pelvic infection, or smoke. A recent study from the M.D. Anderson Cancer Center revealed a sixfold increase in the risk of small bowel complications for patients who smoked more than one pack of cigarettes per day (12% vs. 2% for nonsmokers).[266]

Mild to moderate apical vaginal ulceration or necrosis occurs in 5% to 10% of patients treated with primary radiation therapy for cervical cancer. This complication

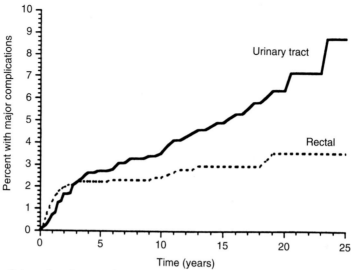

Fig. 28-20 Rates of major rectal and urinary tract complications in 1784 patients treated with radiation therapy for International Federation of Gynecology and Obstetrics stage IB carcinoma of the uterine cervix. (From Eifel PJ, Levenback C, Wharton JT, et al. *Int J Radiat Oncol Biol Phys* 1995;32:1289-1300.)

usually occurs within 12 months after the completion of radiation therapy, rarely progresses to fistula formation, and usually heals within 1 to 6 months with appropriate local care, including use of vaginal estrogen cream or 50% H$_2$O$_2$ douches (depending on severity). The true incidence of vaginal shortening and its influence on sexual dysfunction is poorly documented. Severe shortening is more common in postmenopausal patients, patients who are less sexually active, and patients with more advanced disease at presentation.

REFERENCES

1. Fajardo LF. *Pathology of Radiation Injury.* New York, NY: Masson; 1982.
2. Eifel PJ, Levenback C, Wharton JT, et al. Time course and incidence of late complications in patients treated with radiation therapy for FIGO stage IB carcinoma of the uterine cervix. *Int J Radiat Oncol Biol Phys* 1995;32:1289-1300.
3. Morice P, Thiam-Ba R, Castaigne D, et al. Fertility results after ovarian transposition for pelvic malignancies treated by external irradiation or brachytherapy. *Hum Reprod* 1998;13:660-663.
4. Mitchell MF, Gershenson DM, Soeters RP, et al. The long-term effects of radiation therapy on patients with ovarian dysgerminoma. *Cancer* 1991;67:1084-1090.
5. American Cancer Society. *Cancer Facts & Figures, 2001.* Atlanta, Ga: American Cancer Society; 2001.
6. Landis SH, Murray T, Bolden S, et al. Cancer statistics, 1999. *CA Cancer J Clin* 1999;49:8-31.
7. Wingo PA, Tong T, Bolden S. Cancer statistics, 1995. *CA Cancer J Clin* 1995;45:8-30.
8. Vizcaino AP, Moreno V, Bosch FX, et al. International trends in the incidence of cervical cancer. I. Adenocarcinoma and adenosquamous cell carcinomas. *Int J Cancer* 1998;75:536-545.
9. Zheng T, Holford TR, Ma Z, et al. The continuing increase in adenocarcinoma of the uterine cervix: a birth cohort phenomenon. *Int J Epidemiol* 1996;25:252-258.
10. Bosch FX, Castellsague X, Munoz N, et al. Male sexual behavior and human papillomavirus DNA: key risk factors for cervical cancer in Spain. *J Natl Cancer Inst* 1996;88:1060-1067.
11. Skegg DCG, Corwin PA, Paul C. Importance of the male factor in cancer of the cervix. *Lancet* 1982;2:581-583.
12. Bosch FX, Manos MM, Munoz N, et al. Prevalence of human papillomavirus in cervical cancer: a worldwide perspective. International Biological Study on Cervical Cancer (IBSCC) Study Group. *J Natl Cancer Inst* 1995;87:796-802.
13. Kessler I. Epidemiological aspects of uterine cervix cancer. In: Lurain JR, Sciarra J, eds. *Gynecology and Obstetrics.* Philadelphia, Pa: JB Lippincott; 1990:1.
14. Scheffner M, Werness BA, Huibregtse JM, et al. The E6 oncoprotein encoded by human papillomavirus types 16 and 18 promotes the degradation of p53. *Cell* 1990;63:1129-1136.
15. Schiffman MH. Recent progress in defining the epidemiology of human papillomavirus infection and cervical neoplasia. *J Natl Cancer Inst* 1992;84:394-398.
16. Roteli-Martins CM, Panetta K, Alves VA, et al. Cigarette smoking and high-risk HPV DNA as predisposing factors for high-grade cervical intraepithelial neoplasia (CIN) in young Brazilian women. *Acta Obstet Gynecol Scand* 1998;77:678-682.
17. Ho GY, Kadish AS, Burk RD, et al. HPV 16 and cigarette smoking as risk factors for high-grade cervical intra-epithelial neoplasia. *Int J Cancer* 1998;78:281-285.
18. Prokopczyk B, Cox JE, Hoffmann D, et al. Identification of tobacco-specific carcinogen in the cervical mucus of smokers and non-smokers. *J Natl Cancer Inst* 1997;89:868-873.
19. Ozsaran AA, Ates T, Dikmen Y, et al. Evaluation of the risk of cervical intraepithelial neoplasia and human papilloma virus infection in renal transplant patients receiving immunosuppressive therapy. *Eur J Gynaecol Oncol* 1999;20:127-130.
20. Beral V, Newton R. Overview of the epidemiology of immunodeficiency-associated cancers. *J Natl Cancer Inst Monogr* 1998;23:1-6.
21. Goedert JJ, Cote TR, Virgo P, et al. Spectrum of AIDS-associated malignant disorders. *Lancet* 1998;351:1833-1839.
22. Maiman M, Fruchter RG, Clark M, et al. Cervical cancer as an AIDS-defining illness. *Obstet Gynecol* 1997;89:76-80.

23. Franceschi S, Dal Maso L, Arniani S, et al. Risk of cancer other than Kaposi's sarcoma and non-Hodgkin's lymphoma in persons with AIDS in Italy. Cancer and AIDS Registry Linkage Study. *Br J Cancer* 1998;78:966-970.

24. Serur E, Fruchter RG, Maiman M, et al. Age, substance abuse, and survival of patients with cervical carcinoma. *Cancer* 1995;75:2530-2538.

25. Stubblefield PG. Oral contraceptives and neoplasia. *J Reprod Med* 1984;29:524-529.

26. Thomas DB, Ray RM. Oral contraceptives and invasive adenocarcinomas and adenosquamous carcinomas of the uterine cervix. The World Health Organization Collaborative Study of Neoplasia and Steroid Contraceptives. *Am J Epidemiol* 1996;144:281-289.

27. Plentl AA, Friedman EA. Lymphatics of the cervix uteri. *Lymphatic System of the Female Genitalia: the Morphologic Basis of Oncologic Diagnosis and Therapy.* Philadelphia, Pa: WB Saunders; 1971:75-115.

28. Papanicolaou G, Traut RF. *The Diagnosis of Uterine Cancer by the Vaginal Smear.* New York, NY: Commonwealth Fund; 1943.

29. Kivlahan C, Ingram E. Papanicolaou smears without endocervical cells. Are they inadequate? *Acta Cytol* 1986;30:258-260.

30. Walton RJ. Editorial: the task force on cervical cancer screening programs. *Can Med Assoc J* 1976;114:981.

31. Miller AB. Control of carcinoma of the cervix by exfoliative cytology screening. In: Coppleson M, ed. *Gynecologic Oncology. Fundamental Principles and Clinical Practice.* Edinburgh, Scotland: Churchill Livingstone; 1981:381.

32. Syrjanen KV, Kataja V, Vyliskoski M, et al. Natural history of cervical human papillomavirus lesions does not substantiate the biologic relevance of the Bethesda system. *Obstet Gynecol* 1992;79:675-682.

33. Richart RM, Barron BA. A follow-up study of patients with cervical dysplasia. *Am J Obstet Gynecol* 1969;105:386-393.

34. Manos MM, Kinney WK, Hurley LB, et al. Identifying women with cervical neoplasia: using human papillomavirus DNA testing for equivocal Papanicolaou results. *JAMA* 1999;281:1605-1610.

35. Kinney WK, Manos MM, Hurley LB, et al. Where's the high-grade cervical neoplasia? The importance of minimally abnormal Papanicolaou diagnoses. *Obstet Gynecol* 1998;91:973-976.

36. Hopkins MP, Roberts JA, Schmidt RW. Cervical adenocarcinoma in situ. *Obstet Gynecol* 1988;71:842-844.

37. Azodi M, Chambers SK, Rutherford TJ, et al. Adenocarcinoma in situ of the cervix: management and outcome. *Gynecol Oncol* 1999;73:348-353.

38. Crowther ME, Lowe DG, Shepherd JH. Verrucous carcinoma of the female genital tract: a review. *Obstet Gynecol Surv* 1998;43:263-280.

39. Randall ME, Anderson WA, Mills SE, et al. Papillary squamous cell carcinoma of the uterine cervix: a clinicopathologic study of nine cases. *Int J Gynecol Pathol* 1986;5:1-10.

40. Hirai Y, Takeshima N, Haga A, et al. A clinicocytopathologic study of adenoma malignum of the uterine cervix. *Gynecol Oncol* 1998;70:219-223.

41. Albores-Saavedra J, Gersell D, Gilks CB, et al. Terminology of endocrine tumors of the uterine cervix: results of a workshop sponsored by the College of American Pathologists and the National Cancer Institute. *Arch Pathol Lab Med* 1997;121:34-39.

42. Abeler VM, Holm R, Nesland JM, et al. Small cell carcinoma of the cervix. A clinicopathologic study of 26 patients. *Cancer* 1994;73:672-677.

43. Morris M, Gershenson DM, Eifel PJ, et al. Treatment of small cell carcinoma of the cervix with cisplatin, doxorubicin, and etoposide. *Gynecol Oncol* 1992;47:62-65.

44. Fleming I, Cooper JS, Henson DE, et al, eds. *AJCC Cancer Staging Manual.* 5th ed. Philadelphia, Pa: Lippincott Williams & Wilkins; 1997:189-194.

45. International Federation of Gynecology and Obstetrics. Staging announcement. FIGO staging of gynecologic cancers; cervical and vulva. *Int J Gynecol Cancer* 1995;5:319.

46. League of Nations Health Organization. Inquiry into the results of radiotherapy in cancer of the uterus. Atlas illustrating the division of cancer of the uterine cervix into four stages according to the anatomo-clinical extent of the growth. Stockholm, Sweden: Kungl Boktryckeriet PA Norstedt & Söner; 1938.

47. Burghardt E, Hofmann HMH, Ebner F, et al. Results of surgical treatment of 1028 cervical cancers studied with volumetry. *Cancer* 1992;70:648-655.

48. Eifel PJ, Moughan J, Owen JB, et al. Patterns of radiotherapy practice for patients with squamous carcinoma of the uterine cervix. A Patterns of Care study. *Int J Radiat Oncol Biol Phys* 1999;43:351-358.

49. Heller PB, Malfetano JH, Bundy BN, et al. Clinical-pathologic study of stage IIB, III, and IVA carcinoma of the cervix: extended diagnostic evaluation for paraaortic node metastasis—a Gynecologic Oncology Group study. *Gynecol Oncol* 1990;38:425-430.

50. Rose PG, Adler LP, Rodriguez M, et al. Positron emission tomography for evaluating para-aortic nodal metastasis in locally advanced cervical cancer before surgical staging: a surgicopathologic study. *J Clin Oncol* 1999;17:41-45.

51. Weiser EB, Bundy BN, Hoskins WJ, et al. Extraperitoneal versus transperitoneal selective paraaortic lymphadenectomy in the pretreatment surgical staging of advanced cervical carcinoma (a Gynecologic Oncology Group study). *Gynecol Oncol* 1981;33:283-289.

52. Possover M, Krause N, Plaul K, et al. Laparoscopic para-aortic and pelvic lymphadenectomy: experience with 150 patients and review of the literature. *Gynecol Oncol* 1998;71:19-28.

53. Hacker NF, Wain GV, Nicklin JL. Resection of bulky positive lymph nodes in patients with cervical carcinoma. *Int J Gynecol Cancer* 1995;5:250-256.

54. Potish RA, Downey GO, Adcock LL, et al. The role of surgical debulking in cancer of the uterine cervix. *Int J Radiat Oncol Biol Phys* 1989;17:979-984.

55. Coleman RL, Burke TW, Morris M, et al. Intra-operative radiographs to confirm the adequacy of lymph node resection in patients with suspicious lymphangiograms. *Gynecol Oncol* 1994;51:362-367.

56. Medl M, Peters-Engl C, Schutz P, et al. First report of lymphatic mapping with isosulfan blue dye and sentinel node biopsy in cervical cancer. *Anticancer Res* 2000;20:1133-1134.

57. Alvarez RD, Potter ME, Soong SJ, et al. Rationale for using pathologic tumor dimensions and nodal status to subclassify surgically treated stage IB cervical cancer patients. *Gynecol Oncol* 1991;43:108-112.

58. Piver MS, Chung WS. Prognostic significance of cervical lesion size and pelvic node metastases in cervical carcinoma. *Obstet Gynecol* 1975;46:507-510.

59. Eifel PJ, Morris M, Wharton JT, et al. The influence of tumor size and morphology on the outcome of patients with FIGO stage IB squamous cell carcinoma of the uterine cervix. *Int J Radiat Oncol Biol Phys* 1994;29:9-16.

60. Fyles AW, Pintilie M, Kirkbride P, et al. Prognostic factors in patients with cervix cancer treated by radiation therapy: results of a multiple regression analysis. *Radiother Oncol* 1995;35:107-117.

61. Mendenhall WM, Thar TL, Bova FJ, et al. Prognostic and treatment factors affecting pelvic control of stage IB and IIA-B carcinoma of the intact uterine cervix treated with radiation therapy alone. *Cancer* 1984;53:2649-2654.

62. Perez CA, Grigsby PW, Nene SM, et al. Effect of tumor size on the prognosis of carcinoma of the uterine cervix treated with irradiation alone. *Cancer* 1992;69:2796-2806.

63. Horiot JC, Pigneux J, Pourquier H, et al. Radiotherapy alone in carcinoma of the intact uterine cervix according to G. H. Fletcher guidelines: a French cooperative study of 1383 cases. *Int J Radiat Oncol Biol Phys* 1988;14:605-611.

64. Lanciano RM, Martz K, Coia LR, et al. Tumor and treatment factors improving outcome in stage III-B cervix cancer. *Int J Radiat Oncol Biol Phys* 1991;20:95-100.

65. Logsdon MD, Eifel PJ. FIGO stage IIIB squamous cell carcinoma of the uterine cervix: an analysis of prognostic factors emphasizing the balance between external beam and intracavitary radiation therapy. *Int J Radiat Oncol Biol Phys* 1999;43:763-775.

66. Sevin BU, Lu Y, Bloch DA, et al. Surgically defined prognostic parameters in patients with early cervical carcinoma. A multivariate survival tree analysis. *Cancer* 1996;78:1438-1446.

67. Hawnaur JM, Johnson RJ, Buckley CH, et al. Staging, volume estimation and assessment of nodal status in carcinoma of the cervix: comparison of magnetic resonance imaging with surgical findings. *Clin Radiol* 1994;49:443-452.

68. Mayr NA, Yuh WT, Zheng J, et al. Tumor size evaluated by pelvic examination compared with 3-D quantitative analysis in the prediction of outcome for cervical cancer. *Int J Radiat Oncol Biol Phys* 1997;39:395-404.

69. Toita T, Kakinohana Y, Shinzato S, et al. Tumor diameter/volume and pelvic node status assessed by magnetic resonance imaging (MRI) for uterine cervical cancer treated with irradiation. *Int J Radiat Oncol Biol Phys* 1999;43:777-782.

70. Inoue T, Okumura M. Prognostic significance of parametrial extension in patients with cervical carcinoma stages IB, IIA, and IIB. A study of 628 cases treated by radical hysterectomy and lymphadenectomy with or without postoperative irradiation. *Cancer* 1984;54:1714-1719.

71. Boyce J, Fruchter R, Nicastri A, et al. Prognostic factors in stage I carcinoma of the cervix. *Gynecol Oncol* 1981;12:154-165.

72. Delgado G, Bundy BN, Fowler WC, et al. A prospective surgical pathological study of stage I squamous carcinoma of the cervix: a Gynecologic Oncology Group study. *Gynecol Oncol* 1989;36:314-320.

73. Zreik TG, Chambers JT, Chambers SK. Parametrial involvement, regardless of nodal status: a poor prognostic factor for cervical cancer. *Obstet Gynecol* 1996;87:741-746.

74. Landoni F, Bocciolone L, Perego P, et al. Cancer of the cervix, FIGO stages IB and IIA: patterns of local growth and paracervical extension. *Int J Gynecol Cancer* 1995;5:329-334.

75. Stehman FB, Bundy BN, Disaia PJ, et al. Carcinoma of the cervix treated with radiation therapy. I. A multivariate analysis of prognostic variables in the Gynecologic Oncology Group. *Cancer* 1991;67:2776-2785.

76. Thoms WW, Eifel PJ, Smith TL, et al. Bulky endocervical carcinomas: a 23-year experience. *Int J Radiat Oncol Biol Phys* 1992;23:491-499.

77. Grimard L, Genest P, Girard A, et al. Prognostic significance of endometrial extension in carcinoma of the cervix. *Gynecol Oncol* 1986;31:301-309.

78. Mitani Y, Yukinari S, Jimi S, et al. Carcinomatous infiltration into the uterine body in carcinoma of the uterine cervix. *Am J Obstet Gynecol* 1964;89:984-989.

79. Noguchi H, Shiozawa I, Kitahara T, et al. Uterine body invasion of carcinoma of the uterine cervix as seen from surgical specimens. *Gynecol Oncol* 1988;30:173-182.

80. Perez CA, Camel HM, Askin F, et al. Endometrial extension of carcinoma of the uterine cervix: a prognostic factor that may modify staging. *Cancer* 1981;48:170-180.

81. Averette HE, Nguyen HN, Donato DM, et al. Radical hysterectomy for invasive cervical cancer. A 25-year prospective experience with the Miami technique. *Cancer* 1993;71:1422-1437.

82. Delgado G, Bundy B, Zaino R, et al. Prospective surgical-pathological study of disease-free interval in patients with stage IB squamous cell carcinoma of the cervix: a Gynecologic Oncology Group study. *Gynecol Oncol* 1990;38:352-357.

83. Peters WA III, Liu PY, Barrett RJ Jr, et al. Concurrent chemotherapy and pelvic radiation therapy compared with pelvic radiation therapy alone as adjuvant therapy after radical surgery in high-risk early-stage cancer of the cervix. *J Clin Oncol* 2000;18:1606-1613.

84. Dawtlatly R, Lavie O, Cross PA, et al. Prognostic factors in surgically-treated stage IB-IIB squamous cell carcinoma of the cervix with positive lymph nodes. *Int J Gynecol Cancer* 1998;8:46-47.

85. Inoue T, Morita K. The prognostic significance of number of positive nodes in cervical carcinoma stages IB, IIA, and IIB. *Cancer* 1990;65:1923-1927.

86. Kamura T, Tsukamoto N, Tsuruchi N, et al. Multivariate analysis of the histopathologic prognostic factors of cervical cancer in patients undergoing radical hysterectomy. *Cancer* 1992;69:181-186.

87. Kristensen GB, Abeler VM, Risberg B, et al. Tumor size, depth of invasion, and grading of the invasive tumor front are the main prognostic factors in early squamous cell cervical carcinoma. *Gynecol Oncol* 1999;74:245-251.

88. Ballon SC, Berman ML, Lagasse LD, et al. Survival after extraperitoneal pelvic and paraaortic lymphadenectomy and radiation therapy in cervical carcinoma. *Obstet Gynecol* 1981;57:90-95.

89. Buchsbaum H. Extrapelvic lymph node metastases in cervical carcinoma. *Am J Obstet Gynecol* 1979;133:814-824.

90. Wharton JT, Jones HWI, Day T, et al. Preirradiation celiotomy and extended field irradiation for invasive carcinoma of the cervix. *Obstet Gynecol* 1977;49:333-338.

91. Piver MS, Barlow JJ, Krishnamsetty R. Five-year survival (with no evidence of disease) in patients with biopsy-confirmed aortic node metastases from cervical carcinoma. *Am J Obstet Gynecol* 1981;139:575-578.

92. Tewfik HH, Buchsbaum HJ, Latourette HB, et al. Para-aortic lymph node irradiation in carcinoma of the cervix after exploratory laparotomy and biopsy-proven positive aortic nodes. *Int J Radiat Oncol Biol Phys* 1982;8:13-18.

93. Komaki R, Mattingly RF, Hoffman RG, et al. Irradiation of para-aortic lymph node metastases from carcinoma of the cervix or endometrium: preliminary results. *Radiology* 1983;147:245-248.

94. Berman ML, Keys H, Creasman W, et al. Survival and patterns of recurrence in cervical cancer metastatic to periaortic lymph nodes (a Gynecologic Oncology Group study). *Gynecol Oncol* 1984;19:8-16.

95. Rubin SC, Brookland R, Mikuta JJ, et al. Para-aortic nodal metastases in early cervical carcinoma: long-term survival following extended-field radiotherapy. *Gynecol Oncol* 1984;18:213-217.

96. Brookland RK, Rubin S, Danoff BF. Extended field irradiation in the treatment of patients with cervical carcinoma involving biopsy proven para-aortic nodes. *Int J Radiat Oncol Biol Phys* 1984;10:1875-1879.

97. Nori D, Valentine E, Hilaris BS. The role of paraaortic node irradiation in the treatment of cancer of the cervix. *Int J Radiat Oncol Biol Phys* 1985;11:1469-1473.

98. Podczaski E, Stryker JA, Kaminski P, et al. Extended-field radiation therapy for carcinoma of the cervix. *Cancer* 1990;66:251-258.

99. Cunningham M, Dunton C, Corn B, et al. Extended-field radiation therapy in early-stage cervical carcinoma: survival and complications. *Gynecol Oncol* 1991;43:51-54.

100. Kim PY, Monk BJ, Chabra S, et al. Cervical cancer with para-aortic metastases: significance of residual paraaortic disease after surgical staging. *Gynecol Oncol* 1998;69:243-247.

101. Boyce JG, Fruchter RG, Nicastri AD, et al. Vascular invasion in stage I carcinoma of the cervix. *Cancer* 1984;53:1175-1180.

102. Comerci B, Bolger BS, Flannelly G, et al. Prognostic factors in surgically treated stage IB-IIB carcinoma of the cervix with negative lymph nodes. *Int J Gynecol Cancer* 1998;8:23-26.

103. Pickel H, Haas J, Lahousen M. Prognostic factors in cervical cancer. *Eur J Obstet Gynecol* 1997;71:209-213.

104. Roman T, Souhami L, Freeman C, et al. High dose rate after-loading intracavitary therapy in carcinoma of the cervix. *Int J Radiat Oncol Biol Phys* 1991;20:921-926.

105. Saigo PE, Cain JM, Kim WS, et al. Prognostic factors in adenocarcinoma of the uterine cervix. *Cancer* 1986;57:1584-1593.

106. Eifel PJ, Burke TW, Delclos L, et al. Early stage I adenocarcinoma of the uterine cervix: treatment results in patients with tumors ≤4 cm in diameter. *Gynecol Oncol* 1991;41:199-205.

107. Matthews CM, Burke TW, Tornos C, et al. Stage I cervical adenocarcinoma: prognostic evaluation of surgically treated patients. *Gynecol Oncol* 1993;49:19-23.

108. Alvarez RD, Soong SJ, Kinney WK, et al. Identification of prognostic factors and risk groups in patients found to have nodal metastasis at the time of radical hysterectomy for early-stage squamous carcinoma of the cervix. *Gynecol Oncol* 1989;35:130-135.

109. Burghardt E, Girardi F, Lahousen M, et al. Patterns of pelvic and paraaortic lymph node involvement in ovarian cancer. *Gynecol Oncol* 1991;40:103-106.

110. Kjorstad KE, Kjolvenstvedt A, Strickert T. The value of complete lymphadenectomy in radical treatment of cancer of the cervix, stage IB. *Cancer* 1984;54:2215-2219.

111. Grigsby PW, Perez CA, Kuske RR, et al. Adenocarcinoma of the uterine cervix: lack of evidence for a poor prognosis. *Radiother Oncol* 1988;12:289-296.

112. Kilgore LC, Soong SJ, Gore H, et al. Analysis of prognostic features in adenocarcinoma of the cervix. *Gynecol Oncol* 1988;31:137-148.

113. Miller BE, Flax SD, Arheart K, et al. The presentation of adenocarcinoma of the uterine cervix. *Cancer* 1993;72:1281-1285.

114. Shingelton HM, Gore H, Bradley DH, et al. Adenocarcinoma of the cervix. I. Clinical evaluation and pathologic features. *Obstet Gynecol* 1981;139:799-813.

115. Waldenstrom AC, Horvath G. Survival of patients with adenocarcinoma of the uterine cervix in western Sweden. *Int J Gynecol Cancer* 1999;9:18-23.

116. Eifel PJ, Burke TW, Morris M, et al. Adenocarcinoma as an independent risk factor for disease recurrence in patients with stage IB cervical carcinoma. *Gynecol Oncol* 1995;59:38-44.

117. Kleine W, Rau K, Schwoeorer D, et al. Prognosis of adenocarcinoma of the cervix uteri: a comparative study. *Gynecol Oncol* 1989;35:145-149.

118. Milsom I, Friberg LG. Primary adenocarcinoma of the uterine cervix. A clinical study. *Cancer* 1983;52:942-947.

119. Landoni F, Maneo A, Colombo A, et al. Randomised study of radical surgery versus radiotherapy for stage Ib-IIa cervical cancer. *Lancet* 1997;350:535-540.

120. Hopkins M, Morley GW. A comparison of adenocarcinoma and squamous cell carcinoma of the cervix. *Obstet Gynecol* 1991;77:912-917.

121. Berek JS, Hacker NS, Fu YS, et al. Adenocarcinoma of the uterine cervix: histologic variables associated with lymph node metastasis and survival. *Obstet Gynecol* 1985;65:46-52.

122. Raju K, Kjorstad KE, Abeler V. Prognostic factors in the treatment of stage IB adenocarcinoma of the cervix. *Int J Gynaecol Obstet* 1991;1:69-74.

123. Sevin BU, Method MW, Nadji M, et al. Efficacy of radical hysterectomy as treatment for patients with small cell carcinoma of the cervix. *Cancer* 1996;77:1489-1493.

124. Hong JH, Tsai CS, Chang JT, et al. The prognostic significance of pre- and posttreatment SCC levels in patients with squamous cell carcinoma of the cervix treated by radiotherapy. *Int J Radiat Oncol Biol Phys* 1998;41:823-830.

125. Lin H, ChangChien CC, Huang EY, et al. The role of pretreatment squamous cell carcinoma antigen in predicting nodal metastasis in early stage cervical cancer. *Acta Obstet Gynecol Scand* 2000;79:140-144.

126. Massuger LF, Koper NP, Thomas CM, et al. Improvement of clinical staging in cervical cancer with serum squamous cell carcinoma antigen and CA 125 determinations. *Gynecol Oncol* 1997;64:473-476.

127. Kainz C, Gitsch G, Tempfer C, et al. Vascular space invasion and inflammatory stromal reaction as prognostic factors in patients with surgically treated cervical cancer stage IB to IIB. *Anticancer Res* 1994;14:2245-2248.

128. Höckel M, Schlenger K, Mitze M, et al. Tumor vascularity—a novel prognostic factor in advanced cancer of the uterine cervix. *Proc Soc Gynecol Oncol* 1995;48.

129. Wiggins DL, Granai CO, Steinhoff MM, et al. Tumor angiogenesis as a prognostic factor in cervical carcinoma. *Gynecol Oncol* 1995;56:353-356.

130. Estape R, Angioli R, Wagman F, et al. Significance of intraperitoneal cytology in patients undergoing radical hysterectomy. *Gynecol Oncol* 1998;68:169-171.

131. Kashimura M, Sugihara K, Toki N, et al. The significance of peritoneal cytology in uterine cervix and endometrial cancer. *Gynecol Oncol* 1997;67:285-290.

132. Takeshima N, Katase K, Hirai Y, et al. Prognostic value of peritoneal cytology in patients with carcinoma of the uterine cervix. *Gynecol Oncol* 1997;64:136-140.

133. Lombard I, Vincent-Salomon A, Validire P, et al. Human papillomavirus genotype as a major determinant of the course of cervical cancer. *Gynecol Oncol* 1998;16:2613-2619.

134. Burger RA, Monk BJ, Kurosaki T, et al. Human papillomavirus type 18: association with poor prognosis in early stage cervical cancer. *J Natl Cancer Inst* 1996;88:1361-1368.

135. Ikenberg H, Wiegering I, Pfisterer J, et al. Human papillomavirus DNA in tumor-free regional lymph nodes: a potential prognostic marker in cervical cancer. *Cancer J Sci Am* 1996;2:28-34.

136. Kobayashi Y, Yoshinouchi M, Tianqi G, et al. Presence of human papilloma virus DNA in pelvic lymph nodes can predict unexpected recurrence of cervical cancer in patients with histologically negative lymph nodes. *Clin Cancer Res* 1998;4:979-983.

137. Tseng CJ, Pao CC, Lin JD, et al. Detection of human papillomavirus types 16 and 18 mRNA in peripheral blood of advanced cervical cancer patients and its association with prognosis. *J Clin Oncol* 1999;17:1391-1396.

138. Park JS, Park DC, Kim CJ, et al. HPV-16-related proteins as the serologic markers in cervical neoplasia. *Gynecol Oncol* 1998;69:47-55.

139. Sigurdsson K, Hrafnkelsson J, Geirsson G, et al. Screening as a prognostic factor in cervical cancer: analysis of survival and prognostic factors based on Icelandic population data, 1964-1988. *Gynecol Oncol* 1991;43:64-70.

140. Dattoli MJ, Gretz HF III, Beller U, et al. Analysis of multiple prognostic factors in patients with stage IB cervical cancer: age as a major determinant. *Int J Radiat Oncol Biol Phys* 1989;17:41-47.

141. Lanciano RM, Won M, Coia L, et al. Pretreatment and treatment factors associated with improved outcome in squamous cell carcinoma of the uterine cervix: a final report of the 1973 and 1978 Patterns of Care studies. *Int J Radiat Oncol Biol Phys* 1991;20:667-676.

142. Rutledge FN, Mitchell MR, Munsell M, et al. Youth as a prognostic factor in carcinoma of the cervix: a matched analysis. *Gynecol Oncol* 1992;44:123-130.

143. Mitchell PA, Waggoner S, Rotmensch J, et al. Cervical cancer in the elderly treated with radiation therapy. *Gynecol Oncol* 1998;71:291-298.

144. Hopkins MP, Morley GW. Stage IB squamous cell cancer of the cervix: clinicopathologic features related to survival. *Am J Obstet Gynecol* 1991;164:1520-1527.

145. Spanos WJ, King A, Keeney E, et al. Age as a prognostic factor in carcinoma of the cervix. *Gynecol Oncol* 1989;35:66-68.

146. Bush R. The significance of anemia in clinical radiation therapy. *Int J Radiat Oncol Biol Phys* 1986;12:2047-2050.

147. Girinski T, Pejovic-Lenfant M, Bourhis J, et al. Prognostic value of hemoglobin concentrations and blood transfusions in advanced carcinoma of the cervix treated by radiation therapy: results of a retrospective study of 386 patients. *Int J Radiat Oncol Biol Phys* 1989;16:37-42.

148. Kapp DS, Fischer D, Gutierrez E, et al. Pretreatment prognostic factors in carcinoma of the uterine cervix: a multivariable analysis of the effect of age, stage, histology and blood counts on survival. *Int J Radiat Oncol Biol Phys* 1983;9:445-455.

149. Brady LW, Plenk HP, Hanley JA, et al. Hyperbaric oxygen therapy for carcinoma of the cervix stages IIB, IIIA, IIIB and IVA: results of a randomized study by the Radiation Therapy Oncology Group. *Int J Radiat Oncol Biol Phys* 1981; 7:990-998.

150. Dische S, Anderson PJ, Sealy R, et al. Carcinoma of the cervix—anaemia, radiotherapy and hyperbaric oxygen. *Br J Radiol* 1983;56:251-255.

151. Dische S, Chassagne D, Hope-Stone HF, et al. A trial of Ro 03-8799 (pimonidazole) in carcinoma of the uterine cervix: an interim report from the Medical Research Council Working Party on Advanced Carcinoma of the Cervix. *Radiother Oncol* 1993;26:93-103.

152. Grigsby PW, Winter K, Wasserman TH, et al. Irradiation with or without misonidazole for patients with stages IIIB and IVA carcinoma of the cervix: final results of RTOG 80-05. Radiation Therapy Oncology Group. *Int J Radiat Oncol Biol Phys* 1999; 44:513-517.

153. Maor MH, Gillespie BW, Peters LJ, et al. Neutron therapy in cervical cancer: results of a phase III RTOG study. *Int J Radiat Oncol Biol Phys* 1988;14:885-891.

154. Overgaard J, Bentzen SM, Kolstad P, et al. Misonidazole combined with radiotherapy in the treatment of carcinoma of the uterine cervix. *Int J Radiat Oncol Biol Phys* 1989;16:1069-1072.

155. Sundfør K, Trope C, Suo Z, et al. Normobaric oxygen treatment during radiotherapy for carcinoma of the uterine cervix. Results from a prospective controlled randomized trial. *Radiother Oncol* 1999;50:157-165.

156. Fyles AW, Milosevic M, Wong R, et al. Oxygenation predicts radiation response and survival in patients with cervix cancer [published erratum appears in *Radiother Oncol* 1999;50:371]. *Radiother Oncol* 1998;48:149-156.

157. Höckel M, Vorndran B, Schlenger K, et al. Tumor oxygenation: a new predictive parameter in locally advanced cancer of the uterine cervix. *Gynecol Oncol* 1993;51:141-149.

158. Sundfør K, Lyng H, Rofstad EK. Tumour hypoxia and vascular density as predictors of metastasis in squamous cell carcinoma of the uterine cervix. *Br J Cancer* 1998;78:822-827.

159. Hernandez E, Heller PB, Whitney C, et al. Thrombocytosis in surgically treated stage IB squamous cell cervical carcinoma (a Gynecologic Oncology Group study). *Gynecol Oncol* 1994;55: 328-332.

160. Chen F, Trapido EJ, Davis K. Differences in stage at presentation of breast and gynecologic cancers among whites, blacks, and Hispanics. *Cancer* 1994;73:2838-2842.

161. Mandelblatt J, Andrews H, Kerner J, et al. Determinants of late stage diagnosis of breast and cervical cancer: the impact of age, race, social class, and hospital type. *Am J Public Health* 1991; 81:646-649.

162. Shelton D, Paturzo D, Flannery J, et al. Race, stage of disease, and survival with cervical cancer. *Ethn Dis* 1992;2:47-54.

163. Mundt AJ, Connell PP, Campbell T, et al. Race and clinical outcome in patients with carcinoma of the uterine cervix treated with radiation therapy. *Gynecol Oncol* 1998;71:151-158.

164. Katz A, Eifel PJ, Moughan J, et al. Socioeconomic characteristics of patients with squamous cell carcinoma of the uterine cervix treated with radiotherapy in the 1992 to 1994 patterns of care study. *Int J Radiat Oncol Biol Phys* 2000;47:443-450.

165. Grigsby PW, Perez CA. Radiotherapy alone for medically inoperable carcinoma of the cervix: stage IA and carcinoma in situ. *Int J Radiat Oncol Biol Phys* 1991;21:375-378.

166. Hamberger AD, Fletcher GH, Wharton JT. Results of treatment of early stage I carcinoma of the uterine cervix with intracavitary radium alone. *Cancer* 1978;41:980-985.

167. Burghardt E, Girardi F, Lahousen M, et al. Microinvasive carcinoma of the uterine cervix (International Federation of Gynecology and Obstetrics stage IA). *Cancer* 1991;67:1037-1045.

168. Morris M, Mitchell MF, Silva EG, et al. Cervical conization as definitive therapy for early invasive squamous carcinoma of the cervix. *Gynecol Oncol* 1993;51:193-196.

169. Kucera H, Enzelberger H, Eppel W, et al. The influence of nicotine abuse and diabetes mellitus on the results of primary irradiation in the treatment of carcinoma of the cervix. *Cancer* 1987;60:1-4.

170. Sedlis A, Bundy BN, Rotman MZ, et al. A randomized trial of pelvic radiation therapy versus no further therapy in selected patients with stage IB carcinoma of the cervix after radical hysterectomy and pelvic lymphadenectomy: a Gynecologic Oncology Group Study. *Gynecol Oncol* 1999;73:177-183.

171. Sardi JE, Giaroli A, Sananes C, et al. Long-term follow-up of the first randomized trial using neoadjuvant chemotherapy in stage Ib squamous carcinoma of the cervix: the final results. *Gynecol Oncol* 1997;67:61-69.

172. Lowrey GC, Mendenhall WM, Million RR. Stage IB or IIA-B carcinoma of the intact uterine cervix treated with irradiation: a multivariate analysis. *Int J Radiat Oncol Biol Phys* 1992;24: 205-210.

173. Durrance FY, Fletcher GH, Rutledge FN. Analysis of central recurrent disease in stages I and II squamous cell carcinomas of the cervix on intact uterus. *Am J Roentgenol* 1969;106:831-838.

174. Mendenhall WM, McCarty PJ, Morgan LS, et al. Stage IB-IIA-B carcinoma of the intact uterine cervix greater than or equal to 6 cm in diameter: is adjuvant extrafascial hysterectomy beneficial? *Int J Radiat Oncol Biol Phys* 1991;21:899-904.

175. Keys H, Bundy B, Stehman F, et al. Adjuvant hysterectomy after radiation therapy reduces detection of local recurrence in "bulky" stage IB cervical cancer without improving survival: results of a prospective randomized GOG trial [abstract]. *Cancer J Sci Am* 1997;3:117 (abstract 22).

176. Keys HM, Bundy BN, Stehman FB, et al. Cisplatin, radiation, and adjuvant hysterectomy for bulky stage IB cervical carcinoma. *N Engl J Med* 1999;340:1154-1161.

177. Morris M, Eifel PJ, Lu J, et al. Pelvic radiation with concurrent chemotherapy compared with pelvic and paraaortic radiation for high-risk cervical cancer. *N Engl J Med* 1999;340:1137-1143.

178. Rose PG, Bundy BN, Watkins J, et al. Concurrent cisplatin-based chemotherapy and radiotherapy for locally advanced cervical cancer. *N Engl J Med* 1999;340:1144-1153.

179. Whitney CW, Sause W, Bundy BN, et al. A randomized comparison of fluorouracil plus cisplatin versus hydroxyurea as an adjunct to radiation therapy in stages IIB-IVA carcinoma of the cervix with negative para-aortic lymph nodes: a Gynecologic Oncology Group and Southwest Oncology Group study. *J Clin Oncol* 1999;17:1339-1348.

180. Thomas G, Dembo A, Ackerman I, et al. A randomized trial of standard versus partially hyperfractionated radiation with or without concurrent 5-fluorouracil in locally advanced cervical cancer. *Gynecol Oncol* 1998;69:137-145.

181. Pearcey RG, Brundage MD, Drouin P, et al. A clinical trial comparing concurrent cisplatin and radiation therapy versus radiation alone for locally advanced squamous cell carcinoma of the cervix carried out by the National Cancer Institute of Canada Clinical Trials Group [abstract]. *Proc Am Soc Clin Oncol* 2000;19:378.

182. Wong LC, Ngan HY, Cheung AN, et al. Chemoradiation and adjuvant chemotherapy in cervical cancer. *J Clin Oncol* 1999; 17:2055-2060.

183. Coia L, Won M, Lanciano R, et al. The Patterns of Care Outcome Study for cancer of the uterine cervix. Results of the second national practice survey. *Cancer* 1990;66:2451-2456.

184. Barillot I, Horiot JC, Pigneux J, et al. Carcinoma of the intact uterine cervix treated with radiotherapy alone: a French cooperative study: update and multivariate analysis of prognostic factors. *Int J Radiat Oncol Biol Phys* 1997;38:969-978.

185. Leibel S, Bauer M, Wasserman T, et al. Radiotherapy with or without misonidazole for patients with stage IIIB or IVA squamous cell carcinoma of the uterine cervix: preliminary report of a Radiation Therapy Oncology Group randomized trial. *Int J Radiat Oncol Biol Phys* 1987;13:541-549.

186. Stehman FB, Bundy BN, Thomas G, et al. Hydroxyurea versus misonidazole with radiation in cervical carcinoma: long-term follow-up of a Gynecologic Oncology Group trial. *J Clin Oncol* 1993;11:1523-1528.

187. Chauvergne J, Rohart J, Héron JF, et al. Essai randomisé de chimiothérapie initiale dans 151 carcinomes du col utérin localement étendus (T2b-N1, T3b, M0). *Bull Cancer* 1990;77:1007-1024.

188. Kumar L, Kaushal R, Nandy M, et al. Chemotherapy followed by radiotherapy versus radiotherapy alone in locally advanced cervical cancer: a randomized study. *Gynecol Oncol* 1994;54:307-315.

189. Leborgne F, Leborgne JH, Doldán R, et al. Induction chemotherapy and radiotherapy of advanced cancer of the cervix: a pilot study and phase III randomized trial. *Int J Radiat Oncol Biol Phys* 1997;37:343-350.

190. Souhami L, Gil R, Allan S, et al. A randomized trial of chemotherapy followed by pelvic radiation therapy in stage IIIB carcinoma of the cervix. *Int J Radiat Oncol Biol Phys* 1991;29:970-997.

191. Sundfør K, Trope CG, Hogberg T, et al. Radiotherapy and neoadjuvant chemotherapy for cervical carcinoma. A randomized multicenter study of sequential cisplatin and 5-fluorouracil and radiotherapy in advanced cervical carcinoma stage 3B and 4A. *Cancer* 1996;77:2371-2378.

192. Tattersall MHN, Larvidhaya V, Vootiprux V, et al. Randomized trial of epirubicin and cisplatin chemotherapy followed by pelvic radiation in locally advanced cervical cancer. *Am J Clin Oncol* 1995;13:444-451.

193. Tattersall MHN, Ramirez C, Coppleson M. A randomized trial comparing platinum-based chemotherapy followed by radiotherapy vs. radiotherapy alone in patients with locally advanced cervical cancer. *Int J Gynecol Cancer* 1992;2:244-251.

194. Rotman M, Pajak M, Choi K, et al. Prophylactic extended-field irradiation of para-aortic lymph nodes in stages IIB and bulky IB and IIA cervical carcinomas. Ten-year treatment results of RTOG 79-20. *JAMA* 1995;274:387-393.

195. Haie C, Pejovic MH, Gerbaulet A, et al. Is prophylactic para-aortic irradiation worthwhile in the treatment of advanced cervical carcinoma? Results of a controlled clinical trial of the EORTC radiotherapy group. *Radiother Oncol* 1988;11:101-112.

196. Grigsby PW, Lu JD, Mutch DG, et al. Twice-daily fractionation of external irradiation with brachytherapy and chemotherapy in carcinoma of the cervix with positive para-aortic lymph nodes: phase II study of the Radiation Therapy Oncology Group 92-10. *Int J Radiat Oncol Biol Phys* 1998;41:817-822.

197. Varia MA, Bundy BN, Deppe G, et al. Cervical carcinoma metastatic to para-aortic nodes: extended field radiation therapy with concomitant 5-fluorouracil and cisplatin chemotherapy: a Gynecologic Oncology Group study. *Int J Radiat Oncol Biol Phys* 1998;42:1015-1023.

198. Malfetano JH, Keys H. Aggressive multimodality treatment for cervical cancer with paraaortic lymph node metastases. *Gynecol Oncol* 1991;42:44-47.

199. Shingleton HM, Soong SJ, Gelder MS, et al. Clinical and histopathologic factors predicting recurrence and survival after pelvic

200. Berek JS, Hacker NF, Lagasse LD. Rectosigmoid colectomy and reanastomosis to facilitate resection of primary and recurrent gynecologic cancer. *Obstet Gynecol* 1984;64:715-720.

201. Hatch KD, Shingleton H, Soong S, et al. Anterior pelvic exenteration. *Gynecol Oncol* 1988;31:205-216.

202. Stanhope CR, Webb MJ, Podratz KC. Pelvic exenteration for recurrent cervical cancer. *Clin Obstet Gynecol* 1990;33:897-909.

203. Höckel M, Baußmann E, Mitze M, et al. Are pelvic side-wall recurrences of cervical cancer biologically different from central relapses? *Cancer* 1994;74:648-655.

204. Mahé MA, Gérard JP, Dubois JB, et al. Intraoperative radiation therapy in recurrent carcinoma of the uterine cervix: report of the French Intraoperative Group on 70 patients. *Int J Radiat Oncol Biol Phys* 1996;34:21-26.

205. Stelzer KJ, Koh WJ, Greer BE, et al. The use of intraoperative radiation therapy in radical salvage for recurrent cervical cancer: outcome and morbidity. *Am J Obstet Gynecol* 1995;172:1881-1888.

206. Deutsch M, Parsons J. Radiotherapy for carcinoma of the cervix recurrent after surgery. *Cancer* 1974;34:2051-2055.

207. Potter ME, Alvarez RD, Gay FL, et al. Optimal therapy for pelvic recurrence after radical hysterectomy for early-stage cervical cancer. *Gynecol Oncol* 1990;37:74-77.

208. Hogan WM, Littman P, Griner L, et al. Results of radiation therapy given after radical hysterectomy. *Cancer* 1982;49:1278-1285.

209. Jobsen JJ, Leer JWH, Cleton FJ, et al. Treatment of locoregional recurrence of carcinoma of the cervix by radiotherapy after primary surgery. *Gynecol Oncol* 1989;33:368-371.

210. Thomas GM, Dembo AJ, Black B, et al. Concurrent radiation and chemotherapy for carcinoma of the cervix recurrent after radical surgery. *Gynecol Oncol* 1987;27:254-260.

211. Ijaz T, Eifel PJ, Burke T, et al. Radiation therapy of pelvic recurrence after radical hysterectomy for cervical carcinoma. *Gynecol Oncol* 1998;70:241-246.

212. Wang CJ, Lai CH, Huang HJ, et al. Recurrent cervical carcinoma after primary radical surgery. *Am J Obstet Gynecol* 1999;181:518-524.

213. Roman L, Morris M, Eifel P, et al. Reasons for inappropriate simple hysterectomy in the presence of invasive cancer of the cervix. *Obstet Gynecol* 1992;79:485-489.

214. Andras EJ, Fletcher G, Rutledge F. Radiotherapy of carcinoma of the cervix following simple hysterectomy. *Am J Obstet Gynecol* 1973;115:647-655.

215. Choi DH, Huh SJ, Nam KH. Radiation therapy results for patients undergoing inappropriate surgery in the presence of invasive cervical carcinoma. *Gynecol Oncol* 1997;65:506-511.

216. Hopkins MP, Peters WA, Anderson W, et al. Invasive cervical cancer treated initially by standard hysterectomy. *Gynecol Oncol* 1990;36:7-12.

217. Roman LD, Morris M, Mitchell MF, et al. Prognostic factors for patients undergoing simple hysterectomy in the presence of invasive cancer of the cervix. *Gynecol Oncol* 1993;50:179-184.

218. Benedet J, Odicino F, Maisonneuve P, et al. Carcinoma of the cervix uteri. *J Epidemiol Biostat* 1998;3:5-34.

219. Alberts DS, Garcia D, Mason-Liddil N. Cisplatin in advanced cancer of the cervix: an update. *Semin Oncol* 1991;18:11-24.

220. Park RC, Thigpen JT. Chemotherapy in advanced and recurrent cervical cancer. A review. *Cancer* 1993;71:1446-1450.

221. Omura GA, Blessing J, Vaccarello L, et al. A randomized trial of cisplatin versus cisplatin + mitolactol versus cisplatin + ifosfamide in advanced squamous cell carcinoma of the cervix by the Gynecologic Oncology Group [abstract]. *Gynecol Oncol* 1996;60:120.

222. Boulware RJ, Caderao JB, Delclos L, et al. Whole pelvis megavoltage irradiation with single doses of 1000 rad to palliate

advanced gynecologic cancers. *Int J Radiat Oncol Biol Phys* 1979; 5:333-338.

223. Spanos WJ, Wasserman T, Meoz R, et al. Palliation of advanced pelvic malignant disease with large fraction pelvic radiation and misonidazole: final report of RTOG phase I/II study. *Int J Radiat Oncol Biol Phys* 1987;13:1479-1482.

224. Spanos WJ, Perez CA, Marcus S, et al. Effect of rest interval on tumor and normal tissue response—a report of phase III study of accelerated split course palliative radiation for advanced pelvic malignancies (RTOG-8502). *Int J Radiat Oncol Biol Phys* 1993;25:399-403.

225. Chao C, Williamson JF, Grigsby PW, et al. Uterosacral space involvement in locally advanced carcinoma of the uterine cervix. *Int J Radiat Oncol Biol Phys* 1998;40:397-403.

226. McIntyre JF, Eifel PJ, Levenback C, et al. Ureteral stricture as a late complication of radiotherapy for stage IB carcinoma of the uterine cervix. *Cancer* 1995;75:836-843.

227. Jhingran A, Eifel PJ. Perioperative and postoperative complications of intracavitary radiation for FIGO stage I-III carcinoma of the cervix. *Int J Radiat Oncol Biol Phys* 2000;46:1177-1183.

228. Schwarz G. An evaluation of the Manchester system of treatment of carcinoma of the cervix. *Am J Roentgenol Radium Ther Nucl Med* 1969;105:579-585.

229. International Commission on Radiation Units and Measurements. *Dose and Volume Specification for Reporting Intracavitary Therapy in Gynecology.* Bethesda, Md: International Commission on Radiation Units and Measurements; 1985.

230. Katz A, Eifel PJ. Quantification and correlation of intracavitary brachytherapy parameters in patients with carcinoma of the cervix. *Int J Radiat Oncol Biol Phys* 2000;48:1417-1425.

231. Hamberger AD, Unal A, Gershenson DM, et al. Analysis of the severe complications of irradiation of carcinoma of the cervix: whole pelvis irradiation and intracavitary radium. *Int J Radiat Oncol Biol Phys* 1983;9:367-371.

232. Montana GS, Fowler WC, Varia MA, et al. Analysis of results of radiation therapy for stage IB carcinoma of the cervix. *Cancer* 1987;60:2195-2200.

233. Perez CA, Grigsby PW, Lockett MA, et al. Radiation therapy morbidity in carcinoma of the uterine cervix: dosimetric and clinical correlation. *Int J Radiat Oncol Biol Phys* 1999;44:855-866.

234. Pourquier H, Delard R, Achille E, et al. A quantified approach to the analysis and prevention of urinary complications in radiotherapeutic treatment of cancer of the cervix. *Int J Radiat Oncol Biol Phys* 1987;13:1025-1033.

235. Schoeppel SL, LaVigne ML, Martel MK, et al. Three-dimensional treatment planning of intracavitary gynecologic implants: analysis of ten cases and implications for dose specification. *Int J Radiat Oncol Biol Phys* 1994;28:277-283.

236. Stuecklschweiger GF, Arian-Schad KS, Poier E, et al. Bladder and rectal dose of gynecologic high-dose-rate implants: comparison of orthogonal radiographic measurements with in vivo and CT-assisted measurements. *Radiology* 1991;181:889-894.

237. Haie-Meder C, Kramar A, Lambin P, et al. Analysis of complications in a prospective randomized trial comparing two brachytherapy low dose rates in cervical carcinoma. *Int J Radiat Oncol Biol Phys* 1994;29:1195-1197.

238. Patel FD, Sharma SC, Neigi PS, et al. Low dose rate vs. high dose rate brachytherapy in the treatment of carcinoma of the uterine cervix: a clinical trial. *Int J Radiat Oncol Biol Phys* 1993;28:335-341.

239. Shigematsu Y, Nishiyama K, Masaki N, et al. Treatment of carcinoma of the uterine cervix by remotely controlled afterloading intracavitary radiotherapy with high-dose rate: a comparative study with a low-dose rate system. *Int J Radiat Oncol Biol Phys* 1983;9:351-356.

240. Akine Y, Arimoto H, Ogino T, et al. High-dose-rate intracavitary irradiation in the treatment of carcinoma of the uterine cervix:

early experience with 84 patients. *Int J Radiat Oncol Biol Phys* 1988;14:893-898.

241. Fu KK, Phillips TL. High-dose-rate versus low-dose-rate intracavitary brachytherapy for carcinoma of the cervix. *Int J Radiat Oncol Biol Phys* 1990;19:791-796.

242. Kapp KS, Stuecklschweiger GF, Kapp DS, et al. Prognostic factors in patients with carcinoma of the uterine cervix treated with external beam irradiation and IR-192 high-dose-rate brachytherapy. *Int J Radiat Oncol Biol Phys* 1998;42:531-540.

243. Newman H, James K, Smith C. Treatment of cancer of the cervix with a high-dose-rate afterloading machine (the Cathetron). *Int J Radiat Oncol Biol Phys* 1983;9:931-937.

244. Petereit DG, Sarkaria JN, Potter DM, et al. High-dose-rate versus low-dose-rate brachytherapy in the treatment of cervical cancer: analysis of tumor recurrence—the University of Wisconsin experience. *Int J Radiat Oncol Biol Phys* 1999;45:1267-1274.

245. Arai T, Nakano T, Morita S, et al. High dose rate remote afterloading intracavitary radiation therapy for cancer of the uterine cervix. *Cancer* 1992;69:175-180.

246. Chen M, Lin F, Hong C, et al. High-dose-rate afterloading technique in the radiation treatment of uterine cervical cancer: 399 cases and 9 years experience. *Int J Radiat Oncol Biol Phys* 1991;20:915-919.

247. Eifel PJ. High dose-rate brachytherapy for carcinoma of the cervix: high tech or high risk? *Int J Radiat Oncol Biol Phys* 1992;24:383-386.

248. Joslin CA, Smith CW, Mallik A. The treatment of cervix cancer using high activity ⁶⁰Co sources. *Br J Radiol* 1972;42:108.

249. Petereit DG, Pearcey R. Literature analysis of high dose rate brachytherapy fractionation schedules in the treatment of cervical cancer: is there an optimal fractionation schedule? *Int J Radiat Oncol Biol Phys* 1999;43:359-366.

250. Utley J, von Essen C, Horn R, et al. High-dose-rate afterloading brachytherapy in carcinoma of the uterine cervix. *Int J Radiat Oncol Biol Phys* 1984;10:2259-2263.

251. Petereit DG, Sarkaria JN, Chappell RJ. Perioperative morbidity and mortality of high-dose-rate gynecologic brachytherapy. *Int J Radiat Oncol Biol Phys* 1998;42:1025-1031.

252. Aristizabal SA, Woolfitt B, Valencia A, et al. Interstitial parametrial implants in carcinoma of the cervix stage II-B. *Int J Radiat Oncol Biol Phys* 1987;13:445-450.

253. Martinez A, Edmundson GK, Cox RS, et al. Combination of external beam irradiation and multiple-site perineal applicator (MUPIT) for treatment of locally advanced or recurrent prostatic, anorectal, and gynecologic malignancies. *Int J Radiat Oncol Biol Phys* 1985;11:391-398.

254. Syed AMN, Puthawala AA, Neblett D, et al. Transperineal interstitial-intracavitary "Syed-Neblett" applicator in the treatment of carcinoma of the uterine cervix. *Endocuriether Hyperther Oncol* 1986;2:1-13.

255. Hughes-Davies L, Silver B, Kapp D. Parametrial interstitial brachytherapy for advanced or recurrent pelvic malignancy: the Harvard/Stanford experience. *Gynecol Oncol* 1995;58:24-27.

256. Monk BJ, Tewari K, Burger RA, et al. A comparison of intracavitary versus interstitial irradiation in the treatment of cervical cancer. *Gynecol Oncol* 1997;67:241-247.

257. Erickson B, Gillin MT. Interstitial implantation of gynecologic malignancies. *J Surg Oncol* 1997;66:285-295.

258. Choi JC, Ingenito AC, Nanda RK, et al. Potential decreased morbidity of interstitial brachytherapy for gynecologic malignancies using laparoscopy: a pilot study. *Gynecol Oncol* 1999;73:210-215.

259. Fyles A, Keane TJ, Barton M, et al. The effect of treatment duration in the local control of cervix cancer. *Radiother Oncol* 1992;25:273-279.

260. Eifel P, Thames H. Has the influence of treatment duration on local control of carcinoma of the cervix been defined? *Int J Radiat Oncol Biol Phys* 1995;32:1527-1529.

261. McNeil C. New standard of care for cervical cancer sets stage for next questions [news]. *J Natl Cancer Inst* 1999;91:500a-501a.

262. Wong L, Choo Y, Choy D, et al. Long-term follow-up of potentiation of radiotherapy by cis-platinum in advanced cervical cancer. *Gynecol Oncol* 1989;35:159-163.

263. Chaney AW, Eifel PJ, Logsdon MD, et al. Mature results of a pilot study of pelvic radiotherapy with concurrent continuous infusion intra-arterial 5-FU for stage IIIB-IVA squamous cell carcinoma of the cervix. *Int J Radiat Oncol Biol Phys* 1999;45: 113-118.

264. Eifel PJ. Chemoradiation for carcinoma of the cervix: advances and opportunities. *Radiat Res* 2000;154:229-236.

265. Lanciano RM, Martz D, Montana GS, et al. Influence of age, prior abdominal surgery, fraction size, and dose on complications after radiation therapy for squamous cell cancer of the uterine cervix. A Patterns of Care Study. *Cancer* 1992;69:2124-2130.

266. Eifel PJ, Jhingran A, Atkinson HN, et al. Correlation of smoking history and other patient characteristics with major complications of pelvic radiation therapy for cervical cancer. *J Clin Oncol* 2002;20:3651-3657.

CHAPTER 29

The Endometrium

Anuja Jhingran and Patricia J. Eifel

Carcinoma of the endometrium is the most common malignancy of the female genital tract in the United States, with an annual incidence of 38,300 cases. Between 5000 and 6600 women in the United States die of this disease each year.[1] However, because patients with endometrial carcinoma characteristically present with early-stage disease, usually with symptoms of postmenopausal bleeding, most cases of the disease are curable. The peak incidence occurs in the 50- to 70-year-old age group, with 75% of all cases occurring in postmenopausal women. Of the known risk factors for endometrial carcinoma, the factor that most increases the risk is chronic estrogen exposure, whether because of use of oral unopposed estrogen or conditions that result in chronic increased or prolonged endogenous estrogen exposure (e.g., estrogen-secreting tumors, low number of births of viable offspring, early menarche, late menopause, and morbid obesity).[2,3] Increased risk also has been associated with hypertension, diabetes mellitus, and long-term tamoxifen use in breast cancer patients.[2] Obesity and comorbid illnesses often complicate treatment.

ANATOMY OF THE UTERUS

The uterus is a hollow muscular organ situated in the midline of the pelvis, extending at right angles from the vagina and lying between the bladder and the rectum. The uterus is divided into the corpus, which constitutes the upper two thirds of the organ, and the cervix, which makes up the lower third. The uterine cavity is lined by a mucous membrane, the endometrium, which is composed of columnar cells forming many tubular glands that extend into the stroma and muscular layers. The muscular layer of the uterus, the myometrium, is made up of smooth muscle fibers, arranged in no definite pattern, that interlace randomly. The uterus is covered by an outer serous coat, the peritoneum, that forms the broad ligaments laterally.

EFFECTS OF RADIATION ON THE NORMAL UTERUS

After irradiation of the female pelvis, cyclical uterine bleeding usually ceases. Irradiation of the pelvis with doses as low as 10 to 20 Gy induces ovarian failure,

which is an important contributor to long-term atrophy of the endometrium. Histologically, irradiation of the pelvis leads to acute necrosis of the tubular glands of the endometrium that is later replaced by atrophy of the stroma and glands.[4]

When intracavitary radiation therapy (ICRT) is used to treat endometrial carcinoma, subacute ulcers of the luminal wall may be seen if the uterus is removed 6 to 8 weeks after therapy. These ulcers are usually focal and probably correspond to areas where radiation sources were in contact with the uterine wall. In time, these lesions are replaced by dense fibrous tissue. Usual doses (40 to 50 Gy) of external-beam radiation generally do not cause significant fibrosis of the myometrium.

Despite the changes in the endometrium after radiation therapy, exposure to cyclical hormones after radiation therapy will often induce uterine bleeding, even after combined external-beam radiation therapy and ICRT. This suggests that many women retain at least some functional endometrium even after high-dose radiation therapy. If the cervical os is obstructed, this bleeding can cause the development of a hematometra. Primary carcinomas of the endometrium occasionally develop in women who have undergone definitive irradiation for cervical cancer; this also suggests that some functional endometrium remains after high-dose radiation therapy.

Successful intrauterine pregnancy is probably not possible after combined external-beam pelvic irradiation and ICRT. However, successful pregnancies have been reported after 25 to 50 Gy of external-beam radiation.[5] Premenarchal treatment of the uterus probably arrests its normal development; pregnancies that occur in women who have undergone such treatment often end in spontaneous miscarriage in the second trimester.[6]

ROUTES OF SPREAD

Endometrial carcinomas usually originate in the endometrial epithelium but may then invade locally to involve the myometrium or uterine cervix or metastasize locally to the ovaries, parametrium, or vagina. The uterus has a rich and complex lymphatic network composed of four lymphatic trunks that emerge from the lateral borders of the corpus (Fig. 29-1).[7] The more

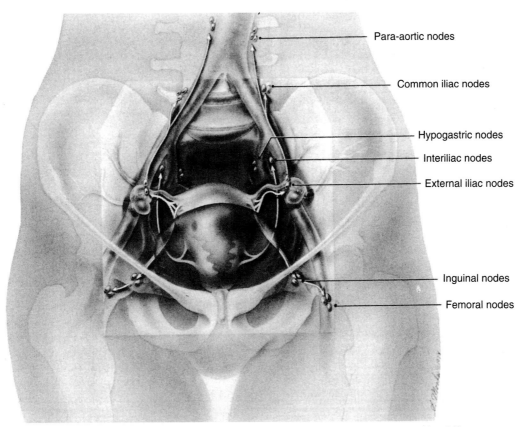

Fig. 29-1 Lymph drainage and lymph node groups of the uterine corpus. Note the difference in drainage between the lower and upper uterine segments. (From Dede JA, Plentl AA, Moore JG. *Surg Gynecol Obstet* 1968;126:533-542.)

superior lymphatic trunks pass through the broad ligament, paralleling the fallopian tube, and drain to the external iliac nodes near the ovary; from there the lymphatic trunks drain into the para-aortic lymph nodes. Lymphatic vessels from the inferior portion of the corpus pass through the broad ligament to the common iliac nodes. Subserosal lymphatics near the junction of the fallopian tube and the uterine body anastomose with lymphatics of the fallopian tube to drain directly to the para-aortic lymph nodes. Lymphatics also pass from the corpus by way of the ovarian pedicle to anastomose with lymphatics of the fallopian tube and empty into the femoral lymph nodes.

Uterine lymphatics interconnect with vessels that drain from the paracervical and paravaginal tissues. Invasion of the lymphatic network of the myometrium in the subserosa and subsequent involvement of the paracervical and paravaginal lymphatics by malignant tumors arising in the uterine corpus is accepted as the cause of posthysterectomy recurrence of cancer in the vaginal vault.

Tumors that penetrate the uterine serosa may directly invade adjacent tissues, such as the bladder, colon, or adnexa, or exfoliate into the abdominal cavity to form implant metastases. Small tumor fragments also may gain access to the peritoneal cavity by traversing the fallopian tubes. Hematogenous dissemination of endometrial carcinoma is uncommon. Sites of distant spread include lung, liver, bone, and brain.

PATHOLOGIC CLASSIFICATION

The International Society of Gynecologic Pathologists has proposed a pathologic classification for endometrial carcinoma (Box 29-1).[8] Aspects of these various cell classifications are discussed briefly in the following paragraphs.

Endometrioid Adenocarcinoma

Endometrial adenocarcinomas are the most common form of carcinoma of the endometrium and account for about 75% to 80% of all cases. These tumors vary from a well-differentiated form with glandular architecture preserved in more than 90% of the tumor (grade 1) to an undifferentiated form with glandular architecture preserved in less than 50% of the tumor (grade 3).

The histopathologic grade of endometrial carcinoma is so important prognostically that grade is part of the

From Zaino RJ. *Pathol Annu* 1995;30:1-28.

BOX 29-1   International Society of Gynecologic Pathologists' Pathologic Classification of Endometrial Carcinoma

Endometrial adenocarcinoma
  Papillary villoglandular
  Secretory
  Ciliated cell
  Adenocarcinoma with squamous differentiation
Mucinous carcinoma
Papillary serous carcinoma
Clear cell carcinoma
Squamous carcinoma
Undifferentiated carcinoma
Mixed types
Miscellaneous carcinoma
Metastatic carcinoma

staging classification (see the section on "Staging" later in this chapter). However, the assignment of the histopathologic grade, especially the distinction between grades 1 and 2, is subject to variation between pathologists. In a study by Taylor and colleagues,[9] two gynecologic pathologists independently reviewed 85 hysterectomy specimens from patients with endometrial carcinoma and had a difference of opinion of at least 1 grade in 26% of the specimens. In view of the uncertain clinical significance of grade-2 pathologic findings, Taylor and colleagues[9] proposed a two-tiered grading system, which would improve both the reproducibility and the prognostic significance of the tumor grade.

Secretory carcinomas account for 2% of all endometrial carcinomas and have a very good outcome. Ciliated cell carcinoma is also uncommon and is often associated with prior estrogen use. The prognosis associated with both of these subtypes is quite good.

About 50% to 60% of cases of endometrial adenocarcinoma show some squamous differentiation. For a tumor to be labeled "adenocarcinoma with squamous differentiation," at least 10% of the tumor must show squamous differentiation. Adenocarcinoma with squamous differentiation represents a continuum of lesions, ranging from adenoacanthoma, which is exceptionally well differentiated and has a benign-looking squamous component, to adenosquamous carcinoma, which is poorly differentiated and has a malignant squamous component.

Mucinous Carcinoma

Mucinous carcinomas, defined as tumors in which at least 50% of the cells are mucinous, can occur in the endometrium and are similar to those that arise from the endocervix. Mucinous carcinomas constitute about 9% of all endometrial carcinomas; the prognosis associated with mucinous carcinomas is similar to that of endometrial adenocarcinomas.

Papillary Serous Carcinoma

First described by Hendrickson and colleagues in 1982,[10] papillary serous carcinoma of the endometrium is morphologically identical to high-grade serous carcinoma of the ovary and represents 10% of all stage I endometrial cancer. Numerous studies have confirmed that papillary serous carcinoma behaves very aggressively. It is associated with frequent deep myometrial invasion and lymphovascular space invasion, a marked tendency for intraperitoneal dissemination, and a poor survival rate compared with other subtypes. Papillary serous carcinomas should be distinguished from other papillary lesions (e.g., villoglandular adenocarcinomas) that are not serous and that have low-grade cytologic features and a relatively good prognosis.

Clear Cell Carcinoma

Clear cell carcinoma represents less than 4% of all cases of endometrial carcinoma and commonly occurs in older black women. Clear cell carcinoma often occurs with papillary serous carcinoma of the uterus and is associated with a poor prognosis. However, the evidence indicates that the prognosis associated with pure clear cell carcinoma is less ominous.[11] It is important to differentiate clear cell carcinoma from grade 1 carcinoma with secretory vacuolization ("secretory carcinoma"), which is associated with an excellent prognosis.

Other Subtypes

Sarcomas arising in the uterus are rare. Pure leiomyosarcomas account for 20% to 30% of all uterine sarcomas; the mean patient age is somewhat younger than for other types of sarcoma. Endometrial stromal sarcomas, which account for 15% to 20% of uterine sarcomas, include benign stromal nodules, low-grade tumors, and high-grade stromal sarcoma. Low-grade tumors (e.g., endolymphatic stromal myosis) tend to recur years after initial surgery both locally and in distant sites. High-grade stromal sarcomas tend to recur within the first 2 years after treatment, most commonly in the pelvis. Carcinosarcoma (müllerian mixed tumor) is the most common sarcoma of the uterus, accounting for more than 50% of all uterine sarcomas. Tumors contain malignant epithelial and sarcomatous elements. Patients with this disease are generally older than 60 years of age. The most common heterologous type is rhabdomyosarcoma, which contains benign epithelial elements and malignant stromal features.

PRETREATMENT EVALUATION

The possibility of endometrial carcinoma should be considered in postmenopausal women with any vaginal bleeding, perimenopausal women with heavy or prolonged vaginal bleeding, and premenopausal women with abnormal bleeding patterns who are obese or oligoovulatory. Although a formal dilatation and curettage was traditionally the standard technique for diagnosis, outpatient endometrial biopsy has now replaced dilatation and curettage in most situations.[12,13] When cervical involvement is suspected, a cervical biopsy should be performed; fractional curettage usually is not very accurate in this situation.[14]

Because endometrial carcinomas are usually surgically staged, the focus of the pretreatment evaluation should be on determining whether the disease is resectable and determining the patient's operative risk. Therefore, in addition to a biopsy, the pretreatment evaluation should include a careful history and physical examination, laboratory studies, and a chest radiograph. Further studies are probably warranted only in patients with abnormal findings on pelvic examination. A serum CA-125 assay should be considered in women with high-risk histologic subtypes, such as papillary serous carcinoma, because the CA-125 level may be predictive of occult extrauterine disease and may be useful as a tumor marker.[15,16]

Computed tomography (CT) is recommended for all patients with high-grade tumors or clinical stage II or higher disease because CT may demonstrate nodal enlargement or extrauterine spread. Contrast-enhanced magnetic resonance imaging (MRI) is not particularly helpful in detecting nodal or peritoneal involvement but has been reported to have an accuracy of 82% in demonstrating the depth of myometrial invasion[17,18] and an accuracy of 90% in demonstrating cervical involvement.[19] In fact, in a meta-analysis, Kinkel and colleagues[20] found that contrast-enhanced MRI was significantly better than nonenhanced MRI or sonography and demonstrated a trend toward better results than CT in assessing myometrial invasion. These authors recommended contrast-enhanced MRI as the "one-stop" examination with the highest efficacy.[20]

Because many women with endometrial cancer are elderly and have comorbid medical conditions, such as obesity, diabetes, and hypertension, the pretreatment evaluation should be individualized on the basis of findings from the medical history and general physical examination.

STAGING

In 1971 the International Federation of Gynecology and Obstetrics (FIGO) adopted a clinical staging system for carcinomas of the uterine corpus, which at that time were often treated with radiation therapy before hysterectomy. The clinical staging system stratified patients with early disease on the basis of a fractional biopsy specimen from the endocervix and the endometrium, the depth of the uterine cavity, and findings on physical examination. However, in the mid-1980s, these techniques for assessment of disease volume and spread were found to yield erroneous findings in as many as one third of patients when compared with histopathologic findings at the time of laparotomy.[21] At the same time, a report by Creasman and colleagues[22] showed that 22% of patients with clinical stage I disease were found to have disease outside the uterus when a surgical staging procedure was performed. Therefore surgeons started doing surgical staging, which led the FIGO in 1989 to design a surgical staging scheme for endometrial cancer.[23] This surgical staging system has since been updated; the most recent update was published in 1997 (Box 29-2).[24]

The FIGO surgical staging system includes important prognostic information about the depth of myometrial infiltration and resolves problems found in the earlier FIGO staging systems, providing more detailed descriptions of tumor grades and for the first time emphasizing the prognostic importance of cytologic grade, particularly for patients with papillary serous adenocarcinomas. However, the FIGO surgical staging system is problematic for several reasons. First, some tumors classified as stage I or II in the clinical staging system are classified as stage III in the surgical staging system, making it impossible to translate from the surgical to the clinical staging system; consequently, current results cannot be related to those of any studies that include patients treated before 1988. Second, the clinical staging system must still be used to categorize disease in patients who are treated with radiation therapy alone or with preoperative external-beam radiation therapy. Third, although surgical staging is mandated, FIGO does not define the extent of the procedure, which varies widely. Fourth, patients with tumor cells in peritoneal washings are classified as having stage III disease even though patients for whom peritoneal fluid is the sole site of extrauterine disease have an excellent prognosis.

PROGNOSTIC FACTORS

In the absence of good prospective randomized studies of adjuvant therapy for endometrial carcinomas, decisions about the need for adjuvant treatment after surgical staging must be based on a thorough understanding of the natural history of the disease and risk factors for recurrence. In particular, the histologic grade and subtype of the carcinoma, the extent of disease in the uterus, and the presence and distribution of extrauterine disease can be used to predict the risk of tumor recurrence in the vagina, pelvis, and abdomen and at distant sites.

Box 29-2   American Joint Committee on Cancer and International Federation of Gynecology and Obstetrics Staging Systems for Cancer of the Corpus Uteri

TNM Categories	FIGO Stage	
TX	—	Primary tumor cannot be assessed
T0	—	No evidence of primary tumor
Tis	—	Carcinoma in situ
T1	I	Tumor confined to corpus uteri
T1a	IA	Tumor limited to endometrium
T1b	IB	Tumor invades up to half of the myometrium
T1c	IC	Tumor invades to more than half of the myometrium
T2	II	Tumor invades cervix but does not extend beyond uterus
T2a	IIA	Endocervical glandular involvement only
T2b	IIB	Cervical stromal invasion
T3	III	Local and/or regional spread as specified in T3a, b, and/or N1 and FIGO IIIA, B, and C below
T3a	IIIA	Tumor involves serosa and/or adnexa (direct extension or metastasis) and/or cancer cells in ascites or peritoneal washings
T3b	IIIB	Vaginal involvement (direct extension or metastasis)
N1	IIIC	Metastasis to the pelvic and/or para-aortic lymph nodes
T4	IVA	Tumor invades bladder mucosa and/or bowel mucosa (Bullous edema is not sufficient to classify a tumor as T4.)
M1	IVB	Distant metastasis. (*Excluding* metastasis to vagina, pelvic serosa, or adnexa. *Including* metastasis to intra-abdominal lymph nodes other than para-aortic, and/or inguinal lymph nodes.)

REGIONAL LYMPH NODES (N)

NX	Regional lymph node(s) cannot be assessed (e.g., previously removed)
N0	No regional lymph node metastasis
N1	Regional lymph node metastasis

DISTANT METASTASIS (M)

MX	Distant metastasis cannot be assessed
M0	No distant metastasis
M1	Distant metastasis

STAGE GROUPING

Stage 0	Tis	N0	M0
Stage IA	T1a	N0	M0
Stage IB	T1b	N0	M0
Stage IC	T1c	N0	M0
Stage IIA	T2a	N0	M0
Stage IIB	T2b	N0	M0
Stage IIIA	T3a	N0	M0
Stage IIIB	T3b	N0	M0
Stage IIIC	T1	N1	M0
	T2	N1	M0
	T3a	N1	M0
	T3b	N1	M0
Stage IVA	T4	Any N	M0
Stage IVB	Any T	Any N	M1

From Fleming I, Cooper JS, Henson DE, et al, eds. *AJCC Cancer Staging Manual.* 5th ed. Philadelphia, Pa: Lippincott Williams & Wilkins; 1997:195-200.

The pathologic stage incorporates many of these risk factors and therefore is prognostic for survival as well as local recurrence.

Age

Younger patients, especially those younger than 60 years, have a significantly better prognosis than older patients.[25-30] However, currently no specific treatment recommendations are based on age.

Histologic Grade

Tumor grade is one of the most sensitive indicators of prognosis. Grade is directly correlated with the depth of myometrial invasion (Table 29-1)[22] and the frequency of lymph node involvement.[22,31-33] In most reports, the 5-year survival rate for patients with grade 1 tumors is at least 90%; for patients with grade 3 tumors, the 5-year survival rate is 65% to 70%.[31,33] Lewis and colleagues[34] reported that the rate of nodal involvement was 5.5% for patients with stage I, grade 1 tumors and 26% for patients with stage I, grade 3 tumors. Several authors have reported that the incidence of deep myometrial invasion in grade 3 tumors is 3 to 4 times the incidence in grade 1 tumors.

Histologic Subtype

Several authors have reported that adenosquamous carcinoma is more malignant than either adenocarcinoma

TABLE 29-1

Correlation Between Tumor Grade and Depth of Myometrial Invasion

Depth of Invasion (% of Tumors)	TUMOR GRADE		
	Grade 1	Grade 2	Grade 3
Endometrium	24	11	7
Inner third	53	45	35
Middle third	12	24	16
Outer third	10	20	42

From Creasman W, Morrow C, Bundy B, et al. *Cancer* 1987;60:2035-2041.

TABLE 29-2

Correlations Between Depth of Myometrial Invasion, Tumor Grade, and Pelvic Node Involvement

Depth of Invasion	NUMBER (%) OF PATIENTS WITH PELVIC NODE INVOLVEMENT		
	Grade 1 (N = 180)	Grade 2 (N = 288)	Grade 3 (N = 153)
Endometrium (N = 86)	0 (0)	1 (3)	0 (0)
Inner third (N = 281)	3 (3)	7 (5)	5 (9)
Middle third (N = 115)	0 (0)	6 (9)	1 (4)
Outer third (N = 139)	2 (11)	11 (19)	22 (34)

From Creasman W, Morrow C, Bundy B, et al. *Cancer* 1987; 60:2035-2041.

or adenoacanthoma, probably because of the malignant squamous elements.[35-37] Patients with adenosquamous carcinoma are best treated as though they have high-grade carcinoma of the uterine corpus.

Papillary serous carcinoma of the endometrium should be treated as an aggressive high-grade tumor because it behaves more like its ovarian counterpart than like a typical endometrioid adenocarcinoma. A recent study by Cirisano and colleagues[38] found that patients with papillary serous or clear cell carcinoma with myometrial invasion less than 2 mm had an estimated 5-year survival rate of 56%, compared with 93% for patients with endometrial adenocarcinoma, and that surgically staged patients had the same outcome as clinically staged patients. Clear cell carcinoma associated with papillary serous carcinoma should be treated as papillary serous carcinoma; however, pure clear cell carcinoma may have a better outcome and could be treated as endometrial carcinoma.[11]

Depth of Myometrial Invasion

The depth of myometrial invasion is one of the most important predictors of lymph node involvement and prognosis (Table 29-2).[22,28,29,39] The depth of myometrial invasion is more strongly associated with lymphatic and extrauterine spread, treatment failure, and relapse than is histologic grade.[40] Therefore, regardless of grade, tumors that have not invaded the myometrium rarely involve lymph nodes and are usually curable with hysterectomy alone (although high-grade tumors will occasionally recur in the vaginal apex). Uterine papillary serous carcinoma may be an exception; this tumor has been reported to behave aggressively in the absence of demonstrable myometrial invasion.[41]

Cervical Invasion

Tumors that involve the cervix are classified by FIGO as stage II. Patients with tumors that involve only endocervical glands (FIGO stage IIA) have a relatively good prognosis, probably similar to that of patients with tumors of comparable grade and depth that are confined to the fundus. Tumors that involve the endocervical stroma are associated with a poorer prognosis, with a higher likelihood of extrauterine involvement and disease recurrence. Presumably, involvement of the cervical stroma gives the tumor access to cervical regional routes of spread, placing pelvic nodes at relatively greater risk. In a small series of surgically staged patients, Fanning and colleagues[42] reported recurrence in 5 of the 8 patients with stage IIB disease and none of the 12 patients with stage IIA disease.

Tumor Size

Schink and colleagues[43] reported a relationship between the size of endometrial primary tumors and rates of lymph node metastasis and survival. The predictive value of tumor size seemed to be independent of the grade or depth of invasion of the endometrial cancer. In cases in which the indications for adjuvant treatment are in a "gray zone," tumor size is one factor that may influence the decision of whether to treat.

Lymph Node Involvement

With the advent of systematic surgical staging, more detailed information is becoming available about the incidence and prognostic importance of various patterns of extrauterine spread. The largest prospective study of surgical staging was conducted by the Gynecologic Oncology Group.[22,44] Reports from this study provide some of the best data available about the relationships between hysterectomy findings, nodal involvement, and outcome (Tables 29-1, 29-2, and 29-3).[22]

TABLE 29-3

Correlations Between Depth of Myometrial Invasion, Tumor Grade, and Para-aortic Node Involvement

	NUMBER (%) OF PATIENTS WITH PARA-AORTIC NODE INVOLVEMENT		
Depth of Invasion	Grade 1 (*N* = 180)	Grade 2 (*N* = 288)	Grade 3 (*N* = 153)
Endometrium (*N* = 86)	0 (0)	1 (3)	0 (0)
Inner third (*N*= 281)	1 (1)	5 (4)	2 (4)
Middle third (*N* = 115)	1 (5)	0 (0)	0 (0)
Outer third (*N* = 139)	1 (6)	8 (14)	15 (23)

From Creasman W, Morrow C, Bundy B, et al. *Cancer* 1987;60:2035-2041.

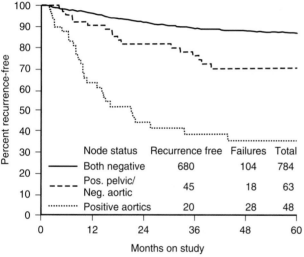

Fig. 29-2 Recurrence-free interval in 784 patients with negative pelvic and para-aortic nodes, 63 patients with positive pelvic but negative para-aortic nodes, and 48 patients with positive para-aortic nodes. (From Morrow C, Bundy B, Kurman R, et al. *Gynecol Oncol* 1991;40:55-65.)

Overall, lymph node metastases were reported in 70 (11%) of 621 evaluable patients.[22] Approximately half of the patients with documented nodal involvement had positive para-aortic nodes, 32% of those with pelvic node metastases also had positive para-aortic nodes, and 12 of 70 patients with regional metastases had only para-aortic node involvement.

A strong correlation exists between lymph node involvement, particularly para-aortic node involvement, and worse prognosis (Fig. 29-2).[39] However, disease that has metastasized to regional nodes seems to be curable in many cases. The Gynecologic Oncology Group

reported a 70% survival rate at 5 years among patients with histologic documentation of pelvic node involvement and no para-aortic node involvement. Although treatment details were not given, it was stated that most patients underwent pelvic irradiation. The survival rate for patients with positive para-aortic nodes in that study was 40%, which is comparable with survival rates in other reports of patients treated with extended-field radiation therapy.[44-47]

Tumor Cells in Peritoneal Washings

Although the presence of tumor cells in peritoneal washings is taken into account in the current FIGO staging system for patients with endometrial carcinoma, the significance of this finding is uncertain. Some investigators have reported a poorer prognosis for patients with tumor cells in peritoneal washings, but these studies have not consistently identified patients with papillary serous carcinomas.[39,48] Other investigators[49,50] have concluded that abnormal peritoneal cytology is not an independent risk factor for recurrence. In a multivariate analysis by Milosevic and colleagues,[49] the conclusion was that although the presence of tumor cells in peritoneal washings was strongly associated with disease recurrence (odds ratio, 4.7; 95% confidence interval, 3.5 to 6.3), this finding was largely due to the association of malignant cytology with other adverse prognostic factors, which dominate the clinical presentation. In the absence of any other adverse features, the true incidence of tumor cells in peritoneal washings is quite low, and this finding would most likely not be an independent predictor for relapse.

Adnexal Metastases and Simultaneous Ovarian Primary Tumors

Although endometrial carcinomas may metastasize to the ovaries, some patients who present with simultaneous disease in the endometrium and ovary actually have multiple primary tumors. In particular, patients who have simultaneous low-grade endometrioid neoplasms with minimal myometrial invasion and early ovarian disease tend to have an excellent prognosis, with survival rates of 80% to 100%, suggesting that these lesions do not represent either metastatic ovarian cancer or metastatic endometrial cancer.[51,52] However, 5% of patients with stage I or occult stage II disease do have adnexal involvement, and this is associated with a fourfold increase in the risk of lymph node involvement and with a worse prognosis.

TREATMENT
Surgery

The mainstay of treatment for adenocarcinoma of the endometrium is surgical removal of the uterus. Although several different surgical procedures have been reported, total abdominal hysterectomy with bilateral salpingo-oophorectomy is widely regarded as preferable for most patients.

Options for evaluation of the regional lymph nodes range from palpation to selective nodal sampling to complete lymphadenectomy. Palpation of the lymph nodes has been shown to be an inaccurate method of determining lymph node status because the size of nodal metastases is often below the threshold permitting clinical detection. In a study of 76 patients with primary endometrial cancer of various histologic types, Girardi and colleagues[53] found that 37% of lymph node metastases were less than 2 mm in diameter and almost 50% were less than 1 cm in diameter. These findings are consistent with those of Creasman and colleagues,[22] who found that fewer than 10% of patients with nodal metastases had grossly positive nodes.

Controversy currently exists in the gynecologic oncology community regarding the proper extent and the therapeutic value of lymphadenectomy. Chuang and colleagues[54] demonstrated that for diagnostic purposes, a limited selective lymphadenectomy in which about 10 nodes were removed accurately reflected the true nodal status. However, the gynecologic oncology community is increasingly performing a complete lymphadenectomy in which 40 to 50 pelvic lymph nodes are retrieved. Some investigators believe that complete lymphadenectomy improves survival,[55-57] whereas others have concluded that lymphadenectomy provides prognostic information only.[26,54,58,59]

Complete lymphadenectomy is associated with higher rates of acute and late complications than are seen with less thorough methods of surgical lymph node evaluation.[39,56] The increased risk of complications is justified, however, if unsuspected disease is detected that would lead to the use of potentially curative pelvic radiation therapy. The risk of complications increases dramatically if pelvic radiation therapy is added after lymphadenectomy.[60,61] Most gynecologic oncologists still recommend pelvic radiation therapy for patients with stage IC, grade 3 disease with negative pelvic lymph nodes.[62] If pelvic radiation therapy is recommended on the basis of known high-risk uterine features, a selective lymphadenectomy in which the para-aortic lymph nodes are also sampled not only leads to a reduction in the risk of radiation therapy complications but also permits determination of the most appropriate radiation fields.

Pelvic lymphadenectomy may indirectly improve the therapeutic ratio by permitting identification of the patients most likely to benefit from adjuvant pelvic irradiation. The patterns of failure for patients with surgically staged disease continue to be defined, and an ongoing trial conducted by the British Research Council in which patients are randomly assigned to pelvic lymph node dissection vs. no lymph node dissection may help determine the importance of surgical staging. At present, treatment of patients with endometrial cancer should be designed to maximize cure rates but also minimize complications.

Adjuvant Radiation Therapy

Despite decades of study, the role of adjuvant radiation therapy (preoperative or postoperative) in the treatment of endometrial cancer has been difficult to define. Historically, patients with early-stage endometrial cancer were treated with radiation therapy delivered using one of a variety of techniques, followed by extrafascial hysterectomy. Supplemental postoperative radiation therapy was added in selected cases on the basis of the pathologic risk factors (e.g., deep myometrial extension, cervical involvement, positive nodes). This was the standard treatment for early-stage endometrial cancer in the United States and other countries by the 1950s, despite a few clinicians who questioned the advantages of selective postoperative irradiation.[63,64]

Later clinicians became more aware of the value of operative findings as a guide to the selection of adjuvant treatment. Because preoperative radiation therapy has never been proven to be more effective than tailored postoperative radiation therapy, the use of preoperative irradiation has declined in favor of initial surgical treatment.[65-67]

Radiation therapy has been shown to reduce the risk of local recurrence, but its effect on survival is unclear. As a result, investigators continue to disagree about the role of adjuvant radiation therapy in the management of endometrial carcinoma.

Several factors have made it difficult to study the value of adjuvant irradiation. Because most newly diagnosed endometrial carcinomas are confined to the uterus, treatment failures after surgery alone are expected in only about 15% of patients. Therefore the margin of improvement achievable with radiation therapy is small, and either large groups of patients or highly selected populations are needed to demonstrate the effects of adjuvant irradiation. The influence of physicians' biases on the selection of patients for adjuvant treatment has limited the value of retrospective studies; in addition, retrospective studies are difficult to compare because of changes over time in the classification systems for staging and grading of endometrial carcinoma. Finally, few randomized trials of adjuvant irradiation have been conducted in patients with endometrial carcinoma, and most of those trials have included mainly patients with low- to intermediate-risk disease, in whom survival differences may not be as apparent. For these reasons, the decision of whether to administer adjuvant irradiation is based primarily on clinicians' understanding of the risk factors for recurrence and the natural history of the disease; their interpretation of data; and their estimates of the risk of complications in each individual case.

Preoperative Radiation Therapy

The primary goal of preoperative intracavitary irradiation is to prevent vaginal recurrences. In early series, overall vaginal recurrence rates after surgery alone were as high as 15% to 25%.[68,69] A few authors have reported much lower vaginal recurrence rates after surgery alone and have suggested that the wide range of reported local recurrence rates may, in part, reflect variations in surgical technique that influence the risk of tumor cell implantation.[70,71]

Most data suggest that in patients with high-risk disease, preoperative irradiation reduces the incidence of vaginal recurrence from 10% to 15% to less than 5%. With preoperative ICRT, the frequency of vaginal recurrence in patients with clinical stage I disease is 0% to 5%.[71-79] However, these results cannot be compared with the recurrence rates of patients not treated with radiation because in nearly all studies, patients were treated with radiation therapy on the basis of a higher risk of recurrence.

In theory, patients with gross tumor involvement of the cervix stand to receive the greatest benefit from preoperative irradiation. In these patients, the preoperative intracavitary technique delivers a greater dose to the paracervical tissues than is possible with postoperative vaginal irradiation. Intrauterine applicators are usually loaded with 35 to 40 mg radium equivalent (RaEq) of cesium and left in place for approximately 72 hours for a total exposure of 3500 to 4000 mg RaEq-hours. Vaginal applicators are loaded to deliver 60 to 70 Gy to the surface of the apical vagina over the same period. After this dose of radiation, hysterectomy can be safely performed within 2 to 3 days.[72,73]

Combined preoperative external-beam radiation therapy and ICRT may be indicated for patients with nonserous tumors that extensively infiltrate the cervix. In this case, the hysterectomy should be delayed until 4 to 6 weeks after irradiation. Alternatively, some surgeons recommend a radical hysterectomy for patients with bulky stage II disease, but the morbidity associated with the more radical surgery is greater, and postoperative radiation therapy may still be necessary.

Postoperative Radiation Therapy

Postoperative pelvic irradiation clearly reduces the risk of pelvic recurrence, but no study has yet determined whether it improves the survival rates of patients with high-risk disease.

In 1980 Aalders and colleagues[29] published a report on a randomized prospective trial of primary surgery and vaginal brachytherapy with and without additional external-beam irradiation in patients with endometrial cancer clinically confined to the uterus. Comprehensive surgical staging was not done, but patients with "proven metastases at surgery" were excluded. A significant reduction in the rate of vaginal and pelvic recurrences was observed in the group that received adjuvant radiation therapy (1.9% vs. 6.9%). These patients also experienced more distant recurrences, and as a result, the overall 5-year survival rate was not improved by the use of external-beam irradiation. Within the subset of patients with deeply invasive grade 3 disease, patients treated with radiation therapy seemed to have a somewhat better survival rate, but the number of patients in this subset was small, and the result was not statistically significant.

In a second prospective randomized trial, Gynecologic Oncology Group study 99,[60] patients with endometrial adenocarcinoma underwent complete surgical staging with pelvic and para-aortic lymph node dissection. Patients with intermediate-risk surgical stage I disease were then randomly assigned to no further therapy or pelvic irradiation with 50.4 Gy. Most patients had relatively low-risk disease features: 80% had grade 1 or 2 disease, and 60% had stage IB disease. Preliminary results published in abstract form in 1998 showed an improvement in the progression-free interval (2-year progression-free survival rates of 96% vs. 88% at 56 months median follow-up, $P = 0.004$) but no significant overall survival benefit with adjuvant radiation therapy. Disease recurred in the pelvis in 3 (2%) of 190 patients treated with adjuvant radiation therapy and in 17 (8%) of 200 patients treated with surgery alone. Full results of this study have yet to be published. Naumann and colleagues[62] surveyed members of the Society of Gynecologic Oncologists to determine the impact of Gynecologic Oncology Group study 99 on their practice. Although 27% of respondents stated that they were less likely to recommend adjuvant radiation therapy as a result of the study, more than 77% reported that they still recommended adjuvant irradiation for patients with high-risk disease, such as stage IC disease and stage IB, grade 3 disease.

A third prospective randomized trial of adjuvant radiation therapy in patients with endometrial carcinoma was conducted in the Netherlands and reported in April 2000 by Creutzberg and colleagues.[80] In this trial, 715 patients with intermediate-risk endometrial carcinoma were randomly assigned after surgery to irradiation with 46 Gy or no irradiation. Nodes considered "suspicious" were sampled. As in the Gynecologic Oncology Group trial 99, most of the patients in the Netherlands trial had relatively low-risk features—90% had grade 1 or 2 disease, and 41% had stage IB disease. The overall survival rates at 5 years were the same in the irradiation and no-irradiation groups (81% vs. 85%); however, 5-year local–regional recurrence rates were 4% in the irradiated group and 14% in the control group (Fig. 29-3).[80] Of the recurrences, 73% were restricted to the vagina. In

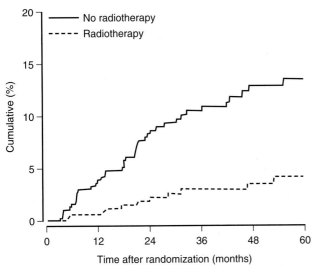

Fig. 29-3 Probability of local–regional (vaginal or pelvic) relapse in patients with intermediate-risk endometrial carcinoma assigned to postoperative radiation therapy or no further treatment. (From Creutzberg CL, van Putten WL, Koper PC, et al. *Lancet* 2000;355:1404-1411.)

patients who did not receive postoperative radiation therapy, 3-year survival rates were 69% after vaginal recurrences and 13% after pelvic or distant relapse (*P* < 0.001).

Influence on survival. In all three of the randomized studies discussed in this section, pelvic radiation therapy clearly reduced the risk of local recurrence; however, too few patients with high-risk disease and too few disease-related deaths were noted to demonstrate or rule out moderate differences in survival between patient subgroups. In the study by Creutzberg and colleagues,[80] grade 3 disease and deep myometrial invasion were both associated with a twofold higher relative risk of local–regional relapse; however, grade 3 disease was the strongest predictor of endometrial-carcinoma-related death. However, only 74 of the 714 patients in the study had grade 3 disease—too few to permit any survival difference to be ruled out in this high-risk population.

Several studies have documented survival rates of 80% to 90% for patients with high-risk disease (e.g., high grade or deeply invasive) treated with postoperative radiation therapy; these findings provide indirect evidence of the treatment's efficacy.[26,58,59,81] Carey and colleagues[26] reported a 5-year relapse-free survival rate of 81% for 157 patients with clinical stage I disease and high-risk features (deep myometrial invasion, grade 3, adenosquamous histology, or cervical involvement). The local recurrence rate was 4%, compared with 29% in a separate group of 28 patients who refused adjuvant treatment. The 70% projected 5-year survival rate reported by the Gynecologic Oncology Group for 63 patients with positive pelvic nodes and negative para-aortic nodes also may provide indirect evidence of a survival benefit of pelvic irradiation in patients with high-risk disease.[39]

Technique and complications. Pelvic irradiation may be delivered using a four-field technique (Fig. 29-4) or anterior and posterior opposed fields with 15- to 20-MV photons. Four fields are usually preferred for patients who have undergone an extensive lymphadenectomy and for patients with wound problems.

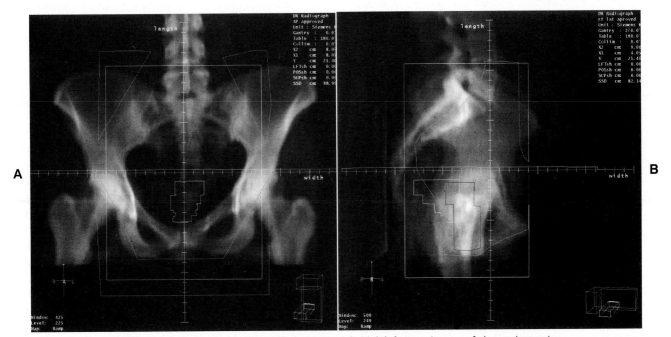

Fig. 29-4 Typical anterior field **(A)** and lateral field **(B)** for carcinoma of the endometrium. The rectum is outlined in yellow and the vagina is outlined on an aquasimulation from computed tomography. (See Color Plate 32, after p. 80, for color reproduction.)

Serious complications are observed in 5% to 15% of all patients who undergo postoperative pelvic irradiation; however, the risk of complications may be greater for patients who have had a staging lymphadenectomy.[61,82,83] The most significant side effects observed are obstruction of the small bowel, fistula formation, proctitis, chronic diarrhea, vaginal stenosis, and insufficiency fractures of bone.

The lateral fields should usually receive less weighting than the anterior and posterior fields (e.g., 50:50:40:40, anteroposterior:posteroanterior:right lateral:left lateral) to reduce the lateral applied dose (a computer plan should be done). Pelvic treatment fields typically extend from the L4 or L5 lumbar vertebra to the mid or lower pubic ramus (a radio-opaque marker is used to verify the presence of at least a 4- to 5-cm margin on the vaginal cuff) (see Fig. 29-4). Prone positioning, bladder distention, and use of a false tabletop have all been reported to decrease the volume of the small bowel within the pelvis. The total treatment dose is usually 40 to 50 Gy at 1.8 to 2.0 Gy/fraction. Extracapsular nodal extension or close margins in patients with cervical disease may warrant an external-beam boost. Possible indications for vaginal vault irradiation are discussed in the section on "Postoperative Vaginal Irradiation" later in this chapter.

Extended-Field Radiation Therapy and Whole-Abdomen Irradiation

Postoperative extended-field radiation therapy is indicated for patients with nonserous endometrial cancer with evidence of extrapelvic disease in the para-aortic nodes only. Five-year survival rates of 30% to 50% have been reported with this treatment (Table 29-4).[39,44-47,84-87] Further studies are needed to determine whether chemotherapy is as effective as extended-field radiation therapy in this setting.

TABLE 29-4

Reported Survival Rates in Patients Treated with Extended-Field Irradiation for Endometrial Carcinoma Metastatic to Para-aortic Lymph Nodes

Study and Reference	Number of Patients	5-Year Survival Rate
Komaki et al[84]	7	60%
Potish[44]	15	40%
Feuer and Calanog[46]	18	50%
Morrow et al[39]	48	37%
Rose et al[45]	17	53%
Corn et al[47]	50	46%
Hicks et al[85]	11	27%
Blythe et al[86]	13	54%
Onda et al[87]	20	75%*

*Patients also received three cycles of cisplatin-containing chemotherapy before radiation therapy.

The upper border of the field should be at the T11 or T12 vertebra to ensure coverage of perirenal nodes that are at risk for direct spread via the tubo-ovarian vessels. Treatment should be delivered with photons of at least 15 MV whenever possible. Four fields may be used, but CT planning should be done to verify that the dose to the kidneys, spinal cord, and para-aortic nodes is below that known to cause complications. The entire field probably cannot be treated with more than 45 to 50.4 Gy at 1.8 Gy/fraction; however, small boost fields may be used to increase the dose to residual gross disease or sites of extracapsular spread to 55 to 60 Gy depending on the volume.

The poor prognosis of uterine papillary serous carcinomas and their tendency to behave as ovarian carcinomas have led radiation oncologists to explore the value of treating these lesions with whole-abdomen radiation therapy (WART). Unfortunately, published reports of WART for uterine papillary serous carcinoma are still largely anecdotal,[88-91] probably because this is a rare disease that has been well recognized for only 10 to 15 years and because it tends to affect elderly women who may not be ideal candidates for aggressive treatment.

Smith and colleagues[91] reported on a series of patients with papillary serous carcinoma treated with WART. The 3-year disease-free survival and overall survival rates were 87% in patients with stage I or II disease but only 32% and 61%, respectively, in patients with stage III or IV disease.[91] Potish[88] reported long-term survival in five (57%) of nine patients who had intraperitoneal spread from uterine papillary serous carcinoma at diagnosis and were treated with WART.

The Gynecologic Oncology Group is comparing WART with chemotherapy (cisplatin and doxorubicin) for patients with stage III or IV disease according to the 1988 FIGO surgical staging system (< 2 cm residual disease).[92] This study will be of particular interest for its comparison of the two treatments in patients with papillary serous tumors, but it will also include patients with nonserous stage III tumors, for whom the risk of intraabdominal dissemination is probably small.

Some authors have recommended WART for patients with FIGO stage III nonserous tumors, but studies of WART in this setting have been retrospective and have included few patients. Smith and colleagues[91] reported 3-year disease-free survival and overall survival rates of 79% and 89%, respectively, after WART in patients with surgical stage III or IV adenocarcinomas of the endometrium. In 1992 the Gynecologic Oncology Group completed a large phase II study of WART in 137 patients with stage I to IV uterine papillary serous carcinoma or clear cell carcinoma and 77 patients with stage III or IV endometrial carcinoma of other histologic subtypes. The results from this study are still being analyzed, but scrutiny of the patterns of failure among patients in whom the pathologic disease features have been carefully reviewed suggests that intraabdominal spread is rare in the case of tumors that have no papillary serous component. This finding suggests that WART is probably not warranted in most cases, even when the cytologic washings contain tumor cells.

WART is usually given using anteroposterior-posteroanterior fields. The photon energy should be based on the thickness of the subcutaneous abdominal tissue. The upper border of the field should be designed under fluoroscopy to give a 1-cm margin on the upper excursion of the diaphragm under quiet respiration. CT assists in treatment planning and is used to verify the position of the kidneys and the borders of the peritoneal cavity. CT studies have shown that the pelvic peritoneum sometimes extends lateral to the anterior iliac crest; therefore use of standard anatomic landmarks can result in underdosage of portions of the peritoneum. Doses of 25 to 30 Gy at 1.5 Gy/fraction are usually tolerated if the patient is treated appropriately with antiemetics and blood counts are followed closely. Posterior two to five half-value layer blocks are most often used to restrict the dose to the kidneys to less than 18 Gy, and liver blocks are most often used to shield the right lobe of the liver after about 25 Gy. Most investigators recommend a boost to the pelvis to bring the total dose to 45 to 50 Gy. Some investigators also boost the dose to the para-aortic nodes and the medial edges of the diaphragm to approximately 42 Gy.

Postoperative Vaginal Irradiation

In selected patients with endometrial carcinoma, vaginal ICRT may be prescribed to prevent vaginal recurrence. The magnitude of the benefit of adjuvant ICRT is difficult to define, however, because criteria for adding external pelvic irradiation differ among physicians and because reported vaginal recurrence rates after hysterectomy alone range from 2% to 20%.

Patients with inner or middle third myometrial invasion and grade 1 to 2 disease have a 3% risk of pelvic and para-aortic nodal involvement[22] and therefore may benefit from vaginal brachytherapy without external-beam radiation therapy whether or not staging lymphadenectomy is done (Table 29-5).* In a few retrospective studies, patients with uterus-confined disease with poor prognostic indicators, such as high-grade disease and deep myometrial penetration, but negative lymph nodes have experienced excellent outcomes after vaginal brachytherapy alone (Table 29-6).[39,55,93,95,96] However, the only prospective trial comparing vaginal brachytherapy with vaginal brachytherapy plus pelvic radiation therapy for such patients suggests an improvement with the addition of external-beam irradiation.[29]

In the delivery of vaginal ICRT, clinicians differ regarding the dose, dose rate, target volume (vaginal length), and type of intracavitary applicators. In general, it is believed that treating the entire vaginal length is unnecessary and may result in excess morbidity from vaginal dysfunction or rectal morbidity. Therefore most clinicians treat only the upper third to half of the vagina. Either colpostats or cylinders can be used to treat the vaginal mucosa, and low-dose-rate (LDR) or fractionated high-dose-rate (HDR) irradiation can be given.

If external-beam radiation therapy is not given, the typical dose delivered with LDR ICRT is 60 to 70 Gy to the vaginal surface over a period of about 72 hours. Some clinicians give additional ICRT to the vaginal cuff after pelvic irradiation, although several reports have failed to document an improved outcome with this approach.[27,97] A typical dose for prophylactic ICRT of the cuff after pelvic irradiation is 30 Gy in 48 hours (LDR) or 15 to 18 Gy in three fractions (HDR) prescribed to the vaginal surface.

*References 39, 55, 56, 59, 93, 94.

TABLE 29-5

Incidence of Pelvic Recurrence After Vaginal Radiation Therapy Alone in Patients with Favorable Prognostic Indicators

Study	Number of Patients	Risk Factors*	Median Follow-up (Years)	Recurrence Rate (%)
NO LYMPHADENECTOMY				
Kucera et al[59]	376	< 2/3, G1	Not stated	0.8
		< 1/3, G1-3	Not stated	0.8
Eltabbakh et al[94]	303	Stage IB, G1-2	8.1	0
LYMPHADENECTOMY				
Morrow et al[39]	49	< 1/3, G1-3	Not stated	0
Orr et al[55]	126	Stage IB, G1-2	3.25	0
		Stage IC, G1		0
Mohan et al[56]	131	Stage IB, G1	8	0

From Greven KM. *Semin Radiat Oncol* 2000;10:29-35.
*< 2/3, Middle third myometrial invasion; < 1/3, inner third myometrial invasion; G, histologic grade.

TABLE 29-6

Incidence of Pelvic Recurrence with Vaginal Brachytherapy Alone After Staging Lymphadenectomy in Patients with Unfavorable Prognostic Indicators

Study	Number of Patients	Risk Factors*	Median Follow-up (Years)	Recurrence Rate (%)
Morrow et al[39]	14	> 1/3 or G3	> 3	0
Fanning et al[95]	18	Stage IC, G3, stage II	2.8	0
Orr et al[55]	60	Stage IC or G3	Not stated	0
MacLeod et al[96]	34	Stage IC or G3, Stage II	6.9	3

From Greven KM. *Semin Radiat Oncol* 2000;10:29-35.
*< 1/3, Inner third myometrial invasion; G, histologic grade.

HDR ICRT has some obvious advantages over LDR ICRT for prophylactic irradiation of the vaginal cuff. Placement of the applicator is simple, requires no sedation, and is an outpatient procedure. The standard geometry of the applicators permits rapid calculation of source dwell times. Also, in this setting, the use of HDR ICRT is less controversial because only a modest dose of radiation is needed to prevent tumor recurrence in the vagina. However, it should be remembered that for most applicator designs, the dose and fraction size at 0.5 cm from the vaginal surface is approximately equivalent to the maximum rectal dose. Dose specification (for LDR or HDR) should always include a calculation of the maximum (i.e., vaginal surface) dose. Sorbe and Smeds,[98] in a prospective study comparing four fractionation schemes, found that the rate of rectal complications exceeded 80% in patients treated with four fractions of 9 Gy prescribed at 10 mm. In recent reports, investigators have recommended several fractionation schemes, including six fractions of 6 Gy,[99] three fractions of 7 Gy,[100] four fractions of 8.5 Gy,[96] and two fractions of 16.2 Gy[101] with dose specified at the vaginal surface. All these investigators have reported vaginal recurrence rates of less than 1.5% among patients with relatively favorable tumors.

Radiation Therapy Alone for Medically or Surgically Inoperable Disease

Even though hysterectomy is the primary treatment for early-stage endometrial cancer, patients with a very high risk of complications after surgery can be treated with radiation therapy alone. Disease-specific survival rates of 75% to 85% and local recurrence rates of 10% to 20% have been reported for patients with clinical stage I or II endometrial carcinoma treated with radiation therapy alone. Prognosis in these patients correlates with clinical stage and histologic grade.[102-108] Brachytherapy alone yields excellent local control in most patients with grade 1 tumors. Patients with large uterine cavities, cervical involvement, or grade 3 tumors should be considered for a course of external-beam irradiation before brachytherapy to treat regional nodes at risk.

When brachytherapy is administered for endometrial carcinoma, it is important to cover the uterine fundus adequately. When the fundus is small, a single intrauterine tandem with increased activity at the tip should broaden the radiation dose distribution in the fundus. However, in patients with larger cavities, Heyman packing or Simon capsules[109-112] can be packed into the uterus to achieve a better distribution to the fundus. Alternatively, a satisfactory dose distribution can sometimes be obtained by placing two tandems in the right and left cornua of the uterus and loading the tandems to achieve the desired distribution (Fig. 29-5). MRI may be helpful in planning treatment. With LDR irradiation, uterine applicators are commonly loaded with 45 to 50 mg RaEq and are left in place for two 72-hour or three 48-hour treatments (or for two 48-hour treatments after 40 to 45 Gy to the whole pelvis). With this approach, reported control rates are high and reported complication rates are low.[104] The vagina does not require as high a dose as it does for cervical cancer unless the cervical stroma is involved. For a clinical stage I tumor, source loadings that yield a vaginal surface dose of 60 to 80 Gy should be sufficient to prevent vaginal recurrence in most patients.

Because most patients with inoperable endometrial carcinoma have multiple medical problems, several groups have recently tried HDR ICRT for these patients.[113-116] In one series, Kucera and colleagues[113] used this approach to treat 228 patients with stage I endometrial carcinoma who were medically inoperable. The overall survival rates at 5 and 10 years were 59.7% and 30.2%, respectively, and the disease-specific survival rates at 5 and 10 years were 85.4% and 75.1%, respectively. Nguyen and Petereit[115] reported good uterine disease control rates (88%) but a high rate of perioperative morbidity and two perioperative deaths in 36 patients treated with HDR brachytherapy for clinical stage I disease.[115,117] Deep vein thrombosis, a possible

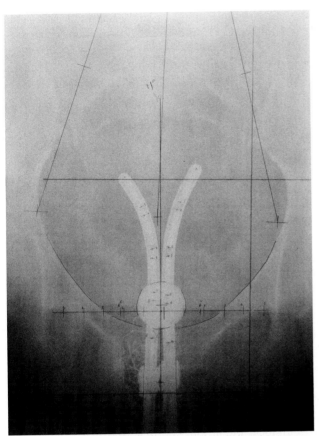

Fig. 29-5 Radiograph showing placement of two tandems in the uterus for the first intracavitary treatment in a patient with inoperable endometrial carcinoma. The loading of the tandem on the right is 10, 5, 10 mg RaEq of cesium, and the loading of the tandem on the left is 10, 10, 5, 5 mg RaEq of cesium. The implants were left in place for 72 hours.

complication of prolonged bed rest during LDR applications, also can be encouraged by prolonged lithotomy positioning for HDR procedures.[115,117] Petereit and colleagues[118] have recommended changes to reduce perioperative morbidity, including using a tandem and a cylinder instead of a tandem and a pair of ovoids to reduce the time patients are in the lithotomy position; use of prophylaxis against deep vein thrombosis; and use of abdominal sonography to visualize the probe in the uterus.[118] Whatever method of brachytherapy is used, patients with inoperable endometrial cancer should be treated only by a dedicated and experienced team in a well-controlled environment with adequate monitoring and emergency medical support.

Treatment of Recurrent Disease

The most common site of vaginal recurrence of endometrial carcinoma is the region of the hysterectomy scar in the apical vagina. Recurrences also may occur suburethrally in the distal anterior vagina. Recurrences at other sites are uncommon.

The mechanism of vaginal recurrence of endometrial carcinoma is not well understood, but at least two possible routes of spread are known: implantation into disturbed sites, principally in the vaginal apex, and spread through the lymphovascular system. The first mechanism is probably most consistent with the relatively high cure rates after aggressive treatment of isolated vaginal recurrences and might explain the wide variation in vaginal recurrence rates reported in different institutions. Several case reports[119,120] of episiotomy scar recurrences in women with cervical cancer (adenocarcinoma or squamous cell carcinoma) who delivered babies vaginally suggests that implantation is a potential mechanism of gynecologic tumor recurrence.

For patients with isolated pelvic recurrence whose initial treatment was hysterectomy alone, 5-year local control rates of 40% to 80% and 5-year survival rates of 30% to 80% can be achieved with radical radiation therapy (Table 29-7).[76,121-133] Survival is correlated with the size, grade, extent, and location of the recurrent tumor; initial myometrial involvement; and the time to recurrence. Greven and Olds[121] found that the size of the recurrence was the most important prognostic factor for local control. In their study, local control was achieved in 6 of 7 patients with tumor bulk less than 2 cm but in only 2 of 10 patients with tumor bulk of 2 cm or greater.[121] If the size and extent of recurrent disease are prognostic for outcome, this would suggest a need for careful follow-up of patients treated with surgery alone.

In the treatment of recurrent disease, a combination of external-beam radiation therapy and brachytherapy is usually indicated; brachytherapy should be tailored to the size, extent, and initial response of the lesion. As is

TABLE 29-7

Survival Rates After Radiation Therapy for Pelvic Recurrences of Endometrial Carcinoma

Study	Time of Observation or Median Follow-up (Years)	Survival Rate (%)
Aalders et al[132]*	3-19	14
Sears et al[123]*	7.5	44
Curran et al[122]*	5	31
Greven and Olds[121]*	3-10	33
Ingersol[130]*	5	48
Kuten et al[129]	5	18
Hart et al[124]	1.25	35% (5 years)
Hoekstra et al[127]	5	44
Reddy et al[76]	5	33
Ackerman et al[125]	5	43
Wylie et al[128]	5	53
Mandell et al[126]*	4	82

*Vaginal recurrences only.

true for primary vaginal cancer, ICRT should not be used to treat endometrial tumors more than 5 mm thick. A variety of interstitial techniques may be indicated depending on the clinical situation. For apical lesions, laparotomy or laparoscopy guidance may be necessary. Combined external-beam radiation therapy and interstitial radiation therapy is usually indicated for distal (usually suburethral) recurrences. The dose is important, and Curran and colleagues[122] reported that patients who received at least 60 Gy had significantly improved survival and pelvic control rates.

UTERINE SARCOMA

Surgery is the primary treatment for all sarcomas arising from the uterus. Total abdominal hysterectomy and bilateral salpingo-oophorectomy is the treatment of choice, although some investigators advocate a more radical surgical approach for low-grade endometrial stromal sarcomas.[134] In general, lymph node dissection and sampling, although it adds information about prognosis, has not improved survival rates. Local failures are common, and most recurrences result from hematogenous dissemination of tumor.

The role of radiation therapy in the management of carcinosarcoma is controversial. Most retrospective reviews of patients with carcinosarcoma have demonstrated a lower rate of pelvic tumor recurrence in patients who received postoperative pelvic irradiation; however, in most cases this has not led to an improvement in survival.[135-146] Potential biases from the small numbers of patients in most studies have made it impossible to determine the efficacy of treatment. The Gynecologic Oncology Group retrospectively evaluated its experience in treating uterine cancer in two studies.[137,138] In both of these studies, the rate of pelvic recurrence was reduced with radiation therapy; however, more cases of distant metastasis were noted in the irradiated group, and therefore overall survival was the same in both groups. The problem with these studies, as with other reviews, was that the tumor stage, grade, and depth of invasion and rates of lymph node involvement were not compared for patients receiving different treatments, making it impossible to determine the efficacy of radiation therapy.

Few studies have separately reported control rates for patients given radiation therapy for leiomyosarcoma, and the numbers of patients are too small to permit evaluation of treatment efficacy.[137,139,140] Patients with close surgical margins may benefit from postoperative irradiation. Because lymph node metastasis from leiomyosarcoma is uncommon, treatment of the operative bed (usually the lower pelvis) may be sufficient in most cases.

Several authors reporting small series of patients with endometrial stromal tumors have commented on the role of radiation therapy, in some cases suggesting that it is effective[147-149] and in others suggesting that it is ineffective.[150] However, reports of radiation therapy for these tumors are little more than anecdotal, and further study is needed to adequately define the role of radiation therapy in this setting.

SUMMARY

Adenocarcinoma of the endometrium occurs predominantly in postmenopausal women, in whom vaginal bleeding is an alarming symptom. For this reason, the diagnosis is often made relatively early and disease control rates are good.

Survival rates of 85% to 90% can be expected for patients with clinical stage I disease. Survival rates for patients with stage II or III disease are significantly lower, approximately 65% and 35%, respectively. In every stage, poorly differentiated (grade 3) and deeply invasive tumors have a less favorable outlook. Regional lymph node metastases occur in a higher proportion of patients than previously suspected. They are much more common in patients with poorly differentiated or advanced lesions involving the cervix or extending beyond the uterus.

An overwhelming amount of data supports the role of radiation therapy in the treatment of patients with endometrial carcinoma. Radiation therapy decreases the frequency of pelvic recurrences and may improve survival rates in high-risk groups of patients.

A possible approach to selecting external-beam or intracavitary treatment for patients in various risk groups is illustrated in Figure 29-6. Patients with grade 1 or 2 disease with no myometrial invasion are unlikely to benefit from adjuvant radiation therapy. Patients with stage IA, grade 3 disease have a low incidence of lymph node involvement, and vaginal brachytherapy alone is probably adequate to ensure optimal local control and minimal sequelae. Patients with stage IB, grade 1 or 2 tumors probably do not need any form of radiation therapy, but patients with stage IB, grade 3 tumors probably benefit from vaginal brachytherapy alone. Patients

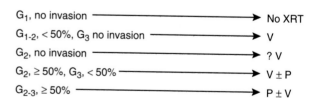

Fig. 29-6 Possible schema for postoperative treatment based on grade and depth of invasion for patients with stage I endometrial carcinoma. However, other prognostic factors, including tumor size and lymph node status, and risk factors for major complications also should be considered in the selection of treatment. *XRT,* Radiation therapy; *V,* vaginal vault radiation therapy; *P,* pelvic radiation therapy; *G,* histologic grade.

most likely to benefit from pelvic irradiation include those with high-grade disease or deep muscle invasion. This is true regardless of whether lymph node sampling has been performed. If patients have had extensive surgical staging or have other risk factors for serious bowel sequelae after pelvic radiation therapy, consideration should be given to treatment with vaginal applicators alone.

REFERENCES

1. Greenlee RT, Hill-Harmon MB, Murray T, et al: Cancer statistics, 2001. *CA Cancer J Clin* 2001;51:15-36.
2. Parazzini F, LaVecchia C. Epidemiology of adenocarcinoma of the cervix. *Gynecol Oncol* 1990;39:40-46.
3. Antunes CM, Stolley PD, Rosenshein NB, et al. Endometrial cancer and estrogen use: report of a large case-control study. *N Engl J Med* 1979;300:9-13.
4. Fajardo LF, Berthrong M, Anderson RE. Female reproductive organs. In: *Radiation Pathology.* New York, NY: Oxford University Press; 2001:289-299.
5. Morice P, Thiam-Ba R, Castaigne D, et al. Fertility results after ovarian transposition for pelvic malignancies treated by external irradiation or brachytherapy. *Hum Reprod* 1998;13:660-663.
6. Mitchell MF, Gershenson DM, Soeters RP, et al. The long-term effects of radiation therapy on patients with ovarian dysgerminoma. *Cancer* 1991;67:1084-1090.
7. Dede JA, Plentl AA, Moore JG. Recurrent endometrial carcinoma. *Surg Gynecol Obstet* 1968;126:533-542.
8. Zaino RJ. Pathologic indicators of prognosis in endometrial adenocarcinoma. Selected aspects emphasizing the Gynecologic Oncology Group experience. *Pathol Annu* 1995;30:1-28.
9. Taylor RR, Zeller J, Lieberman RW, et al. An analysis of two versus three grades for endometrial carcinoma. *Gynecol Oncol* 1999;74:3-6.
10. Hendrickson M, Ross M, Eifel P, et al. Uterine papillary serous carcinoma. A highly malignant form of endometrial adenocarcinoma. *Am J Surg Pathol* 1982;6:93-108.
11. Carcangiu ML, Chambers JT. Early pathologic stage clear cell carcinoma and uterine papillary serous carcinoma of the endometrium: comparison of clinicopathologic features and survival. *Int J Gynecol Pathol* 1995;14:30-38.
12. Greenwood SM, Wright DJ. Evaluation of the office endometrial biopsy in the detection of endometrial carcinoma and atypical hyperplasia. *Cancer* 1979;43:1474-1478.
13. Koss LG, Schreiber K, Moussouris H, et al. Endometrial carcinoma and its precursors: detection and screening. *Clin Obstet Gynecol* 1982;25:49-61.
14. Mannel RS, Berman ML, Walker JL, et al. Management of endometrial cancer with suspected cervical involvement. *Obstet Gynecol* 1990;75:1016-1022.
15. Rose PG, Sommers RM, Reale FR, et al. Serial serum CA-125 measurements for evaluation of recurrence in patients with endometrial carcinoma. *Obstet Gynecol* 1994;84:12-16.
16. Patsner B, Mann WJ. Use of serum CA-125 in monitoring patients with uterine sarcoma. A preliminary report. *Cancer* 1988; 62:1355-1358.
17. Frei KA, Kinkel K, Bonel HM, et al. Prediction of deep myometrial invasion in patients with endometrial cancer: clinical utility of contrast-enhanced MR imaging—a meta-analysis and Bayesian analysis. *Radiology* 2000;216:444-449.
18. Hricak H, Stern JL, Fisher MR, et al. Endometrial carcinoma staging by MR imaging. *Radiology* 1987;162:297-305.
19. Seki H, Takano T, Sakai K. Value of dynamic MR imaging in assessing endometrial carcinoma involvement of the cervix. *AJR Am J Roentgenol* 2000;175:171-176.
20. Kinkel K, Kaji Y, Yu KK, et al. Radiologic staging in patients with endometrial cancer: a meta-analysis. *Radiology* 1999;212:711-718.
21. Cowles TA, Magrina JF, Masterson BJ, et al. Comparison of clinical and surgical-staging in patients with endometrial carcinoma. *Obstet Gynecol* 1985;66:413-416.
22. Creasman W, Morrow C, Bundy B, et al. Surgical pathologic spread patterns of endometrial cancer. A Gynecologic Oncology Group Study. *Cancer* 1987;60:2035-2041.
23. International Federation of Gynecology and Obstetrics. Corpus cancer staging. *Int J Gynaecol Obstet* 1989;28:190.
24. Fleming I, Cooper JS, Henson DE, et al, eds. *AJCC Cancer Staging Manual.* 5th ed. Philadelphia, Pa: Lippincott Williams & Wilkins; 1997:195-200.
25. Greven KM, Corn BW. Endometrial cancer. *Curr Probl Cancer* 1997;21:65-127.
26. Carey MS, O'Connell GJ, Johanson CR, et al. Good outcome associated with a standardized treatment protocol using selective postoperative radiation in patients with clinical stage I adenocarcinoma of the endometrium. *Gynecol Oncol* 1995;57:138-144.
27. Irwin C, Levin W, Fyles A, et al. The role of adjuvant radiotherapy in carcinoma of the endometrium—results in 550 patients with pathologic stage I disease. *Gynecol Oncol* 1998;70:247-254.
28. Grigsby PW, Perez CA, Kuten A, et al. Clinical stage I endometrial cancer: prognostic factors for local control and distant metastasis and implications of the new FIGO surgical staging system. *Int J Radiat Oncol Biol Phys* 1992;22:905-911.
29. Aalders J, Abeler V, Kolstad P, et al. Postoperative external irradiation and prognostic parameters in stage I endometrial carcinoma. *Obstet Gynecol* 1980;56:419-427.
30. Rose PG. Endometrial carcinoma [published erratum appears in *N Engl J Med* 1997;336:1335]. *N Engl J Med* 1996;335:640-649.
31. Wharton JT, Mikuta JJ, Mettlin C, et al. Risk factors and current management in carcinoma of the endometrium. *Surg Gynecol Obstet* 1986;162:515-520.
32. Sutton GP, Geisler HE, Stehman FB, et al. Features associated with survival and disease-free survival in early endometrial cancer. *Am J Obstet Gynecol* 1989;160:1385-1391.
33. Chambers SK, Kapp DS, Peschel RE, et al. Prognostic factors and sites of failure in FIGO stage I, grade 3 endometrial carcinoma. *Gynecol Oncol* 1987;27:180-188.
34. Lewis BV, Stallworthy JA, Cowdell R. Adenocarcinoma of the body of the uterus. *J Obstet Gynaecol Br Commonw* 1970;77:343-348.
35. Silverberg SG, Bolin MG, DeGiorgi LS. Adenoacanthoma and mixed adenosquamous carcinoma of the endometrium. A clinicopathologic study. *Cancer* 1972;30:1307-1314.
36. Ng AB, Reagan JW, Storaasli JP, et al. Mixed adenosquamous carcinoma of the endometrium. *Am J Clin Pathol* 1973;59:765-781.
37. Zaino RJ, Kurman R, Herbold D, et al. The significance of squamous differentiation in endometrial carcinoma. A Gynecologic Oncology Group Study. *Cancer* 1991;68:2293-2302.
38. Cirisano FD Jr, Robboy SJ, Dodge RK, et al. The outcome of stage I-II clinically and surgically staged papillary serous and clear cell endometrial cancers when compared with endometrioid carcinoma. *Gynecol Oncol* 2000;77:55-65.
39. Morrow C, Bundy B, Kurman R, et al. Relationship between surgical-pathological risk factors and outcome in clinical stage I and II carcinoma of the endometrium: a Gynecologic Oncology Group Study. *Gynecol Oncol* 1991;40:55-65.
40. Zaino RJ, Kurman RJ, Diana KL, et al. Pathologic models to predict outcome for women with endometrial adenocarcinoma: the importance of the distinction between surgical stage and clinical stage—a Gynecologic Oncology Group study [published erratum appears in *Cancer* 1997;79:422]. *Cancer* 1996;77:1115-1121.
41. Silva EG, Jenkins R. Serous carcinoma in endometrial polyps. *Mod Pathol* 1990;3:120-128.

42. Fanning J, Alvarez PM, Tsukada Y, et al. Prognostic significance of the extent of cervical involvement by endometrial cancer. *Gynecol Oncol* 1991;40:46-47.

43. Schink JC, Rademaker AW, Miller DS, et al. Tumor size in endometrial cancer. *Cancer* 1991;67:2791-2794.

44. Potish RA. Radiation therapy of periaortic node metastases in cancer of the uterine cervix and endometrium. *Radiology* 1987;165:567-570.

45. Rose P, Cha S, Tak W, et al. Radiation therapy for surgically proven para-aortic node metastasis in endometrial carcinoma. *Int J Radiat Oncol Biol Phys* 1992;24:229-233.

46. Feuer G, Calanog A. Endometrial carcinoma. Treatment of positive paraaortic nodes. *Gynecol Oncol* 1987;27:104-109.

47. Corn BR, Lanciano K, Greven D, et al. Endometrial cancer with para-aortic adenopathy: patterns of failure and opportunities for cure. *Int J Radiat Oncol Biol Phys* 1992;24:223-227.

48. Turner DA, Gershenson DM, Atkinson N, et al. The prognostic significance of peritoneal cytology for stage I endometrial cancer. *Obstet Gynecol* 1989;74:775-780.

49. Milosevic MF, Dembo AJ, Thomas GM. The clinical significance of malignant peritoneal cytology in stage I endometrial carcinoma. *Int J Gynecol Cancer* 1992;2:225-235.

50. Grimshaw RN, Tupper C, Fraser RC, et al. Prognostic value of peritoneal cytology in endometrial carcinoma. *Gynecol Oncol* 1990;36:97-100.

51. Eifel P, Hendrickson M, Ross J, et al. Simultaneous presentation of carcinoma involving the ovary and the uterine corpus. *Cancer* 1982;50:163-170.

52. Pearl ML, Johnston CM, Frank TS, et al. Synchronous dual primary ovarian and endometrial carcinomas. *Int J Gynaecol Obstet* 1993;43:305-312.

53. Girardi F, Petru E, Heydarfadai M, et al. Pelvic lymphadenectomy in the surgical treatment of endometrial cancer. *Gynecol Oncol* 1993;49:177-180.

54. Chuang L, Burke TW, Tornos C, et al. Staging laparotomy for endometrial carcinoma: assessment of retroperitoneal lymph nodes. *Gynecol Oncol* 1995;58:189-193.

55. Orr JW Jr, Holimon JL, Orr PF. Stage I corpus cancer: is teletherapy necessary? *Am J Obstet Gynecol* 1997;176:777-788.

56. Mohan DS, Samuels MA, Selim MA, et al. Long-term outcomes of therapeutic pelvic lymphadenectomy for stage I endometrial adenocarcinoma. *Gynecol Oncol* 1998;70:165-171.

57. Kilgore LC, Partridge EE, Alvarez RD, et al. Adenocarcinoma of the endometrium: survival comparisons of patients with and without pelvic node sampling. *Gynecol Oncol* 1995;56:29-33.

58. Piver MS, Hempling RE. A prospective trial of postoperative vaginal radium/cesium for grade 1-2 less than 50% myometrial invasion and pelvic radiation therapy for grade 3 or deep myometrial invasion in surgical stage I endometrial adenocarcinoma. *Cancer* 1990;66:1133-1138.

59. Kucera H, Vavra N, Weghaupt K. Benefit of external irradiation in pathologic stage I endometrial carcinoma: a prospective clinical trial of 605 patients who received postoperative vaginal irradiation and additional pelvic irradiation in the presence of unfavorable prognostic factors. *Gynecol Oncol* 1990;38:99-104.

60. Roberts JA, Brunetto VI, Keys HM, et al. A phase III randomized study of surgery vs surgery plus adjunctive radiation therapy in intermediate-risk endometrial adenocarcinoma (GOG No. 99) [abstract]. *Gynecol Oncol* 1998;68:135.

61. Lewandowski G, Torrisi J, Potkul RK, et al. Hysterectomy with extended surgical staging and radiotherapy versus hysterectomy alone and radiotherapy in stage I endometrial cancer: a comparison of complication rates. *Gynecol Oncol* 1990;36:401-404.

62. Naumann RW, Higgins RV, Hall JB. The use of adjuvant radiation therapy by members of the Society of Gynecologic Oncologists. *Gynecol Oncol* 1999;75:4-9.

63. Javert C, Douglas R. Treatment of endometrial adenocarcinoma. *Am J Roentgenol* 1956;75:580.

64. Keller D, Kempson FL, Levine G, et al. Management of the patient with early endometrial carcinoma. *Cancer* 1974;33:1108-1116.

65. Maggino T, Romagnolo C, Landoni F, et al. An analysis of approaches to the management of endometrial cancer in North America: a CTF study. *Gynecol Oncol* 1998;68:274-279.

66. Partridge EE, Shingleton HM, Menck HR. The National Cancer Data Base report on endometrial cancer. *J Surg Oncol* 1996;61:111-123.

67. Society of Gynecologic Oncologists. Practice guidelines: uterine corpus—sarcomas. Society of Gynecologic Oncologists Clinical Practice Guidelines. *Oncology (Huntingt)* 1998;12:284-286.

68. Jones HW. Treatment of adenocarcinoma of the endometrium. *Obstet Gynecol Surv* 1975;30:147-169.

69. Rutledge FN, Tan SK, Fletcher GH. Vaginal metastases from adenocarcinoma of the corpus uteri. *Am J Obstet Gynecol* 1958;75:167-174.

70. Lewis GC, Mortel R, Slack NH. Adenocarcinoma of the body of the uterus. *J Obstet Gynaecol Br Commw* 1977;77:342-348.

71. Eifel PJ, Ross J, Hendrickson M, et al. Adenocarcinoma of the endometrium. Analysis of 256 cases with disease limited to the uterine corpus: treatment options. *Cancer* 1983;52:1026-1031.

72. Underwood PB, Lutz MH, Kreutner A, et al. Carcinoma of the endometrium: radiation followed immediately by operation. *Am J Obstet Gynecol* 1977;128:86-95.

73. Ohlsen JD, Johnson GH, Stewart JR, et al. Combined therapy for endometrial carcinoma: preoperative intracavitary irradiation followed promptly by hysterectomy. *Cancer* 1977;39:659-664.

74. Bean HA, Bryant AJS, Carmichael JA, et al. Carcinoma of the endometrium in Saskatchewan: 1966 to 1971. *Gynecol Oncol* 1978;6:503-514.

75. Piver MS, Yazigi R, Blumenson L, et al. A prospective trial comparing hysterectomy, hysterectomy plus vaginal radium, and uterine radium plus hysterectomy in stage I endometrial carcinoma. *Obstet Gynecol* 1979;54:85-89.

76. Reddy S, Lee MS, Hendrickson FR. Pattern of recurrences in endometrial carcinoma and their management. *Radiology* 1979;133:737-740.

77. Sause WT, Fuller DB, Smith WG, et al. Analysis of preoperative intracavitary cesium application vs postoperative external beam radiation in stage I endometrial carcinoma. *Int J Radiat Oncol Biol Phys* 1990;18:1013-1019.

78. Grigsby PW, Perez CA, Kuten A, et al. Clinical stage I endometrial cancer: results of adjuvant irradiation and patterns of failure. *Int J Radiat Oncol Biol Phys* 1991;21:379-385.

79. Calais G, Vitu L, Descamps P, et al. Preoperative or postoperative brachytherapy for patients with endometrial carcinoma stage I and II. *Int J Radiat Oncol Biol Phys* 1990;19:523-527.

80. Creutzberg CL, van Putten WL, Koper PC, et al. Surgery and postoperative radiotherapy versus surgery alone for patients with stage-1 endometrial carcinoma: multicentre randomised trial. PORTEC Study Group. Post Operative Radiation Therapy in Endometrial Carcinoma. *Lancet* 2000;355:1404-1411.

81. Marchetti DL, Caglar H, Driscoll DL, et al. Pelvic radiation in stage I endometrial adenocarcinoma with high-risk attributes. *Gynecol Oncol* 1990;37:51-54.

82. Greven KM, Lanciano RM, Herbert SH, et al. Analysis of complications in patients with endometrial carcinoma receiving adjuvant irradiation. *Int J Radiat Oncol Biol Phys* 1991;21:919-923.

83. Corn BW, Lanciano RM, Greven KM, et al. Impact of improved irradiation technique, age and lymph node sampling on the severe complication rate of surgically staged endometrial cancer patients: a multivariate analysis. *J Clin Oncol* 1994;12:510-515.

84. Komaki R, Mattingly RF, Hoffman RG, et al. Irradiation of para-aortic lymph node metastases from carcinoma of the cervix or endometrium. Preliminary results. *Radiology* 1983;147:245-248.

85. Hicks ML, Piver MS, Puretz JL, et al. Survival in patients with paraaortic lymph node metastases from endometrial adenocarcinoma clinically limited to the uterus. *Int J Radiat Oncol Biol Phys* 1993;26:607-611.

86. Blythe JG, Edwards E, Heimbecker P. Paraaortic lymph node biopsy: a twenty-year study. *Am J Obstet Gynecol* 1997;176:1157-1162.

87. Onda T, Yoshikawa H, Mizutani K, et al. Treatment of node-positive endometrial cancer with complete node dissection, chemotherapy and radiation therapy. *Br J Cancer* 1997;75:1836-1841.

88. Potish RA. Abdominal radiotherapy for cancer of the uterine cervix and endometrium. *Int J Radiat Oncol Biol Phys* 1989;16:1453-1458.

89. Mallipeddi P, Kapp DS, Teng NNH. Long-term survival with adjuvant whole abdominopelvic irradiation for uterine papillary serous carcinoma. *Cancer* 1993;71:3076-3081.

90. Grice J, Ek M, Greer B, et al. Uterine papillary serous carcinoma: evaluation of long-term survival in surgically staged patients. *Gynecol Oncol* 1998;69:69-73.

91. Smith RS, Kapp DS, Chen Q, et al. Treatment of high-risk uterine cancer with whole abdominopelvic radiation therapy. *Int J Radiat Oncol Biol Phys* 2000;48:767-778.

92. Randall ME, Spirtos NM, Dvoretsky P. Whole abdominal radiotherapy versus combination chemotherapy with doxorubicin and cisplatin in advanced endometrial carcinoma (phase III): Gynecologic Oncology Group Study No. 122. *J Natl Cancer Inst Monogr* 1995;19:13-15.

93. Greven KM. Tailoring radiation to the extent of disease for uterine-confined endometrial cancer. *Semin Radiat Oncol* 2000;10:29-35.

94. Eltabbakh GH, Piver MS, Hempling RE, et al. Excellent long-term survival and absence of vaginal recurrences in 332 patients with low-risk stage I endometrial adenocarcinoma treated with hysterectomy and vaginal brachytherapy without formal staging lymph node sampling: report of a prospective trial. *Int J Radiat Oncol Biol Phys* 1997;38:373-380.

95. Fanning J, Nanavati PJ, Hilgers RD. Surgical staging and high dose rate brachytherapy for endometrial cancer: limiting external radiotherapy to node-positive tumors. *Obstet Gynecol* 1996;87:1041-1044.

96. MacLeod C, Fowler A, Duval P, et al. High-dose-rate brachytherapy alone post-hysterectomy for endometrial cancer. *Int J Radiat Oncol Biol Phys* 1998;42:1033-1039.

97. Greven KM, D'Agostino RB Jr, Lanciano RM, et al. Is there a role for a brachytherapy vaginal cuff boost in the adjuvant management of patients with uterine-confined endometrial cancer? *Int J Radiat Oncol Biol Phys* 1998;42:101-104.

98. Sorbe BG, Smeds AC. Postoperative vaginal irradiation with high dose rate after loading technique in endometrial carcinoma stage I. *Int J Radiat Oncol Biol Phys* 1990;18:305-314.

99. Thomas H, Pickerine GL, Dunn P, et al. Treating the vaginal vault in carcinoma of the endometrium using the Buchler afterloading system. *Br J Radiol* 1991;64:1044-1048.

100. Weiss E, Hirnle P, Arnold-Bofinger H, et al. Adjuvant vaginal high-dose-rate afterloading alone in endometrial carcinoma: patterns of relapse and side effects following low-dose therapy. *Gynecol Oncol* 1998;71:72-76.

101. Noyes WR, Bastin K, Edwards SA, et al. Postoperative vaginal cuff irradiation using high dose rate remote afterloading: a phase II clinical protocol. *Int J Radiat Oncol Biol Phys* 1995;32:1439-1443.

102. Grigsby P, Kuske R, Perez C, et al. Medically inoperable stage I adenocarcinoma of the endometrium treated with radiotherapy alone. *Int J Radiat Oncol Biol Phys* 1987;13:483-488.

103. Jones D, Stout R. Results of intracavitary radium treatment for adenocarcinoma of the body of the uterus. *Clin Radiol* 1986;37:169-171.

104. Kupelian PA, Eifel PJ, Tornos C, et al. Treatment of endometrial carcinoma with radiation therapy alone. *Int J Radiat Oncol Biol Phys* 1993;27:817-824.

105. Landgren R, Fletcher G, Delclos L, et al. Irradiation of endometrial cancer in patients with medical contraindication to surgery or with unresectable lesions. *Am J Roentgenol* 1976;126:148-154.

106. Lehoczky O, Bosze P, Ungar L, et al. Stage I endometrial carcinoma: treatment of nonoperable patients with intracavitary radiation therapy alone. *Gynecol Oncol* 1991;43:211-216.

107. Rose PG, Baker S, Kern M, et al. Primary radiation therapy for endometrial carcinoma: a case controlled study. *Int J Radiat Oncol Biol Phys* 1993;27:585-590.

108. Rouanet P, Dubois JB, Gely S, et al. Exclusive radiation therapy in endometrial carcinoma. *Int J Radiat Oncol Biol Phys* 1993;26:223-228.

109. Heyman J. The so-called Stockholm method and the results of treatment of uterine cancer at the Radiummhemmet. *Acta Radiol* 1935;22:129.

110. Luk KH, Castro JR, Meyler TS. 137Cs afterloading intrauterine packing for stage I and stage II adenocarcinoma of the endometrium. *Radiology* 1978;129:229-231

111. Chao CK, Grigsby PW, Perez CA, et al. Brachytherapy-related complications for medically inoperable stage I endometrial carcinoma. *Int J Radiat Oncol Biol Phys* 1995;31:37-42.

112. Grigsby PW. The role of radiotherapy in endometrial carcinoma. *Ann Acad Med Singapore* 1996;25:437-440.

113. Kucera H, Knocke TH, Kucera E, et al. Treatment of endometrial carcinoma with high-dose-rate brachytherapy alone in medically inoperable stage I patients. *Acta Obstet Gynecol Scand* 1998;77:1008-1012.

114. Nguyen C, Souhami L, Roman TN, et al. High-dose-rate brachytherapy as the primary treatment of medically inoperable stage I-II endometrial carcinoma. *Gynecol Oncol* 1995;59:370-375.

115. Nguyen TV, Petereit DG. High-dose-rate brachytherapy for medically inoperable stage I endometrial cancer. *Gynecol Oncol* 1998;71:196-203.

116. Knocke TH, Kucera H, Weidinger B, et al. Primary treatment of endometrial carcinoma with high-dose-rate brachytherapy: results of 12 years of experience with 280 patients. *Int J Radiat Oncol Biol Phys* 1997;37:359-365.

117. Petereit DG, Pearcey R. Literature analysis of high dose rate brachytherapy fractionation schedules in the treatment of cervical cancer: is there an optimal fractionation schedule? *Int J Radiat Oncol Biol Phys* 1999;43:359-366.

118. Petereit DG, Sarkaria JN, Chappell RJ. Perioperative morbidity and mortality of high-dose-rate gynecologic brachytherapy. *Int J Radiat Oncol Biol Phys* 1998;42:1025-1031.

119. Cliby WA, Dodson MK, Podratz KC. Cervical cancer complicated by pregnancy: episiotomy site recurrences following vaginal delivery. *Obstet Gynecol* 1994;84:179-182.

120. Copeland LJ, Saul PB, Sniege N. Cervical adenocarcinoma: tumor implantation in the episiotomy sites of two patients. *Gynecol Oncol* 1987;28:230-235.

121. Greven K, Olds W. Isolated vaginal recurrences of endometrial adenocarcinoma and their management. *Cancer* 1987;60:419-421.

122. Curran WJ, Whittington R, Peters AJ, et al. Vaginal recurrences of endometrial carcinoma: the prognostic value of staging by a primary vaginal carcinoma system. *Int J Radiat Oncol Biol Phys* 1988;15:803-808.

123. Sears JD, Greven KM, Hoen HM, et al. Prognostic factors and treatment outcome for patients with locally recurrent endometrial cancer. *Cancer* 1994;74:1303-1308.

124. Hart KB, Han I, Shamsa F, et al. Radiation therapy for endometrial cancer in patients treated for postoperative recurrence. *Int J Radiat Oncol Biol Phys* 1998;41:7-11.

125. Ackerman I, Malone S, Thomas G, et al. Endometrial carcinoma—relative effectiveness of adjuvant irradiation vs therapy reserved for relapse. *Gynecol Oncol* 1996;60:177-183.

126. Mandell LR, Nori D, Hilaris B. Recurrent stage I endometrial carcinoma: results of treatment and prognostic factors. *Int J Radiat Oncol Biol Phys* 1985;11:1103-1109.

127. Hoekstra CJ, Koper PC, van Putten WL. Recurrent endometrial adenocarcinoma after surgery alone: prognostic factors and treatment. *Radiother Oncol* 1993;27:164-166.

128. Wylie J, Irwin C, Pintilie M, et al. Results of radical radiotherapy for recurrent endometrial cancer. *Gynecol Oncol* 2000; 77:66-72.

129. Kuten A, Grigsby PW, Perez CA, et al. Results of radiotherapy in recurrent endometrial carcinoma: a retrospective analysis of 51 patients. *Int J Radiat Oncol Biol Phys* 1989;17:29-34.

130. Ingersol FM. Vaginal recurrences of carcinoma of the corpus—management and prevention. *Am J Surg* 1971;121:473-477.

131. Greven KM. Interstitial radiation for recurrent cervix or endometrial cancer in the suburethral region. *Int J Radiat Oncol Biol Phys* 1998;41:831-834.

132. Aalders JG, Abeler V, Kolstad P. Recurrent adenocarcinoma of the endometrium: a clinical and histopathological study of 379 patients. *Gynecol Oncol* 1984;17:85-103.

133. Badib AO, Kurohara SS, Beitia AA, et al. Recurrent cancer of the corpus uteri: techniques and results of treatment. *Am J Roentgenol* 1969;105:596-602.

134. DiSaia PJ, Castro JR, Rutledge FN. Mixed mesodermal sarcoma of the uterus. *Am J Roentgenol Radium Ther Nucl Med* 1973; 117:632-636.

135. Echt G, Jepson J, Steel J, et al. Treatment of uterine sarcomas. *Cancer* 1990;66:35-39.

136. George M, Pejovic MH, Kramar A. Uterine sarcomas: prognostic factors and treatment modalities—study on 209 patients. *Gynecol Oncol* 1986;24:58-67.

137. Hornback NB, Omura G, Major FJ. Observations on the use of adjuvant radiation therapy in patients with stage I and II uterine sarcoma. *Int J Radiat Oncol Biol Phys* 1986;12:2127-2130.

138. Larson B, Silfverswärd C, Nilsson B, et al. Mixed Müllerian tumours of the uterus—prognostic factors: a clinical and histopathologic study of 147 cases. *Radiother Oncol* 1990;17:123-132.

139. Major FJ, Blessing JA, Silverberg SG, et al. Prognostic factors in early-stage uterine sarcoma. *Cancer* 1993;71:1702-1709.

140. Moskovic E, Macsweeney E, Law M, et al. Survival, patterns of spread and prognostic factors in uterine sarcoma: a study of 76 patients. *Br J Radiol* 1993;66:1009-1015.

141. Salazar OM, Dunne ME. The role of radiation therapy in the management of uterine sarcomas. *Int J Radiat Oncol Biol Phys* 1980;6:899-902.

142. Sorbe B. Radiotherapy and/or chemotherapy as adjuvant treatment of uterine sarcomas. *Gynecol Oncol* 1985;20:281-289.

143. Wheelock JB, Krebs HB, Schneider V, et al. Uterine sarcoma: analysis of prognostic variables in 71 cases. *Am J Obstet Gynecol* 1985;151:1016-1022.

144. Gerszten K, Faul C, Kounelis S, et al. The impact of adjuvant radiotherapy on carcinosarcoma of the uterus. *Gynecol Oncol* 1998;68:8-13.

145. Ferrer F, Sabater S, Farrus B, et al. Impact of radiotherapy on local control and survival in uterine sarcomas: a retrospective study from the Grup Oncologic Catala-Occita. *Int J Radiat Oncol Biol Phys* 1999;44:47-52.

146. Chauveinc L, Deniaud E, Plancher C, et al. Uterine sarcomas: the Curie Institut experience. Prognosis factors and adjuvant treatments. *Gynecol Oncol* 1999;72:232-237.

147. Rose PG, Boutselis JG, Sachs L. Adjuvant therapy for stage I uterine sarcoma. *Am J Obstet Gynecol* 1987;156:660-662.

148. Larson B, Silfverswärd C, Nilsson B, et al. Endometrial stromal sarcoma of the uterus. A clinical and histopathological study. The Radiumhemmet series 1936-1981. *Eur J Obstet Gynecol Reprod Biol* 1990;35:239-249.

149. Berchuck A, Rubin SC, Hoskins WJ, et al. Treatment of endometrial stromal tumors. *Gynecol Oncol* 1990;36:60-65.

150. DeFusco PA, Gaffey TA, Malkasian GD, et al. Endometrial stromal sarcoma: review of Mayo Clinic experience, 1945-1980. *Gynecol Oncol* 1989;35:8-14.

CHAPTER 30

The Vulva and Vagina

Patricia J. Eifel

EFFECTS OF RADIATION ON THE NORMAL VULVA AND VAGINA
Effects on the Vulva

The external vulva and perineal skin respond to radiation therapy in a manner similar to how other skin responds. Acutely, a brisk erythema may develop with epilation of the pubic hair; as the dose of radiation is increased, patchy or confluent desquamation may occur. The acute skin reaction usually heals within 2 to 3 weeks after the completion of radiation therapy.

Hyperpigmentation and epilation may resolve more slowly, and permanent perineal epilation can occur after high doses (more than 40 to 50 Gy). Over time, the vulvar skin may become atrophic and telangiectasia may develop, particularly if the vulva has received more than 50 to 60 Gy. Diminished estrogen levels may increase the severity of vulvar atrophy. The effects of vulvar radiation therapy on sexual function and satisfaction have not been comprehensively studied.

Effects on the Vagina

The effects of pelvic radiation therapy on vaginal function are related to the dose of radiation, the amount of vaginal mucosa treated to a high cumulative dose, the extent of tissue destruction by tumor, and the care given after irradiation (including estrogen support). Patient factors such as age, menopausal status, and sexual activity also play a role. The vagina is often said to tolerate very high doses of radiation, but these comments usually refer to the relatively low incidence of major side effects involving adjacent organs (bladder, urethra, and rectum) after vaginal intracavitary irradiation. The effect of radiation on these structures is discussed later in this chapter and in Chapter 28.

The influence of radiation therapy on vaginal function, and specifically on sexual function, is much less well documented. Preliminary studies suggest that women who have been treated for cervical or endometrial carcinoma tend to have gradual shortening of the vagina during the first few years after treatment.[1] This is associated with a tendency for treated women to be less sexually active and to report a decrease in sexual satisfaction. However, the specific causes for this decreased sexual activity and satisfaction are not well established.

Typically, definitive treatment of carcinoma of the cervix results in a maximum total dose of 100 to 140 Gy to the apical vagina. Acutely, this treatment causes edema and congestion of the vaginal mucosa.[2] Superficial erosion may appear in the first few months. Over several years, the upper vagina and cervix may become scarred and agglutinated, obscuring the cervical os. These changes may progress over many years and probably accelerate if estrogen support is withdrawn or if the patient is sexually inactive. In some cases, severe foreshortening of the vagina occurs, compromising satisfying sexual intercourse. Severe narrowing and foreshortening of the vagina occurs more commonly in women who are treated when they are postmenopausal.[3] This finding may reflect less consistent use of estrogen replacement therapy, less frequent sexual intercourse, and poorer compliance with recommended use of vaginal dilators.[4]

EPIDEMIOLOGY OF VULVAR AND VAGINAL CANCER

Invasive carcinomas of the vulva and vagina are rare neoplasms, affecting only about 4% and 2% of women with gynecologic tumors, respectively.[5,6] These types of cancer tend to affect elderly women; the median age of women diagnosed with vulvar or vaginal cancer is 65 to 70 years, and the incidence peaks in women more than 70 years old.[6,7]

Evidence that human papillomavirus (HPV) may play a role in the pathogenesis of cervical cancer has led investigators to look for HPV deoxyribonucleic acid (DNA) in vulvar and vaginal neoplasms. Ikenberg and colleagues[8] found HPV DNA in 10 of 18 cases of vaginal cancer. Invasive vaginal carcinoma has also been associated with chronic irritant vaginitis, particularly that type caused by chronic use of a vaginal pessary.[9] It has been suggested that the squamous metaplasia that occurs during healing of mucosal abrasions may encourage HPV infections that, under appropriate conditions, lead to neoplastic transformation.[10]

Although 80% to 90% of vulvar intraepithelial neoplasia (VIN) lesions contain HPV, only 30% to 50% of invasive vulvar carcinomas are associated with evidence of HPV infection.[11,12] Women with HPV-positive tumors tend to be relatively young and have risk factors similar to those associated with cervical cancer.[11,13,14] Some investigators have found a higher rate of *p53* mutations in women with HPV-negative tumors, suggesting that inactivation of *p53* is important in patients with HPV-positive or HPV-negative tumors.[15]

In the early 1970s, an increase in the rate of a rare form of clear cell adenocarcinoma of the vagina and cervix was found to be associated with maternal ingestion of diethylstilbestrol (DES) during pregnancy.[16] The peak number of DES-associated adenocarcinomas occurred in 1975; the incidence then declined as public awareness led to a decrease in the use of DES to prevent miscarriage.[17] The peak risk period for development of adenocarcinoma of the vagina and cervix in women exposed to DES in utero was between the ages of 15 and 22 years. Newly reported cases are now rare in the cohort of exposed women, most of whom are now more than 40 years old. As yet, no clear evidence exists that DES-exposed women are at risk for malignancies other than clear cell carcinoma.[18]

NATURAL HISTORY AND PATTERN OF SPREAD
Vulvar Cancer

About two thirds of vulvar squamous carcinomas involve the labia majora or minora.[19,20] A smaller percentage arise in the clitoris or gynecologic perineum. About 10% are multifocal or too extensive to permit identification of a site of origin. From the site of origin, carcinomas of the vulva can extend to invade the vagina, urethra, or anus; advanced vulvar carcinoma can invade adjacent pelvic bones, particularly the pubis.

The vulva is richly supplied with lymphatic vessels that often cross the midline. As a result, the risk of regional spread is significant for any vulvar carcinoma that has invaded to a depth of more than 1 mm.[19,21] The primary site of lymphatic drainage is to the superficial inguinal nodes. Although carcinomas of the clitoris and Bartholin's gland occasionally spread directly to the deep femoral and even obturator lymph nodes, these nodal groups are rarely involved without evidence of superficial inguinal metastases.[20,22] Despite the extensive anastomosis of lymphatics in the region, metastasis of vulvar carcinoma to contralateral lymph nodes is uncommon in patients with well-lateralized T1 lesions.[23]

The most common site of hematogenous metastasis from vulvar cancer is the lung. Advanced cancer can also spread to bone, liver, and other sites.

Vaginal Cancer

Vaginal cancer arises more often in the upper third of the vagina but may also originate in the middle or lower third; a fairly even distribution of lesions is evident, arising on the anterior, posterior, and lateral walls.[24-27] About 60% of primary apical vaginal cancer is diagnosed in women who have undergone hysterectomy. This is probably a result of the International Federation of Gynecology and Obstetrics (FIGO) convention that classifies any tumor involving both the cervix and vagina as a cervical cancer.

Vaginal cancer spreads laterally to involve the paravaginal tissues and may become fixed to pelvic-wall structures. Although vaginal cancer can invade the adjacent urethra, bladder, or rectum, fewer than 10% of cases involve the mucosa of these structures at presentation.[5,25,27,28]

The vagina, like the vulva, is richly supplied with mucosal and submucosal lymphatics.[29] Nearly all of the pelvic lymph nodes may serve as primary sites of lymphatic drainage from vaginal tumors; the specific nodes at risk depend on the primary tumor location. The drainage of apical vaginal tumors is similar to that of cervical cancer, with initial regional spread primarily to the obturator and hypogastric nodes. The lymphatics of the posterior wall anastomose with those of the anterior rectal wall, draining to the superior and inferior gluteal nodes. Tumors involving the lower third of the vagina drain either to the pelvic nodes or by way of the vulvar lymphatics to the inguinofemoral lymph nodes. Although few data have been collected concerning the risk of regional spread of vaginal cancer, available studies suggest that at least 25% of patients with stage II vaginal cancer have pelvic node metastases.[30,31]

The most common site of hematogenous metastasis from vaginal cancer is the lung. Advanced cancer can also spread to bone, liver, and other sites.

PATHOLOGY

VIN and vaginal intraepithelial neoplasia (VAIN) share many of the clinical and histologic features of cervical intraepithelial neoplasia, although VIN and VAIN tend to occur in older women. Histologically, these lesions are characterized by disruption of the normal epithelial architecture with varying degrees of cytoplasmic and nuclear maturation.[13,32] About 4% of patients treated for VIN subsequently develop an invasive cancer.[33]

Paget's disease of the vulva is a very rare intraepithelial lesion of the epidermis and skin adnexa that typically presents in postmenopausal white women as a pruritic, red, sharply demarcated lesion on the labia majora. Histologically, it is characterized by large, pale, mucopolysaccharide-rich cells that probably arise from primitive epithelial progenitor cells.[34] About 5% to 10% of newly diagnosed Paget's lesions are associated with underlying adenocarcinoma arising in the vulva or a distant site.[35]

More than 90% of invasive vulvar tumors and 80% to 90% of primary vaginal malignancies are squamous cell carcinomas.[5-7] Invasive vulvar carcinomas are most commonly well-differentiated keratinizing squamous carcinomas; HPV-positive tumors often have a wartlike or basaloid growth pattern. Histologically, invasive vaginal carcinomas are similar to squamous tumors from other sites. They are usually well to moderately differentiated and may or may not exhibit prominent keratin formation. Verrucous carcinoma is a rare variant of squamous cell carcinoma that presents as a warty, fungating mass in the vulva or vagina.[36,37] This well-differentiated lesion rarely metastasizes but can be highly infiltrative and locally destructive.

Although they are very rare, primary small-cell anaplastic carcinomas can arise in the vulva or vagina. These tumors resemble neuroendocrine, small-cell anaplastic carcinomas of the lung or cervix, may be admixed with areas of squamous carcinoma or adenocarcinoma, and tend to behave aggressively, with frequent recurrence and distant metastasis.[38-40]

When adenocarcinoma occurs in the vagina, metastasis or local extension from other sites must be ruled out. Except for clear cell carcinomas associated with in utero DES exposure, most primary adenocarcinomas of the vagina occur in postmenopausal women. Adenocarcinomas account for fewer than 5% to 10% of vaginal cancer cases and can demonstrate a variety of müllerian histologic patterns. They may arise in foci of adenosis or endometriosis.[41] Adenocarcinomas of the vagina can arise in or around Bartholin's gland. Rarely, these tumors have an adenoid cystic pattern.[42]

Malignant melanomas of the vulva and vagina represent fewer than 5% of primary neoplasms in these sites.[43,44] A poorer prognosis is associated with deep invasion, ulceration, clinical amelanosis, and older age.[45] Chung and colleagues[46] and Tasseron and colleagues[47] proposed a modification of the Clark classification system (a method of classifying malignant cutaneous melanomas on the basis of level of invasion) that is often used to categorize vulvar melanomas.[46,47] Primary vaginal melanomas usually originate in the lower third of the vagina and tend to have a poorer prognosis than vulvar melanomas (for vaginal melanomas, 5-year survival rates are only 15% to 20% despite aggressive treatment).[48,49]

About 1% to 2% of vulvovaginal malignancies are soft-tissue sarcomas. Leiomyosarcomas are most common, followed by a variety of other histologic subtypes. Risk factors for local recurrence and metastasis are similar to those reported for primary sarcomas arising at other sites and include large size, close surgical margins, and high grade.[50,51] Embryonal rhabdomyosarcoma (sarcoma botryoides) occurs in these sites, particularly in children less than 6 years of age, and is usually treated with chemotherapy combined with surgery or radiation therapy.[52] (Rhabdomyosarcoma is discussed further in Chapter 36.)

DIAGNOSIS, CLINICAL EVALUATION, AND STAGING

Carcinomas involving the vulva and vagina are classified according to FIGO guidelines. Cases are classified as vaginal carcinomas only when "the primary site of the growth is in the vagina."[5] Any tumor that has extended from the vulva to involve the vagina should be classified as a primary vulvar cancer, and any tumor that involves the area of the external cervical os should be classified as a cervical carcinoma.

Patients with invasive vulvar carcinoma usually present with pruritus or a mass; patients with VIN, however, may be asymptomatic at diagnosis.[53,54] Advanced vulvar lesions may be extremely painful. Patients with primary vaginal carcinoma usually present with abnormal vaginal bleeding but may also have pain (including dyspareunia), discharge, or a mass.

All patients with invasive disease should be evaluated with a careful physical examination including a detailed pelvic examination, chest radiography, a complete blood count, and a biochemical profile. In some cases, colposcopy may be needed to rule out a concurrent cervical cancer. Cystoscopy should be performed in patients with tumors near the bladder or urethra, and proctoscopy should be performed in patients with tumors near the anus or rectum. Computed tomography (CT) or magnetic resonance imaging (MRI) scans should be done to evaluate deep inguinal and pelvic lymph nodes, localize the kidneys, and rule out hydronephrosis. MRI may also be very helpful in delineating the distribution of disease in patients with locally advanced vaginal cancer, although the results cannot be used to alter the clinical stage assigned to the lesion.

The FIGO staging system for carcinoma of the vulva was changed from a clinical to a surgical staging system in 1988 and depends on "thorough histopathologic evaluation of the operative specimen (vulva and lymph nodes)." The staging system was revised again in 1994 to create a separate stage IA for tumors that invade no more than 1 mm (Box 30-1).[6,55] Today, many locally advanced vulvar lesions are being treated with initial radiation or chemoradiation; consequently, the absence of a complete surgical specimen may interfere with accurate staging, particularly of the inguinal lymph nodes. FIGO has yet to address this problem.

The FIGO rules for clinical staging of patients with carcinoma of the vagina (Table 30-1)[57] are the same as those for clinical staging of patients with cervical cancer. The categories are also similar, although the differentiation of stage I from stage II tends to be quite subjective because it is often impossible to accurately assess the presence or absence of subvaginal involvement by clinical examination alone. Perez and colleagues[28] recommend a modification of the FIGO system that distinguishes tumors that infiltrate the parametrium (stage IIB) from tumors with

---

BOX 30-1　American Joint Committee on Cancer Staging System for Cancer of the Vulva

PRIMARY TUMOR (T)

TX　Primary tumor cannot be assessed
T0　No evidence of primary tumor
Tis　Carcinoma in situ (preinvasive carcinoma)
T1　Tumor confined to the vulva or vulva and
　　perineum, 2 cm or less in greatest dimension
　　T1a　Tumor confined to the vulva or vulva and
　　　　perineum, 2 cm or less in greatest
　　　　dimension, and with stromal invasion no
　　　　greater than 1 mm*
　　T1b　Tumor confined to the vulva or vulva and
　　　　perineum, 2 cm or less in greatest
　　　　dimension, and with stromal invasion
　　　　greater than 1 mm*
T2　Tumor confined to the vulva or vulva and
　　perineum, more than 2 cm in greatest dimension
T3　Tumor of any size with adjacent spread to the
　　lower urethra and/or vagina or anus
T4　Tumor invades any of the following: upper
　　urethral mucosa, bladder mucosa, rectal mucosa,
　　or is fixed to the pubic bone

REGIONAL LYMPH NODES (N)

NX　Regional lymph nodes cannot be assessed
N0　No regional lymph node metastasis
N1　Unilateral regional lymph node metastasis
N2　Bilateral regional lymph node metastasis

DISTANT METASTASIS (M)

MX　Distant metastases cannot be assessed
M0　No distant metastasis
M1　Distant metastasis (including pelvic lymph node
　　metastasis)

STAGE GROUPING (AJCC + INTERNATIONAL FEDERATION OF GYNECOLOGY AND OBSTETRICS)

Stage 0	Tis	N0	M0
Stage IA	T1a	N0	M0
Stage IB	T1b	N0	M0
Stage II	T2	N0	M0
Stage III	T1	N1	M0
	T2	N1	M0
	T3	N0	M0
	T3	N1	M0
Stage IVA	T1	N2	M0
	T2	N2	M0
	T3	N2	M0
	T4	Any N	M0
Stage IVB	Any T	Any N	M1

From Fleming I, Cooper JS, Henson DE, et al, eds. *AJCC Cancer Staging Manual.* 5th ed. Philadelphia, Pa: Lippincott Williams & Wilkins; 1997:181-184.

*The depth of invasion is defined as the measurement of the tumor from the epithelial-stromal junction of the adjacent most superficial dermal papilla to the deepest point of invasion.

TABLE 30-1

International Federation of Gynecology and Obstetrics Clinical Staging System for Carcinoma of the Vagina

Stage 0	Carcinoma in situ, intraepithelial carcinoma.
Stage I	The carcinoma is limited to the vaginal wall.
Stage II	The carcinoma has involved the subvaginal tissues but has not extended onto the pelvic wall.
Stage III	The carcinoma has extended onto the pelvic wall.
Stage IV	The carcinoma has extended beyond the true pelvis or has clinically involved the mucosa of the bladder or rectum. Bullous edema as such does not permit a case to be allotted to stage IV.
Stage IVA	Spread of the growth to adjacent organs and/or direct extension beyond the true pelvis.
Stage IVB	Spread to distant organs.

From Shepherd J, Sideri M, Benedet J, et al. *J Epidemiol Biostat* 1998;3:103-109.

paravaginal submucosal extension only (stage IIA). However, this system fails to clearly define what is meant by parametrium, particularly for women who have no uterus.

The American Joint Committee on Cancer (AJCC) suggests a tumor-nodes-metastasis (TNM) staging system that allows alteration of stage assignment according to the presence of regional lymph node involvement. This system has not gained acceptance because patients rarely have surgical treatment for vaginal cancer because the stage groupings are inconsistent with accepted FIGO staging criteria and no accepted guidelines are available for determination of regional involvement.

PROGNOSTIC FACTORS
Vulvar Cancer

In patients with vulvar carcinoma, outcomes and the risk of regional metastasis are strongly correlated with tumor size, depth of invasion, tumor thickness, and the presence or absence of lymphovascular space invasion.[58-61] More than 75% of patients with lymphovascular space invasion have positive inguinal nodes.[21,59,62] Various conclusions have been drawn about the prognostic importance of tumor grade and patient age.[21,59,62-65]

The presence or absence of inguinal lymph node involvement has traditionally been considered to be one of the strongest predictors of prognosis. In a 1991 review of 586 patients entered in two Gynecologic Oncology Group (GOG) trials,[66] the authors reported 5-year survival rates of 91% for patients with negative inguinal lymph nodes and 75%, 36%, and 24%, respectively, for patients with one or two, three or four, or five or six positive nodes. However, more than half of the patients with positive nodes did not receive postoperative radiation therapy, which is currently considered standard treatment. For patients who were treated with radiation therapy in a GOG randomized trial published by Homesley and colleagues,[67] no clear difference in outcome was found between patients with one versus two or more positive lymph nodes (Fig. 30-1). In a study by van der Velden and colleagues,[68] findings of extracapsular extension or more than two positive lymph nodes were important predictors of recurrence. However, even though some patients in that study underwent irradiation of the pelvis and inguinal nodes, the impact of radiation therapy was not analyzed. Origoni and colleagues[69] also reported a correlation between extracapsular extension and recurrence.

The very poor 5-year survival rates reported for patients with positive pelvic lymph nodes (23% in the GOG trial)[67] led FIGO to categorize such disease as stage IV.

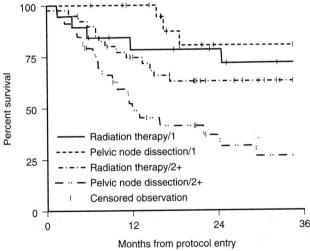

Fig. 30-1 Results of a Gynecologic Oncology Group randomized trial in patients who underwent radical vulvectomy and inguinal node dissection and were found to have inguinal lymph node metastases. Patients were randomly assigned intraoperatively to additional pelvic lymph node dissection (after frozen section diagnosis of inguinal metastases) or postoperative radiation therapy to the pelvis and inguinal nodes. Survival was found to be related to treatment and the number of positive inguinal nodes. (From Homesley HD, Bundy BN, Sedlis A, et al. *Obstet Gynecol* 1986;68:733.)

However, these patients were usually treated with surgery alone; because patients treated with radiation therapy rarely undergo pelvic lymph node dissection, the curability of patients with pelvic node metastases is unknown.

Heaps and colleagues[60] reported a correlation between the tumor-free margin in vulvar excision specimens and the incidence of local failure. They saw no local recurrences in 91 cases in which the uninvolved margin was 8 mm or larger in the fixed specimen (equivalent to about 10 mm in fresh tissue). In contrast, 18 (50%) of 36 patients who had margins smaller than 8 mm experienced a local recurrence.

Vaginal Cancer

Outcome in patients with vaginal cancer is correlated strongly with tumor stage.[24,25,28,70,71] Several investigators have also reported a correlation between outcome and tumor size (measured in centimeters or as the percentage of vaginal wall involved).[24,25,27] Infiltrating, necrotic lesions tend to have a poorer prognosis than exophytic tumors.[28] Tumors that involve the entire vagina tend to have a poor prognosis; however, attempts to correlate the site of vaginal tumors with outcome have yielded variable results.[24,25,28,70,71] Investigators also disagree about the influence of histologic grade and type (e.g., squamous cell carcinoma vs. adenocarcinoma) on outcome.[24,25,31,72,73]

TREATMENT OF VULVAR CANCER
Treatment of Preinvasive Disease

Small VIN lesions are treated with local excision. More extensive VIN can be treated with carbon dioxide (CO_2) laser vaporization. However, careful inspection and biopsies to rule out invasive disease should be done before laser treatment. Extensive disease may require wide local excision or excision of the superficial skin of the vulva (skinning vulvectomy). Although the morbidity of excision may be greater than that of laser vaporization, the ability to examine the surgical specimen is a relative advantage of surgical excision. VIN is often a multicentric disease, and local recurrences often occur even after extensive surgical resection.[74]

Surgical Treatment of Invasive Carcinoma

Minimally invasive vulvar tumors that infiltrate less than 1 mm from the most superficial basement membrane have a very low risk of regional metastasis (< 1%) and can be treated with wide local excision only.[19,21,75] In the most recent modification of its staging system, FIGO subclassified these early lesions in a new stage IA category.[6]

Any tumor that invades more than 1 mm from the most superficial basement membrane requires treatment aimed at both the local tumor and the regional nodes.

Surgical management of vulvar cancer has evolved away from the highly morbid radical en bloc resections that were traditional 20 years ago and toward increasingly individualized, tissue-sparing procedures. In the early 1980s, Hacker and colleagues[76] demonstrated that vulvar resection and inguinal lymphadenectomies could be performed through separate incisions without compromising cure rates and with much less morbidity.

More recently, most surgeons have accepted wide local excision combined with inguinal node dissection as the treatment of choice for early invasive vulvar lesions. The excision should extend down to the inferior fascia of the urogenital diaphragm, and an effort should be made to obtain a tumor-free margin of at least 1 to 2 cm unless doing so would compromise major organ function.[77] Although wide local excision of very large T2 lesions may require near-total vulvectomy, surgery for smaller tumors can be more limited without increasing the risk of local recurrence.[75,78-82] This is particularly advantageous for patients with lesions on the lateral or posterior vulva because the clitoris can be preserved, thus reducing the psychosexual morbidity of treatment. When lesions are close to the urethra, the distal half of the urethra can usually be resected without loss of continence.[77] Although ultraradical surgery combining vulvectomy, exenteration, and lymphadenectomy was once recommended for patients with locally advanced disease involving the urethra or anus, today most of these cases are managed with organ-sparing treatments that include combinations of radiation therapy, surgery, and chemotherapy.

The inguinal nodes must receive some form of treatment if more than 1 mm of stromal invasion is present in the vulvar specimen. Even 2 to 3 mm of invasion is associated with a 10% to 15% risk of inguinal metastasis. Prevention of regional recurrence is critical to the curative management of vulvar cancer because in almost all cases inguinal recurrence leads to death from disease. The standard treatment for the inguinal nodes is a radical lymphadenectomy that removes both the superficial and deep inguinofemoral nodes. The contralateral groin need not be dissected if the primary lesion is a well-lateralized T1 tumor. However, if the primary lesion approaches the midline or involves the anterior labia minora, bilateral dissections should be done.[77] At one time, pelvic node resection was performed for all patients with invasive vulvar cancer. Eventually this procedure was limited to patients with positive inguinal nodes; with the current standard practice of administering radiation therapy to all patients with regional disease, the morbidity of pelvic node dissection is rarely justified.[77,83]

Unfortunately, serious acute and subacute complications of radical inguinal lymphadenectomy are common despite the use of separate groin incisions.[84-87] These include wound complications, chronic lymphedema, and thrombotic complications; the perioperative mortality rate is 2% to 5%.[67,75,79,82] The complication rate

is significantly less when a more limited, superficial inguinal node dissection is performed. Although some surgeons advocate use of this less radical procedure, a 5% to 7% groin recurrence rate has been reported even after negative superficial inguinal dissection.[88,89] Because the implications of groin recurrence are so grave, some surgeons believe that even this low rate is unacceptable. Recently, several groups have explored the use of lymphatic mapping and sentinel lymph node biopsy of the inguinal nodes. Although this technique may ultimately improve the accuracy of more limited regional dissection, data are currently insufficient to justify using this technique to tailor regional treatment. The role of radiation therapy in the management of regional disease is discussed in the next section.

Five-year disease-specific survival rates of approximately 98% and 85% can be expected for patients treated with surgery for stage I (T1 N0 M0) and stage II (T2 N0 M0) disease, respectively.[66]

Postoperative Radiation Therapy

Twenty years ago, vulvar cancer was rarely treated with radiation. Today, radiation therapy is known to improve the survival rate of patients with regional metastases and permit organ preservation in patients with locally advanced disease. Prospective trials have confirmed the importance of radiation therapy in the management of local–regionally advanced disease, but they have also demonstrated that special skill and excellent cooperation are necessary for effective multimodality care of patients with local–regional metastases.

Postoperative radiation therapy is usually indicated in the following situations: more than one positive inguinal node, one grossly positive inguinal node or extracapsular extension of nodal disease, small tumors in patients with medical problems that prohibit radical inguinofemoral lymph node dissection, and a vulvar resection margin of less than 8 to 10 mm.

In 1986 Homesley and colleagues[67] published the results of a randomized, prospective study that evaluated the role of postoperative radiation therapy in patients who had inguinal lymph node metastases. After radical vulvectomy and inguinal lymphadenectomy, patients found to have inguinal metastases were randomly assigned intraoperatively to undergo additional pelvic lymph node dissection or postoperative radiation therapy. Radiation was delivered by means of anteroposterior-posteroanterior fields including the pelvic and inguinal nodes but not the vulva. The trial was closed after 114 eligible patients had been entered because an interim analysis revealed a significant survival advantage for the radiation therapy arm ($P = 0.03$). Subset analysis suggested that patients with clinically positive or multiple histologically positive groin nodes derived the greatest benefit (see Fig. 30-1). Only three groin recurrences were evident in the 59 patients treated with radiation (8%), compared with 13 in the 55 patients treated with surgery alone (24%) (*P* = 0.02). Although the authors detected no difference in the rates of pelvic recurrence, competing risks may have compromised this comparison. This study changed the standard of care for carcinoma of the vulva and remains one of the most important trials dealing with this rare disease. Unfortunately, the preliminary analysis published in 1986 has never been updated to reflect the findings after longer follow-up of these patients.

Referrals for postoperative radiation therapy for treatment of local disease occur most often when the surgeon is unable to obtain an adequate tumor-free margin without compromising anal or urethral function. Patients with deeply invasive lesions, particularly those with lymphovascular space invasion, may also have inadequate margins and may benefit from postoperative irradiation.

Although local recurrences are often controlled with additional surgery, Faul and colleagues[89a] reported an overall 5-year survival rate of only 40% for 47 patients who had an isolated vulvar recurrence after definitive therapy. In an earlier paper, these authors had demonstrated a local recurrence rate of only 16% when patients who had close or positive surgical margins were treated with radiation versus 58% if no radiation therapy was given.[90] The reduction in the rate of recurrence was significant regardless of whether patients had only close (≤ 8 mm) margins (*P* = 0.04) or frankly positive margins (*P* = 0.05). Patients who also have indications for regional treatment usually are treated at least initially through opposing anterior and posterior photon fields. Using a narrower posterior photon field and supplementing the lateral inguinal nodes with electrons (Fig. 30-2) can minimize the dose to the femoral heads. In some cases, patients may be positioned with separated legs or in a full "frog-leg" position to reduce the skin reaction on the upper medial thighs. However, the anterior vulvar skin usually receives less than the target dose when the patient is in this position unless bolus is applied during treatment. Thermoluminescence dosimetry may be helpful in selected cases. However, the frog-leg position is somewhat more difficult to reproduce on a daily basis. An appositional electron beam can be used to boost the dose to the vulva. The electron energy is usually selected by examining the patient in the treatment position. A bolus may be required if low-energy electrons are used. Although interstitial implants are occasionally used to treat deep tissues at risk for recurrence, the more homogeneous dose delivered to the skin surface with an electron beam usually makes this a safer approach for superficial tumors.

Prophylactic Inguinal Irradiation

The benefit of postoperative radiation therapy documented in the trial by Homesley and colleagues[67]

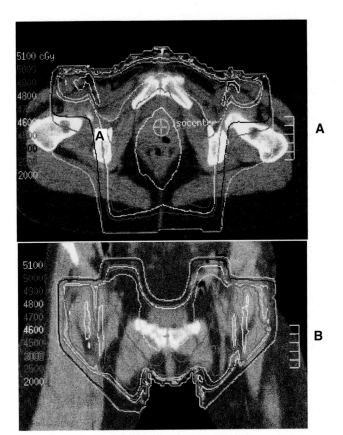

Fig. 30-2 Transverse (**A**) and coronal (**B**) views of the distribution of radiation dose in a patient treated for vulvar carcinoma. A wide 6-MV anterior field encompassed the vulva and the inguinal, external iliac, and internal iliac lymph nodes. A narrower 18-MV posterior field excluded the femoral neck and part of the femoral head. The dose to the lateral inguinal lymph nodes was supplemented using electron fields matched to the lateral borders of the posterior field. A central block in the superior portion of the field reduced the amount of small bowel and rectum in the treatment fields. A modified frog-leg position reduced the skin dose in this patient, who had a posterior lesion. (See Color Plate 33, after p. 80, for color reproduction.)

suggested that radiation therapy might also be used to sterilize potential microscopic disease in clinically negative lymph nodes and avoid the morbidity of inguinal lymphadenectomy. The GOG attempted to test this hypothesis in a trial in which patients with clinically negative nodes were randomly assigned to receive inguinal node irradiation or radical lymphadenectomy (followed by inguinopelvic irradiation in patients with positive nodes) after resection of the primary tumor.[87] An interim analysis, performed after entry of only 58 patients, demonstrated a significantly higher rate of inguinal recurrence and death in the irradiated group. The authors concluded that lymphadenectomy was the superior treatment and closed the trial.

However, this study has been criticized for several reasons. First, in patients treated with radiation therapy alone, only the inguinal nodes were treated, whereas in patients found to have positive pelvic nodes at lymphadenectomy, both the inguinal and pelvic nodes were treated. Second, patients were considered eligible if their groins were believed to be clinically negative for disease. However, this decision was based on clinical examination only, which might have missed large inguinal metastases that would now be detected on routine tomographic scans. Finally, patients who received radiation therapy alone were treated by means of anterior fields with the dose prescribed to a depth of 3 cm; most patients were treated with a combination of 4- to 6-MV photons and 9- to 12-MeV electrons. An analysis of the five postradiation recurrences in the GOG study demonstrated that the inguinal nodes probably received less than the prescribed dose in all of these patients, in several cases by 30% or more.[91] A review of femoral anatomy in 50 other cases demonstrated a mean depth to the femoral vessels of 6.1 cm (range, 2.0 to 8.5 cm).

The Homesley trial demonstrates that microscopic regional disease can be controlled with radiation therapy, and several retrospective studies suggest that radiation therapy can be effective in controlling microscopic disease in patients with clinically negative groin nodes.[67,85,92] Concurrent chemoradiation therapy may be even more effective, although it should be considered investigational in this setting.[93] However, the GOG experience also clearly demonstrates the importance of careful technique that ensures delivery of an adequate dose to the nodes at risk. Tomographic imaging should always be done to rule out lymphadenopathy that may require a combined-modality approach. CT-based treatment planning is strongly recommended, and treatment usually should include at least the distal pelvic nodes (see Fig. 30-2).

Initial Radiation Therapy for Local–Regionally Advanced Disease

Anecdotal reports of dramatic responses of very advanced vulvar cancer to preoperative radiation therapy[94-98] first suggested that radiation therapy might play a role in the initial management of patients with such lesions. In several of these cases, no residual disease was found in the vulvectomy specimen after modest doses of radiation (40 to 55 Gy). However, interest in the use of radiation therapy as a primary treatment modality for patients with advanced vulvar cancer remained lukewarm until studies of gastrointestinal (particularly anal) and head and neck malignancies suggested that concurrent chemotherapy and radiation therapy might be very effective treatment for carcinomas in other sites. More recently, the results of prospective trials of chemoradiation therapy for cervical cancer have fueled interest in this approach.[99-112]

Most studies of chemoradiation therapy for locally advanced or recurrent vulvar cancer have used combinations of cisplatin, 5-fluorouracil (5-FU), and mitomycin C with radiation therapy (Table 30-2). Although the studies have been small, most investigators have been impressed by relatively high complete response rates in patients who usually have very advanced disease.

TABLE 30-2

Concurrent Chemoradiation Therapy for Patients with Locally Advanced or Recurrent Carcinoma of the Vulva

Study and Reference	Number of Patients	Chemotherapy Drugs	RT Dose (Gy)	Patients with Recurrent or Persistent Local Disease After RT ± Surgery (%)	Follow-up (in Months)
Moore et al[99]	73	5-FU + CDDP	47.6	15 (21%)	22-72
Cunningham et al[100]	14	5-FU + CDDP	45-50	4 (29%)	7-81
Landoni et al[101]	58	5-FU + Mito	54	13 (22%)	4-48
Lupi et al[102]	31	5-FU + Mito	54	7 (23%)	22-73
Wahlen et al[103]	19	5-FU + Mito	45-50	1 (5%)	3-70
Eifel et al[104]	12	5-FU + CDDP	40-50	5 (42%)	17-30
Koh et al[105]	20	5-FU ± CDDP or Mito	30-54	9 (45%)	1-75
Russell et al[106]	25	5-FU ± CDDP	47-72	6 (24%)	4-52
Scheistroen and Trope[107]	42	Bleomycin	45	39 (93%)	7-60
Berek et al[108]	12	5-FU + CDDP	44-54	0	7-60
Thomas et al[109]	24	5-FU ± Mito	44-60	10 (42%)	5-43
Evans et al[110]	4	5-FU + Mito	25-70	2 (50%)	20-29
Levin et al[111]	6	5-FU + Mito	18-60	0	1-25
Iversen[112]	15	Bleomycin	15-40	11 (73%)*	4

RT, Radiation therapy; *5-FU*, 5-fluorouracil; *CDDP*, cisplatin; *Mito*, mitomycin C.
*Most patients had unresectable, stage IV lesions.

Although these results are encouraging, it is important to remember that the median age of patients with vulvar cancer is 65 to 70 years. The chemoradiation schedules that have been used successfully in studies of carcinomas that primarily affect younger patients may be less well tolerated by these older women. Although it is probably reasonable to consider treatment with chemoradiation for relatively robust patients with high-risk disease, the need for concurrent chemotherapy has not been rigorously proven in patients with vulvar cancer. Aggressive multimodality regimens should be used with particular caution in patients who have concurrent medical problems or diminished performance status.

Management of Acute Radiation-Induced Side Effects

Radical radiation therapy requires delivery of a relatively high dose of radiation to sensitive skin and mucosa. Most patients develop confluent moist desquamation by the fourth or fifth week of treatment. Despite this, it is rarely necessary or helpful to interrupt treatment. At the beginning of treatment, patients should be warned to expect about 3 weeks of significant discomfort and assured that the pain nearly always resolves within 2 to 3 weeks after the completion of treatment. They should be instructed carefully regarding local care and should be encouraged to wear loose-fitting garments (e.g., boxer shorts and sweat pants) and avoid trauma to the skin. Sitz baths with lukewarm water or aluminum acetate solution (Domeboro's solution) help keep the area clean and, combined with analgesics, reduce patients' discomfort. Patients who develop brisk erythema before the fifteenth treatment nearly always have a superinfection, usually caused by *Candida* species. Treatment of the infection should be started immediately, usually with oral agents, which tend to be better tolerated and more practical than topical agents.

Treatment of Metastatic Vulvar Cancer

Objective responses to chemotherapy in patients with metastatic vulvar cancer have been reported but are infrequent; even phase II studies of cisplatin have been discouraging.[113,114] The ability to deliver aggressive chemotherapy is often compromised by patients' poor performance status. Palliative radiation therapy and supportive care to control pain and local infection can relieve the discomfort of progressive local disease.

TREATMENT OF VAGINAL CANCER
Treatment of Preinvasive Disease

Carcinoma in situ of the vagina (VAIN 3) can be treated with local excision if the lesion is small; larger lesions are often treated with laser ablation after careful colposcopic examination and biopsies to rule out invasion. Rarely, extensive lesions are treated with total vaginectomy and vaginal reconstruction. However, intracavitary radiation therapy is also effective treatment for extensive disease; recurrence rates after treatment of the vaginal surface to a dose of 60 to 80 Gy (low dose rate) are approximately 10% to 15%.[24,25,28] Perez and colleagues[28] emphasize the importance of treating the entire vaginal surface to prevent marginal recurrences. Several authors have reported using fractionated high-dose-rate intracavitary treatment for VAIN 3. However, because the entire vagina must be treated, conservative fractionation schedules are recommended to minimize the risk of adhesive vaginitis and rectal complications.[115,116]

Treatment of Invasive Disease

Radiation therapy is the treatment of choice for most patients with invasive vaginal cancer. The proximity of the bladder and rectum often preclude organ-sparing surgical resection of even relatively small lesions. However, early tumors of the upper posterior vagina can sometimes be treated with radical hysterectomy and partial vaginectomy or, if the patient has no uterus, radical upper vaginectomy.[27] Radical surgery (usually pelvic exenteration) is also indicated for most patients who have had prior radiation therapy. For selected patients with stage IVA disease, pelvic exenteration with vaginal reconstruction may be the treatment of choice, particularly if a rectovaginal or vesicovaginal fistula is present.[30,117,118]

Although radiation therapy can be very effective treatment for invasive vaginal cancer, optimal management of this rare disease requires a detailed understanding of the relevant anatomy and of the natural history of vaginal cancer. The radiation oncologist must also be skilled in the selection and use of a variety of external-beam and brachytherapy techniques. Some of the factors that must be considered before treatment is selected are whether the tumor is located in the proximal, middle, or distal vagina; whether the tumor is on the anterior, posterior, or lateral wall; the thickness of the lesion; the size of the lesion; whether the patient has had a hysterectomy; whether the lesion has been partially or grossly resected and the location of any suspect margins; fixation to the pelvic wall or invasion of the bladder, urethra, or rectum; the presence of regional metastases; and the response to initial external-beam irradiation. As a result, treatment tends to be highly individualized.

Selected patients with small, very superficial tumors can be treated with brachytherapy alone. Perez and colleagues[28] and Chyle and colleagues[24] reported pelvic disease control rates of 88% and 87%, respectively, for small lesions treated with intracavitary radiation therapy alone. Treatment with intracavitary radiation therapy alone is most appropriate for very small apical lesions because the upper vagina can tolerate a vaginal surface dose of 90 to 100 Gy (or higher if the uterus is still in place). For patients who have had a hysterectomy, an examination under anesthesia or vaginal sonography may be needed to determine the thickness of apical lesions. For lesions of the middle or lower third of the vagina, the preferred treatment is a surface dose of 65 to 70 Gy with intracavitary brachytherapy and added a single-plane interstitial implant to increase the tumor dose to 80 to 85 Gy. This reduces the total vaginal dose and the volume of rectum treated to a high dose.

If the lesion is palpable, and particularly if it is more than 2 to 3 mm thick, the pelvic nodes should be treated because the risk of regional disease is significant and the likelihood of successful salvage therapy after recurrence is small. For tumors confined to the proximal half of the vagina, external fields should include the true pelvis and the tumor (marked with radio-opaque seeds) with at least a 4-cm distal margin. Treatment may be delivered by means of anteroposterior-posteroanterior fields or four fields. However, if the posterior vaginal wall is involved, the entire sacrum should be included to cover the perirectal nodes. If the tumor approaches or involves the distal third of the vagina, the medial inguinal nodes should be included in the field. More generous inguinal coverage may be indicated if inguinal metastases are present or if the lesion is deeply invasive and is centered in the distal vagina. If the introitus is included in the field, the morbidity of treatment can be reduced dramatically by treating the patient in a frog-leg position.

Brachytherapy should be tailored to the volume and distribution of the tumor and its response to external-beam irradiation. Apical tumors that are less than 3 to 4 mm thick after external irradiation may be treated with a vaginal cylinder. For more distal tumors, a combination of intracavitary and interstitial brachytherapy, which reduces the total vaginal dose and the volume of rectum treated to a high dose, may be more appropriate. When the uterus is intact, tumors high in the posterior fornix can often be treated with a tandem and ovoids.

Interstitial implants can be inserted freehand (Fig. 30-3) or with an interstitial template. Freehand placement of implants permits better control of the position of needles but requires considerable experience. Vaginal implants may also be positioned using a perineal template. The parallel needle positions acquired with templates produce a very homogeneous dose, but the template interferes somewhat with the brachytherapist's ability to appreciate the position of needles relative to the tumor and other structures. In the case of tumors involving the vaginal apex in patients who have had a hysterectomy, implants can often be effectively placed using a template with laparoscopic or laparotomy guidance.

Although brachytherapy is an important tool in the treatment of vaginal cancer, it should be used only if the entire tumor can be encompassed with an adequate margin.[28,119,120] Even very small tumors will probably

recur if a portion of the tumor receives less than 60 to 70 Gy. Apical tumors that have indistinct margins, deeply invasive tumors that involve the rectovaginal septum, and tumors that are close to the iliac vessels are particularly difficult to cover with brachytherapy. Chyle and colleagues[24] suggested that some tumors may be better treated with external-beam irradiation alone using carefully designed shrinking fields. They reported three vaginal recurrences (11%) in 28 patients with stage II disease treated with external-beam irradiation alone, compared with 12 recurrences (21%) in 58 patients treated with combined external-beam irradiation and brachytherapy. Perez and colleagues[28] reported local recurrence rates of 34% to 44% for patients with stage II disease treated in most cases with a combination of external-beam irradiation and brachytherapy.

Three-dimensional conformal therapy may improve the ability to deliver high doses to the tumor with external-beam therapy alone. However, tightly conformed fields should not be used without careful consideration of possible movement of the target. Although distal vaginal tumors may be relatively stable, the apical vagina can move 4 to 5 cm or more with changes in bladder filling.

Efforts to correlate outcome with the total dose of radiation delivered to the tumor have yielded variable results.[24,28,69,120] This may be because the tumor's size, extent, and initial response to irradiation often influence the dose of radiation and the ability to deliver brachytherapy. When good brachytherapy coverage of the tumor can be accomplished, an effort should be made to treat the tumor to a dose of 75 to 85 Gy. When brachytherapy is not possible, patients may be treated with external-beam irradiation alone using shrinking pelvic fields to deliver a tumor dose of 60 to 66 Gy. However, radiation oncologists who do not feel comfortable with the specialized techniques used to treat these rare tumors should consider referring patients to a specialist. Treatment should be completed in less than 6 to 7 weeks.[119]

Overall, 5-year disease-specific survival rates for patients with invasive vaginal cancer treated with definitive irradiation range from 75% to 95% for stage I disease, 50% to 80% for stage II disease, 30% to 50% for stage III disease, and 15% to 30% for stage IVA disease.*

Probably because of the intimate association of the vagina with bladder and rectum, complication rates tend to be somewhat higher for vaginal cancer than for cervical cancer treated with definitive irradiation.[25,28,68,72,121] Chyle and colleagues[24] reported a 19% incidence of major complications at 20 years (the crude complication rate was 13%) for 301 patients treated with definitive irradiation, similar to the rates reported in smaller series. Vaginal morbidity has not been systematically

---

*References 24, 25, 28, 71, 119, 120.

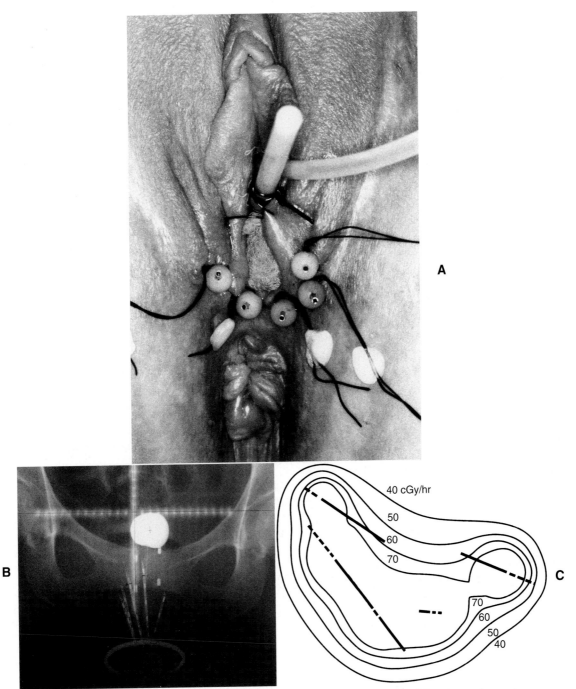

Fig. 30-3 Interstitial implant in a patient with squamous carcinoma involving the vagina and perineal vulva. The implant was used to boost the radiation dose to a 1-cm area of residual thickening after an excellent response to concurrent chemotherapy and external-beam irradiation. Because of its close proximity to the anus and rectum, the tumor was not believed to be amenable to surgical resection. **A,** Five needles were inserted transperineally using a freehand technique. **B,** A 3-cm–diameter cylinder and a small amount of packing were placed in the vagina to displace uninvolved vagina. **C,** Dose distribution in a transverse plane through the center of the implant.

reported but is probably influenced by the initial tumor extent, secondary infection, the age and menopausal status of the patient, and the dose and volume of tissue irradiated.

Role of Chemotherapy

Reports of chemoradiation in patients with vaginal cancer are anecdotal; it is unlikely that prospective randomized trials comparing radiation alone with chemoradiation will be feasible for patients with this rare cancer. However, because vaginal cancer is similar to cervical cancer in its epidemiology and natural history, it is probably reasonable to extrapolate from the randomized trials in cervical cancer[122-125] the use of concurrent cisplatin-based chemotherapy for selected patients with high-risk disease.

Cisplatin-containing chemotherapy is sometimes used to treat patients with metastatic or recurrent vaginal cancer, but reported response rates to chemotherapy are poor.[113,126]

REFERENCES

1. Bruner DW, Lanciano R, Keegan M, et al. Vaginal stenosis and sexual function following intracavitary radiation for the treatment of cervical and endometrial carcinoma. *Int J Radiat Oncol Biol Phys* 1993;27:825-830.
2. Fajardo LF. *Pathology of Radiation Injury.* New York, NY: Masson; 1982.
3. Eifel PJ, Levenback C, Wharton JT, et al. Time course and incidence of late complications in patients treated with radiation therapy for FIGO stage IB carcinoma of the uterine cervix. *Int J Radiat Oncol Biol Phys* 1995;32:1289-1300.
4. Robinson JW, Faris PD, Scott CB. Psychoeducational group increases vaginal dilation for younger women and reduces sexual fears for women of all ages with gynecological carcinoma treated with radiotherapy. *Int J Radiat Oncol Biol Phys* 1999;44:497-506.
5. Beller U, Sideri M, Maisonneuve P, et al. Carcinoma of the vagina. *J Epidemiol Biostat* 2001;6:141-152.
6. Beller U, Sideri M, Maisonneuve P, et al. Carcinoma of the vulva. *J Epidemiol Biostat* 2001;6:155-173.
7. Creasman WT, Phillips JL, Menck HR. The National Cancer Data Base report on cancer of the vagina. *Cancer* 1998;83:1033-1040.
8. Ikenberg H, Runge M, Göppinger A, et al. Human papillomavirus DNA in invasive carcinoma of the vagina. *Obstet Gynecol* 1990;76:432-438.
9. Merino MJ. Vaginal cancer: the role of infectious and environmental factors. *Am J Obstet Gynecol* 1991;165:1255-1262.
10. Hoffman MS, DeCesare SL, Roberts WS, et al. Upper vaginectomy for in situ and occult, superficially invasive carcinoma of the vagina. *Am J Obstet Gynecol* 1992;166:30-33.
11. Bloss JD, Liao SY, Wilczynski SP, et al. Clinical and histologic features of vulvar carcinomas analyzed for human papillomavirus status: evidence that squamous cell carcinoma of the vulva has more than one etiology. *Hum Pathol* 1991;22:711-718.
12. Crum CP. Carcinoma of the vulva: epidemiology and pathogenesis. *Obstet Gynecol* 1992;79:448-454.
13. Crum CP, McLachlin CM, Tate JE, et al. Pathobiology of vulvar squamous neoplasia. *Curr Opin Obstet Gynecol* 1997;9:63-69.
14. Hørding U, Junge J, Daugaard S, et al. Vulvar squamous cell carcinoma and papillomaviruses: indications for two different etiologies. *Gynecol Oncol* 1994;52:241-246.
15. Lee YY, Wilczynski SP, Chumakov A, et al. Carcinoma of the vulva: HPV and p53 mutations. *Oncogene* 1994;9:1655-1659.
16. Herbst AL, Ulfelder H, Poskanzer DC. Adenocarcinoma of the vagina: an association of maternal stilbestrol therapy with tumor appearing in young women. *N Engl J Med* 1971;284:878-881.
17. Herbst AL, Anderson S, Hubby MM, et al. Risk factors for the development of diethylstilbestrol associated clear cell adenocarcinoma: a case-control study. *Am J Obstet Gynecol* 1986;154:814-822.
18. Hatch EE, Palmer JR, Titus-Ernstoff L, et al. Cancer risk in women exposed to diethylstilbestrol in utero. *JAMA* 1998;280:630-634.
19. Andreasson B, Nyboe J. Predictive factors with reference to low-risk of metastases in squamous cell carcinoma in the vulvar region. *Gynecol Oncol* 1985;21:196-206.
20. Plentl AA, Friedman EA. Clinical significance of the vulvar lymphatics. In: *Lymphatic System of Female Genitalia.* Philadelphia, Pa: WB Saunders; 1971:27.
21. Binder SW, Huang I, Fu YS, et al. Risk factors for the development of lymph node metastasis in vulvar squamous carcinoma. *Gynecol Oncol* 1990;37:9-16.
22. DiSaia PJ, Creasman WT, Rich WM. An alternative approach to early cancer of the vulva. *Am J Obstet Gynecol* 1979;133:825-832.
23. Berek JS, Hacker NF. *Practical Gynecologic Oncology.* Baltimore, Md: Williams and Wilkins; 1994.
24. Chyle V, Zagars GK, Wheeler JA, et al. Definitive radiotherapy for carcinoma of the vagina: outcome and prognostic factors. *Int J Radiat Oncol Biol Phys* 1996;35:891-905.
25. Kirkbride P, Fyles A, Rawlings GA, et al. Carcinoma of the vagina—experience at the Princess Margaret Hospital (1974-1989). *Gynecol Oncol* 1995;56:435-443.
26. Plentl AA, Friedman EA. Clinical significance of the vaginal lymphatics. In: *Lymphatic System of Female Genitalia.* Philadelphia, Pa: WB Saunders; 1971:57.
27. Stock RG, Chen ASJ, Seski J. A 30-year experience in the management of primary carcinoma of the vagina: analysis of prognostic factors and treatment modalities. *Gynecol Oncol* 1995;56:45-52.
28. Perez CA, Grigsby PW, Garipagaoglu M, et al. Factors affecting long-term outcome of irradiation in carcinoma of the vagina. *Int J Radiat Oncol Biol Phys* 1999;44:37-45.
29. Plentl AA, Friedman EA. Lymphatics of the vagina. In: *Lymphatic System of Female Genitalia.* Philadelphia, Pa: WB Saunders; 1971:51.
30. Al-Kurdi M, Monaghan JM. Thirty-two years experience in management of primary tumours of the vagina. *Br J Obstet Gynecol* 1981;88:1145-1150.
31. Davis KP, Stanhope CR, Garton GR, et al. Invasive vaginal carcinoma: analysis of early-stage disease. *Gynecol Oncol* 1991;42:131-136.
32. Wilkinson EJ. The 1989 presidential address. International Society for the Study of Vulvar Disease. *J Reprod Med* 1990;35:981-991.
33. Buscema J, Woodruff JD. Progressive histobiologic alterations in the development of vulvar cancer. *Am J Obstet Gynecol* 1980;138:146-150.
34. Koss LG, Brockunier A Jr. Ultrastructural aspects of Paget's disease of the vulva. *Arch Pathol* 1969;87:592-600.
35. Fanning J, Lambert HC, Hale TM, et al. Paget's disease of the vulva: prevalence of associated vulvar adenocarcinoma, invasive Paget's disease, and recurrence after surgical excision. *Am J Obstet Gynecol* 1999;180:24-27.
36. Isaacs JH. Verrucous carcinoma of the female genital tract. *Gynecol Oncol* 1976;4:259-269.
37. Japaze H, Van Dinh T, Woodruff JD. Verrucous carcinoma of the vulva: study of 24 cases. *Obstet Gynecol* 1982;60:462-466.
38. Gil-Moreno A, Garcia-Jimenez A, Gonzalez-Bosquet J, et al. Merkel cell carcinoma of the vulva. *Gynecol Oncol* 1997;64:526-532.
39. Joseph RE, Enghardt MH, Doering DL, et al. Small cell neuroendocrine carcinoma of the vagina. *Cancer* 1992;70:784-789.
40. Miliauskas JR, Leong AS. Small cell (neuroendocrine) carcinoma of the vagina. *Histopathology* 1992;21:371-374.
41. Yaghsezian H, Palazzo JP, Finkel GC, et al. Primary vaginal adenocarcinoma of the intestinal type associated with adenosis. *Gynecol Oncol* 1992;45:62-65.
42. Leuchter RS, Hacker NF, Voet RL, et al. Primary carcinoma of the Bartholin gland: a report of 14 cases and review of the literature. *Obstet Gynecol* 1982;60:361-368.
43. Raber G, Mempel V, Jackisch C, et al. Malignant melanoma of the vulva. Report of 89 patients. *Cancer* 1996;78:2353-2358.

44. Weinstock MA. Malignant melanoma of the vulva and vagina in the United States: patterns of incidence and population-based estimates of survival. *Am J Obstet Gynecol* 1994;171:1225-1230.

45. Ragnarsson-Olding BK, Nilsson BR, Kanter-Lewensohn LR, et al. Malignant melanoma of the vulva in a nationwide, 25-year study of 219 Swedish females: predictors of survival. *Cancer* 1999;86:1285-1293.

46. Chung AF, Woodruff JM, Lewis JL Jr. Malignant melanoma of the vulva: a report of 44 cases. *Obstet Gynecol* 1975;45:638-646.

47. Tasseron EWK, van der Esch EP, Hart AAM, et al. A clinicopathological study of 30 melanomas of the vulva. *Gynecol Oncol* 1992;46:170-175.

48. Buchanan DJ, Schlaerth J, Kurosaki T. Primary vaginal melanoma: thirteen-year disease-free survival after wide local excision and review of recent literature. *Am J Obstet Gynecol* 1998;178:1177-1184.

49. Ragnarsson-Olding B, Johansson H, Rutqvist LE, et al. Malignant melanoma of the vagina. *Cancer* 1993;71:1893-1897.

50. Curtin JP, Saigo P, Slucher B, et al. Soft-tissue sarcoma of the vagina and vulva: a clinicopathologic study. *Obstet Gynecol* 1995;86:269-272.

51. Nirenberg A, Östör AG, Slavin J, et al. Primary vulvar sarcomas. *Int J Gynecol Pathol* 1995;14:55-62.

52. Andrassy RJ, Wiener ES, Raney RB, et al. Progress in the surgical management of vaginal rhabdomyosarcoma: a 25-year review from the Intergroup Rhabdomyosarcoma Study Group. *J Pediatr Surg* 1999;34:731-734.

53. Bernstein SG, Kovacs BR, Townsend DE, et al. Vulvar carcinoma in situ. *Obstet Gynecol* 1983;61:304-307.

54. Friedrich EG Jr, Wilkinson EJ, Fu YS. Carcinoma in situ of the vulva: a continuing challenge. *Am J Obstet Gynecol* 1980;136:830-843.

55. Benedet JL, Bender H, Jones H III, et al. FIGO staging classifications and clinical practice guidelines in the management of gynecologic cancers. FIGO Committee on Gynecologic Oncology. *Int J Gynaecol Obstet* 2000;70:209-262.

56. Fleming ID, Cooper JS, Henson DE, et al, eds. *AJCC Cancer Staging Manual*. 5th ed. Philadelphia, Pa: Lippincott Williams & Wilkins; 1997:181-184.

57. Shepherd J, Sideri M, Benedet J, et al. Carcinoma of the vagina. *J Epidemiol Biostat* 1998;3:103-109.

58. Boyce J, Fruchter RG, Kasambilides E, et al. Prognostic factors in carcinoma of the vulva. *Gynecol Oncol* 1985;20:364-377.

59. Homesley HD, Bundy BN, Sedlis A, et al. Prognostic factors for groin node metastasis in squamous cell carcinoma of the vulva (a Gynecologic Oncology Group study). *Gynecol Oncol* 1993;49:279-283.

60. Heaps JM, Fu YS, Montz FJ, et al. Surgical-pathologic variables predictive of local recurrence in squamous cell carcinoma of the vulva. *Gynecol Oncol* 1990;38:309-314.

61. Husseinzadeh N, Wesseler T, Schellhas H, et al. Significance of lymphoplasmocytic infiltration around tumor cell in the prediction of regional lymph node metastases in patients with invasive squamous cell carcinoma of the vulva: a clinicopathologic study. *Gynecol Oncol* 1989;34:200-205.

62. Husseinzadeh N, Wesseler T, Schneider D, et al. Prognostic factors and the significance of cytologic grading in invasive squamous cell carcinoma of the vulva: a clinicopathologic study. *Gynecol Oncol* 1990;36:192-199.

63. Sedlis A, Homesley H, Bundy BN, et al. Positive groin lymph nodes in superficial squamous cell vulvar cancer. A Gynecologic Oncology Group study. *Am J Obstet Gynecol* 1987;156:1159-1164.

64. Kürzl R, Messerer D. Prognostic factors in squamous cell carcinoma of the vulva: a multivariate analysis. *Gynecol Oncol* 1989;32:143-150.

65. Pinto AP, Signorello LB, Crum CP, et al. Squamous cell carcinoma of the vulva in Brazil: prognostic importance of host and viral variables. *Gynecol Oncol* 1999;74:61-67.

66. Homesley HD, Bundy BN, Sedlis A, et al. Assessment of current International Federation of Gynecology and Obstetrics staging of vulvar carcinoma relative to prognostic factors for survival (a Gynecologic Oncology Group study). *Am J Obstet Gynecol* 1991;164:997-1003.

67. Homesley HD, Bundy BN, Sedlis A, et al. Radiation therapy versus pelvic node resection for carcinoma of the vulva with positive groin nodes. *Obstet Gynecol* 1986;68:733-740.

68. van der Velden J, Lindert ACM, Lammes FB, et al. Extracapsular growth of lymph node metastases in squamous cell carcinoma of the vulva. The impact on recurrence and survival. *Cancer* 1995;75:2885-2890.

69. Origoni M, Sideri M, Garsia S, et al. Prognostic value of pathological patterns of lymph node positivity in squamous cell carcinoma of the vulva stage III and IVA FIGO. *Gynecol Oncol* 1992;45:313-316.

70. Eddy GL, Marks RD, Miller MC, et al. Primary invasive vaginal carcinoma. *Am J Obstet Gynecol* 1991;165:292-296.

71. Kucera H, Vavra N. Radiation management of primary carcinoma of the vagina: clinical and histopathological variables associated with survival. *Gynecol Oncol* 1991;40:12-16.

72. Peters W, Kumar N, Morley G. Carcinoma of the vagina. Factors influencing outcome. *Cancer* 1985;55:892-897.

73. Vavra N, Seifert M, Kucera H, et al. Radiotherapy of primary vaginal carcinoma and effects of histological and clinical factors on the prognosis [in German]. *Strahlenther Onkol* 1991;167:1-6.

74. Kuppers V, Stiller M, Somville T, et al. Risk factors for recurrent VIN. Role of multifocality and grade of disease. *J Reprod Med* 1997;42:140-144.

75. Hacker NF, Berek JS, Lagasse LD, et al. Individualization of treatment for stage I squamous cell vulvar carcinoma. *Obstet Gynecol* 1984;63:155-162.

76. Hacker NF, Leuchter RS, Berek JS, et al. Radical vulvectomy and bilateral inguinal lymphadenectomy through separate groin incisions. *Obstet Gynecol* 1981;58:574-579.

77. Hacker NF. Vulvar cancer. In: Berek JS, Hacker NF, eds. *Practical Gynecologic Oncology*. Philadelphia, Pa: Lippincott Williams & Wilkins; 2000:553.

78. Burke TW, Stringer CA, Gershenson DM, et al. Radical wide excision and selective inguinal node dissection for squamous cell carcinoma of the vulva. *Gynecol Oncol* 1990;38:328-332.

79. Farias-Eisner R, Cirisano FD, Grouse D, et al. Conservative and individualized surgery for early squamous carcinoma of the vulva: the treatment of choice for stage I and II (T1-2 N0-1 M0) disease. *Gynecol Oncol* 1994;53:55-58.

80. Iversen T, Abeler V, Aalders J. Individualized treatment of stage I carcinoma of the vulva. *Obstet Gynecol* 1981;57:85-89.

81. Lin JY, DuBeshter B, Angel C, et al. Morbidity and recurrence with modifications of radical vulvectomy and groin dissection. *Gynecol Oncol* 1992;47:80-86.

82. Magrina JF, Gonzalez-Bosquet J, Weaver AL, et al. Primary squamous cell cancer of the vulva: radical versus modified radical vulvar surgery. *Gynecol Oncol* 1998;71:116-121.

83. Hacker NF, Berek JS, Lagasse LD, et al. Management of regional lymph nodes and their prognostic influence in vulvar cancer. *Obstet Gynecol* 1983;61:408-412.

84. Morley GW. Infiltrative carcinoma of the vulva: results of surgical treatment. *Am J Obstet Gynecol* 1976;124:874-888.

85. Petereit DG, Mehta MP, Buchler DA, et al. A retrospective review of nodal treatment for vulvar cancer. *Am J Clin Oncol* 1993;16:38-42.

86. Podratz KC, Symmonds RE, Taylor WF. Carcinoma of the vulva: analysis of treatment failures. *Am J Obstet Gynecol* 1982;143:340-351.

87. Stehman FB, Bundy BN, Thomas G, et al. Groin dissection versus groin radiation in carcinoma of the vulva: a Gynecologic Oncology Group study. *Int J Radiat Oncol Biol Phys* 1992;24:389-396.

88. Burke TW, Levenback C, Coleman RL, et al. Surgical therapy of T1 and T2 vulvar carcinoma: further experience with radical wide excision and selective inguinal lymphadenectomy. *Gynecol Oncol* 1995;57:215-220.

89. Stehman FB, Bundy BN, Dvoretsky PM, et al. Early stage I carcinoma of the vulva treated with ipsilateral superficial inguinal lymphadenectomy and modified radical hemivulvectomy: a prospective study of the Gynecologic Oncology Group. *Obstet Gynecol* 1992;79:490-497.

89a. Faul C, Mirmow D, Gerszten K, et al. Isolated local recurrence in carcinoma of the vulva: prognosis and implications for treatment. *Int J Gynecol Cancer* 1998;8:409-414.

90. Faul CM, Mirmow D, Huang Q, et al. Adjuvant radiation for vulvar carcinoma: improved local control. *Int J Radiat Oncol Biol Phys* 1997;38:381-389.

91. Koh WJ, Chiu M, Stelzer KJ, et al. Femoral vessel depth and the implications for groin node radiation. *Int J Radiat Oncol Biol Phys* 1993;27:969-974.

92. Henderson RH, Parsons JT, Morgan L, et al. Elective ilioinguinal lymph node irradiation. *Int J Radiat Oncol Biol Phys* 1984;10:811-819.

93. Leiserowitz GS, Russell AH, Kinney WK, et al. Prophylactic chemoradiation of inguinofemoral lymph nodes in patients with locally extensive vulvar cancer. *Gynecol Oncol* 1997;66:509-514.

94. Acosta AA, Given FT, Frazier AB, et al. Preoperative radiation therapy in the management of squamous cell carcinoma of the vulva: preliminary report. *Am J Obstet Gynecol* 1978;132:198-206.

95. Boronow RC. Combined therapy as an alternative to exenteration for locally advanced vulvo-vaginal cancer: rationale and results. *Cancer* 1982;49:1085-1091.

96. Fairey RN, MacKay PA, Benedet JL, et al. Radiation treatment of carcinoma of the vulva, 1950-1980. *Am J Obstet Gynecol* 1985;151:591-597.

97. Hacker NF, Berek JS, Juillard GJF, et al. Preoperative radiation therapy for locally advanced vulvar cancer. *Cancer* 1984; 54:2056-2061.

98. Jafari K, Magalotti M. Radiation therapy in carcinoma of the vulva. *Cancer* 1981;47:686-691.

99. Moore DH, Thomas GM, Montana GS, et al. Preoperative chemoradiation for advanced vulvar cancer: a phase II study of the Gynecologic Oncology Group. *Int J Radiat Oncol Biol Phys* 1998;42:79-85.

100. Cunningham MJ, Goyer RP, Gibbons SK, et al. Primary radiation, cisplatin, and 5-fluorouracil for advanced squamous carcinoma of the vulva. *Gynecol Oncol* 1997;66:258-261.

101. Landoni F, Maneo A, Zanetta G, et al. Concurrent preoperative chemotherapy with 5-fluorouracil and mitomycin C and radiotherapy (FUMIR) followed by limited surgery in locally advanced and recurrent vulvar carcinoma. *Gynecol Oncol* 1996;61:321-327.

102. Lupi G, Raspagliesi F, Zucali R, et al. Combined preoperative chemoradiotherapy followed by radical surgery in locally advanced vulvar carcinoma. A pilot study. *Cancer* 1996; 77:1472-1478.

103. Wahlen SA, Slater JD, Wagner RJ, et al. Concurrent radiation therapy and chemotherapy in the treatment of primary squamous cell carcinoma of the vulva. *Cancer* 1995;75:2289-2294.

104. Eifel PJ, Morris M, Burke TW, et al. Prolonged continuous infusion cisplatinum and 5-fluorouracil with radiation for locally advanced or recurrent carcinoma of the vulva. *Gynecol Oncol* 1995;59:51-56.

105. Koh WJ, Wallace HJ, Greer BE, et al. Combined radiotherapy and chemotherapy in the management of local-regionally advanced vulvar cancer. *Int J Radiat Oncol Biol Phys* 1993;26:809-816.

106. Russell AH, Mesic JB, Scudder SA, et al. Synchronous radiation and cytotoxic chemotherapy for locally advanced or recurrent squamous cancer of the vulva. *Gynecol Oncol* 1992;47:14-20.

107. Scheistroen M, Trope C. Combined bleomycin and irradiation in preoperative treatment of advanced squamous cell carcinoma of the vulva. *Acta Oncol* 1992;32:657.

108. Berek JS, Heaps JM, Fu YS, et al. Concurrent cisplatin and 5-fluorouracil chemotherapy and radiation therapy for advanced-stage squamous carcinoma of the vulva. *Gynecol Oncol* 1991;42:197-201.

109. Thomas G, Dembo A, DePetrillo A, et al. Concurrent radiation and chemotherapy in vulvar carcinoma. *Gynecol Oncol* 1989;34:263-267.

110. Evans LS, Kersh CR, Constable WC, et al. Concomitant 5-fluorouracil, mitomycin-C, and radiotherapy for advanced gynecologic malignancies. *Int J Radiat Oncol Biol Phys* 1988; 15:901-906.

111. Levin W, Goldberg G, Altaras M, et al. The use of concomitant chemotherapy and radiotherapy prior to surgery in advanced stage carcinoma of the vulva. *Gynecol Oncol* 1986;25:20-25.

112. Iversen T. Irradiation and bleomycin in the treatment of inoperable vulval carcinoma. *Acta Obstet Gynecol Scand* 1982;61:195-197.

113. Slayton R, Blessing J, Beecham J, et al. Phase II trial of etoposide in the management of advanced or recurrent squamous cell carcinoma of the vulva and carcinoma of the vagina. *Cancer Treatment Reports* 1987;71:869-870.

114. Thigpen JT, Blessing JA, Homesley H, et al. Phase II trials of cisplatin and piperazinedione in advanced or recurrent squamous cell carcinoma of the vulva: a Gynecologic Oncology Group study. *Gynecol Oncol* 1986;23:358-363.

115. MacLeod C, Fowler A, Dalrymple C, et al. High-dose-rate brachytherapy in the management of high-grade intraepithelial neoplasia of the vagina. *Gynecol Oncol* 1997;65:74-77.

116. Ogino I, Kitamura T, Okajima H, et al. High-dose-rate intracavitary brachytherapy in the management of cervical and vaginal intraepithelial neoplasia. *Int J Radiat Oncol Biol Phys* 1998;40:881-887.

117. Benson C, Soisson AP, Carlson J, et al. Neovaginal reconstruction with a rectus abdominis myocutaneous flap. *Obstet Gynecol* 1993;81:871-875.

118. Berek JS, Hacker NF, Lagasse LD. Rectosigmoid colectomy and reanastamosis to facilitate resection of primary and recurrent gynecologic cancer. *Obstet Gynecol* 1984;64:715-720.

119. Lee WR, Marcus RB, Sombeck MD, et al. Radiotherapy alone for carcinoma of the vagina: the importance of overall treatment time. *Int J Radiat Oncol Biol Phys* 1994;29:983-988.

120. Spirtos NM, Doshi BP, Kapp DS, et al. Radiation therapy for primary squamous cell carcinoma of the vagina: Stanford University experience. *Gynecol Oncol* 1989;35:20-29.

121. Eddy GL, Jenrette JM, Creasman WT. Effect of radiotherapeutic technique on local control in primary vaginal carcinoma. *Int J Gynecol Cancer* 1993;3:399-404.

122. Eifel PJ. Concurrent chemotherapy and radiation: a major advance for women with cervical cancer. *J Clin Oncol* 1999;17:1334-1335.

123. Keys HM, Bundy BN, Stehman FB, et al. Cisplatin, radiation, and adjuvant hysterectomy for bulky stage IB cervical carcinoma. *N Engl J Med* 1999;340:1154-1161.

124. Morris M, Eifel PJ, Lu J, et al. Pelvic radiation with concurrent chemotherapy compared with pelvic and paraaortic radiation for high-risk cervical cancer. *N Engl J Med* 1999;340:1137-1143.

125. Rose PG, Bundy BN, Watkins EB, et al. Concurrent cisplatin-based chemotherapy and radiotherapy for locally advanced cervical cancer. *N Engl J Med* 1999;340:1144-1153.

126. Thigpen JT, Blessing JA, Homesley HD, et al. Phase II trial of cisplatin in advanced or recurrent cancer of the vagina: a Gynecologic Oncology Group study. *Gynecol Oncol* 1986; 23:101-104.

CHAPTER 31

The Ovary

Gillian M. Thomas

ANATOMY AND PHYSIOLOGY

The ovaries are almond-shaped glands located close to the lateral pelvic walls and suspended by the mesovarium of the broad ligament of the uterus. In prepubertal females, the surface of the ovary is covered by a smooth layer of ovarian surface epithelium that gives the surface a dull, grayish appearance, contrasting with the shiny surface of the adjacent peritoneal mesovarium with which it is continuous. After puberty, the surface becomes progressively scarred and distorted because of the repeated rupture of ovarian follicles and discharge of oocytes that are part of ovulation. Maturation of ovarian follicles results in the production of both female hormones and ova.

At puberty, the ovaries contain about 300,000 primordial follicles. These primitive follicles, 20 μm in diameter, consist of an oocyte arrested in prophase of the first meiotic division, surrounded by a single layer of specialized stromal cells, the granulosa cells (Fig. 31-1). During each menstrual cycle, under the influence of follicle-stimulating hormone and luteinizing hormone,

several hundred follicles develop.[1] In each of these follicles, the granulosa cells and surrounding theca cells multiply, leading to formation of the graafian follicle, which reaches 2 cm in diameter before ovulation. The granulosa and theca cells are responsible for the cyclic production of estradiol and progesterone.[2] Also during each menstrual cycle, the oocyte in the dominant follicle is stimulated to complete meiotic division and mature into the ovum, which is shed at ovulation. The unsuccessful follicles and their oocytes degenerate and are reabsorbed.

When the ovaries become depleted of primordial follicles, such as occurs naturally at menopause or as a result of radiation therapy or alkylating chemotherapy, ovulation and production of estradiol and progesterone cease. Because proliferation of the granulosa and theca cells depends on the presence of oocytes, estradiol production in females depends on oogenesis to a far greater degree than testosterone production in males depends on spermatogenesis (see Chapter 26). The oocytes in primitive follicles are more sensitive to radiation damage than are

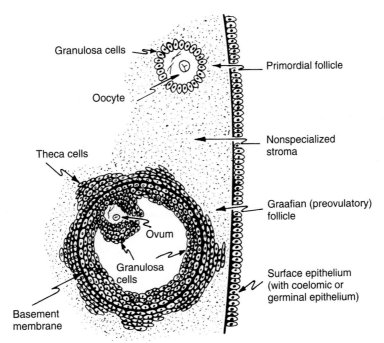

Fig. 31-1 Schematic diagram of a section of the ovary showing functional structures and the tissues from which neoplasms arise.

the ova in mature follicles; the oocytes in graafian follicles may also be more radiosensitive than ova.

RESPONSE OF THE NORMAL OVARY TO IRRADIATION

The radiation dose necessary to induce ovarian failure is age dependent.[3] In women younger than 40 years, doses in excess of 5 Gy (5 to 10 Gy) are required to produce permanent cessation of menses in more than 95% of women; in women older than 40 years, a dose of 3.75 Gy produces amenorrhea in almost 100% of women.[4] Doses of 1.25 to 5 Gy produced permanent amenorrhea in 14 (58%) of 24 women younger than 40 years, whereas doses of 1.25 to 3.75 Gy produced permanent amenorrhea in 18 (78%) of 23 women older than 40 years. Cole[1] used radiation-induced ovarian ablation for the treatment of breast cancer in 235 women. Usually a single treatment of 4.5 Gy was administered to the pelvis. Permanent amenorrhea was induced in 67% (39 of 58) of the women younger than 40 years of age, 90% (70 of 78) of the women age 40 to 44 years, 96% (71 of 74) of the women age 45 to 49 years, and 100% (25 of 25) of the women older than 49 years. Stillman and colleagues[2] reported the effects on ovarian function of abdominal irradiation for childhood malignancies. Most of the 182 girls in this study were prepubertal at diagnosis, but all were more than 14 years old at the time of the study and had been followed for a minimum of 6 years. Primary or secondary amenorrhea and elevated pituitary gonadotropin levels occurred in 68% (17 of 25) of the girls who had both ovaries included in the radiation field (estimated ovarian doses of 12 to 50 Gy); 14% (5 of 35) of the girls who had at least one ovary at the edge of the radiation field (estimated ovarian doses of 0.9 to 10 Gy); and none of the girls who had at least one ovary outside the treatment field (0 of 34, estimated ovarian doses of 0.05 to 1.5 Gy) or who had not received abdominal irradiation (0 of 88).[2]

These findings indicate that ovarian function can be ablated with low doses of radiation. However, in young women, oogenesis is not quite as sensitive to internal scatter radiation as is spermatogenesis in males, and ovarian function can often be preserved by shielding the ovaries from the primary radiation beam or, as practiced in Hodgkin's disease and some cases of cervical carcinoma, by oophoropexy to move the ovaries away from the radiation field.

When nonsurgical ablation of ovarian estrogen production is therapeutically desirable, as in the management of breast cancer, it can be effected in almost 100% of women with a dose of 10 to 15 Gy in four or five fractions. An opposing pair of fields is used, 15 cm wide by 10 cm high, with the inferior border 1 cm below the top of the pubic symphysis.

Cancer therapy in young women (surgery, radiation therapy, chemotherapy, or any combination of these)

may result in unavoidable permanent ablation of ovarian function. Provided that the tumor is not hormonally responsive, hormone replacement therapy is often of benefit in reversing menopausal symptoms and reducing the degree of osteoporosis and cardiovascular disease that may ensue.

CARCINOMA OF THE OVARY

A wide variety of tumors can affect the ovary. A working classification of ovarian neoplasms is presented in Box 31-1. This chapter emphasizes malignant tumors that can be treated successfully with radiation therapy or a combination of radiation therapy and other treatment.

BOX 31-1 Working Classification of Ovarian Neoplasms*

EPITHELIAL TUMORS (85% TO 95%)
Types
1. Serous (tubal type, accounts for approximately 50% of epithelial carcinomas)
2. Mucinous (cervical type, 10%)
3. Endometrioid (endometrial type, 20%)
4. Clear cell (4%)
5. Unclassified/undifferentiated (15%)
Differentiation
1. Benign: cystadenoma
2. Borderline malignancy/low malignant potential (applies mainly to serous and mucinous types)
3. Malignant: cystadenocarcinoma, grades 1, 2, and 3

STROMAL TUMORS
Specialized Stroma: Sex Cord Stromal Tumors (4% to 8%)
1. Granulosa cell–theca cell (estrogen-producing, about 3% to 6% of malignant ovarian tumors)
2. Sertoli-Leydig cell (virilizing, rare)
Nonspecialized Stroma: Mixed Mesodermal Tumor, Lymphoma, Leiomyosarcoma, and others.

GERM CELL TUMORS (2% TO 4%)
Dysgerminoma (1% to 2%)
Embryonic Differentiation
1. Benign cystic teratoma
2. Malignant teratoma (AFP, β-HCG negative)
Extraembryonic Differentiation
1. Endodermal sinus tumor/embryonal carcinoma (AFP positive)
2. Choriocarcinoma (rare, β-HCG positive)

SECONDARY (METASTATIC) CARCINOMAS

AFP, α-Fetoprotein; β-HCG, β-human chorionic gonadotropin.
*Percentages are the approximate frequency of primary malignancies in adults.

Epidemiology

In the United States, ovarian cancer is the leading cause of cancer death from gynecologic malignancies and is the fifth most common cause of cancer death in women.[5] The incidence of ovarian cancer increases with age, with a peak in the eighth decade.[6] The peak incidence is 57 cases per 100,000 women in the 70- to 74-year age group; the median age at diagnosis is 63 years.[7]

Epidemiologic studies have identified several factors important in the carcinogenesis of ovarian cancer. Numerous studies have identified parity, multiple births, history of breast-feeding, and use of oral contraceptives as being protective against the development of ovarian cancer.[8-10] The relationships between each of these factors and ovarian cancer incidence support a recent hypothesis that the development of ovarian cancer is related to incessant ovulation.[11,12] It is postulated that ovarian cancer may develop from an aberrant repair process of the surface epithelium during each ovulation cycle; if this is the case, then factors that result in a decreased number of ovulatory cycles may decrease the risk of ovarian cancer.

An individual patient's risk of developing ovarian cancer also depends on both familial and genetic factors. The lifetime risk for a woman in the general population is 1.6%, but this risk rises to approximately 5% if a single other first-degree family member is affected and to 7% if two relatives are affected.[13] Familial ovarian cancer has been linked to at least three distinct genotypes. The incidence of familial ovarian cancer is unclear, but it is estimated that 1% to 5% of all patients with epithelial ovarian cancer have familial ovarian cancer. Women with the hereditary ovarian cancer syndromes may have a lifetime probability of developing ovarian cancer of as high as 50%.[14]

Pathology

Epithelial tumors account for 90% of all ovarian malignancies. Two thirds of epithelial ovarian tumors, including a range from borderline malignancies through markedly undifferentiated tumors, are frankly malignant. The borderline malignancies have cytologic features of malignancy and can metastasize, although they are characterized by an absence of destructive stromal invasion. The most common type of epithelial ovarian cancer arises from the ovarian surface epithelium. As the epithelium becomes malignant, it exhibits a variety of müllerian-type differentiations. The types of epithelial tumors are listed in Box 31-1 in order of decreasing frequency. In cystadenocarcinomas, the degree of histologic differentiation (grade) is an important predictor of clinical behavior, metastatic potential, and lethality; this is particularly true in serous tumors.

Patterns of Spread

Epithelial ovarian tumors arise from the surface epithelium and eventually penetrate the ovarian capsule. Once the ovarian capsule is penetrated, malignant cells seem to exfoliate into the peritoneal cavity. Tumor cells circulate with the normal circulation of the peritoneal fluid and may implant and grow on any surface in the peritoneal cavity. In addition, tumor cells may obstruct lymphatics, resulting in ascites. Growth of ovarian cancer in the peritoneal cavity may cause matted loops of bowel, resulting in adhesions and mechanical obstruction.

Lymphatic spread may occur, most commonly to the para-aortic and pelvic nodes. The incidence of nodal metastases seems to be related to the stage of disease. Most patients with advanced ovarian cancer may have involvement of pelvic and para-aortic nodes.[15] Only about 15% of patients have extraabdominal disease at the time of first relapse; in most patients, recurrent or persistent disease is intraabdominal.

Surgical Staging

Staging of ovarian cancer is based on findings at surgical exploration and pathologic examination of the surgical specimens. The 1997 revision of the American Joint Committee on Cancer (AJCC) and International Federation of Gynecology and Obstetrics (FIGO) staging system is shown in Box 31-2.[16] Because postoperative therapy is often based on the disease stage and other prognostic factors, meticulous surgical staging is recommended, including, when possible, a vertical abdominal incision, multiple cytologic washings, intact tumor removal, complete abdominal exploration, removal of the ovaries, uterus and tubes, omentectomy, lymph node sampling, and random peritoneal biopsies. When surgical staging is incomplete, the extent of disease may be significantly underestimated: in a study of systematic restaging in 100 patients believed to have stage I or II disease after initial surgical staging, 31 patients (31%) were found to have more advanced disease than initially diagnosed, and 23 (77%) of these 31 patients were found to actually have stage III disease.[17]

In this era when most patients with ovarian cancer are treated with combination chemotherapy regardless of the stage or extent of disease, it could be argued that the detection of occult or microscopic residual disease will not change treatment recommendations for individual patients. However, careful surgical staging is an essential part of maximal removal of tumor, an important aspect of therapy and prognosis.

Prognostic Factors

The most important independent prognostic factors in ovarian cancer are tumor stage, volume of residual disease, and tumor grade.

BOX 31-2 **American Joint Committee on Cancer and International Federation of Gynecology and Obstetrics Staging Systems for Cancer of the Ovary**

AJCC	FIGO	
PRIMARY TUMOR (T)		
TX	—	Primary tumor cannot be assessed
T0	—	No evidence of primary tumor
T1	I	Tumor limited to ovaries (one or both)
T1a	IA	Tumor limited to one ovary; capsule intact, no tumor on ovarian surface. No malignant cells in ascites or peritoneal washings*
T1b	IB	Tumor limited to both ovaries; capsules intact, no tumor on ovarian surface. No malignant cells in ascites or peritoneal washings*
T1c	IC	Tumor limited to one or both ovaries with any of the following: capsule ruptured, tumor on ovarian surface, malignant cells in ascites or peritoneal washings
T2	II	Tumor involves one or both ovaries with pelvic extension
T2a	IIA	Extension and/or implants on uterus and/or tube(s). No malignant cells in ascites or peritoneal washings
T2b	IIB	Extension to other pelvic tissues. No malignant cells in ascites or peritoneal washings
T2c	IIC	Pelvic extension (2a or 2b) with malignant cells in ascites or peritoneal washings
T3 and/ or N1	III	Tumor involves one or both ovaries with microscopically confirmed peritoneal metastasis outside the pelvis and/or regional lymph node metastasis†

AJCC	FIGO	
T3a	IIIA	Microscopic peritoneal metastasis beyond pelvis
T3b	IIIB	Macroscopic peritoneal metastasis beyond pelvis 2 cm or less in greatest dimension
T3c and/ or N1	IIIC	Peritoneal metastasis beyond pelvis more than 2 cm in greatest dimension and/or regional lymph node metastasis
M1	IV	Distant metastasis (excludes peritoneal metastasis)

REGIONAL LYMPH NODES (N)

NX		Regional lymph node(s) cannot be assessed
N0		No regional lymph node metastasis
N1		Regional lymph node metastasis

DISTANT METASTASIS (M)

MX		Distant metastasis cannot be assessed
M0		No distant metastasis
M1		Distant metastasis (excludes peritoneal metastasis)

STAGE GROUPING

Stage IA	T1a	N0	M0
Stage IB	T1b	N0	M0
Stage IC	T1c	N0	M0
Stage IIA	T2a	N0	M0
Stage IIB	T2b	N0	M0
Stage IIC	T2c	N0	M0
Stage IIIA	T3a	N0	M0
Stage IIIB	T3b	N0	M0
Stage IIIC	T3c	N0	M0
	Any T	N1	M0
Stage IV	Any T	Any N	M1

From Fleming I, Cooper JS, Henson DE, et al., eds. *AJCC Cancer Staging Manual.* 5th ed. Philadelphia, Pa: Lippincott Williams & Wilkins; 1997:201-206.

*The presence of nonmalignant ascites is not classified. The presence of ascites does not affect staging unless malignant cells are present.
†Liver capsule metastases are T3/stage III, liver parenchymal metastasis, M1/stage IV. Pleural effusion must have positive cytology for M1/stage IV.

The twenty-third FIGO Annual Report on the Results of Treatment in Gynecological Cancer presented survival results by stage of disease for patients treated between 1990 and 1992. Overall survival rates were 82% for patients with stage I disease, 59% for patients with stage II disease, and 25% for patients with stage III disease. For the entire patient population, the overall survival rate was 42%.

Many studies have shown that the volume of tumor remaining at the completion of the surgery is a significant prognostic factor for survival in both patients treated with radiation therapy and patients treated with chemotherapy.[18-24] Evidence also exists to suggest that the number of residual masses is an important prognostic factor. These findings have resulted in a viewpoint that cytoreductive surgery with maximum tumor reduction has a beneficial effect on outcome.

A multivariate analysis of patients treated at the University of Toronto has confirmed that in addition to tumor stage and residual tumor remaining after surgery, tumor grade and patient age are important independent prognostic factors, whereas histopathologic subtype is less important and may be correlated with other prognostic factors. A multifactorial classification of patients with small-volume or no macroscopic residual disease has been developed and validated in sequential patient cohorts treated at the University of Toronto[24-28] (Figs. 31-2 and 31-3). In this population a combination of stage, residuum, and tumor grade clearly stratified patients into subgroups with widely disparate outcomes after treatment with radiation therapy. This type of classification has been validated by other investigators.[29-31]

Clinical Evaluation

The presenting symptoms of ovarian cancer are often vague and indistinct. The most common symptoms are abdominal discomfort, abdominal pain, and abdominal distention. Gastrointestinal symptoms are relatively common and may include change in bowel habits, nausea or dyspepsia, or early satiety. Unfortunately, 75% to 85% of patients have disease disseminated throughout the peritoneal cavity at presentation.

Because no reliable procedures currently exist for the early detection of ovarian cancer,[32-34] early-stage disease is usually diagnosed after detection of an asymptomatic adnexal mass on routine pelvic examination. However,

the majority of adnexal masses, particularly in premenopausal women, are not malignant.

Abdominal ultrasonography, computed tomography, and magnetic resonance imaging are often used to evaluate both early and advanced disease. Although imaging may aid in ruling out the possibility of hepatic metastases, the extent of intraperitoneal disease is best evaluated at surgery.

The most useful serum marker for ovarian cancer is CA-125. Eighty percent to 85% of patients with epithelial ovarian cancer have elevated CA-125 levels (> 35 U/ml).[35] More than 85% of patients with the serous subtype of epithelial ovarian cancer will have elevations of CA-125, but elevations occur less often in those with mucinous tumors. In postmenopausal women with asymptomatic pelvic masses, a CA-125 level of greater than 65 U/ml has a sensitivity of 97% and a specificity of 78% in the diagnosis of ovarian cancer.[36] However, in premenopausal women, nonmalignant conditions, including endometriosis, fibroids, and pelvic inflammatory disease, may produce elevations of serum CA-125, lowering the specificity of the test. Thus the finding of an elevated CA-125 level in patients older than 50 years is

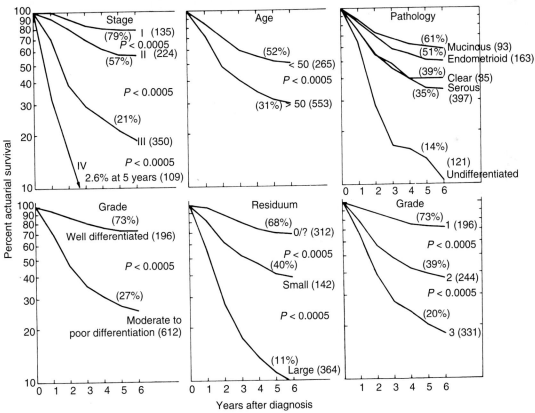

Fig. 31-2 Survival curves of 818 patients with epithelial carcinoma of the ovary treated at the Princess Margaret Hospital between 1971 and 1978 classified according to disease stage, age at diagnosis, histologic subtype, degree of differentiation, amount of residual disease, and grade. The percentage in parentheses above each curve is the 5-year survival rate; the number in parentheses after each curve is the number of patients in the corresponding group.

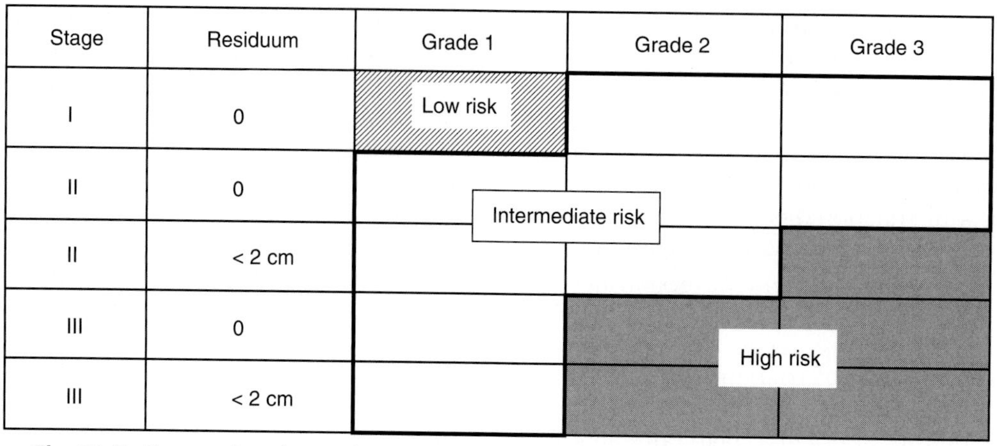

Stage	Residuum	Grade 1	Grade 2	Grade 3
I	0	Low risk		
II	0		Intermediate risk	
II	< 2 cm			High risk
III	0		High risk	
III	< 2 cm			

Fig. 31-3 Prognostic subgroupings according to stage, residuum, and grade in patients with stages I to III ovarian cancer with little or no residual disease. Abdominopelvic irradiation is recommended as the sole postoperative treatment in the intermediate-risk group. (From Carey M, Dembo AJ, Fyles AW, et al. *Int J Gynecol Cancer* 1993;3:24-35.)

suggestive of epithelial ovarian cancer and should prompt surgical exploration.

Treatment

In the past, treatment for ovarian cancer was selected on the basis of tumor stage and clinical-pathologic features. Postsurgical adjuvant therapy included pelvic or whole-abdominal radiation therapy, intraperitoneal colloid therapy, chemotherapy, administration of biological response modifiers, or combinations of these treatments. Today, most patients with ovarian cancer in the United States are treated with primary cytoreductive surgery and, when adjuvant therapy is indicated, combination chemotherapy. However, radiation therapy remains useful in the treatment of certain patient subgroups, as is discussed throughout the "Treatment" section of this chapter.

Surgery

Except in certain subsets of patients with stage I disease, the standard surgical approach to the management of epithelial ovarian cancer is a staging laparotomy with a bilateral salpingo-oophorectomy, a hysterectomy, and surgical cytoreduction of intraperitoneal tumor masses. At many centers, routine para-aortic and pelvic lymph node dissection is performed if this surgery, along with optimal debulking, will render the patient free of residual macroscopic disease.

As stated in the section on "Prognostic Factors" earlier in this chapter, the volume of tumor remaining at the completion of the surgery and the number of residual masses are significant prognostic factors for outcome. Thus most surgeons accept that attempts should be made to minimize the tumor residuum at the time of surgery. It is now recognized that the amount of residual

disease should be treated as a continuum for prognostic purposes, and most investigators now believe that optimal residuum is defined as the largest diameter of the largest residual lesion being less than 1 cm.

Hoskins and colleagues[37] studied the frequency with which optimal primary cytoreduction could be achieved. On average, optimal cytoreduction could be achieved in only about one third of patients.[37] Furthermore, the ultimate value of primary cytoreduction must be interpreted cautiously because even reduction to 1 g of residual tumor leaves approximately 10^9 tumor cells. Usually the most effective chemotherapy currently available will reduce the number of residual cells by about three logs. The number of residual cells will be increased by any tumor proliferation that occurs during chemotherapy and by any resistance that develops as the result of mutations as the tumor ages. Thus cure is unlikely even if all gross tumor is removed. The better outcome of patients with optimal cytoreductive surgery has previously been attributed to the therapeutic effect of surgery, but it could be that patients in whom optimal cytoreductive surgery is possible have biologically less aggressive or more responsive disease. However, because cure is rarely achieved in patients who have a residuum greater than 1 cm, it is usually worthwhile to attempt optimal cytoreduction before treatment is begun, in the hope that this will increase the chance of cure. Among patients with optimal cytoreduction, long-term survival is better for those having no macroscopic residual disease than it is for those having small-volume macroscopic residual disease.

Adjuvant Therapy for Early-Stage Disease

Only 10% to 15% of patients with epithelial ovarian cancer are diagnosed with stage I or II disease after careful staging laparotomy. These patients have a much better prognosis than do patients with advanced disease and constitute approximately one third of the patients with epithelial ovarian cancer who are eventually cured.

Several methodologic factors have hampered a precise understanding of the possible contribution of adjuvant therapy to the treatment of patients with stage I or II disease. These include the relative infrequency of the presentation, underestimates of disease extent during the time when laparotomies were performed less carefully, and lack of understanding of prognostic factors for early-stage disease. Because the prognosis for patients with stage I or II disease is relatively good, the conduct of phase III randomized controlled trials of postoperative adjuvant therapy in this subgroup is hampered by both the anticipated low event rate and the small numbers of patients. To date, no controlled study has established a curative advantage for any postoperative therapy. Decisions about postoperative therapy for patients with stage I or II disease therefore are based not on established benefit but rather on individual patients' predicted risk of relapse as determined by pathologic predictive factors and the physician's practice.

Patients with stage I disease with grade 1 (or sometimes grade 2) differentiation have a 5-year survival rate in excess of 90%.[26,38] Findings from several studies[38,39] support the current practice of advising that no postoperative adjuvant therapy be given to this subgroup. For patients with stage I, grade 2 or 3 disease, the risk of relapse may be as high as 30%. Because of this risk, most physicians in North America would recommend immediate postoperative adjuvant therapy of some type. In Europe, however, arguments have been put forward in favor of withholding adjuvant therapy in patients with high-grade stage I disease. These arguments are based on a randomized trial in which patients were assigned to receive immediate postoperative cisplatin chemotherapy or the same therapy given only at relapse.[39] The overall survival rates at 4 years were similar for the two groups.[39]

External-beam radiation therapy. Clinical trials have evaluated the impact of postoperative radiation therapy on the survival of patients with early-stage epithelial ovarian cancer. In a Gynecologic Oncology Group (GOG) study,[40] patients with stage I disease were randomly assigned after surgery to observation, pelvic radiation therapy, or melphalan. The results of this study were interpreted as inconclusive because surgical staging was not required and a significant proportion of patients were eliminated from the analysis.[40] A study in Toronto compared postoperative pelvic irradiation with observation in patients with stage I or II or asymptomatic stage III disease and failed to demonstrate the superiority of either approach; in this study, as in the GOG study, comprehensive staging was not mandated.[41] Pelvic irradiation did reduce the number of pelvic relapses but, because of an increased rate of recurrence in the upper abdomen in this subgroup, did not improve survival.[41]

No study has rigorously examined the role of abdominopelvic irradiation in stage I disease. A retrospective comparison of pelvic radiation therapy and no treatment[42] showed a statistically insignificant reduction in relapse risk with irradiation only for patients with grade 2 and 3 disease and patients with densely adherent tumors (a subset of patients in which disease may be more correctly classified and treated as stage II).

Intraperitoneal radiocolloid therapy. Because ovarian cancer tends to spread through the coelom, the intraperitoneal installation of radiocolloids, which theoretically deliver high doses of radiation to the peritoneal surfaces, is intuitively attractive for the treatment of early-stage disease. Colloids labeled with radioactive isotopes of phosphorus (^{32}P) or gold (^{198}Au) have been used. ^{198}Au is no longer available for use in North America because it poses a greater radiation hazard to people who come in contact with treated patients. No randomized trials have examined the benefits of ^{32}P versus observation-only in early-stage disease; however, several randomized trials have compared ^{32}P with various chemotherapeutic agents (Table 31-1).[43]

When ^{32}P was compared with single-agent cisplatin in the Norwegian Radium Hospital study,[44] 5-year disease-free survival rates for patients with stage I disease were 86% for patients treated with ^{32}P and 83% for patients treated with cisplatin. A small subgroup of patients with adhesions too extensive to permit treatment with ^{32}P were treated with whole-abdominal irradiation, and their 5-year disease-free survival rate was 95%. Because the incidence of late bowel obstructions requiring surgery was higher in the group treated with ^{32}P (4%) than in the cisplatin group, the authors concluded that cisplatin was the treatment of choice despite the fact that no benefit was found with respect to median survival, time to relapse, or proportion relapsing.

A similar study performed in Italy[39] compared ^{32}P with single-agent cisplatin in patients with stage IC ovarian cancer. Disease-free survival was longer in the cisplatin group; however, no difference was evident in 5-year overall survival rates (81% for cisplatin vs. 79% for ^{32}P).

The GOG conducted a trial of ^{32}P versus three cycles of cisplatin and cyclophosphamide in patients with unfavorable early-stage disease. No differences in survival were observed, but the authors concluded that chemotherapy was the preferred alternative because ^{32}P was associated with a higher incidence of bowel toxicity.[45]

A therapeutic value for ^{32}P has not been established. Because of the variable and unpredictable radiation dose distribution to peritoneal surfaces and the lack of penetration of this pure beta-emitter into tissues, it is unclear that ^{32}P would provide adequate radiation therapy to the entire peritoneal cavity or adequately penetrate the retroperitoneal nodes. If radiation therapy is to be used in ovarian cancer, it is better delivered with external-beam techniques, which provide a uniform and

TABLE 31-1

Five-Year Disease-Free and Overall Survival Rates in Prospective Randomized Trials Comparing ^{32}P Radiocolloid Therapy with Various Chemotherapy Agents in Patients with Early-Stage Ovarian Cancer

Series	Criteria for High Risk	Number of Patients	Study Design	5-Year Disease-Free Survival (%)	5-Year Overall Survival (%)
National Cancer Institute of Canada	IA, IB, G3; IC-III, OpD	257	Pelvic RT + ^{32}P vs. pelvic RT + melphalan vs. whole-abdomen RT	— — —	66 61 62
Gynecologic Oncology Group	IA, IB, G3; IC-II OpD	141	^{32}P vs. melphalan	80 80	78 81
Norwegian Radium Hospital	I-III OpD	340	CDDP vs. ^{32}P	75 81	— —
Italian Interregional Cooperative Group of Gynaecologic Oncology	IC	161	CDDP vs. ^{32}P	95 65	81 79

Modified from Cardenes H, Randall ME. *Semin Radiat Oncol* 2000;10:61-70.
OpD, Optimally debulked; *RT,* radiation therapy; *CDDP,* cisplatin.

predictable radiation dose to the peritoneal cavity and adequately irradiate the entire abdominal contents.

Chemotherapy. Several randomized trials examining the role of chemotherapy in early-stage ovarian cancer are ongoing or have been completed. A study conducted by the Italian Interregional Cooperative Group of Gynaecologic Oncology[39] studied patients with stage IA or IB, grade 2 and 3 tumors. Patients were randomly assigned to immediate cisplatin or to observation, with cisplatin given only at relapse. Although the use of immediate cisplatin improved the disease-free survival rate by approximately 20% compared with the rate in the observation group, overall survival rates with the two treatments were similar (85% for immediate cisplatin vs. 86% for observation), suggesting that platinum-based chemotherapy given at the time of relapse is as effective as immediate treatment of all patients. Other trials comparing observation to single-agent carboplatin[46] or carboplatin in combination with other chemotherapeutic agents are under way.

The GOG, in its protocol 157, is comparing three cycles of adjuvant carboplatin and paclitaxel versus six cycles of a similar regimen. This study will be open to patients considered to be at high risk for relapse, including patients with stage IC, IIA, IIB, or IIC disease with no macroscopic residual disease and patients with stage IA or IB high-grade or clear cell tumors.

General recommendations. The optimal postoperative treatment for patients with high-risk early-stage epithelial ovarian cancer remains to be established. Appropriate treatment options at this time include pelvic irradiation, platinum-based chemotherapy, and paclitaxel-based chemotherapy. Because no form of adjuvant therapy has been shown to provide a survival advantage compared with observation, observation alone can also be considered.

Postoperative Whole-Abdominal and Pelvic Irradiation

The identification of several chemotherapeutic agents with significant activity against advanced ovarian cancer has led to extremely limited use of radiation therapy as definitive postoperative therapy in epithelial ovarian cancer. Nevertheless, the evidence is incontrovertible for the efficacy of radiation therapy in certain subsets of patients.

Extensive experience with the platinum compounds, discovered in the late 1970s, and paclitaxel, introduced in the 1990s, has demonstrated that these drugs may prolong survival times. However, it is unclear whether these drugs produce significant improvements in survival rates. Most patients treated with platinum- or paclitaxel-based chemotherapy still have a relapse of their disease that leads to death.

Response rates to radiation therapy, even in chemotherapy-resistant ovarian cancer, are very high.[47-50] Although most physicians avoid recommending radiation therapy because of concern that it may impair bone marrow reserve—a crucial issue in patients being treated with hematotoxic chemotherapy agents—given the efficacy of radiation therapy, it seems premature to discard this modality from the definitive treatment armamentarium for ovarian cancer.

This discussion reviews the evidence supporting the contribution of radiation therapy to the cure of ovarian cancer and suggest specific patient subgroups in whom definitive postoperative adjuvant whole-abdominal plus pelvic irradiation (hereafter referred to as abdominopelvic irradiation) may have efficacy equivalent to that of chemotherapy.[51,52]

Evidence of efficacy. In ovarian cancer, the dominant route of dissemination is throughout the abdominal cavity, and tumors tend to remain confined to the abdominal cavity for extended periods; at first relapse, regardless of therapy, tumor is confined to the abdominal cavity in approximately 85% of patients.[53,54] Thus in radiation therapy for ovarian cancer, techniques that encompass the whole peritoneal cavity rather than just the pelvis or lower abdomen are likely to have the greatest curative potential.

Several studies have compared abdominopelvic irradiation with pelvic radiation therapy alone or pelvic radiation therapy combined with single-agent alkylating chemotherapy.[52,55] These studies have demonstrated a superior outcome with abdominopelvic irradiation for patients with minimal residual disease after primary surgery.

Substantial evidence is available from five trials to support the curative potential of abdominopelvic irradiation in patients with advanced ovarian cancer (Table 31-2).[25,29,52,56-58] Many retrospective analyses of outcomes in patients treated with abdominopelvic irradiation include patients in whom no residual disease was apparent. In these series, some patients were undoubtedly cured by surgery alone, and thus the magnitude of additional benefit conferred by the radiation therapy is not clear. However, all patients included in the trials summarized in Table 31-2 had known macroscopic residual disease at the time of irradiation. The cure rates were determined by the stage at presentation and the volume of residual disease after surgery. For the four studies with follow-up of more than 10 years (which should permit accurate estimates of the true cure rate because 90% of recurrences develop within 5 years of treatment), the outcomes were similar: Between 38% and 62% of patients with residual disease

smaller than 2 cm were cured after abdominopelvic irradiation. Among patients with stage II disease, the cure rate was higher for patients in whom the pelvis was treated to a higher dose than was the upper abdomen. For patients with residual disease in excess of 2 cm, the probability of cure ranged from 0% to 14%.

Although these studies provide strong evidence that abdominopelvic irradiation can cure patients with small-volume residual ovarian cancer, certain questions have been raised about interpretation of the results. Because aggressive cytoreductive surgery and comprehensive staging were not used in many of these studies, the presence and volume of residual disease may have been either underestimated or overestimated. However, the finding of similar long-term disease-free survival rates in patients with known small-volume macroscopic residual disease after surgery constitutes strong evidence that radiation therapy is curative in selected patients with ovarian cancer.

Selection of patients. In the past three decades, through studies begun at the Princess Margaret Hospital and The University of Texas M.D. Anderson Cancer Center, patients with all stages and extents of ovarian cancer have been treated with abdominopelvic irradiation.[41,59,60] Using data from these studies, Dembo and colleagues[26] performed a detailed multivariate analysis of pathologic prognostic factors and defined the patient and tumor factors that predict a favorable outcome after the administration of this treatment. These authors classified patients with small-volume or no residual ovarian cancer into three groups defined in terms of the risk of recurrence after surgery alone: low, intermediate, and high risk (Fig. 31-4; see also Fig. 31-3).[26] This classification of patients into risk groups has been validated by three other groups of investigators in New Haven,[27] Denmark,[30] and Germany.[31]

The low-risk group is composed of patients with stage I, grade 1 ovarian cancer without evidence of dense adherence or ascites. Multifactorial analysis of prognostic

---

TABLE 31-2

Outcomes After Abdominopelvic Irradiation in Patients with Residual Disease After Surgery

| Study | Study Endpoint | VOLUME OF RESIDUAL DISEASE BEFORE IRRADIATION | |
		< 2 cm	> 2 cm
Dembo, 1985[25]	10-year relapse-free survival rate, %	38	6
Martinez et al, 1985[57]	15-year failure-free survival rate, %	50	14
Fuller et al, 1987[52]	10-year relapse-free survival rate, %	62	0
Wesier et al, 1988[58]	10-year overall survival rate, %	42	10
Goldberg and Peschel, 1988[29]	Surviving fraction at 6 years	0.41	—*

Modified from Ozols RF, Rubin SC, Thomas G, et al. Epithelial ovarian cancer. In: Hoskins WJ, Perez CA, Young RC, eds. *Principles and Practice of Gynecologic Oncology.* 2nd ed. Philadelphia, Pa: Lippincott-Raven; 1997:919-986.
*No patient had residual disease measuring more than 2 cm.

Stage	Residuum	Grade 1	Grade 2	Grade 3
I	0	96 ± 2% (n = 80)	78 ± 5 (71)	62 ± 8 (39)
II	0	91 ± 4 (45)	73 ± 7 (46)	52 ± 7 (47)
II	< 2 cm	No relapses (5)	78 ± 14 (9)	21 ± 11 (14)
III	0	63 ± 14 (15)	26 ± 14 (12)	29 ± 11 (20)
III	< 2 cm	88 ± 12 (8)	45 ± 11 (20)	39 ± 10 (27)

Fig. 31-4 Five-year relapse-free survival rates (± standard deviation) in patients with ovarian cancer according to stage, residuum, and grade. The numbers in parentheses indicate the number of patients in each cell. Low-risk subgroups are indicated by hatched lines; intermediate-risk subgroups are indicated by unshaded boxes enclosed in bold lines; and high-risk subgroups are indicated by shaded boxes. (Fourteen patients without specific grade assignments were excluded.) (From Carey M, Dembo AJ, Fyles AW, et al. *Int J Gynecol Cancer* 1993;3:24-35.)

factors determined that these patients have such a good survival rate after surgery alone (96% ± 2%) that no postoperative therapy is warranted.[26]

In patients with stage II or III disease, the amount and site of residual disease and the tumor grade are strong determinants of the success of abdominopelvic irradiation. Given the restrictions on the dose that can be safely delivered to the upper abdomen and pelvis, abdominopelvic irradiation should be used only in patients with no macroscopic disease in the upper abdomen and with small-volume macroscopic (0 to 2 cm) residual disease in the pelvis.

The intermediate-risk group consists of patients with stage I disease with grade 2 or 3 lesions or dense adherence or ascites; stage II disease, except grade 3 lesions with residual tumor after surgery; and stage III, grade 1 disease with no macroscopic residual tumor or with macroscopic residual tumor measuring less than 2 cm and located in the pelvis. The patients in the intermediate-risk category constitute about one third of the total patient population with ovarian cancer. It is in this intermediate-risk group that abdominopelvic irradiation is most appropriate as the sole postoperative treatment method. With the use of this approach, more than 67% of intermediate-risk patients were alive and disease-free 10 years after treatment, with minimal late morbidity.[23,61]

Patients in the high-risk group have a 10-year recurrence-free rate of approximately 20% after treatment with abdominopelvic irradiation alone after surgery.[23] Although these high-risk patients are now largely treated with cisplatin- or paclitaxel-based chemotherapy, one study has suggested that among high-risk patients who have undergone optimal cytoreduction, cisplatin-based combination chemotherapy followed by abdominopelvic irradiation may significantly improve median survival times and relapse-free survival rates over those that have been achieved among historical controls treated with radiation therapy alone.[62]

A recent study from Australia[63] examined the outcome of 58 patients fulfilling Dembo's definition of intermediate risk.[26] These patients were treated with abdominopelvic irradiation after cytoreductive surgery, and their reported relapse-free and overall survival rates—52% and 55% at 5 years—were similar to those reported by Dembo and colleagues. The consistency of these reports supports a conclusion of a significant curative benefit for abdominopelvic irradiation in patients defined as having intermediate-risk disease by this prognostic classification system. Radiation therapy should therefore still be considered a rational choice of therapy for a large proportion of patients with optimally cytoreduced ovarian cancer.

Treatment technique. The irradiated volume and the total dose are critical determinants of the therapeutic benefit of abdominopelvic irradiation.

Treatment must include the entire peritoneal cavity. Originally, coverage of the peritoneal cavity was accomplished by using a "moving strip" technique developed at the M.D. Anderson Cancer Center.[64,65] However, today the open-field technique is generally preferred because it is simpler, takes less time (6 vs. 10 to 13 weeks), and is associated with less morbidity.[57,64,66] Two randomized studies have compared the moving strip and open-field techniques and have shown them to be equally effective with respect to tumor control.[66,67] In general, parallel opposing portals with a beam energy sufficient to ensure dosage variation of no greater than

5% should be used. Simulator and portal films are required to ensure that the margins are outside the peritoneal reflection laterally and that the treatment portal is above the level of the diaphragm on expiration. The field margins should be outside the iliac wings and below the level of the obturator foramina to ensure adequate coverage of the pelvic floor.

Preliminary results from a randomized study by the National Cancer Institute of Canada suggest that survival is significantly reduced when the peritoneal surfaces were inadequately encompassed by the radiation field. An analysis of several series in which radiation therapy was administered to patients with stage I to III ovarian cancer also showed the prognostic importance of the adequacy of peritoneal coverage.[68]

Tumor doses limited to 22 to 30 Gy result in acceptable rates of side effects. Treatment is generally delivered in daily fractions of 1 to 1.2 Gy, with both fields treated each day. Appropriate renal shielding posteriorly should be used to limit the renal dose to 18 to 20 Gy. Generally a boost dose is given to the pelvis in 1.8- to 2-Gy fractions to bring the total pelvic dose to 45 to 50 Gy. However, it may be best to limit this practice to patients with residual disease confined to the pelvis; in patients with residual macroscopic disease at other sites, boost doses to the sites of distant metastases may be most appropriate. Some investigators have advocated routinely delivering a boost dose to the para-aortic lymph nodes and the medial domes of the diaphragm,[60] although this technique has not been used routinely at the University of Toronto. One randomized study[69] compared two doses of abdominopelvic irradiation in patients with intermediate-risk ovarian cancer: 22.5 Gy in 22 fractions and 27.5 Gy in 27 fractions. No significant difference in overall survival rate was found between the two groups (83% in the low-dose group and 72% in the high-dose group). Similarly, no difference was found in patterns of relapse, hematologic complications, or late complications between the two groups. Thus at least within this dose range, no advantage to using the higher dose of radiation is evident. Within this dose range, hepatic shielding is not required.

Detractors from the role of abdominopelvic irradiation in ovarian cancer have argued that the doses that can be used safely are ineffective in sterilizing residual disease. However, although Fletcher's seminal work suggested that 50 Gy is required to produce a 90% probability of control of microscopic residual disease,[70] more recent radiobiologic modeling[71] based on data from the clinical literature in multiple tumor sites has demonstrated that the dose-response curve for control of subclinical metastases of ovarian cancer present after surgery is in fact different than previously believed. The model suggests that although microscopic disease was previously assumed to imply a tumor burden of 10^8 or 10^9 residual clonogenic cells in all patients, in all

probability the residual tumor burden is actually heterogeneous, ranging from a single cell to 10^8 or 10^9 cells, with many patients having residual tumor burdens near the small end of the range. One implication of this model is that in many patients (i.e., those with lower residual tumor burden), disease control and reduction in the risk of recurrence can be achieved with radiation doses lower than 45 to 50 Gy. In fact, available data regarding abdominopelvic irradiation for control of subclinical ovarian cancer indicate that doses of 22 to 25 Gy in 1-Gy fractions yield a reduction in the rate of metastasis of 38% to 40%.[52,72,73]

The model of heterogeneity of residual tumor cell burden in ovarian cancer helps explain the efficacy and limitations of conventional radiation therapy in ovarian cancer. It explains why the radiation doses used to date, although lower than the 50-Gy dose once believed necessary for disease control, have led to cure in a substantial proportion of patients. Because tolerance limits the dose that can be delivered to the upper abdomen compared with the pelvis, only patients with microscopic upper abdominal disease and a small macroscopic pelvic residuum may be cured with abdominopelvic irradiation.

Side effects. Abdominopelvic irradiation is associated with both acute and chronic side effects. The acute effects usually resolve within 2 to 3 weeks after completion of treatment. Patients commonly report fatigue, which increases during the course of radiation therapy. Gastrointestinal side effects are also common; most patients experience some degree of nausea or anorexia. Fortunately, nausea is often well relieved by the new antinausea agents such as ondansetron. Approximately 75% of patients experience diarrhea with or without abdominal cramping. Acute hematologic toxicity is modest. In a randomized trial from the University of Toronto[69] in which patients were assigned to one of two abdominal doses of radiation—22.5 Gy in 22 fractions or 27.5 Gy in 27 fractions—five patients in the low-dose group and seven in the high-dose group had white cell counts of less than 2×10^9/L at the completion of radiation therapy, and three patients in each arm had grade 3 thrombocytopenia (Table 31-3).[69]

A review of nearly 600 patients treated with abdominopelvic irradiation[74] showed that 10% could not complete treatment, with the most commonly cited reason being myelosuppression. Radiation therapy should be interrupted for thrombocytopenia (platelet count < 50,000/μl [50 × 10^9/L]) or neutropenia (neutrophil count < 1000/μl [1 × 10^9/L]).

The late effects of abdominopelvic irradiation include asymptomatic basal pneumonitis or fibrosis, which is detectable in 15% to 20% of patients on radiography. This results from the necessity of including 1 to 2 cm of the inferior lung field in the radiation portal to ensure adequate coverage of the hemidiaphragm. Eleven of 125 patients in the University of Toronto randomized study of two doses

TABLE 31-3		
Acute and Chronic Side Effects of Abdominopelvic Irradiation in the University of Toronto Randomized Trial of Low-Dose (22.5 Gy) vs. High-Dose (27.5 Gy) Treatment		
Side Effect	Low-Dose Group	High-Dose Group
ACUTE EFFECTS		
WBC count, median	2.7	2.6
(range) ($\times 10^9$/L)	(1.1-4.1)	(1.4-5.2)
Platelet count, median	134	121
(range) ($\times 10^9$/L)	(46-224)	(43-268)
LATE EFFECTS (NUMBER OF PATIENTS)		
Bowel		
Grade 1 or 2	13	10
Grade 3	2	0
Hepatic		
Grade 1 or 2	32	29
Grade 3	0	1
Lung		
Grade 1 or 2	7	4
Bladder		
Grade 1	2	0
Grade 3	1	1

From Fyles AW, Thomas GM, Pintilie M, et al. *Int J Radiat Oncol Biol Phys* 1998;41:543-549.
WBC, White blood cell.

of radiation had radiographic evidence of pneumonitis, although only two patients, both in the high-dose group, had associated symptoms.[69] With upper-abdominal doses of 22 to 25 Gy in 22 to 25 fractions, about 50% of patients will develop a transient elevation of the alkaline phosphatase level a few months after radiation therapy. A rising alkaline phosphatase level in this setting does not usually signify recurrence in the liver.[25]

Late gastrointestinal complications are the complications of greatest concern to most investigators. The frequency and severity of late gastrointestinal side effects depend on the total dose of radiation, the dose per fraction, and the extent and number of previous operations.[75,76] The risk of late complications seems to be increased if lymph node sampling was performed as part of the initial operation.[77] The risk of serious bowel complications may be minimized if the technical principles outlined in the section on "Treatment Technique" earlier in this chapter are followed.

Generally, about 10% to 15% of patients report some diarrhea or persistent bloating related to particular dietary intolerance, but frank malabsorption is extremely rare. Obstruction requiring surgical correction is much more rare than is usually appreciated. In four studies including a total of almost 1100 patients, 5.6% of the patients required bowel surgery for late radiation-related complications (the rates for the individual studies ranged from 1.4% to 14%).[25,29,78,79] In these collected series, four patients (< 0.5%) died as a result of radiation-induced bowel damage.

No cases have been reported of second malignancy as a result of abdominopelvic irradiation. This is in distinct contrast to the findings of Travis and colleagues[80] regarding patients with ovarian cancer treated with platinum-based chemotherapy. The relative risk of leukemia among 28,971 patients who received platinum-based chemotherapy was 4.0 (95% confidence interval of 1.4 to 11.4). The relative risks for treatment with carboplatin and cisplatin were 6.5 and 3.3, respectively.

Abdominopelvic Irradiation vs. Chemotherapy

The relative effectiveness of abdominopelvic irradiation and combination platinum-based chemotherapy as adjuvant treatment in patients with small-volume or no macroscopic residual ovarian cancer after surgery has often been debated. A review of the current literature does not resolve which of these two treatments is preferable.

The GOG in the United States and the National Cancer Institute of Canada both conducted studies that compared abdominopelvic irradiation and platinum-based chemotherapy. Both studies failed to accrue sufficient numbers of patients to permit valid comparisons of the two treatments, probably because of physician biases and the disparate nature of the treatments.

Numerous nonrandomized studies of radiation therapy or chemotherapy for ovarian cancer have been reported, but for multiple reasons, valid comparisons between these studies are not possible. The radiation therapy series tend to be older and thus tend not to have included rigorous staging or aggressive cytoreductive surgery, in contrast with the practice in the recent chemotherapy studies. In the radiation therapy studies, the extent of disease may have been underestimated, and thus the efficacy of irradiation may have been underestimated. On the other hand, patients in the radiation therapy series who had minimal macroscopic residual disease after surgery that did not include extensive cytoreduction may have had a more favorable prognosis than patients in the chemotherapy series who had minimal macroscopic disease after more aggressive debulking surgery. Further complicating comparisons of the radiation therapy and chemotherapy series is the introduction of newer diagnostic techniques and more accurate staging methods, which may have changed the stage distribution of ovarian cancer.

Long-term overall survival rates and progression-free survival rates have now been reported for patients with advanced ovarian cancer treated with cisplatin-based chemotherapy. In the largest reported series, the disease-free survival rate at 4 years was 35%.[81] It would be expected that 10% to 15% more patients would relapse with longer follow-up. Overall survival rates reported for abdominopelvic irradiation in optimal stage III disease are approximately 30% to 35%.[26] These findings seem to indicate that radiation therapy and cisplatin-based chemotherapy produce similar outcomes in patients with ovarian cancer. However, given the limitations outlined in the preceding paragraph, this conclusion is problematic.

It is clear that radiation therapy is effective in the management of ovarian cancer, and it is also clear that when radiation therapy is used as the primary postoperative therapy, optimal results require strict adherence to the criteria for selecting patients and the technical aspects of radiation delivery. The similarity of the long-term survival rates for patients treated with platinum-containing chemotherapy and patients treated with radiation therapy should stimulate renewed interest in the use of radiation therapy in ovarian cancer. Many investigators were quick to discard radiation therapy from the treatment armamentarium once cisplatin's activity was recognized. However, given that the long-term results with cisplatin have been less than satisfactory, radiation therapy deserves continued study. No precedent is evident in any solid tumor for discarding from the treatment armamentarium a single agent with the level of activity seen with radiation therapy in the treatment of ovarian cancer.

No reports have been published of comparisons between abdominopelvic irradiation and the newer chemotherapy agents that have been shown to be active against ovarian cancer. Prospective randomized trials have demonstrated that cisplatin plus paclitaxel improves the survival of patients with advanced ovarian cancer compared with cisplatin plus cyclophosphamide, the previous standard.[82,83] The chemotherapy regimen of choice for all patients with ovarian cancer is now a combination of paclitaxel with either cisplatin or carboplatin.

Further explorations of the role of radiation therapy as primary postoperative adjuvant therapy in epithelial ovarian cancer—either radiation therapy as a single agent or radiation therapy as part of concurrent or sequential combined-modality therapy—are justified. However, at the moment, such studies have low priority. Current issues being explored with regard to optimizing chemotherapy include the dose intensity of the platinum compounds, prolongation of the number of treatment courses, and newer multidrug combinations containing other drugs with identified activity against ovarian cancer (e.g., gemcitabine, topotecan, and docetaxel). In addition, comparisons of intraperitoneal versus intravenous therapy are being conducted.[84]

Consolidation or Salvage Radiation Therapy After Chemotherapy

A strong theoretical basis is evident for the use of sequential multimodality therapy in patients with ovarian cancer. If no cross-resistance occurs between surgery, chemotherapy, and radiation therapy and if these modalities can be combined with acceptable toxicity without diminishment of their individual efficacies, then sequential multimodality therapy would be a means of increasing the total cytoreductive capacity of treatment.

Fuks and colleagues[85] in 1978 were among the first to propose the use of sequential multimodality therapy. Their regimen consisted of cisplatin-based chemotherapy followed by cytoreductive surgery and then abdomino-pelvic irradiation in patients with advanced disease.[85] Since that time, numerous reports of sequential multimodality therapy have appeared.

In 1993 Thomas[86] published a review of 28 studies that examined the role of radiation therapy for either consolidation of results after surgery and chemotherapy or as salvage treatment for residual disease in patients with ovarian cancer (Table 31-4).[86-98] The studies included a total of 713 patients. The review did not provide definitive conclusions about the value of this treatment because most of the studies were single-arm trials without appropriate controls. The balance of the evidence, however, was against a significant curative benefit for radiation therapy used as either salvage or consolidation treatment (see Table 31-4).[86-98]

The failure of this review to detect a benefit from salvage or consolidation radiation therapy may indicate that sequential therapy is indeed not beneficial. On the

---

TABLE 31-4

Results of Consolidation or Salvage Radiation Therapy for Patients with No Residual Disease or Only Microscopic Residual Disease After Surgery and Chemotherapy

Study and Reference	NUMBER SURVIVING/ NUMBER AT RISK	
	No Residual Disease (Consolidation)	Microscopic (< 5 mm) Residual Disease (Salvage)
Chiara et al, 1991[89]	6/9	5/11
Greiner et al, 1984[90]	14/15	5/9*
Reddy et al, 1989[91]	—	4/5
Kuten et al, 1988[92]	5/5	12/18
Solomon et al, 1988[93]	—	4/12
Kong et al, 1988[88]	—	3/5
Rosen et al, 1986[94]	4/4	3/4
Haie et al, 1989[95]	14/23	—
Kersh et al, 1988[96]	1/4	10/15
Goldhirsch et al, 1988[97]	19/24	—
Menczer et al, 1986[98]	9/10†	—
Morgan et al, 1988[87]	—	8/8*

From Thomas GM. *Gynecol Oncol* 1993;51:97-103.

*1 cm residuum.

†Result interpreted as negative by authors.

other hand, methodologic reasons may account for the findings; most of the studies were observational, without appropriate controls, and patient selection was often inappropriate, with inclusion of patients with large-volume residual disease after chemotherapy, patients who had undergone many previous operations, patients who had received protracted chemotherapy and had demonstrated chemoresistance, patients with poor bone marrow reserve, and patients with extensive adhesions.

The Swedish/Norwegian Ovarian Cancer Study Group conducted a multicenter study of sequential combined-modality therapy that closed in April 1993. Seven hundred forty-one patients were randomly assigned to receive or not receive consolidation radiation therapy after four courses of cisplatin and doxorubicin followed by second-look surgery. Ninety-eight patients had microscopic or no macroscopic residual disease and were randomly assigned to receive whole-abdominal radiation therapy, continued chemotherapy with cisplatin and doxorubicin to a total of 10 courses, or observation only. Although the patient groups were relatively small and follow-up was early at the last analysis in July 1994, a significant improvement in survival was reported for patients receiving whole-abdominal radiation therapy. For patients with macroscopic residual disease, no difference in survival was evident between whole-abdominal irradiation and further chemotherapy. Preliminary analyses suggest only mild or moderate reactions to the radiation.

Selection of patients. In studies that reported the amount of residual disease, survival clearly depended on the tumor residuum before radiation therapy. For 473 patients in the 28 series, sufficient information was available to permit calculation of the amount of residual disease. Among these patients, survival rates were 76% (86 of 113) in patients with no residuum, 49% (77 of 158) in patients with microscopic residual disease or residuum less than 5 mm, and 17% (34/202) in patients with macroscopic residual disease.[86] The survival rate for patients with macroscopic disease is probably no different from that achieved with primary surgery and chemotherapy. This finding suggests that salvage radiation therapy is inappropriate for most patients with more than microscopic residual disease after chemotherapy.

It is unclear whether the better survival rates among patients with microscopic or no residual disease are attributable to the abdominopelvic irradiation or rather to the inherently better prognosis of those patients. The observed outcomes are compatible with the variability of already known prognostic factors in ovarian cancer, including patient age, tumor grade, and previous response to chemotherapy; therefore an unequivocal treatment benefit for radiation therapy cannot be established. However, the suggestion of better results among patients with microscopic or no residual disease (see Table 31-4) implies that at least some possible benefit may accrue to these patients and that future randomized, controlled studies should examine the value of consolidation radiation therapy in these patients.

Although most reported studies of consolidation radiation therapy have included too few patients to allow meaningful analyses of possible prognostic and treatment factors that contribute to the observed outcomes, the data of Schray and colleagues[99] are valuable because of the method of analysis and presentation. In a multivariate analysis of prognostic factors for disease-free survival, these authors established that the following factors are significant: tumor grade (70% survival for grades I and II vs. 10% for grades III and IV) and initial residuum before chemotherapy (50% survival for ≤2 cm vs. 14% for > 2 cm). Schray and colleagues[99] also examined the prognostic impact of the amount of residual disease at the time of radiation therapy. Three of five patients with microscopic disease remained disease free after radiation therapy, whereas only five of 21 patients with macroscopic disease that had been debulked to microscopic amounts before consolidation radiation therapy remained disease free. Finally, Schray and colleagues[99] examined the prognostic impact of the number of favorable factors (i.e., amount of residual disease before chemotherapy, amount of residual disease before radiation therapy, and tumor grade). Rates of freedom from disease after radiation therapy were 0% (0 of 17) for patients with none of the favorable factors, 29% (4 of 14) for patients with one favorable factor, 53% (8 of 15) for patients with three favorable factors, and 67% (4 of 6) for patients with four favorable factors.[99]

Appropriate selection of patients for studies of consolidation or salvage radiation therapy should be guided by this information. Radiation therapy is likely to improve cure rates in patients with no macroscopic disease after chemotherapy. However, it is doubtful that radiation therapy would be beneficial for patients requiring further resection of chemoresistant disease before consideration of the use of radiation therapy.[25,26,100,101]

Because radiation therapy is not curative in patients with larger volumes of residual disease, it is unlikely (because of many biological factors that may be operative, including accelerated clonogen proliferation) that salvage radiation therapy would be of curative benefit in patients with large-volume disease who have already undergone extensive surgery (including secondary debulking and chemotherapy, to which resistance may have already been demonstrated).

Altered-fractionation schedules. Altered fractionation schedules are currently being investigated as a potential means of increasing the biologically effective dose of consolidation radiation therapy and reducing its toxicity. The protracted course of antineoplastic therapy involved in sequential multimodality treatment may allow accelerated clonogen proliferation and thus contribute to treatment failure. This theoretical concern, along with the desire to reduce the toxicity of therapy, is the basis for explorations of hyperfractionated regimens.

Morgan and colleagues[87] treated 15 patients with stage III disease and known residual disease after cisplatin-based chemotherapy with 30.4 Gy given in 0.8-Gy fractions twice daily plus a boost of 15 to 19 Gy to the pelvis. All patients completed the planned treatment course, although two required a break because of thrombocytopenia. No episodes of small bowel obstruction occurred. Kong and colleagues[88] performed a similar study of sequential chemotherapy and radiation therapy with a radiation dose of 30 Gy in twice-daily 1-Gy fractions. In that study, only one of 23 patients so treated did not complete the planned therapy. Six patients with gross residual disease were also given a limited-field boost of 15 Gy in 15 fractions after the 30-Gy whole-abdomen dose, but none achieved control of disease and five required surgery for small bowel obstruction attributed to radiation damage. Among the 17 patients who did not receive the boost dose, five developed bowel obstructions, but all were attributed to tumor recurrence and not irradiation. Randall and colleagues[102] published the results of a GOG phase II trial of three cycles of cisplatin plus cyclophosphamide followed by hyperfractionated abdominopelvic irradiation (0.8 Gy per fraction twice daily to a total dose of 30.4 Gy) in patients with optimal stage III disease. This regimen was "well tolerated" and thought to be a "promising management option in selected patients."

Complications. Many studies of abdominopelvic irradiation after chemotherapy have reported complication rates higher than those reported for radiation therapy alone. This may be the result of the use of high radiation doses, protracted chemotherapy, and multiple abdominal operations.[103] Because the benefit of abdominopelvic irradiation after chemotherapy is equivocal and confined probably to a small subset of patients, the risk of complications is a major consideration. This risk can be minimized by restricting the radiation dose in patients who have undergone second-look operations. At present, no reports are available on the use of whole-abdominal irradiation after taxane-based chemotherapy. Concern regarding the use of radiation therapy after taxanes includes concerns about both renal function and possible chemotherapy or radiation recall phenomena.

General recommendations. In summary, it would seem that radiation therapy as consolidative treatment should be confined to patients with negative or microscopic disease at second-look laparotomy, prechemotherapy tumor bulk minimally larger than that of patients with optimally cytoreduced disease, chemotherapy limited to six courses with effective agents that are least toxic to the bone marrow, and radiation therapy delivered with a dose and technique ensuring acceptable complication rates or designed to explore the possible theoretical benefits of hyperfractionated irradiation at somewhat higher than conventionally accepted doses.

Palliation

Recurrent or persistent ovarian cancer after first-line chemotherapy is incurable. Patients with recurrent or persistent disease are often symptomatic, with generalized or localized abdominal symptoms from intraperitoneal disease. Usually, second-, third-, or fourth-line chemotherapy is used in attempts to prolong life and palliate symptoms. Few specific findings are available to permit evaluation of the quality of life or degree of symptom palliation achieved with this approach. Reported response rates range from 10% to 43%, and a variety of side effects have been reported.[47,79,104-112]

Radiation therapy as a palliative modality in ovarian cancer is often neglected but may be very useful if the sole or dominant site of symptomatic disease can be safely encompassed within a radiation field. In such situations (e.g., a fixed pelvic mass eroding the vaginal mucosa and causing bleeding, pain, or bowel or bladder dysfunction in the absence of obvious symptomatic peritoneal disease), local irradiation often produces tumor regression or relief from symptoms. Similarly, radiation therapy may be used to treat localized masses elsewhere in the abdomen, such as the retroperitoneal nodes. Palliative irradiation may also be useful for extra-abdominal disease, particularly supraclavicular or inguinal node masses and bone or brain metastases. Radiation therapy may also be beneficial for the acute relief of painful hepatomegaly resulting from capsular distention.

Limited data are available in the literature concerning the palliative efficacy of radiation therapy in these settings.[47,48,113] Investigators at the M.D. Anderson Cancer Center treated patients with large-single-fraction therapy (1 to 3 fractions of 10 Gy, with fractions delivered 4 weeks apart) and reported overall response rates of 55% in patients treated for pain and 71% in patients treated for bleeding.[113] However, six of the 42 treated patients developed severe radiation-induced bowel injury, which may have been attributable to the large fractions used.[113] Another report of palliative radiation therapy for recurrent ovarian cancer after initial management with cisplatin-containing regimens documented that radiation therapy produced a mean symptom-free interval of 8.5 months in a group of patients with a median survival of 19.5 months.[48]

Corn and colleagues[47] reported the use of fractionated palliative irradiation at 47 sites in 33 patients with symptomatic recurrence of ovarian cancer after front-line cisplatin-based chemotherapy. Palliative responses occurred in 79% of the patients, and complete palliative responses occurred in 51%. The median duration of palliation was 4 months; in 90% of cases, palliation lasted until death. Ninety percent of patients treated for vaginal bleeding and 85% of patients treated for rectal bleeding had their bleeding controlled; 83% of patients treated for pain experienced pain relief. A range of radiation doses was used, but it is unclear whether patients with better performance status received the higher doses. Palliation was more likely among patients with higher Karnofsky performance status and among patients who received a biologically effective dose of irradiation of at least 44 Gy, where the biological effective dose was calculated as (total dose {1+[fractional dose ÷ (alpha/beta)]}), where alpha/beta was set at 10.[47] Too few patients were in this study to permit a multivariate analysis of factors predictive of the observed palliative responses, and thus recommendations regarding the optimal palliative dose cannot be made from the finding in this study. The fractionation schemes used did not allow the construction of a full dose-response curve. However, it is clear from this study that durable palliation can be achieved with local radiation therapy for ovarian cancer that recurs after cisplatin-based chemotherapy, particularly for patients with good performance status.

Future Directions

Clearly, studies are required to explore the integration of radiation therapy with newer cytotoxic agents in the treatment of ovarian cancer, with particular attention paid to the use of concurrent chemotherapy and radiation therapy.

Evidence is clear from studies of other tumors sensitive to radiation therapy—including carcinomas of the anal canal, esophagus, rectum, head and neck, vulva, and cervix[113-118]—that the use of concurrent chemotherapy and radiation therapy may improve local control and survival. Despite the limitations on the radiation dose imposed by the large treatment volume and the need for inclusion of the upper abdomen, concurrent chemotherapy and radiation therapy for epithelial ovarian cancer needs to be explored. In vitro evidence confirms that low doses of radiation therapy can sensitize cisplatin-resistant ovarian cancer cell lines to cisplatin.[119] This suggests a potential clinical role for radiation therapy in treating platinum-resistant ovarian cancer.

A phase I study in 11 patients with stage III or IV ovarian cancer confirmed the feasibility of abdominopelvic irradiation to a dose of 20 Gy with intraperitoneal cisplatin after debulking surgery.[120] Because hematologic and gastrointestinal toxic effects were significant, the use of colony-stimulating growth factors was recommended for future prospective trials.[120] The use of abdominopelvic irradiation in conjunction with low-dose weekly cisplatin (15 mg/m²) has been explored in patients with advanced endometrial cancer and found to be feasible.[121] A similar study[122] has been reported in chemotherapy-refractory ovarian cancer: patients received 30 Gy of abdominopelvic irradiation in 30 fractions with 5 mg/m² of weekly cisplatin. The projected 5- and 10-year survival rates from that study were 44% and 35%, respectively. Thus despite the current focus on exploration of multiple combinations of newer chemotherapeutic agents, studies to explore the integration of radiation therapy with these newer agents are vitally necessary. The taxane compounds, use of which is becoming standard in all stages of ovarian cancer, are not only effective cytotoxic agents but also in vitro radiation sensitizers.[123] Thus concurrent paclitaxel with abdominopelvic irradiation needs to be explored.

Management of Borderline Epithelial Ovarian Tumors

Within the subgroup of ovarian tumors known as *borderline tumors*, natural history and histologic features are better understood for the serous subtype than for the less common subtypes.

Most patients with stage I borderline ovarian malignancies are treated with total hysterectomy and bilateral oophorectomy without postoperative adjuvant therapy. Five-year survival rates with this approach range from 90% to 100%. When patients wish to preserve fertility, conservative therapy consisting of just a unilateral oophorectomy can be used. Although recurrence rates are higher after conservative surgery than after total hysterectomy and bilateral oophorectomy (15% vs. 5%), the higher recurrence rates are not associated with measurable differences in long-term survival, possibly because of the long natural history of ovarian cancer or because bilaterality does not confer a worse prognosis.

Only one prospective randomized trial of adjuvant therapy for stage I borderline ovarian cancer has been done.[124] After complete surgery, patients were randomly assigned to observation, pelvic irradiation, or oral melphalan. Only 1 patient had a recurrence. This study and the excellent overall results of nonrandomized studies in the literature show that adjuvant therapy is not necessary for stage I borderline tumors.

Approximately 20% of patients with borderline epithelial ovarian tumors present with stage III or IV disease. Metastatic borderline tumors are lethal in one third to one half of cases, although the clinical course is often protracted over many years.[125] The significance of peritoneal implants in advanced disease is uncertain. The suggestion has been made that invasive implants carry a worse prognosis than noninvasive implants.[126,127] Noninvasive implants may be not true metastases but rather autochthonous extraovarian neoplasia, treatment of which would be different from treatment of invasive disease.

Kaern and colleagues[128] used cellular deoxyribonucleic acid (DNA) content to identify patients with borderline ovarian tumors with an unfavorable prognosis. Among patients over the age of 60 years with advanced mucinous or serous tumors, the 15-year survival rate was 75% in patients with diploid tumors and 20% in patients with aneuploid tumors. Other investigators subsequently confirmed the prognostic significance of aneuploidy in borderline tumors of the ovary.[129,130]

Although patients with aneuploid tumors are recognized as having a high risk of relapse, presently no evidence is available to show that these patients benefit from any type of adjuvant therapy. Various adjuvant postsurgical therapies have been evaluated, including single-agent alkylating drugs and platinum-based chemotherapy, but their value has not been established.[131] Patients have also been treated with external-beam irradiation, intraperitoneal radioactive colloid therapy, and combined-modality therapies. Second-look laparotomies and clinical observations have demonstrated responses to both chemotherapy and radiation therapy.[132] However, it is impossible to determine whether these therapies offer prolongation of either disease-free survival or overall survival. Although 5-year survival rates for patients with advanced-stage borderline tumors range from 64% to 96%,[131] patients continue to die of disease over time, and mortality rates climb to 30% to 50%.[125] The practice at the University of Toronto in general has been to treat patients with metastatic borderline tumors in the same way as patients with low-grade invasive carcinoma of comparable stage and residual tumor volume. The rarity of metastatic borderline tumors and their long natural history make randomized studies of therapy extremely difficult.

GRANULOSA CELL TUMORS

Granulosa cell tumors are diagnosed as unilateral nonmetastatic tumors in more than 80% of cases.[133,134] Granulosa cell tumors spread to contiguous structures and extend through the peritoneum. Metastasis to lymph nodes, liver, or beyond the abdomen is extremely rare at diagnosis.

Malignant behavior occurs in 25% to 50% of pure granulosa cell and mixed granulosa cell–theca cell tumors. Because granulosa-cell tumors often produce estrogen, a high proportion of patients have endometrial hyperplasia, and about 10% have coexisting endometrial carcinoma.

Metastases and bilaterality are good predictors of disease relapse and probably dense adherence as well. Data in the literature are conflicting with regard to whether the following factors predict relapse in nonmetastatic granulosa cell tumors: cyst size greater than 15 cm, age greater than 40 years, high mitotic rate, atypia, and diffuse pattern.[135-138] Rupture, capsular penetration, and capillary space invasion seem to be nonprognostic in the absence of tumor spread.

Granulosa cell tumors have a propensity for late recurrence after primary therapy, with more than half of deaths occurring more than 5 years after diagnosis. Less than 10% of patients with surgical stage I disease have recurrence, whereas 30% or more of patients with more advanced stage disease have recurrence. More than 70% of patients who develop recurrent disease will die of granulosa cell tumor. Stenwig and colleagues[134] reported a mean interval to recurrence of 8.9 years (range, 1 to 22 years).[139]

The effect of adjuvant therapy in stage I disease is not evaluable. This may be because the disease is rare and has a long natural history. Published reports often span decades of experience during which radiation therapy was applied sporadically and usually with small-volume techniques. In nonrandomized studies of stage I disease, the relapse rate was relatively low regardless of whether postoperative radiation therapy was used.[134,140]

Patients with more extensive disease have usually been treated with surgical resection and postoperative radiation therapy and chemotherapy. Although some patients treated with this approach have remained disease-free, others have experienced recurrent disease, often with a protracted clinical course, which makes it impossible to determine the relative benefits of surgery and radiation therapy.[140]

It is reasonable to offer abdominopelvic irradiation (as in epithelial ovarian cancer; see the section on "Postoperative Whole-Abdominal and Pelvic Irradiation" earlier in this chapter) to patients with bilateral, metastatic, high-risk nonmetastatic, or recurrent granulosa cell tumors provided that the residual tumor bulk is not large. The published experience with chemotherapy is relatively sparse. Certain multidrug regimens may be more effective than single alkylating agents or the combinations of dactinomycin, fluorouracil, and cyclophosphamide; doxorubicin and cisplatin; or doxorubicin, cisplatin, and cyclophosphamide.[141-145] In a GOG study in which vincristine, dactinomycin, and cyclophosphamide were used in patients with advanced or recurrent granulosa cell tumors, only a 20% partial response rate was observed.[146] The highest activity has been reported for the combination of cisplatin, vinblastine, and bleomycin.[147-149] Other investigators are currently using combinations of bleomycin, etoposide, and cisplatin or, more recently, paclitaxel and a platinum drug.

DYSGERMINOMA

Dysgerminoma differs from the epithelial ovarian malignancies in many respects. It mainly occurs in much younger patients (85% of patients are less than 29 years of age at diagnosis); its principal mode of dissemination is nodal rather than transperitoneal; and it is extremely sensitive to radiation therapy, with radio-sensitivity resembling that of the equivalent male tumor, seminoma of the testis.[150,151] About 75% of patients have disease confined to one ovary at the time of diagnosis.

Because dysgerminoma has been shown to be curable with chemotherapy and radiation therapy, management of this disease has changed appreciably over the past two decades.[151] It has been recommended that a laparotomy procedure similar to that required for epithelial ovarian tumors be performed in patients with dysgerminoma, with careful palpation and possible biopsy of retroperitoneal lymph nodes where the ovarian vessels originate from the renal artery and vein. Cytologic examination of peritoneal fluid and omental biopsy are also recommended.

Three large series in the literature have examined the results of conservative surgery without postoperative radiation therapy in 145 patients with stage I dysgerminoma.[150,152,153] Conservative surgery consisted of unilateral oophorectomy only, with or without ipsilateral salpingectomy. The other ovary, tube, and uterus were not removed. Surgical staging was apparently not performed routinely in these series, but the 10-year survival rate for these patients was 91%—similar to survival rates achieved using more aggressive initial and complete surgery followed by radiation therapy. Approximately 25% of patients with stage I disease had a recurrence after surgery, but most of these patients had their disease successfully controlled with radiation therapy, chemotherapy, or further surgery, bringing the 10-year survival rate to the reported 91%.

As the efficacy of chemotherapy against dysgerminoma becomes recognized, investigators are advising unilateral adnexectomy even in the case of minor involvement of the opposite ovary or nodal or peritoneal metastases. One series showed that the use of cisplatin, vinblastine, and bleomycin chemotherapy in these situations resulted in eradication of disease in the contralateral ovary and apparent cure, with preservation of child-bearing capacity.[154]

Baseline investigations after surgery should include chest radiography, bipedal lymphangiography, abdominal computed tomography, and estimation of the levels of the serum tumor markers α-fetoprotein and β-human chorionic gonadotropin. If a conservative surgical approach has been used, close postoperative monitoring for at least 2 years with chest radiography, abdominal computed tomography, and tumor marker evaluations is desirable. The objective of close monitoring is to detect recurrences before they become large, permitting treatment with curative intent with either chemotherapy or radiation therapy.

Data in the literature are conflicting regarding the prognostic importance of primary tumor size in stage IA disease. Some suggestion has been made that the risk of recurrence after conservative surgery may be related to the size of the primary tumor, but the evidence is insufficient to be persuasive against the use of conservative approaches, even in patients with large primary tumors. It is likely that if careful surveillance is adopted after conservative surgery, relapse will be detected early and treated effectively with salvage therapy.[152,155]

The management of stage IB and higher-stage dysgerminoma is controversial. For patients who do not wish to maintain fertility and for patients with disease in the abdominopelvic cavity, it is clear that radiation therapy is indicated and is generally curative. Because of the exquisite radiosensitivity of this tumor, it is unnecessary to exceed doses of 25 Gy in 20 to 25 fractions to the whole abdomen, with possible boosts of 10 Gy to sites of bulky residual disease. Prophylactic mediastinal irradiation is not advocated in stage III disease because extra-abdominal nodal relapse is very rare without uncontrolled abdominal disease, and mediastinal radiation therapy may reduce marrow reserves and prevent the effective use of salvage chemotherapy.[156]

For patients with stage II or III disease who wish to maintain fertility and for patients with supradiaphragmatic or visceral disease, combination chemotherapy is the treatment of choice.[157] Accumulated data from three series show resumption of menses after unilateral oophorectomy and chemotherapy with the combination of cisplatin, vinblastine, and bleomycin in 19 of 20 patients, with two subsequent successful pregnancies.[158] The optimal choice of drugs and duration of therapy have not been determined, although the two most commonly used regimens are vincristine, doxorubicin, and cyclophosphamide and cisplatin, vinblastine, and bleomycin. The latter combination has been used successfully for salvage therapy in patients with relapse after doxorubicin and cyclophosphamide and thus may be more effective. More recent data suggest that the combination of bleomycin, etoposide, and cisplatin cures most patients with recurrent or metastatic dysgerminoma regardless of its bulk.[159,160] This combination has been found to be less toxic than cisplatin, vinblastine, and bleomycin. However, it is important that methods be developed for stratifying dysgerminomas on the basis of risk of recurrence so that chemotherapy regimens can be more effectively tailored to the risk level.

Like testicular seminomas, dysgerminomas may regress slowly and incompletely after chemotherapy but usually do not represent residual disease unless they are enlarging. Consolidation radiation therapy after chemotherapy is not recommended unless a clear sign of progressive disease is evident after chemotherapy. For the rare patient in whom chemotherapy fails to control the disease and who is no longer considered curable, radiation therapy may provide excellent palliation.

REFERENCES

1. Cole MP. Suppression of ovarian function in primary breast cancer. In: Forrest APM, Kunkler PB, eds. *Prognostic Factors in Breast Cancer*. Edinburgh, Scotland: E and S Livingston; 1968.
2. Stillman RJ, Schinfield JS, Schiff I, et al. Ovarian failure in long-term survivors of childhood malignancy. *Am J Obstet Gynecol* 1981;139:62-66.
3. Fajardo LF, Berthrong M, Anderson RE. Female reproductive organs. In: *Radiation Pathology*. New York, NY: Oxford University Press; 2001:289-300.
4. Peck WS, McGreer JT, Kretzschmar NR, et al. Castration of the female by irradiation: the results in 334 patients. *Radiology* 1940; 34:176-186.
5. Greenlee RT, Hill-Harmon MB, Murray T, et al. Cancer statistics, 2001. *CA Cancer J Clin* 2001;51:15-36.
6. Yancik R, Ries LG, Yates JW. Ovarian cancer in the elderly: an analysis of Surveillance, Epidemiology and End Results program data. *Am J Obstet Gynecol* 1986;154:639-647.
7. Yancik R. Ovarian cancer. Age contrasts in incidence, histology, disease stage at diagnosis, and mortality. *Cancer* 1993;71: 517-523.
8. Greene MH, Clark JW, Blayney DW. The epidemiology of ovarian cancer. *Semin Oncol* 1984;11:209-226.
9. Cramer DW, Hutchison GB, Welch WR, et al. Factors affecting the association of oral contraceptives and ovarian cancer. *N Engl J Med* 1982;307:1047-1051.
10. Hartge P, Schiffman MH, Hoover R, et al. A case-control study of epithelial ovarian cancer. *Am J Obstet Gynecol* 1989;161:10-16.
11. Casagrande JT, Louie EW, Pike MC, et al. "Incessant ovulation" and ovarian cancer. *Lancet* 1979;2(8135):170-173.
12. Fathalla MF. Incessant ovulation—a factor in ovarian neoplasia? *Lancet* 1971;2(7716):163.
13. Schildkraut JM, Thompson WD. Familial ovarian cancer: a population-based case-control study. *Am J Epidemiol* 1988; 128: 456-466.
14. Lynch HT, Fitzsimmons ML, Conway TA, et al. Hereditary carcinoma of the ovary and associated cancers: a study of two families. *Gynecol Oncol* 1990;36:48-55.
15. Bergman F. Carcinoma of the ovary: a clinicopathological study of 86 autopsied cases with special reference to mode of spread. *Acta Obstet Gynecol Scand* 1966;45:211-231.
16. Fleming ID, Cooper JS, Henson DE, et al, eds. *AJCC Cancer Staging Manual*. 5th ed. Philadelphia, Pa: Lippincott Williams & Wilkins; 1997:201-206.
17. Young RC, Decker DG, Wharton JT, et al. Staging laparotomy in early ovarian cancer. *JAMA* 1983;250:3072-3076.
18. Hacker NF, Berek JS, Lagasse LD, et al. Primary cytoreductive surgery for epithelial ovarian cancer. *Obstet Gynecol* 1983;61: 413-420.
19. Delgado G, Oram DH, Petrelli EG. Stage III epithelial ovarian cancer: the role of maximal surgical reduction. *Gynecol Oncol* 1984;18:293-298.
20. Conte PF, Sertoli MR, Bruzzone M, et al. Cisplatin, methotrexate and 5-FU combination chemotherapy for advanced ovarian cancer. *Gynecol Oncol* 1985;20:290-297.
21. Posado JG, Marantz AB, Yeung KY, et al. The cyclophosphamide, hexamethylmelamine, 5-FU regimen in the treatment of advanced and recurrent ovarian cancer. *Gynecol Oncol* 1985;20: 21-31.
22. Louie KG, Ozols RF, Meyers CE, et al. Long term results of a cisplatin containing combination chemotherapy regimen for the treatment of advanced ovarian carcinoma. *J Clin Oncol* 1986;4: 1579-1585.
23. Redman JR, Petroni GR, Saigo PE, et al. Prognostic factors in advanced ovarian cancer. *J Clin Oncol* 1986;4:515-523.
24. Hainsworth JD, Grosh WW, Burnett LS, et al. Advanced ovarian cancer: long term results of treatment with intensive cisplatin-based chemotherapy of brief duration. *Ann Intern Med* 1988;108: 165-170.
25. Dembo AJ. Abdominopelvic radiotherapy in ovarian cancer: a 10-year experience. *Cancer* 1985;55:2285-2290.
26. Carey MS, Dembo AJ, Fyles AW, et al. Testing the validity of a prognostic classification in patients with surgically optimal ovarian carcinoma: a 15-year review. *Int J Gynecol Cancer* 1993; 3:24-35.
27. Gershenson DM, Copeland LJ, Wharton JT, et al. Prognosis of surgically determined complete responders in advanced ovarian cancer. *Cancer* 1985;55:1129-1135.
28. Greco FA, Hande KR, Jones HW, et al. Advanced ovarian cancer: long-term follow up after brief intensive chemotherapy [abstract]. *Proc Am Soc Clin Oncol* 1984:166.
29. Goldberg N, Peschel RE. Postoperative abdominopelvic radiation therapy for ovarian cancer. *Int J Radiat Oncol Biol Phys* 1988;14:425-429.
30. Sell A, Bertelsen K, Andersen JE, et al. Randomized study of whole abdomen irradiation versus pelvic irradiation plus cyclophosphamide in treatment of early ovarian cancer. *Gynecol Oncol* 1990;37:367-373.
31. Lindner H, Willich H, Atzinger A. Primary adjuvant whole abdominal irradiation in ovarian carcinoma. *Int J Radiat Oncol Biol Phys* 1990;19:1203-1206.
32. Lynch HT, Kimberling W, Albano WA, et al. Hereditary nonpolyposis colorectal cancer (Lynch syndromes I and II). Clinical description of resource. *Cancer* 1985;56(pt 1):934-938.
33. Mackey SE, Creasman WT. Ovarian cancer screening. *J Clin Oncol* 1995;13:783-793.
34. Schapira MM, Matchar DB, Young MJ. The effectiveness of ovarian cancer screening. A decision analysis model. *Ann Intern Med* 1993;118:838-843.
35. Niloff JM, Bast RC Jr, Schaetzl EM, et al. Predictive value of CA 125 antigen levels in second-look procedures for ovarian cancer. *Am J Obstet Gynecol* 1985;151:981-986.
36. Malkasian GD Jr, Knapp RC, Lavin PT, et al. Preoperative evaluation of serum CA-125 levels in premenopausal and postmenopausal patients with pelvic masses: discrimination of benign from malignant disease. *Am J Obstet Gynecol* 1988;159: 341-346.
37. Hoskins WJ, Bundy BN, Thigpen JT, et al. The influence of cytoreductive surgery on recurrence free interval and survival in small-volume stage III epithelial ovarian cancer: a Gynecologic Oncology Group study. *Gynecol Oncol* 1992;47:159-166.
38. Young RC, Walton LA, Ellenberg SS, et al. Adjuvant therapy in stage I and stage II epithelial ovarian cancer. Results of two prospective randomized trials. *N Engl J Med* 1990;322:1021-1027.
39. Bolis G, Colombo N, Pecorelli S, et al. Adjuvant treatment for early epithelial ovarian cancer: results of two randomised clinical trials comparing cisplatin to no further treatment or chromic phosphate (32P). *Ann Oncol* 1995;6:887-893.
40. Hreschyshyn MM, Park RC, Blessing JA, et al. The role of adjuvant therapy in stage I ovarian cancer. *Am J Obstet Gynecol* 1980;138:139-145.
41. Dembo AJ, Bush RS, Beale FA, et al. The Princess Margaret Hospital study of ovarian cancer: stage I, II and asymptomatic III presentations. *Cancer Treat Rep* 1979;63:249-254.
42. Dembo AJ, Davy M, Stenwig AE, et al. Prognostic factors in patients with stage I epithelial ovarian cancer. *Obstet Gynecol* 1990;75:263-273.
43. Cardenes H, Randall ME. Integrating radiation therapy in the curative management of ovarian cancer: current issues and future directions. *Semin Radiat Oncol* 2000;10:61-70.
44. Vergote IB, Vergote-De Vos LN, Abeler VM, et al. Randomized trial comparing cisplatin with radioactive phosphorus or whole-abdomen irradiation as adjuvant treatment of ovarian cancer. *Cancer* 1992;69:741-749.

45. Young RC, Walton L, Randall M, et al. Randomized clinical trial of adjuvant treatment of women with early (FIGO I-IIA high risk) ovarian cancer. A GOG study [abstract]. *Proc Am Soc Clin Oncol* 1999;18:357a. Abstract 1376.

46. Vergote IB, Trope C. Is adjuvant therapy effective in early-stage ovarian cancer? *Int J Gynecol Cancer* 1995;5(suppl):13.

47. Corn BW, Lanciano RM, Boente M, et al. Recurrent ovarian cancer: effective radiotherapeutic palliation after chemotherapy failure. *Cancer* 1994;74:2979-2983.

48. May LF, Belinson JL, Roland TA. Palliative benefit of radiation therapy in advanced ovarian cancer. *Gynecol Oncol* 1990; 37:408-411.

49. Davidson SA, Rubin SC, Mychalczak B, et al. Limited-field radiotherapy as salvage treatment of localized persistent or recurrent epithelial ovarian cancer. *Gynecol Oncol* 1993;51:349-354.

50. Suzuki S, Fujiwara K, Yamauchi H, et al. Efficacy of radiation therapy for chemoresistant epithelial ovarian cancer [abstract]. 6th Biennial Meeting IGCS. Fukuoka, Japan: Blackwell Science; 1997:81. Abstract P191.

51. Dubois JB, Joyeux H, Solassol CL, et al. Les tumeurs epitheliales de l'ovaire: resultats therapeutiques a propos de 165 stades II et III. *Gynecology Obstetrics Biology Reprod* 1979;14:627-632.

52. Fuller DB, Sause WT, Plenk HP, et al. Analysis of postoperative radiation therapy in stage I through III epithelial ovarian carcinoma. *J Clin Oncol* 1987;5:897-905.

53. Piver MS, Barlow JJ, Lele SB. Incidence of subclinical metastasis in stage I and II ovarian carcinomas. *Obstet Gynecol* 1978; 52:100-104.

54. Rosenoff SH, Young RC, Anderson T, et al. Peritoneoscopy: a valuable staging tool in ovarian carcinoma. *Ann Intern Med* 1975;83:37-41.

55. Dembo A, Bush R, Beale F, et al. Ovarian carcinoma: improved survival following abdominopelvic irradiation in patients with a completed pelvic operation. *Am J Obstet Gynecol* 1979; 134:793-800.

56. Ozols RF, Rubin SC, Thomas G, et al. Epithelial ovarian cancer. In: Hoskins WJ, Perez CA, Young RC, eds. *Principles and Practice of Gynecologic Oncology.* 2nd ed. Philadelphia, Pa: Lippincott-Raven; 1997:919-986.

57. Martinez A, Schray MF, Howes AE, et al. Postoperative radiation therapy for epithelial ovarian cancer: the curative role based on a 24-year experience. *J Clin Oncol* 1985;3:901-911.

58. Weiser EB, Burke TW, Heller PB, et al. Determinants of survival of patients with epithelial ovarian carcinoma following whole abdominal irradiation (WAR). *Gynecol Oncol* 1988;30:201-208.

59. Bush RS, Allt WEC, Beale FA, et al. Treatment of epithelial carcinoma of the ovary: operation, irradiation and chemotherapy. *Am J Obstet Gynecol* 1977;127:692-704.

60. Delclos L, Smith JP. Ovarian cancer, with special regard to types of radiotherapy. *Natl Cancer Inst Monogr* 1975;42:129-135.

61. Klaassen D, Shelley W, Starreveld A, et al. Early stage ovarian cancer: a randomized clinical trial comparing whole abdominal radiotherapy, melphalan, and intraperitoneal chromic phosphate: a National Cancer Institute of Canada Clinical Trials Group report. *J Clin Oncol* 1988;6:1254-1263.

62. Ledermann JA, Dembo AJ, Sturgeon JFG, et al. Outcome of patients with unfavorable optimally cytoreduced ovarian cancer treated with chemotherapy and whole abdominal radiation. *Gynecol Oncol* 1991;41:30-35.

63. Hruby G, Bull CA, Langlands AO, et al. WART revisited: the treatment of epithelial ovarian cancer by whole abdominal radiotherapy. *Australas Radiol* 1997;41:276-280.

64. Dembo AJ, Van Dyk J, Japp B, et al. Whole abdominal irradiation by a moving-strip technique for patients with ovarian cancer. *Int J Radiat Oncol Biol Phys* 1979;5:1933-1942.

65. Delclos L, Braun EJ, Herrera JR, et al. Whole abdominal irradiation by ^{60}Co moving-strip technique. *Radiology* 1963;81:632-641.

66. Fazekas JT, Maier JG. Irradiation of ovarian carcinomas: a prospective comparison of the open-field and moving-strip techniques. *Am J Roentgenol* 1974;120:118-123.

67. Dembo AJ, Bush RS, Beale FA, et al. A randomised clinical trial of moving strip versus open field whole abdominal irradiation in patients with invasive epithelial cancer of ovary [abstract]. *Int J Radiat Oncol Biol Phys* 1983;9(suppl 1):97.

68. Lanciano RM, Randall M. Update on the role of radiotherapy in ovarian cancer. *Semin Oncol* 1991;18:233-247.

69. Fyles AW, Thomas GM, Pintilie M, et al. A randomized study of two doses of abdominopelvic radiation therapy for patients with optimally debulked stage I, II, and III ovarian cancer. *Int J Radiat Oncol Biol Phys* 1998;41:543-549.

70. Fletcher GH. Clinical dose-response curves of human malignant epithelial tumours. *Br J Radiol* 1973;46:1-12.

71. Marks LB. A standard dose of radiation for "microscopic disease" is not appropriate. *Cancer* 1990;66:2498-2502.

72. Dembo AJ. Radiotherapeutic management of ovarian cancer. *Semin Oncol* 1984;11:238-250.

73. Withers HR, Peters LJ, Taylor JMG. Dose-response relationship for radiation therapy of subclinical disease. *Int J Radiat Oncol Biol Phys* 1995;31:353-359.

74. Fyles AW, Dembo AJ, Bush RS, et al. Analysis of complications in patients treated with abdomino-pelvic radiation therapy for ovarian carcinoma. *Int J Radiat Oncol Biol Phys* 1992;22:847-851.

75. Perez CA, Lorba A, Zivnuska F, et al. 60Co moving strip technique in the management of carcinoma of the ovary: analysis of tumor control and morbidity. *Int J Radiat Oncol Biol Phys* 1978;4:379-388.

76. Schray MF, Martinez A, Howes AE. Toxicity of open field whole abdominal irradiation as primary post-operative treatment in gynecological malignancy. *Int J Radiat Oncol Biol Phys* 1988;16:397-403.

77. van Bunnigen B, Bouma J, Kooijman C, et al. Total abdominal irradiation in stage I and II carcinoma of the ovary. *Radiother Oncol* 1988;11:305-310.

78. Dietl J, Marzusch K. Ovarian surface epithelium and human ovarian cancer. *Gynecol Obstet Invest* 1993;35:129-135.

79. Einzig AI, Wiernik PH, Sasloff J, et al. Phase II study and long-term follow up of patients treated with taxol for advanced ovarian adenocarcinoma. *J Clin Oncol* 1992;10:1748-1753.

80. Travis LB, Holowaty EJ, Bergfeldt K, et al. Risk of leukemia after platinum-based chemotherapy for ovarian cancer. *N Engl J Med* 1999;340:351-357.

81. Omura GA, Bundy BN, Berek JS, et al. Randomized trial of cyclophosphamide plus cisplatin with or without doxorubicin in ovarian carcinoma: a Gynecologic Oncology Group study. *J Clin Oncol* 1989;7:457-465.

82. McGuire WP, Hoskins WJ, Brady MF, et al. A phase III trial comparing cisplatin/cytoxan (PC) and cisplatin/taxol (PI) in advanced ovarian cancer (AOC). *Proc Am Soc Clin Oncol* 1993: 12;255. Abstract 808.

83. McGuire WP, Hoskins WJ, Brady MF, et al. Taxol and cisplatin (TP) improves outcome in advanced ovarian cancer (AOC) as compared to cytoxan and cisplatin (CP). *Proc Am Soc Clin Oncol* 1995;14:771.

84. Alberts DS, Liu Y, Hannigan EV, et al. Intraperitoneal cisplatin plus intravenous cyclophosphamide versus intravenous cisplatin plus intravenous cyclophosphamide for stage III ovarian cancer. *N Engl J Med* 1996;335:1950-1955.

85. Fuks Z, Rizel S, Anteby SO, et al. Current concepts in cancer: ovary–treatment for stages III and IV. The multimodal approach to the treatment of stage III ovarian carcinoma.. *Int J Radiat Oncol Biol Phys* 1982;8:903-908.

86. Thomas GM. Is there a role for consolidation or salvage radiotherapy after chemotherapy in advanced epithelial ovarian cancer? *Gynecol Oncol* 1993;51:97-103.

87. Morgan L, Chafe W, Mendenhall W, et al. Hyperfractionation of whole-abdomen radiation therapy: salvage treatment of persistent ovarian carcinoma following chemotherapy. *Gynecol Oncol* 1988;31:122-134.

88. Kong JS, Peters LJ, Wharton JT, et al. Hyperfractionated split-course whole abdominal radiotherapy for ovarian carcinoma: tolerance and toxicity. *Int J Radiat Oncol Biol Phys* 1988;14:737-743.

89. Chiara S, Orsatti M, Franzone P, et al. Abdominopelvic radiotherapy following surgery and chemotherapy in advanced ovarian cancer. *Clin Oncol (R Coll Radiol)* 1991;3:340-344.

90. Greiner R, Goldhirsch A, Davis BW, et al. Whole-abdomen radiation in patients with advanced ovarian carcinoma after surgery, chemotherapy and second-look laparotomy. *J Cancer Res Clin Oncol* 1984;107:94-98.

91. Reddy S, Hartsell W, Graham J, et al. Whole abdomen radiation therapy in ovarian carcinoma: its role as a salvage therapeutic modality. *Gynecol Oncol* 1989;35:307-313.

92. Kuten A, Stein M, Steiner M, et al. Whole abdominal irradiation following chemotherapy in advanced ovarian carcinoma. *Int J Radiat Oncol Biol Phys* 1988;14:273-279.

93. Solomon HJ, Atkinson KH, Coppleson JVM, et al. Ovarian carcinoma: abdominopelvic irradiation following reexploration. *Gynecol Oncol* 1988;31:396-401.

94. Rosen EM, Goldberg ID, Rose C, et al. Sequential multi-agent chemotherapy and whole abdominal irradiation for stage III ovarian carcinoma. *Radiother Oncol* 1986;7:223-232.

95. Haie C, Pejovic-Lenfant MH, George M, et al. Whole abdominal irradiation following chemotherapy in patients with minimal residual disease after second look surgery in ovarian carcinoma. *Int J Radiat Oncol Biol Phys* 1989;17:15-19.

96. Kersh CR, Randall ME, Constable WC, et al. Whole abdominal radiotherapy following cytoreductive surgery and chemotherapy in ovarian carcinoma. *Gynecol Oncol* 1988;31:113-120.

97. Goldhirsch A, Greiner R, Dreher E, et al. Treatment of advanced ovarian cancer with surgery, chemotherapy and consolidation of response by whole-abdominal radiotherapy. *Cancer* 1988;62:40-47.

98. Menczer J, Modan M, Brenner J, et al. Abdominopelvic irradiation for stage II-IV ovarian carcinoma patients with limited or no residual disease at second-look laparotomy after completion of cisplatinum-based chemotherapy. *Gynecol Oncol* 1986;24:149-154.

99. Schray MF, Martinez A, Howes AE, et al. Advanced epithelial ovarian cancer: salvage whole abdominal irradiation for patients with recurrent or persistent disease after combination chemotherapy. *J Clin Oncol* 1988;6:1433-1439.

100. Dembo AJ, Bush RS. Current concepts in cancer: ovary—treatment of stages III and IV. Choice of postoperative therapy based on prognostic factors. *Int J Radiat Oncol Biol Phys* 1982;8:893-897.

101. Dembo AJ, Bush RS, Brown TC. Clinicopathological correlates in ovarian cancer. *Bull Cancer* 1982;69:292-298.

102. Randall ME, Barrett RJ, Spirtos NM, et al. Chemotherapy, early surgical reassessment, and hyperfractionated abdominal radiotherapy in stage III ovarian cancer: results of a Gynecologic Oncology Group study. *Int J Radiat Oncol Biol Phys* 1996;34:139-147.

103. Whelan TJ, Dembo AJ, Bush RS, et al. Complications of whole abdominal and pelvic radiotherapy following chemotherapy for advanced ovarian cancer. *Int J Radiat Oncol Biol Phys* 1992;22:853-858.

104. Hatch KD, Beecham JB, Blessing JA, et al. Responsiveness of patients with advanced ovarian carcinoma to tamoxifen. A Gynecologic Oncology Group study of second-line therapy in 105 patients. *Cancer* 1991;68:269-271.

105. Markman M, Hakes T, Reichman B, et al. Ifosfamide and mesna in previously treated advanced epithelial ovarian cancer: activity in platinum-resistant disease. *J Clin Oncol* 1992;10:243-248.

106. Markman M, Rothman R, Hakes T, et al. Second-line platinum therapy in patients with ovarian cancer previously treated with cisplatin. *J Clin Oncol* 1991;9:389-393.

107. McGuire WP, Rowinsky EK, Rosenshein NB, et al. Taxol: a unique antineoplastic agent with significant activity in advanced ovarian epithelial neoplasms. *Ann Intern Med* 1989;111:273-279.

108. Moore DH, Fowler WC, Jones CP, et al. Hexamethylmelamine chemotherapy for persistent or recurrent epithelial ovarian cancer. *Am J Obstet Gynecol* 1991;165:573-576.

109. Reed E, Jacob J, Ozols RF, et al. 5-Fluorouracil (5-FU) and leucovorin in platinum-refractory advanced stage ovarian carcinoma. *Gynecol Oncol* 1992;46:326-329.

110. Rosen GF, Lurain JR, Newton M. Hexamethylmelamine in ovarian cancer after failure of cisplatin based multiple-agent chemotherapy. *Gynecol Oncol* 1987;27:173-179.

111. Thigpen JT, Vance RB, Khansur T. Second-line chemotherapy for recurrent carcinoma of the ovary. *Cancer* 1993;71:1559-1564.

112. Vergote I, Himmelmann A, Frankendal B, et al. Hexamethylmelamine as a second-line therapy in platinum-resistant ovarian cancer. *Gynecol Oncol* 1992;47:282-286.

113. Adelson MD, Wharton JT, Delclos L, et al. Palliative radiotherapy for ovarian cancer. *Int J Radiat Oncol Biol Phys* 1987;13:17-21.

114. Rose PG, Bundy BN, Watkins EB, et al. Concurrent cisplatin-based chemoradiation in locally advanced cervical cancer. *N Engl J Med* 1999;340:1144-1153.

115. Keys HM, Bundy BN, Stehman FB, et al. Cisplatin, radiation and adjuvant hysterectomy compared with radiation and adjuvant hysterectomy for bulky stage IB cervical carcinoma. *N Engl J Med* 1999;340:1154-1161.

116. Whitney CW, Sause W, Bundy BN, et al. A randomized comparison of fluorouracil plus cisplatin versus hydroxyurea as an adjunct to radiation therapy in stages IIB-IVA carcinoma of the cervix with negative para-aortic lymph nodes. A Gynecologic Oncology Group and Southwest Oncology Group study. *J Clin Oncol* 1999;17:1339-1348.

117. Peters III WA, Liu PY, Barrett RJ, et al. Cisplatin and 5-fluorouracil plus radiation therapy are superior to radiation therapy as adjunctive in high-risk early-stage carcinoma of the cervix after radical hysterectomy and pelvic lymphadenectomy: report of a phase III intergroup study [abstract]. In: *Program of the 30th Annual Conference, Society of Gynecologic Oncologists.* San Francisco, Calif: Academic Press; 1999:443.

118. Morris M, Eifel PJ, Lu J, et al. Pelvic radiation with concurrent chemotherapy versus pelvic and para-aortic radiation for high-risk cervical cancer. A randomized Radiation Therapy Oncology Group clinical trial. *N Engl J Med* 1999;340:1137-1143.

119. Silver DF, Wheeless CR, Dubin NH. Radiotherapy as a cisplatin-sensitizer in a resistant ovarian carcinoma cell line. *Cancer* 1996;77:1850-1853.

120. King LA, Downey GO, Potish RA, et al. Concomitant whole-abdominal radiation and intraperitoneal chemotherapy in advanced ovarian carcinoma: a pilot study. *Cancer* 1991;67:2867-2871.

121. Reisinger SA, Asbury R, Liao SY, et al. A phase I study of weekly cisplatin and whole abdominal radiation for the treatment of stage III and IV endometrial carcinoma: a Gynecologic Oncology Group pilot study. *Gynecol Oncol* 1996;63:299-303.

122. Cmelak AJ, Kapp DS. Long-term survival with whole abdominopelvic irradiation in platinum-refractory persistent or recurrent ovarian cancer. *Gynecol Oncol* 1997;65:453-460.

123. Steren A, Sevin B, Perras J, et al. Taxol as a radiation sensitizer: a flow cytometric study. *Gynecol Oncol* 1993;50:89-93.

124. Creasman WT, Park R, Norris H, et al. Stage I borderline ovarian tumors. *Obstet Gynecol* 1982;59:93-96.

125. Colgan TJ, Norris HJ. Ovarian epithelial tumors of low malignant potential: a review. *Int J Radiat Oncol Biol Phys* 1982;8:219-226.

126. Bell DA, Weinstock MA, Scully RE. Peritoneal implants of ovarian serous borderline tumors. *Cancer* 1988;62:2212-2222.

127. McCaughey WTE, Kirk ME, Lester W, et al. Peritoneal epithelial lesions associated with proliferative serous tumors of ovary. *Histopathology* 1984;8:195-208.

128. Kaern J, Trope C, Kjorstad KE, et al. Cellular DNA content as a new prognostic tool in patients with borderline tumors of the ovary. *Gynecol Oncol* 1990;38:452-457.

129. Drescher CW, Flint A, Hopkins M, et al. Prognostic significance of DNA content and nuclear morphology in borderline ovarian tumors. *Gynecol Oncol* 1993;36:242-246.

130. Padberg BC, Arps H, Franke U, et al. DNA cytophotometry and prognosis in ovarian tumors of borderline malignancy. *Cancer* 1992;69:2510-2514.

131. Chambers JT. Borderline ovarian tumors: a review of treatment. *Yale J Biol Med* 1989;62:351-356.

132. Gershenson DM, Silva EG. Serous ovarian tumors of low malignant potential with peritoneal implants. *Cancer* 1990;65:578-585.

133. Norris HJ, Taylor HB. Prognosis of granulosa-theca tumors of the ovary. *Cancer* 1968;21:255-263.

134. Stenwig JT, Hazekamp JT, Beecham JB. Granulosa cell tumors of the ovary: a clinicopathological study of 118 cases with long term follow-up. *Gynecol Oncol* 1979;136-152.

135. Bompas E, Freyer G, Vitrey D, et al. Granulosa cell tumour: review of the literature [in French]. *Bull Cancer* 2000;87:709-714.

136. Fujimoto T, Sakuragi N, Okuyama K, et al. Histopathological prognostic factors of adult granulosa cell tumors of the ovary. *Acta Obstet Gynecol Scand* 2001;80:1069-1074.

137. Juric G, Zarkovic N, Nola M, et al. The value of cell proliferation and angiogenesis in the prognostic assessment of ovarian granulosa cell tumors. *Tumori* 2001;87:47-53.

138. Miller BE, Barron BA, Wan JY, et al. Prognostic factors in adult granulosa cell tumor of the ovary. *Cancer* 1997;79:1951-1955.

139. Evans AT, Gaffey TA, Malkasian GD, et al. Clinicopathologic review of 118 granulosa and 82 theca cell tumors. *Obstet Gynecol* 1980;55:231-238.

140. Kalavathi N. Granulosa cell tumour: hormonal aspects and radiosensitivity. *Clin Radiol* 1971;22:524-527.

141. Schwartz PE, Smith JP. Treatment of ovarian stromal tumors. *Am J Obstet Gynecol* 1976;125:402-411.

142. Jacobs AJ, Deppe G, Cohen CJ. Combination chemotherapy of ovarian granulosa cell tumor with cisplatinum and doxorubicin. *Gynecol Oncol* 1982;14:294-297.

143. Camlibel F, Caputo TA. Chemotherapy of granulosa cell tumors. *Am J Obstet Gynecol* 1983;145:763-765.

144. Neville AJ, Gilchrist KW, Davis TE. The chemotherapy of granulosa cell tumors of the ovary: experience of the Wisconsin Clinical Cancer Center. *Med Pediatr Oncol* 1984;12:397-400.

145. Pectasides D, Alevizakos N, Athanassiou AE. Cisplatin-containing regimen in advanced or recurrent granulosa cell tumours of the ovary. *Ann Oncol* 1992;3:316-318.

146. Slayton RE. Management of germ cell and stromal tumors of the ovary. *Semin Oncol* 1984;11:299-313.

147. Colombo N, Sessa C, Landoni F, et al. Cisplatin, vinblastine, and bleomycin combination chemotherapy in metastatic granulosa cell tumor of the ovary. *Obstet Gynecol* 1986;67:265-268.

148. Chiara S, Merlini L, Campora E, et al. Cisplatin-based chemotherapy in recurrent or high risk ovarian granulosa cell tumor patients. *Eur J Gynaecol Oncol* 1993;14:314-317.

149. Zambetti M, Escobedo A, Pilotti S, et al. Cisplatin/vinblastine/bleomycin combination chemotherapy in advanced or recurrent granulosa cell tumors of the ovary. *Gynecol Oncol* 1990;36:317-320.

150. Asadourian LA, Taylor HB. Dysgerminoma: an analysis of 105 cases. *Obstet Gynecol* 1969;33:370-379.

151. De Palo G, Pilotti S, Kenda R, et al. Natural history of dysgerminoma. *Am J Obstet Gynecol* 1982;143:799-807.

152. Gordon A, Lipton D, Woodruff JD. Dysgerminoma: a review of 158 cases from the Emil Novak Ovarian Tumor Registry. *Obstet Gynecol* 1981;58:497-504.

153. Malkasian GD Jr, Symmonds RE. Treatment of the unilateral encapsulated ovarian dysgerminoma. *Obstet Gynecol* 1964;90:379-382.

154. Bianchi UA, Sartori E, Favalli G, et al. New trends in the treatment of ovarian dysgerminoma [abstract]. *Gynecol Oncol* 1986;23:246.

155. Krepart G, Smith JP, Rutledge F, et al. The treatment of dysgerminoma of the ovary. *Cancer* 1978;41:986-990.

156. Thomas GM, Dembo AJ, Hacker HF, et al. Current concepts of therapy for dysgerminoma of the ovary. *Obstet Gynecol* 1987;70:268-275.

157. Einhorn LH, Williams SD. Chemotherapy of disseminated seminoma. *Cancer Clinical Trials* 1980;3:307-313.

158. Taylor MH, Depetrillo AD, Turner AR. Vinblastine, bleomycin and cisplatin in malignant germ cell tumors of the ovary. *Cancer* 1985;56:1341-1349.

159. Gershenson DM, Morris M, Cangir A, et al. Treatment of malignant germ cell tumors of the ovary with bleomycin, etoposide, and cisplatin. *J Clin Oncol* 1990;8:715-720.

160. Williams SD, Blessing JA, Hatch KD, et al. Chemotherapy of advanced dysgerminoma: trials of the Gynecologic Oncology Group. *J Clin Oncol* 1991;9:1950-1955.

PART X

Central Nervous System

CHAPTER 32

The Brain and Spinal Cord

Larry E. Kun

TOLERANCE OF THE CENTRAL NERVOUS SYSTEM TO IRRADIATION

The central nervous system (CNS) is increasingly being recognized as a relatively sensitive, often dose-limiting tissue in curative radiation therapy for both CNS and adjacent neoplasms.[1] Radiation injury has been documented on the basis of clinical signs, imaging findings, and histopathologic correlations.[2-6] CNS effects are more pronounced in children and seem to be inversely related to age, with the youngest children having the greatest CNS sensitivity. Of further concern is that numerous chemotherapy agents are associated with unique or enhanced sequelae when given in conjunction with radiation therapy.[7]

Studies of laboratory models of cerebral and spinal cord changes have helped to clarify the pathophysiology of radiation-induced neural damage and to associate the extent of damage with time, dose, delivery, and volume.[8-10] For example, Caveness[11] reported a detailed investigation of the clinical, histologic, and physiologic findings in primates after irradiation comparable with that used clinically. In that study, a single fraction of 20 Gy was uniformly fatal by week 26; this dose produced increased intracranial pressure and ventriculomegaly with scattered necrotic foci most dramatically affecting the brainstem. A single fraction of 15 Gy produced discrete microfoci of white matter necrosis by 26 weeks, with coalescing areas of white matter necrosis present by 56 weeks. Pathologic findings were less pronounced in animals killed 78 weeks after irradiation, suggesting that some recovery had taken place. No clinical or histologic abnormalities were noted after whole-brain irradiation with a single fraction of 10 Gy or with 40 Gy delivered in 20 fractions over 4 weeks.

In experiments more relevant to clinical radiation therapy, delivering 60 Gy to the whole brain in fractions of 2 Gy over a period of 6 weeks caused papilledema and anorexia in pubertal monkeys, but no overt clinical findings were apparent in adult primates. Histologically, the adult brains showed discrete microfoci of white matter necrosis with calcifications by 26 weeks; healing of the degenerative foci along with increased microcalcifications was noted by 52 weeks. The radiation-induced changes were quantitatively greater in younger animals. After 80 Gy delivered in 40 fractions, confluent areas of necrosis appeared in the cerebral hemispheres of younger animals by 32 weeks, progressive necrosis was noted at 52 weeks, and coalescent necrotic regions and atrophy were noted by 78 weeks.

Caveness' findings at lower dose levels are similar to the mineralizing microangiopathy seen in children with acute leukemia treated with cranial irradiation (24 Gy) and methotrexate.[12] Small coalescent foci of necrosis related to microvascular changes may account for the clinically silent lacunar lesions noted in magnetic resonance imaging (MRI) studies in long-term survivors of childhood brain tumors.[13]

Postirradiation CNS effects are typically divided temporally into acute, subacute, and late reactions. Fractionated irradiation rarely produces clinically apparent acute changes, even when the total dose approaches 70 to 80 Gy.[14] Anecdotal reports of transient exaggeration of neurologic signs have been related theoretically to perilesional or intralesional edema that develops at the beginning of irradiation.[15-17] Young and colleagues[18] noted abrupt neurologic deterioration in 50% of patients who were given large (7.5- to 10-Gy) fractions for the treatment of symptomatic cerebral metastases; these investigators attributed this effect to the radiation therapy. Although no similar phenomena were noted in studies by the Radiation Therapy Oncology Group (RTOG) in which 6-Gy fractions were administered, this finding may have been related to the more consistent use of corticosteroids by the RTOG.[16]

Subacute CNS effects are rather common. Jones[19] noted transient, self-limited paresthesias with neck flexion (Lhermitte's sign) that lasted for 1 to 2 months after spinal cord irradiation. These paresthesias, which occur in 15% to 25% of patients after mantle irradiation for Hodgkin's disease, are believed to be secondary to transient demyelination. Comparable transitory neurologic changes, termed the somnolent syndrome, occur after cranial irradiation such as that given for acute leukemia; mild encephalopathy or focal neurologic changes can appear after the treatment of intracranial tumors.[20,21] The cranial syndrome is believed to stem from a transient demyelinating event and is the result of the effects of radiation on the replicating oligodendrocytes.[8] MRI can detect specific dose-related changes in gray and white matter within several weeks of conventionally fractionated irradiation.[22] It is important to bear in mind the potential for self-limited neurologic deterioration, most often during the second month after irradiation, because both clinical and radiologic changes can sometimes mimic tumor progression.[23,24]

Late reactions of the normal brain are the dose-limiting toxicities for radiation treatment. Clinical manifestations of focal neurologic deficits, encephalopathy, or neuropsychological dysfunction accompany various morphologic findings such as atrophy, calcifications, diffuse white matter degeneration, and focal necrosis. Permanent or progressive myelopathy can result from spinal cord irradiation. Late changes in hypothalamic-pituitary function manifest as specific radiation-induced endocrine deficits.

Postirradiation Cerebral Necrosis

Postirradiation cerebral necrosis, the most direct effect of CNS irradiation, is believed to result from direct effects of radiation on both the replicating glial cell compartments and the capillary endothelial cells.[8,9] The theoretical relationship between primary glial cells (i.e., type II astrocytes and oligodendrocytes) and vascular endothelial components is shown in Figure 32-1.[8,25-29] Clinical signs of postirradiation cerebral necrosis are noted 6 to 36 months after therapy.[15,16,30] Cerebral changes often mimic residual or recurrent tumor, with mass effect, enhancement, or cyst formation evident on computed tomography (CT) scans; these changes occur at or near the site of the primary tumor (i.e., the high-dose volume for intracranial neoplasms).[31]

Cerebral necrosis unrelated to intraparenchymal neoplasms has been described in reviews by Kramer and colleagues[32] and Sheline and colleagues.[16] This necrosis has been noted after therapy for extracranial tumors (predominantly those of the skin and paranasal sinuses) and for noninvasive pituitary tumors or craniopharyngiomas. Postirradiation necrosis is a dose-related phenomenon with a relative threshold radiation dose of 50 to 55 Gy if treatment is given in a conventional fractionation schedule (1.8- to 2-Gy fractions given once a day).[16,30,33,34] Marks and colleagues[30] reported the occurrence of necrosis in 5% of 139 patients with intracranial tumors treated with conventional fractionation to doses higher than 45 Gy; six of the seven patients that had necrosis were given total doses in excess of 63 Gy.

The dose-time relationship is critical in determining CNS tolerance, with fraction size the dominant factor among patients receiving doses of 60 to 63 Gy. Necrosis in patients who receive less than 60 Gy has generally

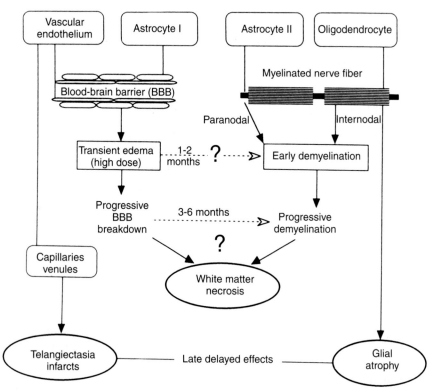

Fig. 32-1 The direct effects of radiation on glial cells (astrocyte II and oligodendrocyte) and the indirect effects secondary to vascular changes, as shown in a scheme developed by van der Kogel. (van der Kogel AJ. Central nervous system radiation injury in small animal models. In: Gutin PH, Leibel SA, Sheline GE, eds. *Radiation Injury to the Nervous System.* New York, NY: Raven Press; 1991:91-112.)

been associated with fractions of greater than 2.5 Gy.[16] Aristazibal and colleagues[33] documented necrosis after treatment for pituitary tumors in 3% of 106 patients given less than 2.2 Gy per day (total dose of about 50 Gy) compared with 15% of 13 patients given doses of greater than 2.2 Gy daily. The influence of fraction size was made apparent in the isoeffect analyses of brain necrosis reported by Sheline and colleagues.[16]

Sheline and colleagues[16] contend that the brain can tolerate a total radiation dose of 50 to 54 Gy given in fractions of 2 Gy once a day. At that dose, cerebral necrosis is estimated to occur in 0.04% to 0.4% of patients. The likelihood of necrosis is higher among patients with primary brain tumors, although the incidence is still estimated to be less than 5% among patients receiving a dose of 55 Gy at 1.8 to 2 Gy per fraction.[34] Tolerance is affected by age, however; both experimental and clinical data indicate that children younger than 2 years can tolerate approximately 10% to 20% less radiation to the brain than those older than 2 years.[11,35,36]

Postirradiation Myelopathy

Postirradiation myelopathy is the spinal cord equivalent of cerebral necrosis. The myelopathy manifests as sensory and motor signs referable to a single cord level, signs that are often clinically indicative of hemisection of the cord (Brown-Séquard syndrome).[37,38] Symptoms occur as early as 6 months after treatment (median of 20 months).[39] The pathophysiology of spinal-cord myelopathy is similar to that of cerebral necrosis, with continued debate concerning the relative importance of vascular endothelial changes (particularly in the spinal cord with end-arterial blood supply to portions of the thoracic cord) and direct effects of the radiation on glial elements.[28,29,40]

The time-dose relationship and tolerance of the spinal cord to irradiation have been analyzed in the context of extraspinal tumors. The thoracic spinal cord seems to be the most sensitive aspect; few instances of lumbar myelopathy have been reported. Phillips and Buschke[41] suggested that the thoracic spine could tolerate a dose as high as 50 Gy given in fractions of 2 Gy once a day. Abbatucci and colleagues[42] observed cervical cord myelopathy after doses of 55 Gy or more. The incidence of myelopathy rises rapidly with increasing doses, approaching 50% at 65 Gy.[29] Multiple clinical trials of large-fraction irradiation for lung cancer have confirmed that the frequency of reactions increases as the fraction size exceeds 2.5 Gy.[43-46] Fraction size also seems to correlate inversely with the latent interval before the development of myelopathy[42]; however, no experimental evidence exists to suggest improved tolerance to fractions less than 2 Gy.[47] The CHART regimen for lung cancer (*Continuous Hyperfractionated, Accelerated Radiation Therapy*) was originally based on a presumed cord tolerance of a low dose per fraction, but that regimen initially was associated with an unacceptable risk of myelopathy.[48,49] In fact, tolerance decreases as the volume or length of cord irradiated increases.[41,42]

Other Late Effects

A unique late effect of cranial irradiation combined with chemotherapy, called leukoencephalopathy, has been observed in children with acute lymphoblastic leukemia, adults with small cell carcinoma of the lung, and patients with primary CNS tumors.[12,50,51] This leukoencephalopathy is a profoundly demyelinating, necrotizing reaction usually noted 4 to 12 months after combined treatment with methotrexate and radiation.[52] Dementia and dysarthria may progress to seizures, ataxia, focal long-tract signs, or death; although most of these symptoms regress after systemic, intrathecal, or intraventricular methotrexate therapy is discontinued, patients are left with permanent neurologic deficits. The occurrence of leukoencephalopathy in patients treated with systemic and intrathecal methotrexate without irradiation and a dose-effect relationship that is more apparent for methotrexate than for radiation suggest that the clinical leukoencephalopathy is more significantly related to the methotrexate than to the radiation.[7] However, white matter changes interpreted as leukoencephalopathy, and so coded in the NCI Common Toxicity criteria, must be distinguished from the clinical syndrome described above.

Decline in intellectual function has been related to cranial irradiation of adults and, particularly, of children.[53-57] Neurocognitive changes in children also correlate significantly with cranial irradiation, young age at diagnosis and therapy, and functional level at the time the irradiation was begun.[53-55,58,59] The occurrence of dose-related neurocognitive alterations suggests a role for continued, if cautious, reduction in the full cranial irradiation dose for patients with medulloblastoma, for example, who exhibit favorable presenting signs.[60] Changes in white matter volume by using MRI segmentation are an objective variable that is closely tied to intellectual function and may permit more detailed studies of the effects of radiation therapy and chemotherapy in the current generation of clinical trials.[61] Intellectual impairment in adults has been noted primarily after intensive chemotherapy and irradiation for the prevention of metastasis from small cell carcinoma of the lung and for treatment of primary CNS lymphomas.[62]

Peripheral nervous system tissue is relatively resistant to irradiation. Acute and subacute symptoms or signs are infrequent; transient cranial nerve neuropathies are noted only with high-dose, single-fraction, high–linear-energy-transfer radiation for pituitary or parasellar tumors.[63] The optic chiasm is often considered a dose-limiting structure when irradiation for suprasellar or adjacent temporal lobe lesions is being planned, with special attention given to limiting the risk of dose-related visual complications.[64] Optic nerve or chiasm injury has been documented in nearly 20% of patients treated with fraction sizes of 2.5 Gy or greater (to total doses of 45 to 50 Gy), compared with 0 of 27 patients and 0 of 500 patients treated with fraction sizes of 1.7 to 2 Gy to the same level.[16,65] Late injury to the brachial plexus observed after the treatment of breast cancer similarly seems to occur largely after high-dose fractions.[66]

CENTRAL NERVOUS SYSTEM NEOPLASMS

Primary tumors of the CNS represent 2% of all cases of cancer in the United States. Approximately 17,200 new cases are diagnosed annually.[67] The incidence of these tumors exceeds that of Hodgkin's disease in adults, and they account for 20% of all cases of childhood cancer. The natural history of tumors of the brain and spinal cord is relatively unusual because aggressive malignant lesions rarely disseminate beyond the neuraxis. Categorizing CNS tumors as benign or malignant is often difficult because histologically low-grade or benign neoplasms are sometimes associated with a poorer prognosis than certain histologically malignant tumors. Rather, it is the potential for local invasiveness or metastasis along the cerebrospinal fluid (CSF) pathways that determines the "malignancy" of CNS tumors. The challenge for both neurosurgeons and radiation oncologists is to remove or devitalize neoplastic tissue in the functionally vital, anatomically confined nervous system.

TUMORS COMMON IN CHILDREN

Brain tumors in children account for one in five cases of childhood cancer. The incidence of primary CNS tumors, particularly the astrocytic lesions, increased in children during the first half of the 1990s; since then, the incidence has leveled off, perhaps because of the added diagnostic sensitivity of MRI.[68] Pediatric brain tumors arise most often in the posterior fossa. Posterior fossa tumors often produce symptoms and signs of increased intracranial pressure because the growing tumor obstructs the flow of CSF through the fourth ventricle. Ataxia often accompanies pressure-related headaches and morning vomiting. Brainstem gliomas cause cranial nerve palsies, ataxia, and long-tract signs, including lateralizing weakness and sensory deficits.

Supratentorial tumors occur in the cerebral hemispheres and the central or deep-seated areas of the thalamus, hypothalamus, suprasellar area, and pineal–third ventricular region. Symptoms are local and include lateralizing neurologic deficits and seizures, which are associated with hemispheric and thalamic tumors; visual and endocrine changes; and specific oculomotor findings, which are associated with tumors of the pineal region.

Primary tumors of the spinal cord account for only 5% of tumors in children. Metastasis to the CNS is uncommon in childhood cancer. Contiguous extradural compression within the spinal canal or at the base of the skull (e.g., in neuroblastoma, rhabdomyosarcoma, or primary bone tumors) is more common than hematogenous metastasis to the brain.

Common primary intracranial tumors diagnosed in children are listed in Table 32-1.[25,26] The histologic classification of pediatric brain tumors has been relatively standardized by the World Health Organization (WHO).[69] The most common tumors are the astrocytic lesions (astrocytomas, malignant gliomas, and brainstem gliomas). Medulloblastoma, which accounts for 20% of all childhood CNS tumors, is part of the broader category of supratentorial primitive neuroectodermal tumors (PNETs) and other embryonal CNS tumors (i.e., cerebral neuroblastoma, ependymoblastoma, and pineoblastoms).[69-71]

Biological findings increasingly define the nature of CNS tumors in children, providing some associations with tumor aggressiveness and outcome. Medulloblastoma, for example, is often associated with *p17* gene deletions; expression of the gene encoding erbB1 (related to epidermal growth factor) and trkC have been reported to be negatively and positively correlated with outcome, respectively.[72,73]

Medulloblastoma

Medulloblastoma represents 20% of childhood brain tumors. Common throughout the pediatric age range, the median age at diagnosis is 6 years, and 25% of tumors occur in children younger than 3 years. Approximately 10% to 20% of medulloblastomas occur in adults,

TABLE 32-1

Relative Incidence of Brain Tumors in Children

Tumor Type	Incidence (%)
INFRATENTORIAL	55
Medulloblastoma	25
Astrocytoma (cerebellum)	15
Brainstem glioma	10
Ependymoma (fourth ventricular region)	6
SUPRATENTORIAL	45
Astrocytoma	23
Malignant glioma (anaplastic astrocytoma, glioblastoma multiforme)	6
Embryonal (primitive neuroectodermal) tumors	4
Ependymoma	3
Craniopharyngioma	6
Pineal region tumors	4
Oligodendroglioma	2

Modified from Duffner PK, Cohen ME, Myers MH, et al. *Neurology* 1986;36:597-601; Childhood Brain Tumor Consortium. *J Neurooncol* 1988;6:9-23.

predominantly in the third to fifth decades. The classic presenting triad of posterior fossa tumors such as medulloblastomas consists of headaches and vomiting (signs of increased intracranial pressure) and ataxia.

Medulloblastoma is by definition a posterior fossa tumor, most often arising in the cerebellar vermis, within the cerebellar hemispheres (typically in adolescents, frequently as the desmoplastic variant) or along the cerebellopontine peduncle. The tumor grows to fill the fifth ventricle and often attaches to the brainstem. Medulloblastoma is the characteristic "seeding" CNS tumor and is associated with subarachnoid dissemination through the CSF; metastasis may be apparent from cytologic findings or from images of radiographic deposits within the intracranial subarachnoid space (along the convexities or within the basal cisterns, sometimes limited to the region of the pituitary stalk) or within the spinal subarachnoid space. Subarachnoid disease is apparent at diagnosis in 20% to 25% of affected children.[13,74] Extraneural disease, usually involving the bone or bone marrow, is an infrequent finding at diagnosis or disease recurrence.[75]

The embryonal CNS tumors represent a group of histologically related neoplasms that occur predominantly in children (Box 32-1).[69] The WHO classification defines the *embryonal tumors* as small, round, blue cell tumors that tend to seed the neuraxis and respond to irradiation and chemotherapy, although the prognosis varies widely. Less common tumors in this category include the *supratentorial PNETs*, the rare, primitive *medulloepithelioma*, and the more recently recognized *atypical/rhabdoid tumor* (see the section on "Tumors in Children Less than

---

BOX 32-1 Embryonal Central Nervous System Tumors*

Medulloblastoma
Central neuroblastoma
Ependymoblastoma
Primitive neuroectodermal tumor (PNET)[†]

ADDITIONAL TUMORS WITH A DISTINCT HISTOLOGY AND DIFFERENT GENETIC PATHWAY OF EVOLUTION
Medulloepithelioma
Atypical teratoid/rhabdoid tumor

PINEAL PARENCHYMAL TUMOR CLASSIFIED CLINICALLY AS AN EMBRYONAL TUMOR
Pineoblastoma

*In the definition proposed by Kleihues and Cavenee,[69] such tumors are "histologically identifiable entities [that] all develop on the background of an undifferentiated round-cell tumor but show a variety of divergent patterns of differentiation."
[†]*PNET* refers to supratentorial tumors; those tumors that occur in the posterior fossa are known as medulloblastomas.

---

3 Years Old" later in this chapter). *Pineoblastoma* is classified separately (see the section on "Pineal Region and Germ Cell Tumors" later in this chapter). The term *posterior fossa PNET* is synonymous with medulloblastoma.[69]

Medulloblastoma is believed to originate from the primitive external granular layer of the developing cerebellum. The tumor is characterized by undifferentiated small, round, blue cells, often including neuroblastic rosettes and with varying degrees of neuronal and glial differentiation. The *desmoplastic* tumors are classically identified by their prominent nodularity and dense areas of reticular fibers.[69] Recently designated histopathogic subsets include *medulloblastoma with extensive nodularity and advanced neuronal differentiation* and *large-cell medulloblastoma*.[73]

Surgery and Staging

Surgery is the initial therapy, with the goal of maximal resection for the sake of both therapy and reestablishing CSF flow. Intraoperative ventriculostomy has replaced the routine initial placement of a ventriculoperitoneal shunt; with current surgical approaches, fewer than 25% of children require postoperative conversion of the temporary ventriculostomy to a permanent ventriculoperitoneal shunt. Gross total resection generally is limited only by substantial invasion of the tumor into the brainstem or infiltration into the peduncle. Gross total or near-total resection (more than 90% of the tumor removed, with < 1.5 cm^2 residual) is achieved in nearly 90% of children more than 3 years old in the United States.[76] The operative mortality should be less than 1% or 2% among children treated with current approaches, and the postoperative morbidity is typically acceptable, with a small proportion of children left with permanent new cranial nerve deficits or marked ataxia.[76,77] The posterior fossa syndrome, marked by severe truncal ataxia, difficulties with speech and swallowing stemming from bulbar effects, and sometimes mutism, seems to be associated with extensive dissection along the lower brainstem; symptoms generally abate considerably over several months after the surgery, although late residual deficits of various severity have been noted.[78]

Postoperative neuraxis staging is standard in defining risk groups and subsequent therapy for medulloblastoma and the other embryonal tumors. Immediate postoperative cranial MRI or CT (preferably done within 1 to 3 days of surgery) defines the postoperative residual effect, which is a more reliable prognostic factor than the operative coding of the extent of resection.[76] Neuraxis staging begins with a contrast-enhanced spinal MRI (preferably more than 10 days after surgery to eliminate the confusion of findings with postoperative debris) and subsequent lumbar CSF cytologic studies; routine bone scanning and bone marrow assessments are standard only in investigational

BOX 32-2 Chang Staging System for Medulloblastoma

PRIMARY TUMOR (T)*

T1 Tumor less than 3 cm in diameter

T2 Tumor at least 3 cm in diameter

T3a Tumor larger than 3 cm in diameter with extension into the aqueduct of Sylvius and/or into foramen of Luschka

T3b Tumor larger than 3 cm in diameter with unequivocal extension into the brainstem

T4 Tumor larger than 3 cm in diameter with extension up past the aqueduct of Sylvius and/or down past the foramen magnum (i.e., beyond the posterior fossa)

DISTANT METASTASIS (M)

M0 No evidence of gross subarachnoid or hematogenous metastasis

M1 Microscopic tumor cells found in cerebrospinal fluid

M2 Gross nodule seedings demonstrating in the cerebellar, cerebral subarachnoid space, or in the third or lateral ventricles

M3 Gross nodular seeding in spinal subarachnoid space

M4 Metastasis outside the cerebrospinal axis

Modified from Chang CH, Housepian EM, Herbert C Jr. An operative staging system and a megavoltage radiotherapeutic technic for cerebellar medulloblastoma. *Radiology* 1969;93:1351-1359.
*The T stage is no longer thought to be prognostically related to outcome.

settings.[13,74] Staging is based on the degree of residual tumor (average risk is defined as the presence of ≤ 1.5 cm^2 of residual tumor) and the presence or absence of subarachnoid or extraneural metastasis (defined according to a modification of the Chang system[79]) (Box 32-2). Most important from the standpoint of planning current therapy is determining whether isolated CSF-cytologic evidence of metastatic disease (M1 disease), imaging evidence of intracranial disease outside the posterior fossa (M2 disease), or imaging evidence of spinal metastasis (M3 disease) is present; extranodal disease is classified as M4.[79] Standard or average-risk disease is defined as total removal or a residual tumor volume of less than 1.5 cm^2 with M0 disease; nearly 60% to 65% of children currently enrolled in U.S. studies at the turn of the century were so classified. The presence of only local residual disease is uncommon in children with high-risk disease; more often, these children have neuraxis dissemination.

Radiation Therapy

Postoperative management currently consists of radiation therapy and chemotherapy.[80] Infants and young children (generally defined as those younger than 3 years) are treated in accordance with developing investigational approaches (see the section on "Tumors in Children Less than 3 Years Old" later in this chapter). The now standard sequence of therapy for children 3 years and younger is to begin radiation therapy within 28 to 31 days of surgery, followed by chemotherapy.[81] Although studies of preirradiation chemotherapy have added significantly to our knowledge of chemosensitivity, randomized trials have shown no benefit from administering chemotherapy before irradiation—and in some instances, results have suggested that this sequence is ultimately detrimental to disease control.[82-85]

Radiation therapy for medulloblastoma is technically demanding and biologically unforgiving. It requires the systematic inclusion of the entire subarachnoid space (craniospinal irradiation [CSI]) followed by a boost to the posterior fossa. One standard technique involving immobilization of patients in the prone position is illustrated in Figure 32-2. Lateral craniocervical fields encompass the intracranial and upper cervical spine regions, with particular attention to including the subfrontal and infratemporal regions (at the cribriform plate in the midline subfrontal area and along the infratemporal regions) (Fig. 32-3).

The conventional dose to the neuraxis in patients given surgery and radiation is 36 Gy (delivered in 1.8-Gy fractions once a day). The progression-free survival rate for patients with localized disease after maximal resection and CSI (36 Gy) is approximately 65% at 5 to 10 years (Table 32-2).[36,86-90] A randomized study of patients with average-risk medulloblastoma conducted by the Pediatric Oncology Group (POG) and Children's Cancer Group (CCG) in the late 1980s established the superiority of a total dose of 36 Gy vs. 23.4 Gy for CSI and the benchmark outcome of more than 90% tumor removal with less than 1.5 cm^2 of residual disease cited above.[86] More recent findings suggest that the combination of reduced-dose CSI (23.4 Gy) and chemotherapy produces disease control rates comparable with or superior to those noted for conventional-dose CSI alone.[91] Large-scale prospective studies are ongoing to document the efficacy of what is now considered the standard treatment for localized medulloblastoma, which is irradiation (CSI dose of 23.4 Gy) followed by cisplatin-containing chemotherapy. Reports of outcome in nonrandomized single-arm trials, further supported by neuropsychological findings from the POG-CCG study noted above, suggest that cognitive function in children with average-risk disease after therapy is superior among those given CSI to 23.4 Gy as opposed to 36 Gy, especially in children 3 to 8.5 years old.[60] Children with metastatic disease at presentation (M1 to M3 disease) require a dose of 36 to 39 Gy to the neuraxis.

Irradiation includes a boost to the posterior fossa region, classically defined as the entire infratentorial

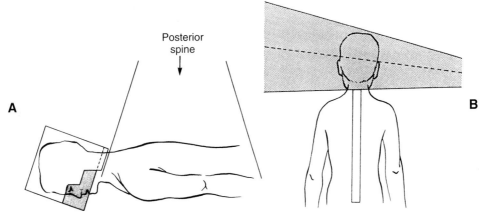

Fig. 32-2 **A,** Classic craniospinal irradiation configurations, with a divergent posterior spinal field matching opposed lateral craniocervical fields. The collimator rotation enabling the craniocervical fields to be matched to the divergence of the posterior spinal field is typically modified at least every five fractions. Field markings for medulloblastoma are determined by the cribriform plate at the orbital level (see Fig. 32-3). **B,** The parallel inferior border from the craniocervical fields is achieved by couch rotation, calculated to achieve a three-dimensional match in the depicted plane.

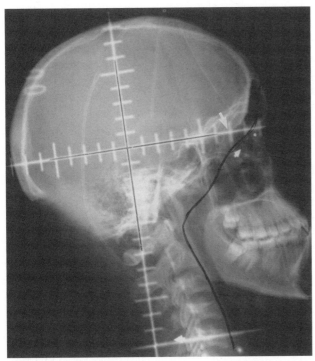

Fig. 32-3 Conventional fluoroscopic image used for simulating the lateral craniocervical fields used in craniospinal irradiation for medulloblastoma (see Fig. 32-2). The *long arrow* indicates the margins along the cribriform plate. The *radiopaque dot* and the *small arrows* indicate the anterior margins of the lateral orbital rims. Divergence rather than a collimator angle is needed when only the subarachnoid space is to be targeted.

volume. The use of opposed lateral posterior fossa fields has been standard, but radiation oncologists are increasingly using a three-dimensional conformal radiation therapy approach[92] to spare the auditory apparatus and,

when possible, the pituitary-hypothalamic region (Fig. 32-4). The cumulative dose delivered to the posterior fossa is typically 54 to 55.8 Gy. A few institutional summaries of patterns of treatment failure for patients with medulloblastoma and descriptions of preliminary experience with target volumes confined to the operative or tumor bed highlight investigational approaches that will be studied prospectively in a planned Children's Oncology Group (COG) study, to begin in 2002.[93,94]

Chemotherapeutic Agents

Several categories of chemotherapeutic agents have shown efficacy in medulloblastoma, namely alkylating agents (e.g., cyclophosphamide or lomustine), platinating agents (e.g., cisplatin. carboplatin), topoisomerase-II inhibitors (e.g., etoposide), and the vinca alkaloids (vincristine). The most common adjuvant treatment for standard or average-risk disease was described by Packer and colleagues[81] and consists of concurrent vincristine during irradiation and postirradiation cycles of lomustine, cisplatin, and vincristine. The addition of concurrent carboplatin or etoposide and high-dose, peripheral stem cell–supporting chemotherapy regimens is being studied in two separate protocols for the treatment of high-risk disease.[95]

Although posterior fossa recurrence previously was regarded as the dominant pattern of failure, more recent studies have indicated that more patients exhibit neuraxis or combined local and disseminated failure. Approaches to the management of disease recurrence are not standardized but often include chemotherapy, further surgery (for localized disease), and the judicious use of further irradiation. Secondary or salvage therapies are rarely successful.

TABLE 32-2

Survival Rates After Craniospinal Irradiation for Medulloblastoma

Study and Reference	Period	Number of Patients	Survival Rates at 5 Years (%)	Survival Rates at 10 Years (%)
Bloom et al, 1969[36]	1950-1964	71	40	30
Berry et al, 1981[87]	1958-1978	122	56	43
Hughes et al, 1986[88]	1977-1985	53	64	42
Bloom et al, 1990[89]	1970-1981	53	53	45
Jenkin et al, 1990[90]	1977-1987	72	71	63
Thomas et al, 2000[86]	1978-1991	(CSI = 36 Gy)	67*	67*
		(CSI = 23 Gy)	52	52

CSI, Craniospinal irradiation.

*Event-free survival rates at 5 and 8 years.

Astrocytoma

Astrocytomas are the most common glial tumors in children, developing in the cerebellum, brainstem, cerebral hemispheres, diencephalon (thalamus, hypothalamus, and third ventricular region, including the optic chiasm), or spinal cord.[96-98] In adults, low-grade tumors occur primarily in the cerebral hemispheres and thalamus; however, malignant astrocytomas far exceed the number of histologically benign lesions beyond the age of 20 years.

The WHO grades astrocytomas as grade I (juvenile pilocytic astrocytoma [JPA]) or grade II (fibrillary astrocytoma or astrocytoma not otherwise specified); high-grade lesions are deemed grade III (anaplastic [malignant] astrocytoma) or grade IV (glioblastoma multiforme).[69] Grossly, the tumors are either solid with discrete or infiltrating margins or cystic. Pilocytic astrocytomas are biologically nonaggressive lesions that are often cystic, occurring predominantly in the cerebellum and diencephalon in children (Fig. 32-5).

The natural history of astrocytomas depends on the age of the patient and the site of origin and histologic classification of the tumor. Pilocytic tumors rarely progress to a more malignant histology; however, fibrillary astrocytomas progress to a more malignant histology in 30% to 50% of cases.[99-101]

Cerebellar Astrocytomas

Cerebellar astrocytomas involve the vermis or hemispheres in 75% of patients; in 25% of children, tumors present as transitional neoplasms that involve the cerebellum and the cerebellar peduncles or adjacent brainstem.[102-105] Cerebellar astrocytomas are classically cystic lesions; the textbook appearance consisting of a large cyst associated with a mural nodule occurs in about one fourth of cases. Grossly, most tumors are either mixed cystic and solid lesions or apparently solid tumors with small cystic components. Histologically, 75% of astrocytomas in this location are JPAs.[102,103,105,106] Debate continues as to whether high-grade gliomas occur in the cerebellum in children; if they do, they are quite uncommon.[107]

Therapy for cerebellar astrocytomas is largely surgical. Reports from institutions indicate that gross total resection is done in 65% to 90% of cases, although this has risen to approximately 85% to 90% in recent series.[96,103,105,106] Resection is more often incomplete among patients with tumors involving the cerebellar peduncles or the brainstem.[103-106] The operative mortality rate should be less than 4%, unlike the rate for patients with medulloblastomas and ependymomas that may invade the adjacent brainstem. Morbidity after radical resection is generally limited in patients with cerebellar astrocytomas.

Recurrence of tumor after radioimaging confirmation of complete surgical removal is uncommon, in the most recent series occurring in less than 10% of patients.[103,105,108,109] Prognosis most closely parallels the extent of resection; multivariate analyses have also identified solid (rather than cystic) lesions, transitional lesions (vs. those confined to the cerebellum), and lesions showing a fibrillary or diffuse histology (vs. JPA) as potentially significant prognostic factors.[103,105,106,110] A direct correlation between the volume of residual tumor and outcome has also been reported.[103]

Indications for radiation therapy are limited in patients with cerebellar astrocytomas. Although radiation therapy has been suggested to be efficacious in those patients with incompletely resected solid lesions, enthusiasm is generally limited for postoperative irradiation for any cerebellar astrocytomas.[108,111] A small subset of tumors, often those that primarily involve the cerebellar peduncle, will recur after initial surgery; the author's approach in the treatment of such tumors is to use irradiation only after tumor progression after a second attempt at resection. In this instance, the clinical target volume should be quite limited and focused on identified areas of residual tumor with a 1-cm margin; standard dose levels are 54 to 55.8 Gy using conventional fractionation.[111]

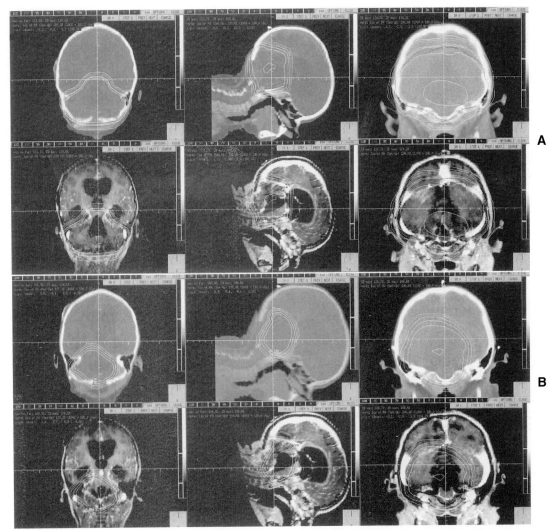

Fig. 32-4 **A,** Treatment plans for a three-dimensional conformal technique demonstrating ideal dose distribution for a six-field, noncoplanar approach targeting the entire posterior fossa. Anatomically, this approach includes the tentorium as it extends superiorly in the posterior clinoid and then inferiorly to define the anterior and superior margins of the posterior fossa. The inferior and posterior margins are defined by the calvarium and the lower margin of foramen magnum. **B,** Three-dimensional conformal dose distribution demonstrating coverage of the primary tumor site (here the operative bed after surgical resection of a medulloblastoma). A multifield, noncoplanar 6-MeV photon approach uses a gross tumor volume that outlines the operative bed, expanded by 2 cm (as modified by anatomic boundaries) to identify the clinical target volume. A 5-mm planning target volume geometrically surrounds the clinical target volume. (See Color Plate 34, after p. 80, for color reproduction.)

Supratentorial Astrocytomas

Supratentorial astrocytomas include diencephalic or central lesions and lesions of the cerebral hemispheres. In children, total resection can be achieved for up to 90% of astrocytomas in the cerebral hemisphere.[96,100,112,113] Diffuse cerebral lesions, including those labeled *gliomatosis cerebri,* can arise in several cerebral lobes with an often low-grade (fibrillary, WHO grade II) histologic appearance but clinically malignant potential. Similarly, thalamic tumors represent a mix of circumscribed JPAs and diffuse, sometimes bithalamic fibrillary tumors; up to 40% of thalamic gliomas are histologically malignant (WHO grade III to IV, anaplastic astrocytoma or glioblastoma).[113-115] Biopsy alone has been the standard surgery for most thalamic astrocytomas because knowledge of the tumor histology is important in guiding therapy.[89,116,117] However, Bernstein and colleagues[118] reported that major resections were performed in up to 33% of patients with circumscribed thalamic tumors; the incidence of major operative morbidity was only 7%.

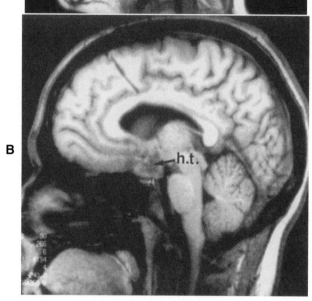

Fig. 32-5 Midline sagittal T1-weighted magnetic resonance imaging scans depicting a hypothalamic/optic-chiasmatic juvenile pilocytic astrocytoma that fills much of the sella and suprasellar region at diagnosis **(A)** and at 2 years after completion of radiation therapy (54 Gy delivered in 30 fractions in a multifield three-dimensional conformal approach) **(B)**. The involution is typical of juvenile pilocytic astrocytomas at this site, including the fairly long interval to reduction. (*h.t.,* Hypothalamic tumor).

A further experience confirmed that limited or aggressive resection may have a role in the treatment of low-grade thalamic gliomas.[119]

The role of radiation therapy in childhood astrocytomas is evolving and now is thought to depend on tumor histology and site, age of the patient, and presence or absence of clinical signs. Several reviews[120] have shown that radiation therapy is efficacious in terms of tumor response, prolonged progression-free interval,

and long-term disease control. A joint CCG-POG prospective trial of postoperative irradiation for incompletely resected astrocytomas was abandoned early in the 1990s because the proportion of children in whom gross total or near-total resection could be achieved had increased substantially and because the wisdom of performing irradiation before symptomatic or radioimaging-documented progression of disease precluded uniform acceptance of irradiation as a randomized option. Preliminary experience in that trial suggested that observation may be appropriate after substantial resection because disease seems to progress in only a minority of such cases 3 to 5 years after surgery[117] (Wisoff, J. Personal communication, 2001). For some patients with central low-grade gliomas (e.g., tectal plate or midbrain, less often hypothalamic or thalamic), cautious observation can identify indolent, stable tumors that may not require immediate intervention if the child is neurologically stable.[98,121] However, such an approach implies a commitment to intervene with surgery, radiation, or both when clinical or radiographic evidence of tumor progression appears.

The systematic use of postoperative irradiation has also been questioned in adults.[116,122-124] Adults more often have sizable peripheral cerebral-hemisphere tumors. Outcome at 5 and 10 years seems to be improved among patients given radiation therapy for incompletely, as opposed to completely, resected tumors.[122-125] A recent trial by the European Organization for Research and Treatment of Cancer (EORTC) to evaluate postoperative observation vs. irradiation for WHO grade I and II hemispheric lesions in adults showed no convincing advantage for either early irradiation or for low-dose (45 Gy) vs. high-dose (60 Gy) therapy.[126]

The effect of radiation therapy is perhaps best documented for central supratentorial lesions. Neurologic improvement has been observed in 80% of patients after irradiation for diencephalic tumors. Objective reduction in the size of supratentorial astrocytomas has been noted in approximately half of the patients studied by prospective CT assessment. Long-term survival in patients with biopsy-proven diencephalic lesions has nearly always required irradiation to therapeutic dose levels.[116] Limited-volume, fractionated irradiation has been reported to control most such lesions, with toxicity apparently being more limited in the pediatric age group.[127]

Optic Pathway Glioma

Tumors of the optic nerves and chiasm are low-grade astrocytomas and occur predominantly in young children, often younger than 3 to 5 years. In 25% to 30% of cases, the tumors are associated with neurofibromatosis.[128] Tumors of the optic nerve often behave as hamartomatous lesions, although up to 50% may extend proximally toward the chiasm. Chiasmatic gliomas present with visual and often with endocrine signs; it is often difficult to distinguish chiasmatic from hypothalamic tumors. In collected reports of 500 cases, 25% of patients with chiasmatic involvement died of tumor-related events.[129,130] In an often-quoted series of 36 children, Hoyt and Baghdassarian[131] indicated that chiasmatic tumors were indolent and nonthreatening. However, later follow-up (at a median of 20 years) documented a 25% tumor-related mortality in a population weighted toward the apparently more benign tumor associated with neurofibromatosis.[132,133]

The efficacy of radiation therapy for tumors of the optic chiasm with or without hypothalamic involvement has been documented in numerous series.[129,134-136] Visual acuity or visual fields are improved in approximately 25% of patients receiving radiation therapy, and neuroimaging shows a reduction in the size of the lesion in these patients.[136,137] Survival rates after irradiation for chiasmatic gliomas reportedly range between 75% and 100% in large series of patients followed for 5 to 10 years.[129,134-136]

Controversy regarding management appropriately surrounds the often benign clinical course of the disease in relation to the potential for treatment-related morbidity with surgery or irradiation. Exophytic JPAs arising in the chiasmatic or hypothalamic region are amenable to incomplete surgical resection[138]; the potential advantage of partial resection lies in delaying more definitive irradiation. Particularly among younger children, a balance between disease progression vs. the potential risk of endocrine and intellectual effects from irradiation has favored a conservative approach.[129,134] Packer and colleagues[139-141] described their experience with chemotherapy, particularly the carboplatin and vincristine regimen. In most young children, previously progressive or symptomatic disease was stabilized with chemotherapy; objective responses were documented in up to 50% of cases, and the median time to disease progression was in excess of 3 years. Initial management with relatively toxicity-free chemotherapy approaches is logical for children with progressive symptomatic chiasmatic or hypothalamic tumors, certainly for those younger than 3 to 5 years and possibly for all children before puberty. Unclear yet is the frequency and durability of disease control among children for whom radiation is begun when their disease progresses during or after chemotherapy. Outside the investigational setting, the treatment of choice remains primary irradiation in children between 5 and 10 years of age because long-term disease control can be achieved in up to 90% of cases.[129,134-136]

Radiation Therapy Technique

Radiation therapy for low-grade astrocytomas uses local target volumes to encompass the typically discrete primary tumor quite narrowly.[127,142,143] Uncommonly, low-grade tumors diffusely infiltrate one or more cerebral lobes, requiring more wide-field or total cranial

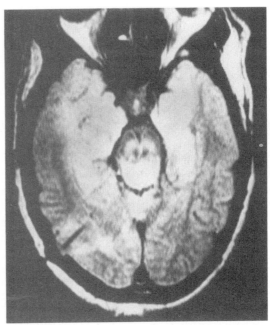

Fig. 32-6 Magnetic resonance imaging scan demonstrating the diffuse, multilobar involvement of a biopsy-proven fibrillary astrocytoma. Although predominantly in the left temporal lobe, the lesion also extends throughout the left parietal, right parietal, and mesencephalic regions. Objective improvement in response to irradiation is often transitory. This type of diffuse cerebral tumor, sometimes called gliomatosis cerebri, is a supratentorial lesion analogous to the more typical diffusely infiltrating pontine glioma.

irradiation (Fig. 32-6). Low-grade, often pilocytic, astrocytomas are associated with multifocal disease or subarachnoid involvement at diagnosis (or, less commonly, at recurrence) in 15% to 20% of patients with childhood astrocytomas.[144-146] Multifocal or metastatic disease is rarely confined to the spinal subarachnoid region; multiple disease sites are almost always apparent on cranial MRI studies, obviating any requirement for spinal imaging or staging in patients with this tumor. Specific histologic subtypes of tumors (i.e., pleomorphic xanthoastrocytoma and meningocerebral astrocytoma) can directly infiltrate the contiguous meninges, but this seems to be associated with an indolent, benign course after surgery alone.[147-149]

Establishing the target volume requires detailed MRI. A 1-cm margin beyond the abnormalities shown on T1- or T2-weighted images seems adequate on the basis of early follow-up data from patients for whom three-dimensionally planned and delivered radiation techniques were used.[127,142,143,150]

A dose-response relationship for astrocytoma has not been well defined. In most series, a radiation dose of approximately 50 Gy delivered in 1.8-Gy, once-daily fractions has proven adequate.[120,129] However, in statistical analyses of rather sizable series of patients, both Albright[116] and Laws[100] and their associates noted an apparent benefit conferred by doses above 40 Gy. Justifying dose levels above 54 to 55 Gy in children is difficult in view of the increase in risk at radiation levels approaching cerebral tolerance. In adults with supratentorial astrocytomas, however, Shaw and colleagues,[125] having shown a dose-response relationship indicating improved survival after at least 53 Gy, recommend levels of 55 to 60 Gy.

Prognosis

Laws and colleagues[100] reviewed the Mayo Clinic experience in 461 patients of all ages with supratentorial astrocytomas treated between 1915 and 1975. The most important correlates of 10- and 15-year survival were age (86% long-term survival in children and adolescents younger than 20 years vs. 33% in those 20 years of age and older) and the degree of tumor involvement, reflected by the neurologic deficit and the extent of resection (37% survival rate in patients after biopsy or limited removal compared with 55% in those after subtotal or total resection). In Shaw's review[125] of the same Mayo experience in adult patients with supratentorial astrocytomas, a role for radiation therapy was clearly indicated for most patients with astrocytomas, with 5- and 10-year survival rates of 68% and 39%, respectively, after at least 53 Gy. Patients treated with less than 53 Gy or no irradiation had a 5-year survival rate of 47% (both groups) and 10-year survival rates of 27% and 11%, respectively. The long-term potential for radiation therapy to control disease specifically in children with hemispheric astrocytomas has been documented in reviews by Bloom[89] and Jenkin[90] and their colleagues, who independently noted that the survival rate reached a plateau between 5 and 15 years after postoperative irradiation. The benefit

of adding radiation after incomplete resection for children with supratentorial hemispheric tumors was made apparent in the Pittsburgh series reported by Pollack and colleagues.[151]

Site-specific survival rates suggest that patients with hypothalamic and chiasmatic astrocytomas enjoy longer survival times than do patients with most other types of supratentorial astrocytomas. In particular, Bloom and colleagues[89] cited 5-year survival rates of 60% to 70% among patients with thalamic or hypothalamic tumors after primary irradiation. Albright and colleagues[116] reported a mean survival duration of 5.1 years after radiation therapy for patients with diencephalic gliomas compared with a mean survival time of less than 1 year for patients who did not undergo irradiation. The virtual lack of tumor progression beyond 5 years after radiation therapy further suggests a role for radiation therapy as a curative modality in the primary management of hypothalamic or chiasmatic tumors.[136,152]

Brainstem Gliomas

Tumors of the brainstem most often involve the pons (70%), followed by the medulla (15% to 20%) and the midbrain (10% to 15%).[153,154] Brainstem gliomas are characterized as either diffusely infiltrating or focal depending on the pattern of involvement; focal tumors are well demarcated, confined to one anatomic segment of the brainstem, and occupy less than half of the brainstem.[155] Most focal tumors are JPAs histologically; they occur more often in the midbrain or medulla but can arise in the pons.[153,156-158] Pontine gliomas are largely diffuse[154,155] (Fig. 32-7). Dorsally exophytic lesions

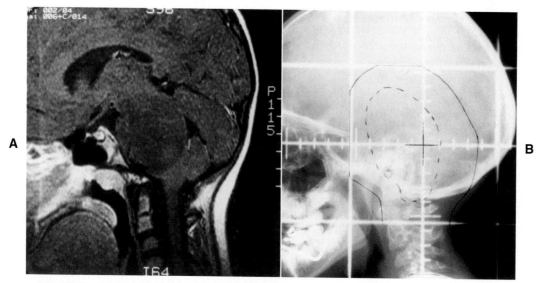

Fig. 32-7 **A,** A sagittal magnetic resonance imaging scan depicting a diffusely infiltrating brainstem glioma involving much of the pons and extending toward the midbrain and the medulla. A typical two-dimensional treatment approach is shown in **B;** use of three-dimensional conformal techniques also may be advantageous.

are relatively benign tumors, generally arising at the pontomedullary junction or from the medulla; histologically, they are JPAs.[156-159] In the past, brainstem tumors have been treated conservatively, with histologic confirmation limited to focal or cystic lesions for which knowledge of the histology or drainage might facilitate treatment.[153,154] Findings from biopsied cases indicate that malignant glioma is present in 40% of patients at diagnosis[154]; the remaining tumors are largely fibrillary astrocytomas.[153,160] At autopsy, however, malignant gliomas are found in more than 80% of cases.[154,160]

Radiation therapy is primarily used for diffusely infiltrating brainstem gliomas. Substantial neurologic improvement occurs in 60% to 70% of patients with diffusely infiltrating pontine gliomas, although long-term survival is limited to 10% to 20% of patients with such gliomas.[154] Dorsally exophytic tumors are usually identified during surgery for a tumor that otherwise fills much of the fourth ventricle. The lesions in more than half of the patients remain indolent after incomplete resection; the 40% or more of tumors that do progress are most often controlled with radiation[157,158] (Fig. 32-8).

Radiation Therapy Technique

Brainstem gliomas tend to infiltrate longitudinally, usually extending beyond the pons to involve the

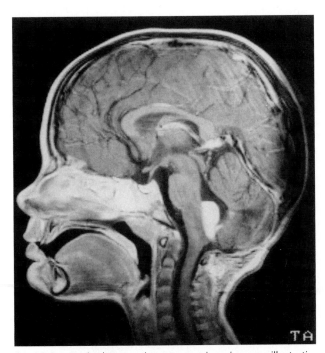

Fig. 32-8 Sagittal magnetic resonance imaging scan illustrating dorsally exophytic brainstem glioma. This discrete, briskly enhancing tumor fills much of the fourth ventricle, attaching along the posterior aspect of the brainstem at the pontomedullary junction. Invasion is often not apparent on imaging; at surgery, however, lesions are often found to blend imperceptibly with the underlying brainstem.

midbrain or medulla and extending peripherally into the cerebellum or medial temporal lobes (see Fig. 32-7). Therefore irradiation is limited to the brainstem and immediately adjacent neural tracts. The infiltrative nature of these tumors can be better appreciated on T2-weighted MRI studies. Clinical target volumes are generally defined with 2-cm margins along the tracts of infiltration (i.e., into the midbrain or medulla, through the peduncles, and into the adjacent cerebellum).[161] Given the poor overall outcome in patients with pontine lesions, many centers continue to use two-dimensional, opposed lateral fields in this setting, again providing a margin around the known tumor extent.

The standard dose for brainstem gliomas is 54 to 56 Gy, given in a conventional fractionation scheme. In a series of trials, hyperfractionated doses given to total doses of 66, 70 to 72, and 76 to 78 Gy indicated no real benefit from the higher doses.[162-164] Most long-term survivors have been adults or children with focal brainstem lesions often outside the pons (i.e., in the midbrain or medulla).[162]

The decade-long experience with hyperfractionated therapy for these tumors has encouraged neurosurgeons, radiation oncologists, and pediatric oncologists to enroll patients in multi-institutional protocols. In one such study, a randomized trial conducted by POG, conventional fractionation to 54 Gy was documented to be as effective as 70 Gy given in twice-daily 1.2-Gy fractions.[165] This trial also documented the apparent negative effect of irradiation in combination with concurrent cisplatin in this setting.[165,166]

Prognosis

The 5-year overall survival rates are 10% to 20% in children with brainstem gliomas and 20% to 30% in adults.[162-164] Median survival after irradiation is only 8 months in patients with classic intrinsic tumors in the pons. Hoffman and colleagues[156,157] initially identified as highly favorable a subset of children in whom exophytic tumors extended into the fourth ventricles. However, it is now known that these tumors are usually JPAs[158]; survival after surgery, with or without radiation, approaches 90% in this selected group.[156-158] Intrinsic pontine tumors, constituting most of the classically identified brainstem gliomas, are usually associated with multiple cranial nerve palsies, diffusely hypodense lesions on CT or MRI studies, and a high-grade histologic appearance indicative of an infiltrating, aggressive neoplasm. Long-term survival in the latter group has consistently been less than 15%. Less common intrinsic tumors that are focal and confined to a segment of the pons or midbrain are associated with slightly better long-term survival rates.[155]

Current chemotherapies have little effect on brainstem gliomas. Adjuvant therapy did not affect outcome in the only published randomized trial.[167]

Ependymomas

Intracranial ependymomas occur predominantly in young children, but they are also seen in older children and adults. Ependymomas also occur as primary spinal cord neoplasms, but this presentation is more common in adults. Posterior fossa ependymomas typically present with the same symptom triad as other posterior fossa tumors in children—headache, vomiting, and ataxia. Associated symptoms include torticollis and lower cranial nerve dysfunction. The median age of children with these tumors is 4 years; however, nearly 30% of infant brain tumors (i.e., those in children younger than 3 years) are ependymomas.[168,169] Infratentorial lesions in younger children may occur more often in girls than in boys. Supratentorial lesions more often present with seizures or focal neurologic abnormalities and are most common in adolescents and adults.

Tumors of the posterior fossa occur predominantly in children; these tumors show a predilection for the fourth ventricle in young children and often involve or originate within the region of the foramen of Luschka[169,170] (Fig. 32-9). Direct extension through the foramen magnum into the upper cervical spinal canal is a characteristic pattern of growth. Ependymomas disseminate into the subarachnoid space in approximately 12% of children.[89,171-174] However, this presentation is more often noted at diagnosis or as a primary site of recurrence in very young children and may be associated with an anaplastic histology; in older children, this

pattern is more common after local recurrence than earlier in the disease.[173,174] Supratentorial tumors often arise in regions adjacent to the ventricular system; growth occurs largely through intraparenchymal extension.[175]

Ependymomas arise from the ependymal cells lining the ventricular system and the central spinal canal. The tumor characteristically includes ependymal rosettes and perivascular pseudorosettes. Ependymomas are differentiated or low-grade lesions; variants include cellular, clear cell, tancytic, and papillary types.[69] In a recent series, 15% to 30% of ependymomas were classified as anaplastic tumors (WHO grade III), marked by increased cellularity and mitotic rate. The tumors are generally well demarcated but can show parenchymal invasion.[69,106] Although ependymomas were regarded by leading neuropathologists in the 1980s as being of little clinical significance, more recently an association has been noted between an anaplastic histology and a less favorable outcome.[176-182] Ependymoblastomas are rare embryonal tumors and are discussed with the other supratentorial PNETs.

Surgery is the initial intervention for most intracranial ependymomas. Even extensive tumors of the fourth ventricle can often be grossly resected; in fact, total resection of even those tumors extending into or arising in the cerebellopontine angle has been achieved.[170,180] The advantage of near-total or total resection is apparent, with considerable improvement in disease control among children in whom complete resection was achieved.[179-181] The price of this control, however, is a

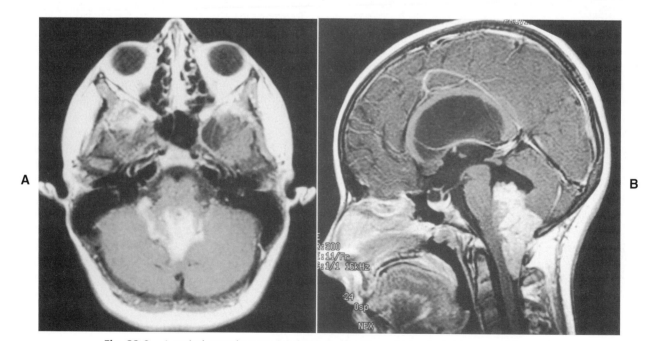

Fig. 32-9 A typical ependymoma involving the fourth ventricle. **A,** Axial computed tomography scan reveals a lesion that fills much of the fourth ventricle and extends through the right foramen of Luschka. **B,** Sagittal magnetic resonance imaging scan shows the tumor extending caudally along the medulla and below the foramen magnum into the upper cervical spinal canal.

significant incidence of new postoperative neurologic deficits, including the posterior fossa syndrome and major new bulbar signs (e.g., palsies of cranial nerves IX and X resulting in difficulty with speech and airway protection), sometimes requiring postoperative tracheostomy or the placement of a feeding tube.[82] Institutional experience generally shows that gross total resection can be accomplished in 50% to 60% of patients with infratentorial ependymoma; however, a total resection rate as high as 90% has been noted recently.[180]

Postoperative irradiation is essentially routine for patients with ependymomas, almost regardless of age, because adjuvant radiation has been shown to increase disease control rates in several major series.[180,182] However, a single experience suggests that disease could be controlled in a certain subgroup of children with supratentorial ependymomas who are treated with total resection alone; in this ongoing COG prospective trial, only a small proportion of patients with such ependymomas are being treated with observation only.[183] For all lesions of the fourth ventricle or cerebellopontine angle, high rates of tumor control have been noted only for patients treated with local postoperative irradiation and radical resection.[179-181,184] Long-term disease control was accomplished in approximately 70% of such children, compared with 20% to 30% of those treated with incomplete resection and similar irradiation.

Ependymomas respond to a variety of chemotherapeutic agents, including cyclophosphamide and vincristine, cisplatin and carboplatin, and etoposide. A randomized trial of adjuvant lomustine, vincristine, and prednisone conducted by the CCG showed no benefit from this chemotherapy.[185] In addition, the initial experience in infants with ependymomas indicated an inverse relationship between the duration of chemotherapy (equivalent to the time of initiating radiation therapy) and disease control, encouraging current institutional and cooperative group trials to limit the use of chemotherapy for this tumor; only for the youngest children (less than 18 months old) has a brief (3 to 4 month) course of chemotherapy been used before irradiation (or second resection and irradiation if measurable disease is apparent at the completion of chemotherapy).[184] For infants, interest in chemotherapy dose escalation continues because of positive preliminary results from the second POG study of infant brain tumors, results that suggested that dose-intensified chemotherapy produced better disease-control rates than did standard chemotherapy.[186] In older children, the usefulness of limited-duration chemoresponsiveness in facilitating second operative resections before radiation is being examined in a current COG trial.

Most clinical experience with ependymomas is based on treatment volumes that, for infratentorial lesions, include the entire posterior fossa and often the upper cervical spinal canal to one to two vertebral levels below the caudal tumor extent. Because recurrent disease is almost always localized to the initial tumor bed and often the site of attachment, and because minimal residual disease is left adjacent to the brainstem or peduncle, current prospective investigations are targeting only the local tumor bed (with margins as tight as 1 cm) using three-dimensional conformal or intensity-modulated radiation therapy[150] (Fig. 32-10). However, findings during an as yet insufficient follow-up period indicate that such limited treatment volumes should be used with caution outside a controlled setting. For supratentorial lesions, a 1- to 2-cm margin around the initial tumor extent is indicated, with potential modifications when the normal brain is reconfigured by tumor resection. Treatment volumes for differentiated and anaplastic ependymomas usually do not differ.[187,188] Previous interest in CSI for anaplastic infratentorial lesions has not continued into contemporary protocols or treatment standards, except in cases in which neuraxis involvement is documented at diagnosis.

Classically, radiation doses of 45 to 54 Gy have been used.[172,179,182] Recently, however, doses of 54 to 55.8 Gy

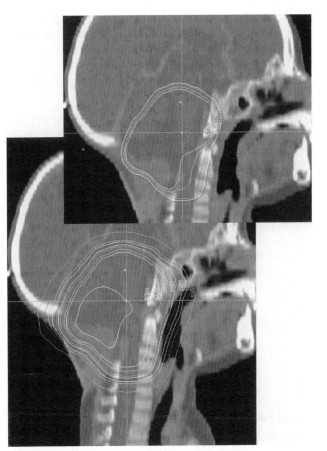

Fig. 32-10 Treatment plan demonstrating isodose volumes for a three-dimensional conformal approach, using multiple noncoplanar 6-MeV photon fields to encompass the tumor within the lower aspect of the posterior fossa and the uppermost spinal canal. The target volume in contemporary protocols more often addresses the tumor bed or surgical bed than the full posterior fossa. (See Color Plate 35, after p. 80, for color reproduction.)

have been reported to achieve superior results and are indicated even after gross total resection.[189,190] Despite apparently encouraging results from a small POG trial of hyperfractionated irradiation (70 Gy given twice daily in 1.2-Gy fractions) for patients with posterior fossa ependymomas, no substantiated role has been established for altered fractionation. The potential value of dose escalation, however, is being explored in trials testing cumulative doses approaching 60 Gy.[150]

Pineal Region and Germ Cell Tumors

A unique group of tumors occur in the pineal region: germ cell tumors, pineal parenchymal tumors, and glial and ependymal tumors (Table 32-3).[69,107,191] Intracranial germ cell tumors occur predominantly in the pineal region, although they can also arise in the anterior third ventricular (suprasellar) region and, less commonly, in thalamic or deep cerebral hemispheric areas.

This unique group of tumors presents with clinically and histologically linked syndromes. Pineal region germinomas occur predominantly in adolescent boys and are associated with multifocal or metastatic disease in the anterior third ventricular region in 10% to 40% of cases.[192-196] Suprasellar (anterior third ventricular) germ cell tumors occur more broadly throughout the pediatric age group and more equally in girls and boys; these tumors are often germinomas but also include other germ cell types. Pineal parenchymal tumors in children are overwhelmingly malignant pineoblastomas, with a considerable proportion occurring in infants and children less than 2 to 3 years old as highly aggressive, widely metastasizing, small, round, blue cell tumors. Pineocytomas are decidedly less common and occur more often in adults.[69,197-199]

Regardless of histology, pineal region tumors typically present with Parinaud's syndrome, consisting of near-light dissociation (pupillary responses are diminished to light but are maintained with attempted accommodation), lack of upward gaze, and incomplete ability to accommodate. Obstructive hydrocephalus is often noted when the tumors occur near the sylvian aqueduct. Suprasellar lesions can also present as hydrocephalus when the growing tumor obstructs the foramen of Monro; diabetes insipidus and visual-field deficits are often also apparent.

Although sometimes debated in the past, it is important to histologically establish the diagnosis of pineal region tumors. Suprasellar lesions have usually been biopsied, both because of their relative accessibility and the broad differential diagnosis that includes astrocytomas of the hypothalamic or chiasmatic region and craniopharyngioma. Germ cell tumors can occasionally be definitively diagnosed on the basis of chemical markers: any significant elevation of the alpha-fetoprotein level in the serum or CSF is diagnostic of a malignant germ cell histiotype (typically embryonal carcinoma, yolk sac tumor, or teratocarcinoma), and marked elevation of β-human chorionic gonadotrophin level (β-HCG; typically over 100 to 1000 mIU/ml) is diagnostic of a choriocarcinoma or malignant mixed germ cell tumors (with choriocarcinomatous elements).[200,201] Moderate elevation of the β-HCG level (50 to 100 mIU/ml) is compatible with a germinoma but cytologic or histologic evidence is required to confirm the diagnosis.[202] Once a diagnosis is established, neuraxis staging (spinal MRI, lumbar CSF cytology) is mandatory for any of the germ cell tumors and pineoblastoma.

An open craniotomy is usually required to biopsy suprasellar tumors.[203] More recently, biopsy has been possible during third ventriculoscopy, often at the time of ventriculoperitoneal shunt insertion or third ventriculostomy. Pineal region tumors can be approached stereotactically, but their challenging location (adjacent to the major draining intracranial veins) has led many neurosurgeons to prefer an open approach. Tumor resection is feasible in the pineal region, although done in only a minority of instances because of the high rate of potential complications. Although insertion of a ventriculoperitoneal shunt is often necessary, the notable incidence of shunt metastasis (with tumor arising

---

TABLE 32-3
Histologic Classification and Relative Incidence of Pineal Region Tumors

Histologic Type*	Relative Frequency†
TUMORS OF GERM CELL ORIGIN	
Germinoma	60% to 80%
Teratoma (differentiated, immature, malignant)	65%
Endodermal sinus tumor	18%
Embryonal carcinoma	7%
Choriocarcinoma	5%
TUMORS OF PINEAL PARENCHYMAL ORIGIN	14%
Pineoblastoma	
Pineocytoma	
TUMORS OF GLIAL ORIGIN	15%
Astrocytoma	
Malignant glioma	
Ganglioglioma (ganglioneuroma)	
Ependymoma	

*Modified from Burger PC, Scheithauer BW, Vogel FS, eds. *Surgical Pathology of the Nervous System and its Coverings*, 3rd ed. New York, NY: Churchill Livingstone; 1991.

†Modified from Burger PC, Scheithauer BW, Vogel FS, eds. *Surgical Pathology of the Nervous System and its Coverings*, 3rd ed. New York, NY: Churchill Livingstone; 1991; Kleihues P, Cavenee WK, eds. *Tumours of the Nervous System*. Lyon, France: IARC Press; 2000.

throughout the peritoneal cavity),[202,203] although low in absolute terms, is relatively more common for this group of tumors than for any other intracranial lesions. Thus performance of a third ventriculostomy, rather than placement of a ventriculoperitoneal shunt, is encouraged for accomplishing internal decompression.

Radiation Therapy Technique

Radiation therapy is highly curative in patients with germinomas in the pineal region, anterior third ventricle, or multiple midline locations.[195,201,204-210] Considerable debate, however, surrounds the appropriate radiation volume for these tumors.[196] Given the recognized incidence of intraventricular and subarachnoid dissemination, craniospinal (or less often full cranial) irradiation has been recommended for both pineal region and suprasellar germinomas.[195,204,211] The outcome in many series indicates that disease is controlled in up to 95% of patients treated with full neuraxis irradiation as a component of their therapy (Table 32-4).[193,196,205,208-215] Local irradiation, variably defined as encompassing the primary tumor site with a margin or the entire third ventricular region, has been associated with long-term disease-free survival rates of more than 80% (see Table 32-4).[193,196,205,208-215] The incidence of neuraxis dissemination varies from less than 10% to 35%.[196,204,209,211,216] No consensus has been reached regarding the appropriate radiation volume because cure rates are relatively high for both local and full-neuraxis irradiation, and the toxic effects associated with the relatively low doses necessary for this disease are exquisitely age-related.[208,210]

Evidence is increasing that 45 Gy delivered to the primary tumor site is adequate to ensure virtually uniform control of pineal region and suprasellar germinomas. Wider-field components (craniospinal or, as done at some institutions, full cranial irradiation) can be limited to doses of 25 Gy.[206,208,209]

Considerable interest has been expressed recently in chemotherapy for intracranial germinomas. Although a high rate of response has been documented, durable control of disease has been achieved in only about half of the patients treated with chemotherapy only, including some of the more rigorous treatment regimens that carry a 5% to 10% rate of toxicity-related death.[212,214,215,217] Notably, CSI is often a successful salvage treatment for germinomas that recur after such therapy.[208]

Early studies conducted by Allen and colleagues[213,218] established that disease control was excellent after combined chemotherapy (with cyclophosphamide or carboplatin) followed by limited-volume, reduced-dose irradiation. Strategies incorporating moderately aggressive chemotherapy and local irradiation (to 30 to 36 Gy for patients showing a good partial or complete response, as shown on imaging studies and by normalization of any elevated markers) or limited-dose CSI (for those with disease dissemination) result in disease control rates exceeding 90%, with limited toxic effects.[210,212,214,217]

TABLE 32-4
Therapy and Outcome in Intracranial Germinomas

| Therapy | RADIATION THERAPY | | Chemotherapy | 5-Year NED Rate (%) | Study and Reference |
	CSI	Local (Gy)			
RT only	+	50-55		85	Shibamoto et al, 1988[211]
	+	45-55		86	Rich et al, 1985[193]
	+	45-59		97	Hardenbergh et al, 1997[209]
	+	45-50		91	Bamberg et al, 1999[212]
	CrI, VtI	45-54		91	Wolden et al, 1995[196]
	0	40-50		87	Calaminus et al, 1994[210]
	0	44		90	Haddock et al, 1997[205]
	+	50		100	Merchant et al, 2000[208]
Chemotherapy + reduced RT	0	30	Cyclophosphamide	91	Allen et al, 1987[213]
	0	40	VP-16/CBCDA; VP-16/ifosfamide	96†	Bouffet et al, 1999[214]
	0	30	(CBCDA or CDDP); vinblastine; bleomycin	92	Calaminus et al, 1994[210]
Chemotherapy only	0	0	CDDP, VP-16, bleomycin	42	Balmaceda et al, 1996[215]

CSI, Craniospinal irradiation (dose levels 24 to 30+ Gy for localized tumors); NED, no evidence of disease; RT, radiation therapy; CrI, full cranial irradiation; VtI, full ventricular volume irradiation (typically to doses of 20 to 36 Gy); CBCDA, carboplatin; CDDP, cisplatin; VP-16, etoposide.
*Includes cases from Rich et al, 1985[193] (CSI or CrI, dose 15 to 44 Gy)
†Event-free survival at 3 years.

Whether such an approach offers any advantage over radiation therapy alone is unclear; prospective trials of this approach are being conducted in Europe and by the COG. It is difficult to improve on the disease control rates produced by primary irradiation, although pre-pubertal patients and those who require CSI before completion of skeletal growth may benefit from a combined-modality approach.

In patients with malignant germ cell tumors (embryonal or yolk sac carcinoma, choricarcinoma), treatment with radiation therapy alone has rarely controlled disease more than 25% to 40% of the time.[203,210] Combined irradiation and chemotherapy seems to be beneficial in such cases, but the chemotherapy must be relatively aggressive and given in doses of 25 to 35 Gy, depending on the response to prior chemotherapy.[219,220]

The application of a stereotactic radiosurgical boost for the more malignant pineal region tumors (including residual malignant tumors with a germ cell histiotype and pineoblastoma) is a reasonable if yet unproven approach. For patients with malignant tumors with a germ cell histiotype that shows evidence of disease on radioimaging (with or without persistently elevated biochemical markers), the addition of a single-fraction boost of 10 to 14 Gy after 45 to 50 Gy is delivered by local external-beam irradiation seems to be effective.

Prognosis

Fairly favorable outcome has recently been observed among patients with pineoblastomas treated with radiation therapy (including CSI) and chemotherapy (including alkylating agents or nitrosoureas in conjunction with vincristine).[221] Disease has been controlled in up to 60% of patients, as compared with the 0% to 10% survival rates for infants treated with prolonged chemotherapy with or without irradiation.[168]

Craniopharyngioma

Craniopharyngiomas are histologically benign tumors derived from squamous cell rests in the region of the pituitary stalk. More than half of these tumors occur in patients younger than 18 years, and craniopharyngiomas represent 3% to 9% of the intracranial tumors of children. The tumor arises as an extra-axial lesion, typically a densely calcified, solid tumor in the suprasellar region with large cystic components (Fig. 32-11). Histologically, such classic adamantine tumors occur in children and adults.[222] Less common are the noncalcified, squamous papillary type, which usually occur in adults.[69,106]

Total surgical resection is usually curative in patients with craniopharyngiomas.[222-229] The decision whether to use surgery or radiation therapy depends on the site of origin and growth of the tumor, which often causes damage to the hypothalamus or optic chiasm and sometimes the adjacent major vessels. Although encapsulated,

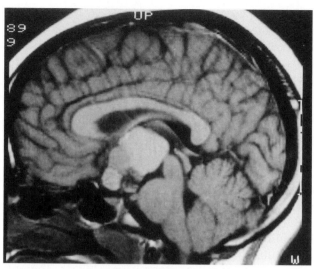

Fig. 32-11 Midline sagittal nonenhanced magnetic resonance imaging scan demonstrates a craniopharyngioma involving the upper aspect of the sella, with a solid component extending into the suprasellar region along the pituitary-hypothalamic stalk. The cystic component is visible superiorly.

the lesion usually adheres to these vital structures, even though it does not actually infiltrate to the level of the tuber cinereum.[223-225] Modern microsurgical techniques allow total resection in up to 75% of cases, with operative mortality rates of l% to 3%.[225,230-232] The incidence of long-term functional deficits may be higher among patients who undergo radical resection than among those treated with irradiation.[226,233-236]

Kramer and colleagues[237,238] established the effectiveness of high-dose irradiation after limited cyst aspiration, initially reporting 5-year survival in nine of 10 patients with later follow-up showing 13- to 15-year survival in six of six children.[239] Subsequent series showed similarly impressive long-term survival data.[228,240-243] Bloom and colleagues[89] updated Kramer's initial findings, reporting a 10-year survival rate of 85% among the children and a 10-year relapse-free survival rate of 80%.[89] Disease control is even better in young adults (92% at 20 years for patients age 16 to 39 years at the time of diagnosis).[243] These latter figures are equal to the best results observed in primary surgical series when corrected to account for cases with incomplete resection.[224,232]

Radiation Therapy Technique

Radiation therapy for craniopharyngioma is designed to narrowly encompass the solid and cystic components of a well-delineated, central neoplasm. Much of the published information involves treatment using coronal arcs of 180 to 220 degrees; three-dimensional conformal or fractionated stereotactic radiation therapy is currently being used to improve dose conformity.[228,240-243]

Craniopharyngiomas show a dose-response relationship. Bloom and colleagues[89,171] noted a superior outcome in response to 50 to 55 Gy compared with the response to less than 50 Gy. Doses of 54 to 55 Gy at 1.8 Gy per fraction are recommended for children. It is not clear that higher doses are necessary or desirable for adults. Doses in excess of 60 Gy are associated with significantly greater toxicity, especially in the visual system, with little improvement in survival.[89,171,244]

Single-fraction radiosurgery has been used, but more broadly in Europe than in the United States.[244,245] Radiosurgery may be appropriate for children with small foci of residual disease, particularly disease that is limited to intrasellar deposits or foci of disease remote from the hypothalamus and chiasm.[244,246]

Prognosis

Excellent long-term survival rates have been noted for patients who undergo total resection or planned limited surgery and irradiation. The proportion of patients in recent series who underwent successful resection approximates 75%.[222-230,232,247] However, even the most vociferous advocates of surgery acknowledge the existence of residual calcifications or apparently viable, radiographically obvious tumor in up to 50% of postoperative CT studies of patients who have undergone gross total resection.[223-225] The rate of disease recurrence after complete resection ranges from 10% to 30%.[222-224,230-232,248] Despite the benign nature of craniopharyngioma, tumor progresses in 70% to 90% of patients after incomplete resection, in the absence of irradiation, at a median of 2 to 3 years.[243,248,249]

Primary irradiation after cyst decompression or partial resection has been associated with progression-free survival rates of 80% to 95% at 5 to 20 years.* Survival rates of 90% to 100% are common among children and adults.

The relative toxicity of primary surgery and irradiation for craniopharyngioma are becoming increasingly apparent. Diabetes insipidus occurs in 75% to 100% of patients after complete surgical resection.[222,230,235,236] Endocrine dysfunction involving other pituitary-hypothalamic hormones has been noted in 40% to 80% of patients after surgery.[235,236] Hypothalamic obesity is apparent in more than 50% of long-term survivors; it is less common among those who undergo limited surgery and irradiation.[235,236] Undesirable personality changes are associated with resections that damage the hypothalamus.

An increased endocrine deficit has been noted among patients whose primary treatment was surgery compared with those who underwent limited resection and irradiation.[235] Up to 25% of children show significant decreases in vision after resection[230,232]; reports of visual complications from radiation therapy have been anecdotal.[244] Overall performance, intellectual function, and memory seem to be equal or better in the population treated by conservative surgery and irradiation than in those treated surgically.[226,234,242,244]

Primitive Neuroectodermal Tumors

In 1973, Hart and Earle[251] described the cerebral PNET as a malignant embryonal tumor that affects children and young adults. The tumor accounts for approximately 3% of supratentorial neoplasms. PNETs are large, often cystic hemispheric tumors characterized histologically by a highly cellular, undifferentiated infiltrate that includes vascular endothelial hyperplasia and necrosis.[69,251,252] In classic descriptions, focal areas of glial or neuronal differentiation constitute less than 5% to 10% of the tumor. The clinically similar cerebral neuroblastoma is distinguished from the Hart/Earle PNET by its degree of neuronal differentiation.[253-255] The specific cerebral PNET encountered in a patient, however, must be distinguished from the broad concept of PNETs advanced by Rorke and colleagues, as discussed earlier in this chapter.[69,70,152,256]

Cerebral PNETs infiltrate widely despite their circumscribed gross appearance. The tumor can also arise multifocally. About one third of cases involve ventricular or spinal subarachnoid dissemination.[250] The more differentiated cerebral neuroblastoma has been observed to be associated with CSF metastasis in an equal proportion of patients at autopsy, although isolated involvement of the subarachnoid space is uncommon.[250,253,255,257]

Recent studies conducted by the CCG have documented the efficacy of combining chemotherapy (the tested regimen included lomustine, prednisone, and vincristine) with CSI for children with cerebral PNETs who are more than 3 or 4 years old.[221,252,256,258-260] Long-term survival approached 60% in this group. For infants and young children, therapeutic approaches are comparable with those used for other embryonal CNS lesions in this age group (see the following section on "Tumors in Children Less than 3 Years Old"). Despite anecdotal reports of disease control after cranial irradiation, CSI is considered standard therapy for supratentorial PNETs, including cerebral neuroblastoma and pineoblastoma.[221,257] The doses and techniques used for supratentorial PNETs are similar to those described for medulloblastoma, with typically a 2-cm margin planned around the tumor bed to define the clinical target volume.

TUMORS IN CHILDREN LESS THAN 3 YEARS OLD

Of pediatric brain tumors, 15% to 20% occur in infants and children younger than 3 years. The most common tumors in this age group are astrocytomas (primarily optic chiasmatic or hypothalamic tumors; cerebellar astrocytomas are uncommon), embryonal tumors (medulloblastoma, PNET, and pineoblastoma), ependymoma,

---

*References 89, 171, 227, 240-244, 247, 248, 250.

and malignant gliomas.[261-263] Tumors occurring almost uniquely in this age group include atypical teratoid/rhabdoid tumors and choroid plexus neoplasms (papillomas and carcinomas).[264-268] Desmoplastic infantile astrocytoma and ganglioglioma are uncommon, and when they do occur, they are typically large tumors that are biologically benign.[269] The operative mortality is relatively high in this age group because of tumor presentations (often sizable, midline or multilobe supratentorial lesions) and the relative lack of elasticity of the still-myelinating brain.

The infant brain is particularly vulnerable to the effects of radiation therapy, particularly with regard to neurocognitive development.[270] Survival rates for patients in this age group with either ependymoma or medulloblastoma are significantly lower than those in other age groups because the tumor in these very young patients is often advanced at presentation and because tumoricidal radiation doses cannot be used.[89,167,171,260,271-273]

The use of prolonged chemotherapy after surgery to delay or obviate the use of radiation therapy for very young children has been studied for nearly 20 years[168,274-280] (Fig. 32-12). Trials of medulloblastoma in infants conducted by the POG, CCG, and International Society of Paediatric Oncology (SIOP) have documented that chemotherapy is effective in only a minority of patients; durable disease control has been achieved in 20% to 30% of patients with chemotherapy alone and in only 35% of those treated with response-defined consolidative irradiation.[168,277-281] Salvage irradiation has achieved a surprising degree of secondary control after progression during chemotherapy, but the dose required to overcome chemotherapy resistance produces late changes in intelligence quotient that make this an ethically unacceptable alternative.[280,282] For infants with ependymoma, earlier intervention with irradiation after prolonged chemotherapy may help

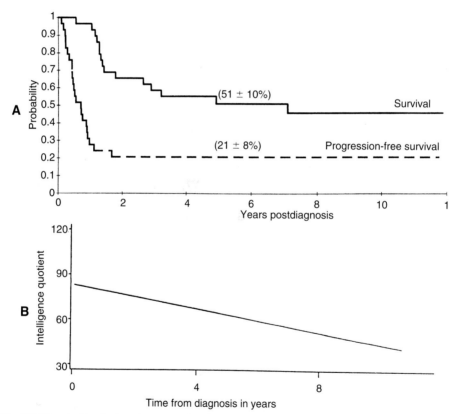

Fig. 32-12 A, Survival and progression-free survival for 29 infants and children aged less than 4 years with medulloblastoma. During the study period (1984-1995), prolonged chemotherapy was used in the hopes of delaying or obviating the substantial neurotoxicity associated with irradiation in such young children. The stable progression-free survival rate after 18 months (21%) reflects the use of irradiation as adjuvant therapy (for those with resected or stable disease during 12 to 24 months of chemotherapy); the 51% overall survival rate at 5 years reflects a high salvage rate from the use of craniospinal irradiation for persistent or progressive disease. **B,** Among the 19 patients who survived for more than 24 months, the high survival rate came at the cost of a steady decline in full-scale intelligence quotient scores, from a pretreatment level approximating 90 to a level just above 60 at 7 years. (From Walter AW, Mulhern RK, Gajjar A, et al. *J Clin Oncol* 1999;17:3720-3728.)

control disease; however, this strategy too seems to work in only a minority of cases.[184] Chemotherapy alone has been an unsuccessful postoperative intervention.[283] Reports of survival among patients with pineoblastoma and atypical teratoid or rhabdoid tumors treated with this approach have been anecdotal.[168,184,221,284]

The current generation of infant brain tumor trials focuses on the judicious use of irradiation. Based on preliminary data in children with recurrent medulloblastoma, the frontline approach in both the Pediatric Brain Tumor Consortium and COG trials is to introduce early, limited-volume three-dimensional conformal radiation therapy to the posterior fossa and primary tumor site alone for patients with M0 medulloblastoma and to the local tumor bed only for those with supratentorial PNETs.[281] For patients with atypical teratoid or rhabdoid tumors, targeted radiation volumes are used after just 2 months of chemotherapy for children 12 months of age and older.[284] For those with ependymomas, the trend is toward immediate postoperative irradiation, at least for patients with tumors that can be grossly resected.[150]

TUMORS COMMON IN ADULTS
Malignant Glioma (Anaplastic Astrocytoma, Glioblastoma Multiforme)

The dominant primary intracranial tumors that occur in adults in terms of both frequency and mortality are the malignant gliomas. These tumors occur in the cerebral hemispheres as sizable, rapidly growing lesions with a characteristic ringlike, enhancing appearance on CT or MRI, with central necrosis, infiltrating margins, and surrounding low-density changes (Fig. 32-13). Malignant gliomas occur in all age groups, but predominate in the fifth and sixth decades, and they account for 35% to 45% of all adult brain tumors.

Histologically, malignant gliomas are heterogeneous neoplasms composed of fibrillary astrocytes; gemistocytes; large, bizarre glial cells; and small anaplastic cells.[69,106] In Kernohan and Sayre's classic categorization[285] of astrocytic neoplasms, which defined these tumors as grade III and grade IV astrocytomas, malignant gliomas were believed to represent progressively dedifferentiated astrocytic tumors marked by a certain degree of pleomorphism, hyperchromaticism, and mitosis. In contemporary neuropathology, malignant gliomas in general are classified as anaplastic astrocytoma or the more malignant glioblastoma multiforme, with the latter identified by the presence of tumor necrosis.[286] Anaplastic astrocytomas account for 10% to 15% of malignant gliomas; more than 85% are glioblastomas.[287]

Malignant gliomas typically infiltrate the adjacent normal brain. Detailed comparisons of imaging and histologic findings have established the anatomy of malignant gliomas. Histologically, the central low-density region seen on neuroimaging studies is a

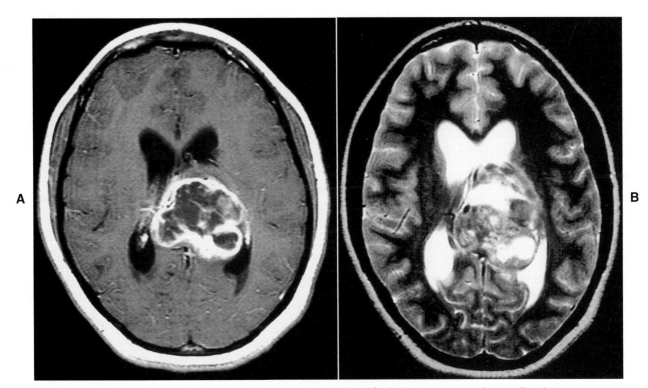

Fig. 32-13 Glioblastoma multiforme arising in the left thalamic region and extending just beyond midline. **A,** Gadolinium-enhanced T1 image shows a ring-enhancing periphery with a dark, necrotic center. **B,** T2-weighted image shows surrounding edematous changes.

necrotic and hypocellular area. The surrounding ring of enhancing tissue is composed of densely cellular tumor. The hypodense area beyond the enhancing tissue seen on CT scans is hypocellular and edematous but infiltrated by small anaplastic T cells.[288] In 50% of cases, scattered tumor cells immediately surrounding the hypodense volume are evident histologically.[289] The often sizable area of increased signal on T2 MR images similarly contains infiltrates of viable T cells.[290] Tumor cells characteristically extend along neural tracts and across the corpus callosum.[289] Distant subarachnoid or subependymal extension occurs in 5% to 9% of patients with malignant gliomas.[291,292]

Surgery for malignant gliomas is usually limited to subtotal resection. Macroscopically, complete removal is achieved in only 10% to 20% of cases.[293-296] The extent of residual tumor visualized on postresection CT scans seems to correlate with outcome, with increased time to progression and survival being associated with smaller residual tumor volumes among both adults and children.[285,297]

Radiation therapy has been the most effective treatment for these aggressive lesions, but generally, it can only delay disease progression or recurrence. Early clinical trials conducted by the Brain Tumor Study Group confirmed the clinical efficacy of irradiation. Median survival increased from 14 weeks after surgery to 36 weeks in patients given postoperative irradiation.[294] The survival rate at 1 year was 24% in patients also treated with radiation therapy, compared with only 3% in patients who had surgery only.[294] One fourth to one half of patients who receive radiation therapy show clinical improvement. Indeed, up to 60% of patients are able to return to work and achieve full function.[298-300]

Despite documented improvement in time to progression and survival, the response to irradiation illustrated on imaging studies is complex and rarely indicative of rapid or significant disease reduction. Essentially all glioblastomas and 65% to 80% of anaplastic astrocytomas recur within 2 to 5 years and result in rapid death, causing malignant gliomas to live up to their reputation of being one of the most aggressive and lethal tumors.[298] Although the anatomy of malignant gliomas suggests that disease extension or metastasis is the source of recurrence, recurrence actually almost always arises from within the central or enhancing portion of the tumor.[301-305] The central tumor is relatively radioresistant, perhaps because of an inherent lack of radiosensitivity or a hypoxic, relatively radioinsensitive necrotic core.[304-305] This pattern of intralesional recurrence has stimulated several lines of clinical investigation to overcome hypoxic cell resistance; considerable interest has also been expressed in exploiting the time-dose relationship to identify an altered fractionation regimen of value in this tumor

system.[287,300] Several trials have also tested modifications in radiation delivery, including physical modalities other than photons and local boost techniques incorporating interstitial brachytherapy or stereotactic radiosurgery.[306-317]

Early trials of radiosensitizers focused on the nitroimidazoles misonidazole and etanidazole.[318] More recent studies have investigated carbogen and nictinamide. Despite some improvement noted from use of these agents with suboptimal irradiation, clinically meaningful benefit was not achieved.[319,320] Longstanding interest in the halogenated pyrimidines (bromodeoxyuridine and iododeoxyuridine) has resulted in several trials of their use with conventional and altered fractionation, but only a marginal benefit has been suggested.[321-324]

The use of irradiation with high–linear-energy-transfer particles has also been examined in clinical trials as a possible way of overcoming the apparent oxygen-related radioresistance of these tumors. However, the use of fast–neutron-beam irradiation generally has produced no significant improvement over conventional photon irradiation.[306,310,325] The rationale for using proton irradiation stems more from the ability to restrict the volume of tissue irradiated than from its being less affected by oxygenation; trials of doses as high as 90 Gy suggest a potential benefit in terms of central tumor control, but no early demonstration of improvement in outcome has been seen.[326]

Stereotactic interstitial implantation of radioactive sources has been done at several European centers since the 1950s. Over the past two decades, prospective studies of temporary stereotactic brain implants using high-activity ^{125}I have evaluated the toxicity and efficacy of volume-limited, high-dose radiation delivery.[307-309] Among selected patients with limited-volume, recurrent malignant gliomas, geometrically planned implantations of radiation sources delivering an average of 60 Gy to the enhancing lesion over 6 days resulted in survival durations of approximately 1 year (for patients with glioblastoma) and 1.5 years (for patients with anaplastic astrocytoma).[307-309,314,327] Results of the Brain Tumor Cooperative Group's prospective, randomized trial suggested that interstitial boost irradiation could be beneficial in appropriately selected cases.[328]

Patients with malignant gliomas who are potentially suitable for local types of therapy (e.g., brachytherapy or radiosurgery) are those with a relatively favorable prognosis, constituting 20% to 40% of cases. The criteria for implantation generally include Karnofsky performance scores above 70, unifocal supratentorial lesions less than 6 cm in the greatest diameter, and no involvement of the midline, corpus callosum, or subependyma.[307,309] A retrospective review of unselected patients treated with standard external brain irradiation revealed that outcome was significantly better among implant-eligible patients with glioblastoma (median survival of 14 months) than among those who were ineligible (median survival of less than 6 months),[329] indicating that any perceived improvement in outcome in patients attributed to the brachytherapy may be artificial. However, both median survival duration and 2- and 3-year survival rates for patients with glioblastoma treated with ^{125}I brachytherapy seem to be superior in single-institution experiences and in comparison with the previously noted findings.[307,309,329] Comparable data for anaplastic astrocytomas are less convincing.[309,329]

Symptomatic local necrosis occurs in 40% to 50% of patients with interstitial implants, and this often requires surgical intervention.[308,309,314,315,320] Interestingly, ultimate survival has been reported to be superior in patients who require a second operation, which presumably reflects the combination-treatment effect.[308]

Stereotactic radiosurgery has been used more recently to achieve a high-dose boost. Patient eligibility criteria are similarly selective, typically including single lesions less than 4 to 5 cm in diameter without subependymal extension and more than 5 mm away from the optic chiasm or brainstem. In the initial U.S. series, which included a high proportion of patients who had undergone limited surgical resection, the median survival was at least equal to that among patients with implants—26 months in those with glioblastoma and more than 36 months in those with anaplastic astrocytoma.[330,331] In a multi-institutional trial of 189 patients, the median survival time was 86 weeks for those with glioblastoma who met all criteria for gamma-knife intervention, compared with 40 weeks for those with more extensive tumors or a less favorable performance score.[311,316,329] The incidence of symptomatic necrosis may be less than that noted in patients with interstitial implants.[260]

Several trials in the United States, Europe, and Japan have assessed modifications in the time-dose relationship.[287,300,326,332-335] Despite an early suggestion that hyperfractionated delivery to higher doses may be beneficial, subsequent studies conducted by the RTOG have shown no substantial benefit from such therapy. A large, randomized dose-escalating trial conducted by the RTOG tested hyperfractionated doses of 64.8 to 81.6 Gy, given in 1.2-Gy fractions twice daily with an interfraction interval of 4 to 8 hours. The results indicated that the ideal dose response occurrred at 72 Gy, although the superiority of this schedule over 60 Gy delivered in conventionally fractionated radiation therapy was inapparent.[332] Indeed, patients who received doses of 75 to 81.6 Gy actually fared less well.[332] Thus without documentation of any reduction in neurotoxicity from hyperfractionated delivery, objective data are few to indicate that the therapeutic ratio and effect of hyperfractionation are greater than those for conventional fractionation.[332,336,337]

Alternative time-dose regimens have included accelerated hyperfractionation (1.5- or 1.6-Gy fractions given twice a day) and accelerated fractionation (1.9- or 2.0-Gy fractions given three times a day), and hypofractionation (fractions of 2.5 to 6 Gy).[320,322,323,334,335] Although the hypofractionation regimens may expedite palliation in patients with advanced or unfavorable conditions, no overall benefit from such regimens has been observed to date.

Chemotherapy has been investigated extensively for the treatment of glioblastomas. As sole adjuvants to surgery, nitrosoureas have been ineffective.[294] When combined with irradiation, nitrosoureas or combinations of agents (e.g., carmustine-hydroxyurea plus procarbazine-teniposide, carmustine-hydroxyurea, vincristine-procarbazine) have been associated with only marginally improved survival times in patients enrolled in prospective studies.[294,299,338] The best results from chemotherapy are noted for penciclovir.[339] However, a recent randomized trial conducted by the Medical Research Council in the United Kingdom of more than 670 patients showed no survival benefit for the patients given penciclovir in addition to standard radiation therapy.[340] A variety of new biological agents are available for the treatment of malignant gliomas, including compounds with specific biological targets (e.g., epidermal growth factor, platelet-derived growth factor) and new antiangiogenesis agents.[341] Studies of local chemotherapy, specifically carmustine-impregnated wafers (Gliadel), have yielded inconclusive results in patients with malignant gliomas, producing an apparent response but having an uncertain value as an adjuvant therapy.[342]

Radiation Therapy Technique

Radiation therapy remains the most effective single agent in prolonging survival in patients with malignant gliomas. It should consist of standard external-beam irradiation with wide local coverage of the neoplasm.[298,302] Anatomic studies of tumor extent, imaging analyses of patterns of recurrence, and clinical trials have shown that the appropriate initial target volume should extend 2 to 3 cm beyond the low-density periphery shown on CT scans or 2 cm beyond the abnormal signal shown on T2-weighted MRI studies.[289,290,302,303,338] Margins of less than 2 cm are theoretically inadequate because of the histologic nature of the tumor[289] and the way in which the initial sites of disease progress.[303]

The use of more limited, high-dose treatment volumes delivered by three-dimensional conformal or proton irradiation may be associated with a relative increase in the peripheral failure rate.[326,343] Central or intralesional disease progression is less common in patients with interstitial implants. Studies of patterns of failure in series of patients treated with brachytherapy have shown that disease recurs primarily in the tumor margin, often within 2 cm of the high-dose implant; the incidence of distant intracranial recurrence is also relatively high.[304,305]

Dose-response data were established early in clinical trials involving patients with malignant gliomas. Specifically, Walker and colleagues[294] showed that median survival improved from 28 weeks for patients given 50 Gy in 25 to 28 fractions to 42 weeks for patients given 60 Gy in the first Brain Tumor Study Group studies (Fig. 32-14).[294] More recently, three-dimensional conformal and proton-based regimens have made it possible to escalate doses to 70 to 90 Gy; however, although central tumor control may be improved, no increase in survival has been yet been found.[326,343] As summarized above, none of the altered fractionation regimens has been shown to improve outcome over that achieved with conventionally fractionated irradiation to 60 to 65 Gy (in 1.8- to 2-Gy fractions given once daily).[333] No data exist to suggest that these recommendations for radiation therapy for adults be adjusted for children; however, the requirement for high-dose irradiation to reasonably large volumes limits the use of this modality in young children with malignant gliomas.

Prognosis

Reports of survival beyond 2 years for adults with glioblastoma remain anecdotal.[344] However, approximately 15% to 25% of patients with anaplastic astrocytoma survive 5 years, with gradually decreasing survival beyond that time noted in most series. Levin and colleagues[339] reported that adjuvant penciclovir chemotherapy is associated with a 35% survival rate at 3 to 5 years in patients with anaplastic lesions; however, similar results seen in other small series have not been substantiated in the recent Medical Research Council trial.[302,340,345] Other factors influencing prognosis include age (survival is progressively better among younger patients, with the best among 18- to 39-year-olds, the next-best among 40- to 59-year-olds, and the worst among those age 60 years or older) and initial

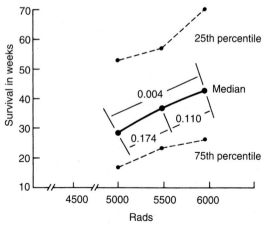

Fig. 32-14 Dose-response analysis for survival in adults with malignant gliomas. (From Walker MD, Green SB, Byar DP, et al. *N Engl J Med* 1980;303:1323-1329.)

performance status.[293,313] Among children with malignant gliomas, the overall progression-free survival rates at 3 to 5 years range from 15% to 20%; in the small subset with completely resected lesions, corresponding survival rates of up to 75% have been reported.[297,346,347]

Oligodendroglioma

Oligodendroglioma is a relatively uncommon tumor that occurs in all age groups. The tumor arises most often in the frontal lobes and occasionally involves the infratentorial or spinal regions. The most common symptom is seizures. The relatively nonaggressive nature of this tumor is indicated by the median survival duration, which is more than 5 years from the onset of symptoms and diagnosis.[348]

Primary surgical resection is the initial therapy for low-grade oligodendrogliomas.[349,350] The role of postoperative irradiation has been poorly defined. In a small retrospective study, Sheline and colleagues[351] noted an improvement in 5-year survival for patients who underwent irradiation as opposed to those who did not (85% vs. 55%, respectively). The survival rate at 10 years was not statistically improved, however. Chin and colleagues[352] noted a progression-free survival rate of 100% at 5 years in 24 patients completing postoperative irradiation. Lindegaard and colleagues[353] noted a benefit from irradiation only among those who had undergone incomplete surgical resection. In a study of a similar group of patients treated in roughly the same period, Reedy and colleagues[354] found no survival advantage from radiation therapy.

In the absence of a prospective trial assessing the efficacy of radiation therapy, it seems justified and prudent to use postoperative irradiation for subtotally resected lesions. Local fields to doses of 50 to 54 Gy approximate the treatment recommended for other low-grade tumors.[98,355]

Although 5-year survival rates in excess of 65% to 90% have been observed in major clinical series, the ultimate survival rate beyond 15 or 20 years was only 30% in two large reviews from an earlier era that examined the pathologic behavior of tumors from more than 500 patients.[348,356] Clearly, late tumor progression and death take place more than 5 to 10 years after diagnosis. Histologic grading is of increasing importance now that a role for penciclovir chemotherapy in the treatment of anaplastic oligodendrogliomas has been established.[357] Long-term survival is higher in patients younger than 40 or 50 years.[356]

Meningioma

Meningiomas are common CNS tumors, most often occurring as intracranial tumors along the convexities or in parasagittal regions. The usually benign meningioma constitutes 15% of adult CNS tumors, with a 2.5:1 female-to-male ratio. The natural history of this tumor was elegantly described in Cushing and Eisenhardt's 1938 monograph,[358] in which they identified the broad dural attachment, or local infiltration, growth along or into the venous sinuses, and osseous invasion or overlying reactive bone formation that typify these lesions. Angioblastic meningiomas seem to be associated with a less favorable outcome than the other so-called benign tumors.[359] Less than 10% of meningiomas are malignant, and these lesions seem to be associated with an unfavorable outcome.[359-361]

Surgery is the primary treatment for most peripherally located intracranial meningiomas. Local tumor recurrence after complete resection occurs in 10% to 20% of cases, related in part to the extent of dural and sinus excision.[359-362]

Symptomatic tumor recurrence or progression occurs in approximately 50% of patients with subtotally excised lesions, most often in patients with meningiomas of the sphenoid ridge and parasellar areas, which represent nearly 30% of all meningiomas (Fig. 32-15).[359,362-364] The efficacy of radiation therapy for incompletely resected meningiomas has been well documented. In particular, Wara and colleagues[365] observed local tumor recurrence in 74% of patients after incomplete resection compared with 29% of patients given postoperative irradiation. Progression-free survival beyond 5 years averages 70% to 90% for patients undergoing incomplete resection and irradiation; disease control rates in excess of 70% to 80% at 8 to 10 years are associated with survival rates exceeding 90%.[366-368] Similar outcomes have been observed among patients who receive radiosurgery either alone or as an adjunct to incomplete surgery.[369-372] Neurologic improvement has been noted in 44% of patients after irradiation for unresected primary lesions.[359] Serial CT studies have confirmed the regression of neoplasms in response to radiation therapy (see Fig. 32-15).[364] In sites such as the optic nerve sheath, operative intervention may be associated with a significant functional deficit. Primary irradiation can improve tumor-related defects in visual acuity and visual fields in these patients.[373]

Radiation Therapy Technique

Because meningiomas are locally infiltrating tumors that produce local tissue changes by means of direct tumor extension or have subclinical, limited multicentricity,[374] local irradiation should include a reasonable margin despite the circumscribed appearance of these tumors on CT scans. Large tumors of the sphenoid ridge

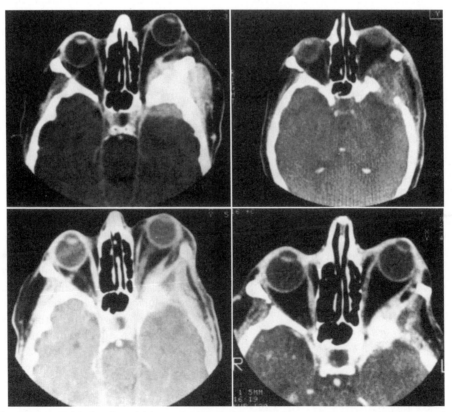

Fig. 32-15 Orbital sphenoidal meningioma. Computed tomography scan demonstrating residual disease after surgery *(top row)* and 2 years after irradiation *(bottom row)*. (From Petty AM, Kun LE, Meyer GA. *J Neurosurg* 1985;62:502-507.)

may extend beyond the cranial vault into the orbit or the facial or cervical regions. Optimal radiologic assessment of tumor extent and the use of wide inferior treatment margins are important in such cases.[364]

Carelia and colleagues[366] were unable to identify a dose-response relationship for meningiomas between 50 and 75 Gy. However, excellent local tumor control has been achieved at doses approaching CNS tolerance, with the recommended treatment being a total dose of 54 to 55 Gy given in 25 to 30 fractions.[359,364,367] The use of radiosurgery as the primary treatment for selected lesions has produced equally positive results; at many centers, radiosurgery is the treatment of first choice for limited-volume lesions that either are difficult to approach surgically or are residual or recurrent after initial resection.[369,371,372,375,376]

Prognosis

The benign nature of meningiomas is confirmed by the limited number of recurrences seen in patients after total surgical resection. After incomplete resection, however, the median time to clinically apparent tumor progression is 4 years after surgery. The median intervals to tumor progression in patients given radiation therapy exceed 5 to 10 years.[364,366,367]

Initial postoperative irradiation for incompletely resected or biopsied meningiomas has achieved excellent local tumor control, as noted in the preceding paragraphs. Indications for initial or delayed radiation therapy remain controversial, although increasing information suggests that incompletely resected lesions along the cavernous sinus and those with malignant histologic features may warrant immediate postoperative irradiation.[360,368,372,375] No apparent decrease in tumor control has been observed in most series of patients who undergo repeat surgery and radiation therapy for disease that recurs after initial incomplete resection.[359,363,367] A more rapid rate of tumor regrowth after subtotal excision has been indicated in children, raising some concern about the advisability of delaying radiotherapeutic intervention in this age group.[377,378]

Identifying the histologic subtype of meningioma[69,361] is important because the local recurrence rate is higher for malignant (anaplastic) meningiomas and because postoperative radiation therapy can effectively control these tumors. For example, Dziuk and colleagues[360] and others[361,363] have reported 15% to 80% differences in 5-year progression-free survival rates related to irradiation. A long-term disease control rate of only 25% at 5 years has been observed for patients who receive single-fraction radiosurgery, largely for recurrent malignant meningiomas.[376]

Primary Malignant Lymphoma of the CNS

Primary malignant lymphoma of the CNS was previously a rare neoplasm, occurring spontaneously in conjunction with immunosuppression. However, the frequency with which it occurs has increased greatly in conjunction with the AIDS epidemic.[379-381] The tumor occurs primarily in the supratentorial region, most often as an isodense, diffusely enhancing lesion involving the basal ganglia or thalamus, the periventricular white matter, or the corpus callosum.[382] Up to 15% to 40% of tumors are multifocal intracranial lesions.[383,384] The CSF contains tumor cells in 10% to 20% of cases; involvement of the ocular vitreous at diagnosis or metachronously is noted in 10% to 25% of cases.[383,385]

The lesion is usually classified as an immunoblastic or lymphoblastic diffuse, large cell, malignant lymphoma, most often of B cell immunophenotype. Systematic evaluation is necessary to differentiate primary lymphoma of the brain from secondary CNS manifestations of malignant lymphoma, although intraparenchymal deposits occur more often with primary tumors than with secondary tumors.

Surgery is limited, often to biopsy alone, but radiation therapy produces a high rate of objective response. Neurologic improvement can be achieved in up to 70% of patients, but median survival has been only 7 to 8 months.[386] Long-term survival after irradiation alone has been limited.[381,383,384,387,388] Chemotherapy has shown increasing efficacy in patients with CNS malignant lymphoma, with rates of objective response often exceeding 50% to 70% in those treated either with regimens including high-dose methotrexate or less often with conventional systemic chemotherapy regimens (e.g., cyclophosphamide, doxorubicin, vincristine, and prednisone).[389-393] The combination of preirradiation chemotherapy and cranial irradiation resulted in median survival times as long as 60 months and 4-year progression-free and overall survival rates of approximately 50% in a moderate-size series from Memorial Sloan-Kettering Cancer Center.[391,394] One drawback to the use of combined methotrexate-irradiation regimens has been their considerable neurotoxicity, which sometimes produces frank dementia, particularly in patients older than 60 years.[390,391]

Radiation Therapy Technique

Given the size, and often the multiplicity, of most primary CNS lymphomas, the minimal target volume is often full cranial irradiation.[384-387] Isolated subarachnoid spinal recurrence after cranial irradiation occurs in 4% to 25% of patients.[98,387] The inability to control the primary tumor within the cranium in a high proportion of patients and the need to coordinate irradiation with chemotherapy have led clinicians away from considerating CSI. This raises a valid argument for avoiding spinal irradiation in deference to the potential benefits conferred by chemotherapy.

A radiation dose-response relationship has been suggested in primary malignant lymphoma of the CNS.

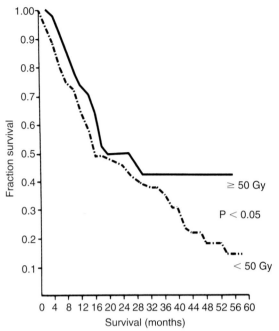

Fig. 32-16 Dose-response analysis for survival among patients with primary cerebral malignant lymphoma after irradiation. (From Murray K, Kun L, Cox J. *J Neurosurg* 1986;65:600-607.)

Murray and colleagues[384] reviewed 198 cases reported in the literature and found a statistically significant improvement in 5-year survival rate for patients given doses of more than 50 Gy (42% vs. 13%) (Fig. 32-16).[384] Recurrence of tumor at the primary site even in patients treated with doses of 50 to 55 Gy led to a major RTOG trial, the results of which failed to demonstrate a significant added benefit from high-dose cranial irradiation.[386] In small series of patients, however, the addition of radiation therapy seems to have prolonged disease control and improved survival relative to the outcome for patients given only chemotherapy.[381,391,394]

Prognosis

Overall survival in patients with primary malignant lymphoma seems to have increased among those treated with combined, sequential chemoradiotherapy; in particular, median survival times have increased severalfold to approximately 4 to 5 years. However, most patients do die of the disease, sometimes as long as 5 years after diagnosis.[391,394]

Carcinoma Metastatic to the Brain

Intracranial metastasis, primarily in the cerebrum, occurs in 10% to 15% of patients with cancer.[395] Of the types of cancer that metastasize preferentially to the brain, cancer of the lung and breast predominate, and gastrointestinal and renal carcinomas are less common. Brain metastasis often occurs at multiple sites; in a classic autopsy series, solitary metastases were found in approximately 40% of cases, two to three lesions in 25% of cases, and four or more foci in 35%.[396]

Treatment of brain metastases is palliative; long-term survival can be achieved in up to 20% of patients with favorable presenting characteristics such as age less than 60 to 65 years, favorable performance status (typically a Karnofsky performance score of at least 70), control of the primary tumor, and absent or controlled extracranial metastasis.[397-399] Corticosteroids alone can transiently reduce symptoms in 60% of patients.[335] However, cranial irradiation achieves more prolonged palliation, with objective improvement in neurologic function in 50% to 70% of patients so treated.[307]

Earlier time-dose studies showed the relative equivalence of the following treatment regimens: 30 to 36 Gy given in 10 to 12 fractions; 20 Gy given in 5 fractions; and 40 Gy given in 15 fractions.[307] The current standard therapy is 30 Gy given in 10 fractions; however, recent randomized trials to assess the benefit of surgery or radiosurgery in selected settings favor 37.5 Gy given in 15 fractions.[400,401]

For patients with a solitary metastasis, the addition of surgical resection or radiosurgery has been associated with significant improvements in survival time (from a median of 15 weeks to a median of 40 weeks in a randomized trial reported by Patchell and colleagues[402]) and in the rate of local control at metastatic sites (from less than 50% for patients treated with cranial irradiation alone to 80% for patients undergoing resection). This increase in survival has been associated with improved functional outcome as well.[402] In several series, the outcome from radiosurgery has been similar to that from operative removal; in all such series, it is the patients with favorable factors (age, performance status, absence of other disease sites) that benefit the most from the addition of local therapy.[371,400,401,403,404] Surgery and radiosurgery seem to achieve equivalent results in most, but not all, such reports.[401,403] Detailed analyses have also shown that the addition of full cranial irradiation improves survival and local tumor control and may be associated with long-term survival in a small but meaningful number of patients undergoing aggressive local therapy.[405] Results for patients with malignant melanoma that has metastasized to the brain have in general paralleled those seen for patients with other carcinomas; however, local therapy may be particularly advantageous for those patients with few metastatic sites and favorable performance status.[403,406]

The treatment selected for patients with brain metastasis depends on the absence or presence of those clinical features consistently associated with improved outcome (i.e., younger than 60 to 65 years, Karnofsky performance score ≥ 70, and the lack of apparent or symptomatic disease at the primary site or other extracranial locations). However, there does seem to be a definite advantage to surgery or radiosurgery for patients with only one metastatic focus; a similar advantage seems to exist for those with only two or three metastatic foci.* In all such patients, and in those with more advanced cranial or extraneural disease, the addition of full cranial irradiation is an important and worthwhile palliative intervention.[397,400,405]

SPINAL CORD TUMORS

Primary tumors of the spinal cord represent 10% to 15% of CNS neoplasms. Extramedullary tumors, including schwannomas and meningiomas, account for nearly half of the lesions in the spinal canal. Primary intramedullary neoplasms are most often gliomas and vascular tumors.

Intramedullary gliomas include ependymomas (60%) and astrocytomas (30%). Ependymomas occur more often in the lumbar region, affecting the conus and cauda equina. Spinal ependymomas are generally low-grade neoplasms; those occurring in the cauda equina are usually well differentiated myxopapillary tumors.[408] The ependymomas tend to develop as discrete lesions, facilitating subtotal or gross total resection.

Gross total resection has led to systemic disease control in recent series with a 5-year follow-up. Aggressive surgery, however, is associated with postoperative neurologic deterioration in 15% of patients.[409] Response to irradiation is well documented, with 75% of patients showing improvement in neurologic status and progression-free survival rates of 70% to 100% at 10 years.[410-412] A local tumor control rate of 80% with no identifiable long-term neurologic toxicity despite doses in excess of 45 Gy indicates that irradiation has a role in the treatment of patients whose spinal tumors are incompletely resected.[412] Patients with tumors of the cauda equina region and conus experience particularly high survival rates after either irradiation or surgical resection.[413,414]

Spinal astrocytomas are more evenly distributed along the length of the spinal cord. These lesions often contain cystic components and most often are low-grade fibrillary tumors. Astrocytomas are more infiltrating than ependymomas, thus limiting surgery to cyst decompression and partial resection.[413] Epstein and colleagues,[415-418] however, described operative techniques that can be used to completely resect many low-grade astrocytomas in children and adults. Aggressive operative intervention is not advantageous for high-grade spinal astrocytomas, however.[410,419,420] In addition, long-term control in patients with spinal astrocytomas treated with irradiation is less predictable than that in patients with ependymomas despite frequent neurologic improvement.[410,412] The disease-free survival rate

at 5 to 10 years ranges from 25% to 60% among patients with spinal astrocytomas.[410,419,420] However, the histologic grade affects outcome, in that patients with low-grade astrocytomas enjoy a short-term (5-year) survival rate of as high as 89% compared with 0% among patients with higher-grade tumors (glioblastoma).[419]

Spinal cord tolerance is an important consideration when reviewing results of patients with intramedullary tumors treated with irradiation.[421] Doses of approximately 50 Gy are recommended for most spinal cord tumors; however, higher doses and the suggestion of a dose-response effect at or above 50 Gy have been reported for localized spinal cord lesions.[422,423]

Extradural metastasis is the most common oncologic diagnosis in patients with spinal cord disease. An estimated 5% of patients who die of cancer have clinical signs of epidural metastases.[424] Extradural involvement usually results from the contiguous extension of a vertebral metastasis, most often in patients with primary cancer of the breast, lung, or prostate. Less common are vertebral metastases from malignant lymphomas and myeloma or carcinomas of the kidney and gastrointestinal tract.

Early evaluation with spinal MRI has been advocated for patients with pain and radiographic evidence of vertebral metastasis without objective neurologic signs.[424,425] The treatment of epidural metastases is controversial, largely with respect to the performance of surgery before irradiation. Conventional procedures have included decompressive laminectomy, at least for patients with rapidly evolving signs or complete block shown by myelography; patients in whom the diagnosis is uncertain or the diagnosis of malignancy is not established require surgical intervention.[327]

Retrospective and prospective studies comparing laminectomy and postoperative irradiation with irradiation alone confirm an apparent advantage to surgical intervention only for patients with nonambulatory symptoms; however, little difference in outcome has been noted in most patients.[424,426-428] Experience with vertebral body resection in selected cases indicates improved neurologic outcome after a more aggressive operative approach.[429-431] Primary irradiation is often the treatment of choice for certain histologic types of tumors known to respond relatively rapidly and for patients with residual functional deficits.

Irradiation for spinal cord compression is considered a radiotherapeutic emergency. Prompt initiation of dexamethasone and high-dose (2- to 4-Gy) fractions are indicated. After 2 or 3 treatments, the dose per fraction and total dose depend on the type of malignancy and clinical status of the patient.

Carcinomatous meningitis or diffuse leptomeningeal infiltration is a relatively uncommon late manifestation of systemic cancer. Primary tumors are usually carcinomas of the breast or lung; small cell lung cancer in particular is often associated with intracranial metastasis.

---

*References 371, 400, 401, 403, 404, 407.

Symptoms and signs referable to the spine predominate in 25% of patients; signs related to spinal root infiltration are often apparent.[432] Treatment consists of cranial or craniospinal irradiation (depending on the histologic findings and coordinated use of chemotherapy), with or without intrathecal or systemic chemotherapy. Responses to treatment are common, but long-term survival results are largely anecdotal.

REFERENCES

1. Schultheiss TE, Kun LE, Ang KK, et al. Radiation response of the central nervous system. *Int J Radiat Oncol Biol Phys* 1995; 31:1093-1112.

2. Fajardo LF, Berthrong M, Anderson RE. Central nervous system and spinal cord. In: *Radiation Pathology*. New York, NY: Oxford University Press; 2001: 351-361.

3. Burger PC, Mahaley MS Jr, Dudka L, et al. The morphologic effects of radiation administered therapeutically for intracranial gliomas: a postmortem study of 25 cases. *Cancer* 1979;44: 1256-1272.

4. Constine LS, Konski A, Ekholm S, et al. Adverse effects of brain irradiation correlated with MR and CT imaging. *Int J Radiat Oncol Biol Phys* 1988;15:319-330.

5. Valk PE, Dillon WP. Radiation injury of the brain. *AJNR Am J Neuroradiol* 1991;12:45-62.

6. Gutin PH. Treatment of radiation necrosis of the brain. In: Gutin PH, Leibel SA, Sheline GE, eds. *Radiation Injury to the Nervous System*. New York, NY: Raven Press; 1991:271-282.

7. DeAngelis LM, Shapiro WR. Drug/radiation interactions and central nervous system injury. In: Gutin PH, Leibel SA, Sheline GE, eds. *Radiation Injury to the Nervous System*. New York, NY: Raven Press; 1991:361-382.

8. Van der Kogel AJ. Central nervous system radiation injury in small animal models. In: Gutin PH, Leibel SA, Sheline GE, eds. *Radiation Injury to the Nervous System*. New York, NY: Raven Press; 1991:91-112.

9. Fike JR, Gobbe GT. Central nervous system radiation injury in large animal models. In: Gutin PH, Leibel SA, Sheline GE, eds. *Radiation Injury to the Nervous System*. New York, NY: Raven Press; 1991:113-136.

10. Ostertag CB. Experimental central nervous system injury from implanted isotopes. In: Gutin PH, Leibel SA, Sheline GE, eds. *Radiation Injury to the Nervous System*. New York, NY: Raven Press; 1991:183-190.

11. Caveness WF. Experimental observations: delayed necrosis in normal monkey brain. In: Gilbert HA, Kagen AR, eds. *Radiation Damage to the Nervous System*. New York, NY: Raven Press; 1980: 1-38.

12. Price RA, Jamieson PA. The central nervous system in childhood leukemia. Subacute leukoencephalopathy. *Cancer* 1975;35(pt 2): 306-318.

13. Fouladi M, Langston J, Mulhern R, et al. Silent lacunar lesions detected by magnetic resonance imaging of children with brain tumors: a late sequela of therapy. *J Clin Oncol* 2000;18:824-831.

14. Salazar OM, Rubin P, Feldstein ML, et al. High dose radiation therapy in the treatment of malignant gliomas: final report. *Int J Radiat Oncol Biol Phys* 1979;5:1733-1740.

15. Kramer S, Lee KF. Complications of radiation therapy: the central nervous system. *Semin Roentgenol* 1974;9:72-83.

16. Sheline GE, Wara WM, Smith V. Therapeutic irradiation and brain injury. *Int J Radiat Oncol Biol Phys* 1980;6:1215-1228.

17. Sheline GE. Irradiation injury of the human brain: a review of clinical experience. In: Gilbert HA, Kagen AR, eds. *Radiation Damage to the Nervous System*. New York, NY: Raven Press; 1980:39-58.

18. Young DF, Posner JB, Chu F, et al. Rapid-course radiation therapy of cerebral metastases: results and complications. *Cancer* 1974; 34:1069-1076.

19. Jones A. Transient radiation myelopathy (with reference to Lhermitte's sign of electrical paresthesia). *Br J Radiol* 1964;37: 727-744.

20. Freeman JE, Johnston PGB, Voke JM. Somnolence after prophylactic cranial irradiation in children with acute lymphoblastic leukaemia. *Br Med J* 1973;4:523-525.

21. Boldrey E, Sheline G. Delayed transitory clinical manifestations after radiation treatment of intracranial tumors. *Acta Radiologica: Therapy, Physics, Biology* 1966;5:5-10.

22. Steen RG, Koury M, Granja CI, et al. Effect of ionizing radiation on the human brain: white matter and gray matter T1 in pediatric brain tumor patients treated with conformal radiation therapy. *Int J Radiat Oncol Biol Phys* 2001;49:79-91.

23. Hoffman WF, Levin VA, Wilson CB. Evaluation of malignant glioma patients during the postirradiation period. *J Neurosurg* 1979;30:624-628.

24. Longee DC, Fiedman HS, Djang NW, et al. Transient late magnetic resonance imaging changes suggesting progression of brain stem glioma: implications for entry criteria for phase II trials. *Neurosurgery* 1988;23:248-253.

25. Duffner PK, Cohen ME, Myers MH, et al. Survival of children with brain tumors: SEER program, 1973-1980. *Neurology* 1986; 36:597-601.

26. Childhood Brain Tumor Consortium. A study of childhood brain tumors based on surgical biopsies from 10 North American institutions: sample description. *J Neurooncol* 1988;6:9-23.

27. Groothuis DR, Wright DC, Ostertag CB. The effect of ^{125}I interstitial radiotherapy on blood-brain barrier function in normal canine brain. *J Neurosurg* 1987;67:895-902.

28. Schultheiss TE, Stephens LC. The pathogenesis of radiation myelopathy: widening the circle. *Int J Radiat Oncol Biol Phys* 1992;23:1089-1091.

29. Schultheiss TE, Stephens LC. Invited review: permanent radiation myelopathy. *Br J Radiol* 1992;65:737-753.

30. Marks JE, Baglan RJ, Prassad SC, et al. Cerebral radionecrosis: incidence and risk in relation to dose, time, fractionation and volume. *Int J Radiat Oncol Biol Phys* 1981;7:242-252.

31. Mikhael MA. Dosimetric considerations in the diagnosis of radiation necrosis of the brain. In: Gilbert HA, Kagen AR, eds. *Radiation Injury to the Nervous System*. New York, NY: Raven Press; 1980:59-92.

32. Kramer S, Southard ME, Mansfield CM. Radiation effect and tolerance of the central nervous system. *Front Radiat Ther Oncol* 1972;6:332-345.

33. Aristizabal S, Caldwell WL, Avila J. The relationship of time-dose fractionation factors to complications in the treatment of pituitary tumors by irradiation. *Int J Radiat Oncol Biol Phys* 1977; 2:667-673.

34. Leibel SA, Sheline GE. Tolerance of the brain and spinal cord to conventional irradiation. In: Gutin PH, Leibel SA, Sheline GE, eds. *Radiation Injury to the Nervous System*. New York, NY: Raven Press; 1991:239-256.

35. Clemente CD, Yamazaki JN, Bennett LR, et al. Brain radiation in newborn rats and differential effects of increased age. *Neurology* 1960;10:669-675.

36. Bloom HJG, Wallace ENK, Henk JM. The treatment and prognosis of medulloblastoma in children. *AJR Am J Roentgenol* 1969; 105:43-62.

37. Boden G. Radiation myelitis of the brain stem. *J Facul Radiolog London* 1950;2:79-94.

38. Pallis CA, Louis S, Morgan RL. Radiation myelopathy. *Brain* 1961; 84:460-479.

39. Schultheiss TE, Higgins EM, el-Mahdi AM. The latent period in clinical radiation myelopathy. *Int J Radiat Oncol Biol Phys* 1984; 10:1109-1115.

40. Myers R, Rogers MA, Hornsey S. A reappraisal of the role of glial and vascular elements in the development of white matter necrosis in irradiated rat spinal cord. *Br J Cancer* 1986;7:221-223.

41. Phillips TL, Buschke F. Radiation tolerance of the thoracic spinal cord. *Am J Roentgenol Rad Ther Nucl Med* 1969;105:659-664.

42. Abbatucci JS, Delozier T, Quint R, et al. Radiation myelopathy of the cervical spinal cord: time, dose and volume factors. *Int J Radiat Oncol Biol Phys* 1978;4:239-248.

43. Hatievoll R, Host H, Kaalhus O. Myelopathy following radiotherapy of bronchial carcinoma with large single fractions: a retrospective study. *Int J Radiat Oncol Biol Phys* 1983;9:41-44.

44. Wara WM, Phillips TL, Sheline GE, et al. Radiation tolerance of the spinal cord. *Cancer* 1975;35:1558-1562.

45. Cohen L, Creditor M. An isoeffect table for radiation tolerance of the human spinal cord. *Int J Radiat Oncol Biol Phys* 1981;7:961-966.

46. Van der Kogel AJ. Radiation tolerance of the rat spinal cord: time-dose relationships. *Radiology* 1977;122:505-509.

47. Ang KK, van der Kogel AJ, van der Schueren E. Lack of evidence for increased tolerance of rat spinal cord with decreasing fraction doses below 2 Gy. *Int J Radiat Oncol Biol Phys* 1985;11:105-110.

48. Dische S, Saunders MI. Continuous, hyperfractionated, accelerated radiotherapy (CHART): an interim report upon late morbidity. *Radiother Oncol* 1989;16:67-74.

49. Dische S. Accelerated treatment and radiation myelitis. *Radiother Oncol* 1991;20:1-2.

50. Norrell H, Wilson CB, Slagel DE, et al. Leukoencephalopathy following the administration of methotrexate into the cerebrospinal fluid in the treatment of primary brain tumors. *Cancer* 1974;33:923-932.

51. Lee JS, Umsawasdi T, Lee Y-Y, et al. Neurotoxicity in long-term survivors of small cell lung cancer. *Int J Radiat Oncol Biol Phys* 1986;12:313-321.

52. Bleyer WA. Neurologic sequelae of methotrexate and ionizing radiation: a new classification. *Cancer Treatment Reports* 1981;65:89-98.

53. Mulhern RK, Ochs J, Kun LE. Changes in intellect associated with cranial radiation therapy. In: Gutin PH, Leibel SA, Sheline GE, eds. *Radiation Injury to the Nervous System*. New York, NY: Raven Press; 1991:325-340.

54. Mulhern RK, Kovnar E, Langston J, et al. Long-term survivors of leukemia treated in infancy: factors associated with neuropsychologic status. *J Clin Oncol* 1992;10:1095-1102.

55. Jannoun L, Bloom HJG. Long-term psychological effects in children treated for intracranial tumors. *Int J Radiat Oncol Biol Phys* 1990;18:747-753.

56. Hochberg FH, Slotnick B. Neuropsychologic impairment in astrocytoma survivors. *Neurology* 1980;30:172-177.

57. Maire J, Coudin B, Guerin J, et al. Neuropsychologic impairment in adults with brain tumors. *Am J Clin Oncol* 1987;10:156-162.

58. Kun LE, Mulhern RK, Crisco JJ. Quality of life in children treated for brain tumors: intellectual, emotional, and academic function. *J Neurosurg* 1983;58:1-6.

59. Radcliffe J, Packer RJ, Atkins TE, et al. Three- and four-year cognitive outcome in children with noncortical brain tumors treated with whole-brain radiotherapy. *Ann Neurol* 1992; 32:551-554.

60. Mulhern RK, Kepner JL, Thomas PRM, et al. Neuropsychological functioning of survivors of childhood medulloblastoma randomized to receive conventional (3,600 cGy/20) or reduced (2,340/13) dose craniospinal irradiation: a Pediatric Oncology Group study. *J Clin Oncol* 1998;16:1723-1728.

61. Mulhern RK, Reddick WE, Palmer SL, et al. Neurocognitive deficits in medulloblastoma survivors and white matter loss. *Ann Neurol* 1999;46:834-841.

62. Craig JB, Jackson DV, Moody D, et al. Prospective evaluation of changes in computed cranial tomography in patients with small cell lung carcinoma treated with chemotherapy and prophylactic cranial irradiation. *J Clin Oncol* 1984;2:1151-1156.

63. Urie MM, Fullerton B, Tatsuzaki H, et al. A dose response analysis of injury to cranial nerves and/or nuclei following proton beam radiation therapy. *Int J Radiat Oncol Biol Phys* 1992;23:27-29.

64. Parsons JT, Bova FJ, Fitzgerald CR, et al. Radiation optic neuropathy after megavoltage external-beam irradiation: analysis of time-dose factors. *Int J Radiat Oncol Biol Phys* 1994;30:755-763.

65. Harris JR, Levene MB. Visual complications following irradiation for pituitary adenomas and craniopharyngiomas. *Radiology* 1976;120:167-171.

66. Svensson H, Westling P, Larsson LG. Radiation-induced lesions of the bronchial plexus correlated to the dose-time-fraction schedule. *Acta Radiol* 1975;14:228-238.

67. Greenlee RT, Hill-Harmon MB, Murray T, et al. Cancer statistics, 2001. *CA Cancer J Clin* 2001;51:15-36.

68. Gurney JG, Davis S, Severson RK, et al. Trends in cancer incidence among children in the U.S. *Cancer* 1996;78:532-541.

69. Kleihues P, Cavenee WK, eds. *Tumours of the Nervous System*. Lyon, France: IARC Press; 2000.

70. Rorke L. The cerebellar medulloblastoma and its relationship to primitive neuroectodermal tumors. *J Neuropathol Exp Neurol* 1983;42:1-15.

71. Hart MN, Earle KM. Primitive neuroectodermal tumors of the brain in children. *Cancer* 1973;32:890-898.

72. Grotzer MA, Janss AJ, Fung JA, et al. TrkC expression predicts good clinical outcome in primitive neuroectodermal brain tumors. *J Clin Oncol* 2000;18:1027-1035.

73. McLendon RE, Friedman HS, Fuchs HE, et al. Diagnostic markers in paediatric medulloblastoma: a Pediatric Oncology Group study. *Histopathology* 1999;34:154-162.

74. Gajjar A, Fouladi M, Walter AW, et al. Comparison of lumbar and shunt cerebrospinal fluid specimens for cytologic detection of leptomeningeal disease in pediatric patients with brain tumors. *J Clin Oncol* 1999;17:1825-1828.

75. Kleinman GM, Hockberg FH, Richardson EP Jr. Systemic metastases from medulloblastoma: report of two cases and review of the literature. *Cancer* 1981;48:2296-2309.

76. Albright AL, Wisoff JH, Zeltzer PM, et al. Effects of medulloblastoma resections on outcome in children: a report from the Children's Cancer Group. *Neurosurgery* 1996;38:265-271.

77. Cochrane DD, Gustavsson B, Poskitt KP, et al. The surgical and natural morbidity of aggressive resection for posterior fossa tumors in childhood. *Pediatr Neurosurg* 1994;20:19-29.

78. Aguiar PH, Plese JP, Ciquini O, et al. Transient mutism following a posterior fossa approach to cerebellar tumors in children: a critical review of the literature. *Childs Nerv Syst* 1995;11:306-310.

79. Chang CH, Housepian EM, Herbert C Jr. An operative staging system and a megavoltage radiotherapeutic technic for cerebellar medulloblastoma. *Radiology* 1969;93:1351-1359.

80. Kun LE, Constine LS. Medulloblastoma: caution regarding new treatment approaches. *Int J Radiat Oncol Biol Phys* 1991;20:897-899.

81. Packer RJ, Sutton LN, Elterman R, et al. Outcome for children with medulloblastoma treated with radiation and cisplatin, CCNU, and vincristine chemotherapy. *J Neurosurg* 1994;81:690-698.

82. Heideman RL, Kovnar EH, Kellie SJ, et al. Preirradiation chemotherapy with carboplatin and etoposide in newly diagnosed embryonal pediatric CNS tumors. *J Clin Oncol* 1995;13:2247-2254.

83. Kovnar EH, Kellie SJ, Horowitz ME, et al. Pre-irradiation cisplatin and etoposide in the treatment of high-risk medulloblastoma and other malignant embryonal tumors of the central nervous system: a phase II study. *J Clin Oncol* 1990;8:330-336.

84. Bailey CC, Gnekow A, Wellek S, et al. Prospective randomized trial of chemotherapy given before radiotherapy in childhood medulloblastoma. International Society of Paediatric Oncology (SIOP) and the (German) Society of Paediatric Oncology (GPO): SIOP II. *Med Pediatr Oncol* 1995;25:166-178.

85. Hartsell WF, Gajjar A, Heideman RL, et al. Patterns of failure in children with medulloblastoma: effects of pre-irradiation chemotherapy. *Int J Radiat Oncol Biol Phys* 1997;39:15-24.

86. Thomas PRM, Deutsch M, Kepner JL, et al. Low-stage medulloblastoma: final analysis of trial comparing standard-dose with reduced-dose neuraxis irradiation. *J Clin Oncol* 2000;18:3004-3011.

87. Berry MP, Jenkin RDT, Keen CW, et al. Radiation treatment for medulloblastoma: a 21-year review. *J Neurosurg* 1981;55:43-51.

88. Hughes EN, Winston K, Cassady JR, et al. Medulloblastoma: results of surgery and radical radiation therapy at the JCRT 1968-1984. *Int J Radiat Oncol Biol Phys* 1986;12:179.

89. Bloom HJG, Glees J, Bell J. The treatment and long-term prognosis of children with intracranial tumors: a study of 610 cases, 1950-1981. *Int J Radiat Oncol Biol Phys* 1990;18:723-745.

90. Jenkin D, Goddard K, Armstrong D, et al. Posterior fossa medulloblastoma in childhood: treatment results and a proposal for a new staging system. *Int J Radiat Oncol Biol Phys* 1990;19:265-274.

91. Packer RJ, Goldwein J, Nicholson HS, et al. Treatment of children with medulloblastomas with reduced-dose craniospinal radiation therapy and adjuvant chemotherapy: a Children's Cancer Group study. *J Clin Oncol* 1999;17:2127-2136.

92. Fukunaga-Johnson N, Sandler HM, Marsh R, et al. The use of 3D conformal radiotherapy (3D CRT) to spare the cochlea in patients with medulloblastoma. *Int J Radiat Oncol Biol Phys* 1998;41:77-82.

93. Merchant TE, Happersett L, Finlay J, et al. Preliminary results of conformal radiation therapy for medulloblastoma. *Neurooncology* 1999;1:177-187.

94. Fukunaga-Johnson N, Lee JH, Sandler HM, et al. Patterns of failure following treatment for medulloblastoma: is it necessary to treat the entire posterior fossa. *Int J Radiat Oncol Biol Phys* 1998;42:143-146.

95. Strother D, Ashley D, Kellie SJ, et al. Feasibility of four consecutive high-dose chemotherapy cycles with stem-cell rescue for patients with newly diagnosed medulloblastoma or supratentorial primitive neuroectodermal tumor after craniospinal radiotherapy: results of a collaborative study. *J Clin Oncol* 2001; 19:2696-2704.

96. Gajjar A, Sanford RA, Heideman R, et al. Low-grade astrocytoma: a decade of experience at St. Jude Children's Research Hospital. *J Clin Oncol* 1997;15:2792-2799.

97. Leibel SA, Sheline GE, Wara WM, et al. The role of radiation therapy in the treatment of astrocytomas. *Cancer* 1975;35:1551-1557.

98. Morantz RA. Radiation therapy in the treatment of cerebral astrocytoma. *Neurosurgery* 1987;20:975-982.

99. Wallner KE, Gonzales MF, Edwards MSB, et al. Treatment results of juvenile pilocytic astrocytoma. *J Neurosurg* 1988;69:171-176.

100. Laws ER, Taylor WF, Clifton MB, et al. Neurosurgical management of low-grade astrocytoma of the cerebral hemispheres. *J Neurosurg* 1984;61:665-673.

101. Krieger MD, Gonzalez-Gomez I, Levy ML, et al. Recurrence patterns and anaplastic change in a long-term study of pilocytic astrocytomas. *Pediatr Neurosurg* 1997;27:1-11.

102. Ilgren EB, Stiller CA. Cerebellar astrocytomas. Clinical characteristics and prognostic indices. *J Neurooncol* 1987;4:293-308.

103. Smoots DW, Geyer JR, Lieberman DM, et al. Predicting disease progression in childhood cerebellar astrocytoma. *Childs Nerv Syst* 14:636-648, 1998.

104. Tomita T, Chou P, Reyes-Mugica M. IV ventricle astrocytomas in childhood: clinicopathological features in 21 cases. *Childs Nerv Syst* 1998;14:537-546.

105. Pencalet P, Maixner W, Sainte-Rose C, et al. Benign cerebellar astrocytomas in children. *J Neurosurg* 1999;90:265-273.

106. Sgouros S, Fineron PW, Hockley AD. Cerebellar astrocytoma of childhood: long-term follow-up. *Childs Nerv Syst* 1995;11:89-96.

107. Burger PC, Scheithauer BW, Vogel FS, eds. *Surgical Pathology of the Nervous System and its Coverings,* 3rd ed. New York, NY: Churchill Livingstone; 1991.

108. Garcia DM, Marks JE, Latifi HR, et al. Childhood cerebellar astrocytomas: is there a role for postoperative irradiation? *Int J Radiat Oncol Biol Phys* 1990;18:815-818.

109. Schneider JH, Raffel C, McComb JG. Benign cerebellar astrocytomas of childhood. *Neurosurgery* 1992;30:58-63.

110. Ilgren EB, Stiller CA. Cerebellar astrocytomas: therapeutic management. *Acta Neurochir* 1986;81:11-26.

111. Larson DA, Wara WM, Edwards MSB. Management of childhood cerebellar astrocytoma. *Int J Radiat Oncol Biol Phys* 1980; 18:971-973.

112. Hirsch J-F, Rose CS, Pierre-Kahn A, et al. Benign astrocytic and oligodendrocytic tumors of the cerebral hemispheres in children. *J Neurosurg* 1989;70:568-572.

113. Hoffman HJ, Soloniuk DS, Humphreys RP, et al. Management and outcome of low-grade astrocytomas of the midline in children: a retrospective review. *Neurosurgery* 1993;33:964-971.

114. Reardon D, Gajjar A, Walter AW, et al. Bithalamic involvement predicts poor outcome among children with thalamic glial tumors. *Pediatr Neurosurg* 1998;29:29-35.

115. Krouwer HGJ, Prados MD. Infiltrative astrocytomas of the thalamus. *J Neurosurg* 1995;82:548-557.

116. Albright AL, Price RA, Guthkelch AN. Diencephalic gliomas of children: a clinicopathologic study. *Cancer* 1985;55:2789-2793.

117. Cairncross JG, Laperriere NJ. Low-grade glioma: to treat or not to treat? *Arch Neurol* 1989;46:1238-1239.

118. Bernstein M, Hoffman HJ, Halliday WC, et al. Thalamic tumors in children: long-term follow-up and treatment guidelines. *J Neurosurg* 1984;61:649-656.

119. Kelly PJ. Stereotactic biopsy and resection of thalamic astrocytomas. *Neurosurgery* 1989;25:185-194.

120. Leibel SA, Sheline GE. Review article: radiation therapy for neoplasms of the brain. *J Neurosurg* 1987;66:1-22.

121. Boydston WR, Sanford RA, Muhlbauer MS, et al. Gliomas of the tectum and periaqueductal region of the mesencephalon. *Pediatr Neurosurg* 1991;17:234-238.

122. Medbery CA, Straus KL, Steinberg SM, et al. Low-grade astrocytomas: treatment results and prognostic variables. *Int J Radiat Oncol Biol Phys* 1988;15:837-841.

123. Whitton AC, Bloom HJG. Low-grade glioma of the cerebral hemispheres in adults: a retrospective analysis of 88 cases. *Int J Radiat Oncol Biol Phys* 1990;18:783-786.

124. Leighton C, Fisher B, Bauman G, et al. Supratentorial low-grade glioma in adults: an analysis of prognostic factors and timing of radiation. *J Clin Oncol* 1997;15:1294-1301.

125. Shaw EG, Daumas-Duport C, Scheithauer BW, et al. Radiation therapy in the management of low-grade supratentorial astrocytomas. *J Neurosurg* 1989;70:853-861.

126. Karim AB, Maat B, Hatlevoll R, et al. A randomized trial of dose-response in radiation therapy of low-grade cerebral glioma: EORTC study 22844. *Int J Radiat Oncol Biol Phys* 1996; 36:549-556.

127. Dunbar SF, Tarbell NJ, Kooy HM, et al. Stereotactic radiotherapy for pediatric and adult brain tumors: preliminary report. *Int J Radiat Oncol Biol Phys* 1994;30:531-539.

128. Listernick R, Louis DN, Packer RJ, et al. Optic pathway gliomas in children with neurofibromatosis 1: consensus statement from the NF1 Optic Pathway Gliomas Task Force. *Ann Neurol* 1997; 41:143-149.

129. Horwich A, Bloom HJG. Optic gliomas: radiation therapy and prognosis. *Int J Radiat Oncol Biol Phys* 1985;11:1067-1079.

130. Alvord EC, Lofton S. Gliomas of the optic nerve or chiasm: outcome by patient's age, tumor site, and treatment. *J Neurosurg* 1988;68:85-98.

131. Hoyt WF, Baghdassarian SA. Optic glioma of childhood: natural history and rationale for conservative management. *Br J Ophthalmol* 1969;53:793-798.

132. Imes RK, Hoyt WF. Childhood chiasmal gliomas: update on the fate of patients in the 1969 San Francisco study. *Br J Ophthalmol* 1986;70:179-182.

133. Wong JYC, Wara W, Sheline GE. Optic gliomas: a reanalysis of the University of California, San Francisco, experience. *Cancer* 1987;60:1847-1855.

134. Jenkin D, Angyalfi S, Becker L, et al. Optic glioma in children: surveillance, resection, or irradiation? *Int Radiat Oncol Biol Phys* 1993;25:215-225.

135. Bataini JP, Delanian S, Ponvert D. Chiasmal gliomas: results of irradiation management in 57 patients and review of literature. *Int J Radiat Oncol Biol Phys* 1991;21:615-623.

136. Tao ML, Barnes PD, Billett AL, et al. Childhood optic chiasm gliomas: radiographic response following radiotherapy and long-term clinical outcome. *Int J Radiat Oncol Biol Phys* 1997;39:579-587.

137. Fletcher WA, Imes RK, Hoyt WF. Chiasmal gliomas: appearance and long-term changes demonstrated by computerized tomography. *J Neurosurg* 1986;65:154-159.

138. Wisoff JH, Abbott R, Epstein F. Surgical management of exophytic chiasmatic-hypothalamic tumors of childhood. *J Neurosurg* 1990;73:661-667.

139. Packer RJ, Lange B, Ater J, et al. Carboplatin and vincristine for recurrent and newly diagnosed low-grade gliomas of childhood. *J Clin Oncol* 1993;11:850-856.

140. Packer RJ, Ater J, Allen J, et al. Carboplatin and vincristine chemotherapy for children with newly diagnosed progressive low-grade gliomas. *J Neurosurg* 1997;86:747-754.

141. Mahoney DH, Cohen ME, Friedman HS, et al. Carboplatin is effective therapy for young children with progressive optic pathway tumors: a Pediatric Oncology Group phase II study. *Neurooncology* 2000;2:213-220.

142. Somaza SC, Kondziolka D, Lunsford LD, et al. Early outcomes after stereotactic radiosurgery for growing pilocytic astrocytomas in children. *Pediatr Neurosurg* 1996;25:109-115.

143. Grabb PA, Lunsford LD, Albright AL, et al. Stereotactic radiosurgery for glial neoplasms of childhood. *Neurosurgery* 1996;38:696-702.

144. Pollack IF, Hurtt M, Pang D, et al. Dissemination of low grade astrocytomas in children. *Cancer* 1994;73:2869-2878.

145. Prados M, Mamelak AN. Metastasizing low grade gliomas in children. Redefining an old disease. *Cancer* 1994;73:2671-2673.

146. Gajjar A, Bhargava R, Jenkins JJ, et al. Low-grade astrocytoma with neuraxis dissemination at diagnosis. *J Neurosurg* 1995;83:67-71.

147. Kepes JJ, Rubinstein LJ, Eng LF. Pleomorphic xanthoastrocytoma: a distinctive meningocerebral glioma of young subjects with relatively favorable prognosis: a study of 12 cases. *Cancer* 1979;44:1839-1852.

148. Taratuto AL, Monges J, Lylyk P, et al. Superficial cerebral astrocytoma attached to dura. *Cancer* 1984;54:2505-2512.

149. Fouladi M, Jenkins J, Burger P, et al. Pleomorphic xanthoastrocytoma (PXA): favorable outcome following complete surgical resection. *Neuro-oncol* 2001;3:184-192.

150. Merchant TE, Zhu Y, Thompson SJ, et al. Preliminary results from a phase II trial of conformal radiation therapy for pediatric patients with localized low-grade astrocytomas and ependymoma. *Int J Radiat Oncol Biol Phys* 2002;52:325-332.

151. Pollack IF, Claassen D, Al-Shboul Q, et al. Low grade gliomas of the cerebral hemispheres in children: an analysis of 71 cases. *J Neurosurg* 1995;82:536-547.

152. McLaurin RL, Breneman J, Aron B. Hypothalamic gliomas: review of 18 cases. *Concepts of Pediatric Neurosurgery* 1987; 7:19.

153. Albright AL, Price RA, Guthkelch AN. Brainstem gliomas of children: a clinicopathologic study. *Cancer* 1983;52:2313-2319.

154. Albright AL, Guthkelch AN, Packer RJ, et al. Prognostic factors in pediatric brainstem gliomas. *J Neurosurg* 1986;65:751-755.

155. Barkovich AJ, Krischer J, Kun LE, et al. Brain stem gliomas: a classification system based on magnetic resonance imaging. *Pediatr Neurosurg* 1990;16:73-83.

156. Hoffman HJ, Becker I, Craven MA. A clinically and pathologically distinct group of benign brainstem gliomas. *Neurosurgery* 1980;7:243-248.

157. Stroink AR, Hoffman HJ, Hendrick EB, et al. Diagnosis and management of pediatric brainstem gliomas. *J Neurosurg* 1986; 65:745-750.

158. Khatib ZA, Heideman RL, Kovnar EH, et al. Predominance of pilocytic histology in dorsally exophytic brain stem tumors. *Pediatr Neurosurg* 1994;20:2-10.

159. Fisher PG, Breiter SN, Carson BS, et al. A clinicopathologic reappraisal of brain stem tumor classification. Identification of pilocytic astrocytoma and fibrillary astrocytoma as distinct entities. *Cancer* 2000;89:1569-1576.

160. Mantravadi RVP, Phatak R, Bellur S, et al. Brainstem gliomas: an autopsy study of 25 cases. *Cancer* 1982;49:1294-1296.

161. Schulz-Ertner D, Debus J, Lohr F, et al. Fractionated stereotactic conformal radiation therapy of brain stem gliomas: outcome and prognostic factors. *Radiother Oncol* 2000;57:215-223.

162. Shrieve DC, Wara WM, Edwards MSB, et al. Hyperfractionated radiation therapy for gliomas of the brainstem in children and in adults. *Int J Radiat Oncol Biol Phys* 1992;24:599-610.

163. Freeman CR, Krischer JP, Sanford RA, et al. Final results of a study of escalating doses of hyperfractionated radiotherapy in brain stem tumors in children: a Pediatric Oncology Group study. *Int J Radiat Oncol Biol Phys* 1993;27:197-206.

164. Freeman CR, Bourgouin PM, Sanford RA, et al. Long term survivors of childhood brain stem gliomas treated with hyperfractionated radiotherapy, clinical characteristics and treatment related toxicities. *Cancer* 1996;77:555-562.

165. Mandell LR, Kadota R, Freeman C, et al. There is no role for hyperfractionated radiotherapy in the management of children with newly diagnosed diffuse intrinsic brainstem tumors: results of a Pediatric Oncology Group phase III trial comparing conventional vs. hyperfractionated radiotherapy. *Int J Radiat Oncol Biol Phys* 1999;43:959-964.

166. Freeman CR, Kepner J, Kun LE, et al. A detrimental effect of a combined chemotherapy-radiotherapy approach in children with diffuse intrinsic brain stem gliomas? *Int J Radiat Oncol Biol Phys* 2000;47:561-564.

167. Tait DM, Thornton-Jones H, Bloom HJG, et al. Adjuvant chemotherapy for medulloblastoma: the first multicenter control trial of the International Society of Paediatric Oncology (SIOP I). *Eur J Cancer Clin Oncol* 1990;26:464-469.

168. Duffner PK, Horowitz ME, Krischer JP, et al. Postoperative chemotherapy and delayed radiation in children less than three years of age with malignant brain tumors. *N Engl J Med* 1993;328:1725-1731.

169. Ilgren EB, Stiller CA, Hughes JT, et al. Ependymomas: a clinical and pathologic study, part 1: biologic features. *Clin Neuropathol* 1984;3:113-121.

170. Sanford RA, Kun LE, Heideman RL, et al. Cerebellar pontine angle ependymoma in infants. *Pediatr Neurosurg* 1997;27:84-91.

171. Bloom HJG. Intracranial tumors: response and resistance to therapeutic endeavors, 1970-1980. *Int J Radiat Oncol Biol Phys* 1982;8:1083-1113.

172. Vanuystel LJ, Bessell EM, Ashley SE, et al. Intracranial ependymoma: long-term results of a policy of surgery and radiotherapy. *Int J Radiat Oncol Biol Phys* 1982;23:313-319.

173. Goldwein JW, Glauser TA, Packet RJ, et al. Recurrent intracranial ependymomas in children: survival, patterns of failure, and prognostic factors. *Cancer* 1990;66:557-563.

174. Rezai AR, Woo HH, Lee M, et al. Disseminated ependymomas of the central nervous system. *J Neurosurg* 1996;85:618-624.

175. Centeno RS, Lee AA, Winter J, et al. Supratentorial ependymomas. Neuroimaging and clinicopathological correlation. *J Neurosurg* 1986;64:209-215.

176. Rawlings CE III, Giangaspero F, Burger PC, et al. Ependymomas: a clinicopathologic study. *Surg Neurol* 1988;29:271-281.

177. Rorke LB. Relationship of morphology of ependymoma in children to prognosis. *Prog Exp Tumor Res* 1987;30:170-174.

178. Ross GW, Rubinstein LJ. Lack of histopathological correlation of malignant ependymomas with postoperative survival. *J Neurosurg* 1989;70:31-36.

179. Rousseau P, Habrand JL, Sarrazin D, et al. Treatment of intracranial ependymomas of children: review of a 15-year experience. *Int J Radiat Oncol Biol Phys* 1994;28:381-386.

180. Pollack IF, Gerszten PC, Martinez AJ, et al. Intracranial ependymomas of childhood: long-term outcome and prognostic factors. *Neurosurgery* 1995;37:655-667.

181. Healey EA, Braners PD, Kupsky WJ, et al. The prognostic significance of postoperative residual tumor in ependymoma. *Neurosurgery* 1991;28:666-672.

182. Nazar GB, Hoffman HJ, Becker LE, et al. Infratentorial ependymomas in childhood: prognostic factors and treatment. *J Neurosurg* 1990;72:408-417.

183. Hukin J, Epstein F, Lefton D, et al. Treatment of intracranial ependymoma by surgery alone. *Pediatr Neurosurg* 1998;29:40-45.

184. Duffner PK, Krischer JP, Sanford RA, et al. Prognostic factors in infants and very young children with intracranial ependymomas. *Pediatr Neurosurg* 1998;28:215-222.

185. Lefkowitz I, Evans A, Sposto R, et al. Adjuvant chemotherapy of childhood posterior fossa (PF) ependymoma: craniospinal irradiation with or without CCNU, vincristine (VCR) and prednisone (P). *Proc Am Soc Clin Oncol* 1989;8:87a.

186. Strother D, Kepner J, Aronin P, et al. Dose-intensive (DI) chemotherapy (CT) prolongs event-free survival (EFS) for very young children with ependymoma (EP). Results of Pediatric Oncology Group (POG) Study 9233. *Proc Am Soc Clin Oncol* 2000;19:585a, 2302.

187. Goldwein JW, Corn BW, Finlay JL, et al. Is craniospinal irradiation required to cure children with malignant (anaplastic) intracranial ependymomas? *Cancer* 1991;67:2766-2771.

188. Merchant TE, Haida T, Wang M-H, et al. Anaplastic ependymoma: treatment of pediatric patients with or without craniospinal radiation therapy. *J Neurosurg* 1997;86:943-949.

189. Kovnar EH, Curran W, Tomita T, et al. Hyperfractionated irradiation for childhood ependymoma: improved local control in subtotally resected tumors [abstract]. Paper presented at: Eighth International Symposium on Pediatric Neuro-Oncology; May 6-9, 1998; Rome, Italy.

190. Aggarwal R, Yeung D, Muhlbauer M, et al. Efficacy and feasibility of stereotactic radiosurgery in the primary management of unfavorable pediatric ependymoma. *Radiother Oncol* 1997;43:269-273.

191. Herrick MK. Pathology of pineal tumors. In: Neuwelt EA, ed. *Diagnosis and Treatment of Pineal Region Tumors.* Baltimore, Md: Williams and Wilkins; 1984:31-60.

192. Glenn OA, Barkovich AJ. Intracranial germ cell tumors: a comprehensive review of proposed embryonic deprivation. *Pediatr Neurosurg* 1996;24:242-251.

193. Rich TA, Cassady JR, Strand RD, et al. Radiation therapy for pineal and suprasellar germ cell tumors. *Cancer* 1985;55:932-940.

194. Ho DM, Lieu H-C. Primary intracranial germ cell tumor. Pathologic study of 51 patients. *Cancer* 1992;70:1577-1584.

195. Dernaley DP, A'Hern RP, Whittaker S, et al. Pineal and CNS germ cell tumors: Royal Marsden Hospital experience 1962-1987. *Int J Radiat Oncol Biol Phys* 1990;18:773-781.

196. Wolden SL, Wara WM, Larson DA, et al. Radiation therapy for primary intracranial germ-cell tumors. *Int J Radiat Oncol Biol Phys* 1995;32:943-949.

197. Borit A, Blackwood W, Mair WGP. The separation of pineocytoma from pineoblastoma. *Cancer* 1980;45:1408-1418.

198. DiSclafani A, Hudgins RJ, Edwards MSB, et al. Pineocytomas. *Cancer* 1989;63:302-304.

199. Schild SE, Scheithauer BW, Schomberg PJ, et al. Pineal parenchymal tumors. Clinical, pathologic, and therapeutic aspects. *Cancer* 1993;72:870-880.

200. Schild SE, Haddock MG, Scheithauer BW, et al. Nongerminomatous germ cell tumors of the brain. *Int J Radiat Oncol Biol Phys* 1996;36:557-563.

201. Shibamoto Y, Takahashi M, Sasai K. Prognosis of intracranial germinoma with syncytiotrophoblastic giant cells treated by radiation therapy. *Int J Radiat Oncol Biol Phys* 1997;37:505-510.

202. Jennings MT, Gelman R, Hochberg F. Intracranial germ-cell tumors: natural history and pathogenesis. *J Neurosurg* 1985;63:155-167.

203. Jenkin D, Berry M, Chan H, et al. Pineal region germinomas in childhood: treatment considerations. *Int J Radiat Oncol Biol Phys* 1990;18:541-545.

204. Sung D, Harisiadis L, Chang CG. Midline pineal tumors and suprasellar germinomas: highly curable by irradiation. *Radiology* 1978;128:745-751.

205. Haddock MG, Schild SE, Scheithauer BE, et al. Radiation therapy for histologically confirmed primary central nervous system germinoma. *Int J Radiat Oncol Biol Phys* 1997;38:915-923.

206. Shibamoto Y, Takahashi M, Abe M. Reducton of the radiation dose for intracranial germinoma: a prospective study. *Br J Cancer* 1994;70:984-989.

207. Shirato H, Nishio M, Sawamura Y, et al. Analysis of long-term treatment of intracranial germinoma. *Int J Radiat Oncol Biol Phys* 1997;37:511-515.

208. Merchant TE, Sherwood SH, Mulhern RM, et al. CNS germinoma: disease control and long-term functional outcome for 12 children treated with craniospinal irradiation. *Int J Radiat Oncol Biol Phys* 2000;46:1171-1176.

209. Hardenbergh PH, Golden J, Billet A, et al. Intracranial germinoma: the case for lower dose radiation therapy. *Int J Radiat Oncol Biol Phys* 1997;39:419-426.

210. Calaminus G, Bamberg M, Baranzelli MC, et al. Intracranial germ cell tumors: a comprehensive update of the European data. *Neuropediatrics* 1994;25:26-32.

211. Shibamoto Y, Abe M, Yamashita J, et al. Treatment results of intracranial germinoma as a function of the irradiation volume. *Int J Radiat Oncol Biol Phys* 1998;15:285-290.

212. Bamberg M, Kortmann R-D, Calaminus G, et al. Radiation therapy for intracranial germinoma: results of the German Cooperative Prospective Trials MAKEI 83/86/89. *J Clin Oncol* 1999;17:2585-2592.

213. Allen JC, Kim JH, Packer RJ. Neoadjuvant chemotherapy for newly diagnosed germ cell tumors of the central nervous system. *J Neurosurg* 1987;67:65-70.

214. Bouffet E, Baranzelli MC, Patte C, et al. Combined treatment modality for intracranial germinomas: results of a multicentre SFOP experience. *Br J Cancer* 1999;79:1199-1204.

215. Balmaceda C, Heller G, Rosenblum M, et al. Chemotherapy without irradiation. A novel approach for newly diagnosed CNS germ cell tumors: results of an international cooperative trial. *J Clin Oncol* 1996;14:2908-2915.

216. Linstadt D, Wara WM, Edwards MSB, et al. Radiotherapy of primary intracranial germinomas: the case against routine

craniospinal irradiation. *Int J Radiat Oncol Biol Phys* 1988;15: 291-297.

217. Buckner JC, Peethambaram PP, Smithson WA, et al. Phase II trial of primary chemotherapy followed by reduced-dose radiation for CNS germ cell tumors. *J Clin Oncol* 1999;17:933-940.

218. Allen JC, DaRosso RC, Donahue B. A phase II trial of preirradiation carboplatin in newly diagnosed germinoma of the central nervous system. *Cancer* 1994;74:940-944.

219. Robertson PL, DaRosso RC, Allen JC. Improved prognosis of intracranial non-germinoma germ cell tumors with multimodality therapy. *J Neurooncol* 1997;32:71-80.

220. Aoyama H, Shirato H, Yoshida H, et al. Retrospective multi-institutional study of radiotherapy for intracranial non-germinomatous germ cell tumors. *Radiother Oncol* 1998;49:55-59.

221. Jakacki RI, Zeltzer PM, Boyett JM, et al. Survival and prognostic factors following radiation and/or chemotherapy for primitive neuroectodermal tumors of the pineal region in infants and children: a report of the Children's Cancer Group. *J Clin Oncol* 1995;13:1377-1383.

222. Adamson TE, Wiestler OD, Kleihues P, et al. Correlation of clinical and pathological features in surgically treated craniopharyngiomas. *J Neurosurg* 1990;73:12-17.

223. Hoffman HJ, De Silva M, Humphreys RP, et al. Aggressive surgical management of craniopharyngiomas in children. *J Neurosurg* 1992;76:47-52.

224. Hoffman HJ. Surgical management of craniopharyngioma. *Pediatr Neurosurg* 1994;21:44-49.

225. Yarsargil MG, Curcic M, Kis S, et al. Total removal of craniopharyngiomas: approaches and long-term results in 144 patients. *J Neurosurg* 1990;73:3-11.

226. Sanford RA. Craniopharyngioma: results of survey of the American Society of Pediatric Neurosurgery. *Pediatr Neurosurg* 1994;21:39-43.

227. Scott RM, Hetelekidis S, Barnes PD, et al. Surgery, radiation, and combination therapy in the treatment of childhood craniopharyngioma—a 20-year experience. *Pediatr Neurosurg* 1994;21:75-81.

228. Wen B-C, Hussey DH, Staples J, et al. A comparison of the roles of surgery and radiation therapy in the management of craniopharyngiomas. *Int J Radiat Oncol Biol Phys* 1989;16:17-24.

229. Sweet WH. History of surgery for craniopharyngiomas. *Pediatr Neurosurg* 1994;21:28-38.

230. Tomita T, McLone DG. Radical resections of childhood craniopharyngiomas. *Pediatr Neurosurg* 1993;19:6-14.

231. Yasargil MC, Curcic M, Kis S, et al. Total removal of craniopharyngiomas: approaches and long-term results in 144 patients. *J Neurosurg* 1990;73:3-11.

232. Tomita T, McLone DG. Radical resections of childhood craniopharyngiomas. *Pediatr Neurosurg* 1993;19:6-14.

233. Fischer EG, Welch K, Shillito J Jr, et al. Craniopharyngiomas in children: long-term effects of conservative surgical procedures combined with radiation therapy. *J Neurosurg* 1990;73:534-540.

234. Fischer EG, Welch K, Shilito J Jr, et al. Craniopharyngiomas in children. Long-term effects of conservative surgical procedures combined with radiation therapy. *J Neurosurg* 1990;73:534-540.

235. Sklar CA. Craniopharyngioma: endocrine sequelae of treatment. *Pediatr Neurosurg* 1994;21:120-123.

236. Curtis J, Daneman D, Hoffman HJ, et al. The endocrine outcome after surgical removal of craniopharyngiomas. *Pediatr Neurosurg* 1994;21:24-27.

237. Kramer S, Southard M, Mansfield CM. Radiotherapy in the management of craniopharyngiomas. *AJR Am J Roentgenol* 1968;103:44-52.

238. Kramer S, McKissock W, Concannon JP. Craniopharyngiomas: treatment by combined surgery and radiation therapy. *J Neurosurg* 1961;18:217-226.

239. Kramer S, Southard M, Mansfield CM. Radiotherapy in the management of craniopharyngiomas: further experience and late results. *Am J Roentgenol Radium Ther Nucl Med* 1968;103:44-52.

240. Regine WF, Kramer S. Pediatric craniopharyngiomas: long-term results of combined treatment with surgery and radiation. *Int J Radiat Oncol Biol Phys* 1992;24:611-617.

241. Brada M, Thomas DGT. Craniopharyngioma revisited. *Int J Radiat Oncol Biol Phys* 1993;27:471-475.

242. Hetelididis S, Barnes PD, Tao ML, et al. Twenty year experience in childhood craniopharyngioma. *Int J Radiat Oncol Biol Phys* 1993;27:189-195.

243. Rajan B, Ashley S, Gorman C, et al. Craniopharyngioma—long term results following limited surgery and radiotherapy. *Radiother Oncol* 1993;26:1-10.

244. Flickinger JC, Lunsford LD, Singer J, et al. Megavoltage external beam irradiation of craniopharyngiomas: analysis of tumor control and morbidity. *Int J Radiat Oncol Biol Phys* 1990;19:117-122.

245. Lunsford LD, Pollack BE, Kondziolka DS, et al. Stereotactic options in the management of craniopharyngioma. *Pediatr Neurosurg* 1994;21:90-97.

246. Backlund E-O, Axelsson B, Bergstrand C-G, et al. Treatment of craniopharyngiomas—the stereotactic approach in a ten to twenty-threes' perspective. Surgical, radiological and ophthalmological aspects. *Acta Neurochir* 1989;99(pt 1):11-19.

247. Baskin DS, Wilson CB. Surgical management of craniopharyngiomas: a review of 74 cases. *J Neurosurg* 1986;65:22-27.

248. Merchant TE, Kiehna EN, Sanford RA, et al. Craniopharyngioma: the St. Jude Children's Research Hospital experience. *Int J Radiat Oncol Biol Phys* 2002;53:533-542.

249. Hoogenhout J, Otten BJ, Kazem I, et al. Surgery and radiation therapy in the management of craniopharyngiomas. *Int J Radiat Oncol Biol Phys* 1984;10:2293-2297.

250. Sung DI, Chang CH, Harisiadis L, et al. Treatment results in craniopharyngiomas. *Cancer* 1981;47:847-852.

251. Hart MN, Earle KM. Primitive neuroectodermal tumors of the brain in children. *Cancer* 1973;32:890-897.

252. Kosnik EJ, Boesel CP, Bau J, et al. Primitive neuroectodermal tumors of the central nervous system in children. *J Neurosurg* 1978;48:741-746.

253. Bennett JP, Rubinstein LJ. The biological behavior of primary cerebral neuroblastoma: a reappraisal of the clinical course in a series of 70 cases. *Ann Neurol* 1984;16:21-27.

254. Cruz-Sanchez FF, Rossi ML, Hughes JT, et al. Differentiation in embryonal neuroepithelial tumors of the central nervous system. *Cancer* 1991;67:965-976.

255. Berger MS, Edwards MSB, Wara WM, et al. Primary cerebral neuroblastoma: long-term follow-up reiew and therapeutic guidelines. *J Neurosurg* 1983;59:418-423.

256. Gaffney CC, Sloane JP, Bradley NJ, et al. Primitive neuroectodermal tumors of the cerebrum: pathology and treatment. *J Neurooncol* 1985;3:23-33.

257. Berger MS, Edwards MSB, LaMasters D, et al. Pediatric brainstem tumors: radiographic, pathological, and clinical correlations. *Neurosurgery* 1983;12:298-302.

258. Horten BC, Rubinstein LJ. Primary cerebral neuroblastoma: a clinicopathological study of 35 cases. *Brain* 1976;99:735-756.

259. Ashwal S, Hinshaw DB Jr, Bedros A. CNS primitive neuroectodermal tumors of childhood. *Med Pediatr Oncol* 1984;12:180-188.

260. Zeltzer PM, Boyett JM, Finlaye JL, et al. Metastasis stage, adjuvant treatment, and residual tumor are prognostic factors for medulloblastoma in children: conclusions from the Children's Cancer Group 921 randomized phase III study. *J Clin Oncol* 1999;17:832-845.

261. Stiller CA, Bunch KJ. Brain and spinal tumors in children aged under two years: incidence and survival in Britain, 1971-1985. *Br J Cancer* 1992;66:S50-S53.

262. Cohen BH, Packer RJ, Siegel KR, et al. Brain tumors in children under 2 years: treatment, survival and long-term prognosis. *Pediatr Neurosurg* 1993;19:171-179.

263. Brown K, Mapstone TB, Oakes WJ. A modern analysis of intracranial tumors of infancy. *Pediatr Neurosurg* 1997;26:25-32.

264. Gilles FH, Sobel EL, Tavare CJ, et al. Age-related changes in diagnoses, histological features, and survival in children with brain tumors: 1930-1979. *Neurosurgery* 1995;37:1056-1068.

265. Rorke LB, Packer RJ, Biegel JA, et al. Central nervous system atypical teratoid/rhabdoid tumors of infancy and childhood: definition of an entity. *J Neurosurg* 1996;85:56-65.

266. Burger PC, Yu I-T, Tihan T, et al. Atypical teratoid/rhabdoid tumor of the central nervous system: a highly malignant tumor of infancy and childhood frequently mistaken for medulloblastoma. A Pediatric Oncology Group study. *Am J Surg Pathol* 1998;22:1083-1092.

267. Pancelet P, Sainte-Rose C, Lellough-Tubiana A, et al. Papillomas and carcinomas of the choroid plexus in children. *J Neurosurg* 1998;88:521-528.

268. Weiss E, Behring B, Behnke J, et al. Treatment of primary malignant rhabdoid tumor of the brain: report of three cases and review of the literature. *Int J Radiat Oncol Biol Phys* 1998;41:1013-1019.

269. Taratuto AL, Monges J, Lylyk P, et al. Superficial cerebral astrocytoma attached to dura: report of six cases in infants. *Cancer* 1984;54:2505-2512.

270. Mulhern RK, Hancock J, Fairclough D, et al. Neuropsychological status of children treated for brain tumors: a critical review and integrative analysis. *Med Pediatr Oncol* 1992;20:181-191.

271. Evans AE, Jenkin RDT, Sposto R, et al. The treatment of medulloblastoma. Results of a prospective randomized trial of radiation therapy with and without CCNU, vincristine, and prednisone. *J Neurosurg* 1990;72:572-582.

272. Deutsch M. Radiotherapy for primary brain tumors in very young children. *Cancer* 1982;50:2785-2789.

273. Jenkin D, Greenberg M, Hoffman H, et al. Brain tumors in children: long-term survival after radiation therapy. *Int J Radiat Oncol Biol Phys* 1995;31:445-451.

274. Allen JC, Helson L, Jereb B. Preradiation chemotherapy for just this minute diagnosed childhood brain tumors: a modified phase II trial. *Cancer* 1983;52:2001-2006.

275. Baram TZ, van Eys J, Dowell RE, et al. Survival and neurologic outcome in infants with medulloblastoma treated with surgery and MOPP chemotherapy: a preliminary report. *Cancer* 1987;60:173-177.

276. Horowitz ME, Mulhern RK, Kun LE, et al. Brain tumors in the very young child: postoperative chemotherapy in combined-modality treatment. *Cancer* 1988;61:428-434.

277. Duffner PK, Horowitz ME, Krischer JP, et al. The treatment of malignant brain tumors in infants and very young children: an update of the Pediatric Oncology Group experience. *Neurooncology* 1999;1:152-161.

278. Geyer JR, Zeltzer PM, Boyett JM, et al. Survival of infants with primitive neuroectodermal tumors or malignant ependymomas of the CNS treated with eight drugs in 1 day: a report from the Children's Cancer Group. *J Clin Oncol* 1994;12:1607-1615.

279. Kuhl J, Beck J, Bode U, et al. Delayed radiation therapy (RT) after postoperative chemotherapy (PCH) in children less than 3 years of age with medulloblastoma. Results of the trial HIT-SKK'87, and preliminary results of the pilot trial HIT-SKK'92. *Med Pediatr Oncol* 1995;25:250.

280. Walter AW, Mulhern RK, Gajjar A, et al. Survival and neurodevelopmental outcome of young children with medulloblastoma at St. Jude Children's Research Hospital. *J Clin Oncol* 1999;17:3720-3728.

281. Dupuis-Girod S, Hartmann O, Benhamou E, et al. Will high dose chemotherapy followed by autologous bone marrow transplantation supplant craniospinal irradiation in young children treated for medulloblastoma? *J Neurooncol* 1996;27:87-98.

282. Gajjar A, Mulhern RK, Heideman RL, et al. Medulloblastoma in very young chilren: outcome of definitive craniospinal irradiation following incomplete response to chemotherapy. *J Clin Oncol* 1994;12:1212-1216.

283. Grill J, Le Deley M-C, Gambarelli D, et al. Postoperative chemotherapy without irradiation for ependymoma in children under 5 years of age: a multicenter trial of the French Society of Pediatric Oncology. *J Clin Oncol* 2001;19:1288-1296.

284. Hilden JM, Watterson J, Longee DC, et al. Central nervous system atypical teratoid tumor/rhabdoid tumor: response to intensive therapy and review of the literature. *J Neurooncol* 1998;40:265-275.

285. Kernohan JW, Sayre GP. *Tumors of the Central Nervous System.* Washington, DC: American Registry of Pathology, Armed Forces Institute of Pathology; 1952.

286. Nelson JS, Taukada Y, Schoenfeld D, et al. Necrosis as a prognostic criterion in malignant supratentorial, astrocytic gliomas. *Cancer* 1983;52:550-554.

287. Werner-Wasik M, Scott CB, Nelson DF, et al. Final report of a phase I/II trial of hyperfractionated and accelerated hyperfractionated radiation therapy with carmustine for adults with supratentorial malignant gliomas. Radiation Therapy Oncology Group study 83-02. *Cancer* 1996;77:1535-1543.

288. Burger PC, Heinz ER, Shibata T, et al. Topographic anatomy and CT correlations in the untreated glioblastoma multiforme. *J Neurosurg* 1988;68:698-704.

289. Halperin EC, Bentel G, Heinz ER, et al. Radiation therapy treatment planning in supratentorial glioblastoma multiforme: an analysis based on postmortem topographic anatomy with CT correlations. *Int J Radiat Oncol Biol Phys* 1989;17:1347-1350.

290. Kelly PJ, Daumas-Duport C, Kispert DB, et al. Imaging-based stereotaxic serial biopsies in untreated intracranial glial neoplasms. *J Neurosurg* 1987;66:865-874.

291. Choucair AK, Levin VA, Gutin PH, et al. Development of multiple lesions during radiation therapy and chemotherapy in patients with gliomas. *J Neurosurg* 1986;65:654-658.

292. Kopelson G, Linggood R. Infratentorial glioblastoma: the role of neuraxis irradiation. *Int J Radiat Oncol Biol Phys* 1982;8:999-1003.

293. Nelson DF, Nelson JS, Davis DR, et al. Survival and prognosis of patients with astrocytoma with atypical or anaplastic features. *J Neurooncol* 1985;3:99-103.

294. Walker MD, Green SB, Byar DP, et al. Randomized comparisons of radiotherapy and nitrosoureas for the treatment of malignant glioma after surgery. *N Engl J Med* 1980;303:1323-1329.

295. Prados MD, Gutin PH, Phillips TL, et al. Highly anaplastic astrocytoma: a review of 357 patients treated between 1977 and 1989. *Int J Radiat Oncol Biol Phys* 1992;23:3-8.

296. Wood JR, Green SB, Shapiro WR. The prognostic importance of tumor size in malignant gliomas: a CT scan study by the Brain Tumor Cooperative Group. *J Clin Oncol* 1988;6:338-343.

297. Wisoff JH, Boyett JM, Berger MS, et al. Current neurosurgical management and the impact of the extent of resection in the treatment of malignant gliomas of childhood: a report of the Children's Cancer Group Trial no. CCG-945. *J Neurosurg* 1998;89:52-59.

298. Garden AS, Maor MH, Yung WKA, et al. Outcome and patterns of failure following limited-volume irradiation for malignant astrocytomas. *Radiother Oncol* 1991;20:99-110.

299. Fine HA, Dear KB, Loeffler JS, et al. Meta-analysis of radiation therapy with and without adjuvant chemotherapy for malignant gliomas in adults. *Cancer* 1993;71:2585-2597.

300. Murray KJ, Nelson DF, Scott C, et al. Quality-adjusted survival analysis of malignant glioma. Patients treated with twice-daily radiation (RT) and carmustine: a report of Radiation Therapy

Oncology Group study 83-02. *Int J Radiat Oncol Biol Phys* 1995;31:453-459.

301. Sneed PK, Gutin PH, Larson DA, et al. Patterns of recurrence of glioblastoma multiforme after external irradiation followed by implant boost. *Int J Radiat Oncol Biol Phys* 1994;29:719-727.

302. Hochberg FH, Pruitt A. Assumptions in the radiotherapy of glioblastoma. *Neurology* 1980;30:907-911.

303. Wallner KE, Galicich JH, Krol G, et al. Patterns of failure following treatment for glioblastoma multiforme and anaplastic astrocytoma. *Int J Radiat Oncol Biol Phys* 1989;16:1405-1409.

304. Loeffler JS, Alexander E III, Hochberg FH, et al. Clinical patterns of failure following stereotactic interstitial irradiation for malignant gliomas. *Int J Radiat Oncol Biol Phys* 1990;19:1455-1462.

305. Agbi CB, Bernstein M, Laperriere N, et al. Patterns of recurrence of malignant astrocytoma following stereotactic interstitial brachytherapy with ^{125}I implants. *Int J Radiat Oncol Biol Phys* 1992;23:321-326.

306. Laramore GE, Diener-West M, Griffin TW, et al. Randomized neutron dose searching study for malignant gliomas of the brain: results of an RTOG study. *Int J Radiat Oncol Biol Phys* 1988;14:1093-1102.

307. Loeffler JS, Alexander E III, Wen PJ, et al. Results of stereotactic brachytherapy used in the initial management of patients with glioblastoma. *J Natl Cancer Inst* 1990;82:1918-1921.

308. Scharfen CO, Sneed PK, Wara WM, et al. High activity 1211 interstitial implant for gliomas. *Int J Radiat Oncol Biol Phys* 1992;24:583-591.

309. Prados MD, Gutin PH, Phillips TL, et al. Interstitial brachytherapy for newly diagnosed patients with malignant gliomas: the UCSF experience. *Int J Radiat Oncol Biol Phys* 1992;24:593-597.

310. Stelzer KJ, Laramore GE, Griffin TW, et al. Fast neutron radiotherapy: the University of Washington experience. *Acta Oncol* 1994;33:275-280.

311. Larson DA, Gutin PH, McDermott M, et al. Gamma knife for glioma: selection factors and survival. *Int J Radiat Oncol Biol Phys* 1996;36:1045-1053.

312. Pickles T, Goodman GB, Rheaume DE, et al. Pion radiation for high grade astrocytoma: results of a randomized study. *Int J Radiat Oncol Biol Phys* 1997;37:491-497.

313. Sneed PK, Prados MD, McDermott MW, et al. Large effect of age on survival of patients with glioblastoma treated with radiotherapy and brachytherapy boost. *Neurosurgery* 1995;36:898-904.

314. Wen PY, Alexander E III, Black PM, et al. Long-term results of stereotactic brachytherapy used in the initial treatment of patients with glioblastomas. *Cancer* 1994;73:3029-3036.

315. Shrieve DC, Alexander E III, Wen PY, et al. Comparison of stereotactic radiosurgery and brachytherapy in the treatment of recurrent glioblastoma multiforme. *Neurosurgery* 1995;36:275-284.

316. Mehta MP, Masciopinto J, Rozental J, et al. Stereotactic radiosurgery for glioblastoma multiforme: report of a prospective study evaluating prognostic factors and analyzing long-term survival advantage. *Int J Radiat Oncol Biol Phys* 1994;30:541-549.

317. Buatti JM, Friedman WA, Bova FJ, et al. Linac radiosurgery for high grade gliomas: the University of Florida experience. *Int J Radiat Oncol Biol Phys* 1995;32:205-210.

318. Nelson DF, Diener-West M, Weinstein AS, et al. A randomized comparison of misonidazole sensitized radiotherapy plus BCNU and radiotherapy plus BCNU for treatment of malignant glioma after surgery: final report of an RTOG study. *Int J Radiat Oncol Biol Phys* 1986;12:1793-1800.

319. Urtusan R, Band P, Chapman JD, et al. Radiation and high-dose metronidazole in supratentorial glioblastomas. *N Engl J Med* 1976;294:1364-1367.

320. Mirabell R, Mornex F, Greiner R, et al. Accelerated radiotherapy, carbogen, and nicotinamide in glioblastoma multiforme: report of European Organization for Research and Treatment of Cancer Trial 22933. *J Clin Oncol* 1999;17:3143-3149.

321. Hegarty TJ, Thornton AF, Diaz RF, et al. Intraarterial bromodeoxyuridine radiosensitization of malignant gliomas. *Int J Radiat Oncol Biol Phys* 1990;19:421-428.

322. Sullivan FJ, Herscher LL, Cook JA, et al. National Cancer Institute (phase II) study of high-grade glioma treated with accelerated hyperfractionated radiation and iododeoxyuridine: results in anaplastic astrocytoma. *Int J Radiat Oncol Biol Phys* 1994;30:583-590.

323. Groves MD, Maor MH, Meyers C, et al. A phase II trial of high-dose bromodeoxyuridine with accelerated fractionation radiotherapy followed by procarbazine, lomustine, and vincristine for glioblastoma multiforme. *Int J Radiat Oncol Biol Phys* 1999;45:127-135.

324. Prados MD, Scott C, Sandler H, et al. A phase 3 randomized study of radiotherapy plus procarbazine, CCNU, vincristine (PCV) with or without BrdU for the treatment of anaplastic astrocytoma: a preliminary report of the Radiation Therapy Oncology Group study 9404. *Int J Radiat Oncol Biol Phys* 1999;45:1109-1115.

325. Saroja KR, Mansell J, Hendrickson FR, et al. Failure of accelerated neutron therapy to control high grade astrocytomas. *Int J Radiat Oncol Biol Phys* 1989;17:1295-1297.

326. Fitzek MM, Thornton AF, Rabinov JD, et al. Accelerated proton/photon irradiaton to 90 cobalt gray equivalent for glioblastoma multiforme: results of a phase II prospective trial. *J Neurosurg* 1999;91:251-260.

327. Leibel SA, Gutin PH, Wara WM, et al. Survival and quality of life after interstitial implantation of removable high-activity 1211 sources for treatment of patients with recurrent malignant gliomas. *Int J Radiat Oncol Biol Phys* 1989;17:1129-1139.

328. Selker RG, Shapiro WR, Green S, et al. A randomized trial of interstitial radiotherapy (IRT) boost for the treatment of newly diagnosed malignant glioma (glioblastoma multiforme, anaplastic astrocytoma, anaplastic oligodendroglioma, malignant mixed glioma): Brain Tumor Cooperative Group study 87-01 [abstract]. Paper presented at: *Forty-fifth Meeting of the Congress of Neurological Surgeons*; October 14-18, 1995; San Francisco.

329. Florell RC, MacDonald DR, Irish W, et al. Selection bias, survival, and brachytherapy for glioma. *J Neurosurg* 1992;76:179-183.

330. Loeffler JSI, Alexander E III, Shea WM, et al. Radiosurgery as part of the initial management of patients with malignant gliomas. *J Clin Oncol* 1992;10:1379-1385.

331. Sankaria JN, Mehta MP, Loeffler JS, et al. Radiosurgery in the initial management of malignant gliomas: survival comparison with the Radiation Therapy Oncology Group recursive partitioning analysis. *Int J Radiat Oncol Biol Phys* 1995;32:931-942.

332. Nelson DF, Curran WJ Jr, Scott C, et al. Hyperfractionated radiation therapy and BIS-chlorethyl nitrosourea in the treatment of malignant glioma: possible advantage observed at 72 Gy in 1.2 Gy bid fractions: report of the Radiation Therapy Oncology Group protocol 8302. *Int J Radiat Oncol Biol Phys* 1993;25:193-207.

333. Fallia C, Olmi P. Hyperfractionated and accelerated radiation therapy in central nervous system tumors (malignant gliomas, pediatric tumors, and brain metastases). *Radiother Oncol* 1997;43:235-246.

334. Brada M, Sharpe G, Rajan B, et al. Modifying radical radiotherapy in high grade gliomas: shortening the treatment through acceleration. *Int J Radiat Oncol Biol Phys* 1999;43:287-292.

335. Levin VA, Maor MH, Thall PF, et al. Phase II study of accelerated fractionation radiation therapy with carboplatin followed by vincristine chemotherapy for the treatment of glioblastoma multiforme. *Int J Radiat Oncol Biol Phys* 1995;33:357-364.

336. Halperin EC. Multiple-fraction-per-day external beam radiotherapy for adults with supratentorial malignant gliomas. *J Neurooncol* 1992;14:255-262.

337. Fulton DS, Urtasun RC, Scott-Brown I, et al. Increasing radiation dose intensity using hyperfractionation on patients with malignant glioma: final report of a prospective phase I-II dose response study. *J Neurooncol* 1992;14:63-72.

338. Shapiro WR, Green SB, Burger PC, et al. Randomized trial of three chemotherapy regimens and two radiotherapy regimens in postoperative treatment of malignant glioma: Brain Tumor Cooperative Group Trial no. 8001. *J Neurosurg* 1989;71:1-9.

339. Levin VA, Silver P, Hannigan J, et al. Superiority of post-radiotherapy adjuvant chemotherapy with CCNU, procarbazine, and vincristine (PCV) over BCNU for anaplastic gliomas: NCOG 6G61 final report. *Int J Radiat Oncol Biol Phys* 1990;18:321-324.

340. Medical Research Council Brain Tumour Working Party. Randomized trial of procarbazine, lomustine, and vincristine in the adjuvant treatment of high-grade astrocytoma: a Medical Research Council Trial. *J Clin Oncol* 2001;19:509-518.

341. del Rowe J, Scott C, Werner-Wasik M, et al. Single-arm, open-label phase II study of intravenously administered Tirapazamine and radiation therapy for glioblastoma multiforme. *J Clin Oncol* 2000;18:1254-1259.

342. Valtonen S, Timonen U, Toivanan P, et al. Interstitial chemotherapy with carmustine-loaded polymers for high-grade gliomas: a randomized double-blind study. *Neurosurgery* 1997;41:44-49.

343. Nakagawa K, Aoki Y, Fujimaki T, et al. High-dose conformal radiotherapy influenced the pattern of failure but did not improve survival in glioblastoma multiforme. *Int J Radiat Oncol Biol Phys* 1998;40:1141-1149.

344. Sheline GE. Radiotherapy for high grade gliomas. *Int J Radiat Oncol Biol Phys* 1990;18:793-803.

345. Yung WKA, Janus TJ, Maor M, et al. Adjuvant chemotherapy with carmustine and cisplatin for patients with malignant gliomas. *J Neurooncol* 1992;12:131-135.

346. Heideman RL, Kuttesch J, Gajjar AJ, et al. Supratentorial malignant gliomas in childhood: a single institution perspective. *Cancer* 1997;80:497-504.

347. Finlay JL, Boyett JM, Yates AJ, et al. Randomized phase III trial in childhood high-grade astrocytoma comparing vincristine, lomustine, and prednisone with the eight-drugs-in-1 regimen. *J Clin Oncol* 1995;13:112-123.

348. Mork SJ, Lindegaard K-F, Halvorsen TB, et al. Oligodendroglioma: incidence and biological behavior in a defined population. *J Neurosurg* 1985;63:881-889.

349. Shaw EG, Scheithauer BW, O'Fallon JR, et al. Oligodendrogliomas: the Mayo Clinic experience. *J Neurosurg* 1992;76:428-434.

350. Shaw EG, Scheithauer BW, O'Fallon JR. Management of supratentorial low-grade gliomas. *Oncology* 1993;7:97-107.

351. Sheline GE, Boldney E, Karisburg P, et al. Therapeutic considerations in tumors affecting the central nervous system: oligodendrogliomas. *Radiology* 1964;82:44-49.

352. Chin HW, Hazel JJ, Kim TH, et al. Oligodendrogliomas. I. a clinical study of cerebral oligodendrogliomas. *Cancer* 1980;45:1458-1466.

353. Lindegaard K-F, Mork SJ, Eide GE, et al. Statistical analysis of clinicopathological features, radiotherapy, and survival in 270 cases of oligodendroglioma. *J Neurosurg* 1987;67:224-230.

354. Reedy PD, Bay JW, Hahn JF. Role of radiation therapy in the treatment of cerebral oligodendroglioma: an analysis of 57 cases and a literature review. *Neurosurgery* 1983;67:224-230.

355. Allison RR, Schulsinger A, Vongtama V, et al. Radiation and chemotherapy improve outcome in oligodendroglioma. *Int J Radiat Oncol Biol Phys* 1997;37:399-403.

356. Ludwig CL, Smith MT, Godfrey AD, et al. A clinicopathological study of 323 patients with oligodendrogliomas. *Ann Neurol* 1986;19:15-21.

357. Cairncross JG, MacDonald DR. Successful chemotherapy for recurrent malignant oligodendroglioma. *Ann Neurol* 1988;23:460-464.

358. Cushing H, Eisenhardt L. *Meningiomas: Their Classification, Regional Behavior, Life History, and Surgical End Results.* Springfield, IL: Charles C Thomas; 1938.

359. Glaholm J, Bloom HJG, Crow JH. The role of radiotherapy in the management of intracranial meningiomas: the Royal Marsden Hospital experience with 186 patients. *Int J Radiat Oncol Biol Phys* 1990;18:755-761.

360. Dziuk T, Woo S, Butler B, et al. Malignant meningioma: an indication for initial aggressive surgery and adjuvant radiotherapy. *J Neurooncol* 1998;37:177-188.

361. Jaaskelainen J, Haltia M, Servo A. Atypical and anaplastic meningiomas: radiology, surgery, radiotherapy, and outcome. *Surg Neurol* 1986;25:233-242.

362. Mirimanoff RO, Rosoretz DE, Linggood RM, et al. Meningioma: analysis of recurrence and progression following neurosurgical resection. *J Neurosurg* 1985;62:18-24.

363. Goldsmith BJ, Wara WM, Wilson CB, et al. Postoperative irradiation for subtotally resected meningiomas. A retrospective analysis of 140 patients treated from 1967 to 1990. *J Neurosurg* 1994;80:195-201.

364. Petty AM, Kun LE, Meyer GA. Radiation therapy for incompletely resected meningiomas. *J Neurosurg* 1985;62:502-507.

365. Wara WM, Sheline GE, Newman H, et al. Radiation therapy of meningiomas. *AJR Am J Roentgenol* 1975;123:453-458.

366. Carelia RJ, Ransohoff J, Newall J. Role of radiation therapy in the management of meningioma. *Neurosurgery* 1982;10:332-339.

367. Forbes AR, Goldberg ID. Radiation therapy in the treatment of meningioma: the Joint Center for Radiation Therapy experience, 1970 to 1982. *J Clin Oncol* 1984;2:1139-1143.

368. Maguire PD, Clough R, Friedman AH, et al. Fractionated external-beam radiation therapy for meningiomas of the cavernous sinus. *Int J Radiat Oncol Biol Phys* 1999;44:75-79.

369. Lunsford L. Contemporary management of meningiomas: radiation therapy as an adjuvant and radiosurgery as an alternative to surgical removal? *J Neurosurg* 1994;80:187-190.

370. Kondziolka D, Flickinger JC, Perez B. Judicious resection and/or radiosurgery for parasagittal meningiomas: outcomes from a multicenter review. *Neurosurgery* 1998;43:405-413.

371. Kondziolka D, Levy EI, Niranjan A, et al. Long-term outcomes after meningioma radiosurgery: physician and patient perspectives. *J Neurosurg* 1999;91:44-50.

372. Shafron DH, Friedman WA, Buatti JM, et al. Linac radiosurgery for benign meningiomas. *Int J Radiat Oncol Biol Phys* 1999;43:321-327.

373. Smith JL, Vuksanovic MM, Yates BM, et al. Radiation therapy for primary optic nerve meningiomas. *J Clin Neuroophthalmol* 1981;1:85-89.

374. Borovich B, Doron Y, Braun J, et al. Recurrence of intracranial meningiomas: the role played by regional multicentricity. Clinical and radiological aspects. *J Neurosurg* 1986;65(pt 2):168-171.

375. Roche P-H, Regis J, Dufour H, et al. Gamma knife radiosurgery in the management of cavernous sinus meningiomas. *J Neurosurg* 2000;93:68-73.

376. Ojemann SG, Sneed PK, Larson DA, et al. Radiosurgery for malignant meningioma: results in 22 patients. *J Neurosurg* 2000;93:62-67.

377. Deen HC Jr, Scheithauer BW, Ebersold MJ. Clinical and pathologic study of meningiomas of the first two decades of life. *J Neurosurg* 1982;56:317-322.

378. Drake JM, Hendrick EB, Becker LE, et al. Intracranial meningiomas in children. *Pediatr Neurosci* 1986;12:134-139.

379. Snow RB, Lavyne MH. Intracranial space-occupying lesions in AIDS patients. *Neurosurgery* 1985;16:148-153.

380. So YT, Beckstead JH, Davis RL. Primary central nervous system lymphoma in AIDS: a clinical and pathologic study. *Ann Neurol* 1986;20:566-S72.

381. Reni M, Ferreri AJ, Garancini MP, et al. Therapeutic management of primary central nervous system lymphoma in immunocompetent patients: results of a critical review of the literature. *Ann Oncol* 1997;8:227-234.

382. Jack CR, Reese DF, Scheithauer BW. Radiographic findings in 32 cases of primary CNS lymphoma. *AJR Am J Roentgenol* 1986; 146:271-276.

383. Hochberg FH, Miller DC. Primary central nervous system lymphoma. *J Neurosurg* 1988;68:835-853.

384. Murray K, Kun L, Cox J. Primary malignant lymphoma of the central nervous system. *J Neurosurg* 1986;65:600-607.

385. Socie G, Piprot-Chauffat C, Schlienger M, et al. Primary lymphoma of the central nervous system: an unresolved therapeutic problem. *Cancer* 1990;65:322-326.

386. Nelson DF, Martz KL, Bonner H, et al. Non-Hodgkin's lymphoma of the brain: can high-dose, large-volume radiation therapy improve survival? Report on a prospective trial by the Radiation Therapy Oncology Group study 8315. *Int J Radiat Oncol Biol Phys* 1992;23:9-17.

387. Loeffler JS, Ervin TJ, Mauch P, et al. Primary lymphomas of the central nervous system: patterns of failure and factors that influence survival. *J Clin Oncol* 1985;3:490-494.

388. Laperriere NJ, Cerezo L, Milosevic MF, et al. Primary lymphoma of brain: results of management of a modern cohort with radiation therapy. *Radiother Oncol* 1997;43:247-252.

389. Glass J, Gruber ML, Cher L, et al. Preirradiation methotrexate chemotherapy of primary central nervous system lymphoma: long-term outcome. *J Neurosurg* 1994;81:188-195.

390. Abrey LE, DeAngelis LM, Yahalom J. Long-term survival in primary CNS lymphoma. *J Clin Oncol* 1998;16:859-863.

391. Abrey LE, Yahalom J, DeAngelis LM. Treatment for primary CNS lymphoma: the next step. *J Clin Oncol* 2000;18: 3144-3150.

392. Schultz C, Scott C, Sherman W, et al. Preirradiation chemotherapy with cyclophosphamide, doxorubicin, vincristine, and dexamethasone for primary CNS lymphomas: initial report of Radiation Therapy Oncology Group Protocol 88-06. *J Clin Oncol* 1996;14:556-564.

393. O'Neill BP, Wang C-H, O'Fallon JR, et al. Primary central nervous system non-Hodgkin's lymphoma (PCNSL): Survival advantages with combined initial therapy? A final report of the North Central Cancer Treatment Group study 86-72-52. *Int J Radiat Oncol Biol Phys* 1999;43:559-563.

394. Ferreri AJM, Reni M, Villa E. Therapeutic management of primary central nervous system lymphoma: lessons from prospective trials. *Ann Oncol* 2000;11:927-937.

395. Posner JB. Management of central nervous system metastases. *Semin Oncol* 1977;4:81-91.

396. Pickren JW, Lopez G, Tsukada Y, et al. Brain metastases: an autopsy study. *Cancer Treatment Symposia* 1983;2:295-313.

397. Gaspar L, Scott C, Rotman M, et al. Recursive partitioning analysis (RPA) of prognostic factors in three Radiation Therapy Oncology Group brain metastases trials. *Int J Radiat Oncol Biol Phys* 1997;37:745-751.

398. Swift PS, Phillips T, Martz K, et al. CT characteristics of patients with brain metastases treated in Radiation Therapy Oncology Group study 79-16. *Int J Radiat Oncol Biol Phys* 1993;25:209-214.

399. Smalley SR, Laws ER Jr, O'Fallon JR, et al. Resection for solitary brain metastasis: role of adjuvant radiation and prognostic variables in 229 patients. *J Neurosurg* 1992;77:531-540.

400. Shaw EG. Radiotherapeutic management of multiple brain metastases: "3000 in 10" whole brain radiation is no longer a "no brainer." *Int J Radiat Oncol Biol Phys* 1999;45:253-254.

401. Auchter RM, Lamond JP, Alexander E III, et al. A multi-institutional outcome and prognostic factor analysis of radiosurgery for resectable single brain metastasis. *Int J Radiat Oncol Biol Phys* 1996;35:27-35.

402. Patchell RA, Tibbs PA, Walsh JW, et al. A randomized trial of surgery in the treatment of single metastases to the brain. *N Engl J Med* 1990;322:494-500.

403. Alexander E III, Moriarty TM, Davis RB, et al. Stereotactic radiosurgery for the definitive, noninvasive treatment of brain metastases. *J Natl Cancer Inst* 1995;87:34-40.

404. Flickinger JC, Kondziolka D, Lunsford LD, et al. A multi-institutional experience with stereotactic radiosurgery for resectable single brain metastasis. *Int J Radiat Oncol Biol Phys* 1994;28:797-802.

405. Smalley SR, Laws ER Jr, O'Fallon JR, et al. Resection for solitary brain metastasis: role of adjuvant radiation and prognostic variables in 229 patients. *J Neurosurg* 1992;77:531-540.

406. Choi KN, Withers HR, Rotman M. Intracranial metastases from melanoma: clinical features and treatment by accelerated fractionation. *Cancer* 1985;56:1-9.

407. Weltman E, Salvajoli JV, Brandt RA, et al. Radiosurgery for brain metastases: a score index for predicting prognosis. *Int J Radiat Oncol Biol Phys* 2000;46:1155-1161.

408. Mork SJ, Loken AC. Ependymoma: a follow-up study of 101 cases. *Cancer* 1977;40:907-915.

409. McCormick PC, Torres R, Post KD, et al. Intramedullary ependymoma of the spinal cord. *J Neurosurg* 1990;72:523-532.

410. Reimer R, Onofrio BM. Astrocytomas of the spinal cord in children and adolescents. *J Neurosurg* 1985;63:669-675.

411. Kopelson G, Linggood RM, Leinman GM, et al. Management of intramedullary spinal cord tumors. *Radiology* 1980;135:473-479.

412. Chun HC, Schmidt-Ulrich RK, Wolfson A, et al. External beam radiotherapy for primary spinal cord tumors. *J Neurooncol* 1990; 9:211-217.

413. Guidetti B, Mercuri S, Vagnozzi R. Long-term results of the surgical treatment of 129 intramedullary spinal gliomas. *J Neurosurg* 1981;54:323-330.

414. Cooper PR, Epstein F. Radical resection of intramedullary spinal cord tumors in adults: recent experience in 29 patients. *J Neurosurg* 1985;63:492-499.

415. Epstein J. Spinal cord astrocytomas of childhood. *Prog Exp Tumor Res* 1987;30:135-153.

416. Epstein FJ, Farmer J-P, Freed D. Adult intramedullary astrocytomas of the spinal cord. *J Neurosurg* 1992;77:355-359.

417. Epstein F, McCleary EL. Intrinsic brain-stem tumors of childhood: surgical indications. *J Neurosurg* 1986;64:11-15.

418. Epstein F. Intraaxial tumors of the cervicomedullary junction in children. *Concepts Pediatr Neurosurg* 1987;7:117.

419. Kopelson G, Linggood RM, Kleinman GM, et al. Management of intramedullary spinal cord tumors. *Radiology* 1980;135:473-479.

420. O'Sullivan C, Jenkin RD, Doherty MA, et al. Spinal cord tumors in children: long-term results of combined surgical and radiation treatment. *J Neurosurg* 1994;81:507-512.

421. Kopelson G. Radiation tolerance of the spinal cord previously damaged by tumor and operation: long term neurological improvement and time-dose-volume relationships after irradiation of intraspinal gliomas. *Int J Radiat Oncol Biol Phys* 1982;8:925-929.

422. Shaw EG, Evans RG, Scheitghauer BW, et al. Radiotherapeutic management of adult intraspinal ependymomas. *Int J Radiat Oncol Biol Phys* 1986;12:323-327.

423. Garcia DM. Primary spinal cord tumors treated with surgery and postoperative irradiation. *Int J Radiat Oncol Biol Phys* 1985;11: 1933-1939.

424. Bryne TN. Spinal cord compression from epidural metastases. *N Engl J Med* 1992;327:614-619.

425. Rodichok LD, Harper GR, Ruckdeschel JC, et al. Early diagnosis of spinal epidural metastases. *Am J Med* 1981;70:1181-1188.

426. Young RF, Post EM, King GA. Treatment of spinal epidural metastases. *J Neurosurg* 1980;53:741-748.

427. Sorensen PS, Borgesen SE, Rohde K, et al. Metastatic epidural spinal cord compression: results of treatment and survival. *Cancer* 1990;65:1502-1508.

428. Latini P, Maranzano E, Ricci S, et al. Role of radiotherapy in metastatic spinal cord compression: preliminary results from a prospective trial. *Radiother Oncol* 1989;15:227-233.

429. Sundaresan N, Galicich JH, Lane JM, et al. Treatment of neoplastic epidural cord compression by vertebral body resection and stabilization. *J Neurosurg* 1985;63:676-684.

430. Siegal T, Seigal T. Surgical decompression of anterior and posterior malignant epidural tumors compressing the spinal cord: a prospective study. *Neurosurgery* 1985;17:424-432.

431. Herbert SH, Solin LJ, Rate WR, et al. The effect of palliative radiation therapy on epidural compression due to metastatic malignant melanoma. *Cancer* 1991;67:2472-2476.

432. Olsen ME, Chernik NL, Posner JB. Infiltration of the leptomeninges by systemic cancer. *Arch Neurol* 1974;30:122-137.

PART XI

Leukemia, Lymphoma, and Hodgkin's Disease

CHAPTER 33

Leukemias and Lymphomas

James D. Cox, Chul S. Ha, and Richard B. Wilder

RESPONSE OF NORMAL HEMATOPOIETIC TISSUES TO IRRADIATION

As noted in Chapter 1, the hematopoietic stem cells are among the most exquisitely radiosensitive cells in the body. Total body irradiation produces profound changes in the bone marrow, changes that are reflected in the peripheral blood at varying intervals after irradiation. Similar doses delivered to whole blood in vitro produce few immediate or delayed effects.[1] The changes in the peripheral blood reflect the effects of radiation on the blood-forming organs, not on the circulating cells themselves. Lymphopenia has been demonstrated after extracorporeal irradiation of the peripheral blood,[2] but doses several orders of magnitude higher than those that cause bone marrow effects are required to have any influence on the other elements of the peripheral blood. The following discussion is confined to the clinically important changes produced by doses and types of ionizing radiation that might be encountered in the clinical setting.

Bone Marrow

A voluminous literature is available concerning the effects of whole-body irradiation in laboratory animals. Thus the single total body irradiation dose that is lethal in 30 days to 50% of a group of laboratory animals, the $LD_{50/30}$, is clearly defined for most mammals. For obvious reasons, little information is available for humans, and most of that comes from accidental exposures in which the dose to the bone marrow has been estimated with a greater or lesser degree of certainty.

Tubiana and colleagues[3-6] have provided the most definitive data from their experiences with using total body irradiation for immunosuppression purposes in the first renal transplantation attempts in Europe between 1959 and 1962. Forty-one patients received total body doses ranging from 1 to 6 Gy in one or two fractions. Patients were maintained in a controlled environment until leukocyte levels returned to normal. The investigators observed that the initial decrease in the peripheral blood counts was more rapid and the nadir was reached sooner with higher doses. They concluded that the LD_{50} in humans is higher than 4.5 Gy.

The larger experience with single-dose or fractionated irradiation followed by bone marrow transplantation[7,8] is somewhat more difficult to interpret because most patients treated with lethal doses followed by bone marrow reconstitution had primary disease processes that affected the bone marrow.[9,10]

Bloom[11] carefully studied the changes in rabbit bone marrow after total body irradiation. Mitosis in the marrow ceased 30 minutes after a dose of 3.5 Gy. Numbers of nucleated red cells had begun to decrease, and more mature forms predominated. The megakaryocytes remained normal in number and appearance at first but disappeared in 2 days. The rather abrupt and nearly simultaneous regeneration of platelets, reticulocytes, and granulocytes suggested a rapid proliferation of a multipotent stem cell with accelerated differentiation during the fourth week after total body irradiation.

Local irradiation of limited amounts of bone marrow is associated with recovery of the marrow that is faster than recovery after total body irradiation. Knospe and colleagues[12] gave single doses of 20, 40, 60, or 100 Gy to the hind limbs of rats and examined the marrow at intervals up to 1 year. Regeneration of the bone marrow began 7 to 14 days after irradiation regardless of the dose, but the degree of cellularity at any time was dose-dependent. During the second and third months after irradiation, sinusoidal disruption and disappearance were noted in all irradiated marrow specimens. This was associated with the maximum decrease in bone marrow cellularity. After 6 months, marrow regeneration was evident only in those animals that received 20 Gy or less, and this recovery followed regeneration of sinusoidal structures. This observation suggests that hematopoietic recovery depends on regeneration of the microcirculation of the bone marrow. Fishburn and colleagues[13] demonstrated that marrow in juvenile rats could repopulate with higher levels of cellularity and after higher radiation doses than could the marrow from adult rodents.

In humans, locally irradiated marrow shows a marked decrease in cellularity after being exposed to 4 Gy over a 3-day period.[14] After a dose of 10 Gy given over 8 days, complete disappearance of normoblasts and early granulocytes occurs, along with a significant reduction in marrow cellularity. Some mature granulocytes persist after a dose of 20 Gy given over 16 days, but megakaryocytes are absent. No suppression of the unirradiated bone marrow is evident. Indeed, Morardet and colleagues[15,16] found regeneration of the marrow to be dependent not only on the absorbed dose but also on the volume of bone marrow irradiated. With lesser volumes irradiated (20% to 30% of the bone marrow), recovery was less complete than when the volume of irradiated marrow was larger (equal to or greater than 60%). They suggested that this difference in regeneration was the result of increased stimulation of hematopoiesis caused by the inability of the unirradiated marrow to achieve sufficient production.

Knowledge of the distribution of active marrow is useful in anticipating the magnitude of the effects of irradiating various sites in clinical practice. The best available information in this regard is the work of Ellis[17] (Table 33-1). Approximately 40% of the active bone marrow in the adult is in the pelvis, and an additional 25% is located in the thoracic and lumbar vertebrae. The significance of this distribution is obvious in the extensive treatment of patients with Hodgkin's disease or follicular lymphomas. In children, a relatively greater amount of active bone marrow is present in the long bones (45% at age 5 years), but this rapidly decreases in adolescence. After age 20, negligible amounts of active bone marrow are present in the long bones.[17,18]

High local doses such as those administered routinely in clinical radiation therapy may produce sufficient bone marrow injury that repopulation never occurs. Sykes and colleagues[19,20] found failure of repopulation in the sternal bone marrow at doses of approximately 30 Gy, but doses up to 25 Gy consistently produced regeneration within 1 month. Total doses in excess of 40 Gy with common fractionation presumably produce bone marrow ablation. The failure of recovery is undoubtedly related to disruption of the microcirculation of the marrow. When the bone marrow is not repopulated, the predominant picture is one of fatty replacement. Despite the inability of the bone marrow to repopulate, it can support the growth of metastatic cancer.[19,20]

The study of bone marrow regeneration after total nodal irradiation for Hodgkin's disease indicates that total doses of 40 Gy or more produce prolonged suppression of marrow that can continue for at least 1 year.[21,22] In 27 patients studied with bone marrow scanning agents, Rubin and colleagues[21,22] reported that 50% showed evidence of partial or complete regeneration at 1 year, and 80% showed regeneration at 2 or 3 years after irradiation. They described redistribution of bone marrow activity in half of the patients studied. Sacks and colleagues[23] used ^{111}In to evaluate the bone marrow of 48 patients, ages 15 to 69 years, given radiation therapy for a variety of malignant disease (three fourths of which were Hodgkin's neoplasms). They found that local marrow regeneration was influenced by the total dose, the age of the patient, and the total amount of bone marrow irradiated. Regeneration was noted in 25 of 31 patients who underwent treatment of bone marrow on both sides of the diaphragm compared with only one of 11 patients who underwent treatment of bone marrow on only one side of the diaphragm. These findings are in keeping with that of greater stimulation of marrow regeneration with larger treatment volumes described by Morardet and colleagues.[15,16]

Changes in the Peripheral Blood After Total Body Irradiation

Normally a delicate balance exists among the life span of the circulating blood cells, the rate of replacement of these cells, and the body's demand for them. Irradiation of hematopoietic tissues upsets this balance by reducing or interrupting the supply of blood cells. Leukopenia, granulocytopenia, anemia, and thrombocytopenia develop at rates that depend on the severity of the damage and the normal life span of the circulating cells. The postirradiation fluctuations of leukocyte counts and the percentages of granulocytes, erythrocytes, and platelets are shown graphically in Figure 37-1. The extreme sensitivity of lymphopoietic tissue manifests early as a rapid lymphocytopenia. The degree to which the short life span of the lymphocyte and its unique characteristic of undergoing interphase death explain this change in peripheral lymphocyte counts is unclear. Granulocyte counts change more slowly. They are little altered by a total body irradiation dose of 0.5 Gy, but they change to a greater degree and more rapidly as the total-body radiation dose increases (see Fig. 37-2).

Platelets

Megakaryocytes, from which platelets are produced, are the least radiosensitive of the myeloid elements. Platelets have a circulating life of 8 to 11 days. Radiation damage to megakaryocytes is reflected in the circulating blood in 2 to 3 days. The nadir of thrombocytopenia is reached approximately 2 weeks after a single large dose of total body irradiation (see Fig. 37-1), and recovery begins

TABLE 33-1

Distribution of Active Bone Marrow in the Adult

Site	Total Red Marrow (%)
Head	13.1
Upper limb girdle	8.3
Sternum	2.3
Ribs	7.9
Vertebrae, cervical	3.4
Vertebrae, thoracic	14.1
Vertebrae, lumbar	10.9
Sacrum	13.9
Lower limb girdle	26.1

From Ellis RE. *Phys Med Biol* 1961;5:255-258.

at about 3 weeks. Unlike their precursors, circulating platelets are resistant to high doses of radiation (75 Gy).[24]

Red Blood Cells

Circulating red blood cells, like other circulating formed elements, are resistant to direct damage by irradiation. The normal red cell has an average circulating life span of 120 days. After total body irradiation, the red cell count decreases more slowly and returns to normal earlier than do the other formed elements. In clinical radiation therapy, anemia rarely results from a course of radiation therapy.

When fractionated low-dose total body irradiation is given over a period of many months or years, an entirely different picture is seen in the peripheral blood. The highly radiosensitive erythropoietic stem cells are not allowed to recover, and anemia develops in addition to leukopenia. The exact dose levels necessary to produce these changes in humans are not known. Total doses above 20 Gy have been achieved with fractionated total body irradiation for chronic lymphocytic leukemia.[25]

Lymph Nodes

A vasculoconnective tissue framework serves as the supporting structure for lymphocytes and lymphoblasts within the lymph nodes. Lymph enters the nodes through sinuses and passes between lymphocytes and macrophages, some of which are phagocytic. Each of the cellular elements (e.g., lymphocytes, macrophages, endothelial cells) exhibits a different radiosensitivity. Thus the cells that constitute the lymphopoietic tissues vary considerably in their sensitivity to ionizing radiation.

The response of the lymphoid tissue in the rabbit is representative of this variation.[26] Within half an hour of delivering an $LD_{50/30}$ dose to rabbits (a total body dose of approximately 8 Gy), nuclear debris appears in the lymph node and rapidly increases to a maximum at 8 hours. Macrophages are not noticeably altered, but they become active phagocytically as the debris appears. Most of the debris is phagocytized in 20 hours (Fig. 33-1). Within 24 hours, the fibrovascular framework and macrophages dominate the picture; hemorrhagic areas

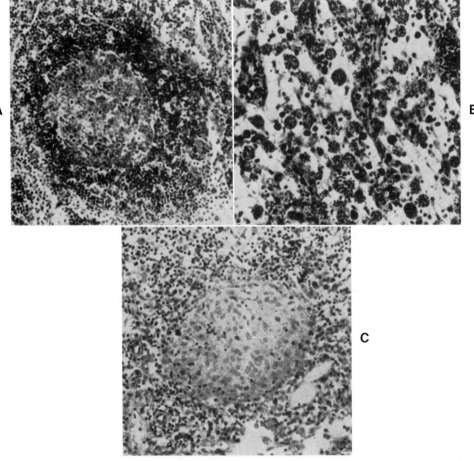

Fig. 33-1 Response of mesenteric lymph node of the rabbit to irradiation. **A,** Normal nodule with active germinal center. (×245) **B,** Seventeen hours after a single dose of 800 roentgens. (×245) **C,** Twenty-four hours after a single dose of 800 roentgens. (×245) (Courtesy United States Atomic Energy Commission.) (From De Bruyn PPH. Lymph node and intestinal tissue. In: Bloom W, ed. *Histopathology of Irradiation.* New York, NY: McGraw-Hill; 1948.)

and perivascular edema can be seen. Approximately 5 days after the single-dose total body irradiation, lymphocytes begin to reappear in the lymph node. Plasma cells are seen about 9 days after irradiation but become less numerous several weeks later. Three weeks after the $LD_{50/30}$ dose, lymphopoiesis is observed in cortical areas, and by 4 months the lymph node looks normal histologically.

With smaller doses, destruction is less complete and the return to normal is more rapid. For example, after 0.5 Gy, the lymph node appears normal in 27 hours. Engeset[27] described the effects of local irradiation with 30 Gy given to the popliteal lymph nodes of rats. The same processes were evident as in the rabbit, but lymphocytic repopulation was evident at 24 hours; by 48 hours the nuclear debris had disappeared. Although recovery was nearly complete 1 week after irradiation, chronic changes appeared after 2 weeks. A gradual increase in connective tissue and progressive decreases in germinal centers and cortical lymphocytes were observed. One year after irradiation, the normal lymph node architecture was almost completely disrupted.

In addition to changing lymphopoietic function, moderately high radiation doses also affect the reticuloendothelial elements. Doses of 20 to 30 Gy diminish their functions, and doses of 65 Gy abolish them.[28] However, even this high dose produced no obstruction to the flow of lymph through the nodes. However, functional changes in reticuloendothelial elements do occur. Several investigators[27,29-32] have evaluated the ability of locally irradiated lymph nodes to remove particulate material (e.g., tumor cells, erythrocytes, charcoal particles, or colloidal gold) infused into the afferent lymphatics. Most of these studies suggest that the barrier function of nodes is reduced. However, these experiments involved the use of a few large fractions and evaluated immediate effects. Correlation of these changes with those expected in the clinical setting are lacking. Transient suppression of lymph-node function undoubtedly occurs in the clinical setting, but with the usual clinical fractionation and moderate or even high total doses, lymph nodes seem to recover rather completely (Fig. 33-2).

Lymphatic vessels are resistant to doses of radiation that are sufficient to produce cutaneous and subcutaneous necrosis in the hind limb of dogs.[33] Nineteen months after conventional x-irradiation (36 Gy in three fractions in 14 days), Sherman and O'Brien[33] demonstrated normal lymphatics in the irradiated zone of animals that had developed extensive soft-tissue necroses. Confirmation of the resistance of lymphatic vessels to irradiation has been provided by Engeset[27] and Lenzi and Bassani.[34] Although irradiation has been implicated as a direct cause of lymphatic obstruction, evidence of obliteration of lymphatic vessels is rarely seen clinically except when the lymph node was known to be involved by cancer or when surgical intervention had interrupted normal lymphatic pathways. In such circumstances, lymphedema may develop as a result of fibrosis or enhancement of postoperative scarring.

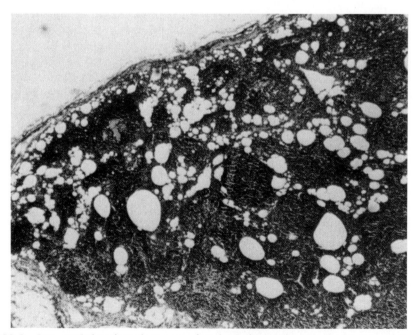

Fig. 33-2 Para-aortic lymph node 3 years after dose of 35 Gy in 4 weeks for metastatic seminoma. The nodal anatomy appears well preserved. The capsular and medullar sinusoids contain lipid droplets from a recent lymphangiogram. An embryonal carcinoma was discovered in the remaining testicle. (×160)

Spleen

The response of the spleen to ionizing radiation is very similar to that of the lymph nodes. The white pulp is similar in structure to lymph nodes, and the red pulp contains the remaining formed elements of whole blood. In humans, lymphopoiesis normally occurs in the white pulp of the spleen. Granulopoiesis occurs in the red pulp of the spleen in rabbits, rats, and mice (and in humans in certain abnormal conditions), thereby providing the opportunity to study the relative radio-sensitivity of lymphopoiesis and granulopoiesis side by side.

Murray[35] described the morphologic changes in the spleen after a total body radiation dose of approximately 8 Gy in the rabbit. As noted above for the bone marrow, mitosis ceases within 30 minutes of this $LD_{50/30}$ dose. By 3 hours, the white pulp retains only a few lymphocytes, and by 8 hours, the reticular cells show nuclear abnormalities, but they do not die. During this same period, destruction becomes evident in all elements of the red pulp except reticular cells and the cells of the circulating blood. Lymphopoiesis is reestablished in about 9 days, erythroblasts and myeloblasts reappear by 14 days, and myelopoiesis becomes hyperactive in about 3 weeks. As a result of the rapid cell loss, the spleen shrinks to half its normal weight within 24 hours. The false impression of reticuloendothelial hyperplasia is the result of the less radiosensitive cells being forced into a smaller volume. After a single dose of 8 Gy, lymphopoiesis is always seen before myelopoiesis, even though the lymphocyte count in the peripheral blood is slower to return to normal than the granulocyte count. Splenic atrophy can occur after irradiation with relatively high total doses (40 Gy),[36] and the consequences are similar to those seen after splenectomy. However, experience with hundreds of patients followed for 10 or more years after treatment with total doses of 30 Gy suggests that functional consequences at this dose level are absent or exceedingly rare.

LEUKEMOGENIC EFFECTS OF IONIZING RADIATION

The principles of mutagenesis and carcinogenesis, including leukemogenesis, can be found in Chapter 1. Susceptibility to the development of leukemia among mammalian species varies widely. Humans and mice are relatively susceptible, whereas rats, rabbits, and guinea pigs are relatively resistant.

Total body irradiation has been demonstrated as a cause of leukemia in humans. The Radiation Effects Research Foundation, formerly the Atomic Bomb Casualty Commission, has carefully followed the residents of Hiroshima who were exposed to a single acute dose of photons and neutrons from a fission bomb. The relative

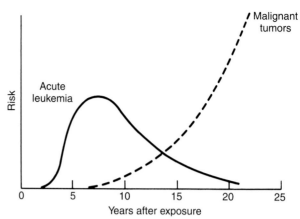

Fig. 33-3 Schematic model of the risk of leukemia and malignant tumors in survivors of the Hiroshima atomic bomb. (Modified from United Nations Scientific Committee on the Effects of Atomic Radiation [UNSCEAR]. Genetic and somatic effects of ionizing radiation. *1986 Report to the General Assembly.* New York, NY; 1986.)

risk of leukemia and several types of cancer (Fig. 33-3) was higher with the greater doses associated with proximity to the hypocenter. Acute granulocytic leukemia was seen within 18 months of exposure. The peak incidence of acute leukemia was seen 5 years after the blast and approached normal levels approximately 15 years later for those younger than 15 years. The risk in older individuals remained above normal more than 25 years after exposure.[37]

An increased risk of leukemia among the pioneers of radiology was suspected as early as 1911.[38] March[39] found an increased risk of death from leukemia among early radiologists as compared with physicians who were not radiologists, and this risk persisted among physicians who died in the 1950s.[40] With more complete understanding of this risk and appropriate rules for radiation protection, the increase in leukemia among radiologists has been eliminated entirely.[41]

Court-Brown and Abbatt[42] described an increased frequency of death from leukemia in a group of patients given irradiation to the spine for ankylosing spondylitis between 1940 and 1954. The work of Court-Brown and Doll[43] has suggested a linear dose-response relationship in radiation leukemogenesis, although the findings of the Radiation Effects Research Foundation[44] have led investigators to suspect a linear-quadratic dose-response relationship.

Levine and Bloomfield[45] provided a comprehensive review of the extensive literature concerning the risk of acute leukemia and myelodysplastic syndromes secondary to treatment for Hodgkin's disease. They concluded that the use of radiation therapy alone, even with large fields, was associated with few or no cases of secondary acute leukemias: "The overwhelming majority of the cases resulted in the setting of chemotherapy use, almost always involving an alkylating agent."[45]

Coltman and Dixon[46] found an increased risk of acute leukemia after treatment of Hodgkin's disease that was related to the age at which the patients were treated. Those who were greater than 40 years of age (153 patients) at the time of treatment had a risk of nearly 20%, compared with lower risks in patients 20 to 39 years of age (376 patients) and an even lower risk for patients who were younger than 20. Intravenous radioactive phosphorus (^{32}P) was thought to be a cause of leukemic evolution after its administration for polycythemia vera. A prospective trial of phlebotomy vs. intravenous ^{32}P administration revealed no difference in the frequency of leukemia after treatment.[47]

TREATMENT OF LEUKEMIA

The natural history of the different types of acute leukemia before effective therapy was developed justified the designations of "acute" or "chronic" at that time. Therapeutic successes over the past 20 years have profoundly altered the natural history in some of these diseases, most notably acute leukemia in children.[48,49] More than half of children with acute leukemia, properly treated, are long-term survivors, free of all evidence of disease and no longer on therapy.[50] A lesser degree of progress has occurred in adults with acute leukemia.[51] Chronic leukemias have proved far more resistant to treatment, but recent results are encouraging.

Radiation therapy has a limited role in the care of patients with leukemia. Its use is confined to palliative treatment. The most common indications for irradiation are urgent ones, including irradiation of the base of the skull for cranial nerve abnormalities due to infiltration of the leptomeninges or involvement of the cauda equina with pain and weakness in the lower extremities. The nature of these leukemic infiltrates is such that imaging studies may be normal. In the presence of manifest leukemia and neurologic abnormalities, irradiation on clinical grounds alone is often palliative. Larger tumor infiltrations may be seen in patients with lymphocytic or myelocytic leukemias. Biopsies of the former may be interpreted as lymphomas and those of the latter may be called *granulocytic sarcomas* (formerly termed *chloromas*). Low total doses such as 20 to 25 Gy are usually sufficient for rapid palliation.[52]

HODGKIN'S DISEASE

Hodgkin's disease is an unusual form of cancer in that the neoplastic cells (Reed-Sternberg cells) account for only a very small portion of the disease process; most of that process results from the wide range of inflammatory cells and fibrous bands that accompany the Reed-Sternberg cells. Hodgkin's disease arises mainly within the lymph nodes, and evidence is accumulating to suggest that most of the Reed-Sternberg cells are of B-cell origin.[53] Considered uniformly fatal 50 years ago, Hodgkin's disease is now considered one of the most curable types of cancer.[54] Areas of active research in Hodgkin's disease include understanding its pathogenesis at the molecular level and minimizing side effects from treatment while maintaining high cure rates. The remainder of this section consists of an overview of the disease, with emphasis on its management.

Pathology and Clinical Presentation

According to the Revised European-American Classification of Lymphoid Neoplasms (REAL), published in 1994, Hodgkin's disease can be classified as either classical Hodgkin's disease or a (nodular) lymphocyte-predominant form. Histologic subtypes of classical Hodgkin's disease proposed at that time were nodular sclerosis, mixed cellularity, lymphocyte depletion, and lymphocyte-rich; the lymphocyte-rich category was considered provisional at that time.[55] The more recent World Health Organization (WHO) classification scheme[56] essentially incorporates the REAL classification; in the WHO scheme, the lymphocyte-rich form is considered a category of classical Hodgkin's disease and the terms *Hodgkin's disease* and *Hodgkin's lymphoma* are considered interchangeable.[56]

Classical Hodgkin's disease can be distinguished from the lymphocyte-predominant form on the basis of morphology and immunophenotype. Morphologically, classical Hodgkin's disease is characterized by the presence of Reed-Sternberg cells or lacunar cells on a background of lymphocytes, histiocytes, eosinophils, and plasma cells. The lymphocyte-predominant form of Hodgkin's disease is characterized by the presence of abundant lymphocytic and histiocytic ("L & H" or "popcorn") cells. Immunophenotypically, the Reed-Sternberg cells in classical Hodgkin's disease express the CD15 and CD30 cell-surface antigens but not CD45; in the lymphocyte-predominant form, the "L&H" or "popcorn" cells do not express CD15 or CD30 but do express CD45. CD20 is also expressed in the lymphocyte-predominant form but is not likely to be expressed in classical Hodgkin's disease.[55]

Classical and lymphocyte-predominant Hodgkin's disease can also be distinguished by their clinical presentations. Classical Hodgkin's disease has a bimodal age distribution, with the first peak around age 20 and the second past age 50, whereas the age at appearance of the lymphocyte-predominant form is not bimodal but rather is between the mid-20s and mid-30s. Classical Hodgkin's disease tends to present with centrally located lesions at stage II or III and in about 40% of cases with constitutional or B symptoms (described further in the following section on "Staging Evaluation"). The lymphocyte-predominant form tends to present with peripheral lesions and at stage I or II, and fewer than 20% of patients have B symptoms at presentation.[57]

Epidemiology and Etiology

The expected number of new cases of Hodgkin's disease in the United States in 2001 is 7400 (3900 male, 3500 female), and the number of deaths is estimated at 1300 (700 male, 600 female).[58] The most common histologic subtype of Hodgkin's disease in the United States and Canada is nodular sclerosis (70%), followed by mixed cellularity (25%), lymphocyte-predominant (5%), lymphocyte-depleted (< 1%), and lymphocyte-rich (incidence yet to be defined); the variations among countries and over time are substantial.[57] Risk factors associated with Hodgkin's disease are family history, higher socioeconomic and educational status, and Epstein-Barr virus infection. Monozygotic twins have a greatly (ninety-ninefold) increased risk of Hodgkin's disease relative to dizygotic twins, suggesting a genetic basis for the disease.[59] Evidence of links between Hodgkin's disease and the Epstein-Barr virus includes the appearance of elevated immunoglobulin G and A (IgG and IgA) antibody titers at least 3 years before the diagnosis of Hodgkin's disease.[60] The detection of the viral genome in the Reed-Sternberg cells by in-situ hybridization also raises the speculation that Epstein-Barr virus may be involved in the development of Hodgkin's disease.[61]

Staging Evaluation

Staging evaluations for Hodgkin's disease should include complete history and physical examination; complete blood count; assessment of electrolytes, erythrocyte sedimentation rate (ESR), β2-microglobulin levels; liver function tests; bilateral bone marrow biopsy and aspiration; chest x-ray; computed tomography (CT) scanning of the neck, chest, abdomen, and pelvis; gallium scanning; and in some cases, lymphangiography.

The most widely accepted staging system for Hodgkin's disease remains the Ann Arbor system[62] as modified at the Cotswolds meeting,[63] although definitions of lymph node regions and interpretations of extralymphatic sites or organs have varied. Some generally accepted definitions of typically involved lymph-node regions are the cervical, axillary, mediastinal, para-aortic, splenic, mesenteric, and ilio-inguino-femoral regions; some authors report involvement of the infraclavicular, hilar, and inguino-femoral areas separately.[64] Other less commonly involved regions are Waldeyer's ring, the epitrochlear or brachial nodes, and the popliteal nodes. The Ann Arbor/American Joint Committee on Cancer system is summarized in Box 33-1.[65] Each stage grouping also includes *A* and *B* categories, with *B* denoting the presence of constitutional symptoms such as unexplained temperatures above 38°C (100.4°F) for 3 or more consecutive days, drenching night sweats, or unexplained weight loss of more than 10% during the 6 months before diagnosis. *A* denotes the absence of such symptoms.[65]

BOX 33-1 Ann Arbor/American Joint Committee on Cancer Staging System for Hodgkin's Disease

STAGE GROUPING

I   Involvement of a single lymph node region (I) or localized involvement of a single extralymphatic organ or site (I_E)

II   Involvement of two or more lymph node regions on the same side of the diaphragm (II) or localized involvement of a single associated extralymphatic organ or site and its regional lymph node(s) with or without involvement of other lymph node regions on the same side of the diaphragm (II_E)

NOTE: the number of lymph node regions involved may be indicated by a subscript (e.g., II_3).

III   Involvement of lymph node regions on both sides of the diaphragm (III), which may also be accompanied by localized involvement of an associated extralymphatic organ or site (IIIE), by involvement of the spleen (III_S), or both (III_{E+S})

IV   Disseminated (multifocal) involvement of one or more extralymphatic organs, with or without associated lymph node involvement, or isolated extralymphatic organ involvement with distant (nonregional) nodal involvement

From Fleming I, Cooper JS, Henson DE, et al, eds. *AJCC Cancer Staging Manual*, 5th ed. Philadelphia, Pa: Lippincott Williams & Wilkins; 1997:285-287.

Treatment of Early-Stage (Selected Stage I and II) Disease

Radiation Therapy

In the early 1920s, Rene Gilbert, a Swiss radiotherapist, recognized the importance of treating contiguous, lymph node–bearing regions that are not clinically involved when radiation is to be used as the only treatment for Hodgkin's disease.[66] Despite this observation, the administration of low doses of radiation to clinically involved sites remained the standard of care over the next four decades. Consequently, Hodgkin's disease was considered incurable. Although Peters reported in 1950 that early-stage Hodgkin's disease could be cured with radiation therapy,[67] physicians remained skeptical. In 1963, Easson's and Russell's landmark article, "The Cure of Hodgkin's Disease," reemphasized that radiation therapy could be curative if administered properly.[68] In the 1960s and 1970s, Henry Kaplan at Stanford University helped to refine radiation therapy techniques and with Saul Rosenberg helped popularize the use of radiation therapy for early-stage disease.[69] This work led to the first-ever decline in the age-adjusted mortality rate for Hodgkin's disease after 1970.[70] Since the 1970s, many patients with early-stage Hodgkin's disease have been treated with subtotal nodal irradiation (also known as extended-field radiation therapy; includes the treatment of the mantle and para-aortic regions and the spleen), and radiation therapy remains the single most effective therapeutic agent.

An extensive study of radiation therapy for clinical stage I or II supradiaphragmatic Hodgkin's disease came from the Princess Margaret Hospital in Toronto, which reported on 250 patients treated between 1978 and 1986 with a median follow-up of 6.3 years. In that study, the actuarial overall survival rate was 83%, the cause-specific survival rate was 90%, and the relapse-free survival (RFS) rate was 72% at 8 years (Fig. 33-4).[71] The local-control rate was 95%, with only two true in-field failures. The criteria for treatment with radiation only were evolving throughout the period of this retrospective analysis; nevertheless, the factors predictive of favorable cause-specific survival were age less than 50 years and an ESR of less than 40, and those predictive of favorable RFS were age less than 50, ESR less than 40, and the lymphocyte-predominant or nodular-sclerosis histologic subtype.[71]

Some of the best-known prognostic factors for Hodgkin's disease were derived from a series of prospective trials carried out by the European Organization for Research and Treatment of Cancer (EORTC). This group classified stages I and II Hodgkin's disease as falling into one of three prognostic categories: very favorable, favorable, and unfavorable. *Very favorable* disease is that which meets all six of the following criteria: (1) clinical stage IA, (2) female sex, (3) age less than 40 years, (4) ESR of less than 50, (5) lymphocyte-predominant or nodular-sclerosis histology, and (6) a mediastinum:thoracic ratio (ratio of the horizontal diameter of the mediastinal tumor to the thoracic diameter measured at the T5-6 interspace) of less than 35%. The presence of any of the following factors connotes *unfavorable* disease: age 50 or

older, B symptoms, ESR of 50 or more, disease at more than three sites, and a mediastinum:thoracic ratio of more than 35%. *Favorable* disease is connoted by clinical stage I or II disease that does not meet the *very favorable* or *unfavorable* criteria. Results from the recent H7 trials of the EORTC indicated that treatment of 165 patients with favorable disease with subtotal nodal irradiation produced an RFS rate of 81% and an overall survival rate of 96% at 6 years.[72]

Despite the high cure rates obtained with radiation therapy alone, some proportion of patients who are cured of Hodgkin's disease will experience some long-term complications resulting from the radiation therapy (described further in the section on Radiation Toxicity later in this chapter and in Chapter 1). Although pulmonary and cardiac complications have been reduced greatly through improvements in techniques and better understanding of how to minimize long-term side effects, the risk of developing a second malignancy still persists, a risk that poses particular problems for young patients who are otherwise cured of the disease.[73-75]

Ongoing attempts to modify treatment for early-stage Hodgkin's disease so as to reduce the adverse effects of radiation or chemotherapy without sacrificing high cure rates are described in the following paragraphs.

Radiation Volume

Attempts to reduce the volume of radiation delivered to patients with early-stage Hodgkin's disease include the recent EORTC H7VF trial, in which 40 patients with very favorable disease were treated with mantle radiation therapy only.[72] At 6 years, the overall survival rate for this group was 96% and the RFS rate was 73%. However, most relapses appeared in the nodal extension area, which would have been covered by irradiation of the para-aortic and spleen areas. The RFS rate of 73% was thought to be too low, and mantle radiation therapy alone has not been used in any subsequent EORTC trial.[76]

The H5 trial of the EORTC involved 237 patients with favorable disease (clinical stage I or clinical stage II without mediastinal disease, age 40 or younger, ESR 70 or less, and lymphocyte-predominant or nodular-sclerosis histology).[77] The 198 patients who had no evidence of disease on laparotomy were randomly assigned to undergo mantle field or mantle plus para-aortic field radiation therapy. No difference was found between the groups in 6-year RFS rate (74% mantle-only vs. 72% mantle-plus para-aortic) or overall survival rate (96% vs. 89%).

The H7 trial also compared radiation with radiation plus chemotherapy with epirubicin, bleomycin, vinblastine, and prednisone (EBVP). Patients with favorable disease were randomly assigned to receive subtotal nodal irradiation (*N* = 165) or six cycles of EBVP followed by involved-field radiation therapy (*N* = 168).[72,76] The RFS rate at 6 years was 81% for the radiation-only group and 92% for the chemotherapy plus radiation

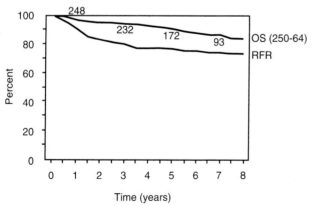

Fig. 33-4   The actuarial overall and relapse-free survival rates for 250 patients with stage I or II supradiaphragmatic Hodgkin's disease treated with radiation at the Princess Margaret Hospital in Toronto, Canada, between 1978 and 1986. (From Gospodarowicz MK, Sutcliffe SB, Clark RM, et al. *Int J Radiat Oncol Biol Phys* 1992;22:859-865.)

group (P = 0.004). The corresponding overall survival rates were 96% and 98% (P = 0.156), a good salvage rate for those who experienced relapse after subtotal nodal irradiation. The current H9F trial is assigning patients with very favorable or favorable disease to undergo six cycles of EBVP followed by (1) no radiation therapy, (2) 20 Gy of involved-field radiation therapy, or (3) 36 Gy of involved-field radiation therapy.[78]

Radiation Dose

In attempts to evaluate whether radiation dose could be reduced for early-stage Hodgkin's disease, Vijayakumar and Myrianthopoulos[79] reviewed the literature and found that the likelihood of in-field recurrence after the treatment of subclinical disease with radiation therapy alone to 27 Gy was only 5%. Seydel and colleagues[80] and Mendenhall and colleagues[81] have also suggested that 20 to 30 Gy is adequate for treating microscopic disease when the only treatment is to be radiation.

For gross disease, Kaplan[82] found a 4.4% recurrence rate after delivery of 35 to 40 Gy; an apparent linear dose-response relationship was noted in this 1966 retrospective review, which included patients with non-Hodgkin's lymphoma,[83] a group in which the recurrence rate after radiation therapy was unusually high,[84] and a group in which some patients were given 2.75 Gy daily to a single anterior or posterior field four days per week.[85] After excluding these patients, Fletcher and Shukovsky[86] observed a sigmoid dose-response relationship for Hodgkin's disease, findings that were subsequently corroborated by several other investigators. In that analysis, administration of 35 Gy resulted in combined in-field and marginal recurrence rates of 5% or less. Vijayakumar and Myrianthopoulos[79] reviewed megavoltage data from treatment of 4117 at-risk sites for Hodgkin's disease and suggested that achieving an in-field control rate of 98% would require 36.9 Gy for disease smaller than 6 cm and 37.4 Gy for disease larger than 6 cm. Brincker and Bentzen[87] later reported that fitting a dose-response curve to the data compiled by Vijayakumar and Myrianthopoulos[79] revealed a plateau in local control at doses greater than 32.5 Gy. In contrast, the Patterns of Care Outcome Study for Hodgkin's disease[88] and studies by Thar and colleagues,[89] Schewe and colleagues,[90] and Sears and colleagues[91] all found no benefit for doses higher than 30 Gy. Part of the discrepancy in these findings may have resulted from failure to distinguish marginal from in-field recurrences.[92] In addition, most of the analyses described above used prescribed dose rather than the minimum dose actually delivered to the tumor.

The German Hodgkin's Lymphoma Study Group, in its HD4 trial, compared relapse-free and overall survival rates after either 40 Gy given as extended-field radiation (subtotal nodal irradiation) or 30 Gy given as extended-field radiation followed by a 10-Gy boost to involved disease sites.[93] Patients had pathologically proven stage IA, IIA, or IIB disease.[93] The 5-year freedom from treatment-failure rate was 82% for those given the boost dose vs. 70% for those given 40 Gy without the boost (P = 0.026). The 5-year overall actuarial survival rate was 97% for the boost group and 93% for the no-boost group (P = 0.067). No true in-field failures were found within the extended-field volume in either group, and thus the authors concluded that 30 Gy was sufficient to control subclinical disease.

Radiation Toxicity

Late complications of mantle irradiation include lung, heart, and thyroid dysfunction; second malignancies; growth abnormalities; and Lhermitte's sign. However, in at least one study,[94] total radiation doses of less than 30.6 Gy, given in 17 fractions, produced a low incidence of late complications. Boivin and colleagues[95] suggested that mediastinal irradiation modestly increases the age-adjusted risk of death from myocardial infarction. At an average follow-up of 9.5 years, Hancock and colleagues[96] reported that mediastinal irradiation to a total dose of less than 30 Gy given in daily doses of 1.5 to 2.75 Gy did not increase the risk of cardiac death but that mediastinal doses of more than 30 Gy increased the relative risk of cardiac death to 3.5. Subcarinal blocking after 30 to 35 Gy reduces the relative risk for cardiac diseases such as congestive heart failure and pancarditis from 5.3 to 1.4 but does not significantly reduce the risk of acute myocardial infarction because the proximal coronary arteries still receive the full dose of radiation. The increased risk of second malignancies from previous irradiation has been well documented.[74,97] The main long-term hazard associated with radiation therapy is the risk of forming solid tumors. The incidence of breast cancer is increased in women who were younger than 30 years at the time of mantle irradiation; the younger the patient and the greater the radiation dose, the higher the relative risk.[98-100] The cumulative risk of developing a solid tumor such as osteosarcoma or carcinoma of the breast, thyroid, lung, stomach or colon is approximately 0.3% to 0.5% per year[101,102] and increases with time, particularly 10 years or more after the irradiation. Irradiated patients also have an increased risk of developing non-Hodgkin's lymphoma[101] but not acute nonlymphocytic leukemia, unlike those who undergo chemotherapy with alkylating agents.[97] Children who undergo radiation therapy can experience growth abnormalities.

Staging Laparotomy

Other evaluations of prognostic factors for early-stage Hodgkin's disease have led to investigations of the value of histologic findings obtained from laparotomy. The EORTC H6F trial, conducted from 1982 to 1988, included 262 patients with favorable clinical stage I or II disease who were randomized to undergo staging laparotomy (with splenectomy) or no laparotomy.[103] Patients who did not have laparotomy (i.e., those who underwent clinical staging) were treated with subtotal nodal irradiation. Patients assigned to the laparotomy group who showed no evidence of disease on laparatomy were treated either with mantle radiation therapy (if the histology was lymphocyte-predominant or nodular-sclerosis) or with mantle and para-aortic radiation therapy (if the histology was mixed-cellularity or lymphocyte-depleted). If the laparotomy findings were positive, the patients were treated with chemotherapy plus radiation therapy as follows: six cycles of either mechlorethamine, vincristine, procarbazine, and prednisone (MOPP) or doxorubicin, bleomycin, vinblastine, and dacarbazine (ABVD), with mantle radiation therapy given between the third and fourth cycles. At a median follow-up of 64 months, the 6-year overall survival rate was 93% for the no-laparotomy group and 89% for the laparotomy group ($P = 0.24$); the corresponding 6-year freedom from progression rates were 78% and 83% ($P = 0.27$). The three treatment-related deaths were all in the laparotomy group. Even though the treatment outcomes were equivalent, the recommendation from this study was to abandon laparotomy because of the accompanying mortality associated with laparotomy and splenectomy.

The University of Texas M.D. Anderson Cancer Center recently reported results from a retrospective analysis of 145 patients with pathologically confirmed stage I or II Hodgkin's disease who were treated with mantle radiation therapy alone.[104] Patients were treated between 1967 and 1991, and the median follow-up was 12.2 years. Four factors (male sex, age 40 years or older, the presence of B symptoms, and having disease at at least three sites) were found to be adverse prognostic factors for progression-free survival. Of the 145 patients studied, 54 had no adverse prognostic factors, 70 had one, and 21 had two adverse prognostic factors. Lower numbers of adverse prognostic factors were associated with better overall survival ($P = 0.006$) and progression-free survival ($P < 0.0001$). Progression-free survival rates were 96% in the absence of any adverse prognostic factors and 57% to 63% in the presence of one or two of these factors.

The prognostic factors obtained from retrospective analyses should be verified by prospective trials, as is currently being done at the Harvard Joint Center for Radiation Therapy.[105] The eligibility criteria for this trial of mantle radiation therapy alone are having pathologic stage IA or IIA, nonbulky upper mediastinal disease (tumor not more than one third of the thoracic diameter) of lymphocyte-predominant or nodular-sclerosis histology (pathologic stage IA disease can be of mixed cellularity). In this trial, laparotomy is not required if the patient presents with stage IA lymphocyte-predominant Hodgkin's disease. Preliminary findings from this trial have been reported,[105] but longer follow-up will be needed to reach definitive conclusions.

Radiation versus Chemotherapy

In a study conducted in Italy, Biti and colleagues[106] evaluated outcome among 89 patients with pathologic stage I or IIA Hodgkin's disease who were randomized to undergo subtotal nodal irradiation or six cycles of MOPP. At a median follow-up of 8 years, the overall survival rate was higher after irradiation than after chemotherapy (93% vs. 56%, $P < 0.001$). Rates of freedom from progression were similar for the two groups (76% vs. 64%). Moreover, azoospermia was documented in 100% of the men in the chemotherapy group compared with 0% of the irradiation group; amenorrhea was documented in 50% of the women in the chemotherapy group and in 10% of the irradiation group. The authors contended that radiation therapy alone should remain the treatment of choice for early-stage Hodgkin's disease with favorable prognostic factors until more effective and less toxic chemotherapy becomes available.

The U.S. National Cancer Institute published a report on 106 patients with pathologically confirmed stage IA, IB, IIA, IIB, or IIIA1 disease who were randomized to receive subtotal or total nodal irradiation or at least six cycles of MOPP (or two additional cycles after a complete response).[107] At a median follow-up of 7.5 years, the projected 10-year disease-free survival rate among those treated with radiation was 60% compared with 86% among those treated with MOPP ($P = 0.009$). The projected 10-year overall survival rate was 76% for the radiation therapy and 92% for the MOPP group ($P = 0.051$). However, these intergroup differences in disease-free and overall survival rates disappeared when patients with bulky mediastinal disease and stage IIIA1 disease were excluded from the analysis. The conclusion was that MOPP was as effective as irradiation in the treatment of selected patients with early-stage Hodgkin's disease. However, survival rates and complications over the long term remain to be seen.

Which chemotherapy agents are most effective in the treatment of early-stage Hodgkin's disease is not clear. Ongoing trials to address these questions include the EORTC H9F trial, in which six cycles of EBVP are followed by randomization between no radiation therapy, 20 Gy, or 36 Gy.[78] The HD10 trial, conducted by the German Hodgkin's Lymphoma Study Group, involves two or four cycles of ABVD followed by randomization between 20 and 30 Gy of involved-field radiation therapy.[108] Another trial of the Stanford V regimen (doxorubicin, vinblastine, mechlorethamine, vincristine, bleomycin, etoposide, and prednisone with granulocyte colony-stimulating factor) with involved-field radiation is also in progress.[109]

Chemotherapy Toxicity

Although current trials are focusing on reducing the dose and volume of radiation in an attempt to reduce radiation-induced toxicity, chemotherapy also has toxic effects. These effects (including those not yet known because of the short follow-up from chemotherapy trials) should be kept in mind when chemotherapy is recommended for patients with favorable stage I or II Hodgkin's disease.

Of interest in this regard are the findings from two large studies comparing radiation therapy and chemotherapy for the treatment of Hodgkin's disease. The first of these studies was a review of 1013 patients with Hodgkin's disease treated at the M.D. Anderson Cancer Center between 1966 and 1987.[110] The median follow-up was more than 5 years (except for patients who were treated with cyclophosphamide, vincristine, procarbazine, and prednisolone alternated with doxorubicin, bleomycin, dacarbazine, lomustine, and prednisone, for whom it was 3 years). At 20 years, the overall and disease-specific survival rates for the entire population were 60% and 76%. Interestingly, the relative hazard ratios for developing acute myelogenous leukemia, non-Hodgkin's lymphoma, or solid tumors were higher for those treated with chemotherapy alone than for those treated with radiation therapy (with or without chemotherapy). This phenomenon was thought to result from the fact that patients who received chemotherapy as part of the combined-modality treatment received less chemotherapy than those patients who were treated with chemotherapy alone. The other study, at the Harvard Joint Center for Radiation Therapy, retrospectively reviewed 794 patients with pathologically confirmed stages IA and IIIB Hodgkin's disease treated between 1969 and 1988.[73] In that study, 489 patients were treated with radiation therapy alone; 158 were treated with radiation therapy and chemotherapy; and the other 147 patients had been treated initially with radiation, experienced relapse, and were then treated with chemotherapy. The 20-year actuarial survival rate was 73%. However, the absolute excess mortality risk from second malignancy and causes other than Hodgkin's disease was higher for those treated with combined-modality therapy than for those treated with radiation only. Although the death rate from Hodgkin's disease declined over time, the risk of death from other causes such as second malignancy and cardiac disease continued to rise. It was projected that the mortality from the second malignancy would surpass that from Hodgkin's disease by 15 to 20 years after treatment. As noted above, the HD10 trial of the German Hodgkin's Lymphoma Study Group is testing the effectiveness of two or four cycles of ABVD, which has proven effective in advanced disease, given with lower-dose, lower-volume radiation therapy (20 or 30 Gy to involved fields) for patients with favorable stage I or II Hodgkin's disease.[108] This approach, it is hoped, will be effective with fewer of the side effects associated with other chemotherapy or radiation therapy regimens.

In summary, subtotal nodal irradiation remains the standard treatment for good-prognosis, early-stage Hodgkin's disease—that is, it has the longest track record. Carefully selected, pathologically staged patients may respond well to mantle irradiation alone. However, the morbidity and mortality associated with laparotomy and splenectomy must be kept in mind. Results from chemotherapy trials, with or without involved-field radiation therapy, are promising, but long-term follow-up is needed, especially in terms of second malignancies and salvage rates.

Treatment of Intermediate-Stage (Unfavorable Stages I and II) and Less-Advanced Stage III Disease

Intermediate-stage disease seems to respond to combination chemotherapy and radiation therapy, although the optimal chemotherapy agents, number of cycles, field sizes, and radiation dose have yet to be identified. Studies that address these and related questions are summarized below. In its H7U trial, the EORTC described outcome for 389 patients with unfavorable disease (patients age 50 or older or who have an ESR of 50 or more, B symptoms, disease at more than three sites, or a mediastinum:thoracic ratio of more than 35%) randomized to receive six cycles of EBVP followed by involved-field radiation therapy or six cycles of alternating MOPP and ABV followed by involved-field radiation therapy.[72] At 6 years, the RFS rates were 94% for the MOPP-ABV group and 79% for the EBVP group and corresponding overall survival rates were 89% and 82%. Given these rather disappointing findings, EBVP has not been used in subsequent trials involving patients with unfavorable disease. Instead, the subsequent H8U trial randomized patients with unfavorable disease into one of three groups: the first was given six alternating cycles of MOPP-ABV followed by involved-field radiation therapy to 36 Gy, the second was given four cycles of MOPP-ABV followed by involved-field radiation therapy to 36 Gy, and the third was given four cycles of MOPP-ABV followed by subtotal nodal irradiation to 36 Gy.[78] The findings from H8U have yet to be published. In the current H9U trial, patients with unfavorable disease are randomized to receive six cycles of ABVD, four cycles of ABVD, or four cycles of bleomycin, etoposide, doxorubicin, cyclophosphamide, vincristine, procarbazine, and prednisone (BEACOPP); all groups receive involved-field radiation therapy to 30 Gy after the chemotherapy.[78]

Preliminary findings are available from an Italian study of 114 patients randomized to undergo four cycles of ABVD followed by either involved-field radiation therapy to 36 Gy or subtotal nodal irradiation to 30 Gy with a 6-Gy boost to the involved sites.[111] Eligible patients could have clinical stage I with bulky disease or stage IB, IIA, or IIEA disease. At 5 years, the complete response rates were 98% for those given involved-field radiation and 100% for those given subtotal nodal irradiation.

Corresponding freedom-from-progression rates were 94% and 95%, and overall survival rates were 96% and 100%. Given the lack of statistical difference in these rates between the two groups, involved-field radiation after four cycles of AVBD was thought to be sufficient.

The German Hodgkin's Lymphoma Study Group HD8 trial also compared outcome for patients at intermediate risk who received two cycles of cyclophosphamide, vincristine, procarbazine, and prednisone (COPP) with two cycles of ABVD followed by either subtotal nodal irradiation (30 Gy followed by a 10-Gy boost) or involved-field radiation therapy (30 Gy followed by a 10-Gy boost). Eligible patients had stage I or II disease with at least one of the following risk factors: bulky mediastinal or extranodal disease, massive splenic involvement, an ESR of 50 or more (or an ESR of 30 or more in combination with B symptoms), or lymph-node involvement in at least three sites; or stage IIIA disease in the absence of any of these risk factors. A total of 1069 patients were randomized. At a median follow-up of 20 months, no difference was apparent between the groups in RFS (93%) or overall survival (98%). The authors concluded that involved-field radiation is sufficient after this chemotherapy regimen.[112]

The German Hodgkin's Lymphoma Study Group HD9 trial involved a comparison of involved-field radiation therapy given after one of three chemotherapy regimens. The first group was given four cycles of COPP and four cycles of ABVD followed by involved-field radiation therapy of 30 Gy to initially bulky disease sites (≥ 5 cm) and 40 Gy to the area of residual disease; the second group was given eight cycles of baseline BEACOPP followed by the same radiation therapy; and the third group was given escalated-dose BEACOPP with granulocyte colony-stimulating factor support followed by the same radiation therapy.[113,114] Eligible patients were age 16 to 65 years, with stage IIB disease with bulky mediastinal disease, extranodal involvement, or massive splenic disease; stage IIIA disease with any of the above risk factors, an ESR of more than 50, or at least three areas of lymph-node involvement; stage IIIB disease; or stage IV disease. This study accrued 1300 patients between 1993 and 1998. At the third interim analysis in February 1998, the 2-year freedom-from-treatment failure rates were 72% for the COPP-ABVD group, 81% for the BEACOPP group, and 89% for the escalated-dose BEACOPP group; corresponding survival rates were 89%, 94%, and 96% (P value was not significant). Freedom from treatment failure was significantly better (P = 0.05) in the escalated-dose BEACOPP group than in the baseline BEACOPP group in this analysis. Notably, the COPP-ABVD treatment was dropped from the trial after the first interim analysis, which was completed in September 1996.

An alternative chemotherapy-plus-radiation therapy protocol being tested for bulky or advanced Hodgkin's disease is the Stanford V program.[109] The treatment protocol involves 12 weeks of intensive chemotherapy followed by 36 Gy of involved-field radiation therapy to sites of bulky (≥ 5 cm) disease and to macroscopic splenic disease. Of the 121 patients accrued, the median age was 27 years and the median follow-up was 4.5 years. The 5-year survival rate for the entire group was 95%, and the failure-free survival rate was 89%. The failure-free survival rate for the 37 patients with stage I or II disease was 100%, and that for the 46 patients with stage III disease and the 38 patients with stage IV disease was 85%. Encouraging results from this trial[115] led to initiation of trial 2496 by the Eastern Cooperative Oncology Group (ECOG) and Southwest Oncology Group (SWOG), in which the Stanford V program will be compared with ABVD chemotherapy.[115]

Treatment of Advanced (Stage IIB, III, or IV) Disease

Chemotherapy, or combined chemotherapy and radiation, has been less successful in controlling Hodgkin's disease that presents at advanced stages than it is for early-stage disease. Multiagent chemotherapy seems more effective than single-agent chemotherapy or radiation alone, but the most effective and least toxic of these regimens has yet to be identified. Recent findings regarding the efficacy of treatments for advanced disease are summarized in the remainder of this section.

One of the earliest large-scale randomized studies comparing the standard MOPP combination with the noncross-resistant ABVD combination for Hodgkin's disease was performed at the Instituto Nazionale Tumori in Milan, where the ABVD combination was initially conceived. Patients with stage IIB, IIIA, or IIIB disease (verified by either laparotomy or laparoscopy) were randomized to receive either three cycles of MOPP followed by radiation therapy followed by three more cycles of MOPP or three cycles of ABVD followed by radiation therapy followed by three more cycles of ABVD.[116] Either subtotal or total nodal irradiation was used according to whether the para-aortic nodes were involved. Patients were accrued to the study between 1974 and 1982. A total of 232 patients were randomized, and the groups were stratified by tumor histology, laparotomy vs. laparoscopy, and disease stage. At 7 years, the ABVD treatment had produced superior rates of freedom from progression (81% vs. 63%, P < 0.002), RFS (88 % vs. 77%, P = 0.06) and overall survival (77% vs. 68%, P = 0.03).

Another trial addressing the question of which chemotherapy regimen is the most effective in advanced Hodgkin's disease was a Cancer and Leukemia Group B (CALGB) study[117] in which patients with stage IIIA2, IIIB, IVA, or IVB disease (including those in first relapse after previous radiation therapy) were randomized to undergo six to eight cycles of either MOPP or ABVD or 12 cycles of alternating MOPP and ABVD. No radiation therapy was given in this study. Laparotomy was performed only if findings on lymphangiography and abdominal CT scanning were equivocal or negative. At 5 years, the failure-free survival rates were 50% for the MOPP-only group, 61% for the ABVD-only group, and 65% for the alternating MOPP-ABVD group; corresponding overall survival rates were 66%, 73%, and 75%. Both the ABVD and the MOPP-ABVD treatments produced higher failure-free survival rates than did MOPP alone ($P = 0.02$), but no differences were found among groups in overall survival rate. The authors concluded that ABVD alone was as effective as MOPP-ABVD and both were superior to MOPP alone; moreover, ABVD alone was less myelotoxic than the MOPP regimens.

Another modification of the MOPP-ABVD combination for advanced disease was tested in an Intergroup trial in which patients were randomized to undergo either sequential MOPP-ABVD chemotherapy or a hybrid MOPP-ABV regimen.[118] Eligibility criteria were the same as those for the CALGB trial noted above (stage IIIA2, IIIB, IVA, or IVB disease or first relapse after radiation therapy). Patients were stratified for age, previous radiation therapy, bulky disease, and performance status. Those assigned to the sequential group were treated with six cycles of MOPP; if complete response (CR) was achieved, they were given three cycles of ABVD. If the first six cycles of MOPP produced a partial response (PR), two more cycles of MOPP were given. If CR or stable disease was attained at that point, patients were then given three cycles of ABVD. Patients assigned to the hybrid-regimen group were given six cycles of the hybrid chemotherapy. If those six cycles produced a CR, patients were given two more cycles of hybrid chemotherapy; if those six cycles produced PR, hybrid chemotherapy was repeated till two cycles beyond CR (to a total of 12 cycles). No radiation therapy was given as a part of this trial. Patients were accrued between January 1987 and July 1989. A total of 691 patients were randomized and analyzed at a median follow-up of 7.3 years. The 8-year failure-free survival rate was 64% for the hybrid chemotherapy group and 54% for the sequential chemotherapy group ($P = 0.01$). The corresponding 8-year overall survival rates were 79% and 71% ($P = 0.02$). Although fewer incidents of acute leukemia and myelodysplasia were documented in the hybrid group than in the sequential group ($P = 0.01$), the hybrid-treatment group developed more grade 4 or 5 leukopenia ($P < 0.001$), neutropenia ($P < 0.001$), and pulmonary toxicity ($P = 0.004$).

Another large-scale comparison of ABVD to a MOPP-ABV hybrid regimen for advanced Hodgkin's disease was the CALGB 8952 trial, which involved the SWOG, the ECOG, and the National Cancer Institute of Canada.[119] A total of 865 patients with a stage III or IV or recurrent disease after radiation therapy alone were accrued and stratified by age, stage, and previous radiation therapy. Chemotherapy was given for up to eight to 10 cycles for those who responded. The CR rate was 71% for the ABVD group and 73% for the MOPP-ABV hybrid group ($P = 0.4$); at 3 years, the corresponding failure-free survival rates were 65% and 67% ($P = 0.3$) and the overall survival rates were 87% and 85% ($P = 0.8$). However, the study was closed in November 1995 because of excessive numbers of treatment-related deaths and second malignancies among the hybrid group (16 deaths and 12 second malignancies in the hybrid group vs. nine deaths [$P = 0.13$] and two second malignancies [$P = 0.006$] in the ABVD group).

Radiation Therapy After Complete Response to Chemotherapy

A SWOG study, published in 1994, explored whether the addition of low-dose radiation after chemotherapy could prevent relapse and improve survival among patients with stage III or IV Hodgkin's disease.[120] Patients with clinical or pathologic stage III or IV disease were given six cycles of nitrogen mustard, vincristine, prednisone, bleomycin, doxorubicin, and procarbazine (MOP-BAP). Patients who achieved a CR were randomly assigned to undergo low-dose involved-field radiation therapy or no further treatment. Radiation doses (all delivered only to initially involved sites) were 20 Gy (in 1.5-Gy fractions) to nodes, 15 Gy (in 1.5-Gy fractions) to liver, 15 Gy (in 1.25-Gy fractions) to spleen, and 10 Gy (in 1-Gy fractions) to lungs. Between 1978 and 1988, 530 eligible patients underwent six cycles of MOP-BAP and 322 achieved CR; among these patients, 278 agreed to participate in the randomization, and 135 were assigned to receive radiation and 143 to receive no further treatment. However, only 104 of the 135 patients in the radiation group actually underwent irradiation, and 130 of the 143 in the no-radiation group actually received no further treatment. Intent-to-treat analysis of these 278 patients showed the 5-year remission-duration estimate to be 79% for the radiation group and 68% for the no-radiation group ($P = 0.09$). However, analysis of the 234 patients who actually received the randomized treatment showed the 5-year remission-duration rates to be 85% for the radiation group and 67% for the no-radiation group ($P = 0.002$). Limiting the analysis to the 169 patients with nodular-sclerosis histology revealed 5-year remission duration rates of 82% for the radiation group and 60% for the no-radiation group ($P = 0.002$). Further limiting the analysis to the 74 patients with nodular-sclerosis histology and bulky disease made a still larger difference in 5-year remission-duration rates: to 76% (radiation group) and 46% (no-radiation group) ($P = 0.006$); analysis of the 95 patients with nodular-sclerosis histology and non-bulky disease revealed 5-year remission-duration rates of 88% (radiation) and 68% (no radiation) ($P = 0.06$).

Notably, bulky disease was defined in this trial as any mass 6 cm or larger. Shortcomings of this study included a change in study design after early problems with accrual and the fact that 16% of the patients did not receive the assigned treatment. Nevertheless, this trial demonstrated a significant benefit for low-dose involved-field radiation therapy, at least for some subsets of patients.

The HD3 trial of the German Hodgkin's Lymphoma Study Group also studied the effectiveness of adjuvant radiation or chemotherapy after a CR to chemotherapy.[121] Patients with clinical or pathologic stage IIIB or IV disease were treated with three cycles of COPP and ABVD chemotherapy. Those who achieved CR were randomized to undergo either involved-field radiation therapy (20 Gy to initially involved areas) or one more cycle of COPP-ABVD. Between 1984 and 1988, 288 patients were accrued, and 171 achieved CR after three cycles of COPP-ABVD. Only 100 of these patients were randomized, 51 to the radiation-therapy group and 49 to the additional-chemotherapy group. The two groups did not differ in freedom from treatment failure or overall survival rates. Interestingly, the relative risk of failure of 21 patients who refused further treatment after a CR to three chemotherapy cycles was 3.67 in comparison with patients given consolidation treatment. Although the number of patients studied was small, these findings underscore the importance of consolidation treatment. Whether more than six cycles of chemotherapy will eliminate the need for consolidation therapy remains to be seen.

A similar study was conducted recently by the Groupe d'Études des Lymphomes de l'Adulte.[122] In their H89 trial, 418 patients with stage IIIB or IV Hodgkin's lymphoma who had achieved a complete or partial response to six cycles of doxorubicin, bleomycin, vinblastine, procarbazine, and prednisone (ABVPP) or a MOPP-ABV hybrid regimen were randomized to undergo either two additional cycles of chemotherapy or extended-field radiation therapy to 30 to 40 Gy. The radiation fields were subtotal nodal (i.e., mantle, para-aortic, and spleen). However, the inverted Y with spleen fields were used if the iliac or inguinal nodes were involved. Although consolidation treatment with radiation seemed to confer a slight advantage over consolidation with chemotherapy in terms of disease-free survival ($P = 0.07$), no difference was found in overall survival rate between those given radiation or chemotherapy consolidation. However, because the radiation fields were substantially larger than the involved fields in this study, the putative increase in toxicity may have negated any benefit achieved by radiation in terms of an improvement in disease-free survival.

Radiation Therapy after Partial Response to Chemotherapy

The EORTC and the Groupe Pierre-et-Marie-Curie performed a randomized trial comparing involved-field radiation therapy and no radiation therapy for patients who achieved a CR to six cycles of MOPP-ABV hybrid chemotherapy for stage III or IV Hodgkin's disease.[123] In this study, 405 patients were evaluable after six cycles of chemotherapy; 240 (59%) had achieved PR, 149 (37%) achieved CR, and 16 (4%) did not respond to the induction chemotherapy. Patients who achieved CR were randomized to undergo radiation or no radiation; the results from that aspect of the study are not yet available. However, findings from those who achieved PR, who were then given involved-field radiation therapy of 30 Gy (with a boost of 4 to 10 Gy as needed) in 1.5- to 2-Gy fractions, are encouraging. At a median follow-up of 43 months, the 5-year progression-free and overall survival rates for the 149 partial responders (122 of whom underwent irradiation) were 75% and 87%, rates similar to those for patients who achieved CR. These results, although preliminary, strongly support the role of radiation therapy for those who achieve PR to induction chemotherapy because prognosis for those patients seems to be as good as that for those who achieved CR to induction chemotherapy.

Predictors of Outcome

The International Prognostic Factors Project recently sought to identify prognostic factors (in addition to Ann Arbor stage) for advanced Hodgkin's disease.[124] Analyzed data were pooled from 5141 patients from 25 centers in Europe and North America. Eligible patients had to be between 15 and 65 years old with advanced Hodgkin's disease that had been treated with at least four planned cycles of "state-of-the-art" combination chemotherapy, with or without radiation therapy. The definition of advanced disease was left to the contributors. Of the 4695 patients analyzed, more than 75% of the patients had been treated with doxorubicin-based regimens, 20% with MOPP or a MOPP-like regimen, and 40% had undergone radiation therapy. Another requirement was that treatment had to have begun before January 1, 1992 to ensure sufficiently long follow-up. The variables at diagnosis examined in relation to the endpoint (freedom from disease progression) were age, sex, tumor histology, Ann Arbor stage, presence of B symptoms, extent of mediastinal involvement, inguinal-node, lung, liver, and bone marrow involvement, hemoglobin level, serum albumin level, ESR, white blood cell and platelet counts, absolute and relative lymphocyte counts, and alkaline phosphatase, lactate dehydrogenase, and creatinine levels. Seven of these factors were identified in a Cox regression model as having independent adverse significance: serum albumin level of less than 4 g/dl, hemoglobin level of less than 10.5 g/dl, male sex, age 45 years or older, stage IV disease, white blood cell count of 15,000/mm³ or more, and lymphocyte count of either less than 600/mm³ or less than 8% of the number of white blood cells. The prognostic score was defined as the number of these adverse variables present at diagnosis. That score predicted the freedom from progression rate as follows:

    0, or no factors (7% of the patients): 84%
    1 (22% of the patients): 77%
    2 (29% of the patients): 67%
    3 (23% of the patients): 60%
    4 (12% of the patients): 51%
    5 or higher (7% of the patients): 42%

Freedom-from-progression rates seemed to reach a plateau after 4 years regardless of prognostic score. Unfortunately, this scoring technique could not identify a subgroup of patients at very high risk of progression.

In summary, for the treatment of intermediate- and advanced-stage Hodgkin's disease, consolidation radiation therapy probably improves at least relapse-free survival after CR to chemotherapy. Radiation therapy is recommended after partial response in most situations. The balance between benefit and risk probably varies with number of involved sites and bulkiness of the disease.

Subdiaphragmatic Disease

About 5% to 12% of the patients with stage I or II Hodgkin's disease present with disease that appears only below the diaphragm. Compared with supradiaphragmatic disease, subdiaphragmatic Hodgkin's disease is more likely to appear in men and at older ages, is less likely to be of nodular-sclerosis histology, and is more likely to be of lymphocyte-predominant histology. Given the relative rarity of this condition, no prospective randomized trials have been conducted, and most of the available information comes from retrospective reports from individual institutions. Reported adverse prognostic factors are central disease (vs. peripheral disease)[125,126]; older age; B symptoms[127]; and low albumin and hemoglobin levels.[128] Laparotomy is no longer thought to be necessary, given the ability to visualize abdominopelvic disease on CT scans, the morbidity associated with splenectomy, and satisfactory treatment outcome without laparotomy.[126] As for treatment, radiation therapy (administered in inverted Y and spleen fields) seems to be adequate when the disease is limited to the inguinofemoral areas. For more centrally located disease (i.e., that in the para-aortic- or iliac-node regions), total nodal irradiation or combined-modality therapy is recommended because of a high incidence of recurrence above the diaphragm. Combined-modality therapy is generally recommended for patients with stage IIB disease; whether those with stage IB disease would also benefit from chemotherapy is less clear. In general, long-term follow-up of patients with subdiaphragmatic Hodgkin's disease shows overall and relapse-free survival rates similar to those that would be expected in supradiaphragmatic Hodgkin's disease.[128]

Lymphocyte-Predominant Hodgkin's Disease

Whether lymphocyte-predominant Hodgkin's disease behaves any differently than does classical Hodgkin's disease remains a matter of debate.

Survival and Relapse-free Rates

In 1988 a group from Stanford published a retrospective analysis of 73 patients with lymphocyte-predominant Hodgkin's disease treated between 1963 and 1985.[129] Of this group, 41 patients had the diffuse subtype and 32 had the nodular subtype. The median follow-up was 9.4 years (range, 0.3 to 23.5 years). Among those with the nodular subtype, RFS rates were 83% at 5 years and 55% at 10 years; the 10-year RFS rate for patients with the diffuse subtype was 92% (P = 0.017). The median time to relapse was 5.2 years for those with the nodular subtype and 3.7 years for those with the diffuse subtype. However, overall survival rates were no different for the two subtypes.

In 1999 investigators at the M.D. Anderson Cancer Center published a retrospective analysis of 70 patients with lymphocyte-predominant Hodgkin's disease treated between 1960 and 1992.[130] Of these 70 patients, 58 had the nodular subtype and 12 had the diffuse subtype; cases with any discernable nodularity were classified as nodular. The median age of the patients was 25 years. Median follow-up for living patients was 12.3 years (range, 3 to 37 years). The overall survival rates for the entire group were 97% at 5 years, 84% at 10 years, and 80% at 15 years; the corresponding RFS rates were 84%, 71%, and 71%. No differences in RFS or overall survival rates were found between patients with the nodular vs. diffuse subtypes.

In 1999 the European Task Force on Lymphoma reported an analysis of 219 patients with lymphocyte-predominant Hodgkin's disease pooled from 17 European and American centers.[131] The median observation time was 6.8 years. Survival and failure-free survival rates were no better among these patients than were stage-comparable results for classical Hodgkin's disease from the German Hodgkin's Lymphoma Study Group trials. Although the actual data were not presented in the Task Force study, no significant differences in patient characteristics or survival results reportedly were observed among the nodular, diffuse, or nodular-plus-diffuse cases of lymphocyte-predominant Hodgkin's disease.[131] Significantly, 27% of the patients with lymphocyte-predominant disease who experienced relapse had multiple relapses, which raises the question of how best to minimize the treatment for lymphocyte-predominant disease in light of good salvage rates and good survival rates after relapse. Moreover, diffuse lymphocyte-predominant Hodgkin's disease seems to be disappearing as a diagnostic entity as more cases are recognized as being lymphocyte-rich classical Hodgkin's disease.[55]

Secondary Malignancies

Another finding from the European Task Force study mentioned above was a 2.9% incidence of non-Hodgkin's lymphoma among patients with lymphocyte-predominant Hodgkin's disease. This finding raises the question of whether patients with this form of the disease are more susceptible to developing non-Hodgkin's lymphoma than are patients with classical Hodgkin's disease.[131] The answer to this question is not straightforward. Analysis of the international database on Hodgkin's disease shows that the risk of developing non-Hodgkin's lymphoma after treatment for Hodgkin's disease continues to increase over a 20-year period, from about 1% at 10 years to a 4% cumulative incidence at 20 years.[75] Bodis and colleagues,[132] in reviewing 325 cases of lymphocyte-predominant Hodgkin's disease, found a 2.5% chance of developing secondary non-Hodgkin's lymphoma. Because lymphocyte-predominant Hodgkin's disease sometimes co-exists with large cell lymphoma even at presentation, it may seem to have a higher chance of transforming into non-Hodgkin's lymphoma.[133] Evaluations of the incidence of non-Hogdkin's lymphoma in the presence of lymphocyte-predominant Hodgkin's disease should focus on actuarial cumulative incidence rather than crude incidence rates.

Response to Chemotherapy

In a study conducted by the Harvard Joint Center for Radiation Therapy, 16 patients with lymphocyte-predominant Hodgkin's disease were given chemotherapy, either as initial treatment or at first relapse.[132] Eight of 12 patients treated with MOPP or MOPP-like regimens achieved "durable" CR, compared with two of six patients treated with ABVD-etoposide, vinblastine, and doxorubicin (EVA) regimens, thus raising the question of whether MOPP was more effective than ABVD-EVA for this disease. Findings from a later M.D. Anderson Cancer Center review suggested that patients treated with radiation therapy alone had better RFS than patients treated with chemotherapy alone or combined chemoradiation therapy.[130] However, data from both studies should be interpreted cautiously because both were retrospective analyses and selection bias was present in terms of who was treated with chemotherapy.

In summary, no conclusive evidence exists to suggest that the lymphocyte-predominant form of Hodgkin's disease behaves any differently than does the classical form. Because the salvage rates for the lymphocyte-predominant form may be better than those for the classical form, even after multiple recurrences, some clinicians may advocate less-intensive treatment for patients with lymphocyte-predominant Hodgkin's disease.

Radiation Therapy Techniques
Mantle Field Irradiation

In mantle field irradiation, the bilateral cervical, supraclavicular, infraclavicular, axillary, mediastinal, and hilar lymphatics are the target volumes (Fig. 33-5, A). Simulations are usually performed with the patient supine with arms akimbo. This position has the advantage of easy reproducibility, although keeping the hands raised rather than at the waist would allow a bit more of the lung parenchyma to be spared through superolateral movement of the axillary lymphatics.[134] The patient's neck is slightly hyperextended so that the mouth block can also block the occipital head without compromising the coverage of the cervical lymphatics.

Equally weighted 6-MV opposed photon fields are usually used for mantle radiation. Lung blocks are shaped superolaterally for adequate coverage of the axillary and infraclavicular lymphatics. Medially, the lung blocks should allow margins adequate to cover the mediastinum and bilateral hila. The inferolateral border of the lung blocks is determined by the lateral-most point of the sixth rib. The inferior border of the mantle fields is placed immediately above the highest point of excursion of the left hemidiaphragm on expiration, unless this placement compromises tumor coverage in the lower mediastinum. If the inferior border is lower than this, field matching with the para-aortic and spleen fields may take place in the spleen, which is undesirable. The left ventricle of the heart is shielded throughout the treatment unless this shielding would compromise tumor coverage. After 25.2 Gy, the inferior field border is raised superiorly to about 2 vertebral bodies below the carina to shield additional heart volume, unless this movement would compromise tumor coverage.[135] An anterior larynx block is placed over the true vocal cords after 19.8 Gy unless it compromises tumor coverage.

Para-aortic– and Spleen-Field Irradiation

Expanding the radiation field to include the para-aortic nodes and spleen (see Fig. 33-5, B) usually involves the use of equally weighted 18-MV opposed photon fields. The superior border of these fields is matched with the inferior border of the mantle fields. The inferior border is usually at the L4-L5 interspace, which would allow coverage of the entire para-aortic lymphatics. The margin left around the spleen should be sufficient to allow splenic excursion with breathing.

Involved-Field Irradiation

The term *involved fields* usually implies treatment of the tumor volumes that were present before chemotherapy, with some additional margins. The exact extent of the fields depends on the location of the initial disease, the extent of residual disease after chemotherapy, and the exposure to adjacent organs such as kidneys,

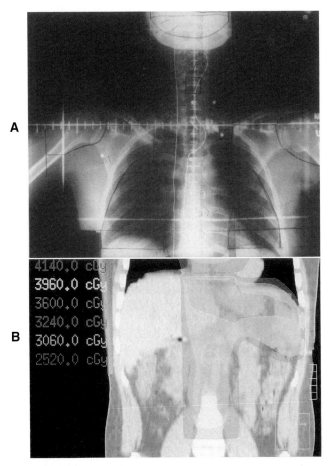

Fig. 33-5 **A**, A typical initial mantle irradiation field for a patient with Hodgkin's disease to be treated with radiation only. **B**, Dosimetry for para-aortic and spleen fields for the patient in **A**. (See Color Plate 36, after p. 80, for color reproduction of Part B.)

heart, and salivary glands. The advantages of higher dose and larger target volume must be balanced against the additional morbidity associated with this technique.

NON-HODGKIN'S LYMPHOMA
Etiology and Epidemiology

Non-Hodgkin's lymphoma is a heterogeneous group of diseases characterized by malignant lymphocytes. The etiology remains unknown, although *Helicobacter pylori* infection, viral infections, chemical and physical agents, congenital and acquired immunodeficiency states, and autoimmune disorders such as Hashimoto's thyroiditis may play roles in the pathogenesis of non-Hodgkin's lymphoma.

In contrast to Hodgkin's disease, incidence and mortality rates for non-Hodgkin's lymphoma have increased over the past three decades.[136] The American Cancer Society estimates that 56,200 people will be diagnosed with and 26,300 will die of non-Hodgkin's lymphoma

in the United States in 2001.[58] It is the fifth most common type of cancer, excluding cutaneous carcinomas, in the United States.

Follicular lymphomas most often present as advanced disease,[137] with adenopathy in 95% of cases and constitutional symptoms in 5% of cases. Diffuse lymphomas present with extranodal disease in approximately 50% of cases and with constitutional symptoms in 15% of cases. Follicular lymphomas occur with equal frequency in men and women, whereas diffuse lymphomas occur more often in men than in women (1.5:1.0).

Bcl-2 gene rearrangement, characterized by the t(14;18)(q32;q21) translocation, is found in up to 90% of follicular lymphomas and between 20% and 30% of diffuse lymphomas.[138] The t(14;18) translocation occurs in follicular lymphomas at two common sites: the major breakpoint region (MBR) and the minor cluster region (mcr). Lopez-Guillermo and colleagues[139] at the M.D. Anderson Cancer Center observed the t(14;18) translocation at MBR and mcr in 71% and 11% of follicular lymphomas, respectively. No breakpoint (germline) was detected in the remaining 18% of follicular lymphomas.

Whether detection of the t(14;18) translocation can be used to predict if a patient will respond to treatment remains controversial. Most groups[140-145] have failed to observe an association between the t(14;18) translocation and response to treatment, possibly because of differing patient characteristics and the lack of a standardized method for polymerase chain reaction analysis. In addition, MBR positivity has been detected in approximately 7% of healthy individuals[146-149] and patients with nonmalignant diseases.[149-151] Undefined mechanisms other than bcl-2 gene rearrangement can lead to elevated bcl-2 protein expression,[152] which blocks programmed cell death (apoptosis).[143] Elevated bcl-2 protein expression may also play a role in resistance to chemotherapy[138,153] and radiation therapy.[154] Some groups[138,143] have reported that elevated bcl-2 protein expression is an independent, unfavorable prognostic factor in non-Hodgkin's lymphoma. p53 protein overexpression may also be an independent, unfavorable prognostic factor through mediation of multidrug resistance.[145] Mantle cell lymphoma is characterized by the t(11;14)(q13;q32) translocation, which involves the *bcl-1* gene.[155,156] The proto-oncogene *c-myc* is expressed in most cases of Burkitt's lymphoma.[157]

Pathology

Non-Hodgkin's lymphoma is essentially of follicular or diffuse histology, although more complex classification systems are currently in use. Although follicular-vs.-diffuse lymphoma diagnoses are reproducible from one pathologist to the next, diagnoses of histologic subtypes within these two categories are not.[158,159] The REAL classification system, proposed by the International

Lymphoma Study Group in 1994,[55] was developed because new lymphoid disease entities had been recognized that were not part of the National Cancer Institute Working Formulation[160] and because a common classification system that could be used internationally was needed.[161] A comparison of the Working Formulation and REAL schemes is presented in Table 33-2.[55,162] Differences in overall survival rate according to REAL

TABLE 33-2

Comparisons of the National Cancer Institute Working Formulation[160] and the Revised European-American Classification of Lymphoid Neoplasms[55] Definitions of Non-Hodgkin's Lymphoma

| Working Formulation | REVISED EUROPEAN-AMERICAN CLASSIFICATION OF LYMPHOID NEOPLASMS (REAL) | |
	B-Cell Neoplasms	T-Cell Neoplasms
LOW GRADE		
Small lymphocytic, consistent with CLL	B-cell CLL/PLL/SLL Marginal zone/MALT Mantle cell	T-cell CLL/PLL LGL ATL/L (chronic and smoldering types)
Small lymphocytic, plasmacytoid	Lymphoplasmacytic- immunocytoma Marginal zone/MALT	
Follicular, predominantly small cleaved cell	Follicle center, follicular, grade I Mantle cell Marginal zone/MALT	
Follicular, mixed small cleaved and large cell	Follicle center, follicular, grade II Marginal zone/MALT	
INTERMEDIATE GRADE		
Follicular, large cell	Follicle center, follicular, grade III	
Diffuse, small cleaved cell	Mantle cell Follicle center, diffuse small cell Marginal zone/MALT	T-cell CLL/PLL LGL ATL/L Angioimmunoblastic
Angiocentric		
Diffuse, mixed small and large cell	Large B-cell lymphoma (rich in T cells) Follicle center, diffuse small cell Lymphoplasmacytoid Marginal zone/MALT Mantle cell	Peripheral T-cell unspecified ATL/L Angioimmunoblastic Angiocentric Intestinal T-cell lymphoma
Diffuse, large cell	Diffuse large B-cell lymphoma	Peripheral T-cell lymphoma ATL/L Angioimmunoblastic Angiocentric Intestinal T-cell
HIGH GRADE		
Large-cell immunoblastic	Diffuse large B-cell lymphoma	Peripheral T-cell unspecified Angioimmunoblastic Angiocentric Intestinal T-cell Angioplastic large cell
Lymphoblastic	Precursor B-lymphoblastic	Precursor T-lymphoblastic
SMALL NONCLEAVED CELL		
Burkitt's	Burkitt's	
Non-Burkitt's	High-grade B-cell, Burkitt-like diffuse large B-cell	

From Shipp MA, Mauch PM, Harris NL. Non-Hodgkin's lymphomas. In DeVita VT, Jr, Hellman S, Rosenberg SA, eds. *Cancer: Principles and Practice of Oncology*, 5th ed. Philadelphia, Pa: Lippincott-Raven; 1997:2165-2220.
CLL, Chronic lymphocytic leukemia; *PLL*, prolymphocytic leukemia; *SLL*, small lymphocytic lymphoma; *MALT*, mucosa-associated lymphoid tissue; *LGL*, large granular lymphocyte leukemia; *ATL/L*, adult T-cell lymphoma/leukemia.

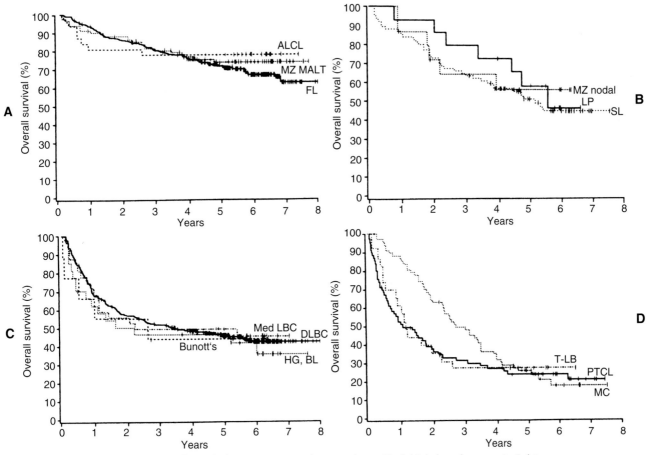

Fig. 33-6 Overall survival rates among subtypes of non-Hodgkin's lymphomas. **A,** Subtypes in which overall survival rates are more than 70% are anaplastic large T/null-cell lymphoma *(ALCL)*, marginal-zone B-cell lymphoma of mucosa-associated lymphoid tissue *(MZ MALT)*, and follicular lymphoma *(FL)*. **B,** Subtypes in which overall survival rates range from 70% to 50% are marginal-zone B-cell lymphoma of nodal type *(MZ nodal)*, lymphoplasmacytoid lymphoma *(LP)*, and small lymphocytic lymphoma *(SL)*. **C,** Subtypes in which overall survival rates range from 49% to 30% are primary mediastinal large B-cell lymphoma *(Med LBC)*, diffuse large B-cell lymphoma *(DLBC)*, high-grade B-cell Burkittlike lymphoma *(HG, BL)*, and Burkitt's lymphoma. **D,** Subtypes in which overall survival rates are less than 30% are precursor T-lymphoblastic lymphoma *(T-LB)*, peripheral T-cell lymphoma *(PTCL)*, and mantle cell lymphoma *(MC)*. (From A clinical evaluation of the International Lymphoma Study Group classification of non-Hodgkin's lymphoma. *Blood* 1997;89:3909-3918.)

category are illustrated in Figure 33-6.[163] The REAL classification was slightly modified recently in the WHO classification scheme.[164]

The incidence of the various types of lymphomas, in decreasing order of frequency, is as follows: large B-cell lymphoma (31%), follicular lymphoma (22%), marginal zone B-cell lymphoma of mucosa-associated lymphoid tissue (MALT) (8%), peripheral T-cell lymphoma (7%), small B-lymphocytic lymphoma (also known as chronic lymphocytic leukemia [CLL]) (7%), mantle cell lymphoma (6%), anaplastic large T/null cell lymphoma (2%), and primary mediastinal large B-cell lymphoma (2%); tumors of uncommon histology constitute the remainder of the non-Hodgkin's lymphomas.[163] One such tumor, monocytoid B-cell lymphoma, is rare. It

occurs in older individuals, involves lymph nodes rather than extranodal tissues, and is similar morphologically and immunologically to MALT lymphoma.[165,166]

Cell surface marker analysis (immunophenotyping) can help in resolving cases that are difficult to diagnose on the basis of morphology.[167] B-cell lineage is suggested by the presence of CD19, CD20, and CD22, and T-cell lineage is suggested by the expression of CD2, CD3, and CD7. Follicular follicle-center lymphomas are characteristically CD5- and CD43-, MALT lymphomas are CD5- and CD10-, mantle cell lymphomas are CD5+ and CD23-, and angiocentric T-cell/natural killer cell lymphomas are CD56+. Although cell surface marker analysis constitutes one piece of the diagnostic puzzle, few cell surface markers are lineage-specific.

Presentation and Staging Work-up
Presenting Sites of Disease

Non-Hodgkin's lymphomas can arise in many different sites, including, in order of decreasing frequency:

Lymph nodes
Gastrointestinal tract
    Stomach
    Small bowel
    Colon and rectum
    Appendix
    Esophagus
Waldeyer's ring
    Nasopharynx
    Palatine tonsil
    Base of tongue
Orbit
Brain
Thyroid
Paranasal sinuses
Testis
Oral cavity
Bone
Breast
Uterus
Bladder
Skin
Lung
Salivary glands

Disease arising at these sites have different etiologic factors, distinct natural histories, and variable responses to treatment.[163,168]

Staging Work-up

Pretreatment evaluation is similar to that for Hodgkin's disease, with the main differences being that gallium scans are not recommended for low-grade lymphomas[169] and lymphangiography is not used for non-Hodgkin's disease. A single photon emission CT gallium scan can sometimes help distinguish a diffuse lymphoma from fibrosis when a residual mass is present after treatment,[170] but its value in initial staging is controversial.[171] Small, single-institution studies suggest that positron emission tomography (PET) scans are more sensitive than gallium scans, particularly for detecting hepatic, splenic, and bone marrow involvement.[171] Unfortunately, few prospective trials have been done to compare gallium and PET scans. PET scans, by detecting increased glycolytic activity in malignant cells, can help distinguish necrotic cells from viable lymphoma[172,173]; they can also reveal sites of bone marrow involvement that are not detected in iliac crest biopsies.[174] Several studies have suggested that PET scans are more sensitive and specific than CT scans.[173,175-177] Consequently, PET scanning may eventually replace some current staging methods.[171]

Ann Arbor Staging System

Although originally developed for Hodgkin's disease, the American Joint Committee on Cancer has adopted the Ann Arbor staging system for non-Hodgkin's lymphoma to avoid confusion (see Box 33-1). In the Ann Arbor staging system, the thymus, appendix, Waldeyer's ring, and Peyer's patches are considered lymphatic sites. However, because of the clinical behavior of lymphomas at these sites, most oncologists refer to the aforementioned sites as extranodal. The Ann Arbor staging system is, by itself, of limited use in predicting the outcome of patients with non-Hodgkin's lymphoma,[178,179] primarily because it fails to address tumor burden.[180] It is more useful when combined with the serum lactate dehydrogenase level, performance status, presence of extranodal sites of disease, and age of the patient. These five factors, which independently predict overall survival, make up the age-adjusted international prognostic index proposed by the International Non-Hodgkin's Lymphoma Prognostic Factors Project (Table 33-3).[181]

Intermediate- and High-Grade Lymphomas

The following section on intermediate- and high-grade lymphomas includes diffuse large B-cell and anaplastic large-cell lymphomas in immunocompetent, nonpregnant patients.

Prognostic Factors

The international prognostic index (see Table 33-3)[181] incorporates the main prognostic factors for intermediate-grade and large-cell immunoblastic lymphomas. (The Zubrod performance scale,[182] which is part of the international prognostic index, is given in Table 33-4.)

TABLE 33-3	
Age-adjusted International Prognostic Index for Non-Hodgkin's Lymphoma*	
Variable	**Adverse Feature**
Lactate dehydrogenase level	> Normal
Ann Arbor stage	III or IV
Zubrod Performance Status	≤ 2
Extranodal involvement†	> 1 site
Age	> 60 years

From A predictive model for aggressive non-Hodgkin's lymphoma: the International Non-Hodgkin's Lymphoma Prognostic Factors Project. *N Engl J Med* 1993;329:987-994.
*Each adverse feature is assigned one point. The sum of the points is the international prognostic index (IPI). An IPI ≤ 2 indicates a good prognosis and an IPI > 2 indicates a poor prognosis.
†Extranodal involvement is only considered in patients age > 60 years.

TABLE 33-4

Zubrod Performance Status Scale

Points	Description
0	Normal activity, asymptomatic
1	Symptomatic but fully ambulatory
2	Symptomatic and in bed 1% to 49% of the day
3	Symptomatic and in bed 50% to 99% of the day
4	100% bedridden
5	Dead

Modified from Stanley KE. *J Natl Cancer Inst* 1980;65:25-32.

Minor shortcomings of the prognostic index are its occasional lack of clarity in distinguishing stage I and II disease from stage III and IV disease and in defining what constitutes an extranodal site.

Patients with intermediate-grade or large-cell immunoblastic lymphomas who have an elevated serum lactate dehydrogenase level and more than one extranodal site of disease are at high risk of developing a recurrence in the central nervous system (CNS), which carries a poor prognosis.[183] Patients with lymphoma involving the testes are also at increased risk of developing CNS involvement.[184]

Radiation Dose-Response Analysis

Before the 1980s, patients with intermediate- and high-grade lymphomas were typically treated with radiation therapy alone. Between 1979 and 1987, four randomized studies[185-188] demonstrated an improvement in 5-year disease-free survival from the addition of cyclophosphamide, vincristine, and prednisone chemotherapy to radiation therapy. Doxorubicin was subsequently found to be active against this disease, giving rise to the current practice of cyclophosphamide, doxorubicin, vincristine, and prednisone (CHOP) chemotherapy[189,190] followed by involved-field radiation therapy.

Stryker and colleagues[191] reported that the mean dose that produced local control in patients treated with radiation therapy alone was 48 Gy compared with 37 Gy in patients treated with both chemotherapy and radiation therapy. Mirza and colleagues[192] have suggested that after a CR to chemotherapy has been achieved, a total radiation dose of only 30 Gy is sufficient. Kamath and colleagues[193] have also suggested that 30 Gy is an adequate dose for large B-cell lymphomas that are initially 6 cm or smaller and completely respond to chemotherapy. Similarly, Wilder and colleagues[194] at the M.D. Anderson Cancer Center observed that 30 Gy is adequate for lymphomas smaller than 3.5 cm that completely respond to a median of three cycles of chemotherapy. In that study, 45 Gy was recommended for lymphomas that were larger than 10 cm before chemotherapy and completely responded to six cycles of chemotherapy.[194] After analyzing a different group of

patients at the M.D. Anderson Cancer Center, Fuller and colleagues[195] also recommended doses of at least 40 Gy for lymphomas that are initially 10 cm or larger and completely respond to chemotherapy. Others have reported that doses of at least 40 Gy seem to be necessary for local control of large B-cell lymphomas that are larger than 6 cm at the start of chemotherapy[193] or that respond only partially to chemotherapy.[193,196,197] The dose-response relationship in the above studies may reflect the presence of a greater residual tumor burden after treatment of bulky lymphomas with induction chemotherapy.[198] Along these lines, data from the M.D. Anderson Cancer Center suggest that resection of more than 80% of bulky lymphomas before chemoradiation may lead to improved survival.[199]

Ann Arbor Stages I and II Disease

Both the SWOG[200] and ECOG[196] randomized trials demonstrated a benefit for involved-field radiation therapy after CHOP induction chemotherapy for patients with clinical stages I and II large B-cell lymphomas. In the SWOG trial,[200] the 5-year disease-free survival rates were 77% for three cycles of CHOP chemotherapy followed by involved-field radiation therapy (40 to 55 Gy) to the prechemotherapy tumor volume. In contrast, 5-year disease-free survival was only 64% for those given eight cycles of CHOP chemotherapy without radiation therapy (*P* = 0.03). Higher doses of radiation (i.e., 45 to 55 Gy) were typically administered if the lymphoma was initially larger than 10 cm or if only a PR was achieved to induction chemotherapy. The 5-year overall survival rates for chemoradiation vs. chemotherapy alone were 82% and 72% (*P* = 0.02). Results from the ECOG trial have only been published in abstract form.[196] In patients who achieved CR to eight cycles of CHOP chemotherapy, the administration of involved-field radiation therapy to the prechemotherapy tumor volume to 30 Gy significantly improved disease-free survival (6-year rates 73% vs. 58%, *P* = 0.03). Overall survival rate among patients given radiation therapy also seemed to improve (6-year rates 84% vs. 70%, *P* = 0.06). When eight cycles of CHOP chemotherapy produced PR and radiation therapy to 40 Gy was administered, the 6-year disease-free and overall survival rates were 54% and 64%. This is an important observation, as it suggests that partial responders to chemotherapy treated with radiation therapy did nearly as well as complete responders treated with chemotherapy alone.

Ann Arbor Stages III and IV Disease

Some groups[201-203] believe that radiation therapy has no role in treating bulky stage III or IV large B-cell lymphomas. However, retrospective studies from Houston, Tex. (M.D. Anderson Cancer Center)[204,205]; Manchester, England[206]; and Milan, Italy[207] suggest that the delivery of involved-field radiation therapy to lymphomas that measure 4 cm or more before induction chemotherapy may improve disease-free and overall survival rates. Moreover, the only prospective randomized study conducted to date demonstrated a benefit for radiation therapy in patients with bulky (defined as larger than 10 cm) stage IV diffuse large B-cell lymphomas.[208] In that study, patients who achieved CR to anthracycline-based chemotherapy were randomized to receive or not receive involved-field radiation therapy to 40 to 50 Gy to initially bulky sites of disease. Radiation therapy produced a significant improvement in disease-free survival (5-year rates 72% vs. 35%, $P < 0.01$) and overall survival (5-year rates 81% vs. 55%, $P < 0.01$).

Low-Grade (Follicular) Lymphomas
Prognostic Factors

Whether the international prognostic index was useful for follicular lymphomas was controversial shortly after its introduction,[209,210] although more recent evidence supports its validity.[163,211,212] Overall and failure-free survival rates for patients with follicular lymphomas are shown in Figure 33-7.[163,168] Outcome for patients with follicular lymphomas varies greatly according to their index scores, as is also the case for patients with diffuse lymphomas.[163,213] Hence, both the histologic diagnosis and the international prognostic index can be used to help choose the treatment to be given to a particular patient.[163,164,211,212]

Molecular markers are currently being examined for their potential use as indicators of disease status and prognosis. For example, groups are studying whether molecular response, as assessed by polymerase chain reaction analysis, can be considered an early endpoint with which to predict long-term disease-free survival.[214] Bertoni and colleagues[144] reported that a molecular CR to chemotherapy was associated with better overall survival. Similarly, Lopez-Guillermo and colleagues[215] suggested that a molecular CR to chemotherapy was associated with improved failure-free survival. This finding was corroborated by Apostolidis and colleagues,[216] who reported that a molecular CR to chemotherapy was associated with a lower risk of relapse and death. Gribben and colleagues[217] found that the reappearance of t(14;18)-positive circulating cells was strongly associated with recurrence of lymphoma after myeloablative therapy. Ha and colleagues[218] and Cox[219] have suggested that a molecular CR is a favorable prognostic sign in patients treated with central lymphatic irradiation.

Radiation Dose-Response Analysis

Arthur and colleagues[220] reported that doses ranging from 20 to 30 Gy produced local control of 27 (100%) of 27 low-grade lymphomas. Sutcliffe and colleagues,[221]

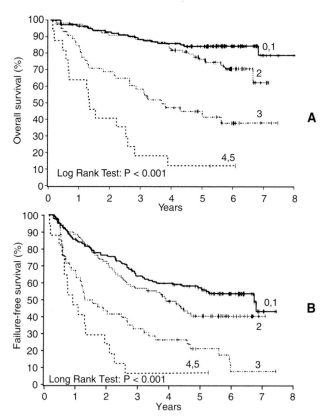

Fig. 33-7 Overall **(A)** and failure-free **(B)** survival rates for patients with follicular lymphomas grouped according to score on the international prognostic index. (From A clinical evaluation of the International Lymphoma Study Group classification of non-Hodgkin's lymphoma. *Blood* 1997;89:3909-3918.)

on the other hand, did not observe a dose-response relationship with doses ranging from 20 Gy to 40 Gy. Cox and colleagues[222] reported that doses of less than 25 Gy produced local control of 83 (90%) of 92 low-grade lymphomas, and doses ranging from 25 Gy to 46 Gy controlled 21 (100%) of 21 lymphomas. Kamath and colleagues[193] have suggested that 30 Gy is sufficient for most low-grade lymphomas except for small-volume disease in the orbit, where 20 to 25 Gy may be sufficient.

Ann Arbor Stages I to III Disease

Whether low-grade lymphomas are curable is unclear because few patients have been followed for 15 years or more.[223] Besa and colleagues[224] at the M.D. Anderson Cancer Center reported recurrences 16 years after involved-field radiation therapy. Although MacManus and Hoppe[223] at Stanford observed no recurrences 14 to 30 years after radiation therapy to one side of the diaphragm, relapses were noted 22 years after total nodal irradiation (Fig. 33-8).

Paryani and colleagues[225] and MacManus and Hoppe[223] at Stanford have reported that total lymphoid irradiation for stage I or II follicular lymphomas does

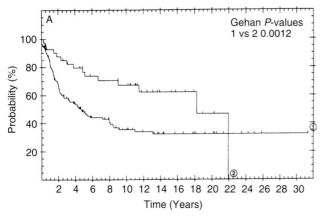

Fig. 33-8 Effect of radiation therapy field size on freedom from relapse in 177 patients with Ann Arbor stage I or II follicular lymphomas. *Curve 1* represents the results of radiation therapy to one side of the diaphragm (136 patients) and *curve 2* represents the results of radiation therapy to both sides of the diaphragm (41 patients). (From MacManus MP, Hoppe RT. *J Clin Oncol* 1996;14:1282-1290.)

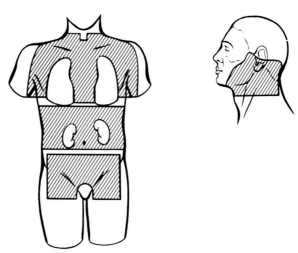

Fig. 33-9 Clinical target volumes in central lymphatic irradiation. Treatment is begun to the region with the greatest tumor burden. The superior-most region shown is irradiated only if Waldeyer's ring or the upper cervical nodes are involved. The daily fraction size is 1.5 Gy for the whole abdomen and 1.8 Gy for the remaining regions.

not significantly improve overall survival compared with involved-field radiation therapy (15-year rates 45% for total nodal irradiation vs. 43% for involved-field irradiation, *P* = 0.19). As a result, at many institutions, patients with stage I or II follicular lymphomas are treated with involved-field radiation therapy.[226-230] However, the Stanford group did note that in patients with stage I or II follicular lymphomas, the delivery of radiation therapy to both sides of the diaphragm improved freedom from relapse (15-year rates 62% vs. 36%, *P* = 0.001; see Fig. 33-8).[223]

The M.D. Anderson Cancer Center is one of the few institutions where central lymphatic irradiation is administered for clinical stage I to III follicular lymphomas. Central lymphatic irradiation differs from total lymphoid irradiation in that all of the mesenteric lymph nodes are included in the clinical target volume (Fig. 33-9). Consequently, wider abdominal and pelvic portals are irradiated than in total lymphoid irradiation. This aggressive treatment is advocated because low-grade lymphomas are less likely to recur with this approach (Fig. 33-10; see Fig. 33-8).[231,232] Central lymphatic irradiation typically consists of opposed, equally weighted mantle, whole abdominal, and whole pelvic fields that are treated in three stages separated by a 4-week break (see Fig. 33-9). Waldeyer's ring is irradiated only if it is involved or if high cervical adenopathy is present that is not adequately covered by the mantle fields.[231] The radiation portals encompassing the bulkiest disease are treated first. Follicular lymphomas up to 2.5 cm in size can be irradiated to 30.0 Gy in 20 fractions over 4 weeks when the abdomen is treated, or to 30.6 Gy in 17 fractions over 3.5 weeks when extraabdominal disease is treated.[193,231,233] When the whole abdomen is irradiated, 1.5-Gy rather than 1.8-Gy fractions are delivered

daily to reduce acute and late toxic reactions. At the M.D. Anderson Cancer Center, gross disease (i.e., disease larger than 2.5 cm) is treated to a cumulative total dose of 40.5 Gy in 27 fractions over 5.5 weeks when abdominal disease is treated, or to 39.6 Gy in 22 fractions over 4.5 weeks when extraabdominal disease is treated.[233] (The radiation therapy technique used for mantle-field irradiation is described in the previous section on "Hodgkin's Disease.") A geometric calculation is performed to determine the skin gap that is required for the mantle and abdominal fields to match in the midfrontal plane. Port films are checked weekly. The lateral borders of the abdominal fields are placed along the periphery of the rib cage to ensure full coverage of the entire abdominal cavity. The inferior border of the abdominal fields is placed at the L4-L5 vertebral interspace. Two half-value layer kidney blocks are included in the posterior field from the start of treatment to keep the dose to the kidneys below 20 Gy.[234] After the administration of 30 Gy to the isocenter, lateral or oblique fields may be required to keep the dose to the kidneys below 20 Gy. Five half-value layer liver blocks are added to the anterior and posterior fields beginning typically at 21.0 Gy. The medial edge of the liver blocks is drawn to ensure adequate coverage of the celiac and para-aortic nodes. Unless the patient is very thin, 18-MV photons are recommended. Patients are treated 5 days per week. For the pelvic fields, a match with the abdominal fields is performed as described above. The lateral borders are placed just medial to the anterior superior iliac spine. The inferior border is usually placed 5 cm below the ischial tuberosities. The genitalia and perineum are shielded by using a block, the superior border of which

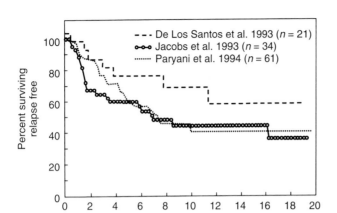

Fig. 33-10 Freedom from relapse in follicular lymphoma treated with either central lymphatic irradiation or total nodal irradiation. The *curve* labeled *De Los Santos et al. 1993* represents patients with stage I-III disease, whereas the *remaining two curves* include only patients with stage III disease. The number of patients in each study is shown in parentheses. (Data from Paryani SB, Hoppe RT, Cox RS, et al. *J Clin Oncol* 1984;2:841-848; Jacobs JP, Murray KJ, Schultz CJ, et al. *J Clin Oncol* 1993;11:233-238; De Los Santos JF, Mendenhall NP, Lynch JW. *Int J Radiat Oncol Biol Phys* 1997;38:3-8.)

is placed just above the pubic symphysis. A clamshell shield can be used for additional shielding of the scrotum. Six-MV photons are recommended for the anterior pelvic field, and 18-MV photons are recommended for the posterior field. For large patients, 18-MV photons can be used for both fields.

De Los Santos and colleagues[232] reported that treatment with central lymphatic irradiation produced 5-year, 10-year, and 15-year freedom-from-relapse rates of 75%, 58%, and 58% for patients with stage I to III follicular lymphomas (see Fig. 33-10). For patients with stage III follicular lymphomas, Jacobs and colleagues[231] observed a 15-year disease-free survival rate of 40% after the administration of either central lymphatic irradiation or total lymphoid irradiation (see Fig. 33-10). Paryani and colleagues[235] also reported a 15-year freedom-from-relapse rate of 40% for patients with stage III follicular lymphomas treated with total lymphoid irradiation (see Fig. 33-10).

Central lymphatic irradiation can also be offered for follicular lymphomas that have recurred after treatment with chemotherapy alone, provided that the bone marrow has never been involved.[236] In such salvage central lymphatic irradiation, liver blocks are used from the start to reduce the risk of hepatitis.[204]

Mahe and colleagues[237] used irradiation of the whole abdomen and pelvis (0.8 Gy twice daily to a total dose of 20.0 Gy over 3 weeks) to treat 22 patients with follicular lymphomas that had recurred subdiaphragmatically after chemotherapy. This approach resulted in 10-year disease-free and overall survival rates of 37% and 45%. As a result, the authors suggested that

abdominopelvic irradiation may be a feasible alternative when bone marrow transplantation is not possible.

Most randomized studies have shown that adding chemotherapy to involved-field radiation therapy results in an improvement in disease-free survival but does not significantly improve overall survival for patients with stage I or II follicular lymphomas.[228] Chemotherapy alone is commonly recommended for patients with stage III follicular lymphomas that are bulky or causing symptoms or organ dysfunction.[238,239] The addition of involved-field radiation therapy does not improve failure-free or overall survival in patients with stage III follicular lymphomas.[240] Hence, the use of combined-modality therapy is controversial in patients with stage I to III follicular lymphomas.[238]

Ann Arbor Stage IV Disease

The timing and type of treatment for stage IV follicular lymphomas are a matter of debate. Twenty-three percent of low-grade lymphomas spontaneously regress, at least partially.[241] Horning and Rosenberg[242] at Stanford observed no overall survival benefit for immediate as opposed to delayed chemotherapy in patients with stage III or IV follicular lymphomas. Similarly, a prospective trial conducted by the National Cancer Institute found no overall survival benefit for immediate vs. delayed treatment.[243] Consequently, most oncologists advocate a watch-and-wait philosophy for previously untreated, smaller than 10 cm, stages III and IV follicular lymphomas that are not causing symptoms or organ dysfunction.[241,244] However, some oncologists recommend immediate treatment with chemotherapy of such patients.[245] Recently, antisense oligonucleotides that inhibit bcl-2 protein expression have been introduced[246] that may sensitize tumor cells to chemotherapy.[247] Rituximab immunotherapy also constitutes a promising approach.[248] Rituximab is a chimeric, anti-CD20 monoclonal antibody.[249] It is the first monoclonal antibody to gain U.S. Food and Drug Administration approval for cancer therapy. Radioimmunotherapy constitutes another promising approach.[250]

Marginal Zone/Mucosa-associated Lymphoid Tissue Lymphoma

Treatment of an *H. pylori* infection with two antimicrobial agents and a potent acid-inhibiting drug or bismuth[251] can produce complete remission in about half of gastric MALT lymphomas.[252] Consequently, this antibiotic-based approach can be offered to patients with localized gastric MALT lymphomas associated with an *H. pylori* infection. In patients with *H. pylori*–negative or antibiotic-resistant gastric MALT lymphomas, involved-field radiation therapy alone is recommended (Fig. 33-11).[253-255] After a median follow-up of 30 months, Yahalom and colleagues[255] reported a

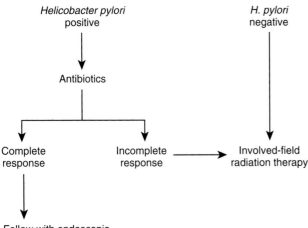

Fig. 33-11 Treatment algorithm for localized gastric mucosa-associated lymphoid tissue *(MALT)* lymphoma.

disease-free survival rate of 94% ± 5% in patients given a median dose of 30 Gy in 20 fractions over 4 weeks.

Zinzani and colleagues[256] reported results from 75 patients with previously untreated stage I_E to I_V nongastrointestinal MALT lymphomas who were given treatment ranging from local administration of interferon-α to surgery and postoperative chemoradiation. The 5-year freedom-from-progression rate for the 47 patients with stage I_E or II_E disease, many of whom underwent involved-field radiation therapy, was 71%. The National Comprehensive Cancer Network Practice Guidelines[257] recommend that stages I_E and II_E, non-gastric and *Heliobacter pylori*–negative or antibiotic-resistant gastric MALT lymphomas be treated with involved-field radiation therapy to 30 to 36 Gy.

Peripheral T-Cell Lymphoma

The incidence of peripheral T-cell lymphomas is increasing particularly rapidly, for reasons that remain unclear.[258] Patients with peripheral T-cell lymphomas tend to be younger than 35 years and have widespread disease at presentation.[259] A complete response to anthracycline-based chemotherapy occurs in only about 45% of cases, and disease-free survival typically is brief (see Fig. 33-6, *D*).[260] Hence, the prognosis for peripheral T-cell lymphoma is poorer than for most other non-Hodgkin's lymphomas (see Fig. 33-6, *D*).[163] Chemotherapy followed by involved-field radiation therapy to initially bulky sites of disease is recommended.

Burkitt's Lymphoma

In adults, Burkitt's lymphomas typically arise in extranodal sites and involve the abdomen (e.g., the cecum and mesentery).[203,261] For patients with stage IV disease,

CNS prophylaxis with chemotherapy, with or without cranial irradiation to a total dose of 24 Gy in 12 fractions over 2.5 weeks, is indicated.[261] In addition, cranial irradiation to a total dose of 24 Gy in 12 fractions over 2.5 weeks can be used to palliate symptoms in patients with a chemorefractory CNS recurrence. Patients with Burkitt's lymphomas have 5-year overall survival rates (30% to 49%) similar to those with high-grade, B-cell Burkittlike lymphomas, diffuse large B-cell lymphomas, and primary mediastinal large B-cell lymphomas (see Fig. 33-6, *C*).[163]

Mantle Cell Lymphoma

Mantle cell lymphoma typically presents as advanced disease that cannot be cured with conventional chemotherapy (see Fig. 33-6, *D*).[155,156,262] Patients at the M.D. Anderson Cancer Center who have mantle cell lymphoma and are less than 60 years old undergo hyper-fractionated cyclophosphamide, vincristine, doxorubicin and dexamethasone chemotherapy alternating with high-dose methotrexate and cytarabine chemotherapy, total body irradiation, and bone marrow transplantation. For previously untreated patients with stage IV disease, this approach produced 3-year event-free and overall survival rates of 72% and 92%, rates that compare favorably with the 28% event-free and 56% overall-survival rates observed for historical controls treated with CHOP-based chemotherapy.[263] Despite the paucity of randomized trials showing a benefit for transplantation, many oncologists advocate an aggressive approach in young patients because the median survival duration after standard, CHOP-like chemotherapy is only 3 years.[264]

Precursor B- and T-Lymphoblastic Lymphoma

Patients with precursor T-lymphoblastic lymphomas tend to be younger than those with precursor B-lymphoblastic lymphomas and more often present with bone marrow involvement.[265] Patients with lymphoblastic lymphomas involving the mediastinum can progress to a leukemic phase that is cytologically indistinguishable from acute lymphoblastic leukemia.[266] Given the natural history of the disease, CNS prophylaxis with intrathecal chemotherapy is indicated. At some institutions, CNS prophylaxis also includes cranial irradiation to a dose of 24 Gy given in 12 fractions over 2.5 weeks.[267,268]

The use of mediastinal irradiation is controversial, with some groups reserving this approach for patients who present with respiratory distress or those who achieve only a PR to chemotherapy.[266,269] Others[270] deliver mediastinal irradiation to all adults with precursor T-lymphoblastic lymphomas that involve the mediastinum in an effort to improve local control.

Mycosis Fungoides

Mycosis fungoides, also known as Sezary syndrome or cutaneous T-cell lymphoma, is a clinicopathologic diagnosis. Staging guidelines from the Mycosis Fungoides Cooperative Group are presented in Table 33-5.[271] Pathologic features include an infiltrate of atypical T lymphocytes with cerebriform nuclei in the epidermis (epidermotropism).[55] These cells may form aggregates known as Pautrier's microabscesses.[272,273] In most cases, malignant T cells express CD2, CD3, CD4, and CD5 but not CD7.[55]

Because of the rarity of mycosis fungoides (only 1000 new cases appear each year in the United States) and the consequent paucity of randomized trials, treatment remains controversial.[274] Total-skin electron-beam radiation therapy has been used to treat patients with mycosis fungoides since 1951.[275] Acute side effects of this therapy include generalized erythema, dry desquamation, and soreness of the hands and feet. The treatment also causes reversible alopecia, loss of fingernails and toenails, decreased ability to sweat for 6 to 12 months, chronically dry skin, and an increased risk of second cutaneous cancer.

The Ontario Cancer Foundation has suggested that total-skin electron-beam radiation therapy is potentially curative in approximately 29% of patients with T1 or T2 mycosis fungoides, provided that no palpable nodal sites are present.[276] The Stanford group has also suggested that total-skin electron-beam radiation therapy is potentially curative in patients with early-stage disease. Hoppe and colleagues[277] reported that in patients with plaques involving less than 25% of the skin surface (i.e., limited-plaque disease), total-skin electron-beam radiation therapy resulted in a 10-year disease-free survival rate of 45%. No recurrences were observed 4 to 10 years after irradiation.

<table>
<tr><td colspan="3">

TABLE 33-5

The Mycosis Fungoides Cooperative Group Staging Guidelines for Cutaneous T-Cell Lymphoma
</td></tr>
<tr><th>Clinical Stage</th><th>T Category (Skin)*</th><th>Palpable Nodal Sites</th></tr>
<tr><td>I</td><td>T0–T1</td><td>0-1</td></tr>
<tr><td>II</td><td>T0–T1</td><td>2-8</td></tr>
<tr><td></td><td>T2</td><td>0-1</td></tr>
<tr><td>III</td><td>T2</td><td>2-8</td></tr>
<tr><td></td><td>T3</td><td>0-8</td></tr>
<tr><td>IV</td><td>T4</td><td>0-8</td></tr>
</table>

From Lamberg SI, Green SB, Byar DP et al. *Ann Intern Med* 1984;100:187-192.

*Primary tumor classification: *T1*, plaques, papules, or eczematous patches involving less than 10% of the skin; *T2*, plaques, papules or eczematous patches involving at least 10% of the skin; *T3*, at least 3 tumors; and *T4*, generalized erythroderma or Sezary syndrome.

Kim and colleagues[278] reported that patients with plaques involving less than 10% of the skin treated with topical mechlorethamine (nitrogen mustard) have achieved life expectancies similar to those of age- and sex-matched control populations. Likewise, Hamminga and colleagues[279] have reported that topical mechlorethamine and total-skin electron-beam radiation therapy are equally effective in the treatment of patients who have plaques involving less than 10% of the skin. Two other groups[280,281] have also suggested that topical mechlorethamine is potentially curative in patients with early-stage mycosis fungoides. The CR rate for patients with limited-plaque disease after topical mechlorethamine in ointment (approximately 55%) is not as high as that after electron-beam radiation therapy (approximately 95%).[272] Nevertheless, such patients can be treated with total-skin electron-beam radiation therapy if disease progresses after topical mechlorethamine, and they achieve the same outcome as if they had initially undergone radiation therapy.[282]

One prospective randomized trial has addressed aggressive vs. conservative treatment in patients with mycosis fungoides. In that trial, no benefit was found in terms of disease-free or overall survival for early, aggressive treatment consisting of cyclophosphamide, doxorubicin, etoposide, and vincristine chemotherapy and total-skin electron-beam radiation therapy compared with a more conservative approach beginning with topical mechlorethamine.[283] Nevertheless, the toxicity of chemotherapy and total-skin electron-beam radiation therapy in that study was considerable.

Localized radiation therapy[284-286] (e.g., 30 Gy in 15 fractions over 3 weeks using a 2-cm margin for visible and palpable disease[287]) and psoralen activated with ultraviolet-A light (PUVA)[288,289] are also effective treatment options for patients with early-stage mycosis fungoides.[273]

Total-skin electron-beam radiation therapy is typically recommended for patients who present with thick plaques or have a recent history of rapid progression of cutaneous disease and are no longer responding to topical mechlorethamine or PUVA.[273] In patients who undergo total-skin electron-beam radiation therapy, overall survival is significantly better when a total dose of 30 Gy or more is delivered in daily 1.5- to 2.0-Gy fractions.[277] Some groups[279,290] have reported that the application of topical mechlorethamine after electron-beam radiation therapy prolongs disease-free survival.

Zackheim[291] and Chinn and colleagues[290] recommend chemotherapy for the initial, palliative management of cutaneous symptoms in patients with lymph-node or visceral metastases, reserving total-skin electron-beam radiation therapy for disease that does not respond to chemotherapy. Progression-free survival after high-dose chemotherapy and autologous stem cell or bone marrow rescue has typically been less than

4 months, although experience with this approach is limited.[292-294]

In summary, most physicians recommend topical mechlorethamine,[278-281,290,295-297] localized radiation therapy,[284-286] or PUVA[288,289] for patients with mycosis fungoides involving less than 10% of the skin. Combination chemotherapy is commonly recommended for patients with lymph-node or visceral metastases.[273,280,291,298]

At the M.D. Anderson Cancer Center, total-skin electron-beam radiation therapy is administered by using a Stanford dual, fixed-angle, six-field technique[299] modified to include a 1.2-cm Lucite scatter plate to reduce the electron energy and improve dose homogeneity.[300] A total dose of 32 Gy is delivered in nine cycles over 8 weeks.[300]

Primary Central Nervous System Lymphoma in Immunocompetent Patients

The mean age at diagnosis of primary CNS lymphoma in immunocompetent patients is 55 years.[301] Most patients present with a focal neurological deficit such as hemiparesis or dysphasia.[302,303] A stereotactic biopsy is recommended for diagnosis.[301] Treatment as part of an established protocol is recommended if possible.[301]

The administration of high-dose systemic chemotherapy before whole-brain irradiation has improved median survival from 12 to 18 months to 30 to 45 months.[303] The trend has been to reduce the dose of whole-brain irradiation in patients undergoing combined-modality therapy because of concerns regarding neurotoxicity.[304,305] The latest protocol being considered by the Radiation Therapy Oncology Group consists of high-dose, intravenous methotrexate induction chemotherapy over 7 weeks with leucovorin rescue. Patients without residual lymphoma undergo whole-brain irradiation in 1.2 Gy fractions twice daily to a dose of 36 Gy in 30 fractions over 3 weeks. The dose of whole-brain irradiation in complete responders is kept relatively low to reduce the risk of late neurotoxicity; patients older than 60 years are at particular risk.[306] The portion of the orbits posterior to the lenses of the eyes should be included in the planning target volume. If slit-lamp examination or vitrectomy reveals involvement of the vitreous humor, the anterior chambers of the eyes should also be included in the radiation therapy fields.[301] Patients with residual lymphoma after induction chemotherapy undergo whole-brain irradiation to 45 Gy in 25 daily 1.8-Gy fractions over 5 weeks. No boost to the primary tumor is planned because it does not reduce the risk of CNS recurrence.[301,306] Four weeks after the completion of radiation therapy, treatment with six cycles of procarbazine, lomustine, and vincristine chemotherapy is initiated. Methotrexate should not be given after whole-brain irradiation because of the potential for supra-additive neurotoxicity.[307] To reduce the risk of late neurotoxicity from methotrexate-based chemotherapy followed by whole-brain irradiation,[306] Freilich and colleagues[308] and Dahlborg and colleagues[309] have treated primary CNS lymphoma initially with chemotherapy alone and reported a median survival of 30 to 41 months. Cognitive function was preserved or improved in patients who remained free of disease.[308,309] Because little published information exists regarding this approach, many oncologists recommend high-dose, methotrexate-based induction chemotherapy followed by whole-brain irradiation as the initial treatment for patients with good performance status. Abrey and colleagues[306] reported a 5-year overall survival rate of 22% with this approach. Disabled patients requiring special care and assistance can simply be treated with a palliative course of whole-brain irradiation.[301]

Acquired Immunodeficiency Syndrome–Related Non-Hodgkin's Lymphoma

At present, no standard therapy exists for acquired immunodeficiency syndrome (AIDS)–related non-Hodgkin's lymphoma. Despite high initial CR rates to chemotherapy, most studies report a median survival of less than 1 year, with approximately half of patients dying of the lymphomas and the others dying of opportunistic infections or other AIDS-related complications.[310]

Extramedullary Plasmacytoma

Extramedullary plasmacytoma is a rare type of cancer characterized by the presence of clonal CD38-positive plasma cells outside the bone marrow.[55] Extramedullary plasmacytomas tend to arise in the mucosa of the head and neck region. The results achieved with radiation therapy at the M.D. Anderson Cancer Center were recently updated by Liebross and colleagues.[311] Radiation therapy resulted in a 5-year local control rate of 95% and a 5-year freedom-from-progression rate of 56%, suggesting that approximately one third of cases diagnosed as extramedullary plasmacytoma may actually have occult malignant cells in the bone marrow outside the radiation therapy fields (i.e., undiagnosed multiple myeloma).

Dose-response analyses have been hampered by small numbers of patients (often fewer than 25) and high local control rates (92% to 100%) in published reports.[311-317] Current practice at the M.D. Anderson Cancer Center consists of the delivery of 45 Gy in 25 fractions over 5 weeks, with the acknowledgment that the optimal dose of radiation remains unclear.

The clinical target volume, like the dose, is controversial. At some institutions, the regional lymph nodes are electively irradiated,[316,317] whereas at other institutions they are not.[313,318] At the M.D. Anderson Cancer Center, the decision regarding elective nodal irradiation is based on the guidelines for a squamous cell carcinoma arising at the same site.[311] For example, regional lymph nodes are electively irradiated for extramedullary plasmacytomas of the oral cavity, oropharynx, or nasopharynx. However, regional lymph nodes are not included in the clinical target volume for extramedullary plasmacytomas of the maxillary sinus or nasal cavity. Radiation therapy results in a median survival of 9.5 years.[311]

REFERENCES

1. Pritchard SL, Rogers PCJ. Rationale and recommendations for the irradiation of blood products. *Crit Rev Oncol Hematol* 1987;7:115-138.
2. Schiffer LM, Chanana AD, Cronkite EP, et al. Extracorporeal irradiation of the blood. *Semin Hematol* 1966;3:154-167.
3. Tubiana M, Carde P, Burgers JMV, et al. Prognostic factors in non-Hodgkin's lymphoma. *Int J Radiat Oncol Biol Phys* 1986;12:503-514.
4. Tubiana M, Frindel E, Croizat H, et al. Effects of radiations on bone marrow. *Pathol Biol* 1979;27:326-334.
5. Tubiana M, Hayat M, Henry-Amar M, et al. Five-year results of the EORTC randomized study of splenectomy and spleen irradiation in clinical stages I and II of Hodgkin's disease. *Eur J Cancer* 1981;17:355-363.
6. Tubiana M, Henry-Amar M, van der Werf-Messing B, et al. A multivariate analysis of prognostic factors in early stage Hodgkin's disease. *Int J Radiat Oncol Biol Phys* 1985;11:23-30.
7. Shank B, Andreeff M, Li D. Cell survival kinetics peripheral blood and bone marrow during total body irradiation for marrow transplantation. *Int J Radiat Oncol Biol Phys* 1983;9:1613-1623.
8. Bortin MM, Gale RP, Rimm AA. Allogeneic bone marrow transplantation for 144 patients with severe aplastic anemia. *JAMA* 1981;245:1132-1139.
9. Champlin RE, Gale RP. Role of bone marrow tranplantation in the treatment of hematologic malignancies and solid tumors: critical review of syngeneic, autologous, and allogeneic transplants. *Cancer Treat Rep* 1984;68:145-161.
10. Santos GW. Bone marrow transplantation in leukemia-current status. *Cancer* 1984;54:2732-2740.
11. Bloom W. *Histopathology of Irradiation from External and Internal Sources.* New York, NY: McGraw-Hill; 1948.
12. Knospe WH, Loeb V, Huguley CM. Bi-weekly chlorambucil treatment of chronic lymphocytic leukemia. *Cancer* 1974;33:355-362.
13. Fishburn RI, Dobelbower RR, Patchefsky AS, et al. The effect of age on the long-term response of bone marrow to local fractionated irradiation. *Cancer* 1975;35:1685-1691.
14. Lehar TJ, Kiely JM, Pease GL, et al. Effect of local irradiation on human bone marrow. *Am J Roentgenol* 1966;96:183-190.
15. Morardet N, Parmentier C, Flamant R. Etude par le fer 59 des effete de la radiothÈrapie Ètendue des hÈmatosarcomes sur l'erythropoiese [in French]. *Biomedicine* 1973;18:228-234.
16. Morardet N. Parmentier C, Hayat M, et al. Effects of radiotherapy on the bone marrow granulocytic stem cells of patients with malignant lymphomas, part II: long-term effects. *Int J Radiat Oncol Biol Phys* 1978;4:853-857.
17. Ellis RE. The distribution of active bone marrow in the adult. *Phys Med Biol* 1961;5:255-258.
18. Atkinson HR. Bone marrow distribution as a factor in estimating radiation to the blood-forming organs: a survey of present knowledge. *J Coll Radiol Aust* 1962;6:149-154.
19. Sykes MP, Chu FC, Saval H, et al. The effects of varying dosages of irradiation upon sternal marrow regeneration. *Radiology* 1964;83:1084-1088.
20. Sykes MP, Savel H, Chu FC, et al. Long-term effects of therapeutic irradiation upon bone marrow. *Cancer* 1964;17:1144-1148.
21. Rubin P, Constine L, Bennett JM. Hodgkin's disease IIB or not to-be using irradiation alone or in combination with chemotherapy? That is the question! *J Clin Oncol* 1986;4:455-457.
22. Rubin P, Landman S, Mayer E, et al. Bone marrow regeneration and extension after extended field irradiation in Hodgkin's disease. *Cancer* 1973;32:699-711.
23. Sacks EL, Goris ML, Glatstein E, et al. Bone marrow regeneration following large field radiation. *Cancer* 1978;42:1057-1065.
24. Greenberg ML, Chanana AD, Cronkite EP, et al. Extracorporeal irradiation of blood in man: radiation resistance of circulating platelets. *Radiat Res* 1968;35:147-154.
25. Del Regato JA. Total body irradiation in the treatment of chronic lymphogenous leukemia: Janeway Lecture, 1973. *Am J Roentgenol Radium Ther Nucl Med* 1974;120:504-520.
26. DeBruyn PPH. Lymph node and intestinal lymphatic tissue. In: Bloom W. ed. *Histopathology of Irradiation.* New York, NY: McGraw-Hill; 1948.
27. Engeset A. Irradiation of lymph nodes and vessels. *Acta Radiol* 1964;229.
28. Teneff S, Stoppani F. L'influenza delle irradiazioni sulle linfoghi-andole e sulfa circolazione linfatica [in French]. *Radiol Med* 1935;22:768-787.
29. Dettman PN, King ER, Zimberg YH. Evaluation of lymph node function following irradiation or surgery. *Am J Roentgenol* 1966;96:711-718.
30. Fisher B, Fisher ER. Barrier functions of lymph node to tumor cells and erythrocytes. Normal nodes. *Cancer* 1967;20(pt 1):1907-1913.
31. Fisher B, Fisher ER. Barrier function of lymph node to tumor cells and erythrocytes. Effect of x-ray, inflammation, sensitization, and tumor growth. *Cancer* 1967;20(pt 2):1914-1919.
32. O'Brien PH, Moss WT, Ujiki GT, et al. Effect of irradiation on tumor-infused lymph nodes. *Radiology* 1970;94:407-411.
33. Sherman JO, O'Brien PH. Effects of ionizing irradiation on normal lymphatic vessels and lymph nodes. *Cancer* 1967;20:1851-1858.
34. Lenzi M, Bassani G. The effect of radiation on the lymph and on the lymph vessels. *Radiology* 1963;80:814-817.
35. Murray RG. The spleen. In: Bloom W, ed. *Histopathology of Irradiation.* New York, NY: McGraw-Hill; 1948.
36. Dailey MO, Coleman CN, Kaplan HS. Radiation-induced splenic atrophy in patients with Hodgkin's disease and non-Hodgkin's lymphomas. *N Engl J Med* 1980;302:215-217.
37. United Nations Scientific Committee on the Effects of Atomic Radiation. *Genetic and Somatic Effects of Ionizing Radiation: 1986 Report to the General Assembly.* New York, NY; 1986.
38. Von Jagic N, Schwarz G, von Siebenrock L. Blutefunde bei Rontgenologen. *Klin Wochenschr* 1911;48:1220-1222.
39. March HC. Leukemia in radiologists in a 20 year period. *Am J Med Sci* 1950;220:282-286.
40. March HC. Leukemia in radiologists, 10 years later. *Am J Med Sci* 1961;242:137-149.
41. Logue JN, Barrick MK, Jessup TG. Mortality of radiologists and pathologists in the radiation registry of physicians. *J Occup Med* 1986;28:91-99.
42. Court-Brown WMC, Abbatt JD. The incidence of leukemia in ankylosing spondylitis treated with x-ray: a preliminary report. *Lancet* 1955;1:1283-1285.
43. Court-Brown WMC, Doll R. Leukemia and aplastic anemia in patients irradiated for ankylosing spondylitis. *M Res Counc Spec Rep Ser* 1957;295.
44. Wakabayashi T, Kato H, Ikeda T, et al. Studies of the mortality of A-bomb survivors, report 7: incidence of cancer in 1959-1978, based on the tumor register, Nagasaki. *Radiat Res* 1983;93(pt 3):112-146.

45. Levine EG, Bloomfield CD. Leukemias and myelodysplastic syndromes secondary to drug, radiation, and environmental exposure. *Semin Oncol* 1992;19:47-84.

46. Coltman CA Jr, Dixon DO. Second malignancies complicating Hodgkin's disease: a Southwest Oncology Group 10-year follow-up. *Cancer Treat Rep* 1982;66:1023-1033.

47. Berk PD, Goldberg JD, Silverstein MN, et al. Increased incidence of acute leukemia in polycythemia vera associated with chlorambucil therapy. *N Engl J Med* 1981;304:441-447.

48. Pinkel D. General Motors Cancer Research Foundation Prizes: Charles F. Kettering Prize: curing children of leukemia. *Cancer* 1987;59:1683-1691.

49. Pinkel D. The ninth annual David Karnofsky Lecture: treatment of acute lymphocytic leukemia. *Cancer* 1979;43:1128-1137.

50. Bleyer WA, Harland S, Coccio P, et al. The staging of childhood acute lymphoblastic leukemia: strategies of the Children's Cancer Study Group and a 3-dimensional technic of multivariate analysis. *Med Pediatr Oncol* 1986;14:271-280.

51. Clarkson BD, Gee T, Mertelsmann R, et al. Current status of treatment of acute leukemia in adults: an overview of the Memorial experience and review of literature. *Crit Rev Oncol Hematol* 1986;4:221-248.

52. Ha CS, Chung WK, Koller CA, et al. Role of radiation therapy to the brain in leukemic patients with cranial nerve plasies in the absence of radiological findings. *Leuk Lymphoma* 1999;32:497-503.

53. Cossman J, Annunziata CM, Barash S, et al. Reed-Sternberg cell genome expression supports a B-cell lineage. *Blood* 1999;94:411-416.

54. Cox J, Ha C. Prevention of diagnostic and treatment-related sequelae in stage I and II Hodgkin's disease. In: Meyer J, ed. *Frontiers of Radiation Therapy and Oncology.* Basel, Switzerland: Karger; 1999:85-97.

55. Harris NL, Jaffe ES, Stein H, et al. A Revised European-American classification of lymphoid neoplasms: a proposal from the International Lymphoma Study Group. *Blood* 1994;84:1361-1392.

56. Harris NL, Jaffe ES, Diebold J, et al. The World Health Organization classification of neoplastic diseases of the haematopoietic and lymphoid tissues: report of the Clinical Advisory Committee Meeting, Airlie House, Va, November 1997. *Hematol J* 2000;1:53-66.

57. Harris NL. The many faces of Hodgkin's disease around the world: what have we learned from its pathology? *Ann Oncol* 1998;9(suppl 5):S45-56.

58. Greenlee RT, Hill-Harmon MB, Murray T, et al. Cancer statistics, 2001. *CA Cancer J Clin* 2001;51:15-36.

59. Mack TM, Cozen W, Shibata DK, et al. Concordance for Hodgkin's disease in identical twins suggesting genetic susceptibility to the young-adult form of the disease. *N Engl J Med* 1995;332:413-418.

60. Mueller N, Evans A, Harris NL, et al. Hodgkin's disease and Epstein-Barr virus. Altered antibody pattern before diagnosis. *N Engl J Med* 1989;320:689-695.

61. Chapman AL, Rickinson AB. Epstein-Barr virus in Hodgkin's disease. *Ann Oncol* 1998;9(suppl 5):S5-16.

62. Carbone P, Kaplan H, Musshoff K. Report of the committee on Hodgkin's disease classification. *Cancer Res* 1971;31:1869-1861.

63. Lister TA, Crowther D, Sutcliffe SB, et al. Report of a committee convened to discuss the evaluation and staging of patients with Hodgkin's disease: Cotswolds meeting [published erratum appears in *J Clin Oncol* 1990;8:1602]. *J Clin Oncol* 1989;7:1630-1636.

64. Kaplan HS, Rosenberg SA. The treatment of Hodgkin's disease. *Med Clin North Am* 1966;50:1591-1610.

65. American Joint Committee on Cancer. Hodgkin's disease. In: Fleming I, Cooper J, Henson D, et al. eds. *AJCC Cancer Staging Manual.* 5th ed. Philadelphia, Pa: Lippincott Williams and Wilkins; 1997:285-287.

66. Gilbert R. Radiotherapy in Hodgkin's disease (malignant granulomatosis): anatomic and clinical foundations; governing principles; results. *Am J Roentgenol Radium Ther Nucl Med* 1939;41:198-241.

67. Peters MV. A study in survivals in Hodgkin's disease treated radiologically. *Am J Roentgenol* 1950;63:299-311.

68. Easson E, Russell M. The cure of Hodgkin's disease. *Br Med J* 1963;1:1704-1707.

69. Rosenberg SA, Kaplan HS, Hoppe RT, et al. The Stanford randomized trials of the treatment of Hodgkin's disease 1967-1980. In: Rosenberg SA, Kaplan HS, eds. *Malignant Lymphomas: Etiology, Immunology, Pathology, Treatment.* New York, NY: Academic Press; 1982:513-522.

70. Devessa S, Silverman D, Young J, et al. Cancer incidence and mortality trends among whites in the United States, 1947-1984. *J Natl Cancer Inst* 1987;79:701-770.

71. Gospodarowicz MK, Sutcliffe SB, Clark RM, et al. Analysis of supradiaphragmatic clinical stage I and II Hodgkin's disease treated with radiation alone. *Int J Radiat Oncol Biol Phys* 1992;22:859-865.

72. Noordijk EM, Carde P, Hagenbeek A, et al. Combination of radiotherapy and chemotherapy is advisable in all patients with clinical stage I-II Hodgkin's disease. Six-year results of the EORTC-GPMC controlled clinical trials H7-VF, H7-F and H7-U [abstract]. *Int J Radiat Oncol Biol Phys* 1997;39:173. Abstract 177.

73. Mauch PM, Kalish LA, Marcus KC, et al. Long-term survival in Hodgkin's disease: relative impact of mortality, second tumors, infection, and cardiovascular disease. *Cancer J Sci Am* 1995;1:33-42.

74. Tucker MA, Coleman CN, Cox RS, et al. Risk of second cancers after treatment for Hodgkin's disease. *N Engl J Med* 1988;318:76-81.

75. Henry-Amar M. Second cancer after the treatment for Hodgkin's disease: a report from the International Database on Hodgkin's disease. *Ann Oncol* 1992;3:117-128.

76. Noordijk EM, Carde P, Mandard AM, et al. Preliminary results of the EORTC-GPMC controlled clinical trial H7 in early-stage Hodgkin's disease. EORTC Lymphoma Cooperative Group and Groupe Pierre-et-Marie-Curie. *Ann Oncol* 1994;5:107-112.

77. Carde P, Burgers JM, Henry-Amar M, et al. Clinical stages I and II Hodgkin's disease: a specifically tailored therapy according to prognostic factors. *J Clin Oncol* 1988;6:239-252.

78. Wolf J, Tesch H, Parsa-Parsi R, et al. Current clinical trials for the treatment of adult Hodgkin's disease: common strategies and perspectives. *Ann Oncol* 1998;9:S79-S82.

79. Vijayakumar S, Myrianthopoulos LC. An updated dose-response analysis in Hodgkin's disease. *Radiother Oncol* 1992;24:1-13.

80. Seydel HG, Bloedorn FG, Wizenberg MJ. Time-dose-volume relationship in Hodgkin's disease. *Radiology* 1967;89:919-922.

81. Mendenhall NP, Rodriguez LL, Moore-Higgs GJ, et al. The optimal dose of radiation in Hodgkin's disease: an analysis of clinical and treatment factors affecting in-field disease control. *Int J Radiat Oncol Biol Phys* 1999;44:551-561.

82. Kaplan HS. Evidence for a tumoricidal dose level in the radiotherapy of Hodgkin's disease. *Cancer Res* 1966;26:1221-1224.

83. Jacobs ML, Marasso FJ. Lymphomas: relationship between dosage and recurrence. *Radiology* 1964;88:106-107.

84. Scott RM, Brizel HE. Time-dose relationships in Hodgkin's disease. *Radiology* 1964;82:1043-1049.

85. Raubitschek A, Glatstein E. The never-ending controversies in Hodgkin's disease. *Int J Radiat Oncol Biol Phys* 1989;17:1115-1117.

86. Fletcher GH, Shukovsky LJ. The interplay of radiocurability and tolerance in the irradiation of human cancers. *J Radiol Electrol* 1975;56:383-400.

87. Brincker H, Brentzen SM. A re-analysis of available dose-response and time-dose data in Hodgkin's disease. *Radiother Oncol* 1994;30:227-230.

88. Hanks GE, Kinzie JJ, White RL, et al. Patterns of care outcome studies: results of the national practice in Hodgkin's disease. *Cancer* 1983;51:569-573.

89. Thar TL, Million RR, Hausner RJ, et al. Hodgkin's disease, stages I and II: relationship of recurrence to size of disease, radiation dose, and number of sites involved. *Cancer* 1979;43:1101-1105.

90. Schewe KL, Reavis J, Kun LE, et al. Total dose, fraction size, and tumor volume in the local control of Hodgkin's disease. *Int J Radiat Oncol Biol Phys* 1988;15:25-28.

91. Sears JD, Greven KM, Ferree CR, et al. Definitive irradiation in the treatment of Hodgkin's disease. Analysis of outcome, prognostic factors, and long-term complications. *Cancer* 1997;79:145-151.

92. Schewe KL, Kun LE, Cox JD. A step toward ending the controversies in Hodgkin's disease. *Int J Radiat Oncol Biol Phys* 1989;17:1123-1124.

93. Duhmke E, Diehl V, Loeffler M, et al. Randomized trial with early-stage Hodgkin's disease testing 30 Gy vs. 40 Gy extended field radiotherapy alone. *Int J Radiat Oncol Biol Phys* 1996;36:305-310.

94. Vlachaki MT, Ha CS, Hagemeister FB, et al. Stage I Hodgkin disease: radiation therapy and chemotherapy at the University of Texas M. D. Anderson Cancer Center, 1996-1997. *Radiology* 1998;208:739-747.

95. Boivin JF, Hutchinson GB, Lubin JH, et al. Coronary artery disease mortality in patients treated for Hodgkin's disease. *Cancer* 1992;69:1241-1247.

96. Hancock SL, Tucker MA, Hoppe RT. Factors affecting late mortality from heart disease after treatment of Hodgkin's disease. *JAMA* 1993;270:1949-1955.

97. Swerdlow A, Douglas A, Vaughan HG, et al. Risk of second primary cancers after Hodgkin's disease by type of treatment: analysis of 2486 patients in the British National Lymphoma Investigation. *BMJ* 1992;304:1137-1143.

98. Hancock S, Tucker M, Hoppe R. Breast cancer after treatment of Hodgkin's disease. *J Natl Cancer Inst* 1993;85:25-31.

99. Aisenberg AC, Finkelstein DM, Doppke KP, et al. High risk of breast carcinoma after irradiation of young women with Hodgkin's disease. *Cancer* 1997;79:1203-1210.

100. Bhatia S, Robison LL, Oberlin O, et al. Breast cancer and other second neoplasms after childhood Hodgkin's disease. *N Engl J Med* 1996;334:745-751.

101. Vlachaki MT, Ha CS, Hagemeister FB, et al. Long-term outcome of treatment for Ann Arbor stage 1 Hodgkin's disease: patterns of failure, late toxicity and second malignancies. *Int J Radiat Oncol Biol Phys* 1997;39:609-616.

102. Nyandoto P, Muhonen T, Joensuu H. Second cancer among long-term survivors from Hodgkin's disease. *Int J Radiat Oncol Biol Phys* 1998;42:373-378.

103. Carde P, Hagenbeek A, Hayat M, et al. Clinical staging versus laparotomy and combined modality with MOPP versus ABVD in early-stage Hodgkin's disease: the H6 twin randomized trials from the European Organization for Research and Treatment of Cancer Lymphoma Cooperative Group. *J Clin Oncol* 1993;11:2258-2272.

104. Liao Z, Ha CS, Vlachaki MT, et al. Mantle irradiation alone for pathologic stage I and II Hodgkin's disease: long-term follow-up and patterns of failure [abstract]. *Int J Radiat Oncol Biol Phys* 1999;45:216. Abstract 134.

105. Jones E, Mauch P. Limited radiation therapy for selected patients with pathological stage IA and IIA Hodgkin's disease. *Semin Radiat Oncol* 1996;6:162-171.

106. Biti GP, Cimino G, Cartoni C, et al. Extended-field radiotherapy is superior to MOPP chemotherapy for the treatment of pathologic stage I-IIA Hodgkin's disease: eight-year update of an Italian prospective randomized study. *J Clin Oncol* 1992; 10:378-382.

107. Longo DL, Glatstein E, Duffey PL, et al. Radiation therapy versus combination chemotherapy in the treatment of early-stage Hodgkin's disease: seven-year results of a prospective randomized trial. *J Clin Oncol* 1991;9:906-917.

108. Jox A, Sieber M, Wolf J, et al. Hodgkin's disease—new treatment strategies toward the cure of patients. *Cancer Treat Rev* 1999;25:169-176.

109. Horning SJ, Hoppe RT, Breslin S, et al. Brief chemotherapy (CT) (Stanford V) and involved field radiotherapy (RT) are highly effective for advanced Hodgkin's disease [abstract]. *Proc Am Soc Clin Oncol* 1998;17:16a.

110. Rodriguez MA, Fuller LM, Zimmerman SO, et al. Hodgkin's disease: study of treatment intensities and incidences of second malignancies. *Ann Oncol* 1993;4:125-131.

111. Santoro A, Bonfante V, et al. Four cycles of ABVD followed by involved field irradiation (IF-RT) is the treatment of choice for early stage Hodgkin's disease (HD): 5-year results of a randomized trial [abstract]. *Eur J Cancer* 1997;33(suppl 8):262s. Abstract 1185.

112. Duhmke E, Sehlen S, Diehl V, et al. Prospective randomized trial in combined modality treatment (CMT) of intermediate risk Hodgkin's disease (IRHD) using extended field (EF) vs. involved field (IF) radiation therapy (RT) [abstract]. *Int J Radiat Oncol Biol Phys* 1999;45(suppl 3):215. Abstract 133.

113. Diehl V, Franklin J, Hasenclever D, et al. BEACOPP: a new regimen for advanced Hodgkin's disease. German Hodgkin's Lymphoma Study Group. *Ann Oncol* 1998;9(suppl 5):S67-S71.

114. Diehl V, Franklin J, Hasenclever D, et al. BEACOPP, a new dose-escalated and accelerated regimen, is at least as effective as COPP/ABVD in patients with advanced-stage Hodgkin's lymphoma: interim report from a trial of the German Hodgkin's Lymphoma Study Group. *J Clin Oncol* 1998;16:3810-3821.

115. Horning SJ, Williams J, Bartlett NL, et al. Assessment of the Stanford V regimen and consolidative radiotherapy for bulky and advanced Hodgkin's disease: Eastern Cooperative Oncology Group pilot study E1492. *J Clin Oncol* 2000;18:972-980.

116. Santoro A, Bonadonna G, Valagussa P, et al. Long-term results of combined chemotherapy-radiotherapy approach in Hodgkin's disease: superiority of ABVD plus radiotherapy versus MOPP plus radiotherapy. *J Clin Oncol* 1987;5:27-37.

117. Canellos GP, Anderson JR, Propert KJ, et al. Chemotherapy of advanced Hodgkin's disease with MOPP, ABVD, or MOPP alternating with ABVD. *N Engl J Med* 1992;327:1478-1484.

118. Glick JH, Young ML, Harrington D, et al. MOPP/ABV hybrid chemotherapy for advanced Hodgkin's disease significantly improves failure-free and overall survival: the 8-year results of the intergroup trial. *J Clin Oncol* 1998;16:19-26.

119. Duggan D, Petroni G, Johnson J, et al. MOPP/ABV versus ABVD for advanced Hodgkin's disease—a preliminary report of CALGB 8952 (with SWOG, ECOG, NCIC) [abstract]. *Proc Am Soc Clin Oncol* 1997;16:12a.

120. Fabian CJ, Mansfield CM, Dahlberg S, et al. Low-dose involved field radiation after chemotherapy in advanced Hodgkin disease. A Southwest Oncology Group randomized study. *Ann Intern Med* 1994;120:903-912.

121. Diehl V, Loeffler M, Pfreundschuh M, et al. Further chemotherapy versus low-dose involved-field radiotherapy as consolidation of complete remission after six cycles of alternating chemotherapy in patients with advanced Hodgkin's disease. German Hodgkin's Lymphoma Study Group (GHSG). *Ann Oncol* 1995;6:901-910.

122. Ferme C, Sebban C, Hennequin C, et al. Comparison of chemotherapy to radiotherapy as consolidation of complete or good partial response after six cycles of chemotherapy for patients

with advanced Hodgkin's disease: results of the groupe d'etudes des lymphomes de l'Adulte H89 trial. *Blood* 2000;95:2246-2252.

123. Raemaekers J, Burgers M, Henry-Amar M, et al. Patients with stage III/IV Hodgkin's disease in partial remission after MOPP/ABV chemotherapy have excellent prognosis after additional involved-field radiotherapy: interim results from the ongoing EORTC-LCG and GPMC phase III trial. The EORTC Lymphoma Cooperative Group and Groupe Pierre-et-Marie-Curie. *Ann Oncol* 1997;8:111-114.

124. Hasenclever D, Diehl V, Armitage JO, et al. A prognostic score for advanced Hodgkin's disease. International Prognostic Factors Project on Advanced Hodgkin's Disease. *N Engl J Med* 1998;339:1506-1514.

125. Krikorian JG, Portlock CS, Mauch PM. Hodgkin's disease presenting below the diaphragm: a review. *J Clin Oncol* 1986; 4:1551-1562.

126. Roos DE, O'Brien PC, Wright J, et al. Treatment of subdiaphragmatic Hodgkin's disease: is radiotherapy alone appropriate only for inguino-femoral presentations? *Int J Radiat Oncol Biol Phys* 1994;28:683-691.

127. Leibenhaut MH, Hoppe RT, Varghese A, et al. Subdiaphragmatic Hodgkin's disease: laparotomy and treatment results in 49 patients. *J Clin Oncol* 1987;5:1050-1055.

128. Liao Z, Ha CS, Fuller LM, et al. Subdiaphragmatic stage I and II Hodgkin's disease: long-term follow-up and prognostic factors. *Int J Radiat Oncol Biol Phys* 1998;41:1047-1056.

129. Regula D, Hoppe R, Weiss L. Nodular and diffuse types of lymphocyte predominance Hodgkin's disease. *N Engl J Med* 1988;318:214-219.

130. Ha CS, Kavadi V, Dimopoulos MA, et al. Hodgkin's disease with lymphocyte predominance: long-term results based on current histopathologic criteria. *Int J Radiat Oncol Biol Phys* 1999;43:329-334.

131. Diehl V, Sextro M, Franklin J, et al. Clinical presentation, course, and prognostic factors in lymphocyte-predominant Hodgkin's disease and lymphocyte-rich classical Hodgkin's disease: report from the European Task Force on Lymphoma Project on Lymphocyte-Predominant Hodgkin's Disease. *J Clin Oncol* 1999; 17:776-783.

132. Bodis S, Kraus M, Pinkus G, et al. Clinical presentation and outcome in lymphocyte-predominant Hodgkin's disease. *J Clin Oncol* 1997;15:3060-3066.

133. Sundeen JT, Cossman J, Jaffe ES. Lymphocyte-predominant Hodgkin's disease nodular subtype with coexistent large cell lymphoma—histological progression or composite malignancy? *Am J Surg Pathol* 1988;12:599-606.

134. Pergolizzi S, Settineri N, Gaeta M, et al. What is the best position of the arms in mantle field for Hodgkin's disease? *Int J Radiat Oncol Biol Phys* 2000;46:119-122.

135. Plowman PN. Radiotherapy considerations in patients with Hodgkin's disease who receive mediastinal radiotherapy and anthracycline-containing chemotherapy. *Clin Oncol* 1998;10: 384-391.

136. Rabkin CS, Devesa SS, Zahm SH, et al. Increasing incidence of non-Hodgkin's lymphoma. *Semin Hematol* 1993;30:286-296.

137. Gupta RK, Lister TA. Current management of follicular lymphoma. *Curr Opin Oncol* 1996;8:360-365.

138. Gascoyne RD, Adomat SA, Krajewski S, et al. Prognostic significance of *bcl-2* protein expression and *bcl-2* gene rearrangement in diffuse aggressive non-Hodgkin's lymphoma. *Blood* 1997;90:244-251.

139. Lopez-Guillermo A, Cabanillas F, McDonnell TI, et al. Correlation of *bcl-2* rearrangement with clinical characteristics and outcome in indolent follicular lymphoma. *Blood* 1999;93:3081-3087.

140. Levine EG, Arthur DC, Frizzera G, et al. Cytogenetic abnormalities predict clinical outcome in non-Hodgkin lymphoma. *Ann Intern Med* 1988;108:14-20.

141. Pezzella F, Jones M, Ralfkiaer E, et al. Evaluation of *bcl-2* protein expression and 14;18 translocation as prognostic markers in follicular lymphoma. *Br J Cancer* 1992;65:87-89.

142. Tilly H, Rossi A, Stamatoullas A, et al. Prognostic value of chromosomal abnormalities in follicular lymphoma. *Blood* 1994;84:1043-1049.

143. Martinka M, Comeau T, Foyle A, et al. Prognostic significance of t(14;18) and *bcl-2* gene expression in follicular small cleaved cell lymphoma and diffuse large cell lymphoma. *Clin Invest Med* 1997;20:364-370.

144. Bertoni F, Bosshard G, Roggero E, et al. Clinical relevance of *bcl-2*(MBR)/J(H) rearrangement detected by polymerase chain reaction in the peripheral blood of patients with follicular lymphoma. *Br J Cancer* 1997;76:36-39.

145. Sun RX, Coste J, Segara C, et al. MBR rearrangement and p-glycoprotein expression are not independent prognostic factors like *p53* protein in malignant lymphoma. *Clin Lab Haematol* 1998;20:87-94.

146. Liu Y, Hernandez AM, Shibata D, et al. *Bcl-2* translocation frequency rises with age in humans. *Proc Natl Acad Sci U S A* 1994;91:8910-8914.

147. Ji W, Qu GZ, Ye P, et al. Frequent detection of *bcl-2/JH* translocations in human blood and organ samples by a quantitative polymerase chain reaction assay. *Cancer Res* 1995;55: 2876-2882.

148. Limpens J, Stad R, Vos C, et al. Lymphoma-associated translocation t(14;18) in blood B-cells of normal individuals. *Blood* 1995;85:2528-2536.

149. Dolken G, Illerhaus G, Hirt C, et al. *bcl-2/JH* rearrangements in circulating B-cells of healthy blood donors and patients with nonmalignant diseases. *J Clin Oncol* 1996;14:1333-1344.

150. Limpens J, de Jong D, van Krieken JH, et al. *bcl-2/JH* rearrangements in benign lymphoid tissues with follicular hyperplasia. *Oncogene* 1991;6:2271-2276.

151. Aster JC, Kobayashi Y, Shiota M, et al. Detection of the t(14;18) at similar frequencies in hyperplastic lymphoid tissues from American and Japanese patients. *Am J Pathol* 1992;141: 291-299.

152. Pezzella F, Tse AG, Cordell JL, et al. Expression of the *bcl-2* oncogene protein is not specific for the 14;18 chromosomal translocation. *Am J Pathol* 1990;137:225-232.

153. Hill ME, MacLennan KA, Cunningham DC, et al. Prognostic significance of *bcl-2* expression and *bcl-2* major breakpoint region rearrangement in diffuse large cell non-Hodgkin's lymphoma: a British National Lymphoma Investigation Study. *Blood* 1996;88:1046-1051.

154. Kariya S, Ogawa Y, Yoshida S, et al. X-irradiation enhances the expression of *bcl-2* in HL-60 cells: the resulting effects on apoptosis and radiosensitivity. *Int J Mol Med* 1999;3:145-152.

155. Garcia-Conde J, Cabanillas F. Mantle cell lymphoma: a lymphoproliferative disorder associated with aberrant function of the cell cycle. *Leukemia* 1996;10(suppl 2):S78-S83.

156. de Boer CJ, van Krieken JH, Schuuring E, et al. *Bcl-1/cyclin D1* in malignant lymphoma. *Ann Oncol* 1997;8(Suppl 2): 109-117.

157. Hutchison RE, Finch C, Kepner J, et al. Burkitt lymphoma is immunophenotypically different from Burkitt-like lymphoma in young persons. *Ann Oncol* 2000;11(suppl 1):35-38.

158. Classification of non-Hodgkin's lymphomas. Reproducibility of major classification systems. NCI non-Hodgkin's Classification Project Writing Committee. *Cancer* 1985;55:91-95.

159. Dick F, Van Lier S, Banks P, et al. Use of the working formulation for non-Hodgkin's lymphoma in epidemiologic studies: agreeement between reported diagnoses and a panel of experienced pathologists. *J Natl Cancer Inst* 1987;78:1137-1144.

160. National Cancer Institute sponsored study of classifications of non-Hodgkin's lymphomas: summary and description of a

working formulation for clinical usage. The Non-Hodgkin's Lymphoma Pathologic Classification Project. *Cancer* 1982;49:2112-2135.

161. Fisher RI, Miller TP, Grogan TM. New REAL clinical entities. *Cancer J Sci Am* 1998;4(suppl 2):S5-12.

162. Shipp MA, Mauch PM, Harris NL. Non-Hodgkin's lymphomas. In: DeVita VT, Jr, Hellman S, Rosenberg SA, eds. *Cancer: Principles and Practice of Oncology.* 5th ed. Philadelphia, Pa: Lippincott-Raven; 1997:2165-2220.

163. No authors listed A clinical evaluation of the International Lymphoma Study Group classification of non-Hodgkin's lymphoma. The Non-Hodgkin's Lymphoma Classification Project. *Blood* 1997;89:3909-3918.

164. Pileri SA, Milani M, Fraternali-Orcioni G, et al. From the REAL classification to the upcoming WHO scheme: a step toward universal categorization of lymphoma entities? *Ann Oncol* 1998;9:607-612.

165. Sheibani K, Sohn CC, Burke JS, et al. Monocytoid B-cell lymphoma: a novel B-cell neoplasm. *Am J Pathol* 1986;124:310-318.

166. Nizze H, Cogliatti SB, von Schilling C, et al. Monocytoid B-cell lymphoma: morphological variants and relationship to low-grade B-cell lymphoma of the mucosa-associated lymphoid tissue. *Histopathology* 1991;18:403-414.

167. Armitage JO, Weisenburger DD. New approach to classifying non-Hodgkin's lymphomas: clinical features of the major histologic subtypes. Non-Hodgkin's Lymphoma Classification Project. *J Clin Oncol* 1998;16:2780-2795.

168. Cox JD. Lymphomas and leukemia. In: Cox JD, ed. *Moss' Radiation Oncology: Rationale, Technique, Results.* 7th ed. St. Louis, Mo: Mosby; 1994:793-826.

169. Gallamini A, Biggi A, Fruttero A, et al. Revisiting the prognostic role of gallium scintigraphy in low-grade non-Hodgkin's lymphoma. *Eur J Nucl Med* 1997;24:1499-1506.

170. Gasparini M, Bombardieri E, Castellani M, et al. Gallium-67 scintigraphy evaluation of therapy in non-Hodgkin's lymphoma. *J Nucl Med* 1998;39:1586-1590.

171. Bangerter M, Griesshammer M, Bergmann L. Progress in medical imaging of lymphoma and Hodgkin's disease. *Curr Opin Oncol* 1999;11:339-342.

172. de Wit M, Bumann D, Beyer W, et al. Whole-body positron emission tomography (PET) for diagnosis of residual mass in patients with lymphoma. *Ann Oncol* 1997;8(Suppl 1):57-60.

173. Jerusalem G, Beguin Y, Fassotte MF, et al. Whole-body positron emission tomography using 18F-fluorodeoxyglucose for post-treatment evaluation in Hodgkin's disease and non-Hodgkin's lymphoma has higher diagnostic and prognostic value than classical computed tomography scan imaging. *Blood* 1999; 94:429-433.

174. Moog F, Bangerter M, Kotzerke J, et al. ^{18}F-fluorodeoxyglucose-positron emission tomography as a new approach to detect lymphomatous bone marrow. *J Clin Oncol* 1998;16:603-609.

175. Moog F, Bangerter M, Diederichs CG, et al. Extranodal malignant lymphoma: detection with FDG PET versus CT. *Radiology* 1998;206:475-481.

176. Stumpe KD, Urbinelli M, Steinert HC, et al. Whole-body positron emission tomography using fluorodeoxyglucose for staging of lymphoma: effectiveness and comparison with computed tomography. *Eur J Nucl Med* 1998;25:721-728.

177. Zinzani PL, Magagnoli M, Chierichetti F, et al. The role of positron emission tomography (PET) in the management of lymphoma patients. *Ann Oncol* 1999;10:1181-1184.

178. Rosenberg SA. Validity of the Ann Arbor staging classification for the non-Hodgkin's lymphomas. *Cancer Treat Rep* 1977; 61:1023-1027.

179. Urba WJ, Duffey PL, Longo DL. Treatment of patients with aggressive lymphomas: an overview. *J Natl Cancer Inst Monogr* 1990;10:29-37.

180. Moore DF Jr, Cabanillas F. Overview of prognostic factors in non-Hodgkin's lymphoma. *Oncology* 1998;12:17-24.

181. No authors listed. A predictive model for aggressive non-Hodgkin's lymphoma: The International Non-Hodgkin's Lymphoma Prognostic Factors Project. *N Engl J Med* 1993;329:987-994.

182. Stanley KE. Prognostic factors for survival in patients with inoperable lung cancer. *J Natl Cancer Inst* 1980;65:25-32.

183. van Besien K, Ha CS, Murphy S. Risk factors, treatment, and outcome of central nervous system recurrence in adults with intermediate-grade and immunoblastic lymphoma. *Blood* 1998; 91:1178-1184.

184. Touroutoglou N, Dimopoulos MA, Younes A, et al. Testicular lymphoma: late relapses and poor outcome despite doxorubicin-based therapy. *J Clin Oncol* 1995;13:1361-1367.

185. Landberg TG, Hakansson LG, Moller TR, et al. CVP-remission maintenance in stage I or II non-Hodgkin's lymphomas. Preliminary results of a randomized study. *Cancer* 1979;44: 831-838.

186. Monfardini S, Banfi A, Bonadonna G, et al. Improved five-year survival after combined radiotherapy-chemotherapy for stage I-II non-Hodgkin's lymphoma. *Int J Radiat Oncol Biol Phys* 1980;6:125-134.

187. Nissen NI, Ersboll J, Hansen HS, et al. A randomized study of radiotherapy versus radiotherapy plus chemotherapy in stage I-II non-Hodgkin's lymphomas. *Cancer* 1983;52:1-7.

188. Somers R, Burgers M, Quasim M, et al. EORTC trial non-Hodgkin's lymphomas. *Eur J Cancer Clin Oncol* 1987;23:283-293.

189. Fisher RI, Gaynor ER, Dahlberg S, et al. Comparison of a standard regimen (CHOP) with three intensive chemotherapy regimens for advanced non-Hodgkin's lymphoma. *N Engl J Med* 1993;328:1002-1006.

190. Fisher RI. Cyclophosphamide, doxorubicin, vincristine, and prednisone versus intensive chemotherapy in non-Hodgkin's lymphoma. *Cancer Chemother Pharmacol* 1997;40:S42-46.

191. Stryker JA, Abt AB, Eyester MA, et al. Histopathologic subclassification of diffuse histiocytic lymphoma and response to therapy. *Radiology* 1982;142:501-506.

192. Mirza MR, Brincker H, Specht L. The integration of radiotherapy into the primary treatment of non-Hodgkin's lymphoma. *Crit Rev Oncol Hematol* 1992;12:217-229.

193. Kamath SS, Marcus RB Jr, Lynch JW, et al. The impact of radiotherapy dose and other treatment-related and clinical factors on in-field control in stage I and II non-Hodgkin's lymphoma. *Int J Radiat Oncol Biol Phys* 1999;44:563-568.

194. Wilder RB, Tucker SL, Ha CS, et al. Dose-response analysis for radiotherapy delivered to patients with intermediate grade and large-cell immunoblastic lymphomas that completely responded to induction, CHOP-based chemotherapy. *Int J Radiat Oncol Biol Phys* 2001;49:17-22.

195. Fuller LM, Krasin MJ, Velasquez WS, et al. Significance of tumor size and radiation dose to local control in stage I-III diffuse large cell lymphoma treated with CHOP-Bleo and radiation. *Int J Radiat Oncol Biol Phys* 1995;31:3-11.

196. Glick JH, Kim KJ, Earle J, et al. An ECOG randomized phase III trial of CHOP vs. CHOP + radiotherapy (XRT) for intermediate grade early stage non-Hodgkin's lymphoma (NHL) (abstract). *Proc Am Soc Clin Oncol* 1995;14:391.

197. Aref A, Narayan S, Tekyi-Mensah S, et al. Value of radiation therapy in the management of chemoresistant intermediate grade non-Hodgkin's lymphoma. *Radiat Oncol Investig* 199;7:186-191.

198. Fletcher GH. Lucy Wortham James Lecture. Subclinical disease. *Cancer* 1984;53:1274-1284.

199. Romaguera JE, Velasquez WS, Silvermintz KB, et al. Surgical debulking is associated with improved survival in stage I-II diffuse large cell lymphoma. *Cancer* 1990;66:267-272.

200. Miller TP, Dahlberg S, Cassady JR, et al. Chemotherapy alone compared with chemotherapy plus radiotherapy for localized

intermediate- and high-grade non-Hodgkin's lymphoma. *N Engl J Med* 1998;339:21-26.

201. Danieu L, Wong G, Koziner B, et al. Predictive model for prognosis in advanced diffuse histiocytic lymphoma. *Cancer Res* 1986;46:5372-5379.

202. Shipp MA, Klatt MM, Yeap B, et al. Patterns of relapse in large-cell lymphoma patients with bulk disease: implications for the use of adjuvant radiation therapy. *J Clin Oncol* 1989;7:613-618.

203. Coiffier B. Treatment of aggressive non-Hodgkin's lymphoma. *Semin Oncol* 1999;26:12-20.

204. Velasquez W, Fuller LM, Oh KK, et al. Combined modality therapy in stage III and stage IIIE diffuse large cell lymphomas. *Cancer* 1984;53:1478-1483.

205. Schlembach PJ, Wilder RB, Tucker SL, et al. Impact of involved field radiotherapy after CHOP-based chemotherapy on stage III-IV, intermediate grade and large-cell immunoblastic lymphomas. *Int J Radiat Oncol Biol Phys* 2000;48:1107-1110.

206. Crowther D. New approaches to the management of patients with non-Hodgkin's lymphoma of high-grade pathology. First Gordon Hamilton-Fairley memorial lecture. *Br J Cancer* 1981;43:417-435.

207. Ferreri AJ, Dell'Oro S, Reni M, et al. Consolidation radiotherapy to bulky or semibulky lesions in the management of stage III-IV diffuse large B cell lymphomas. *Oncology* 2000;58:219-226.

208. Aviles A, Delgado S, Jesus Nambo M, et al. Adjuvant radiotherapy to sites of previous bulky disease in patients stage IV diffuse large cell lymphoma. *Int J Radiat Oncol Biol Phys* 1994;30:799-803.

209. Aviles A. The International Index is not useful in the classification of low-grade lymphoma. *J Clin Oncol* 1994;12:2766-2768.

210. Lopez-Guillermo A, Montserrat E, Bosch F, et al. Applicability of the International Index for aggressive lymphomas to patients with low-grade lymphoma. *J Clin Oncol* 1994;12:1343-1348.

211. Foussard C, Desablens B, Sensebe L, et al. Is the International Prognostic Index for aggressive lymphomas useful for low-grade lymphoma patients? Applicability to stage III-IV patients. The GOELAMS Group, France. *Ann Oncol* 1997;8:49-52.

212. Decaudin D, Lepage E, Brousse N, et al. Low-grade stage III-IV follicular lymphoma: multivariate analysis of prognostic factors in 484 patients—a study of the groupe d'Etude des lymphomes de l'Adulte. *J Clin Oncol* 1999;17:2499-2505.

213. Wilder RB, Rodriguez MA, Medeiros LJ, et al. International prognostic index-based outcomes for diffuse large B-cell lymphomas. *Cancer* 2002;94:3083-3088.

214. Cabanillas F. Can we cure indolent lymphomas? *Clin Cancer Res* 1997;3:2655-2659.

215. Lopez-Guillermo A, Cabanillas F, McLaughlin P, et al. Molecular response assessed by PCR is the most important factor predicting failure-free survival in indolent follicular lymphoma: update of the MDACC series. *Ann Oncol* 2000;11:137-140.

216. Apostolidis J, Gupta RK, Grenzelias D, et al. High-dose therapy with autologous bone marrow support as consolidation of remission in follicular lymphoma: long-term clinical and molecular follow-up. *J Clin Oncol* 2000;18:527-536.

217. Gribben JG, Neuberg D, Barber M, et al. Detection of residual lymphoma cells by polymerase chain reaction in peripheral blood is significantly less predictive for relapse than detection in bone marrow. *Blood* 1994;83:3800-3807.

218. Ha CS, Tucker SL, Lee M-S, et al. The significance of molecular response of follicular lymphoma to central lymphatic irradiation as measured by polymerase chain reaction for t(14;18)(q32;q21). *Int J Radiat Oncol Biol Phys* 2001;49:727-732.

219. Cox JD. Cure and follicular lymphoma. *Int J Radiat Oncol Biol Phys* 1997;38:1-2.

220. Arthur K. Follicular lymphoma—a review of 58 cases. *Clin Radiol* 1968;19:347-350.

221. Sutcliffe SB, Gospodarowicz MK, Bush RS, et al. Role of radiation therapy in localized non-Hodgkin's lymphoma. *Radiother Oncol* 1985;4:211-223.

222. Cox JD, Koehl RH, Turner WM, et al. Irradiation in the local control of malignant lymphoreticular tumors (non-Hodgkin's malignant lymphoma). *Radiology* 1974;112:179-185.

223. MacManus MP, Hoppe RT. Is radiotherapy curative for stage I and II low grade follicular lymphoma? Results of a long-term follow-up study of patients treated at Stanford University. *J Clin Oncol* 1996;14:1282-1290.

224. Besa PC, McClaughlin PW, Cox JD, et al. Long-term assessment of patterns of treatment failure and survival in patients with stage I or II follicular lymphoma. *Cancer* 1995;75:2361-2367.

225. Paryani SB, Hoppe RT, Cox RS, et al. Analysis of non-Hodgkin's lymphomas with nodular and favorable histologies, stages I and II. *Cancer* 1983;52:2300-2307.

226. Sutcliffe SB, Gospodarowicz MK, Bergsagel DE, et al. Prognostic groups for management of localized Hodgkin's disease. *J Clin Oncol* 1985;3:393-401.

227. Pendlebury S, el Awadi M, Ashley S, et al. Radiotherapy results in early stage low grade nodal non-Hodgkin's lymphoma. *Radiother Oncol* 1995;36:167-171.

228. MacManus MP, Hoppe RT. Overview of treatment of localized low-grade lymphomas. *Hematol Oncol Clin North Am* 1997;11:901-918.

229. Gospodarowicz MK, Lippuner T, Pintilie M, et al. Stage I and II follicular lymphoma: longterm outcome and patterns of failure following treatment with involved field radiation therapy alone. *Int J Radiat Oncol Biol Phys* 1999;45:217.

230. Tsang RW, Gospodarowicz MG, Bezjak A, et al. Staging and management of localized non-Hodgkin's lymphomas: variations among experts in radiation oncology. *Int J Radiat Oncol Biol Phys* 1999;45:389.

231. Jacobs JP, Murray KJ, Schultz CJ, et al. Central lymphatic irradiation for stage III nodular malignant lymphoma: long-term results. *J Clin Oncol* 1993;11:233-238.

232. De Los Santos JF, Mendenhall NP, Lynch JW. Is comprehensive lymphatic irradiation for low-grade non-Hodgkin's lymphoma curative therapy? Long-term experience at a single institution. *Int J Radiat Oncol Biol Phys* 1997;38:3-8.

233. Bush RS, Gospodarowicz M. The place of radiation therapy in the management of patients with localized non-Hodgkin's lymphoma. In: Rosenberg SA, Kaplan HS, eds. *Malignant Lymphomas: Etiology, Immunology, Pathology, Treatment.* New York, NY: Academic Press; 1982:485-502.

234. Thompson PL, Mackay IR, Robson GSM, et al. Late radiation nephritis after gastric x-irradiation for peptic ulcer. *Quarterly J Med, New Series* 1971;40:145-157.

235. Paryani SB, Hoppe RT, Cox RS, et al. The role of radiation therapy in the management of stage III follicular lymphomas. *J Clin Oncol* 1984;2:841-848.

236. Ha CS, Tucker SL, Blanco AI, et al. Salvage central lymphatic irradiation in follicular lymphomas following failure of chemotherapy: a feasibility study. *Int J Radiat Oncol Biol Phys* 1999;45:1207-1212.

237. Mahe M, Bourdin S, Le Pourhiet-Le Mevel A, et al. Salvage extended-field irradiation in follicular non-Hodgkin's lymphoma after failure of chemotherapy. *Int J Radiat Oncol Biol Phys* 2000;47:735-738.

238. Hiddemann W, Unterhalt M, Buske C, et al. Treatment of follicular follicle centre lymphomas: current status and future perspectives. *J Intern Med Suppl* 1997;740:55-62.

239. Peterson BA. Current treatment of follicular low-grade lymphomas. *Semin Oncol* 1999;26:2-11.

240. Kong JS, Ha CS, Wilder RB, et al. Stage III follicular lymphoma: long-term follow-up and patterns of failure. *Int J Radiat Oncol Biol Phys* 2002 (in press).

241. Rosenberg SA. The low-grade non-Hodgkin's lymphomas: challenges and opportunities. *J Clin Oncol* 1985;3:299-310.

242. Horning SJ, Rosenberg SA. The natural history of initially untreated low-grade non-Hodgkin's lymphomas. *N Engl J Med* 1984;311:1471-1475.

243. Young RC, Longo DL, Glatstein E, et al. The treatment of indolent lymphomas: watchful waiting v. aggressive combined modality treatment. *Semin Hematol* 1988;25:11-16.

244. Portlock CS, Rosenberg SA. No initial therapy for stage III and IV non-Hodgkin's lymphomas of favorable histologic types. *Ann Intern Med* 1979;90:10-13.

245. Cabanillas FF. Management of patients with low-grade follicular lymphoma. *Am J Clin Oncol* 1989;12:81-87.

246. Cotter FE. Antisense therapy of hematologic malignancies. *Semin Hematol* 1999;36:9-14.

247. Pich A, Rancourt C. A role for intracellular immunization in chemosensitization of tumor cells? *Gene Ther* 1999;6:1202-1209.

248. Bendandi M, Longo DL. Biologic therapy for lymphoma. *Curr Opin Oncol* 1999;11:343-350.

249. McLaughlin P, White CA, Grillo-Lopez AJ, et al. Clinical status and optimal use of rituximab for B-cell lymphomas. *Oncology* 1998;12:1763-1769.

250. Knox SJ, Meredith RF. Clinical radioimmunotherapy. *Semin Radiat Oncol* 2000;10:73-93.

251. Unge P. Eradication therapy of *Helicobacter pylori*. A review. Report from a workshop organized by the Swedish and Norwegian Medical Products Agencies, September 1995. *J Gastroenterol* 1998;33:57-61.

252. Steinbach G, Ford R, Glober G, et al. Antibiotic treatment of gastric lymphoma of mucosa-associated lymphoid tissue. An uncontrolled trial. *Ann Intern Med* 1999;131:88-95.

253. Taal BG, Burgers JM, van Heerde P, et al. The clinical spectrum and treatment of primary non-Hodgkin's lymphoma of the stomach. *Ann Oncol* 1993;4:839-846.

254. Schechter NR, Portlock CS, Yahalom J. Treatment of mucosa-associated lymphoid tissue lymphoma of the stomach with radiation alone. *J Clin Oncol* 1998;16:1916-1921.

255. Yahalom J, Schecter NR, Gonzales M, et al. Effective treatment of MALT lymphoma of the stomach with radiation alone. *Ann Oncol* 1999;10(suppl 3):135.

256. Zinzani PL, Magagnoli M, Galieni P, et al. Nongastrointestinal low-grade mucosa-associated lymphoid tissue lymphoma: analysis of 75 patients. *J Clin Oncol* 1999;17:1254.

257. No authors listed. NCCN preliminary non-Hodgkin's lymphoma practice guidelines. *Oncology* 1997;11:281-246.

258. Morgan G, Vornanen M, Puitinen J, et al. Changing trends in the incidence of non-Hodgkin's lymphoma in Europe Biomed Study Group. *Ann Oncol* 1997;8:49-54.

259. Melnyk A, Rodriguez A, Pugh WC, et al. Evaluation of the Revised European-American Lymphoma classification confirms the clinical relevance of immunophenotype in 560 cases of aggressive non-Hodgkin's lymphoma. *Blood* 1997;89:4514-4520.

260. Lopez-Guillermo A, Cid J, Salar A, et al. Peripheral T-cell lymphomas: initial features, natural history, and prognostic factors in a series of 174 patients diagnosed according to the REAL classification. *Ann Oncol* 1998;9:849-855.

261. Ostronoff M, Soussain C, Zambon E, et al. Burkitt's lymphoma in adults: a retrospective study of 46 cases. *Nouv Rev Fr Hematol* 1992;34:389-397.

262. Meusers P, Hense J, Brittinger G. Mantle cell lymphoma: diagnostic criteria, clinical aspects and therapeutic problems. *Leukemia* 1997;11:S60-64.

263. Khouri IF, Romaguera J, Kantarjian H, et al. Hyper-CVAD and high-dose methotrexate/cytarabine followed by stem-cell transplantation: an active regimen for aggressive mantle-cell lymphoma. *J Clin Oncol* 1998;16:3803-3809.

264. Morrison VA, Peterson BA. High-dose therapy and transplantation in non-Hodgkin's lymphoma. *Semin Oncol* 1999;26:84-98.

265. Soslow RA, Baergen RN, Warnke RA. B-lineage lymphoblastic lymphoma is a clinicopathologic entity distinct from other histologically similar aggressive lymphomas with blastic morphology. *Cancer* 1999;85:2648-2654.

266. Weinstein HJ, Vance ZB, Jaffe N, et al. Improved prognosis for patients with mediastinal lymphoblastic lymphoma. *Blood* 1979;53:687-694.

267. Coleman CN, Picozzi VJ. Jr, Cox RS, et al. Treatment of lymphoblastic lymphoma in adults. *J Clin Oncol* 1986;4:1628-1637.

268. Colgan JP, Andersen J, Habermann TM, et al. Long-term maintenance and central nervous system prophylaxis in lymphoblastic non-Hodgkin's lymphoma. *Leuk Lymphoma* 1994;15:291-296.

269. Levitt LJ, Aisenberg AC, Harris NL, et al. Primary non-Hodgkin's lymphoma of the mediastinum. *Cancer* 1982;50:2486-2492.

270. Levine AM, Forman SJ, Meyer PR, et al. Successful therapy of convoluted T-lymphoblastic lymphoma in the adult. *Blood* 1983;61:92-98.

271. Lamberg SI, Green SB, Byar DP, et al. Clinical staging for cutaneous T-cell lymphoma. *Ann Intern Med* 1984;100:187-192.

272. Diamandidou E, Cohen PR, Kurzrock R. Mycosis fungoides and Sezary syndrome. *Blood* 1996;88:2385-2409.

273. Kim YH, Hoppe RT. Mycosis fungoides and the Sezary syndrome. *Semin Oncol* 1999;26:276-289.

274. Duncan K, Heald P. Cutaneous T-cell lymphoma: centuries of controversy. *Semin Cutan Med Surg* 1998;17:133-140.

275. Lo TC, Salzman FA, Moschella SL, et al. Whole body surface electron irradiation in the treatment of mycosis fungoides. *Radiology* 1979;130:453-457.

276. Tadros AA, Tepperman BS, Hryniuk WM, et al. Total skin electron irradiation for mycosis fungoides: failure analysis and prognostic factors. *Int J Radiat Oncol Biol Phys* 1983;9:1279-1287.

277. Hoppe RT, Cox RS, Fuks Z, et al. Electron-beam therapy for mycosis fungoides: the Stanford University experience. *Cancer Treat Rep* 1979;63:691-700.

278. Kim YH, Jensen RA, Watanabe GL, et al. Clinical stage IA (limited patch and plaque) mycosis fungoides: a long-term outcome analysis. *Arch Dermatol* 1996;132:1309-1313.

279. Hamminga B, Noordijk EM, van Vloten WA. Treatment of mycosis fungoides: total-skin electron-beam irradiation vs topical mechlorethamine therapy. *Arch Dermatol* 1982;118:150-153.

280. Zachariae H, Thestrup-Pedersen K, Sogaard H. Topical nitrogen mustard in early mycosis fungoides. A 12-year experience. *Acta Derm Venereol* 1985;65:53-58.

281. Vonderheid EC, Tan ET, Kantor AF, et al. Long-term efficacy, curative potential, and carcinogenicity of topical mechlorethamine in cutaneous T cell lymphoma. *J Am Acad Dermatol* 1989;20:416-428.

282. Hoppe RT. The management of mycosis fungoides at Stanford-standard and innovative treatment programmes. *Leukemia* 1991;5:46-48.

283. Kaye FJ, Bunn PA, Steinberg SM, et al. A randomized trial comparing combination electron beam radiation and chemotherapy with topical therapy in the initial treatment of mycosis fungoides. *N Engl J Med* 1989;321:1784-1790.

284. Lo TCM, Salzman FA, Costey GE, et al. Megavolt electron irradiation for localized mycosis fungoides. *Acta Radiol Oncol* 1981;20:71-74.

285. Wilson LD, Kacinski BM, Jones GW. Local superficial radiotherapy in the management of minimal stage IA cutaneous T-cell lymphoma. *Int J Radiat Oncol Biol Phys* 1998;40:109-115.

286. Micaily B, Miyamoto C, Kantor G. Radiotherapy for unilesional mycosis fungoides. *Int J Radiat Oncol Biol Phys* 1998;42:361-364.

287. Cotter GW, Baglan RJ, Wasserman TH, et al. Palliative radiation treatment of cutaneous mycosis fungoides-A dose response. *Int J Radiat Oncol Biol Phys* 1983;9:1477-1480.

288. Herrmann JJ, Roenigk HH Jr, Hurria A, et al. Treatment of mycosis fungoides with photochemotherapy (PUVA): long-term follow-up. *Acad Dermatol* 1995;33:234-242.

289. Watson A. Photochemotherapy for mycosis fungoides: current status. *Australas J Dermatol* 1997;38:9-11.

290. Chinn DM, Chow S, Kim YH, et al. Total skin electron beam therapy with or without adjuvant topical nitrogen mustard or nitrogen mustard alone as initial treatment of T2 and T3 mycosis fungoides. *Int J Radiat Oncol Biol Phys* 1999;43:951-958.

291. Zackheim HS. Treatment of cutaneous T-cell lymphoma. *Semin Dermatol* 1994;13:207-215.

292. Ferra C, Servitje O, Petriz L, et al. Autologous haematopoietic progenitor transplantation in advanced mycosis fungoides. *Br J Dermatol* 1999;140:1188-1189.

293. Marcus R, Burrows NP, Roberts SO, et al. Erythrodermic mycosis fungoides treated with total body irradiation and autologous bone marrow transplantation. *Clin Exp Dermatol* 1995;20:73-75.

294. Bigler RD, Crilly P, Micaily B, et al. Autologous bone marrow transplantation for advanced stage mycosis fungoides. *Bone Marrow Transplant* 1991;7:133-137.

295. Hoppe RT, Abel EA, Deneau DG, et al. Mycosis fungoides: management with topical nitrogen mustard. *J Clin Oncol* 1987;5:1796-1803.

296. Ramsay DL, Halperin PS, Zeleniuch-Jacquotte A. Topical mechlorethamine for early stage mycosis fungoides. *J Am Acad Dermatol* 1988;19:684-691.

297. Kemme DJ, Bunn PA Jr. State of the art therapy of mycosis fungoides and Sezary syndrome. *Oncology* 1992;6:31-42; discussion 44, 47-38.

298. Wilson LD, Kacinski BM, Edelson RL, et al. Cutaneous T-cell lymphomas. In: DeVita VT Jr, Hellman S, Rosenberg SA, eds. *Cancer: Principles and Practice of Oncology.* 5th ed. Philadelphia, Pa: Lippincott-Raven; 1997:2220-2232.

299. Hoppe RT, Fuks Z, Bagshaw MA. Radiation therapy in the management of cutaneous T-cell lymphoma. *Cancer Treat Rep* 1979;63:625-632.

300. Antolak JA, Cundiff JH, Ha CS. Utilization of thermoluminescent dosimetry in total skin electron beam radiotherapy of mycosis fungoides. *Int J Radiat Oncol Biol Phys* 1998;40:101-108.

301. Newton HB, Fine HA. NCCN clinical practice guidelines for non-immunosuppresed primary CNS lymphoma. *Oncology* 1999;13:153-160.

302. Fine HA, Mayer RJ. Primary central nervous system lymphoma. *Ann Intern Med* 1993;119:1093-1104.

303. Deangelis LM. Current management of primary central nervous system lymphoma. *Oncology* 1995;9:63-71.

304. Nelson DF. Radiotherapy in the treatment of primary central nervous system lymphoma (PCNSL). *J Neurooncol* 1999; 43:241-247.

305. Roman DD, Sperduto PW. Neuropsychological effects of cranial radiation: current knowledge and future directions. *Int J Radiat Oncol Biol Phys* 1995;31:983-998.

306. Abrey LE, DeAngelis LM, Yahalom J. Long-term survival in primary CNS lymphoma. *J Clin Oncol* 1998;16:859-863.

307. Delattre JY, Shapiro WR, Posner JB. Acute effects of low-dose cranial irradiation on regional capillary permeability in experimental brain tumors. *J Neurol Sci* 1989;90:147-153.

308. Freilich RJ, Delattre JY, Monjour A, et al. Chemotherapy without radiation therapy as initial treatment for primary CNS lymphoma in older patients. *Neurology* 1996;46:435-439.

309. Dahlborg SA, Henner WD, Crossen JR, et al. Non-AIDS primary CNS lymphoma: first example of a durable response in a primary brain tumor using enhanced chemotherapy delivery without cognitive loss and without radiotherapy. *Cancer J Sci Am* 1996;2:166-174.

310. DeMario MD, Liebowitz DN. Lymphomas in the immunocompromised patient. *Semin Oncol* 1998;25:492-502.

311. Liebross RH, Ha CS, Cox JD, et al. Clinical course of solitary extramedullary plasmacytoma. *Radiother Oncol* 1999;52:245-249.

312. Bush SE, Goffinet DR, Bagshaw MA. Extramedullary plasmacytoma of the head and neck. *Radiology* 1981;140:801-805.

313. Knowling MA, Harwood AR, Bergsagel DE. Comparison of extramedullary plasmacytomas with solitary and multiple plasma cell tumors of bone. *J Clin Oncol* 1983;1:255-262.

314. Wasserman TH. Diagnosis and management of plasmacytomas. *Oncology* 1987;1:37-41.

315. Brinch L, Hannisdal E, Abrahamsen AF, et al. Extramedullary plasmacytoma and solitary plasmacytoma of the head and neck. *Eur J Haematol* 1990;44:131-134.

316. Mayr NA, Wen BC, Hussey DH. et al. The role of radiation therapy in the treatment of solitary plasmacytomas. *Radiother Oncol* 1990;17:293-303.

317. Bolek TW, Marcus RB Jr, Mendenhall NP. Solitary plasmacytoma of bone and soft tissue. *Int J Radiat Oncol Biol Phys* 1996;36:329-333.

318. Susnerwala SS, Shanks JH, Banerjee SS, et al. Extramedullary plasmacytoma of the head and neck region: clinicopathological correlation in 25 cases. *Br J Cancer* 1997;75:921-927.

PART XII

Musculoskeletal System

CHAPTER 34

The Bone

Naomi R. Schechter and Valerae O. Lewis

Bone tumors represent less than 0.5% of all primary tumors, and bone destruction is their sine qua non. This discussion of primary malignant tumors of bone will stress the role of radiation therapy, but some brief comments on diagnostic imaging of bone tumors are given as well.

Although bone tumors disseminate almost exclusively via the blood, radiation fields must be designed to spare soft tissue in the areas of lymphatic drainage to reduce the risk of late lymphedema. In combined-modality therapy, it is essential that the orthopedic surgeon and the diagnostic radiologist, together with the radiation and medical oncologists, be involved in any treatment decision from the outset.

RESPONSE OF NORMAL BONE TO IRRADIATION

Bone is almost twice as dense as soft tissue, with an effective atomic number approaching 14. However, in the range of machine energies currently in use, photon radiation is absorbed primarily by means of the Compton process, which is essentially independent of the atomic number of the attenuating tissues. Although bone absorption of particle radiation with high linear energy transfer is greater than that of photons, this is significant only when neutron irradiation is used in osteogenic and other skeletal sarcomas. It is important to distinguish between the relative radiosensitivity of growing cartilage and bone in a child and the relative radioresistance of mature bone and cartilage in the adult. Arrested growth can be seen in children, for whom the $TD_{5/5}$ (tolerance dose; the dose at which the risk of injury is 5% at 5 years) is 10 Gy and the $TD_{50/5}$ (50% chance of injury) is 30 Gy, whereas the corresponding values for necrosis and fracture in the adult are a $TD_{5/5}$ of 60 Gy and a $TD_{50/5}$ of 100 Gy given with conventional fractionation. The threshold for radiographic changes in normal adult bone is about 50 Gy given over 5 weeks, with the changes being manifested at least 2 years after the irradiation, although in the dose ranges used clinically, these radiographically demonstrated changes in trabecular pattern and cortical thickening are usually not significant. It is highly likely, however, that if concomitant or sequential multiple-agent chemotherapy

is given with the radiation, these $TD_{5/5}$ and $TD_{50/5}$ guidelines should be modified downward.

Radiation Effects on Bone Growth

The anatomy and physiology of the growth plate was well described in a 1995 report of a late effects consensus conference. Much of the early work was performed by Kember and colleagues.[1,2] In summary, ossification centers develop within the cartilage of a fetus or growing child. Some bones (such as the wrist, ankle, and zygoma) develop from a single ossification center. Others (such as the femur) develop from one point in the center and one or more others in the epiphyseal end. The growth plate is a column of cells that remains between the secondary epiphysis and metaphysis until after puberty, when it fuses. The growth plate consists of three layers: reserve cells, proliferative cells, and hypertrophic cells. As the cells mature, they progress down the column. When they reach a certain distance from the top of the growth plate, calcium is released and ossification occurs. In rodents, nearly all of the cells in the proliferative zone are dividing.[1,3] In humans, the growth rate is fastest at birth, slower during childhood (cell-cycle time of approximately 20 to 30 days at age 5 to 8 years), and then faster again during puberty.[2]

This proliferative zone is sensitive to radiation therapy and its fractionation.[4,5] In mice, irradiated osteoblasts demonstrate decreased cell proliferation and a dose-dependent, sustained reduction in collagen production relative to control cells[6]; in irradiated tibia, bone growth is reduced in a dose-dependent manner.[7] The roles of hyperfractionation and accelerated hyperfractionation in these models are under investigation.[4,5,8]

In children, irradiation of the axial skeleton can cause height abnormalities (especially in children aged less than 6 years or children aged 11 to 13 years given more than 33 to 35 Gy),[9-11] partial irradiation of vertebral bodies can cause scoliosis,[12-14] and hip irradiation can cause slipped capital femoral epiphysis (especially in children younger than 4 years given more than 25 Gy)[15] and avascular necrosis (especially in children given more than 30 Gy, steroids, or concomitant chemotherapy).[16,17] Ultimately, stature depends on patient age at time of treatment, total dose of radiation, volume treated,[10] and growth hormone supply (which may be reduced secondary to cranial irradiation).[18]

Kroll and colleagues[19] reviewed the records of 236 patients who had been given radiation for malignant disease during childhood; some degree of bone deformity was seen in 40%, more commonly when radiation was administered before 2 years of age. When tumor control requires the irradiation of growing epiphyseal cartilage, the recommendations of the late effects consensus conference are to avoid dose gradients across vertebral bodies (especially laterally), to use relatively small fraction sizes (1.8 Gy or less), and to make sure that the patient and family are aware of the various risks of bone irradiation. Furthermore, early identification and treatment of bone abnormalities are essential. For example, patients with spinal curvatures of more than 20 degrees may benefit from brace support. Patients with mild leg length discrepancies may benefit from shoe lifts; patients with severe leg length discrepancies may need amputation. Patients with severe epiphyseal widening or mild epiphyseal slippage may benefit from surgical pinning; patients with severe epiphyseal slippage (more than 60 degrees) may need osteotomy and osteoplasty.[16]

Amifostine may confer some protection.[20-22] To determine the relative benefits of sparing longitudinal bone growth by fractionation alone vs. pretreatment with amifostine, Damron and colleagues[21] randomized 24 weanling 4-week-old male Sprague-Dawley rats to receive fractionated radiation therapy alone ($N = 12$) or amifostine pretreatment ($N = 12$). The distal femur and proximal tibia in the right leg of each animal were exposed to 17.5 Gy total in three to five fractions with the contralateral leg used as a control. The use of amifostine for radioprotection when the rats received radiation in five fractions significantly reduced the femoral and overall percentage growth arrest and limb length discrepancy compared with rats that received only the five fractions. Anticipated growth loss from a single 17.5-Gy radiation dose was reduced by 30.8% in the femur, 20.3% in the tibia, and 25.7% overall in the total limb.

In another study, Damron and colleagues[22] found a directly proportional relationship between amifostine dose and its protective effects on the growth plate. They exposed 36 weanling Sprague-Dawley rats to a single dose of 17.5 Gy to the right knee, again with the contralateral limb used as a nonirradiated control. Six groups of six rats were each given amifostine intraperitoneally 20 minutes before radiation exposure at the following doses: 0, 50, 100, 150, 200, or 250 mg/kg. Six weeks after treatment, the rats were killed and the lower limbs were disarticulated, skeletonized, radiographed, and measured. Statistically significant dose-related differences were observed between amifostine dosage groups for mean right-sided growth, growth loss, and limb length discrepancy. The mean amount of right-sided growth recovered by amifostine administration

increased from 14% at 50 mg/kg to 57% at 250 mg/kg. Growth loss and limb discrepancy were significantly reduced in proportion to increasing amifostine doses.[22]

Cranial and total-body irradiation (TBI) in young patients can cause hormone deficiencies affecting both stature and bone density.[18,23-27] Short height and osteopenia are likely multifactorial, but it is notable that growth-hormone deficiency is the most common endocrine deficiency observed after cranial irradiation.[26,28] TBI alone causes height loss.

Clement-de Boers and colleagues[29] noted that among patients who in childhood had undergone bone marrow transplant (BMT) after chemotherapy and TBI with 7.5 Gy or more, final height was compromised because of blunted growth in puberty, but patients who had not undergone TBI suffered no height loss. Thyroid function and adrenal function were normal in all patients, and no growth-hormone deficiency was detected.

When cranial irradiation is added to TBI, especially single-fraction TBI, the effects on height are even worse. Cohen and colleagues[25] reviewed the cases of 181 patients who had BMT before puberty and had reached their final height. Previous cranial irradiation plus single-dose TBI caused the greatest negative effect on final height. Fractionation of TBI reduced this effect significantly, and conditioning with busulfan and cyclophosphamide seemed to eliminate it. Girls did better than boys, and the younger the person was at time of BMT, the greater the loss in height. Nevertheless, most patients (140 of 181) reached an adult height that was within the normal range of the general population. As Murray and colleagues[30] reported, the clinical picture for adults with growth-hormone deficiency resulting from primary hypothalamic-pituitary disease during childhood is similar to that described for long-term survivors of childhood cancer: increased fat mass and reductions in lean mass, strength, exercise tolerance, bone mineral density, and quality of life.

Arikoski and colleagues[26] found that for survivors of childhood acute lymphoblastic leukemia, both male sex and a history of cranial irradiation were associated with low lumbar and femoral bone-marrow densities. Plasma insulin-like growth factor-I (IGF-I) and its growth-hormone-dependent binding protein (IGFBP-3) are of no diagnostic value for growth-hormone deficiency after TBI. Brauner and colleagues[31] interpreted the presence of normal or high IGF-I levels despite low growth-hormone peaks to suggest that bone irradiation induces lesions that cause resistance to IGF-I.

The production of growth hormone may improve over time on its own (years after BMT), but early growth-hormone replacement has shown benefit.[23,24] Hovi and colleagues[24] found that 3 years of growth-hormone treatment, begun 2 to 6 years after BMT, yielded an increase in mean height standard-deviation score of 0.4, whereas untreated patients suffered a decrease in standard-deviation score of 0.8 during the corresponding time ($P = 0.009$). Other hormonal problems, such as gonadal failure, also may contribute to growth impairment. The importance of early hormone replacement therapy cannot be overemphasized.[32]

Clinically relevant effects of radiation therapy on the dental and craniofacial development of children include malocclusion, reduced mobility of the temporomandibular joint, growth retardation, and osteoradionecrosis.[33] Malocclusion and reduced mobility of the temporomandibular joint can cause muscle pain and headaches,[33] in part from treatment-induced inflammation and eventual fibrosis of the joint.[33] Qualitative changes, such as regularly spaced lines in the enamel and dentine of the teeth, have been found to correspond with cycles of chemotherapy. Qualitative and quantitative changes, such as true dental hypoplasia, have been associated with TBI.[34] Children treated with cranial irradiation before 5 years of age exhibit a reduced growth of the mandible, the mandible being 4 times more radiosensitive than the maxilla.[35]

Radiation-induced alterations of factors related to bone remodeling and wound healing have a potential role in the pathogenesis of osteoradionecrosis.[36] Ashamalla and colleagues[37] found hyperbaric oxygen could be safely used to prevent and treat radiation-induced bone and soft tissue complications in children. In mice, radiation effects on bone growth can be significantly reduced by hyperbaric oxygen after 10 or 20 Gy but not after 30 Gy. At 30 Gy, basic fibroblast growth factor (bFGF, or FGF2) still significantly reduces the degree of bone shortening, but hyperbaric oxygen provides no added benefit to the FGF2 therapy.[6] Rodent studies suggest that recombinant human bone morphogenic protein-2 in soluble collagen type-1 carrier delivered to an irradiated bone defect (3 mm, calvarial) can increase new bone formation (34% ± 14% of the defect area within 21 days, as compared with 7% ± 2% for type-1 collagen carrier alone and 5% ± 2% if untreated; untreated, unirradiated bone defects show a spontaneous osseous regeneration of 90% ± 7% of the defect area within 21 days).[38]

Rapidly reproducing bone marrow cells are highly radiosensitive. The effects on regenerative potential vary with the volume irradiated. Management of the hematopoietic effects of radiation therapy includes surveillance, antibiotic therapy, blood product transfusion, and occasionally hematopoietic growth factors, BMT, or reinfusion of peripheral blood stem cells.[39]

Ding and colleagues[40] studied the bone marrow protectant effects of acidic-FGF (aFGF, or FGF1) and bFGF (FGF2) given within a day of radiation therapy. The radioprotectant effect of these drugs in rodents treated with a single dose of TBI was characterized by a dose-modification factor of 1.15. In fractionated systems, FGF2 seems to be more effective than FGF1 (respective

dose-modification factors of 1.22 and 1.04). FGF1 given 24 and 4 hours before irradiation with an otherwise lethal dose of TBI improves the repopulation of hematopoietic progenitor cells of bone marrow; this effect is not associated with an increase in the S-phase fraction or detectable circulating levels of the cytokines interleukin-3, tumor necrosis factor alpha (TNF-α), or granulocyte-macrophage colony-stimulating factor, suggesting that other mechanisms of protection are responsible. A protective effect exists even if FGF1 is given 24 hours after radiation therapy.[41] FGF2, given 24 and 4 hours before the first dose of fractionated TBI, aids in the recovery of bone marrow hematopoietic cells and peripheral white blood cells, red blood cells, and platelets.[40,42]

In rodents, neither the rate of tumor growth or metastasis nor the radiosensitivity of tumors seems to be altered by treatment with FGF1 or FGF2.[40,43,44] When radiation therapy is used alone, prophylactic use of hematopoietic growth factors has not been justified.[45] Using laser Doppler flow measurements of blood flow in rodent tibia, Okunieff and colleagues[7,44,46] studied whether the angiogenic effect of FGF2 would counteract the chronic antiangiogenic effect of radiation on bone growth. They found that chronic radiation bone toxicity was associated with decreased perfusion, without elevation of circulating or soft-tissue TNF-β or TNF-α.[7] Radiation toxicity to rodent bone (30 Gy in a single fraction to the hind limb) is alleviated by bFGF therapy, even if begun up to 5 weeks after the irradiation. Okunieff and colleagues[46] postulated that the increased laser Doppler flow of the contralateral nonirradiated tibia was due to circulating angiogenesis factors that are elevated to compensate for the radiation-induced antiangiogenesis.

RADIATION THERAPY IN THE PREVENTION OF HETEROTOPIC BONE FORMATION

Heterotopic ossification (HO) is thought to occur when, in sites of surgery or other trauma, pluripotent mesenchymal cells inappropriately differentiate into osteoblastic stem cells.[47-52] HO is particularly problematic when it occurs near joints, because in advanced form it can limit motion and cause significant pain.[53-55] After total hip arthroplasty, HO can occur in more than one third of the cases.[56] The risk is particularly high (approximately 50%) after open reduction–internal fixation for acetabular fractures.[57] Risk factors for HO include being male and having a history of previous postoperative HO in the ipsilateral or contralateral hip.[48,58-63] Other factors that can increase the risk of HO include prior trauma or operation, hypertrophic osteoarthritis, diffuse idiopathic skeletal hyperostosis, ankylosing spondylitis, and Paget's disease.[47,48,58,61,64-68]

For pelvic HO, Brooker's grading system is useful.[58] In that system, class I HO is characterized by the presence of islands of bone within the soft tissue around the hip, class II by bone spurs from the pelvis or proximal end of the femur that leave at least 1 cm between opposing bone surfaces, class III by bone spurs from the pelvis or proximal end of the femur that reduce the space between opposing bone surfaces to less than 1 cm, and class IV by apparent bone ankylosis.[58]

The best management is prevention.[69-71] Treatment options for the prevention of HO include the use of nonsteroidal antiinflammatory drugs and radiation therapy (such as a single 7-Gy postoperative dose).[70-80] The drugs may seem a safer option, but gastrointestinal and hematologic side effects can be serious, particularly for patients who are taking steroids or anticoagulants and patients with postoperative ileus or peptic ulcer disease.[78,81] Side effects from nonsteroidal antiinflammatory agents prevent more than one third of such patients from completing a 2-week treatment course (starting on postoperative day 1).[82,83] These drugs also can cause problems with the stability of noncemented components because of their interference with the ingrowth of bone.[84,85]

Significant acute or subacute adverse effects of a 7-Gy postoperative radiation dose are rare, as are second malignancies.[81] For the treatment of advanced HO, reoperation may be necessary, followed by a single 7-Gy radiation therapy dose.[81] The best time to give postoperative radiation therapy is within the first 72 hours after surgery.*

Preoperative and postoperative radiation therapy for the prevention of HO have been compared, and although neither has proven to be better than the other, postoperative treatment has been favored because of the belief that the rapidly dividing postoperative cells are more radiosensitive than their preoperative counterparts.[89,94-96] The field for postoperative radiation therapy need include only the soft tissue plane around the neck of the implant to be treated. For example, Lo and colleagues[70] treated a 5 to 6 cm × 14 cm field with a 25-degree collimator angle, without custom blocking. Patient selection precludes definitive evaluation of the success of radiation therapy; however, modern series with a 7-Gy postoperative dose report failure rates of 5% to 16%.† Lo[81] regards successful radiation therapy as that which can reduce HO within the radiation field within the first 6 months after surgery to 15% or less.

Induction of Secondary Tumors by Radiation

Some patients have a genetic predisposition to the development of secondary tumors.[98,99] Wong and colleagues[98] reported on 1604 patients with retinoblastoma who survived at least 1 year after diagnosis; the

incidence of subsequent cancer was elevated only among the 961 patients with hereditary retinoblastoma, of whom 190 cases of cancer were diagnosed vs. the 6.3 expected in the general population (relative risk, 30; 95% confidence interval [CI], 26 to 47). The cumulative incidence (± standard error) of a second cancer at 50 years after diagnosis was 51.0% (± 6.2%) for hereditary retinoblastoma and 5.0% (± 3.0%) for nonhereditary retinoblastoma.[98]

Radiation therapy can further increase the risk of secondary malignancies. Radiation doses as small as 10 mGy received by a fetus in utero lead to an increase in the risk of childhood cancer, with an excess absolute risk coefficient at this level of exposure of approximately 6%/Gy.[100]

The most common secondary bone tumor after local field irradiation is sarcoma, the incidence of which seems to be dose-dependent (at least at high doses).[98,101-105] The accumulation of skeletal doses from ^{226}Ra and ^{225}Ra by radial dial painters has been proven to be an important predictor of risk of death from bone sarcoma; the risk is even greater in those exposed before skeletal growth is complete.[101,102,106]

In the retinoblastoma series discussed above,[98] 114 of the 190 cancer diagnoses after irradiation were sarcomas, and those sarcomas were of diverse histologic types. For soft tissue sarcomas, the relative risk values showed a stepwise increase at all dose categories and were statistically significant at 10 to 29.9 Gy and at 30 to 59.9 Gy. A radiation risk for all sarcomas combined was evident at doses above 5 Gy, rising to a 10.7-fold increase at doses of 60 Gy or greater ($P < 0.05$).[98]

Tucker and colleagues[99] reviewed the cases of 64 patients in whom bone cancer developed after childhood cancer and compared these cases with 209 matched controls who had survived cancer in childhood but who did not have bone cancer later. Patients who had had radiation therapy had 2.7 times the risk of those who had not (95% CI, 1.0 to 7.7), and a sharp dose-response gradient was evident, reaching a fortyfold higher risk after doses to the bone of more than 60 Gy.

After adjustment for radiation therapy, treatment with alkylating agents was also linked to bone cancer (relative risk, 4.7; 95% CI, 1.0 to 22.3), with the risk increasing as cumulative drug exposure rose.[99] In a review by Kuttesch and colleagues[103] of 266 Ewing's sarcoma survivors, the median latency to the diagnosis of the second malignancy was 7.6 years (range, 3.5 to 25.7 years). The estimated cumulative incidence rate at 20 years for any second malignancy was 9.2% (standard deviation, 2.7%) and that for secondary sarcoma was 6.5% (standard deviation, 2.4%). The cumulative incidence rate of secondary sarcoma depended on the radiation dose ($P = 0.002$); no secondary sarcomas developed among patients who had received less than 48 Gy, whereas the absolute risk of secondary sarcoma

---

*References 52, 64, 69, 70, 79, 86-93.
†References 70, 72, 79, 91, 92, 97.

was 130 cases per 10,000 person-years of observation among patients who had received 60 Gy or more.[103]

Hematologic tumors (such as leukemia) and solid secondary tumors (such as osteosarcoma) can develop after TBI.[107-110] As Niethammer and Mayer[108] reported, different types of secondary cancer occur at various times after BMT; lymphoproliferative disease can occur during the first year, leukemias and myelodysplastic syndromes after several years, and solid tumors even later. The incidence of second neoplasias after BMT seems to be higher in children than in adults.[108] When corrected for competing risks, TBI increases the risk of cancer in rhesus monkeys by a factor of 8.[109]

The risk of leukemia after irradiation of the pelvis is relatively small.[111-114] Of a cohort of 110,000 women with invasive cancer of the uterine corpus who survived at least 1 year after the initial cancer (assembled from nine population-based cancer registries), the leukemia risk associated with partial-body radiation therapy for uterine corpus cancer was small—about 14 excess cases per 10,000 women followed for 10 years.[113] The quoted risk for acute myelogenous leukemia in patients with prostate cancer treated with radiation therapy is 0.1% at 10 years.[114]

The risk of leukemia after radioactive iodine treatment is small as well. De Vathaire and colleagues[115] studied 1771 patients treated for a thyroid cancer in two institutions. None of these patients had been treated with external radiotherapy and 1497 had received [131]I. After a mean follow-up of 10 years, no case of leukemia was observed, compared with 2.5 expected according to the coefficients derived from Japanese atomic bomb survivors ($P = 0.1$).[115]

[89]Sr has been associated with cases of leukemia in patients with metastatic prostate cancer, but the exact risk is unknown and needs to be investigated.[116]

BONE IMAGING

Accurate diagnosis of bone tumors requires a multimodality approach with clinical-radiologic-pathologic correlation.[117,118] Appropriate diagnostic and staging evaluation should be performed before biopsy.[117] Plain radiographs can help determine tumor morphology, including patterns of bone destruction (geographic, moth-eaten, or permeated); lesion margins (from sclerotic rim to ill-defined margin), internal characteristics of the lesion (nonmatrix-producing tumors, non-mineralized matrix-producing tumors, mineralized matrix-producing tumors); type of host bone response (medullary or periosteal); location (femur, tibia, humerus, etc.), site (metaphysis, diaphysis, or epiphysis), and position (central, eccentric, or periosteal) of the lesion in the skeletal system and in the individual bone; soft tissue involvement; and number of lesions.[117]

A skeletal survey is necessary to distinguish plasmacytoma from multiple myeloma.[119] Plain radiographs

also can help identify radiation-induced bone changes such as osteoradionecrosis (with its characteristically ill-defined cortical destruction) and radiation-induced sarcoma (with its characteristically aggressive pattern of bone destruction).[120] Computed tomography (CT) and magnetic resonance imaging (MRI) are useful for determining the extent of bone tumors.[121] CT is particularly useful for the assessment of cortical invasion, periosteal reaction, soft tissue or lesion matrix calcification or ossification, and fracture fragment positioning or configuration, especially in complex anatomical sites such as the spine, pelvis, and hindfoot.[117,118] MRI is useful for evaluating the extent of soft tissue involvement before treatment and the follow-up of primary bone tumors after treatment.[122]

In contrast to CT and MRI, which evaluate anatomy, are bone scans, which evaluate local osteoblastic activity. Thus bone scans are useful for screening asymptomatic high-risk patients and documenting the osteoblastic response necessary for concentration of therapeutic radionuclides such as ^{89}Sr or [153]Sm-lexidronam.[118,123,124] Gallium scans are useful for evaluating both primary and metastatic lesions of malignant fibrous histiocytoma when the tumor invades the skeletal system.[125] Positron emission tomography may prove useful for ruling out osseous metastases, but further investigation is warranted.[126]

PRIMARY MALIGNANT TUMORS OF BONE
Plasmacytoma

Solitary plasmacytoma of bone is a rare presentation of plasma cell dyscrasia. Solitary plasmacytomas of bone constitute approximately 2% of all cases of myeloma and 70% of all plasmacytomas.[127] Solitary plasmacytomas of bone have been considered to be an early manifestation of multiple myeloma[128-130]; however, diagnostic criteria have been established to define solitary plasmacytoma of the bone as a distinct entity. According to the strictest of these criteria, solitary plasmacytoma of bone can be considered a distinct entity if no other skeletal lesions are radiographically evident, if bone marrow is free of plasma cells, and if results from serum and urine protein electrophoresis are negative. Unfortunately, the diagnostic criteria vary considerably in the literature.[128,131-133] These criteria have included histologically confirmed solitary lesion on skeletal survey (with or without a soft tissue mass), bone marrow plasmacytosis level of less than 10% or of less than 5%, serum and urine electrophoresis findings that are positive, negative, or become negative after treatment of the lesion.[127,129,131,134-138] These different diagnostic criteria not only make comparisons among studies difficult, but, as Liebross and colleagues[138] have suggested, this variation may be a factor in the different time courses that have been reported for the lesions to progress to systemic disease.

Like multiple myeloma, solitary plasmacytoma of bone is more common in men, with a reported ratio of 3:1. Although multiple myeloma is most common in the sixth and seventh decade, solitary plasmacytoma of bone presents at younger ages.[127,128] The most common locations for solitary plasmacytomas of bone are in the long bones, pelvis, and spine. In a review of 46 patients with solitary plasmacytomas of bone, Frassica and colleagues[131] found that 54% had lesions in the spine.

Pain is the most common symptom, and other symptoms tend to reflect the location of the tumor. Lesions in the spine may present with neurologic compromise. The neurologic changes are usually accompanied by lumbar or thoracic pain of several months' duration.

Solitary plasmacytomas of bone are exquisitely radiosensitive and their response to radiation is rapid. In their series of 37 patients with plasmacytoma (27 with solitary plasmacytomas of bone), Bolek and colleagues[130] found that radiation therapy effectively achieved local control. In that study, only one patient with solitary plasmacytomas of bone developed local failure. Within 15 years, however, all of the solitary plasmacytomas of bone had progressed to multiple myeloma. Liebross and colleagues[138] found that local megavoltage radiation (median dose, 50 Gy; range, 30 to 70 Gy) achieved effective local control in 96% of their patients with solitary plasmacytomas of bone. No late toxic effects were found. Of their patients, 29 (51%) developed multiple myeloma. No radiation dose-response relationship was found for local control or subsequent progression to multiple myeloma.[138] In another study of 16 patients with solitary plasmacytosis, however, Mill and Griffith,[133] did find a dose-response relationship between radiation dose and progression of solitary plasmacytoma of bone to multiple myeloma. They found that patients given more than 50 Gy to their lesions had less likelihood of developing multiple myeloma.

Although local control of the solitary plasmacytoma is quite good after radiation therapy, the question arises of whether the use of local radiation is addressing the entire clinical picture. Most series show local control rates of more than 90%, but more than 50% of cases progress to multiple myeloma. The question thus arises as to whether radiation is achieving satisfactory disease control. Aviles and colleagues,[139] in attempting to address this question, examined the role of adjuvant chemotherapy after radiation therapy in patients with solitary plasmacytoma. After a median follow-up of 8.9 years, disease-free and overall survival rates were improved among the patients treated with combined therapy: 22 of the patients in the combined-treatment group remained alive and free of disease compared with only 13 patients given radiation only.[139] However, the groups in that study were too small to draw definitive conclusions regarding adjuvant chemotherapy.

Another small study by Mayr and colleagues[140] produced results concordant with those of Aviles; none of five patients with solitary plasmacytomas of bone who received adjuvant chemotherapy progressed to multiple myeloma compared with 9 of 12 patients (75%) who did not receive chemotherapy. However, in a series of 32 cases of solitary plasmacytomas of bone, Holland and colleagues[129] reported that adjuvant chemotherapy did not affect the incidence of conversion but did seem to delay conversion to myeloma. These studies, taken together, suggest that combined-modality therapy for solitary plasmacytoma of bone warrants further investigation. Radiation therapy provides an excellent treatment option for local control.

Chondrosarcomas

Chondrosarcomas were first described in 1943 by Lichtenstein and Jaffe[141] as sarcomas whose tumor cells are associated with a cartilaginous matrix. Although chondrosarcomas are the second most common primary tumor of bone, they are nonetheless uncommon. According to the Mayo Clinic, less than 9.2% of the malignant tumors in their series were chondrosarcomas.[128]

Lesions are referred to as central, peripheral, primary, or secondary depending on where in the bone they originate or whether they originate from preexisting lesions. However, this classification bears no relation to overall prognosis. Central chondrosarcomas arise within the medullary canal, and peripheral chondrosarcomas originate from the cortex of the bone. Primary chondrosarcomas that arise de novo tend to be central and constitute approximately 75% of all chondrosarcomas.[142] Secondary chondrosarcomas constitute approximately 25% of all lesions, tend to be peripheral, and arise from preexisting benign cartilage lesions. The most common preexisting lesions from which secondary chondrosarcomas arise are enchondromas. However, chondrosarcomas also can arise from Paget's disease, fibrous dysplasia, unicameral bone cysts, irradiated bone, chondromyxoid fibromas, chondroblastomas, and synovial chondromatosis.

Malignant transformation of solitary enchondromas is thought to occur in less than 3% of cases. In multiple enchondromatosis (Ollier's disease), Maffucci's syndrome (endochondromatosis with hemangiomas), and hereditary multiple exostoses, the incidence of transformation is higher.

Primarily a tumor of adulthood, chondrosarcomas are most common in the fourth to seventh decades. They tend to have a slight male predominance. Chondrosarcomas are rare in children,[143-145] although secondary chondrosarcomas tend to occur at a considerably earlier age than primary lesions.[146] Local swelling and pain are the most common presenting symptoms. Pain is considered to be an indication of growth of a lesion and often heralds malignant transformation of a preexisting lesion of the bone to a secondary chondrosarcoma. Progressive pain, pain at rest, and nocturnal pain are all harbingers of malignancy. Pathologic fracture occurs in 3% to 8% of patients with chondrosarcoma.[147,148]

Although chondrosarcomas can arise in any bone in the body, they occur most commonly in the pelvis, hip girdle, and shoulder girdle. In the long bones of the body, these lesions tend to be metaphyseal and extend into the diaphysis. Epiphyseal involvement is rare. Chondrosarcomas have a characteristic appearance on radiography, appearing as poorly marginated destructive lesions of bone with areas of randomly distributed calcifications. Areas of lucency surrounding the matrix calcification are suggestive of malignancy. Endosteal scalloping is common, and cortical destruction is also an indication of malignancy. New periosteal bone is rarely seen. CT (which is quite sensitive for revealing subtle cortical disruption) and MRI can provide valuable information concerning the extent of the tumor and its relationship to the surrounding anatomy.

The natural history of conventional chondrosarcomas is one of relatively slow growth and low metastatic potential. However, dedifferentiated lesions, high-grade lesions, and mesenchymal lesions are often characterized by aggressive local growth and early metastatic spread. Dahlin and Beabout[149] in 1971 defined dedifferentiated chondrosarcomas as a distinct clinical entity characterized by low-grade cartilage lesions juxtaposed to high-grade nonchondroid sarcoma. Such lesions account for 6% of all chondrosarcomas. Their behavior and treatment is based on their high-grade sarcoma component.

The prognosis for patients with chondrosarcoma depends on the histologic grade and clinical characteristics of the disease. Tumor size and anatomic site influence survival rates, for they often dictate treatment and adequacy of surgical resection. The definitive treatment for chondrosarcoma is wide surgical resection. After adequate surgical treatment, survival rates are 80% to 90% for patients with grade I disease, 50% to 80% for grade II disease, and 40% for grade III disease.[142] Inadequate surgical margins are associated with a high likelihood of local recurrence, with reported rates as high as 75% to 92%.[148,150,151]

As is true for other types of sarcoma, a direct relationship exists between the stage of the disease and the prognosis. Metastasis at the time of initial presentation is the most powerful determinant of long-term survival.[152] Chondrosarcomas tend to metastasize to lung and rarely to soft tissues and bone. Because these lesions tend to metastasize late in the course of the disease, 5-year survival statistics may not be appropriate for determining the natural history of and overall prognosis for metastatic disease.

Wide surgical resection necessitates reconstruction of the skeletal defect. The options for intercalary reconstruction include the use of allografts, vascularized autografts (i.e., vascularized fibula), or prostheses. If joint reconstruction is needed, the options are allograft-prosthetic composites, arthrodesis, osteoarticular allografts, and endoprosthetic reconstruction. Given the morbidity of these procedures, some clinicians advocate intralesional surgery with adjuvant therapy for low-grade chondrosarcomas to preserve joint anatomy and function. Several studies of patients with low-grade chondrosarcomas that have been treated with intralesional excision and adjuvant therapy have demonstrated no compromise in clinical outcome.[153-155]

Chondrosarcomas are considered to be relatively radioresistant.[128,152] However, recent reports suggest that local control of lesions in the cervical spine and base of the skull can be obtained with proton beam and three-dimensional conformal treatment techniques.[156-160] In one series by Rosenberg and colleagues,[160] chondrosarcoma located at the base of the skull was treated with high-dose postoperative fractionated precision radiation therapy at doses of 64.2 to 79.6 Gy; 5- and 10-year local control rates were 99% and 98%, respectively, and 5- to 10-year survival rates were 99%. Hug and colleagues[158] gave high-dose proton radiation therapy postoperatively to patients with residual tumor after surgical resection and observed an actuarial 5-year survival of 100%, with toxic effects noted in only 7% of the patients. Munzenrider and Liebsch[161] found proton therapy to be "ideal for treating skull base and cervical spine tumors, for the dose can be focused while sparing the brain, brain stem, cervical cord, and optic nerves." Thus wide surgical resection remains the definitive treatment, but both proton-beam and three-dimensional conformational radiation therapy may offer promising results when used in the adjuvant setting or for inaccessible lesions. Long-term (15- to 20-year) follow-up studies are still needed, however.

Primary Malignant Lymphoma of Bone

Lymphoma of bone is a rare entity that was first identified by Oberling[162] in 1928. However, it was not until 1939, when Parker and Jackson[163] reported on their series of "reticulum cell sarcoma," that lymphoma of the bone was recognized as a distinct clinical entity. Multiple terms, including reticulum cell sarcoma, malignant lymphoma of bone, primary skeletal lymphoma, and osteolymphoma, have been used to describe the disease. Primary lymphoma of bone, as it is most commonly referred to, constitutes approximately 0.2% of all bone tumors and 5% of all extranodal lymphomas.[164,165] Primary lymphoma of bone was initially described as a malignant lymphoid infiltrate within bone, with or without cortical invasion or soft tissue extension but without concurrent involvement of regional lymph nodes or distant viscera.[166,167] Recently, some authors have expanded the definition to permit lymph node involvement but have stipulated a 6-month time frame between the appearance of the primary focus and the emergence of nodal involvement.[168,169]

Primary lymphoma of bone occurs in males and females in a ratio of 1.8:1 and can occur at any age.[128,170-173] The sites most commonly affected are the long bones. Pain is the most common presenting symptom, and pathologic fracture has been observed in 20% to 30% of cases.[174] Although radiography can help establish the diagnosis, no pathognomonic radiographic features have been noted. Radiographically, these lesions tend to be permeative and located in the metaphyses or diaphyses of long bones (Fig. 34-1, *A* and *B*). Phillips and colleagues[175] evaluated characteristic radiographic findings and found that pathologic fracture, layered periosteal new bone, broken periosteal new bone, cortical breakthrough, soft tissue mass, and soft tissue swelling were the most helpful criteria in establishing the prognosis of the lesion.[175] CT and MRI can assess the extent of the lesion and the presence of an associated soft tissue mass (see Fig. 34-1, *C* and *D*).

The importance of a complete staging work-up cannot be overemphasized. Such a work-up consists of radiography of the bone involved, a bone scan, and CT of the abdomen and pelvis. Before CT became widely available for abdominal and pelvic evaluation, patients with primary lymphoma of bone underwent staging laparotomies to exclude other possible primary sites; many extraosseous lesions may have been missed in such patients. Currently, CT scanning of the abdomen and pelvis can facilitate a more precise assessment of extraosseous disease and has therefore become an integral part of the evaluation of primary lymphoma of bone. Bone scans are used to evaluate the skeleton for evidence of multifocal disease (see Fig. 34-1, *E*). Many investigators have described cases in which lesions that were initially considered to represent primary bone lymphoma were subsequently found to represent systemic disease after a more careful staging analysis.[176]

Treatment of primary lymphoma of bone remains controversial. Surgery is currently used primarily as a diagnostic aid or in the treatment of pathologic fractures. Some authors have recommended radiation therapy for the treatment of localized disease[177] and chemotherapy for patients with more extensive disease.[173] These authors have proposed that radiation be used for Ann Arbor stage 1E disease and that combination therapy be used for higher-stage disease. Recently, combined-modality therapy has been advocated for all stages of disease, given the high distant relapse rates observed after treatment with radiation therapy only.[166,168,178,179] Combined-modality therapy in adults has now been shown to yield survival superior to that produced by radiation alone.

With the use of combined-modality therapy, the prognosis for patients with primary lymphoma of bone is generally considered to be good. Bacci and colleagues[180] found that 88% of patients treated with chemotherapy and radiation were continuously disease-free after a median follow-up of 87 months. Ferreri and colleagues[168] observed that patients with primary lymphoma of bone treated with chemotherapy and whole-bone radiation to a dose of 40 Gy, followed by a boost to a total dose of 45 Gy to areas of bulk disease, had a lower local relapse rate (88% to 90%) and a more favorable 5-year survival rate (40% to 63%) than did patients treated with radiation alone. The studies of Dubey and colleagues[172] suggest that radiation doses of about 46 Gy provide optimal local control and, when combined with chemotherapy, improved long-term survival.

Children also may present with solitary osseous involvement of lymphoma. In pediatric cases, it is not clear if such a presentation represents primary lymphoma of bone or an early manifestation of systemic disease.[177,181] Typically, children with disease considered to be at high risk of relapse have been treated with more aggressive therapy. Loeffler and colleagues[182] reported an 8-year actuarial survival rate of 90% for children with primary lymphoma of bone who were treated with combination therapy. However, they also reported in the same study the development of two cases of secondary sarcoma in the radiation field among the 11 children in whom the original disease had been successfully treated.

In an attempt to reduce the incidence of side effects and the risk of secondary malignancies while maintaining similar control of the primary disease, some authors have investigated less intensive regimens. In a series of 31 patients, Suryanarayan and colleagues[177] found that patients who were treated with only 9 weeks of chemotherapy and no radiation (two thirds of the total population) had a projected 5-year survival rate of 100% and an event-free survival rate of 95%. Although long-term follow-up is still required, these results led the authors to conclude that primary lymphoma of bone in children can be treated successfully with shorter-duration chemotherapy regimens and without radiation. The reason for the differences in outcome observed between children and adults is unclear. However, until prospective randomized clinical trials have been performed, combined-modality therapy should be considered the treatment of choice for adults with primary lymphoma of bone.

Chordoma

Chordomas are rare malignant tumors that arise from the remnants of the notochord. Chordomas represent approximately 1% of all malignant bone tumors. They display a predilection for the ends of the spinal cord; approximately 40% to 60% of lesions are located in the sacrococcygeal region of the spine, 15% to 20% are

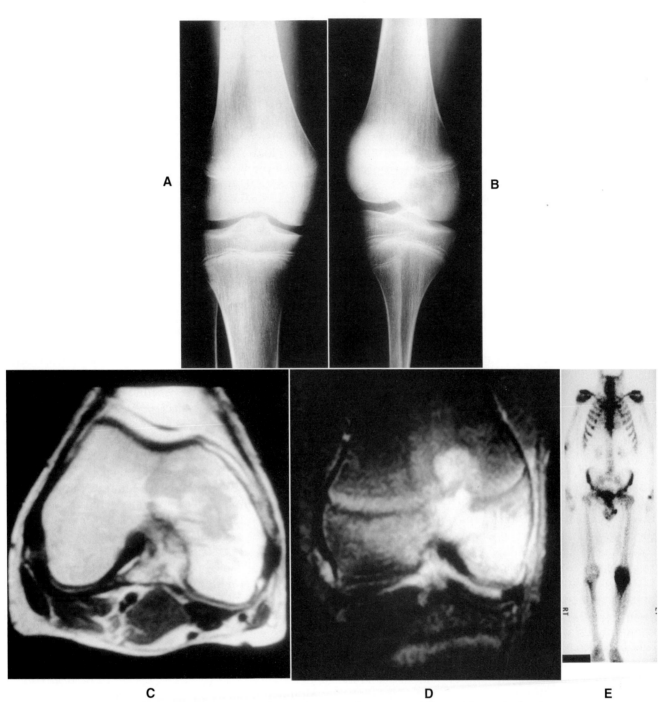

Fig. 34-1 **A** and **B,** Plain films of the right knee of a 13-year-old boy with pain in that knee for 3 to 4 months reveal a poorly circumscribed lytic lesion in the medial femoral condyle crossing the growth plate. **C,** Axial T1-weighted MR image of the right knee shows a poorly circumscribed lesion in the medial condyle extending to the trochlea. The lesion itself shows a gross decrease in signal intensity. **D,** Proton-weighted MR image shows a poorly defined lesion with decreased signal intensity in the medial femoral condyle. **E,** Bone scan shows increased uptake about the right distal femur. A biopsy revealed malignant lymphoma of large B-cell type, most consistent with primary large B-cell lymphoma of bone.

located in the thoracic, lumbar, and cervical spine, and approximately 40% are located at the base of the skull.

Chordomas are uncommon in patients younger than 30 years. They do, however, occur in a broad age range and are most common in the fifth to seventh decades.

Chordomas generally affect men more often than women, with reported ratios of 1.2:1 to 2:1. In the Mayo Clinic series, approximately 64% of 356 patients with chordomas were male,[128] whereas Bjornsson and colleagues[147] reported that 48% of their 40 patients were male.

Chordomas are indolent lesions, and it is not uncommon for symptoms to be present for several years before diagnosis.[147] Symptoms are related to the location and size of the tumor and thus are varied. Headaches, increased intracranial pressure, or cranial nerve symptoms are often associated with cranial tumors. Pain, neurologic deficits, or symptoms similar to those resulting from a herniated disc can be produced by vertebral tumors. Pain, neurologic compromise, and bowel or bladder dysfunction can result from sacral or sacrococcygeal tumors.

Radiographic features of chordomas also depend on their location. Because these lesions originate from the remnants of the notochord, they appear at the midline. In sacral and sacrococcygeal tumors, bony destruction is central and irregular. A soft tissue mass is usually present anteriorly, and calcification within the soft tissue mass is common. CT and MRI are helpful because routine radiography often fails to adequately delineate sacral lesions. CT can be used to delineate the lesion, assess the extent of peripheral reactive sclerosis, and define the degree and extension of the calcifications.[183] MRI can delineate soft tissue mass extension, longitudinal extension of tumors, and sacral root involvement.[184,185] Chordomas that arise in the mobile spine generally arise within the vertebral bodies, but extension into the posterior elements is common. Vertebral destruction is associated with peripheral sclerosis, and reactive new bone is often observed. Multiple contiguous vertebral involvement can be seen. Cranial lesions are almost always associated with radiographic changes. Destruction of the clivus or sella turcica and bony destruction in the spheno-occipital and hypophyseal regions are often readily apparent. MRI of these regions facilitates visualization of soft tissue extension.

Although chordomas are slow-growing malignant tumors, their prognosis is guarded. Most often, death occurs not from distant metastasis but rather from local extension of the tumor. In a series of 40 patients with chordoma described by Bjornsson and colleagues,[186] the long-term survival rate was 37% even though only 5% of patients developed lung metastases. Patient age and tumor location are important prognostic factors, with age less than 40 years and proximal vertebral lesions associated with improved long-term survival.[187,188]

Depending on the location of the lesion, treatment and prognosis vary. Wide or complete excision is the treatment of choice. However, wide excision is not feasible for all tumors. Kaiser and colleagues[189] reported that the recurrence rate among tumors that had been entered during surgery was approximately 3 times higher than that for tumors that had not been compromised at the time of surgery.

Radiation has been advocated as an adjuvant treatment when surgical margins are positive for residual disease.[156,187,190-192] Both conventional fractionated high-dose and proton-photon-beam therapy have been used for postoperative treatment.[190,193-195] Munzenrider and Liebsch[161] suggested that charged-particle beams were ideal for treating skull-base and cervical chordomas because such beams can deliver precise high-dose radiation to localized areas of disease while sparing surrounding normal tissues. These techniques have proved particularly useful in spinal and cranial lesions. al-Mefty and colleagues[190] concluded that proton-photon therapy effectively controlled tumors after radical surgery, but follow-up in this study was short. Borba and colleagues[193] and Habrand and colleagues[196] have both advocated proton-photon therapy for children; and Borba and colleagues reported a 68% 5-year actuarial survival rate and a 63% disease-free survival rate in their series of four pediatric patients with intracranial chordomas. Conventional therapy consisting of high-dose fractionated radiation therapy has produced comparable results. Romero and colleagues[197] demonstrated that the prognosis for patients given a postoperative radiation dose of 48 Gy was better than that for patients given doses of less than 40 Gy. Their study suggested that high-dose postoperative radiation may increase the disease-free interval for patients with microscopic residual disease. Klekamp and Samii[198] found that patients treated with postoperative radiation doses of 60 to 70 Gy had a significantly longer recurrence-free interval than did patients who had suboptimal excision and no radiation therapy.

These results suggest that radiation therapy, with either proton-photon or conventional high-dose beams, is a valuable adjuvant treatment option for patients with incompletely resected disease. However, when possible, wide surgical resection should remain the definitive treatment of choice. As emphasized by Catton and colleagues,[191] radiation therapy may play an important role in controlling microscopic disease and affording palliative pain control, but it rarely cures gross residual disease.

Malignant Fibrous Histiocytoma

Although formerly thought to be similar in character and radioresponsiveness to osteosarcoma or fibrosarcoma, malignant fibrous histiocytoma of bone has been recently reported to be a distinct clinicopathologic entity.[199,200] It may even be clinicopathologically distinct from soft tissue malignant fibrous histiocytoma.[199] Histologically, malignant fibrous histiocytoma of bone has areas of fibrogenic differentiation (often in a storiform pattern) or areas of histiocytes and anaplastic giant cells.[200-203] It can usually be classified as either storiform-pleomorphic (63%) or histiocytic (19%) based on the predominance of one of the patterns.[199]

This high-grade bone tumor (presenting at grade 2 in 1% of cases, grade 3 in 27%, and grade 4 in 72%) is seen with fairly equal frequency in men and women, and it likewise occurs with fairly equal frequency through the second to eighth decades of life, although most patients are older than 40 years.[199,204] The most common clinical symptom on presentation is pain at an average duration of 6 months (range, 1 week to 2 years), with or without swelling or a mass; other symptoms and signs include limping, deformity, joint stiffness, and proptosis.[199,204] Approximately half of patients present with tumors at the ends of the long bones of the lower extremities; in a series of 81 patients described by Nishida and colleagues,[199] the most common sites were around the knee joint (29%) and around the pelvis and pelvic girdle, including the proximal femur (22%). The most common site of metastasis is the lung (82%).[204]

Malignant fibrous histiocytoma of bone can occur in response to irradiation, but it more often arises spontaneously; in the Nishida series,[199] 13 of 81 patients had a history of previous irradiation for a variety of primary tumors. Radiographically, the tumor appears aggressive, with a permeative pattern of bone destruction, ill-defined lesion margins, and a wide zone of transition from normal to abnormal bone[199] (Fig. 34-2). In the Nishida series,[199] 13 patients had radiographs available for review; 62% of the lesions were purely osteolytic, 38% were mixed osteolytic and sclerotic, 38% caused a periosteal reaction, 85% were associated with cortical destruction and an extraosseous soft tissue mass, 92% showed no matrix calcification, none were exclusively epiphyseal in location, and a few were associated with pathologic fracture.[199] Most patients described in the literature have been treated surgically, either with wide local excision or amputation.[199,201,204]

The prognosis for malignant fibrous histiocytoma is best for tumors treated with wide and radical procedures with negative margins. Reported 1-year local recurrence-free survival rates are 100% after amputation or disarticulation and 72.4% after limb-salvage procedures; the 1-, 5-, and 10-year disease-free survival rates are 72.8%, 66.5%, and 60.9% if adequate margins are taken, compared with 59.8%, 48.3%, and 26.4% if not.[199]

Patients with localized extremity lesions seem to do better than those with axial skeleton lesions (with 2-, 5-, and 10-year disease-free survival rates of 67.4%, 62.0%, and 52.3%, compared with 71.4%, 52.1%, and 27.8%, respectively), and postoperative radiation therapy seems to improve the prognosis for tumors excised with inadequate margins (2-, 5-, and 10-year disease-free survival rates of 61.5%, 61.5%, and 41.0%, compared with 58.3%, 35.0%, and 11.7%, respectively), but the differences among these numbers are not statistically significant.[199]

Radiation alone may cure patients; in the Nishida series,[199] five of eight patients with localized malignant fibrous histiocytoma of bone treated primarily with radiation therapy were alive at last follow-up, and four of those five were without disease. Likewise, in a series from the Istituto Ortopedico Rizzoli in Italy, eight patients received radiation as the primary treatment; a clinical cure was obtained in three and significant palliation in one.[201] Bacci and colleagues[205] reported on the use of neoadjuvant chemotherapy (high-dose methotrexate, cisplatin, and doxorubicin) in 22 patients with nonmetastatic malignant fibrous histiocytoma of bone and found that limb salvage was possible in 20 of those patients. The histologic response to chemotherapy was graded as 90%, and at an average follow-up of 40 months, 15 patients remained continuously disease-free and 7 had relapse with metastases. No local recurrences were observed.[205]

Hemangioendothelioma

Hemangioendothelioma, a rare tumor thought to be of vascular origin, is seen in equal frequency through the second to sixth decades of life, more often in men than in women.[206,207] Most of these tumors are thought to be benign or low grade, but they can be locally aggressive.[206,207] Malignant lesions do occur and are often called hemangiosarcomas.[208] Radiologically, tumors appear as (often multiple) osteolytic lesions in the metaphysis or epiphysis of long bones or in the pelvis.[206,207] In the more malignant type, cortical erosion can be detected, and advanced lesions can create a honeycomb appearance with bone expansion; periosteal reactions are rare.[206,207]

The differential diagnosis includes metastatic carcinoma and myeloma, although single bone involvement suggests hemangioendothelioma.[209] Histologically, epithelioid hemangioendothelioma is typified by solid cell nests or cords of epithelial-like cells and prominent endothelial-lined vascular spaces surrounded by proliferating tumor cells.[206] They also may have intravascular papillary-like projections with epithelial or histiocyte-like cells.[209] Wide surgical excision is the treatment of choice, and amputation should be considered for multifocal disease. Radiation therapy should be considered when these tumors appear in weight-bearing bones or vertebral bodies or are widely distributed in the skeleton or foot.[206,210-213] With 45 to 50 Gy given over 4.5 to 5 weeks, at least 75% of such patients should have complete disappearance of pain.[214]

Giant Cell Tumor of Bone

Giant cell tumors of bone have been described as the most challenging benign tumors of bone.[152] They constitute approximately 5% of all primary bone tumors and 21% of all benign tumors of bone.[128] These tumors have a slight female predominance, with a female-to-male

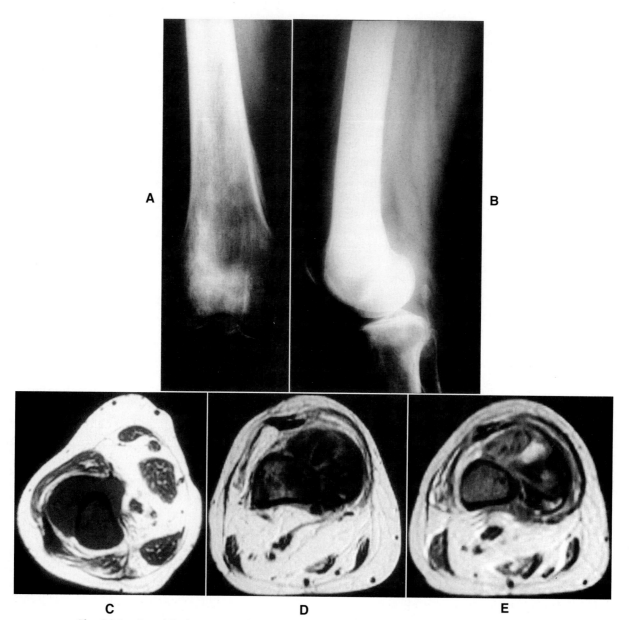

Fig. 34-2 **A** and **B,** Anteroposterior and lateral radiographs of the distal femur and proximal tibia of a 64-year-old woman with recently developed pain and swelling indicate an ill-defined lytic lesion in the distal femur. **C,** Axial T1-weighted MR image through the thigh shows a large, soft-tissue mass about the femur that extends laterally. The mass and marrow are of low density. **D,** Axial T2-weighted MR image shows a very large, heterogeneous soft-tissue mass located medially that appears to be within the knee joint. **E,** Additional gadolinium-enhanced images through the distal femur confirm the large size and heterogeneity of the soft tissue mass.

ratio of 1.3:1.[215,216] Most commonly appearing in the third decade of life, less than 5% of giant cell tumors occur in skeletally immature patients.[217,218] In a Mayo Clinic series, 84% of giant cell tumors occurred in patients older than 19 years.[128]

Most giant cell tumors are found in the epiphyses of long bones, but they may extend into the metaphyses as well. In several published series,[219-224] only 1.2% of giant cell tumors were found to involve the metaphysis or diaphysis without epiphyseal involvement. Approximately 50% were located about the knee (distal femur

and proximal tibia), with the proximal humerus and distal radius being the third and fourth most common sites.

Pain and swelling are the most common presenting symptoms. The incidence of pathologic fracture can range from 11% to 37%.[220,225,226] Soft tissue extension is common. Radiographically, these lesions are eccentrically located, are lytic, have narrow zones of transition, and tend to be juxta-articular. The lesions lack peripheral sclerosis and surrounding periosteal reaction. Giant cell tumors can appear quite aggressive and are characterized by extensive local bony destruction, cortical breakthrough,

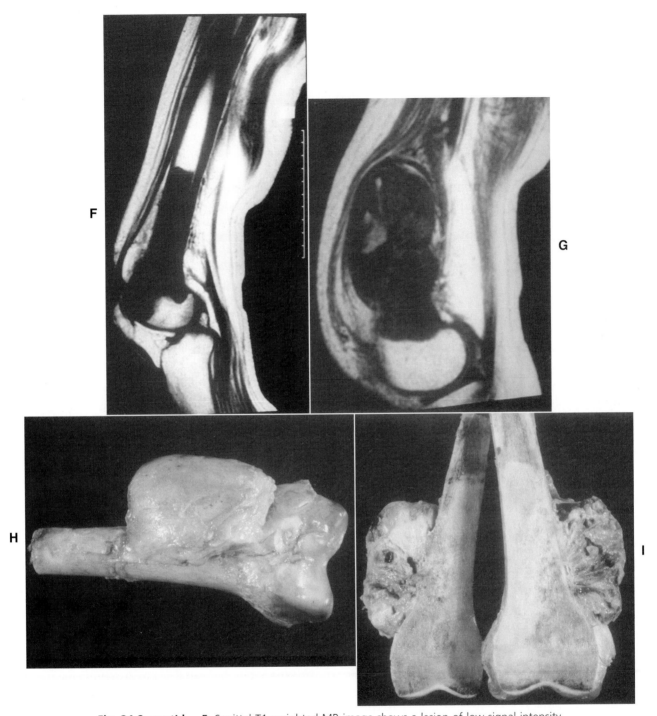

Fig. 34-2, cont'd   F, Sagittal T1-weighted MR image shows a lesion of low signal intensity extending from the distal femur to the femoral diaphysis. **G,** Sagittal T1-weighted MR image shows a very large soft-tissue mass located laterally in addition to the intramedullary lesion extending from the distal femur to the femoral diaphysis. **H and I,** Photographs of the gross specimen without the surrounding soft tissue/muscle. The soft tissue mass seems to be growing off the lateral femoral cortex and condyle. The specimen was identified as a high-grade malignant fibrous histiocytoma with minimal necrosis.

and soft tissue expansion. Campanacci and colleagues[220] proposed a grading system for giant cell tumors that was based on their radiographic appearance. The Campanacci system is similar to that proposed by Ennecking[227] for benign bone tumors. No correlation has been found between these grading systems and prognosis.

The natural history of giant cell tumors varies widely and can include local bony destruction, local metastasis,

metastasis to the lung, metastasis to lymph nodes (rare), or malignant transformation. Approximately 3% of giant cell tumors will metastasize to the lung. These metastases appear as 'clusters' of giant cell tumors located within the lung.[228-232] Lung metastases appear an average of 3 to 5 years after the initial diagnosis of the primary lesion. The significance of these metastases is unclear; reports have been made of multiple unresectable lung lesions that remain stable and some that spontaneously regress.[228,233-237] Thus long-term follow-up is important for patients with metastatic disease.

Spontaneous malignant transformation of giant cell tumor is relatively uncommon. Dahlin[128] defined malignant transformation as a sarcoma associated with a typical giant cell tumor at presentation or as a sarcoma arising at the site of a preexisting giant cell tumor. Malignant transformation can occur as long as 25 years after the initial presentation.[238,239] Many authors have hypothesized that malignant transformation of giant cell tumors may be caused by, or at least associated with, radiation therapy.[128,152,240,241]

Treatment of giant cell tumor has ranged from simple curettage to wide en bloc resection. Wide en bloc resection results in the lowest recurrence rate but also necessitates prosthetic reconstruction and is associated with considerable surgical and functional morbidity. In contrast, simple curettage with minimal surgical and functional morbidity produced recurrence rates as high as 30% in some series.[226,242-244] Recently, several authors have treated giant cell tumors with simple curettage and high-speed burring of the cavity followed by reconstruction with insertion of polymethylmethacrylate or a bone graft and have described a decrease of local recurrence rates of 20% to 25%.[245,246] Adjuvant therapies with phenol, argon laser, or cryotherapy to the curetted cavity, followed by packing with polymethylmethacrylate, have further reduced recurrence rates to 2% to 10%.[247-252]

Radiation therapy has been used as a primary or adjunct therapy for giant cell tumors. Historically, these lesions were considered to be radioresistant, but more recent findings suggest that they may be radiosensitive.[253] Radiation is generally not recommended in the orthopedic literature as a primary or adjunctive treatment for lesions of the axial skeleton[241] because of concerns regarding malignant transformation. However, these concerns are based on studies done when giant cell tumors were treated with orthovoltage radiation. In these studies, patients were given several orthovoltage treatments, resulting in a high cumulative dose and high dose to the bone. Megavoltage radiation, at doses of 40 to 70 Gy, limits the dose to the bone while still preventing tumor progression. Because malignant transformation seems to depend on dose, lower rates of transformation have been observed when modern radiation therapeutic techniques are used. Thus megavoltage treatments have become the preferred radiation regimen.[253-257]

Radiation therapy has been proposed to treat patients who cannot undergo surgery for medical reasons or whose tumors are in locations not amenable to operative treatment, or when a potential for significant morbidity from tumor relapse or subsequent surgery exists.[255,258] Chakravarti and colleagues[254] concluded that giant cell tumors of bone can be effectively treated with megavoltage radiation with clinical results that are comparable to those observed after curettage and adjuvant treatment. A series by Nair and Jyothirmayi[259] also suggested that treatment with radiation at doses of 40 to 60 Gy, given in 15 to 30 fractions, also produced results comparable to those from surgical treatment. Nair and Jyothirmayi[259] concluded that radiation was effective in producing local control without major complications or risk of malignant transformation. Even though both studies described no malignant transformation, median follow-up times were only 9.9 years and 48 months, respectively. The median time for malignant transformation is thought to be approximately 10 years.

In summary, operative treatment consisting of curettage and reconstruction with methylmethacrylate or bone grafting combined with adjuvant therapy remains the standard of care for giant cell tumor. However, radiation therapy may offer an alternative treatment option for inaccessible giant cell tumors, tumors of the axial skeleton, and tumors in individuals who are not candidates for surgery.

Eosinophilic Granuloma

Eosinophilic granuloma is a solitary or multifocal osseous lesion that is part of a spectrum known as Langerhans cell histiocytosis or, in earlier days, histiocytosis X. Langerhans cell histiocytosis consists of a systemic fulminant form (Letterer-Siwe disease), a chronic disseminated form (Hand-Schüller-Christian disease), and a localized form limited to bone or lung (eosinophilic granuloma).[260] Most patients (60% to 80%) with Langerhans cell histiocytosis have the localized form, but they can develop disseminated disease. If dissemination is going to occur, it most commonly does so during the first year after presentation.[261] We now know that mononuclear cells of the dendritic line, found in the epidermis but derived from bone marrow precursors, are the primary proliferative element. These cells, known as Langerhans cells, characteristically contain cytoplasmic organelles called Birbeck granules. Older lesions may appear dominantly fibrotic and be misdiagnosed as chronic osteomyelitis.[260]

The age incidence for single lesions peaks between 5 and 10 years, with most lesions occurring in patients under the age of 20. Almost all series note a predominance in boys over girls, with a ratio of 2:1. Although their appearance on skeletal surveys can vary depending on the bones involved, the lesions are usually lytic and

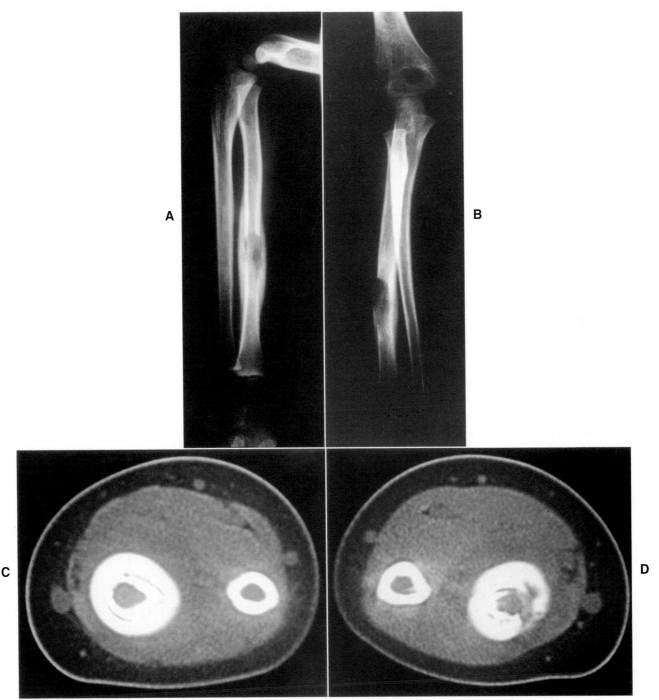

Fig. 34-3 **A,** Anteroposterior radiograph of the right forearm of a 4-year-old boy with pain of several months' duration and no history of significant trauma shows a lytic lesion within the midshaft of the radius with significant periosteal reaction about the lesion. A fracture may be present within this lesion. Significant periosteal reaction is noted. **B,** Lateral radiograph shows a large lytic lesion within the distal radius. **C,** Computed tomography (CT) scan through the midforearm shows significant periosteal reaction around the radius, with "onion-skin" layering. **D,** CT scan through the diaphyseal portion of the radius shows circumferential periosteal reaction as well as the absence of radial cortex and thinning of the periosteal reaction. The final diagnosis was eosinophilic granuloma.

rounded, often having a scalloped outline (Fig. 34-3). 99Tc bone scanning fails to demonstrate the lesion in approximately one third of cases, and a skeleton survey remains the procedure of choice.[262] Aggressive surgical

curettage is an acceptable method of treatment for many lesions, although total removal of the lesion is not always necessary.[263] Even biopsy with or without curettage can initiate healing, and some lesions simply resolve spontaneously over months to years. Intralesional corticosteroid treatment has been reported to be effective, convenient, and safe for control of local disease.[264] Systemic disease is often treated with chemotherapy, including vinblastine and etoposide.[264-267] When localized lesions are symptomatic or occur in weight-bearing bones or critical sites of the head and neck such as the orbit, mastoid, or mandible, radiation therapy is the treatment of choice.[268]

Eosinophilic granulomas are exquisitely radiosensitive, and most authors favor doses in the range of 6 to 8 Gy, given in three or four fractions, using fields that include any soft-tissue extension. Some reports describe the use of larger radiation doses (e.g., 10 to 15 Gy) for adults and for patients whose disease includes a soft-tissue component.[268-271] In-field recurrences are rare after radiation therapy, unless the extent of soft-tissue involvement is underestimated.[268,270] In a study from the University of California at Los Angeles,[270] 35 (88%) of 40 bone lesions were controlled by radiation, but when soft tissues were involved, the rate of control dropped to 11 (69%) of 16. Interestingly, all in-field recurrences occurred in adults who had involvement of multiple bones and soft-tissue extension.[270] If a lesion thought to be eosinophilic granuloma fails to resolve after retreatment with an additional 10 to 15 Gy, the initial diagnosis should be reconsidered, especially if the lesion is solitary and in the femur, pelvis, or vertebral bodies.

RADIATION THERAPY IN THE TREATMENT OF METASTATIC BONE DISEASE

Bone metastases can cause pain secondary to periosteal stretching, mechanical damage, nerve entrapment, and muscle spasm.[272] Metastases are most often lytic because of direct resorption of bone or indirect stimulation of osteoclast activity, a mechanism that may be inhibited by the use of bisphosphonates.[273] Bone metastases also can stimulate destructive peritumoral osteoblastic activity, which is visible on bone scanning.[274] Bone metastases must be distinguished from radiation-induced changes such as radiation osteitis (spongy destruction in weight-bearing areas such as the ileosacral joint, without a pathologic soft tissue mass)[275] and insufficiency fractures in irradiated pelvises, which show a typical symmetric uptake pattern on bone scintigraphy.[276] Other diseases in the differential diagnosis include degenerative disk disease, osteoporosis, and spondylosis (Figs. 34-4 and 34-5).

Radiation therapy for palliation of symptoms yields complete pain relief in approximately 50% of patients and partial pain relief in an additional 40%.[277,278] The incidence of pain relief is higher for patients with prostate or breast primary tumors than in patients with primary tumors in the lung or elsewhere.[277] A prognostic factor for prostate cancer patients with bone

metastases is the rate of increase in the number of bone metastases as estimated by serial bone scans.[279] Prognostic factors for breast cancer patients with bone metastases include serum lactate dehydrogenase level, age, and performance status; if the metastases are limited to the axial bones, then multivariate analysis indicates that maintenance chemohormonal therapy and an age of more than 55 years are good prognostic factors.[280]

In general, the time to pain relief is on the order of weeks, with 96% of patients who eventually experience minimal relief doing so within the first 4 weeks of treatment, whereas nearly 50% of those who achieve complete relief do so for the first time more than 4 weeks after treatment. The treatment effect lasts for several months (median 12 weeks for complete relief, median 23 weeks for partial relief).[277] For this reason, it is important to aggressively manage symptoms while awaiting response to therapy; persistent or recurrent pain after therapy may be caused by bony instability or fracture before reossification occurs, necessitating surgical intervention.[281,282]

Pathologic fracture is a real risk with bone metastases. The rate is approximately 8% after radiation therapy.[277,283] Some recommend prophylactic surgical stabilization, such as use of an intramedullary rod, when more than 50% of the cortex is involved because the risk of fracture is high (near 50%) under those conditions.[284-286] A brief fractionated course of radiation therapy (e.g., 30 Gy given in 10 fractions) is routinely given after surgery.[274] Lytic lesions in long weight-bearing bones such as the femur may require use of crutches or a walker or limb immobilization until the bone heals.[274]

With regard to local radiation therapy, the benefit of fractionated vs. single-dose radiation therapy remains controversial, although most North American physicians still use fractionated schedules.[287-298] The most common fractionation scheme in the United States is 30 Gy, given in 10 fractions.[299] In 1982 the Radiation Therapy Oncology Group (RTOG) reported that among more than 1000 patients (266 with solitary metastases and 750 with multiple osseous metastases), the low-dose, short-course schedules seemed to be as effective as high-dose, long-course schedules; however, in 1985, Peter Blitzer[278] reanalyzed the data and found that evaluating the percentage of patients with "complete combined relief" (where success means that both pain and narcotic use fall to zero) revealed a trend favoring protracted programs (40.5 Gy in 15 2.7-Gy fractions and 30 Gy in 10 3-Gy fractions). For patients with solitary metastases, complete combined relief occurred in 55% of patients (38 of 69) treated with 15 2.7-Gy fractions compared with only 37% (25 of 68) treated with 5 4-Gy fractions. For those with multiple metastases, complete combined relief occurred in 46% of patients (72 of 158)

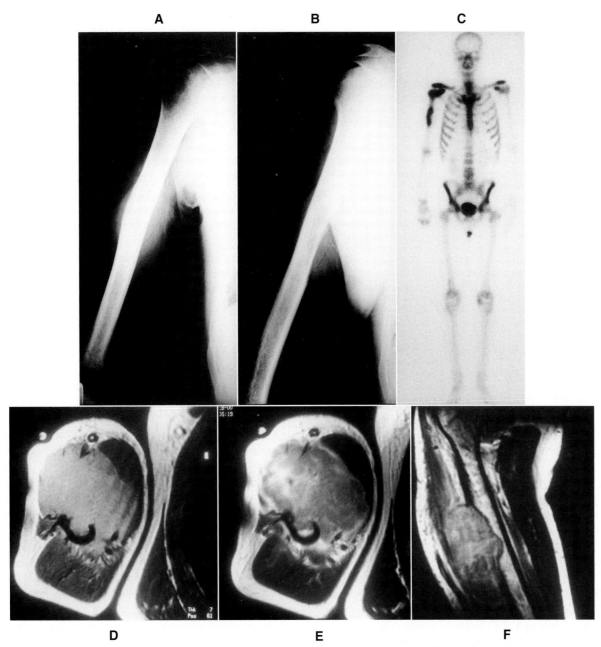

Fig. 34-4 **A** and **B,** Two views of the humerus of a 55-year-old man with an enlarging mass in the right arm suggest a large soft tissue mass at the midshaft of the humerus with slight scalloping of the bone. **C,** Bone scan shows significantly increased uptake in the proximal, diaphyseal portion of the humerus. **D,** Axial T2-weighted magnetic resonance imaging (MRI) scan shows a 6-cm homogeneous mass encompassing the anterior portion of the arm and displacing the deltoid, with some anterior cortical erosion of the humerus. **E,** Axial T2-weighted gadolinium-enhanced MRI through the arm shows peripheral and lateral enhancement and displacement of the biceps muscle. The medial neurovascular bundle of the mass is visible posteriorly. **F,** Coronal T1-weighted sagittal MRI shows a large soft tissue mass with cortical erosion. Most of the mass resides in the soft tissue and extends the length of the mid-diaphyseal portion of the humerus. A biopsy revealed a metastatic moderately differentiated adenocarcinoma.

treated with 10 3-Gy fractions compared with only 36% (48 of 135) treated with 5 3-Gy fractions, 40% (59 of 147) treated with 5 4-Gy fractions, and 28% (39 of 137) treated with 5 5-Gy fractions. Multivariate analysis of the solitary and multiple metastasis groups together showed the number of fractions to be associated with complete combined relief ($P = 0.0003$), but not the dose per fraction ($P > 0.10$).[278]

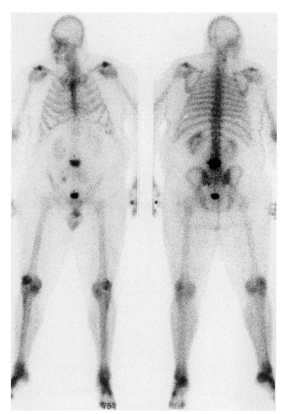

Fig. 34-5 Bone scan of a patient with prostate cancer shows metastatic disease involving the L4 vertebral body and probably the right sacroiliac joint.

At the M.D. Anderson Cancer Center, we treat bone metastases with 30 Gy given in 10 3-Gy fractions. Other institutions support the use of single-dose or short-course local-field radiation therapy as an equally effective, more convenient option.[290,293,294,300-304] In a prospective randomized trial of 270 patients, N = 2, Hoskin and colleagues[294] demonstrated a dose-response relationship with single-dose radiation therapy: at 4 weeks, 8 Gy provided a higher probability of pain relief than 4 Gy, although the ability of single-dose radiation therapy to provide pain relief in this study (27% to 35% complete relief and 58% to 88% partial relief) was less than that in the RTOG trials of fractionated treatment.[290] Similarly, Uppelschoten and colleagues[283] found that 6-Gy single-dose local field irradiation provided partial pain relief in 88% of patients with painful bony metastases and complete relief in 39%. When the treatment was given to the vertebrae, in-field spinal cord compression developed in 9% of patients; when given to the pelvis or femur, in-field fractures developed in 8%.[283] This experience is similar to the 8% risk of fracture after fractionated radiation therapy noted in the RTOG series.[277] These findings require further confirmation, but they suggest that 6- to 8-Gy single-dose radiation therapy may prove to be a useful alternative to fractionated regimens such as 10 3-Gy fractions, although trends have been found favoring the more protracted schedules

in terms of pain relief and recalcification.[277,283,290,294,303-305] In a large phase III Dutch trial in which 1171 patients were randomly assigned to receive either 8 Gy in one fraction (N = 585) or six fractions of 4 Gy (N = 586), 4 times more retreatments were necessary in the single-dose group.[306]

Studies of hemibody irradiation (HBI) confirm the superiority of fractionated radiation for durable palliation. For single-fraction HBI, the RTOG 7810 trial showed doses of 6 Gy for upper-body HBI and 8 Gy for lower-body HBI to be the most effective and least toxic.[307] Zelefsky and colleagues[308] at Memorial Sloan-Kettering Cancer Center compared fractionated HBI (25 to 30 Gy in 9 or 10 fractions) to 6-Gy (upper body HBI) or 8-Gy (lower body HBI) single doses. The need for retreatment was far less in the fractionated group (13%; 2 of 15) than in the single-dose group (71%; 10 of 14) (P = 0.001). The palliation also lasted longer in the fractionated group (8.5 vs. 2.8 months).[308]

The major dose-limiting toxic effect of HBI is hematologic (thromboleukopenia). The major nonhematologic side effects are gastrointestinal, which can be alleviated by premedication with ondansetron or other antiemetic agents.[309,310] An advantage of HBI is the speed of relief; most patients have significant relief of pain within 2 weeks of completing fractionated HBI and within 72 hours of completing single-dose HBI.[307,308,311,312] Considering the relatively short life span of patients with widespread bony metastases, the duration of pain relief from HBI is excellent as well; in the series described by Algara and colleagues,[312] the mean duration of response to single-fraction HBI (6 Gy for upper HBI and 8 Gy for lower HBI) was 101 days, or 70% of the expected life span. The RTOG also has investigated the use of single-dose HBI (again, 6 Gy for upper and 8 Gy for lower body) after local-field fractionated radiation therapy (10 3-Gy fractions) to delay the development of new sites of disease (RTOG 8206; phase III; N = 499). Although toxicity rates were higher in the group given HBI than in those given fractionated radiation, that toxicity was reversible and was balanced by a doubling in the time to the appearance of new disease (from 6.3 to 12.6 months).[313]

An alternative to HBI for the management of micrometastatic disease is the use of radioisotopes such as ^{89}Sr.[314] ^{89}Sr (Metastron), with a half-life of 50.6 days and maximum energy of 1.4 MeV, is a popular radiopharmaceutical for the treatment of bone metastases, with overall response rates as high as 80% for patients with prostate or breast cancer.[315-319] Relief begins in 1 to 3 weeks, peaks at 6 weeks, and lasts for a mean of 12 months.[320] Radioisotopes are particularly useful when patients (with adequate marrow reserve and no evidence of impending spinal cord compression) have bone scan evidence of metastatic bony disease on both sides of the diaphragm.[320,321] ^{89}Sr is less toxic to marrow than its predecessor ^{32}P, although multiple or sequential high doses should be used with caution because of myelotoxicity.[315] The bone-to-marrow uptake ratio for ^{89}Sr is 10:1, and the retention time varies greatly (e.g., 11% to 88% at 3 months) depending on the degree of metastatic bony involvement.[322-325] Up to 22% of patients are pain-free at 3 months.[320] The optimum palliative dose is 40 mCi/kg (1.5 MBq/kg).[318] With hematologic surveillance, repeated treatment is an option, with the efficacy potentially the same as that achieved with the first dose.[326] Low-dose concomitant platinum therapy has been used to further improve the pain control achieved with ^{89}Sr alone.[327,328]

^{153}Sm-lexidronam is another bone-seeking radiopharmaceutical licensed for use in the United States.[329] The relative advantage of ^{153}Sm-lexidronam is its short half-life (46.3 hours) and low energy (mean beta-particle energies of 810 keV [20%], 710 keV [50%], and 640 keV [30%]; mean gamma photon energy of 103 keV).[330,331] Pain relief from ^{153}Sm-lexidronam is prompt, with significant pain improvement as early as the first week after drug administration.[332] Pain relief occurs in most patients (61% to 90%) and lasts at least 3 or 4 months.[332-339] Repeated administrations are possible with careful monitoring of white blood cell and platelet counts; with a standard dose of 1.0 mCi/kg, nadir reportedly occurs in 3 to 5 weeks and recovery is within 5 to 8 weeks of drug administration.[336]

Hortobagyi and colleagues[340] described a phase III study of 382 women with stage IV breast cancer and at least one lytic bone lesion who were given cytotoxic chemotherapy. These women significantly benefited from intravenous administration of the bisphosphonate pamidronate disodium (90 mg given as a 2-hour monthly infusion for 12 cycles). Pamidronate is already the treatment of choice for patients with tumor-induced hypercalcemia.[341] Compared with placebo, pamidronate reduces the median time to the occurrence of first skeletal complications (13.1 vs. 7.0 months, $P = 0.005$), the proportion of patients in whom any skeletal complication occurs (43% vs. 56%, $P = 0.008$), the increase in bone pain ($P = 0.046$), and the deterioration of performance status ($P = 0.027$).[340]

The definition of skeletal complications included both the occurrence of an event and the need for therapeutic action or symptom control (e.g., pathologic fractures, surgery for fracture or impending fracture, radiation, spinal cord compression, and hypercalcemia).[340,342] Pamidronate's mechanism of action includes inhibition of osteoclast activity, perhaps most importantly by prevention of the attachment of osteoclast precursor cells to bone.[341] This may be accomplished by pamidronate's binding to hydroxyapatite crystals, making it more difficult for osteoclasts to recognize exposed unmineralized bone surfaces.[343] Pamidronate also may be directly toxic to osteoclasts.[343] Oral bisphosphonates such as clodronate disodium are

under investigation; their biodistribution and adverse effects (especially gastrointestinal effects) need to be further evaluated.[343,344] In one study, clodronate therapy had to be discontinued in 3% of patients because of adverse gastrointestinal side effects.[344]

REFERENCES

1. Kember N. Cell population kinetics of bone growth in long bones. *Clin Orthop* 1971;76:213-230.
2. Kember N, Sissons H. Quantitative histology of the human growth plate. *J Bone Joint Surg* 1976;58B:426-435.
3. Walker K, Kember N. Cell kinetics of growth cartilage in the rat tibia. I. Measurements in young rats. *Cell Tissue Kinetics* 1972;5:401-408.
4. Eifel PJ. Decreased bone growth arrest in weanling rats with multiple radiation fractions per day. *Int J Radiat Oncol Biol Phys* 1988;15:141-145.
5. Alheit H, Baumann M, Thames HD, et al. Fractionation effect on radiation-induced growth retardation of tibia in rabbits and rats. *Acta Oncol* 1998;37:151-158.
6. Wang X, Ding I, Xie H, et al. Hyperbaric oxygen and basic fibroblast growth factor promote growth of irradiated bone. *Int J Radiat Oncol Biol Phys* 1998;40:189-196.
7. Okunieff P, Wang X, Rubin P, et al. Radiation-induced changes in bone perfusion and angiogenesis. *Int J Radiat Oncol Biol Phys* 1998;42:885-889.
8. Wechsler-Jentzsch K, Huepfel H, Schmidt W, et al. Failure of hyperfractionated radiotherapy to reduce bone growth arrest in rats. *Int J Radiat Oncol Biol Phys* 1993;26:427-431.
9. Probert JC, Parker BR. The effects of radiation therapy on bone growth. *Radiology* 1975;114:155-162.
10. Willman K, Cox R, Donaldson S. Radiation induced height impairment in pediatric Hodgkin's disease. *Int J Radiat Oncol Biol Phys* 1994;28:85-92.
11. Neuhauser EB, Wittenborg MH, Berman CZ. Irradiation effects of roentgen therapy on the growing spine. *Radiology* 1952;59:637-649.
12. Riseborough E, Grabias S, Burton R, et al. Skeletal alterations following irradiation for Wilm's tumor. *J Bone Joint Surg* 1976;58:526-536.
13. Willich E, Kuttig H, Pfeil G, et al. Wirbelsaulenveranderungen nach bestrahlung wegen wilmstumor im kleinkindesalter. Retrospektive interdisziplinare langzeitstudie an 82 kindern. *Strahlenther Onkol* 1990;166:815-821.
14. Heaston D, Libshitz H, Chan R. Skeletal effects of megavoltage irradiation in survivors of Wilm's tumor. *Am J Roentgenol* 1979;133:389-395.
15. Silverman C, Thomas P, McAlister W, et al. Slipped capital femoral epiphysis in irradiated children: dose volume and age relationships. *Int J Radiat Oncol Biol Phys* 1981;7:1357-1363.
16. Eifel PJ, Donaldson SS, Thomas PR. Response of growing bone to irradiation: a proposed late effects scoring system. *Int J Radiat Oncol Biol Phys* 1995;31:1301-1307.
17. Libshitz H, Edeikin B. Radiotherapy changes of the pediatric hip. *Am J Roentgenol* 1981;137:585-588.
18. Cohen A, van Lint MT, Uderzo C, et al. Growth in patients after allogeneic bone marrow transplant for hematological diseases in childhood. *Bone Marrow Transplant* 1995;15:343-348.
19. Kroll SS, Woo SY, Santin A, et al. Long-term effects of radiotherapy administered in childhood for the treatment of malignant diseases. *Ann Surg Oncol* 1994;1:473-479.
20. Tamurian RM, Damron TA, Spadaro JA. Sparing radiation-induced damage to the physis by radioprotectant drugs: laboratory analysis in a rat model. *J Orthop Res* 1999;17:286-292.
21. Damron TA, Spadaro JA, Tamurian RM, et al. Sparing of radiation-induced damage to the physis: fractionation alone compared

to amifostine pretreatment. *Int J Radiat Oncol Biol Phys* 2000; 47:1067-1071.

22. Damron TA, Spadaro JA, Margulies B, et al. Dose response of amifostine in protection of growth plate function from irradiation effects. *Int J Cancer* 2000;90:73-79.

23. Holm K, Nysom K, Rasmussen MH, et al. Growth, growth hormone and final height after BMT. Possible recovery of irradiation-induced growth hormone insufficiency. *Bone Marrow Transplant* 1996;18:163-170.

24. Hovi L, Saarinen-Pihkala UM, Vettenranta K, et al. Growth in children with poor-risk neuroblastoma after regimens with or without total body irradiation in preparation for autologous bone marrow transplantation. *Bone Marrow Transplant* 1999; 24:1131-1136.

25. Cohen A, Rovelli A, Bakker B, et al. Final height of patients who underwent bone marrow transplantation for hematological disorders during childhood: a study by the Working Party for Late Effects-EBMT. *Blood* 1999;93:4109-4115.

26. Arikoski P, Komulainen J, Voutilainen R, et al. Reduced bone mineral density in long-term survivors of childhood acute lymphoblastic leukemia. *J Pediatr Hematol Oncol* 1998;20:234-240.

27. Fletcher BD, Crom DB, Krance RA, et al. Radiation-induced bone abnormalities after bone marrow transplantation for childhood leukemia. *Radiology* 1994;191:231-235.

28. Barr JD, Barr MS, Lemley TJ, et al. Percutaneous vertebroplasty for pain relief and spinal stabilization. *Spine* 2000;25:923-928.

29. Clement-De Boers A, Oostdijk W, Van Weel-Sipman MH, et al. Final height and hormonal function after bone marrow transplantation in children. *J Pediatr* 1996;129:544-550.

30. Murray RD, Brennan BM, Rahim A, et al. Survivors of childhood cancer: long-term endocrine and metabolic problems dwarf the growth disturbance. *Acta Paediatr Suppl* 1999;88:5-12.

31. Brauner R, Adan L, Souberbielle JC, et al. Contribution of growth hormone deficiency to the growth failure that follows bone marrow transplantation. *J Pediatr* 1997;130:785-792.

32. Locatelli F, Giorgiani G, Pession A, et al. Late effects in children after bone marrow transplantation: a review. *Haematologica* 1993;78:319-328.

33. Dahllof G, Rozell B, Forsberg CM, et al. Histologic changes in dental morphology induced by high dose chemotherapy and total body irradiation. *Oral Surg Oral Med Oral Pathol* 1994; 77:56-60.

34. Dahllof G, Krekmanova L, Kopp S, et al. Craniomandibular dysfunction in children treated with total-body irradiation and bone marrow transplantation. *Acta Odontol Scand* 1994;52:99-105.

35. Dahllof G. Craniofacial growth in children treated for malignant diseases. *Acta Odontol Scand* 1998;56:378-382.

36. Gal TJ, Munoz-Antonia T, Muro-Cacho CA, et al. Radiation effects on osteoblasts in vitro: a potential role in osteoradionecrosis. *Arch Otolaryngol Head Neck Surg* 2000;126:1124-1128.

37. Ashamalla HL, Thom SR, Goldwein JW. Hyperbaric oxygen therapy for the treatment of radiation-induced sequelae in children. The University of Pennsylvania experience. *Cancer* 1996;77: 2407-2412.

38. Wurzler KK, DeWeese TL, Sebald W, et al. Radiation-induced impairment of bone healing can be overcome by recombinant human bone morphogenetic protein-2. *J Craniofac Surg* 1998; 9:131-137.

39. Coquard R. Late effects of ionizing radiations on the bone marrow. *Cancer Radiother* 1997;1:792-800.

40. Ding I, Wu T, Matsubara H, et al. Acidic fibroblast growth factor (FGF1) increases survival and haematopoietic recovery in total body irradiated C3H/HeNCr mice. *Cytokine* 1997;9:59-65.

41. Ding I, Huang K, Wang X, et al. Radioprotection of hematopoietic tissue by fibroblast growth factors in fractionated radiation experiments. *Acta Oncol* 1997;36:337-340.

42. Okunieff P, Mester M, Wang J, et al. In vivo radioprotective effects of angiogenic growth factors on the small bowel of C3H mice. *Radiat Res* 1998;150:204-211.

43. Ding I, Huang K, Snyder ML, et al. Tumor growth and tumor radiosensitivity in mice given myeloprotective doses of fibroblast growth factors. *J Natl Cancer Inst* 1996;88:1399-1404.

44. Okunieff P, Abraham EH, Moini M, et al. Basic fibroblast growth factor radioprotects bone marrow and not RIF1 tumor. *Acta Oncol* 1995;34:435-438.

45. Janssens P, Mitine C, Beauduin M, et al. Is there potential for granulocyte or granulocyte-macrophage colony stimulating factors in radiotherapy? *Eur J Cancer* 1994;30A:642-645.

46. Okunieff P, Wang X, Li M, et al. Chronic radiation bone toxicity is associated with decreased perfusion without elevation of circulating or soft tissue TGF beta or TNF alpha. *Adv Exp Med Biol* 1998;454:325-333.

47. Jowsey J, Coventry MB, Robins PR. Heterotopic ossification: theoretical consideration, possible etiologic factors, and a clinical review of total hip arthroplasty patients exhibiting this phenomenon, in the hip. Presented at the Fifth Open Scientific Meeting of the Hip Society, St. Louis, Mo, 1977.

48. Ritter MA, Vaughan RB. Ectopic ossification after total hip arthroplasty: predisposing factors, frequency, and effect on results. *J Bone Joint Surg Am* 1977;59:345-351.

49. Nollen AJ, Sloof TJ. Para-articular ossification after total hip replacement. *Acta Orthop Scand* 1973;44:230-241.

50. Buring K. On the origin of cells in heterotopic bone formation. *Clin Orthop* 1975;110:293-301.

51. Chalmers J, Grary DH, Rush J. Observations on the induction of bone in soft tissue. *J Bone Joint Surg Br* 1975;57:36-45.

52. Parkinson JR, Evarts CM, Hubbard LF. Radiation therapy in the prevention of heterotopic ossification after total hip arthroplasty, in the hip. Presented at the Tenth Open Scientific Meeting of the Hip Society, St. Louis, Mo, 1982.

53. Garland DW. A clinical perspective on common forms of acquired heterotopic ossification. *Clin Orthop* 1991;263:13-29.

54. Stover SL, Niemann KM, Tulloss JR. Experience with surgical resection of heterotopic bone in spinal cord injury patients. *Clin Orthop* 1991;263:71-77.

55. Fingeroth RJ, Ahmed AQ. Single dose 6 Gy prophylaxis for heterotopic ossification after total hip arthroplasty. *Clin Orthop* 1995;317:131-140.

56. Nollen AJ, van Douveren FQ. Ectopic ossification in hip arthroplasty: a retrospective study of predisposing factors in 637 cases. *Acta Orthop Scand* 1993;64:185-187.

57. McLaren AC. Prophylaxis with indomethacin for heterotopic bone. After open reduction of fractures of the acetabulum. *J Bone Joint Surg Am* 1990;72:245-247.

58. Brooker AF, Bowerman JW, Robinson RA. Ectopic ossification following total hip replacement: incidence and a method of classification. *J Bone Joint Surg Am* 1973;55:1629-1632.

59. DeLee J, Ferrari A, Charnley J. Ectopic bone formation following low friction arthroplasty of the hip. *Clin Orthop* 1976;121:53-59.

60. Kjaergaard-Andersen P, Hougaard K, Linde F. Heterotopic bone formation after total hip arthroplasty in patients with primary or secondary coxarthrosis. *Orthopedics* 1990;13:1211-1217.

61. Ahrengart L, Lindgren U. Functional significance of heterotopic bone formation after total hip arthroplasty. *J Arthroplasty* 1989;4:125-131.

62. Lazansky MG. Complications revisited: the debit side of total hip replacement. *Clin Orthop* 1973;95:96-103.

63. Sodemann B, Persson PE, Nilsson OS. Nonsteroid anti-inflammatory drugs prevent the recurrence of heterotopic ossification after excision. *Arch Orthop Trauma Surg* 1990;109:53-56.

64. Ayers DC, Evarts CM, Parkinson JR. The prevention of heterotopic ossification in high-risk patients by low-dose radiation therapy after total hip arthroplasty. *J Bone Joint Surg Am* 1986;68: 1423-1430.

65. Evans EB, Smith JR. Bone and joint changes following burns: a roentgenographic study. Preliminary report. *J Bone Joint Surg Am* 1959;41:785-799.

66. Bisla RS, Ranawat CS, Inglis AE. Total hip replacement in patients with ankylosing spondylitis with involvement of the hip. *J Bone Joint Surg Am* 1976;58:233-238.

67. Ahrengart L, Lindgren U. Heterotopic bone after hip arthroplasty. Defining the patient at risk. *Clin Orthop* 1993;293:153-159.

68. Han CD, Choi CH, Suh CO. Prevention of heterotopic bone formation after total hip arthroplasty using 600 rad in single dose in high risk patient. *Yonsei Med J* 1997;38:96-100.

69. Coventry MB, Scanlon PW. The use of radiation to discourage ectopic bone: a nine-year study in surgery about the hip. *J Bone Joint Surg Am* 1981;63:201-208.

70. Lo TC, Healy WL, Covall DJ. Heterotopic bone formation after hip surgery: prevention with single-dose postoperative hip irradiation. *Radiology* 1988;168:851-854.

71. Lo TC, Seckel BR, Salzman FA. Single-dose electron beam irradiation in treatment and prevention of keloids and hypertrophic scars. *Radiother Oncol* 1990;19:267-272.

72. Knelles D, Barthel T, Karrer A. Prevention of heterotopic ossification after total hip replacement: a prospective, randomised study using acetylsalicylic acid, indomethacin, and fractional or single-dose irradiation. *J Bone Joint Surg Am* 1997;79:596-602.

73. Elmstedt E, Lindhilm TS, Nilsson OS. Effect of ibuprofen on heterotopic ossification after hip replacement. *Acta Orthop Scand* 1985;56:25-27.

74. Pagnani MJ, Pellicci PM, Salvati EA. Effect of aspirin on heterotopic ossification after total hip arthroplasty in men who have osteoarthritis. *J Bone Joint Surg Am* 1991;73:924-929.

75. Ritter MA, Gioe TJ. The effect of indomethacin on paraarticular ectopic ossification following total hip arthroplasty. *Clin Orthop* 1982;167:113-117.

76. Spry NA, Dally MJ, Benjamin B, et al. Heterotopic bone formation affecting the hip joint is preventable in high risk patients by post-operative radiation. *Australas Radiol* 1995;39:379-383.

77. Moore KD, Goss K, Anglen JO. Indomethacin versus radiation therapy for prophylaxis against heterotopic ossification in acetabular fractures: a randomised, prospective study. *J Bone Joint Surg Br* 1998;80:259-263.

78. Lewallen DG. Heterotopic ossification following total hip arthroplasty. *Instr Course Lect* 1995;44:287-292.

79. Healy WL, Lo TC, DeSimone AA, et al. Single-dose irradiation for the prevention of heterotopic ossification after total hip arthroplasty. A comparison of doses of five hundred and fifty and seven hundred centigray. *J Bone Joint Surg Am* 1995;77:590-595.

80. Heyd R, Strassmann G, Kirchner J, et al. Postoperative radiotherapy in the prevention of heterotopic ossification after endoprosthetic hip joint replacement. *Strahlenther Onkol* 1996;172:543-552.

81. Lo TC. Radiation therapy for heterotopic ossification. *Semin Radiat Oncol* 1999;9:163-170.

82. Kjaersgaard-Andersen P, Ritter MA. Prevention of formation of heterotopic bone after total hip arthroplasty. *J Bone Joint Surg Am* 1991;73:942-947.

83. Cella JP, Salvati EA, Sculco TP. Indomethacin for the prevention of heterotopic ossification following total hip arthroplasty: effectiveness, contraindications, and adverse effects. *J Arthroplasty* 1988;3:229-234.

84. Trancik T, Mills W, Vinson N. The effect of indomethacin, aspirin, and ibuprofen on bone ingrowth into a porous-coated implant. *Clin Orthop* 1989;249:113-121.

85. Maloney WJ, Krushell RJ, Jasty M. Incidence of heterotopic ossification after total hip replacement: effect of the type of fixation of the femoral component. *J Bone Joint Surg Am* 1991;73:191-193.

86. Brunner R, Morscher E, Hunig R. Para-articular ossification in total hip replacement: an indication for irradiation therapy. *Arch Orthop Trauma Surg* 1987;106:102-107.

87. MacLennan I, Keys HM, Evarts CM. Usefulness of postoperative hip irradiation in the prevention of heterotopic bone formation in a high risk group of patients. *Int J Radiat Oncol Biol Phys* 1984;10:49-53.

88. Kennedy WF, Gruen TA, Chessin H. Radiation therapy to prevent heterotopic ossification after cementless total hip arthroplasty. *Clin Orthop* 1991;262:185-191.

89. Seegenschmiedt MH, Keilholz L, Martus P, et al. Prevention of heterotopic ossification about the hip: final results of two randomized trials in 410 patients using either preoperative or postoperative radiation therapy. *Int J Radiat Oncol Biol Phys* 1997;39:161-171.

90. Evarts CM, Ayers DC, Puzas JE. Prevention of heterotopic bone formation in high-risk patients by postoperative irradiation, in the hip. Presented at the Fourteenth Open Scientific Meeting of the Hip Society, St. Louis, Mo, 1987.

91. Healy WL, Lo TC, Covall DJ. Single-dose radiation therapy for prevention of heterotopic ossification after total hip arthroplasty. *J Arthroplasty* 1990;5:369-375.

92. Childs HA III, Cole T, Falkenberg E, et al. A prospective evaluation of the timing of postoperative radiotherapy for preventing heterotopic ossification following traumatic acetabular fractures. *Int J Radiat Oncol Biol Phys* 2000;47:1347-1352.

93. Arnold M, Stas P, Kummermehr J, et al. Radiation-induced impairment of bone healing in the rat femur: effects of radiation dose, sequence and interval between surgery and irradiation. *Radiother Oncol* 1998;48:259-265.

94. Pellegrini VDJ, Gregoritch SJ. Preoperative irradiation for prevention of heterotopic ossification following total hip arthroplasty. *J Bone Joint Surg Am* 1996;78:870-881.

95. Craven PL, Urist MR. Osteogenesis by radioisotope labelled cell populations in implants of bone matrix under the influence of ionizing radiation. *Clin Orthop* 1971;76:231-233.

96. van Leeuwen WM, Deckers P, de Lange WJ. Preoperative irradiation for prophylaxis of ectopic ossification after hip arthroplasty. a randomized study in 62 hips. *Acta Orthop Scand* 1998;69:116-118.

97. Blount LH, Thomas BJ, Tran L. Postoperative irradiation for the prevention of heterotopic bone: analysis of different dose schedules and shielding considerations. *Int J Radiat Oncol Biol Phys* 1990;19:809-811.

98. Wong FL, Boice JD Jr, Abramson DH, et al. Cancer incidence after retinoblastoma. Radiation dose and sarcoma risk. *JAMA* 1997;278:1262-1267.

99. Tucker MA, D'Angio GJ, Boice JD. Bone sarcomas linked to radiotherapy and chemotherapy in children. *N Engl J Med* 1987;317:588-593.

100. Doll R, Wakeford R. Risk of childhood cancer from fetal irradiation. *Br J Radiol* 1997;70:130-139.

101. Carnes BA, Groer PG, Kotek TJ. Radium dial workers: issues concerning dose response and modeling. *Radiat Res* 1997;147:707-714.

102. Gossner W. Pathology of radium-induced bone tumors: new aspects of histopathology and histogenesis. *Radiat Res* 1999;152:S12-15.

103. Kuttesch JF Jr, Wexler LH, Marcus RB, et al. Second malignancies after Ewing's sarcoma: radiation dose-dependency of secondary sarcomas. *J Clin Oncol* 1996;14:2818-2825.

104. Le Vu B, de Vathaire F, Shamsaldin A, et al. Radiation dose, chemotherapy and risk of osteosarcoma after solid tumours during childhood. *Int J Cancer* 1998;77:370-377.

105. Nekolla EA, Kreisheimer M, Kellerer AM, et al. Induction of malignant bone tumors in radium-224 patients: risk estimates based on the improved dosimetry [published erratum in *Radiat Res* 2000;153:848]. *Radiat Res* 2000;153:93-103.

106. Fry SA. Studies of U.S. radium dial workers: an epidemiological classic. *Radiat Res* 1998;150:S21-S29.

107. Greenberger JS, Anderson J, Berry LA, et al. Effects of irradiation of CBA/CA mice on hematopoietic stem cells and stromal cells in long-term bone marrow cultures. *Leukemia* 1996;10:514-527.

108. Niethammer D, Mayer E. Long-term survivors: an overview on late effects, sequelae and second neoplasias. *Bone Marrow Transplant* 1998;21:S61-63.

109. Broerse JJ, Bartstra RW, van Bekkum DW, et al. The carcinogenic risk of high dose total body irradiation in non-human primates. *Radiother Oncol* 2000;54:247-253.

110. Kirova YM, Rafi H, Voisin MC, et al. Radiation-induced bone sarcoma following total body irradiation: role of additional radiation on localized areas. *Bone Marrow Transplant* 2000; 25:1011-1013.

111. Kleinerman RA, Littlefield LG, Tarone RE, et al. Chromosome aberrations in lymphocytes from women irradiated for benign and malignant gynecological disease. *Radiat Res* 1994;139:40-46.

112. Kleinerman RA, Boice JD Jr, Storm HH, et al. Second primary cancer after treatment for cervical cancer. An international cancer registries study. *Cancer* 1995;76:442-452.

113. Curtis RE, Boice JD Jr, Stovall M, et al. Relationship of leukemia risk to radiation dose following cancer of the uterine corpus. *J Natl Cancer Inst* 1994;86:1315-1324.

114. Gershkevitsh E, Rosenberg I, Dearnaley DP, et al. Bone marrow doses and leukaemia risk in radiotherapy of prostate cancer. *Radiother Oncol* 1999;53:189-197.

115. de Vathaire F, Schlumberger M, Delisle MJ, et al. Leukaemias and cancers following iodine-131 administration for thyroid cancer. *Br J Cancer* 1997;75:734-739.

116. Kossman SE, Weiss MA. Acute myelogenous leukemia after exposure to strontium-89 for the treatment of adenocarcinoma of the prostate. *Cancer* 2000;88:620-624.

117. Priolo F, Cerase A. The current role of radiography in the assessment of skeletal tumors and tumor-like lesions. *Eur J Radiol* 1998;27(suppl 1):S77-85.

118. Pomeranz SJ, Pretorius HT, Ramsingh PS. Bone scintigraphy and multimodality imaging in bone neoplasia: strategies for imaging in the new health care climate. *Semin Nucl Med* 1994; 24:188-207.

119. Jackson A, Scarffe JH. Upper humeral cortical thickness as an indicator of osteopenia: diagnostic significance in solitary myeloma of bone. *Skeletal Radiol* 1991;20:363-367.

120. Mitchell MJ, Logan PM. Radiation-induced changes in bone. *Radiographics* 1998;18:1125-1136.

121. Panicek DM, Gatsonis C, Rosenthal DI, et al. CT and MR imaging in the local staging of primary malignant musculoskeletal neoplasms: report of the Radiology Diagnostic Oncology Group. *Radiology* 1997;202:237-246.

122. Balzarini L, Sicilia A, Ceglia E, et al. Magnetic resonance in primary bone tumors: a review of 10 years of activities. *Radiol Med (Torino)* 1996;91:344-347.

123. Thomann KH, Dul MW. Bone scintigraphy: a review of the procedure and its applications. *Optom Vis Sci* 1994;71:502-507.

124. Donohoe KJ. Selected topics in orthopedic nuclear medicine. *Orthop Clin North Am* 1998;29:85-101.

125. Lin WY, Kao CH, Hsu CY, et al. The role of Tc-99m MDP and Ga-67 imaging in the clinical evaluation of malignant fibrous histiocytoma. *Clin Nucl Med* 1994;19:996-1000.

126. Focacci C, Lattanzi R, Iadeluca ML, et al. Nuclear medicine in primary bone tumors. *Eur J Radiol* 1998;27(suppl 1):S123-131.

127. Hernandez JA, Land KJ, McKenna RW. Leukemias, myeloma, and other lymphoreticular neoplasms. *Cancer* 1995;75:381-394.

128. Unni KK. *Dahlin's Bone Tumors: General Aspects and Data on 11,087 Cases.* 5th ed. New York, NY: Lippincott-Raven; 1996:463.

129. Holland J, Trenkner DA, Wasserman TH, et al. Plasmacytoma. Treatment results and conversion to myeloma. *Cancer* 1992; 69:1513-1517.

130. Bolek TW, Marcus RB, Mendenhall NP. Solitary plasmacytoma of bone and soft tissue. *Int J Radiat Oncol Biol Phys* 1996;36: 329-333.

131. Frassica DA, Frassica FJ, Schray MF, et al. Solitary plasmacytoma of bone: Mayo Clinic experience. *Int J Radiat Oncol Biol Phys* 1989;16:43-48.

132. Lewanski CR, Bates T, Bowen J, et al. Solitary bone plasmacytoma: management of isolated local relapse following radiotherapy. *Clin Oncol* 1999;11:348-351.

133. Mill WB, Griffith R. The role of radiation therapy in the management of plasma cell tumors. *Cancer* 1980;45:647-652.

134. Bullough PG. Cartilage-forming tumors and tumor-like conditions. In: *Bullough and Vigorita's Orthopaedic Pathology.* 3rd ed. London: Mosby-Wolfe; 1997:357-365.

135. Chang MY, Shih LY, Dunn P, et al. Solitary plasmacytoma of bone. *J Formos Med Assoc* 1994;93:397-402.

136. Dimopoulos MA, Goldstein J, Fuller L, et al. Curability of solitary bone plasmacytoma. *J Clin Oncol* 1992;10:587-590.

137. Greenberg P, Parker RG, Fu YS, et al. The treatment of solitary plasmacytoma of bone and extramedullary plasmacytoma. *Am J Clin Oncol* 1987;10:199-204.

138. Liebross RH, Ha CS, Cox JD, et al. Solitary bone plasmacytoma: outcome and prognostic factors following radiotherapy. *Int J Radiat Oncol Biol Phys* 1998;41:1063-1067.

139. Aviles A, Huerta-Guzman J, Delgado S, et al. Improved outcome in solitary bone plasmacytomata with combined therapy. *Hematol Oncol* 1996;14:111-117.

140. Mayr NA, Wen BC, Hussey DH, et al. The role of radiation therapy in the treatment of solitary plasmacytomas. *Radiother Oncol* 1990; 17:293-303.

141. Lichtenstein L, Jaffe HL. Chondrosarcomas of bone. *Am J Pathol* 1943;19:553-589.

142. Marcove RC, Mike V, Hutter RV, et al. Chondrosarcoma of the pelvis and upper end of the femur. An analysis of factors influencing survival time in one hundred and thirteen cases. *J Bone Joint Surg* 1972;54:561-572.

143. Aprin H, Riseborough EJ, Hall JE. Chondrosarcoma in children and adolescents. *Clin Orthop* 1982;166:226-232.

144. Young CL, Sim FH, Unni KK, et al. Case report 559. Chondrosarcoma of the proximal humeral epiphysis. *Skeletal Radiol* 1989;18:403-405.

145. Young CL, Sim FH, Unni KK, et al. Chondrosarcoma of bone in children. *Cancer* 1990;66:1641-1648.

146. Mirra JM, Gold R, Downs J, et al. A new histological approach to the differentiation of enchondroma from chondrosarcoma of bones: a clinicopathologic analysis of 51 cases. *Clin Orthop* 1985;201:214-237.

147. Bjornsson J, McLeod RA, Unni KK, et al. Primary chondrosarcoma of long bones and limb girdles. *Cancer* 1998;83:2105-2119.

148. Pritchard DJ, Lunke RJ, Taylor WF, et al. Chondrosarcoma: a clinicopathologic and statistical analysis. *Cancer* 1980;45: 149-157.

149. Dahlin DC, Beabout JW. Dedifferentiation of low-grade chondrosarcomas. *Cancer* 1971;28:461-466.

150. Gitelis S, Bertoni F, Picci P, et al. Chondrosarcoma of bone. The experience at the Istituto Ortopedico Rizzoli. *J Bone Joint Surg Am* 1981;63:1248-1257.

151. Lee FY, Mankin HJ, Fondren G, et al. Chondrosarcoma of bone: an assessment of outcome. *J Bone Joint Surg Am* 1999;81: 326-338.

152. Simon MA, Springfield D, eds. *Surgery for Bone and Soft-Tissue Sarcomas.* Vol. 1. New York, NY: Lippincott Williams & Wilkins; 1998:756.

153. Bauer HC, Brosjo O, Kreicbergs A, et al. Low risk of recurrence of enchondroma and low-grade chondrosarcoma in extremities. 80 patients followed for 2-25 years. *Acta Orthop Scand* 1995;66: 283-288.

154. Marcove RC, Stovell PB, Huvos AG, et al. The use of cryosurgery in the treatment of low and medium grade chondrosarcoma. A preliminary report. *Clin Orthop* 1977;122:147-156.

155. Schreuder HW, Pruszczynski M, Veth RP, et al. Treatment of benign and low-grade malignant intramedullary chondroid tumours with curettage and cryosurgery. *Eur J Surg Oncol* 1998;24:120-126.

156. Debus J, Haberer T, Schulz-Ertner D, et al. Carbon ion irradiation of skull base tumors at GSI. First clinical results and future perspectives. *Strahlenther Onkol* 2000;176:211-216.

157. Gripp S, Pape H, Schmitt G. Chondrosarcoma of the larynx: the role of radiotherapy revisited—a case report and review of the literature. *Cancer* 1998;82:108-115.

158. Hug EB, Loredo LN, Slater JD, et al. Proton radiation therapy for chordomas and chondrosarcomas of the skull base. *J Neurosurg* 1999;91:432-439.

159. Muthukumar N, Kondziolka D, Lunsford LD, et al. Stereotactic radiosurgery for chordoma and chondrosarcoma: further experiences. *Int J Radiat Oncol Biol Phys* 1998;41:387-392.

160. Rosenberg AE, Nielsen GP, Keel SB, et al. Chondrosarcoma of the base of the skull: a clinicopathologic study of 200 cases with emphasis on its distinction from chordoma. *Am J Surg Pathol* 1999;23:1370-1378.

161. Munzenrider JE, Liebsch NJ. Proton therapy for tumors of the skull base. *Strahlenther Onkol* 1999;175:57-63.

162. Oberling C. Les reticulosarcomes at les reticuloendotheliosarcomes de la moelle osseuse sarcomes d'Ewing. *Bull Assoc Fr Etude Cancer (Paris)* 1928;17:259-296.

163. Parker JW, Jackson H. Primary reticulum cell sarcoma of bone. *Surg Gynecol Obstet* 1939;68:45-53.

164. Freeman C, Berg JW, Cutler SJ. Occurrence and prognosis of extranodal lymphomas. *Cancer* 1972;29:252-260.

165. Rudders RA, Ross ME, DeLellis RA. Primary extranodal lymphoma: response to treatment and factors influencing prognosis. *Cancer* 1978;42:406-416.

166. Boston HC, Dahlin DC, Ivins JC, et al. Malignant lymphoma (so-called reticulum cell sarcoma) of bone. *Cancer* 1974;34:1131-1137.

167. Pettit CK, Zukerberg LR, Gray MH, et al. Primary lymphoma of bone. *Am J Surg Pathol* 1990;14:329-334.

168. Ferreri AJ, Reni M, Ceresoli GL, et al. Therapeutic management with adriamycin-containing chemotherapy and radiotherapy of monostotic and polyostotic primary non-Hodgkin's lymphoma of bone in adults. *Cancer Invest* 1998;16:554-561.

169. Shoji H, Miller TR. Primary reticulum cell sarcoma of bone. Significance of clinical features upon the prognosis. *Cancer* 1971;28:1234-1244.

170. Baar J, Burkes RL, Bell R, et al. Primary non-Hodgkin's lymphoma of bone. *Cancer* 1994;73:1194-1199.

171. Chin HW, McGuire MH, Block M, et al. Primary lymphoma of bone. *Nebr Med J* 1990;75:303-306.

172. Dubey P, Ha CS, Besa PC, et al. Localized primary malignant lymphoma of bone. *Int J Radiat Oncol Biol Phys* 1997;37:1087-1093.

173. Nishiyama N, Nakatani S, Inoue K, et al. Primary lymphoma of bone originating in a rib. *Jpn J Thorac Cardiovasc Surg* 2000;48:180-183.

174. Heyning FH, Hogendoorn PC, Kramer MH, et al. Primary non-Hodgkin's lymphoma of bone: a clinicopathological investigation of 60 cases. *Leukemia* 1999;13:2094-2098.

175. Phillips WC, Kattapuram SV, Doseretz DE, et al. Primary lymphoma of bone: relationship of radiographic appearance and prognosis. *Radiology* 1982;144:285-290.

176. Jones D, Kraus MD, Dorfman DM. Lymphoma presenting as a solitary bone lesion. *Am J Clin Pathol* 1999;111:171-178.

177. Suryanarayan K, Shuster JJ, Donaldson SS, et al. Treatment of localized primary non-Hodgkin's lymphoma of bone in children: a Pediatric Oncology Group study. *J Clin Oncol* 1999;17:456-459.

178. Wang CC, Fleischli DJ. Primary reticulum cell sarcoma of bone. With emphasis on radiation therapy. *Cancer* 1968;22:994-998.

179. Wang CC. Treatment of primary reticulum-cell sarcoma of bone by irradiation. *N Engl J Med* 1968;278:1331-1332.

180. Bacci G, Picci P, Bertoni F, et al. Primary non-Hodgkin's lymphoma of bone: results in 15 patients treated by radiotherapy combined with systemic chemotherapy. *Cancer Treat Rep* 1982;66:1859-1862.

181. Link MP, Shuster JJ, Donaldson SS, et al. Treatment of children and young adults with early-stage non-Hodgkin's lymphoma. *N Engl J Med* 1997;337:1259-1266.

182. Loeffler JS, Tarbell NJ, Kozakewich H, et al. Primary lymphoma of bone in children: analysis of treatment results with adriamycin, prednisone, Oncovin (APO), and local radiation therapy. *J Clin Oncol* 1986;4:496-501.

183. Meyer JE, Lepke RA, Lindfors KK, et al. Chordomas: their CT appearance in the cervical, thoracic and lumbar spine. *Radiology* 1984;153:693-696.

184. Hudson TM, Galceran M. Radiology of sacrococcygeal chordoma. Difficulties in detecting soft tissue extension. *Clin Orthop* 1983;175:237-242.

185. Rosenthal DI, Scott JA, Mankin HJ, et al. Sacrococcygeal chordoma: magnetic resonance imaging and computed tomography. *AJR Am J Roentgenol* 1985;145:143-147.

186. Bjornsson J, Wold LE, Ebersold MJ, et al. Chordoma of the mobile spine. A clinicopathologic analysis of 40 patients. *Cancer* 1993;71:735-740.

187. Cheng EY, Ozerdemoglu RA, Transfeldt EE, et al. Lumbosacral chordoma. Prognostic factors and treatment. *Spine* 1999;24:1639-1645.

188. Mitchell A, Scheithauer BW, Unni KK, et al. Chordoma and chondroid neoplasms of the spheno-occiput. An immunohistochemical study of 41 cases with prognostic and nosologic implications. *Cancer* 1993;72:2943-2949.

189. Kaiser TE, Pritchard DJ, Unni KK. Clinicopathologic study of sacrococcygeal chordoma. *Cancer* 1984;53:2574-2578.

190. al-Mefty O, Borba LA. Skull base chordomas: a management challenge. *J Neurosurg* 1997;86:182-189.

191. Catton C, O'Sullivan B, Bell R, et al. Chordoma: long-term follow-up after radical photon irradiation. *Radiother Oncol* 1996;41:67-72.

192. Slater JM, Slater JD, Archambeau JO. Proton therapy for cranial base tumors. *J Craniofac Surg* 1995;6:24-26.

193. Borba LA, Al-Mefty O, Mrak RE, et al. Cranial chordomas in children and adolescents. *J Neurosurg* 1996;84:584-591.

194. Logroscino CA, Astolfi S, Sacchettoni G. Chordoma: long-term evaluation of 15 cases treated surgically. *Chir Organi Mov* 1998;83:87-103.

195. Schoenthaler R, Castro JR, Petti PL, et al. Charged particle irradiation of sacral chordomas. *Int J Radiat Oncol Biol Phys* 1993;26:291-298.

196. Habrand JL, Mammar H, Ferrand R, et al. Proton beam therapy (PT) in the management of CNS tumors in childhood. *Strahlenther Onkol* 1999;175:91-94.

197. Romero J, Cardenes H, la Torre A, et al. Chordoma: results of radiation therapy in eighteen patients. *Radiother Oncol* 1993;29:27-32.

198. Klekamp J, Samii M. Spinal chordomas—results of treatment over a 17-year period. *Acta Neurochir (Wien)* 1996;138:514-519.

199. Nishida J, Sim FH, Wenger DE, et al. Malignant fibrous histiocytoma of bone. A clinicopathologic study of 81 patients. *Cancer* 1997;79:482-493.

200. Dahlin DC, Unni KK, Matsuno T. Malignant (fibrous) histiocytoma of bone—fact or fancy? *Cancer* 1977;39:1508-1516.

201. Capanna R, Bertoni F, Bacchini P. Fibrous histiocytoma of bone. *Cancer* 1984;76:177-187.

202. Huvos AG, Heilweil M, Bretsky SS. The pathology of malignant fibrous histiocytoma of bone: a study of 130 patients. *Am J Surg Pathol* 1985;9:853-871.

203. Dahlin DC, Unni KK. *Bone Tumors: General Aspects and Data on 8,542 Cases.* 4th ed. Springfield, Mass: Charles C. Thomas; 1986:357-365.

204. Weiss SW, Enzinger FM. Malignant fibrous histiocytoma, an analysis of 200 cases. *Cancer* 1978;41:2250-2266.

205. Bacci G, Avella M, Picci P. Primary chemotherapy and delayed surgery for malignant fibrous histiocytoma of bone in the extremity. *Tumors* 1990;76:537-542.

206. Wold LE, Unni KK, Beabout JW, et al. Hemangioendothelial sarcoma of bone. *Am J Surg Pathol* 1982;6:59-70.

207. Campanacci M, Boriani S, Giunti A. Hemangioendothelioma of bone. *Cancer* 1980;46:804-814.

208. Dorfman HD, Steiner GC, Jaffe HL. Vascular tumors of bone. *Hum Pathol* 1971;2:349-376.

209. Tillman RM, Choong PF, Beabout JW, et al. Epithelioid hemangioendothelioma of bone. *Orthopedics* 1997;20:177-180.

210. Larsson SE, Lorentzon R, Boquist L. Malignant hemangioendothelioma of bone. *J Bone Joint Surg* 1975;57A:84-89.

211. Glenn JN, Reckling FW, Mantz FA. Malignant hemangioendothelioma in a lumbar vertebra: a rare tumor in an unusual location. *J Bone Joint Surg* 1974;56A:1279-1282.

212. Garcia-Moral CA. Malignant hemangioendothelioma of bone. Review of world literature and report of two cases. *Clin Orthop* 1972;82:70-79.

213. Welles L, Dorfman H, Valentine ES, et al. Low grade malignant hemangioendothelioma of bone: a disease potentially curable with radiotherapy. *Med Pediatr Oncol* 1994;23:144-148.

214. Faria SL, Schlupp WR, Chiminazzo H. Radiotherapy in the treatment of vertebral hemangiomas. *Int J Radiat Oncol Biol Phys* 1985;11:387-390.

215. Frassica FJ, Sanjay BK, Unni KK, et al. Benign giant cell tumor. *Orthopedics* 1993;16:1179-1183.

216. Schajowicz F, Granato DB, McDonald DJ, et al. Clinical and radiographic features of atypical giant cell tumors of bone. *Br J Radiol* 1991;64:877-889.

217. Kransdorf MJ, Sweet DE, Buetow PC, et al. Giant cell tumor in skeletally immature patients. *Radiology* 1992;184:233-237.

218. Picci P, Manfrini M, Zucchi V, et al. Giant cell tumor of bone in skeletally immature patients. *J Bone Joint Surg* 1983;65:486-490.

219. Bogumill GB, Schultz MA, Johnson LC. Giant cell tumor: a metaphyseal lesion. *J Bone Joint Surg* 1972;54:1558.

220. Campanacci M, Giunti A, Olmi R. Metaphyseal and diaphyseal localization of giant cell tumors. *Chir Organi Mov* 1975;62:29-34.

221. Fain JS, Unni KK, Beabout JW, et al. Nonepiphyseal giant cell tumor of the long bones. Clinical, radiologic, and pathologic study. *Cancer* 1993;71:3514-3519.

222. Peison B, Feigenbaum J. Metaphyseal giant cell tumor in a girl of 14. *Radiology* 1976;118:145-146.

223. Sherman M, Fabricus R. Giant cell tumors in metaphysis of a child. *J Bone Joint Surg Am* 1961;43:1225-1229.

224. Wilkerson JA, Cracchiolo A. Giant cell tumor of the tibial diaphysis. *J Bone Joint Surg Am* 1969;51:1205-1209.

225. Hudson TM, Schiebler M, Springfield DS, et al. Radiology of giant cell tumors of bone: computed tomography, arthro-tomography, and scintigraphy. *Skeletal Radiol* 1984;11:85-95.

226. McDonald DJ, Sim FH, McLeod RA, et al. Giant cell tumor of bone. *J Bone Joint Surg Am* 1986;68:235-242.

227. Enneking WF. *Musculoskeletal Tumor Surgery.* Vol. 1. New York, NY: Churchill Livingstone, 1983.

228. Bertoni F, Present D, Sudanese A, et al. Giant cell tumor of bone with pulmonary metastases. Six case reports and a review of the literature. *Clin Orthop* 1988;237:275-285.

229. Maloney WJ, Vaughan LM, Jones HH, et al. Benign metastasizing giant cell tumor of bone. Report of three cases and review of the literature. *Clin Orthop* 1989;243:208-215.

230. Szyfelbein WM, Schiller AL. Cytologic diagnosis of giant cell tumor of bone metastatic to lung. A case report. *Acta Cytol* 1979;23:460-464.

231. Connell D, Munk PL, Lee MJ, et al. Giant cell tumor of bone with selective metastases to mediastinal lymph nodes. *Skeletal Radiol* 1998;27:341-345.

232. Tubbs WS, Brown LR, Beabout JW, et al. Benign giant cell tumor of bone with pulmonary metastases: clinical findings and radiologic appearance of metastases in 13 cases. *AJR Am J Roentgenol* 1992;158:331-334.

233. Mirra JM, Ulich T, Magidson J, et al. A case of probable benign pulmonary "metastases" or implants arising from a giant cell tumor of bone. *Clin Orthop* 1982;46:245-254.

234. Nojima T, Takeda N, Matsuno T, et al. Case report 869. Benign metastasizing giant cell tumor of bone. *Skeletal Radiol* 1994;23:583-585.

235. Rock MG, Pritchard DJ, Unni KK. Metastases from histologically benign giant cell tumor of bone. *J Bone Joint Surg Am* 1984;66:269-274.

236. Cheng JC, Johnston JO. Giant cell tumor of bone. Prognosis and treatment of pulmonary metastases. *Clin Orthop* 1997;338:205-214.

237. Kay RM, Eckardt JJ, Seeger LL, et al. Pulmonary metastasis of benign giant cell tumor of bone. Six histologically confirmed cases, including one of spontaneous regression. *Clin Orthop* 1994;302:219-230.

238. Gitelis S, Wang JW, Quast M, et al. Recurrence of a giant cell tumor with malignant transformation to a fibrosarcoma twenty-five years after primary treatment. A case report. *J Bone Joint Surg Am* 1989;71:757-761.

239. Mori Y, Tsuchiya H, Karita M, et al. Malignant transformation of a giant cell tumor 25 years after initial treatment. *Clin Orthop* 2000;381:185-191.

240. Nascimento AG, Huvos AG, Marcove RC. Primary malignant giant cell tumor of bone: a study of eight cases and review of the literature. *Cancer* 1979;44:1393-1402.

241. Rock MG, Sim FH, Unni KK, et al. Secondary malignant giant cell tumor of bone. Clinicopathological assessment of nineteen patients. *J Bone Joint Surg Am* 1986;68:1073-1079.

242. Dahlin DC, Cupps RE, Johnson EW. Giant cell tumor: a study of 195 cases. *Cancer* 1970;25:1061-1070.

243. Goldenberg RR, Campbell CJ, Bonfiglio M. Giant cell tumor of bone. An analysis of two hundred and eighteen cases. *J Bone Joint Surg Am* 1970;52:619-664.

244. Kreicbergs A, Lonnqvist PA, Nilsson B. Curettage of benign lesions of bone. Factors related to recurrence. *Int Orthop* 1985;8:287-293.

245. Blackley HR, Wunder JS, Davis AM, et al. Treatment of giant cell tumors of long bones with curettage and bone-grafting. *J Bone Joint Surg Am* 1999;81:811-820.

246. Leeson MC, Lippitt SB. Thermal aspects of the use of polymethylmethacrylate in large metaphyseal defects in bone. A clinical review and laboratory study. *Clin Orthop* 1993;295:239-245.

247. Gitelis S, Mallin BA, Piasecki P, et al. Intralesional excision compared with en bloc resection for giant cell tumors of bone. *J Bone Joint Surg Am* 1993;75:1648-1655.

248. Malawer MM, Bickels J, Meller I, et al. Cryosurgery in the treatment of giant cell tumor. A long-term followup study. *Clin Orthop* 1999;359:176-188.

249. Marcove RC, Sheth DS, Brien EW, et al. Conservative surgery for giant cell tumors of the sacrum. The role of cryosurgery as a supplement to curettage and partial excision. *Cancer* 1994;74:1253-1260.

250. O'Donnell RJ, Springfield DS, Motwani HK, et al. Recurrence of giant cell tumors of the long bones after curettage and packing with cement. *J Bone Joint Surg Am* 1994;76:1827-1833.

251. Persson BM, Wouters HW. Curettage and acrylic cementation in surgery of giant cell tumors of bone. *Clin Orthop* 1976; 120:125-133.

252. Pogrel MA. The management of lesions of the jaws with liquid nitrogen cryotherapy. *J Calif Dent Assoc* 1995;23:54-57.

253. Bennett CJ Jr, Marcus RB Jr, Million RR, et al. Radiation therapy for giant cell tumor of bone. *Int J Radiat Oncol Biol Phys* 1993;26:299-304.

254. Chakravarti A, Spiro IJ, Hug EB, et al. Megavoltage radiation therapy for axial and inoperable giant cell tumor of bone. *J Bone Joint Surg Am* 1999;81:1566-1573.

255. Malone S, O'Sullivan B, Catton C, et al. Long-term follow-up of efficacy and safety of megavoltage radiotherapy in high-risk giant cell tumors of bone. *Int J Radiat Oncol Biol Phys* 1995;33:689-694.

256. Seider MJ, Rich TA, Ayala AG, et al. Giant cell tumors of bone: treatment with radiation therapy. *Radiology* 1986;161:537-540.

257. Suit H, Spiro I. Radiation treatment of benign mesenchymal disease. *Semin Radiat Oncol* 1999;9:171-178.

258. Schwartz LH, Okunieff PG, Rosenberg A. Radiation therapy in the treatment of difficult giant cell tumors. *Int J Radiat Oncol Biol Phys* 1989;17:1085-1088.

259. Nair MK, Jyothirmayi R. Radiation therapy in the treatment of giant cell tumor of bone. *Int J Radiat Oncol Biol Phys* 1999; 43:1065-1069.

260. Stull MA, Kransdorf MJ, Devaney KO. Langerhans cell histiocytosis of bone. *Radiographics* 1992;12:801-823.

261. Schajowicz F, Slullitel J. Eosinophilic granuloma of bone and its relationship to Hand-Schuller-Christian and Letterer-Siwe syndromes. *J Bone Joint Surg* 1973;55:545-565.

262. Siddqui AR, Tashjian JH, Lazarus K. Nuclear medicine studies and evaluation of skeletal lesions in children with histiocytosis X. *Radiology* 1981;140:287-289.

263. Hartman KS. A review of 114 cases with oral involvement. *Oral Surg Oral Med Oral Pathol Oral Radiol Endod* 1980;49:38-54.

264. Egeler RM, Thompson RCJ, Voute PA, et al. Intralesional infiltration of corticosteroids in localized Langerhans cell histiocytosis. *J Pediatr Orthop* 1992;12:811-814.

265. Cline MJ. The histiocytic malignancies. In: Haskell CM, ed. *Cancer Treatment.* 2nd ed. Philadelphia, Pa: Saunders; 1987: 843-850.

266. Raney RB Jr. Chemotherapy for children with aggressive fibromatosis and Langerhans' cell histiocytosis. *Clin Orthop* 1991; 262:58-63.

267. Ishii E, Matsuzaki A, Okamura J, et al. Treatment of Langerhans cell histiocytosis in children with etoposide. *Am J Clin Oncol* 1992;15:515-517.

268. Anonsen CK, Donaldson SS. Langerhans' cell histiocytosis of the head and neck. *Laryngoscope* 1987;97:537-542.

269. Pereslegin IA, Ustinova VF, Podlyaschuk EL. Radiotherapy for eosinophilic granuloma of bone. *Int J Radiat Oncol Biol Phys* 1981;7:317-321.

270. Selch MT, Parker RG. Radiation therapy in the management of Langerhan's cell histiocytosis. *Med Pediatr Oncol* 1990;18:97-102.

271. Greenberger JS, Cassady JR, Jaffe N. Radiation therapy in patients with histiocytosis: management of diabetes insipidus and bone lesions. *Int J Rad Oncol Biol Phys* 1979;5:1749-1755.

272. Montebello JF, Hartson-Eaton M. The palliation of osseous metastasis with ^{32}P or ^{89}Sr compared with external beam and hemibody irradiation: a historical perspective. *Cancer Invest* 1989;7:139-160.

273. Garrett IR. Bone destruction in cancer. *Semin Oncol* 1993;20:4-9.

274. Hoegler D. Radiotherapy for palliation of symptoms in incurable cancer. *Curr Probl Cancer* 1997;21:129-183.

275. Holler U, Petersein A, Golder W, et al. Radiation-induced osteonecrosis of the pelvic bones vs. bone metastases—a difficult differential diagnosis. *Aktuelle Radiol* 1998;8:196-197.

276. Martinez Caballero A, Moreno Yubero A, Caballero Carpena O, et al. Bone metastasis versus insufficiency fractures due to pelvic radiotherapy for gynecologic neoplasm. *Rev Esp Med Nucl* 1999; 18:292-297.

277. Tong D, Gillick L, Hendrickson FR. The palliation of symptomatic osseous metastases: final results of the RTOG. *Cancer* 1982;50:893-899.

278. Blitzer PH. Reanalysis of the RTOG study of palliation of symptomatic osseous metastasis. *Cancer* 1985;55:1468-1472.

279. Ohmori K, Matsui H, Yasuda T, et al. Evaluation of the prognosis of cancer patients with metastatic bone tumors based on serial bone scintigrams. *Jpn J Clin Oncol* 1997;27:263-267.

280. Yoden E, Murakami M, Kuroda Y, et al. Clinical results and prognostic factors of radiotherapy for bone metastases from breast cancer. *Nippon Igaku Hoshasen Gakkai Zasshi* 1999;59:27-33.

281. Janjan NA. Radiation for bone metastases: conventional techniques and the role of systemic radiopharmaceuticals. *Cancer* 1997;80:1628-1645.

282. Mercadante S. Malignant bone pain: pathophysiology and treatment. *Pain* 1997;69:1-18.

283. Uppelschoten JM, Wanders SL, de Jong JM. Single-dose radiotherapy (6 Gy): palliation in painful bone metastases. *Radiother Oncol* 1995;36:198-202.

284. Parrish F, Murray JA. Surgical treatment for secondary neoplastic fractures. *J Bone Joint Surg Am* 1970;52:665-686.

285. Fiedler M. Prophylactic internal fixation of secondary neoplastic deposits of long bones. *Br J Med* 1973;1:341-343.

286. Schmidt RG. Management of extremity metastatic bone cancer. *Curr Probl Cancer* 1995;19:125-184.

287. Rose CM, Kagan R. The final report of the export panel for the Radiation Oncology Bone Metastase Work Group of the American College of Radiology. *Int J Radiat Oncol Biol Phys* 1998;40:1117-1124.

288. Mandoliti G, Polico C, Capirci C, et al. Radiation therapy of bone metastases in the elderly: a multicentric survey of the Italian Geriatric Radiation Oncology Group. *Rays* 1997;22:57-60.

289. Rasmusson B, Vejborg I, Jensen AB, et al. Irradiation of bone metastases in breast cancer patients: a randomized study with 1 year follow-up. *Radiother Oncol* 1995;34:179-184.

290. Niewald M, Tkocz HJ, Abel U, et al. Rapid course radiation therapy vs. more standard treatment: a randomized trial for bone metastases. *Int J Radiat Oncol Biol Phys* 1996;36:1085-1089.

291. Booth M, Summers J, Williams MV. Audit reduces the reluctance to use single fractions for painful bone metastases. *Clin Oncol (R Coll Radiol)* 1993;5:15-18.

292. Chander SS, Sarin R. Single fraction radiotherapy for bone metastases: are all questions answered? *Radiother Oncol* 1999;52: 191-193.

293. Price P, Hoskin PJ, Easton D. Prospective randomized trial of single and multi-fraction radiotherapy schedules in the treatment of painful bony metastases. *Radiother Oncol* 1986;6:247-255.

294. Hoskin PJ, Price P, Easton D. A prospective randomized trial of 4 Gy or 8 Gy single doses in the treatment of metastatic bone pain. *Radiother Oncol* 1992;23:74-78.

295. Stevens G, Firth I. Patterns of fractionation for palliation of bone metastases. *Australas Radiol* 1995;39:31-35.

296. Roos DE. Continuing reluctance to use single fractions of radiotherapy for metastatic bone pain: an Australian and New Zealand practice survey and literature review. *Radiother Oncol* 2000;56: 315-322.

297. Bremer M, Rades D, Blach M, et al. Effectiveness of hypofractionated radiotherapy in painful bone metastases. Two prospective studies with 1×4 Gy and 4×4 Gy. *Strahlenther Onkol* 1999; 175:382-386.

298. Chow E, Danjoux C, Wong R, et al. Palliation of bone metastases: a survey of patterns of practice among Canadian radiation oncologists. *Radiother Oncol* 2000;56:305-314.

299. Coia LR, Hanks GE, Martz K. Practice patterns of palliative care for the United States 1984-1985. *Int J Radiat Biol Phys* 1988; 14:1261-1269.

300. Madsen EL. Painful bone metastasis: efficacy of radiotherapy assessed by the patients. A randomized trial comparing 4 Gy × 6 versus 10 Gy × 2. *Int J Radiat Oncol Biol Phys* 1983;9: 1775-1779.

301. Okawa T, Kita M, Goto M. Randomized prospective clinical study of small, large and twice-a-day fraction radiotherapy for painful bone metastases. *Radiother Oncol* 1988;13:99-104.

302. Gaze MN, Kelly CG, Kerr GR, et al. Pain relief and quality of life following radiotherapy for bone metastases: a randomised trial of two fractionation schedules. *Radiother Oncol* 1997; 45:109-116.

303. Arcangeli G, Giovinazzo G, Saracino B, et al. Radiation therapy in the management of symptomatic bone metastases: the effect of total dose and histology on pain relief and response duration. *Int J Radiat Oncol Biol Phys* 1998;42:1119-1126.

304. Nielsen OS, Bentzen SM, Sandberg E, et al. Randomized trial of single dose versus fractionated palliative radiotherapy of bone metastases. *Radiother Oncol* 1998;47:233-240.

305. Koswig S, Budach V. Remineralization and pain relief in bone metastases after different radiotherapy fractions (10 times 3 Gy vs. 1 time 8 Gy). A prospective study. *Strahlenther Onkol* 1999; 175:500-508.

306. Steenland E, Leer JW, van Houwelingen H, et al. The effect of a single fraction compared to multiple fractions on painful bone metastases: a global analysis of the Dutch Bone Metastasis Study [published erratum in *Radiother Oncol* 1999;53:167]. *Radiother Oncol* 1999;52:101-109.

307. Salazar OM, Rubin P, Hendrickson FR. Single dose half body irradiation for palliation of multiple bone metastases from solid tumors. *Cancer* 1986;58:29-36.

308. Zelefsky MJ, Scher HI, Forman JD. Palliative hemiskeletal irradiation for widespread metastatic prostate cancer: a comparison of single dose and fractionated regimens. *Int J Radiat Oncol Biol Phys* 1989;17:1281-1285.

309. Scarantino CW, Caplan R, Rotman M, et al. A phase I/II study to evaluate the effect of fractionated hemibody irradiation in the treatment of osseous metastases—RTOG 88-22. *Int J Radiat Oncol Biol Phys* 1996;36:37-48.

310. Priestman TJ. Clinical studies with ondansetron in the control of radiation-induced emesis. *Eur J Cancer* 1989;25:S29-S33.

311. Hayashi S, Hoshi H, Iida T, et al. Multi-fractionated wide-field radiation therapy for palliation of multiple symptomatic bone metastases from solid tumors. *Radiat Med* 1999;17:411-416.

312. Algara M, Valls A, Ruiz V, et al. Half-body irradiation. Palliative efficacy and predictive factors of response in 78 procedures. *Med Clin (Barc)* 1994;103:85-88.

313. Poulter CA, Cosmatos D, Rubin P. A report of RTOG 8206: a phase III study of whether the addition of single dose hemibody irradiation is more effective than local field irradiation alone in the treatment of symptomatic osseous metastases. *Int J Radiat Oncol Biol Phys* 1992;23:207-214.

314. Quilty PM, Kirk D, Bolger JJ, et al. A comparison of the palliative effects of strontium-89 and external beam radiotherapy in metastatic prostate cancer. *Radiother Oncol* 1994;31:33-40.

315. Porter AT, McEwan AJB. Strontium-89 as an adjuvant to external beam radiation improves pain relief and delays disease progression in advanced prostate cancer: results of a randomized controlled trial. *Semin Oncol* 1993;20:38-43.

316. Porter AT, McEwan AJB, Powe JE. Results of a randomized phase-III trial to evaluate the efficacy of strontium-89 adjuvant to local field external beam irradiation in the management of

endocrine resistant metastatic prostate cancer. *Int J Radiat Oncol Biol Phys* 1993;25:805-813.

317. Robinson RG, Preston DF, Spicer JA, et al. Radionuclide therapy of intractable bone pain: emphasis on strontium-89. *Semin Nucl Med* 1992;22:28-32.

318. Robinson RG, Spicer JA, Blake GM. Strontium-89: treatment results and kinetics in patients with painful metastatic prostate and breast cancer in bone. *Radiographics* 1989;9:271-281.

319. Lee BC, Shav-Tal Y, Peled A, et al. A hematopoietic organ-specific 49-kD nuclear antigen: predominance in immature normal and tumor granulocytes and detection in hematopoietic precursor cells. *Blood* 1996;87:2283-2291.

320. Baumrucker S. Palliation of painful bone metastases: strontium-89. *Am J Hosp Palliat Care* 1998;15:113-115.

321. Brundage MD, Crook JM, Lukka H. Use of strontium-89 in endocrine-refractory prostate cancer metastatic to bone. Provincial Genitourinary Cancer Disease Site Group. *Cancer Prev Control* 1998;2:79-87.

322. Blake GM, Gray JM, Zivanovic MA. Strontium-89 radionuclide therapy: a dosimetric study using impulse response function analysis. *Br J Radiol* 1987;60:685-692.

323. Blake GM, Zivanovic MA. Sr-89 therapy: strontium kinetics in disseminated carcinoma of the prostate. *Eur J Nucl Med* 1986; 12:447-454.

324. Blake GM, Zivanovic MA, McEwan AJ. Sr-89 radionuclide therapy: dosimetry and hematologic toxicity in two patients with metastasizing prostatic carcinoma. *Eur J Nucl Med* 1987;13:41-46.

325. Breen SL, Powe JE, Porter AT. Dose estimation in strontium-89 radiotherapy of metastatic prostatic carcinoma. *J Nucl Med* 1992;33:1316-1323.

326. Pons F, Herranz R, Garcia A, et al. Strontium-89 for palliation of pain from bone metastases in patients with prostate and breast cancer. *Eur J Nucl Med* 1997;24:1210-1214.

327. Sciuto R, Festa A, Tofani A, et al. Platinum compounds as radiosensitizers in strontium-89 metabolic radiotherapy. *Clin Ter* 1998;149:43-47.

328. Sciuto R, Maini CL, Tofani A, et al. Radiosensitization with low-dose carboplatin enhances pain palliation in radioisotope therapy with strontium-89. *Nucl Med Commun* 1996;17: 799-804.

329. McEwan AJ. Use of radionuclides for the palliation of bone metastases. *Semin Radiat Oncol* 2000;10:103-114.

330. Singh A, Holmes RA, Farhanghi M. Human pharmacokinetics of samarium-153 EDTMP in metastatic cancer. *J Nucl Med* 1989;30:1814-1818.

331. Heggie JCP. Radiation absorbed dose calculations for samarium-153-EDTMP localized in bone. *J Nucl Med* 1991;32:840-844.

332. Serafini AN, Houston SJ, Resche I. Palliation of pain associated with metastatic bone cancer using samarium-153 lexidronam: a double-blind placebo-controlled clinical trial. *J Clin Oncol* 1998; 16:1574-1581.

333. Eary JF, Collins C, Appelbaum FR. Sm-153 EDTMP treatment of hormone refractory prostate carcinoma. *J Nucl Med* 1990;31: 755, Abstract 203.

334. Turner JH, Claringbold PG. A phase II study of treatment of painful multifocal skeletal metastases with single and repeated dose samarium-153 ethylenediaminetetramethylene phosphonate. *Eur J Cancer* 1991;27:1084-1086.

335. Bayouth JE, Macey DJ, Kasi LP, et al. Dosimetry and toxicity of samarium-153 EDTMP administered for bone pain due to skeletal metastases. *J Nucl Med* 1994;35:63-69.

336. Collins C, Eary JF, Donaldson G, et al. Samarium-153-EDTMP in bone metastases of hormone refractory prostate carcinoma: a phase I/II trial. *J Nucl Med* 1993;34:1839-1844.

337. Serafini AN. Current status of systemic intravenous radiopharmaceuticals for the treatment of painful metastatic bone disease. *Int J Radiat Oncol Biol Phys* 1994;30:1187-1194.

338. Farhanghi M, Holmes RA, Volkert WA, et al. Samarium-153-EDTMP: pharmacokinetic, toxicity and pain response using an escalating dose schedule in treatment of metastatic bone cancer. *J Nucl Med* 1992;33:1451-1458.

339. van Rensburg AJ, Alberts AS, Louw WK. Quantifying the radiation dosage to individual skeletal lesions treated with samarium-153 EDTMP. *J Nucl Med* 1998;39:2110-2115.

340. Hortobagyi GN, Theriault RL, Porter L, et al. Efficacy of pamidronate in reducing skeletal complications in patients with breast cancer and lytic bone metastases. Protocol 19 Aredia Breast Cancer Study Group. *N Engl J Med* 1996; 335:1785-1791.

341. Coukell AJ, Markham A. Pamidronate. A review of its use in the management of osteolytic bone metastases, tumour-induced hypercalcaemia and Paget's disease of bone. *Drugs Aging* 1998; 12:149-168.

342. Hillner BE, Ingle JN, Berenson JR, et al. American Society of Clinical Oncology guideline on the role of bisphosphonates in breast cancer. American Society of Clinical Oncology Bisphosphonates Expert Panel. *J Clin Oncol* 2000;18: 1378-1391.

343. Diener KM. Bisphosphonates for controlling pain from metastatic bone disease. *Am J Health Syst Pharm* 1996; 53: 1917-1927.

344. Serkies K, Jereczek-Fossa B, Badzio A, et al. Clodronate in the management of bone metastases: a clinical study of 91 patients. *Neoplasma* 1999;46:317-322.

CHAPTER 35

The Soft Tissue

Matthew T. Ballo and Gunar K. Zagars

By convention, the term *soft tissue* refers to all of the nonepithelial, nonreticuloendothelial extraskeletal tissues of the body, including the fibrous connective tissue, adipose tissue, muscle (skeletal and smooth), blood and lymph vessels, and peripheral nerve sheaths. Neoplasms arising within and consisting of soft tissue elements are called *soft-tissue tumors*. Despite their histopathologic diversity, these tumors share many pathobiological features, justifying their inclusion in one oncotaxonomic group.

Broadly speaking, soft-tissue tumors can be classified according to their clinical behavior as benign, borderline, or malignant. Benign tumors (e.g., lipoma, neurofibroma, leiomyoma) closely resemble their normal tissue of origin, show little if any local invasion, have no metastatic propensity, and rarely recur after excision. Borderline lesions (e.g., desmoid tumor, dermatofibrosarcoma protuberans) are locally invasive and have a significant tendency to recur after excision, and some types occasionally metastasize. Malignant soft-tissue tumors—soft-tissue sarcomas (STSs)—are locally invasive and have a high propensity toward hematogenous metastasis. Although many sarcomas have a benign histogenetic counterpart (e.g., liposarcoma-lipoma, leiomyosarcoma-leiomyoma, fibrosarcoma-fibroma), transformation of soft-tissue tumors from benign to malignant forms is extremely rare, and most sarcomas arise without known precursor lesions. Moreover, because the benign tumors are easily cured by resection, radiation therapy has little role in their management. Thus this chapter deals only with sarcomas and selected intermediate soft-tissue tumors.

EPIDEMIOLOGY AND ETIOLOGY

Approximately 8700 new cases and 4400 deaths are caused by STS in the United States each year. However, STS is rare and accounts for less than 1% of all new non–skin-cancer diagnoses.[1] The median patient age at presentation varies from 40 to 60 years, although these tumors can occur at any age from infancy on.[1-5] Males are slightly more commonly affected than females, but this sex difference is small.[2] No racial predilection has been found.[5]

Etiologic factors for STS are poorly defined. Although patients sometimes report antecedent trauma to the site of their sarcoma (e.g., prior surgery or reaction to a foreign body[6-8]), it is generally believed that trauma serves to bring the patient's attention to the lesion rather than having any causative role. Chronic lymphedema of the upper extremity as a sequela of breast cancer management is associated with the development of lymphangiosarcoma (this phenomenon is known as the Stewart-Treves syndrome).[9] Postirradiation sarcoma is a well-recognized potential complication of radiation therapy. The diagnosis of radiation-induced sarcoma requires that the sarcoma arise in a previously irradiated site and that a latency of at least a few years occur.[10] With an incidence of 0.03% to 0.22% and a median latency period of 10 years, radiation-induced sarcomas have been difficult to characterize.[11] However, they usually present in an advanced stage, are high grade, metastasize early, respond poorly to therapy, and are fatal. Malignant fibrous histiocytoma (MFH) is the most commonly diagnosed radiation-induced sarcoma, followed by angiosarcoma.[12,13] Postirradiation liposarcoma has not been reported.[5] The etiologic significance of exposure to phenoxyacetic acid herbicides (e.g., Agent Orange) remains controversial, though most reports do support at least a weak association.[14-16]

In keeping with the concept that oncogenes are responsible for carcinogenesis in general, evidence is mounting for genetic etiologic factors in selected STSs. Several sarcomas occur in well-defined hereditary settings. Neurofibromatosis I (von Recklinghausen's disease), inherited as an autosomal dominant defect that consists of a mutation that causes a lack of function in the neurofibromin gene, is characterized by the development of multiple benign neurofibromas and by a high incidence of malignant peripheral nerve sheath tumor (also known as malignant schwannoma, neurogenic sarcoma, or neurofibrosarcoma).[17] Optic glioma, astrocytoma, and pheochromocytoma also occur in these patients. Neurofibromatosis II (hereditary acoustic neuroma), an autosomal dominant disorder defined by a mutant merlin protein, is characterized by the development of acoustic neuroma and is associated with meningioma, glioma, and schwannoma.[5] Hereditary retinoblastoma—also an autosomal dominant disease, with a mutation that causes a lack of function in the retinoblastoma gene—is associated with an increased risk of bone and soft-tissue sarcomas.[18] Gardner's syndrome, an autosomal dominant variant of hereditary polyposis coli, is associated with desmoid tumors and rarely with fibrosarcoma or liposarcoma.[5] Finally, among those conditions heralding a hereditary predisposition to sarcoma is the Li-Fraumeni syndrome, which is inherited as an autosomal dominant trait with incomplete penetrance and is caused by a mutation that causes a lack of function in the *p53* gene. This disorder manifests a high incidence of a variety of tumors, among them MFH, rhabdomyosarcoma, osteosarcoma, and breast cancer occurring in patients younger than typical.[19,20] Genetic factors are further implicated by the finding of characteristic chromosome translocations in some sarcomas. Consistent translocations have been described in myxoid liposarcoma (t[12;16]), clear-cell sarcoma (t[12;22]), alveolar rhabdomyosarcoma (t[2;13]), synovial sarcoma (t[X;18]), and Ewing's sarcoma (t[11;22]).[21]

PATHOLOGY

The pathologic classification of STSs is based on the type of tissue comprising the tumor, that is, on its histologic appearance.[5,22,23] For many STSs, this histologic classification also implies a specific histogenesis or cell type of origin—for example, leiomyosarcoma from smooth muscle, liposarcoma from fat, angiosarcoma from lymph or blood vessels, or rhabdomyosarcoma from skeletal muscle. For some STSs, the histologic classification does not imply a well-defined cell of origin—for example, MFH, alveolar soft-part sarcoma, or synovial sarcoma.

Currently, some 25 major categories of STSs are recognized, and when subcategories are considered, some 60 types have been described.[5,24] Complicating this taxonomy is the use of some 300 synonyms for these 60 types of STS.[24] The more common types are MFH (20% to 30% of cases), liposarcoma (10% to 20%), synovial sarcoma (5% to 10%), rhabdomyosarcoma (5% to 10%), leiomyosarcoma (5% to 10%), malignant peripheral nerve sheath tumor (malignant schwannoma) (5% to 10%), and fibrosarcoma (5% to 10%).[5,24-26] These tumors account for approximately 70% to 80% of all STSs.

Accurate recognition of STS type requires expertise in the pathology of these tumors. Even then, the rate of agreement among pathologists on histologic type is only about 70%.[27,28] In difficult cases, the use of immunocytochemistry or electron microscopy might be helpful.[29] Although no marker pattern is diagnostic of a particular tumor, the following markers can aid in diagnosis[5,21]:

Vimentin, a cytoskeletal protein normally present in mesenchymal tissue but absent in epithelia, is present in most STSs, but may occasionally occur in adenocarcinomas.

Desmin, an integral part of the cytoskeleton of cardiac, skeletal, and smooth muscle, is present in most rhabdomyosarcomas but occurs in only one half of leiomyosarcomas and is occasionally expressed in Ewing's sarcoma, liposarcoma, and MFH.

Cytokeratin, characteristic of epithelia, is classical for the diagnosis of carcinoma but has been found in some epithelioid sarcomas, synovial sarcomas, and other STSs.

S-100 protein, a "brain-specific" protein, is present in nearly all melanomas and clear-cell sarcomas, but is also found in many malignant nerve sheath tumors and in some carcinomas.

In addition to classifying an STS according to its type, the pathologist must assign a grade—an estimate of the degree of the tumor's virulence based on its histologic appearance. Features typically assessed for grading are cellular differentiation, cellular pleomorphism, degree of cellularity, mitotic activity, necrosis, and invasiveness.[30] Both three-tier[27,31-33] and four-tier[34] grading schemes have been proposed. The American Joint Committee on Cancer (AJCC) staging system recommends a four-tier system (Box 35-1),[35] but a three-tier system of low, intermediate, and high grade seems to be the most widely used.

Unfortunately, the grading of STSs remains largely subjective and is extremely controversial. Different investigators have found different pathologic features to be significant as grading criteria. Some found degree of cellularity to be significant[31,36] and others not[28,32]; some found degree of differentiation to be significant,[28] and others not[31,36]; pleomorphism was significant according to some,[31,36] but not to others[28]; likewise, necrosis was found to be significant by some,[28,31] but not by others.[36] Most investigators have found mitotic rate to be a significant factor.[28,31,36] In the face of this uncertainty, it might seem surprising that all of the various grading systems seem to predict the metastatic potential of STSs.[28,31-34,36,37]

An alternative to tumor grading on an individual basis is the use of histotype as an indicator of grade.[5] Histologic grading is based on multivariate analyses that include nonhistologic features such as tumor size and site (superficial vs. deep) in the statistical model. These studies have found that most of the "classical" histopathologic indicators of grade lose independent prognostic significance.[22,26] For many years we have used a purely histologic grading classification (Box 35-2), which correlates well with prognosis.[22,38-41] Recent advances in understanding molecular markers suggest that objective measures of tumor virulence may emerge.[42-44] Meanwhile, every effort should be made to grade each individual patient's tumor because grade, however assigned, remains the strongest predictor of outcome.

PRESENTATION, NATURAL HISTORY, AND PROGNOSIS

Although STSs can arise in any part of the body, the most common site is an extremity, especially a lower extremity (Table 35-1).[3,45-47] Most STSs arise within

---

BOX 35-1   American Joint Committee on Cancer Staging System for Soft-Tissue Sarcomas

PRIMARY TUMOR (T)

TX	Primary tumor cannot be assessed
T0	No evidence of primary tumor
T1	Tumor 5 cm or less in greatest dimension
T1a	Superficial tumor
T1b	Deep tumor
T2	Tumor more than 5 cm in greatest dimension
T2a	Superficial tumor
T2b	Deep tumor

REGIONAL LYMPH NODES (N)

NX	Regional lymph nodes cannot be assessed
N0	No regional lymph node metastases
N1	Regional lymph node metastases

DISTANT METASTASES (M)

MX	Distant metastases cannot be assessed
M0	No distant metastases
M1	Distant metastases

HISTOPATHOLOGIC GRADE

GX	Grade cannot be assessed
G1	Well differentiated
G2	Moderately differentiated
G3	Poorly differentiated
G4	Undifferentiated

STAGE GROUPING

Stage I				
A	G1-2	T1a-1b	N0	M0
B	G1-2	T2a	N0	M0
Stage II				
A	G1-2	T2b	N0	M0
B	G3-4	T1a-1b	N0	M0
C	G3-4	T2a	N0	M0
Stage III	G3-4	T2b	N0	M0
Stage IV	Any G	Any T	N1	M0
	Any G	Any T	N0	M1

From Fleming ID, Cooper JS, Henson DE, et al, eds. *AJCC Cancer Staging Manual.* 5th ed. Philadelphia, Pa: Lippincott Williams & Wilkins; 1997:149-156.

BOX 35-2   Malignancy Grouping of Specific Types of Soft-Tissue Sarcoma*

GROUP 1

Locally recurring soft-tissue neoplasms with no or very
    little metastatic potential
Desmoid tumor
Atypical lipomatous tumor
Dermatofibrosarcoma protuberans

GROUP 2

Sarcomas of intermediate aggressiveness
    (but with metastatic capability)
Myxoid liposarcoma
Extraskeletal myxoid chondrosarcoma
Myxoid malignant fibrous histiocytoma
Hemangiopericytoma

GROUP 3

Aggressive sarcomas
Malignant fibrous histiocytoma
Synovial sarcoma
Pleomorphic liposarcoma
Cellular myxoid liposarcoma
Dedifferentiated liposarcoma
Angiosarcoma
Leiomyosarcoma
Malignant peripheral nerve sheath tumor
    (malignant schwannoma)
Rhabdomyosarcoma (all types)
Alveolar soft-part sarcoma
Extraskeletal osteosarcoma
Extraskeletal Ewing's sarcoma
Malignant melanoma of soft parts (clear-cell sarcoma)
Epithelioid sarcoma

Modified from Evans HL. *Hematol Oncol Clin North Am* 1995;9:653-656.
*Including locally recurring nonmetastasizing neoplasms.

---

muscle, but they also can arise in intermuscular planes, subcutaneous tissue, fat, nerves, veins, and other tissues. Although any type of STS can arise in any site, some types have a predilection for particular sites; for example, liposarcoma is the most common retroperitoneal STS, synovial sarcoma tends to arise near (but not within) joints, and myxoid liposarcoma favors the upper medial thigh. Usually the patient notes a painless mass, although pain can occur if the lesion impinges on neurovascular structures. Typical are a 4-month delay between the onset of symptoms and presentation to a physician and a 1-month delay between presentation and diagnosis.[3]

The tumor's growth rate depends on its histologic subtype and grade; local spread is directed along the pathways of least resistance. Growth begins radially, pushing surrounding tissues into a well-delineated

TABLE 35-1

Anatomic Sites of 6286 Soft-Tissue Sarcomas

Study and Reference	Lower Extremity	Upper Extremity	Head and Neck	Trunk*
Abbas et al[45]	81	42	24	90
Potter et al[46]	152	59	12	84
Torosian et al[47]	208	81	21	182
Lawrence et al[3]	2110	594	406	1440
M.D. Anderson Cancer Center 1965-1987	240	136	66	158
TOTALS	2891 (46%)	912 (15%)	529 (8%)	1954 (31%)

*Approximately 50% were retroperitoneal.

compression zone. Beyond this area of compressed normal tissue lies a reactive zone characterized by edema, neovascularity, and inflammatory infiltrate. The combination of these two zones creates a "pseudocapsule," sometimes prompting inexperienced surgeons to perform a "shell-out" procedure.[48] The pseudocapsule invariably contains numerous points of microscopic tumor penetration,[30] and local failure is common if no additional treatment is given.

As STSs grow, they typically respect the major intermuscular septa and remain confined to the compartment of origin. Extracompartmental extension may occur after surgical manipulation but is typically found late because local extension occurs through perforating vascular channels.[48] Most STSs grow along the direction of muscle bundles or along aponeurotic sheaths in the vicinity of their origin. In extremity STSs, this pattern of growth dictates generous longitudinal margins for surgery and radiation but permits relatively narrow transverse margins.

Several histologic subtypes are characterized by unique local growth patterns. Desmoid tumor[49] and epithelioid sarcoma[50] both lack the well-defined pseudocapsule described above, making delineation and complete surgical resection difficult. Malignant peripheral nerve sheath tumors are also difficult to resect completely because of their propensity for local extension along major nerve trunks. Finally, angiosarcoma of the skin has a striking tendency for presentation with widespread dermal involvement that is often underappreciated clinically.[51]

Metastasis

Lymph node metastases from STSs are uncommon, occurring in fewer than 10% of patients at any time during the disease.[25,52] In a review of experience at Massachusetts General Hospital, Mazeron and Suit[25] reported that the incidence of STS metastases was 5.9% in 323 patients. This finding was consistent with their evaluation of pooled data from published reports on more than 2000 patients, in which the crude incidence of lymph node metastases was 3.9%. When combining the pooled data with their own institutional experience, these investigators found that histologic subtype, grade, and size were the most important determinants of lymph node metastasis. Lymph node involvement was highest for the clear-cell (27.5%), epithelioid (20%), synovial-cell (13.7%), angiosarcoma (11.4%), and rhabdomyosarcoma (14.8%) subtypes. No lymph node metastases occurred in the 63 patients with grade 1 lesions, compared with incidences of 2% and 12% among the 118 and 142 patients with grade 2 and grade 3 lesions, respectively. Tumor diameter of less than 5 cm was associated with a 3% incidence of lymph node involvement, compared with 15% for lesions of 5 cm or larger.

Hematogenous metastasis is a common and serious event in patients with STS. The lung is the most common site of metastasis, but lesions can appear in bone and, especially in the case of retroperitoneal STS, in the liver. Metastases are detected in 20% to 25% of patients at the time of initial presentation.[3] New metastases develop within 5 years of local treatment in most patients,[53-55] and the incidence of these metastases is closely correlated with tumor grade and size. Each of these factors, grade and size, is a highly significant and independent determinant of metastatic relapse.

The importance of grade in predicting metastases has been illustrated in several reports. Lindberg and colleagues,[56] reporting on 300 patients, found metastasis rates of 5%, 28%, and 43% for grades 1, 2, and 3 tumors, respectively. Trojani and colleagues[27] reviewed the experience of 155 patients and reported metastasis-free survival rates of 69%, 46%, and 16% at 5 years for those with grades 1, 2, and 3 lesions, respectively. Markhede and colleagues[36] described similar findings using a four-tier system applied to 97 patients; the metastasis rate was 0%, 30%, 34%, and 60% for grade 1, 2, 3, and 4 lesions, respectively.

The influence of tumor size is illustrated in a report by Lindberg and colleagues,[56] who found that tumors less than 5 cm in largest dimension had a metastasis rate of 13%, compared with a metastasis rate of 35% for tumors exceeding 5 cm. Although 5 cm is generally accepted as the boundary between "large" and "small" STS and is the basis of the AJCC "T" classification system,[35] the relationship between size and metastatic propensity is more or less continuous. The continuity of this relationship is illustrated by our data on synovial sarcoma,[41] showing that the actuarial 10-year incidence of metastatic relapse was 0%, 35%, 61%, and 100% for tumors of less than 2 cm, 2 to 5 cm, 5 to 10 cm, and more than 10 cm, respectively. The independent effects of grade and tumor size on metastatic propensity are illustrated in our study on MFH.[39] Pleomorphic MFH, a high-grade STS according to our system of classification (see Box 35-2),[22] had 10-year metastasis rates of 23% and 51% for tumors of up to 5 cm and greater than 5 cm, respectively; myxoid MFH, an intermediate-grade STS, had 10-year metastasis rates of 4% and 22% for tumors of up to 5 cm and larger than 5 cm, respectively. Although grade was an important determinant of metastasis, tumor size was also important in each grade group.

The only factor other than grade and size that regularly correlates with metastatic relapse is tumor depth, with lesions superficial to the deep fascia displaying a significantly lower metastatic propensity than similar lesions located deep in the fascia.[44,57-59] This feature is incorporated in the current AJCC staging system (see Box 35-1).[35] Such factors as patient age and sex have an uncertain effect on metastatic propensity.[5,36,60,61] Likewise, the significance of tumor primary site as an independent determinant of outcome is uncertain. Although STSs arising in the head and neck or in the retroperitoneum are associated with a significantly poorer outcome than are STSs at other sites,[62-64] this phenomenon is generally believed to reflect the anatomic constraints on radical resection of head and neck lesions and the large size of retroperitoneal tumors, rather than any intrinsic virulence of lesions arising in these sites. Because patient survival is largely determined by whether metastasis develops, the prognostic factors for survival are the same as those for metastatic relapse.

Local Recurrence

Because of their infiltrative growth pattern, STSs have a marked tendency to recur locally, especially after conservative excision. Even after more radical treatment, local recurrence remains a potential problem. After definitive treatment, whether by radical surgery alone or by combined conservation surgery and radiation, local relapse occurs in 15% to 25% of cases. The major prognostic factors for local recurrence are resection margins positive for disease and a history of prior recurrence; tumor grade

and size have little influence on the likelihood of local recurrence.[36,46,58,59,65-69] Thus low- or intermediate-grade tumors (such as desmoids, dermatofibrosarcoma protuberans, or myxoid MFH) have the same propensity for local recurrence as high-grade lesions (such as pleomorphic MFH or synovial sarcoma).

Retroperitoneal STSs are notorious for their recurrence rates, which exceed 80% and even 90% in some series because of the anatomic impossibility of achieving adequate resection margins.[62,70,71] It is important to realize that the prognostic factors for local recurrence (prior local recurrence, disease in the resection margin) are different from those for metastatic relapse (tumor grade, size of primary lesion, and depth of invasion).

STAGING

The AJCC staging system (see Box 35-1) uses three known prognostic factors: tumor size, tumor grade, and tumor depth. This system applies to all STSs except for Kaposi's sarcoma, dermatofibrosarcoma protuberans, and desmoid tumor. Also excluded are sarcomas arising within the confines of the dura mater, including the brain, and sarcomas arising within parenchymatous organs or hollow viscera. Depth is defined in relation to the superficial muscular fascia. Any tumor involving the superficial muscular fascia and retroperitoneal disease are considered deep. The validity of this clinicopathologic staging system and its ability to predict relapse (in the form of distant metastasis) and tumor-related mortality have been confirmed.[59,72,73] It should be noted that the AJCC's use of tumor grade in assigning tumor stage in STSs is almost unique among the group's staging systems, highlighting the importance of grade as a determinant of outcome for patients who have this cancer.

Diagnostic and Staging Work-up

Virtually all new, enlarging, or symptomatic soft-tissue masses should be regarded as potential sarcomas. A timely and correctly performed biopsy is an important early step in evaluation. Four biopsy techniques are available: incisional biopsy, excisional biopsy, core-needle biopsy, and fine-needle aspiration. Excisional biopsy—removal of the entire grossly evident lesion without a margin—invariably passes through the apparent plane of the pseudocapsule ("shell out"), often contaminates surrounding tissue, complicates subsequent surgical management, and should not be performed.[74-76] Incisional biopsy—the removal of a wedge of tumor—is generally the most appropriate method but should be performed by an oncologic surgeon. The incision should be located so that the tumor can be excised easily during the definitive surgical procedure; the incision also should be placed directly over the tumor to avoid tunneling through tissue. The incision should be longitudinal for extremity lesions, and hemostasis must be meticulous.[74,77] A poorly planned or executed biopsy procedure can significantly reduce the chances for local control and increase the number and complexity of surgical procedures required.[78,79] The less-invasive biopsy procedures—core-needle biopsy and fine-needle aspiration—have been criticized because of the small amounts of tissue obtained, but in experienced hands they have been shown to be successful. Core-needle biopsy, which retrieves a thin sliver of tissue, usually by using a Tru-Cut needle, has been shown to allow the correct histopathologic type and grade to be assigned to approximately 90% of STSs.[80] In our practice, core-needle biopsy is the preferred initial biopsy technique and can be guided by computed tomography (CT) scan, if appropriate. This technique has the potential to eliminate inappropriate biopsy incision placement and to decrease the incidence of wound healing complications.[81]

Less certain is the role of fine-needle aspiration in the initial diagnostic work-up because even experienced cytopathologists are often unable to assign a grade or histopathologic type to samples obtained this way.[5,36,82] However, fine-needle aspiration is useful in documenting relapse in established cases of STS.

A thorough assessment of the AJCC staging features and of relevant patient factors is crucial to the formulation of an optimal treatment strategy for a patient with STS. Clinical findings are usually disappointingly nonspecific, and radiologic imaging studies are indispensible.[83] The primary imaging studies for evaluating STS are CT scanning and magnetic resonance imaging (MRI), supplemented by plain radiography, ultrasonography, and angiography when appropriate.

The optimal modality for evaluating a primary tumor varies with the tumor type, its location, and the features of interest.[83] In general, MRI is the modality of choice for evaluating the extent of STSs because it can delineate tumor margins and neurovascular structures and can provide images in several planes. In direct comparisons, preoperative MRI has been found to be superior to CT scanning for assessing tumor resectability[84] and for distinguishing muscle from tumor.[85,86] However, CT scanning provides better visualization of fatty tumors and tumor calcification and permits a better assessment of tissue-bone interfaces than MRI.[87] For the radiation oncologist, CT has the advantage of providing scout images from which the tumor can be related to bony landmarks.

Possible uses of positron emission tomography (PET)[88] and radionuclide imaging with novel radionuclides[89] are areas of active research. In a recent prospective evaluation of 30 suspected malignant masses, PET scans were performed and the tumors categorized as either benign or one of three malignant grades. All 12 of the high-grade lesions were correctly identified by the PET scan characteristics. The low-grade lesions, on the other hand, could not be distinguished from the benign lesions.[88] Although present research is in its early phase, both PET scanning and radionuclide imaging may become increasingly important, particularly in evaluating the response of STSs to nonsurgical treatment.[89,90]

Because STSs have a marked propensity for metastasis to the lungs, all patients with intermediate- or high-grade tumors who have normal chest x-ray images require a CT scan of the chest.[91] Patients with retroperitoneal STS should be evaluated for hepatic metastases by means of CT scanning. Because myxoid liposarcoma metastasizes preferentially to retroperitoneal soft tissues,[40] patients who have this type of STS should undergo CT scanning of the abdomen. Patients with alveolar soft-part sarcoma should undergo a radionuclide brain scan because of this sarcoma's peculiar tendency to metastasize to the brain.[92] The low incidence of regional nodal metastases suggests that specific evaluation of lymph nodes is unnecessary, although radionuclide sentinel node mapping[93] may have a place for patients with epithelioid or clear-cell sarcoma (melanoma of soft parts). In practice, the regional nodes are often included in the imaging studies of the primary tumor and further investigation is not needed.

TREATMENT
Surgery

Surgical resection remains the mainstay of treatment for most patients with localized STS. Except for select sarcomas, such as the "round-cell" types (extraskeletal Ewing's, malignant peripheral neuroectodermal tumor, embryonal and alveolar rhabdomyosarcoma, and neuroblastoma), which can be successfully treated with a combination of radiation and chemical agents, most STSs cannot be reliably eradicated without resection of gross disease. Historical experience with limited excision has demonstrated a high incidence of residual microscopic and even gross tumor[75] and an incidence of local recurrence as high as 90%.* The infiltrative nature of these tumors often dictates the use of radical surgical procedures.

In an attempt to rationalize surgery for STS, Enneking and colleagues[48] presented a classification of surgical procedures. Notably, this system was developed for lesions of the extremity; true "radical" resection is rarely possible for lesions arising in the head and neck, trunk wall, mediastinum, or retroperitoneum. The Enneking classification has two surgical procedures—local excision or amputation—and four surgical margins—intralesional, marginal, wide, or radical. The resulting eight combinations of terms describe the type of surgical procedure possible and the relationship between the plane of dissection, the lesion, its pseudocapsule, and surrounding normal tissues (Table 35-2). An amputation, for example, can range from a radical procedure, in which the level of amputation passes proximal to the origin of the muscles containing the lesion, to a debulking procedure, in which the level of amputation actually passes through the lesion

---

*References 45, 48, 53, 55, 94, 95.

TABLE 35-2

Four Surgical Margins and Related Procedures

Surgical Margins and Related Procedures	Definition
RADICAL MARGIN	An aggressive procedure removing the entire anatomic compartment involved by tumor, including neurovascular structures.
Radical amputation	Amputation is proximal to the origin of the muscles adjacent to the lesion, usually above the joint proximal to the tumor.
Radical compartment resection	All compartmental muscles are removed from origin to insertion.
WIDE MARGIN	Removal of the lesion and the surrounding reactive zone with a cuff of normal tissue included.
Wide amputation	The level of amputation is within normal tissue outside the reactive zone.
Wide local excision	A rim of normal tissue surrounds the plane of dissection, but no attempt is made to remove the entire muscle.
Myectomy	The involved muscle is removed only from origin to insertion.
MARGINAL MARGIN	The plane of dissection passes through the pseudocapsular-reactive zone. This is usually associated with positive microscopic margins.
Marginal amputation	The level of amputation passes through the reactive zone.
Marginal excision (excisional biopsy or "shell out")	This method is appropriate for benign lesions only.
INTRALESIONAL MARGIN	This diagnostic procedure consists of resection inside the pseudocapsule. It is invariably associated with positive microscopic margins.
Debulking amputation	The level of amputation passes through the lesion.
Incisional biopsy or intralesional debulking	This is the preferred diagnostic procedure.

Modified from Enneking WF, Spanier SS, Malawer MM. *Cancer* 1981;47:1005-1022.

itself. A local procedure can be equally radical in that the entire compartment containing the lesion is removed, or it may be incisional, wherein only a small portion of the lesion is removed for diagnostic purposes.

The terms *wide* or *marginal* reflect margins as outlined in Table 35-2. In practice, the terms *amputation, radical compartmental resection* (monobloc soft-part resection),[96] and *wide local excision* describe the majority of therapeutic surgical procedures performed for STS. The use of this terminology, however, is no substitute for pathologic assessment and designation of the final margin as positive or negative for disease.

As indicated, unsatisfactory early experience with limited excision resulted in the adoption of radical resection—radical monobloc soft-part resection, radical compartment resection, and amputation—as the standard surgical procedures for STS. Table 35-3 summarizes the local control rates achieved with radical surgery as the sole treatment.* In general, local recurrence occurs in 10% to 25% of patients depending on the surgical series. Amputation achieves local control in more than 90% of patients,[36,66,67,99] whereas radical nonamputative resection achieves local control in 75% to 85% of

TABLE 35-3

Local Recurrence Rates After Radical Surgical Procedures Alone

Study and Reference	Number of Patients	Number of Primary Amputations (%)	5-Year Local Recurrence Rate (%)
Cantin et al[55]	653	Not available	29
Abbas et al[45]	143	51 (36)	26
Simon et al[97]	45	23 (51)	17
Markhede et al[36]	97	15 (15)	22
Shiu et al[98]	297	139 (47)	18
Berlin et al[66]	54	29 (54)	17

patients.* Thus radical surgery alone can achieve high rates of local control. However, this salutary effect comes with significant morbidity and a rate of primary amputation of 50% in some series (Table 35-3). Moreover, the expected survival time for patients treated with amputation has often been inferior to that for patients treated with less radical resection because patients who undergo amputation generally have large, high-grade lesions and a high incidence of

*References 36, 45, 55, 66, 97, 98.

*References 36, 48, 59, 66, 67, 99, 100.

micrometastatic disease.[99] The high local control rate attendant to amputation has never been shown to be reflected in overall survival. Finally, the use of truly radical surgery is anatomically limited to extremity tumors and is rarely applicable to nonextremity sites.

Recognizing these problems, many investigators have explored the combination of conservative surgery and radiation therapy. Other surgical oncologists, however, have sought to redefine the selection criteria for tumors that might be adequately managed using less radical surgery—myectomy or function-sparing wide local excision—as the sole treatment.[53,82,100] The results of both approaches are considered next.

Adjuvant Radiation Therapy

Although radical surgery alone provides satisfactory local control, it does so at the expense of significant functional deficits and is rarely applicable to nonextremity tumors. By the 1960s it was known that complete responses could be attained when radiation therapy was used alone for gross disease,[101] dispelling the long-held belief that STSs were highly resistant to radiation. Clinical research then turned to combining limited (conservative or conservation) surgical excision with adjuvant radiation therapy. Suit and colleagues[102] reported initial success using this technique at The University of Texas M.D. Anderson Cancer Center in the early 1970s.

Lindberg and colleagues[56] updated this experience, reviewing 300 patients with STS treated by conservative surgical resection (either excisional biopsy or wide local excision) and postoperative radiation. No patient was treated for gross disease, and radiation doses ranged from 60 to 75 Gy. The 5-year overall survival and local control rates of 61% and 78% were comparable to those attained by radical surgery alone but without causing a loss of limb function. The ultimate limb preservation rate of 84% is consistent with the 83%,[103] 84%,[60] 87%,[104] and 90%[99] rates reported by colleagues applying similar conservation techniques.

The only randomized trial comparing radical amputation with limb-sparing surgery plus radiation therapy was performed by the National Cancer Institute (NCI).[105] In that trial, 43 adult patients with high-grade STS of an extremity were prospectively randomized in a 2-to-1 fashion to receive limb-sparing surgery plus radiation therapy (27 patients) or radical amputation (16 patients). Both randomization groups received doxorubicin, cyclophosphamide, and high-dose methotrexate chemotherapy. Patients in the limb-sparing group received 50 Gy to the entire anatomic area at risk, with a boost to the tumor bed of an additional 10 to 20 Gy. At a median follow-up time of 56 months, four local recurrences had occurred in the group given limb-sparing surgery plus radiation therapy, but no local recurrences occurred in the amputation group ($P = 0.06$). Despite the slight difference in the incidence of local failure, no differences were found in disease-free or overall survival.

Conservation Surgery Plus Radiation Therapy

In an attempt to further define the role of radiation therapy, two prospective randomized trials (Table 35-4) compared conservation surgery plus radiation therapy with conservation surgery alone.[106-108] The first trial,[106] from Memorial Sloan-Kettering Cancer Center, randomized patients with extremity or superficial trunk STS to undergo either conservation surgery alone (86 patients) or conservation surgery plus brachytherapy (78 patients). The brachytherapy was performed using catheters afterloaded with ^{192}Ir to deliver 42 to 45 Gy over 4 to 6 days. After a median follow-up time of 76 months, the 5-year actuarial local control rate was 82% in the conservation surgery plus brachytherapy group compared with 69% in the conservation surgery–only group ($P = 0.04$). The positive effect of

---

TABLE 35-4

Randomized Trials Comparing Conservation Surgery Plus Radiation Therapy with Conservation Surgery Alone

Study and Reference/ Tumor Grade	Treatment	Number of Patients	Local Failure Rate (%)	P Value	Median Follow-up Time	Radiation Dose and Technique
Yang et al[108]						
High-grade lesions	RT	44	0 (0)	0.003	9.6 yr	63 Gy EBRT
	No RT	47	9 (22)			
Low-grade lesions	RT	26	1 (4)	0.016	9.9 yr	63 Gy EBRT
	No RT	24	8 (37)			
Pisters et al[106]						
High-grade lesions	RT	56	5 (11)	0.0025	6.3 yr	42-45 Gy
	No RT	63	19 (34)			brachytherapy
Low-grade lesions	RT	22	8 (33)	0.49	6.3 yr	42-45 Gy
	No RT	23	6 (24)			brachytherapy

RT, Radiation therapy; *EBRT*, external-beam radiation therapy.

adjuvant radiation therapy was limited to the 119 patients who had high-grade lesions and was not apparent in the 45 patients who had low-grade disease. Differences in the treatment effect could have resulted from small patient numbers,[106] particularly among those expected to be at the highest risk of local recurrence (only 9 of 45 patients who had both low-grade disease and positive margins were randomized), or radiobiological reasons (cells in slow-growing low-grade tumors might not have been given an opportunity to traverse radiosensitive phases of the cell cycle during the implantation period).[107]

The second trial,[108] from the NCI, randomized patients with extremity STS to limb-sparing surgery alone (71 patients) or limb-sparing surgery plus external-beam radiation therapy (70 patients). The radiation consisted of 45 Gy (1.80 Gy/fraction) to wide fields and then an 18-Gy boost to the tumor bed defined by surgical clips. At a median follow-up time of 115 months, 17 failures had occurred in the surgery-only group, compared with one failure in the surgery-plus-radiation group ($P = 0.0001$). Unlike the Memorial Sloan-Kettering Cancer Center experience, in this study radiation therapy improved local control of both the 91 high-grade tumors and the 50 low-grade tumors. This discrepancy suggests a radiobiological difference in the sensitivity of STSs to brachytherapy and external-beam radiation, but it also might simply reflect the fact that a higher number of low-grade tumors in the NCI series were at high risk of local recurrence (that is, 21 of 50 patients had both low-grade disease and close or positive margins).

Numerous experiences in which conservation surgery has been followed by radiation therapy have been published; overall, this approach has been found to result in local control for 80% to 90% of patients who have extremity or nonretroperitoneal truncal STS (Table 35-5). *These results are comparable to those achieved using radical surgery alone (see Table 35-3).

The most consistently identified prognostic factors for local recurrence after conservation surgery and radiation therapy are resection margins positive for microscopic disease[59,67,68,111,114] and prior local recurrence.[39,59,69,113] Retroperitoneal STSs are notorious for local recurrence because of anatomic constraints precluding complete resection and normal tissue tolerances limiting the permissible radiation doses.[62,70,71,115,116] Similar constraints hamper local control in the head and neck region.[117] Less consistently reported factors that might influence local control include radiation dose (Table 35-6)[†] or field size[60,99] and tumor histologic subtype.[40,68,113] Factors that do not correlate with local control when using the combined-modality treatment approach are tumor size and grade and depth with respect to the superficial fascia (superficial vs. deep).[‡]

Traditionally, radiation has been applied postoperatively (see Table 35-5). This sequencing has the advantage of (1) allowing the radiation therapy dose and field size to be tailored to fit the surgical findings (e.g., margin status, tumor histologic subtype and grade); (2) eliminating delay in complete resection of the primary lesion; and (3) possibly eliminating the need for radiation therapy altogether in select cases. However, preoperative radiation has its advantages, too: (1) It requires smaller field sizes and lower radiation doses; (2) it eliminates any delay between incomplete surgical resection and the start of radiation therapy; (3) it treats a fully oxygenated tumor and limits the dissemination of viable tumor cells at the time of resection; and (4) it increases resectability by eliminating peripheral microscopic tumor extension.

---

*References 56, 60, 61, 67, 69, 95, 99, 103, 106, 108-113.
†References 60, 67, 69, 95, 99, 111, 113, 118.
‡References 40, 41, 59, 67, 69, 73, 99, 103, 106.

TABLE 35-5

Local Control Rates After Postoperative Radiation Therapy

Study and Reference	Number of Patients	Follow-up Time	Evaluation Period	Local Control Rate
Lindberg et al[56]	300	2 yr (minimum)	5 yr	78%
Leibel et al[95]	29	2 yr (minimum)	Crude	90%
Potter et al[61]	123	3.2 yr (median)	Crude	92%
Abbatucci et al[109]	113	Not stated	5 yr	86%
Bell et al[67]	100	1.2 yr (median)	Crude	72%
Pao et al[99]	50	5.8 yr (median)	Crude	78%
Dinges et al[69]	93	Not stated	5 yr	82%
Keus et al[103]	117	7.4 yr (median)	5 yr	81%
Suit et al[110]	150	Not stated	5 yr	87%
Fein et al[111]	67	2.6 yr (median)	5 yr	87%
Mundt et al[60]	50	3.6 yr (median)	5 yr	76%
Pisters et al[106]	78	6.3 yr (median)	5 yr	82%
Cheng et al[112]	64	5.3 yr (mean)	5 yr	91%
Yang et al[108]	70	9.6 yr (median)	10 yr	98%
Pollack et al[113]	165	8.1 yr (median)	5 yr	81%

TABLE 35-6

Radiation Dose-Response Data for Microscopic Disease

Study and Reference	Median Dose	Dose Range	Dose Response
Leibel et al[95]	—	50-75 Gy	NS
Bell et al[67]*	—	24-60 Gy	NS
Pao et al[99]	60 Gy (mean)	45-69 Gy	NS
Robinson et al[118]†	—	40-75 Gy	NS
Dinges et al[69]	59 Gy	45-72 Gy	> 65 Gy
Fein et al[111]‡	60.4 Gy	39.6-71 Gy	> 62.5 Gy
Mundt et al[60]	—	50-68 Gy	> 60 Gy
Pollack et al[113]	59.4 Gy (mean)	44-75 Gy	NS

NS, No statistically significant association found.

*Fraction size varied from 2 to 8 Gy.

†Fraction size varied from 1.25 Gy twice a day to 4.4 Gy once a day.

‡Some patients received an interstitial boost of 10 to 20 Gy (median, 16 Gy).

Preoperative Radiation

The potential for smaller radiation volumes in the preoperative setting was confirmed by Nielson and colleagues,[119] who reported on a series of 26 patients who had undergone both preoperative irradiation and independent repeat simulation after undergoing definitive surgery. The target volume in the postoperative simulation included the entire surgical cavity and drain sites rather than gross tumor only, as it had in the preoperative simulation. The size of the preoperative radiation field and the number of joints included were significantly smaller than in the postoperative setting.

The potential effectiveness of a lower radiation dose also makes preoperative radiation more attractive than postoperative radiation. Although never definitively proven, the notion that tumors in surgically undisturbed tissues respond better to radiation, perhaps by virtue of their greater oxygenation, is hallowed by long tradition, going back to the work of Fletcher in the 1960s.[120] It is therefore generally accepted that 50 Gy delivered preoperatively has the same effect on microscopic tumor as 60 to 70 Gy delivered postoperatively.

Several authors have suggested that local control might be optimized through the selective use of preoperative or postoperative radiation therapy.[38,110,113,121,122] The tumor status at the time of presentation, therefore, should guide the timing of radiation therapy. We reviewed the experience of 128 patients given preoperative radiation therapy to a median dose of 50 Gy before excision or reexcision at the M.D. Anderson Cancer Center (the preoperative group) and 165 patients given postoperative radiation therapy to a median dose of 64 Gy after definitive excision (the postoperative group).[113] When comparing the 10-year rates of local control, treatment approach had no effect (82% preoperative vs. 81% postoperative); however, disease status at the time of presentation had a significant effect. For patients initially presenting with gross disease and given primary preoperative radiation therapy, the local control rate was 88% at 10 years, compared with 67% for similar patients who received postoperative radiation (*P* = 0.01). In contrast, for patients presenting at the M.D. Anderson Cancer Center after undergoing excisional biopsy elsewhere (i.e., those who had no gross disease), the 10-year local control rates favored a strategy of immediate reexcision and then radiation therapy (91% postoperative vs. 72% preoperative, *P* = 0.02). We concluded that patients presenting with gross disease were best served by preoperative therapy, whereas patients presenting after resection in which margins are positive or uncertain for disease are best treated with reresection and postoperative radiation. Several investigators have reported their experience with preoperative radiation, and local control rates are on the order of 85% (Table 35-7).*

It is not clear whether the two approaches yield any real difference in local control. However, resection margins containing tumor cells are particularly ominous for the patient treated with preoperative radiation. Tanabe and colleagues[114] reviewed 95 consecutive patients with

---

*References 38, 60, 69, 110, 112, 113, 123.

TABLE 35-7

Local Control Rates After Preoperative Radiation Therapy

Study and Reference	Number of Patients	Follow-up Time	Evaluation Period	Local Control Rate
Willet et al[123]	27	1.4 yr (mean)	Crude	100%
Barkley et al[38]	110	Not stated	Crude	90%
Suit et al[110]	160	Not stated	5 yr	92%
Dinges et al[69]	9	Not stated	5 yr	89%
Mundt et al[60]	7	3.6 yr (median)	5 yr	88%
Cheng et al[112]	48	5.3 yr (mean)	5 yr	83%
Pollack et al[113]	128	8.1 yr (median)	5 yr	82%

intermediate- or high-grade extremity STS who received preoperative radiation therapy (median dose, 50 Gy) and then limb-sparing surgery. The final microscopic margin was positive for disease in 24 patients and no additional radiation therapy was delivered. The 5-year rate of local control was 91% for margin-negative tumors and 62% for margin-positive tumors ($P = 0.005$). Multivariate analysis showed that positive surgical margins and intraoperative tumor violation independently predicted an increased risk of local failure.

No satisfactory strategy has been developed for tumors found to have positive margins at surgery after preoperative irradiation. Potential approaches include the use of intraoperative boost radiation, a brachytherapy boost, and an external-beam boost. All of these approaches suffer from the theoretical disadvantage that they represent split-course irradiation.

Eliminating radiation therapy for patients who clearly do not benefit from it is desirable, although identifying these patients is difficult. Tumor size has consistently been shown to be unrelated to the probability of local control,[39-41,59,67-69,111,114] but interest has been renewed in managing lesions less than 5 cm in largest diameter with surgery alone. In a retrospective review of 174 patients with STS of the extremity and a median follow-up time of 48 months, Geer and colleagues[100] reported that surgery alone yielded a local recurrence rate of only 11% for patients with small high-grade lesions and 7% for those with small low-grade lesions. The favorable overall 5-year survival rate of 94% for all patients and the lack of benefit from adjuvant radiation therapy or chemotherapy led the authors to conclude that small lesions should not be included in adjuvant therapy trials. In contrast, another review of patients with small high-grade extremity lesions revealed 5-year local failure and overall survival rates of 18% and 83%, respectively.[73] Because of the median follow-up time in this study (76 months), the authors stressed the importance of long-term follow-up and reemphasized the importance of adjuvant therapy. Thus it is still not clear which patients with T1 tumors can be treated effectively with conservation surgery alone; it would seem prudent to approach all such cases with combined surgery and radiation until prospective randomized trials can delin-

eate which patients can be spared the potential toxicity of combined-modality treatment.

Brachytherapy

As an alternative to external-beam radiation, brachytherapy has the advantage of delivering a high dose of radiation to a limited volume of tissue while accelerating the time in which the total dose can be delivered. Although the procedure is less expensive than external-beam irradiation[124] and the patient can usually return to "normal" activity in a relatively short period, clinical experience with this strategy is still relatively limited (Table 35-8).[106,125,126] After wide local excision and placement of metal clips to outline the areas at risk, afterloaded catheters are used to place single-plane implants of ^{192}Ir. The target volume is defined as the surgical bed plus a margin of approximately 2 cm.[107] The surgical scar and drain sites are not included. The catheters are loaded 6 or more days after surgery because wound complications increase if catheters are loaded within 5 days.[127] The minimum dose is 42 to 45 Gy delivered over 4 to 6 days. The skin dose should be kept below 20 Gy.

The target volume for brachytherapy remains a topic of controversy. It is at odds with the aim of external-beam therapy, which stresses the importance of wide radiation margins. Some brachytherapy reports have substantiated this concern. Habrand and colleagues,[125] from the Institut Gustave Roussy, reviewed the experience of 48 patients treated by iridium implantation with a 2- to 3-cm margin around the surgical bed. They reported local failure in 16 patients (33%); 14 of the failures (88%) occurred in the margins. Another concern with brachytherapy is its apparent ineffectiveness compared with external-beam radiation therapy for low-grade tumors. Prospective randomized trials will be needed to delineate the relative places of brachytherapy and teletherapy as adjuvants to the surgical resection of STSs.

The importance of local control and its relationship to overall survival remains controversial. In retrospective analyses, local recurrence has consistently been shown to be associated with an increased incidence of metastatic relapse and decreased rates of overall survival[55,78,128-130]; however, a causal relationship cannot be assumed. Local

TABLE 35-8
Surgery and Brachytherapy for Soft-Tissue Sarcoma

Study and Reference	Dose of Iridium-192	Number of Patients	Local Control Rate
Habrand et al[125]	25-72 Gy over 2-19 days* (median, 60 Gy)	48	67%
Pisters et al[106]	42-45 Gy over 4-5 days	78	82%
Chaudhary et al[126]	29-50 Gy (median, 30 Gy)	33	75%

*Dose range included four patients receiving external-beam radiation therapy.

recurrence may simply represent aggressive disease, with distant metastases occurring at the time of initial presentation rather than at the time of local recurrence. The NCI and Memorial Sloan-Kettering Cancer Center randomized trials discussed above showed statistically different local control rates without differences in overall survival. Although these trials suggested a lack of survival benefit through improved local control, their power was insufficient to prove no difference.

Several retrospective studies have attempted to address this controversy further. Gustafson and colleagues[131] reviewed the experience of 375 patients with STS of the extremity and trunk wall. Of the 128 patients who developed distant metastases, 63 had local failure and 65 did not. The timing of the metastases and the distribution of clinicopathologic factors were similar in the two groups, supporting the conclusion that local control was of minor importance as a determinant of metastatic failure. Similarly, Heslin and colleagues[132] reviewed 168 patients with primary, high-grade, deep, and large (≥ 5 cm) extremity STS. There were 21 (13%) local recurrences. The time to the development of distant metastases from the date of initial presentation was no different for patients with and without local failure.

Further elucidation of this problem awaits additional study, perhaps using local recurrence as a time-dependent variable in a multivariate regression analysis.[106,129,130] Although the influence of local recurrence on metastatic outcome remains uncertain, the importance of local control should not be underestimated. At the very least, local control secures the primary site, avoiding further potentially debilitating local treatment; it also might have a salutary effect on metastatic dissemination.

RADIATION THERAPY TECHNIQUES

Radiation therapy techniques for STSs vary depending on the location and size of the tumor and on the extent of prior surgery. The diversity in clinical situations encountered with these tumors requires a corresponding diversity in technical approaches, which can include the use of photons, electrons, compensating filters, wedge filters, three-dimensional treatment planning, intensity-modulated radiation therapy, and brachytherapy, all supplemented by a variety of positioning and immobilization devices. In the face of this technical diversity, the choice of an appropriate approach for an individual patient can be perplexing because no data demonstrate the superiority of one technique over another. Treatment planning is, therefore, based on general principles applicable to most clinical situations.

Postoperative external-beam radiation will be considered first. Treatment should not begin before the surgical wound has healed completely and usually commences 4 to 6 weeks after the operation.

Volume Considerations

The requisite postoperative radiation volume remains controversial, but it is universally accepted that the surgical bed plus a variable margin judged to be at risk of harboring occult tumor should constitute the treatment volume.

Controversy surrounds the optimal width for this margin of normal tissue. Traditionally, margins of 5 to 7 cm for most tumors,[56] or 5 to 10 cm for small lesions and 10 to 15 cm for large lesions,[110,122,133] have been recommended. Few studies report the outcome according to radiation margin; two reports found that margins exceeding 5 cm were superior to narrower ones, but that margins greater than 10 cm were not apparently beneficial.[60,99] Thus we usually use a 5-to 7-cm margin, as originally proposed by Lindberg.[56]

The radiation margin referred to is in the direction of the involved muscle compartment—the direction of potential spread of sarcoma—not in a direction perpendicular to it. For extremity sarcomas, this is the longitudinal direction, parallel to the limb. The radiation margin perpendicular to the path of least resistance is usually 2 to 3 cm, and it could hardly be larger without treating the whole circumference of the extremity. Drain holes and surgical scars are usually included in the radiation volume. For sarcomas at sites other than an extremity, these margin recommendations often cannot be achieved and lesser margins are used.

The need for large radiation volumes, particularly the need to treat scars and drain holes, has been called into question by proponents of brachytherapy, who typically treat a 2- to 3-cm proximal-distal, 1- to 2-cm lateral, and 1.5- to 3-cm thick volume without irradiating the scar or drain holes.[106,107] It is possible that the phenomenon of marginal recurrence has been overemphasized; in our experience, only about 20% of local recurrences are at the edge of or just beyond the radiation field.[39-41] Nevertheless, until this issue is resolved, we continue to recommend the modest 5- to 7-cm longitudinal margin.

Diagnostic imaging, by means of either MRI or CT scan both before and after surgery, is crucial to the delineation of an appropriate target volume. Further, a radiation therapy planning CT scan is indispensable in most situations, and centers that cannot perform such scans should not be irradiating patients who have STS.

General principles and some data[102,134] dictate consideration of the following issues regarding radiation volume. The whole circumference of an extremity should never be treated to more than 50 Gy, and a generous strip of unirradiated tissue should remain to allow lymphatic drainage. At least half the cross section of a weight-bearing bone should be spared, if possible, and the entire cavity of a major joint should be irradiated only if absolutely necessary. Likewise, attempts should be made to spare major tendons, such as the patellar and Achilles tendons. Finally, organ tolerance must be respected when irradiating intrathoracic or retroperitoneal STSs. Lesions of the hand and foot can be irradiated with an acceptable outcome if attention is paid to technical details.[135]

Dose

Having defined the radiation volume, attention turns to the selection of an appropriate dose. This too is controversial. As summarized in Table 35-6, no agreement has been reached on a dose-response relation within the range of 60 to 70 Gy, but most authors recommend a total dose of at least 60 Gy. Our current practice, based more on general principles than on unequivocal data, calls for postoperative radiation of 60 Gy at 2 Gy/fraction for tumors with margins negative for microscopic disease; when the resection margin is positive, the dose is raised to 64 to 66 Gy.

To minimize the risk of complications, a shrinking-field approach is used: The initial large volume is treated to 50 Gy; the next 10 Gy is given in an area of "conedown" to the surgical bed (outlined by surgical clips or defined by the scar), plus a 1- to 2-cm margin. If a further boost is given, it is usually directed to the tumor bed itself. The definition of radiation volume for preoperative radiation proceeds along the same lines. We recommend the same 5- to 7-cm margin longitudinally and a 2- to 30-cm margin laterally. The dose for preoperative radiation is 50 Gy at 2 Gy/fraction, and no field reductions are made routinely.[110,113] Once the volume and dose are decided upon, detailed planning proceeds to delineate patient positioning, immobilization, and beam geometry.

Most tumors arising in an extremity can be irradiated by using parallel opposed beams, with the extremity suitably positioned and with the use of custom blocking (Figs. 35-1 and 35-2). In general, extremity lesions are best treated with 4- to 6-MeV photon beams, supplemented by electron field boosts as appropriate. The use of high-energy beams might be appropriate, but care

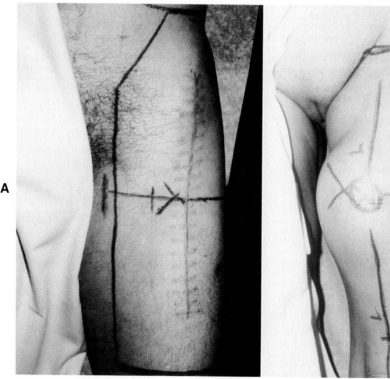

Fig. 35-1 Radiation therapy fields used for treatment of thigh soft-tissue sarcoma. **A,** A 53-year-old man underwent wide local excision in December 1980 for a 9 × 7 × 4-cm tumor within the proximal rectus femoris muscle. Pathologic examination confirmed malignant fibrous histiocytoma and resection margins negative for disease. Parallel opposed anteriorly weighted 6-MV photon fields were used to deliver 50 Gy over 5 weeks. An additional 10 Gy was given through an appositional electron beam over the scar and surgical bed. The patient was alive with no evidence of disease as of January 1998. **B,** A 75-year-old woman underwent incisional biopsy of a rapidly enlarging medial thigh mass in March 1984. Pathologic examination confirmed malignant fibrous histiocytoma. After seven cycles of cisplatin, vindesine, dacarbazine, and doxorubicin chemotherapy, preoperative radiation was delivered to a dose of 50 Gy over 5 weeks using opposed oblique fields of 6-MV photons. The leg was abducted, laterally rotated, and flexed during treatment.

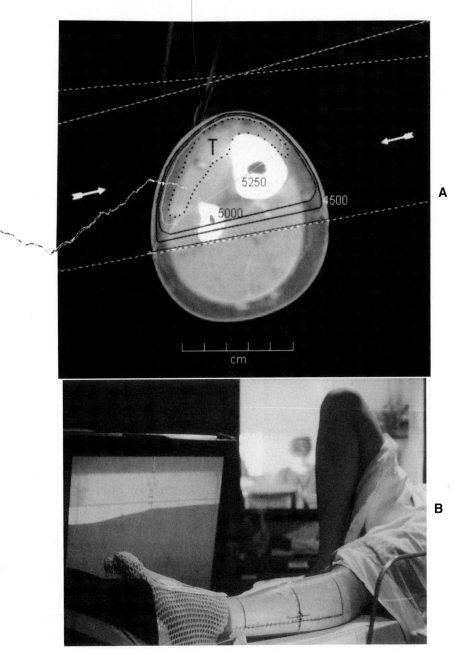

Fig. 35-2 A 24-year-old woman underwent excisional biopsy at a referring institution in November 1999 for a slowly enlarging mass measuring 4 × 5 cm located anterior to the left tibia. Pathologic examination confirmed epithelioid sarcoma. Physical and radiologic examination revealed gross residual disease measuring 1.5 × 2 cm. **A,** Preoperative radiation was delivered to a dose of 50 Gy over 5 weeks using left posterior and right anterior oblique fields of ^{60}Co without wedges. **B,** The patient was positioned to avoid irradiation of the contralateral leg. Immobilization and a three-point laser line set-up were used for daily reproducibility.

must be taken not to underdose superficial regions. In this regard, we still find the cobalt beam useful for lesions of the hands and feet and for superficially located lesions. The upper extremity is often best treated in an abducted position so that it is away from the trunk, but such a set-up can prevent the performance of a planning CT scan in the treatment position. Lesions of the upper inner thigh are best treated with the extremity in a "frog-leg" position so that the radiation is directed away from the contralateral thigh and the genitalia. Lesions of the buttock or posterior thigh are best approached with the patient in a prone position and with a wedge-pair field arrangement. Superficial trunk lesions can be treated using a pair of tangents or an appositional electron beam.

Retroperitoneal tumors pose a significant therapeutic problem, and the utility of radiation is questionable. We prefer preoperative irradiation because the maximum dose achievable rarely exceeds 50.4 Gy (1.8 Gy/fraction). Parallel opposed fields, often oblique, commonly cover the lesion while sparing adjacent organs. Occasionally a more complex set-up is necessary, and three-dimensional conformal techniques may be valuable. In any event, the radiation margin for these tumors tends to be smaller than that for extremity tumors. The deep location of these tumors dictates the use of high-energy photons (10 to 20 MV).

Lesions of the head and neck are often amenable to three-dimensional or intensity-modulated therapy because their daily set-up is highly reproducible and radiation volumes tend to be small. These volumes must be defined sharply to avoid critical structures. Similar high-precision techniques are indispensable for paravertebral tumors.

The technique of brachytherapy involves the placement of a single-plane implant in the surgical bed.[107,136-138] After excision of the tumor, the surgical bed is outlined with radio-opaque clips, and brachytherapy afterloading parallel catheters, spaced 1 cm apart, are inserted percutaneously into the target site. Orthogonal radiographs provide three-dimensional data for calculating the prescribed dose, which is specified at 1 cm from the plane of the implant. For adjuvant irradiation with brachytherapy alone, a dose of 45 to 50 Gy over 4 to 6 days is commonly prescribed.[107,136] The catheters are not loaded with radionuclide until at least the sixth day after surgery to allow some wound healing and thereby reduce the risk of wound complications.[127]

COMPLICATIONS

A variety of complications can follow the use of combined surgery and radiation. Among the complications that might occur are fibrosis and induration, wound breakdown, decreased range of joint motion, edema, cutaneous telangiectasia, joint contracture, cutaneous ulceration, peripheral neuropathy, osteonecrosis, bone fracture, and various internal organ dysfunctions, depending on the treatment site. Attributing complications to radiation or to surgery is difficult because both modalities can contribute to the genesis of any particular sequela. In practice, complications developing months or years after treatment are ascribed to radiation. Significant late complications—requiring surgical management or interfering with function—occur in 8% to 15% of patients irradiated postoperatively.[39-41,56,61,67,111] Most complications are evident by 5 years, but a small proportion occur beyond this time.[39,135]

Patients should be counseled that an irradiated area remains at risk for complications indefinitely and that activities that pose a significant risk of trauma to the treated site need to be avoided. Although it has been difficult to prove, the incidence of radiation complications seems to correlate with dose and volume irradiated and with anatomic site treated. Doses exceeding 65 Gy seem to increase complications,[55,134] as do radiation field sizes exceeding 35 cm.[134]

Irradiating the whole circumference of an extremity to doses beyond 50 Gy is fraught with risks. One study reported that 6 of 18 patients in whom the whole circumference of an extremity was irradiated required amputation because of severe complications, including edema.[102] It is also well documented that the distal lower extremity tolerates treatment less well than does the upper extremity. In our experience with patients treated for STS of the distal extremities, the overall incidence of complications was higher for those with tumors of the foot and ankle; 2 of 33 patients underwent amputation in one series we studied, whereas no patients with a tumor of the wrist or hand required amputation because of a complication.[135]

As indicated earlier, treatment planning should aim for the following features to minimize the risk of complications: A generous strip of tissue should be spared to avoid irradiating the whole circumference of an extremity; at least half the cross section of a weight-bearing bone should be spared; treatment of the whole of a major joint cavity should be avoided; treatment of major tendons should be avoided; and the tolerance of other organs should be considered when treating intrathoracic, abdominal, and pelvic STSs. Physical therapy to maintain joint mobility in the face of radiation-related muscle wasting and shortening may prevent or ameliorate functional deficits.[134] Quality-of-life assessments have failed to reveal any significant differences between patients treated with amputation and those undergoing conservation surgery and radiation.[139,140] This finding probably reflects humans' remarkable ability to adjust to adversity; it is hardly plausible that life without a limb is just as good as life with one.

Radiation delivered preoperatively carries a significant risk of wound complications after surgery. Bujko and colleagues[141] reported on 202 patients treated with preoperative irradiation and conservation surgery. Of these patients, 143 were given a postoperative boost by either an interstitial implant or external-beam radiation. The overall wound complication rate was 37%: wound dehiscence occurred in 24% of patients, infection in 6%, seroma in 3.5%, skin graft breakdown in 3%, and hematoma in 0.5%. Reoperation was required in 17% of cases, and six patients (3%) required amputation as a result of wound healing problems. Multivariate analysis showed that tumor in the lower extremity, increasing patient age, and postoperative boost using an interstitial implant were predictive of increased risk of wound morbidity. The authors suggested that gentle handling of tissues during the operation, meticulous hemostasis, avoidance of closure under tension, and elimination of dead space through the use of drains and rotation flaps might decrease wound complication rates.

Retrospective analyses[112,113] and one randomized trial[142] have documented that wound complications are more common after preoperative than postoperative radiation. Our experience is typical of these differences. Only 20 of 338 patients (6%) who underwent conservation surgery at the M.D. Anderson Cancer Center with planned postoperative radiation developed significant wound complications, whereas 14 of 130 patients (25%) who received radiation first developed such complications. Evidence exists to suggest that the appropriate use of vascularized tissue transfer can reduce complication rates after preoperative irradiation.[143] Although the radiation dose and volume are smaller in preoperative irradiation than in postoperative irradiation, the incidences of late sequelae are approximately the same.[112,113]

RADIATION THERAPY ALONE

The role of radiation therapy in the management of STS has generally been that of controlling residual microscopic disease after conservation surgical resection. In a limited number of cases, however, radiation has been applied as primary therapy for gross disease, with local control reported in up to a third of patients (Table 35-9).[144-146]

Windeyer and colleagues[101] reviewed the experience of patients with fibrosarcoma, including detailed data about their clinical responses to doses of radiation ranging from 60 to 85 Gy. Among the 22 patients given radiation therapy alone for either unresectable gross primary tumors or surgical recurrences, the clinical complete response rate was 64%. An additional 5 patients (23%) had a partial response, and in 3 the disease remained unchanged. Among the 14 patients achieving a complete response, 6 developed subsequent recurrence.

Tepper and Suit[144] studied 51 patients treated for gross disease after tumor biopsy or postsurgical tumor recurrence. The 5-year overall survival and local control rates were 25% and 33%, respectively. For the 36 patients treated with doses greater than 64 Gy, the local control rate was 43%. The trend was toward better local control when the lesions were smaller than 5 cm (87%) than it was when they measured 5 to 10 cm (53%) or were larger than 10 cm (30%).

Similar results were reported by Slater and colleagues[146] in a review of 72 patients treated with photons alone (57 patients) or photons combined with neutrons (15 patients). The overall 5-year local control rate was 29%, although control was obtained in 11 (42%) of the 27 patients treated with doses of 65 Gy or higher. In addition, the median duration of local control was 21 months in the group given doses higher than 65 Gy as compared with 13 months in the group given lower doses. Thus definitive radiation therapy may have a role in patients with distant metastases for whom the only alternative means of controlling the primary tumor would be radical amputation.

CHEMOTHERAPY

Although the need for effective systemic therapy for patients with high-grade large STSs is evident, the role of adjuvant chemotherapy in the management of localized STS remains controversial.[147,148] Numerous trials have compared doxorubicin chemotherapy alone with observation (Table 35-10)[149-158] or have compared combination chemotherapy with observation (Table 35-11).[159-168] The results of these trials are mixed, and the trials have been subject to much criticism because of small patient numbers, long accrual times, and high ineligibility rates. In addition, the patients included often had cancer of mixed histologic subtypes or grades and tumor locations.

In an effort to overcome these limitations, Zalupski and colleagues[169] performed a meta-analysis of the published data, finding that disease-free and overall survival at 10 years were improved by the use of doxorubicin-based chemotherapy. The analysis was subsequently repeated[170] using the raw patient data updated by the individual investigators of each trial. This meta-analysis included 1568 patients from 14 trials, with a median follow-up time of 9.4 years. Adjuvant chemotherapy was found to significantly improve both local relapse-free survival rate (81% vs. 75%, $P = 0.016$) and recurrence-free survival rate (55% vs. 45%, $P = 0.0001$). However, the use of adjuvant chemotherapy conferred no improvement in overall survival (54% vs. 50%, $P = 0.12$).

The results of any meta-analysis, however, must be interpreted with caution because they can only be as good as the results of the individual trials included.[147] For example, in this large meta-analysis, tumor histologic subtype and grade were reviewed in only 59% and 25% of patients, respectively.[170] In addition, both the European Organization for Research and Treatment of Cancer (EORTC)[161] and the Scandinavian Sarcoma Group (SSG)[154] trials, two of the largest, had poor patient compliance with chemotherapy and very high rates of patient ineligibility. Finally, because the majority of patients' tumors (58%) were located in an extremity and because patients with recurrent disease were excluded, it is unclear whether the results can be applied to nonextremity sarcomas or to patients presenting with recurrent disease.

TABLE 35-9

Local Control of Gross Disease with Radiation Therapy Alone

Study and Reference	Number of Patients	Local Control Rate
Tepper and Suit[144]	51	33%
Dewer et al[145]	25	20%
Slater et al[146]	72	29%

TABLE 35-10

Trials Comparing Adjuvant Doxorubicin to Observation for Resectable Soft-Tissue Sarcomas

Study and Reference	N	Median Follow-up Time (Months)	Treatment	Local–Regional Control Rate	Disease-Free Survival Rate	Overall Survival Rate	Sites
IGSC[149-153]	80	54	450 mg/m^2 doxorubicin (cumulative dose)	—	67%	68%	All
	88		Observation	—	59%	62%	
Scandinavian Sarcoma Group[154]	77	40	60 mg/m^2 doxorubicin q4wk for 9 cycles	92%	62%	75%	All
	77		Observation	92%	56%	70%	
Rizzoli (Bologna)[155,156]	24	27.6	450 mg/m^2 doxorubicin (cumulative dose)	96%	79%*	—	Ext
	35		Observation	91%	54%	—	
UCLA[157]	57	28	90 mg/m^2 doxorubicin for 5 cycles	96%	58%	84%	Ext
	62		Observation	89%	54%	80%	
Gynecologic Oncology Group[158]	75	—	60 mg/m^2 doxorubicin q3wk for 8 cycles	—	59%	60%	Uterine
	81		Observation	—	47%	52%	

IGSC, Intergroup Sarcoma Study Group; *UCLA*, University of California-Los Angeles; *Ext*, extremity.
*$P < 0.05$.

The meta-analysis did confirm that local control can be improved through the use of systemic chemotherapy (27% reduction in the risk of local recurrence, absolute benefit 6%). The NCI trial[164,165] and the EORTC trial[161] had shown improvements in local control resulting from doxorubicin alone and combination chemotherapy, respectively (details of the combination therapy are given in Table 35-11). Within the EORTC trial, however, the benefit was limited to head, neck, and trunk lesions, whereas only extremity lesions were included in the NCI trial. These findings suggest that the combination of chemotherapy and radiation deserves investigation as a strategy to improve local control.

The only completed trial examining modern chemotherapy for STS in an appropriately high-risk cohort of patients was conducted by the Italian Cooperative Group trial (Rizzoli [Bologna], see Table 35-11); results have been published only in abstract form.[159,160] In that study, 104 patients who had localized extremity or limb girdle, high-grade (3 or 4), deeply seated, and either primary tumors larger than 5 cm or recurrent lesions of any size were randomized to observation or five cycles of epirubicin, ifosfamide, mesna, and granulocyte colony-stimulating factor. After a median follow-up time of 24 months, combination chemotherapy seemed to have improved the rates of disease-free and overall survival. Formal reports of this trial are awaited.

Given the uncertainties surrounding the effectiveness of adjuvant chemotherapy, patients with large high-grade sarcomas should be enrolled in established chemotherapy trials. At present no role has been definitively established for adjuvant chemotherapy in localized STS.

MANAGEMENT OF RECURRENT DISEASE

The management of relapsed STS is determined by the site of relapse. Isolated local recurrence is managed according to the principles outlined above. If the recurrence occurs after prior resection alone (without adjuvant radiation) and the lesion is amenable to wide local resection, this treatment should be combined with adjuvant radiation in virtually all cases. The optimal management strategy for local recurrence in patients treated with prior surgery and irradiation is unclear; further wide resection, radical soft-part resection, and amputation have all been used.[39,56,133]

Adjuvant brachytherapy seems to have a role in this setting. Two studies looked at a total of 66 patients who

TABLE 35-11

Trials Comparing Adjuvant Combination Chemotherapy to Observation for Resectable Soft-Tissue Sarcomas

Study and Reference	N	Median Follow-up Time	Treatment	Local–Regional Control Rate	Disease-Free Survival Rate	Overall Survival Rate	Sites
Rizzoli (Bologna)[159,160]	53	24 mo	Epirubicin, ifosfamide, mesna, G-CSF	—	64%*	83%*	Ext
	51		Observation	—	45%	65%	
EORTC[161]	145	80 mo	CyVADIC for 8 cycles	83%*†	56%*	63%	All
	172		Observation	69%	43%	56%	
Foundation Bergonie (Bordeaux)[162]	31	52.4 mo	CyVADIC for 9 cycles	97%	87%*	87%*	All
	28		Observation	82%	54%	37%	
M.D. Anderson Cancer Center[163]	20	120 mo	VAC-VAdC	90%	55%*	65%	Ext
	23		Observation	65%	35%	57%	
NCI-Extremity[164,165]	37	7.1 yr	AC-MTX	97%*	75%*	82%	
	28		Observation	86%	54%	60%	
NCI-Head & Neck, Breast, and Trunk[166]	17	35 mo	AC-MTX	—	77%	68%	
	14		Observation	—	49%	58%	
NCI-Retroperitoneum[167]	8	29 mo	AC-MTX	—	50%	47%	
	7		Observation	—	86%	100%	
Mayo[168]	30	64.3 mo	VADIC/VAdC	53%	88%	82%	All
	31		Observation	52%	68%	82%	

EORTC, European Organization for the Research and Treatment of Cancer; *NCI*, National Cancer Institute; *G-CSF*, granulocyte colony-stimulating factor; *A*, Adriamycin (doxorubicin); *V*, vincristine; *Ad*, actinomycin D; *Cy* and *C*, cyclophosphamide; *MTX*, methotrexate; *DIC*, dacarbazine; *Ext*, extremity.

*$P < 0.05$.

†Reduction in local recurrence was significant in head, neck, and trunk soft-tissue sarcomas only.

had isolated local recurrences after surgery and external-beam radiation to doses of 45 to 70 Gy; they reported that re-resection plus interstitial irradiation to doses of 45 to 50 Gy achieved local control in 68%[138] and 52%[137] of patients, with an acceptable incidence of complications. Patients who develop metastatic relapse are generally given chemotherapy, but their long-term survival rate is poor (approximately 10% at 10 years after metastatic relapse[39]). Nevertheless, there is a role for resection of metastases (metastasectomy) in select situations, especially in patients who have isolated lung metastases, for whom a 3-year survival rate of 40% after resection has been reported.[46]

SPECIAL ANATOMIC SITES

At many sites, including the retroperitoneum, head and neck, and hand and foot, anatomic constraints often preclude wide local excision, and the tolerance of normal structures often limits the delivery of appropriate doses of radiation. For STS arising in these locations, local control remains a formidable challenge.

Retroperitoneum

Retroperitoneal STSs are distinguished by bulky presentation, fixation to vital structures, and local recurrence, even after complete surgical resection (Fig. 35-3). The predominant histologic subtype is liposarcoma; leiomyosarcoma is the second most common histologic subtype, and other subtypes also have been described.[62,167,171] At the time of surgical resection, only 55% of patients will be found to have grossly resectable disease, and of these, 80% will require the removal of adjacent organs; in some 25% debulking resection is possible, and in approximately 20% the tumor will be deemed unresectable.[62,70,167,171]

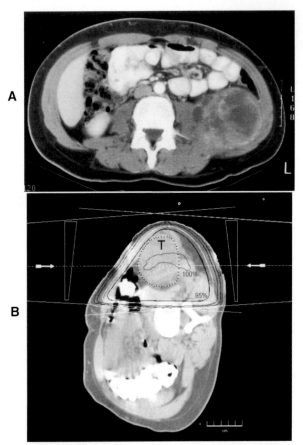

Fig. 35-3 A 28-year-old woman with neurofibromatosis developed left flank pain in May 1998 and was found to have a large retroperitoneal mass displacing the kidney. Pathologic examination of a computed tomography (CT)–guided fine-needle aspiration biopsy specimen confirmed high-grade neurogenic sarcoma. **A,** Diagnostic CT scan showing an 8 × 8-cm retroperitoneal mass with areas of enhancement and necrosis. **B,** The simulation and the treatment were done with the patient in the left lateral decubitus position to spare as much bowel as possible. Using lateral parallel opposed 6-MV photon fields, a tumor dose of 50 Gy was delivered over 5 weeks before surgery, with concurrent doxorubicin chemotherapy. Complete surgical resection was followed by 15 Gy intraoperative electron-beam radiation therapy. The patient was alive with bone metastases in the sacrum at the most recent follow-up.

The extent of surgical resection remains the most important predictor of long-term survival. Patients undergoing complete gross resection have a 10-year survival rate of approximately 45%, compared with an 8% survival for patients in whom only debulking is possible.[62,171] Further, patients in whom partial resection is achieved have a 5-year survival rate of approximately 25%, compared with a 9% survival rate among those in whom no resection is done.[62] It is unclear whether these results reflect a true benefit of resection or merely pathobiological features that favor resectability.

Even after complete gross resection, local recurrence is common, occurring in up to 90% of patients if they survive to 10 years.[62] The use of adjuvant radiation therapy has met with limited success in improving local control. Fein and colleagues[115] reviewed the experience of 21 patients treated with surgical resection and radiation. Only one patient had surgical margins that were microscopically negative for disease. The mean radiation dose was 54 Gy. The 2-year rates of local control and overall survival were 72% and 69%, respectively. Local control seemed to be improved by doses greater than 55.2 Gy. Tepper and colleagues[71] similarly reported a modest dose-related response, with improvements in local control seen for doses greater than 60 Gy. Local control might also be improved through the use of an intraoperative radiation therapy boost. In another randomized trial from the NCI,[116] 35 patients with resected retroperitoneal STS were randomized to undergo 20 Gy as an intraoperative boost in combination with 35 to 40 Gy postoperative external-beam radiation therapy (15 patients) or 50 to 55 Gy postoperative external-beam radiation therapy alone. After a median follow-up time of 8 years, the overall survival rates were similar, but local control was better in those patients given the intraoperative boost (60% vs. 20%, $P < 0.05$). However, the overall intra-abdominal relapse rates were similar in the two groups. The incidence of radiation-related peripheral neuropathy was higher in the intraoperative-boost group, but the incidence of radiation-related enteritis was lower. Efforts to improve survival through the use of adjuvant chemotherapy have been unsuccessful. In a small randomized trial reported by the NCI,[167] the 2-year actuarial survival rate was worse in eight patients given doxorubicin-based chemotherapy than in seven patients who were only observed (100% vs. 47%, $P = 0.06$). The initial treatment for all 15 patients was complete surgical resection.

Currently, most patients with retroperitoneal STS are destined to live with their disease and undergo palliative resections as dictated by their symptoms.

Head and Neck

Among STSs affecting the head and neck, the most commonly reported histologic subtype is malignant fibrous histiocytoma.[63,117,172] Overall survival consistently decreases as tumor grade increases, whereas surgical margins positive for microscopic disease are prognostic for local recurrence.[64,172,173] Although head and neck STSs are rare and heterogeneous in presentation, local control rates after conservative resection and radiation therapy have consistently been 65% to 75%.[64,117,173,174] Adjuvant radiation therapy has a significant role in the management of head and neck STSs in view of the difficulty in achieving resection margins that are free of disease. Adjuvant radiation plays a particularly important role in the management of angiosarcoma arising in the skin of the scalp.[175]

Distal Extremities

For STSs arising in the hand, wrist, foot, and ankle, anatomic constraints make it difficult to perform wide local excision and still preserve function. In addition, there is an unsubstantiated belief that these anatomic locations tolerate radiation therapy poorly.[176] An early experience with surgical management alone for STS of the hand and foot resulted in local failure in only 7 of 50 patients (14%); however, radical or limited amputation was required in 74% to achieve this result.[176] Five of the seven local failures occurred in the patients who underwent wide local excision alone. This high amputation rate contrasts with the 24% rate reported by Talbert and colleagues[135] after conservative surgery and radiation therapy in 78 patients with wrist, hand, ankle, or foot STSs. Reasons for amputation included salvage after

recurrent disease in 13 patients and complications in 6. After a median follow-up time of 7.9 years, the actuarial 5- and 10-year local control rates were 80% and 74%, respectively. The 69% overall survival rate at 10 years compared favorably to that obtained using radical surgery, yet a normal or fairly normal extremity was retained in more than two thirds of patients. Clearly, amputation will be necessary to treat a small percentage of primary distal extremity STS; however, a conservative approach has been shown to be successful in most cases.

When irradiating the hand or foot, one must be aware of the unusual acute radiation reaction that can affect the palm or sole; in our experience, patients often develop an edematous, painful, and erythematous response by the fifth week (Fig. 35-4). Although uncomfortable and alarming, this reaction heals within approximately

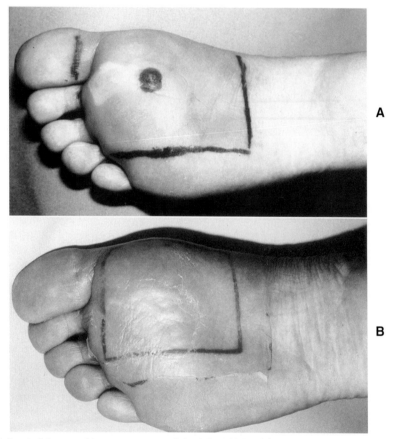

A

B

Fig. 35-4 A 24-year-old man presented in July 1983 with an 8-year history of a slowly enlarging lesion on the plantar aspect of the right foot. Physical examination revealed a 4.5 × 3-cm mass. Pathologic examination of an excisional biopsy specimen confirmed extraosseous Ewing's sarcoma. He received two courses of chemotherapy (cyclophosphamide, vincristine, doxorubicin, and dacarbazine) and was then referred for radiation therapy. **A,** The patient was positioned prone with his foot on a pillow. A single appositional 12-MeV electron beam delivered 50 Gy over 5 weeks, with a small margin around the primary tumor. An additional 10 Gy was delivered using 9-MeV electrons. The dose was prescribed to the 90% isodose line, and skin dose was maximized through the use of wax bolus. **B,** After delivery of 50 Gy, significant erythema and blistering was apparent. It resolved completely within 1 month. No evidence of disease was present as of January 1994.

1 month, and its development is probably related to the unusual anatomic tethering of skin to underlying tissue in these locations.

SELECTED TUMOR TYPES

The following section describes the more common variants of STS and those of special interest to radiation oncologists.

Malignant Fibrous Histiocytoma

MFH is now the most commonly diagnosed STS. The term represents a pleomorphic high-grade STS characterized microscopically by plump spindle cells arranged in a cartwheel or storiform pattern around slit-like vessels (Fig. 35-5).[5,177] Although numerous histologic subtypes of MFH have been described, only myxoid change, characteristic of myxoid MFH, seems to be of prognostic value. Myxoid MFH is categorized as intermediate grade; other variants (storiform-pleomorphic, giant-cell, and inflammatory) are considered high grade.[22] Zagars and colleagues[39] reviewed the experience of 271 patients with MFH treated with conservative surgery and radiation. The overall survival rates at 5, 10, and 15 years of 68%, 60%, and 46%, respectively, were similar to those reported by others.[178,179]

Determinants of metastatic relapse and overall survival were histologic variant (myxoid vs. nonmyxoid) and tumor size. The 10-year overall survival and metastatic relapse rates were 75% and 13%, respectively, for myxoid tumors, compared with 56% and 40%, respectively, for the nonmyxoid tumors. Patients with nonmyxoid tumors larger than 5 cm in diameter fared significantly worse than those with tumors measuring 5 cm or less. In contrast, a 10-cm diameter seemed to be a better discriminator of metastatic potential within the myxoid variants. The 10-year metastatic rate for myxoid tumors larger than 10 cm was 44%, compared with 8% for smaller lesions.

Adverse determinants of local control included prior local recurrence (42% of those with a prior local recurrence experienced another one vs. 22% of patients in whom no prior local recurrence had occurred; $P < 0.01$) and margins microscopically positive for disease (39% of patients with positive margins experienced local failure vs. 17% of others; $P = 0.01$). Tumor site (extremity vs. nonextremity), location (distal vs. proximal), size ($\leq$ 5 cm vs. > 5 cm), and histologic variant (myxoid vs. nonmyxoid) were not associated with the likelihood of local control. Thus it is important to distinguish the myxoid variant from its much more common nonmyxoid counterpart. Both subtypes are equally aggressive locally, but myxoid MFH has significantly less metastatic potential than the nonmyxoid variant.

Synovial Sarcoma

Synovial sarcoma is a high-grade STS characterized by a predilection for the para-articular regions of the extremities in adolescents and young adults. It often presents in close association with tendon sheaths, bursae, and joint capsules, although it does not arise from synovial structures.[5] Microscopically, distinct epithelial and spindle-cell components can be seen in varying proportions. This pattern creates a morphologic spectrum between two histologic variants, biphasic and monophasic synovial sarcoma. Further subclassification into biphasic, monophasic fibrous, monophasic epithelial, and poorly differentiated synovial sarcoma has been described,[5] although the prognostic value of these distinctions has been questioned.[22]

In a study of 85 patients who had synovial sarcoma treated with conservative resection and radiation, Mullen and Zagars[41] reported 5-, 10-, and 15-year overall survival rates of 76%, 63%, and 57%, respectively. The 10-year metastasis rate was 48%, with mortality resulting almost entirely from metastatic relapse. Multivariate analysis showed that small tumor size, young patient age ($\leq$ 20 years), and female sex independently predicted favorable overall survival. As has been described by others,[180] the survival probability correlated particularly closely with tumor size. The distinction of biphasic versus monophasic histology was not a significant determinant of outcome. Ten-year survival rates showed a clear relationship to tumor size (for lesions $\leq$ 2 cm, the 10-year survival rate was 90%; for tumors > 2 but $\leq$ 5 cm in diameter, the rate was 72%; for those > 5 but $\leq$ 10 cm across, the rate was 57%; and for those > 10 cm in diameter, the rate was 15% [$P < 0.0001$]). Adjuvant chemotherapy was not shown to affect overall

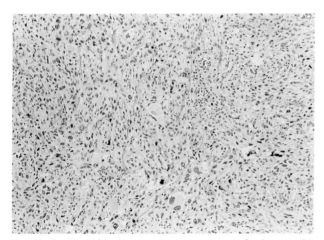

Fig. 35-5 Typical microscopic appearance of pleomorphic malignant fibrous histiocytoma (×100). This is often characterized by a storiform pattern and a mixture of bizarre-appearing plump fibroblastic cells, giant cells containing multiple hyperchromatic irregular nuclei, and increased mitotic activity. (Courtesy A.K. Raymond, M.D.)

survival favorably; however, the high metastatic propensity highlights the need for effective systemic therapy. The 5- and 10-year local control rates of 14% and 20%, respectively, were comparable to those reported by others.[181]

Liposarcoma

The pathobiological characteristics of liposarcoma are variable, ranging from low-grade, nonmetastasizing to highly aggressive ones with a propensity for local and metastatic recurrence. Behavior can be judged by the microscopic appearance of the primary by estimating the degree of differentiation.[182] Enzinger and Weiss[5] suggested a five-tiered classification system; that system was subsequently modified by Evans[183] to three histologic variants with distinct clinical behaviors: (a) the low-grade well-differentiated liposarcoma (also known as atypical lipomatous tumor), (b) the intermediate-grade myxoid liposarcoma, and (c) the high-grade pleomorphic liposarcoma. A fourth variant known as dedifferentiated liposarcoma represents the coexistence of well-differentiated liposarcoma with a poorly differentiated, nonlipogenic spindle-cell element (usually MFH) within the same neoplasm. This variant usually occurs in the setting of multiply recurrent well-differentiated liposarcoma and is included in the high-grade category because of its metastatic potential.[183]

Liposarcoma commonly occurs in the thigh and retroperitoneum, although the tumor can arise anywhere. Certain histologic variants seem to have a predilection for specific anatomic locations: myxoid liposarcoma and pleomorphic sarcoma arise within the upper thigh, whereas well-differentiated and dedifferentiated liposarcoma arise within the retroperitoneum.[40,183] Myxoid liposarcoma has an unusual proclivity for soft tissue (particularly retroperitoneal) rather than pulmonary metastases.[40,183,184] This histologic variant is also uniformly associated with the t(12;16) chromosome translocation.[185] Liposarcoma is one of the few STSs that has not been reported as a radiation-induced sarcoma.[5] A review of our experience with conservative surgery and radiation therapy in 112 patients who had liposarcoma confirmed its wide spectrum of clinical behavior. The overall survival rates at 5, 10, and 15 years were 79%, 69%, and 61%, respectively, but survival was highly dependent on histologic variant. The actuarial 10-year overall survival rates for the well-differentiated, myxoid, and pleomorphic variants were 87%, 76%, and 39%, respectively; the rates of metastasis in these same groups were 0%, 22%, and 41%, respectively. In multivariate analysis, factors predictive of decreased overall survival were pleomorphic histologic variant (vs. myxoid) and tumor size greater than 5 cm. In contrast to other STS, for which local control seems to be independent of histologic variant, the subcategory of liposarcoma type seems to predict the probability of local control.[40,184] We found a local recurrence rate of 37% for patients who had pleomorphic liposarcomas, in contrast to 8% and 7% for those who had the well-differentiated and myxoid variants, respectively.[40]

Desmoid Tumor

Desmoid tumor, also known as aggressive fibromatosis, is a locally invasive tumor with no metastatic potential. Microscopically, these tumors are characterized by spindle-shaped cells in a collagenous matrix lacking the pleomorphic, atypical, or hyperchromatic nuclei of malignancy (Fig. 35-6).[5] One of the major determinants of local control after surgical management is the status of the resection margins.[186-189] In a review of 118 patients from our institution,[190] a local recurrence rate of 54% was attained by surgery alone when the microscopic margins contained cancer cells; local recurrences dropped to 27% if the resection margins were negative for disease ($P = 0.003$). In a second group of 46 patients whose desmoid tumors were managed with gross total resection and radiation therapy, the prognostic significance of microscopically positive margins was lost. Postsurgical treatment recommendations are observation in cases of completely resected disease and radiation to 50 Gy in cases of microscopic residual disease. In certain situations in which recurrence might compromise functional and cosmetic outcome, postoperative radiation therapy is recommended regardless of the margin status. In a separate analysis of 23 patients[191] treated for gross disease with radiation alone, the rate of local control was 69%, comparable to that reported by others.[189,192,193] Our data suggested a modest dose-related response for doses greater than 50 Gy. Beyond doses of 56 Gy, complications increased significantly, prompting our final recommendation of 56 Gy for control of gross disease.[191]

Dermatofibrosarcoma Protuberans

Dermatofibrosarcoma protuberans is an uncommon, low-grade cutaneous STS characterized by aggressive local behavior but little metastatic potential. Microscopically, the tumor may be recognized by slender fibroblasts arranged in a storiform pattern.[5] Similar to the desmoid, dermatofibrosarcoma protuberans tumors are locally infiltrative, with control determined primarily by the adequacy of the surgical resection. Wide local resection with at least a 3-cm margin, including the underlying fascia, has generally been the recommended treatment.[194] Local recurrence rates of 10% to 20%, however, can still be expected.[195-197] Mohs micrographic surgical excision has been associated with a less than 10% rate of recurrence,[198] but it is labor-intensive,

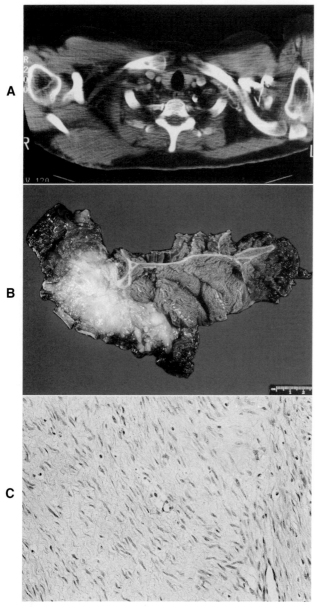

Fig. 35-6 A 38-year-old man presented in August 1995 with a right posterior shoulder mass that had enlarged slowly over a 5-year time span. **A,** Computed tomography scan (shown) and magnetic resonance imaging scan revealed a 7.5 × 7.5 × 3.5-cm mass arising from the musculature of the right upper back, with invasion of the supraspinatus muscle and subcutaneous fatty tissue. No definite bone abnormality was noted. **B,** Grossly the tumor abutted the scapula, and resection required near total scapulectomy. The tumor had a firm consistency and a coarsely trabecular appearance when sectioned. **C,** Pathologic examination revealed elongated slender spindle-shaped cells of uniform appearance and abundant surrounding collagen consistent with desmoid tumor (×200). Microscopically no bone invasion was seen, however; margins were close and postoperative radiation therapy was recommended. Oblique parallel opposed 6-MV photon fields were used to deliver 50 Gy over 5 weeks. No evidence of disease was present as of September 1999. (**C** Courtesy A.K. Raymond, M.D.)

results in significant tissue defects, and is difficult to perform on larger or recurrent lesions.

More limited surgical resection combined with radiation therapy may be used when complete surgical resection of the lesion would be difficult. Ballo and colleagues[198] reported only one local recurrence among 19 patients, 10 of whom had already experienced at least one prior recurrence and 6 of whom had positive microscopic margins. Suit and colleagues[199] reported three local recurrences among 15 patients, 5 of whom had experienced prior relapse and 12 of whom had positive microscopic margins.

Current recommendations are complete resection plus observation if margins are negative and radiation therapy of 50 to 60 Gy if the margins are close (< 2 to 3 cm) or positive for disease. Adjuvant radiation therapy also may be indicated in situations where complete resection would entail significant cosmetic or functional deficits.

Hemangiopericytoma

Hemangiopericytoma is an uncommon STS derived from vascular pericytes[5] that is of interest to radiation oncologists by virtue of its radiosensitivity. These tumors most commonly arise in the pelvis, thigh, or head and neck.[200-202] They are highly vascular, like glomus tumors. Histologic grading is difficult, but a high mitosis rate seems to correlate with metastatic potential. Highly mitotic tumors are associated with a less than 50% 5-year survival rate.[200,201]

The radiosensitivity of hemangiopericytomas is indicated by the achievement of local control in approximately 50% of patients irradiated for gross tumor to doses of 50 to 55 Gy.[203,204] These same reports show a local control rate exceeding 90% when radiation is given as an adjuvant to resection. Radiation is indicated for unresectable disease and as an adjuvant for high-grade tumors. In the adjuvant setting, the high vascularity of these tumors suggests that preoperative radiation might be more effective than postoperative radiation; although to our knowledge, this theory has not been tested.

REFERENCES

1. Greenlee RT, Hill-Harmon MB, Murray T, et al. Cancer statistics, 2001. *CA Cancer J Clin* 2001;15-36.
2. Pollock RE, Karnell LH, Menck HR, et al. The National Cancer Data Base report on soft tissue sarcomas. *Cancer* 1996;78:2247-2257.
3. Lawrence W, Donegan WL, Natarajan N, et al. Adult soft tissue sarcomas: a pattern of care survey of the American College of Surgeons. *Ann Surg* 1987;205:349-359.
4. Rydholm A, Berg NO, Gullberg B, et al. Epidemiology of soft-tissue sarcoma in the locomotor system. *Acta Path Microbiol Immunol Scand [A]* 1984;92:363-374.
5. Enzinger FM, Weiss SW. *Soft Tissue Tumors*, 3rd ed. St. Louis, Mo: Mosby; 1995.
6. Inoshita T, Youngberg GA. Malignant fibrous histiocytoma arising in previous surgical sites: a report of two cases. *Cancer* 1984; 53:176-183.

7. Jennings TA, Peterson L, Axiotis CA, et al. Angiosarcoma associated with foreign body material: a report of three cases. *Cancer* 1988;62:2436-2444.

8. Lindeman G, McKay MJ, Taubman KL, et al. Malignant fibrous histiocytoma developing in bone 44 years after shrapnel trauma. *Cancer* 1990;66:2229-2232.

9. Stewart FW, Treves N. Lymphangiosarcoma in postmastectomy lymphedema: a report of six cases in elephantiasis chirurgica. *Cancer* 1948;1:64-81.

10. Cahan WG, Woodard HQ, Higinbotham NL, et al. Sarcoma arising in irradiated bone: report of eleven cases. *Cancer* 1948;1:3-29.

11. Robinson E, Neugut AI, Wylie P. Clinical aspects of postirradiation sarcomas. *J Natl Cancer Inst* 1988;80:233-240.

12. Laskin WB, Silverman TA, Enzinger FM. Postirradiation soft tissue sarcomas: an analysis of 53 cases. *Cancer* 1988;62:2330-2340.

13. Patel SG, See ACH, Williamson PA, et al. Radiation induced sarcoma of the head and neck. *Head Neck* 1999;21:346-354.

14. Hardell L, Eriksson M. The association between soft tissue sarcomas and exposure to phenoxyacetic acids: a new case-referent study. *Cancer* 1988;62:652-656.

15. Wingren G, Fredrikson M, Brage HN, et al. Soft tissue sarcoma and occupational exposure. *Cancer* 1990;66:806-811.

16. Dich J, Zahm SH, Hanberg A, et al. Pesticides and cancer. *Cancer Causes Control* 1997;8:420-443.

17. Hosoi K. Multiple neurofibromatosis (von Recklinghausen's disease) with special reference to malignant transformation. *Arch Surg* 1931;22:258-281.

18. Wong FL, Boice JD, Abramson DH, et al. Cancer incidence after retinoblastoma: radiation dose and sarcoma risk. *JAMA* 1997;278:1262-1267.

19. Li FP, Fraumeni JF. Soft-tissue sarcomas, breast cancer, and other neoplasms: a familial syndrome? *Ann Intern Med* 1969;71:747-752.

20. Li FP, Fraumeni JF, Mulvihill JJ, et al. A cancer syndrome in twenty-four kindreds. *Cancer Res* 1988;48:5358-5362.

21. Fisher C. Current aspects of the pathology of soft tissue sarcomas. *Semin Radiat Oncol* 1999;9:315-327.

22. Evans HL. Classification and grading of soft-tissue sarcomas. *Hematol Oncol Clin North Am* 1995;9:653-656.

23. Recommendations for the reporting of soft tissue sarcomas. *Mod Pathol* 1998;11:1257-1261.

24. Hajdu SI. *Pathology of Soft Tumors*. Philadelphia, Pa: Lea & Febiger; 1979.

25. Mazeron J, Suit HD. Lymph nodes as sites of metastases from sarcomas of soft tissue. *Cancer* 1987;60:1800-1808.

26. Hashimoto H, Daimaru Y, Takeshita S, et al. Prognostic significance of histologic parameters of soft tissue sarcomas. *Cancer* 1992;70:2816-2822.

27. Trojani M, Contesso G, Coindre JM, et al. Soft-tissue sarcomas of adults: study of pathological prognostic variable and definition of a histopathological grading system. *Int J Cancer* 1984;33:37-42.

28. Coindre JM, Trojani M, Contesso G, et al. Reproducibility of a histopathologic grading system for adult soft tissue sarcoma. *Cancer* 1986;58:306-309.

29. Leyvraz S, Costa J. Issues in the pathology of sarcomas of the soft tissue and bone. *Semin Oncol* 1989;16:273-280.

30. Broders AC, Hargrave R, Meyerding HW. Pathological features of soft tissue fibrosarcoma with special reference to the grading of its malignancy. *Surg Gynecol Obstet* 1939;69:267-280.

31. Costa J, Wesley RA, Glatstein E, et al. The grading of soft tissue sarcomas: results of a clinicohistolopathologic correlation in a series of 163 cases. *Cancer* 1984;53:530-541.

32. Van Unnik JAM, Coindre JM, Contesso C, et al. Grading of soft tissue sarcomas: experience of the EORTC Soft Tissue and Bone Sarcoma Group. *Eur J Cancer* 1993;29A:2089-2093.

33. Myhre-Jensen O, Kaae S, Hjollund Madsen E, et al. Histological grading in soft-tissue tumours. *Acta Path Microbiol Immunol Scand [A]* 1983;91:145-150.

34. Angervall L, Kindblom L, Rydholm A, et al. The diagnosis and prognosis of soft tissue tumors. *Semin Diagn Pathol* 1986;3:240-258.

35. Fleming ID, Cooper JS, Henson DE, et al, eds. *AJCC Cancer Staging Manual*, 5th ed. Philadelphia, Pa: Lippincott Williams & Wilkins; 1997:149-156.

36. Markhede G, Angervall L, Stener B. A multivariate analysis of the prognosis after surgical treatment of malignant soft-tissue tumors. *Cancer* 1982;49:1721-1733.

37. Guillou L, Coindre JM, Bonichon F, et al. Comparative study of the National Cancer Institute and French Federation of Cancer Centers sarcoma group grading systems in a population of 410 adult patients with soft tissue sarcoma. *J Clin Oncol* 1997;15:350-362.

38. Barkley HT, Martin RG, Romsdahl MM, et al. Treatment of soft tissue sarcomas by preoperative irradiation and conservative surgical resection. *Int J Radiat Oncol Biol Phys* 1988;14:693-699.

39. Zagars GK, Mullen JR, Pollack A. Malignant fibrous histiocytoma: outcome and prognostic factors following conservative surgery and radiotherapy. *Int J Radiat Oncol Biol Phys* 1996;34:683-694.

40. Zagars GK, Goswitz MS, Pollack A. Liposarcoma: outcome and prognostic factors following conservation surgery and radiation therapy. *Int J Radiat Oncol Biol Phys* 1996;36:311-319.

41. Mullen JR, Zagars GK. Synovial sarcoma outcome following conservation surgery and radiotherapy. *Radiother Oncol* 1994;33:23-30.

42. Pollock RE. Molecular determinants of soft tissue sarcoma proliferation. *Semin Surg Oncol* 1994;10:315-322.

43. El-Naggar AK, Ayala AG, Abdul-Karim FW, et al. Synovial sarcoma: a DNA flow cytometry study. *Cancer* 1990;65:2295-2300.

44. Pisters PWT, Pollock RE. Staging and prognostic factors in soft tissue sarcoma. *Semin Radiat Oncol* 1999;9:307-314.

45. Abbas JS, Holyoke ED, Moore R, et al. The surgical treatment and outcome of soft-tissue sarcoma. *Arch Surg* 1981;116:765-769.

46. Potter DA, Glenn J, Kinsella T, et al. Patterns of recurrence in patients with high-grade soft-tissue sarcomas. *J Clin Oncol* 1985;3:353-366.

47. Torosian MH, Friedrich C, Godbold J, et al. Soft-tissue sarcoma: initial characteristics and prognostic factors in patients with and without metastatic disease. *Semin Surg Oncol* 1988;4:13-19.

48. Enneking WF, Spanier SS, Malawer MM. The effect of the anatomic setting on the results of surgical procedures for soft parts sarcoma of the thigh. *Cancer* 1981;47:1005-1022.

49. Hunt RT, Morgan MC, Ackerman LV. Principles in the management of extra-abdominal desmoids. *Cancer* 1960;20:825-836.

50. Batsakis JG. Epithelioid sarcoma. *Ann Otol Rhinol Laryngol* 1989;98:659-660.

51. Rosai J, Sumner HW, Kostianovsky M, et al. Angiosarcoma of the skin: a clinicopathologic and fine structural study. *Hum Pathol* 1976;7:83-109.

52. Fong Y, Coit DG, Woodruff JM, et al. Lymph node metastasis from soft tissue sarcoma in adults. Analysis of data from a prospective database of 1772 sarcoma patients. *Ann Surg* 1993; 217:72-77.

53. Rydholm A, Rööser B. Surgical margins for soft-tissue sarcoma. *J Bone Joint Surg* 1987;69A:1074-1078.

54. Dewer JA, Duncan W. A retrospective study of the role of radiotherapy in treatment of soft tissue sarcoma. *Clin Radiol* 1985;36:629-632.

55. Cantin J, McNeer GP, Chu FC, et al. The problem of local recurrence after treatment of soft tissue sarcoma. *Ann Surg* 1968;168:47-53.

56. Lindberg RD, Martin RG, Romsdahl MM, et al. Conservative surgery and postoperative radiotherapy in 300 adults with soft-tissue sarcomas. *Cancer* 1981;47:2391-2397.

57. Tsujimoto M, Aozasa D, Ueda K, et al. Multivariate analysis for histologic prognostic factors in soft tissue sarcomas. *Cancer* 1988; 62:994-998.

58. Collin C, Godbold J, Hajdu S, et al. Localized extremity soft tissue sarcomas: an analysis of factors affecting survival. *J Clin Oncol* 1987;5:601-612.

59. Pisters PWT, Leung DHY, Woodruff J, et al. Analysis of prognostic factors in 1041 patients with localized soft tissue sarcomas of the extremities. *J Clin Oncol* 1996;14:1679-1689.

60. Mundt AJ, Awan A, Sibley GS, et al. Conservative surgery and adjuvant radiation therapy in the management of adult soft tissue sarcoma of the extremities: clinical and radiobiological results. *Int J Radiat Oncol Biol Phys* 1995;32:977-985.

61. Potter DA, Kinsella T, Glatstein E, et al. High-grade soft tissue sarcomas of the extremities. *Cancer* 1986;58:190-205.

62. Storm FK, Eilber FR, Mirra J, et al. Retroperitoneal sarcomas: a reappraisal of treatment. *J Surg Oncol* 1981;17:1-7.

63. Willers H, Hug EB, Spiro IJ, et al. Adult soft tissue sarcomas of the head and neck treated by radiation and surgery or radiation alone: patterns of failure and prognostic factors. *Int J Radiat Oncol Biol Phys* 1995;33:585-593.

64. Tran LM, Mark R, Meier R, et al. Sarcomas of the head and neck. *Cancer* 1992;70:169-177.

65. Singer S, Corson JM, Demetri GD, et al. Prognostic factors predictive of survival for truncal and retroperitoneal soft-tissue sarcoma. *Ann Surg* 1995;221:185-195.

66. Berlin O, Stener B, Angervall L, et al. Surgery for soft tissue sarcoma in the extremities. *Acta Orthop Scand* 1990;61:475-486.

67. Bell RS, O'Sullivan B, Liu FF, et al. The surgical margin in soft-tissue sarcoma. *J Bone Joint Surg* 1989;71A:370-375.

68. Herbert SH, Corn BW, Solin LJ, et al. Limb-preserving treatment for soft tissue sarcomas of the extremities: the significance of surgical margins. *Cancer* 1993;72:1230-1238.

69. Dinges S, Budach V, Budach W, et al. Local recurrences of soft tissue sarcomas in adults: a retrospective analysis of prognostic factors in 102 cases after surgery and radiation therapy. *Eur J Cancer* 1994;30A:1636-1642.

70. Karakousis CP, Velez AF, Emrich LJ. Management of retroperitoneal sarcomas and patient survival. *Am J Surg* 1985;150:376-380.

71. Tepper JE, Suit HD, Wood WC, et al. Radiation therapy of retroperitoneal soft tissue sarcomas. *Int J Radiat Oncol Biol Phys* 1984;10:825-830.

72. Gaynor JJ, Tan CC, Casper ES, et al. Refinement of clinicopathologic staging for localized soft tissue sarcoma of the extremity: a study of 423 adults. *J Clin Oncol* 1992;10:1317-1329.

73. Fleming JB, Berman RB, Cheng S, et al. Long-term outcome of patients with American Joint Committee on Cancer stage IIB extremity soft tissue sarcomas. *J Clin Oncol* 1999;17:2772-2780.

74. Rosenberg SA, Glatstein EJ. Perspectives on the role of surgery and radiation therapy in treatment of soft tissue sarcomas of the extremities. *Semin Oncol* 1981;8:190-200.

75. Guiliano AE, Eilber FR. The rationale for planned reoperation after unplanned total excision of soft-tissue sarcomas. *J Clin Oncol* 1985;3:1344-1348.

76. Karakousis CP, Driscoll DL. Treatment and local control of primary extremity soft tissue sarcomas. *J Surg Oncol* 1999;71:155-161.

77. Romsdahl MM. Open biopsy of sarcomas. In: Ryan JR, Baker LO, eds. *Recent Concepts in Sarcoma Treatment.* Dordrecht: Kluwer Academic; 1987:69-75.

78. Gustafson P, Dreinhöfer KE, Rydholm A. Soft tissue sarcoma should be treated at a tumor center: a comparison of quality of surgery in 375 patients. *Acta Orthop Scand* 1994;65:47-50.

79. Rööser B, Rydholm A, Alvegård T. Centralization of soft tissue sarcoma: status in Sweden in 1982. *Acta Orthop Scand* 1987; 58:641-644.

80. Ball ABS, Fisher C, Pittam M, et al. Diagnosis of soft tissue tumours by Tru-cut biopsy. *Br J Surg* 1990;77:756-758.

81. Ayala AG, Ro JY, Fanning CV, et al. Core needle biopsy and fine needle aspiration in the diagnosis of bone and soft-tissue lesions. *Hematol Oncol Clin North Am* 1995;9:633-651.

82. Rydholm A, Gustafson P, Rööser B, et al. Limb-sparing surgery without radiotherapy based on anatomic location of soft tissue sarcoma. *J Clin Oncol* 1991;9:1757-1765.

83. Manaster BJ. Musculoskeletal oncologic imaging. *Int J Radiat Oncol Biol Phys* 1991;21:1643-1651.

84. Bland KI, McCoy DM, Kinard RE, et al. Application of magnetic resonance imaging and computer tomography as an adjunct to the surgical management of soft tissue sarcomas. *Ann Surg* 1987;205:473-481.

85. Chang AE, Matory YL, Dwyer AJ, et al. Magnetic resonance imaging versus computed tomography in the evaluation of soft tissue tumors of the extremities. *Ann Surg* 1987;205:340-348.

86. Petasnick JP, Turner DA, Charter JR, et al. Soft-tissue masses of the locomotor system: comparison of MR imaging with CT. *Radiology* 1986;160:125-133.

87. Kransdorf MJ, Moser RP, Jelinek J, et al. Soft tissue masses: diagnosis using MR imaging. *AJR Am J Roentgenol* 1989;153-158.

88. Lucas JD, O'Doherty MJ, Cronin BF, et al. Prospective evaluation of soft tissue masses and sarcomas using fluorodeoxyglucose positron emission tomography. *Br J Surg* 1999;86:550-556.

89. Nishizawa K, Okunieff P, Elmaleh D, et al. Blood flow of human soft tissue sarcomas measured by thallium-201 scanning: prediction of tumor response to radiation. *Int J Radiat Oncol Biol Phys* 1991;20:593-597.

90. Ramanna L, Waxman A, Binney G, et al. Thallium-201 scintigraphy in bone sarcoma: comparison with gallium-67 and technetium-MDP in the evaluation of chemotherapeutic response. *J Nucl Med* 1990;31:567-572.

91. Pass HI, Dwyer A, Makuch R, et al. Detection of pulmonary metastases in patients with osteogenic and soft tissue sarcomas: the superiority of CT scans compared with conventional tomograms using dynamic analysis. *J Clin Oncol* 1985;3:1261-1265.

92. Lieberman PH, Brennan MF, Kimmel M, et al. Alveolar soft-part sarcoma: a clinicopathologic study of half a century. *Cancer* 1989; 63:63-70.

93. Morton DL, Ollila DW. Critical review of the sentinel node hypothesis. *Surgery* 1999;126:815-819.

94. Gerner RE, Moore GE, Pickren JW. Soft tissue sarcomas. *Ann Surg* 1975;181:803-808.

95. Leibel SA, Tranbaugh RF, Wara WM, et al. Soft tissue sarcomas of the extremities: survival and patterns of failure with conservative surgery and postoperative irradiation compared to surgery alone. *Cancer* 1982;50:1076-1083.

96. Bowden L, Booher RJ. The principles and techniques of resection of soft parts for sarcoma. *Surgery* 1958;44:963-977.

97. Simon MA, Enneking WF. The management of soft-tissue sarcomas of the extremities. *J Bone Joint Surg* 1976;58A:317-327.

98. Shiu MH, Castro EB, Hajdu SI, et al. Surgical treatment of 297 soft tissue sarcomas of the lower extremity. *Ann Surg* 1975; 182:597-602.

99. Pao WJ, Pilepich MV. Postoperative radiotherapy in the treatment of extremity soft tissue sarcomas. *Int J Radiat Oncol Biol Phys* 1990;19:907-911.

100. Geer RJ, Woodruff J, Casper ES, et al. Management of small soft-tissue sarcoma of the extremity in adults. *Arch Surg* 1992; 127:1285-1289.

101. Windeyer B, Dische S, Mansfield CM. The place of radiotherapy in the management of fibrosarcoma of the soft tissues. *Clin Radiol* 1966;17:32-40.

102. Suit HD, Russell WO, Martin RG. Management of patients with sarcoma of soft tissue in an extremity. *Cancer* 1973;31:1274-1255.

103. Keus RB, Rutgers EJT, Ho GH, et al. Limb-sparing therapy of extremity soft tissue sarcomas: treatment outcome and long-term functional results. *Eur J Cancer* 1994;30A:1459-1463.

104. Brandt TA, Parsons JT, Marcus RB, et al. Preoperative irradiation for soft tissue sarcomas of the trunk and extremities in adults. *Int J Radiat Oncol Biol Phys* 1990;19:899-906.

105. Rosenberg SA, Tepper J, Glatstein E, et al. The treatment of soft-tissue sarcomas of the extremities: prospective randomized evaluations of (1) limb-sparing surgery plus radiation therapy compared with amputation and (2) the role of adjuvant chemotherapy. *Ann Surg* 1982;196:305-315.

106. Pisters PWT, Harrison LB, Leung DHY, et al. Long-term results of a prospective randomized trial of adjuvant brachytherapy in soft tissue sarcoma. *J Clin Oncol* 1996;14:859-868.

107. Harrison LB, Franzese F, Gaynor JJ, et al. Long-term results of a prospective randomized trial of adjuvant brachytherapy in the management of completely resected soft tissue sarcomas of the extremity and superficial trunk. *Int J Radiat Oncol Biol Phys* 1993;27:259-265.

108. Yang JC, Chang AE, Baker AR, et al. Randomized prospective study of the benefit of adjuvant radiation therapy in the treatment of soft tissue sarcomas of the extremity. *J Clin Oncol* 1998;16:197-203.

109. Abbatucci JS, Boulier N, De Ranieri J, et al. Local control and survival in soft tissue sarcomas of the limbs, trunk walls and head and neck: a study of 113 cases. *Int J Radiat Oncol Biol Phys* 1986;12:579-586.

110. Suit HD, Spiro IJ. The role of radiation in patients with soft tissue sarcomas. *Cancer Control* 1994;1:592-598.

111. Fein DA, Lee WR, Lanciano RM, et al. Management of extremity soft tissue sarcomas with limb-sparing surgery and postoperative irradiation: do total dose, overall treatment time, and the surgery-radiotherapy interval impact on local control? *Int J Radiat Oncol Biol Phys* 1995;32:969-976.

112. Cheng EY, Dusenbery KE, Winters MR, et al. Soft tissue sarcomas: preoperative versus postoperative radiotherapy. *J Surg Oncol* 1996;61:90-99.

113. Pollack A, Zagars GK, Goswitz MS, et al. Preoperative radiotherapy in the treatment of soft tissue sarcomas: a matter of presentation. *Int J Radiat Oncol Biol Phys* 1998;42:563-572.

114. Tanabe KK, Pollock RE, Ellis LM, et al. Influence of surgical margins on outcome in patients with preoperatively irradiated extremity soft tissue sarcomas. *Cancer* 1994;73:1652-1659.

115. Fein DA, Corn BW, Lanciano RM, et al. Management of retroperitoneal sarcomas: does dose escalation impact on locoregional control? *Int J Radiat Oncol Biol Phys* 1995;31:129-134.

116. Sindelar WF, Kinsella TJ, Chen PW, et al. Intraoperative radiotherapy in retroperitoneal sarcomas: final results of a prospective, randomized, clinical trial. *Arch Surg* 1993;128:402-410.

117. Krause DH, Dubner S, Harrison LB, et al. Prognostic factors for recurrence and survival in head and neck soft tissue sarcomas. *Cancer* 1994;74:697-702.

118. Robinson M, Barr L, Fisher C, et al. Treatment of soft tissue sarcomas with surgery and radiotherapy. *Radiother Oncol* 1990;18:221-233.

119. Nielsen OS, Cummings B, O'Sullivan B, et al. Preoperative and postoperative irradiation of soft tissue sarcoma: effect of radiation field size. *Int J Radiat Oncol Biol Phys* 1991;21:1595-1599.

120. Fletcher GH. The evolution of the basic concepts underlying the practice of radiotherapy from 1949 to 1977. *Radiology* 1978;127:3-19.

121. Atkinson L, Garvan JM, Newton NC. Behavior and management of soft connective tissue sarcomas. *Cancer* 1963;16:1552-1562.

122. Suit HD, Mankin HJ, Wood WC, et al. Preoperative, intraoperative, and postoperative radiation in the treatment of primary soft tissue sarcoma. *Cancer* 1985;55:2659-2667.

123. Willett CG, Schiller AL, Suit HD, et al. The histologic response of soft tissue sarcoma to radiation therapy. *Cancer* 1987;60:1500-1504.

124. Janjan NA, Yasko AW, Reece GP, et al. Comparison of charges related to radiotherapy for soft-tissue sarcomas treated by preoperative external-beam irradiation versus interstitial implantation. *Ann Surg Oncol* 1994;1:415-422.

125. Habrand JL, Gerbaulet A, Pejovic MH, et al. Twenty years experience of interstitial iridium brachytherapy in the management of soft tissue sarcomas. *Int J Radiat Oncol Biol Phys* 1991;20:405-411.

126. Chaudhary AJ, Laskar S, Badhwar R. Interstitial brachytherapy in soft tissue sarcomas: the Tata Memorial Hospital experience. *Strahlenther Onkol* 1998;174:522-528.

127. Ormsby MV, Hilaris BS, Nori D, et al. Wound complications of adjuvant radiation therapy in patients with soft-tissue sarcomas. *Ann Surg* 1989;210:93-99.

128. Lewis JJ, Leung D, Heslin M, et al. Association of local recurrence with subsequent survival in extremity soft tissue sarcoma. *J Clin Oncol* 1997;15:646-652.

129. Emrich LJ, Ruka W, Driscoll DL, et al. The effect of local recurrence on survival time in adult high-grade soft tissue sarcomas. *J Clin Epidemiol* 1989;42:105-110.

130. Stotter AT, A'Hern RP, Fisher C, et al. The influence of local recurrence of extremity soft tissue sarcoma on metastasis and survival. *Cancer* 1990;65:1119-1129.

131. Gustafson P, Rööser B, Rydholm A. Is local recurrence of minor importance for metastases in soft tissue sarcoma? *Cancer* 1991;67:2083-2086.

132. Heslin MJ, Woodruff J, Brennan MF. Prognostic significance of a positive microscopic margin in high-risk extremity soft tissue sarcoma: implications for management. *J Clin Oncol* 1996;14:473-478.

133. Suit HD, Mankin HJ, Wood WC, et al. Treatment of the patient with stage M0 soft tissue sarcoma. *J Clin Oncol* 1988;6:854-862.

134. Stinson SF, DeLaney TF, Greenberg J, et al. Acute and long-term effects on limb function of combined modality limb sparing therapy for extremity soft tissue sarcomas. *Int J Radiat Oncol Biol Phys* 1991;21:1493-1499.

135. Talbert ML, Zagars GK, Sherman NE, et al. Conservative surgery and radiation therapy for soft tissue sarcomas of the wrist, hand, ankle, and foot. *Cancer* 1990;66:2482-2491.

136. Shiu MH, Hilaris BS, Harrison LB, et al. Brachytherapy and function-saving resection of soft tissue sarcoma arising in the limb. *Int J Radiat Oncol Biol Phys* 1991;21:1485-1492.

137. Pearlstone DB, Janjan NA, Feig BW, et al. Re-resection with brachytherapy for locally recurrent soft tissue sarcoma arising in a previously radiated field. *Cancer J Sci Am* 1999;5:25-33.

138. Nori D, Shupak K, Shiu MH, et al. Role of brachytherapy in recurrent extremity sarcoma in patients treated with prior surgery and irradiation. *Int J Radiat Oncol Biol Phys* 1991;20:1229-1233.

139. Sugarbaker PH, Barofsky I, Rosenberg SA, et al. Quality of life assessment of patients in extremity sarcoma clinical trials. *Surgery* 1982;91:17-23.

140. Weddington WW, Segraves KB, Simon MA. Psychological outcome of extremity sarcoma survivors undergoing amputation or limb salvage. *J Clin Oncol* 1985;3:1393-1399.

141. Bujko K, Suit HD, Springfield DS, et al. Wound healing after preoperative radiation for sarcoma of soft tissues. *Surg Gynecol Obstet* 1993;176:124-134.

142. O'Sullivan B, Davis A, Canadian Sarcoma Group, et al. Effect on radiotherapy field sizes in a recently completed Canadian Sarcoma Group and NCI Canada Clinical Trials Group randomized trial comparing pre-operative and post-operative radiotherapy in extremity soft tissue sarcoma (abstract 176). *Int J Radiat Oncol Biol Phys* 1999;45(suppl):238-239.

143. Bell RS, Mahoney J, O'Sullivan B, et al. Wound healing complications in soft tissue sarcoma management: comparison of three treatment protocols. *J Surg Oncol* 1991;46:190-197.

144. Tepper JE, Suit HD. Radiation therapy alone for sarcoma of soft tissue. *Cancer* 1985;56:475-479.

145. Dewer JA, Duncan W. A retrospective study of the role of radiotherapy in the treatment of soft tissue sarcoma. *Clin Radiol* 1985;36:629-632.

146. Slater JD, McNeese MD, Peters LJ. Radiation therapy for unresectable soft tissue sarcomas. *Int J Radiat Oncol Biol Phys* 1986;12:1729-1734.

147. Verweij J, Seynaeve C. The reason for confining the use of adjuvant chemotherapy in soft tissue sarcoma to the investigational setting. *Semin Radiat Oncol* 1999;9:352-359.

148. Benjamin RS. Evidence for using adjuvant chemotherapy as standard treatment of soft tissue sarcoma. *Semin Radiat Oncol* 1999;9:349-351.

149. Antman K, Ryan L, Borden E, et al. Pooled results from three randomized adjuvant studies of doxorubicin versus observation in soft tissue sarcoma: 10 year results and review of the literature. In: Salmon S, ed. *Adjuvant Therapy of Cancer VI.* Philadelphia, Pa: WB Saunders; 1990:529-543.

150. Baker LH. Adjuvant therapy for soft tissue sarcomas. In: Ryan JR, Baker LO, eds. *Recent Concepts in Sarcoma Treatment.* Dordrecht: Kluwer Academic; 1988:131-136.

151. Wilson RE, Wood WC, Lerner HL, et al. Doxorubicin chemotherapy in the treatment of soft-tissue sarcoma. *Arch Surg* 1986;121:1354-1359.

152. Lerner HJ, Amato DA, Savlov ED, et al. Eastern Cooperative Oncology Group: a comparison of adjuvant doxorubicin and observation for patients with localized soft tissue sarcoma. *J Clin Oncol* 1987;5:613-617.

153. Antman K, Suit H, Amato D, et al. Preliminary results of a randomized trial of adjuvant doxorubicin for sarcomas: lack of apparent difference between treatment groups. *J Clin Oncol* 1984;2:601-608.

154. Alvegård TA, Sigurdsson H, Mouridsen H, et al. Adjuvant chemotherapy with doxorubicin in high-grade soft tissue sarcoma: a randomized trial of the Scandinavian Sarcoma Group. *J Clin Oncol* 1989;7:1504-1513.

155. Gherlinzoni F, Bacci G, Picci P, et al. A randomized trial for the treatment of high-grade soft-tissue sarcomas of the extremities: preliminary observations. *J Clin Oncol* 1986;4:552-558.

156. Picci P, Bacci G, Gherlinzoni F, et al. Results of a randomized trial for the treatment of localized soft tissue tumors (STS) of the extremities in adult patients. In: Ryan JR, Baker LO, eds. *Recent Concepts in Sarcoma Treatment.* Dordrecht: Kluwer Academic; 1988:144-148.

157. Eilber FR, Giuliano AE, Huth JF, et al. A randomized prospective trial using postoperative adjuvant chemotherapy (Adriamycin) in high-grade extremity soft-tissue sarcomas. *Am J Clin Oncol* 1988;11:39-45.

158. Omura GA, Blessing JA, Major F, et al. A randomized clinical trial of adjuvant Adriamycin in uterine sarcomas: a Gynecologic Oncology Group study. *J Clin Oncol* 1985;3:1240-1245.

159. Frustaci S, Gherlinzoni F, De Paoli A, et al. Preliminary results of an adjuvant randomized trial on high risk extremity soft tissue sarcomas (STS): the interim analysis (abstract). *Proc Am Soc Clin Oncol* 1997;16:496a.

160. Picci P, Frustaci S, De Paoli A, et al. Localized high-grade soft tissue sarcomas of the extremities in adults: preliminary results of the Italian Cooperative study (abstract). *Sarcoma* 1998;1:194.

161. Bramwell V, Rouesse J, Steward W, et al. Adjuvant CYVADIC chemotherapy for adult soft tissue sarcoma—reduced local recurrence but no improvement in survival: a study of the European Organization for Research and Treatment of Cancer Soft Tissue and Bone Group. *J Clin Oncol* 1994;12:1137-1149.

162. Ravaud A, Binh Bui N, Coindre J, et al. Adjuvant chemotherapy with CyVADIC in high risk soft tissue sarcoma: a randomized prospective trial. In: Salmon S, ed. *Adjuvant Therapy of Cancer VI.* Philadelphia, Pa: WB Saunders; 1990:556-566.

163. Benjamin RS, Terjanian TO, Fenoglio CJ, et al. The importance of combination chemotherapy for adjuvant treatment of high-risk patients with soft-tissue sarcomas of the extremity. In: Salmon S, ed. *Adjuvant Therapy of Cancer V.* Orlando, Fla: Grune & Stratton; 1987:735-744.

164. Rosenberg SA, Tepper J, Glatstein E, et al. Prospective randomized evaluation of adjuvant chemotherapy in adults with soft tissue sarcomas of the extremities. *Cancer* 1983;52:424-434.

165. Chang AE, Kinsella T, Glatstein E, et al. Adjuvant chemotherapy for patients with high-grade soft-tissue sarcomas of the extremity. *J Clin Oncol* 1988;6:1491-1500.

166. Glenn J, Kinsella T, Glatstein E, et al. A randomized, prospective trial of adjuvant chemotherapy in adults with soft tissue sarcomas of the head and neck, breast, and trunk. *Cancer* 1985;55:1206-1214.

167. Glenn J, Sindelar WF, Kinsella T, et al. Results of multimodality therapy of resectable soft-tissue sarcomas of the retroperitoneum. *Surgery* 1985;97:316-325.

168. Edmonson JH, Fleming TR, Ivins JC, et al. Randomized study of systemic chemotherapy following complete excision of nonosseous sarcomas. *J Clin Oncol* 1984;2:1390-1396.

169. Zalupski MM, Ryan JR, Hussein ME, et al. Defining the role of adjuvant chemotherapy for patients with soft tissue sarcoma of the extremities. In: Salmon SE, ed. *Adjuvant Therapy of Cancer VII.* Philadelphia, Pa: JB Lippincott; 1983:385-392.

170. Tierney JF, Stewart LA, Parmar MKB. Adjuvant chemotherapy for localised resectable soft-tissue sarcoma of adults: meta-analysis of individual data. *Lancet* 1997;350:1647-1654.

171. Jaques DP, Coit DG, Hajdu SI, et al. Management of primary and recurrent soft-tissue sarcoma of the retroperitoneum. *Ann Surg* 1990;212:51-59.

172. Le QX, Fu KK, Kroll S, et al. Prognostic factors in adult soft-tissue sarcomas of the head and neck. *Int J Radiat Oncol Biol Phys* 1997;37:975-984.

173. Weber RS, Benjamin RS, Peters LJ, et al. Soft tissue sarcomas of the head and neck in adolescents and adults. *Am J Surg* 1986;152:386-392.

174. McKenna WG, Barnes MM, Kinsella TJ, et al. Combined modality treatment of adult soft tissue sarcomas of the head and neck. *Int J Radiat Oncol Biol Phys* 1987;13:1127-1133.

175. Morrison WH, Byers RM, Garden AS, et al. Cutaneous angiosarcoma of the head and neck. *Cancer* 1995;76:319-327.

176. Owens JC, Shiu MH, Smith R, et al. Soft tissue sarcomas of the hand and foot. *Cancer* 1985;55:2010-2018.

177. Fletcher CDM. Pleomorphic malignant fibrous histiocytoma: fact or fiction? A critical reappraisal based on 159 tumors diagnosed as pleomorphic sarcoma. *Am J Surg Pathol* 1992;16:213-228.

178. Rööser B, Willén H, Gustafson P, et al. Malignant fibrous histiocytoma of soft tissue: a population-based epidemiologic and prognostic study of 137 patients. *Cancer* 1991;67:499-505.

179. Fagundes HM, Lai PP, Dehner LP, et al. Postoperative radiotherapy for malignant fibrous histiocytoma. *Int J Radiat Oncol Biol Phys* 1992;23:615-619.

180. Wright PH, Sim FH, Soule EH, et al. Synovial sarcoma. *J Bone Joint Surg* 1982;64A:112-122.

181. Rööser B, Willén H, Hugoson A, et al. Prognostic factors in synovial sarcoma. *Cancer* 1989;63:2182-2185.

182. Chang HR, Hajdu SI, Collin C, et al. The prognostic value of histologic subtypes in primary extremity liposarcoma. *Cancer* 1989;64:1514-1520.

183. Evans HL. Liposarcoma: a study of 55 cases with a reassessment of its classification. *Am J Surg Pathol* 1979;3:507-523.

184. Cheng EY, Springfield DS, Mankin HJ. Frequent incidence of extrapulmonary sites of initial metastasis in patients with liposarcoma. *Cancer* 1995;75:1120-1127.

185. Knight JC, Renwick PJ, Cin PD, et al. Translocation t(12;16) (q13;p11) in myxoid liposarcoma and round cell liposarcoma: molecular and cytogenetic analysis. *Cancer Res* 1995; 55:24-27.

186. Pritchard DJ, Nascimento AG, Petersen IA. Local control of extra-abdominal desmoid tumors. *J Bone Joint Surg Am* 1996;78:848-854.

187. McKinnon JG, Neifeld JP, Kay S, et al. Management of desmoid tumors. *Surg Gynecol Obstet* 1989;169:104-106.

188. Goy BW, Lee SP, Eilber F, et al. The role of adjuvant radiotherapy in the treatment of resectable desmoid tumors. *Int J Radiat Oncol Biol Phys* 1997;39:659-665.

189. Spear MA, Jennings LC, Mankin HJ, et al. Individualizing management of aggressive fibromatosis. *Int J Radiat Oncol Biol Phys* 1998;40:637-645.

190. Ballo MT, Zagars GK, Pollack A, et al. Desmoid tumor: prognostic factors and outcome after surgery, radiation therapy, or combined surgery and radiation therapy. *J Clin Oncol* 1999;17: 158-167.

191. Ballo MT, Zagars GK, Pollack A. Radiation therapy in the management of desmoid tumors. *Int J Radiat Oncol Biol Phys* 1998;42:1007-1014.

192. Schmitt G, Mills EED, Levin V, et al. Radiotherapy of aggressive fibromatosis. *Eur J Cancer* 1992;28A:832-835.

193. Kamath SS, Parsons JT, Marcus RB, et al. Radiotherapy for local control of aggressive fibromatosis. *Int J Radiat Oncol Biol Phys* 1996;36:325-328.

194. Bendix-Hansen K, Myhre-Jensen O, Kaae S. Dermatofibrosarcoma protuberans: a clinico-pathological study of nineteen cases and a review of world literature. *Scand J Plast Reconstr Surg* 1983; 17:247-252.

195. McPeak C, Cruz T, Nicastri A. Dermatofibrosarcoma protuberans: an analysis of 86 cases—five with metastases. *Ann Surg* 1967;166:803-816.

196. Roses DF, Valensi Q, LaTrenta G, et al. Surgical treatment of dermatofibrosarcoma protuberans. *Surg Gynecol Obstet* 1986; 162: 449-452.

197. Gloster HM, Harris KR, Roenigk RK. A comparison between Mohs micrographic surgery and wide surgical excision for the treatment of dermatofibrosarcoma protuberans. *J Am Acad Dermatol* 1996;35:82-87.

198. Ballo MT, Zagars GK, Pisters P, et al. The role of radiation therapy in the management of dermatofibrosarcoma protuberans. *Int J Radiat Oncol Biol Phys* 1998;40:823-827.

199. Suit H, Mankin HJ, Efrid J, et al. Radiation in management of patients with dermatofibrosarcoma protuberans. *J Clin Oncol* 1996;14:2365-2369.

200. McMaster MJ, Soule EH, Ivins JC. Hemangiopericytoma: a clinicopathologic study and long-term followup of 60 patients. *Cancer* 1975;36:2232-2244.

201. Enzinger FM, Smith BH. Hemangiopericytoma: an analysis of 106 cases. *Hum Pathol* 1976;7:61-82.

202. Smullens SN, Scotti DJ, Osterholm JL, et al. Preoperative embolization of retroperitoneal hemangiopericytomas as an aid in their removal. *Cancer* 1982;50:1870-1875.

203. Mira JG, Chu FC, Fortner JG. The role of radiotherapy in the management of malignant hemangiopericytoma. *Cancer* 1977; 39:1254-1259.

204. Jha N, McNeese M, Barkley HT, et al. Does radiotherapy have a role in hemangiopericytoma management? Report of 14 new cases and a review of the literature. *Int J Radiat Oncol Biol Phys* 1987;13:1399-1402.

PART XIII

Childhood Cancer

CHAPTER 36

Childhood Cancer

Larry E. Kun

Approximately 9000 new cases of childhood cancer occur annually in the United States. Cancer is the second most common cause of death in children less than 18 years old. The most common pediatric malignant diseases are listed in Table 36-1. Two categories of tumors account for half of all cases of childhood cancer: acute leukemias and central nervous system (CNS) tumors. Many of the other common neoplasms are broadly classified as small round cell tumors, reflecting the basic histologic features of neuroblastoma, malignant lymphoma, Hodgkin's disease, rhabdomyosarcoma, Ewing's sarcoma, and retinoblastoma.[1]

Pediatric cancer is relatively sensitive to radiation therapy and chemotherapy. Combinations of surgery and radiation therapy with multiagent chemotherapy since the 1960s have resulted in sharply increased survival rates for children with most types of cancer. Controlled clinical trials have sought to define the roles of complementary treatment modalities and newer therapeutic interventions while seeking to optimize disease control and minimize late sequelae. Given the risks of radiation therapy, particularly for young children, it is essential to clearly identify those children for whom radiation therapy is truly important for both local–regional disease control and survival. The advent of more sophisticated, image-guided radiation techniques has been particularly advantageous in pediatric oncology, and in several disease settings, these techniques have increased the role for radiation therapy in childhood cancer treatment.

NORMAL TISSUE EFFECTS

Radiation therapy in children requires a delicate balance between efficacy and radiation-related late toxic effects. Acute radiation effects are similar to those occurring in adults; however, the heightened toxicity of combined chemoradiation therapy must be borne in mind because multiagent chemotherapy is often used either in sequence or concurrently with irradiation.

It is incumbent on the radiation oncology community to recognize the functional consequences of childhood cancer and its therapies. Of 142 children followed for 6 to 21 years after successful cancer management during the 1950s and 1960s, Li and Stone[2] described major physical defects in 52%, but virtually all survivors were living "fully active lives." More recent series similarly indicate physical abnormalities in most long-term survivors, 40% of whom show functional deficits after childhood cancer therapy.[3] Data from long-term survivors of Wilms' tumor treated before 1 year of age confirm the frequency of significant, largely musculoskeletal changes but the relative lack of life-threatening or disabling problems.[2,4,5]

Growth disturbances are unique effects of cancer therapy in growing children and have been noted in approximately 40% of long-term survivors.[2,4,6] Scoliosis, for example, had been noted as a consequence of inhomogeneous vertebral irradiation.[7] Vertebral growth changes after current radiation techniques are identifiable although clinically insignificant at dose levels below 35 Gy.[4,8] Reduction in vertebral height after

TABLE 36-1
Cancer in Children

Cancer Type	Percentage Occurring in Children	Predominant Age at Occurrence
Acute leukemia	31.0	2-8 years
Acute lymphoblastic leukemia	21.0	2 years, then stable
Other	10.0	2-18 years
Central nervous system	19.0	Varies with histology
Malignant lymphoma	8.0	Varies with type
Hodgkin's disease	6.0	Increases with age
Neuroblastoma	8.0	0-3 years
Wilms' tumor	6.0	< 5 years
Soft tissue sarcomas	5.0	< 5 years > 10-12 years
Bone sarcomas	5.0	Increases with age > 10 years
Retinoblastoma	2.5	0-2 years
Germ cell tumors	2.5	< 1 year; > 8-10 years
Liver tumors	2.5	4 years

radiation therapy at dose levels of at least 24 Gy is most apparent in children treated before 6 years of age or during the adolescent growth spurt.[8] Changes in soft-tissue development often exceed changes in developing bone after modern radiation therapy. Muscular hypoplasia, for example, is common, resulting in functional or aesthetic alterations depending on the region irradiated (Fig. 36-1).[9]

Radiation changes in long bones include reduction in bone length resulting from treatment of epiphyseal growth centers.[6] The apparent threshold for significant changes in bone length is age-related; changes can be anticipated after doses as low as 10 to 15 Gy in very young children (younger than 3 years) and more than 25 Gy in children beyond 3 to 5 years of age. Growth deficits are proportional to the amount of potential growth related to the irradiated epiphysis at the time of treatment. In the head and neck region, doses as low as 18 Gy are associated with observable defects in skull or facial bone development.[10] Orbital growth is altered after surgery plus irradiation for retinoblastoma.[10]

Alterations in growth also occur as a result of radiation-related endocrine dysfunction. Growth hormone deficiency has been noted in more than 50% of children who have undergone irradiation of the pituitary-hypothalamic region.[11,12] A dose effect is apparent, with growth hormone deficits after doses above 35 to 40 Gy in children treated for primary brain tumors and sarcomas of the head and neck region.[12-14] After 24 Gy of

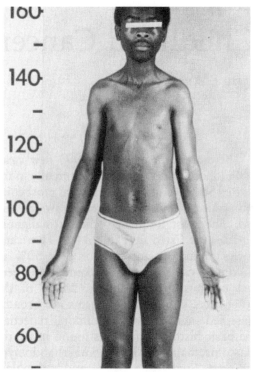

Fig. 36-1 Muscular hypoplasia after mantle irradiation in childhood.

preventive cranial irradiation for acute lymphoblastic leukemia (ALL), subtle growth hormone deficits become apparent as the child undergoes the pubertal growth spurt.[13,15] In girls, even low radiation doses (18 to 24 Gy for ALL) have been associated with early onset of puberty.[16] Hypothyroidism also occurs relatively often after cranial irradiation; when the thyroid region is included within the radiation volume, clinical or chemical evidence of decreased thyroid function is apparent in 10% to 25% of children after doses of 18 to 26 Gy (e.g., for ALL or Hodgkin's disease) and in more than 50% of children after doses exceeding 25 to 30 Gy (e.g., for medulloblastoma, sarcoma, or Hodgkin's disease).[17-20] Complicating matters are recent findings indicating that up to 50% of children with brain tumors have preexisting hormonal deficits before undergoing irradiation.[21]

Other radiation-related somatic changes include late pulmonary deficits. These are caused primarily by diminished thoracic and lung parenchymal volumes after low-dose irradiation (15 Gy) in young children with Wilms' tumor and after carmustine as a component of multimodality therapy in children with brain tumors.[22,23]

The identification of CNS changes after cranial irradiation in conjunction with intrathecal or intravenous chemotherapy in ALL has led to relatively limited use of preventive cranial irradiation in this setting. A subacute syndrome of somnolence, often associated with nausea, irritability, or low-grade fever, has been documented in approximately 50% of children 4 to 8 weeks after cranial irradiation to 18 to 24 Gy.[24,25] Cerebral atrophy and mineralizing microangiopathy are identifiable on computed tomography (CT) or magnetic resonance imaging (MRI) studies after treatment with cranial irradiation or chemotherapy.[26-29] Leukoencephalopathy is a more profound, sometimes fatal entity histologically identified as focal coagulative necrosis of the white matter.[30] The clinical syndrome includes lethargy, seizures, perceptual changes, and cerebellar dysfunction. The imaging diagnosis is based on characteristic diffuse white matter changes (Fig. 36-2). Although leukoencephalopathy is independently related to cranial irradiation and to methotrexate (predominately systemic but also intrathecal), its incidence is highest among patients treated with high-dose or prolonged intravenous methotrexate after cranial irradiation.[31,32]

Neuropsychological alterations have been well documented in survivors of ALL. Eiser[33] initially described significant deterioration of the intelligence quotient (IQ) in children treated with cranial irradiation. Several subsequent studies[34-37] have confirmed IQ declines related to cranial irradiation and to methotrexate administration.[36] Treatment before 3 to 4 years of age has, in general, been associated with a greater risk of neuropsychological deficits.[38,39]

Reproductive and genetic effects of abdominal irradiation include an increased risk of perinatal mortality

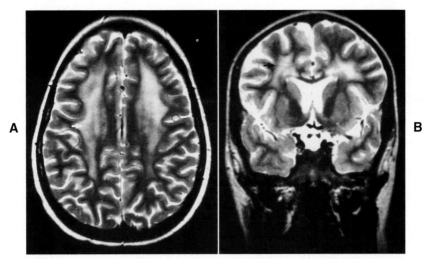

Fig. 36-2 T2-weighted magnetic resonance images (**A,** transverse section; **B,** coronal section) reveal extensive white matter changes (*arrow*) characteristic of leukoencephalopathy in an 11-year-old child given high-dose methotrexate without irradiation for acute lymphoblastic leukemia. The imaging findings were associated with the onset of generalized seizures and lassitude, all of which improved over the ensuing 6 to 8 months.

and low-birth-weight infants; no excess of congenital malformations or early malignancies in first-generation offspring has been described.[40-42]

Perhaps the single most important issue affecting the risk-benefit ratio for radiation therapy in children is the frequency of secondary tumors. After orthovoltage irradiation, Li and colleagues[43] reported a 10-year actuarial incidence of treatment-related second neoplasms approaching 14%. Although related both to alkylating agents and radiation therapy, 90% of the tumors in Li's initial study occurred within the radiation fields. The frequency of secondary tumors after megavoltage irradiation approximates 4% to 7% at 20 years.[44,45] Secondary cancer is more common in girls than in boys, reflecting an incidence of radiation-related breast cancer of as much as 20% after the second decade after irradiation for pediatric Hodgkin's disease.[44,46]

Some findings suggest that certain disease entities, including Ewing's sarcoma, are associated with a higher incidence of secondary cancer, especially sarcomas.[47,48] An increased incidence of both spontaneous and treatment-related neoplasms is apparent in children with genetically determined disorders such as neurofibromatosis, xeroderma pigmentosum, and Gorlin's or basal cell nevus syndrome.[49-54] The highest risk of secondary cancer is in children with the genetic form of retinoblastoma. In this group of young children with known familial disease or spontaneous bilateral disease, the chance of secondary tumors, largely but not entirely radiation-related bone sarcomas, has been reported to be 25% to 40% by 20 years after treatment and up to 50% by 50 years after irradiation (compared with only 5% in patients with similarly treated but spontaneous, unilateral retinoblastoma).[44,55] Fully one third of

second malignant neoplasms after radiation therapy identified in the Late Effects Study Group[44] occurred in patients with genetic disorders.[56-60]

In considering the added benefit of irradiation in disease control, one must always consider the potential for functional limitations and even death that follow therapeutic interventions in this often vulnerable age group.[44] As the role for technically sophisticated radiation therapy is reexamined and often expanded, it is important to neither discount the importance of local–regional control, often best achieved with irradiation, nor ignore the late consequences of irradiation in young and developing children.

ACUTE LEUKEMIAS
Clinical and Biological Features

Acute leukemias are the most common types of cancer in children. ALL in particular represents 80% of pediatric leukemias and about 20% of all cases of childhood cancer. The most common presenting symptoms and signs relate to bone marrow replacement and include fever and neutropenia, petechiae or hemorrhage associated with thrombocytopenia, fatigue related to anemia, and bone and joint pain. The incidence of ALL peaks between 2 and 8 years of age.

ALL is a systemic disease. Clinical features predictive of a relatively poor prognosis include age younger than 1 year or older than 9 years, white blood cell count higher than 50,000, and T-cell or mature B-cell immunophenotype (vs. the more favorable B-cell progenitor immunophenotype).[61,62]

Immunologic studies identify a B-cell lineage in about 85% of ALL cases; 60% have surface B-cell differentiation antigens (early pre–B-cell, associated with a relatively favorable prognosis), 20% have intracellular immunoglobulin heavy chains (pre–B-cell), and 1% have actual surface immunoglobulin (B-cell). T-cell characteristics are present in 15% of ALL cases, classically associated with age older than 10 years, high white blood cell count, and mediastinal lymphadenopathy.[63] Leukocyte immunophenotype is determined by using monoclonal antibodies to lineage-specific clusters-of-differentiation molecular markers.[61,62] Therapy and outcome are defined by the immunophenotype, with modern risk-adapted regimens producing excellent outcomes in patients with B-lineage or T-lineage ALL.[61,62,64-66]

Cytogenetic features have also been found to affect the prognosis of ALL. Hyperdiploidy and the presence of the *TEL-AML1* fusion gene correlate strongly with a favorable outcome among children 1 to 9 years old; in contrast, the presence of the *BCR-ABL* fusion gene or the Philadelphia chromosome in ALL identifies a high-risk patient cohort.[61,62,67,68] The poor prognosis for children with ALL who are less than 1 year old is associated with the relatively specific *MLL* gene rearrangement characteristic of the disease in this age group.[69-71]

In addition to the clinical and biological features associated with outcome in ALL, early response to therapy is highly predictive of disease control. Conversely, the presence of residual disease (whether evident clinically or only by molecular analysis [defined as minimal residual disease]) early during induction therapy or at completion of the induction regimen is associated with a high risk of subsequent relapse.[68,72,73]

Acute myelogenous and myelomonocytic leukemias represent about 15% of childhood leukemias. Recent results show improvement in outcome in these leukemias, although not to the impressive level now associated with ALL.[74,75]

Meningeal Leukemia
Preventive Therapy for Occult Disease

The concept of prolonged multiagent chemotherapy for curative treatment of ALL was introduced in the mid-1960s.[76,77] The basic strategy of induction therapy followed by consolidation chemotherapy produced durable hematologic remissions while highlighting the problem of meningeal (CNS) leukemia. In early trials in which no specific CNS therapy was used, the incidence of initial meningeal failure was as high as 70%.[78] A prospective randomized trial at St. Jude Children's Research Hospital[79] confirmed the utility of preventive craniospinal irradiation (CSI) (24 Gy in 15 to 16 fractions) early during hematologic remission, reducing the incidence of CNS relapse from 67% to 4%.

Subsequent studies showed that cranial irradiation combined with intrathecal methotrexate was as effective

as CSI and was associated with less hematologic suppression.[76,77] Sequential studies by the Pediatric Oncology Group (POG), Children's Cancer Group (CCG), and European researchers, in addition to several large single-institution trials in the United States, have shown that systemic methotrexate with repeated intrathecal instillations of methotrexate alone or in combination with cytarabine and hydrocortisone results in a CNS failure rate of less than 5% in children with B-lineage ALL or T-cell disease plus a white blood count of less than 50,000 to 100,000.[61,62,66,80-87]

The current treatment regimens for ALL incorporate induction, intensification (or consolidation; this phase often uses moderate- to high-dose systemic methotrexate), and continuation therapy for a total of 2.5 years after remission. In conjunction with repeated intrathecal chemotherapy, the more intensive methotrexate-based regimens have improved the control of hematologic and non-CNS extramedullary (e.g., testicular) disease.[85,86,88] The higher-risk patients do have a greater incidence of CNS relapse when treated without cranial irradiation, and the Berlin-Frankfurt-Munster group has continued to recommend somewhat less intensive methotrexate regimens than are typical in the United States, in combination with 12 Gy of cranial irradiation.[84,88] Unclear at this time is where the balance between avoiding radiation-associated sequelae and avoiding methotrexate-related neurologic effects (seizures and white matter alterations occurred at an alarming rate in several recent U.S. studies) will ultimately put the threshold for cases requiring preventive cranial irradiation.[89]

Recent series in Italy and the Netherlands and an ongoing study at St. Jude Children's Research Hospital have sought to obviate cranial irradiation for all ALL cases without CNS involvement at diagnosis.[84,87,90] In comparison to the Italian and Dutch chemotherapy-only studies with similar systemic and intrathecal components, the Berlin-Frankfurt-Munster trials for children with very high-risk disease (defined as T-cell disease presenting with a blood cell count of more than 100,000) have shown significantly superior results with the addition of 12 Gy of preventive cranial irradiation. The event-free survival rates in the Berlin-Frankfurt-Munster trials were twice the rates in Dutch and German chemotherapy-only studies; and the incidence of CNS failure was one fifth that noted without cranial irradiation.[82-85,87,90]

Technique of Cranial Irradiation

Preventive cranial irradiation in the United States is currently restricted to children or adolescents with T-cell ALL and a white blood cell count of more than 50,000 to 100,000. The technique used must assure adequate coverage of the entire intracranial subarachnoid space. Treatment demands careful attention to margins at the base of the skull, particularly the region of the cribriform plate and the temporal fossa (Fig. 36-3). The target

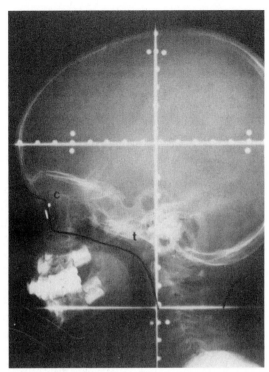

Fig. 36-3 Cranial irradiation field for preventive therapy in acute lymphoblastic leukemia. The field includes the cribriform plate *(c)* of the subfrontal region and the temporal fossa *(t)* at the base of the skull.

volume includes the posterior retina and orbital apex, requiring specific techniques to block the anterior half of the eye (and lens). A lower margin at the bottom of the second cervical vertebra has become standard, assuring clearance at the base of the skull (see Fig. 36-3). The radiation field around the calvarium should be sufficient to assure full dose delivery at the subarachnoid space, typically 5 to 10 mm beyond the skull.

The currently used total dose for the small cohort requiring preventive cranial irradiation is 18 Gy (most often given as once-daily 1.5-Gy fractions); this dose was recently reduced to 12 Gy in selected studies in Europe and the United States.[84,85]

Treatment of Overt Disease

Meningeal leukemia is documented at diagnosis in approximately 5% of ALL cases.[91-94] CNS disease is defined by the presence of leukemic cells and at least five white blood cells per ml in the cerebrospinal fluid (CSF). CNS-2 disease, with blasts but fewer than five white blood cells in the CSF, has been identified as a potentially negative prognostic factor and has consistently been managed with somewhat augmented intrathecal chemotherapy.[83,87,90,92,95] Most current clinical trials incorporate cranial irradiation (12 or 18 Gy) for children with CNS involvement at diagnosis, with ongoing studies further testing the role of chemotherapy alone in this setting.[61,82,88]

CNS relapse after initial remission requires careful integration of radiation therapy and chemotherapy. Early studies using CSI for overt CNS relapse were marked by frequent second CNS relapses.[79] Subsequent studies confirmed consistent CNS control after clearance of malignant cells from the CSF with intrathecal chemotherapy and prompt initiation of CSI.[96-99] Reports of successful management of CNS relapse without adequate CSI are limited.[100,101] The most recent POG and European reports indicate a role for intensive chemotherapy lasting 6 to 12 months followed by CSI (cranial irradiation to 24 to 25 Gy and spinal irradiation to 15 Gy).[99,102,103] Among patients who sustain late CNS relapse (i.e., relapse more than 18 months after initial remission), a secondary event-free survival rate of 83% at 4 years has been reported.[102] An ongoing trial by the Children's Oncology Group (COG) will study whether irradiation in patients with late CNS relapse can be limited to only cranial therapy (18 Gy). For children with early CNS relapse, an approach of systemic chemotherapy with CSI results in an only 46% event-free survival rate at 4 years, indicating a continuing requirement for CSI and perhaps a need for bone marrow transplantation in that setting.[102]

Technique of Craniospinal Irradiation

The target volume for CSI includes the same intracranial volume described above for cranial irradiation plus the spinal subarachnoid space. The lower margin must extend below S2 to encompass the caudal limit of the thecal sac. Lateral craniocervical fields adjoining a posterior spinal field are most often used. Minimizing inhomogeneity at the field junction requires correcting for divergence (see Fig. 32-2). The lateral craniocervical fields are angled at the gantry to establish parallel, nondivergent beams at the level of the orbital rim; in addition, the collimators are angled to parallel the cephalad divergence of the entering posterior spinal field. Correction for caudal divergence of the entering lateral craniocervical fields can be achieved by angling the treatment pedestal; alternatively, this divergence can be corrected to meet in the midplane by using a calculated 5- to 10-mm gap at the lateral cervical region to match the projection of the light fields at the midplane posteriorly. It is good practice to change the junction by 1 to 2 cm at least once during CSI with the spinal doses recommended for ALL. Both immobilization and reproducibility can be improved by using a prone position with a custom-made device to ensure appropriate patient positioning.

Testicular Leukemia

With current chemotherapy regimens, the occurrence of testicular relapse of ALL has become anecdotal.[62,90] In instances of testicular involvement at relapse, bilateral testicular irradiation to 20 to 25 Gy has been uniformly successful in achieving local disease control, with the ultimate outcome dependent on the timing of testicular failure.[104-106] Electron-beam irradiation is simplest and appropriate in this setting.

Prognosis

Studies in which current therapies are used report 70% to 80% overall rates of continuous complete remission for children (i.e., those older than 2 years) with ALL.* Even children with high-risk disease factors treated with current regimens enjoy long-term disease control and survival at rates of 70% or more.[62,65,66,90] The major challenge remaining in ALL is in achieving a leukemia-free survival rate of more than 50% among infants (i.e., those less than 2 years old) and in the limited cohort of patients with specific biologically unfavorable presentations (e.g., Philadelphia-chromosome–positive ALL), for whom bone marrow transplantation has become the standard early in remission.[61,68]

WILMS' TUMOR

Wilms' tumor is a malignant renal tumor occurring predominantly in young children. The tumor is believed to arise from embryonic nephrogenic rests. Nearly 70% of Wilms' tumors occur in children younger than 4 years. A palpable or visible abdominal mass is usually the only presenting sign. Abdominal pain or hematuria occurs in less than one fourth of patients.

Wilms' tumor has been associated with genitourinary anomalies (e.g., cryptorchidism or hypospadias) and somatic malformations (most commonly hemihypertrophy or aniridia). Approximately 10% of children show abnormalities in the *WT-1* gene (11p13 deletion) associated with the WAGR syndrome (*W*ilms' tumor, *a*niridia, *g*enitourinary abnormalities, and mental *r*etardation).[108] The Beckwith-Wiedemann syndrome includes exophthalmos, macroglossia, and gigantism often in association with Wilms' tumor.[109]

It is important to distinguish between Wilms' tumor and mesoblastic nephroma, a mesenchymal hamartoma occurring in infancy. Fully 25% of mesoblastic nephromas are diagnosed in newborns.[110,111] Mesoblastic nephroma has a benign course after resection.

Wilms' tumors comprise epithelial components, including primitive tubules and glomeruli, mixed with areas of mesenchymal tumor, including fibrous, smooth, and skeletal muscle elements. Nephrogenic rests are present in 40% of cases. A single focus of intralobar rests is usually associated with Wilms' tumor in the WAGR syndrome. The finding of several foci of intralobar rests (or nephroblastomatosis) in unilateral Wilms' tumor is associated with metachronous disease in the remaining kidney.[108,111-113] Perilobar nephrogenic rests are more common than intralobar rests in the general pediatric population and are multifocal and often bilateral.

The National Wilms' Tumor Study (NWTS) has identified striking correlations between histology and prognosis. In 85% of cases, tumors contain only differentiated epithelial or mesenchymal elements. Such tumors have a favorable prognosis. Histologic findings associated with an unfavorable prognosis are noted in 12% to 15% of patients. Anaplastic Wilms' tumor is noted in 5% of cases; it is rare in infants, but accounts for 13% of tumors in children older than 5 years.[112,114-116] Lymph node metastasis and hematogenous dissemination are more common in anaplastic tumors.[112,114,115]

Clear cell sarcoma of the kidney is technically distinct from Wilms' tumor but shares a common clinical presentation and age distribution. The clear cell tumors metastasize preferentially to bone and brain.[112,117] Rhabdoid tumors are highly aggressive lesions occurring primarily in the kidney (but also in other visceral or CNS sites) in very young children.[112,118] Rhabdoid tumors metastasize widely to liver, lungs, and bone. Brain tumors arise independently in infants with renal rhabdoid tumors, associated with a chromosome 22 deletion and the *INI1* gene.[119-121] Rhabdoid tumors are truly independent of Wilms' tumors.

Prognostic factors identified in the report of Garcia and colleagues[122] in 1963 led to the first suggestions for staging of Wilms' tumor. Cassady and colleagues[123] proposed a tumor-nodes-metastasis (TNM) system built on Garcia's data, correlating prognosis with tumor size, capsular invasion, lymph node involvement, and distant metastasis. The NWTS initially used groups I to IV (and V for bilateral disease) based on tumor extension and resectability. Analysis of the first 2 trials conducted by the NWTS (NWTS-1 and NWTS-2) indicated the importance of lymph node metastasis.[112,115] The current NWTS staging system shown in Table 36-2 is based on histologic evidence of resection margins, infiltrative characteristics of the lesion, and the presence of lymph node metastasis.[124,125]

With nephrectomy and postoperative abdominal irradiation, Gross and Neuhauser[126] reported a disease-free survival rate of 47% among 38 patients with Wilms' tumor by 1950. Farber[127] later described a 70% survival rate with the addition of dactinomycin. However, subsequent studies including the NWTS-1 trial found that disease-free survival with adjuvant dactinomycin only slightly exceeded the 50% rate established with surgery and irradiation alone.[115,123] The improved survival noted by Farber[127] largely reflected the ability of dactinomycin and pulmonary irradiation to salvage nearly 50% of patients with lung metastases.

Prospective trials have proven the efficacy of surgery and combination chemotherapy using vincristine and

---

*References 62, 65, 66, 84, 85, 87, 88, 103, 107.

TABLE 36-2

National Wilms' Tumor Study Staging System for Wilms' Tumor

Stage	Description
I	Tumor limited to kidney and completely resected.
	Renal capsule intact or infiltrated but not penetrated; renal sinus invaded < 2 mm; vessels of renal sinus not involved; tumor not ruptured or biopsied (fine-needle aspiration allowed); and no evidence of tumor at or beyond the margins of resection.
II	Tumor extends beyond kidney but completely resected.
	Renal sinus invaded > 2 mm; vessels of renal sinus or outside the renal parenchyma involved; and/or tumor biopsied (except fine-needle aspiration) or spillage confined to the flank and does not involve peritoneal surface. No evidence of tumor at or beyond the margins of resection.
III	Residual nonhematogenous tumor confined to the abdomen.
	Abdominopelvic lymph nodes involved; tumor penetrates peritoneal surface; tumor implants on peritoneal surface; gross or microscopic residual tumor after surgery; tumor incompletely resected because of local infiltration into vital structures; and/or tumor spillage not confined to flank.
IV	Hematogenous metastases (lung, liver, bone, brain, etc.); and/or lymph node metastases outside the abdominopelvic region. "CT only" lung metastases do not mandate stage IV.
V	Bilateral renal involvement at diagnosis. Each side staged according to above criteria.

From the National Wilms' Tumor Study. (Available at: http://www.nwts.org.)
CT, Computed tomography.

dactinomycin, or vincristine alone in early-stage disease, for patients with differentiated Wilms' tumor.[115,124,128,129]

Radiation Therapy
Indications for Abdominal Irradiation

Routine postoperative irradiation has been effective in virtually eliminating abdominal recurrences of Wilms' tumor.[32,123,130] With increasingly effective chemotherapy, however, abdominal irradiation can be omitted in some groups.[131,132]

The indications for abdominal irradiation relate directly to disease extent and inversely to the intensity of chemotherapy. Results of the NWTS-1 and NWTS-2 trials for patients with early-stage disease (intrarenal stage I) confirmed this relationship, indicating that postoperative abdominal irradiation could be avoided when using effective chemotherapy for what is now considered stage I differentiated Wilms' tumor.[124,134] With more intensive chemotherapy, anaplastic stage I tumors also do not require postoperative irradiation. Stage I clear cell sarcomas are treated with local irradiation after chemotherapy.[132]

For stage II disease (i.e., microscopic residual disease without lymph node involvement), the third NWTS trial (NWTS-3) included a comparison of 20 Gy of tumor bed irradiation plus chemotherapy versus chemotherapy alone (vincristine and dactinomycin, with or without doxorubicin) and found a 2-year relapse-free survival rate of 88% with chemotherapy for favorable-histology tumors and 92% with the addition of radiation therapy. Abdominal failure occurred in only 3% of cases without irradiation; protocols now obviate irradiation for differentiated stage II disease while requiring it for tumors with anaplastic changes or unfavorable histologic types.[116,131,132,134]

Breslow and colleagues[115,135] described tumor factors that were associated with abdominal failure in the early NWTS trials. Statistically significant factors include abdominal spread (defined as contiguous disease extension into the peritoneum or other abdominal organs, usually associated with macroscopic residual abdominal tumor), operative rupture (either locally into the tumor bed or diffusely through the peritoneum), lymph node metastasis, and unfavorable histologic type. In the NWTS-2 trial, abdominal tumor recurrences occurred in 20% of cases with unfavorable histologic types.[133]

All patients with stage III disease (macroscopic residual abdominal disease, lymph node metastasis, or diffuse peritoneal tumor spillage) require postoperative irradiation.[124,133] However, for stage III disease exclusive of diffuse peritoneal spillage, no evidence exists to suggest that whole abdominal irradiation is necessary. Local tumor bed irradiation is indicated for this group, including the para-aortic lymph nodes.

No obvious radiation therapy dose-response relationship for Wilms' tumor has been apparent. The NWTS-1 trial showed an equal frequency of abdominal failure after doses of 18 to 20 Gy, 20 to 24 Gy, and 24 to 40 Gy.[131-133] In the NWTS-3 trial, patients with stage III disease were randomly assigned to receive 10.8 or 20 Gy after surgery. An investigator option to boost the dose to areas of gross residual disease to 20 Gy in the 10.8-Gy group was used in only 2% of cases. With 10.8 Gy and three-drug chemotherapy, abdominal failure occurred in only 4% of cases; with two drugs, the 10.8-Gy dose was inadequate, allowing an 11% abdominal recurrence rate.[131] Similar single-institution results have established a local dose of 10 to 12 Gy as the standard for stage III disease with favorable histology.[136,137] Most investigators use a 10-Gy boost dose to sites of overt disease, identified arbitrarily in the NWTS schema as residual disease measuring at least 3 cm in diameter. (One of the more common indications for a boost dose is residual disease in the inferior vena cava.[138]) For anaplastic Wilms' tumor and rhabdoid tumor in particular, radiation doses of 20 to 30 Gy were used in the NWTS-2, -3, and -4 trials, but the current protocol (NTWS-5) does not prescribe different doses on the basis of histology, although the rationale for this is not readily apparent.

Preoperative irradiation was tested in the earlier European International Society of Pediatric Oncology (SIOP) trials.[6] However, preoperative irradiation has not been used extensively in the United States because of concerns regarding the certainty of diagnosis and the potential loss of information regarding both tumor stage and histology.[132,134]

Technique of Abdominal Irradiation

Treatment fields for local irradiation encompass the preoperative tumor bed and adjacent para-aortic lymph nodes. In practice, treatment fields extend from the diaphragm to a level below the primary tumor as typically defined by CT. The lateral aspect of the treatment field tangentially includes the abdominal wall; the medial border extends beyond the contralateral vertebral margin to include the para-aortic lymph node chain. Opposed anterior and posterior fields are used. The dose levels are defined in the previous paragraphs.

For patients requiring whole abdominal irradiation, the treatment volume must include the entire peritoneal cavity. The upper margins include the diaphragm bilaterally; the inferior margin is usually defined at the midobturator level, blocking the acetabular and femoral head regions. The dose to the remaining (contralateral) kidney should be minimized; in cases where dose levels in excess of 10.8 Gy are indicated, the dose to any substantial portion of the remaining kidney should not exceed 10 to 12 Gy. When treating bilateral Wilms' tumor, maximal reduction in the remaining functioning renal substance should be confirmed by a dose-volume histogram.

For patients with bilateral tumors or metastatic disease, the need for abdominal irradiation is defined by the local extent of disease in each affected kidney.

Pulmonary Irradiation

The ability to achieve durable disease-free survival in patients with pulmonary metastasis from Wilms' tumor followed the introduction of combined chemotherapy (dactinomycin) and lung irradiation.[123,127,139] Ultimate disease control after metastatic failure in the lungs was seen in approximately 50% of patients in earlier series.[140-143] The findings indicated the necessity to treat the entire lung volume rather than limited fields.[144,145]

The likelihood of disease control after metastasis is inversely related to the intensity of the initial chemotherapy regimen. This can be seen most easily in terms of *secondary* disease-free survival (i.e., control of

posttreatment recurrences) in the first three NWTS studies: 51% in the NWTS-1, 40% in the NWTS-2, and 34% in the NWTS-3.[142] At the same time, overall survival consistently improved over the three NWTS studies, indicating that the proportion of patients developing metastasis progressively diminished but that the ability to salvage treatment failures also diminished.

Approximately 12% of patients with Wilms' tumor have pulmonary metastasis at diagnosis. Treatment including pulmonary irradiation and chemotherapy has resulted in disease control in 75% of stage IV (lung metastasis) cases with favorable histology.[142,145,146] However, a subset analysis of the NWTS-3 trial showed no apparent benefit from the addition of lung irradiation for those with lung metastases evident only on CT (i.e., normal plain x-ray films of the chest); the relapse-free survival rate was 85% with or without thoracic irradiation.[147] The United Kingdom Children's Cancer Study Group First Wilms' Tumor Study, in contrast, showed a less favorable 65% disease control rate in patients with metastatic disease who did not receive thoracic irradiation, thus suggesting that thoracic irradiation does have a role.[129]

Prognosis

In recent series, disease-free survival rates for all stages combined approach 90%. For those with tumors of favorable histology, the NWTS-3 trial showed 4-year survival rates of 96%, 92%, and 86% for stages I, II, and III, respectively.[124] The relapse-free survival rate for patients with nonmetastatic favorable-histology Wilms' tumor was 88%.[124,125] Age over 4 years, large primary tumor size, and lymph node metastasis are prognostically negative factors.[125] Recent information on anaplastic Wilms' tumor shows an improvement in survival for patients with anaplastic tumors; children with tumors that have only focal anaplastic changes have better survival rates than children whose tumors have diffuse anaplasia.[116,117,148]

The use of doxorubicin-containing chemotherapy and irradiation for treatment of clear cell sarcoma produce results that approach those for Wilms' tumors of favorable histology.[124,148,149]

NEUROBLASTOMA

Neuroblastoma is a primitive neuronal tumor of sympathetic nervous tissue. These classic "small, round, blue cell" tumors are derived from primative neural crest cells. Described as enigmatic, neuroblastoma has been associated with spontaneous regression, maturation, or both; it also has a particular age-dependent prognosis, with persistently high mortality rates among children more than 1 year old.[150-152] A spectrum of cellular maturation is noted among tumors described as ganglioneuroblastoma (with features of immature, undifferentiated neuroblasts and mature ganglion cells) and ganglioneuroma (composed entirely of mature cellular elements, some of which are presumed to represent spontaneous maturation from earlier occult neuroblastoma).

The median age at diagnosis of neuroblastoma is 21 months; 30% of neuroblastoma cases are diagnosed in infants less than 1 year old and 80% in children less than 4 years old. The primary tumor site is most often in the abdomen, including the adrenal medulla, celiac axis, or paravertebral ganglia. Posterior mediastinal tumors account for 15% of cases, and 10% arise in the cervical sympathetic chain.

Neuroblastoma typically spreads to bone marrow, liver, and bone; 60% of children more than 1 year of age have identifiable hematogenous metastasis at diagnosis. Local disease extension occurs most notably in paravertebral locations, with tumor infiltrating through the neural foramina and spreading within the contiguous spinal canal as so-called dumbbell tumors. Lymph node metastasis has been reported in 33% to 48% of cases.[153,154]

A special pattern of metastatic neuroblastoma (stage 4S) associated with a high frequency of spontaneous cellular maturation or regression has been described.[152,155] Infants with stage 4S disease have small primary tumors and metastatic involvement confined to the liver, skin, or bone marrow and are known to have a good prognosis with observation only or very limited therapy.[156-158]

The clinicopathologic prognostic scheme defined by Shimada includes patient age, the mitosis-karyorrhexis index (MKI), proportion of differentiated neuroblasts, and stromal pattern.[159] Favorable-prognosis cases in this system are defined as follows: stroma-rich without a nodular pattern in patients of all ages; stroma-poor, differentiated, and an MKI of less than 100 in patients 1.5 to 5 years old; or stroma-poor and an MKI of greater than 2000 in patients less than 1.5 years old. Unfavorable-prognosis cases have converse defining characteristics.[159]

Among the biological variables predictive of therapeutic response and outcome in neuroblastoma, the most important is *N-myc* amplification, present in 25% of patients at diagnosis (5% to 10% of those with local–regional disease and 30% to 40% with disseminated disease).[160-162] Loss of heterozygosity at chromosome 1, an allelic loss at 1p36, correlates with *N-myc* amplification.[163] Other prognostic biological characteristics include *bcl-2* gene expression, a negative indicator correlated with unfavorable histology and *N-myc* amplification; TRK nerve growth factor expression, a positive indicator correlated with very young age and limited stage; and P-glycoprotein expression, a positive indicator.[164-166]

Staging

Several staging systems have been used for neuroblastoma. Of the systems most commonly used in the past,

the Evans-D'Angio and POG systems are based, respectively, on anatomic extent and on extent, degree of resection, and nodal involvement (Table 36-3[167-169]). The new International Neuroblastoma Staging System (INSS) was recently revised to better define the midline (i.e., INSS stage 3 was redefined to require disease extending across the width of the vertebral column). The use of stage 4S was also limited to infants less than 1 year old.[170] As noted earlier in this section, the latter special category refers to cases with local stage 1 or 2 primary lesions and metastases limited to the skin, liver, and bone marrow (specifically excluding those with imaging evidence of osseous disease).[152]

The complex interactions of clinical factors (e.g., stage and age), biology (e.g., *N-myc* amplification and, for infants, deoxyribonucleic acid [DNA] ploidy), and histology currently define low-, intermediate-, and high-risk presentations for risk-related protocol therapy in trials conducted by the COG.[171] Localized neuroblastoma generally has a very favorable prognosis after surgery, with or without chemotherapy.[161,172-177]

Surgery, Observation, Chemotherapy, and a Limited Role for Radiation Therapy

Most cases of localized neuroblastoma are managed by surgery alone, with disease-free survival rates of 85% to 90% and overall survival rates approaching 95%.[161,172,173,175-177] No proven benefit exists for adjuvant irradiation or chemotherapy.[175,177] Almost identical disease control rates can be achieved for patients with extracapsular but node-negative presentations (INSS stage 2A) after surgery (used either as primary treatment or adjuvant treatment after chemotherapy for sizable primary lesions) using relatively nonintensive chemotherapy.[178] Researchers from Memorial-Sloan Kettering Cancer Center reported similar disease-free and overall survival rates after using observation and limited additional surgery, essentially without cytotoxic chemotherapy, in a cohort of moderate size.[175] When used, chemotherapeutic regimens include cyclophosphamide, doxorubicin, cisplatin, and either etoposide or teniposide. The incidence of local failure is less than 10% after adjuvant chemotherapy.[178]

The areas of controversy with regard to use of radiation therapy focus on locally advanced or regional stage disease. INSS stage 2B includes patients with unilateral primary tumors and ipsilateral nodal metastasis. The impact of nodal involvement has been somewhat unclear; several early reports have indicated an adverse effect.[158,179] Whether more consistent use of regional irradiation would eliminate any effect of nodal extension was speculated on in series reported several years ago.[154] In a POG prospective randomized trial of postoperative chemotherapy with or without irradiation (24 to 30 Gy in 16 to 20 fractions) in children more than

TABLE 36-3

Staging Systems for Neuroblastomas

Evans and Colleagues[167]	Pediatric Oncology Group[169]	International Staging System[168]
STAGE I Tumor confined to the organ or structure of origin.	**STAGE A** Complete gross resection of primary tumor, with or without microscopic residual disease. Intracavitary lymph nodes that are not adhered to or removed in continuity with primary tumor are histologically free of tumor (nodes adhered to or within tumor resection may be positive for tumor without upstaging patient to stage C). If primary tumor in abdomen or pelvis, liver histologically free of tumor.	**STAGE 1** Localized tumor confined to the area of origin; complete gross excision, with or without microscopic residual disease; identifiable ipsilateral and contralateral lymph nodes negative microscopically.
STAGE II Tumor extending in continuity beyond the origin or structure of origin but not crossing the midline. Regional lymph nodes on the ipsilateral side may be involved.	**STAGE B** Gross unresected primary tumor. Nodes and liver same as stage A.	**STAGE 2A** Unilateral tumor with incomplete gross excision; identifiable ipsilateral and contralateral lymph nodes negative microscopically. **STAGE 2B** Unilateral tumor with complete or incomplete gross excision; positive ipsilateral regional lymph nodes; and identifiable contralateral lymph nodes negative microscopically.
STAGE III Tumor extending in continuity beyond the midline. Regional lymph nodes may be involved bilaterally.	**STAGE C** Complete or incomplete resection of primary tumor. Intracavitary nodes that are not adhered to primary tumor, are histologically positive for tumor. Liver as in stage A.	**STAGE 3** Tumor infiltrating across the midline with or without regional lymph node involvement; or unilateral tumor with contralateral regional lymph node involvement; or midline tumor with bilateral regional lymph node involvement.
STAGE IV Remote disease involving the skeleton, bone marrow, soft tissue, distant lymph node groups, and so on (see stage IV-S below).	**STAGE D** Any dissemination of disease beyond intracavitary nodes, i.e., extracavitary nodes, liver, skin, bone marrow, or bone.	**STAGE 4** Dissemination of tumor to distant lymph nodes, bone, bone marrow, liver, and/or other organs (except as defined in stage 4S).
STAGE IV-S Patients who would otherwise be stage I or stage II but who have remote disease confined to liver, skin, or bone marrow (without radiographic evidence of bone metastases on complete skeletal survey).		**STAGE 4S** Localized primary tumor as defined (see p. 921).

1 year old with stage C neuroblastoma, children with local tumor extent comparable with INSS stage 3 or Evans-D'Angio stage III who received radiation therapy had superior rates of complete response (76% with irradiation vs. 56% with chemotherapy only), event-free survival (59% vs. 32%), and overall survival (73% vs. 41%) than comparably staged children who had chemotherapy only. The mediastinal and supraclavicular nodal regions received doses of 24 and 18 Gy, respectively.[180] A subsequent POG trial in stage C cases used dose-intensive chemotherapy and second-look surgery, reserving irradiation for those with residual local–regional disease after the second-look surgery.[181] The overall results were said to be comparable with the earlier study group that received radiation but showed a poor outcome (< 10% event-free survival) for those with *N-myc* amplification.[181] Experience with treating residual, nonmetastatic neuroblastoma in children more than 1 year old either with observation and surgery or with nonmyeloablative chemotherapy has generally been interpreted to indicate that limited indications for irradiation exist in children with less than metastatic disease at diagnosis.[173-177,182] The use of intraoperative irradiation has also been explored in selected settings, often for regional consolidation therapy in children who initially had stage 4 disease and responded to chemotherapy.[183,184]

For children older than 1 or 2 years presenting with stage 4 disease, long-term disease control rates generally range from 20% to 40%.[113,171,185,186] The degree of progress over the past decade is unclear. The use of high-dose, myeloablative chemotherapy (with autologous marrow or peripheral stem cell reconstitution), sometimes combined with total body irradiation, has resulted in survival rates approximating 40% in some series. Concurrent CCG trials found that intensive chemotherapy produced better 4-year event-free survival rates than did conventional chemotherapy (40% vs. 19%, respectively).[171,185,186] A benefit from primary tumor resection in patients with stage 4 disease has been supported in recent analyses.[187,188] However, a benefit from local or regional irradiation in stage 4 disease has never been proven, although patterns of failure analyses have shown local–regional disease recurrence in up to one third of children with stage 4 disease.[182,189] The use of 18 to 21 Gy (typically 0.15 Gy per fraction, delivered once or twice daily) to local–regional sites of residual disease before high-dose chemotherapy and total body irradiation has been studied. Institutional and cooperative group experiences suggest that this regimen is tolerable and effective.[182,189-192] For patients with evidence of residual disease on images obtained before planned ablative chemotherapy, regional irradiation seems to be beneficial. Total body irradiation regimens typically involve 12 Gy given in fractions of 0.2 Gy once or twice daily or 0.12 Gy twice a day.[190,192]

For infants with stage 2B or 3 disease, less aggressive (i.e., no myeloablative) chemotherapy has resulted in disease control rates of more than 90%.[193,194] The DNA index has been an important prognostic variable, with inferior outcome among infants with diploid patterns. Those with stage 4 disease have survival rates of 75% to 80% after modern chemotherapy.[180,195] It is uncommon to require irradiation in this age group.

Infants presenting with stage 4S disease represent a small group with a relatively favorable prognosis.[152] Survival rates approach 90% with limited intervention such as limited-intensity chemotherapy. A significant minority of patients will present with urgent respiratory compromise resulting from massive hepatomegaly; recent series indicate up to two thirds of cases requiring any form of therapy will need hepatic irradiation.[157] Typical hepatic irradiation regimens deliver a total of 4.5 Gy, given in three consecutive daily 1.5-Gy fractions to the entire liver.[157]

Neuroblastoma often presents in paravertebral locations, both intrathoracic and intra-abdominal. The so-called dumbbell pattern, with direct extension through the neural foramina into the epidural compartment of the spinal canal, is relatively common. Current therapy for paravertebral neuroblastoma is most often chemotherapy alone, with occasional indications for laminectomy or irradiation at presentation.[161,196] For patients presenting with progressive abdominal disease or disseminated osseous disease, palliative irradiation is highly effective. Local doses of 21 to 30 Gy using conventional or accelerated fractionation often produce immediate relief of bone pain or improvement in bulky retroperitoneal disease. Radiolabeled meta-iodobenzyl-guanidine has been shown to be effective against diffuse, symptomatic bone metastases.[158,197,198]

RHABDOMYOSARCOMA

Rhabdomyosarcoma is a primitive tumor of skeletal muscle origin accounting for more than 70% of childhood soft tissue sarcomas. The most common sites of origin are the head and neck (40%), the genitourinary tract (20% to 25%), the extremities (15% to 20%), and the trunk (15% to 20%). Children younger than 6 years more commonly have tumors of the head and neck and genitourinary tract (especially vaginal, bladder, and prostatic tumors) compared with adolescents, who more often have tumors of the extremities, trunk (thorax, retroperitoneum, or perineum), and paratesticular regions.

Ultrastructural studies of rhabdomyosarcoma often reveal the striated muscle origin. In the Intergroup Rhabdomyosarcoma Study Group (IRS) studies in the United States,[199] embryonal rhabdomyosarcoma has been the most common histologic subtype; alveolar rhabdomyosarcoma has been the second most common subtype; and undifferentiated sarcomas and peripheral neuroepitheliomas (also called peripheral primitive neuroectodermal tumors or extraosseous Ewing's sarcoma) have accounted for the remaining tumors. The histologic subtypes are associated with various clinical and biological findings. Embryonal rhabdomyosarcoma, which accounts for 55% of cases, occurs primarily in children younger than 8 years and at head and neck or genitourinary sites; the tumor is associated with loss of heterozygosity at chromosome 11 (11p15). Alveolar rhabdomyosarcoma, which accounts for 20% of cases, is more common in adolescents, originating in extremity or truncal sites; a specific t(2;13)(q35;q14) translocation marks this entity. Botryoid rhabdomyosarcoma, which accounts for 5% of cases, is an exophytic growth, marked histologically by a subepithelial cambium layer of dense cellularity; the tumor occurs predominantly in infants as bladder or vaginal lesions and less commonly in young children within the nasopharynx. Other uncommon subtypes of rhabdomyosarcoma include undifferentiated and pleomorphic sarcomas. Extraosseous Ewing's sarcoma (or peripheral primitive neuroectodermal tumor) is considered a separate entity, initially identified by the IRS Group but now managed and reported with osseous Ewing's tumors.[200-206]

Uncommon lesions related to rhabdomyosarcoma include ectomesenchymomas (rhabdomyosarcoma with neuronal differentiation) and Triton tumors (malignant peripheral nerve sheath tumors with rhabdomyosarcoma components).[202-204,206]

The natural history of rhabdomyosarcoma is of local tissue infiltration, regional lymph node involvement, and hematogeneous dissemination. The tumor notoriously spreads along soft tissue planes. Primary tumors in the nasopharynx (and nasal cavity), paranasal sinuses, middle ear, and infratemporal or pterygoid fossa are grouped as parameningeal lesions; they share a tendency to involve the adjacent base of the skull by direct bone erosion or infiltration along cranial nerves (Fig. 34-4).[207]

Rhabdomyosarcoma is typically an invasive tumor, presenting as local–regional disease in 83% of cases and as overt metastases in 17%.[199,208,209] Lymph node metastasis has been documented in 15% of children at diagnosis; primary tumors were in the prostate in 40%, paratesticular region in 25%, extremities in 12%, head or neck (excluding orbit, where no node-positive cases were reported in IRS-II) in 7%, and trunk in 5%.[208,209]

The initial IRS studies (IRS-I, -II, and -III) used postoperative disease extent to define stage groups (Table 36-4).[209-211] The postoperative staging of children with rhabdomyosarcoma in these studies indicated that 15% had localized, completely resected tumors (group I) and 18% had metastatic disease (group IV).[212,213] Half of all tumors could not be completely resected (group III), and 15% to 20% of patients had microscopic local or regional residual disease after grossly complete resection (group II).[212,213]

Although these results confirmed the prognostic value of the grouping system, individual tumor factors (i.e., primary site, size, invasiveness, and lymph node metastasis) more accurately predicted outcome.[211,214] The current *preoperative* IRS staging system is therefore based on primary site, tumor extent (local invasiveness and size), and the presence or absence of regional lymph node metastasis or distant metastasis (Table 36-5).[209,210] The system is easily simplified by noting nonmetastatic tumors in favorable sites as stage I, localized tumors up

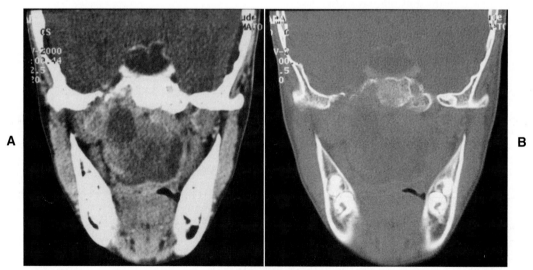

Fig. 36-4   Primary parameningeal rhabdomyosarcoma of the nasopharynx. **A,** Direct computed tomography (CT) with contrast outlines a sizable, complex tumor that fills the nasopharynx and extends through the base of the skull to involve the region of the right cavernous sinus. **B,** CT at bone window setting shows the extent of destruction of the right sphenoid.

TABLE 36-4

Surgical-Pathologic Grouping System Used in Intergroup Rhabdomyosarcoma Study Group Trials

Group	Criteria
I	Localized disease, completely resected: A. Confined to the muscle or organ of origin B. Infiltration outside organ or muscle of origin; regional lymph nodes not involved
II	Compromised or regional resection of three types, including the following: A. Grossly resected tumors with microscopic residual B. Regional disease, completely resected, in which lymph nodes may be involved and/or extension of tumor into an adjacent organ may be present C. Regional disease with involved lymph nodes, macroscopically resected but with evidence of microscopic residual disease
III	Incomplete resection or biopsy with macroscopic residual disease
IV	Distant metastases present at diagnosis

From Lawrence W Jr, Anderson JR, Gehan EA, et al. *Cancer* 1997;80:1165-1170.

to 5 cm in diameter in other sites as stage II, size above 5 cm or the presence of lymph node metastasis as stage III, and hematogenous dissemination as stage IV. The IRS-IV study used stage to determine chemotherapy regimen and group to determine radiation regimen.

Radiation Therapy
Central Role in Treatment

Therapy for rhabdomyosarcoma includes surgery and chemotherapy for essentially all presentations; irradiation is indicated for microscopic (group II) or overt (group III) local–regional disease and sites of metastatic involvement (group IV). Earlier studies of surgery alone documented limited disease control after radical surgery at selected sites—a 45% disease-free survival rate for patients with orbital tumors and up to 70% disease-free survival rates for patients with limited bladder lesions outside the trigone.[215,216] Therapy in North America almost uniformly follows the guidelines of the IRS protocols.

Rhabdomyosarcoma was initially thought to respond poorly to irradiation. Reports by Cassady and colleagues,[217] Edland,[218] and Nelson[219] in the 1960s established the efficacy of radiation therapy, describing local tumor control after wide-field irradiation to dose levels of 50 to 60 Gy. For orbital tumors, primary irradiation achieved local tumor control in 90% of cases, although

TABLE 36-5

Preoperative Staging System Used by the Intergroup Rhabdomyosarcoma Study Group

Stage	Sites	Invasiveness*	Size	Lymph Nodes†	Distant Metastases‡
I	Orbit, head and neck (except parameningeal) Genitourinary tract (except bladder or prostate)	T1 or T2	a (< 5 cm) or b (≥ 5 cm)	N0 or N1 or N2	M0
II	Bladder or prostate Extremity Head and neck parameningeal Other (including trunk, retroperitoneum, and so on)	T1 or T2	a (< 5 cm)	N0 or NX	M0
III	Bladder or prostate Extremity Head and neck parameningeal Other (including trunk, retroperitoneum, and so on)	T1 or T2	a (< 5 cm) b (≥ 5 cm)	N1 N0 or N1 or NX	M0
IV	All	T1 or T2	a (< 5 cm) or b (≥ 5 cm)	N0 or N1	M1

Modified from Lawrence W Jr, Anderson JR, Gehan EA, et al. *Cancer* 1997;80:1165-1170.
*T1, confined to anatomic site of origin; T2, extension and/or fixation to the surrounding tissue
†N0, regional lymph nodes not clinically involved; N1, regional lymph nodes clinically involved by neoplasm; NX, clinical status of regional lymph nodes unknown (especially with sites that preclude lymph node evaluation)
‡M0, no distant metastasis; M1, metastasis present.

survival was limited to 66% because of hematogenous metastases.[220]

The addition of chemotherapy has improved both local tumor control and survival. Jereb and colleagues[221] reported a 2-year disease-free survival rate of 82% for patients with localized disease treated with chemotherapy versus 47% for patients treated without chemotherapy.

Combining chemotherapy and irradiation with less radical surgery has proved feasible in many cases. Initial chemotherapy followed by surgery and response-directed irradiation has proven effective for a significant proportion of lesions that are not easily and completely resectable at presentation.[222-226]

For children with localized rhabdomyosarcoma (group I), the addition of radiation therapy did not improve overall disease control in the initial IRS studies.[213,227] The failure-free survival rate with late follow-up of the IRS-I through -III trials was only 79% in a recent update from Wolden and colleagues.[228] Most group I lesions are relatively limited in size, are often located in the extremities, are unusually small bladder lesions, or are located in nonparameningeal sites in the head or neck. Findings regarding local control without irradiation indicated higher rates of local failure for tumors larger than 5 cm, with alveolar or undifferentiated histology, and at sites other than the genitourinary tract. In group I cases with alveolar or undifferentiated histology in the IRS-I and -II trials, the addition of radiation therapy significantly enhanced local tumor control (73% vs. 44%) and overall survival (82% vs. 52%).[228] For embryonal tumors, a trend toward improved failure-free survival was not statistically significant; no difference in overall survival was apparent.[228] In current trials, a reduced radiation dose (36 to 41.4 Gy) is recommended for children with unfavorable histology and group I (localized, resected) disease.

For patients with group II disease (microscopic residual disease only), dose levels of 36 to 40 Gy produce durable local control in more than 90% of cases.[199,229-231] For those with group III tumors (representing up to two thirds of local–regional presentations), dose levels of 45 Gy (selectively used in children younger than 6 years with tumors smaller than 5 cm) to 50 Gy (in conventional fractions, typically 1.8 Gy, occasionally reduced to 1.5 Gy, once daily) produce an 80% likelihood of local tumor control (Table 36-6).[232] The rate of local–regional failure is 15% for tumors originating within the head and neck or genitourinary region and no larger than 10 cm; for lesions originating in the chest, pelvis, trunk, or extremities or for primary lesions larger than 10 cm at other, more favorable sites, the rate of local–regional failure is significantly higher, at 35%.[232]

The importance of radiation therapy is apparent from the high rate of local recurrence among the most

TABLE 36-6

Protocol-Required Total Radiation Dose for Group III Rhabdomyosarcoma Patients and Corresponding Local Failure Rates*

Patient Age	Tumor Size	Dose	Local Failure Rate (%)
< 6 years	< 5 cm	40-45 Gy	16
	≥ 5 cm	45-50 Gy	23
≥ 6 years	< 5 cm	45-50 Gy	14
	≥ 5 cm	50-55 Gy	26

From Wharam MD, Hanfelt JJ, Tefft MC, et al. *Int J Radiat Oncol Biol Phys* 1997;38:797-804.
*Special pelvic sites excluded.

favorable orbital tumors when the primary treatment is chemotherapy. The SIOP experience indicates a local failure rate of 45% without irradiation compared with 10% with irradiation in the IRS experience.[232-234] A comparative analysis of parameningeal rhabdomyosarcoma trials from the IRS, SIOP, and German and Italian cooperative studies indicated significantly superior 5-year event-free survival and overall survival rates in the IRS experience (71% event-free survival and 74% overall survival), where radiation therapy (median dose 53 Gy) was used systematically, compared with the SIOP experience (36% event-free survival and 55% overall survival), where irradiation was limited to children older than 5 years with signs of intracranial extension, or the German (47% and 47%, respectively) or Italian (39% and 39%, respectively) experiences, where radiation therapy was either delayed for 3 months or limited to a median dose of 45 to 46 Gy with no central quality control.[233]

Orbital rhabdomyosarcoma is generally approached with biopsy and irradiation as group III disease; a minority of patients (group II) undergo initial resection, usually short of exenteration, and irradiation. The target volume typically includes the entire orbit, although more limited radiation therapy may be appropriate for anterior lesions. Disease control and survival rates exceed 90% with approaches that include irradiation as local therapy.[232,233,235] More than 80% of patients experience cataracts after radiation therapy for orbital rhabdomyosarcoma, and reduced vision has been documented in 70% of cases.[236] Surgery for symptomatic sequelae of primary radiation therapy or disease recurrence is required in approximately 15% of cases with long-term follow-up.[236] Xerophthalmia occurs less often than might be expected, but posttherapy orbital hypoplasia has been documented in a majority of surviving children.[236]

Parameningeal rhabdomyosarcoma often demonstrates overt extension into the base of the skull, manifesting as cranial nerve palsy, base of skull erosion on CT or MRI, or direct intracranial extension.[61,237,238] The initial IRS experience demonstrating a 35% rate of meningeal (largely extradural rather than subarachnoid) extension has subsequently been reduced to rates of less than 15% or 20% for local or marginal failures with wide local radiation volumes (including margins of 2 cm above the skull base for signs of cranial nerve or bone erosion, and wider margins around sites of overt intracranial extension on neuroimaging).[61,232,238,239] Tumors at other head and neck sites have a very favorable outcome with primary irradiation or irradiation combined with judicious surgery.[232,240]

For bladder and prostate rhabdomyosarcoma, therapy in earlier IRS studies involved a change from primary surgery to primary chemotherapy and selected, delayed irradiation, resulting in disease control with bladder preservation in only 25% of children in the IRS-I and -II trials.[223-225,241] More recent experience with early use of local irradiation (usually about 45 Gy at week 20) in the IRS-III trial has achieved 80% disease-free survival and 60% preservation of bladder control.[241] Use of partial cystectomy for lesions away from the bladder trigone, often in conjunction with radiation therapy, has been particularly successful.[223] Combined-modality therapy has produced favorable functional outcome.[242]

Paratesticular rhabdomyosarcoma has been among the most favorable presentations, although in recent IRS trials, the use of less aggressive chemotherapy when assessment of para-aortic nodes has been done only with imaging resulted in a higher rate of failure.[61,202,243] The less common vaginal rhabdomyosarcoma has been successfully managed with brachytherapy.[244]

Rhabdomyosarcoma originating in the extremities and trunk (including thorax, abdomen/retroperitoneum, pelvis, and perineum) is common in adolescents and frequently has an alveolar histology. Treatment generally includes induction chemotherapy followed by primary irradiation or delayed resection, the latter best followed by dose-adjusted irradiation depending on the extent of resection.*

Technique

Radiation therapy can be initiated at diagnosis or after induction chemotherapy. No data exist to suggest that delaying radiation therapy for up to 4 months is deleterious except for tumors at parameningeal sites. For patients with intracranial extension of parameningeal tumors, it is important to initiate irradiation at the very start of combined-modality therapy.

The radiation technique used should ensure broad coverage of the primary tumor, with 2-cm margins beyond the preoperative, prechemotherapy tumor volume in most instances. For tumors in areas where

abdominal or pelvic viscera present problems with radiation tolerance, margins may be limited to 1 cm. For tumors at parameningeal sites, it is important to identify 2-cm dosimetric margins in all three dimensions. The advantage of three-dimensional conformal techniques is just beginning to be apparent.[247] Treatment of regional lymph nodes is indicated primarily for patients with proven nodal involvement; however, the high incidence of lymph node metastasis in extremity tumors of alveolar or undifferentiated histology warrants consideration of adjacent lymph node irradiation in this setting.[232,248]

The established dose level of 40 Gy for microscopic residual disease (IRS group II) provides local tumor control in 95% to 98% of cases.[249,250] However, limited data suggest that doses less than 40 Gy may be adequate for microscopic residual disease after initial surgery.[230] For macroscopic residual disease, the IRS reports indicate that 50 Gy produces excellent disease control in most settings; however, review data substantiate a higher local failure rate with large tumors or unfavorable histologic types, findings that argue for consideration of higher dose levels in such settings.[232] Hyperfractionated irradiation to dose levels of 59.4 Gy (0.11 Gy twice a day) has produced outcomes rather similar to those with conventionally fractionated irradiation, although the final results of the IRS-V randomized trial testing hyperfractionated delivery are not yet available.[231,251]

Flamant and colleagues[244] reported disease control and excellent functional preservation in 15 of 17 patients with vaginal rhabdomyosarcoma treated with an individualized technique of intracavitary irradiation.

Prognosis

The IRS trials have resulted in continual improvements in outcome, with 5-year survival rates for patients with rhabdomyosarcoma increasing from 56% (IRS-I) to 63% (IRS-II) to 72% (IRS-III).[199,232] Outcome depends on tumor site and histology, extent of local disease, and lymph node involvement.

RETINOBLASTOMA

Retinoblastoma is a malignant embryonal neoplasm arising in the retina during fetal life or early childhood. The tumor is unilateral in two thirds of patients and bilateral in one third of patients. More than 90% of these tumors occur before age 4 years; the median age is 8 months for patients with bilateral retinoblastoma and 26 months for those with unilateral disease. Diagnosis in children typically is made on the basis of leukokoria (white eye reflex, in which the retinal tumor reflects light), strabismus, or glaucoma.

A family history of retinoblastoma is present in 10% of patients. Retinoblastoma is the classic genetically

---

*References 224, 229, 231, 232, 245, 246.

inherited pediatric cancer; genetic studies of the disease have not only confirmed Knudson's "two-hit hypothesis" of cancer development but provided the evidence for the discovery of cancer suppressor genes.[252] Retinoblastoma results from the loss or mutation of both copies of the *RB1* gene, located at 13q14.[55,253,254]

Retinoblastoma arises from the inner nuclear layer of the retina. Histologically, the tumor comprises small, uniform neuroectodermal cells with various degrees of photoreceptor differentiation. Tumor cells grow through the retinal layers, often infiltrating into the surrounding choroid or the vitreous. Lesions with pronounced late choroidal involvement may extend extrasclerally along the emissary vessels. Tumor cells gain access to the optic nerve by direct infiltration at the optic disk or by extension along the central vessels. Lesions that involve the optic nerve can be associated with diffuse subarachnoid involvement, an uncommon late manifestation of the disease. Even with negative surgical margins, however, tumors that infiltrate through the lamina cribrosa (i.e., into the optic nerve proper) have been associated with an increased risk of orbital recurrence or metastatic disease.[255]

Staging for retinoblastoma has classically been based on Reese's system (Box 36-1).[256] Groups are defined by the number, size, and location of intraocular tumors and indicate the suitability of a tumor for less than

---

BOX 36-1   Reese-Ellsworth Staging System for Retinoblastoma

GROUP I (VERY FAVORABLE)
a. Solitary tumor, less than 4 dd*, at or behind the equator
b. Multiple tumors, none over 4 dd, all at or behind the equator

GROUP II (FAVORABLE)
a. Solitary lesion, 4-10 dd, at or behind the equator
b. Multiple tumors, 4-10 dd, behind the equator

GROUP III (DOUBTFUL)
a. Any lesion anterior to the equator
b. Solitary lesions larger than 10 dd behind the equator

GROUP IV (UNFAVORABLE)
a. Multiple tumors, some larger than 10 dd
b. Any lesion extending anteriorly to the ora serrata

GROUP V (VERY UNFAVORABLE)
a. Massive tumors involving over half the retina
b. Vitreous seeding

From Reese AB. *Tumors of the Eye.* 3rd ed. Hagerstown, Md: Harper & Row; 1976.
**dd*, Disk diameter (1 dd = 1.6 mm).

---

exenterative treatment (i.e., radiation therapy, cryotherapy, or photocoagulation).

Radiation Therapy

Treatment for retinoblastoma has been determined largely by the presence or absence of advanced ocular disease at diagnosis. Enucleation alone is appropriate for many unilateral tumors, which are often sufficiently advanced to obviate consideration of eye-preserving local therapies. For children older than 2 or 3 years in whom the genetic form of disease can reasonably be excluded if the presentation is unilateral, one can consider focal therapy alone (more often photocoagulation or cryotherapy, but also brachytherapy or, in some institutions, focal external beam irradiation).[257] The use of standard, full ocular radiation techniques for sporadic cases of unilateral disease has been documented; the combination of chemotherapy and more focal irradiation in this setting has been used infrequently.[258]

For patients with bilateral retinoblastoma, at least one eye shows group V disease in more than 90% of instances. The principle of therapy is to preserve the eye in any case in which there is a reasonable expectation that functional vision might result. In practice, most children with bilateral disease begin treatment with chemotherapy, followed by local measures including focal surgical approaches (cryotherapy for anterior lesions or photocoagulation for more posterior areas) and irradiation (focal brachytherapy plaques or external-beam irradiation, depending on the extent of disease after chemotherapy).[259-262]

External-beam irradiation has been used with considerable success for moderate to advanced intraocular disease; findings over the past four decades have documented disease control in 70% to 80% of cases with group I to III disease. Cassady and colleagues[263] reported a 73% disease control rate, with good to fair vision, among 120 patients treated with external-beam irradiation between 1954 and 1963; both orthovoltage and megavoltage (22.5-MV) x-ray techniques were used during this period. In the 1980s, Schipper reported from Utrecht that tumor was controlled and vision preserved in 33 (94%) of 35 patients with group I to III disease by using an anatomically precise lateral linear accelerator technique with ocular fixation and a narrowly defined target volume (Fig. 36-5).[264] With more advanced ocular disease, Schipper and colleagues[265] described ocular preservation in 11 (79%) of 14 patients with group IV disease but 0 of 5 patients with group V disease. The Utrecht irradiation technique has also achieved disease control in a limited number of cases with vitreous seeding and otherwise limited tumor extent.[265,266]

The use of chemotherapy has resulted in primary tumor control in only a very limited subset of cases but

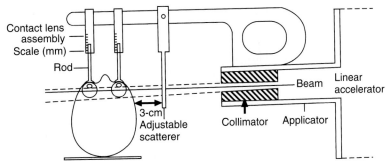

Fig. 36-5 Diagram of a treatment approach for retinoblastoma involving opposed lateral fields, here closely calibrated to identify the posterior margin of the optic lens, with a fixed correlation between the central ray of the photon beam (defining the anterior coronal plane) and the anterior position of the eye (here affixed to the head of the accelerator by a suction contact). Current approaches include opposed lateral beams such as those shown here or three-dimensional conformal configurations. (Technique described in Schipper J, Tan KE, van Peperzeel HA. *Radiother Oncol* 1985;3:117-132.)

has achieved substantial reductions in the extent of ocular disease, facilitating apparently successful use of local treatment modalities in most cases.[259-262] Objective responses to alkylating agents (especially cyclophosphamide, ifosfamide, and cisplatin), etoposide, vincristine, and doxorubicin have been seen.[260,267] One goal of initial chemotherapy approaches has been to limit the use of external-beam irradiation because of the relatively high rate of secondary cancer in children with the genetic form of disease (bilateral or multifocal disease) and late orbital deformities after irradiation in this very young population.[10,45,185,260-262] More focal types of therapy, such as focal surgical or radiotherapeutic interventions, have shown excellent rates of disease control in ocular disease without vitreous seeding.[10,185,258,260-262] For advanced cases with massive intraocular or vitreous disease, initial chemotherapy followed by external-beam irradiation in responding patients has allowed ocular preservation in some cases that would otherwise have required enucleation.[259-262,268,269] Close ophthalmologic observation during initial chemotherapy is critical to maximize local "salvage" approaches.

Local irradiation techniques have included ^{60}Co applicators and more recently the use of ^{192}Ir or ^{125}I. The high rate of recurrence after focal radiation therapy only had limited enthusiasm for brachytherapy in cases with bilateral presentations; however, renewed interest in this modality has been shown in conjunction with chemotherapy.[257]

When irradiation is used as the primary therapy, cryotherapy or photocoagulation may be needed for local sites of apparent disease persistence or as adjuvant therapy for tumors extending anteriorly within the globe.[265]

Visual acuity after irradiation depends on tumor size and location. In 22 eyes with tumor control, Egbert and colleagues[270] reported visual acuity of better than 20/40 in five, up to 20/100 in five, 20/200 to hand movements in nine, and no vision in three eyes. Poor visual results correlate primarily with tumor involvement of the macular region.[257,270] Deterioration in visual status and the need for enucleation may result infrequently from late effects of therapy rather than tumor recurrence; late effects include vitreous hemorrhage, retinopathy, and ischemic optic nerve neuropathy.[257,270]

Orbital irradiation is indicated postoperatively for documented scleral extension of tumor, extraocular disease, or tumor infiltration of the optic nerve beyond the lamina cribrosa.[271] Cranial irradiation or CSI has been used in patients with microscopic extension of retinoblastoma to the cut end of the optic nerve or CNS involvement at diagnosis. Long-term disease control in this setting has been rare.[57,267]

Radiation Therapy Technique

The anterior field margin for lateral photon irradiation is placed just behind the lens, in practice, 7 to 9 mm posterior to the anterior surface of the eye.[264] With three-dimensional conformal radiation approaches, multifield, noncoplanar configurations may offer an advantage in full-retinal disease control, with relative sparing of the optic lens and in most circumstances with avoiding irradiation to the contralateral eye when appropriate.[255] Use of a single anterior electron field or multiple obliqued electron fields may achieve uniform retinal irradiation, with rates of later cataractogenesis and ocular effects similar to those produced by the three-dimensional approaches.[255,272]

Sedation is usually necessary to ensure the accuracy of daily positioning and immobilization. Schipper[264] has detailed an exquisite radiation therapy technique using a globe-fixing contact lens mechanically attached to the linear accelerator gantry to ensure both ocular immobilization and proper field placement on a daily basis.

No firm radiation dose-response data have been published for retinoblastoma. The report of Cassady and colleagues[263] of the early Columbia experience showed equal tumor control rates with doses of 35 to 40 Gy and doses of more than 40 Gy delivered in hypofractionated regimens (3.33- to 4-Gy fractions delivered three times a week). Schipper and colleagues[265] also used three fractions per week, delivering 45 Gy in 15 treatments. The rate of tumor control and visual preservation seems to approach a balance at 40 to 50 Gy, suggesting that a fractionated regimen of 2 Gy, given four to five times weekly to a total dose of 40 to 45 Gy, is effective. Whether dose levels can be successfully reduced in the setting of adjuvant or, more often, "salvage" irradiation after initial response to or progression after chemotherapy remains uncertain.[259,260]

Prognosis

The survival rate after treatment of retinoblastoma is excellent, with more than 90% survival rates documented for all stages.[258-261,265,273,274] Even in patients with advanced (group V) disease, survival rates of 70% to 90% have been reported in long-term series from North America and Europe.[57,275,276] It is noteworthy that advanced, frequently extraocular extension of disease at diagnosis limits results in developing countries to half that level.[277]

No evidence exists to suggest that conservative primary therapy has increased the risk of subsequent hematogenous metastasis or death. Overall survival rates in patients with advanced bilateral disease are virtually identical after bilateral enucleation (92%) and initial bilateral irradiation with delayed enucleation for disease recurrence (88%).[275] Death from retinoblastoma in patients with group I to IV disease has been rare.[259-261]

LIVER NEOPLASMS

Primary tumors of the liver are rare in children. Hepatoblastoma is the most common malignant liver neoplasm in children up to age 5 years, after which hepatocellular carcinoma becomes the most common. Hepatoblastoma is a tumor type that occurs as part of the Beckwith-Wiedemann syndrome.[278] Hepatoblastoma is often a unifocal tumor. Histologically, it is identified as an epithelial tumor (with fetal or embryonal components) or a mixed lesion (also including mesenchymal components).[279]

Hepatocellular carcinoma occurs in children older than 5 years; as in adults, it is associated with hepatitis-B surface antigen.[280] Both hepatoblastoma and hepatocellular carcinoma present as abdominal masses, usually associated with elevated serum alpha-fetoprotein levels.

Hepatic tumors have been managed primarily by surgical resection, with major series showing 50% to 65% of such tumors to be potentially resectable at diagnosis.[281-283] Among 48 cases reported by Giacomantonio and colleagues,[282] 16 patients underwent gross surgical resection; 11 of these 16 patients survived without recurrence, seven of nine after surgery alone and four of seven after preoperative chemotherapy and tumor removal. Operative mortality rates are approximately 2% to 10%.[282-284]

Preoperative irradiation has been described anecdotally; recent studies[281,285,286] have emphasized tumor regression with chemotherapy (dactinomycin, cyclophosphamide, vincristine, and fluorouracil; and more recently, doxorubicin, and cisplatin) before attempted resection. Among patients with residual disease after surgery, responses to radiation therapy, chemotherapy, or both have been documented, and a suggestion in the series by Habrand and colleagues[287] was made that radiation doses of 24 to 45 Gy can successfully control limited postoperative residual disease.

REFERENCES

1. Donaldson SS. Patterns of failure in childhood solid tumors. *Cancer Treat Symp* 1983;2:267-283.
2. Li FP, Stone R. Survivors of cancer in childhood. *Ann Intern Med* 1976;84:551-553.
3. Garre ML, Gandus S, Cesana B, et al. Health status of long-term survivors after cancer in childhood. Results of an uninstitutional study in Italy. *Am J Pediatr Hematol Oncol* 1994;16:143-152.
4. Thomas PR, Griffith KD, Fineberg BB, et al. Late effects of treatment for Wilms' tumor. *Int J Radiat Oncol Biol Phys* 1983;9:651-657.
5. Taylor RE. Morbidity from abdominal radiotherapy in the First United Kingdom Children's Cancer Study Group Wilms' Tumour Study. United Kingdom Children's Cancer Study Group. *Clin Oncol (R Coll Radiol)* 1997;9:381-384.
6. Jereb B, Burgers JM, Tournade MF, et al. Radiotherapy in the SIOP (International Society of Pediatric Oncology) nephroblastoma studies: a review. *Med Pediatr Oncol* 1994;22:221-227.
7. Riseborough EJ, Grabias SL, Burton RI, et al. Skeletal alterations following irradiation for Wilms' tumor: with particular reference to scoliosis and kyphosis. *J Bone Joint Surg Am* 1976;58:526-536.
8. Probert JC, Parker BR. The effects of radiation therapy on bone growth. *Radiology* 1975;114:155-162.
9. Oliver JH, Gluck G, Gledhill RB, et al. Musculoskeletal deformities following treatment of Wilms' tumour. *Can Med Assoc J* 1978;119:459-464.
10. Kaste SC, Chen G, Fontanesi J, et al. Orbital development in long-term survivors of retinoblastoma. *J Clin Oncol* 1997;15:1183-1189.
11. Shalet SM, Beardwell CG, Morris-Jones PH, et al. Pituitary function after treatment of intracranial tumours in children. *Lancet* 1975;2:104-107.
12. Shalet SM, Beardwell CG, Aarons BM, et al. Growth impairment in children treated for brain tumours. *Arch Dis Child* 1978;53:491-494.
13. Swift PG, Kearney PJ, Dalton RG, et al. Growth and hormonal status of children treated for acute lymphoblastic leukaemia. *Arch Dis Child* 1978;53:890-894.
14. Lustig RH, Rose SR, Burghen GA, et al. Hypothalamic obesity caused by cranial insult in children: altered glucose and insulin dynamics and reversal by a somatostatin agonist. *J Pediatr* 1999;135:162-168.

15. Shalet SM, Beardwell CG, Twomey JA, et al. Endocrine function following the treatment of acute leukemia in childhood. *J Pediatr* 1977;90:920-923.

16. Kaleita TA, Reaman GH, MacLean WE, et al. Neurodevelopmental outcome of infants with acute lymphoblastic leukemia: a Children's Cancer Group report. *Cancer* 1999;85:1859-1865.

17. Samaan NA, Vieto R, Schultz PN, et al. Hypothalamic, pituitary and thyroid dysfunction after radiotherapy to the head and neck. *Int J Radiat Oncol Biol Phys* 1982;8:1857-1867.

18. Robison LL, Nesbit ME, Sather HN. Thyroid abnormalities in long-term survivors of childhood acute lymphoblastic leukemia [abstract]. *Pediatr Res* 1985;19:266.

19. Oberfield SE, Allen JC, Pollack J, et al. Long-term endocrine sequelae after treatment of medulloblastoma: prospective study of growth and thyroid function. *J Pediatr* 1986;108:219-223.

20. Constine LS, Donaldson SS, McDougall IR, et al. Thyroid dysfunction after radiotherapy in children with Hodgkin's disease. *Cancer* 1984;53:878-883.

21. Merchant TE, Kushner BH, Sheldon JM, et al. Effect of low-dose radiation therapy when combined with surgical resection for Ewing sarcoma. *Med Pediatr Oncol* 1999;33:65-70.

22. Wohl ME, Griscom NT, Traggis DG, et al. Effects of therapeutic irradiation delivered in early childhood upon subsequent lung function. *Pediatrics* 1975;55:507-516.

23. Jakacki RI, Schramm CM, Donahue BR, et al. Restrictive lung disease following treatment for malignant brain tumors: a potential late effect of craniospinal irradiation. *J Clin Oncol* 1995; 13:1478-1485.

24. Freeman JE, Johnston PG, Voke JM. Somnolence after prophylactic cranial irradiation in children with acute lymphoblastic leukaemia. *Br Med J* 1973;4:523-525.

25. Bleyer WA. Neurologic sequelae of methotrexate and ionizing radiation: a new classification. *Cancer Treatment Reports* 1981; 65:89-98.

26. Price RA, Birdwell DA. The central nervous system in childhood leukemia. Mineralizing microangiopathy and dystrophic calcification. *Cancer* 1978;42(pt 3):717-728.

27. Peylan-Ramu N, Poplack DG, Pizzo PA, et al. Abnormal CT scans of the brain in asymptomatic children with acute lymphocytic leukemia after prophylactic treatment of the central nervous system with radiation and intrathecal chemotherapy. *N Engl J Med* 1978;298:815-818.

28. Riccardi R, Brouwers P, Di Chiro G, et al. Abnormal computed tomography brain scans in children with acute lymphoblastic leukemia: serial long-term follow-up. *J Clin Oncol* 1985;3:12-18.

29. Ochs JJ, Parvey LS, Whitaker JN, et al. Serial cranial computed-tomography scans in children with leukemia given two different forms of central nervous system therapy. *J Clin Oncol* 1983;1:793-798.

30. Price RA, Jamieson PA. The central nervous system in childhood leukemia. Subacute leukoencephalopathy. *Cancer* 1975;35(pt 2): 306-318.

31. Aur RJ, Simone JV, Verzosa MS, et al. Childhood acute lymphocytic leukemia: study VIII. *Cancer* 1978;42:2123-2134.

32. Bleyer WA, Griffin TW. White matter necrosis, mineralizing microangiopathy, and intellectual abilities in survivors of childhood leukemia: associations with CNS irradiation and methotrexate therapy. In: Gilbert HA, Kagan AR, eds. *Radiation Damage to the Nervous System.* New York, NY: Raven Press; 1980: 155-174.

33. Eiser C. Intellectual abilities among survivors of childhood leukaemia as a function of CNS irradiation. *Arch Dis Child* 1978;53:391-395.

34. Meadows AT, Gordon J, Massari DJ, et al. Declines in IQ scores and cognitive dysfunctions in children with acute lymphocytic leukaemia treated with cranial irradiation. *Lancet* 1981;2: 1015-1018.

35. Rowland JH, Glidewell OJ, Sibley RF, et al. Effects of different forms of central nervous system prophylaxis on neuropsychologic function in childhood leukemia. *J Clin Oncol* 1984;2:1327-1335.

36. Williams JM, Davis KS. Central nervous system prophylactic treatment for childhood leukemia: neuropsychological outcome studies. *Cancer Treat Rev* 1986;13:113-127.

37. Whitt JK, Wells RJ, Lauria MM, et al. Cranial radiation in childhood acute lymphocytic leukemia. Neuropsychologic sequelae. *Am J Dis Child* 1984;138:730-736.

38. Jannoun L. Are cognitive and educational development affected by age at which prophylactic therapy is given in acute lymphoblastic leukaemia? *Arch Dis Child* 1983;58:953-958.

39. Walter AW, Hancock ML, Pui CH, et al. Secondary brain tumors in children treated for acute lymphoblastic leukemia at St Jude Children's Research Hospital. *J Clin Oncol* 1998;16:3761-3767.

40. Li FP, Gimbrere K, Gelber RD. Adverse pregnancy outcome after radiotherapy for childhood Wilms' tumors [abstract]. *Proc Am Soc Clin Oncol* 1986;5:202.

41. Li FP, Fine W, Jaffe N, et al. Offspring of patients treated for cancer in childhood. *J Natl Cancer Inst* 1979;62:1193-1197.

42. Green DM, Fine WE, Li FP. Offspring of patients treated for unilateral Wilms' tumor in childhood. *Cancer* 1982;49: 2285-2288.

43. Li FP, Cassady JR, Jaffe N. Risk of second tumors in survivors of childhood cancer. *Cancer* 1975;35:1230-1235.

44. Hudson MM, Jones D, Boyett J, et al. Late mortality of long-term survivors of childhood cancer. *J Clin Oncol* 1997;15:2205-2213.

45. Wong FL, Boice JD Jr, Abramson DH, et al. Cancer incidence after retinoblastoma. Radiation dose and sarcoma risk. *JAMA* 1997; 278:1262-1267.

46. Beaty O III, Hudson MM, Greenwald C, et al. Subsequent malignancies in children and adolescents after treatment for Hodgkin's disease. *J Clin Oncol* 1995;13:603-609.

47. Tucker MA, D'Angio GJ, Boice JD Jr, et al. Bone sarcomas linked to radiotherapy and chemotherapy in children. *N Engl J Med* 1987;317:588-593.

48. Kuttesch JF Jr, Wexler LH, Marcus RB, et al. Second malignancies after Ewing's sarcoma: radiation dose-dependency of secondary sarcomas. *J Clin Oncol* 1996;14:2818-2825.

49. Garber JE, Goldstein AM, Kantor AF, et al. Follow-up study of twenty-four families with Li-Fraumeni syndrome. *Cancer Res* 1991;51:6094-6097.

50. Riccardi VM. Von Recklinghausen neurofibromatosis. *N Engl J Med* 1981;305:1617-1627.

51. Listernick R, Charrow J, Greenwald M, et al. Natural history of optic pathway tumors in children with neurofibromatosis type 1: a longitudinal study. *J Pediatr* 1994;125:63-66.

52. Matsui I, Tanimura M, Kobayashi N, et al. Neurofibromatosis type 1 and childhood cancer. *Cancer* 1993;72:2746-2754.

53. Kraemer KH, Lee MM, Scotto J. Xeroderma pigmentosum. Cutaneous, ocular, and neurologic abnormalities in 830 published cases. *Arch Dermatol* 1987;123:241-250.

54. Swift M, Morrell D, Massey RB, et al. Incidence of cancer in 161 families affected by ataxia-telangiectasia. *N Engl J Med* 1991; 325:1831-1836.

55. Eng C, Li FP, Abramson DH, et al. Mortality from second tumors among long-term survivors of retinoblastoma. *J Natl Cancer Inst* 1993;85:1121-1128.

56. Abramson DH, Ellsworth RM, Zimmerman LE. Nonocular cancer in retinoblastoma survivors. *Transact Am Acad Ophthalmol Otolaryngol* 1976;81:454-457.

57. Rubin CM, Robison LL, Cameron JD, et al. Intraocular retinoblastoma group V: an analysis of prognostic factors. *J Clin Oncol* 1985;3:680-685.

58. Lueder GT, Judisch F, O'Gorman TW. Second nonocular tumors in survivors of heritable retinoblastoma. *Arch Ophthalmol* 1986;104:372-373.

59. Abramson DH, Ellsworth RM, Kitchin FD, et al. Second nonocular tumors in retinoblastoma survivors. Are they radiation-induced? *Ophthalmol* 1984;91:1351-1355.

60. Sagerman RH, Cassady JR, Tretter P, et al. Radiation induced neoplasia following external beam therapy for children with retinoblastoma. *Am J Roentgenol Radium Ther Nucl Med* 1969; 105:529-535.

61. Raney RB Jr, Tefft M, Newton WA, et al. Improved prognosis with intensive treatment of children with cranial soft tissue sarcomas arising in nonorbital parameningeal sites. A report from the Intergroup Rhabdomyosarcoma Study. *Cancer* 1987;59:147-155.

62. Pui CH. Childhood leukemias. *N Engl J Med* 1995;332:1618-1630.

63. Crist WM, Grossi CE, Pullen DJ, et al. Immunologic markers in childhood acute lymphocytic leukemia. *Semin Oncol* 1985;12:105-121.

64. Pui CH, Behm FG, Crist WM. Clinical and biologic relevance of immunologic marker studies in childhood acute lymphoblastic leukemia. *Blood* 1993;82:343-362.

65. Reiter A, Schrappe M, Ludwig WD, et al. Chemotherapy in 998 unselected childhood acute lymphoblastic leukemia patients. Results and conclusions of the multicenter trial ALL-BFM 86. *Blood* 1994;84:3122-3133.

66. Schorin MA, Blattner S, Gelber RD, et al. Treatment of childhood acute lymphoblastic leukemia: results of Dana-Farber Cancer Institute/Children's Hospital Acute Lymphoblastic Leukemia Consortium Protocol 85-01. *J Clin Oncol* 1994;12:740-747.

67. Rubnitz JE, Downing JR, Pui CH, et al. TEL gene rearrangement in acute lymphoblastic leukemia: a new genetic marker with prognostic significance. *J Clin Oncol* 1997;15:1150-1157.

68. Ribeiro RC, Broniscer A, Rivera GK, et al. Philadelphia chromosome-positive acute lymphoblastic leukemia in children: durable responses to chemotherapy associated with low initial white blood cell counts. *Leukemia* 1997;11:1493-1496.

69. Behm FG, Raimondi SC, Frestedt JL, et al. Rearrangement of the MLL gene confers a poor prognosis in childhood acute lymphoblastic leukemia, regardless of presenting age. *Blood* 1996; 87:2870-2877.

70. Pui CH, Kane JR, Crist WM. Biology and treatment of infant leukemias. *Leukemia* 1995;9:762-769.

71. Reaman G, Zeltzer P, Bleyer WA, et al. Acute lymphoblastic leukemia in infants less than one year of age: a cumulative experience of the Children's Cancer Study Group. *J Clin Oncol* 1985; 3:1513-1521.

72. Gajjar A, Ribeiro R, Hancock ML, et al. Persistence of circulating blasts after 1 week of multiagent chemotherapy confers a poor prognosis in childhood acute lymphoblastic leukemia. *Blood* 1995;86:1292-1295.

73. Cave H, van der Werff ten Bosch J, Suciu S, et al. Clinical significance of minimal residual disease in childhood acute lymphoblastic leukemia. European Organization for Research and Treatment of Cancer—Childhood Leukemia Cooperative Group. *N Engl J Med* 1998;339:591-598.

74. Wells RJ, Woods WG, Buckley JD, et al. Treatment of newly diagnosed children and adolescents with acute myeloid leukemia: a Children's Cancer Group study. *J Clin Oncol* 1994;12:2367-2377.

75. Creutzig U, Ritter J, Riehm H, et al. Improved treatment results in childhood acute myelogenous leukemia: a report of the German cooperative study AML-BFM-78. *Blood* 1985;65: 298-304.

76. Aur RJ, Simone JV, Hustu HO, et al. Cessation of therapy during complete remission of childhood acute lymphocytic leukemia. *N Engl J Med* 1974;291:1230-1234.

77. Aur RJ, Hustu HO, Verzosa MS, et al. Comparison of two methods of preventing central nervous system leukemia. *Blood* 1973;42:349-357.

78. Pinkel D. Pattern of failure in acute lymphocytic leukemia. *Can Treat Sympos* 1983;2:259-266.

79. Hustu HO, Aur RJ. Extramedullary leukaemia. *Clin Haematol* 1978;7:313-337.

80. Bleyer WA, Poplack DG. Prophylaxis and treatment of leukemia in the central nervous system and other sanctuaries. *Semin Oncol* 1985;12:131-148.

81. Sullivan MP, Chen T, Dyment PG, et al. Equivalence of intrathecal chemotherapy and radiotherapy as central nervous system prophylaxis in children with acute lymphatic leukemia: a Pediatric Oncology Group study. *Blood* 1982;60:948-958.

82. Laver JH, Barredo JC, Amylon M, et al. Effects of cranial radiation in children with high risk T cell acute lymphoblastic leukemia: a Pediatric Oncology Group report. *Leukemia* 2000;14:369-373.

83. Pui CH, Mahmoud HH, Rivera GK, et al. Early intensification of intrathecal chemotherapy virtually eliminates central nervous system relapse in children with acute lymphoblastic leukemia. *Blood* 1998;92:411-415.

84. Conter V, Schrappe M, Arico M, et al. Role of cranial radiotherapy for childhood T-cell acute lymphoblastic leukemia with high WBC count and good response to prednisone. Associazione Italiana Ematologia Oncologia Pediatrica and the Berlin-Frankfurt-Munster groups. *J Clin Oncol* 1997;15:2786-2791.

85. Nachman J, Sather HN, Cherlow JM, et al. Response of children with high-risk acute lymphoblastic leukemia treated with and without cranial irradiation: a report from the Children's Cancer Group. *J Clin Oncol* 1998;16:920-930.

86. Freeman AI, Boyett JM, Glicksman AS, et al. Intermediate-dose methotrexate versus cranial irradiation in childhood acute lymphoblastic leukemia: a ten-year follow-up. *Med Pediatr Oncol* 1997;28:98-107.

87. Kamps WA, Bokkerink JP, Hahlen K, et al. Intensive treatment of children with acute lymphoblastic leukemia according to ALL-BFM-86 without cranial radiotherapy: results of Dutch Childhood Leukemia Study Group Protocol ALL-7 (1988-1991). *Blood* 1999;94:1226-1236.

88. Schrappe M, Reiter A, Henze G, et al. Prevention of CNS recurrence in childhood ALL: results with reduced radiotherapy combined with CNS-directed chemotherapy in four consecutive ALL-BFM trials. *Klin Padiatr* 1998;210:192-199.

89. Mahoney DH Jr, Shuster JJ, Nitschke R, et al. Acute neurotoxicity in children with B-precursor acute lymphoid leukemia: an association with intermediate-dose intravenous methotrexate and intrathecal triple therapy—a Pediatric Oncology Group study. *J Clin Oncol* 1998;16:1712-1722.

90. Pui CH, Boyett JM, Rivera GK, et al. Long-term results of Total Therapy studies 11, 12 and 13A for childhood acute lymphoblastic leukemia at St Jude Children's Research Hospital. *Leukemia* 2000;14:2286-2294.

91. Rivera GK, Mauer AM. Controversies in the management of childhood acute lymphoblastic leukemia: treatment intensification, CNS leukemia, and prognostic factors. *Semin Hematol* 1987; 24:12-26.

92. Mahmoud HH, Rivera GK, Hancock ML, et al. Low leukocyte counts with blast cells in cerebrospinal fluid of children with newly diagnosed acute lymphoblastic leukemia. *N Engl J Med* 1993;329:314-319.

93. Cherlow JM, Sather H, Steinherz P, et al. Craniospinal irradiation for acute lymphoblastic leukemia with central nervous system disease at diagnosis: a report from the Children's Cancer Group. *Int J Radiat Oncol Biol Phys* 1996;36:19-27.

94. Kun LE. CNS disease at diagnosis: a continuing challenge in childhood lymphoblastic leukemia. *Int J Radiat Oncol Biol Phys* 1996;36:257-259.

95. Gilchrist GS, Tubergen DG, Sather HN, et al. Low numbers of CSF blasts at diagnosis do not predict for the development of CNS leukemia in children with intermediate-risk acute lymphoblastic leukemia: a Children's Cancer Group report. *J Clin Oncol* 1994; 12:2594-2600.

96. Kun LE, Camitta BM, Mulhern RK, et al. Treatment of meningeal relapse in childhood acute lymphoblastic leukemia. I. Results of craniospinal irradiation. *J Clin Oncol* 1984;2:359-364.

97. Kumar P, Mulhern RK, Regine WF, et al. A prospective neurocognitive evaluation of children treated with additional chemotherapy and craniospinal irradiation following isolated central nervous system relapse in acute lymphoblastic leukemia. *Int J Radiat Oncol Biol Phys* 1995;31:561-566.

98. Ribeiro RC, Rivera GK, Hudson M, et al. An intensive re-treatment protocol for children with an isolated CNS relapse of acute lymphoblastic leukemia. *J Clin Oncol* 1995;13:333-338.

99. Winick NJ, Smith SD, Shuster J, et al. Treatment of CNS relapse in children with acute lymphoblastic leukemia: a Pediatric Oncology Group study. *J Clin Oncol* 1993;11:271-278.

100. Buhrer C, Hartmann R, Fengler R, et al. Importance of effective central nervous system therapy in isolated bone marrow relapse of childhood acute lymphoblastic leukemia. BFM (Berlin-Frankfurt-Munster) Relapse Study Group. *Blood* 1994;83:3468-3472.

101. Land VJ, Thomas PR, Boyett JM, et al. Comparison of maintenance treatment regimens for first central nervous system relapse in children with acute lymphocytic leukemia. A Pediatric Oncology Group study. *Cancer* 1985;56:81-87.

102. Ritchey AK, Pollock BH, Lauer SJ, et al. Improved survival of children with isolated CNS relapse of acute lymphoblastic leukemia: a Pediatric Oncology Group study. *J Clin Oncol* 1999; 17:3745-3752.

103. van den BH, Odink AE, Behrendt H. Delayed craniospinal irradiation for a first isolated central nervous relapse of acute lymphoblastic leukemia: report on 14 cases. *Med Pediatr Oncol* 2000;34:402-406.

104. Wofford MM, Smith SD, Shuster JJ, et al. Treatment of occult or late overt testicular relapse in children with acute lymphoblastic leukemia: a Pediatric Oncology Group study. *J Clin Oncol* 1992;10:624-630.

105. Finklestein JZ, Miller DR, Feusner J, et al. Treatment of overt isolated testicular relapse in children on therapy for acute lymphoblastic leukemia. A report from the Children's Cancer Group. *Cancer* 1994;73:219-223.

106. Buchanan GR, Boyett JM, Pollock BH, et al. Improved treatment results in boys with overt testicular relapse during or shortly after initial therapy for acute lymphoblastic leukemia. A Pediatric Oncology Group study. *Cancer* 1991;68:48-55.

107. Mahoney DH Jr, Shuster JJ, Nitschke R, et al. Intensification with intermediate-dose intravenous methotrexate is effective therapy for children with lower-risk B-precursor acute lymphoblastic leukemia: a Pediatric Oncology Group study. *J Clin Oncol* 2000;18:1285-1294.

108. Huff V, Miwa H, Haber DA, et al. Evidence for WT1 as a Wilms' tumor (WT) gene: intragenic germinal deletion in bilateral WT. *Am J Hum Genet* 1991;48:997-1003.

109. Breslow NE, Beckwith JB. Epidemiological features of Wilms' tumor: results of the National Wilms' Tumor Study. *J Natl Cancer Inst* 1982;68:429-436.

110. Howell CG, Otherson HB, Kiviat NE, et al. Therapy and outcome in 51 children with mesoblastic nephroma: a report of the National Wilms' Tumor Study. *J Pediatr Surg* 1982;7: 826-831.

111. Beckwith JB, Kiviat NB, Bonadio JF. Nephrogenic rests, nephroblastomatosis, and the pathogenesis of Wilms' tumor. *Pediatr Pathol* 1990;10:1-36.

112. Beckwith JB, Palmer NF. Histopathology and prognosis of Wilms' tumors: results from the First National Wilms' Tumor Study. *Cancer* 1978;41:1937-1948.

113. Bowman LC, Hancock ML, Santana VM, et al. Impact of intensified therapy on clinical outcome in infants and children with neuroblastoma: the St. Jude Children's Research Hospital experience, 1962 to 1988. *J Clin Oncol* 1991;9:1599-1608.

114. Bonadio JF, Storer B, Norkool P. Anaplastic Wilms' tumor: clinical and pathologic studies. *J Clin Oncol* 1985;3:513-520.

115. Breslow N, Churchill G, Beckwith JB, et al. Prognosis for Wilms' tumor patients with nonmetastatic disease at diagnosis—results of the Second National Wilms' Tumor Study. *J Clin Oncol* 1985;3:521-531.

116. Green DM, Beckwith JB, Breslow NE, et al. Treatment of children with stages II to IV anaplastic Wilms' tumor: a report from the National Wilms' Tumor Study Group. *J Clin Oncol* 1994;12: 2126-2131.

117. Beckwith JB, Larson E. Case 7. Clear cell sarcoma of kidney. *Pediatric Pathology* 1989;9:211-218.

118. Weeks DA, Beckwith JB, Mierau GW, et al. Rhabdoid tumor of kidney. A report of 111 cases from the National Wilms' Tumor Study Pathology Center. *Am J Surg Pathol* 1989;13:439-458.

119. Bonnin JM, Rubinstein LJ, Palmer NF, et al. The association of embryonal tumors originating in the kidney and in the brain. A report of seven cases. *Cancer* 1984;54:2137-2146.

120. Rorke LB, Packer R, Biegel J. Central nervous system atypical teratoid/rhabdoid tumors of infancy and childhood. *J Neurooncol* 1995;24:21-28.

121. Biegel JA, Rorke LB, Packer RJ, et al. Monosomy 22 in rhabdoid or atypical tumors of the brain. *J Neurosurg* 1990;73:710-714.

122. Garcia M, Douglass C, Schlosser JV. Classification and prognosis in Wilms' tumor. *Radiology* 1963;80:574-580.

123. Cassady JR, Tefft M, Filler RM, et al. Considerations in the radiation therapy of Wilms' tumor. *Cancer* 1973;32:598-608.

124. D'Angio GJ, Breslow N, Beckwith JB, et al. Treatment of Wilms' tumor. Results of the Third National Wilms' Tumor Study. *Cancer* 1989;64:349-360.

125. Breslow N, Sharples K, Beckwith JB, et al. Prognostic factors in nonmetastatic, favorable histology Wilms' tumor. Results of the Third National Wilms' Tumor Study. *Cancer* 1991;68:2345-2353.

126. Gross RE, Neuhauser EBD. Treatment of mixed tumors of the kidney in childhood. *Pediatrics* 1950;6:843.

127. Farber S. Chemotherapy in the treatment of leukemia and Wilms' tumor. *JAMA* 1966;198:826-836.

128. Tournade MF, Com-Nougue C, de Kraker J, et al. Optimal duration of preoperative therapy in unilateral and nonmetastatic Wilms' tumor in children older than 6 months: results of the Ninth International Society of Pediatric Oncology Wilms' Tumor Trial and Study. *J Clin Oncol* 2001;19:488-500.

129. Pritchard J, Imeson J, Barnes J, et al. Results of the United Kingdom Children's Cancer Study Group First Wilms' Tumor Study. *J Clin Oncol* 1995;13:124-133.

130. D'Angio GJ, Breslow NE. Treatment of Wilms' tumor: results of the National Wilms' Tumor Study. *Cancer* 1989;64:349-360.

131. Thomas PR, Tefft M, Compaan PJ, et al. Results of two radiation therapy randomizations in the Third National Wilms' Tumor Study. *Cancer* 1991;68:1703-1707.

132. Thomas PR. Wilms' tumor: changing role of radiation therapy. *Semin Radiat Oncol* 1997;7:204-211.

133. Thomas PR, Tefft M, Farewell VT, et al. Abdominal relapses in irradiated Second National Wilms' Tumor Study patients. *J Clin Oncol* 1984;2:1098-1101.

134. Burgers JM, Tournade MF, Bey P, et al. Abdominal recurrences in Wilms' tumours: a report from the SIOP Wilms' Tumour Trials and Studies. *Radiother Oncol* 1986;5:175-182.

135. Breslow NE, Palmer NF, Hill LR, et al. Wilms' tumor: prognostic factors for patients without metastases at diagnosis: results of the National Wilms' Tumor Study. *Cancer* 1978;41:1577-1589.

136. Tobin RL, Fontanesi J, Kun LE, et al. Wilms' tumor: reduced-dose radiotherapy in advanced-stage Wilms' tumor with favorable histology. *Int J Radiat Oncol Biol Phys* 1990;19:867-871.

137. Flentje M, Weirich A, Graf N, et al. Abdominal irradiation in unilateral nephroblastoma and its impact on local control and survival. *Int J Radiat Oncol Biol Phys* 1998;40:163-169.

138. Ritchey ML, Kelalis PP, Haase GM, et al. Preoperative therapy for intracaval and atrial extension of Wilms' tumor. *Cancer* 1993;71:4104-4110.

139. Green DM, Jaffe N. The role of chemotherapy in the treatment of Wilms' tumor. *Cancer* 1979;44:52-57.

140. Reference deleted in proofs.

141. Reference deleted in proofs.

142. Breslow NE, Churchill G, Nesmith B, et al. Clinicopathologic features and prognosis for Wilms' tumor patients with metastases at diagnosis. *Cancer* 1986;58:2501-2511.

143. Green DM, Breslow NE, Evans I, et al. Treatment of children with stage IV favorable histology Wilms' tumor: a report from the National Wilms' Tumor Study Group. *Med Pediatr Oncol* 1996;26:147-152.

144. Monson KJ, Brand WN, Boggs JD. Results of small-field irradiation of apparent solitary metastasis from Wilms' tumor. *Radiology* 1972;104:157-160.

145. Macklis RM, Oltikar A, Sallan SE. Wilms' tumor patients with pulmonary metastases. *Int J Radiat Oncol Biol Phys* 1991; 21: 1187-1193.

146. de Kraker J, Lemerle J, Voute PA, et al. Wilms' tumor with pulmonary metastases at diagnosis: the significance of primary chemotherapy. International Society of Pediatric Oncology Nephroblastoma Trial and Study Committee. *J Clin Oncol* 1990;8:1187-1190.

147. Green DM, Fernbach DJ, Norkool P, et al. The treatment of Wilms' tumor patients with pulmonary metastases detected only with computed tomography: a report from the National Wilms' Tumor Study. *J Clin Oncol* 1991;9:1776-1781.

148. Corey SJ, Andersen JW, Vawter GF, et al. Improved survival for children with anaplastic Wilms' tumors. *Cancer* 1991; 68:970-974.

149. Green DM, Breslow NE, Beckwith JB, et al. Treatment of children with clear-cell sarcoma of the kidney: a report from the National Wilms' Tumor Study Group. *J Clin Oncol* 1994;12: 2132-2137.

150. Brodeur GM, Azar C, Brother M, et al. Neuroblastoma. Effect of genetic factors on prognosis and treatment. *Cancer* 1992; 70:1685-1694.

151. De Bernardi B, Pianca C, Boni L, et al. Disseminated neuroblastoma (stage IV and IV-S) in the first year of life. Outcome related to age and stage. Italian Cooperative Group on Neuroblastoma. *Cancer* 1992;70:1625-1633.

152. van Noesel MM, Hahlen K, Hakvoort-Cammel FG, et al. Neuroblastoma 4S: a heterogeneous disease with variable risk factors and treatment strategies. *Cancer* 1997;80:834-843.

153. Hayes FA, Green A, Hustu HO, et al. Surgicopathologic staging of neuroblastoma: prognostic significance of regional lymph node metastases. *J Pediatr* 1983;102:59-62.

154. Rosen EM, Cassady JR, Kretschmar C, et al. Influence of local–regional lymph node metastases on prognosis in neuroblastoma. *Med Pediatr Oncol* 1984;12:260-263.

155. D'Angio GJ, Evans AE, Koop CE. Special pattern of widespread neuroblastoma with a favourable prognosis. *Lancet* 1971; 1:1046-1049.

156. Spunt SL, Poquette CA, Hurt YS, et al. Prognostic factors for children and adolescents with surgically resected nonrhabdomyosarcoma soft tissue sarcoma: an analysis of 121 patients treated at St. Jude Children's Research Hospital. *J Clin Oncol* 1999;17:3697-3705.

157. Nickerson HJ, Matthay KK, Seeger RC, et al. Favorable biology and outcome of stage IV-S neuroblastoma with supportive care or minimal therapy: a Children's Cancer Group study. *J Clin Oncol* 2000;18:477-486.

158. Matthay KK. Stage 4S neuroblastoma: what makes it special? *J Clin Oncol* 1998;16:2003-2006.

159. Shimada H, Chatten J, Newton WA Jr, et al. Histopathologic prognostic factors in neuroblastic tumors: definition of subtypes of ganglioneuroblastoma and an age-linked classification of neuroblastomas. *J Natl Cancer Inst* 1984;73:405-416.

160. Brodeur GM, Hayes FA, Green AA, et al. Consistent N-myc copy number in simultaneous or consecutive neuroblastoma samples from sixty individual patients. *Cancer Res* 1987; 47:4248-4253.

161. Rubie H, Hartmann O, Michon J, et al. N-Myc gene amplification is a major prognostic factor in localized neuroblastoma: results of the French NBL 90 study. Neuroblastoma Study Group of the Société Française d'Oncologie Pediatrique. *J Clin Oncol* 1997;15:1171-1182.

162. Perez CA, Matthay KK, Atkinson JB, et al. Biologic variables in the outcome of stages I and II neuroblastoma treated with surgery as primary therapy: a Children's Cancer Group study. *J Clin Oncol* 2000;18:18-26.

163. Caron H, van Sluis P, van Hoeve M, et al. Allelic loss of chromosome 1p36 in neuroblastoma is of preferential maternal origin and correlates with N-myc amplification. *Nat Genet* 1993;4:187-190.

164. Castle VP, Heidelberger KP, Bromberg J, et al. Expression of the apoptosis-suppressing protein Bcl-2 in neuroblastoma is associated with unfavorable histology and N-myc amplification. *Am J Pathol* 1993;143:1543-1550.

165. Nakagawara A, Arima-Nakagawara M, Scavarda NJ, et al. Association between high levels of expression of the TRK gene and favorable outcome in human neuroblastoma. *N Engl J Med* 1993;328:847-854.

166. Chan HS, Haddad G, Thorner PS, et al. P-glycoprotein expression as a predictor of the outcome of therapy for neuroblastoma. *N Engl J Med* 1991;325:1608-1614.

167. Evans AE, D'Angio GJ, Randolph J. A proposed staging for children with neuroblastoma. Children's Cancer Study Group A. *Cancer* 1971;27:374-378.

168. Brodeur GM, Castleberry R. Neuroblastoma. In: Pizzo PA, Poplack DG, eds. *Principles and Practice of Pediatric Oncology.* Philadelphia, Pa: Lippincott-Raven; 1997:7610-798.

169. Brodeur GM, Seeger RC, Barrett A, et al. International criteria for diagnosis, staging, and response to treatment in patients with neuroblastoma. *J Clin Oncol* 1988;6:1874-1881.

170. Brodeur GM, Pritchard J, Berthold F, et al. Revisions of the international criteria for neuroblastoma diagnosis, staging, and response to treatment. *J Clin Oncol* 1993;11:1466-1477.

171. Matthay KK. Intensification of therapy using hematopoietic stem-cell support for high-risk neuroblastoma. *Pediatr Transplant* 1999;3(suppl 1):72-77.

172. Nitschke R, Smith EI, Shochat S, et al. Localized neuroblastoma treated by surgery: a Pediatric Oncology Group Study. *J Clin Oncol* 1988;6:1271-1279.

173. Matthay KK, Sather HN, Seeger RC, et al. Excellent outcome of stage II neuroblastoma is independent of residual disease and radiation therapy. *J Clin Oncol* 1989;7:236-244.

174. Rubie H, Michon J, Plantaz D, et al. Unresectable localized neuroblastoma: improved survival after primary chemotherapy including carboplatin-etoposide. Neuroblastoma Study Group of the Société Française d'Oncologie Pediatrique (SFOP). *Br J Cancer* 1998;77:2310-2317.

175. Kushner BH, Cheung NK, LaQuaglia MP, et al. Survival from locally invasive or widespread neuroblastoma without cytotoxic therapy. *J Clin Oncol* 1996;14:373-381.

176. Garaventa A, De Bernardi B, Pianca C, et al. Localized but unresectable neuroblastoma: treatment and outcome of 145 cases. Italian Cooperative Group for Neuroblastoma. *J Clin Oncol* 1993;11:1770-1779.

177. De Bernardi B, Conte M, Mancini A, et al. Localized resectable neuroblastoma: results of the second study of the Italian Cooperative Group for Neuroblastoma. *J Clin Oncol* 1995;13: 884-893.

178. Nitschke R, Smith EI, Altshuler G, et al. Postoperative treatment of nonmetastatic visible residual neuroblastoma: a Pediatric Oncology Group study. *J Clin Oncol* 1991;9:1181-1188.

179. Ninane J, Pritchard J, Morris Jones PH, et al. Stage II neuroblastoma. Adverse prognostic significance of lymph node involvement. *Arch Dis Child* 1982;57:438-442.

180. Castleberry RP, Kun LE, Shuster JJ, et al. Radiotherapy improves the outlook for patients older than 1 year with Pediatric Oncology Group stage C neuroblastoma. *J Clin Oncol* 1991;9:789-795.

181. Strother D. Treatment of Pediatric Oncology Group stage C neuroblastoma: a preliminary POG report [abstract]. *Proceedings of the American Society of Clinical Oncology* 1993;12:1422.

182. Wolden SL, Gollamudi SV, Kushner BH, et al. Local control with multimodality therapy for stage 4 neuroblastoma. *Int J Radiat Oncol Biol Phys* 2000;46:969-974.

183. Haas-Kogan DA, Fisch BM, Wara WM, et al. Intraoperative radiation therapy for high-risk pediatric neuroblastoma. *Int J Radiat Oncol Biol Phys* 2000;47:985-992.

184. Leavey PJ, Odom LF, Poole M, et al. Intra-operative radiation therapy in pediatric neuroblastoma. *Med Pediatr Oncol* 1997;28:424-428.

185. Matthay KK, Villablanca JG, Seeger RC, et al. Treatment of high-risk neuroblastoma with intensive chemotherapy, radiotherapy, autologous bone marrow transplantation, and 13-cis-retinoic acid. Children's Cancer Group. *N Engl J Med* 1999;341:1165-1173.

186. Frappaz D, Michon J, Coze C, et al. LMCE3 treatment strategy: results in 99 consecutively diagnosed stage 4 neuroblastomas in children older than 1 year at diagnosis. *J Clin Oncol* 2000; 18:468-476.

187. La Quaglia MP, Kushner BH, Heller G, et al. Stage 4 neuroblastoma diagnosed at more than 1 year of age: gross total resection and clinical outcome. *J Pediatr Surg* 1994;29:1162-1165.

188. Ikeda H, August CS, Goldwein JW, et al. Sites of relapse in patients with neuroblastoma following bone marrow transplantation in relation to preparatory "debulking" treatments. *J Pediatr Surg* 1992;27:1438-1441.

189. Matthay KK, Atkinson JB, Stram DO, et al. Patterns of relapse after autologous purged bone marrow transplantation for neuroblastoma: a Children's Cancer Group pilot study. *J Clin Oncol* 1993;11:2226-2233.

190. McCowage GB, Vowels MR, Shaw PJ, et al. Autologous bone marrow transplantation for advanced neuroblastoma using teniposide, doxorubicin, melphalan, cisplatin, and total-body irradiation. *J Clin Oncol* 1995;13:2789-2795.

191. Lindsley K. Wilms' tumor and neuroblastoma. In: Leibel S, Phillips T, eds. *Textbook of Radiation Oncology*. Philadelphia, Pa: WB Saunders; 1998:994-1012.

192. Stram DO, Matthay KK, O'Leary M, et al. Consolidation chemoradiotherapy and autologous bone marrow transplantation versus continued chemotherapy for metastatic neuroblastoma: a report of two concurrent Children's Cancer Group studies. *J Clin Oncol* 1996;14:2417-2426.

193. Look AT, Hayes FA, Mitschke R, et al. Cellular DNA content as a predictor of response to chemotherapy in infants with unresectable neuroblastoma. *N Engl J Med* 1984;311:231-235.

194. Look AT, Hayes FA, Shuster JJ, et al. Clinical relevance of tumor cell ploidy and N-myc gene amplification in childhood neuroblastoma: a Pediatric Oncology Group study. *J Clin Oncol* 1991; 9:581-591.

195. Katzenstein HM, Bowman LC, Brodeur GM, et al. Prognostic significance of age, MYCN oncogene amplification, tumor cell ploidy, and histology in 110 infants with stage D(S) neuroblastoma: the Pediatric Oncology Group experience—a Pediatric Oncology Group study. *J Clin Oncol* 1998;16:2007-2017.

196. De Bernardi B, Pianca C, Pistamiglio P, et al. Neuroblastoma with symptomatic spinal cord compression at diagnosis: treatment and results with 76 cases. *J Clin Oncol* 2001;19:183-190.

197. Sisson JC, Shapoiro B, Hutchinson RJ, et al. Survival of patients with neuroblastoma treated with ^{125}I MIBG. *Am J Clin Oncol* 1996;19:144-148.

198. Matthay KK, DeSantes K, Kasegawa B, et al. Phase I dose escalation of ^{131}I-metaiodobenzylguanidine with autologous bone marrow support in refractory neuroblastoma. *J Clin Oncol* 1998;16:229-236.

199. Crist W, Gehan EA, Ragab AH, et al. The Third Intergroup Rhabdomyosarcoma Study. *J Clin Oncol* 1995;13:610-630.

200. Scrable H, Cavenee W, Ghavimi F, et al. A model for embryonal rhabdomyosarcoma tumorigenesis that involves genome imprinting. *Proc Natl Acad Sci USA* 1989;86:7480-7484.

201. Douglass EC, Shapiro DN, Valentine M, et al. Alveolar rhabdomyosarcoma with the t(2;13): cytogenetic findings and clinicopathologic correlations. *Med Pediatr Oncol* 1993;21:83-87.

202. Wexler LH, Helman LJ. Rhabdomyosarcoma and the undifferentiated sarcomas. In: Pizzo PA, Poplack DG, eds. *Principles and Practice of Pediatric Oncology*. Philadelphia, Pa: Lippincott-Raven; 1997:799-829.

203. Asmar L, Gehan EA, Newton WA, et al. Agreement among and within groups of pathologists in the classification of rhabdomyosarcoma and related childhood sarcomas. Report of an international study of four pathology classifications. *Cancer* 1994;74:2579-2588.

204. Newton WA Jr, Soule EH, Hamoudi AB, et al. Histopathology of childhood sarcomas, Intergroup Rhabdomyosarcoma Studies I and II: clinicopathologic correlation. *J Clin Oncol* 1988;6:67-75.

205. Tsokos M, Webber BL, Parham DM, et al. Rhabdomyosarcoma. A new classification scheme related to prognosis. *Arch Pathol Lab Med* 1992;116:847-855.

206. Arndt CA, Crist WM. Common musculoskeletal tumors of childhood and adolescence. *N Engl J Med* 1999;341:342-352.

207. Raney RB, Meza, J, Anderson JR, et al. Treatment of children and adolescents with localized parameningeal sarcoma: experience of the Intergroup Rhabdomyosarcoma Study Group protocols IRS-II through -IV, 1978-1997. *Med Pediatr Oncol* 2002;38: 22-32.

208. Raney RB Jr, Tefft M, Maurer HM, et al. Disease patterns and survival rate in children with metastatic soft-tissue sarcoma. A report from the Intergroup Rhabdomyosarcoma Study (IRS)-I. *Cancer* 1988;62:1257-1266.

209. Lawrence W Jr, Anderson JR, Gehan EA, et al. Pretreatment TNM staging of childhood rhabdomyosarcoma: a report of the Intergroup Rhabdomyosarcoma Study Group. Children's Cancer Study Group. Pediatric Oncology Group. *Cancer* 1997;80:1165-1170.

210. Lawrence W Jr, Hays DM, Heyn R, et al. Lymphatic metastases with childhood rhabdomyosarcoma. A report from the Intergroup Rhabdomyosarcoma Study. *Cancer* 1987;60: 910-915.

211. Pedrick TJ, Donaldson SS, Cox RS. Rhabdomyosarcoma: the Stanford experience using a TNM staging system. *J Clin Oncol* 1986;4:370-378.

212. Crist WM, Garnsey L, Beltangady MS, et al. Prognosis in children with rhabdomyosarcoma: a report of the Intergroup Rhabdomyosarcoma Studies I and II. Intergroup Rhabdomyosarcoma Committee. *J Clin Oncol* 1990;8:443-452.

213. Maurer HM, Gehan EA, Beltangady M, et al. The Intergroup Rhabdomyosarcoma Study-II. *Cancer* 1993;71:1904-1922.

214. Rodary C, Gehan EA, Flamant F, et al. Prognostic factors in 951 nonmetastatic rhabdomyosarcoma in children: a report from the International Rhabdomyosarcoma Workshop. *Med Pediatr Oncol* 1991;19:89-95.

215. Jones IS, Reese AB, Kraut J. Orbital rhabdomyosarcoma. An analysis of 62 cases. *Am J Ophthalmol* 1966;61:721-736.

216. Tefft M, Jaffe N. Proceedings: sarcoma of the bladder and prostate in children. Rationale for the role of radiation therapy

based on a review of the literature and a report of fourteen additional patients. *Cancer* 1973;32:1161-1177.

217. Cassady JR, Sagerman RH, Tretter P, et al. Radiation therapy for rhabdomyosarcoma. *Radiology* 1968;91:116-120.

218. Edland RW. Embryonal rhabdomyosarcoma. *AJR Am J Roentgenol Radium Ther Nucl Med* 1965;93:671.

219. Nelson AJ III. Embryonal rhabdomyosarcoma. Report of twenty-four cases and study of the effectiveness of radiation therapy upon the primary tumor. *Cancer* 1968;22:64-68.

220. Sagerman RH, Tretter P, Ellsworth RM. The treatment of orbital rhabdomyosarcoma of children with primary radiation therapy. *Am J Roentgenol Radium Ther Nucl Med* 1972;114:31-34.

221. Jereb B, Cham W, Lattin P, et al. Local control of embryonal rhabdomyosarcoma in children by radiation therapy when combined with concomitant chemotherapy. *Int J Radiat Oncol Biol Phys* 1976;1:217-225.

222. Hays DM, Lawrence W Jr, Crist WM, et al. Partial cystectomy in the management of rhabdomyosarcoma of the bladder: a report from the Intergroup Rhabdomyosarcoma Study. *J Pediatr Surg* 1990;25:719-723.

223. Hays DM, Raney RB, Wharam MD, et al. Children with vesical rhabdomyosarcoma (RMS) treated by partial cystectomy with neoadjuvant or adjuvant chemotherapy, with or without radiotherapy. A report from the Intergroup Rhabdomyosarcoma Study (IRS) Committee. *J Pediatr Hematol Oncol* 1995;17:46-52.

224. Raney RB Jr, Gehan EA, Hays DM, et al. Primary chemotherapy with or without radiation therapy and/or surgery for children with localized sarcoma of the bladder, prostate, vagina, uterus, and cervix. A comparison of the results in Intergroup Rhabdomyosarcoma Studies I and II. *Cancer* 1990;66:2072-2081.

225. Martelli H, Oberlin O, Rey A, et al. Conservative treatment for girls with nonmetastatic rhabdomyosarcoma of the genital tract: a report from the Study Committee of the International Society of Pediatric Oncology. *J Clin Oncol* 1999;17:2117-2122.

226. Breneman JC, Wiener ES. Issues in the local control of rhabdomyosarcoma. *Med Pediatr Oncol* 2000;35:104-109.

227. Maurer HM, Beltangady M, Gehan EA, et al. The Intergroup Rhabdomyosarcoma Study-I. A final report. *Cancer* 1988;61:209-220.

228. Wolden SL, Anderson JR, Crist WM, et al. Indications for radiotherapy and chemotherapy after complete resection in rhabdomyosarcoma: a report from the Intergroup Rhabdomyosarcoma Studies I to III. *J Clin Oncol* 1999;17:3468-3475.

229. Regine WF, Fontanesi J, Kumar P, et al. Local tumor control in rhabdomyosarcoma following low-dose irradiation: comparison of group II and select group III patients. *Int J Radiat Oncol Biol Phys* 1995;31:485-491.

230. Mandell L, Ghavimi F, Peretz T, et al. Radiocurability of microscopic disease in childhood rhabdomyosarcoma with radiation doses less than 4,000 cGy. *J Clin Oncol* 1990;8:1536-1542.

231. Regine WF, Fontanesi J, Kumar P, et al. A phase II trial evaluating selective use of altered radiation dose and fractionation in patients with unresectable rhabdomyosarcoma. *Int J Radiat Oncol Biol Phys* 1995;31:799-805.

232. Wharam MD, Hanfelt JJ, Tefft MC, et al. Radiation therapy for rhabdomyosarcoma: local failure risk for clinical group III patients on Intergroup Rhabdomyosarcoma Study II. *Int J Radiat Oncol Biol Phys* 1997;38:797-804.

233. Oberlin O, Rey A, Anderson J, et al. Treatment of orbital rhabdomyosarcoma: survival and late effects of treatment—results of an international workshop. *J Clin Oncol* 2001;19:197-204.

234. Kodet R, Newton WA Jr, Hamoudi AB, et al. Orbital rhabdomyosarcomas and related tumors in childhood: relationship of morphology to prognosis—an Intergroup Rhabdomyosarcoma Study. *Med Pediatr Oncol* 1997;29:51-60.

235. Fiorillo A, Migliorati R, Vassallo P, et al. Radiation late effects in children treated for orbital rhabdomyosarcoma. *Radiother Oncol* 1999;53:143-148.

236. Raney RB, Anderson JR, Kollath J, et al. Late effects of therapy in 94 patients with localized rhabdomyosarcoma of the orbit: report from the Intergroup Rhabdomyosarcoma Study (IRS)-III, 1984-1991. *Med Pediatr Oncol* 2000;34:413-420.

237. Tarbell NJ. Extent of bone erosion predicts survival in non-orbital rhabdomyosarcoma of the head and neck in children [abstract]. *Proceedings of the American Society of Clinical Oncology* 1987;6:222a.

238. Mandell LR, Massey V, Ghavimi F. The influence of extensive bone erosion on local control in non-orbital rhabdomyosarcoma of the head and neck. *Int J Radiat Oncol Biol Phys* 1989;17:649-653.

239. Tefft M, Fernandez C, Donaldson M, et al. Incidence of meningeal involvement by rhabdomyosarcoma of the head and neck in children: a report of the Intergroup Rhabdomyosarcoma Study (IRS). *Cancer* 1978;42:253-258.

240. Raney RB, Asmar L, Vassilopoulou-Sellin R, et al. Late complications of therapy in 213 children with localized, nonorbital soft-tissue sarcoma of the head and neck: a descriptive report from the Intergroup Rhabdomyosarcoma Studies (IRS)-II and - III. IRS Group of the Children's Cancer Group and the Pediatric Oncology Group. *Med Pediatr Oncol* 1999;33:362-371.

241. Heyn R, Newton WA, Raney RB, et al. Preservation of the bladder in patients with rhabdomyosarcoma. *J Clin Oncol* 1997;15:69-75.

242. Raney B Jr, Heyn R, Hays DM, et al. Sequelae of treatment in 109 patients followed for 5 to 15 years after diagnosis of sarcoma of the bladder and prostate. A report from the Intergroup Rhabdomyosarcoma Study Committee. *Cancer* 1993;71:2387-2394.

243. Wiener ES, Lawrence W, Hays D, et al. Retroperitoneal node biopsy in paratesticular rhabdomyosarcoma. *J Pediatr Surg* 1994;29:171-177.

244. Flamant F, Gerbaulet A, Nihoul-Fekete C, et al. Long-term sequelae of conservative treatment by surgery, brachytherapy, and chemotherapy for vulval and vaginal rhabdomyosarcoma in children. *J Clin Oncol* 1990;8:1847-1853.

245. Heyn R, Beltangady M, Hays D, et al. Results of intensive therapy in children with localized alveolar extremity rhabdomyosarcoma: a report from the Intergroup Rhabdomyosarcoma Study. *J Clin Oncol* 1989;7:200-207.

246. Ghavimi F, Mandell LR, Heller G, et al. Prognosis in childhood rhabdomyosarcoma of the extremity. *Cancer* 1989;64:2233-2237.

247. Merchant TE. Conformal therapy for pediatric sarcomas. *Semin Radiat Oncol* 1997;7:236-245.

248. Donaldson SS. The value of adjuvant chemotherapy in the management of sarcomas in children. *Cancer* 1985;55:2184-2197.

249. Tefft M, Wharam M, Gehan E. Local and regional control by radiation of rhabdomyosarcoma in IRS-II (abstract 83). *Int J Radiat Oncol Biol Phys* 1988;15(Suppl 1):159.

250. Kun L. Treatment factors affecting local control in childhood rhabdomyosarcoma [abstract]. *Proceed Am Soc Clin Oncol* 1986;5:207a.

251. Donaldson SS, Asmar L, Breneman J, et al. Hyperfractionated radiation in children with rhabdomyosarcoma—results of an Intergroup Rhabdomyosarcoma Pilot Study. *Int J Radiat Oncol Biol Phys* 1995;32:903-911.

252. Knudson AG Jr. Mutation and cancer: statistical study of retinoblastoma. *Proc Natl Acad Sci USA* 1971;68:820-823.

253. Gallie BL. Retinoblastoma gene mutations in human cancer. *N Engl J Med* 1994;330:786-787.

254. Moll AC, Imhof SM, Bouter LM, et al. Second primary tumors in patients with retinoblastoma. A review of the literature. *Ophthalmic Genet* 1997;18:27-34.

255. Steenbakkers RJ, Altschuler MD, D'Angio GJ, et al. Optimized lens-sparing treatment of retinoblastoma with electron beams. *Int J Radiat Oncol Biol Phys* 1997;39:589-594.

256. Reese AB. *Tumors of the Eye.* 3rd ed. Hagerstown, MD: Harper and Row; 1976.

257. Hernandez JC, Brady LW, Shields JA, et al. External beam radiation for retinoblastoma: results, patterns of failure, and a proposal for treatment guidelines. *Int J Radiat Oncol Biol Phys* 1996;35:125-132.

258. Pradhan DG, Sandridge AL, Mullaney P, et al. Radiation therapy for retinoblastoma: a retrospective review of 120 patients. *Int J Radiat Oncol Biol Phys* 1997;39:3-13.

259. Shields CL, Shields JA, Needle M, et al. Combined chemoreduction and adjuvant treatment for intraocular retinoblastoma. *Ophthalmology* 1997;104:2101-2111.

260. Friedman DL, Himelstein B, Shields CL, et al. Chemoreduction and local ophthalmic therapy for intraocular retinoblastoma. *J Clin Oncol* 2000;18:12-17.

261. Murphree AL, Villablanca JG, Deegan WF III, et al. Chemotherapy plus local treatment in the management of intraocular retinoblastoma. *Arch Ophthalmol* 1996;114:1348-1356.

262. Gallie BL, Budning A, DeBoer G, et al. Chemotherapy with focal therapy can cure intraocular retinoblastoma without radiotherapy. *Arch Ophthalmol* 1996;114:1321-1328.

263. Cassady JR, Sagerman RH, Tretter P, et al. Radiation therapy in retinoblastoma. An analysis of 230 cases. *Radiology* 1969;93:405-409.

264. Schipper J. An accurate and simple method for megavoltage radiation therapy of retinoblastoma. *Radiother Oncol* 1983;1:31-41.

265. Schipper J, Tan KE, van Peperzeel HA. Treatment of retinoblastoma by precision megavoltage radiation therapy. *Radiother Oncol* 1985;3:117-132.

266. Freeman CR, Esseltine DL, Whitehead VM, et al. Retinoblastoma: the case for radiotherapy and for adjuvant chemotherapy. *Cancer* 1980;46:1913-1918.

267. Pratt CB, Crom DB, Howarth C. The use of chemotherapy for extraocular retinoblastoma. *Med Pediatr Oncol* 1985;13:330-333.

268. Madreperla SA, Hungerford JL, Doughty D, et al. Treatment of retinoblastoma vitreous base seeding. *Ophthalmology* 1998;105:120-124.

269. Reference deleted in proofs.

270. Egbert PR, Donaldson SS, Moazed K, et al. Visual results and ocular complications following radiotherapy for retinoblastoma. *Arch Ophthalmol* 1978;96:1826-1830.

271. Khelfaoui F, Validire P, Auperin A, et al. Histopathologic risk factors in retinoblastoma: a retrospective study of 172 patients treated in a single institution. *Cancer* 1996;77:1206-1213.

272. Merchant TE, Gould CJ, Hilton NE, et al. Ocular preservation after 36-Gy external beam radiation therapy for retinoblastoma. *J Pediatr Hematol Oncol* 2002;24:246-249.

273. Howarth C, Meyer D, Hustu HO, et al. Stage-related combined modality treatment of retinoblastoma. Results of a prospective study. *Cancer* 1980;45:851-858.

274. Czyzewski EA, Goldman S, Mundt AJ, et al. Radiation therapy for consolidation of metastatic or recurrent sarcomas in children treated with intensive chemotherapy and stem cell rescue. A feasibility study. *Int J Radiat Oncol Biol Phys* 1999;44:569-577.

275. Abramson DH, Ellsworth RM, Tretter P, et al. Simultaneous bilateral radiation for advanced bilateral retinoblastoma. *Arch Ophthalmol* 1981;99:1763-1766.

276. Rubin CM, Robison LL, Cameron JD, et al. Intraocular retinoblastoma group V: an analysis of prognostic factors. *J Clin Oncol* 1985;3:680-685.

277. Gaitan-Yanguas M. Retinoblastoma: analysis of 235 cases. *Int J Radiat Oncol Biol Phys* 1978;4:359-365.

278. Sotelo-Avila C, Gonzalez-Crussi F, Fowler JW. Complete and incomplete forms of Beckwith-Wiedemann syndrome: their oncogenic potential. *J Pediatr* 1980;96:47-50.

279. Lack EE, Neave C, Vawter GF. Hepatoblastoma. A clinical and pathologic study of 54 cases. *Am J Surg Pathol* 1982;6:693-705.

280. Ohaki Y, Misugi K, Sasaki Y, et al. Hepatitis B surface antigen positive hepatocellular carcinoma in children. Report of a case and review of the literature. *Cancer* 1983;51:822-828.

281. Gauthier F, Valayer J, Thai BL, et al. Hepatoblastoma and hepatocarcinoma in children: analysis of a series of 29 cases. *J Pediatr Surg* 1986;21:424-429.

282. Giacomantonio M, Ein SH, Mancer K. Thirty years of experience with pediatric primary malignant liver tumors. *J Pediatr Surg* 1984;19:523.

283. Price JB Jr, Schullinger JN, Santulli TV. Major hepatic resections for neoplasia in children. *Arch Surg* 1982;117:1139-1141.

284. Tagge EP, Tagge DU, Reyes J, et al. Resection, including transplantation, for hepatoblastoma and hepatocellular carcinoma: impact on survival. *J Pediatr Surg* 1992;27:292-296.

285. Weinblatt ME, Siegel SE, Siegel MM, et al. Preoperative chemotherapy for unresectable primary hepatic malignancies in children. *Cancer* 1982;50:1061-1064.

286. Ortega JA, Krailo MD, Haas JE, et al. Effective treatment of unresectable or metastatic hepatoblastoma with cisplatin and continuous infusion doxorubicin chemotherapy: a report from the Children's Cancer Study Group. *J Clin Oncol* 1991;9:2167-2176.

287. Habrand JL, Nehme D, Kalifa C, et al. Is there a place for radiation therapy in the management of hepatoblastomas and hepatocellular carcinomas in children? *Int J Radiat Oncol Biol Phys* 1992;23:525-531.

PART XIV

Special Considerations

CHAPTER 37

Radiation Therapy for Bone Marrow or Stem Cell Transplantation

Colleen A. Lawton

HISTORY OF TOTAL BODY IRRADIATION FOR MARROW OR STEM CELL TRANSPLANTATION

Total body irradiation has played a pivotal role in bone marrow transplantation since the first successful transplants were performed in mice in the 1950s.[1] It was noted then that following supralethal doses of total body irradiation with the infusion of compatible bone marrow allowed cells to maintain viability. After this preliminary work, similar studies were performed with canines[2] and primates.[3] In this early transplantation era, it was shown that total body irradiation of animals had a profound effect on the immune system, but administration of appropriate types and quantities of bone marrow could lead to repair of the damage produced by the radiation. This preliminary animal research quickly led to the exploration of bone marrow transplantation in humans.

Bone marrow transplantation in humans dates back to the late 1950s, when Thomas and colleagues[4] performed bone marrow infusion on a handful of patients who were suffering from fatal diseases, mostly leukemias. Thomas's early work provided several important insights into bone marrow transplantation. That work involved the first successful infusions of bone marrow into humans without significant clinical problems such as pulmonary emboli. Subsequently, Thomas's group showed that it was the radiation rather than the 'chemotherapy' (as it was known in the late 1950s) that produced sufficient immunosuppression for the infused marrow to be accepted. Finally, they proved that the doses of total body irradiation necessary to adequately suppress the patient's immune system to allow successful engraftment were well above the generally accepted median lethal dose for humans.

With this early work, both autologous (between host and self) and syngeneic (between identical siblings) bone marrow transplantations were well under way. Unfortunately, allogeneic transplantation (transplantation between two persons who are not identical twins) was significantly hindered in its initial development because of problems with nonengraftment.[5] Once this problem was overcome, as a result of better understanding of the histocompatibility antigens, the next hurdle was the serious and potentially lethal sequelae of transplantation now recognized as graft-versus-host disease, in which the donor graft attacks the host's organs. A suggestion of this process had been seen in rodent models,[6] but a real understanding of it in the human system did not occur until 1975, when Thomas and colleagues[7] described the disease and developed a grading system for it. With the advent of drugs such as methotrexate and cyclosporine, physicians were able to control this lethal complication,[8] allowing allogeneic bone marrow transplantation to flourish.

Most transplants today are allogeneic and are given after a conditioning regimen of chemotherapy (usually cyclophosphamide) to destroy the normal bone marrow followed by external-beam irradiation of the entire body. This combination effectively kills tumor cells and suppresses the host immune system at lower doses than would be necessary if either modality was used alone. Thus total body irradiation remains an important part of the transplantation strategy.

RESPONSE OF NORMAL BONE MARROW TO TOTAL BODY IRRADIATION

It is readily apparent that total body irradiation, alone or in conjunction with bone marrow transplantation, affects virtually every organ system, depending on the dose and fractionation. This section focuses on the effects of irradiation on normal bone marrow and other hematopoietic tissues. Additional details are given in Chapters 1 and 33.

The effects of total body irradiation on experimental animals have been well documented;. the $LD_{50/30}$ (the single dose that is lethal at 30 days to 50% of the experimental animals tested) is well defined for most mammals. However, little such information is available regarding total body irradiation in humans except in cases of accidental exposure, where retrospective estimations of dose made the findings less reliable.[9]

Tubiana and colleagues[10] have provided some unique information regarding the effects of total body irradiation on humans. They used total body irradiation for immunosuppression in 41 patients undergoing kidney transplants. After irradiation with 1 to 6 Gy, given in one or two fractions, patients were maintained in "aseptic" rooms and given a controlled diet until their leukocyte levels returned to normal. Despite these precautions, two patients who received 6 Gy died within a month after the transplantation, with aplasia resulting from the irradiation being the most likely cause of death. Seven of 17 patients given between 3.5 and 4.5 Gy in one or two sessions died within 40 days after the transplantation. Four of those deaths most likely were the result of aplasia or infection enhanced by the aplasia resulting from the irradiation.

Figure 37-1 illustrates the changes in amounts of peripheral blood elements in patients from this series. The investigators observed that the initial decrease in peripheral blood counts was more rapid and the nadir was reached sooner after higher radiation doses, as illustrated in Figure 37-2, for granulocyte counts. They concluded that the median lethal dose in humans must be greater than the previous estimate of 4.5 Gy, a conclusion substantiated by observations of the victims of the Chernobyl nuclear reactor accident.

Even when large amounts of bone marrow are exposed to high doses of radiation, marrow recovery can occur provided that a significant portion of the bone marrow is shielded.[11] However, Sykes and colleagues[12] showed that 30 Gy given at 10 Gy a week seems to be the dose beyond which bone marrow regeneration does not occur. After being given irradiation to local sites of involvement at doses of 30 Gy or more for localized breast carcinoma, sternal biopsies showed little or no marrow regeneration in 54 of their 56 cases (96.5%).

Response of Peripheral Blood

The work of Tubiana and colleagues[10] showed that total body irradiation has a profound and dose-dependent effect on peripheral blood counts. Figure 37-1 shows that significant doses of total body irradiation, such as those used in association with marrow or stem cell transplantation, produce leukopenia, granulocytopenia, anemia, and thrombocytopenia. As discussed in the following paragraphs, the magnitude of the respective cytopenias depends not only on the dose of radiation but also on the inherent radiosensitivity of the circulating cells and their precursors and on the normal life span of the circulating cells.

Leukocytes

Being the most radiosensitive of the peripheral blood cells, lymphocyte counts drop dramatically soon after total body irradiation.[13] Lymphoid precursors are also highly radiosensitive; the time required for recovery of recirculating lymphocytes depends on the dose, and the process is known to require weeks or even months in rodents. Granulocytes and their precursors are less radiosensitive, and therefore granulocyte counts fall 1 to 2 days after total body irradiation (see Fig. 37-1).[10] Significant granulocyte regeneration usually does not occur until approximately 20 to 25 days after total body irradiation.

Platelets

Circulating platelets are relatively radioresistant.[14] Given their normal circulating life span of 8 to 11 days, the drop in peripheral platelet counts is delayed relative to that of the other myeloid cells. The platelet precursor cells, the megakaryocytes, are the least radiosensitive of

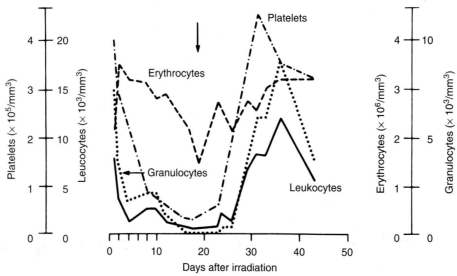

Fig. 37-1 Changes in relative amounts of peripheral blood elements in humans after total body irradiation with 4.3 Gy in two fractions. Day 0 is the first day of irradiation. (From Tubiana M, Frindel E, Croizat H, et al. *Pathol Biol* (Paris) 1979;27:326-334.)

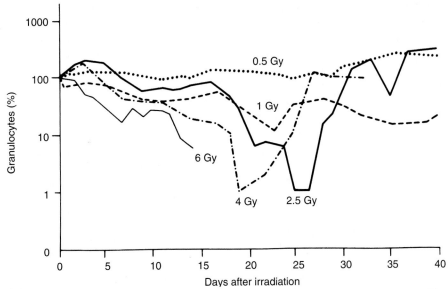

Fig. 37-2   Comparison of changes in circulating granulocytes in five patients given total body irradiation in single doses ranging from 0.5 to 6 Gy. Levels are expressed as percent of preirradiation granulocyte counts. (From Tubiana M, Frindel E, Croizat H, et al. *Pathol Biol* (Paris) 1979;27:326-334.)

the myeloid elements[13]; measurable damage reflected in the peripheral blood counts appears approximately 2 to 3 days after total body irradiation. The nadir lasts approximately 2 to 3 weeks.

Erythrocytes

Red blood cells have the longest circulating life span of the peripheral blood cells (120 days), and in the mature, circulating form are resistant to direct damage from irradiation. After total body irradiation in preparation for bone marrow transplantation, the erythrocyte counts drop the slowest and recover the fastest of all the circulating cell types (see Fig. 37-1). In this way the total body irradiation given for marrow or stem cell transplantation is unlike the fractionated low doses of total body irradiation given over periods of months to years for chronic lymphocytic leukemia, from which erythropoietic stem cells do not completely recover.[15]

Effects on the Spleen

The white pulp of the spleen is structurally similar to lymph nodes, and the response of the spleen to ionizing radiation is similar to that of the lymph nodes (see Chapter 33). In humans, lymphocyte maturation takes place largely in the white pulp of the spleen and in the lymph nodes.

Extensive experience with splenic irradiation in patients with early-stage Hodgkin's disease has revealed no significant clinical effect of the radiation. To our knowledge, no reports have been made that suggest a clinically significant change in the spleen after local irradiation for Hodgkin's disease or after total body irradiation in conjunction with marrow or stem cell transplantation.

TYPES OF TRANSPLANTS

Cells to be used for transplantation can be obtained in one of two ways. In the traditional bone marrow harvest, the patient is anesthetized and multiple marrow samples are collected by needle aspiration from the iliac crest or occasionally from the sternum. In the more recent and now more common procedure, donors are given cytokines, with or without chemotherapy, to stimulate the production and release of stem cells from the marrow into the peripheral blood ("stem cell mobilization"). Stem cells are then removed from the peripheral blood by apheresis, and the remaining blood is returned to the donor.

The relationship of the donor to the recipient defines the type of marrow or stem cell transplant—autologous, syngeneic, or allogeneic. Each type is described briefly in the following paragraphs.

Autologous Transplants

In autologous transplants, the donor is also the recipient. In this procedure, stem cells are harvested from the patient and frozen, after which the patient undergoes a conditioning regimen involving ablative chemotherapy with or without irradiation. Once the conditioning regimen has been completed, the frozen stem cells are thawed and reinfused. If the stem cells are thought to be contaminated by malignant cells, they may be purged before being reinfused. This process involves exposing the isolated stem cells to agents such as monoclonal antibodies in an attempt to remove any neoplastic cells.

Syngeneic Transplants

Syngeneic transplantation takes place between genetically identical twins. As noted earlier in this chapter, some of the first successful transplants in humans were syngeneic. This type of transplant is rarely used, for the obvious reason that few patients have genetically identical twins.

Allogeneic Transplants

Allogeneic marrow or stem cell transplantation takes place between two nonidentical individuals of the same species (for example, two humans) and can be subdivided into two broad categories, namely related and unrelated. Related allogeneic bone marrow transplantation occurs between two genetically related individuals. Such transplants are further categorized according to the degree of human leukocyte antigen (HLA) matching. A completely matched donor and recipient transplant occurs between HLA-identical siblings, whereas a mismatched related transplant occurs between relatives who match at only three, four, or five of the six major HLA loci. The donor can be a parent, aunt, cousin, or any of a number of relatives having the appropriate HLA type.

Unrelated allogeneic marrow or stem cell transplantation takes place between two genetically unrelated people. Success with this type of transplant requires that the donor and recipient share most, if not all, of the six major HLA loci.

USES OF MARROW OR STEM CELL TRANSPLANTATION

The use of marrow or stem cell transplantation has been increasing over time (Fig. 37-3) as success rates continue to improve, especially for leukemias and lymphomas. Most of the marrow or stem cell transplants to date have been performed in patients with leukemia.[16] Initially, transplantation was considered only for acute leukemias in refractory phases or after multiple relapses,[17] but currently many patients with high-risk acute leukemias are referred for transplant during their first remission. Such patients include children with Philadelphia chromosome-positive acute lymphocytic leukemia and adults with acute leukemia with high-risk features.[18,19]

Patients with chronic leukemia did not routinely undergo transplantation in the early years because the natural history of the disease allowed many patients to live for years before they succumbed to the disease. But as bone marrow transplantation became safer, it was considered and used successfully for patients with chronic leukemias (especially chronic granulocytic leukemia).[20-22] Today adult patients with chronic myelogenous leukemia (CML) routinely undergo transplantation while they are in early chronic-phase disease if an appropriate donor can be found.[22-24]

Lymphomas make up the other major disease category for which transplantation is performed. Both Hodgkin's and non-Hodgkin's lymphomas have been successfully treated with autologous, syngeneic, or allogeneic bone marrow transplantation.[25,26] Today most patients with lymphomas are treated with standard chemotherapy, irradiation, or both, and are considered for marrow or stem cell transplantation only if the disease proves refractory to these therapies. Experimentally, peripheral blood stem cell infusions may be used to enhance marrow recovery after intensive chemotherapy. Some reports, though, suggest that autologous marrow or stem cell transplantation is appropriate as front-line therapy in patients with certain aggressive lymphomas.[27-29]

Other uses of bone marrow transplantation are for noncancerous but otherwise fatal conditions, such as

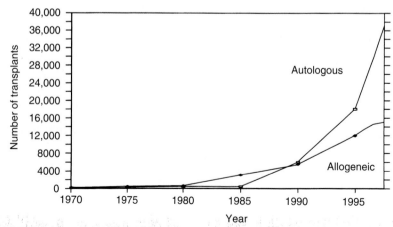

Fig. 37-3 Numbers of patients undergoing allogeneic and autologous blood and marrow transplant worldwide, 1970 to 1998. (Courtesy International Bone Marrow Transplant Tumor Registry.)

severe aplastic anemia and some congenital immuno-deficiency disorders,[18,30-33] and for some solid tumors. The most successful transplants for treating solid tumors have been done for children with neuroblastoma[34] or Ewing's sarcoma.[35-37] Transplants for solid tumors in adults, especially autologous transplants for breast cancer, have been studied extensively but remain controversial.[38-43]

ROLES OF TOTAL BODY IRRADIATION IN MARROW OR STEM CELL TRANSPLANTATION AND TECHNIQUES FOR ITS DELIVERY

Total body irradiation serves two different but important functions in preparation for marrow or stem cell transplantation. The first of these functions is to suppress the immune system; in fact, total body irradiation was first used in humans expressly for this purpose.[4] The second function is to kill tumor cells. For cancer patients, this role can be as important as immunosuppression.

Techniques for the delivery of total body irradiation have evolved in North America since Heublein[44] published the first description of a dedicated unit in 1932. In that unit, four beds were placed in a single room with an x-ray machine at one end, and four patients could be treated simultaneously. The exposure rate varied from 1.26 roentgens/hr for patients in the closer beds to 0.68 roentgen/hr for those in the more distant beds. This technique was quite progressive for its time, but today's techniques are very different.

Kim and colleagues[45] and, subsequently, Van Dyk[46] described the various techniques for delivery of total body irradiation in use at several major centers across North America. From these reports, it is clear that several different techniques can successfully deliver uniform total body irradiation (i.e., ± 10% dose homogeneity) through the use of single or opposing cobalt sources or single or opposing low-energy liner accelerators. Several centers also use high-energy linear accelerators, but use of such equipment requires careful attention to superficial doses.[47-49] The position of the patient during treatment also varies; although no one position is inherently better than another, dose uniformity is easier to obtain when the patient is treated while lying down or standing. Opposed lateral techniques can be combined with anteroposterior-posteroanterior techniques to improve dose homogeneity and to make selective organ shielding easier.[44,50-52]

Today treatment stands for total body irradiation can be purchased and customized to fit a transplantation center's needs. Use of such stands (one of which is shown in Fig. 37-4) allows safe, effective, and uniform dose delivery in combination with effective partial organ shielding. When the appropriate energy range of x-rays is determined and dose uniformity is obtained, the next two issues to be addressed are dose rate and fractionation.

Many reports suggest that lower dose rates produce the largest therapeutic gains, because the repair capacity of bone marrow stem cells and malignant hematopoietic cells is more limited than that of other cells in mammals.[50,53-56] Clinical data in support of the use of low dose rates can be found in an International Bone Marrow Transplant Registry report by Weiner and colleagues,[57] which described a statistically significant difference in the incidence of interstitial pneumonitis between the use of very low dose rates (up to 0.03 Gy/min) vs. higher ones. These findings led some transplant centers to continue to use low dose rates to deliver total body irradiation. However, other evidence suggests that the therapeutic gain from the use of lower dose rates is limited and that the use of higher dose rates (e.g., 0.2 to 0.3 Gy/min) is safe.[49,58,59] The most common dose rates in use today range from 0.05 to 0.2 Gy/min.

The value of fractionation in total body irradiation is somewhat clearer. When total body irradiation was initially performed, the usual dose was 8 to 10 Gy, given as a single fraction at low dose rates (up to 5 Gy/min).[7] It was subsequently shown that fractionating the irradiation not only allowed higher total doses to be given safely but also improved long-term survival.[60,61]

Next, Shank and colleagues[62] introduced the concept of hyperfractionated irradiation as a way of decreasing the incidence of pneumonitis and allowing even higher total doses to be delivered. Doses above 12 Gy seemed to be necessary for transplants from siblings who were less than fully HLA matched.[63,64] To date, Thomas and colleagues[22] have pushed the fractionated dose the farthest—to 15.75 Gy, given in seven once-daily fractions over 7 days. Although this method allowed better control of CML, the associated toxicity was unacceptably high, resulting in worse overall survival than could be obtained with the more conventional dose of 12 Gy, given in six fractions over 6 days. Thus it seems that the dose limit of total body irradiation has been reached even with fractionation. Today the most common fractionation schedule used in the United States is 12 Gy in six fractions, given either once a day over 6 days or twice a day over 3 days.

Selective organ shielding has been used by several centers across the United States in an effort to decrease the toxicity associated with marrow or stem cell transplantation, especially toxicity to the lung.[49,62] One technique for selective shielding of the lungs is to use thin lead shields (Fig. 37-5, *A*), with the goal of attenuating the dose only enough to account for the difference in density between the lung and soft tissues. Another option is to use thicker lung blocks (see Fig. 37-5, *B*), with the goal of reducing the dose to the lung by a substantial amount (e.g., 50% or 60% of the total dose).[49] The thicker lung blocks are used most often at centers that use more than the standard dose of 12 Gy in six fractions. Shielding that is customized to fit each patient allows delivery of higher total doses to be delivered by means of total body irradiation. Selective

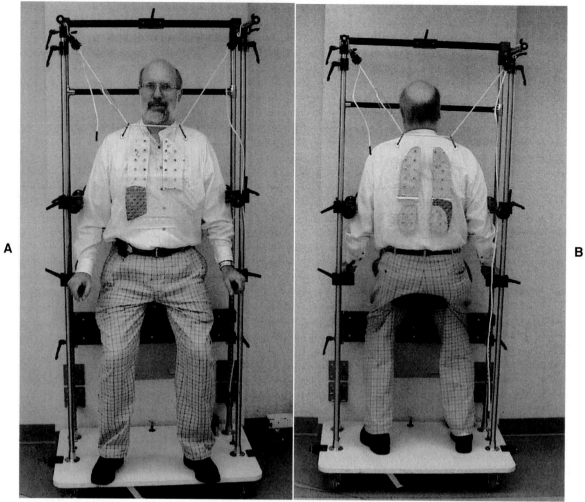

Fig. 37-4 Stand for total body irradiation designed by Mick-Radio Nuclear, New York, NY, and used at the Medical College of Wisconsin. Note the partial transmission blocks.

shielding designed specifically for the liver and kidneys has been developed at the Medical College of Wisconsin (see Fig. 37-5, *B*). Use of these customized shields has reduced the incidence of long-term toxic effects after total body irradiation.[49,51]

OTHER TYPES OF IRRADIATION USED WITH MARROW OR STEM CELL TRANSPLANTATION

Localized irradiation can be used in conjunction with marrow or stem cell transplantation, with or without total body irradiation. Specific uses have varied widely, but the most common focus on three goals: treating tumor in the spleen, treating tumor in the central nervous system, and boosting the radiation dose to areas of local disease.

Irradiation of the Spleen

Before the development of bone marrow transplantation for CML in the late 1970s and early 1980s, splenectomy

was often used in an attempt to reduce tumor burden and prevent relapse and blastic transformation.[65,66] Since then several investigators have noted that splenectomy, with its associated morbidity, could be avoided by giving low doses of radiation to the spleen in conjunction with total body irradiation and bone marrow transplantation.[52,65-69] Results from some randomized trials[68] have suggested a disease-free survival advantage from the use of splenic irradiation for some patients with CML. Usual boost doses to the spleen, given in conjunction with total body irradiation for marrow or stem cell transplantation, are approximately 5 to 6 Gy given over 2 or 3 days in two or three fractions.

Irradiation of the Central Nervous System

Central nervous system irradiation as part of the treatment of acute leukemia is not a new concept. Children with high-risk acute lymphocytic leukemia routinely have been treated with cranial and sometimes spinal irradiation, either as prophylaxis against the development of

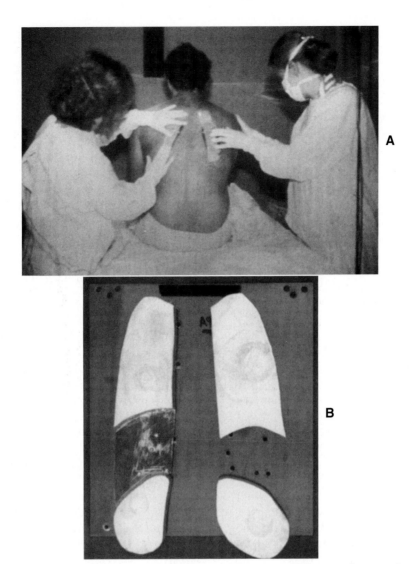

Fig. 37-5 **A,** Thin lead shields are used to correct for density differences between lung and soft tissue. **B,** Lung, liver, and kidney blocks used in total body irradiation at the Medical College of Wisconsin for significant shielding of those organs. (**A** Courtesy Nancy Tarbell, M.D., Harvard Medical School, Department of Radiation Oncology.)

disease in the central nervous system or as treatment of known central nervous system involvement.[70] This therapy is not without sequelae, but when the treatment is therapeutic, often there is little choice.

When the central nervous system is irradiated in conjunction with marrow or stem cell transplantation, doses vary widely, depending mostly on whether total body irradiation is part of the transplantation strategy. If the central nervous system is irradiated in conjunction with the usual doses of total body irradiation (12 Gy in six fractions), then the boost doses are usually about 9 to 12 Gy, given in daily 1.5- to 2-Gy fractions. Doses for central nervous system irradiation for marrow or stem cell transplantation without total body irradiation can be much higher (24 to 30 Gy, given in a fractionated course).

Boost Doses for Local Disease

In conjunction with marrow or stem cell transplantation, boosting the radiation dose to areas of local disease with external-beam therapy has been performed not only for hematologic forms of cancer such as leukemias and lymphomas but also for solid tumors such as neuroblastomas in children. Boost doses also have been used for breast cancer patients undergoing autologous marrow or stem cell transplantation. Doses vary widely depending on the type of tumor as well as the type of transplant and whether total body irradiation will be used with the transplant. In patients with leukemias and lymphomas who are undergoing allogeneic bone marrow transplantation, boost doses of approximately 10 to 20 Gy (fractionated) are used before the total body irradiation.[18,26] Higher doses can be used after transplantation, especially for lymphomas in which residual bulky disease is present. Doses appropriate to the type of tumor are used when total body irradiation is not used.

SEQUELAE OF TOTAL BODY IRRADIATION AND MARROW OR STEM CELL TRANSPLANTATION

Sequelae caused solely by total body irradiation are somewhat difficult to identify, because that irradiation is given in conjunction with conditioning chemotherapy—which is also toxic—and the transplant procedure. Therefore the acute and late sequelae of total body irradiation with marrow or stem cell transplantation will be discussed briefly below with the understanding that many of these sequelae have multiple causes.

Acute Toxic Effects

The major life-threatening acute toxicity of total body irradiation at doses that are used for marrow or stem cell transplantation is to the hematopoietic system. The effects of the usual doses of total body irradiation on peripheral blood counts are so dramatic that death would result if stem cell support (or transplantation) were not performed.[11] However, because marrow or stem cell transplantation is an integral part of the procedure, the hematopoietic toxicity of total body irradiation is not a problem in this context.

Gastrointestinal toxic effects from total body irradiation are expected, and nausea and vomiting are common, typically beginning within the first hour after irradiation begins and lasting up to 48 hours after the final dose. Antiemetics such as ondansetron and granisetron can reduce nausea and vomiting considerably but cannot eliminate them completely.[69] Diarrhea is also common after total body irradiation and is aggravated by the antibiotics and chemotherapy that are part of the transplantation process.

The parotid glands are acutely sensitive to radiation (as discussed in detail in Chapter 6), and parotitis is experienced by most patients who undergo total body irradiation. Parotitis presents as acute swelling of the parotid glands with associated jaw or facial pain. Parotitis can be treated effectively with steroids, which are commonly used during transplantation. Left untreated, parotitis subsides in 2 to 3 days.

Skin erythema or tanning is common after total body irradiation at the usual 12-Gy dose level. This effect is transient, and dry or moist desquamation is rare. Oral mucositis also is common in total body irradiation, but it is intimately associated with the conditioning chemotherapy. Conditioning chemotherapy, particularly with cyclophosphamide,[7,71] is known to cause mucositis, but the total body irradiation certainly increases its severity.

Most patients experience alopecia within 7 to 14 days after receiving total body irradiation[72]; although chemotherapy plays a role in hair loss, irradiation alone can cause it as well. The alopecia is usually complete but reversible, and significant regrowth of hair generally occurs within 3 to 6 months after the end of the treatment.

Significant damage to vital organs can occur as an acute effect of total body irradiation; in this chapter, damage to specific organs is discussed in the following section on long-term effects.

Long-Term Effects
Hepatotoxicity

Venoocclusive disease of the liver is a significant and often life-threatening complication of marrow or stem cell transplantation; it can occur after conditioning with either total body irradiation, chemotherapy, or both.[73-75] This disease, which was first described as a clinicopathologic entity in 1977, presents as hepatic dysfunction that usually develops within 3 weeks after marrow transplantation.[75] Characteristic features include ascites and hepatomegaly associated with abdominal pain and weight gain. Histologic changes include concentric subintimal thickening and luminal narrowing in the terminal hepatic venules or small sublobular veins. Venoocclusive disease of the liver is fatal in approximately one third of those affected.[75]

The development of venoocclusive disease of the liver depends on many factors, the most notable of which are the presence of underlying liver disease, the patient's age, and the conditioning regimen used.[75] Venoocclusive disease does not seem to be related to graft-versus-host disease. Data from at least one institution do suggest a relationship between the dose of total body irradiation and the incidence of venoocclusive disease[49]; thus at doses greater than 12 Gy in six fractions, the use of partial organ shielding should be considered.

Pulmonary Toxicity

Interstitial pneumonia or pneumonitis is a frequent complication of total body irradiation.[76] Interstitial pneumonitis has been documented in up to 50% of all patients who have undergone transplantation, and approximately half of those cases are fatal.[77] Although pulmonary pathogens have been recovered in many cases, the pneumonitis seems to be of idiopathic origin in between 30% and 40% of patients experiencing this effect after stem cell transplantation.[78] Interstitial pneumonitis usually presents as a fever, nonproductive cough, and some shortness of breath within 90 days after total body irradiation. Histopathologic findings include lung edema, fibrosis, variable cellular infiltrates, and alveolar exudates.

Unquestionably, the radiation dose delivered to the lungs during total body irradiation participates in the development of pneumonitis, especially idiopathic pneumonitis. The radiation dose, dose rate, and fractionation schedule all seem to be related to the incidence of pneumonitis.[57,79] Keane and colleagues[76] compared the incidence of interstitial pneumonitis at centers where total body irradiation was delivered as a single 10-Gy dose and those where the dose was lower (4 to 9.5 Gy). They found that the incidence of pneumonitis, of either infectious or idiopathic origin, was much lower when lower doses were used. The use of low dose rates also seems to be associated with a decrease in the incidence of interstitial pneumonitis.[79]

In addition to total dose and dose rate, fractionation seems to affect the incidence of interstitial pneumonitis. Shank and colleagues[62] showed that fractionating the irradiation significantly decreased the incidence of interstitial pneumonitis from 70% for a single dose to 33% for the regimen of 13.2 Gy given in 11 fractions over 4 days. This beneficial effect of fractionation on the incidence of interstitial pneumonitis has been shown elsewhere as well.[60,80]

In an effort to clarify the effect of bone marrow transplantation including total body irradiation on lung function, researchers at some centers have used pulmonary function tests at selected intervals after transplantation.[81-83] Results from one such study indicate that the incidence of pneumonitis is associated not only with the conditioning regimen used but also with preexisting lung damage.[82] Results from a large study of pulmonary function after conditioning that included total body irradiation at the Medical College of Wisconsin[84] indicate that patients who survive for 100 days after a bone marrow transplant show an initial decline in pulmonary function but subsequently recover unless other factors such as infection or significant graft-versus-host disease are present. Radiation dose to the lung also affected pulmonary function, specifically forced vital capacity.[84]

Thus total body irradiation certainly plays a role in the development of interstitial pneumonitis after bone marrow transplantation, but it is only one of several contributory factors. For patients who are to be treated with total body irradiation at doses that exceed the usual 12 Gy given in six fractions, the use of selective partial lung shielding should be seriously considered so as to minimize the incidence of pneumonitis.[84,85]

Cardiotoxicity

Cardiac damage has been reported to follow marrow or stem cell transplantation, but cardiac effects generally are related more to the chemotherapy than to the irradiation.[86-89] Cyclophosphamide, in particular, is a significant cardiotoxin, especially in high doses, and some centers recommend that total body irradiation be used so that the dose of cyclophosphamide can be reduced.[87] Cardiac toxicity can be expressed as cardiomyopathy,

pericarditis, or both. The mortality rate among affected patients is approximately 10%.[87,89]

Renal Toxicity

Unlike cardiotoxicity, renal toxicity associated with bone marrow transplantation seems to be strongly related to the total body irradiation rather than the chemotherapy.[90-93] The clinical presentation of the renal damage is consistent with radiation nephritis and includes increased serum creatinine levels, decreased glomerular filtration rates, anemia, and hypertension, all occurring approximately 6 to 20 months after bone marrow transplantation.[91] Even the histologic appearance of the renal injury resembles radiation damage. However, because the total doses of radiation are rather low relative to the amount of renal damage produced, the cause of the damage probably depends on radiation but also on other factors. In a European study of 75 patients, Mirabell and colleagues[94] found the incidence of renal injury associated with bone marrow transplantation is not only related to the total radiation dose but may also be related to the dose per fraction. Selective renal shielding during total body irradiation can significantly decrease the incidence of renal toxicity.[51]

Cataracts

Cataracts can develop in patients who undergo marrow or stem cell transplantation. The incidence of cataract development in patients conditioned with chemotherapy only is 15% to 20%.[95] The previous use of single-dose total body irradiation in conjunction with bone marrow transplantation resulted in a much higher incidence of cataracts (approximately 80% at 5 years after transplantation).[96] Fortunately, this risk can be greatly reduced (to the levels associated with chemotherapy only) by using fractionated radiation.[97-100] Moreover, if cataracts do develop and impair the patient's vision, they can be surgically corrected.

Effects on Gonadal Function and Fertility

Radiation-induced infertility is a problem for patients who undergo marrow or stem cell transplantation. Ninety-five percent of males will have azoospermia after total body irradiation. More than 95% of postmenarchal females will become amenorrheic after bone marrow transplantation, but a few will resume menstruation. The potential for recovery is age-dependent. Approximately 80% of females who are premenarchal at the time of the transplant will ultimately achieve menarche after transplantation; also, postmenarchal females who are less than 18 years old are very likely to recover sufficient ovarian function to resume menstration.[101,102] Patients should be informed that loss of fertility is quite likely but that cases of childbearing and fathering of children have been documented after transplantation.[103,104]

Effects on Growth and Development

Total body irradiation delivered to prepubertal patients is known to produce problems with growth and development.[81,101,105-108] Data from the University of California at San Francisco[107] show that when prepubertal patients with leukemia are given total body irradiation in preparation for transplant, 80% to 90% will have diminished growth, 17% will have delayed or arrested puberty, and 100% will have minor abnormalities in the intelligence quotient at 1 year, with recovery within approximately 3 years. However, at least one study has shown that growth retardation was equivalent among children whose conditioning regimen consisted of only chemotherapy (with busulfan and cyclophosphamide) and those given a conditioning regimen of cyclophosphamide and total body irradiation.[109] In a more recent study, children with acute myeloid leukemia whose conditioning regimen consisted of busulfan and cyclophosphamide also showed abnormal gonadotropin levels, with the abnormality being more prominent in girls than in boys.[110]

Thyroid Dysfunction

Total body irradiation, whether given as a single or fractionated dose, also can cause thyroid dysfunction, which itself can affect growth and development in children. Usually the hypothyroidism is mild and transient, and resolves spontaneously.[111,112] However, the incidence of hypothyroidism does increase over time after irradiation, and hypothyroidism can occur late; consequently, thyroid function should be followed up for several years after total body irradiation.

Secondary Malignancies

Secondary malignancies are not uncommon after marrow or stem cell transplantation. Witherspoon and colleagues[113] have reported that the age-adjusted incidence of secondary malignancies after transplantation is 6.7 times that of primary cancer in the general population. The secondary malignancies can be caused not only by total body irradiation but also by chemotherapy and by additional localized radiation given in preparation for transplantation.[114] Secondary malignancies appearing after bone marrow transplantation tend to be one of two types—B-cell lymphoproliferative disorders, including non-Hodgkin's lymphomas, and other solid tumors.

B-cell lymphoproliferative disorders can occur under conditions of prolonged immunosuppression other than those associated with transplantation, but they are becoming increasingly common among bone marrow transplant patients because of mismatched transplants and T-cell depletion.[115,116] These B-cell disorders seem to be related to the Epstein-Barr virus; when the virus infects B lymphocytes in immunocompromised patients, the cells can proliferate uncontrollably, with extensive infiltration, organ damage (possibly fatal), or conversion to aggressive, usually fatal lymphoma.[30] Fortunately, the risk of developing lymphoproliferative disorders is low (0.6%), and total body irradiation in the conditioning regimen does not seem to be a causative factor.[116] Although secondary leukemias can appear after bone marrow transplantation, their incidence is low compared with those of lymphomas and solid tumors.[113]

An association has been noted between conditioning regimens containing total body irradiation and the occurrence of secondary solid tumors in both humans and dogs.[113,117] In the Witherspoon and colleagues series,[113] 13 of the 35 cases of secondary cancer that appeared after bone marrow transplantation were solid tumors.

Although a risk of secondary malignancies is associated with undergoing marrow or stem cell transplantation, patients undergoing this procedure usually have lethal diseases for which transplantation offers the possibility of cure. In this context, the risk of second malignancies, although high, may be acceptable.

Psychological Effects

Psychological effects are an important aspect of the late sequelae of total body irradiation as well as the transplantation process. Given the gravity of the diseases being treated and the intensity of the treatment, some psychological morbidity would be expected. A prospective, quantitative psychosocial evaluation of 31 adults who underwent bone marrow transplantation was conducted by Leigh and colleagues in the United Kingdom.[118] In that study, the incidence of psychosocial morbidity (measured with standardized psychological measurement tools) was 54%; moreover, morbidity was still present at 6 to 9 months after the transplantation, but the type of transplant was unrelated to the occurrence of morbidity. Patients with CML faired worse in terms of psychosocial morbidity after transplant than did patients with other diseases, probably because they had no experience with intense hematologic therapy before undergoing the transplantation.[118] With regard to pediatric patients, a retrospective review of 73 children who had undergone allogeneic transplants showed that most patients (about 75%) reported having few psychosocial problems after the transplant.[108] Finally, cancer patients who received adjuvant psychosocial therapy after diagnosis in another study[119] generally showed less psychological morbidity than patients who did not. Thus it is possible that psychological intervention would be helpful to at least some patients undergoing transplantation, and such intervention should be considered.[119]

CONCLUSIONS

Because the morbidity associated with the use of total body irradiation in marrow or stem cell transplantation is fairly significant, one might ask, why use total body irradiation at all? According to Shank,[120] total body irradiation for cancer treatment has several theoretical advantages over chemotherapy with regard to cytoreduction: "sanctuary sites" such as the testes are not spared, the dose is homogeneous throughout the body and independent of blood supply, radiation has no known cross-resistance with other agents, the effective dose is not affected by detoxification or excretion, and the dose distribution can be adjusted by using partial tissue blocks for radiosensitive normal tissues (e.g., lung) or by boosting the dose to radioresistant areas.

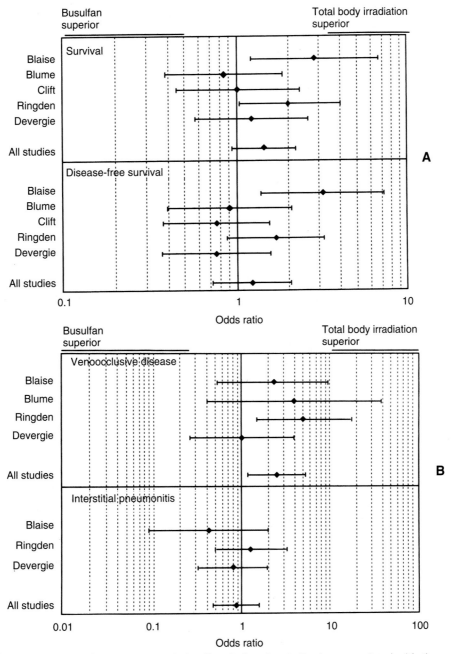

Fig. 37-6 Results from a meta-analysis of survival and complications associated with the use of regimens that include busulfan plus cyclophosphamide vs. regimens that include total body irradiation as conditioning for bone marrow transplantation. **A,** Survival and disease-free survival are not statistically different; yet a trend favoring the use of total body irradiation is evident. **B,** Patients conditioned for transplant with busulfan plus cyclophosphamide have a higher rate of venoocclusive disease (and perhaps interstitial pneumonitis) than do patients conditioned with regimens that included total body irradiation. (From Hartman AR, Williams SF, Dillon JJ. *Bone Marrow Transplant* 1998;22:439-443.)

With these advantages in mind, it would make sense to use total body irradiation for immunosuppression in circumstances in which the alternative (busulfan and cyclophosphamide) is not as effective, such as for transplantation of T-cell–depleted material. Outcomes of bone marrow transplants with and without total body irradiation for acute leukemia have been studied by investigators from France as well as from Japan. In the study from France, Blaise and colleagues[121] showed a statistically significant improvement in disease-free survival for patients with acute myeloid leukemia who underwent total body irradiation. In the study from Japan,[122] 81 patients underwent total body irradiation and 42 did not, and a survival advantage favored those who underwent total body irradiation.

Finally, a recent meta-analysis comparing busulfan plus cyclophosphamide vs. total body irradiation as conditioning regimens indicated that the chemotherapy-based conditioning regimen produced a higher incidence of venoocclusive disease of the liver and suggested that overall survival and disease-free survival rates were higher among those given total body irradiation (Fig. 37-6).[123]

The aforementioned evidence supports the continued use of total body irradiation in preparation for marrow or stem cell transplantation in selected patients. Further investigation of dose rates and fractionation schedules is needed to minimize the toxic effects of total body irradiation while maximizing its effectiveness.

REFERENCES

1. Odell TF, Tausche FG, Lindsley DL, et al. Homotransplantation of functional erythropoietic elements in rat following total-body irradiation. *Ann N Y Acad Sci* 1957;64:811-825.
2. Alpen EL, Baum SJ. Acute radiation protection of dogs by bone marrow auto transfusions. Presented at: meeting of the Radiation Research Society; May 13-15, 1957: Rochester, NY.
3. Crouch BG, Overman RR. Whole-body radiation protection in primates. *Fed Proc* 1957;16:27.
4. Thomas ED, Lochte HL Jr, Lu WC, et al. Intravenous infusion of bone marrow in patients receiving radiation and chemotherapy. *N Engl J Med* 1957;257:491-496.
5. Bortin MM. A compendium of reported human bone marrow transplants. *Transplantation* 1970;9:571-587.
6. Trentin JJ. Mortality and skin transplantability in x-irradiated mice receiving isologous, homologous or heterologous bone marrow. *Proc Soc Exp Biol Med* 1956;92:688-693.
7. Thomas ED, Storb R, Clift RA, et al. Bone-marrow transplantation (second of two parts). *N Engl J Med* 1975;292:895-902.
8. Storb R, Deeg HJ, Thomas ED, et al. Marrow transplantation for chronic myelocytic leukemia: a controlled trial of cyclosporine versus methotrexate for prophylaxis of graft-versus-host disease. *Blood* 1985;66:698-702.
9. Champlin R. Symposium: treatment for victims of nuclear accidents: the role of bone marrow transplantation. *Radiat Res* 1988; 113:205-210.
10. Tubiana M, Frindel E, Croizat H, et al. Effects of radiations on bone marrow. *Pathol Biol* (Paris) 1979;27:326-334.
11. Rubin P, Landman S, Mayer E, et al. Bone marrow regeneration and extension after extended field irradiation in Hodgkin's disease. *Cancer* 1973;32:699-711.
12. Sykes HP, Chu FCH, Wilkerson WG. Local bone marrow changes secondary to therapeutic irradiation. *Radiology* 1960;75:919-929.
13. Fajardo LF, Berthrong M, Anderson RE. Radiation and host defense mechanisms. In: *Radiation Pathology*. New York, NY: Oxford University Press; 2001:87-96.
14. Greenberg ML, Chanana AD, Cronkite EP, et al. Extracorporeal irradiation of blood in man: radiation resistance of circulating platelets. *Radiat Res* 1968;35:147-154.
15. Del Regato JA. Total body irradiation in the treatment of chronic lymphogenous leukemia: Janeway Lecture, 1973. *Am J Roentgenol Radium Ther Nucl Med* 1974;120:504-520.
16. Horowitz MM, Loberiza FR, Bredeson CN, et al. Transplant registries: guiding clinical decisions and improving outcomes. *Oncology* (Huntingt) 2001;15:649-659.
17. Thomas ED, Buckner CD, Banaji M, et al. One hundred patients with acute leukemia treated by chemotherapy, total body irradiation, and allogeneic marrow transplantation. *Blood* 1977;49: 511-533.
18. Ash RC, Casper JT, Chitambar CR, et al. Successful allogeneic transplantation of T-cell-depleted bone marrow from closely HLA-matched unrelated donors. *N Engl J Med* 1990;322:485-494.
19. Tallman MS, Kopecky KJ, Amos D, et al. Analysis of prognostic factors for the outcome of marrow transplantation or further chemotherapy for patients with acute nonlymphocytic leukemia in first remission. *J Clin Oncol* 1989;17:326-337.
20. Doney K, Buckner D, Sales GE, et al. Treatment of chronic granulocytic leukemia by chemotherapy, total body irradiation and allogeneic bone marrow transplantation. *Exp Hematol* 1978;6: 738-747.
21. Fefer A, Cheever MA, Thomas ED, et al. Disappearance of Ph[1]-positive cells in four patients with chronic granulocytic leukemia after chemotherapy, irradiation and marrow transplantation from an identical twin. *N Engl J Med* 1979;300:333-337.
22. Thomas ED. Total body irradiation regimens for marrow grafting. *Int J Radiat Oncol Biol Phys* 1990;19:1285-1288.
23. Gratwohl A, Hermans J, Niederwieser D, et al. Bone marrow transplantation for chronic myeloid leukemia: long-term results. Chronic Leukemia Working Party of the European Group for Bone Marrow Transplantation. *Bone Marrow Transplant* 1993;12:509-516.
24. Jones RJ. Biology and treatment of chronic myeloid leukemia. *Curr Opin Oncol* 1997;9:3-7.
25. Carella AM, Congiu AM, Gaozza E, et al. High-dose chemotherapy with autologous bone marrow transplantation in 50 advanced resistant Hodgkin's disease patients: an Italian study group report. *J Clin Oncol* 1988;6:1411-1416.
26. Lundberg JH, Hansen RM, Chitambar CR, et al. Allogeneic bone marrow transplantation for relapsed and refractory lymphoma using genotypically HLA-identical and alternative donors. *J Clin Oncol* 1991;9:1848-1859.
27. Gulati SC, Shank B, Black P, et al. Autologous bone marrow transplantation for patients with poor-prognosis lymphoma. *J Clin Oncol* 1988;6:1303-1313.
28. Freedman AS, Takvorian E, Neuberg D, et al. Autologous bone marrow transplantation in poor-prognosis intermediate-grade and high-grade B-cell non-Hodgkin's lymphoma in first remission: a pilot study. *J Clin Oncol* 1993;11:931-936.
29. Gianni AM, Bregni M, Siena S, et al. High-dose chemotherapy and autologous bone marrow transplantation compared with MACOP-B in aggressive B-cell lymphoma. *N Engl J Med* 1997; 336:1290-1297.
30. Good RA. Bone marrow transplantation symposium: bone marrow transplantation for immunodeficiency disease. *Am J Med Sci* 1987;294:68-74.
31. Ramsay NKC, Kim T, Nesbit ME, et al. Total lymphoid irradiation and cyclophosphamide as preparation for bone marrow transplantation in severe aplastic anemia. *Blood* 1980;55:344-346.

32. Bacigalupo A, Oneto R, Bruno B, et al. Current results of bone marrow transplantation in patients with acquired severe aplastic anemia. Report of the European Group for blood and marrow transplantation. *Acta Haematol* 2000;103:19-25.

33. Margolis DA, Casper JT. Alternative-donor hematopoietic stem-cell transplantation for severe aplastic anemia. *Semin Hematol* 2000;37:43-55.

34. Halperin EC, Constine LS, Tarbell NJ, et al (eds). *Pediatric Radiation Oncology*, 3rd ed. Philadelphia, Pa: Lippincott Williams & Wilkins; 1999:163-202.

35. Marcus RB, Graham-Pole JR, Springfield DS, et al. High-risk Ewing's sarcoma: end-intensification using autologous bone marrow transplantation. *Int J Radiat Oncol Biol Phys* 1988;15:53-59.

36. Ladenstein R, Laset C, Pinkerton R, et al. Impact of megatherapy in children with high-risk Ewing's tumors in complete remission: a report from EBMT Solid Tumour registry. *Bone Marrow Transplant* 1995;15:697-705.

37. Ladenstein R, Gadner H, Hartmann O, et al. The European experience with megadose therapy and autologous bone marrow transplantation in solid tumors with poor prognosis (Ewing sarcoma, germ cell tumors and brain tumors). *Wien Med Wochenschr* 1995;145:55-57.

38. Bonadonna G, Gianni AM. High-dose chemotherapy and autologous bone marrow transplant for adjuvant treatment of poor-risk breast cancer. *Oncol J Club* 1990;2:3-11.

39. Peters WP, Shpall EJ, Jones RB, et al. High-dose combination alkylating agents with bone marrow support as initial treatment for metastatic breast cancer. *J Clin Oncol* 1988;6:1368-1376.

40. Shea T, Bitran J, Abboud C, et al. Multi-center study with multiple cycles of PBSC supported high-dose therapy for stage IV breast cancer [abstract]. *Proc Am Soc Clin Oncol* 2000;19:59a. Abstract 230.

41. Klein JL, Dansey R, Karanes C, et al. High-dose chemotherapy (STAMP 1) and peripheral blood progenitor cell transplantation following Adriamycin induction chemotherapy for high-risk primary and locally advanced breast cancer [abstract]. *Proc Am Soc Clin Oncol* 2000;19:60a. Abstract 234.

42. Sundaram S, Lancaster D, Silva J, et al. Oral capecitabine is an active and well tolerated primary palliative treatment in patients with metastatic breast cancer who progress after high dose chemotherapy and autologous stem cell support [abstract]. *Proc Am Soc Clin Oncol* 2000;19:58a. Abstract 223.

43. Martinelli G, Cinieri S, Ferrucci P, et al. Multiple high-dose chemotherapy with docetaxel, epirubicin and cyclophosphamide for high risk breast cancer: clinical results of a phase II study [abstract]. *Proc Am Soc Clin Oncol* 2000;19:56a. Abstract 218.

44. Heublein AC. A preliminary report on continuous irradiation of the entire body. *Radiology* 1932;18:1051-1062.

45. Kim TH, Khan FM, Galvin JM. A report of the work party: comparison of total body irradiation techniques for bone marrow transplantation. *Int J Radiat Oncol Biol Phys* 1980;6:779-784.

46. Van Dyk J. Magna field irradiation: physical considerations. *Int J Radiat Oncol Biol Phys* 1983;9:915.

47. Findley DO, Skov DD, Blume KG. Total body irradiation with a 10 MV linear accelerator in conjunction with bone marrow transplantation. *Int J Radiat Oncol Biol Phys* 1980;6:695-702.

48. Glasgow GP, Mill WB, Phillips GL II, et al. Comparative ^{60}CO total body irradiation (220 cm SAD*) and 25-meV total body irradiation (370 cm SAD) dosimetry. *Int J Radiat Oncol Biol Phys* 1980;6:1243-1250.

49. Lawton CA, Barber-Derus SW, Murray KJ, et al. Technical modifications in hyperfractionated total body irradiation for T-lymphocyte-depleted bone marrow transplant. *Int J Radiat Oncol Biol Phys* 1989;17:319-322.

50. Kolb HJ, Rieder I, Bodenberger U, et al. Dose rate and dose fractionation studies in total body irradiation of dogs. *Pathol Biol* (Paris) 1979;27:370-372.

51. Lawton CA, Barber-Derus SW, Murray KJ, et al. Influence of renal shielding on the incidence of late renal dysfunction associated with bone marrow transplantation in adult patients. *Int J Radiat Oncol Biol Phys* 1992;23:681-686.

52. Lapidot T, Singer TS, Salomon O, et al. Booster irradiation to the spleen following total body irradiation: a new immunosuppressive approach for allogeneic bone marrow transplantation. *J Immunol* 1988;141:2619-2624.

53. Krebs JS, Jones DCL. The LD$_{50}$ and the survival of bone-marrow colony forming cells in mice: effect of rate of exposure to ionizing radiation. *Radiat Res* 1972;5:374-380.

54. Lichter AS, Tracy D, Lam WC, et al. Total body irradiation in bone marrow transplantation: the influence of fractionation and delay of marrow infusion. *Int J Radiat Oncol Biol Phys* 1980;6:301-309.

55. Peters LJ, Withers HR, Cundiff JH, et al. Radiobiological considerations in the use of total body irradiation for bone-marrow transplantation. *Radiology* 1979;131:243-247.

56. Travis EL, Peters LJ, McNeill J, et al. Effect of dose-rate on total body irradiation: lethality and pathologic findings. *Radiother Oncol* 1985;4:341-351.

57. Weiner RS, Bortin MM, Gale RP, et al. Interstitial pneumonitis after bone marrow transplantation. *Ann Intern Med* 1986; 104:168-175.

58. Kim TH, McGlave RB, Ramsay N, et al. Comparison of two total body irradiation regimens in allogeneic bone marrow transplantation for acute non-lymphoblastic leukemia in first remission. *Int J Radiat Oncol Biol Phys* 1990;19:889-897.

59. Song CW, Kim TH, Khan FM, et al. Radiobiological basis of total body irradiation with different dose rate and fractionation: repair capacity of hemopoietic cells. *Int J Radiat Oncol Biol Phys* 1981; 7:1695-1701.

60. Cosset JM, Baume D, Pico JL, et al. Single dose versus hyperfractionated total body irradiation before allogeneic bone marrow transplantation: a nonrandomized comparative study of 54 patients at the Institut Gustave-Roussy. *Radiother Oncol* 1989; 15:151-160.

61. Deeg HJ, Storb R, Longton G, et al. Single dose or fractionated total body irradiation and autologous marrow transplantation in dogs: effects of exposure rate, fraction size, and fractionation interval on acute and delayed toxicity. *Int J Radiat Oncol Biol Phys* 1988;15:647-653.

62. Shank B, Hopfan S, Kim JH, et al. Hyperfractionated total body irradiation for bone marrow transplantation. I. Early results in leukemia patients. *Int J Radiat Oncol Biol Phys* 1981;7:1109-1115.

63. Soderling CCB, Song CW, Blazar BR, et al. A correlation between conditioning and engraftment in recipients of MHC-mismatched T-cell-depleted murine bone marrow transplants. *J Immunol* 1985; 135:941-946.

64. Trigg ME, Billing R, Sondel PM, et al. Clinical trial depleting T lymphocytes from donor marrow for matched and mismatched allogeneic bone marrow transplants. *Cancer Treat Rep* 1985; 69:377-386.

65. Clift RA, Buckner CD, Thomas FD, et al. Treatment of chronic granulocytic leukaemia in chronic phase by allogeneic marrow transplantation. *Lancet* 1982;ii(8299):621-623.

66. Goldman JM, Baughan AS, McCarthy DM, et al. Marrow transplantation for patients in the chronic phase of chronic granulocytic leukaemia. *Lancet* 1982;ii(8299):623-625.

67. Gratwohl A, Hermans J, Biezen AV, et al. No advantage for patients who receive splenic irradiation before bone marrow transplantation for chronic myeloid leukemia. *Bone Marrow Transplant* 1992;10:147-152.

68. Gratwohl A, Hermans J, Biezen AV, et al. Splenic irradiation before bone marrow transplantation for chronic myeloid leukemia [abstract]. *Bone Marrow Transplant* 1996;17(suppl 1):S61.

69. Spitzer TR, Friedman CJ, Bushnell W, et al. Double-blind randomized, parallel group study on the efficacy and safety of oral

granisetron and oral ondansetron in the prophylaxis of nausea and vomiting in patients receiving hyperfractionated total body irradiation. *Bone Marrow Transplant* 2000;26:203-210.

70. Halberg FE, Kramer JH, Moore IM, et al. Prophylactic cranial irradiation dose effects on late cognitive function in children treated for acute lymphoblastic leukemia. *Int J Radiat Oncol Biol Phys* 1992;22:13-16.

71. Thomas ED, Storb R, Clift RA, et al. Bone-marrow transplantation. *N Engl J Med* 1975;292:832-843.

72. Thomas ED, Sanders JE, Flournoy N, et al. Marrow transplantation for patients with acute lymphoblastic leukemia in remission. *Blood* 1979;54:468-476.

73. Ganem G, Saint-Marc Girardin MF, Kuentz M, et al. Venocclusive disease of the liver after allogeneic bone marrow transplantation in man. *Int J Radiat Oncol Biol Phys* 1988;14:879-884.

74. Jones RJ, Lee KSK, Beschorner WE, et al. Venocclusive disease of the liver following bone marrow transplantation. *Transplantation* 1987;44:778-783.

75. Shulman HM, McDonald GB, Matthews D, et al. An analysis of hepatic venocclusive disease and centrilobular hepatic degeneration following bone marrow transplantation. *Gastroenterology* 1980;79:1178-1191.

76. Keane TJ, Van Dyk J, Rider WD. Idiopathic interstitial pneumonia following bone marrow transplantation: the relationship with total body irradiation. *Int J Radiat Oncol Biol Phys* 1981;7:1365-1370.

77. Gluckman E, Devergie A, Dutreix A, et al. Total body irradiation in bone marrow transplantation. *Pathol Biol* (Paris) 1979;27:349-352.

78. Neiman PE, Reeves W, Ray G, et al. A prospective analysis of interstitial pneumonia and opportunistic viral infection among recipients of allogeneic bone marrow grafts. *J Infect Dis* 1977;136:754-767.

79. Bortin MM, Kay HEM, Gale RP, et al. Factors associated with interstitial pneumonitis after bone marrow transplantation for acute leukaemia. *Lancet* 1982;1:437-439.

80. Latini P, Aristei C, Aversa F, et al. Lung damage following bone marrow transplantation after hyperfractionated total body irradiation. *Radiother Oncol* 1991;22:127-132.

81. Deeg HJ. Acute and delayed toxicities of total body irradiation. *Int J Radiat Oncol Biol Phys* 1983;9:1933-1939.

82. Springmeyer SC, Silvestri R, Kosanke R, et al. Pulmonary function after marrow transplantation. *J Supramol Struct* 1980;4:40.

83. Tait RC, Burnett AK, Robertson AG, et al. Subclinical pulmonary function defects following autologous and allogeneic bone marrow transplantation: relationship to total body irradiation and graft-versus-host disease. *Int J Radiat Oncol Biol Phys* 1991;20:1219-1227.

84. Gore EM, Lawton CA, Ash RC, et al. Pulmonary function changes in long-term survivors of bone marrow transplantation. *Int J Radiat Oncol Biol Phys* 1996;36:67-75.

85. Labar B, Bogdanic V, Nemet D, et al. Total body irradiation with or without lung shielding for allogeneic bone marrow transplantation. *Bone Marrow Transplant* 1992;9:343-347.

86. Braverman AC, Antin JH, Plappert MT, et al. Cyclophosphamide cardiotoxicity in bone marrow transplantation: a prospective evaluation of new dosing regimens. *J Clin Oncol* 1991;9:1215-1223.

87. Cazin B, Gorin NC, Laporte JP, et al. Cardiac complications after bone marrow transplantation: a report on a series of 63 consecutive transplantations. *Cancer* 1986;57:2061-2069.

88. Lele SS, Durrant STS, Atherton JJ, et al. Demonstration of late cardiotoxicity following bone marrow transplantation by assessment of exercise diastolic filling characteristics. *Bone Marrow Transplant* 1996;17:1113-1118.

89. Hertenstein B, Stefanic M, Schmeiser T, et al. Cardiac toxicity of bone marrow transplantation: predictive value of cardiologic evaluation before transplant. *J Clin Oncol* 1994;12:998-1004.

90. Juckett M, Perry EH, Daniels BS, et al. Hemolytic uremic syndrome following bone marrow transplantation. *Bone Marrow Transplant* 1991;7:405-409.

91. Lawton CA, Cohen EP, Barber-Derus SW, et al. Late renal dysfunction in adult survivors of bone marrow transplantation. *Cancer* 1991;67:2795-2800.

92. Tarbell NJ, Guinan EC, Niemeyer C, et al. Late onset of renal dysfunction in survivors of bone marrow transplantation. *Int J Radiat Oncol Biol Phys* 1988;15:99-104.

93. Van Why SK, Friedman AL, Wei LJ, et al. Renal insufficiency after bone marrow transplantation in children. *Bone Marrow Transplant* 1991;7:383-388.

94. Mirabell R, Bieri S, Mermillod B, et al. Renal toxicity after allogenic bone marrow transplantation: the combined effects of total-body irradiation and graft-versus-host disease. *J Clin Oncol* 1996;14:579-585.

95. Bray LC, Carey PJ, Proctor SJ, et al. Ocular complications of bone marrow transplantation. *Br J Ophthalmol* 1991;75:611-614.

96. Gordon KB, Char DH, Sagerman R. Late effects of radiation on the eye and ocular adnexa. *Int J Radiat Biol Oncol Phys* 1995;31:1123-1139.

97. Deeg HJ, Flournoy N, Sullivan KM, et al. Cataracts after total body irradiation and marrow transplantation: a sparing effect of dose fractionation. *Int J Radiat Oncol Biol Phys* 1984;10:957-964.

98. Benyunes MC, Sullivan KM, et al. Cataracts after bone marrow transplantation: long/term follow-up of adults treated with fractionated total body irradiation. *Int J Radiat Oncol Biol Phys* 1995;32:661-670.

99. Belkacemi Y, Labopin M, Vernant JP, et al. Cataracts after total body irradiation and bone marrow transplantation in patients with acute leukemia in complete remission: a study of the European group for blood and marrow transplantation. *Int J Radiat Oncol Biol Phys* 1998;41:659-668.

100. Zierhut D, Lohr F, Schraube P, et al. Cataract incidence after total body irradiation. *Int J Radiat Oncol Biol Phys* 2000;46:131-135.

101. Spinelli S, Chiodi S, Bacigalupo A, et al. Ovarian recovery after total body irradiation and allogenic bone marrow transplantation: long-term follow-up of 79 females. *Bone Marrow Transplant* 1994;14:373-380.

102. Mertens AC, Ramsay NKC, Kouris S, et al. Patterns of gonadal dysfunction following bone marrow transplantation. *Bone Marrow Transplant* 1998;22:345-350.

103. Giri N, Vowels MR, Barr AL, et al. Successful pregnancy after total body irradiation and bone marrow transplantation for acute leukaemia. *Bone Marrow Transplant* 1992;10:93-95.

104. Gulati SC, Van Poznak C. Pregnancy after bone marrow transplantation. *J Clin Oncol* 1998;16:1978-1985.

105. Sanders J. Effects of cyclophosphamide and total body irradiation on ovarian and testicular function [abstract]. *Exp Hematol* 1982;10(suppl 11):49.

106. Sanders JE, Pritchard S, Mahoney P, et al. Growth and development following marrow transplantation for leukemia. *Blood* 1986;68:1129-1135.

107. Chou RH, Wong GB, Kramer JH, et al. Toxicities of total-body irradiation for pediatric bone marrow transplantation. *Int J Radiat Oncol Biol Phys* 1996;34:843-851.

108. Matthes-Martin S, Lamche M, Ladenstein R, et al. Organ toxicity and quality of life after allogeneic bone marrow transplantation in pediatric patients: a single centre retrospective analysis. *Bone Marrow Transplant* 1999;23:1049-1053.

109. Wingard JR, Plotnick LP, Freemer CS, et al. Growth in children after bone marrow transplantation: busulfan plus cyclophosphamide versus cyclophosphamide plus total body irradiation. *Blood* 1992;79:1068-1073.

110. Afify Z, Shaw P, Clavano-Harding A, et al. Growth and endocrine function in children with acute myeloid leukemia

after bone marrow transplantation using busulfan/cyclophosphamide. *Bone Marrow Transplant* 2000;25:1087-1092.

111. Boulad F, Bromley M, Black P, et al. Thyroid dysfunction following bone marrow transplantation using hyperfractionated radiation. *Bone Marrow Transplant* 1995;15:71.

112. Kauppila M, Koskinen P, Irjala K, et al. Long-term effects of allogeneic bone marrow transplantation (BMT) on pituitary, gonad, thyroid and adrenal function in adults. *Bone Marrow Transplant* 1998;22:331-337.

113. Witherspoon RP, Fisher LD, Schoch G, et al. Secondary cancers after bone marrow transplantation for leukemia or aplastic anemia. *N Engl J Med* 1989;321:784-789.

114. Kirova Y, Rafi H, Voisin M-C, et al. Radiation-induced bone sarcoma following total body irradiation: role of additional radiation on localized areas. *Bone Marrow Transplant* 2000;25:1011-1013.

115. Shapiro RS, McClain K, Frizzera G, et al. Epstein-Barr virus-associated B cell lymphoproliferative disorders following bone marrow transplantation. *Blood* 1988;71:1234-1243.

116. Zutter MM, Martin PJ, Sale GE, et al. Epstein-Barr virus lymphoproliferation after bone marrow transplantation. *Blood* 1988;72:520-529.

117. Deeg HJ, Storb R, Prentice R, et al. Increased cancer risk in canine radiation chimeras. *Blood* 1980;55:233-239.

118. Leigh S, Wilson KCM, Burns R, et al. Psychosocial morbidity in bone marrow transplant recipients: a prospective study. *Bone Marrow Transplant* 1995;16:635-640.

119. Greer S, Moorey S, Baruch JD, et al. Adjuvant psychological therapy for patients with cancer: a prospective randomized trial. *BMJ* 1992;304:675-679.

120. Shank B. Total body irradiation for marrow or stem-cell transplantation. *Cancer Invest* 1998;16:397-404.

121. Blaise D, Maraninchi D, Archimbaud E, et al. Allogeneic bone marrow transplantation for acute myeloid leukemia in first remission: a randomized trial of a busulfan-cytoxan versus cytoxan-total body irradiation as preparative regimen: a report from the Group d'Etudes de la Greefe de Moelle Osseuse. *Blood* 1992;79:2578-2582.

122. Inoue T, Ikeda H, Yamazaki H, et al. Role of total body irradiation as based on the comparison of preparation regimens for allogeneic bone marrow transplantation for acute leukemia in first complete remission. *Strahlenther Onkol* 1993;169:250-255.

123. Hartman AR, Williams SF, Dillon JJ. Survival, disease-free survival and adverse effects of conditioning for allogeneic bone marrow transplantation with busulfan/cyclophosphamide vs total body irradiation: a meta-analysis. *Bone Marrow Transplant* 1998;22:439-443.

Additional Reading

Thomas ED. Bone marrow transplantation: past experiences and future prospects. *Semin Oncol* 1992;19:3-6.

CHAPTER 38

Palliative Care

Nora A. Janjan, Marc E. Delclos, Matthew T. Ballo, and
Christopher H. Crane

Over the past 10 years, 11 million cases of cancer have been diagnosed, and 5 million people have died from the disease. Approximately half of the patients diagnosed with cancer will develop metastatic disease. More than 70% of all cancer patients develop symptoms from either their primary or metastatic disease.[1-4] A decrease in the total number of cancer deaths in 1997 compared with 1996 was not sustained in 1998—there were 955 more cancer-related deaths than in 1997.[5] In the United States, cancer is the second most common cause of death, accounting for 23% of all deaths in 1998, and is the leading cause of death among women age 40 to 79 years. In 2001 it is estimated that 1,268,000 new cases of cancer will be diagnosed, and 553,400 patients will die of the disease, which is more than 1500 people a day. Cancer of the lung, prostate, breast, and rectum constitute more than 50% of all cancer deaths.

Palliation represents a large component of cancer treatment and includes the use of therapeutic and supportive care measures. Unlike other aspects of cancer therapy, tumor control and survival are not the only endpoints of success in palliative care. Quality of life is now recognized as an endpoint secondary in importance only to survival.[6,7] The goal of palliative care is to effectively and efficiently relieve symptoms and to maintain maximum quality of life for the duration of the patient's life.[2-4,8-13] Effective palliation of cancer-related pain can enhance quality of life by improving functional and emotional well-being. The effectiveness of palliative therapy is measured in terms of the percentage of patients who continue to experience persistent or recurrent symptoms and whether those symptoms can be relieved by using other therapeutic modalities.[12,14,15] Like other aspects of cancer care, effective palliative care also requires a multidisciplinary approach.[16,17]

SCOPE AND SOCIOECONOMIC COSTS OF PALLIATIVE CARE
Debilitation and Financial Burden

The debility that results from cancer and cancer treatment is an important socioeconomic issue. Among more than 9700 community-based Medicare beneficiaries surveyed in a study by Stafford and Cyr,[18] the 1647 people who had cancer reported having poorer health, more limitations on the activities of daily living, and greater use of health care resources than those who did not have cancer. Cancer patients reported difficulty walking (38%), getting out of a chair (21%), completing heavy housework (34%), and shopping (17%). Poorer health was noted more often among patients with lung, breast, prostate, or colon cancer. Having lung, bladder, or prostate cancer was predictive of increased health care use, and lung cancer was most often associated with limitation in activities of daily living.

Even though the decrease in functional capacity among cancer patients is generally not as prolonged as that among patients with other chronic diseases (e.g., arthritis, stroke, or emphysema), the annual health care costs for cancer patients are higher than the health care costs for those with other chronic diseases.[19] The mean annual Medicare reimbursement for lung cancer was more than twice that for colon, breast, or prostate cancer. Assuming that not all of the people in the Medicare review who had cancer had active disease at the time of the analysis, the proportion of cancer patients who are functionally impaired and using more health care resources would be even greater if only those with active disease were included in the analysis.

Approximately 300,000 patients in the United States receive palliative radiation therapy each year, at a total annual cost of $900 million. By way of comparison, about 100,000 patients receive curative radiation therapy, at a total annual cost of $1.1 billion.[20] The National Institutes of Health estimates that the overall cost of cancer in 2000 was $180.2 billion, including $60 billion in direct medical costs, $15 billion resulting from lost productivity due to illness, and $105.2 billion resulting from lost productivity due to death.[5] Because health care costs are a key economic and political issue, such analyses are increasingly important. The goal for the medical community is to develop palliative care strategies that cost-effectively relieve suffering, increase personal independence, and prevent complications that may be caused by the disease and its treatment.

It is important to recognize that terminal illnesses impose substantial burdens, economic and otherwise, on patients and those who care for them. In a study by Emanuel and colleagues,[21] 988 terminally ill patients and 893 caregivers from six randomly selected cities across the United States were interviewed, and transportation, nursing care, personal care, and financial needs were evaluated. The leading causes of terminal illness were cancer (51.8%), heart disease (18%), and chronic obstructive pulmonary disease (10.9%). The mean age of the participants was 66.5 years (range, 22 to 109 years), and 59.4% were at least 65 years old. Among these patients, 50.2% experienced substantial pain, 70.9% had shortness of breath after walking one block or less, 35.5% had urinary or fecal incontinence, 16.8% had symptoms of depression, and 17.5% were bedridden for more than half of every day. In the 6 months before the study, 66.5% had been hospitalized, 22.3% of whom were in intensive care units and 36.8% of whom had undergone a surgical procedure. Overall, 35% of patients had substantial health care needs that consumed more than 10% of their household income; 16% of families had to take out a loan, spend their savings, or work an additional job to cover medical costs. Patients with substantial health care needs were more likely to consider euthanasia. In addition, administering care significantly affected the lives of more than 35% of caregivers.

End-of-Life Care

Of the families included in the study by Emanuel and colleagues,[21] only 28% felt burdened by the illness if the attending physician was involved in administering terminal care, compared with 42% of families whose physicians were not involved in this level of care ($P = 0.005$). However, physicians are rarely trained in how to administer end-of-life care. On average, medical textbooks devote only 2% of their total page count to end-of-life care.[22] In a review of the 50 top-selling textbooks from multiple medical specialties, only 24% of textbooks—and only 38% of oncology textbooks—had helpful information on end-of-life care.

Difficulties in providing adequate end-of-life care also were reflected in findings from another report of physical symptoms among 350 hospice inpatients with cancer.[23] In that study, the mean number of symptoms per patient actually increased from 6 on admission to 10 during the course of hospice care.[23] The mean number of symptoms correlated directly with the patients' performance status; patients with seven symptoms had performance status scores of 10 to 20, those with six symptoms had scores of 30 to 50, and those with four symptoms had scores of 60 or higher (a higher score indicates better functioning). Among patients with performance scores of 10 to 20, 94% had anorexia, 47% had edema, and 50% had dyspnea. In contrast, these symptoms occurred in only 29%, 16%, and 10% (respectively) of patients with a performance status score of 60 or more. Finally, in this study, pain was reportedly treated in 65% of patients at admission and in 88% of patients at the time of death.[23]

Pain Treatment

Barriers to effective pain treatment include lack of assessment, patients' reluctance to report pain and to use analgesics, and physicians' reluctance to prescribe opioids.[1,16,17,24,25] In a study of hospital inpatients referred to a pain service,[16] the mean pain score on a visual analogue scale (on which 10 is the worst pain imaginable) was 5.2 at presentation; 56% of the patients in this study had pain scores of 5 or higher, and 20% had pain scores of 8 or higher. All patients had previously used opioids, and 41 were receiving opioids at the time of consultation. Within 24 hours of consulting the pain service, the mean pain score had dropped to 2.7 ($P < 0.05$).[16]

Similar findings were noted among 108 patients referred to an outpatient multidisciplinary bone metastases clinic.[17] The median age of that population (27% of whom were working full or part time) was 55 years, and 69% of the patients were younger than 65 years. The time since diagnosis of the primary tumor ranged from 2 weeks to 23 years (median, 22 months), and metastased had been diagnosed in 30% of patients within the past 6 months. Pain was the presenting symptom in 74% of patients at diagnosis. The patients' average pain was rated as moderate to severe by 79% of patients and severe by 21%; the patients' worst pain was rated as severe by 78% and intolerable by 22%. Only 45% of patients experienced good relief from prescribed analgesics, and 23% indicated that the prescribed analgesics were ineffective.[17]

Extended life spans and improvements in screening techniques have greatly increased the number of diagnosed cases of the four most common types of cancer—lung, breast, prostate, and colorectal. All of these tumors have high rates of metastatic spread to bone and to visceral structures, which can cause pain.[5,26,27] Musculoskeletal pain can occasionally also reflect an undiagnosed malignancy. In a study of 491 patients with new or recurring experiences of bone pain who had no known underlying malignancy, 4% of the entire group and 9% of those who were 50 years of age or older had definite evidence of metastasis.[28,29] The pain was diffuse in 57% of patients, was localized to the back in 52%, to the hips or pelvis in 16%, and to the extremities in 15%. Malignancies subsequently were diagnosed in the lung in 32% of patients and in the prostate in 16% of patients.

Prostate Cancer

Prostate cancer is the second leading cause of cancer death among men,[5,30,31] and pain will develop during the course of the disease in 75% of cases.[32] Radiographically detectable bone metastases will develop in 20% of patients with stage A2 (T1b) or B (T2) disease, 40% of patients with stage C (T3) disease, and 62% of patients with stage D1 (T4) disease presentations.[33-37]

In the 1970s only 50% of prostate tumors were confined to the prostate gland at diagnosis, and metastases were present in 30% of cases at diagnosis. In a population-based study of prostate cancer in which routine screening was not performed and only palliative intervention was provided, associations were noted among patients with regard to disease-specific death rate, stage of disease, and tumor differentiation.[29,33] Of 719 new cases, 45% were diagnosed incidentally, only 31% had organ-confined disease, and 35% of patients had bone metastases at diagnosis. Symptoms at diagnosis included prostatism (42%), bone pain (12%), and fatigue (9%). The median age at diagnosis was 75 years. Age at diagnosis, however, did not influence disease-specific survival rates. Prostate cancer was the cause of death in 62% of these patients, and the disease-specific survival rates at 1, 5, and 10 years were 80%, 38%, and 17%, respectively.

Even today, when patients who present with symptoms are referred to a urologist, only 70% have disease that is confined to the prostate gland; among patients undergoing prostatectomy, only 50% are confirmed to have disease that is confined to the prostate gland. Although routine screening with digital rectal examination and prostate-specific antigen measurements can detect more than 90% of cases, only 70% are confirmed on pathologic examination as being confined to the gland.

The risk of subsequent development of distant metastasis is significantly lower when the primary tumor is controlled by treatment than when it is not. For example, survival rates after an isolated recurrence of prostate cancer are influenced by the initial stage of the disease and the disease-free interval between initial treatment and recurrence.[34,36,37] In more than 70% of cases of locally recurrent prostate cancer, radiation can control symptoms such as hematuria, urinary outflow obstruction, ureteral obstruction, and lower extremity edema.[36] With or without local recurrence, the survival rate is compromised by the presence of distant metastases. The survival rates at 5 years and 10 years after pelvic recurrence of prostate cancer are 50% and 22%, respectively. When distant metastases are present, the survival rate at 5 years is 20% and that at 10 years is less than 5%.[34,37]

PROGNOSTIC FACTORS AFFECTING PALLIATIVE CARE
Metastasis

Prognosis in many types of cancer is influenced by the overall metastatic burden and the number and location of sites involved by disease. The site of the primary disease and the presence of a solitary metastatic site are predictive of more prolonged survival.[38-42] The presence of bone metastasis is predictive for progression of disease to other sites as well; bone metastasis is the most common cause of cancer-related pain.[*]

The median duration of survival is a critical factor in evaluating the effects of palliative therapy and in determining the appropriate type of palliative therapy. When metastases are found in the lung, liver, or central nervous system in addition to the bone, the prognosis is especially poor. After bone metastasis is diagnosed, median survival duration is 12 months for patients with breast cancer, 6 months for patients with prostate cancer, and 3 months for patients with lung cancer. For patients with breast cancer, the median survival duration is 48 months if metastases are confined to the skeletal system, but it decreases to only 9 months if visceral metastasis is also present.[26,27] For patients with prostate cancer, the distribution of bone metastases as well as the simple fact of their presence has prognostic significance. Survival times are significantly longer when the metastases are restricted to the pelvis and lumbar spine and longer also among patients in whom salvage hormonal therapy induces a response.[34,35,43] However, any metastatic involvement outside the pelvis and lumbar spine shortens survival time regardless of the effect of salvage hormonal therapy.

In one study, a bone scan index was formulated on the basis of proportions of tumor involvement in individual bones, and that index was then examined in relation to known prognostic factors and survival in patients with androgen-independent prostate cancer.[44] In multivariate proportional hazards analyses, only bone scan index, age, hemoglobin level, and lactate dehydrogenase level were associated with survival. Survival durations were 18.3 months for patients with a bone scan index of less than 1.4%, 15.5 months for those with an index of 1.4% to 5.1%, and 8.1 months for those with an index of more than 5.1%.

Quality of Life

Quality-of-life measurements can enhance the prognostic information derived from the Karnofsky performance status score and extent of disease and aid in predicting survival. Physical symptoms such as pain, dry mouth, constipation, change in taste, lack of appetite and energy, bloating, nausea, vomiting, weight loss, and drowsiness or dizziness portend a poor prognosis.[38] In one study of 208 patients with terminal cancer (median survival duration, 15 weeks), shorter survival time was independently associated with the following factors: primary site (lung cancer vs. breast or gastrointestinal cancer), the presence of liver metastases or comorbid conditions, weight loss of more than 8 kg in the previous 6 months, and clinical estimation by the treating physician of a survival duration of less than 2 months.[45]

---

*References 5, 26, 27, 33, 35-37, 43.

Laboratory assessments, including serum albumin levels of less than 35 g/L, lymphocyte counts of less than 1×10^9/L, and lactate dehydrogenase levels of more than 618 U/L also were associated with poor prognosis. After these independent factors were accounted for in the analysis, other factors such as performance status, symptoms other than nausea and vomiting, tumor burden, and socioeconomic characteristics did not independently influence the prognosis.[45]

Estimating Survival Duration

It is important to consider issues regarding the estimation of prognosis when developing a palliative care plan. Some of these issues can affect analgesic management. Many physicians will only prescribe opiate analgesics after patients are thought to have less than 6 months to live or after palliative radiation therapy fails to induce a response.[1,25,46] This practice results in substantial undertreatment of cancer-related pain. First, it is difficult for physicians to make an accurate prognosis. In a review of five studies involving a total of 468 patients considered to have less than 6 months to live, physicians could accurately predict survival duration only about half of the time (range, 22% to 70% of the time). In these studies, the actual median survival duration was 3.5 weeks (range, 2 to 5 weeks) compared with the median survival of 6 weeks (range, 4.5 to 8 weeks) estimated by the physicians.[47] Second, patients should not have to suffer with symptoms just because their physicians believe that they may live for more than 6 months.

Some of the uncertainties involved in making a prognosis were overcome in the Study to Understand Prognoses and Preferences for Outcomes and Risks of Treatments.[48] This study first retrospectively evaluated the prognoses of 4301 patients and developed a model with which to predict survival duration based on the outcome of that evaluation. The model was then prospectively tested with 4028 new patients.[49] Next the model was applied by physicians in 1757 cases to estimate the likelihood that a patient would survive for 2 months or for 6 months. Among the cases analyzed were 406 patients with advanced colon cancer, 764 patients with lung cancer, and 594 patients with multiple organ system failure with malignancy. The physicians' estimates fell within 7.5% of those generated by the model; model estimates were always within 3% of the actual survival duration, and the physicians' estimates were within 9% of the actual survival duration. Although the physicians' estimates of prognosis were generally accurate, the patients themselves tended to overestimate their survival duration. However, once patients acknowledged that they had at least a 10% chance of dying within 6 months, they were more likely to choose palliative care over therapeutic care. Despite this finding and despite efforts to educate physicians and patients about palliative care options and about end-of-life issues, many patients in that study continued to receive ineffective or inappropriate cancer treatments.[47]

PALLIATIVE VERSUS CURATIVE CARE: PHILOSOPHICAL AND ECONOMIC DIFFERENCES IN APPROACH

Most of the cost of cancer care is incurred in the final months of the patient's life. For several reasons, only a small percentage of patients with extensive disease receive innovative therapies as part of a clinical trial. With regard to administration of palliative therapy, cancer is treated as a chronic disease, and cancer symptoms are controlled in two ways—by direct treatment of the symptoms (e.g., giving the patient opioids for pain) and by treating the cause of the symptoms, the cancer. The goal of the latter method is to shrink the tumor as much as possible and thereby reduce symptoms.

In this context, cancer treatment does not always produce a sufficient improvement in survival duration; it only serves to maintain comfort. Physicians must communicate to patients and their families the outcomes that can reasonably be achieved through the use of palliative care and begin discussions of end-of-life issues. There is a growing recognition that physicians must be better trained in end-of-life issues, including hospice care, so that they can discuss these issues knowledgeably and compassionately.

Keeping the goals of palliative care in mind, palliative therapy should target symptomatic areas or areas at which morbidity caused by disease progression is likely to occur. Aggressive therapy should be reserved for patients with an extended survival prognosis, to maintain functional integrity (e.g., surgical stabilization of a pathologic fracture), or for those in a clinical trial. Therapies that cause morbidity and provide little to no palliative benefit should not be administered.

The role of systemic agents (e.g., chemotherapy drugs, hormones, bisphosphonates, and radiopharmaceuticals, given alone or in combination with localized irradiation) in palliative care has not been clearly defined. Interest has increased in palliative chemotherapy with agents such as gemcitabine that provide little or no increase in survival duration but do relieve cancer-related symptoms.[50,51] In general, many of the other agents, when used to treat bone metastases, do not provide a level of pain relief comparable with localized irradiation.

Although palliation constitutes a large part of radiation therapy practice, radiation is generally underused in palliative care. At The University of Texas M.D. Anderson Cancer Center, about 25% of all radiation treatments are administered with palliative intent, and this has been the pattern of practice for more than 40 years.[52] Consistent with practices in the United States, approximately 25% of patients in Sweden to whom radiation therapy was administered received radiation with palliative intent; however, only 10% of all Swedish cancer patients were given any radiation at all.[53] Because symptoms of metastases will develop in more than half of patients who have prostate, breast, or lung cancer, palliative radiation therapy is being greatly underused.

Treatment Modalities

Many types of clinical problems require palliative care, and identifying the most appropriate multidisciplinary approach to treatment can be challenging. Among patients with bone metastases, for example, several different clinical problems, such as pathologic fracture and spinal cord compression, can occur and will require different multidisciplinary interventions. Among the issues that need to be addressed are how therapies can be combined to achieve additive or synergistic effects and how to treat visceral and bone metastases. In regard to combining therapies for palliative care, just as is true for curative therapies, studies are needed to evaluate the effectiveness of the combination of radiation (external-beam radiation and radiopharmaceuticals) with chemotherapy, hormonal therapy, and bisphosphonates. Cost-benefit considerations also are important. A Trans-Canada study, for example, found that the combination of localized irradiation and the radioisotope ^{89}Sr was more cost-effective than radiation alone.[54-56]

Specific to radiation therapy, studies of the costs and benefits of single-fraction radiation, radiopharmaceuticals, and systemic therapies need to be pursued. Although abbreviated radiation courses may result in cost savings, the patients' responses to these modalities must be critically analyzed. Such analyses must account for the type of primary tumor, location and extent of metastases, and prognosis. Ineffective palliative therapy given by any means is especially costly because unrelieved pain and disability can result in the continued need for analgesics, extended functional limitation, and the need for systemic therapies and surgery.[57,58]

Bisphosphonates

Much controversy exists surrounding the cost-benefit ratio associated with using bisphosphonates to treat bone metastases. One study showed that the cost of pamidronate exceeded the cost savings realized from preventing the adverse events.[59] The projected net cost of preventing an adverse skeletal-related event was $3940 with chemotherapy and $9390 with hormonal therapy.[59] The cost/unit benefit was $108,200 with chemotherapy and $305,300 with hormonal therapy per quality-adjusted year.

A cost-analysis study conducted in Canada showed similar findings[60]: Over a 12-month period, the total cost in the pamidronate group was 44% higher than in the placebo group. Without surgical intervention,

pamidronate increased costs by $31,600/quality-adjusted life year. Surgical intervention, which was required by 6% of the study group in addition to the pamidronate, increased the total cost of palliative care by $13,300/quality-adjusted life year. Based on the number of breast cancer patients that would meet clinical indications for receiving pamidronate, the added cost for bisphosphonates would exceed $10 million (Canadian currency)/year in Ontario. Studies are clearly needed to show how the use of bisphosphonates in combination with other therapeutic modalities can be optimized to improve the overall cost profile of this family of drugs.

Radiation

Radiation therapy is highly cost-effective when compared with analgesic therapy. The cost of radiation therapy was evaluated in 66 patients who received palliative radiation totaling 30 Gy in 10 fractions (72%) or 20 Gy in 5 fractions (28%).[61] Pain scores decreased about 4 points (0 to 10 scale) after radiation therapy, from a median level of 5.58 points before treatment to 1.55 points after treatment.[61] Likewise, incident-related pain with movement decreased 5 points, from 7.32 points before treatment to 1.94 points after treatment. The estimated cost of radiation therapy ranged from $1200 to $2500/patient. With durable pain relief for 9 months, the estimated cost of analgesics over the same period would have totaled $9000 to $36,000. In this study, a brief course of radiation therapy proved to significantly reduce pain and was cost-effective when compared with the continued need for analgesics. This is a particularly important consideration for the treatment of hospice patients.

Chemotherapy versus Bisphosphonates

Despite these concerns, bisphosphonates have been recommended for breast cancer patients who have lytic bone metastases and who are undergoing chemotherapy or hormonal therapy. In a report of more than 700 breast cancer patients randomly assigned to receive chemotherapy either alone or with bisphosphonates,[62,63] bone metastases were first diagnosed 18 months before study entry, and in about 70% of patients, bone was the only site of metastatic disease. This study demonstrated that the development of skeletal complications was delayed by the bisphosphonates; with chemotherapy alone, skeletal complications occurred at 7.0 months, whereas with systemic chemotherapy plus bisphosphonates skeletal complications occurred at 12 months. With chemotherapy alone, the proportion of skeletal complications was 56%, whereas with systemic chemotherapy plus bisphosphonates the proportion was 43%.[62,63] With hormonal therapy alone, skeletal complications occurred at 7.0 months, compared with 10 months with hormonal therapy plus bisphosphonates.[64] The proportion of skeletal complications was reduced by 67% with hormonal therapy alone and by 56% with the combination therapy.

In both studies, the occurrence of nonvertebral pathologic fractures, surgery or radiation therapy, bone pain, and hypercalcemia were all substantially reduced with bisphosphonates. However, no survival advantage was observed in the bisphosphonate group; the median survival duration was 37 months. With extended follow-up, 78% of patients in both the bisphosphonate and placebo groups died because of progression of breast cancer before completing 24 months of treatment, with a median survival duration of about 18 months.[65]

In these trials, bisphosphonates were used to increase response to systemic therapy, because these drugs delayed the development of skeletal complications and decreased the number of patients referred for palliative radiation therapy, or in some cases delayed the need for palliative radiation therapy. Radiation therapy in these studies was given only for the appearance of symptomatic progressive disease while bisphosphonates and systemic therapy were being administered. Although statistically significant improvements were observed, less than half of the original cohort of breast cancer patients completed the first year of the trial and less than one third continued the randomized therapy for 2 years.[62-68]

Reasons for discontinuing therapy included the occurrence of adverse events, poor response to therapy, or refusal by nearly half of the patients to continue treatment.[65] Almost half of these patients developed a skeletal event while being given bisphosphonates. Although a benefit from bisphonate use was shown, research is needed to determine the optimal schedule of administration for bisphosphonates and how these drugs can best be combined with other modalities in consideration of the cost-benefit issues.[69]

Research Questions Yet to Be Answered

The need for further research on bisphosphonates is best demonstrated by intriguing results of a study of bisphosphonates with adjuvant systemic therapy for breast cancer. This prospective randomized trial involved more than 300 patients who had immunohistochemical evidence of at least one tumor cell in a bone marrow aspirate.[70] More than 80% of patients had T1 or T2 disease, almost 50% had node-negative disease, and more than 70% had estrogen receptor-positive tumors; 81% of patients were given adjuvant systemic chemotherapy, hormonal therapy, or a combination. Substantial decreases in the occurrence of distant metastases (13% vs. 29%), bone metastases (8% vs. 17%), and visceral metastases (8% vs. 19%) were observed among patients who received adjuvant bisphosphonate therapy, resulting in a substantial increase in survival rate (96% vs. 85%).

The effects of bisphosphonates on apoptosis, adhesion molecules, and proteases are thought to play a role in the development of visceral metastases. When combined with cytotoxic agents that suppress cell proliferation, however, bisphosphonates interfere with tumor cell adhesion and invasion.[70] These factors raise many questions.

It is not known how long bisphosphonates should be infused or whether another type of administration, such as pulsed therapy, would be more effective. Another consideration is whether the schedule of administration should be different for adjuvant vs. palliative treatment. It also is not known whether other bone-targeting therapies, such as radiopharmaceuticals, or more cost-effective approaches would improve response over that produced by an adjuvant or palliative combination of chemotherapy plus hormonal therapy.

Evaluating Outcomes of Palliative Therapy

The findings of the studies discussed above demonstrate two key points regarding evaluation of the outcomes of palliative therapy. First, palliative therapy for symptomatic metastases often does not provide a significant survival benefit, even if the same approach improves survival when given in the adjuvant setting. Physicians must not confuse what can be accomplished with adjuvant therapy with what can be accomplished with palliative therapy. The goal of palliative therapy, whether administered in an oncologic or hospice practice, is the prompt and cost-effective relief of symptoms with little treatment-related morbidity. In most cases, radiation therapy can be given efficiently, with few side effects, and at a relatively low cost compared with systemic therapies. Second, almost one third of patients will develop distant metastases despite receiving adjuvant systemic chemotherapy plus hormonal therapy.

In one study of patients with T1 breast cancer, the frequencies of first distant metastases were 1% to 2%/month in those with node-negative disease, 2% to 4%/month in those with one to three positive nodes, and 3% to 6%/month in those with more than three positive nodes.[71] From this finding and from the assumption that mortality is reduced by 30% with adjuvant chemotherapy, patients with T1 disease would potentially have a higher rate of distant metastases with neoadjuvant chemotherapy (1% to 4% for each month that surgery is delayed).[71] Novel approaches are needed to increase the effectiveness of adjuvant therapies to prevent disease recurrence. Clearly defined approaches are needed to treat advanced and metastatic cancer as a chronic disease.

SYMPTOM RELIEF IN LOCALLY ADVANCED OR METASTATIC DISEASE

Most patients with cancer have symptoms, and those symptoms must be controlled regardless of whether treatment is administered with curative or palliative intent. Radiation oncologists need to be knowledgeable about the management of cancer-related pain, because controlling pain facilitates the ability to create radiation-field simulations and administer palliative therapy. The Joint Commission on Accreditation of Healthcare Organizations issued a new set of standards for the assessment and management of pain; these standards went into effect on January 1, 2001. The standards state that all patients have the right to appropriate assessment and management of pain and that patients should be taught that pain management is a part of treatment.

The results of a survey of Radiation Therapy Oncology Group (RTOG) physicians showed that 83% believed that most cancer patients with pain were undermedicated.[46] In their practice, 40% of the physicians surveyed reported that pain management was of poor or fair quality, and 23% said they would not use opioid analgesics until the patient's estimated survival duration was 6 months or less. Seventy-seven percent of physicians cited poor pain assessment as a barrier to adequate pain management, 60% cited the reluctance of patients to report pain, 72% cited the reluctance of patients to take analgesics, and 40% cited the reluctance of the physicians to prescribe opioids. For 72% of the RTOG physicians, the prescription of opioid analgesics was prompted by the failure to respond to palliative radiation therapy.[46] These results proved to be not substantially different from the responses to the same survey among Eastern Cooperative Oncology Group physicians 7 years earlier,[25] before publication of the Agency for Health Care Policy and Research's Cancer Pain Management Guidelines.[2,13]

As stated previously in this chapter, one of the barriers to effective pain management as observed by physicians is a lack of knowledge about assessing symptoms and determining treatment.[1,25] In addition, patients must be encouraged to report symptoms such as pain. Objective signs of acute pain, such as tachycardia, sweating, and facial grimacing, often are absent in chronic pain syndromes. The patients should be reassured that their pain can be controlled and that pain management is an integral part of cancer therapy. Patients who become fatigued because of pain often cannot tolerate the side effects of antineoplastic therapy. A clear history that identifies factors that could be related to the pain and a careful physical and neurologic examination should be performed to help direct diagnostic studies. Because more than 70% of the pain that is experienced by cancer patients is related to the disease, diagnostic evaluations should be performed frequently.

Pain Categories

Cancer pain can be divided into two broad categories: somatic or visceral pain and neuropathic pain. These categories of pain differ in etiology, symptoms, and response to analgesics and palliative radiation. Somatic or visceral pain arises from direct stimulation of afferent nerves caused by tumor infiltration of skin, soft tissue, or viscera.[2,72,73] Somatic pain is often described as well-localized dull or aching discomfort. Visceral pain tends to be poorly localized and is often referred to a dermatomic area remote from the source of pain. Common causes of somatic pain include bone metastases; liver metastases that result in capsular distention and biliary, bowel, or ureteral obstruction; and distention of normal skin or soft tissue structures from an expanding tumor mass (Box 38-1).[74] In general, somatic or visceral pain can be controlled with palliative antineoplastic treatment and conventional analgesics.

Neuropathic pain develops after injury to or chronic compression of nerves. Common causes of neuropathic pain include tumor invasion of a nerve plexus, spinal nerve root compression, herpes zoster infection, or surgical interruption of intercostal nerves (by thoracotomy or mastectomy). Neuropathic pain is described as sharp, burning, or shooting and often is associated with paresthesias and dysesthesias. Response to conventional analgesics is usually poor, but antidepressant or anticonvulsant medications may be helpful. Radiation therapy is one of the most effective—and often the only—therapeutic option for relieving pain caused by nerve compression or infiltration by a malignant tumor. Examples of neuropathic pain syndromes commonly encountered in radiation therapy include superior sulcus ("Pancoast") tumor, otalgia from head and neck cancer, brachial plexopathy in breast cancer, and epidural metastases. Among patients predicted to have an extended survival time, neuropathic pain often can be best relieved by a high-dose, extended course of radiation therapy in an attempt to secure durable pain relief.

Pharmacologic Principles
Tolerance and Addiction

Knowledge concerning appropriate use of analgesics is essential for any physician caring for cancer patients. The choice of an analgesic drug must be individualized. Too often, this choice is influenced by unfounded fears in both patient and physician about tolerance, addiction, and respiratory depression rather than by the level of pain experienced.[2,3,24,75-78] Tolerance is defined as the need to increase the dose of a drug to achieve the same analgesic effect. Tolerance is a normal physiologic response to opioids and is characterized by a decrease in the duration of the analgesic effect. The dose may be increased, occasionally to enormous levels, because there is no upper limit on the prescribed dose for strong opioids such as morphine. If tolerance develops, an alternative opioid may be used; adjuvant analgesics, such as nonsteroidal antiinflammatory drugs, may be given; or these interventions may be combined.

BOX 38-1   Specific Pain Syndromes in Patients with Cancer

PAIN SYNDROMES ASSOCIATED WITH DIRECT TUMOR INFILTRATION

Tumor Infiltration of Bone
  Base of skull syndromes—metastases to:
    Jugular foramen
    Clivus
    Sphenoid sinus
  Vertebral body syndromes—metastases to:
    C2
    C7, T1
    L1
  Sacral syndrome
Tumor Infiltration of Nerve
  Peripheral neuropathy
  Plexopathy
    Brachial
    Lumbar
    Sacral
  Nerve root
    Leptomeningeal metastases
  Spinal cord
    Epidural spinal cord compression
    Intramedullary metastasis

PAIN SYNDROMES ASSOCIATED WITH CANCER THERAPY

Postsurgery Syndromes
  Postthoracotomy syndrome: intercostal nerve injury
  Postmastectomy syndrome: intercostal brachial radial nerve injury
  Postradical neck dissection syndrome: cervical plexus injury
  Phantom limb syndrome
Postchemotherapy Syndromes
  Peripheral neuropathy
  Aseptic necrosis of the femoral head
  Steroid pseudorheumatism
  Posttherapeutic neuralgia
Postirradiation Syndromes
  Radiation fibrosis of brachial and lumbar plexus
  Radiation myelopathy
  Radiation-induced second primary tumors
  Radiation necrosis of bone

PAIN SYNDROMES NOT ASSOCIATED WITH CANCER OR CANCER THERAPY

Cervical and lumbar osteoarthritis
Thoracic and abdominal aneurysms
Diabetic neuropathy
Myofascial pain syndromes
Migraine and tension headaches

From Foley KM, Arbelt E. Management of cancer pain. In: DeVita VT, Hellman S, Rosenberg SA, eds. *Cancer: Principles and Practice of Oncology.* 3rd ed. Philadelphia, Pa: JB Lippincott, 1989; 2:2064-2087.

In contrast to tolerance, physical dependence is a normal physiologic response that occurs in response to the administration of steroids, some antihypertensive agents, and analgesics. Physical dependence becomes obvious when opioids are discontinued, and it is manifested through withdrawal symptoms, such as diaphoresis, nausea, and vomiting. Analgesics must be discontinued in the same way as steroids are, by slow tapering of the dose. Withdrawal symptoms can be prevented or treated by administering a dose of analgesic of about 25% of the previous daily dose. The onset of withdrawal symptoms is related to the half-life of the drug being used; symptoms of withdrawal may begin 6 to 12 hours after morphine is discontinued, whereas these symptoms may be delayed for several days if methadone is prescribed.

Psychological dependence (addiction) is an abnormal behavioral condition characterized by an overwhelming involvement in the acquisition and use of a drug for reasons other than pain relief.[2,72,73] Addiction is rare among patients who receive opioids for control of cancer pain. Tolerance and physical dependence are predictable pharmacologic effects of chronic narcotic administration, and they are distinct from addiction. Patients and their families should be counseled about the rarity of addiction when opioids are prescribed for legitimate medical indications.

Opioid pseudoaddiction describes behavior that mimics psychological dependence that occurs as a consequence of inadequate treatment of cancer pain. Pseudoaddiction may result from inadequate analgesic dosing schedules ("as needed" prescriptions) during periods of continuous pain, the use of dosing intervals that are greater than the duration of action of the prescribed analgesic, or the use of prescribed analgesics that are too weak to address the level of pain.[76] Unlike true addiction, pseudoaddictive behavior resolves once the pain is adequately managed.

Fear of addiction limits the use of narcotic analgesics in clinical practice. In addition, the unsubstantiated concerns of the past regarding physician prescription records and regulatory issues present an additional barrier to effective pain management. Federal and state laws affirm the essential medical value of controlled substances for cancer patients with intractable pain.

Patients and physicians should be reassured that the rates of addiction and abuse have not increased even though the medical use of opioid analgesics has increased since the publication of pain guidelines. From 1990 to 1996, the medical use of morphine increased by 59%, fentanyl by 1168%, oxycodone by 23%, and hydromorphone by 19%. During the same time, the use of meperidine decreased by 35%.[79] Although the incidence of drug abuse increased 6.6%, the proportion of abuse cases related to opioids decreased from 5.1% to 3.8%. Reports of abuse of meperidine decreased by 39%, abuse of oxycodone by 29%, abuse of fentanyl by 59%, and abuse of hydromorphone by 15%; abuse associated with morphine increased by 3%. Therefore the trend of increasing medical use of opioid analgesics to treat pain did not seem to contribute to the abuse of opioid analgesics.

Approaches for Prescribing Analgesics

The World Health Organization has advocated the use of a three-step approach in prescribing analgesics. (This approach is discussed at length in Chapters 22 and 23.) The approach is indexed to the patient's self-report of the inten-sity of the pain as mild, moderate, or severe.[80] The schedule of administration and the type of analgesic are then based on the frequency and severity of the pain. If the pain is constant, a long-acting analgesic should be prescribed. Long-acting analgesics can be administered orally every 8 or every 12 hours depending on the pain cycle. Transdermal fentanyl, which is administered as a patch, is an alternative means of continuous analgesic administration; patches can be replaced every 48 to 72 hours.

A short-acting opioid also should be prescribed as supplemental treatment for breakthrough pain until the next dose of a long-acting analgesic is given. Breakthrough pain is an incident-related symptom event; for example, it can be brought on by walking or undergoing a diagnostic procedure or by an inadequate dose or schedule of administration of the long-acting analgesic.[73,81] Short-acting analgesics also can be used alone for intermittent pain.

Moderate to severe pain can be treated with opioid analgesics around the clock, either alone or in combination with a nonsteroidal antiinflammatory agent (Table 38-1).[3] In accordance with the course of the disease and response to treatment, analgesic needs may increase or decrease for any individual patient. Patients and families should be given information about how to titrate analgesics so that the patient's pain can be controlled around the clock and the patient can enjoy normal activities and sleep patterns.

Analgesics that are complexed with acetaminophen or aspirin should be avoided because of possible renal and hepatic toxic effects. Nonsteroidal antiinflammatory agents also have serious potential side effects, including gastrointestinal bleeding, renal toxicity, and inhibition of platelets. Although these agents can be effective as co-analgesics, the possibility of toxic reactions persists. Analgesics should be given orally whenever possible, because intramuscular injections can cause discomfort, infection or bruising at the injection site, and irregular drug absorption. In addition, analgesics should be administered around the clock rather than as needed to avoid cycles of pain. Higher doses of analgesics are needed to *treat* pain as opposed to *preventing* pain. Analgesic side effects, such as constipation, should be anticipated and treated.

More than 90% of cancer-related pain can be controlled. A variety of alternative long- and short-acting opioid analgesics and routes of administration have become available. When oral administration is not possible, rectal suppositories can be used as an alternative or as a breakthrough analgesic.[81] (A list of oral and rectal opioid analgesics and their characteristics is shown in Table 38-2.)[81] Giving opioids in oral form also has the advantage of their being directly absorbed into the bloodstream from the oral mucosa, thereby avoiding the first-pass effect (in which drug metabolism begins as the drug passes through the gut mucosa and liver). If the oral mucosa is intact but the patient cannot swallow, morphine can be delivered sublingually, at an absorption rate of about 22%. Another product, a lozenge that contains fentanyl, provides pain relief within minutes of administration and lasts for 1 to 2 hours. Other means, such as a nerve block or an epidural catheter that administers opioids directly to the spine, should be considered if the pain or analgesic side effects are poorly controlled.[82-84] A common example is a celiac axis block for pain resulting from pancreatic cancer.

Clinical Considerations
Choice of Palliative Modalities

Curative therapy attempts to render the patient free of disease. This approach can be applied in the treatment of either primary or metastatic disease. The prognosis for a patient who is rendered disease-free after resection of a single liver metastasis from rectal cancer is better than that for a patient with extensive, inoperable lung cancer who does not have metastatic disease. Unlike curative therapy, in which a high total dose of radiation is administered to eradicate a tumor, palliation radiation therapy usually involves use of a hypofractionated schedule. Typical hypofractionated radiation schedules for palliative therapy are 2.5-Gy fractions given over a 3-week period for a total dose of 35 Gy; 20 Gy given over a 1-week period; and a single dose of 4 to 8 Gy. In the United States, the most common schedule involves giving 30 Gy in 10 fractions over 2 weeks.[12,85-93] The dose fractionation schedule used depends on prognosis, volume, and irradiation target site.

Treatment with palliative intent is intended to control the symptoms of disease when the disease cannot be

---

TABLE 38-1
Classes of Analgesic Agents Used to Treat Cancer Pain

Drug Classes and Names	Usual Doses for Adults
GROUP I: NONNARCOTIC ANALGESICS (NONSTEROIDAL ANTIINFLAMMATORY DRUGS)	
Commonly Used Drugs	
Acetylsalicylic acid (aspirin)	500-1000 mg q 4-6 hr po
Acetaminophen	500-1000 mg q 4-6 hr po
Indomethacin	25-50 mg tid po
Naprosyn	500 mg; then 250 mg q 6-8 hr po
Ibuprofen (Motrin, others)	200-400 mg q 4-6 hr po
Ketoprofen (Orudis)	25-50 mg q 4-6 hr po
Ketorolac (Toradol)	30-60 mg
GROUP II: NARCOTIC AGONISTS AND ANTAGONISTS	
Agonists	
Morphine and congeners	
Morphine*	15-30 mg q 3-4 hr po
Hydromorphone	4-8 mg q 3-4 hr po
Codeine	30-60 mg q 3-4 hr po
Oxycodone*	15-30 mg q 3-4 hr po
Levorphanol	2-3 mg q 3-4 hr po
Meperidine and congeners	
Meperidine (Demerol)	Not recommended
Methadone and congeners	
Propoxyphene (Darvon)	65-130 mg q 4-6 hr
Methadone (Dolophine)	5-10 mg q 4-8 hr
Transdermal fentanyl (Duragesic)	25-100 μg/hr q 3 days

Drug Classes and Names	Usual Doses for Adults
Partial Agonists and Agonist–Antagonists	
Pentazocine	None are recommended for chronic dosing in cancer patients
Buprenorphine	
Nalbuphine	
Butorphanol	
GROUP III: ADJUVANT ANALGESIC DRUGS	
Anticonvulsants	
Phenytoin (Dilantin)	100-300 mg tid po
Carbamazepine (Tegretol)	200-600 mg qid po
Phenothiazines	
Methotrimeprazine (Levoprome)	15 mg q 4-6 hr im
Tricyclic Antidepressants	
Amitriptyline	10-150 mg/day po
Desipramine	25-150 mg/day po
Nortriptyline	25-150 mg/day po
Steroids	
Dexamethasone	4 mg qid po
Antihistamines	
Hydroxyzine (Vistaril)	25 mg q 4-6 hr po
Stimulants (Including Amphetamines)	
Amphetamine	2.5-10 mg po
Ritalin	5-10 mg po
Caffeine	100-200 mg/day
Mexiletine	150 mg bid/tid po

Modified from Jacox A, Carr DB, Payne R. *N Engl J Med* 1994; 330:651-655.
*Morphine/oxycodone can be given as an immediate release formulation, or as a sustained release preparation.

TABLE 38-2
Dosages and Characteristics of Rectal and Oral Opioids

Opioid	Dosage Form	Time to Peak Level	Duration of Action
Morphine	Oral tablets	1.1 hr	< 6 hr
Morphine	Controlled release	5.4 hr	8-12 hr
Morphine	Rectal solution	5 hr	6 hr
Morphine	Rectal suppositories	1.1 hr	< 6 hr
Hydromorphone	Rectal suppositories	1 hr	4-6 hr

From Lipman AG. New and alternative noninvasive opioid dosage forms and routes of administration. In: Berger A, Portenoy RK, Weissman DE, eds. *Principles and Practice of Supportive Oncology*, Update 2000;3:1-8.

---

eradicated. Effective antineoplastic therapy provides the greatest palliative benefit for locally advanced or metastatic cancer in any organ. Radiation can be used alone or in combination with other antineoplastic therapies. The symptoms most commonly relieved by radiation therapy are pain, bleeding, and obstruction. The palliative interventions recommended depend on the patient's clinical status, burden of disease, and the site of symptoms. For either locally advanced or metastatic disease, these factors are indexed to the relative effectiveness, durability, and morbidity of each palliative intervention. Prognosis represents the single most important factor in choosing a palliative therapy.

Several clinical, prognostic, and therapeutic factors must be considered in developing a treatment regimen for a course of palliative radiation therapy. Clinical status is accounted for in the treatment set-up and in the number of treatments prescribed. The radiation dose-fractionation schedule and technique also should take into account the integration of other therapies. Many radiation therapy options exist for tumors that cause localized symptoms. Brachytherapy and conformal and intensity-modulated radiation therapy can be used to better localize radiation dose and reduce side effects, especially in a previously irradiated area.[53,58,86,93-95]

Reirradiation

Issues regarding reirradiation are especially important in palliative therapy. Experimental data suggest that acute-responding tissues recover from radiation injury in a few months and can tolerate another full course of radiation therapy. However, the variability in recovery from radiation among late-reacting tissues is considerable.[96] The heart, bladder, and kidney do not seem to recover from any late radiation effects. But the skin, mucosa, lung, and spinal cord do recover from subclinical radiation injury. This recovery depends on the organ irradiated, the size of the initial dose of radiation, and the interval between doses of radiation. Clinical correlates exist and limited toxic reactions have generally been reported with reirradiation.[97]

Symptomatic Site Location

In choosing palliative care, the location of the symptomatic site is more important than the state or type of tumor at that site. In general, radiation portals are used to palliate bronchial obstruction, whether caused by a primary lung cancer, recurrent breast cancer, or metastatic melanoma. The number of radiation fractions prescribed for treatment with palliative intent depends more on prognosis than on primary histology. Common sites palliated by radiation, either alone or in combination with other treatments, include tumor involvement of the lung, pelvis, skin and subcutaneous tissues, brain, and bone. Symptoms resulting from cancer in these sites include pain, bleeding, visceral obstruction, and lymphovascular obstruction.

Normal Tissue Tolerance

The limited radiation tolerance of normal tissues, such as the spinal cord, that are adjacent to a bone metastasis makes it impossible to administer a radiation dose that is large enough to eradicate a measurable volume of tumor. Palliative radiation should produce sufficient tumor regression from critical structures to relieve symptoms for the duration of the patient's life.

Symptoms that recur after palliative radiation most commonly result from localized regrowth of tumor. Control of cancer-related pain with the use of analgesics is imperative to allow comfort during and while awaiting response to therapeutic interventions. Pain represents a sensitive measure of disease activity. Close follow-up should be performed after any palliative therapeutic intervention to ensure control of cancer and treatment-related pain and to initiate diagnostic studies to identify progressive or recurrent disease.

BONE METASTASES

Although metastasis can occur at any site, more than half of the time palliative therapy is prescribed to relieve symptoms of bone metastases.[1-4] In 1993, about 800,000 patients in the United States were estimated to have metastatic disease, and metastases to bone were the most common.[92] Metastatic involvement of a solitary bony site or of only the bones is rare, occurring in less than 10% of patients. Among hospitalized patients, severe pain was experienced by more than 50% of patients with bone metastases.[4] One of the most important goals in the treatment of bone metastases is to relieve suffering and return the patient to independent function.[52,93] The location of the metastasis, however, can influence the degree of pain relief that can be achieved by palliative interventions.

Metastases to weight-bearing bones and bones involved in ambulation and activities of daily living are less likely to respond completely to palliative interventions. Pain relief can be achieved with radiation therapy in 73% of patients with spine metastases, 88% with limb lesions, 67% with pelvic metastases, and 75% with metastases to other parts of the skeleton.[14] Bone metastases from prostate or breast cancer involve the axial skeleton more than 80% of the time because of the predilection of these tumors to involve the red marrow. Metastatic invasion of the bone cortex rarely happens without red marrow involvement.[98-109] For this reason, the spine, pelvis, and ribs generally are involved before metastases become evident in the skull, femora, humeri, scapulae and sternum. The mechanisms involved in the metastatic spread of cancer to the bone are complex. The predilection of specific types of tumors to metastasize to bone is not well understood.

Bone is unique because it is continuously remodeled by local and systemic growth factors. The process involved in bone remodeling includes an increase in osteoclast activity followed by the appearance and proliferation of osteoblast precursors, which lay down new bone as they mature.[102-109] Tumors can release osteoclastic stimulatory factors either locally or systematically. These factors include the parathyroid hormone-related protein, transforming growth factor-alpha, transforming growth factor-beta, prostaglandins, and cytokines.[110] Tumors also can indirectly stimulate bone loss through the activation of immune mechanisms that release cytokines, including tumor necrosis factor and interleukin-1.

Metastases to bone result from a synergistic relationship between the cancer cell and the bone that results in increased bone resorption resulting from release of mediators from the cancer cells or leukocytes. Factors released during bone resorption promote growth of the cancer through activation of proliferation-associated oncogenes. The relationship between bone invasion and bone pain is unknown. Pain may result from the stimulation of nerve endings by the release of factors such as prostaglandins, bradykinin, histamine, or substance P in areas of bone involvement.[107] A mass effect from stretching of the periosteum, pathologic fracture, or direct tumor growth into adjacent nerves and tissues may explain the appearance of pain from larger metastatic deposits.

Multidisciplinary evaluation of patients with metastatic disease to the bone allows comprehensive management of the associated symptoms, determination of the risk of pathologic fracture, and coordination of the administration of a wide range of available antineoplastic therapies.[12,108,109] Bone scans are the most sensitive and specific method of detecting bone metastases, but magnetic resonance imaging (MRI) is the best available technique for evaluating neoplastic invasion of the bone marrow, vertebrae, central nervous system, and peripheral nerves.[43,98-100,110] Metastases to bone and other areas rarely fail to be detected when radiographic diagnosis is pursued. When radiographic confirmation of malignancy is equivocal, bone biopsy should be considered.[101-103]

Symptom Management

Bone metastases can be treated with localized or systemic therapies or a combination of both.[93,86,102,107,111]

Because localized radiation treats only a localized symptomatic site of disease, often it is used in coordination with systemic therapies such as chemotherapy, hormonal therapy, and bisphosphonates. Radiopharmaceuticals are another systemic option for treating diffuse symptomatic bone metastases. Because the radiation is deposited directly at the involved area in the bone, radiopharmaceuticals such as ^{89}Sr also can be used to treat bone metastases when symptoms recur in a previously irradiated site.[54-56,112-123] Radiopharmaceuticals also can be used as an adjuvant to localized external-beam irradiation and reduce the development of other symptomatic sites of disease.

Radiation Schedules: The RTOG Trial

Experience with palliative radiation for bone metastases comes mainly from a prospective clinical trial conducted by the RTOG to compare a variety of treatment schedules.[124,125] To account for prognosis, patients were stratified on the basis of whether they had solitary or multiple sites of bone metastasis. Initial analysis of the results led to the conclusion that low-dose, short-course treatment schedules were as effective as high-dose, protracted treatment programs.[124] For patients with solitary bone metastases, no difference in pain relief was noted after a dose of 20 Gy given in 4-Gy fractions than after a dose of 40.5 Gy given in 2.7-Gy fractions (Table 38-3).[124] Pain relapsed in 57% of patients at a median of 15 weeks after completion of therapy at each dose level. For patients with multiple bone metastases, the following dose schedules were compared: 30 Gy at 3 Gy/fraction, 15 Gy at 3 Gy/fraction, 20 Gy at 4 Gy/fraction, and 25 Gy at 5 Gy/fraction. No difference was identified in the rates of pain relief between these treatment schedules. Partial pain relief was achieved in 83% of the patients, and complete relief was achieved in 53% of patients. More than 50% of these patients developed recurrent pain; the fracture rate was 8%; and the median

TABLE 38-3

Percentage of Patients Responding to Radiation

Patient Group and Total Dose (Gy)	Dose/Fraction (Gy)	Tumor Dose at 2 Gy/Fraction	NUMBER OF WEEKS AFTER RADIATION THERAPY			
			< 2	2-4	4-12	12-20
SOLITARY METASTASES						
40.5	2.7	42.9	7%	29%	53%	77%
20.0	4	23.3	16%	50%	66%	82%
MULTIPLE METASTASES						
30.0	3	32.5	19%	48%	73%	84%
15.0	3	16.2	34%	70%	84%	93%
20.0	4	23.3	28%	53%	75%	88%
25.0	5	31.25	22%	41%	72%	80%

Data from Tong D, Gillick L, Hendrickson FR. *Cancer* 1982;50:893-899.

duration of pain control was 12 weeks for all radiation schedules used to treat multiple bone metastases. Prognostic factors for response included the initial pain score and site of the primary tumor.

Reanalysis of results. A subsequent reanalysis of the results from this RTOG study included use of a different definition of complete pain relief (absence of pain and cessation of the use of narcotics).[125] When this definition was used, pain relief was found to be related to both the number of fractions and the total dose of radiation.[125] Complete pain relief was achieved in 55% of patients with solitary bone metastases who received 40.5 Gy at 2.7 Gy/fraction as compared with 37% of patients who received a total dose of 20 Gy at 4 Gy/fraction (Table 38-4).[125] A similar relationship was observed upon reanalysis for patients with multiple bone metastases. Complete pain relief was achieved in 46% of patients who received 30 Gy at 3 Gy/fraction compared with 28% of patients treated to 25 Gy in 5-Gy fractions. In most cases, the interval to response was 4 weeks for both complete and minimal relief of symptoms.

Three important issues can be identified from this experience. First, the results of the reanalysis demonstrated the importance of defining response to therapy. Second, the revised definitions of response showed that the total radiation dose did influence the degree to which pain was relieved (see Table 38-4), that is, higher radiation doses resulted in higher rates of pain relief. (These results also correspond well to those of another study of patients with breast, prostate, or lung cancer in which patients treated with total doses of 40 Gy or more had higher rates of complete pain relief [63% to 71%] than did those treated with less than 40 Gy [44% to 62%].[14]) Third, the amount of time needed to experience pain relief after radiation therapy was fairly long (see Table 38-3); only half of the patients who eventually responded showed relief of symptoms at 2 to 4 weeks

after radiation therapy,[124,125] thus underscoring the need for continued analgesic support after completion of radiation therapy. Accomplishment of maximum relief consistently took 12 to 20 weeks after radiation therapy, a period that may reflect the time needed for reossification. Radiographic evidence of recalcification is observed in about one fourth of such cases, and 70% of the time, recalcification is evident within 6 months of completing radiation and other palliative therapies.[106-109] Therefore determining the time to response as well as defining the parameters of response are critical to an evaluation of outcome. The total dose of radiation also may be a significant factor for complete pain relief.

Similar issues were observed when pretreatment pain characteristics were used to determine the efficacy of palliative radiation.[39,72,73,126] Among patients who had a life expectancy of only a few months, fewer than 25% had a complete response to palliative radiation. (A complete response was defined as becoming pain-free within 28 days after the start of treatment, with "stable" use of analgesics.) A partial response was achieved in 35% of patients, and 42% had no response to palliative radiation. Pretreatment evidence of neuropathic pain was the only significant prognostic or clinical variable that predicted failure to respond to palliative radiation, and severe neurogenic symptoms were present in 33% of patients treated.[39,72,73,126]

Other Schedules

A variety of radiation therapy schedules have been evaluated in palliative therapy for bone metastases. One trial compared 30 Gy given in 10 fractions to 15 Gy given in 3 fractions at 2 fractions/week to 217 patients with breast cancer.[127] No difference was observed in pain scores, analgesic use, treatment side effects, or survival. At 12 months of follow-up, about 70% of patients had little or no limitation on activity.[127]

TABLE 38-4

Dose Response Evaluation From Reanalysis of the Radiation Therapy Oncology Group Bone Metastases Protocol

Patient Group	Dose/Fraction (Gy)	Total Dose (Gy)	Tumor Dose at 2 Gy/Fraction	Complete Response Rate*	P Value
SOLITARY BONE METASTASES					
	2.7	40.5	42.9	55%	< 0.0003
	4.0	20.0	23.3	37%	
MULTIPLE BONE METASTASES					
	3.0	30	32.5	46%	< 0.0003
	3.0	15.0	16.2	36%	
	4.0	20.0	23.3	40%	
	5.0	25.0	31.25	28%	

Data from Blitzer PH. *Cancer* 1985;55:1468-1472.
*Excludes the use of analgesics and accounts for retreatment.

Consistent with other reports, the survival rates were 45% at 3 months, 33% at 6 months, and only 20% at 1 year.

Response to Treatment

Response to treatment may be the most important prognostic factor in bone metastases. A prospective randomized trial compared 30 Gy given in 2-Gy fractions to 20 Gy given in 4-Gy fractions among 100 patients with a median follow-up of 12 months.[128] The primary tumor was located in the breast in 43% of patients, lung in 24%, and prostate in 14%. The pelvis (31%), vertebrae (30%), and ribs (20%) were the most common sites treated. These characteristics were equally distributed between the study groups.

The biologically effective doses were 28 Gy_{10} and 36 Gy_{10} for the two treatment groups. No significant differences were observed between the groups in frequency of pain relief, duration of pain relief, mobility, or pathologic fractures.[128] The mean interval from the completion of radiation to pain relief was approximately 10 days for both groups. The mean duration of pain relief was 245 days in each group, and it lasted for up to 84% of the remaining survival time. Importantly, responders had a highly significant ($P < 0.0001$) improvement in the duration of relief. Other factors (in addition to radiation schedule) that influenced overall survival rate were primary tumor site ($P < 0.0001$), performance status ($P < 0.0001$), age ($P < 0.03$), and biologically effective dose ($P < 0.04$).

The importance of the relationship between pain control and survival was noted unexpectedly in a trial comparing best medical management of pain with placement of an intrathecal catheter for pain control in patients with locally advanced and recurrent cancer. Most of the patients in this trial, preliminary results of which were presented at the 2001 meeting of the American Society of Clinical Oncology, had lung or ovarian cancer. Improvements in pain control were associated with a significant survival benefit among patients with the intrathecal catheters. It is possible that survival may be linked to improved mobility afforded by pain control. It is not known whether pain, through its effects on sleep and other functions, also affects cytokine release and other immunologic variables that may ultimately affect survival. This is an area of active research.

Whether a dose-response relationship exists in the treatment of bone metastases is unknown. The published results do not control for histology, type (blastic or lytic), or location of the metastases or type of pain (i.e., neuropathic, mechanical, or somatic), and many of the older reports do not include validated pain surveys or account for use of analgesics. The definition and duration of response is variable.[85,129,130] It is often unclear how many patients who had been assigned to a high-dose group actually completed therapy and how many who had been assigned to a low-dose group actually received a high dose of radiation as a result of retreatment.[85] Three reports suggest the existence of a dose-response relationship in the treatment of bone metastases.[125,131,132]

The RTOG study[124,125] also demonstrated that level of pain also correlated with prognosis in patients with multiple bone metastases. This survival difference may be an important observation, because unrelieved pain and the resultant sequelae of immobility can contribute to mortality as well as morbidity.* Larger data sets that include prognostic factors in multivariate analysis are required to determine the effect of pain and the response to therapy on quality of life and survival.

Further research may determine that the radiation dose schedules should be specific to the primary tumor, the site of metastases, and the type of pain if response is to be maximized. Regardless of the radiation therapy schedule used, retreatment should be considered at the first sign of symptom progression in order to achieve the maximum and most durable level of palliation. Pain management should be optimized in light of reports of its relationship to survival. Future research should target level of pain relief and the cost-effectiveness of treatment.

Single- versus Multiple-Fraction Radiation

Although equal rates of response have been observed for single vs. several radiation fractions, future analyses should evaluate survival and durability of response. Criteria need to be established to determine which clinical presentation is best treated with single-fraction therapy vs. multiple-fraction therapy.[130,133] Most importantly, these analyses should assess the efficacy and costs of treating symptoms that recur in an irradiated field.

Single-fraction radiation is used extensively in Europe and is the subject of an RTOG trial. Because it is convenient, cost-effective, and can be repeated, single-fraction radiation is of special interest in the palliative-care setting. In the United States, however, the efficacy of this treatment continues to raise concern. The cost and convenience benefits from a shorter course of radiation may be lost through the continued need for analgesics.

A cost-effectiveness comparison was conducted among 1171 patients who were randomly assigned to receive radiation at 8 Gy in one fraction or 24 Gy in six fractions.[134] The two treatment groups were equivalent in terms of palliation, including use of analgesics; however, 25% of the 8-Gy group required retreatment compared with 7% of the 24-Gy multifraction group. A cost analysis showed that treatment in the 8-Gy group cost $1734 (European currency) as compared with $2305 (European currency) for those in the multifraction group, representing a 25% cost difference. However, when the costs of retreatment were included in the analysis, the cost difference was reduced to only 8%,

---

*References 18, 19, 34, 35, 37, 38, 40, 126.

although an economic advantage continued to exist because of the savings in radiation therapy capacity.

Many issues must be evaluated before single-fraction radiation can be advocated for the treatment of all bone metastases; close follow-up is needed to determine which patients treated in this way will require retreatment.[130,133] Discussions regarding radiation dose fractionation must further be considered in the context of multidisciplinary treatment. These and other issues are reviewed in the following section.

A single, large radiation fraction is reportedly as effective in relieving pain as is radiation delivered in several smaller doses. Radiobiologically, a single 8-Gy fraction would produce the same side effects in late-reacting tissues as those produced by 18 Gy given in nine 2-Gy fractions.[135] The radiobiologically equivalent dose to the tumor of a single 8-Gy fraction would be 12 Gy if 2-Gy fractions were used. The most common dose fractionation schedule used for palliative radiation in the United States is 30 Gy given in 10 fractions. Radiobiologically, this is equivalent to 36 Gy at 2 Gy/fraction for late-reacting tissues and 32.5 Gy to the tumor.

When single-dose vs. multiple-dose schedules from several studies were compared, no difference was reported in either how quickly symptoms resolved or the duration of pain relief.[12,89-92,133,136-142] In each case, symptom relief lasted 3 months in 70% of patients, 6 months in 37%, and 12 months in 20%. As was true in the RTOG study, about 69% of patients responded at 4 weeks, and response rates reached a plateau in 80% of patients at 8 weeks.[124,125,136-142] Complete response rates after a single 8-Gy fraction totaled 15% at 2 weeks, 23% at 4 weeks, 28% at 8 weeks, and 39% at 12 weeks after radiation.

The Bone Pain Trial Working Party[138] conducted a trial among 765 patients with skeletal metastases, comparing a single 8-Gy fraction to either 20 Gy given in 5 fractions or 30 Gy given in 10 fractions. Pain severity and analgesic requirements were recorded before treatment, 2 weeks after treatment, and at 1, 2, 3, 4, 5, 6, 8, 10, and 12 months of follow-up. Pain relief was the primary endpoint.

In all three groups, pain management with analgesics before radiation therapy had been inadequate. Consistent with other findings, 70% of patients in this study had moderate to severe pain when they presented for radiation therapy despite the fact that 70% were taking opioid analgesics. No difference was identified in the time to first improvement in pain, time to complete pain relief, time to pain recurrence, risk of spinal cord compression or pathologic fracture, nausea or vomiting, or analgesic requirements between the single-dose vs. multiple-dose radiation schedules.

Overall, 57% of patients experienced a complete response to radiation. At 6 and 12 months of follow-up, however, about 55% of patients still required opioid analgesics. Retreatment was twice as common in the single-dose 8-Gy group (23% vs. 10%), although this difference did not influence overall pain relief. The authors felt that physicians were more likely to administer retreatment after a single 8-Gy course of radiation than after a multiple-fraction course of therapy.

Reirradiation for persistent or recurrent pain is often precluded when higher radiation doses are administered. Because the radiobiological dose from a single dose is relatively low, reirradiation is generally possible.[15,136-142] Although reirradiation was necessary in 25% of the patients in the Bone Pain Trial who received a single 8-Gy radiation fraction, all of those patients reportedly responded to the second dose of radiation. By comparison, when a single 4-Gy fraction was compared with a single 8-Gy fraction, the rate of response was slightly lower and fewer acute radiation-induced reactions were noted in the lower-dose group, but a greater proportion of patients required reirradiation.[141] When reirradiation was accounted for, the overall rate of response was equivalent for the 8-Gy and 4-Gy groups.

Reirradiation with a single 4-Gy fraction also yields a 74% response rate, including a 31% complete response rate.[136] Pain relief also was achieved in 46% of patients who did not initially respond to a single 4- or 8-Gy fraction. Patients who had a previous complete response to therapy were more likely to respond to reirradiation when compared with the group that previously experienced a partial response (85% vs. 67%).

A shorter radiation therapy schedule, like the use of single fractions, is advantageous for patients with poor prognostic factors. First, it is easier for patients with a poor performance status to complete therapy. Second, response rates are equal for single- and multiple-fraction therapy at 3 months because the median survival duration is less than 6 months in patients with poor prognostic factors.[12,87,92,139-143] The option of retreatment after a single fraction of radiation also may be an advantage among patients with good prognostic factors in terms of periodically reducing tumor burden and controlling symptoms in noncritical anatomic sites. Higher radiation doses that provide more durable pain relief are considered warranted for patients with good prognostic factors who require treatment over the spine and other critical sites.[14,86,93,144-150]

Survival Duration

The projected survival duration is the critical issue in determining the optimal radiation dose and schedule for palliative radiation. In one study,[88] only 12 of 245 patients were alive at the time of analysis, with approximately 50% alive at 6 months, 25% at 1 year, 8% at 2 years, and 3% at 3 years after palliative radiation. For patients with breast cancer in that study, the corresponding survival rates after palliative radiation were 60%, 44%, 20%, and 7%; for patients with prostate cancer, the survival rates were 60% at 6 months, 24% at 1 year, and 0% at 2 years.[88] In the RTOG trial, the median survival duration for patients with solitary bone metastases was 36 weeks; for those with multiple bone metastases, it was 24 weeks.[124,125]

It may not matter that the response to radiation therapy is optimized either through a more protracted course, if a dose response relationship exists, or through retreatment.[61,85] Consideration must be given to patient mobility and access, convenience, and cost-effectiveness. Clearly, a durable and significant response from radiation, not the schedule of administration, is the key issue in palliative radiation.

Morbidity

Pathologic fracture and spinal cord compression are significant consequences of bone metastasis. Pain that persists or recurs after palliative radiation should be evaluated to exclude as its cause progression of disease, extension of disease outside the radiation portal (resulting in referred pain), and bone fracture. Reduced cortical strength can cause compression, stress, or microfractures. Plain radiographs have a 91% concordance rate in detecting after-treatment disease progression and fractures, in comparison to the 57% specificity rate of bone scans performed after radiation therapy.[108]

Pathologic Fractures

Pathologic fractures occur in 8% to 30% of patients with bone metastases.[151-156] Proximal long bones are involved more commonly than distal bones; consequently, 50% of pathologic fractures occur in the femur, and 15% occur in the humerus (Fig. 38-1). The femoral neck and head are the most common locations for pathologic fracture because of the propensity for metastases

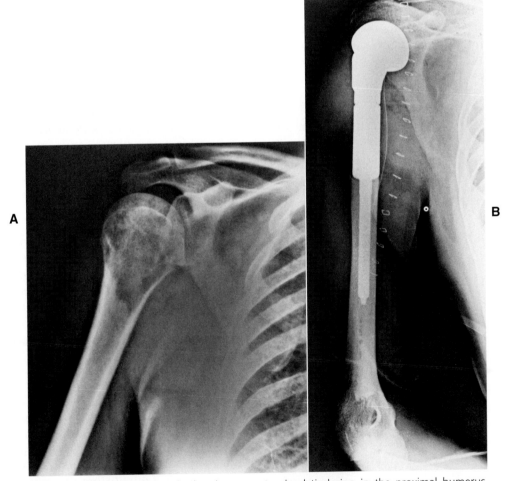

Fig. 38-1 A, Plain radiograph showing an extensive lytic lesion in the proximal humerus. B, Prophylactic internal fixation was performed to prevent pathologic fracture. The patient, who experienced pain primarily in the hip, would have been put on crutches to reduce stress on the involved femur. A bone scan and x-ray films obtained to exclude other sites of metastatic involvement identified this lesion in the humerus. The humerus would certainly have fractured if all of the patient's weight had been displaced to the upper extremities with crutches.

to involve proximal bones and because of the stress of weight placed on this part of the femur. More than 80% of pathologic fractures occur in patients with breast (50%), kidney, lung, or thyroid cancer.

Approximately 10% to 30% of pathologic fractures that occur in long bones where a metastatic lesion is present will require surgical intervention. Clinically, the outcome for patients with a pathologic fracture resulting from a bone metastasis after surgical repair is comparable to that of patients sustaining a traumatic fracture.[152-154] Prognosis is generally poor if hypercalcemia is present and if parenteral narcotics are required to control pain from other sites of bone metastases. In such cases, the decision for surgical intervention should be based on the severity of the symptoms associated with the fracture.[152] As shown in Figure 38-2, postoperative radiation is often given after surgical fixation of a pathologic fracture to reduce the risk of progressive disease in the bone that could lead to instability of the internal fixation.[157]

Treatment of pathologic fracture or impending fracture depends on the bone involved and the patient's clinical status. Indications for surgical intervention of pathologic fracture or impending fracture include an expected survival duration of more than 6 weeks, the ability to accomplish internal stability of the fracture

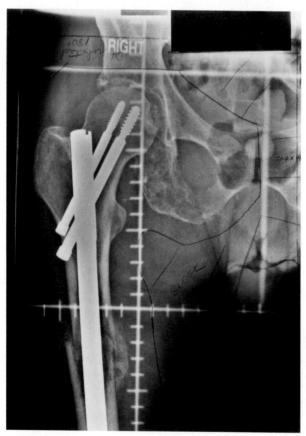

Fig. 38-2 Typical radiation portal after fixation of a pathologic fracture of the femur. Radiation is given to treat residual disease around the internal fixation device, pubis, and acetabulum.

site, and the absence of coexistent conditions that would preclude early mobilization (metastasis involving weight-bearing bones and lytic lesions more than 2 or 3 cm in size or metastases that destroy more than 50% of the cortex).[152-156] It is unclear whether osteolytic metastases are more likely to lead to fracture than are osteoblastic lesions because osteoblastic lesions, by definition, have an osteolytic component that facilitates the formation of new bone.

Spinal Cord Compression

The vertebral column is the site of metastatic tumors in 40% of patients who die of cancer. Approximately 70% of vertebral metastases involve the thoracic spine, 20% the lumbosacral region, and 10% the cervical spine. The average time from the original diagnosis of cancer to the development of metastatic spinal disease is 30 months. The development of spinal cord compression is associated with a poor overall prognosis, and the median survival duration among these patients is 7 months, with a 36% probability of a 1-year survival. After the diagnosis of epidural spinal cord compression, the median survival duration is 5 months. Once epidural spinal cord compression is diagnosed, the mean survival duration is 14 months for patients with breast cancer, 12 months for prostate cancer, 6 months for malignant melanoma, and 3 months for lung cancer.[5,144,151]

Symptoms. Pain is the initial symptom in approximately 90% of patients with spinal cord compression. Paraparesis or paraplegia occurs in more than 60% of cases, sensory loss in 70% to 80%, and bladder or bowel disturbances in 14% to 77%.[88,144-150] The extent of the epidural mass influences prognosis, because a complete spinal block results in greater residual neurologic impairment than a partial block.

Weakness can signal the rapid progression of symptoms, and 30% of patients with weakness become paraplegic within 1 week. Rapid development of weakness, defined as weakness occurring less than 2 months after the appearance of spinal cord compression, most commonly occurs in lung cancer, whereas in breast and prostate cancer, weakness can progress more slowly. Neurologic deficits can develop within a few hours in up to 20% of patients with spinal cord compression.[144-150,158,159] The severity of weakness at presentation is the most important predictor of recovery of function; 90% of patients who are ambulatory at presentation will be ambulatory after treatment. Only 13% of patients who are paraplegic will regain function, particularly if paraplegia had been present for more than 24 hours before the initiation of therapy. Over 30% of patients who develop spinal cord compression are alive 1 year later, and 50% of them will remain ambulatory with appropriate therapy.

Pain might be present for days or months before neurologic dysfunction appears. Unlike degenerative joint disease, which primarily occurs in the low cervical and low lumbar regions, pain caused by epidural spinal cord compression can occur anywhere in the spinal axis and is aggravated by recumbency. The most common site for epidural metastases is the thorax, followed by the lumbar region and then the cervical region. Lung and breast cancer tends to metastasize to the thoracic spine, but colon and pelvic tumors have a predilection for the lumbosacral region.[157]

Back pain in any cancer patient, especially those with known metastatic involvement of the vertebral bodies, should raise the suspicion of spinal cord compression. The risk of spinal cord compression exceeds 60% among patients with back pain and plain-film evidence of vertebral collapse from metastatic cancer.[144-150,157-165]

Epidural spinal cord disease has been documented in 17% of asymptomatic patients who have an abnormal bone scan but normal plain films; 47% of asymptomatic patients with vertebral metastases noted both on bone scan and plain films also will have associated epidural disease.[158] Symptomatic patients with a normal vertebral contour and osteoblastic changes on plain film and bone scan also should be evaluated for spinal cord compression (Fig. 38-3).

Radiographic determination. Radiographic determination of the involved spinal levels is critical to radiation treatment planning. Clinical assessment of the location of epidural spinal cord compression is incorrect in 33% of cases.[144-146] Plain-film radiographs will show involvement of more than one spinal level in about one third of patients. On such films, destruction of the pedicles is commonly indicative of spine metastases. In contrast, computed tomography (CT) scans show that the initial anatomic location of metastases is in the posterior portion of the vertebral body and that destruction of the pedicles occurs only in combination with involvement of the vertebral body (Fig. 38-4).[162] Osteoblastic bony expansion, common in both prostate and breast cancer, can result in spinal cord compromise as well as osteolytic vertebral compression fractures.[161]

If the results of MRI, tomographic studies, and surgical findings are included, more than 85% of patients will have evidence of multiple sites of vertebral involvement.[144-150,158,162,166,167] Multiple sites of epidural involvement also are common; 10% to 38% of epidural metastases involve multiple noncontiguous spinal levels.[157] Findings from 337 patients evaluated between 1985 and 1993 were reviewed to assess the

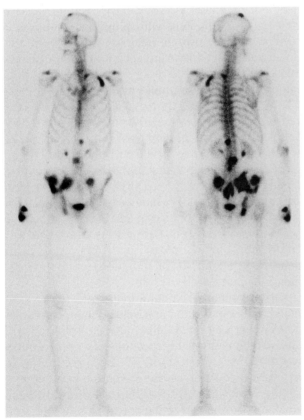

Fig. 38-3 Bone scan demonstrating multifocal metastatic disease. Involvement of weight-bearing areas such as the pelvis and lower lumbar area significantly affects mobility.

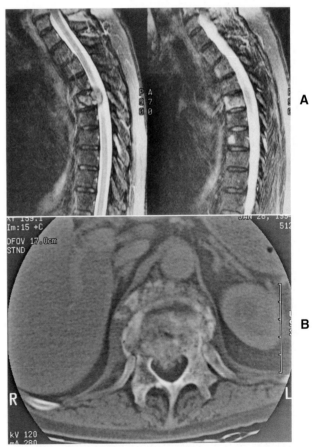

Fig. 38-4 A, Sagittal magnetic resonance image of the thoracic spine showing involvement of the posterior aspect of the vertebral body resulting in partial spinal cord compression. B, Axial computed tomography scan showing direct impingement on the spinal cord.

benefit of complete spinal imaging.[166] When the entire spine was evaluated radiographically, 32% of patients had multiple sites of epidural involvement; when imaging was limited to the symptomatic site, multiple areas of epidural tumor spread were detected in only 18% of cases. Although failure to image the cervical spine would have missed only 1% of epidural tumor deposits, this percentage increased to 21% if either the thoracic or lumbar regions were not fully imaged. The presence of multiple epidural tumor deposits was an independent prognostic factor for poorer survival. Secondary epidural tumor deposits were included 93% of the time within the radiation portals.

Treatment. Treatment for spinal cord compression includes emergent corticosteriods, radiation therapy, neurosurgical intervention, or a combination thereof. Radiation therapy is the treatment of choice in most cases (Fig. 38-5).[95,157,168] Functional outcome depends on the level of symptoms at the time radiation is administered. The outcome of 166 patients who presented to a cancer center with spinal cord compression confirmed on MRI was reviewed in terms of performance and neurologic status.[168] More than half of the patients had prostate or breast cancer, and 13% had lung cancer. The thoracic spine was most commonly involved, either alone (57%) or in combination with lesions in the lumbar region (11%). Multiple levels of epidural involvement were documented in 28% of patients. Symptoms included back pain in 122, limb weakness in 128, sensory loss in 90, and sphincter disturbance in 53 patients. More than 50% of the patients had moderate to major neurologic disturbances.

Radiation therapy was given to 92% of patients. Median survival duration from confirmation of spinal cord compression was 82 days (range, 1 to 349 days). Performance status improved in 16% of patients, and neurologic status improved in only 20% of cases. In 55% to 60% of patients, performance and neurologic status remained the same, and 25% were worse after treatment.[168] Thirty-two percent of patients died in the hospital. Most of the remaining 68% returned home; only 11% were sent to another hospital, 4% to a rehabilitation center, and 5% to a hospice. Pretreatment performance and neurologic status proved to be highly predictive of outcome. Hence, because disability and pain continue even after treatment, ongoing medical intervention is needed to assist in home care efforts.

Importance of early treatment. Spinal cord compression resulting from metastatic tumor can be prevented or effectively treated when diagnosed early.* The most common radiation therapy schedule for spinal cord compression and carcinomatous plexopathy is 30 Gy in 10 fractions; pain relief can be accomplished in 73% of patients thus treated.[158,159]

Although more prolonged courses of radiation have been given for spinal cord compression, a short course was evaluated in a patient group with a poor overall prognosis.[169] Among the 53 patients treated, 11 had lung cancer, 11 prostate cancer, 9 had gastrointestinal cancer, 5 had renal cell cancer, and 3 had breast cancer. Pain was present in 96% of patients and motor weakness was present in 84%; 41% were unable to walk, and 12% were paraplegic. Radiation therapy consisted of a single 8-Gy fraction; a second 8-Gy fraction was given after 1 week to patients whose tumors responded or stabilized.[169] The median field size was 136 cm^2, and all patients treated to the upper abdomen were premedicated. Pain relief was accomplished in 67% of patients, and motor function improved in 63%.

Early diagnosis and therapy were very important in predicting response to radiation therapy; only 38% of nonambulatory patients and 44% of those with bladder incontinence improved, but ability to ambulate and maintain continence was preserved in 91% and 98% of patients, respectively.[169] The median survival duration was 5 months; 30% survived for 1 year. Survival was significantly better among ambulatory than among nonambulatory patients. For patients with spinal cord compression and poor prognostic factors, a short course of radiation seemed to provide efficient and effective palliation.

In the treatment of epidural spinal cord compression, a statistically significant improvement in functional outcome has been reported for laminectomy plus radiation relative to either modality used alone for certain clinical presentations. Laminectomy has been recommended for prompt reduction of tumor volume in attempts to provide rapid relief from compression injury of the spinal cord and stabilize the spinal axis.[95] The rate of

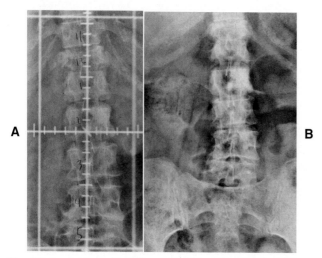

Fig. 38-5 **A,** Typical radiation portal for treatment of multifocal disease involvement of the vertebral bodies and epidural region. **B,** Blastic lesions can be seen in the pedicles, especially at L2.

---

*References 95, 144-150, 157, 158, 162, 168.

tumor regression after radiation therapy is too slow in such cases to effect recovery of lost neurologic function.

Several studies have indicated that the use of radiation to treat a partial spinal cord block resulted in 64% of patients regaining ambulation, 33% achieving normalization of sphincter tone, and 72% becoming pain-free, with a median survival duration of 9 months.[147-150] With a complete spinal cord block, only 27% of patients will show improvement in motor function after radiation therapy alone, and 42% will continue to have pain. Therefore surgical intervention should be considered among patients presenting with a complete spinal cord block. In paraparetic patients who undergo laminectomy plus irradiation, 82% regain the ability to walk, 68% have improved sphincter function, and 88% have relief of pain.

Laminectomy for vertebral and epidural metastases also is indicated for tumor progression in a previously irradiated area, for cases in which the spine is stabilized, for paraplegic patients with limited disease and good probability of survival, and for establishing a diagnosis.[144-150] Adjuvant radiation therapy is often given to treat microscopic residual disease after neurosurgical intervention in patients who have not previously undergone irradiation. Surgical restoration of the vertebral alignment may be required because of neurologic compromise and pain caused by progressive vertebral collapse. Vertebral collapse may occur as a result of cancer or vertebral instability after cancer therapy (Fig. 38-6). Appropriate diagnostic studies and interventions should be pursued, because neurologic compromise and pain

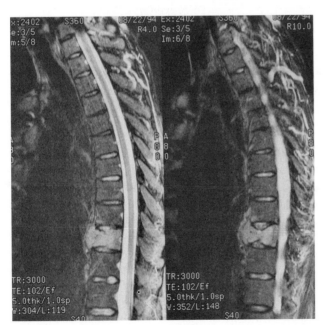

Fig. 38-6 Sagittal magnetic resonance images shows normal spinal cord but recurrent tumor extending from the vertebral body. Specialized treatment planning is needed to ensure that adequate radiation doses are delivered to the involved region.

from vertebral instability can be as devastating as that from epidural spinal cord metastases.[149,163]

Paravertebral masses are most commonly associated with lung cancer and are rare in prostate cancer.[164,165] Approximately 20% of patients with epidural spinal cord compression will have an associated paravertebral mass. Surgical resection combined with radiation therapy has been suggested to improve functional outcome when a paravertebral mass is associated with spinal cord compression because radiation alone is less effective for large tumor burdens.

Radiation Tolerance of the Spinal Cord

The potential for developing radiation myelitis from total radiation doses that exceed 40 Gy at 2 Gy/fraction represents the limiting factor in the treatment of large tumor burdens near or involving the spinal canal. Moreover, the length of the spinal cord that needs to be irradiated substantially affects the radiation tolerance of the spinal cord.[170-172] Histopathologic changes observed after experimental fractionated irradiation of the spinal cord include white matter necrosis, massive hemorrhage, and segmental parenchymal atrophy; these changes are consistently associated with abnormal neurologic signs.[172] Other pathologic responses involve focal fiber loss and white matter vacuolation. Other experimental findings have shown that the time course and the extent of long-term recovery from radiation depend on the specific type and age of the tissue.[170,172]

Radiation tolerance of the spinal cord, like that of other tissues, is based on the dose per fraction, total dose, and volume of tissue treated. The most important of these factors is the isodose per fraction. Clinical and experimental experience have failed to demonstrate any difference in radiosensitivity in different segments of the spinal cord.[170,173] The risk of radiation myelitis in the cervicothoracic spine is less than 5% when a 60-Gy radiation dose is given in 1.72-Gy fractions or when 50 Gy is given in daily 2-Gy fractions. Among patients who have received chemotherapy or have had spinal injury, the total dose to the spinal cord is generally limited to 40 Gy given in 2-Gy fractions to minimize the risk of irreversible radiation injury to the spinal cord.

In addition to isodose, the total dose is also extremely important in defining the radiation tolerance of the spinal cord. A steep curve based on total radiation dose predicts the risk of developing radiation myelopathy; a small increase in total radiation dose can result in a large increase in the risk of radiation myelopathy.[170,172] However, estimates from a linear-quadratic model[173] suggest that no progressive myelopathies would be produced from doses of 60 Gy in 2-Gy fractions to the spinal cord. Concerns have been raised that the conservative limit of radiation dose to the spinal cord has compromised tumor control. With conventional fractionation of 1.8 to

2 Gy, the incidence of myelitis at 5 years was 0.2% after 45 Gy and 1% to 5% after 60 Gy.[173] These determinations from a linear-quadratic model have correlated well with clinical findings.

Retreatment of a previously irradiated segment of the spinal cord places the patient at high risk of radiation-induced myelopathy, because other neurologic pathways cannot compensate for an injury to a specific level of the spinal cord. Within 6 months, repair of spinal tissue is about 30%. If 50 Gy was administered initially, this percentage of repair would represent 85% of the tolerance dose to the spinal cord.[96,172] Allowing 1 to 2 years between radiation doses for repair, the tolerance dose to the spinal cord is determined to be about 135% of that with reirradiation. Therefore a total dose of 75 to 81 Gy, given in two radiation courses with conventional fractionation spaced 1 to 2 years apart, should not result in substantial injury. The use of conformal or intensity-modulated radiation therapy techniques, in combination with spinal cord recovery, provide another option for reirradiation.[95] If the patient cannot be treated surgically, reirradiation may be the only viable option for maintaining neurologic integrity for the remainder of the patient's life (see Fig. 38-6). Given the limited overall prognosis, the risk of long-term radiation injury is small.

The radiation tolerance of the spinal cord also can be compromised by prior injury. Vasogenic edema of the spinal cord and nerve roots can be caused by compression injury, along with venous hemorrhage, loss of myelin, and ischemia. Synthesis of prostaglandin E$_2$, which increases in the presence of vasogenic edema, can be inhibited by steroids or nonsteroidal antiinflammatory agents.[157,170,172] Radiation can cause two forms of injury—white matter damage and vasculopathy. White matter damage is associated with diffuse demyelination and swollen axons that can be focally necrotic and have associated glial reaction. Vascular damage has been shown experimentally to be age-dependent and can result in vascular necrosis.

Types of Injury

Six major types of injury have been shown experimentally to result from radiation to the spinal column; five occur in the spinal cord and one in the dorsal root ganglia. The most severe spinal lesions, all of which are caused by vascular damage and result in neurologic dysfunction, include white matter necrosis, hemorrhage, and segmental parenchymal atrophy. The two less severe forms of spinal lesion include focal fiber loss and scattered white matter vacuolation caused by damage to glial cells, axons, the vasculature, or a combination of these. Less severe sequelae occur after lower total doses of radiation and are less likely to result in neurologic dysfunction. In dorsal root ganglia, radiation damage causes the formation of intracytoplasmic vacuoles and loss of neurons and satellite cells that could affect sensory function.

These injuries are distinct from the demyelination of the posterior columns associated with the self-limiting Lhermitte's syndrome.[172] Meningeal thickening and fibrosis also can be observed after radiation, but the clinical significance of these conditions is unknown. Ependymal and nerve root damage from radiation is rare.

Experimental findings that high doses of steroids are more effective than lower doses in reversing edema and improving neurologic function are consistent with findings from clinical trials, including a well-designed randomized trial in which radiation therapy was given either with high-dose corticosteroids or with placebo.[157] In that trial, the group that received corticosteroids was more likely to retain or regain ambulation than was the group that received placebo. Pain relief also was more rapid and complete with high-dose steroids (initial bolus of 100 mg followed by 4 mg of dexamethasone 4 times a day for the duration of radiation therapy) among patients suspected of having spinal cord compression.

Persistent or recurrent pain after radiation therapy for vertebral metastases should be investigated to exclude the possibility of progressive disease inside or outside the radiation portal, or mechanical spinal instability caused by a vertebral compression fracture (Fig. 38-7). Radiation-induced neural injury generally does not result in pain. Compression fractures that occur shortly after completion of radiation therapy are related more to bone insufficiency with tumor-cell kill than to the effects of radiation. Radiation-related changes in the bone marrow that appear on MRI scans after radiation therapy

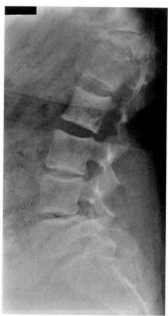

Fig. 38-7 Compression fraction of the 12th thoracic vertebral body in a patient who had previously experienced a pain-free interval after palliative radiation. Vertebral weakness and rapid tumor regression resulted in the compression fracture, which caused recurrent back pain because of spinal instability.

can be distinguished from those characteristic of progressive disease.* Trials are underway in which bone mineral density evaluations are being used to determine the response of lytic bone lesions to therapeutic radiation.[176]

Clinical and radiographic evidence suggests that leptomeningeal carcinomatosis also should be considered in the diagnostic evaluation of persistent or recurrent pain. Leptomeningeal carcinomatosis occurs more often than expected. For example, only half of the cases of leptomeningeal carcinomatosis occurring with breast cancer will be diagnosed before the patients die.[144,150,158,177,178] At least three cerebrospinal fluid samples are necessary to exclude the possibility of leptomeningeal disease, because the initial cytologic analysis fails to show tumor cells in 10% to 40% of cases.[177] MRI can identify leptomeningeal disease among patients with normal findings on cerebrospinal fluid cytology, and MRI is sensitive and specific in locating regions of nodular leptomeningeal involvement. Except for nodular leptomeningeal involvement, where localized radiation therapy may have some benefit as an adjuvant treatment, intrathecal chemotherapy is generally the treatment of choice.[178]

Treating Disseminated Bone Metastases

Other therapeutic approaches, including wide-field radiation therapy, systemic radionuclides, and bisphosphonates, have been used to treat disseminated bone metastases. Both approaches are useful in augmenting the therapeutic effect of localized radiation and in preventing the progression of asymptomatic bone lesions. Although it is not usually a significant consideration in localized irradiation, adequate bone marrow reserve is required for wide-field radiation therapy and systemic radionuclides. Bone marrow scans can be performed to determine the volume of functioning marrow and to assess the feasibility of using these techniques.[98,102,113,114,117]

Wide-Field (Hemibody) Radiation Therapy

Hemibody irradiation, with 6- to 10-Gy radiation doses given in a single fraction to the upper, middle, or lower body, has been used to treat diffuse bone metastases. Response rates are consistently reported to be more than 70%, and 20% or more of patients experience complete relief of pain. Among patients with prostate cancer, the overall response rate is 80% (30% having complete relief of pain); the mean duration of pain relief is 15 weeks, and the mean survival duration is 25 weeks.[178-181] The overall response rate for all types of primary tumors is 80%. About half of the patients who receive hemibody irradiation experience relief of pain within 48 hours of treatment. More than half of the patients so treated do not require further palliative

irradiation for recurrent bone pain over the remainder of their lives.

An RTOG study demonstrated that hemibody irradiation reduced the time to disease progression and decreased the need for subsequent palliative radiation therapy of bone metastases at 1 year of follow-up when compared with local-field irradiation alone.[180] These results are consistent with the experiences of others using hemibody irradiation.[179-181] Median survival duration after hemibody irradiation was substantially better among patients who presented with a good performance status score; approximately 90% of patients experiencing complete response and 70% of those showing partial response had a good to excellent performance status before radiation therapy. Prior systemic therapy does not influence response to wide-field radiation therapy. In one study, patients given hemibody irradiation for symptomatic bone metastases refractory to chemotherapy and hormonal therapy had complete response rates of 70% and partial response rates of 24%.[181] Symptoms were palliated in 88% of cases when a previously treated area was reirradiated. Significant toxicity was observed in less than 10% of patients, whereas 50% experienced stabilization of disease at 1 year. With current strategies, the acute toxic effects associated with hemibody irradiation are manageable. Premedication prevents nausea, and partial shielding minimizes the dose to the lung and thus the risk of radiation pneumonitis. Acute hematologic depression is limited.

Because of the potential for toxic effects to visceral structures and the difficulties in treatment set-up, hemibody irradiation is not routinely used to palliate multifocal bone metastases. Hemibody irradiation may have permanent effects on bone marrow reserve, which can be problematic if subsequent chemotherapy is needed. For these reasons, radiopharmaceuticals, which cause no systemic toxic effects other than affecting blood counts, have gained popularity over hemibody irradiation for treating multifocal bone metastases. However, radiopharmaceuticals are most useful for blastic bone lesions, and hemibody irradiation may be an important palliative option among patients with diffuse lytic bone metastases that are refractory to other therapies.

Radiopharmaceuticals

The most common radiopharmaceuticals used in the treatment of bone metastases are ^{89}Sr and ^{153}Sm. Many reports show that radiopharmaceuticals provide effective palliation of pain lasting up to 6 months in 60% to 80% of patients with breast or prostate cancer.[54-56,112,117-123,182,183] Improvements in functional status and quality of life have been observed, and about 20% of patients have complete resolution of pain.

Strontium-89. Pain control has been reported to be superior among patients with disseminated prostate cancer treated with both ^{89}Sr and localized irradiation

---

*References 98-100, 162, 166, 167, 174, 175.

compared with localized irradiation alone.[54-56] [89]Sr combines with the calcium component of hydroxyapatite in osteoblastic lesions. Because the activity of ^{89}Sr is limited to bone, its use is contraindicated when epidural disease is associated with vertebral metastases. Myelotoxicity, expressed as a 25% decline in initial platelet and white blood cell counts, is usually transient and is the only substantial toxic effect associated with [89]Sr.[54,114,117]

Several clinical trials have shown ^{89}Sr to be effective and easily administered in an outpatient setting. Because the radiation dose absorbed by the bone marrow after a dose of ^{89}Sr is 2 to 50 times less than the dose delivered to osteoblastic lesions, the radiation dose that can be delivered to metastatic bone lesions via ^{89}Sr can range from 3 Gy to more than 300 Gy.

Clinical response to ^{89}Sr, which is comparable to response to wide-field radiation therapy, has been documented in both subjective and objective terms. Subjective response, defined as symptomatic improvement in a validated survey, has been reported by more than 80% of prostate cancer patients. Evidence of objective response, documented as reductions in alkaline and acid phosphatase levels, also were associated with a decrease in uptake by metastatic lesions on sequential bone scans.[54-56,112,117-123,183] Prior therapies for prostate cancer, including localized radiation therapy and systemic chemotherapy or hormone therapy, do not influence the toxicity of or the clinical response to [89]Sr. As an adjuvant to localized external-beam radiation for treatment of metastatic prostate cancer, ^{89}Sr can improve pain relief and delay progression of disease. At 3 months' follow-up, almost twice as many patients treated with ^{89}Sr were reported to be pain-free when compared with patients treated with localized external-beam radiation.[54-56] Analgesics were no longer required by 17% of patients treated with ^{89}Sr, whereas only 2% of the patients treated with localized external-beam radiation alone were able to discontinue analgesics. Quality-of-life assessments demonstrated increased physical activity along with improved pain relief after ^{89}Sr was administered in conjunction with localized external-beam radiation. A cost-benefit analysis has suggested that the administration of ^{89}Sr results in reductions in the cost of hospitalization for tertiary care.[54-56]

Samarium-153 and other radiopharmaceuticals. Several other radiopharmaceuticals available for treatment of disseminated bone metastases include [153]Sm, gallium nitrate, ^{32}P, and [186]Re.[54-56,112,117-123,182,183] The therapeutic mechanism of action of radiopharmaceuticals reflects their physical and biological half-lives in the bone lesion, their mean energy, and the delivered dose. Table 38-5[182] summarizes some of the physical characteristics and clinical data for various radionuclides. [32]P and ^{89}Sr emit pure beta rays (little penetration in tissue), whereas [186]Re and [153]Sm emit both beta rays and relatively high-energy gamma-ray photons (103 to 159 KeV) that penetrate tissue for some distance.

Because [153]Sm has a gamma-ray component, the distribution of the radiation dose can be imaged directly. Scans generated after injection of [153]Sm are comparable with diagnostic scans obtained with technetium 99m; both show that mean skeletal uptake is more than 50% of the dose.[121] Nonskeletal sites receive negligible radiation doses, and unabsorbed radiation is cleared within 6 to 8 hours of administration.[120] In a double-blind placebo-controlled clinical trial, [153]Sm was shown to be effective in palliating painful bone metastases in patients with breast cancer.[116] Pain relief occurred within 1 week and was maintained for at least 16 weeks after administration. Approximately 65% of patients responded within the first 4 weeks, and 43% had relief of pain of at least 16 weeks' duration. No substantial toxic effects to the bone marrow have been observed. Recommended doses range from 1.0 to 1.5 mCi/kg. Multiple administrations are possible in about one third of cases.[123]

The mechanism of action of [186]Re, which concentrates selectively in bone, is similar to that of technetium diphosphonate 99m, which is used in diagnostic bone

---

TABLE 38-5

Characteristics of Radiopharmaceuticals Used to Treat Bone Metastases

Radioisotope	Radiation Type	Half-life (days)	Typical Response Rate (%)	Typical Time to Response (days)	Typical Duration of Response (months)	Extent of Myelo-suppression
Phosphorus 32	↑ Energy beta	14	78	14	1.5-11.3	3+
Strontium 89	↓ Energy beta	50	70-80	7-20	≤ 6	1+
Samarium 153	Beta/gamma	2	65	7-21	3-4	3+
Rhenium 186	Beta/gamma	4	80	7-21	2	1+
Tin 117m	Beta/gamma	14	—	—	—	?
Iodine 131	↓ Energy beta	8	72	—	≤ 2	0 to +1

From Friedland J. *Urol Clin North Am* 1999;26:391-402.

scans. This characteristic allows direct imaging of the deposition of ^{186}Re in bone metastases. The metastatic lesion receives tens of gray of radiation after administration of ^{186}Re, whereas the radiation dose to the marrow is limited to 0.75 Gy.[112,183,184] Thrombocytopenia seems to be the dose-limiting toxicity. Similar to reports of the use of ^{89}Sr in patients with prostate cancer, decreases in prostate-specific antigen levels also have been observed after the administration of ^{186}Re.[184]

^{32}P has been used for more than 30 years to treat bone metastases; 77% of patients with prostate cancer experience substantial pain relief.[112] The rates and durations of response observed with ^{32}P are similar to those observed with wide-field radiation and ^{89}Sr. However, the main disadvantage of ^{32}P is severe hematologic toxicity, which develops in about 30% of patients.

Marrow suppression resulting from radioisotopes is caused by either penetrating gamma-radiation or the long half-life of the radioisotope. For example, ^{89}Sr produces transient cytopenia because it has a fairly long half-life (51 days), even though it emits a beta particle of low penetrance and low energy (1.46 MeV) (see Table 38-5).[182] Hematologic toxicity is more pronounced in patients who begin treatment with platelet counts of less than 6×10^4, white blood cell counts of less than 2.5×10^3, or more than 30% involvement of the red marrow-bearing bone.[114,117] Compromise of red marrow-bearing bone can be a consequence of tumor or prior radiation or chemotherapy.

Comparative trials. Comparative clinical trials are necessary to determine whether any difference exists in the onset and pattern of response of ^{153}Sm, ^{89}Sr, and other radiopharmaceuticals. Clinical experience with ^{186}Re and other radiopharmaceuticals is still limited, and these agents are in various stages of clinical investigation.[54-56,112,117-123,182-184] Several strategies have been proposed to enhance the therapeutic effectiveness of these and other agents, including further dose-intensity studies, adjunctive administration of biphosphonates, and concurrent administration with chemotherapy.[118] Although bone marrow toxicity is limited with the doses of radiopharmaceuticals currently administered (either alone or in combination with other agents), future dose-intensity studies may require temporary hematologic support with colony-stimulating factors.

Sequential x-rays and bone scans after hormonal and radiopharmaceutical therapy for breast or prostate cancer demonstrate an osteoblastic response that reflects remodeling of the bone in osteolytic osseous metastases.[108,109] Approximately one third of patients will have evidence of increased tracer uptake (flare) on bone scans obtained 8 to 16 weeks after treatment. Of these patients, 72% will respond to the treatment. By comparison, only 36% of those with little or no flare will respond to treatment.

The advantages of radiopharmaceuticals include ease of administration, low toxicity, and potential for reuse. Future clinical studies will examine the use of radiopharmaceuticals earlier in the course of metastatic disease and in combination with other therapies. For example, ^{89}Sr has been combined with several other chemotherapeutic agents in the treatment of prostate cancer, and early reports suggest synergistic effects in both analgesia and cytotoxicity.[183] Other areas in which research is needed are dose and schedule of administration and selection of the radiopharmaceutical that will provide the optimal response based on tumor type and other factors.

BRAIN METASTASES

Radiation is used to relieve the symptoms of headache, seizure, nausea, vomiting, and neurologic dysfunction associated with brain metastases. Surgery, either alone or in combination with radiation, is often performed for a solitary brain metastasis if the patient's performance status is good and if the cancer burden is otherwise limited. Radiation is generally given over 2 to 3 weeks in daily fractions of 2.5 to 3 Gy. Total radiation doses range from 25 Gy (given after resection) to 30 Gy (given for unresectable disease that carries a poor prognosis) (Fig. 38-8).[185]

Reirradiation of brain tumors and brain metastases is common. The role of radiosurgery was evaluated in an RTOG study of 156 cases of recurrent brain tumor and brain metastasis.[186] Patients with recurrent brain tumors constituted 36% of the group, and these patients had had a median prior radiation dose of 60 Gy. The remaining 64% of patients had recurrent brain metastases, and their median prior radiation dose was 30 Gy. The maximum tolerated dose for tumors 2 cm or smaller was 24 Gy; that for 2 to 3-cm tumors was 18 Gy; and that for 3 to 4-cm tumors was 15 Gy.[186] Tumor size was associated with a significant increase in the risk of grade 3 or higher neurotoxicity. Tumors between 2 and 4 cm in diameter were 7 to 16 times more likely to be associated with grade 3 or higher neurotoxicity. The incidence of radiation-induced necrosis in this study was 5% at 6 months, 8% at 12 months, 9% at 19 months, and 11% at 24 months. In another study,[97] patients with recurrent brain metastases treated with a linear accelerator instead of a gamma knife had 2.8 times the risk of progression within the radiosurgical target volume. This finding was not related to patient group, because 61% of patients with recurrent brain tumors, compared with 30% of patients with brain metastases, were treated with the gamma knife.[97]

External-beam radiation therapy has been used to re-treat patients with persistent symptoms caused by brain metastases who are not candidates for radiosurgery. Generally, if symptoms recur within 3 to 4 months of administration of radiation, reirradiation is

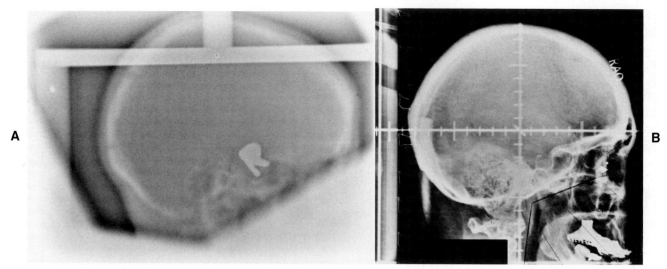

Fig. 38-8 **A,** A typical radiation portal used to treat brain metastases. **B,** A simulation film obtained to encompass the base of the skull.

unlikely to be effective. However, additional therapy may benefit patients who develop recurrent neurologic symptoms 6 to 9 months later and who have a Karnofsky performance status score of more than 50. With steroid administration and reirradiation, response rates of 60% have been reported. Generally, a total dose of 25 to 30 Gy is prescribed in 2- to 2.5-Gy fractions.[97] The risk of late toxicity depends on the total cumulative dose, volume of tumor reirradiated, and interval between the first and second course of radiation.[96] A 14% risk of necrosis exists when a dose of 86 Gy or more is given in 2-Gy fractions.

Reirradiation with external-beam radiation therapy for recurrent gliomas was investigated in 24 patients who had previously received a median radiation dose of 60 Gy.[97] With reirradiation, the total cumulative dose was limited to 92 Gy; reirradiation was given in 1.5-Gy fractions in combination with oral lomustine (130 mg/m^2 every 6 weeks). The response rate was 57%, and two patients survived more than 5 years. Median time to progression and overall survival duration were 8 and 14 months, respectively. No substantial neurologic toxicity was reported from use of this approach.[97]

Brachytherapy also has been used to treat recurrent brain tumors. This technique has been applied in select patient groups, namely those with good neurologic function and whose tumors are well-defined and located within 5 cm of midline.[97] The primary complication has been necrosis, which necessitated reoperation in 49% of patients. Median survival duration among patients with glioblastoma multiforme was 54 weeks.[97]

Prognosis also has been linked to scores on the Mini-Mental Status Examination before and after palliative radiation for brain metastases. In an RTOG study, 445 patients with brain metastases were given 1.6 Gy twice daily to a total dose of 54.4 Gy, or a radiation therapy regimen totaling 30 Gy given in 10 fractions to the entire brain. The average score before irradiation was 26.5 (range, 11 to 30); 16% of the patients had scores of less than 23 before irradiation, indicating possible dementia.[187] Median survival during treatment was 4.2 months, and 37% of patients were alive at 6 months. On multivariate analysis, the pretreatment Mini-Mental Status score and Karnofsky performance score were predictive of outcome. Survival rates of 81% at 6 months and 66% at 1 year were observed for patients whose Mini-Mental Status scores before and after irradiation were higher than 23. Death from brain metastases was associated with decline in Mini-Mental Status score and site of the primary tumor (breast vs. lung). Overall, a 30-Gy radiation dose administered over 2 weeks proved to be an effective treatment for brain metastases, and no substantial advantage was observed with a more prolonged course of therapy.

LUNG TUMORS OR METASTASES

Involvement of the lung and mediastinum, whether by a locally advanced primary tumor or metastases from elsewhere, can result in a variety of symptoms, some of them emergent, and often requires palliative intervention.[188] Pain can result from tumor invasion of the ribs and nerve roots of the chest wall (Fig. 38-9). Vertebral involvement can be associated with spinal cord compression. Obstructive pneumonitis and hemoptysis can result from bronchial obstruction. Mediastinal infiltration can cause superior vena cava syndrome.

All of these clinical presentations can be palliated with external-beam radiation that encompasses disease evident on diagnostic images and that treats pain referred

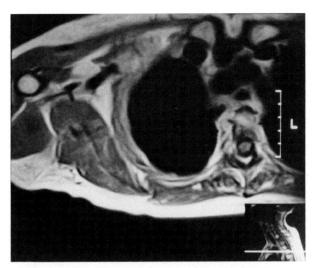

Fig. 38-9 Axial computed tomography scan showing tumor masses invading the chest wall.

along involved nerve roots. A schedule of 30 Gy of radiation delivered in 10 fractions over 2 to 3 weeks is typically prescribed for treatment of previously unirradiated sites. Using such a palliative radiation schedule in 65 patients with non–small cell lung cancer resulted in decreased hemoptysis in 79% of patients, decreased arm or shoulder pain in 56%, decreased chest-wall pain in 53%, decreased cough in 49%, and decreased dyspnea in 39%.[189] However, reductions in fatigue (experienced by 22% of patients) and loss of appetite (experienced by 11%) were minimal. Decreases in dyspnea strongly correlated with radiographic evidence of response.[189] Although palliative radiation is effective, most patients will have residual symptoms that require medical management.

If the tumor site has been previously irradiated, radiation therapy techniques that exclude critical anatomic structures such as the spinal cord are used. A review of more than 1500 cases of lung cancer treated from 1982 to 1997 revealed that 23 patients underwent reirradiation for relief of symptoms.[190] Median duration of follow-up was 3.2 months (range, 0 to 17.5 months). Consistent with other published reports, hemoptysis decreased or resolved in all 6 patients with that symptom, 4 of 5 patients had reduced pain, 9 of 15 had reduced coughing, and 11 of 15 had decreased dyspnea.[190] The risk of radiation pneumonitis associated with such treatments can be decreased by using narrow margins around the radiation portal.

Other approaches, such as brachytherapy, can be used when the symptomatic site is well localized and accessible. In these cases, large doses of radiation can be delivered within a few minutes by a high-dose-rate brachytherapy unit.[94,181] Brachytherapy can be used as a boost to external-beam radiation therapy or to re-treat a previously irradiated area. Precise details of techniques and radiation doses vary, but most schedules involve giving 6 to 10 Gy every 1 to 2 weeks for up to three fractions or a single

fraction of 10 to 20 Gy. Overall symptom response rates range between 70% and 90%, and palliation is durable in 60% of patients.[181] Relief of specific symptoms included hemoptysis in 54% of patients, cough in 94%, dyspnea in 86%, and pulmonary collapse in 51%.[94]

Patients with recurrent symptoms can be treated with another round of brachytherapy or with other methods. The incidence of radiation bronchitis and stenosis among such patients was 17%, and fatal hemoptysis occurred in 5.5%. Tumors of the right main-stem bronchus and the right upper-lobe bronchus seem to be more susceptible to development of fatal hemorrhage than left-sided lesions.

Symptoms of dyspnea should be addressed medically while a response to radiation therapy is awaited. Oxygen therapy, maintenance of adequate hemoglobin levels, and opioids are effective treatments for dyspnea; respiratory depression will not occur if the patients have been previously treated with opioids. Although benzodiazepines often are used, such agents have been found to be ineffective in four of five randomized trials.[191]

Brachytherapy also has been used in the treatment of esophageal cancer. Relief of dysphagia in several reports ranges between 70% and 85%.[94] A combination of a short course of external-beam radiation (30 Gy in 10 fractions) plus brachytherapy as a boost relieves dysphagia for 3 to 6 months. Relative contraindications include a tumor length of 10 cm or more, extension to the gastroesophageal junction or cardia, skip lesions, extensive extraesophageal spread, macroscopic regional adenopathy, tracheoesophageal fistula, cervical esophageal involvement, or stenosis that cannot be bypassed.[94]

HEAD AND NECK TUMORS

Palliation of locally advanced head and neck malignancies often requires a more protracted radiation schedule because of the sensitivity of the structures, such as the arytenoids and cervical spinal cord, in the radiation field. List and colleagues[192] evaluated quality-of-life variables before and during chemoradiation for locally advanced head and neck cancer and at 3-month intervals after treatment. Severe treatment-related toxic effects led to declines in all quality-of-life and functional domains. By 12 months, marked improvement was observed, although up to one third of patients continued to experience difficulty swallowing, hoarseness, and mouth or throat pain, all of which were present at levels comparable to those before treatment. Substantial increases in dry mouth (58% vs. 17%), inability to distinguish tastes (32% vs. 8%), and the need for a soft-food diet (82% vs. 42%) were documented after chemoradiation. The pretreatment quality-of-life level was the best predictor of quality of life, regardless of residual side effects or functional impairment.

Aggressive management of treatment-related side effects can improve tolerance of head and neck irradiation.

In a study by Janjan and colleagues,[193] symptoms of head and neck irradiation were effectively controlled by using a specific pain management regimen that included opioid analgesics. With this regimen, the incidence of pain lasting more than 12 hours/day decreased by 35%, and the incidence of mean weight loss of more than 5 kg decreased by 41%. Moderate to severe pain during the first week of radiation therapy was noted in 15% of patients in this study. Significant improvements in symptom control were observed from the use of opioid analgesics over the use of traditional codeine elixirs to control symptoms. Pain intensity decreased by 11% by the third week of radiation therapy, by 24% during the fifth week, and by 26% during the seventh week. At the completion of radiation therapy, pain intensity at its worst was mild in 43% of patients, moderate in 23% of patients, and severe in 6%. The frequency of the pain was occasional in 46% of patients, most of the day in 17%, and always in 6%.

Late radiation effects are of particular concern in reirradiation of recurrent head and neck cancer. In a recent assessment of the total biological effect of the retreatment of recurrent nasopharyngeal cancer,[194] the severity of damage during the initial course of radiation was the major determinant of complications associated with retreatment. Repair of normal tissues was evident because the tolerated doses were higher than expected for a single course of radiation.[194] The complication-free survival rate at 5 years was actually lower in the retreatment group (48%) than in a group initially treated with a single course of radiation (81%). A 20% risk of complications at 5 years would occur with a total biologically equivalent dose of 143 Gy_3 (where Gy_3 indicates an alpha/beta ratio of 3) with retreatment or 111 Gy_3 among patients treated with a single course.

PELVIC DISEASE

Locally advanced or metastatic disease in the pelvis often presents as hemorrhage and visceral, lymphovascular, or nerve root obstruction. Treatment may require emergent radiation therapy or surgery. Hemorrhage is commonly associated with tumors involving the rectum and genitourinary tracts. As is true for tumors in the lung, radiation is an effective means of stopping active bleeding. Colorectal cancer is often diagnosed among patients with unexplained bleeding.

Colorectal tumor involvement also can produce obstruction, often requiring the placement of a stent to maintain the integrity of the visceral lumen while the radiation is being given.[188,195] Occasionally, a diverting colostomy will be required to bypass intestinal obstruction or the formation of a fistula. If these procedures are not performed, intestinal colic can be palliated quickly with opioids, but anticholinergics such as scopolamine, atropine, and loperamide decrease peristalsis in the smooth muscle of the intestinal tract.[195,196] Intestinal obstruction also can produce nausea and vomiting, which can be palliated with nasogastric decompression and pharmacologic agents. Octreotide, an analogue of somatostatin, reduces gastrointestinal secretions, motility, and splanchnic blood flow; has a proabsorptive effect on water and ions; and may inhibit the secretion of vasoactive intestinal peptides. These actions help to disrupt the cycle of distention-intestinal secretion-peristalsis and bleeding.[196,197]

Because colorectal tumors tend to be locally advanced, radiation therapy is given preoperatively with conventional fractionation if little or no metastatic disease is evident. This regimen is intended to stop bleeding, render the tumor operable, and provide a chance for cure. For extensive metastatic disease, 30 to 35 Gy of radiation can be given over 2 to 3 weeks to palliate symptoms of bleeding and obstruction. In two studies, 35 Gy in 14 fractions, 30 Gy in 10 fractions, and 30 Gy in 6 fractions were given twice weekly for 3 weeks for this purpose.[198,199] A diverting colostomy was required in 16% of patients before radiation therapy. No substantial treatment-related toxic effects were observed. Regardless of whether radiation was given in conventional or hypofractionated schedules or with or without infusional fluorouracil, symptoms from the primary tumor resolved in 94% of cases, and the endoscopic complete response rate was 36%.

The colostomy-free survival rate was 87% among patients who underwent palliative chemoradiation and 51% among patients who received preoperative chemoradiation. When surgery was performed, the 2-year survival rate was 46%, compared with 11% after palliative chemoradiation. Control of symptomatic pelvic disease was not substantially different between the two treatments (81% for palliative chemoradiation and 91% for preoperative chemoradiation).[198] Predictors of control of pelvic disease included the severity of pelvic pain at presentation, a biologically equivalent radiation dose of less than 35 Gy at 2 Gy/fraction, and poor tumor differentiation. Poor tumor differentiation and selection for palliative chemoradiation were predictive of a worse overall survival.

Tumors involving the cervix can hemorrhage and require emergent radiation therapy. Superficial x-rays applied directly to the bleeding cervix through a cone can treat the bleeding site and do not compromise later irradiation of other pelvic structures.[188] Usually cone therapy involves radiation doses of between 5 and 10 Gy given in 1 to 3 applications. Brachytherapy also can be used to treat gynecologic tumors, especially those in the vagina, cervix, and endometrium.

Bladder cancer or tumors that secondarily invade the bladder also can result in significant bleeding that can be palliated by external-beam radiation therapy. Urinary obstruction is common in locally advanced pelvic cancer, especially tumors of the prostate and cervix.

Occasionally, placement of a urinary stent or a urostomy or nephrostomy will be required until radiation-induced tumor regression is sufficient to reestablish the integrity of the urinary tract.[188] As is true for the bowel and gynecologic tracts, formation of vesical fistulae, either from the tumor itself or from tumor regression, remains a concern.

In one recent study,[200] palliative radiation administered as 35 Gy in 10 fractions or 21 Gy in 3 fractions was evaluated among 272 patients with bladder cancer. At a follow-up of at least 3 months, 71% of those who received 35 Gy and 64% of those who received 21 Gy achieved symptomatic improvement.[200] No difference in the radiation schedules was noted in terms of efficacy, toxicity, or survival. The overall survival rate was approximately 77% at 3 months, 35% at 12 months, and 19% at 24 months.

The pelvic lymph nodes and major blood vessels can become obstructed by tumor. This condition occurs most often when tumors arise in pelvic structures but also can occur with pelvic metastases from breast and other types of cancer.[188] Lymphovascular obstruction results in painful edema that is refractory to diuretic and other therapies. Severe obstruction can lead to fluid and electrolyte imbalances. Pelvic irradiation can relieve lymphovascular obstruction by causing tumor regression.

Pelvic tumors also can invade the sacral plexus and result in intractable pain. Such tumors proceed along nerve roots and can invade the sacrum as well. Pain caused by visceral obstruction, lymphovascular obstruction, or both often responds more rapidly to palliative radiation than does the neuropathic pain arising from sacral plexus involvement. Other radiation therapy approaches such as brachytherapy are of limited effectiveness when the cancer persists or recurs after external-beam radiation; pain management techniques are often required to control pain associated with sacral plexus involvement.

Reirradiation of the pelvis for symptomatic recurrence has generally been well tolerated, although data are limited. Care must be taken to exclude the intestines from the radiation portals given the risk of late small-bowel toxicity. Although data on treatment volume are limited, the cumulative radiation dose, reirradiation dose, and time interval between courses were not found to be related to late toxicity.[96]

SKIN AND SUBCUTANEOUS-TISSUE INVOLVEMENT

Tumors can cause ulceration of the skin and subcutaneous tissues that is often painful and distressing because of constant drainage as well as creating the potential for the development of sepsis in immunocompromised patients. Localized radiation can be used to destroy tumor and allow reepithelialization of the skin.

Electron-beam radiation therapy is generally used because it can better target the skin and subcutaneous tissues while avoiding irradiation of underlying normal structures. Although 10 radiation treatments are usually given, the course of radiation can be abbreviated further and can be administered over 1 to 5 days. Occasionally, skin and subcutaneous lesions are treated with brachytherapy, in which the radioactive sources are placed in a mold that sits on top of the tumor and treatment is delivered over a few minutes (for high-dose-rate therapy) or over a few days (for low-dose-rate therapy).

CONCLUSIONS
Diagnostic Recommendations

Pain that persists after palliative radiation should be evaluated to exclude progression of disease in the treated area; extension of disease outside the radiation portal, which can cause referred pain; and bone fracture. Reduced cortical strength can result in compression, stress, or microfractures. Plain radiographs often clearly delineate lytic changes and fractures after radiation therapy.

Therapeutic Recommendations

Radiation therapy remains an important modality in palliative care. Several clinical, prognostic, and therapeutic factors must be considered in choosing the optimal regimen. Adequate management of cancer-related pain is important both during and after palliative irradiation. For locally advanced and metastatic cancer, efficient and effective palliative treatment is imperative to relieve symptoms, improve function, and minimize disease-related morbidity.

More specific prognostic criteria are needed to identify the appropriate treatment regimen for bone metastases. A staging system for metastatic disease affecting the skeleton should take into consideration performance status, type and extent of bone and visceral involvement, time to disease progression, and primary tumor site and should account for prior failed therapies as well. Because only the bone is treated, external-beam radiation or radiopharmaceuticals continue to be considered localized therapies for systemic disease. The response to and outcomes after radiation therapy must be specifically defined relative to the irradiated and unirradiated sites of disease, and other antineoplastic and supportive care therapies should be administered as needed.

Radiation therapy is an important means of treating localized symptoms related to tumor involvement because it provides a wide range of therapeutic options. Radiobiological principles, the radiation tolerance of adjacent normal tissues, and the patient's clinical condition influence selection of the radiation technique, dose, and fraction size. However, the optimal dose and treatment schedule is not fully defined. Further study is necessary to integrate validated pain scores, use of analgesics, prognostic factors, and radiobiological principles to better define the most efficient and efficacious treatment schedule according to the clinical presentation.

Palliative irradiation should be integrated into multidisciplinary therapeutic approaches because of the need to treat associated symptoms and other underlying medical problems. Antineoplastic therapy can induce tumor regression, relieve cancer-related symptoms, and maintain functional integrity. Control of cancer-related pain through the use of analgesics is imperative to provide comfort during radiation therapy and while awaiting response to that therapy. Pain represents a sensitive measure of disease activity. Close follow-up should be performed to ensure control of cancer and treatment-related pain and to identify progressive or recurrent disease.

REFERENCES

1. Cleeland CS, Gonin R, Hatfield AK, et al. Pain and its treatment in outpatients with metastatic cancer. *N Engl J Med* 1994;330: 592-596.
2. Jacox AK, Carr DB, Payne R, eds. *Management of Cancer Pain. Clinical Practice Guideline No. 9.* Rockville, Md: Agency for Health Care Policy and Research; 1994 (AHCPR publication 94-0592).
3. Jacox A, Carr DB, Payne R. New clinical practice guidelines for the management of pain in patients with cancer. *N Engl J Med* 1994; 330:651-655.
4. Brescia FJ, Portenoy RK, Ryan M, et al. Pain, opioid use, and survival in hospitalized patients with advanced cancer. *J Clin Oncol* 1992;10:149-155.
5. Greenlee RT, Hill-Harmon MB, Murray T, et al. Cancer statistics, 2001. *CA Cancer J Clin* 2001;51:15-36.
6. Anonymous. Outcomes of cancer treatment for technology assessment and cancer treatment guidelines. American Society of Clinical Oncology. *J Clin Oncol* 1996;14:671-679.
7. Cassel EJ. The nature of suffering and the goals of medicine. *N Engl J Med* 1982;306:639-645.
8. Porzsolt F. Goals of palliative cancer therapy: scope of the problem. *Cancer Treat Rev* 1993;19(suppl A):3-14.
9. Rubens RD. Approaches to palliation and its evaluation. *Cancer Treat Rev* 1993;19(suppl A):67-71.
10. Porzsolt F, Tannock I. Goals of palliative cancer therapy. *J Clin Oncol* 1993;11:378-381.
11. Cella DF, Tulsky DS. Quality of life in cancer: definition, purpose, and method of measurement. *Cancer Invest* 1993;11:327-336.
12. Janjan NA. Radiation for bone metastases-conventional techniques and the role of systemic radiopharmaceuticals. *Cancer* 1997;80:1628-1645.
13. Liu L, Meers K, Capurso A, et al. The impact of radiation therapy on quality of life in patients with cancer. *Cancer Practice* 1998; 6:237-242.
14. Arcangeli G, Micheli A, Arcangeli F, et al. The responsiveness of bone metastases to radiotherapy: the effect of site, histology and radiation dose on pain relief. *Radiother Oncol* 1989;14:95-101.
15. Mithal NP, Needham PR, Hoskin PJ. Retreatment with radiotherapy for painful bone metastases. *Int J Radiat Oncol Biol Phys* 1994;29:1011-1014.
16. Manfredi PL, Chandler S, Pigazzi A, et al. Outcomes of cancer pain consultations. *Cancer* 2000;89:920-924.
17. Janjan NA, Payne R, Gillis T, et al. Presenting symptoms in patients referred to a multidisciplinary clinic for bone metastases. *J Pain Symptom Manage* 1998;16:171-178.
18. Stafford RS, Cyr PL. The impact of cancer on the physical function of the elderly and their utilization of health care. *Cancer* 1997;80:1973-1980.
19. Cohen HJ. Cancer and the functional status of the elderly. *Cancer* 1997;80:1883-1886.
20. Hanks GE. The crisis in health care costs in the United States: some implications for radiation oncology. *Int J Radiat Oncol Biol Phys* 1992;23:203-206.
21. Emanuel EJ, Fairclough DL, Slutsman J, et al. Understanding economic and other burdens of terminal illness: the experience of patients and their caregivers. *Ann Intern Med* 2000;132:451-459.
22. Rabow MW, Hardie GE, Fair JM, et al. End of life care content in 50 textbooks from multiple specialties. *JAMA* 2000;283:771-778.
23. Morita T, Tsunoda J, Inoue S, et al. Contributing factors to physical symptoms in terminally ill cancer patients. *J Pain Symptom Manage* 1999;18:338-346.
24. Pargeon KL, Hailey BJ. Barriers to effective cancer pain management: a review of the literature. *J Pain Symptom Manage* 1999;18: 358-368.
25. Von Roenn JH, Cleeland CS, Gonin R, et al. Physicians attitudes and practice in cancer pain management: a survey from the Eastern Cooperative Oncology Group. *Ann Intern Med* 1993;119:121-126.
26. Sherry MM, Greco FA, Johnson DH, et al. Breast cancer with skeletal metastases at initial diagnosis-distinctive clinical characteristics and favorable prognosis. *Cancer* 1986;58:178-182.
27. Sherry MM, Greco FA, Johnson DH, et al. Metastatic breast cancer confined to the skeletal system. *Am J Med* 1986;81:381-386.
28. Jacobson AF. Musculoskeletal pain as an indicator of occult malignancy. *Arch Intern Med* 1997;157:105-109.
29. Vuorinen E. Pain as an early symptom in cancer. *Clin J Pain* 1993; 9:272-278.
30. Pienta KJ, Esper PS. Risk factors for prostate cancer. *Ann Intern Med* 1993;118:793-833.
31. Abbas F, Scardino PT. The natural history of clinical prostate carcinoma. *Cancer* 1997;80:827-833.
32. Chisholm GD, Rana A, Howard GCW. Management options for painful carcinoma of the prostate. *Semin Oncol* 1993; 20(suppl 2):34-37.
33. Borre M, Nerstrom B, Overgaard J. The natural history of prostate carcinoma based on a Danish population treated with no intent to cure. *Cancer* 1997;80:917-928.
34. Soloway MS, Hardeman SW, Hickey D, et al. Stratification of patients with metastatic prostate cancer based on extent of disease on initial bone scan. *Cancer* 1988;61:195-202.
35. Yamashita K, Denno K, Ueda T, et al. Prognostic significance of bone metastases in patients with metastatic prostate cancer. *Cancer* 1993;71:1297-1302.
36. Perez CA, Cosmatos D, Garcia DM, et al. Irradiation in relapsing carcinoma of the prostate. *Cancer* 1993;71:1110-1122.
37. Lai PP, Perez CA, Lockett MA. Prognostic significance of pelvic recurrence and distant metastases in prostate carcinoma following definitive radiotherapy. *Int J Radiat Oncol Biol Phys* 1992;24:423-430.
38. Chang VT, Thaler HT, Polyak TA, et al. Quality of life and survival-the role of multidimensional symptom assessment. *Cancer* 1998;83:173-179.
39. Grabowski CM, Unger JA, Potish RA. Factors predictive of completion of treatment and survival after palliative radiation therapy. *Radiology* 1992;184:329-332.
40. Reuben DB, Mor V, Hiris J. Clinical symptoms and length of survival in patients with terminal cancer. *Arch Int Med* 1988;148: 1586-1591.
41. Fielding LP, Henson DE. Multiple prognostic factors and outcome analysis in patients with cancer-communication from the American Joint Committee on Cancer. *Cancer* 1993;71:2426-2429.
42. Portenoy RK, Miransky J, Thaler HT, et al. Pain in ambulatory patients with lung or colon cancer. *Cancer* 1992;70:1616-1624.

43. Knudson G, Grinis G, Lopez-Majano V, et al. Bone scan as a stratification variable in advanced prostate cancer. *Cancer* 1991; 68:316-320.

44. Sabbatini P, Larson SM, Kremer A, et al. Prognostic significance of extent of disease in bone in patients with androgen-independent prostate cancer. *J Clin Oncol* 1999;17:948-957.

45. Vigano A, Bruera E, Jhangri GS, et al. Clinical survival predictors in patients with advanced cancer. *Arch Intern Med* 2000;160:861-868.

46. Cleeland CS, Janjan NA, Scott CB, et al. Cancer pain management by radiotherapists: a survey of Radiation Oncology Group physicians. *Int J Radiat Oncol Biol Phys* 2000;47:203-208.

47. Lamont EB, Christakis NA. Some elements of prognosis in terminal cancer. *Oncology* 1999;13:1165-1170.

48. No authors listed. SUPPORT: Study to understand prognoses and preferences for outcomes and risks of treatments. Study design. *J Clin Epidemiol* 1990;43:1S-123S.

49. Zhong Z, Lynn J. Review of the Lamont/Christakis article. *Oncology* 1999;13:1172-1173.

50. Archer VR, Billingham LJ, Cullen MH. Palliative chemotherapy: no longer a contradiction in terms. *The Oncologist* 1999;4:470-477.

51. Oh WK, Kantoff PW. Treatment of locally advanced prostate cancer: is chemotherapy the next step? *J Clin Oncol* 1999;17: 3664-3675.

52. Janjan NA. An emerging respect for palliative care in radiation oncology. *J Palliat Med* 1998;1:83-88.

53. SBU-The Swedish Council on Technology Assessment in Health Care. *Acta Oncologica* 1997;35(suppl 6, vol 1):89-97.

54. Porter AT, Ben-Josef E. Strontium 89 in the treatment of bony metastases. In: DeVita VT, Hellman S, Rosenberg SA, eds. *Important Advances in Oncology*. Philadelphia, Pa: JB Lippincott; 1995:87-94.

55. Porter AT, McEwan AJB, Powe JE, et al. Results of a randomized Phase III trial to evaluate the efficacy of Strontium 89 adjuvant to local field external beam irradiation in the management of endocrine resistant metastatic prostate cancer. *Int J Radiat Oncol Biol Phys* 1993;25:805-813.

56. Porter AT, McEwan AJB. Strontium 89 as an adjuvant to external beam radiation improves pain relief and delays in disease progression in advanced prostate cancer: results of a randomized controlled trial. *Semin Oncol* 1993;20:38-43.

57. Dale RG, Jones B. Radiobiologically based assessments of the net costs of fractionated radiotherapy. *Int J Radiat Oncol Biol Phys* 1996;36:739-746.

58. Janjan NA. Radiotherapeutic approaches to cancer pain management. *Highlights Oncol Prac* 1997;14:103-113.

59. Hillner BE, Weeks JC, Desch CE, et al. Pamidronate in prevention of bone complications in metastatic breast cancer: a cost-effectiveness analysis. *J Clin Oncol* 2000;18:72-79.

60. Dranitsaris G, Hsu T. Cost utility analysis of prophylactic pamidronate for the prevention of skeletal related events in patients with advanced breast cancer. *Support Care Cancer* 1999; 7:271-279.

61. Macklis RM, Cornelli H, Lasher J. Brief courses of palliative radiotherapy for metastatic bone pain. *Am J Clin Oncol* 1998; 21:617-622.

62. Hortobagyi GN, Theriault RL, Porter L, et al. Efficacy of pamidronate in reducing skeletal complications with breast cancer and lytic bone metastases. *N Engl J Med* 1996;335:1785-1791.

63. Hortobagyi GN, Theriault RL, Lipton A, et al. Long-term prevention of skeletal complications of metastatic breast cancer with pamidronate. *J Clin Oncol* 1998;16:2038-2044.

64. Theriault RL, Lipton A, Hortobagyi GN, et al. Pamidronate reduces skeletal morbidity in women with advanced breast cancer and lytic bone lesions: a randomized, placebo-controlled trial—Protocol 18 Aredia Breast Cancer Study Group. *J Clin Oncol* 1999; 17:846-854.

65. Lipton A, Theriault RL, Hortobagyi GN, et al. Pamidronate prevents skeletal complications and is effective palliative treatment in women with breast carcinoma and osteolytic bone metastases. *Cancer* 2000;88:1082-1090.

66. Body JJ, Bartl R, Burckhardt P, et al. Current use of bisphosphonates in oncology. *J Clin Oncol* 1998;16:3890-3899.

67. Bloomfield DJ. Should bisphosphonates be part of the standard therapy of patients with multiple myeloma or bone metastases from other cancers? An evidence-based review. *J Clin Oncol* 1998; 16:1218-1225.

68. Lipton A. Bisphosphonates and breast cancer. *Cancer* 1997;80: 1668-1673.

69. Hillner BE. The role of bisphosphonates in metastatic breast cancer. *Semin Radiat Oncol* 2000;10:250-253.

70. Diel IJ, Solomayer EF, Costa SD, et al. Reduction in new metastases in breast cancer with adjuvant clodronate treatment. *N Engl J Med* 1998;339:357-363.

71. Thames HD, Buchholz TA, Smith CD. Frequency of first metastatic events in breast cancer: implications for sequencing of systemic and local-regional treatment. *J Clin Oncol* 1999;17: 2649-2658.

72. Kelly JB, Payne R. Pain syndromes in the cancer patient. *Neurologic Clinics* 1991;9:937-953.

73. Portenoy RK. Cancer pain management. *Semin Oncol* 1993;20: 19-35.

74. Foley KM, Arbelt E. Management of cancer pain. In: DeVita VT, Hellman S, Rosenberg SA, eds. *Cancer: Principles and Practice of Oncology*. 3rd ed. Philadelphia, Pa: JB Lippincott; 1989: Vol. 2, pp. 2064-2087.

75. Paice JA, Toy C, Shott S. Barriers to cancer pain relief: fear of tolerance and addiction. *J Pain Symptom Manage* 1998;16:1-9.

76. Weissman, DE. Doctors, opioids, and the law: the effect of controlled substances regulations on cancer pain management. *Semin Oncol* 1993;20(2 suppl 1):53-58.

77. Hill CS. The barriers to adequate pain management with opioid analgesics. *Semin Oncol* 1993;20(2 suppl 1):1-5.

78. Lebovits AH, Florence I, Bathina R, et al. Pain knowledge and attitudes of healthcare providers: practice characteristic differences. *Clin J Pain* 1997;13:237-243.

79. Joranson DE, Ryan KM, Gilson AM, et al. Trends in medical use and abuse of opioid analgesics. *JAMA* 2000;283:1710-1714.

80. World Health Organization. *Cancer Pain Relief*. Geneva, Switzerland:World Health Organization; 1986.

81. Lipman AG. New and alternative noninvasive opioid dosage forms and routes of administration. In: Berger A, Portenoy RK, Weissman DE, eds. *Principles and Practice of Supportive Oncology*, Update 2000;3:1-8.

82. Hassenbusch SJ, Portenoy RK. Current practices in intraspinal therapy–a survey of clinical trends and decision making. *J Pain Symptom Manage* 2000;20:S4-S11.

83. Bennett G, Serafini M, Burchiel K, et al. Evidence-based review of the literature on intrathecal delivery of pain medication. *J Pain Symptom Manage* 2000;20:S12-S36.

84. Bennett G, Burchiel K, Buchser E, et al. Clinical guidelines for intraspinal infusion: report of an expert panel. *J Pain Symptom Manage* 2000;20:S37-S43.

85. Ratanatharathorn V, Powers WE, Moss WT, et al. Bone metastases: review and critical analysis of random allocation trials of local field treatment. *Int J Radiation Oncol Biol Phys* 1999;44:1-18.

86. Awan AM, Weichselbaum RR. Palliative radiotherapy. *Hematol Oncol Clin North Am* 1990;4:1169-1181.

87. Bates T, Yarnold JR, Blitzer P, et al. Bone metastases consensus statement. *Int J Radiat Oncol Biol Phys* 1992;23:215-216.

88. Bates T. A review of local radiotherapy in the treatment of bone metastases and cord compression. *Int J Radiat Oncol Biol Phys* 1992;23:217-221.

89. Niewald M, Tkocz HJ, Abel U, et al. Rapid course radiation therapy vs. more standard treatment: a randomized trial for bone metastases. *Int J Radiat Oncol Biol Phys* 1996;36:1085-1089.

90. Gaze MN, Kelly CG, Kerr GR, et al. Pain relief and quality of life following radiotherapy for bone metastases: a randomised trial of two fractionation schedules. *Radiother Oncol* 1997;45:109-116.

91. Ben-Josef E, Shamsa F, Williams AO, et al. Radiotherapeutic management of osseous metastases: a survey of current patterns of care. *Int J Radiat Oncol Biol Phys* 1998;40:915-921.

92. Rose CM, Kagan AR. The final report of the expert panel for the Radiation Oncology Bone Metastasis Work Group of the American College of Radiology. *Int J Radiat Oncol Biol Phys* 1998; 40:1117-1124.

93. Powers WE, Ratanatharathorn V. Palliation of bone metastases. In: Perez CA, Brady LW, eds. *Principles and Practice of Radiation Oncology*. 3rd ed. Philadelphia, Pa: Lippincott Raven; 1998: 2199-2219.

94. Shasha D, Harrison LB. The role of brachytherapy for palliation. *Semin Radiat Oncol* 2000;10:221-239.

95. Bilsky MH, Lis E, Raizer J, et al. The diagnosis and treatment of metastatic spinal tumor. *The Oncologist* 1999;4:459-469.

96. Nieder C, Milas L, Ang KK. Tissue tolerance to reirradiation. *Semin Radiat Oncol* 2000;10:200-209.

97. Morris DE. Clinical experience with retreatment for palliation. *Semin Radiat Oncol* 2000;10:210-221.

98. Steiner RM, Mitchell DG, Rao VM, et al. Magnetic resonance imaging of diffuse bone marrow disease. *Radiol Clin North Am* 1993;31:383-409.

99. Algra PR, Bloem JL, Tissing H, et al. Detection of vertebral metastases: comparison between MR imaging and bone scintigraphy. *Radiographics* 1991;11:219-232.

100. Le Bihan DJ. Differentiation of benign versus pathologic compression fractures with diffusion-weighted MR imaging: a closer step toward the "holy grail" of tissue characterization? *Radiology* 1998;207:305-307.

101. Albright JA, Gillespie, TE, Butaud TR. Treatment of bone metastases. *Semin Oncol* 1980;7:418-433.

102. Nielsen OS, Munro AJ, Tannock IF. Bone metastases: pathophysiology and management policy. *J Clin Oncol* 1991;9:509-524.

103. Hendrix RW, Rogers LF, Davis TM Jr. Cortical bone metastases. *Radiology* 1991;181:409-413.

104. Garrett IR. Bone destruction in cancer. *Semin Oncol* 1993; 20(suppl 2):4-9.

105. Orr FW, Kostenuik P, Sanchez-Sweatman OH, et al. Mechanisms involved in the metastasis of cancer to bone. *Breast Cancer Res Treat* 1993;25:151-163.

106. Ford HT, Yarnold JR. Radiation therapy—pain relief and recalcification. In: Stoll BA, Parbhoo S, eds. *Bone Metastases: Monitoring and Treatment*. New York, NY: Raven; 1983:343-354.

107. Mercadante S. Malignant bone pain: pathophysiology and treatment. *Pain* 1997;69:1-18.

108. Hortobagyi GN, Libshitz HI, Seabold JE. Osseous metastases of breast cancer-clinical, biochemical, radiographic, and scintigraphic evaluation of response to therapy. *Cancer* 1984;53: 577-582.

109. Vogel CL, Schoenfelder J, Shemano I, et al. Worsening bone scan in the evaluation of antitumor response during hormonal therapy of breast cancer. *J Clin Oncol* 1995;13:1123-1128.

110. Pluijm G, Lowik C, Papapoulos S. Tumour progression and angiogenesis in bone metastasis from breast cancer: new approaches to an old problem. *Cancer Treat Rev* 2000;26:11-27.

111. Conte PF, Latreille J, Mauriac L, et al. Delay in progression of bone metastases in breast cancer patients treated with intravenous pamidronate: results from a multinational randomized controlled trial. *J Clin Oncol* 1996;14:2552-2559.

112. Holmes RA. Radiopharmaceuticals in clinical trials. *Semin Oncol* 1993;20:22-26.

113. Robinson RG, Preston DF, Baxter KG, et al. Clinical experience with Strontium 89 in prostatic and breast cancer patients. *Semin Oncol* 1993;20:44-48.

114. Robinson RG, Preston DF, Schiefelbein M, et al. Strontium 89 therapy for the palliation of pain due to osseous metastases. *JAMA* 1995;274:420-424.

115. Krishnamurthy GT, Swailem FM, Srivastava SC, et al. Tin-117m(4+)DTPA: pharmacokinetics and imaging characteristics in patients with metastatic bone pain. *J Nucl Med* 1997;38: 230-237.

116. Serafini AN, Houston SJ, Resche I, et al. Palliation of pain associated with metastatic bone cancer using samarium-153 lexidronam: a double-blind placebo-controlled clinical trial. *J Clin Oncol* 1998;16:1574-1581.

117. Rogers CL, Speiser BL, Ram PC, et al. Efficacy and toxicity of intravenous strontium-89 for symptomatic osseous metastases. *J Brachytherapy International* 1998;14:133-142.

118. Sciuto R, Maini CL, Tofani A, et al. Radiosensitization with low-dose carboplatin enhances pain palliation in radioisotope therapy with strontium-89. *Nucl Med Commun* 1996;17:799-804.

119. Bolger JJ, Dearnaley DP, Kirk D, et al. Strontium-89 [metastron] versus external beam radiotherapy in patient with painful bone metastases secondary to prostatic cancer: preliminary report of a multicenter trial. *Semin in Oncol* 1993;20:32-33.

120. Eary JF, Collins C, Stabin M, et al. Samarium 153-EDTMP biodistribution and dosimetry estimation. *J Nucl Med* 1993;34:1031-1036.

121. Bayouth JE, Macey DJ, Kasi LP, et al. Doimetry and toxicity of samarium-153-EDTMP administered for bone pain due to skeletal metastases. *J Nucl Med* 1994;35:63-69.

122. McEwan AJB, Amyotte GA, McGowan DG, et al. A retrospective analysis of the cost-effectiveness of treatment with metastron in patients with prostate cancer metastatic to bone. *Eur Urol* 1994;26:26-31.

123. Alberts AS, Smit BJ, Louw WKA, et al. Dose response relationship and multiple dose efficacy and toxicity of samarium-153-EDTMP in metastatic cancer to bone. *Radiother Oncol* 1997; 43:175-179.

124. Tong D, Gillick L, Hendrickson FR. The palliation of symptomatic osseous metastases: final results of the study by the Radiation Therapy Oncology Group. *Cancer* 1982;50:893-899.

125. Blitzer PH. Reanalysis of the RTOG study of the palliation of symptomatic osseous metastasis. *Cancer* 1985;55:1468-1472.

126. Rutten EHJM, Crul BJP, van der Toorn PPG, et al. Pain characteristics help to predict the analgesic efficacy of radiotherapy for the treatment of cancer pain. *Pain* 1997;69:131-135.

127. Rasmusson B, Vejborg I, Jensen AB, et al. Irradiation of bone metastases in breast cancer patients: a randomized study with 1 year follow-up. *Radiother Oncol* 1995;34:179-184.

128. Niewald M, Tkocz HJ, Abel U, et al. Rapid course radiation therapy vs. more standard treatment: a randomized trial for bone metastases. *Int J Radiat Oncol Biol Phys* 1996;36:1085-1089.

129. Dawson R, Currow D, Stevens G, et al. Radiotherapy for bone metastases: a critical appraisal of outcome measures. *J Pain Symptom Manage* 1999;17:208-218.

130. Chandler SS, Sarin R. Single fraction radiotherapy for bone metastases: are all questions answered? *Radiother Oncol* 1999; 52:191-193.

131. Gillick LS, Goldberg S. Technical Report No 185R. *Final Analysis of RTOG Protocol No. 74-02*. Boston: Department of Biostatistics, Sidney Farber Cancer Institute; 1981.

132. Jeremic B, Shibamoto Y, Adimovic L, et al. A randomized trial of three single-dose radiation therapy regimens in the treatment of metastatic bone pain. *Int J Radiat Oncol Biol Phys* 1998; 42:161-167.

133. Nielsen OS. Palliative radiotherapy of bone metastases: there is now evidence for the use of single fractions. *Radiother Oncol* 1999;52:95-96.

134. Steenland E, Leer JW, van Houwelingen H, et al. The effect of a single fraction compared to multiple fractions on painful bone

metastases: a global analysis of the Dutch Bone Metastasis Study. *Radiother Oncol* 1999;52:101-109.

135. Barton M. Tables of equivalent dose in 2 Gy fractions: a simple application of the linear quadratic formula. *Int J Radiat Oncol Biol Phys* 1995;31:371-378.

136. Jeremic B, Shibamoto Y, Igrutinovic I. Single 4 Gy re-irradiation for painful bone metastasis following single fraction radiotherapy. *Radiother Oncol* 1999;52:123-127.

137. Nielsen OS, Bentzen SM, Sandberg E, et al. Randomized trial of single dose versus fractionated palliative radiotherapy of bone metastases. *Radiother Oncol* 1998;47:233-240.

138. Bone Pain Trial Working Party. 8 Gy single fraction radiotherapy for the treatment of metastatic skeletal pain: randomised comparison with a multifraction schedule over 12 months of patient follow-up. *Radiother Oncol* 1999;52:111-121.

139. Barak F, Werner A, Walach N, et al. The palliative efficacy of a single high dose of radiation in treatment of symptomatic osseous metastases. *Int J Radiat Oncol Biol Phys* 1987;13:1233-1235.

140. Cole DJ. A randomized trial of a single treatment versus conventional fractionation in the palliative radiotherapy of painful bone metastases. *Clin Oncol* 1989;1:59-62.

141. Hoskin PJ, Price P, Easton D, et al. A prospective randomised trial of 4 Gy or 8 Gy single doses in the treatment of metastatic bone pain. *Radiother Oncol* 1992;23:74-78.

142. Price P, Hoskin PJ, Easton D, et al. Prospective randomised trial of single and multifraction radiotherapy schedules in the treatment of painful bone metastases. *Radiother Oncol* 1986; 6:247-255.

143. Madsen EL. Painful bone metastasis: efficacy of radiotherapy assessed by the patients: a randomized trial compairing 4 Gy × 6 versus 10 Gy x 2. *Int J Radiat Oncol Biol Phys* 1983;9:1775-1779.

144. Boogerd W, van der Sande JJ. Diagnosis and treatment of spinal cord compression in malignant disease. *Cancer Treat Reviews* 1993;19:129-150.

145. Byrne TN. Spinal cord compression from epidural metastases. *New Engl J Med* 1992;327:614-619.

146. Grant R, Papadopoulos SM, Greenberg HS. Metastatic epidural spinal cord compression. *Neurol Clin* 1991;9:825-841.

147. Maranzano E, Latini P, Checcaglini F, et al. Radiation therapy in metastatic spinal cord compression–a prospective analysis of 105 consecutive patients. *Cancer* 1991;67:1311-1317.

148. Janjan NA. Radiotherapeutic management of spinal metastases. *J Pain Symptom Manage* 1996;1:47-56.

149. Loblaw DA, Laperriere NJ. Emergency treatment of malignant extradural spinal cord compression: an evidence-based guideline. *J Clin Oncol* 1998;16:1613-1624.

150. Boogerd W. Central nervous system metastasis in breast cancer. *Radiother Oncol* 1996;40:5-22.

151. Paterson AHG. Bone metastases in breast cancer, prostate cancer and myeloma. *Bone* 1987;8(suppl 1):17-22.

152. Bunting RW, Boublik M, Blevins FT, et al. Functional outcome of pathologic fracture secondary to malignant disease in a rehabilitation hospital. *Cancer* 1992;69:98-102.

153. Townsend PW, Smalley SR, Cozad SC, et al. Role of postoperative radiation therapy after stabilization of fractures caused by metastatic disease. *Int J Radiat Oncol Biol Phys* 1995;31:43-49.

154. Heisterberg L, Johansen TS. Treatment of pathologic fractures. *Acta Orthop Scand* 1979;50:787-790.

155. Fidler M. Incidence of fracture through metastases in long bones. *Acta Orthop Scand* 1981;52:623-627.

156. Oda MAS, Schurman DJ. Monitoring of pathological fracture. In: Stoll BA, Parbhoo S, eds. *Bone Metastases: Monitoring and Treatment*. New York, NY: Raven; 1983:271-288.

157. Quinn JA, De Angelis LM. Neurologic emergencies in the cancer patient. *Semin Oncol* 2000;27:311-321.

158. Boogerd W, van der Sande JJ, Kroger R. Early diagnosis and treatment of spinal metastases in breast cancer: a prospective study. *J Neurol Neurosurg Psychiatry* 1992;55:1188-1193.

159. Turner S, Marosszeky B, Timms I, et al. Malignant spinal cord compression: a prospective evaluation. *Int J Radiat Oncol Biol Phys* 1993;26:141-146.

160. Peteet J, Tay V, Cohen G, MacIntyre J. Pain characteristics and treatment in an outpatient cancer population. *Cancer* 1985;57:1259-1265.

161. Wada E, Yamamoto T, Furuno M, et al. Spinal cord compression secondary to osteoblastic metastasis. *Spine* 1993;18:1380-1381.

162. Algra PR, Heimans JJ, Valk J, et al. Do metastases in vertebrae begin in the body or the pedicles?—imaging study in 45 patients. *AJR Am J Roentgenol* 1992;158:1275-1279.

163. Landmann C, Hunig R, Gratzi O. The role of laminectomy in the combined treatment of metastatic spinal cord compression. *Int J Radiat Oncol Biol Phys* 1992;24:627-631.

164. Kim RY, Smith JW, Spencer SA, et al. Malignant epidural spinal cord compression associated with a paravertebral mass: its radiotherapeutic outcome on radiosensitivity. *Int J Radiat Oncol Biol Phys* 1993;27:1079-1083.

165. Bach F, Agerlin N, Sorensen JB, et al. Metastatic spinal cord compression secondary to lung cancer. *J Clin Oncol* 1992;10:1781-1787.

166. Schiff D, O'Neill BP, Wang CH, et al. Neuroimaging and treatment implications of patients with multiple epidural spinal metastases. *Cancer* 1998;83:1593-1601.

167. Saip P, Tenekeci N, Aydiner A, et al. Response evaluation of bone metastases in breast cancer: value of magnetic resonance imaging. *Cancer Invest* 1999;17:575-580.

168. Cowap J, Hardy JR, A'Hearn R. Outcome of malignant spinal cord compression at a cancer center: implications for palliative care services. *J Pain Symptom Manage* 2000;19:257-264.

169. Maranzano E, Latini P, Perrucci E, et al. Short-course radiotherapy [8 Gy x 2] in metastatic spinal cord compression: an effective and feasible treatment. *Int J Radiat Oncol Biol Phys* 1997;38:1037-1044.

170. Jeremic B, Djuric L, Mijatovic L. Incidence of radiation myelitis of the cervical spinal cord at doses of 5500 cGy or greater. *Cancer* 1991;68:2138-2141.

171. Wen PY, Blanchard KL, Block CC, et al. Development of Lhermitte's sign after bone marrow transplantation. *Cancer* 1992;69:2262-2266.

172. Powers BE, Thames HD, Gillette SM, et al. Volume effects in the irradiated canine spinal cord: do they exist when the probability of injury is low? *Radiother Oncol* 1998;46:297-306.

173. Fowler JF, Bentzen SM, Bond SJ, et al. Clinical radiation doses for spinal cord: the 1998 international questionnaire. *Radiother Oncol* 2000;55:295-300.

174. Sugimura H, Kisanuki A, Tamura S, et al. Magnetic resonance imaging of bone marrow changes after irradiation. *Invest Radiol* 1994;29:35-41.

175. Yankelevitz DF, Henschke C, Knapp PH, et al. Effect of radiation therapy on thoracic and lumbar bone marrow: evaluation with MR imaging. *Am J Roentgenol* 1991;157:87-92.

176. Shapiro CL, Keating J, Angell JE, et al. Monitoring therapeutic response in skeletal metastases using dual-energy x-ray absorptiometry: a prospective feasibility study in breast cancer patients. *Cancer Invest* 1999;17:566-574.

177. Bach F, Bjerregaard B, Soletormos G, et al. Diagnostic value of cerebrospinal fluid cytology in comparison with tumor marker activity in central nervous system metastases secondary to breast cancer. *Cancer* 1993;72:2376-2382.

178. Russi EG, Pergolizzi S, Gaeta M, et al. Palliative radiotherapy in lumbosacral carcinomatous neuropathy. *Radiother Oncol* 1993; 26:172-173.

179. Salazar OM, Rubin P, Hendrickson FR, et al. Single-dose half-body irradiation for palliation of multiple bone metastases from solid tumors—final Radiation Therapy Oncology Group Report. *Cancer* 1986;58:29-36.

180. Poulter CA, Cosmatos D, Rubin P, et al. A report of RTOG 8206: A phase III study of whether the addition of single dose hemi-body irradiation to standard fractionated local field irradiation is more effective than local field irradiation alone in the treatment of symptomatic osseous metastases. *Int J Radiat Oncol Biol Phys* 1992;23:207-214.

181. Barton R, Kirkbride P. Special techniques in palliative radiation oncology. *J Palliative Med* 2000;3:75-83.

182. Friedland J. Local and systemic radiation for palliation of metastatic disease. *Urol Clin North Am* 1999;26:391-402.

183. Silberstein EB. Systemic radiopharmaceutical therapy of painful osteoblastic metastases. *Semin Radiat Oncol* 2000;10:240-249.

184. De Klerk JMH, Zonnenberg BA, van het Schip AD, et al. Dose escalation study of rhenium-186 hydroxyethylidene disphosphonate in patients with metastatic prostate cancer. *Eur J Nucl Med* 1994;21:1114-1120.

185. Kagan AR. Palliation of brain and spinal cord metastases. In: Perez CA, Brady LW, eds. *Principles and Practice of Radiation Oncology*. 3rd ed. Philadelphia, Pa: Lippincott Raven; 1998: 2187-2198.

186. Shaw E, Scott C, Souhami L, et al. Single dose radiosurgical treatment of recurrent previously irradiated primary brain tumors and brain metastases: final report of RTOG Protocol 90-05. *Int J Radiat Oncol Biol Phys* 2000;47:291-298.

187. Murray KJ, Scott C, Zachariah B, et al. Importance of the mini-mental status examination in the treatment of patients with brain metastases: a report from the Radiation Therapy Oncology Group Protocol 91-04. *Int J Radiat Oncol Biol Phys* 2000;48:59-64.

188. Kagan AR. Palliation of visceral recurrences and metastases. In: Perez CA, Brady LW, eds. *Principles and Practice of Radiation Oncology*, 3rd ed. Philadelphia, Pa: Lippincott Raven; 1998:2219-2226.

189. Langenduk JA, ten Velde GPM, Aaronson NK, et al. Quality of life after palliative radiotherapy in non-small cell lung cancer: a prospective study. *Int J Radiat Oncol Biol Phys* 2000;47:149-155.

190. Gressen EL, Werner-Waski M, Cohn J, et al. Thoracic reirradiation for symptomatic relief after prior radiotherapeutic management for lung cancer. *Am J Clin Oncol* 2000;23:160-163.

191. Ripamonti C. Management of dyspnea in advanced cancer patients. *Support Care Cancer* 1999;7:233-243.

192. List MA, Siston A, Haraf D, et al. Quality of life and performance in advanced head and neck cancer patients on concomitant chemoradiotherapy: a prospective examination. *J Clin Oncol* 1999;17:1020-1028.

193. Janjan NA, Weissman DE, Pahule A. Improved pain management during radiation therapy for head and neck carcinoma. *Int J Radiat Oncol Biol Phys* 1992;23:647-652.

194. Lee AWM, Foo W, Law SCK, et al. Total biological effect on late reactive tissues following reirradiation for recurrent nasopharyngeal carcinoma. *Int J Radiat Oncol Biol Phys* 2000;46:865-872.

195. Mancini I, Bruera E. Constipation in advanced cancer patients. *Support Care Cancer* 1998;6:356-364.

196. Rousseau P. Management of malignant bowel obstruction in advanced cancer: a brief review. *J Palliative Med* 1998;1:65-72.

197. Gagnon B, Mancini I, Pereira J, et al. Palliative management of bleeding events in advanced cancer patients. *J Palliative Care* 1998;14:50-54.

198. Crane CH, Janjan NA, Abbruzzese JL, et al. Effective pelvic symptom control using initial chemoradiation without colostomy in metastatic rectal cancer. *Int J Radiat Oncol Biol Phys* 2001; 49:107-116.

199. Janjan NA, Breslin T, Lenzi R, et al. Avoidance of colostomy placement in advanced colorectal cancer with twice weekly hypofractionated radiation plus continuous infusion 5-fluorouracil. *J Pain Symptom Manage* 2000;20:266-272.

200. Duchesne GM, Bolger JJ, Griffiths GO, et al. A randomized trial of hypofractionated schedules of palliative radiotherapy in the management of bladder carcinoma: results of medical research council trial BA09. *Int J Radiat Oncol Biol Phys* 2000; 47:379-388.

CHAPTER 39

Clinical Applications of New Modalities

Craig W. Stevens

Cancer treatment is changing rapidly in several ways. Technical innovations have allowed three-dimensional conformal radiation therapy (CRT) and intensity-modulated radiation therapy (IMRT) to become widespread. Stereotactic radiosurgery will expand beyond the cranium to the lung and other sites. Patient/tumor positioning will become more precise with the use of real-time portal imaging and sonography, respiratory gating, and megavoltage computed tomography (CT). The use of proton and other exotic particle therapy may further improve radiation dose delivery.

Functional imaging will be integrated into treatment planning. This integration is already beginning with ^{18}F-fludeoxyglucose (FDG) positron emission tomography (PET) scanning and has the potential to involve assessments of hypoxia, cell surface markers, protein synthesis, blood flow, cell proliferation, apoptosis, and many other processes.

Molecular oncology also is rapidly advancing. As recently as a few years ago, the most interesting new therapies involved taxanes or topoisomerase inhibitors. Although important, these agents simply represented new classes of cytotoxic chemotherapy—new agents that exploit minor differences between tumor and normal tissue to produce cytotoxic effects. In contrast, the next generation of *molecular chemotherapy* will target critical molecular events in the carcinogenic process and will be advanced through rational drug development processes. Targets for this approach include growth factors (and their receptors), signal transduction cascades, cell cycle control, angiogenesis, and immune responses. Some agents to be used in molecular chemotherapy can be applied relatively indiscriminately to a given tumor type, such as the use of farnesyl transferase inhibitors to target *ras* protein signaling in lung cancer. Others such as Herceptin therapy against *HER-2/neu* will require molecular assessment of individual tumors before therapy is begun. Thus molecular staging may become as important as the physical staging done today. Eventually, molecular imaging of each patient's tumor may allow therapy to be tailored to each patient.

The number of classes of therapies will also increase. Gene therapy will include viruses and specific oligonucleotides. Clinical application of antibodies and other protein-based therapies will increase. Immunotherapy will likely be used to improve antitumor immune response and may range from tumor vaccines to cytokine-based gene therapy.

As the molecular consequences of therapy for cancer continue to be revealed, new protectors will be developed to further improve the therapeutic index. Amifostine is currently in clinical trials. Promising new agents include keratinocyte growth factor (KGF) and combinations of pentoxifylline and vitamin E.

The ability of clinicians to maintain a current knowledge of the oncologic literature requires a substantial understanding of molecular biology, immunology, cancer biology, physics, and imaging. The oncology team will grow to include a wide array of experts in imaging, interventional radiology, molecular oncology and immunology. Ultimately, it will be the task of these physicians to integrate all this information to make sound decisions for our patients. The reader of this chapter is encouraged to follow the literature closely and supplement it with MEDLINE searches to keep up to date on current protocols (i.e., by following the protocol lists by means of the Physician's Data Query at http://cancernet.nci.nih.gov/pdq.htm).

NEW TECHNOLOGY

The goals of improved treatment planning and the use of exotic particle therapy are to improve the therapeutic ratio by reducing the toxicity of radiation therapy while ensuring that effective doses are delivered to the tumor.

Three-Dimensional Conformal or Intensity-Modulated Radiation Therapy

The ability to conform radiation dose distributions to include tumor but spare normal tissue is the hallmark of modern radiation therapy. Three-dimensional CRT was originally described soon after the development of CT scanning.[1,2] Most of the practical implementation aspects have been developed at Memorial Sloan-Kettering Cancer Center,[3] the University of Michigan,[4] the University of Washington,[5] and the University of North Carolina.[6]

Modern treatment planning requires high-resolution CT scanning to accurately map tumor and normal anatomic structures while the patient lies immobilized in the treatment position. Using three-dimensional reconstructed images, treatment portals are then designed to treat the entire tumor volume while avoiding normal tissue to the greatest extent possible. This often, but not necessarily, involves the use of noncoplanar beams that have been custom-blocked, wedged, and appropriately weighted. Advanced software to optimize beam weightings has been developed in a few centers but is not generally available. This technique has been implemented for use in most disease sites and has, for the most part, replaced traditional two-dimensional approaches for all but palliative cases. Conformal radiation therapy produces dose distributions that compare favorably with those of brachytherapy,[7] and in carefully selected patients has efficacy[8] similar to that of brachytherapy. Although brachytherapy offers slightly better dose distribution, brachytherapy is much more difficult to learn, and its clinical effectiveness depends greatly on the skills of the operator.

The most extensive experience with three-dimensional CRT has been in the treatment of prostate cancer, and several excellent reviews of this application have been published.[9,10] Investigators have found that, compared with patients treated with two-dimensional techniques, patients treated with three-dimensional CRT techniques had a higher local control rate and a lower complication rate.[11,12] The 5-year actuarial risk of developing grade 3 late gastrointestinal toxic effects was approximately 0.75%, and that of developing grade 3 late genitourinary toxic effects was approximately 3%[8,13]; these values are significantly lower than the risk of similar toxic effects associated with conventional beam arrangements. These improvements have allowed dose escalation to almost 80 Gy with acceptable toxicity. The best approach to three-dimensional CRT is IMRT because this method provides the most homogeneous dose distribution within the prostate and the lowest critical organ doses.[14] Although the costs of initial work-up and treatment are higher with IMRT/three-dimensional CRT than with standard therapy, the long-term costs are similar because three-dimensional CRT offers improved rates of toxicity and disease-free survival.[15]

Several potential pitfalls have been described in the three-dimensional CRT process. First, the existence of a learning curve for three-dimensional CRT implies that initial plans for implementing this technique will be generated slowly and that training time for physicians, physicists, dosimetrists, and radiation therapists will be needed. It is recommended that training begin on a tumor site for which much published literature exists, such as the prostate. *International Commission on Radiation Units and Measurement Reports 50* and *62* describe the standard nomenclature for prescribing, recording, and reporting photon-beam data pertinent to three-dimensional CRT.[16,17]

A second potential problem can arise when the anatomy shown by CT scans is assumed to be correct simply because much detail is visible. Clinicians must remember that the images do not show or account for tumor motion, although such motion might have been apparent during fluoroscopy. This failure of CT to recognize tumor motion is particularly important for thoracic and abdominal tumors, in which gating may be required.[18] Potential inconsistencies in set-up and patient positioning, penumbral effects, and tissue nonhomogeneity must be accounted for in the planning margins. The main goal of three-dimensional CRT is to better define structures and not necessarily to narrow the treatment margins. A third potential problem is that although expansion of gross tumor volumes to planning target volumes is relatively simple with most planning systems, the uniformly symmetric expansion of margins involved in three-dimensional CRT is not logical in all cases (e.g., brain tumors are unlikely to be located outside the skull).

Despite these few caveats, three-dimensional CRT is a very powerful tool that allows normal tissue to be spared and, where needed, radiation dosage to be escalated. Clinically significant sparing of normal tissue with three-dimensional CRT techniques has been demonstrated for parotids,[19] pediatric tumors,[20] brain,[21] and many other tumors. In addition, three-dimensional CRT can be used to treat recurrent tumors more safely than could be done using traditional techniques.[22] Three-dimensional CRT is being developed for non–small cell lung carcinoma (NSCLC), which can improve the normal tissue dose-volume histogram,[23] but is best achieved if clinically uninvolved nodes are not irradiated.[24] Whether this is a good idea awaits clinical trials.

Stereotactic Radiosurgery

Radiosurgery is a technique to deliver very large radiation fractions to a small volume of tissue with precise immobilization. The technique was first described by Leksell in 1949.[25] The main features that distinguish radiosurgery from standard external-beam radiation therapy are as follows: (1) treatment volumes are small; (2) single (or a few) large fractions are delivered with the intent of obliterating all living tissue with the high-dose region; (3) a large number of fields, or arcs, are used to spread entrance and exit doses over a large volume; and (4) set-up typically requires a head frame/halo for very precise (approximately 1 mm or less) set-up, although this type of precision is difficult to achieve in extracranial sites.

To date, most radiosurgery targets have been intracranial because the precise patient positioning needed to limit the toxicity associated with this technique is possible with the use of head frames. Radiosurgery has been used successfully to treat a variety of intracranial diseases, including arteriovenous malformations, acoustic neuromas, meningiomas, gliomas, and brain metastases. Glomus tumors and nasopharyngeal and paranasal sinus tumors have also been treated by using halo immobilization.

Recently, radiosurgery techniques have been applied to extracranial sites, most often in the lung and liver for the treatment of metastases.[26-28] The main problem that arises with extracranial radiosurgery is that patient immobilization is much less precise, with set-up uncertainty in the range of 3 to 5 mm, than it is for intracranial radiosurgery. Fortunately, these extracranial sites can usually afford the larger treatment margins because of the inherent redundancy of the organ tissues involved. This technique will become important as more early-stage lung cancer is detected through CT screening[29] and may be applicable to a variety of other tumors for which current treatments are associated with very high rates of local failure, such as pancreatic cancer.

Protons and Other Exotic Particles

Another approach to improving isodose distribution is through the use of particles with Bragg peaks; examples of such particles include protons, pions, and helium nuclei. These particles cause most of their ionizations at an energy-dependent depth with almost no exit dose. The entrance doses tend to be approximately 70% to 80% of the target dose, depending on the size of the target and on the depth. Although the dosimetry associated with the technique is very efficient, these particles are very expensive to deliver. Very-high-energy accelerators are needed to generate clinically useful beams (100 to 800 MeV for protons), which are also very difficult to bend and shape. Some diseases such as tumors of the eye are clearly best treated with protons.[30,31]

As can be seen in Color Plate 37, after p. 80, the high-dose region of IMRT and proton plans are very similar and conform quite well to the planning target volumes. Standard photon dose distributions (see Color Plate 37, *A* and *B*) are clearly inferior to those generated either by photon IMRT or by protons. However, compared with proton treatment, IMRT photon treatment exposes a much greater body volume to modest doses because of the exit dose from the photon beams. These differences are likely to be important in cases in which tumors are near regions with low radiation tolerance (e.g., lung, kidney, or previously treated volumes) and for younger patients who have many years in which to develop second malignancies that may require further radiation therapy. Clinical trials will be needed to determine whether these differences merit the use of proton therapy despite its higher cost.

Radiation Protectors

Another approach to decreasing the toxicity associated with radiation treatment is to use compounds that protect normal tissues from the effects of such treatment. Two strategies for radioprotection are discussed below.

Amifostine

Amifostine (WR-2721) is an organic thiophosphate compound that was initially developed during World War II to protect soldiers from the acute effects of battlefield irradiation. WR-2721 is rapidly dephosphorylated to WR-1065 by alkaline phosphatase in endothelial cells, and all of the radioprotective effects can be attributed to the WR-1065 metabolite.[32] Several excellent recent reviews of amifostine have been published.[33,34] Amifostine protects bone marrow from the effects of hemibody irradiation,[35] cyclophosphamide,[36] cisplatin,[37] mitomycin C,[38] and paclitaxel.[39] The agent also helps prevent the salivary dysfunction associated with radioiodine therapy for patients with thyroid carcinoma.[40] In fact, amifostine accumulates in the salivary glands[41] and has been shown to decrease the levels of xerostomia in patients irradiated for head and neck cancer. Amifostine also reduces the nephrotoxicity[42] and neurotoxicity caused by cisplatin. This agent also reduces the acute mucositis from irradiation of the head and neck[43] but is poorly tolerated if given twice per day. Table 39-1 demonstrates that amifostine can reduce both grade 4 toxicity and the duration of the use of a feeding tube in patients receiving radiation therapy alone for head and neck cancer. The major and dose-limiting toxicities of this agent are emesis, hypotension, and malaise.[44] Despite its protective effects on normal tissue, amifostine does not protect tumors from the effects of chemotherapy or radiation therapy and thus may well have a useful role in cancer therapy.

Keratinocyte Growth Factor

KGF is a mitogen for many epithelial tissues. Thus theoretically then, it could be used to increase the cellularity of normal mucosa such as the esophagus before or during radiation therapy and so reduce toxicity. However, KGF could be applied in this manner only if tumor cells did not respond to KGF. Interestingly, KGF does not seem to stimulate growth of colon carcinoma cells, even though the receptor for KGF is present on the surface of colon carcinoma cells[45]; furthermore, pretreatment or rodents with KGF significantly improved the survival rate after either radiation therapy or chemotherapy.[46] However, the concentration of KGF receptor correlates with the depth of invasion in endometrial carcinoma,[47] and KGF stimulates cell division in breast cancer[48]; thus it is unlikely that KGF can be used to increase normal cellular proliferation (and so reduce toxicity) in all disease sites. The application of KGF to patients undergoing radiation therapy is under active clinical investigation.

Molecular Targets

Unlike the trial-and-error approach used to discover traditional chemotherapeutic agents, modern drug

TABLE 39-1

Acute Mucosal Reactions and Duration of Use of a Feeding Tube in Patients Treated with Amifostine

	Amifostine			Control			
MUCOSITIS							
Maximum grade	2	3	4	2	3	4	
WHO*	1	10	1	1	3	8	($P < 0.02$) (Mantel-Haenszel)
RTOG*	4	7	1	1	11	0	(NS)
Mean duration of "at least grade 3" (WHO), days	25.1 (6.21 SE)			49.2 (8.33 SE)			($P < 0.03$) (t-test)
FEEDING TUBE (DURATION OF USE, MONTHS)							
Median	0.8			2.3			
Mean	1			2.5			($P < 0.01$) (t-test)

From Bourhis J, De Crevoisier R, Abdulkarim B, et al. *Int J Radiat Oncol Biol Phys* 2000;46:1105-1108.
WHO, World Health Organization; *RTOG,* Radiation Therapy Oncology Group; *NS,* not significant; *SE,* standard error.
*One patient in each group could not be evaluated for this item.

discovery is more of a rational development process that takes advantage of a better understanding of the molecular differences between normal and neoplastic tissue or that targets pathways that are critical to maintaining cell survival (e.g., replacement of wild-type *p53*, leading to apoptosis of malignant cells but not adjacent normal cells). The number of potential therapeutic targets is constantly increasing, and the agents described below have been selected as examples. With so many new targets and drugs to test, it will be difficult to choose which to study first. However, clinical scientists are obliged to study those agents and targets most likely to benefit their patients rather than those most likely to attract funding for research.

Hypoxia

The radiation dosage required by hypoxic cells is three times the dosage required by aerobic cells to achieve an equivalent level of killing by ionizing irradiation. The oxygen concentration curve for the oxygen effect is quite steep, such that most of the radiosensitization from oxygen occurs by the time an oxygen pressure of 10 mm Hg has been obtained. Tumor hypoxia is thought to be one of the principal culprits in radiation therapy failure. In 1955, Thomlinson and Gray reported the first evidence of hypoxia in human tumors[49]; these researchers found gradients of viable and necrotic cells radially situated near blood vessels in human lung metastases. The viable cells were closest to the vessels, which are a source of oxygen, whereas the necrotic cells were the most distant (more than 150 µm) from the blood vessels. As tumors enlarge to a radius that exceeds this distance, many of their cells die; but between the aerobic and anoxic

regions is a zone of hypoxic but viable (and radio-resistant) cells. Radiation-induced death of aerobic cells should make oxygen available to previously hypoxic cells, resulting in reoxygenation of tumors. Both tumor hypoxia and tumor reoxygenation after radiation therapy have been measured in animal models and humans.[50-53]

It is now possible to accurately quantify oxygen within human tumors in situ. Workers have shown that hypoxia was present in carcinoma of the uterine cervix and that this hypoxia was independent of stage and grade of tumor[54] but correlated with vascular density and necrosis.[55] Hypoxia was present in the tumor periphery, which is typically believed to be well oxygenated, and in the central regions of tumor. Similar results have been found in patients with carcinoma of the breast[56] and head and neck.[57] None of these studies attempted to determine the relationship between these findings and clinical outcome after treatment. However, other studies have shown that hypoxia is an independent predictor of outcome in tumors of the cervix (both primary[58] and recurrent[59]), head and neck,[60] and brain.

Specific toxins have been developed to kill hypoxic cells. These toxins have varied widely (e.g., *Clostridium*-based gene therapy and gene therapy driven by hypoxia-inducible promoters[61]), but the hypoxic-cell toxin most used in the clinic is tirapazamine (TPZ).[62,63] TPZ is a benzotriazine di-N-oxide that, under hypoxic conditions, is rapidly metabolized to a toxic intermediate by P_{450} reductase.[64] TPZ-induced cytotoxicity depends on the rate of drug metabolism, the oxygen concentration, the ability of target cells to repair DNA damage,[65] and the free radical scavenging capabilities of the target cells.

TPZ is an excellent radiosensitizer for use with large, single radiation fractions[66] and for fractionated radiation therapy, providing a dose-modifying factor of 1.5 to 3.0.[67] TPZ also significantly increases the tumor cytotoxicity of cisplatin,[68] carboplatin, cyclophosphamide,[69] doxorubicin, etoposide, fluorouracil, and paclitaxel. Among these drugs, fluorouracil was the only agent noted to have mildly increased systemic toxicity when used after pretreatment with TPZ. The activities of cyclophosphamide, doxorubicin, etoposide, and paclitaxel were enhanced most when TPZ was given 24 hours before the chemotherapeutic agent.[70] TPZ increases the toxic effects of both hyperthermia and radioimmunotherapy.[71]

A recently completed phase III study compared the outcome of 466 patients with very advanced (stage IIB or IV) NSCLC who were randomly assigned to receive, with palliative intent, either cisplatin alone or cisplatin plus TPZ.[72] The results showed a significant increase in the median survival time for patients given TPZ (34.6 vs. 27.7 weeks; P = 0.0078) (Fig. 39-1). It is not clear that this use of TPZ will cure more patients with advanced lung cancer, but the results suggest that such treatment in combination with surgery or radiation therapy could be useful in earlier-stage disease. Toxicity was similar in both treatment groups. Multiple radiation-TPZ or chemoradiation-TPZ trials are under way for lung, cervix, and head and neck cancer. The major effects of toxicity of TPZ are muscle cramping, vomiting, and fatigue.[73]

Unfortunately, hypoxia may cause problems other than increased radioresistance or chemoresistance. Brizel and colleagues demonstrated that hypoxia correlated strongly with survival time and the development of distant metastases in patients with poorly differentiated soft tissue sarcoma,[74] suggesting that hypoxia may be a marker for tumor aggressiveness in addition to radiation

therapy failure. The authors' own preliminary observations in patients with stage T1 or T2 clinical N0 NSCLC tumors suggest that hypoxia predicts for the presence of unsuspected intrathoracic metastases. These data suggest that, compared with patients with nonhypoxic tumors, patients with hypoxic tumors might require more aggressive systemic treatment. Hypoxia has been proposed to be the major selective factor for determining whether cells acquire mutations and deletions of *p53*.[75] Thus although preliminary results are heartening, it must be remembered that, if the principal effect of hypoxia is to select for metastasis-prone or apoptosis-resistant cells, better systemic therapy will still be required for hypoxic tumors regardless of the use of TPZ.

Signal Transduction Cascades

One of the most important differences between tumors and normal cells is the uncontrolled division of tumor cells, which is caused by accumulated changes to normal cell signaling pathways for growth and apoptosis. Workers have hypothesized that if these changes can be corrected or blocked, then tumor cells might become more sensitive to treatment or might simply die. Therefore much research has been performed to better understand cell growth, cell cycle control, and apoptosis to guide the design of molecular therapies. Several examples are discussed below and in the section on "Immunotherapy" (Herceptin and C225) later in this chapter.

Farnesyltransferase Inhibitors

Ras oncogenes are activated by point mutations in many types of human cancer, such as 7% to 80% of cases of colorectal cancer, 25% to 87% of cases of pancreatic cancer, and 25% to 48% of cases of NSCLC.[76] The *ras* proteins serve as intermediaries between many

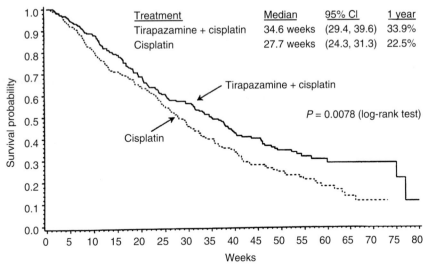

Treatment	Median	95% CI	1 year
Tirapazamine + cisplatin	34.6 weeks	(29.4, 39.6)	33.9%
Cisplatin	27.7 weeks	(24.3, 31.3)	22.5%

P = 0.0078 (log-rank test)

Fig. 39-1 Time to disease progression in 466 patients with non–small cell lung carcinoma treated with cisplatin alone or cisplatin plus tirapazamine. (From von Pawel J, von Roemeling R, Gatzemeier U, et al. *J Clin Oncol* 2000;18:1351-1359.)

cell surface receptors and intracellular kinases and are a subgroup of G-proteins that use guanosine triphosphate to regulate activation of these downstream kinases. Point mutations in the guanosine triphosphate binding site lead to constitutive activation of *ras* and fool the cell into acting as though mitogenic signals are being delivered to the extracellular surface of the plasma membrane. *Ras* proteins must be present on the intracellular surface of the plasma membrane to be active and must be prenylated (either by farnesylation or geranyl-geranylation) to be transported to the membrane. The prenylation step is therefore a possible target to inactivate *ras* signaling. Various small molecules have also been developed to block the downstream effects of *ras* activation, such as the mitogen-activated protein kinase activation,[77,78] but are beyond the scope of this chapter.

Activation of the *ras* oncogene is associated with an increase in radioresistance in some systems,[79] and blocking ras prenylation can also radiosensitize tumor cells.[80] Upstream oncogenic effects (e.g., upregulation of growth factor receptors) can also be blocked by inhibiting *ras* prenylation.[81] Other known effects of *ras* signaling pathways include vascular endothelial growth factor upregulation in response to hypoxia.[82] These findings suggest that clinical use of farnesyltransferase inhibitors concurrently with radiation therapy could increase local tumor control, at least for those tumors known to harbor *ras* mutations.

p53 Gene Therapy

Gene therapy has the potential to correct genetic alterations in malignant cells (i.e., gene replacement therapy), target tumor cells with toxic genes (i.e., cytotoxic gene therapy), improve tolerance to therapy (by improving detoxification of chemotherapy via bone marrow progenitors), conduct immunotherapy (by delivering cytokines or other immunostimulatory molecules to tumors in situ), or purge bone marrow of neoplastic cells (e.g., by treating bone marrow with cytotoxic adenovirus with high affinity for epithelial cells).[83] Gene therapy generally has three components: (1) a gene of interest (e.g., *p53*); (2) a promoter element, either constitutively active or organ-specific (e.g., the prostate-specific antigen promoter), to control gene expression; and (3) a viral vector with high affinity for the target cell population (e.g., adenovirus for epithelial cells, herpesvirus for neural/glial cells, or lentivirus for bone marrow cells). Alternatively, gene therapy can involve an antisense approach using small oligonucleotides that are complementary to a specific mutation (usually to down-regulate dominantly acting oncogenes).

The original concept of gene replacement therapy involves the replacement of genes, usually tumor suppressor genes,[84] whose function has been lost during oncogenesis. The major advantage of this approach is that the transgene would be relatively nontoxic to adjacent normal tissues because these tissues already contain the endogenous copies. The major disadvantage is that maximum effect can occur only if every tumor cell is transduced. Gene replacement therapy is best used in combination with other types of therapy, both local and systemic. The paradigm for this approach is the *p53* gene, which is described below.

Radiation therapy can be used in a variety of ways to improve the effects of gene therapy.[85] First, radiation therapy is synergistic with the cell killing mechanism of many gene therapy strategies. The high spatial conformality of both intratumoral gene therapy injections and radiation therapy can cooperate to produce a desired effect. Second, radiation-inducible promoters have been developed that can increase transgene production in areas of high radiation dosage. This strategy has the potential to become more useful after better systemically injected vectors are developed. Third, gene therapy vectors can be developed to produce high levels of radiosensitizers at the site of intratumoral injection, thereby potentially decreasing the required radiation dosage. Fourth, radiation may actually increase the amount of vector that enters target cells, at least for some cell types.[86]

Alterations in the *p53* gene are present in approximately 50% of types of human cancer and are the most common mutations in human malignancy. The wild-type p53 protein is itself a tumor suppressor gene important for apoptosis, cell cycle checkpoints, and genomic stability. A wide array of point mutations causes *p53* stabilization but results in a protein that can no longer function properly in one or more cellular pathways. Proper *p53* regulation occurs by the interaction of this protein with its negative regulator MDM-2 and by phosphorylation and acetylation at many sites. It seemed likely, then, that replacement of wild-type *p53* in tumor cells might restore apoptosis and make tumor cells more sensitive to therapy, particularly if very high intracellular *p53* protein levels could be achieved.

Gene therapy with *p53* has been successfully performed using retroviral[87] and adenoviral vectors.[88] Preclinical studies also suggest that liposome-encapsulated *p53* can act systemically and reduce the incidence of metastases, at least in some model systems.[89] Retroviral *p53* is well tolerated by patients and can have some benefit[90]; however, adenoviral vectors are currently preferred because they can be produced in high titer, they easily infect epithelial cells, and they do not require cell division to produce transgene. In addition, adenoviral *p53* can dramatically increase wild-type *p53* levels in human tumors and result in marked growth delay,[91] restoration of cell cycle checkpoints, apoptosis, and radiosensitization.[92] By down-regulating vascular endothelial growth factor[93] and neovascularization, adenoviral *p53* also greatly inhibits tumor angiogenesis.[94]

p53 gene therapy enhances the effect of cisplatin,[95] paclitaxel,[96] and radiation therapy and is at least additive with fluorouracil, methotrexate, and etoposide.[97] Furthermore, drugs that increase *p53* stability can also augment *Ad-p53* effects in vivo.[98] Controversy exists as to whether *p53* gene therapy induces a bystander effect by which nontransduced cells are killed. Reported potential mechanisms include suppression of angiogenesis and production of *fas*-ligand. These effects may be tumor-specific.

Preclinical trials of *p53* gene therapy have demonstrated efficacy in many types of human cancer such as pancreatic,[99] head and neck,[91] prostate,[100] and lung.[95] Therapeutic effects can be demonstrated even in tumors with wild-type *p53*, likely because a very large amount of normal protein can overcome presumed mutations downstream of *p53*.

Several preliminary human trials have been performed using *Ad-p53*. In metastatic lung cancer, intratumoral *Ad-p53* injections are well tolerated and can reduce tumor size.[101] Unfortunately, this therapy does not affect tumors that have not been injected with virus. Antiviral immune response does not seem to reduce the efficacy of subsequent intratumoral injections. In a recent clinical study that showed great promise,[102] 13 evaluable patients with unresectable NSCLC who were not candidates for chemotherapy were treated with radiation therapy (60 Gy) and three intratumoral injections of *Ad-p53* every 2 weeks during radiation therapy. Three months after completing therapy, the biopsy specimens of eight of the 11 surviving patients were pathologically negative for malignancy. In contrast, a similar group of patients who were treated with 60 Gy alone had a pathologically negative rate of less than 20%.[103]

Another approach to *Ad-p53*-based gene therapy is to use the natural affinity of adenovirus for epithelial cells as an agent to purge bone marrow before reinfusion.[104] Topical application of *Ad-p53* can also cause regression of premalignant lesions and may be useful for chemoprevention.[105] In addition, *Ad-p53* may be useful after surgical resection in patients with advanced head and neck cancer.[106]

Six to 10 ml of resuspended *Ad-p53* can be safely injected into tumors, under the guidance of CT or bronchoscopy,[107] with adenoviral doses as high as 10^{11} plaque-forming units (approximately 10^{12} viral particles).[108] Major toxic effects of *Ad-p53* treatment are fever, myalgias, and pain/bleeding at the injection site.

These data suggest that substantial improvements in local control may be possible by combining gene therapy with radiation therapy, and chemotherapy may further augment cell killing. However, *Ad-p53* gene therapy has no systemic effect on micrometastases, and thus its application is limited to tumor types with high local failure rates such as lung, brain, and pancreas and possibly to locally recurrent disease that requires reirradiation.

Also, some cells that escape *Ad-p53*-induced cell killing can become resistant to further killing by *Ad-p53* alone,[109] although the mechanism for this effect is not clear. Treatment through intratumoral injection also requires skilled endoscopists and radiologists to safely deliver multiple viral doses. *Ad-p53* gene therapy is thus likely to play a greater role in future treatment of cancer and, it is hoped, will improve survival in some patients with advanced cancer.

Angiogenesis Inhibitors

Angiogenesis is a complex process by which new blood vessels are generated and existing blood vessels remodeled.[110,111] Such blood vessel alteration is normally required for wound healing and for normal embryonic development. Angiogenesis is co-opted by tumor cells in response to nutrient/oxygen depletion caused by uncontrolled cell growth and metabolism. Because Thomlinson and Gray[49] demonstrated that viable tumor cells can be found only within about 150 µm from arterioles, it is clear that angiogenesis is required for tumors to become macroscopic. More than 40 antiangiogenic agents are currently being reviewed by the United States Food and Drug Administration. Three of the agents that are farthest along in the approval process are discussed in this section.

Angiostatin was originally purified as a 38-kDa cleavage fragment of plasminogen[112] and has been shown to strongly block endothelial cell proliferation. Granulocyte-macrophage colony-stimulating factor can stimulate macrophages to produce metalloelastase, which converts plasminogen into angiostatin.[113] If given systemically to rodents bearing any of a variety of human tumor xenografts, angiostatin induces a marked regression of tumors and no detectable metastases. Tumors regress to small nodules and, if angiogenesis blockade is maintained, do not grow back.[114] Angiostatin can also induce apoptosis of endothelial cells, decrease the motility of these cells without slowing their rate of proliferation,[115] and block the ability of tumor cells to invade normal tissue.[116] In addition, angiostatin blocks the effects of angiogenin, basic fibroblast growth factor, and vascular endothelial growth factor on endothelial cells.[117]

Endostatin is a 20-kDa cleavage fragment from collagen XVIII[118] and is another small peptide that induces tumor dormancy in rodent models by blocking angiogenesis. At least in some model systems, endostatin and angiostatin are synergistic.[119] Radiation therapy is synergistic with angiostatin[120] in the killing of tumor cells in rodent models of lung, prostate, and head and neck carcinoma and glioblastoma. No data regarding synergy between cytotoxic chemotherapy and angiostatin have been published.

Endostatin and angiostatin are relatively nontoxic, and repeated administration does not seem to cause impairment in wound healing.[121] Angiostatin and endostatin can be delivered by gene therapy, which can result in prolonged tumor dormancy[122]; however, it is not clear whether delivery through gene therapy produces outcomes superior to those produced by systemic administration of these agents.

Thalidomide is another agent capable of blocking angiogenesis but with the consequence of tumor hypoxia.[123] This toxicity can be overcome by the concurrent use of the hypoxic-cell toxin tirapazamine, and this regimen reduces lung metastases in experimental systems. Thalidomide exerts its antiangiogenic effects by downregulating integrins (components of the extracellular matrix important for adhesion of epithelial cells to the matrix), and by blocking the effects of basic fibroblast growth factor.[124] Thalidomide has shown considerable activity against multiple myeloma[125] and renal cell carcinoma; slight activity against gliomas; and no effect as a single agent against breast cancer, ovarian cancer, or melanoma.[126]

Angiogenesis blockade has great potential in the treatment of human cancer. The nontoxic nature of these compounds makes them ideal agents for chemoprevention as well. In more advanced disease, antiangiogenic agents may be synergistic with radiation therapy and chemotherapy and can produce a state of long-term dormancy. Using tumor dormancy as an endpoint is perhaps somewhat counterintuitive; however, if the goal of therapy is to ensure that patients do not die of cancer (or of complications resulting from treatment), producing long-term dormancy rather than a "cure" of disease might be a reasonable and realistic goal.

Cyclooxygenase-2 Inhibitors

Another interesting class of agents comprises inhibitors of cyclooxygenase-2 (COX-2), is an inducible enzyme that is important for local prostaglandin production. Although COX-2 was initially thought to play a role in carcinogenesis because of the observation that patients taking daily aspirin therapy (a very nonspecific COX-2 inhibitor) had a lower incidence of colorectal cancer,[127] workers later found that this effect resulted from COX-2 inhibition and that COX-2 was often induced in a variety of types of human cancer.[128] COX-2 inhibitors block angiogenesis and promote apoptosis.[129] These agents also can be used as radiosensitizers in vivo with no apparent increase in normal tissue toxicity, at least in animal model systems.[130] Clinical trials of combinations of COX-2 inhibitors, chemotherapy, and radiation therapy for colorectal and lung cancer are under way.

Immunotherapy

Immunotherapy can kill tumor cells systemically by reactivating the host's antitumor immunity. Several examples of immunotherapy and the potential role of these agents in combination with radiation therapy are discussed in the following section. More detailed analysis of individual aspects of immunotherapy is provided in excellent published reviews of immunology and immunotherapy,[131] dendritic cell therapy,[132,133] cytokine gene therapy,[134] paracrine effects of cytokines,[135] the importance of human leukocyte antigen molecules in the immune response,[136] tumor antigens,[137] and cancer vaccines.[138] Two approaches to immunotherapy are discussed below.

Vaccine Therapy

Several investigators have hypothesized that poor antitumor immunity arises because of ineffective antigen presentation, and variety of animal studies[139-141] suggest that this hypothesis is correct. To test this hypothesis in humans, 17 patients with metastatic renal cell carcinoma were enrolled in a clinical trial designed as follows:[142] patients underwent resection of at least 1 specimen of gross tumor. Dendritic cells obtained from peripheral blood monocytes were fused with purified epithelial cells from the tumor and irradiated, and the fused cells were returned to the patient by subcutaneous injection every 6 weeks. Of the 17 patients, seven patients responded. Of the four patients who had a complete response, three patients remained disease-free for as long as 21 months. Of the 17 patients, 11 developed an immune response to autologous tumor cells. Three patients experienced no toxic effects other than fever. Thus vaccination with tumor cell:dendritic cell hybrids can be effective and nontoxic. However, no data are available on how best to combine this approach with standard therapy.

Antibody Therapy

To be effective, tumor antigens should be present on the target cell surface in high concentration, should not be shed, and should have limited expression on normal cells. For instance, although prostate-specific antigen is present at high concentrations on most prostate carcinoma cells and although its expression is limited to the prostate, prostate-specific antigen is shed into the serum in large amounts, making it a less-than-ideal target for antibody therapy. Good candidates for use as antibody therapy include viral antigens (e.g., human papillomavirus for cervical carcinoma and hepatitis B for hepatocellular carcinoma), cell surface receptors (CD20 for B-cell tumors and c-ErbB-2 for several epithelial tumors), and tumor-associated/differentiation-associated antigens (carcinoembryonic antigen for certain types of adenocarcinoma and the melanoma antigen MAGE for certain types of testicular carcinoma). Antitumor antibodies must have a high binding constant and must be "humanized" as much as possible to reduce the host response to the antibody. Antitumor antibodies can also be radiolabeled and used in trace amounts for diagnostic studies or at a higher concentration (or with different isotopes) to improve the therapeutic effect. Several antitumor antibody therapies have been developed over the past several years (and more are likely to be developed), and a complete description of their use and potential efficacy is beyond the scope of this chapter.

IDEC-C2B8 (Rituximab, Genentech) is an anti-CD20 chimeric mouse/human antibody that has potential utility in all B-cell lymphomas that express CD20. This agent mediates complement- and antibody-dependent cell-mediated cytotoxicity and has direct antiproliferative effects against malignant B-cell lines in vitro.[143] Initial phase I/II studies in patients with otherwise chemotherapy-refractory low-grade lymphomas demonstrated response rates of about 50%.[143-145] Toxicity was quite limited, with fever and chills being self-limited and most pronounced during the first few cycles, and only about 10% of the toxic reactions reported were grade 3. Human antichimeric antibodies were very rarely detected. The likelihood of tumor response was highly consistent with follicular histology, with the ability to sustain a high serum level of antibody after the first infusion, and with a longer duration of remission after prior chemotherapy.[142] Serum antibody levels were higher in patients who responded to the drug and in patients with smaller tumors.[145] Recurrences of disease tended to be CD20-negative. These data suggest that aggressive treatment with Rituximab at initial presentation might result in better rates of long-term survival.

Administering Rituximab in combination with standard chemotherapeutic regimen combining cyclophosphamide, doxorubicin, vincristine, and prednisone (CHOP) to patients with low-grade B-cell lymphoma resulted in a 95% response rate (38 of 40 patients).[146] Twenty-two patients had a complete response, and seven of eight patients with the bcl-2 (t[14;18]) translocation had complete responses as confirmed by polymerase chain reaction assay. This combination of immunotherapy and chemotherapy was well tolerated, but a randomized trial is needed to identify a survival advantage. Monoclonal antibodies can also be radiolabeled.[147,148] This increases response rates to the 60% to 70% range[149] when used as a single agent in refractory disease. Rituximab is also active in cutaneous B-cell lymphoma,[150] and intratumoral injection can significantly reduce lesion size (Fig. 39-2). Whether Rituximab would add to the effects of total nodal irradiation is unknown.

Antibodies to epidermal growth factor receptor (EGFR) have also been developed for therapeutic use in the treatment of those tumor types in which EGFR is overexpressed, such as breast, ovarian, bladder, head and neck, and prostate carcinoma.[151] Combination immunotherapy may also be effective, since antibodies to EGFR and HER-2/neu are at least additive in their cytotoxic effects[152] and with other kinase inhibitors.[153] C225 is also synergistic with the effects of radiation,[154] topotecan,[155] and possibly cisplatin.[156] Interestingly,

several small molecules that block EGFR function (e.g., PD153035[157]) also are cytotoxic and increase the efficacy of C225. Clinical trials combining radiation therapy and C225 are under way.

In summary, immunotherapy holds great promise for patients with cancer. If the host immune response can be enhanced to address micrometastases, then aggressive local therapy, even in patients with very advanced cancer, may result in cure. A better understanding of immunotherapy, and how to best integrate it with standard therapy, is likely to significantly improve outcomes for patients with cancer.

COMBINED-MODALITY THERAPY: THE NEXT GENERATION

The integration of biological therapies with standard combined-modality therapy will present several challenges. First, many of these agents have minimal systemic toxicity, so the classic study design (i.e., phase I, II, and III) has little meaning. Intermediate markers of efficacy will become important and will require routine monitoring of target molecule downstream effects (e.g., decreased ras protein or activity for antisense compounds). Unfortunately, most of this monitoring will require assessment of tumor tissue, and perhaps normal tissue as well, by biopsy during therapy. Advances in molecular imaging will undoubtedly reduce the need for invasive monitoring of drug effects, but this change will not occur soon enough for many patients entering clinical trials now.

Second, the timing of various components of therapy will be critical. For example, administration of agents that cause cell cycle blockade in the (radiosensitive) G_2/M phase must be timed so that the cell cycle blockade actually occurs during the administration of radiation therapy, as has been demonstrated quite elegantly by Yuhchyau Chen and colleagues at the University of Rochester.[158,159] Several cancer cell lines were pretreated with various concentrations of either docetaxel or paclitaxel. Radiosensitization was found to be directly dependent on the amount of cell cycle synchronization and radiation therapy delivered during the G_2/M phase. This radiosensitization could be achieved at taxane concentrations much lower than those required for direct cytotoxic effects. Thrice-weekly low-dose taxane treatment has been associated with little toxicity and a response rate that is much better than that for standard radiation therapy.

Third, the combination or combinations of biological agents eventually integrated into cancer therapy will require careful preclinical validation. For example, it is not clear whether cellular pathways need to be blocked at many points or whether better responses could be obtained by instead blocking several pathways. Immunotherapy may work better if the tumor bed (and

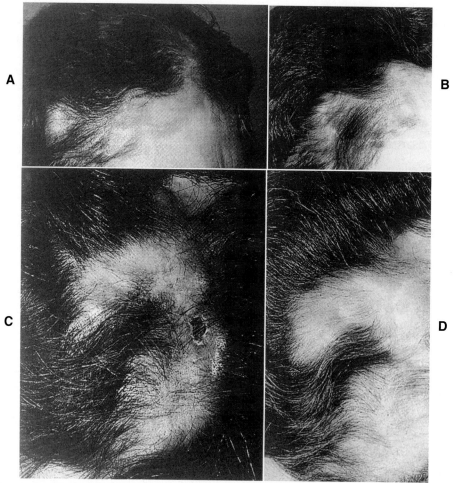

Fig. 39-2   Clinical aspect of cutaneous B-cell tumor nodules before treatment (**A** and **C**) and after nine intralesional injections of Rituximab (**B** and **D**). Note the marked reduction of the size of the treated lesions. (From Hainzerling L, Drummer R, Kempf W. *Arch Dermatol* 2000; 136:374-378.)

infiltrating immunocytes) are not irradiated, or cell death from irradiation may enhance the immune response. The answer to such questions may well be tumor type-specific or even patient-specific; if so, improvements in molecular diagnostics will be needed.

Molecular Diagnostics/Functional Imaging

As is emphasized in the previous sections, rapid advances are under way in developing molecular therapies to interrupt cellular processes important for tumor growth and metastases. Today, assessment of both the appropriateness of therapy (e.g., ensuring the presence of EGFR before administering C225 therapy) and of the molecular effects of therapy usually requires tumor tissue for analysis. Ideally, noninvasive imaging techniques will eventually replace biopsy. Toward that end, any antibody used for therapy can be radiolabeled with radionuclides that are appropriate for imaging

(e.g., ^{99m}Tc or ^{111}In) and for administration to patients subjected to single photon emission computed tomography (SPECT) imaging.

Radiolabeled Ligands

ProstaScint (CYT-356)[160] scanning uses an ^{111}In-labeled monoclonal antibody specific for a glycoprotein that is found primarily on the cell membrane of prostate tissue. The assay is effective in pretreatment staging[161] and in the detection of recurrences of prostate cancer after radical prostatectomy.[162] This assay is also effective in staging prostate cancer that is prostate-specific antigen–negative. ProstaScint seems approximately as sensitive as routine bone scanning in detecting osseous metastases and can also detect tumor in regional lymphatics.

Other potential agents for molecular staging are small molecules such as octreotide,[163] which binds specifically to the somatostatin receptor. This agent, initially developed because several neuroendocrine tumors display high levels of the somatostatin receptor, has been used clinically since the late 1980s. Radioimmunotherapy began soon thereafter.[164] However, elevated somatostatin receptor levels have been found in lung carcinoma and high-grade gliomas, suggesting a possible role for octreotide in the staging of these diseases as well.

Positron Emission Tomography

PET is a novel nuclear medicine study that is similar to SPECT scanning and allows imaging of radiolabeled tracers. The most commonly used imaging agent is FDG, which is discussed in the following section as a paradigm.[165] PET with [18]FDG dates to the late 1970s, when the principal application of interest using this technique was normal brain metabolism.[166] However, interest soon turned to tumor metabolism.[167]

The sensitivity of this technique for the detection of malignant lesions is almost 90%, and the positive predictive value is 95%; therefore whole-body FDG-PET is promising both in determining the nature of a localized lesion and in defining the systemic extent of malignant disease.[168] FDG-PET is an excellent staging tool. For example, when the PET-predicted stage was compared with histopathologically confirmed stage in a series of 87 patients with NSCLC, 86% of the cases were accurately staged with PET, 2% were understaged, and 12% were overstaged. This inaccuracy resulted in an overall sensitivity of 82%, an overall specificity of 86%, a positive predictive value for regional lymph node metastases of 47%, and a negative predictive value for regional lymph nodal metastases of 97% among patients whose cancer was otherwise clinically categorized as stage I disease.[165] Interestingly, overall glucose uptake is another strong predictor of outcome for these patients with early-stage disease.[169] FDG-PET is more sensitive than ^{131}I for monitoring thyroid carcinoma.[170] In fact, FDG-PET is the single best test for staging NSCLC.[171] Unfortunately, current PET resolution is 5 mm at best, so findings of PET studies must be compared and coregistered with anatomic images such as those generated by CT.

FDG-PET also has great potential use in radiation therapy treatment planning. Provided that the primary tumor has good FDG uptake, negative findings in the regional lymphatics may allow lower radiation doses to be safely used. In medically inoperable T1 or T2 NSCLC tumors, FDG-PET may allow the mediastinum to be omitted from the radiation field with more confidence. FDG-PET will also be efficient at assessing regional lymph nodes in patients with seemingly early-stage disease.

PET has the potential to image several cellular processes other than glucose metabolism. Amino acids or lipids can be monitored using ^{11}C,[172] and [15]O can be used to monitor blood flow and oxygen consumption.[173] Chemotherapy uptake can also be monitored.[174]

Thus the use of PET scanning will increase dramatically in the near future; it will help better accomplish triage of patients for treatment, and it will allow more appropriate treatment of their disease.

Hypoxic Imaging

Hypoxia is an important predictor of outcome and metastasis but is very difficult to measure. Noninvasive measurements of hypoxia have been developed to expand the knowledge of hypoxia to tumor sites not accessible by needle electrode and to allow serial measurements in patients after therapy (e.g., with radiation or with TPZ). Hypoxia-specific diagnostic agents such as EF-5 (2-[2-nitro-1-H-imidazol-1-yl]-N-[2,2,3,3,3-pentafluoropropyl] acetamide)[175] and pimonidazole[176] may eventually be applied more widely than cumbersome polarographic techniques. The recent ability to label the hypoxia marker 2-(2-nitroimidazol-1[H]-yl)-N-(3-fluoropropyl)acetamide (EF-1) with FDG[177] may allow PET imaging of hypoxic tumors. ^{99m}Tc-labeled misonidazole using SPECT, as well as ^{18}F-misonidazole[178] using PET scanning techniques, are also entering the clinic. Studies of these agents will define the role of hypoxia as a predictor of outcome or metastases in a wide array of types of human cancer and may be important as part of the initial work-up for patients enrolled in TPZ trials.

Genomics

The study of downstream effects of molecular therapy will be greatly augmented by the use of genomic screening. Complementary DNA (cDNA) microarray technology can assess levels of gene expression in a few cells microdissected from a tumor specimen. cDNA is then subjected to reverse transcriptase-polymerase chain reaction assay, and gene expression is compared with either standards or normal tissue. Although this technique allows thousands of markers[179,180] to be assessed simultaneously, screening large numbers of markers makes analysis of prognostic factors quite difficult. Bioinformatics techniques to address such large data sets are still under development.[181] The extreme sensitivity of the assay also requires that tumor cells be purified from underlying normal tissue and, owing to intratumoral heterogeneity, may even require cell purification from several regions of the tumor. However, cDNA microarrays offer the potential to rapidly screen individual tumors and to tailor therapy accordingly.

CONCLUSIONS

The armamentarium of therapies in the war on cancer is growing rapidly. Costly basic science research is producing results that will likely have significant effects on clinical radiation oncology. Several points now need emphasis.

The first of these points is that an understanding of molecular biology and molecular oncology is critical to the rational application of modern therapies. Although training programs have for many years relegated the field of radiobiology to a minor or peripheral role in cancer therapy, this attitude must change, and change quickly, if we are to properly combine radiation therapy with molecular therapies. Second, new radiation therapy techniques (e.g., dose escalation, treatment planning techniques, twice-daily fractionation) are important, but their role in improving outcome is likely to be smaller than that of molecular approaches. In fact, molecular approaches to reducing or reversing radiation therapy-induced toxicity are now entering the clinic. Third, cancer treatment will become much more complex and individualized. The roles of diagnostic and interventional radiology, pathology, endoscopy, and immunology are all likely to increase. The best cancer care will be delivered at centers with well-integrated, experienced, multidisciplinary teams. Fourth, hundreds of new agents are now becoming available for clinical use, and prioritizing their use will be difficult. Unfortunately, much of the prioritization is likely to be based on drug company funding rather than on the potential efficacy of the drugs.

The meaning of the term *combined-modality therapy* will probably be very different from its meaning in the past. Newer combined-modality therapies will likely produce less toxicity and, it is hoped, better outcome. It will probably take years to optimize therapies for many types of cancer. However, with so many promising approaches, the outlook for cancer survival is now brighter than ever.

REFERENCES

1. McShan DL, Silverman A, Lanza DM, et al. A computerized three-dimensional treatment planning system utilizing interactive colour graphics. *Br J Radiol* 1979;52:478-481.
2. Reinstein LE, McShan D, Webber BM, et al. A computer-assisted three-dimensional treatment planning system. *Radiology* 1978;127:259-264.
3. Mohan R, Barest G, Brewster LJ, et al. A comprehensive three-dimensional radiation treatment planning system. *Int J Radiat Oncol Biol Phys* 1988;15:481-495.
4. Ten Haken RK, Lawrence TS, McShan DL, et al. Technical considerations in the use of 3D beam arrangements in the abdomen. *Radiother Oncol* 1991;22:19-28.
5. Kalet IJ, Jacky JP. A research-oriented treatment planning program system. *Comput Programs Biomed* 1982;14:85-98.
6. Rosenman J, Sailer SL, Sherouse GW, et al. Virtual simulation: initial clinical results. *Int J Radiat Oncol Biol Phys* 1991;20:843-851.
7. Hsu IC, Pickett B, Shinohara K, et al. Normal tissue dosimetric comparison between HDR prostate implant boost and conformal external beam radiotherapy boost: potential for dose escalation. *Int J Radiat Oncol Biol Phys* 2000;46:851-858.
8. Zelefsky MJ, Cowen D, Fuks Z, et al. Long term tolerance of high dose three-dimensional conformal radiotherapy in patients with localized prostate carcinoma. *Cancer* 1999;85:2460-2468.
9. Hanks GE. Conformal radiotherapy for prostate cancer. *Ann Med* 2000;32:57-63.
10. Verhey LJ. Comparison of three-dimensional conformal radiation therapy and intensity-modulated radiation therapy systems. *Semin Radiat Oncol* 1999;9:78-98.
11. Perez CA, Michalski JM, Purdy JA, et al. Three-dimensional conformal therapy or standard irradiation in localized carcinoma of prostate: preliminary results of a nonrandomized comparison. *Int J Radiat Oncol Biol Phys* 2000;47:629-637.
12. Michalski JM, Purdy JA, Winter K, et al. Preliminary report of toxicity following 3D radiation therapy for prostate cancer on 3DOG/RTOG 9406. *Int J Radiat Oncol Biol Phys* 2000;46:391-402.
13. Dearnaley DP, Khoo VS, Norman AR, et al. Comparison of radiation side-effects of conformal and conventional radiotherapy in prostate cancer: a randomised trial. *Lancet* 1999;353:267-272.
14. Oh CE, Antes K, Darby M, et al. Comparison of 2D conventional, 3D conformal, and intensity-modulated treatment planning techniques for patients with prostate cancer with regard to target-dose homogeneity and dose to critical, uninvolved structures. *Med Dosim* 1999;24:255-263.
15. Horwitz EM, Hanlon AL, Pinover WH, et al. The cost effectiveness of 3D conformal radiation therapy compared with conventional techniques for patients with clinically localized prostate cancer. *Int J Radiat Oncol Biol Phys* 1999;45:1219-1225.
16. International Commission on Radiation Units and Measurement. Prescribing, recording and reporting photon beam therapy. Bethesda, Maryland: ICRU Report 50; 1993.
17. International Commission on Radiation Units and Measurement. Prescribing, recording and reporting photon beam therapy. Bethesda, Md: ICRU Report 62(suppl); 1999. Supplement to ICRU Report 50.
18. Ramsey CR, Scaperoth D, Arwood D, et al. Clinical efficacy of respiratory gated conformal radiation therapy. *Med Dosim* 1999; 24:115-119.
19. Eisbruch A, Dawson LA, Kim HM, et al. Conformal and intensity modulated irradiation of head and neck cancer: the potential for improved target irradiation, salivary gland function, and quality of life. *Acta Otorhinolaryngol Belg* 1999;53:271-275.
20. Fuss M, Hug EB, Schaefer RA, et al. Proton radiation therapy (PRT) for pediatric optic pathway gliomas: comparison with 3D planned conventional photons and a standard photon technique. *Int J Radiat Oncol Biol Phys* 1999;45:1117-1126.
21. Perks JR, Jalali R, Cosgrove VP, et al. Optimization of stereotactically-guided conformal treatment planning of sellar and parasellar tumors, based on normal brain dose volume histograms. *Int J Radiat Oncol Biol Phys* 1999;45:507-513.
22. De Neve W, De Gersem W, Derycke S, et al. Clinical delivery of intensity modulated conformal radiotherapy for relapsed or second-primary head and neck cancer using a multileaf collimator with dynamic control. *Radiother Oncol* 1999;50:301-314.
23. Graham MV, Purdy JA, Emami B, et al. Clinical dose-volume histogram analysis for pneumonitis after 3D treatment for non-small cell lung cancer (NSCLC). *Int J Radiat Oncol Biol Phys* 1999; 45:323-329.
24. McGibney C, Holmberg O, McClean B, et al. Dose escalation of chart in non–small cell lung cancer: is three-dimensional conformal radiation therapy really necessary? *Int J Radiat Oncol Biol Phys* 1999;45:339-350.
25. Leksell L. A stereotaxic apparatus for intracerebral surgery. *Acta Chir Scand* 1949;99:229-233.
26. Blomgren H, Lax I, Naslund I, et al. Stereotactic high dose fraction radiation therapy of extracranial tumors using an accelerator. Clinical experience of the first thirty-one patients. *Acta Oncol* 1995;34:861-870.
27. Tokuuye K, Sumi M, Ikeda H, et al. Technical considerations for fractionated stereotactic radiotherapy of hepatocellular carcinoma. *Jpn J Clin Oncol* 1997;27:170-173.
28. Cardinale RM, Wu Q, Benedict SH, et al. Determining the optimal block margin on the planning target volume for extracranial

stereotactic radiotherapy. *Int J Radiat Oncol Biol Phys* 1999; 45:515-520.

29. Henschke CI, McCauley DI, Yankelevitz DF, et al. Early Lung Cancer Action Project: overall design and findings from baseline screening. *Lancet* 1999;354:99-105.

30. Munzenrider JE. Proton therapy for uveal melanomas and other eye lesions. *Strahlenther Onkol* 1999;175:68-73.

31. Lomax AJ, Bortfeld T, Goitein G, et al. A treatment planning intercomparison of proton and intensity modulated photon radiotherapy. *Radiother Oncol* 1999;51:257-271.

32. Mori T, Watanabe M, Horikawa M, et al. WR-2721, its derivatives and their radioprotective effects on mammalian cells in culture. *Int J Radiat Biol Relat Stud Phys Chem Med* 1983;44:41-53.

33. Capizzi RL. Recent developments and emerging options: the role of amifostine as a broad-spectrum cytoprotective agent. *Semin Oncol* 1999;26:1-2.

34. Werner-Wasik M. Future development of amifostine as a radioprotectant. *Semin Oncol* 1999;26:129-134.

35. Constine LS, Zagars G, Rubin P, et al. Protection by WR-2721 of human bone marrow function following irradiation. *Int J Radiat Oncol Biol Phys* 1986;12:1505-1508.

36. Glover D, Glick JH, Weiler C, et al. WR-2721 protects against the hematologic toxicity of cyclophosphamide: a controlled phase II trial. *J Clin Oncol* 1986;4:584-588.

37. Glover D, Glick JH, Weiler C, et al. Phase I/II trials of WR-2721 and cis-platinum. *Int J Radiat Oncol Biol Phys* 1986;12:1509-1512.

38. Poplin EA, LoRusso P, Lokich JJ, et al. Randomized clinical trial of mitomycin-C with or without pretreatment with WR-2721 in patients with advanced colorectal cancer. *Cancer Chemother Pharmacol* 1994;33:415-419.

39. Taylor CW, Wang LM, List AF, et al. Amifostine protects normal tissues from paclitaxel toxicity while cytotoxicity against tumour cells is maintained. *Eur J Cancer* 1997;33:1693-1698.

40. Bohuslavizki KH, Brenner W, Klutmann S, et al. Radioprotection of salivary glands by amifostine in high-dose radioiodine therapy. *J Nucl Med* 1998;39:1237-1242.

41. Takahashi I, Nagai T, Miyaishi K, et al. Clinical study of the radioprotective effects of Amifostine (YM-08310, WR-2721) on chronic radiation injury. *Int J Radiat Oncol Biol Phys* 1986;12:935-938.

42. Capizzi RL. Amifostine reduces the incidence of cumulative nephrotoxicity from cisplatin: laboratory and clinical aspects. *Semin Oncol* 1999; 26:72-81.

43. Bourhis J, De Crevoisier R, Abdulkarim B, et al. A randomized study of very accelerated radiotherapy with and without amifostine in head and neck squamous cell carcinoma. *Int J Radiat Oncol Biol Phys* 2000;46:1105-1108.

44. Kligerman MM, Turrisi AT III, Urtasun RC, et al. Final report on phase I trial of WR-2721 before protracted fractionated radiation therapy. *Int J Radiat Oncol Biol Phys* 1988;14:1119-1122.

45. Otte JM, Schmitz F, Banasiewicz T, et al. Expression of keratinocyte growth factor and its receptor in colorectal cancer. *Eur J Clin Invest* 2000;30:222-229.

46. Farrell CL, Bready JV, Rex KL, et al. Keratinocyte growth factor protects mice from chemotherapy and radiation-induced gastrointestinal injury and mortality. *Cancer Res* 1998;58:933-939.

47. Visco V, Carico E, Marchese C, et al. Expression of keratinocyte growth factor receptor compared with that of epidermal growth factor receptor and erbB-2 in endometrial adenocarcinoma. *Int J Oncol* 1999;15:431-435.

48. Zhang Y, Sugimoto Y, Kulp SK, et al. Estrogen-induced keratinocyte growth factor mRNA expression in normal and cancerous human breast cells. *Oncol Rep* 1998;5:577-583.

49. Thomlinson RH, Gray LJ. This histologic structure of some human lung cancers and the possible implications of radiotherapy. *Br J Cancer* 1955;9:537-549.

50. Badib AO, Webster JH. Changes in tumor oxygen tension during radiation therapy. *Acta Radiol* 1969;8:247-257.

51. Cater DB, Silver IA. Quantitative measurements of oxygen tension in normal tissues and in the tumors of patients before and after radiotherapy. *Acta Radiol* 1960;53:233-256.

52. Lartigau E, Vitu L, Haie-Meder C, et al. Feasibility of measuring oxygen tension in uterine cervix carcinoma. *Eur J Cancer* 1992; 28A:1354-1357.

53. Pappova N, Siracka E, Vacek A, et al. Oxygen tension and prediction of the radiation response. Polarographic study in human breast cancer. *Neoplasma* 1982;29:669-674.

54. Hocke M, Schlenger K, Knoop C, et al. Oxygenation of carcinomas of the uterine cervix: evaluation by computerized O_2 tension measurements. *Cancer Res* 1991;51:6098-6102.

55. Lyng H, Sundfor K, Rofstad EK. Oxygen tension in human tumours measured with polarographic needle electrodes and its relationship to vascular density, necrosis and hypoxia. *Radiother Oncol* 1997;44:163-169.

56. Vaupel P, Schlenger K, Knoop C, et al. Oxygenation of human tumors: evaluation of tissue oxygen distribution in breast cancers by computerized O_2 tension measurements. *Cancer Res* 1991;51:3316-3322.

57. Fleckenstein W, Jungblut JR, Suckfull M. Distribution of oxygen pressure in the peripheral and centre of malignant head and neck tumors. In: Ehrly AM, Hauss J, Huch R, eds. *Clinical Oxygen Pressure Measurement II.* Berlin: Blackwell Ueberreuter Wissenschaft; 1990:81-90.

58. Knocke TH, Weitmann HD, Feldmann HJ, et al. Intratumoral pO_2-measurements as predictive assay in the treatment of carcinoma of the uterine cervix. *Radiother Oncol* 1999;53:99-104.

59. Hockel M, Schlenger K, Hockel S, et al. Tumor hypoxia in pelvic recurrences of cervical cancer. *Int J Cancer* 1998;79:365-369.

60. Brizel DM, Dodge RK, Clough RW, et al. Oxygenation of head and neck cancer: changes during radiotherapy and impact on treatment outcome. *Radiother Oncol* 1999;53:113-117.

61. Dachs GU, Patterson AV, Firth JD, et al. Targeting gene expression to hypoxic tumor cells. *Nat Med* 1997;3:515-520.

62. Zeman EM, Brown JM, Lemmon MJ, et al. SR-4233: a new bioreductive agent with high selective toxicity for hypoxic mammalian cells. *Int J Radiat Oncol Biol Phys* 1986;12:1239-1242.

63. Brown JM. The hypoxic cell: a target for selective cancer therapy—eighteenth Bruce F. Cain Memorial Award lecture. *Cancer Res* 1999;59:5863-5870.

64. Patterson AV, Barham HM, Chinje EC, et al. Importance of P450 reductase activity in determining sensitivity of breast tumour cells to the bioreductive drug, tirapazamine (SR 4233). *Br J Cancer* 1995;72:1144-1150.

65. Biedermann KA, Wang J, Graham RP, et al. SR 4233 cytotoxicity and metabolism in DNA repair-competent and repair-deficient cell cultures. *Br J Cancer* 1991;63:358-362.

66. Zeman EM, Hirst VK, Lemmon MJ, et al. Enhancement of radiation-induced tumor cell killing by the hypoxic cell toxin SR 4233. *Radiother Oncol* 1988;12:209-218.

67. Brown JM, Lemmon MJ. Potentiation by the hypoxic cytotoxin SR 4233 of cell killing produced by fractionated irradiation of mouse tumors. *Cancer Res* 1990;50:7745-7749.

68. Dorie MJ, Brown JM. Tumor-specific, schedule-dependent interaction between tirapazamine (SR 4233) and cisplatin. *Cancer Res* 1993;53:4633-4636.

69. Langmuir VK, Rooker JA, Osen M, et al. Synergistic interaction between tirapazamine and cyclophosphamide in human breast cancer xenografts. *Cancer Res* 1994;54:2845-2847.

70. Dorie MJ, Brown JM. Modification of the antitumor activity of chemotherapeutic drugs by the hypoxic cytotoxic agent tirapazamine. *Cancer Chemother Pharmacol* 1997;39:361-366.

71. Wilder RB, Langmuir VK, Mendonca HL, et al. Local hyperthermia and SR 4233 enhance the antitumor effects of radioimmunotherapy in nude mice with human colonic adenocarcinoma xenografts. *Cancer Res* 1993;53:3022-3027.

72. von Pawel J, von Roemeling R, Gatzemeier U, et al. Tirapazamine plus cisplatin versus cisplatin in advanced non-small-cell lung cancer: a report of the international CATAPULT I (Cisplatin and Tirapazamine in Subjects with Advanced Previously Untreated Non–Small-Cell Lung Tumors) study group. *J Clin Oncol* 2000; 18:1351-1359.

73. Treat J, Johnson E, Langer C, et al. Tirapazamine with cisplatin in patients with advanced non–small-cell lung cancer: a phase II study. *J Clin Oncol* 1998;16:3524-3527.

74. Brizel DM, Scully SP, Harrelson JM, et al. Tumor oxygenation predicts for the likelihood of distant metastases in human soft tissue sarcoma. *Cancer Res* 1996;56:941-943.

75. Graeber TG, Osmanian C, Jacks T, et al. Hypoxia-mediated selection of cells with diminished apoptotic potential in solid tumours. *Nature* 1996;379:88-91.

76. Minamoto T, Mai M, Ronai Z. K-*ras* mutation: early detection in molecular diagnosis and risk assessment of colorectal, pancreas, and lung cancers–a review. *Cancer Detect Prev* 2000;24:1-12.

77. de Gunzburg J. Proteins of the *ras* pathway as novel potential anticancer therapeutic targets. *Cell Biol Toxicol* 1999;15:345-358.

78. Pincus MR, Brandt-Rauf PW, Michl J, et al. *ras-p21*–induced cell transformation: unique signal transduction pathways and implications for the design of new chemotherapeutic agents. *Cancer Invest* 2000;18:39-50.

79. McKenna WG, Weiss MC, Endlich B, et al. Synergistic effect of the *v-myc* oncogene with H-ras on radioresistance. *Cancer Res* 1990;50:97-102.

80. Bernhard EJ, McKenna WG, Hamilton AD, et al. Inhibiting ras prenylation increases the radiosensitivity of human tumor cell lines with activating mutations of *ras* oncogenes. *Cancer Res* 1998;58:1754-1761.

81. Cohen-Jonathan E, Monteil S, Toulas C, et al. Farnesylated protein is involved in radioresistance induced by the 24 kD basic fibroblast growth factor isoform in HeLa cells [abstract]. *Proc Am Assoc Cancer Res* 1997;38:300a.

82. Feldkamp MM, Lau N, Rak J, et al. Normoxic and hypoxic regulation of vascular endothelial growth factor (VEGF) by astrocytoma cells is mediated by Ras. *Int J Cancer* 1999;81:118-124.

83. Gomez-Navarro J, Curiel DT, Douglas JT. Gene therapy for cancer. *Eur J Cancer* 1999;35:2039-2057.

84. Roth JA. Restoration of tumour suppressor gene expression for cancer. *Forum* 1998;8:368-376.

85. Chmura SJ, Advani SJ, Kufe DW, et al. Strategies for enhancing viral-based gene therapy using ionizing radiation. *Radiat Oncol Invest* 1999;7:261-269.

86. Zeng M, Cerniglia GJ, Eck S, et al. High-efficiency stable gene transfer of adenovirus into mammalian cells using ionizing radiation. *Hum Gene Ther* 1997;8:1025-1032.

87. Fujiwara T, Cai DW, Georges RN, et al. Therapeutic effect of a retroviral wild-type *p53* expression vector in an orthotopic lung cancer model. *J Natl Cancer Inst* 1994;86:1458-1462.

88. Wills KN, Maneval DC, Menzel P, et al. Development and characterization of recombinant adenoviruses encoding human *p53* for gene therapy of cancer. *Hum Gene Ther* 1994;5:1079-1088.

89. Lesoon-Wood LA, Kim WH, Kleinman HK, et al. Systemic gene therapy with *p53* reduces growth and metastases of a malignant human breast cancer in nude mice. *Hum Gene Ther* 1995;6: 395-405.

90. Roth JA, Nguyen D, Lawrence DD, et al. Retrovirus-mediated wild-type *p53* gene transfer to tumors of patients with lung cancer. *Nat Med* 1996;2:985-991.

91. Liu TJ, Zhang WW, Taylor DL, et al. Growth suppression of human head and neck cancer cells by the introduction of a wild-type *p53* gene via a recombinant adenovirus. *Cancer Res* 1994;54:3662-3667.

92. Chang EH, Jang YJ, Hao Z, et al. Restoration of the G1 checkpoint and the apoptotic pathway mediated by wild-type *p53* sensitizes squamous cell carcinoma of the head and neck to radiotherapy. *Arch Otolaryngol* 1997;123:507-512.

93. Bouvet M, Ellis LM, Nishizaki M, et al. Adenovirus-mediated wild-type *p53* gene transfer down-regulates vascular endothelial growth factor expression and inhibits angiogenesis in human colon cancer. *Cancer Res* 1998;58:2288-2292.

94. Riccioni T, Cirielli C, Wang X, et al. Adenovirus-mediated wild-type *p53* overexpression inhibits endothelial cell differentiation in vitro and angiogenesis in vivo. *Gene Ther* 1998;5:747-754.

95. Nguyen DM, Spitz FR, Yen N, et al. Gene therapy for lung cancer: enhancement of tumor suppression by a combination of sequential systemic cisplatin and adenovirus-mediated *p53* gene transfer. *J Thorac Cardiovasc Surg* 1996;112:1372-1376; discussion 1376-1377.

96. Nielsen LL, Lipari P, Dell J, et al. Adenovirus-mediated *p53* gene therapy and paclitaxel have synergistic efficacy in models of human head and neck, ovarian, prostate, and breast cancer. *Clin Cancer Res* 1998;4:835-846.

97. Gurnani M, Lipari P, Dell J, et al. Adenovirus-mediated *p53* gene therapy has greater efficacy when combined with chemotherapy against human head and neck, ovarian, prostate, and breast cancer. *Cancer Chemother Pharmacol* 1999;44:143-151.

98. Kataoka M, Schumacher G, Cristiano RJ, et al. An agent that increases tumor suppressor transgene product coupled with systemic transgene delivery inhibits growth of metastatic lung cancer in vivo. *Cancer Res* 1998;58:4761-4765.

99. Bouvet M, Bold RJ, Lee J, et al. Adenovirus-mediated wild-type *p53* tumor suppressor gene therapy induces apoptosis and suppresses growth of human pancreatic cancer. *Ann Surg Oncol* 1998;5:681-688.

100. Yang C, Cirielli C, Capogrossi MC, et al. Adenovirus-mediated wild-type *p53* expression induces apoptosis and suppresses tumorigenesis of prostatic tumor cells. *Cancer Res* 1995;55:4210-4213.

101. Roth JA, Swisher SG, Merritt JA, et al. Gene therapy for non–small cell lung cancer: a preliminary report of a phase I trial of adenoviral *p53* gene replacement. *Semin Oncol* 1998;25:33-37.

102. Swisher S, Roth JA, Komaki R, et al. A phase II trial of adevoviral mediated *p53* gene transfer (RPR/INGN 201) in conjuction with radiation therapy in patients with localized non–small cell lung cancer (NSCLC) [abstract]. *Proc Am Soc Clin Oncol* 2000; 19:461a.

103. Le Chevalier T, Arriagada R, Quoix E, et al. Radiotherapy alone versus combined chemotherapy and radiotherapy in nonresectable non-small-cell lung cancer: first analysis of a randomized trial in 353 patients. *J Natl Cancer Inst* 1991;83: 417-423.

104. Seth P, Brinkmann U, Schwartz GN, et al. Adenovirus-mediated gene transfer to human breast tumor cells: an approach for cancer gene therapy and bone marrow purging. *Cancer Res* 1996; 56:1346-1351.

105. Eicher SA, Clayman GL, Liu TJ, et al. Evaluation of topical gene therapy for head and neck squamous cell carcinoma in an organotypic model. *Clin Cancer Res* 1996;2:1659-1664.

106. Clayman GL, Frank DK, Bruso PA, et al. Adenovirus-mediated wild-type *p53* gene transfer as a surgical adjuvant in advanced head and neck cancers. *Clin Cancer Res* 1999;5:1715-1722.

107. Kauczor HU, Schuler M, Heussel CP, et al. CT-guided intratumoral gene therapy in non–small-cell lung cancer. *Eur Radiol* 1999;9: 292-296.

108. Swisher SG, Roth JA, Nemunaitis J, et al. Adenovirus-mediated *p53* gene transfer in advanced non–small-cell lung cancer. *J Natl Cancer Inst* 1999;91:763-771.

109. Vinyals A, Peinado MA, Gonzalez-Garrigues M, et al. Failure of wild-type *p53* gene therapy in human cancer cells expressing a mutant *p53* protein. *Gene Ther* 1999;6:22-33.

110. Hagedorn M, Bikfalvi A. Target molecules for anti-angiogenic therapy: from basic research to clinical trials. *Crit Rev Oncol Hematol* 2000;34:89-110.

111. Griffioen AW, Molema G. Angiogenesis: potentials for pharmacologic intervention in the treatment of cancer, cardiovascular diseases, and chronic inflammation. *Pharmacol Rev* 2000; 52:237-268.

112. O'Reilly MS, Holmgren L, Shing Y, et al. Angiostatin: a novel angiogenesis inhibitor that mediates the suppression of metastases by a Lewis lung carcinoma. *Cell* 1994;79:315-328.

113. Dong Z, Yoneda J, Kumar R, et al. Angiostatin-mediated suppression of cancer metastases by primary neoplasms engineered to produce granulocyte/macrophage colony-stimulating factor. *J Exp Med* 1998;188:755-763.

114. O'Reilly MS, Holmgren L, Chen C, et al. Angiostatin induces and sustains dormancy of human primary tumors in mice. *Nat Med* 1996;2:689-692.

115. Claesson-Welsh L, Welsh M, Ito N, et al. Angiostatin induces endothelial cell apoptosis and activation of focal adhesion kinase independently of the integrin-binding motif RGD. *Proc Natl Acad Sci U S A* 1998;95:5579-5583.

116. Stack MS, Gately S, Bafetti LM, et al. Angiostatin inhibits endothelial and melanoma cellular invasion by blocking matrix-enhanced plasminogen activation. *Biochem J* 1999;340:77-84.

117. Kim JH, Kim JC, Shin SH, et al. The inhibitory effects of recombinant plasminogen kringle 1-3 on the neovascularization of rabbit cornea induced by angiogenin, bFGF, and VEGF. *Exp Mol Med* 1999;31:203-209.

118. O'Reilly MS, Boehm T, Shing Y, et al. Endostatin: an endogenous inhibitor of angiogenesis and tumor growth. *Cell* 1997; 88:277-285.

119. Yokoyama Y, Dhanabal M, Griffioen AW, et al. Synergy between angiostatin and endostatin: inhibition of ovarian cancer growth. *Cancer Res* 2000;60:2190-2196.

120. Mauceri HJ, Hanna NN, Beckett MA, et al. Combined effects of angiostatin and ionizing radiation in antitumour therapy. *Nature* 1998;394:287-293.

121. Berger AC, Feldman AL, Gnant MF, et al. The angiogenesis inhibitor, endostatin, does not affect murine cutaneous wound healing. *J Surg Res* 2000;91:26-31.

122. Nguyen JT, Wu P, Clouse ME, et al. Adeno-associated virus-mediated delivery of antiangiogenic factors as an antitumor strategy. *Cancer Res* 1998;58:5673-5677.

123. Minchinton AI, Fryer KH, Wendt KR, et al. The effect of thalidomide on experimental tumors and metastases. *Anticancer Drugs* 1996;7:339-343.

124. McCarty MF. Thalidomide may impede cell migration in primates by down-regulating integrin beta-chains: potential therapeutic utility in solid malignancies, proliferative retinopathy, inflammatory disorders, neointimal hyperplasia, and osteoporosis. *Med Hypotheses* 1997;49:123-131.

125. Barlogie B. Thalidomide (T) in the management of multiple myeloma (MM): the Arkansas experience in >300 patients with single agent and combination chemotherapy [abstract]. *Proc Am Soc Clin Oncol* 2000;19:9a.

126. Eisen T, Boshoff C, Mak I, et al. Continuous low dose thalidomide: a phase II study in advanced melanoma, renal cell, ovarian and breast cancer. *Br J Cancer* 2000;82:812-817.

127. Thun MJ, Namboodiri MM, Heath CW Jr. Aspirin use and reduced risk of fatal colon cancer. *N Engl J Med* 1991;325:1593-1596.

128. Fujita T, Matsui M, Takaku K, et al. Size- and invasion-dependent increase in cyclooxygenase 2 levels in human colorectal carcinomas. *Cancer Res* 1998;58:4823-4826.

129. Seed MP, Freemantle CN, Alam CA, et al. Apoptosis induction and inhibition of colon-26 tumour growth and angiogenesis: findings on COX-1 and COX-2 inhibitors in vitro and in vivo and topical diclofenac in hyaluronan. *Adv Exp Med Biol* 1997;433:339-342.

130. Kishi K, Petersen S, Petersen C, et al. Preferential enhancement of tumor radioresponse by a cyclooxygenase-2 inhibitor. *Cancer Res* 2000;60:1326-1331.

131. Bremers AJ, Parmiani G. Immunology and immunotherapy of human cancer: present concepts and clinical developments. *Crit Rev Oncol Hematol* 2000;34:1-25.

132. Fong L, Engleman EG. Dendritic cells in cancer immunotherapy. *Ann Rev Immunol* 2000;18:245-273.

133. Morse MA, Lyelry HK. VIII. Immuno-modulation-28. Dendritic cell-based immunization for cancer therapy. *Adv Exp Med Biol* 2000;465:335-346.

134. Simons JW, Mikhak B. Ex-vivo gene therapy using cytokine-transduced tumor vaccines: molecular and clinical pharmacology. *Semin Oncol* 1998;25:661-676.

135. Pardoll DM. Paracrine cytokine adjuvants in cancer immunotherapy. *Ann Rev Immunol* 1995;13:399-415.

136. Tait BD. HLA class I expression on human cancer cells. Implications for effective immunotherapy. *Hum Immunol* 2000; 61:158-165.

137. Wang RF, Rosenberg SA. Human tumor antigens for cancer vaccine development. *Immunol Rev* 1999;170:85-100.

138. Chamberlain RS. Prospects for the therapeutic use of anticancer vaccines. *Drugs* 1999;57:309-325.

139. Gong Y, Chen D, Kashiwabe M, et al. Induction of antitumor activity by immunization with fusions of dendritic and carcinoma cells. *Nat Med* 1997;3:558-561.

140. Kugler A, Seseke F, Thelen P, et al. Autologous and allogeneic hybrid cell vaccine in patients with metastatic renal cell carcinoma. *Br J Urol* 1998;82:487-493.

141. Bancereau J, Steinman RM. Dendritic cells and the control of immunity. *Nature* 1998;392:245-252.

142. Kugler A, Stuhler G, Walden P, et al. Regression of human metastatic renal cell carcinoma after vaccination with tumor cell-dendritic cell hybrids. *Nat Med* 2000;6:322-325.

143. Maloney DG, Grillo-Lopez AJ, White CA, et al. IDEC-C2B8 (Rituximab) anti-CD20 monoclonal antibody therapy in patients with relapsed low-grade non-Hodgkin's lymphoma. *Blood* 1997;90:2188-2195.

144. Tobinai K, Kobayashi Y, Narabayashi M, et al. Feasibility and pharmacokinetic study of a chimeric anti-CD20 monoclonal antibody (IDEC-C2B8, rituximab) in relapsed B-cell lymphoma. The IDEC-C2B8 Study Group. *Ann Oncol* 1998;9:527-534.

145. McLaughlin P, Grillo-Lopez AJ, Link BK, et al. Rituximab chimeric anti-CD20 monoclonal antibody therapy for relapsed indolent lymphoma: half of patients respond to a four-dose treatment program. *J Clin Oncol* 1998;16:2825-2833.

146. Czuczman MS, Grillo-Lopez AJ, White CA, et al. Treatment of patients with low-grade B-cell lymphoma with the combination of chimeric anti-CD20 monoclonal antibody and CHOP chemotherapy. *J Clin Oncol* 1999;17:268-276.

147. Behr TM, Wormann B, Gramatzki M. Low- versus high-dose radioimmunotherapy with humanized anti-CD22 or chimeric anti-CD20 antibodies in a broad spectrum of B cell-associated malignancies. *Clin Cancer Res* 1999;5:3304s-3314s.

148. Wiseman GA, White CA, Witzig TE, et al. Radioimmunotherapy of relapsed non-Hodgkin's lymphoma with zevalin, a 90Y-labeled anti-CD20 monoclonal antibody. *Clin Cancer Res* 1999; 5:3281s-3286s.

149. Witzig TE, White CA, Wiseman GA, et al. Phase I/II trial of IDEC-Y2B8 radioimmunotherapy for treatment of relapsed or refractory CD20(+) B-cell non-Hodgkin's lymphoma. *J Clin Oncol* 1999;17:3793-3803.

150. Hainzerling L, Dummer R, Kempf W, et al. Intralesional therapy with anti-CD20 monoclonal antibody rituximab in primary cutaneous B-cell lymphoma. *Arch Dermatol* 2000;136: 374-378.

151. Goldstein NI, Prewett M, Zuklys K, et al. Biological efficacy of a chimeric antibody to the epidermal growth factor receptor in a human tumor xenograft model. *Clin Cancer Res* 1995;1: 1311-1318.

152. Ye D, Mendelsohn J, Fan Z. Augmentation of a humanized anti-HER2 mAb 4D5 induced growth inhibition by a human-mouse chimeric anti-EGF receptor mAb C225. *Oncogene* 1999;18: 731-738.

153. Tortora G, Caputo R, Pomatico G, et al. Cooperative inhibitory effect of novel mixed backbone oligonucleotide targeting protein kinase A in combination with docetaxel and anti-epidermal growth factor-receptor antibody on human breast cancer cell growth. *Clin Cancer Res* 1999;5:875-881.

154. Milas L, Mason K, Hunter N, et al. In vivo enhancement of tumor radioresponse by C225 antiepidermal growth factor receptor antibody. *Clin Cancer Res* 2000;6:701-708.

155. Ciardiello F, Bianco R, Damiano V, et al. Antitumor activity of sequential treatment with topotecan and anti-epidermal growth factor receptor monoclonal antibody C225. *Clin Cancer Res* 1999;5:909-916.

156. Baselga J, Pfister D, Cooper MR, et al. Phase I studies of anti-epidermal growth factor receptor chimeric antibody C225 alone and in combination with cisplatin. *J Clin Oncol* 2000; 18:904-916.

157. Bos M, Mendelsohn J, Kim YM, et al. PD153035, a tyrosine kinase inhibitor, prevents epidermal growth factor receptor activation and inhibits growth of cancer cells in a receptor number-dependent manner. *Clin Cancer Res* 1997;3:2099-2106.

158. Keng P, Chen Y, Okunieff P. Comparative analysis of docetaxel and paclitaxel: cell cycle and radiosensitization effect in human cancer cell lines [abstract]. *Proc Am Soc Clin Oncol* 2000; 19:662a.

159. Chen Y, Pandya K, Feins R, et al. Pulsed paclitaxel radiosensitization for thoracic malignancy: a clinical trial design based on pre-clinical research of human lung cancer cells [abstract]. *Proc Am Soc Clin Oncol* 2000;19:514a.

160. Lopes AD, Davis WL, Rosenstraus MJ, et al. Immunohistochemical and pharmacokinetic characterization of the site-specific immunoconjugate CYT-356 derived from antiprostate monoclonal antibody 7E11-C5. *Cancer Res* 1990; 50:6423-6429.

161. Murphy GP, Maguire RT, Rogers B, et al. Comparison of serum PSMA, PSA levels with results of Cytogen-356 ProstaScint scanning in prostatic cancer patients. *Prostate* 1997;33:281-285.

162. Kahn D, Williams RD, Manyak MJ, et al. 111Indium-capromab pendetide in the evaluation of patients with residual or recurrent prostate cancer after radical prostatectomy. The ProstaScint Study Group. *J Urol* 1998;159:2041-2046; discussion 2046-2047.

163. Krenning EP, Bakker WH, Breeman WA, et al. Localisation of endocrine-related tumours with radioiodinated analogue of somatostatin. *Lancet* 1989;1:242-244.

164. Lamberts SW, Hofland LJ, van Koetsveld PM, et al. Parallel in vivo and in vitro detection of functional somatostatin receptors in human endocrine pancreatic tumors: consequences with regard to diagnosis, localization, and therapy. *J Clin Endocrinol Metab* 1990;71:566-574.

165. Farrell MA, McAdams HP, Herndon JE, et al. Non-small cell lung cancer: FDG PET for nodal staging in patients with stage I disease. *Radiology* 2000;215:886-890.

166. Phelps ME, Huang SC, Hoffman EJ, et al. Tomographic measurement of local cerebral glucose metabolic rate in humans with [^{18}F]2-fluoro-2-deoxy-D-glucose: validation of method. *Ann Neurol* 1979;6:371-388.

167. Nolop KB, Rhodes CG, Brudin LH, et al. Glucose utilization in vivo by human pulmonary neoplasms. *Cancer* 1987;60:2682-2689.

168. Hoh CK, Hawkins RA, Glaspy JA, et al. Cancer detection with whole-body PET using 2-[^{18}F]fluoro-2-deoxy-D-glucose. *J Comput Assist Tomogr* 1993;17:582-589.

169. Vansteenkiste JF, Stroobants SG, Dupont PJ, et al. Prognostic importance of the standardized uptake value on [^{18}F]-fluoro-2-deoxy-glucose-positron emission tomography scan in non-small cell lung cancer: an analysis of 125 cases. Leuven Lung Cancer Group. *J Clin Oncol* 1999;17:3201-3206.

170. Alnafisi NS, Driedger AA, Coates G, et al. FDG PET of recurrent or metastatic 131I-negative papillary thyroid carcinoma. *J Nucl Med* 2000;41:1010-1015.

171. Marom EM, McAdams HP, Erasmus JJ, et al. Staging non–small cell lung cancer with whole-body PET. *Radiology* 1999;212: 803-809.

172. Wu F, Orlefors H, Bergstrom M, et al. Uptake of 14C- and 11C-labeled glutamate, glutamine and aspartate in vitro and in vivo. *Anticancer Res* 2000;20:251-256.

173. Taniguchi H, Koyama H, Masuyama M, et al. Angiotensin-II–induced hypertension chemotherapy: evaluation of hepatic blood flow with oxygen-15 PET. *J Nucl Med* 1996;37:1522-1523.

174. Dimitrakopoulou-Strauss A, Strauss LG, Schlag P, et al. Intravenous and intra-arterial oxygen-15-labeled water and fluorine-18-labeled fluorouracil in patients with liver metastases from colorectal carcinoma. *J Nucl Med* 1998;39:465-473.

175. Evans SM, Bergeron M, Ferriero DM, et al. Imaging hypoxia in diseased tissues. *Adv Exp Med Biol* 1997;428:595-603.

176. Raleigh JA, Chou SC, Arteel GE, et al. Comparisons among pimonidazole binding, oxygen electrode measurements, and radiation response in C3H mouse tumors. *Radiat Res* 1999;151:580-589.

177. Evans SM, Kachur AV, Shiue CY, et al. Noninvasive detection of tumor hypoxia using the 2-nitroimidazole [18F]EF1. *J Nucl Med* 2000;41:327-336.

178. Yang DJ, Wallace S, Cherif A, et al. Development of F-18-labeled fluoroerythronitroimidazole as a PET agent for imaging tumor hypoxia. *Radiology* 1995;194:795-800.

179. Cole KA, Drizman DB, Emmert-Buck MR. The genetics of cancer—a 3D model. *Nat Genet* 1999;21:38-41.

180. Duggan DJ, Bittner M, Chen Y, et al. Expression profiling using cDNA microarrays. *Nat Genet* 1999;21:10-14.

181. Bassett DE Jr, Eisen MB, Boguski MS. Gene expression informatics—it's all in your mine. *Nat Genet* 1999;21:51-55.

Index

Note: Pages followed by an f indicate figures; by a t indicate tables; by a b indicate boxes.